KV-420-658

5/78 £75.00

THE LEUZ INDEX OF PLASTIC SURGERY 1921 A.D. to 1946 A.D.

THE McDOWELL INDEXES OF PLASTIC SURGICAL LITERATURE

Edited By

FRANK McDOWELL, M.D., Sc.D.

Professor of Surgery, University of Hawaii
Professor of Clinical Surgery, Stanford University
Editor-in-Chief, *Plastic and Reconstructive Surgery*

VOLUME III

THE LEUZ INDEX OF PLASTIC SURGERY 1921 A.D. to 1946 A.D.

Compiled
By

Christopher A. Leuz, M.D.

The Williams and Wilkins Co./Baltimore

THIS SERIES OF INDEXES IS SPONSORED BY THE EDUCATIONAL FOUNDATION OF THE AMERICAN SOCIETY OF PLASTIC AND RECONSTRUCTIVE SURGEONS, INC.

Copyright ©, 1977
THE WILLIAMS & WILKINS COMPANY
428 E. Preston Street
Baltimore, Md. 21202, U.S.A.

All rights reserved. This book is protected by copyright. No part of this book may be reproduced in any form or by any means, including photocopying, or utilized by any information storage and retrieval system without written permission from the copyright owner.

Made in the United States of America

Library of Congress Cataloging in Publication Data

Leuz, Christopher A
The Leuz index of plastic surgery, 1921 A.D. to 1946 A.D.

(The McDowell indexes of plastic surgical literature; v. 3)
1. Surgery, Plastic—Indexes. I. Title. II. Title: Index of plastic surgery, 1921 A.D. to 1946 A.D. III. Series. [DNLM: 1. Surgery, Plastic—Bibliography. 2. Surgery, Plastic—Indexes. ZW0600 M138 v. 3]
Z6667.P5M33 vol. 3 [RD118] 617'.95'016s
ISBN 0-683-05763-4 [617'.95'016] 76-44288

Composed and printed at the
WAVERLY PRESS, INC.
Mt. Royal and Guilford Aves.
Baltimore, Md. 21202, U.S.A.

EDITOR'S FOREWORD

This is the third volume of five, which will comprise a total index of the plastic surgical literature of the world from the beginning of time until now.

Volume I, the Zeis Index (900 B.C. to 1863 A.D.), was issued early in 1977 and has been highly successful. Volume II, the Patterson Index (1864 A.D. to 1920 A.D.), is being prepared now and should be ready for publication late in 1978. This Volume III, the Leuz Index (1921 A.D. to 1946 A.D.), is the largest of the five. Volume IV, the Ivy Index (1946 A.D. to 1971 A.D.), was issued in 1971 as "The 25-Year Index of Plastic and Reconstructive Surgery." (The recent renaming of it is appropriate, because Dr. Ivy personally compiled the index cards for 23 of the 25 years covered by that index.) Volume V, the Honolulu Index (1971 A.D. to 1976 A.D.), is now in press.

The five volumes constitute a matched set which will take up about 9 linear inches on your desk, fitting nicely between small bookends. They are the most valuable tool imaginable for the working plastic surgeon and for investigators and scholars in this field. To paraphrase Santayana, "the penalty for those who do not know what has been tried in plastic surgery is that they will have to repeat it." The diligent use of these five volumes will not only keep you informed as to the best procedure developed to date for the patient at hand, but will also help you to avoid the thousands of mistakes that have been made in the past. Instead of having to start on "square one" and find out by trial and error every time, you can stand on the shoulders of all your predecessors and start where they finished. Plastic surgeons are the only specialists in all of medicine to have such a valuable resource.

As noted in the foreword of Volume I, an invitation was issued in the June 1971 issue of the *Journal* for colleagues to help in the compilation and publication of this series. Among those who answered was Dr. Christopher A. Leuz, then a Resident in Plastic Surgery on the service of Dr. Ralph Blocksma at the Butterworth Hospital and the Blodgett Memorial Hospital in Grand Rapids, Michigan. After considerable correspondence with Dr. Leuz, and consultation with Dr. Blocksma, I chose Dr. Leuz to do this third volume. Though he was young at the time for an undertaking of this magnitude, it became evident that he was a thorough and fine scholar who had the tenacity of purpose to see it through. The choice was one of the best ones I have ever made.

In 1974 Dr. Leuz finished his residency and finished compiling this index on 44,000 cards. He and Mrs. Leuz then departed for Belgium, and later went to Zaire. About 15 months after his departure the cards were flown to Honolulu where the entire index was disassembled, gone through card-by-card for final editing, and then reassembled. Some categories were added, some were taken out, and all of the entries under each subject (and under each author) were arranged chronologically. The editorial assistants for the *Journal*, Mary McDowell, Kitty Dabney, and Barbara Kramer, were of great help in this. In general, however, the credit for the completeness and the good features of this index should go to Dr. and Mrs. Leuz, the blame for any shortcomings or mistakes should be placed on me.

Now, let us hear something about Dr. Leuz. He has been much too modest to write anything about himself, but Dr. Blocksma furnished us with the following.

"Chris Leuz put forth a prodigious effort in compiling this volume. I am sure that he initiated the project by using his own sparse financial resources, and later he was helped by our office and by the Butterworth Hospital Research Committee. His wife, Lois, is a nurse and she entered into the project wholeheartedly with him, often working well into the night and through weekends to complete it.

"As you see from his *curriculum vitae,* he did his internship in 1964–65 at Butterworth Hospital and from 1965 to 1968 he served as a medical missionary in Vietnam, taking his whole family into the interior during the height of the Vietnam War. He went as a conscientious objector. I visited him in Vietnam in 1968 at the height of that conflict, and I was amazed to find that he and Lois were serving both sides for medical care in a jungle location not far from Da Nang. As I recall, they were finally forced to evacuate their home and "hospital" when it was caught in the crossfire between the Viet Cong and the South Vietnamese.

"He returned to Grand Rapids in 1968 where he completed a residency in general surgery in 1972 and plastic surgery in 1974. He passed his written examinations immediately afterward, and then proceeded to Brussels, Belgium, for study in tropical medicine. There he received the DMT degree in tropical medicine; his wife also received her degree in that field, passing the examinations which were given in the French language.

"This dedicated family then elected to go as medical missionaries to Kimpese in the Republic of Zaire, where he is working in plastic surgery and also doing some ophthalmic surgery. It must be obvious that only a person with his intense dedication and fine ability would have been able and willing to successfully put together this massive bibliography."

In addition to thanking Dr. and Mrs. Leuz for this *tour de force,* I would like to thank all of the officers and members of the Educational Foundation of the American Society of Plastic and Reconstructive Surgeons. They have sponsored this Master Series of Indexes and have done so much to help us get it published.

Frank McDowell, M.D., Sc.D.

Honolulu, Hawaii

AUTHOR'S PREFACE

It is hoped that this volume will help the researcher or the student (each of us falls into one or both of these categories) to more quickly gain the information that he desires. Perhaps it will also enable the inquirer to become more familiar with the failures of the previous generation of physicians, so that these failures are no longer repeated from generation to generation. With our present rate of expansion of medical knowledge, we can no longer afford the luxury of learning from our own mistakes.

The sole source for this index has been the *Index Medicus,* and the format used is that of the *Index Medicus*. More than two hundred subject headings related to plastic surgery were researched to obtain the list of articles included in this volume. Each of these articles was then categorized by the names of the authors and as much as possible into three other general areas: the anatomical location, the pathological process, and the corrective procedure utilized. The articles chosen for inclusion in this volume were, in my opinion, those relating to the mainstream of plastic surgery. Someone else, I'm sure, would have included categories differing from the ones that I chose. For this shortcoming in the volume I, alone, take responsibility.

Many people helped in the preparation of this index. Particularly, I want to thank the Research Committee of Butterworth Hospital in Grand Rapids, Michigan, for their financial support—without which this index could not have been compiled at this time. The librarians, Miss Elaine Dechow of Butterworth Hospital and Mr. V. Peter Skuja of Blodgett Memorial Hospital in Grand Rapids, were of great assistance to me. The encouragement of Dr. Frank McDowell, Editor of *Plastic and Reconstructive Surgery,* and of Dr. Ralph Blocksma, my former chief, was greatly appreciated. Finally, I want to thank my wife, Lois Gross Leuz, for her assistance in typing and filing in articles and for the incalculable moral support which she gave to me during the more than two years that we worked on this index.

Christopher A. Leuz, M.D.

Kimpese, Republique du Zaire

NOTES ON THE USE OF THIS INDEX

In general, this index follows the format of *Index Medicus* and is easy to use. It is a subject and author index, not a title index. The subjects and authors are interdigitated throughout in alphabetical manner.

Within each subject category the individual entries are arranged chronologically—so that the user can quickly ascertain the chronological development of any procedure(s) year-by-year.

To keep the book from being impossibly large and inordinately expensive, it has been necessary to limit duplication or triplication of entries—and to file most of them under a single subject heading (plus under the name of the first author). Thus a paper on the skin grafting of a burned hand will probably not be found under "skin grafting," again under "burns," and again under "hands," but under only one of these three. The user must, therefore, exercise a modicum of ingenuity and think of the various headings where the entry he desires could be located. To help him in the search, he will find in the back of the volume a complete "List of Subject Headings." The liberal use of this list will make the search very much easier.

A

ABALOS, J. B. AND NATALE, A. M.: Artificial vagina—plastic surgery; Abalos' method. Rev. de chir. *7:*551-557, Dec '28

ABASCAL, H.: Fomentobiol (vaccine broth) in burns; 5 cases. Cron. med.-quir. de la Habana *59:*411-413, Oct '33

ABASCAL, H.: Keloid in Negro race. Cron. med.-quir. de la Habana *59:*145-155, April '33

ABBOTT, A. C.: Dupuytren's contracture; review of literature and report of new technique in surgical treatment; preliminary statement. Canad. M. A. J. *20:*250-253, March '29

ABBOTT, A. C.: Protruding ear and its surgical treatment. Manitoba M. Rev. *26:*335-339, June '46

ABBOTT, L. C.: Reconstructive orthopedic surgery (tendon transplantation and arthrodesis of wrist) for disabilities resulting from irreparable injuries to radial nerve. J. Nerv. and Ment. Dis. *99:*466-474, May '44

ABBOTT, L. C. *et al:* Use of penicillin therapy in conjunction with free bone grafting in infected areas. Surg. Gynec. and Obst. *83:*101-106, July '46

ABBOTT, L. C. AND GILL, G. G.: Use of cancellous bone grafts in orthopedic surgery. Brunn, Med.-Surg. Tributes, pp. 1-11, '42

ABBOTT, M. D. AND GEPFERT, J. R.: Topical use of medicated (with sulfanilamide, sulfonamide) human plasma. U. S. Nav. M. Bull. *42:*193-194, Jan '44

ABBOTT, T. R. (see SCHWARTZ, A. B.) Nov '36

ABBOTT, T. R. (see SCHWARTZ, A. B.) March '46

ABBOTT, W. D. (see MICHAEL, P.) Oct '43

ABBOTT, W. E. *et al:* Metabolic alterations following thermal burns; effect of treatment with whole blood and electrolyte (salt) solution or with plasma following experimental burn. Surgery *17:*794-804, June '45

ABBOTT, W. E. *et al:* Metabolic alterations following thermal burns; use of whole blood and electrolyte solution (salt) in treatment of burned patients. Ann. Surg. *122:*678-692, Oct '45

ABDANSKI, A.: Cancer of lower lip in child 9 years old. Rev. de chir., Paris *52:*557-559, July '33

Abdomen, Defect of

Skin flap cover for projecting intestine. STEINBERG, M. E. Ann. Surg. *83:*123-125, Jan '26

Morphological genesis of cleft of abdomen and bladder (ectopia vesicae). STERNBERG, H. Urol and Cutan. Rev. *31:*475-479, Aug '27

Abdomen, Defect of—Cont.

Congenital absence of abdominal wall. FLETCHER, W. M. A., M. J. Australia *1:* 435-436, April 7, '28

Gastroschisis in new-born; 2 cases. KLEINER, B. Monatschr. f. Geburtsh. u. Gynak. *84:*281-293, March '30

Congenital absence of part of abdominal wall. GAMBLE, H. A. South. M. J. *25:*771-772, July '32

Gastro-enteroschisis; case. KRAUSS, F. Deutsche med. Wchnschr. *62:*258, Feb 14, '36

Pathogenesis of cleft formation of anterior wall of abdomen (gastroschisis); rare case. LIPPMANN, O. Zentrabl. f. Gynak. *61:*516-524, Feb 27, '37

Agenesis of abdominal wall in infant. CAUSSADE, L. *et al*. Rev. med. de Nancy *66:*262-265, March 15, '38

Deformities of ventral line of abdominal closure; umbilical hernia and gastroschisis. PÜTZ, T. Geburtsh. u. Frauenh. *1:*663-671, Oct '39

Gastroschisis, rare teratologic condition in new-born; case. BERNSTEIN, P. Arch. Pediat. *57:*505-513, '40

Gastrothoracoschisis (fetal eventration) with clinical symptoms of uterine rupture. ARANYI, S. Zentralbl. f. Gynak. *66:*1757-1762, Oct 31, '42

Gastroschisis, with case report. WATKINS, D. E. Virginia M. Monthly *70:*42-44, Jan '43

Gastrothoracoschisis; rare case of fetal maldevelopment. GHOSH, P. K. Calcutta M. J. *41:*10-12, Jan '44

Congenital defect of abdominal wall in newborn (gastroschisis). JOHNS, F. S. Ann. Surg. *123:*886-899, May '46

Abdominal Flap

Abdominal flap to cover defect after mammectomy. SOUPAULT, R. Presse med. *31:*177-178, Feb 24, '23 (illus.)

Abdominal skin flap after amputation of breast. HEIDENHAIN, L. Zentralbl. f. Gynak. *47:*2649-2650, Nov 29, '24

One stage tubed abdominal flaps; single pedicle tubes. SHAW, D. T. AND PAYNE, R. L., Jr. Surg. Gynec. and Obst. *83:*205-209, Aug '46

Abdominoplasty

Operations for pendulous breast and pendulous abdomen. KÜSTER, H. Monatschr. f. Geburtsh. u. Gynak. *73:*316-341, June '26

Plastic operations for pendulous abdomen and pendulous breast; a survey. FRIST, J. Med. Klin. *23:*1269-1271, Aug 19, '27

Abdominoplasty – Cont.

Esthetic surgery of pendulous breast, abdomen and arms in female. THOREK, M. Illinois M. J. *58:*48-57, July '30

Nasenplastik und sonstige Gesichtsplastik. Nebst einem Anhang über Mammaplastik und . . . Körperplastik, by Jacques Joseph. C. Kabitsch, Leipzig, 1931

Pendulous abdomen, surgical treatment. FLESCH-THEBESIUS, M. AND WEINSHEIMER, K. Chirurg *3:*841–846, Oct 1, '31

Chirurgie réparatrice: Plastique et esthétique de la poitrine, des seins, et de l'abdomen, by L. Dartigues. Lépine, Paris, 1936

Advances in plastic surgery (abdomen). HABERLAND, H. F. O. Zentralbl. f. Chir. *63:*154-156, Jan 18, '36

Pendulous abdomen, surgical therapy. IGARZABAL, J. E. Semana med. *1:*1361-1365, June 16, '38 comment by Goni Moreno *2:*52-53, July 7, '38 reply by Igarzabal *2:*152-153, July 21, '38

(comment on article by Igarzabel on pendulous abdomen). GONI MORENO, I. Semana med. *2:*52-53, July 7, '38

Chirurgie plastique abdominale; cure chirurgicale de ptose cutanée abdominale, ventre en tablier, by Charles Claoué. Maloine, Paris, 1940

Plastic Surgery of the Breast and Abdominal Wall, by Max Thorek. C C Thomas Co., Springfield, Ill., 1942

Circular dermolipectomy of trunk in obesity. SOMALO, M. Arq. de cir. clin. e exper. *6:*540-543, April–June '42

Cruciform ventral dermolipectomy; swallow-shaped incision. SOMALO, M. Prensa med. argent. *33:*75-83, Jan 11, '46

ABDULAEV, G. G.: Kankrov operation in therapy of dacryocystitis. Sovet. vestnik oftal. *8:*710-711, '36

ABDULAEV, G. G.: Surgical therapy of cicatricial trachoma. Sovet. vestnik oftal. *8:*712-715, '36

ABELS, Bird-face (opisthogenia). Wien. med. Wchnschr. *77:*1208, Sept 3, '27

ABELSON, J. M.: Orthodontics as aid in repairing congenital cleft palate. Am. J. Orthodontics *25:*154-158, Feb '39

ABERCROMBIE, P. H.: Salivary fistula communicating with external auditory meatus. J. Laryng. and Otol. *45:*474-476, July '30

ABERNATHY, S.: Malignant melanoma of skin. Memphis M. J. *19:*54-58, April '44

ABERNETHY, D. A.: Hypertelorism in several generations. Arch. Dis. Childhood *2:*361-365, Dec '27

ABERNETHY, D. A.: Primary double epithelioma of face; case. Brit. J. Surg. *16:*687-689, April '29

ABOULKER, H. AND GOZLAN, A.: Naso-orbital epitheliomas; 10 cases. Ann. d'oto-laryng., pp. 381-398, April '31

ABRAHAMSON, R. H. (see BURMAN, M.) Nov '43

ABRAJANOFF, A. A.: Freedom in plastic surgery. Vestnik khir. (no. 35-36) *12:*10-19, '28

ABRAMOVIČS, H.: Megalosyndactylia; case. Munchen. med. Wchnschr. *76:*921, May 31, '29

ABRAMSON, B. P.: Transfusion of blood stabilized with magnesium sulfate in experimental shock.

ABRAMSON, P. D.: Treatment of cleft lip and palate. Tri-State M. J. *14:*2559, Nov '41

ABREU E LIMA, A.: Congenital vaginal absence; surgical therapy of case. Ann. brasil. de gynec. *7:*478-484, June '39

ACHARD, C.: Poisoning from use of picric acid in burn therapy. Rev. gen. de clin. et de therap. *41:*65-68, Jan 29, '27

ACHARD, P.: Vertical fractures of mandibular ramus; cases. Rev. de stomatol. *36:*321-326, May '34

ACKERMAN, A. A. (see FIELD, H. J.) March '36

ACKERMAN, L. V. (see BURFORD, W. N. *et al*) July '44

ACKERMAN, L. V. (see BURFORD, W. N.) Sept '45

ACKMAN, D. AND WILSON, G.: Sulfathiazole (sulfanilamide derivative) emulsion; further experience in burns. Canad. M. A. J. *47:*1-7, July '42

ACKMAN, D. *et al:* Report on management of burns with sulfathiazole emulsion, using occlusive compression dressing. Ann. Surg. *119:*161-177, Feb '44

Acne

Subcutaneous division of sebaceous glands in treatment of acne vulgaris. MONCORPS, C. Munchen. med. Wchnschr. *76:*997-998, June 14, '29

Cryotherapy (slush method using carbon dioxide snow) for acne. DOBES, W. L. AND KEIL, H. Arch. Dermat. and Syph. *42:*547-558, Oct '40

Treatment of acne vulgaris with comedos by monoterminal electrodesiccation. NOMLAND, R. Arch. Dermat. and Syph. *48:*302-304, Sept '43

Superfluous hair and acne-cause and cure. KAUFMAN, S. M. Hygeia *24:*272, Apr '46

Surgical cure of acne rosacea and rhino-

Acne—Cont.
phyma with skin grafting. MACOMBER, D. W. Rocky Mountain M. J. *43:*466-467, June '46

Acne Scars

Treatment of acne-keloid of nape of neck by diathermo-coagulation; cases. RAVAUT, P. AND FILLIOL, L. Bull. Soc. franc. de dermat. et syph. *35:*942-946, Dec '28
Correction of cicatrices from smallpox and acne necrotica. HALLE, M. Fortschr. d. Therap. *8:*505-506, Aug 25, '32
Cyrotherapy (with mixture containing carbon dioxide snow) for acne and its scars. KARP, F. L. *et al.* Arch. Dermat. and Syph. *39:*995-998, June '39
Evaluation of cryotherapy of post-acne scars. HOLLANDER, L. AND SHELTON, J. M. Pennsylvania M. J. *45:*226-228, Dec '41
Failure with cryotherapy (using carbon dioxide slush) in treatment of acne scars. FRIEDLANDER, H. M. Arch. Dermat. and Syph. *46:*734-736, Nov '42
Rhinophyma and hypertrophic acne; treatment by means of cold (high frequency) knife. IBARRA PEREZ, R. Vida nueva *52:*231-236, Nov '43
Disseminated keloid acne; case. MERCADAL PEYRI, J. Actas dermo-sif. *35:*839-849, May '44
Formula for cryotherapy (with carbon dioxide slush) for acne and postacne scarring. ZUGERMAN, I. Arch. Dermat. and Syph. *54:*209-210, Aug '46

ACQUAVIVA, (see GIRAUDEAU) July '35
ADAIR, F. E. (see PACK, G. T.) Jan '39
ADAIR, F. E. (see SPIES, J. W. *et al*) March '34
ADAIR, F. E.: Epitheliomas of hand; types and treatment. S. Clin. North America *13:*423-430, April '33
ADAIR, F. E.: Melanoma treatment; 400 cases. Surg., Gynec. and Obst. *62:*406-409, Feb (no. 2A) '36
ADAIR, F. E. AND HERRMANN, J. B.: Unusual metastatic manifestations of breast cancer: metastasis to mandible, with report of 5 cases. Surg. Gynec. and Obst. *83:*289-295, Sept '46
ADAIR, F. E.; PACK, G. T. AND NICHOLSON, M. E.: Differential diagnosis of subungual melanomas; 4 cases. Bull. Assoc. franc. p. l'etude du cancer *19:*549-566, July '30
ADAMEK, G. (see DEMEL, R.) 1929
ADAMS, B. D.: Device for fixation of hands and arms for certain operative cases. New England J. Med. *210:*423, Feb 22, '34
ADAMS, B. S.: Extension treatment for fractures of fingers. Journal-Lancet *51:*283-284, May 1, '31
ADAMS, B. S.: Finger fractures and hand. Minnesota Med. *12:*515-520, Sept '29
ADAMS, E. H.: Urinary obstruction caused by distended sigmoid associated with imperforate anus. Atlantic M. J. *31:*311-312, Feb '28
ADAMS, F.: Exstrophy of bladder and its therapy. Arch. f. klin. Chir. *205:*695, '44
ADAMS, H. D.: Dupuytren's contracture. Lahey Clin. Bull. *2:*75-78, Jan '41
ADAMS, H. D.: Dupuytren's contracture. S. Clin. North America *22:*899-906, June '42
ADAMS, H. D.: Surgical management of radiation ulceration (grafting). Lahey Clin. Bull. *2:*203-206, Jan '42
ADAMS, J. C.: Unusual amputation of finger and tendon. U. S. Nav. M. Bull. *27:*379-380, April '29
ADAMS, J. L. AND GRAVES, J. Q.: Surgical shock. New Orleans M. and S. J. *76:*291-295, Dec '23
ADAMS, R. C. (see LUNDY, J. S. *et al*) Aug '44
ADAMS, R. C.: Regional anesthesia for operations about neck. Anesthesiology *2:*515-529, Sept '41
ADAMS, R. C.: Shock, blood transfusion and supportive treatment. Mil. Surgeon *89:*34-41, July '41
ADAMS, W. M.: Acute lacerations of face. Mississippi Doctor *17:*139-142, Aug '39
ADAMS, W. M.: Care of military and civilian injuries; internal wiring fixation of facial fractures. Am. J. Orthodontics (Oral Surg. Sect.) *29:*111-130, Feb '43
ADAMS, W. M.: Congenital absence of vagina and its construction. Memphis M. J. *18:*3-5, Jan '43
ADAMS, W. M.: Construction of artificial vagina. Surg., Gynec. and Obst. *76:*746-751, June '43
ADAMS, W. M.: Facial fractures; internal wiring fixation. Surgery *12:*523-540, Oct '42
ADAMS, W. M.: Facial fractures; treatment by wiring fixation. Mississippi Doctor *19:*427-435, Feb '42
ADAMS, W. M.: Free transplantation of nipples and areolae in breast hypertrophy. Surgery *15:*186-195, Jan '44
ADAMS, W. M.: Local burn treatment, with special reference to sulfadiazine (sulfanilamide derivative). Memphis M. J. *17:*5-8, Jan '42
ADAMS, W. M.: Operation for congenital eyelid ptosis; case. Memphis M. J. *10:*16, April '35
ADAMS, W. M.: Reconstructive surgery (face).

Mississippi Doctor *15:*23-28, Feb '38

Adams, W. M.: Results achieved with plastic surgery. Memphis M. J. *13:*3-6, Jan '38

Adams, W. M.: Treatment of facial fractures (description of extra-oral fixation appliance). J. Tennessee M. A. *35:*469-475, Dec '42

Adams, W. M. and Crawford, J. K.: Sulfadiazine (sulfanilamide derivative) in burns. South. Surgeon *11:*324-340, May '42

Adams, W. R.: Bone grafting. Surg., Gynec. and Obst. *36:*97-98, Jan '23 (illus.)

Addison, O. L.: Cleft-palate, some pitfalls in operation. Lancet *1:*818-819, April 18, '25

Addison, P. I.: Treatment of nonunion and loss of substance in fracture of edentulous mandible. J. Am. Dent. A. *25:*1081-1084, July '38

Adkins, G. E.: Nasal septal deformities. New Orleans M. and S. J. *86:*102-105, Aug '33

Adler, A.: Plastic operation for unusually extensive gynecomastia. Zentralbl. f. Chir. *64:*889-893, April 10, '37

Adler, D.: Emergency plastic surgery. Arq. de cir. clin. e exper. *6:*651-653, April–June '42

Adler, D.: Grafts and inclusions in nasal surgery. Rev. brasil. de oto-rino-laring. *8:*679-682, Nov-Dec '40

Adler, D.: Plastic surgery, concept and tendencies in North America. Arq. de cir. clin. e exper. *6:*695-702, April–June '42

Adler, D.: Plastic surgery; conception and tendencies in North America. Hospital, Rio de Janeiro *20:*643-650, Oct '41

Adler, D.: Plastic surgery of nose. Rev. med. brasil. *2:*67-82, Feb '39

Adler, D.: Refrigerated cartilage for use in plastic surgery. Arq. de cir. clin. e exper. *6:*608-611, April–June '42

Adler, E.: Peripheral facial paralysis, based upon 50 observations. Acta med. orient. *2:*1-9, Dec '42–Jan '43

Adler, H.: Technic of plastic operation for saddle nose. Arch. f. klin. Chir. *160:*780-781, '30

Adler, H. J.: Intranasal plastic operation of deformed end of nose. Acta oto-laryng. *10:*130-134, '26

Adler, S.: New method for slowly healing ulcers. Gyogyaszat *77:*376-377, June 20, '37

Adson, A. W. (see Pulford, D. S.) June '26

Adson, A. W.: Surgical treatment of facial paralysis. Arch. Otolaryng. *2:*217-249, Sept '25 also: Tr. Sect. Laryng. Otol. and Rhin., A. M. A., pp. 187-211, '25

Adson, A. W.: Surgical treatment of peripheral nerve injuries. J. Kansas M. Soc. *37:*497, Dec '36

Adson, A. W. and Ott, W. O.: Preservation of facial nerve in radical treatment of parotid tumors. Arch. Surg. *6:*739-746, May '23 (illus.)

Afanaseva, A. V.: Comparative evaluation of methods for amputation of fingers. Vestnik khir. *42:*232-239, '36

Affonso, J.: Congenital fistula of penile urethra; case in boy 9 years old. Arq. de cir. e ortop. *2:*81-83, Sept '34

Afonso, J.: Zeno method of burn therapy by immobilization in plaster cast. Arq. brasil. de cir. e ortop. *6:*302-309, Sept-Dec '38

Agafonov, F. A.: Treatment of inflammation of hand. Sovet. vrach. zhur., pp 544-546, April 15 '36

Agatston, S. A.: Resection of levator palpebrae muscle by conjunctival route; simplified technic. Arch. Ophth. *27:*994-996, May '42

Agnantis, C.: Palpebrosuperciliary autoplasty; case. Ann. d'ocul. *167:*226-229, March '30

Agostinelli, E.: Phalloplasty; technic of skin grafting in avulsion of skin of penis and scrotum; review of literature and report of case. Policlinico (sez. prat.) *46:*1303-1306, July 17, '39

Agrifoglio, M.: Carpometacarpal dislocation; case. Arch. di ortop. *46:*615-628, June 30, '30

Aguerre, J. A. Jr.: Pharyngolaryngeal burns and scalds; prognosis, complications and therapy. Arch. de pediat. d. Uruguay *5:*181-190, May '34

Aguilar, H. and Zavaleta, D.: Therapy of cancer of eyelid by evisceration followed by plastic surgery; case. Hosp. argent. *4:*506-512, Jan 15, '34

Aguilar, H. D.: Grave burns, with special reference to hypoproteinemia. Prensa med. argent. *31:*1446-1449, Aug 2, '44

Aguilera, V. M.: Wounds of the neck. Arch. Soc. cirujanos hosp. *13:*3-11, June '43

Aguirre, J. A. (see Ivanissevich, O. *et al*) April '39

Ahlberg, A.: Solitary enchondromas of hand bones; 3 cases treated surgically. Acta chir. Scandinav. *89:*75-80, '43

Ahlswede, E.: Digestion of keloids, cicatrices and buboes with pepsin-hydrochloric acid. Arch. Dermat. and Syph. *3:*142, Feb '21

Aievoli, E.: Infections of hand. Riforma med. *41:*36, Jan 12, '25

Aikawa, T.: Circulating blood volume and operative trauma; experimental studies. Arch. f. klin. Chir. *181:*330-336, '34

Aimes, A.: Subcutaneous rupture of tendon of long extensor of thumb; case. Progres med., pp. 1533-1534, Oct 3, '36

Aimes, A.: Surgical therapy of chronic nontuberculous arthropathies. Progres med., pp. 1433-1437, Sept 15, '34

Ainslie, J. P.: Modern burn treatment. M. J. Australia *2:*339-340, Oct 10, '42

Ainsworth-Davis, J. C.: Preservation of function in burnt hand (including description of steering wheel apparatus). Brit. M. J. *1:*724,

June 13, '42
AIRD, I.: Ear-pit (congenital aural and preauricular fistula). Edinburgh M. J. *53:*498–507, Sept '46
AIRD, I.: Surgery of peripheral nerve injury. Post-Grad. M. J. *22:*225–254, Sept '46
AITKEN, G. T.: Lessons learned from review of cases of hand wounds evacuated from South Pacific. Am. Acad. Orthop. Surgeons, Lect., pp. 202–208, '44
AJO, A.: Plastic surgery of eyelids. Nord. med. *15:*2437–2440, Sept 5, '42
AKERMAN, J.: Obstetrical shock. South. M. J. *19:*134–136, Feb '26
AKERMAN, N.: Therapy of dislocation fractures of zygoma. Acta chir. Scandinav. *80:*359–364, '38
AKHVLEDYANI, A. V.: Baldwin's operation in case of complete absence of vagina. J. akush. i zhensk. boliez. *39:*912–916, '28
AKS, L. V.: Therapy of badly consolidated and nonconsolidated jaw fractures. Ortop. i travmatol. (no. 1) *13:*30–35, '39
AKS, L. V.: Feeding and care of patients with maxillofacial wounds. Ortop. i. travmatol. (no. 1) *14:*90–96, '40
AKSELRUD, S. S.: Polydactylia and oligophalangia. Ortop. i travmatol. (no. 4) *11:*66–75, '37
ALAJOUANINE, T., MAIRE, R., AND GUILLAUME, J.: Dupuytren's contracture localized to 2 last fingers of left hand and accompanied by Bernard-Horner ocular sympathetic syndrome of same side, observed 15 years after lesion of cubital nerve of opposite side. Rev. neurol. *2:*679–683, Dec '30
ALANTAR, I. H.: Acrocephalosyndactylia (Apert syndrome) in new-born infant; case. Arch. de med. d. enf. *40:*171–172, March '37
ALARCON, C. J. AND GENATIOS, T.: Dermoepidermal grafts in therapy of ulcers of legs. Rev. san. y asist. social *8:*783–796, Aug '43
ALBAN, H. (see SIMON, H. E.) Dec '45
ALBANESE, A.: Changes in nerve implants. Arch. ital. di chir. *4:*215–228, Nov '21 (illus.) abstr: J.A.M.A. *78:*250, Jan 21, '22
ALBANESE, A.: Treatment of Volkmann's ischemic paralysis; case. Rinasc. med. *6:*181–183, April 15, '29
ALBANESE, A. R.: Cervical sympathectomy in therapy of facial paralysis. Prensa med. argent. *31:*415–417, March 1, '44
ALBEE, F. H.: Bone drilling in resistant chronic ulcers; new principle. Am. J. Surg. *54:*605–608, Dec '41
ALBEE, F. H.: Bone graft; reconstructive surgery. Internat. clinics *2:*225–236, June '25
ALBEE, F. H.: Certain fundamental laws underlying surgical use of bone graft. Ann. Surg. *74:*196, Aug '21
ALBEE, F. H.: Formation of radius congenitally absent; condition 7 years after implantation of bone graft. Ann. Surg. *87:*105–110, Jan '28
ALBEE, F. H.: Fundamentals in bone transplantation, experiences in 3,000 bone graft operations. J.A.M.A. *81:*1429–1432, Oct 27, '23
ALBEE, F. H.: Principles for bone transplanting. Nederlandsch Tijdschr. v. Geneesk. *1:*2230–2233, May 26, '23
ALBEE, F. H.: Reconstructive surgery. Cir. ortop. y traumatol., Habana *6:*153–155, Oct–Dec '38
ALBEE, F. H.: Symposium on surgical treatment of chronic arthritis; present status of arthroplasty. New York State J. Med. *39:*2118–2125, Nov 15, '39
ALBEE, F. H.: Ununited fracture of lower jaw with or without loss of bone. S. Clin. N. America *3:*301–341, April '23 (illus.)
ALBEE, F. H.: Various uses of bone transplants. Proc. Roy. Soc. Med. (Sect. Orthop.) *23:*31–36, April '30
ALBEE, FRED H., AND KUSHNER, ALEXANDER: *Bone Graft Surgery in Disease, Injury, and Deformity.* Appleton-Century Co., New York, 1940
ALBERT, B.: Hand injuries. Rozhl. v chir. a gynaek. (cast chir.) *14:*3–19, '35
ALBERT, F.: Treatment of facial paralysis by excision of cervical sympathetic ganglion; case. Liege med. *22:*592–599, April 28, '29
ALBERT, F.: Treatment of cuts of flexor tendons of fingers by tendinous graft. Liege med. *23:*1069–1077, Aug 10, '30 also: Ann. Soc. med.-chir. de Liege *63:*18–21, Sept '30
ALBERT, R.: Resection of superior cervical sympathetic ganglion for facial paralysis; case. J. de chir. et ann. Soc. belge de chir. *27:*285–291, '28
ALBERTENGO, J. B. (see BABBINI, R. J. *et al*) Oct '41
ALBERTI, V.: Surgical therapy of rhinophyma; case. Rassegna internaz. di clin. e terap. *12:*1050–1060, Nov 15, '31
ALBORNOZ, I. (see CARTELLI, N.) May–June '37
ALBRIGHT, H. L.: Cancer of face, especially in region of eye; method of treatment. Am. J. Surg. *33:*176–179, Aug '36
ALCAINO, A. AND RODRÍGUEZ, D. M.: West's dacryocystorhinostomy in 300 cases. Arch. de oftal. hispano-am. *31:*65–79, Feb '31
ALCAINO, Q. A.: Rhinology and plastic surgery of nasal pyramid. Rev. otorrinolaring. *4:*73–123, Sept '44
ALDEN, B. F.: Combined satchel handle or tubed pedicle and large delayed whole skin pedicle flaps in case of plastic surgery of face, neck and chest. Surg., Gynec. and Obst. *41:*493–496, Oct '25
ALDERS, N.: Nature, diagnosis, clinical aspects,

pathogenesis and treatment of obstetric shock. Wien. klin. Wchnschr. *43:*1562–1565, Dec 18, '30

Aldred-Brown, G. R. P.: Finger traps for banjo splint. Brit. M. J. *1:*652, Apr 27, '46

Aldrich, R. H.: Burn therapy with compound of aniline dyes (acrio-violet and brilliant green). New England J. Med. *217:*911–914, Dec 2, '37

Aldrich, R. H.: Compound of aniline dyes (acriviolet and brilliant green) in burns. Maine M. J. *28:*5–7, Jan '37

Aldrich, R. H.: Critical survey of burn therapy. J. Maine M. A. *33:*21–30, Feb '42

Aldrich, R. H.: Major and minor burns. M. Clin. North America *27:*1229–1246, Sept '43

Aldrich, R. H.: Role of infection in burns Px č gentian violet. New England J. Med. *208:*299–309, Feb 9, '33

Aldrich, R. H.: Story of burns, treatment of burns. Am. J. Nursing *33:*851–855, Sept '33

Aldunate Phillips, E.: Pedicle grafts. Arch. Soc. cirujanos hosp. *15:*758–764, Dec '45

Aleksiewicz, J.: New nasal prosthesis (celluloid). Polska gaz. lek. *9:*214–216, March 16, '30

Aleman: Fracture of lower jaw; prosthetic treatment. Cluj. med. *10:*378–395, Aug 1, '29

Aleman, O.: Successful operation for prognathism. Hygiea *84:*239–240, March 31, '22 (illus.)

Alesen, L. A.: Traumatic shock and hemorrhage. California and West. Med. *58:*265–269, May '43

Alessandrini: Diathermosurgery for furunculosis. Rev. med. de Chile *67:*1348–1352, Dec '39

Alessandrini, I.: Extraoral device for immobilization of mandibular fractures. Rev. med. de Chile *70:*298–299, April '42

Alessandrini, I.; Corte, P. and Vargas, R.: Facial prosthesis. Bol. Soc. de cir., Chile *9:*450–451, Dec 23, '31

Alexander, C. S.: Tarsectomy in incomplete eyelid ptosis. Texas State J. Med. *30:*511–514, Dec '34

Alexander, E. Jr. (see Lamon, J. D. Jr.) Feb '45

Alexander, G.: Plastic correction of protruding ears. Wien. klin. Wchnschr. *41:*1217–1218, Aug 23, '28

Alexander, G.: Technic of plastic operations on ear. Ztsch. f. Hals-, Nasen-u. Ohrenh. *21:*6–10, May 10, '28

Alexander, G. F.: Lip-graft operation for trichiasis of eyelid. Tr. Ophth. Soc. U. Kingdom *52:*162–169, '32

Alexander, G. J.: Deviated nasal septums and their correction in young children. J. Ophth., Otol. and Laryng. *32:*325–337, Oct '28

Alexander, H. H. Jr.: Burns and compound fractures; review of their closed treatment. Indust. Med. *12:*434–436, July '43

Alexander, R. J.: Correction of facial paralysis. (muscle transplant.) Rocky Mountain M. J. *38:*713–716, Sept '41

Alexandrow, G. N.: Unusual case of absence of phalanges and wrist bones. Zentralbl. f. Chir. *63:*1110–1111, May 9, '36

Alexeeff, O. A. (see Bytchkoff, V. S.) 1929

Alexenco, V. (see Bart, C. *et al*) June '40

Alferow, M. W.: Artificial vagina formation by Kirschner-Wagner operation; case. Zentralbl. f. Gynak. *57:*884–885, April 15, '33

Alfredo, J.: Cheiloplasty by Estlander technic. Rev. med. de Pernambuco *5:*233–237, June '35

Alfredo, J.: Correction of collapse of ala nasi; 2 cases. Rev. oto-laring. de Sao Paulo *2:*207–210, May–June '34

Alfredo, J.: Facial plastic surgery; cases. Rev. med. de Pernambuco *4:*277–301, Dec '34

Alfredo, J.: Medicolegal aspects of plastic surgery. Rev. med. de Pernambuco *14:*173–180, Aug '44

Alfredo, J.: Modern plastic surgery (face). Rev. med. de Pernambuco *6:*109–118, April '36

Alfredo, J.: Partial rhinomyoplasty. Brasil-med. *43:*1564–1567, Dec 21, '29

Alfredo, J.: Plastic surgery applied to war wounds of face. Rev. med. de Pernambuco *13:*1–10, Jan '43

Alfredo, J.: Social importance of facial surgery. Rev. med. de Pernambuco *6:*317–320, Sept '36

Alfredo, J.: Therapy of collapse of nostril. Rev. med. de Pernambuco *5:*22–26, Jan '35

Alglave, P.: Dermo-epidermic grafts. J. de chir. *29:*659–667, June '27

Alhaique, A.: Plastic surgery (of keloids). Rinasc. med. *9:*25–27, Jan 15, '32

Alhswede, E. H.: Pepsin-hydrochloric acid treatment of keloids, further indications. Arch. Dermat. and Syph. *3:*648, May '21

Alich, S.: Free graft in reparation of extensive axillary wound after burns. Turk tib cem. mec *4:*183–187, '38

Aljama, V.: Stenosing tenosynovitis of flexors; treated cases. (hand) Rev. espan. cir., traumatol. y ortop. *1:*373–374, Nov '44

Alkiewicz, J.: Contracture of middle fingers as new occupational deformation in milkers; case. Dermat. Wchnschr. *107:*1233–1234, Oct 15, '38

Alkio, V. V.: Treatment of stenosis of lacrimal ducts by insertion of spiral shaped cannula.

Duodecim *51:*1076, '35; *52:*51, '36 Abstr: Klin. Monatsbl. f. Augenh. *96:*319–324, March '36
ALLBRITTEN, F. F. Jr.: Surgical repair of deep branch of radial nerve. Surg., Gynec. and Obst. *82:*305–310, March '46
ALLDREDGE, R. H. (see THOMPSON, T. C.) Oct '44
ALLEN, A. G. AND NORTHFIELD, D. W. C.: Facial paralysis; intraoral splint. Lancet *2:*172–173, Aug 5, '44
ALLEN, A. G. AND NORTHFIELD, D. W. C.: Intraoral splint for facial palsy. Brit. Dent. J. *79:*213–215, Oct 19, '45
ALLEN, A. M.: Physiologic and pharmacologic aspects of burn therapy. Indust. Med. *8:*480–482, Nov '39
ALLEN, B. (see DRUSS, J. G.) March '40
ALLEN, C. I. (see MCCLURE, R. D.) May '35
ALLEN, C. R. (see SLOCUM, H. C.) July '45
ALLEN, E. P. (see CAMP, J. D.) Feb '40
ALLEN, E. V. AND GHORMLEY, R. K.: Lymphedema of extremities; etiology, classification and treatment; report of 300 cases. Ann. Int. Med. *9:*516–539, Nov '35
ALLEN, F. M.: Shock and refrigeration; newer developments. J. Internat. Coll. Surgeons *8:*438–452, Sept–Oct, '45
ALLEN, F. M.: Theory and therapy of shock; excessive fluid administration. Am. J. Surg. *61:*79–92, July '43
ALLEN, F. M.: Theory and therapy of shock; reduced temperatures. Am. J. Surg. *60:*335–348, June '43
ALLEN, F. M.: Theory and therapy of shock; varied fluid injections. Am. J. Surg. *62:*80–104, Oct '43
ALLEN, F. M.: Treatment of surgical shock. Dia med. *17:*996–1000, Sept 3, '45
ALLEN, F. M.: Treatment of surgical shock and embolism. J. Internat. Coll. Surgeons *7:*423–434, Nov–Dec '44
ALLEN, F. M., CROSSMAN, L. W. AND SAFFORD, F. K. Jr.: Reduced temperature in burn therapy. New York State J. Med. *43:*951–952, May 15, '43
ALLEN, F. M. B.: Case of hypertelorism without mental defect. Arch. Dis. Childhood *1:*171–174, June '26
ALLEN, H. S. (see MASON, M. L.) Jan '41
ALLEN, H. S. (see MASON, M. L.) 1942
ALLEN, H. S.: Treatment of superficial injuries and burns of hand. J.A.M.A. *116:*1370–1373, March 29, '41
ALLEN, H. S. AND KOCH, S. L.: Severe burns. Surg., Gynec. and Obst. *74:*914–924, May '42
ALLEN, J. G. *et al:* Sulfathiazole (sulfanilamide preparation) ointment in burns. Arch. Surg. *44:*819–828, May '42
ALLEN, J. W. (see CAMERON, G. R. *et al*) Aug '43
ALLEN, J. W.; BURGESS, F. AND CAMERON, G. R.: Toxic effects of propamidine therapy in burns. J. Path. and Bact. *56:*217–223, April '44
ALLEN, V. K.: Rectal herniation with intrasphincteric repair. Clinics *3:*1014–1022, Dec '44
ALLENDE, C. I.: Grave wounds of hands; biologic therapy. Bol. y trab., Acad. argent. de cir. *24:*714–720, Aug 21, '40
ALLENDE, C. T. (see ALURRALDE, M.) May–June '23
ALLENDE, G.: Ankylosis of jaw following smallpox; case. Bol. y trab. de la Soc. de cir. de Buenos Aires *14:*951–959, Nov 26, '30
ALLENDE, G.: Chondrosarcoma of fingers; case. Rev. ortop. y tramatol. *6:*71–81, July '36
ALLISON, W. L.: Peripheral nerve lesions of the hand. Texas State J. Med. *20:*46–51, May '24
ALM, T. J. (see EVANS, E. I.) July '44
ALMOYNA, C. M.: Traumatic shock, physiopathology and therapy. Medicina, Madrid (pt. I) *11:*518–527, June '43
ALONSO, J. M.: Fractures of upper jaws. Ann. d'oto-laryng., pp. 1062–1070, Oct '35
ALONSO, J. M.: Surgical therapy of cancer of hypopharnyx. An. Fac. de med. de Montevideo *28:*812–818, '43
ALONSO, J. M.: Therapy of cancer of larynx. An. de oto-rino-laring. d. Uruguay *9:*215–232, '39
ALONSO, J. M. AND QUINTELA, U.: Spontaneous reconstruction of lower maxilla after total surgical removal; case. An. de oto-rino-laring. d. Uruguay *1:*72–76, '31
ALRICH, E. M. AND LEHMAN, E. P.: Effect of plaster confinement applied at varying intervals after burning. Surgery *15:*899–907, June '44
ALTAVISTA, A. E.: Thyroglossal fistula due to persistence of thyroglossal tract; cases. Rev. otorrinolaring. d. litoral *1:*232–241, March '42
ALTEMEIER, W. A.: Hemorrhage complicating cutaneous burn (zinc peroxide therapy). Cincinnati J. Med. *23:*176–178, June '42
ALTEMEIER, W. A. AND CARTER, B.N.: Infected burns with hemorrhage. Ann. Surg. *115:*1118–1124, June '42
ALTERI: Surgical therapy of cancer of jaws. Morgagni *77:*1199–1201, Nov 10, '35
ALTMAN, H. AND TROTT, R. H.: Muscle transplant for paralysis of radial nerve. J. Bone and Joint Surg. *28:*440–446, July '46
ALTRUDA, J. B.: New instrument for taking skin grafts. M. J. and Rec. *133:*348, April 1, '31
ALTSCHUL, R. (see DE ANGELIS, E.) 1930

ALTUKHOV, P. P.: Cheap method of burn therapy. Sovet. med. (no. 6) *8:*27–28, '44
ALURRALDE, M. AND ALLENDE, C. T.: Anastomosis of facial nerve to correct contracture. Rev. Assoc. med. argent. *36:*259–266, May–June '23 (illus.) abstr: J. A. M. A. *81:*1730, Nov 17, '23
ALVAREZ, G. (see GAREISO, A.) Jan '37
ALVAREZ, G.: Progressive hemiatrophies combined with scleroderma; pathogenic study. Arch. argent. de pediat. *21:*83–94, Feb '44
ALVAREZ GRAU, J. (see APOLO, E.) 1939
ALVAREZ-ZAMORA, R. (see CAMPOS MARTIN, R. *et al*) April '43
ALVARO, M. E. AND SAMPAIO DORIA, A.: Congenital fistula of lacrimal gland, with report of case. Rev. oto-neuro-oftal. *12:*283–290, Nov '37
ALVARO, M. E. AND SAMPAIO DORIA, A.: Congenital lacrimal fistula. Cong. argent. de oftal. (1936) *2:*583–590, '38
ALVES, E.: Burn therapy. Hora med., Rio de Janeiro *2:*45–51, Aug '44
ALVES, O.: Costal graft and ivory inclusions in reconstruction of saddle nose by transsupraciliary route. Rev. oto-laring. de Sao Paulo (no. 5, bis) *4:*843–863, Sept–Oct '36
ALVES, O.: Marble inclusion by trans-superciliary route in saddle nose. Arq. de cir. clin. e exper. *6:*512–517, April–June '42
ALVES, O.: Marble implantation by transsuperciliary route in saddle nose; case. Rev. brasil. de oto-rino-laring. *7:*347–350, July–Aug '39
ALVES, O.: Nasal prosthesis to hide deformity; case. Rev. oto-laring. de Sao Paulo (no. 5, bis) *4:*873–877, Sept–Oct '36
ALVES, O.: Orbital prosthesis after Riedel operation in frontal sinusitis; case. Arq. de cir. clin. e exper. *6:*322–323, April–June '42
ALVES, O.: Partial rhinoplasty after destruction of nose by syphilis; case. Rev. oto-laring. de Sao Paulo (no. 5, bis) *4:*865–871, Sept–Oct '36
ALVES, O.: Plastic surgery of nasal deformities. Arq. de cir. clin. e exper. *6:*320–322, April–June '42
ALVES, O.: Surgical therapy of protruding ears. Arq. de cir. clin. e exper. *6:*517–519, April–June '42
ALVES, O.: Traumatic fracture of nasal septum and its therapy.Rev. oto-laring. de Sao Paulo *6:*373–378, Sept–Oct '38
ALVIS, B. Y.: Minor surgery of eyelids. Tr. Indiana Acad. Ophth. and Otolarng. *28:*78–93, '44
ALVIS, B. Y.: Operations for correction of ptosis of eyelids. Tr. Indiana Acad. Ophth. and Otolaryng. *28:*97–115, '44
AMADO, C. F.: Convalescent serum in treatment of grave burns of children; 2 cases. Semana med. *1:*1696–1698, June 2, '32
AMADON, P. D.: Electrocoagulation of melanomas and its dangers. Surg., Gynec. and Obst. *56:*943–946, May '33
AMARAL, O. AND VIEIRA FILHO, O.: Early care of facial wounds. Rev. med. brasil. *13:*111–116, July '42
AMARANTE, R. C. L. (see DE SANSON, R. D.) March '43
AMBROS, Z.: Autoplastic and heteroplastic bone grafts. Chir. narz. ruchu *10:*345–356, '37
AMELIN: Plastic closure of salivary fistula with transposed skin flaps. Khirurgiya, no. 6, pp. 43–44, '45
AMELINE, A.: Use of solution of sodium chloride, bicarbonate and thiosulfate in prevention of surgical shock. Presse med. *54:*174–175, March 16, '46
AMERICAN BOARD OF PLASTIC SURGERY, INC.: J.A.M.A. *117:*752–753, Aug 30, '41
AMERSBACH, K.: Deviation of septum with insufficient nasal respiration as indication for submucous resection; preliminary report. Arch. f. Ohren-, Nasen-u. Kehl Kopfh. *143:*241–245, '37
AMERSBACH, R. (see GLAESMER, E.) July '27
AMERSBACH, R. (see GLAESMER, E.) Sept '28
AMERSBACH, R.: Rules and experiences in operative treatment of pendulous breast. Schweiz. med. Wchnschr. *60:*974–976, Oct 11, '30
AMIES, A. (see DENEHY, W. J.) Feb '33
AMIES, A. AND BAGHEL, D.: Prosthetic appliance for atresia palati in edentulous patient. M. J. Australia *2:*600–601, Oct 31, '36
AMSLER, M.: Dacryocystorhinostomy. Schweiz. med. Wchnschr. *66:*1268–1270, Dec 12, '36
AMSLER, M.: Dacryocystorhinostomy for obstruction. Ophthalmologica *107:*50–51, Jan–Feb '44
ANAGNOSTIDIS, N.: Histologic study of effect of local application of certain medicaments in third degree burns. Deutsche Ztschr. f. Chir. *252:*248–256, '39
ANAND, H. L.: Correcting spastic entropion of upper lid following total tarsectomy, by transplanting a shaving from concha auriculae. Indian J. Ophth. *1:*20–23, Jan '40
ANARDI, T.: Deep branchiogenous cysts in right side of neck. Tumori *12:*217–225, '26

Anatomy

Anatomie medico-chirurgicale, Fascicles 2 and 3, La Face, by PHILIPPE B. BELLOCQ. Masson et Cie, Paris, 1926
La revisión de la morfología arterial en las regiones anatómicas que atañen a la oto-rino-laringología, by PEDRO BELOU. La Sociedad Argentina de Oto-rino-laringología, Buenos Aires, 1939

Anatomy – Cont.
Surgical Anatomy of the Head and Neck, by John F. Barnhill. Wm. Wood and Co., New York, 1937. Second Edition (with William J. Mellinger), 1940
The Human Face, by Max Picard (translated from the German by G. Endore). Cassell and Co., London, 1942
Anatomy of the Head and Neck, by Robert T. Hill. Lea and Febiger Co., Phila., 1946

Andersen, Poul Fogh: Harelip and cleft palate. Nord. med. *19:*1597–1598, Sept 25, '43
Andersen, Poul Fogh: Harelip and cleft palate; 1,000 patients submitted to operation. Acta chir. Scandinav. *94:*213–242, '46
Andersen, Poul Fogh: *Inheritance of Harelip and Cleft Palate*. Nyt Nordisk Forlag Arnold Busck, Copenhagen, 1942
Andersen, Poul Fogh: Surgical therapy of harelip and cleft palate in Denmark. Ugesk. f. Laeger *101:*1187–1193, Oct 12, '39
Andersen, V. F.: Surgical therapy of harelip in Denmark; results of 4 years of using Veau method. Plast. chir. *1:*35–38, '39
Anderson, B. G.: Jaw fractures. Connecticut M. J. *6:*799–805, Oct '42
Anderson, C. B. C. and Douglas, J. P.: Burns due to explosion. J. Roy. Army M. Corps *70:*168–177, March '38
Anderson, C. M.: Congenital occlusion of choana. J. A. M. A. *109:*1788–1792, Nov 27, '37
Anderson, C. M.: Congenital occlusion of choana. Tr. Sect. Laryng., Otol. and Rhin., J.A.M.A., pp. 83–97, '37
Anderson, C. M.: Further observations on prevention with insulin-glucose in shock. Anesth. and Analg. *1:*346–353, Nov–Dec '28
Anderson, C. M.: Use of glucose and insulin in prevention of surgical shock. California and West. Med. *27:*56–61, July '27
Anderson, E. R.: Clinical aspects of branchial fistulas, with case report of bilateral complete fistulas. Minnesota Med. *25:*789–795, Oct '42
Anderson, G. M.: Maintenance of facial form after removal of right half of mandible. Internat. J. Orthodontia *17:*860–864, Sept '31
Anderson, G. V. W.: Artificial vagina. East African M. J. *12:*377–378, March '36
Anderson, N. P.: Epithelioma of lip; case from Postgraduate Hospital, New York City. Physical Therap. *46:*350–352, July '28
Anderson, T. F. and Roberts, M. A. W.: Treatment of ulcers with skin grafts. East African M. J. *9:*79–83, June '32
Anderson, W. D.: Dislocations of thumb. M. Press *208:*158, Sept 2, '42
Anderson, W. S.: Full thickness skin grafts in injured fingers; 2 cases. Memphis M. J. *17:*23–24, Feb '42
Andersson, O. J.: Practical and easily prepared finger splint. Svenska lak.-tidning. *32:*1776–1777, Dec 20, '35
Andina, F.: Plastic closure of tissue defects in region of lower leg. Zentralbl. f. Chir. *70:*682, May 8, '43
Andina, M.: Technical points suggesting dacryocystorhinostomy. Rev. cubana de oft. *1:*424–426, Nov '29
Andre, R. H.: Treatment of shock in urologic surgery. S. Clin. North America *20:*431–438, April '40
Andreasen, A.: Section of flexor tendons of middle finger of left hand through palmar wound; primary suture and cure. J. Bone and Joint Surg. *14:*700–701, July '32
Andreassen, M.: Operative treatment of hypertrophy of breast; description of new method. Ugesk. f. laeger *103:*608–613, May 8, '41
Andreesen, R.: Manifestations of fatigue (necrosis and pseudarthrosis) of carpal scaphoid bone caused by chronic trauma (work with pneumatic tools). Fortschr. a. d. Geb. d. Rontgenstrahlen *60:*253–263, Oct '39
Andren, G.: Radium treatment of haemangiomata, lymphangiomata and naevi pigmentosi. Experiences from "Radium-hemmet," 1909–1924. Acta radiol. *8:*1–45, '27
Andreon, E.: Perisynovial phlegmons in hand; cases. Arch. urug. de med., cir. y especialid. *17:*80–83, July '40
Andreon, E.: Therapy of acute hand infections. Arch. urug. de med., cir. y especialid. *14:*567–575, June '39
Andreucci, A.: Ectrodactylia and syndactylia; case. Monitore zool. ital. *27:*289–296, Dec 30, '26
Andrews, E.: Surgical shock. Northwest Med. *34:*122–126, April '35
Andrews, G. C. and Kelly, R. J.: Treatment of vascular nevi by injection of sclerosing solutions. Arch. Dermat. and Syph. *26:*92–94, July '32
Andresen, V.: "Norwegian system" of functional orthopedics of jaw deformities. Ztschr. f. Stomatol. *35:*664–678, May 28, '37
Andrievskiy, B. Y.: Clinical application of salt solutions in shock. Novy khir. arkhiv *37:*580–588, '37
Andrus, W. De W. (see Dingwall, J. A. III) 1944
Andrus, W. De W. (see Dingwall, J. A. III) Sept '44
Andrus, W. De W.: Present concepts of origin and treatment of traumatic shock; collective review. Internat. Abstr. Surg. *75:*161–175, '42; in Surg., Gynec. and Obst. Aug '42

ANDRUS, W. DE W. AND DINGWALL, J. A. III.: Sulfonamide-impregnated membranes; further experience. Ann. Surg. *119:*694-699, May '44

ANDRUS, W. DE W., NICKEL, W. F., AND SCHMELKES, F. C.: Burn therapy; chemotherapeutic membranes containing sulfanilamide, sulfonamide, with and without azochloramid, hypochlorite derivative. Arch. Surg. *46:*1-8, Jan '43

Anesthesia

General versus local anesthesia in operations on nose and throat. WATSON, W. R. New York M. J. *113:*444, March 16, '21

Blocking nerve for lower jaw surgery. DE VRIES, J. J. Nederlandsch Tijdschr. f. Geneesk. *1:*197-200, Jan 14, '22

Plastic surgery of head, face and neck, local anesthesia in operations upon head, face and neck. TIECK, G. J. E. *et al.* Am. J. Surg. *36:*29-42, Feb '22 (illus.)

New local anesthetic for nose and throat work. BULSON, A. E. JR. Ann. Otol. Rhinol. and Laryngol. *31:*131-136, March '22

General anesthesia in submucous and other nasal operations. POE, J. G. Am. J. Surg. (Anesthesia supp.) *37:*56-57, April '23

Anesthesia and shock. DE WAELE, H. Compt. rend. Soc. de biol. *91:*909-910, Oct 24, '24

Block anesthesia in nasal surgery. PARSONS, J. G. Northwest Med. *24:*223-227, May '25

Reposition of dislocated mandible under local anesthesia. KULENKAMPFF, D. Munchen. med. Wchnschr. *72:*2229, Dec 25, '25

Reposition of dislocated mandible in local anesthesia. HÖRHAMMER, C. Munchen. med. Wchnschr. *73:*446-447, March 12, '26

Local anaesthesia in submucous resection of nasal septum. STURM, F. P. Brit. M. J. *1:*720, April 16, '27

Local anaesthesia in submucous resection of nasal septum. MCKELVIE, B. Brit. M. J. *1:*920, May 21, '27

Essential facts in connection with use of local anesthesia in nose and throat surgery. GATEWOOD, W. L. Virginia M. Monthly *54:*163-166, June '27

Rectal anesthesia in facial surgery. JACOD, M. Ann. d. mal. de l'oreille, du larynx *46:*583-586, June '27

Topical application of cocaine in nose. HOWARD, E. F. New Orleans M. and S. J. *80:*162-167, Sept '27

New methods of anesthetizing jaws and face. LINDEMANN, A. Narkose u. Anaesth. *1:*3-16, Jan 15, '28

Anesthesia – Cont.

Simplified maxillary anesthesia. HARTSTEIN, S. D. Am. Dent. Surgeon *48:*90, Feb '28

Accidents in conduction anesthesia of sphenopalatine ganglion; 4 cases. ULLMANN, S. Ztschr. f. Hals-, Nasen-u. Ohrenh. *21:*587-595, May 10, '28

Resection under local anesthesia of lower part of jaw, with integrity of nasal membrane; case. HEYNINX, A. Ann. d. mal. de l'oreille, du larynx *47:*996, Nov '28

Morphine-scopolamine narco-anaesthesia in nasal surgery. THACKER NEVILLE, W. S. Proc. Roy. Soc. Med. (Sect. Laryng.) *22:*61-64, Sept '29

Neotonocain (procaine preparation) in surgery of fingers. STEOPOE, V. Romania med. *7:*245, Nov 15, '29

Depth of action of percaine solution by application to mucous membrane of nose in surgical anesthesia. BIRKHOLZ. Klin. Wchnschr. *9:*72, Jan 11, '30

General anesthesia for nasal surgery. FORBES, S. B. South. M. J. *23:*305-308, April '30

Anesthesia in operations on face and neck. GUISEZ, J. Ann. d. mal. de l'orcillc, du larynx *49:*516-524, May '30

Novacain (procaine hydrochloride) applied topically as local anesthetic in nasal surgery; preliminary report. NEFF, E. AND DIMOND, W. B. Ann. Otol., Rhin. and Laryng. *39:*593-594, June '30

Plastic surgery of nose by Italian method under general ether anesthesia by peritoneal route with J. B. Abalos' technic; case. NATALE, A. M. AND BARBERIS, J. C. Rev. med. del Rosario *20:*487-489, Oct '30

Freezing of facial nerve in treatment of harelip. GOETZE, O. Zentralbl. f. Chir. *58:*927-930, April 11, '31

Intrapharyngeal nitrous oxide insufflation in staphylorrhaphy. NYST, P. M. E. P. Nederl. tijdschr. v. geneesk. *75:*2059-2061, April 18, '31

Local anesthesia in nasal septal surgery. SONNTAG, A. Ztschr. f. Laryng., Rhin. *21:*32-36, June '31

Deep block anesthesia of second and third divisions of fifth nerve. BROWN, J. B. Surg., Gynec. and Obst. *53:*832-835, Dec '31

Deep block anesthesia of second and third divisions of fifth nerve. BROWN, J. B. Internat. J. Orthodontia *18:*193-199, Feb '32

Anesthetization in burns. LAQUEUR, B. Therap. d. Gegenw. *73:*144, March '32

Plastic preparation of nose; preliminary report on new local anesthetic. STRAATSMA,

Anesthesia – Cont.
C. R., M. J. and Rec. *135:*399–400, April 20, '32
Inhalation anesthesia with chlorylene (trichloroethylene) in plastic surgery of face. KELLER, P. Dermat. Wchnschr. *95:*973–985, July 2, '32
Cleft palate repair, with notes on administration of anesthetics. MITCHELL, A. AND MACKENZIE, J. R. Brit. J. Surg. *20:*214–219, Oct '32
Regional anesthesia with solution of procaine hydrochloride and epinephrine in surgery of fingers. DE ROUGEMONT, J. AND CARCASSONNE, F. Presse med. *41:*218–220, Feb 8, '33
Rectal anesthesia with tribrom-ethanol in cervicofacial surgery; indications, technic, results and experimental studies. MOULONGUET, A. AND LEROUX-ROBERT, J. Ann. d'oto-laryng., pp. 283–304, March '34
Cleft lip repair under bilateral infra-orbital nerve block at infra-orbital foramina. NYI, P. C. Chinese M. J. *48:*373–384, April '34
Rectal anesthesia with mixture of ether, tribromethanol and oil in cervicofacial surgery. JACOD, M. Lyon chir. *32:*35–42, Jan–Feb '35
Method of local anesthesia for intranasal operations. LANE, F. F., U. S. Nav. M. Bull. *33:*55–59, Jan '35
Local anesthesia with procaine hydrochloride as anesthesia of choice in operations on upper maxilla. AUBRY, M. Presse med. *43:*592, April 10, '35
Anesthesia in plastic surgery of nose. ERCZY, M. Orvosi hetil. *79:*641–643, June 8, '35
Rectal anesthesia with mixture of ether, tribromethanol and oil in cervicofacial surgery. JACOD, M. Ann. d'oto-laryng., pp. 802–808, July '35
Regional anesthesia of breast with procaine hydrochloride in plastic surgery. BRETECHE, *et al.* Bull. med., Paris *49:*685–686, Oct 5, '35
Simplified method of local anesthesia for removal of sebaceous cysts. HAVENS, F. Z., S. Clin. North America *15:*1230–1232, Oct '35
Technic of local anesthesia for total extirpation of parotid gland. FINOCHIETTO, R. AND DICKMANN, G. H. Semana med. *2:*1349–1352, Nov 7, '35
Local anesthesia in total excision of parotid. GUTIERREZ, A. Rev. de cir. de Buenos Aires *15:*288–292, May '36
Potassium bromide as anesthetic in facial orbital surgery. KHRAMELASHVILI, N. G. Sovet. vrach. zhur., pp. 667–678, May 15, '36

Anesthesia – Cont.
Necrosis of finger tips following use of local anesthetic in operation for contracture; study of epinephrine toxicity. HANKE, H. Chirurg *8:*684–687, Sept 1, '36
Endotracheal anesthesia supplementing avertin (tribrom-ethanol) in cleft palate operations. LEIGH, M. D. AND FITZGERALD, R. R. Canad. M. A. J. *35:*427–428, Oct '36
Injection anesthesia for submucous resection. LIEBERMANN, T. Budapesti orvosi ujsag *34:*831–832, Oct 1, '36
Selection of anesthetic in cases of jaw fracture. WEISENGREEN, H. H., J. Bone and Joint Surg. *18:*1005–1007, Oct '36
Local anesthesia in plastic surgery of vagina. DE ARAGON, E. R. Vida nueva *39:*272–275, April 15, '37
Anesthesia (endotracheal oxygen-ether vapor) for harelip and cleft palate operations on babies. AYRE, P. Brit. J. Surg. *25:*131–132, July '37
Avertin (tribrom-ethanol) in reduction of facial fractures. FENNELLY, W. A., J. Am. Dent. A. *24:*1089–1104, July '37
Discussion on choice and technic of anesthetics for nasal surgery. LAYTON, T. B. *et al.* J. Laryng. and Otol. *52:*501–512, July '37
Endotracheal anesthesia for babies with cleft palate. AYRE, P. Anesth. and Analg. *16:*330–333, Nov–Dec '37
Injection anesthesia for submucous resection. LIEBERMANN, T. Ztschr. f. Hals, Nasen-u. Ohrenh. *41:*290, '37
Intranasal procaine anesthesia in nasal surgery. LEAMER, B. V., U. S. Nav. M. Bull. *36:*498–499, Oct '38
Anesthesia of inferior maxillary nerve by way of zygoma in jaw surgery. POPESCU, G. AND PRICORIU, S. Rev. san. mil., Bucuresti *37:*873–875, Oct '38
Blocking and forming of nose in child aged 4. DUJARDIN, E. Ugesk. f. laeger *101:*211–212, Feb 16, '39
Surgical treatment under regional anesthesia for harelip. GINESTET, G. AND GINESTET, F. Rev. de stomatol. *31:*212, April '29
Reduction of blocked temporomaxillary luxation under regional transmasseteric anesthesia. LEBOURG, L. Presse med. *47:*872, May 31, '39
Nerve trunk anesthesia of nasal cavity. GATTI-MANACINI. Arch. ital. di otol. *51:*495–512, Oct '39
Methods for producing local anesthesia for intranasal operations. LILLIE, H. I. *et al.* Ann. Otol., Rhin. and Laryng. *49:*38–51, March '40

Anesthesia – Cont.
Local anesthesia of distal half of forearm and of hand. FINOCHIETTO, R. AND ZAVALETA, D. E. Rev. med. y cien. afines *2:*295-297, May 30, '40
Anesthesia for faciomaxillary surgery. MUSHIN, W. W. Post-Grad. M. J. *16:*245-246, July '40
Preanesthetic medication with special consideration of problems in maxillofacial surgery. LYMAN, E. E. Mil. Surgeon *88:*57-62, Jan '41
Procaine hydrochloride truncular anesthesia of nerves of nasal lobule; technic. MAGGIOROTTI, U. Boll. d. mal. d. orecchio, d. gola, d. naso *59:*17-18, Jan '41
Regional anesthesia of head and neck. MOUSEL, L. H. Anesthesiology *2:*61-73, Jan '41
Procaine hydrochloride block of phrenic nerve in therapy of postoperative complications, with report of case of autoplastic repair of face. PENIDO BURNIER, E. M. Rev. med.-cir. do Brasil *49:*53-68, Feb '41
Anesthesia for harelip surgery during infancy. SPAID, J. D., J. Indiana M. A. *34:*143-145, March '41
General anesthesia for jaw casualties. HAUGEN, F. P. Mil. Surgeon *89:*70-80, July '41
Regional anesthesia for operations about neck. ADAMS, R. C. Anesthesiology *2:*515-529, Sept '41
Problem of anesthesia in surgery of temporomaxillary joint. MONDADORI, E. C. F. An. paulist. de med. e cir. *42:*227-230, Sept '41
Review of local anesthesia in maxillofacial cases. O'HARA, D. M. Mil. Surgeon *89:*652-656, Oct '41
Intratracheal anesthesia for surgery of head. THORSON, J. A., J. Iowa M. Soc. *31:*465-472, Oct '41
Anesthesia for surgery about head. EVERSOLE, U. H., J.A.M.A. *117:*1760-1764, Nov 22, '41
Branchial plexus block anesthesia (procaine hydrochloride) in operations on upper extremity. PATRICK, J. Tr. Roy. Med.-Chir. Soc. Glasgow, pp. 39-45, '40-'41; in Glasgow M. J. Nov '41
General anesthesia in treatment of maxillofacial cases. FISCHER, T. E. Mil. Surgeon *89:*877-892, Dec '41
Postural instillation; method of inducing local anesthesia. MOFFETT, A. J., J. Laryng. and Otol. *56:*429-436, Dec '41
Block of branches of trigeminal nerve for surgery. PLAZA, F. L. Jorn. neuro-psiquiat. panam., actas (1939) *2:*104-112, '41
Protection of surgeon against anesthetic gases while performing plastic surgery on cleft palate. REBELO NETO, J. Arq. de cir. clin. e exper. *6:*641-645, April-June '42
Choice of anesthesia for maxillofacial surgery in war and civilian injuries. MARVIN, F. W. Am. J. Orthodontics (Oral Surg. Sect) *28:*254-257, May '42
Nasal surgery – local anesthesia; technic and practical considerations. HOOVER, W. B., S. Clin. North America *22:*661-673, June '42
Practical points in anesthesia at maxillofacial unit. HUNTER, J. T. Anesth. and Analg. *21:*223-228, July-Aug '42
Problems of anesthesia in plastic surgery. GORDON, R. A. Anesthesiology *3:*507-513, Sept '42
Shock and anesthesia. HARKINS, H. N. Anesth. and Analg. *21:*273-279, Sept-Oct '42
Burns and explosions in anesthesia. EHLERS, G. Deutsche Ztschr. f. Chir. *255:*485-522, '42
Brachial plexus block anesthesia of upper extremities. GRISWOLD, R. A. AND WOODSON, W. H. Am. J. Surg. *59:*439-443, Feb '43
Trichloroethylene anesthesia in plastic surgery. GORDON, R. A. AND SHACKLETON, R. P. W. Brit. M. J. *1:*380-381, March 27, '43
Nitrous oxide-oxygen anesthesia; endotracheal technic in oromaxillofacial surgery. TYLER, E. A. Anesth. and Analg. *22:*177-179, May-June '43
Anatomic considerations in local anesthesia of jaws. PHILLIPS, W. H., J. Oral Surg. *1:*112-121, April '43
Twilight sleep in plastic surgery. FINE, A. Eye, Ear, Nose and Throat Monthly *22:*342-343, Sept '43
Intravenous novocain (procaine hydrochloride) for analgesia in burns; preliminary report. GORDON, R. A. Canad. M. A. J. *49:*478-481, Dec '43
Topical use of medicated (with sulfanilamide, sulfonamide) human plasma in burns. ABBOTT, M. D. AND GEPFERT, J. R. U. S. Nav. M. Bull. *42:*193-194, Jan '44
Local regional anesthesia in nose and throat operations. MARTIN, G. E., J. Laryng. and Otol. *59:*38-43, Jan '44
Economy in use of cocaine, by Moffett method of postural instillation. CLARKE, L. T., J. Roy. Army M. Corps. *82:*135-137, March '44
Anesthesia in otorhinolaryngology. CULLEN, S. C. Tr. Am. Acad. Ophth. (1943) *48:*240-247, March-April '44
Extranasal block anesthesia for submucous

Anesthesia – Cont.
resection. FRED, G. B. Ann. Otol., Rhin. and Laryng. *53:*127–132, March '44
Anesthesia in fractures of jaws. SHACKLETON, R. P. W. Lancet *1:*396–398, March 25, '44
Principles of anesthesia in plastic surgery. APGAR, V., S. Clin. North America *24:*474–479, April '44
Regional anesthesia of nose. DALE, H. W. L. Lancet *1:*562–563, April 29, '44
Postural instillation (for induction of local anesthesia); added note. MOFFETT, A. J., J. Laryng. and Otol. *59:*151–153, April '44
Ethyl chloride spray for freezing donor area for skin grafting. GASTON, J. H., J. M. A. Georgia *33:*151, May '44
Brachial plexus block anesthesia; improved technic. MURPHEY, D. R. JR. Ann. Surg. *119:*935–943, June '44
Monocaine hydrochloride; clinical experiences and technic of administration in rhinoplasty. BERSON, M. I. Anesth. and Analg. *23:*189–195, Sept–Oct '44
Anesthesia by procaine hydrochloride block of cervical plexus in neck surgery. FINOCHIETTO, R. Prensa med. argent. *31:*1757–1760, Sept 6, '44
Local anesthesia in burn therapy. RIVAS DIEZ, B. AND DELRIO, J. M. A. Bol. y trab., Acad. argent. de cir. *28:*1182–1192, Nov 22, '44
Anesthesia (topical anesthesia and administration of pentothal sodium, barbital derivative, before intratracheal use of nitrous oxide and oxygen) for oral surgery in presence of cautery and diathermy. ELLIOT, H. L. AND ARROWOOD, J. G. Anesthesiology *6:*32–38, Jan '45
Anesthesia for patient in burn therapy. PAPPER, E. M. Surgery *17:*116–121, Jan '45
Orotracheal anesthesia for cheiloplasty. SLOCUM, H. C. AND ALLEN, C. R. Anesthesiology *6:*355–358, July '45
Preanesthetic sedation in plastic surgery. ARESPACOCHAGA, F. E. Semana med. *2:*375–376, Sept 6, '45
Local anesthesia with nupercaine in reconstructive surgery. PARINA, G. A. Khirurgiya, no. 1, pp. 25–27, '45
Anesthesia in maxillofacial surgical unit with British Liberation Army. THORNTON, H. L. AND ROWBOTHAM, S. Anesthesiology *6:*580–596, Nov '45
Anesthesia of recent injuries of jaw and face. ROCHE, G. K. T. Anesthesiology *7:*233–254, May '46
Vinesthene (vinyl ether) anesthesia for repair of harelip and cleft palate. DAPLYN, P. F. L. Brit. M. J. *2:*117–119, July 27, '46
Anesthetic management in reconstructive surgery of mandible. PAPPER, E. M. AND ROVENSTINE, E. A. Am. J. Orthodontics (Oral Surg. Sect.) *32:*433–438, Jul '46
Precise technic of local anesthesia in rhinoplasties. MALBEC, E. F., J. Internat. Coll. Surgeons *9:*495–505, Jul–Aug '46 also: Prensa med. argent. *33:*1594–1601, Aug 2, '46
Anesthesia in Plastic Surgery Unit Canadian Army Overseas. GORDON, R. A. Bull. Acad. Med., Toronto *19:*233–237, Aug '46
Anesthesia during surgical therapy of cleft palate. LOMBARD, P. Presse med. *54:*566, Aug 31, '46
Anesthesia for oropharyngeal surgery. PERNWORTH, P. H. Anesth. and Analg. *25:*200–203, Sept–Oct '46

Anesthesia Complications

Ocular complications from local anesthesia in resection of upper jaw. DORON, G. Zentralbl. f. Chir. *54:*2966–2969, Nov 19, '27
Necrotic ulcer from cocaine-epinephrine injections; 2 cases. QUINTARELLI, L. Ann. di med. nav. *1:*67–75, Jan–Feb '27
Tetany following use of cocaine and epinepherine in nasal surgery; observations and treatment; preliminary report. ROBERTS, S. E. Tr. Sect. Laryng., Otol. and Rhin., A. M. A., pp. 22–30, '29
Acute pulmonary edema in course of local anesthesia for deviation of nasal septum; case. VAN DEN BOSSCHE, P. Ann. d. mal. de l'oreille, du larynx *49:*983–995, Oct '30
Complications of local anesthesia in surgery of nasal septum. ZIEGLER, E. Ztschr. f. Hals-, Nasen-u. Ohrenh. *32:*476–479, '33
Extensive cerebral changes in case of "sudden" death following plastic transfer of skin or neck under local anesthesia. CAMMERMEYER, J. Acta path. et microbiol. Scandinav. *15:*307–329, '38
Accidents to septum in anesthesia with novocain (procaine hydrochloride) in nose. LEDERER, L. Arch. f. Ohren-, Nasen-u. Kehlkopfh. *150:*162–167, '41

ANGIELOWICZ, (see FRIEDEL, C. *et al*) July '37
ANGLESIO, B.: Plastic surgery of thumb and of thenar region. Boll. e mem. Soc. piemontese di chir. *6:*64–72, '36
ANGULO, A. W. (see ELY, J. O.) Feb '43
ANNECCHINO, A.: Macrodactyly; case. Pediatria *49:*162–166, March '41

Annovazzi, G.: Sixteen years maintenance of autoplastic bone graft; case. Clin. chir. *31:*1051–1081, Oct '28

Anokhin, P. K. (see Grashchenkov, N. I. P.) 1942

Anselmo, J. J. (see Martinez Cordoba, F. *et al*) Aug '43

Anson, B. J. (see Mason, M. L. *et al*) Jan '40

Anson, B. J. (see McCormack, L. J. *et al*) Jan '45

Anson, B. J. and Ashley, F. L.: Midpalmar compartment, associated spaces and limiting layers. Anat. Rec. *78:*389–407, Nov 25, '40

Antelava, N. V.: Plastic operations for covering cutaneous defects following soft tissue wounds. Khirurgiya, no. 6, pp. 40–43, '45

Antonetti, H.: Grave postoperative hemorrhages; pathogenesis of late hemorrhages and their treatment by shock. Presse med. *39:*1766–1768, Dec 2, '31

Antonioli, G. M. (see Serafini, G.) 1926

Antonioli, G. M.: Facial paralysis treated by spino-facial anastomosis; 2 cases. Gior. d. r. Accad. di med. di Torino *33:*80–88, Feb '27

Antonioli, G. M.: Clinical and histological study of Dupuytren's contracture. Ann. ital. di chir. *6:*1011–1037, Oct '27

Antonioli, G. M. (see Serafini, G.) Jan–March '28

Antonioli, G. M.: Surgery of traumatic facial paralysis. Clin. chir. *31:*81–104, Feb '28

Antos, R. J.; Dworkin, R. M. and Green, H. D.: Shock associated with deep muscle burns. Proc. Soc. Exper. Biol. and Med. *57:*11–13, Oct '44

Anus

Cicatricial contracture of buttocks nearly occluding anus; plastic operation on buttocks. Ashhurst, A. P. C., S. Clin. N. America *2:*77–79, Feb '22 (illus.)

Annular stricture of rectum and anus; treatment by tunnel skin graft; preliminary report. Keller, W. L. Am. J. Surg. *20:*28–32, April '33

Plastic surgery of anal canal after unsuccessful Whitehead operation. Fischer, A. W. Zentralbl. f. Chir. *61:*157–159, Jan 20, '34

Plastic repair of patulous anus by means of fascia lata strips. Cato, E. Australian and New Zealand J. Surg. *4:*315–317, Jan '35

Plastic surgery of anus; using fatty flap of bulbocavernosus muscle, in therapy of incontinence of feces, following transplantation of vestibular anus; case. Holtermann, C. Zentralbl. f. Gynak. *63:*60–66, Jan 7, '39

Congenital vaginal and anal atresia. Sigwart, W. Geburtsh. u. Frauneh. *2:*628–635, Dec '40

Anus—Cont.

Results with fascia plastic operation for incontinence of anus. Stone, H. G. and McLanahan, S. Ann. Surg. *114:*73–77, July '41

Utilization of pedicle skin grafts in correction of cicatricial stenosis of anus. Cole, W. H. and Greeley, P. W. Surgery *12:*349–354, Sept '42

New operation for atresia ani vaginalis. Murdoch, R. L. Tr. Am. Proct. Soc. (1941) *42:*274–285, '42

Radical operation for intractable pruritis ani (skin transplantation). Young, F. and Scott, W. J. M. Surgery *13:*911–915, June '43

Plastic use of skin in simple anal stricture; reconstruction of anal lining; pilonidal disease. Martin, E. G. Clinics *3:*1011–1013, Dec '44

Operative treatment of anal stricture (modification of Young operation). Joseph, E. S. Acta med. orient. *4:*312–313, Sept '45

Atresia, surgical therapy of case of anal. Malucelli, O. An. paulist. de med. e cir. *51:*193–197, Mar '46

Therapy of anus atresia. Harrenstein, R.J. Nederl. tijdschr. v. geneesk. *90:*698–700, June 22, '46

Malformation of anus and rectum. Rosenblatt, M. S. and May, A. Surg., Gynec. and Obst. *83:*499–506, Oct '46

Anus, Imperforate

Persistent cloaca with imperforate anus as a cause of foetal ascites. Cruickshank, J. N. Brit. M. J. *2:*980, Dec 10, '21

Imperforate anus; case report. Wathen, J. R. Kentucky M. J. *19:*827, Dec '21

Imperforate anus; report of case. Brunemeier, E. H. China M. J. *37:*748–749, Sept '23

Embryologic study of case of exstrophy of bladder with umbilical hernia and aplasia of anus and rectum. Garcia, C. L. Semana med. *1:*347–355, Feb 22, '23 (illus.)

Treatment of imperforate anus. Desmarest, E. and Ebrard, D. Arch. de med. d. enf. *29:*96–101, Feb '26

Imperforate anus; surgical treatment of cases of maldevelopment of terminal bowel and anus. Fitchet, S. M. Boston M. and S. J. *195:*25–31, July 1, '26

Imperforate anus; case. Garrido-Lestache, J. Pediatria espan. *15:*273–275, Sept '26

Surgical treatment of congenital anal atre-

Anus, Imperforate—Cont.
sia. KUTTER, A. Beitr. z. klin. Chir. *138:*756-763, '26
Congenital case of recto-urethral fistula with imperforate anus. DOTTI, S. Gazz. med. lomb. *86:*41-44, March 25, '27
Imperforate anus; case. MUKERJI, S. N. Indian M. Gazz. *62:*521-522, Sept '27
Surgical treatment of imperforate anus; with report of case. BELL, L. P. Am. J. Obst. and Gynec. *14:*603-608, Nov '27
Unusual developmental abnormalities (including imperforate anus). (epispadias). THOMAS, A. K. Brit. M. J. *2:*985-986, Nov 26, '27
Urinary obstruction caused by distended sigmoid associated with imperforate anus. ADAMS, E. H. Atlantic M. J. *31:*311-312, Feb '28
Imperforate anus; case. MAN, I. Indian M. Gaz. *43:*81-82, Feb '28
Complete imperforation of anus in new-born; operation. GALY-GASPARROU, *et al.* Bull. Soc. d'obst. et de gynec. *17:*335, March '28
Imperforate anus with persistent cloacal duct. KILFOY, E. J. Ann. Surg. *91:*151-154, Jan '30
Imperforate anus. BROWN, C. F. China M. J. *43:*274-277, March '29
Vaginal fistula with anal atresia; case. VECCHIONE, F. Gazz. internaz. med.-chir. *37:*255-260, April 30, '29
Imperforate anus, with exit through prostatic urethra; 3 cases. HELWIG, F. C. Am. J. Dis. Child. *38:*559-561, Sept '29
Late results of imperforate anus operation. SATANOWSKY, S. Arch. argent. de pediat. *4:*25-29, Jan '33
Imperforate anus. CURTIS, G. M. AND KREDEL, F. E. Ohio State M. J. *29:*183-184, March '33
Imperforate anus with communication between rectal ampulla and bladder; case. MARRIQ, AND FAURE, MME. Bull. Soc. med.-chir. de l'Indochine *13:*150-151, Feb-March '35
Congenital anorectal imperforation; case. RUEDA MAGRO, G. Rev. med. veracruzana *15:*1544-1546, July 1, '35
Ectopia vesicae, imperforate rectum and anus, true hermaphroditism and other anomalies. POTTER, A. H. Am. J. Surg. *31:*172-178, Jan '36
Imperforate anus, plastic repair. ROSENAK, I. Zentralbl. f. Chir. *63:*2235-2238, Sept 19, '36
Imperforate anus, bowel opening into urethra; hypospadias; presentation of new

Anus, Imperforate—Cont.
plastic methods. YOUNG, H. H., J.A.M.A. *107:*1448-1451, Oct 31, '36
Use of prepuce to epithelialize tract in treatment of imperforate anus. DAVISON, T. C. South. Surgeon *7:*68-70, Feb '38
Therapy of imperforate anus in new-born infants. PETIT, P. Semaine d. hop. de Paris *16:*38-42, Feb '40
Imperforate anus in 12 year-old girl; case. GRAF, W. J., J. Med. *21:*82-83, April '40
Two-stage operation for imperforate anus. LISTON, J. J. Brit. M. J. *1:*852, May 25, '40
Imperforate anus, intrinsic congenital malformations. STRODE, J. E. Proc. Staff Meet. Clin., Honolulu *7:*1-7, March (pt. 2) '41
Two cases of imperforate anus. MCCREADY, I. A. J. Brit. M. J. *1:*290, Feb 26, '44

ANZILOTTI, G.: Precancer lesion of lip. Riforma med. *38:*411-413, May 1, '22
ANZINGER, F. P.: Congenital absence of right ear with cleft of left upper eyelid. Ohio State M. J. *19:*869-870, Dec '23
APERT: Acrocephalosyndactylia. Bull. et mem. Soc. med. d. hop. de Par. *47:*1669-1672, Dec 7, '23
APERT, E.: Hereditary contracture of palmar fascia; efficiency of radium emanation. Bull. et mem. Soc. med. d. hop. de Paris *49:*1502-1505, Nov 27, '25 abstr: J.A.M.A. *86:*380, Jan 30, '26
APERT, AND REGNAULT, F.: Acrocephalic dysostosis; study of cranium of patient with acrocephalosyndactylia. Bull. et mem. Soc. med. d. hop. de Paris *53:*832-835, July 1, '29
APERT, E. *et al:* Acrocephalosyndactylia. Bull. et mem. Soc. med. d. hop. de Par. *47:*1672-1675, Dec 7, '23

Apert's Syndrome

Acrocephalosyndactylia. APERT. Bull. et mem. Soc. med. d. hop. de Par. *47:*1669-1672, Dec 7, '23
Acrocephalosyndactylia. APERT, *et al.* Bull. et mem. Soc. med. d. hop. de Par. *47:*1672-1675, Dec 7, '23
Acrocephaly associated with syndactylism, with report of case. LANGMANN, A. G. Arch. Pediat. *41:*699-706, Oct '24
Acrocephalosyndactylia. DE BRUIN, J. Nederl. Tijdschr. v. Geneesk. *2:*2380-2393, Nov 28, '25 also: Acta Paediat. *5:*280-293, '26 abstr: J.A.M.A. *86:*456, Feb 6, '26
Acrocephalosyndactylia; case. DE TONI, G. Pediatria *34:*1305-1309, Dec 1, '26
Syndactylia with acrocephaly; case. BIANCHINI, A. Radiol. med. *14:*1-12, Jan '27

Apert's Syndrome—Cont.
Combined acrocephaly and syndactylism occurring in mother and daughter; case report. WEECH, A. A. Bull. Johns Hopkins Hosp. *40:*73–76, Feb '27
Acrocephalosyndactylia; 2 cases. REUSS, A. Wien. med. Wchnschr. *77:*1208, Sept 3, '27
Acrocephalosyndactylia; clinical study with description of recent case (roentgen examination by Prof. Lars Edling). WIGERT, V. Svenska Lak.-Sallsk. Handl. *53:*91–112, '27
Roentgen ray findings in case of acrocephaly with syndactylia. ROVIDA, F. Gass. med. lomb. *87:*49–56, April 10, '28
Acrocephaly with associated syndactylism. BOSTOCK, J., M. J. Australia *1:*572–574, May 12, '28
Acrocephalosyndactylia with postneurotic atrophy of optic nerves. BUSSOLA, E. Riv. oto-neuro-oft. *5:*503–520, Nov–Dec '28
Acrocephalosyndactylia and ocular hypertelorism; 2 cases. JANSEN, M. Nederl. Tijdschr. v. Geneesk. *2:*5864–5867, Nov 24, '28
Acrocephalosyndactylia; case. BONABA, J. AND BAUZÁ, J. A. Rev. de med., Rosairo *3:*419–424, Dec '28
Dysostosis with acrocephalosyndactylia; case. LESNÉ, E. *et al*. Bull. Soc. de pediat. de Paris *26:*488–495, Dec '28
Acrocephalosyndactylia; case. ROMAGNA MANOIA, A. Riv. di antropol. *28:*165–188, '28–'29
Acrocephalosyndactylia in brother and sister. CHRISTIANSEN, T. Hospitalstid. *72:*178–184, Feb 14, '29
Acrocephalosyndactylia in brother and sister. NORVIG, J. Hospitalstid. *72:*165–178, Feb 14, '29
Acrocephalic dysostosis; study of cranium of patient with acrocephalosyndactylia. APERT, AND REGNAULT, F. Bull. et mem. Soc. med. d. hop. de Paris *52:*832–835, July 1, '29
Acrocephalosyndactylia; 2 cases. CAUSSADE, L. AND NICOLAS. Paris med. *2:*399–402, Nov 2, '29
Acrocephalosyndactylia, a general malformation of bony system. EDLING, L. Acta radiol., supp. 3, pars 2, pp. 70–71, '29
Pathogenic theories in typical case of acrocephalosyndactylia; case. VALENTINI, P. Clin. pediat. *13:*211–222, March '31
Acrocephalosyndactylia; case. FLINKER, A. Virchows Arch. f. path. Anat. *280:*546–553, '31
Acrocephalosyndactylism; case. JOHNSTONE, G. G. Lancet *2:*15–16, July 2, '32

Apert's Syndrome—Cont.
Acrocephalosyndactylia (Apert syndrome). PLUCIŃSKI, K. Ginek. polska *11:*661–676, July–Sept '32
Hereditary craniofacial dysostosis and its relations with acrocephalosyndactylia. CROUZON, O. Bull. et mem. Soc. med. d. hop. de Paris *48:*1568–1574, Dec 12, '32
Unusual familial developmental disturbance of face, (acrocephalosyndactylia, craniofacial dystosis and hypertelorism). CHOTZEN, F. Monatschr. f. Kinderh. *55:*97–122, '32
General skeletal changes in acrocephalosyndactylia. WIGERT, V. Acta psychiat. et neurol. *7:*701–718, '32
Acrocephalosyndactylia, microcephaly, ptosis of eyelids and infantillism; addition of acute spasmodic paraplegia. EUZIÈRE, J. *et al*. Arch. Soc. d. sc. med. et biol. de Montpellier *14:*110–119, March '33
Acrocephalosyndactylia (Apert syndrome) in congenital syphilitic; case. ROCH. Bull. et mem. Soc. med. d. hop. de Paris *49:*513–518, April 17, '33
Anomalies of eye and orbit in acrocephalosyndactylia (Apert syndrome). WAARDENBURG, P. J. Maandschr. v. kindergeneesk. *3:*196–212, Feb '34
Oxycephalosyndactylia; case. DE CASTRO, A. Rev. neurol. *1:*359–367, March '34
Peculiar form of craniofacial malformation (acrocephalosyndactylia with facial asymmetry and ophthalmoplegia); case. KREINDLER, A. AND SCHACHTER, M. Paris med. *2:*102–105, Aug 4, '34
Question of double malformations; acrocephalosyndactylia and dysencephalia splanchnocystica. GRUBER, G. B. Beitr. z. path. Anat. u. z. allg. Path. *93:*459–476, '34
Acrocephalosyndactylia (Apert syndrome); case. NOVIS FILHO, A. Brasil-med. *49:*28–32, Jan 12, '35
Congenital craniofacial aplasia and malformation of toes (Apert syndrome); case. GUÉRIN, R. J. de med. de Bordeaux *112:*171–173, March 10, '35
Cranial deformities due to premature synosteoses of sutures with particular reference to Crouzon's disease (craniofacial dysostoses) and Apert syndrome (acrocephaly and syndactylia). MASTROMARINO, A. Arch. di ortop. *51:*233–304, June 30, '35
Acrocephalosyndactylia (Apert syndrome) in new-born infant; case. ALANTAR, I. H. Arch. de med. d. enf. *40:*171–172, March '37
Etiologic study of multiple congenital malformations, with report of case of acrocephalosyndactylia. BERARIU, A. Rev. pediat. si

Apert's Syndrome – Cont.
puericult. *1:*314–318, May–Aug '37
Acrocephalosyndactylia; evolution of case. CAUSSADE, L. *et al.* Rev. med. de Nancy *65:*576–586, July 1, '37
Genesis of genopathic syndrome (Bardet-Biedl acrocephalosyndactylia). POOL, F. L. Wien. Arch. f. inn. Med. *31:*187–200, '37
Etiology of acrocephalosyndactylia. SCHWARZWELLER, F. Ztschr. f. menschl. Vererb.-u. Konstitutionslehre *20:*341–349, '37
Pneumatization of bones of face in Crouzon's disease, Apert's syndrome and oxycephaly; 13 cases. DE GUNTEN, P. Schweiz. med. Wchnschr. *68:*268–270, March 12, '38
Acrocephalosyndactylia; case. SITTIG, O. AND BAUMRUCK, K. O. Med. Klin. *34:*502–505, April 14, '38
Acrocephalosyndactylia of Apert; case report and brief review of literature. ASENCIO CAMACHO, F. Bol. Asoc. med. de Puerto Rico *30:*309–314, Aug '38
Acrocephalosyndactylia (Apert syndrome); case. GAREISO, A. *et al.* Rev. med. latino-am. *23:*1245–1265, Aug '38
Acrocephalosyndactyly; case. ROUDINESCO, MME. Bull. et mem. Soc. med. d. hop. de Paris *56:*624–627, Nov 25, '40
Acrocephalosyndactylia with cleft hand in one of a pair of uniovular twins. GOLL, H. AND KAHLICK-KOENNER, D. M. Ztschr. f. menschl. Vererb.-u. Konstitutionslehre *24:*516–535, '40
Genetics of acrocephalosyndactylia. FERRIMAN, D. Proc. Internat. Genet. Cong. (1939) *7:*120, '41

APETROSYAN, K. A.: Plastic reconstruction of fingers by means of transplantation of toes. Ortop. i travmatol. (no. 1) *13:*74–78, '39
APFELBACH, G. L. (see FOX, T. A.) Oct '40
APGAR, V.: Principles of anesthesia in plastic surgery. S. Clin. North America *24:*474–479, April '44
APOLO, E.: Importance of immobilization in plastic surgery of harelip. An. de oto-rino-laring. d. Uruguay *9:*207–214, '39
APOLO, E.: Nasal deformity in harelip; anatomic study. Arq. de cir. clin. e exper. *6:*339–343, April–June '42
APOLO, E.: Nasal deformity in harelip; surgical problem. Arq. de cir. clin. e. exper. *6:*645–651, April–June '42
APOLO, E. AND ALVAREZ GRAU, J.: Therapy of harelip and of velopalatine fissures. An. de oto-rino-laring. d. Uruguay *9:*102–109, '39
APPELMANS, M. (see VAN DER STRAETEN) July '34
APPELMANS, M.: Radium treatment of epitheliomas of eyelids. Rev. belge sc. med. *2:*829–840, Dec '30
APPLE, C. W. (see ARMBRECHT, E. C.) Jan '43
APPLEBAUM, A. AND MARMELSTEIN, M.: Congenital bilateral anopthalmos vera with unilateral polydactyly and cleft palate; case. Arch. Ophth. *29:*258–265, Feb '43
APRILE, H.: Fractures of lower jaw; therapy. Rev. med. y cien. afines *1:*62–64, May 30, '39
ARAI, A.: Plastic surgery for atresia of anterior portion of nose, case. Oto-rhino-laryng. *9:*605, July '36
ARANDES, R. (see PIULACHS, P.) March '43
ARANYI, S.: Gastrothoracoschiasis (fetal eventration) with clinical symptoms of uterine rupture. Zentralbl. f. Gynak. *66:*1757–1762, Oct 31, '42
ARAUJO, D. G. AND BERTI, A.: Living graft of eyebrows in leprosy. Rev. brasil. de leprol. (num. espec.) *8:*7–13, '40
ARÁUZ, S. AND GAMES, F.: Posttraumatic frontal sinusitis; recovery after replacement of bone segment of frontal bone displaced by accident; case. Rev. Asoc. med. argent. *46:*509–510, July '32
ARBUCKLE, M. F.: Comparison of results obtained by surgery and radiation therapy in cancer of larynx. South. M. J. *32:*1008–1014, Oct '39
ARBUCKLE, M. F.: String method of removing tight ring from swollen finger. Mil. Surgeon *90:*184, Feb '42
ARCE, J.; IVANISSEVICH, O. AND FERRARI, R. C.: Hand injuries caused by breadmaking machine; cases of industrial accidents. Bol. Inst. de clin. quir. *5:*13–46, '29
ARCHAMBAULT, L. AND FROMM, N. K.: Progressive facial hemiatrophy; 3 cases. Arch. Neurol. and Psychiat. *27:*529–584, March '32
ARCHER, V. W. (see WOODWARD, F. D.) Dec '40
ARCELIN, F.: Radiotherapy of epithelioma of eyelids; aesthetic results. Lyon med. *149:*289–292, March 6, '32
ARCONE, R. (see RAFFO, J. M.) July '37
ARDOINO, A.: Perifemoral sympathectomy associated with dermoepidermal grafts in therapy of varicose ulcers; 7 cases. Policlinico (sez. prat.) *44:*1265–1267, June 28, '37
AREL, F.: Periarterial sympathectomy and Thiersch graft in therapy of varicose veins. Turk tib cem. mec. *3:*394–395, '37
ARELLANO, E. R.: Dental cyst in patient operated for harelip; case. Cron. med. mex. *29:*337–342, Aug '30
ARENAS, N. AND BOLLA, I.: Congenital absence of vagina; creation of artificial vagina by au-

toplastic procedure. Semana med. *1:*841–845, April 4, '40

Arenas, N. and Pepe, A. L.: Elephantiasis of vulva and of left leg; results of surgical therapy. Semana med. *2:*664–673, Sept 21, '39

Arespacochaga, F. E.: Preanesthetic sedation in plastic surgery. Semana med. *2:*375–376, Sept 6, '45

Arespacochaga, F. E.: Plastic surgical contribution to emergency surgery. Dia med. *16:*626–630, June 12, '44

Arespacochaga, F. L.: Free skin grafts; clinical and technical study. Dia med. *17:*186–188, March 5, '45

Arezzi, G.: Transplantation of ureters into sigmoid and cystectomy in radical therapy of exstrophy; late results in case. Arch. ital. di urol. *16:*384–405, Dec '39

Arganaraz, R.; Sibbald, D. and Courtis, B.: Dacryocystorhinostomy by nasal route (West operation) and its results. Cong. argent. de oftal. (1936) *2:*491–496, '38

Argil, G.: Surgical shock. Medicina, Mexico *22:*259–268, June 25, '42

Arguelles Lopez, R.: Tendon transplantation, in therapy of inveterate radial paralysis. Rev. clin. espan. *2:*319–323, April 1, '41

Arie, G. (see Prudente, A.) April–June '42

Aries, L. J. (see Davis, L.) Dec '37

Arkin, V.: Modification of Maher's operation for entropion. Klin. Monatsbl. f. Augenh. *77:*677–680, Nov '26

Arlotta, A. and Lari, G. L.: Frequency of fractures of lower jaw due to rebound from blow of fist. Stomatol. *28:*1073–1079, Dec '30

Armbrecht, E. C.: Cleft lip and cleft palate. West Virginia M. J. *28:*59–64, Feb '32

Armbrecht, E. C.: Jaw fractures. Internat. J. Orthodontia *22:*957–975, Sept '36

Armbrecht, E. C. and Apple, C. W.: Tumors of maxilla. Am. J. Orthodontics (Oral Surg. Sect.) *29:*60–64, Jan '43

Armour, J. C. (see Coloviras, G. J. Jr. *et al*) Dec '42

Armstrong, B. and Jarman, T. F.: Method of dealing with chronic osteomyelitis by saucerization followed by skin grafting. J. Bone and Joint Surg. *18:*387–396, April '36

Armstrong, H. G.: Cysts and fistulae; thyroglossal; with notes of case. St. Michael's Hosp. M. Bull. *3:*90–93, Dec '28

Armstrong, H. G.: Hand injuries. St. Michael's Hosp. M. Bull. *4:*54–73, June '30

Armstrong, T.M.: Lexer operation for ptosis of eyelids. Tr. Ophth. Soc. Australia (1940) *2:*84–85, '41

Arnaud, M.: Therapy of Volkmann syndrome. Marseille-med. *1:*229–232, Feb 15, '34

Arnheim, E. E.: Cervicomediastinal lymphangioma (cystic hygroma); 2 cases in infants. J. Mt. Sinai Hosp. *10:*404–410, Sept–Oct '43

Arnold, A.C.: Cutaneous horn of upper lip. M. J. Australia *1:*662, June 13, '42

Arnold, G.: Serious mutilation of palate due to tonsillectomy. Monatschr. f. Ohrenh. *76:*377–381, Aug '42

Arnold, G. E.: Unusual case of submucosal cleft palate in conjunction with deformity of soft palate and nasal speech. Arch. f. Ohren-, Nasen-u. Kehlkopfh. *147:*173–176, '40

Arnoldi, W.: Cystic tumors of anterior nares due to embryonal maldevelopment; 3 cases. Ztschr. f. Laryng., Rhin. *18:*58–69, '29

Arnolds, A.: Plastic operation for web-like dermatogenous contractures of large joints. Zentralbl. f. Chir. *55:*838–840, April 7, '28

Arnulf, G. (see Freidel, C. *et al*) July '37

Aron, M. (see Simon, R.) July '22

Aronovich, G. D.: Gunshot wounds of maxillofacial region with spinal complications. Am. Rev. Soviet Med. *1:*344–350, April '44 also: Khirurgiya, no. 1, pp. 14–22, '43

Aronowicz. (see L'Hirondel, C.) July '35

Aronsson, H.: So-called late rupture of extensor pollicis longus tendon after fracture of radius. Nord. med. (Hygiea) *2:*1985–1987, June 30, '39

Aronstein, E.: Roentgen epilation. Radiology *32:*95–96, Jan '39

Arraiza, D. (see Juaristi, V.) April '27

Arrivat: Burn therapy by practitioner. Rev. gen. de clin. et de therap. *52:*293–296, April 30, '38

Arrowood, J. G. (see Elliot, H. L.) Jan '45

Arsenio Plaza: Epinephrine in treatment of burns. Siglo med. *70:*560–562, Dec 9, '22 abstr: J.A.M.A. *80:*438, Feb 10, '23

Arteries

Collateral circulation in hand after cutting radial and ulnar arteries at wrist. Lawrence, H. W. Indust. Med. *6:*410–411, July '37

Traumatic aneurysm of ulnar artery; case. McLaughlin, C. W. Jr. U. S. Nav. M. Bull. *42:*428–430, Feb '44

Arthritis

Snapping finger in polyarthritis. Helweg, J. Ugesk. f. Laeger *86:*546–547, July 17, '24 abstr: J.A.M.A. *83:*1042, Sept 27, '24

Snapping finger in polyarthritis. Helweg, J. Klin. Wchnschr. *3:*2383–2384, Dec 23, '24 abstr: J.A.M.A. *84:*560, Feb 14, '25

Arthritis – Cont.
Surgical treatment of arthritis. NIENY, K. Zentralbl. f. Chir. *54:*3218–3219, Dec 10, '27
Scope of surgery in treatment of chronic rheumatoid and osteo-arthritis. PAGE, C. M. Brit. M. J. *1:*343–345, March 3, '28
Treatment of suppurative arthritis of fingers by resection of joint. ISELIN, M. Union med. du Canada *57:*385–393, July '28
Conservative and operative treatment of arthritis deformans. GOETZE, O. Med. Welt *5:*81–83, Jan 17, '31
Surgery in certain types of arthritis. CHOLLETT, B. G. AND BERSHON, A. L. Ohio State M. J. *27:*205–209, March '31
Surgical treatment of chronic arthritis. MEYERDING, H. W., J.A.M.A. *97:*751–757, Sept 12, '31
Surgical therapy of articular rheumatism. MASSART, R. Bull. et mem. Soc. de med. de Paris *137:*385–395, May 27, '33
Surgical therapy of rheumatic arthritis. MASSART, R. J. de med. de Paris *52:*644–646, Nov 2, '33
Surgical treatment of arthritic joints. McBRIDE, E. D. Southwestern Med. *17:*321–323, Oct '33
Surgical therapy of chronic nontuberculous arthropathies. AIMES, A. Progres med., pp. 1433–1437, Sept 15, '34
Surgical therapy in articular rheumatism. MASSART, R. AND VIDAL-NAQUET, G. Monde med., Paris *44:*971–977, Nov 1, '34
What to expect of surgical therapy in chronic rheumatism. MASSART, R. AND VIDAL-NAQUET, G. J. de med. de Paris *55:*69–71, Jan 24, '35
Surgical therapy of chronic rheumatism; indications and results. WEISSENBACH, R. J. Monde med., Paris *45:*40–52, Jan 1–15, '35
Modern surgical therapy of chronic progressive rheumatism. WEISSENBACH, R. J. Hopital *23:*287–289, April (B) '35
Surgery of arthritis. CAMPBELL, W. C. South. Surgeon *4:*353–371, Oct '35
Surgical treatment of chronic arthritis. KRIDA, A. Hygeia *13:*1117–1119, Dec '35
Surgical treatment of arthritis. McBRIDE, E. D. Southwestern Med. *20:*346–349, Sept '36
Dangers of surgical interventions on joints in course of evolute period of chronic polyarthritis. COSTE, F. *et al.* Presse med. *45:*729–730, May 15, '37
Principles of orthopedic and surgical treatment in rheumatoid arthritis. FISHER, A. G. T., J. Bone and Joint Surg. *19:*657–666, July '37
Surgical procedures in treatment of arthritis. HUDSON, R. T. Kentucky M. J. *35:*373–375, Aug '37

Arthritis – Cont.
Orthopedic surgery in treatment of rheumatism and rheumatoid arthritis. TIPPETT, G. O. Practitioner *139:*271–278, Sept '37
Surgical indications in rheumatoid arthritis. POILLEUX, F. Gax. med. de France *44:*923–925, Nov 1, '37
Surgical reconstruction of rheumatoid cripple. WILSON, P. D., M. Clin. North America *21:*1623–1639, Nov '37
Opera-glass hand in chronic arthritis; "la main en lorgnette" of Marie and Leri. NELSON, L. S., J. Bone and Joint Surg. *20:*1045–1049, Oct '38
Therapy of arthritis from point of view of surgeon. SIMON, R. Strasbourg med. *98:*484–488, Dec 5, '38
Author's experience with orthopedicosurgical therapy of chronic primary polyarthritis. MOCCIA, G. Arch. ital. di chir. *53:*124–134, '38
Orthopedicosurgical therapy of chronic rheumatism. MAROTTOLI, O. R. An. de cir. *5:*137–145, June '39
Orthopedic and surgical aspects of chronic rheumatism. FISHER, A. G. T. Practitioner *143:*286–296, Sept '39
Symposium on surgical treatment of chronic arthritis; present status of arthroplasty. ALBEE, F. H. New York State J. Med. *39:*2118–2125, Nov 15, '39
Surgical treatment of chronic arthritis. SELIG, S. New York State J. Med. *39:*2114–2117, Nov 15, '39
Surgical therapy of arthritis. DICKSON, F. D. Ann. Surg. *113:*869–876, May '41
Principles of orthopedic treatment of rheumatoid arthritis. BELL, B. T. Pennsylvania M. J. *44:*1304–1305, July '41
Procedures in chronic rheumatoid disease. WETHERBY, M. Journal-Lancet *61:*414–417, Oct '41
Useful surgical procedures for rheumatoid arthritis involving joints of upper extremity. SMITH-PETERSEN, M. N. *et al.* Arch. Surg. *46:*764–770, May '43
Splint for control of ulnar deviation of fingers in rheumatoid arthritis. BODENHAM, D. C. Lancet *2:*354–355, Sept 18, '43
Nylon fabric arthroplasty of carpometacarpal joint of thumb. BURMAN, M. Bull. Hosp. Joint Dis. *4:*74–78, Oct '43
Role of surgery in chronic arthritic patient (Nathan Lewis Hatfield lecture). COLONNA, P. C. Clinics *2:*955–965, Dec '43
Surgical therapy of chronic rheumatism. FERRE, R. L. Rev. Asoc. med. argent. *58:*324–330, May 30, '44

ARTHUR, H. R.: Branchial fistula; case. Brit. J. Surg. *29:*440–441, April '42
ARWINE, J. T.: Successful treatment of postoperative facial paralysis. M. Bull., Vet. Admin. *8:*404, May '32
ARTZ, L.: Burns from chlorosulphonic acid in industrial plant. Dermat. Wchnschr. *97:*995–997, July 8, '33
ARTZ, L.: Methods of burn therapy. Wien. klin. Wchnschr. *48:*644–647, May 18, '35
ARTZ, L. AND FUHS, H.: Radiotherapy of cancer of lips. Wien. klin. Wchnschr. *45:*15–18, Jan 1, '32
ARTZ, L. AND FUHS, H.: Radium therapy of cancer of lips, with especial consideration of permanent results. Wien. klin. Wchnschr. *46:*706–708, June 9, '33
ASBECK, C. (see NIEDEN, H.) 1931
ASBECK, F.: Therapy of "Knuckle pads" with carbon dioxide snow. Dermat. Wchnschr. *110:*457–461, June 1, '40
ASBELL, M. B.: Analysis of 115 cases fractured jaw. Am. J. Orthodontics *25:*282–289, March '39
ASBURY, M.K. (see BENEDICT, W. L.) June '29
ASCHAN, P. E.: Plastic surgery of war wounds. Deut. Militarazt *9:*142, March '44
ASCHAN, P. E.: Plastic surgery in treatment of war wounds. Nord. med. (Finska lak.-sallsk. handl.) *22:*933-939, May 19, 1944
ASCHER, K. W.: Free homeoplastic skin grafting; comment on Deucher and Ochsner's article. Arch. f. klin. Chir. *137:*198, '25
ASCHER, K. W.: Reconstruction of destroyed lacrimal excretory apparatus. Med. Klin. *25:*749-750, May 10, '29

Ascher Syndrome

Ascher syndrome (blepharochalasis, double upper lip and goiter), with report of case. GALLINO, J. A. AND CORA ELISEHT, F. Prensa med. argent. *32:*2423-2426, Dec 7, '45

ASENCIO CAMACHO, F.: Acrocephalosyndactylia of Apert; case report and brief review of literature. Bol. Asoc. med. de Puerto Rico *30:*309–314, Aug '38
ASHBURY, H. H.: Therapy of keloids. Urol. and Cutan. Rev. *42:*441-444, June '38
ASHE, W. F. JR. AND ROBERTS, L. B.: Experimental human burns; partial report. War Med. *7:*82–83, Feb '45
ASHER, R. (see KATZ, L. N. *et al*) May '43
ASHHURST, A. P. C.: Cicatricial contracture of buttocks nearly occluding anus; plastic operation on buttocks. S. Clin. N. America *2:*77–79, Feb '22 (illus.)
ASHHURST, A. P. C.: Recurrent unilateral subluxation of mandible; excision of interarticular cartilage in cases of snapping jaw. Ann. Surg. *73:*712, June '21
ASHHURST, A. P. C.: Rupture of tendon of extensor longus pollicis following a Colles' fracture. Ann. Surg. *78:*398–400, Sept '23
ASHLEY, F.: Foreskins as skin grafts. Ann. Surg. *106:*252–256, Aug '37
ASHLEY, F. L. (see ANSON, B. J.) Nov '40
ASHWORTH, C. T. (see MUIRHEAD, E. E. *et al*) June '42
ASHWORTH, C. T. (see MUIRHEAD, E. E. *et al*) July '42
ASHWORTH, C. T.: Pathogenesis and treatment of shock. Tri-State M. J. *13:*2735–2738, April '41
ASHWORTH, H. S.: Adjustable, non-solid appliance for nasal restoration, attached to upper denture. Brit. Dent. J. *80:*157-160, March 1, '46
ASIS Y GARCÍA DE LA CAMACHA: New technic for surgical therapy of pendulous breast. Actas Soc. de cir. de Madrid *3:*35–42, Oct–Dec '34
ASIS, R.: Total loss of pavilion of ear and its plastic repair; technic in case. Actas Soc. de cir. de Madrid *5:*131-136, Jan–Mar '46
ASKALONOVA, T. M. AND ZAKHAROV, A. P.: Correction of eyelid ptosis by means of buried sutures. Vestnik oftal. (no. 6) *14:*64–66, '39
ASPINALL, A.: Complete separation of facial bones from base of skull. M. J. Australia *1:*292–294, March 17, '23 (illus.)
ASPINALL, A.: Hand injuries. M. J. Australia *2:*529–532, Oct 7, '39
ASPINALL, A. J.: Repair of facial defects. J. Coll. Surgeons, Australasia *1:*230–232, Nov '28
ASRATYAN, E. A.: Shock; new method for treatment. Am. Rev. Soviet Med. *2:*37–43, Oct '44
ASSALI, J. (see ROUDIL, G.) Jan '35
ASTLEY, G. M.: Therapy of decubitus ulcers. Am. J. Surg. *50:*734–737, Dec '40
ASTRAKHANSKIY, V. A.: Method of homoplastic bone grafts. Sovet. khir. *4:*202-209, '33
ASTRAKHANSKIY, V. A.: Plastic method in construction of artificial vagina. Sovet. khir., no. 9, pp. 497–500, '36
ASTRUP, T. (see VOLKERT, M.) 1943
ASTRUP, T. (see VOLKER, M.) July '44
ATANASIU, I. (see GILORTEANU, I.) July-Aug '39
ATANOV, V. A.: Injuries of tendons in glass workers and their treatment. Khirurgiya, no. 1, pp. 46–53, '39
ATKINS, H. J. B.: Burn therapy. Guy's Hosp. Gaz. *54:*320–324, Nov 2, '40

ATKINS, H. J. B.: War surgery; management of burns. Brit. M. J. *1:*704, June 6, '42; 729, June 13 '42

ATKINSON, D. T.: Corrective surgery of eyelids and nose. J. Ophth., Otol. and Laryng. *32:*73–82, March '28

ATKINSON, D. T.: Evolution of submucous resection with new technic. Laryngoscope *37:*132–136, Feb '27

ATKINSON, D. T.: Recent nasal fractures. Eye, Ear, Nose and Throat Monthly *10:*147–148, May '31

ATLAS, L. N.: Role of second thoracic spinal segment in preganglionic sympathetic innervation of human hand; surgical implications. Ann. Surg. *114:*456–461, Sept '41

ATTWATER, H. L. AND HUGHES, J. R.: Repair of fistula of penile urethra. Lancet *2:*569–570, Sept 3, '38

AUBARET: So-called lacrymal or senile ectropion of lower eyelid, and its treatment. Medecine *7:*261–262, Jan '26

AUBINEAU, E.: Congenital entropion; 2 cases. Ann. d'ocul. *165:*161–169, March '28

AUBONE, J. (see CORA ELISEHT, F.) Nov–Dec '38

AUBONE, J. C.: Immediate therapy of surgical perforations of nasal septum. Rev. Asoc. med. argent. *50:*669–671, May–June '37

AUBONE, J. C.: New surgical technic for correcting septal perforation in nose. Rev. Asoc. med. argent. *55:*288–290, April 15–30, '41

AUBRIOT, P: Endonasal surgery and terrain. Rev. med. de l'est *60:*269–277, April 15, '32

AUBRY, M.: Local anesthesia with procaine hydrochloride as anesthesia of choice in operations on upper maxilla. Presse med. *43:*592, April 10, '35

AUBRY, M. AND FREIDEL, C.: *Chirurgie de la face et de la région maxillo-faciale.* Masson et Cie, Paris, 1942

AUBRY, M.: Skin autoplasty by Hungarian method. Semaine d. hop. Paris *21:*488–491, May 14, '45

AUBRY, M.: Surgical therapy of laryngopharyngeal cancer. Ann. d'oto-laryng., pp. 905–908, Nov–Dec '39

AUBRY, M.: Synthetic resins as tissue implants. Ann. d'oto-laryng. *13:*10–13, Jan–Feb '46

AUBRY, M. AND BOURDON, E.: Retro-auricular route of access to temporomaxillary joint. Ann. d'oto-laryng. *12:*465–476, Oct–Dec '45

AUBRY, M. AND DUCOURTIOUX, M: Restoration of ala nasi following its excision for cancer. Ann. d'oto-Laryng., pp. 89–92, July–Sept '44

AUCHINCLOSS, H.: New operation for elephantiasis. Porto Rico J. Pub. Health and Trop. Med. *6:*149, Dec '30

Auchincloss Operation

Auchincloss operation in elephantiasis; preliminary report. TORGERSON, W. R. Porto Rico J. Pub. Health and Trop. Med. *6:*411–418, June '31

Case report of 12 Auchincloss or modified Auchincloss operations for filariasis elephantiasis; preliminary report. DEL TORO, J. *et al.* Porto Rico J. Pub. Health and Trop. Med. *7:*3–10, Sept '31

AUD, G.: Corrective rhinoplasty. Kentucky M. J. *21:*105–110, Feb '23

AUDOUIN, J., AND NEVEU, J.: *Technique de la parotidectomie totale avec conservation du nerf facial.* Maloine, Paris, 1941

AUDRY, M. (see DECOURT, J. *et al*) March–April '41

AUERBACH, H. (see JARDENI, J.) Aug '37

AUFDERHEIDE, P. J.: Treatment of fractures of maxilla, mandible and other bones of face. J. Am. Dent. A. *21:*950–961, June '34

AUFRANC, O. E. (see SMITH-PETERSEN, M. N. *et al*) May '43

AUFRICHT, G. (see ESSER, J. F. S.) 1922

AUFRICHT, G.: Combined nasal plastic and chin plastic; correction of microgenia by osteocartilaginous transplant from large hump nose. Am. J. Surg. *25:*292–296, Aug '34

AUFRICHT, G.: Dental molding compound cast and adhesive strapping in rhinoplastic procedure. Arch. Otolaryng. *32:*333–338, Aug '40

AUFRICHT, G.: Evaluation of pedicle flaps versus skin grafts in reconstruction of surface defects and scar contractures of chin, cheeks and neck. Surgery *15:*75–84, Jan '44

AUFRICHT, G.: Hints and surgical details in rhinoplasty. Laryngoscope *53:*317–335, May '43

AUFRICHT, G.: Immediate transplantation on defects of ear and nose due to accident; 2 cases. Arch. Otolaryng. *17:*769–773, June '33

AUFRICHT, G.: Medical progress; recent developments in plastic surgery. New York Med. (no. 8) *2:*17–20, April 20, '46

AUFRICHT, G.: Modern surgery (plastic); achievements and possibilities. M. Rec. *146:*310–313, Oct 6, '37

AUGÉ, A. AND COTSAFTIS, G. G.: Angioma of lower lip reduced by injections of quinine urethane. Arch. Soc. d. sc. med. et biol. de Montpellier *9:*84–86, Feb '28

AURÉGAN: Extrabuccal apparatus for immobilization in therapy of fractures of lower jaw. Bull. et mem. Soc. d. chirurgiens de Paris *25:*192–197, March 17, '33

AUSEMS, A. W.: Spontaneous correction of harelip. Nederlandsch Tijdschr. v. Geneesk. *2:*1942, Nov 10, '23

AUSTIN, E. R.: Congenital fistula of external ear; case. Proc. Staff Meet. Clin., Honolulu *10:*1-4, Jan '44

AUSTIN, E. R.: Projecting auricle (lop ear); case corrected by surgery (New-Erich method). Proc. Staff Meet. Clin., Honolulu *9:*45-48, May '43

AUSTIN, LOUIE T. (with John B. Erich): *Traumatic Injuries of Facial Bones*. W. B. Saunders Co., Phila., 1944

AUSTIN, T. R.: Mechanism and treatment of surgical shock. U. S. Nav. M. Bull. *35:*426-434, Oct '37

AUSTIN, W. E.: Macrodactyly; case. Canad. M. A. J. *45:*148, Aug '41

AUSTREGESILO, A.; PORTUGAL, J. R. AND GUSMAO, D.: Progressive facial hemiatrophy; total hemiatrophy; case. Arch. brasil, de med. *33:*387-408, Nov-Dec '43

AUVRAY: Phlegmon of hand with acute metastatic osteomyelitis of femur, followed by spontaneous fracture at this point; operation; fatal case. Bull. et mem. Soc. nat. de chir. *54:*592-598, April 28, '28

AVENT, C. H. JR.: Anatomy and pathology of hand infections. Memphis M. J. *15:*140-142, Sept '40

AVERBAKH, M. AND IVANOVA, MME.: Plastic dacryocystorhinostomy in 1200 cases. Ann. d'ocul. *172:*913-936, Nov '35

AVIZONIS, V.: Denig operation for burns of eyes. Medicina, Kaunas *19:*309-315, April '38

AVRAMOVICI, A.: Spontaneous cure of cancer of lip. Lyon chir. *24:*257-268, May-June '27

AXHAUSEN, G.: Arthroplasty of jaws. Munchen. med. Wchnschr. *88:*776-779, July 11, '41

AXHAUSEN, G.: Basic principles of therapy of gunshot wounds of face in military surgery. Ztschr. f. Stomatol. *37:*436-440, April 28, '39

AXHAUSEN, G.: Bone transplantation in major resections of lower jaw; case of osteofibroma. Chirurg *12:*442-444, Aug 1, '40

AXHAUSEN, G.: Correction of acquired asymmetry caused by osteomyelitis of lower jaw. Deutsche Ztschr. f. Chir. *248:*533-551, '37

AXHAUSEN, G.: Corrective osteotomy of maxilla. Deutsche Ztschr. f. Chir. *248:*515-522, '37

AXHAUSEN, G.: Exposure of temporomaxillary joint. Chirurg *3:*713-716, Aug 15, '31

AXHAUSEN, G.: Free transplantation of bone with periosteum in jaw surgery; 2 cases of excision of tumors. Chirurg *1:*23-30, Nov 2, '28

AXHAUSEN, G.: Implantation of bone into lower jaw. Deutsche Ztschr. f. Chir. *227:*368-385, '30

AXHAUSEN, G.: Jaw resection; plastic and prosthetic surgery. Fortschr. d. Zahnh. *6:*917-952, Nov '30

AXHAUSEN, G.: Pathology and therapy of temporomandibular joint. Fortschr. d. Zahnh. *7:*199-215, March '31

AXHAUSEN, G.: Perforation of palate due to suction attachment of dental plate. Deutsche Zahn-, Mund-u. Kieferh. *1:*343-348, '34

AXHAUSEN, G.: Plastic correction after unsatisfactory healing following operation for harelip. Chirurg *11:*321-334, May 1, '39

AXHAUSEN, G.: Plastic surgery of breast. Med. Klin. *22:*1437-1440, Sept 17, '26

AXHAUSEN, G.: Principles of plastic operation (Langenbeck-Axhausen) of cleft palate. (Reply to Veau). J. de chir. *49:*47-53, Jan '37

AXHAUSEN, G.: (Reply to Veau's comments on Axhausen's book.) Deutsche Ztschr. f. Chir. *247:*582-589, '36

AXHAUSEN, G.: Speech function following 300 palate operations. Zentralbl. f. Chir. *69:*770, May 9, '42

AXHAUSEN, G.: Surgery of cleft lip, jaw and palate. Chirurg *10:*1-10, Jan 1, '38

AXHAUSEN, G.: Surgical therapy of war wounds of jaws and face. Chirurg *11:*801-807, Dec 1, '39

AXHAUSEN, G.: Tardy rupture of tendon with fracture of radius. Beitr. z. klin. Chir. *133:*78-88, '25

AXHAUSEN, G.: Tasks and accomplishments of maxillary surgery. Deutsche med. Wchnschr. *58:*401-404, March 11, '32

AXHAUSEN, G.: Technic and results of plastic surgery of the palate. Zentralbl. f. Chir. *62:*2211-2215, Sept 14, '35

AXHAUSEN, G.: Technic of plastic surgery of cleft palate. Chirurg *8:*299-313, April 15, '36

AXHAUSEN, G.: *Technik und Ergebnisse der Gaumenplastik*. Georg Thieme, Stuttgart, 1936

AXHAUSEN, G.: Question of traumatic cleft palate. Deutsche Zahn-, Mund-u. Kieferh. *1:*340-342, '34

Axhausen Operation (See also Von-Langenbeck-Axhausen Operation)

Bone transplantation by Axhausen's method in case of pseudoarthrosis of lower jaw resulting from defective healing. NISSEN, R. Deutsche Ztschr. f. Chir. *229:*140-142, '30

Operative treatment of tumors of jaw by Axhausen method of bone transplantation. KLEINSCHMIDT, O. Arch. f. klin. Chir. *164:*205-212, '31

Results of bridge plastic (Axhausen) operation for cleft palate in 45 cases. IMMENKAMP, A. Deutsche Ztschr. f. Chir. *249:*326-336, '37

Lahey plastic repair using bipedicled flap. Bol. y trab., Soc. argent. de cirujanos *4:*292-293, '43 also: Rev. Asoc. med. argent. *57:*495, July 30, '43
BAILEY, H.: Branchial fistula. Clin. J. *56:*619, Dec 28, '27
BAILEY, H.: Case of true congenital thyroglossal fistula. Proc. Roy. Soc. Med. (Clin. Sect.) *17:*6-7, Jan '25
BAILEY, H.: Clinical aspects of branchial cysts. Brit. J. Surg. *10:*565-572, April '23 (illus.)
BAILEY, H.: Clinical aspects of branchial fistula. Brit. J. Surg. *21:*173-182, Oct '33
BAILEY, H.: Cystic hygroma. Clin. J. *66:*242-244, June '37
BAILEY, H.: Cystic hygroma (of neck). J. Internat. Coll. Surgeons *2:*31-33, Jan-April '39
BAILEY, H.: Diagnosis of branchial cyst, with note upon its removal. Brit. M. J. *1:*940-941, June 2, '28
BAILEY, H.: Hand infections; dry after-treatment. Lancet *2:*189-190, Aug 16, '41
BAILEY, H.: Ischemic contracture, treatment by transplantation of internal epicondyle. Brit. J. Surg. *16:*335-337, Oct '28
BAILEY, H. AND DRISCOLL, W. P.: Shock in pregnant and puerperal woman. Am. J. Obst. and Gynec. *11:*287-304, March '26
BAILEY, H.: Similarity of certain tuberculous cervical abscesses and branchial cysts. Brit. J. Tuberc. *25:*167-170, Oct '31
BAILEY, H.: Thyroglossal cysts and fistulae. Brit. J. Surg. *12:*579-589, Jan '25
BAILEY, H.: Treatment of parotid tumors with special reference to total parotidectomy. Brit. J. Surg. *28:*337-346, Jan '41
BAILEY, L. (see BALLANCE, C. *et al*) Jan '26
BAILEY, O. T. AND FORD, R.: Tissue reactions induced by series of fibrogen plastics implanted in abdominal wall of guinea pigs. Arch. Path. *42:*535-542, Nov '46
BAILEY, W. AND KISKADDEN, W.: Treatment of birthmarks. California and West. Med. *59:*265-268, Nov '43
BAILLEUL, AND REGNER: Graft of osseous tissue using bouillon and paste of living bone. Bull. et mem. Soc. d. chirurgiens de Paris *27:*414-418, July 5, '35
BAIOCCHI, P.: Structure and reabsorption of parchment; histology, sterilization and bacteriologic control. Folia med. *24:*1068-1084, Oct 15, '38
BAIRD, C. L.: Review of current literature on classification, etiology and treatment of shock. Mil. Surgeon *89:*24-34, July '41
BAIRD, J. M. (see CLAY, G. E.) 1936
BAIRD, J. M. (see CLAY, G. E.) Oct '36
BAIRD, J. P.: Treatment of cleft lip and palate. J. Tennessee M. A. *17:*257-264, Dec '24
BAJEU, G. (see BOLINTINEANU, G.) Jan '32
BAKÁCS, G.: Surgical aspects of progressive unilateral facial atrophy. Orvosi hetil. *78:*590-593, June 30, '34
BAKER, G. S.: Cranioplasty with tantalum plate in postwar period. S. Clinics North America *26:*841-845, Aug '46
BAKER, H.: Hemiatrophy of a face with eye complications. Proc. Roy. Soc. Med. *32:*364-365, Feb '39
BAKER, J. M. (see COAKLEY, W. A.) Aug '44
BAKER, J. W. (see MASON, J. T.) Oct '31
BAKER, R. D.: Untoward effects of various substances recommended in burn therapy; experimental tests on rats. Arch. Surg. *48:*300-304, April '44
BAKER, W. B. AND VONACHEN, H. A.: Provitamin A ointment in burns. Indust. Med. *6:*584-589, Nov '37

Baker Operation

Use of modified Baker anchorage in naval dental service for fractured jaw. DARNALL, W. L., U. S. Nav. M. Bull. *19:*42-45, July '23 (illus.)

BAKES, F. P.: Present status of speech training of patients who wear speech correction appliances. Am. J. Orthodontics (Oral Surg. Sec.) *32:*718-723, Nov '46
BAKHMUTOVA, E. A.: Therapy of maxillary fractures according to Ivy. Sovet. med. (no. 4) *4:*38-39, '40
BAKKAL, T. S.: Plastic surgery with tissue pedicles (Filatov's method). Vestnik Khir. (no. 25) *9:*144-146, '27
BAKODY, J. T.: Tantalum cranioplasty. Ohio State M. J. *42:*29-33, Jan '46
BAKRY, M.: Easy and successful operation for over-eversion of eyelids. Bull. Ophth. Soc. Egypt *22:*20-23, '29
BAKRY, M.: Multiple fibromata of eyelid and forehead; removal; case. Bull. Ophth. Soc. Egypt *22:*78, '29
BAKUSHINSKIY, R. N.: Therapy of cicatricial contracture of hand and fingers after burns. Ortop. i travmatol. (no. 2) *12:*76-83, '38
BALABAN, M.: Burn therapy. Dia med. *15:*24-25; 33-35, Jan 11, '43
BALACCO, F.: Importance of suture of lacrimal sac and nasal mucosa in dacryocystorhinostomy. Boll. d'ocul. *18:*876-880, Nov '39
BALAKHOVSKIY, S. D.; KLIMENKOVA, L. A. AND CHERKASSOV, F. M.: Question of local vitamin deficiency; therapy of burns with vitaderm (carotene preparation). Novy khir. arkhiv *36:*49-64, '36

BALCH, F. G. JR.: Traumatic shock. J. Maine M. A. *30:*216–218, Sept '39
BÂLCU, S. (see NASTA, T. *et al*) March–April '34
BALDENWECK: Correction of frontal depression by inclusion of celluloid; case. Ann. d. mal. de l'oreille, du larynx *47:*757, Aug '28
BALDENWECK, L.: Submucous resection. Medecine *12:*75–79, Jan '31
BALDINO, S.: Correction of trachomatous entropion of upper eyelid. Rassegna ital. d'ottal. *4:*212–217, March–April '35
BALDRIDGE, R. R. (see MACFEE, W. F.) March '30
BALDRIDGE, R. R. (see MACFEE, W. F.) Aug '34
BALDWIN, J. F.: Restoration of vermilion border in certain operation. Am. J. Surg. *22:*232, Nov '33

Baldwin Operation

Congenital absence of vagina, accompanied by marked nervous symptoms; Baldwin's operation and removal of ovarian tissue. WRIGHT, T. Am. J. Surg. *36:*114–115, May '22
Artificial vagina made by Baldwin's method for congenital defect in vagina. RABINOWITSCH, K. N. Zentralbl. f. Gynak *50:*1851–1864, July 10, '26 abstr: J.A.M.A. *87:*1081, Sept 25, '26
Functions of isolated fascia of jejunum tenue used in operation for artificial vagina by Baldwin's method. VAKAR, A. A. Russk. Klin. *7:*19–34, Jan '27
Formation of artificial vagina by Baldwin method with Constantini's modification. TICHONOVICH, A. J. Akush. i Zhensk. Boliez. *38:*301–305, May–June '27
Baldwin operation for formation of artificial vagina; report of 6 cases. JUDIN, S. Surg., Gynec. and Obst. *44:*530–539, April (pt. 1) '27
Baldwin operation with Constantini's modification for artificial vagina; case. LAMPRECHT, V. L., J. akush. i zhensk. boliez. *39:*916–918, '28
Baldwin operation in case of complete absence of vagina. AKHVLEDYANI, A. V., J. akush. i zhensk. boliez. *39:*912–916, '28
Artificial vagina formation by Baldwin's method. GAMBAROW, G. Monatschr. f. Geburtsh. u. Gynak. *78:*106–108, Jan '28
Intestinal obstruction simulated by segregated closed loop of bowel; case following Baldwin operation for artificial vagina. QUIGLEY, R. A. Northwest Med. *28:*122–123, March '29
Function of isolated section of small intestine

Baldwin Operation – Cont.

three and one-half years after Baldwin's operation (artificial vagina.) VAKAR, A. A. Russk. klin. *12:*565–575, Oct–Nov '29
Primary carcinoma of vagina following Baldwin reconstruction operation for congenital absence of vagina. RITCHIE, R. N. Am. J. Obst. and Gynec. *18:*794–799, Dec '29
Baldwin operation for formation of vagina closely resembling normal one, from vagina septa (bipartite vagina). FRANKENBERG, B. E. Zentralbl. f. Chir. *57:*2792–2796, Nov 8, '30
Baldwin operation for artificial vagina; 7 cases. GITELSON, U. E., J. akush. i zhensk. boliez. *41:*467–476, '30
Baldwin operation in case of congenital absence of vagina. TCHARKVIANI, I. I., J. akush. i zhensk. boliez. *41:*477–481, '30
Formation of artificial vagina; contribution to 25th anniversary of Baldwin operation. RABINOVITCH, C. N. Am. J. Surg. *13:*480–483, Sept '31
Baldwin operation in congenital absence of vagina; result after 11 years. BROHEE, G., J. de chir. et ann. Soc. belge de chir. *(32–30):*13–16, Jan '33
Baldwin operation in congenital absence of vagina; result after 11 years. BROHEE, G. Scalpel *86:*825–829, June 3, '33
Baldwin operation for artificial vagina. SCHEPETINSKY, A. Monatschr. f. Geburtsh. u. Gynak. *95:*270–273, Oct '33
Colpoplasty by modified Baldwin technic for congenital absence of vagina; case. COSTANTINI, AND FERRARI. Mem. Acad. de chir. *62:*1213–1215, Oct 28, '36
Formation of artificial vagina according to Baldwin technic. LEBEDEV, V. F. Sovet. khir., no. 2, pp. 351–354, '36
Baldwin operation in case of pseudohermaphroditism and vulviform hypospadias. CABANES, E. AND XICLUNA, R. Algerie med. *43:*333–336, July '39
Case of genital aplasia; artificial vagina successfully constructed by Baldwin operation. BODENHEIMER, M. AND GOLDMAN, M. L., J. Mt. Sinai Hosp. *7:*310–315, Jan–Feb '41
Congenital absence of vagina treated successfully by Baldwin technic. O'NEILL, T. Brit. M. J. *2:*746–747, Dec 11, '43

Baldwin-Mori Operation

Baldwin-Mori operation for artificial vagina; case. GUTIÉRREZ, A. Bol. y trab. de la Soc. de cir. de Buenos Aires *17:*739–742, Aug 2, '33
Baldwin-Mori operation for artificial vagina;

Baldwin-Mori Operation—Cont.

case. GRIDNEW, A. Gynec. et obst. *34:*312-314, Oct '36

Evaluation of formation of artificial vagina by Baldwin-Mori operation. GRIDNEV, A. Arch. f. Gynak. *162:*397-402, '36

Baldwin-Mori operation for congenital absence of vagina. HORTOLOMEI, N. Rev. de chir., Bucuresti *42:*136-138, Jan-Feb '39

Artificial vagina; plastic surgery according to Baldwin-Mori. CONSTANTINESCU, M. AND COVALI, N. Rev. de chir., Bucuresti *43:*296-298, March-April '40

Creation of artificial vagina by Baldwin-Mori operation. GONI MORENO, I. Bol. y trab., Acad. argent. de cir. *24:*453-460, July 3, '40

Artificial vagina; Baldwin-Mori procedure; surgical technic. GONI MORENO, I. Prensa med. argent. *27:*2579-2583, Dec 11, '40

BALESDENT, E.: Plaster casts in local burn therapy. Hospital, Rio de Janeiro *21:*753-768, May '42

BALKIN, S. G. (see WALDRON, C. W.) Feb '42

BALKIN, S. G. (see WALDRON, C. W. *et al*) July '43

BALKIN, S. G.: Fractures of malar-zygomatic compound. Journal-Lancet *62:*267-270, July '42

BALKIN, S. G. AND WALDRON, C. W.: Bilateral fracture of condyles of edentulous mandible with marked retrusion displacement; case. J. Oral Surg. *2:*58-63, Jan '44

BALKIN, S. G.; DOWMAN, C. E. AND KLEMPERER, W. W.: Managment of extensive defects in craniocerebral injuries. J.A.M.A. *128:*70-72, May 12, '45

BALKOW, E.: Artificial vagina formation from sigmoid. Ztschr. f. Geburtsh. u. Gynak. *112:*256-260, '36

BALKOW, E.: Plastic replacement of vagina with portion of sigmoid flexure (Ruge operation) after Wertheim operation for total extirpation; case. Deutsche med. Wchnschr. *62:*586-588, April 10, '36

BALL, J. M.: Skin-grafting in acute symblepharon (eyelids). Lancet *1:*863, April 24, '26

BALLANCE, C.: Experiments in which central endo of divided cervical sympathetic nerve was anastomosed to peripheral end of divided facial nerve and to peripheral end of divided hypoglossal nerve. Arch. Neurol. and Psychiat. *25:*1-28, Jan '31

BALLANCE, C.: Facial nerve anastomosis in paralysis. J. Egyptian M. A. *12:*63-68, May '29

BALLANCE, C.: Operative treatment of facial palsy, with observations on prepared nerve graft. Proc. Roy. Soc. Med. *27:*1367-1372, Aug '34 also: J. Laryng. and Otol. *49:*709-718, Nov '34

BALLANCE, C.: Operative treatment of facial paralysis; with account of animal experiments. Brit. M. J. *1:*787-788, April 30, '32

BALLANCE, C.: Results of nerve anastomosis; preliminary remarks: lateral implantation of 2 ends of divided nerve into neighbouring uninjured nerve. Brit. J. Surg. *11:*327-346, Oct '23 (illus.)

BALLANCE, C.: Surgical treatment of paralysis of face, vocal cords, and diaphragm. Tr. Roy. Med.-Chir. Soc., Glasgow *21:*90-102, '27

BALLANCE, C. AND DUEL, A. B.: Operative treatment of facial palsy by introduction of nerve grafts into fallopian canal and by other intratemporal methods. Arch. Otolaryng. *15:*1-70, Jan '32

BALLANCE, C. AND DUEL, A. B.: Operative treatment of facial palsy by introduction of nerve grafts into fallopian canal and by other intratemporal methods. Tr. Am. Otol. Soc. *21:*288-295, '31

BALLANCE, C. *et al:* Results of suturing divided nerves (particularly in horses). Proc. Roy. Soc. Med. *27:*1207-1210, July '34

BALLANCE, C.; COLLEDGE, L. AND BAILEY, L.: Further results of nerve anastomosis. Brit. J. Surg. *13:*535-558, Jan '26

Ballance-Duel Operation (See also Duel-Ballance Operation)

Surgical treatment of facial palsy; Ballance-Duel method. DUEL, A. B. Laryngoscope *42:*579-587, Aug '32

Clinical experiences in surgical treatment of facial palsy by autoplastic grafts; Ballance-Duel method. DUEL, A. B. Arch. Otolaryng. *16:*767-788, Dec '32

Modification of Ballance-Duel technic in treatment of facial paralysis. SULLIVAN, J. A. Tr. Am. Acad. Ophth. *41:*282-299, '36

Repair of facial nerve lesion by Ballance-Duel graft. MCARTHUR, G. A. D., M. J. Australia *2:*1123-1124, Dec 31, '38

Intratemporal repair of facial nerve for facial paralysis (Ballance-Duel operation). CASSIDY, W. A. Nebraska M. J. *25:*47-50, Feb '40

Surgical therapy of otogenic facial paralysis according to Ballance-Duel and Bunnell; 35 cases. KETTEL, K. Nord. med. (Hospitalstid.) *24:*1783-1795, Oct 6, '44

BALLIN, M.: Method of cranioplasty using as a graft one-half the thickness of bony part of rib. Surg., Gynec. and Obst. *33:*79, July '21

BALOD, K.: Simple method for preparing dacryocystorhinostomy needles. Klin. Monatsbl. f. Augenh. *108:*626, Sept–Oct '42

BALOGH, K.: New mouth retractor for oral surgery. Ztschr. f. Stomatol. *40:*669–671, Sept 11, '42

BALON, L. R.: Plastic reconstruction of soft tissues of face during period of secondary suture. Khirurgiya, no. 3, pp. 30–31, '44

BALSINGER, W. E.: Intranasal correction of hump and hooked noses. Am. J. Surg. *36:*184–186, Aug '22 (illus.)

BALTIN, M. M. AND SVYADOSHCH, B. I.: Roentgen diagnosis of blunt and gunshot injuries to orbit. Vestnik oftal. *18:*306–311, '41

BALTIN, W.: Tannin therapy of burns of all degrees. Monatschr. f. Unfallh. *49:*65–80, March '42

BALTODANO BRICENO, E.: Use of ambrine (paraffin dressing) in burns. Med. de los ninos *36:*300–304, Oct '35

BALTZELL, N. A.: Tannic acid treatment in burns. J. Florida M. A. *15:*597–599, June '29

BALYEAT, F. S.: Depressed fractures of zygoma. California and West. Med. *37:*315, Nov '32

BALZA, J. (see CRAMER, F. E. K.) Jan '41

BAMES, H. O.: Cartilage transplants in facial surgery. Rev. de chir. structive, pp. 281–285, June '36

BAMES, H. O.: Commonest deformities of face presenting themselves for correction, and their correctibility. Rev. de chir. structive, pp. 219–232, March '36

BAMES, H. O.: Correction of abnormally large breasts. Southwestern Med. *25:*10–13, Jan '41

BAMES, H. O.: Correction of pendulous breasts. Am. J. Surg. *10:*80–83, Oct '30

BAMES, H. O.: Eliminating facial scars. M. J. and Rec. *131:*348–350, April 2, '30

BAMES, H. O.: Esthetic surgery. California and West. Med. *33:*588–591, Aug '30

BAMES, H. O.: Plastic reconstruction of breast deformities. Rev. de chir. structive, pp. 293–297, June '36

BAMES, H. O.: Plastic repair of facial deformations. Bol. y trab. de la Soc. de cir. de Buenos Aires *22:*116–119, May 4, '38

BAMES, H. O.: Plastic surgery of breast hypertrophy; technic. Bol. Soc. de cir. de Rosario *5:*18–20, May '38

BAMES, H. O.: Plastic surgical advances in Latin America. Tr. Am. Soc. Plastic and Reconstructive Surg. *12:*43–45, '43

BAMES, H. O.: Problems of plastic surgery and surgery of the breast in particular. Dia med. *10:*907–908, Sept 5, '38

BAMES, H. O.: Reconstruction for breast hypertrophy. California and West. Med. *48:*341–343, May '38

BAMES, H. O.: Reconstruction of nasal lobule, using skin graft. An. de cir. *4:*224–229, Sept '38

BAMES, H. O.: Review of plastic operations of breast. M. Rec. *143:*273–274, April 1, '36

BAMES, H. O.: Strategy in solution of problems in reconstructive surgery. Tr. Am. Soc. Plastic and Reconstructive Surg. *12:*17–21, '43

BAMES, H. O.: Surgical sculpturing. J. Coll. Surgeons, Australasia *3:*104–109, July '30

BAMES, H. O.: Transplantation of nipple, most complicated form of pedicle graft. Rev. de chir. structive, pp. 93–96, June '37

BAMES, H. O.: Truth and fallacies of face peeling and face lifting. M. J. and Rec. *126:*86–87, July 20, '27

BAMES, O.: Plastic surgery. Rev. med. peruana *10:*249–256, May '38

BANCROFT, F. W.: Cutaneous burns. New England J. Med. *202:*811–822, April 24, '30

BANCROFT, F. W.: Emergency care of burns and other injuries. New York State J. Med. *42:*361–368, Feb 15, '42

BANCROFT, F. W. AND ROGERS, C. S.: Late treatment of burns. Tr. South S. A. *40:*73–81, '27

BANCROFT, F. W. AND ROGERS, C. S.: Late burn treatment. Arch. Surg. *16:*979–999, May '28

BANCROFT, F. W. AND ROGERS, C. S.: Treatment of cutaneous burns. Ann. Surg. *84:*1–18, July '26

BANCROFT, F. W.; STANLEY-BROWN, M. AND TAYLOR, R. F.: Modified Kondoleon operation for sclerosed leg with ulceration (grafts.) Ann. Surg. *111:*874–891, May '40

Bandages

Leukoplast for bandaging burns. SMIRNOV, V. I. Khirurgiya, no. 1, pp. 54–59, '39

BANET, V.: Interpretation of suture of tendons. An. de cir. *4:*352–354, May '32

BANET, V. AND BOLAÑOS, J. M.: Branchial cyst with dermic steatonecrosis; case. Bol. Liga contra el cancer *8:*97–104, April '33

BANGERTER, A.: Instruments to facilitate mucosal suture in dacryocystorhinostomy. Ophthalmologica *104:*171–174, Sept '42

BANGERTER, J.: Implantation of ureters into large intestine in treatment of epispadias. Schweiz. med. Wchnschr. *65:*747–748, Aug 17, '35

BANISTER, J. B. (see MCINDOE, A. H.) June '38

BANISTER, J. B. AND MCINDOE, A. H.: Congenital absence of vagina, treated by means of indwelling skin-graft. Proc. Roy. Soc. Med. *31:*1055–1056, July '38

Banjo Splint

Modification of banjo splint for finger fractures. WILSON, C. S. Canad. M. A. J. *46:*585-586, June '42

BANKOFF, GEORGE: *Plastic Surgery*. Medical Publications, London, 1944.
BANKOFF, G.: Surgical treatment of elephantiasis. J. Trop. Med. *47:*49-53, Oct-Nov '44
BANKS, A. G.: Avulsion of scalp. Brit. M. J. *2:*893-894, Nov 17, '28
BANNICK, E. G.: Symposium on acute burns; medical care. Proc. Staff. Meet., Mayo Clin. *8:*123-126, Feb 22, '33
BARAJAS VILCHES, F.: Fistula auris congenita; surgical therapy; 2 cases. Rev. med. de Canarias *1:*243-244, June '32
BARAJAS Y DE VILCHES, J. M.: Complete congenital branchial fistula. Siglo med. *84:*85-86, July 27, '29
BARAKIN, M. (see DE MUNTER, L.) April '37
BARANGER, J.: Two grafts on flexor tendons. J. de med. de Bordeaux *109:*203-204, March 10, '32
BÁRÁNY, R.: Successful surgical treatment of large suppurative cyst of second branchial cleft; case. Acta oto-laryng. *14:*556-559, '30
BARASCH (see OLIVIER, G.) July '46
BARATA, E.: Osteogenic tumor of mandible; case. Brasil-med. *59:*244-247, July 7-14, '45
BARBAGLIA, V.: Etiology and pathogenesis of multiple keloid. Gior. ital. di dermat. e sifil. *69:*1573-1596, Dec '28
BARBARA, G. (see Sézary, A. *et al*) Feb '33
BARBARO: Treatment of cleft palate with sutures; case. Bull. et mem. Soc. nat. de chir. *56:*1186-1195, Nov 15, '30
BARBER, C. G.: Skin transplantation by injection; effect on healing of granulating wounds. Arch. Surg. *43:*21-31, July '41
BARBER, H. W.: Etiology and treatment of common diseases of face and scalp (acne). Guy's Hosp. Gaz. *53:*397-399, Dec 16, '39 *53:*381, Dec 2, '39
BARBER, R. F.: Industrial diseases and accidents of hand (also infections). New York State J. Med. *36:*1736-1740, Nov 15, '36
BARBERA, G.: Behavior of skin grafts under experimental avitaminosis. C. Bull. War Med. *4:*211-212, Dec '43
BARBERA, S.: Relation between nasal occlusion and development of paranasal sinuses, with special reference to 2 cases of congenital occlusion of choanae. Oto-rino-laring. ital. *6:*563-576, Dec '36
BARBERIS, J. C. (see NATALE, A. M.) Oct '30
BARBERIS, J. C.: External masculine pseudohermaphroditism with mistake in sex; surgical therapy of case. Bol. Soc. de cir. de Rosario *5:*125-150, June '38
BARBERIS, J. C.: Fractures of lower jaw; therapy by extension; case. Bol. Soc. de cir. de Rosario *5:*478-484, Nov '38
BARBERIS, J. C.: Skin grafts in surgical correction of defective cicatrix of hand causing contracture; 2 cases. Bol. Soc. de cir. de Rosario *5:*469-477, Nov '38
BARBEROUSSE: Dupuy-Dutemps and Bourguet technic in dacryocystotomy. Bull. Soc. d'opht. de Paris, p. 226, March '31
BARBIERI, P. (see PORRIT, A. E.) Oct '44
BARBIERI PALMIERI, C.: Blue scar formation; 2 cases. Boll. Soc. med.-chir. Modena *42:*613-618, '41-'42
BARBIZET (see ROYER) July '45
BARCAT, J. R.: Therapy of penal and penoscrotal hypospadias; supplementary notes on Ombredanne operation. J. de chir. *58:*418-426, '41-'42
BARCELONE, R. D. (see BABBINI, R. J. *et al*) Oct '41
BARDELLI, L.: New technic of operation for eyelid ptosis. Boll. d'ocul. *8:*289-301, April '29
BARDANZELLU, T.: Nida method of correcting ptosis of upper eyelid. Rassegna ital. d'ottal. *8:*449-453, July-Aug '39
BARDANZELLU, T.: New method of surgical therapy of subcutaneous angiomas of face. Arch. di ottal. *39:*520-543, Nov-Dec '32

Bardet-Biedl Syndrome

Genesis of genopathic syndrome (Bardet-Biedl acrocephalosyndactylia). POOL, F. L. Wien. Arch. f. inn. Med. *31:*187-200, '37

BARDON, J.: Case of exstrophy of bladder in woman aged 39. J. d'urol. *16:*384-389, Nov '23
BARDONNET (see COTTE, G.) 1944
BARENBOYM, S. (see ZENO, L.) 1937

Barg Operation

Barg operation (eyelids) according to data of Trachoma Institute in Turkmenistan. Vestnik oftal. (no. 2) *15:*46-48, '39

BARGE, P.: Congenital cyst of right lateral cervical region developed from lateral vestiges of "cervical sinus." Ann. d'anat. path. *15:*1025-1031, Dec '38
BARISON, F.: Cure of Dupuytren's contracture associated with diabetes by roentgen irradiation of hypophysis; case. Gior. di psichiat. e di neuropat. *60:*45-64, '32
BARKAN, H. (see BARKAN, O.) Nov '24
BARKAN, H. (see RODIN, F. H.) March '35
BARKAN, O. AND BARKAN, H.: Treatment of

lime burn of eye. J.A.M.A. *83:*1567–1569, Nov 15, '24

BARKER, C.: New nasal septal chisel. J.A.M.A. *79:*216, July 15, '22 (illus.)

BARKER, C. B.: Surgical treatment of ectropion and entropion. J. Oklahoma M. A. *31:*418–420, Dec '38

BARKER, D. E.: Improved method for experimental grafting. Arch. Path. *32:*425–428, Sept '41

BARKER, D. E.: War wounds of spinal cord; surgical treatment of decubitus ulcers. J.A.M.A. *129:*160, Sept 8, '45

BARKER, D. E.; ELKINS, C. W. AND POER, D. H.: Methods of closure of decubitus ulcers in paralyzed patient. Ann. Surg. *123:*523–530, Apr '46

BARKER, D. E.; ELKINS, C. W. AND POER, D. H.: Methods of closure of decubitus ulcers in paralyzed patient. Tr. South. S. A. (1945) *57:*54–61, '46

BARKER, N. W. AND HINES, E. A. JR.: Arterial occlusion in hands and fingers associated with repeated trauma. Proc. Staff Meet., Mayo Clin. *19:*345–349, June 28, '44

BARKHASH, S. A.: Placenta as plastic material in eye surgery. Vestnik oftal. *17:*758–761, '40

BARLING, S.: Tannic acid in burns. Birmingham M. Rev. *3:*58–61, March '28 also: Clin. J. *57:*277–281, June 13, '28

BARMAK, M. AND CONCILIO, L.: Grave burns. Rev. Assoc. paulista de med. *16:*306–315, May '40

BARMAN, J. M.: Counterstroke electrocoagulation of buccal mucosa during treatment of facial lesions. Rev. argent. dermatosif. *28:*191–192, June '44

BARMAN, J. M.: Diathermal depilation in therapy of hypertrichosis. Rev. med. de Rosario *35:*703–709, Aug '45

BARMONDIERE: Burn therapy. Prat. med. franc. *6:*258–260, June (B) '27

BARNARD, M. A.: Forum on therapy of wartime injuries; shock. New York State J. Med. *43:*228–230, Feb 1, '43

BARNES, C. K.: Spontaneous rupture of extensor pollicis longus. J.A.M.A. *87:*663, Aug 28, '26

BARNES, J. M.: Burn therapy. (hands) Brit. M. J. *1:*408–410, April 3, '43

BARNES, J. M. AND ROSSITER, R. J.: Tannic acid toxicity in burn therapy. Lancet *2:*218–222, Aug 21, '43

BARNES, J. P.: Review of modern burn treatment. Arch. Surg. *27:*527–544, Sept '33

BARNES, R.; BACSICH, P. AND WYBURN, G. M.: Histologic study of predegenerated autograft (ulnar). Brit. J. Surg. *33:*130–135, Oct '45

BARNES, R. *et al:* Fate of peripheral nerve homografts in man. Brit. J. Surg. *34:*34–41, July '46

BARNETT, L. A. (see HAMILTON, J. E.) Dec '43

BARNEVILLE (see VERRIÈRE) Feb '34

BARNHILL, JOHN F.: *Surgical Anatomy of the Head and Neck*. Wm. Wood and Co., New York, 1937. Second Edition (with William J. Mellinger), 1940.

BÁRON, A.: Importance of spongiosa in bone transplantation. Zentralbl. f. Chir. *53:*2332–2341, Sept 11, '26

BARON C.: Burn therapy. Kentucky M. J. *31:*579, Dec '33

BARR, H. B. (see COLBY, F.) Nov '32

BARRABIA VARALLA, A.: Sulfonamides; local use in burns. Semana med. *2:*568–569, Sept 2, '43

BARRAQUER FERRE, L.: Facial paralysis; diagnosis and therapy. Med. clin., Barcelona *1:*334–338, Nov '43

BARRAYA. (see MOURE, P.) Jan '34

BARRET, M.: Tannic acid in burns. Clinique, Paris *31:*135–138, May (A) '36

BARRETO NETO, M. (see PINHEIRO, J.) 1943

BARRETT, J. H.: Rhinoplastic correction of common deformities. Texas State J. Med. *41:*315–318, Oct '45

BARRON, J. B. (see JACOBSEN, H. H.) May '43

BARROS LIMA: Plastic repair of face by means of skin transplantation; case. Arq. de cir. e ortop. *1:*386–394, June '34

BARROUX, R. (see CHARBONNEL) Jan–Apr '41

BARROW, S. C.: Treatment of X-ray burn. Radiology *4:*54, Jan '25

BARROWS, D. N.: Artificial vagina; Kirschner-Wagner operation. Am. J. Obst. and Gynec. *31:*156–158, Jan '36

BARRY, T. (see PASSE, E. R. G.) April '41

BARSKY, A. J. (see SHEEHAN, J. E.) 1931

BARSKY, A. J.: Indications and limitations of plastic surgery. Radiol. Rev. and Mississippi Valley M. J. *59:*95–98, May '37

BARSKY, A. J.: Molded bone graft. Surgery *18:*755–763, Dec '45

BARSKY, A. J.: New instruments for nasal reconstructive surgery. Arch. Otolaryng. *22:*487–490, Oct '35

BARSKY, A. J.: New method for repair of small loss of alar rim. Arch. Otolaryng. *39:*325–326, April '44

BARSKY, A. J.: *Plastic Surgery*. W. B. Saunders Co., Phila., 1938

BARSKY, A. J.: Plastic surgery for general practitioner (grafts). Radiol. Rev. and Mississippi Valley M. J. *59:*13–15, Jan '37

BARSKY, A. J.: Plastic surgical repair of unusual dermatologic conditions. S. Clin. North America *19:*459–466, April '39

BARSKY, A. J.: Psychology of patient undergoing plastic surgery. Am. J. Surg. *65:*238–243, Aug '44

BARSKY, A. J.: Use of one flap to restore extensive losses of middle third of face. Ann. Surg. *118:*988–999, Dec '43

BARSKY, A. J.: Use of one flap to restore extensive losses of middle third of face. Tr. Am. Soc. Plastic and Reconstructive Surg. *12:*29–41, '43

BART, C.; ALEXENCO, V. AND STOLERU, D.: Burn therapy with infra-red light. Rev. stiint. med. *29:*490–495, June '40

BARTHÉLEMY, M.: Normet's citrated solution in shock. Bull. et mem. Soc. nat. de chir. *55:*1050–1052, July 20, '29

BARTLETT, E. I.: Technique of complete operation on breast. Surg., Gynec. and Obst. *52:*71–78, Jan '31

BARTOLI, O.: Influence of nervous system on transplantation of homoplastic grafts of striated muscular tissue. Policlinico (sez. chir.) *37:*361–370, Aug '30

BARTOLI, O.: Neurotization of homoplastic grafts of striated muscle. Arch. ed atti d. Soc. ital. di chir. *36:*1170, '30

BARTON, D. (see PICK, F.) Oct '43

BARTON, J. F.: After effects of nasal septal operation on children. Tr. Pacific Coast Oto-Ophth. Soc. *23:*172–177, '38

BARUCH, D.: Traumatic shock due to war wound. J. de chir. *23:*354–372, April '24

BARUK, H. (see LECHELLE, P. *et al*) May '27

BASAVILBASO, J.: Endonasal plastic surgery. Prensa med. argent. *13:*23–25, June 10, '26

BASAVILBASO, J.: Ivory in alloplasty of nasal fossae. Prensa med. argent. *13:*597–598, Nov 30, '26 also: Rev. de especialid. *1:*564–567, '26

BASS, H. H.: Precancerous lesions of oral cavity and their treatment. Internat. J. Med and Surg. *40:*321–323, Aug '27

BASS, Y. M. AND ZHOLONDZ, A. M.: Primary skin graft in fresh injuries of hand and fingers. Sovet. khir. (nos. 3–4) *6:*350–357, '34

BASSI, P.: Surgical therapy of tendon wounds; experimental study. Ann. ital. di chir. *18:*33–48, Jan–Feb '39

BASTERRA, J.: Technic of extranasal dacryocystorhinostomy. Arch. de oftal. hispano-am. *36:*208–216, April '36

BASTERRA, J.: Technic of extranasal dacryocystorhinostomy. Cron. med., Valencia *39:*354–363, May 15, '35

BASTIANELLI, P.: Cleft palate and harelip treated by mobilization of 2 triangular osseous segments from cleft palate. Boll. d. mal. d. orecchio, d. gola. e d. naso *49:*137–153, May '31

BASTOS, E.: Thyroglossal fistulae. Rev. oto-laring. de Sao Paulo *3:*227–238, May–June '35

BASTOS ANSART, M.: Factors of success and failure in tendon transplantation. Rev. de cir. de Buenos Aires *13:*657–673, Nov '34

BASTOS ANSART, M.: Factors in success and failure of tendon transplants; especially in therapy of sequels of poliomyelitis. Bol. y trab. de la Soc. de cir. de Buenos Aires *18:*848–868, Sept 12, '34

BASTOS ANSART, M.: Problems in plastic surgery. Rev. med. de Barcelona *8:*18–35, July '27 also: Arch. de med., cir. y espec. *27:*356–365, Sept 24, '27

BASTOS ANSART, M.: Successful and unsuccessful tendon transplants. Cir. ortop. y traumatol., Madrid *1:*5–26, '36

BASTUG, K. Ö. (see LÜTFÜ, Ö.) Dec '36

BASZERRA, J.: End-results in dacryocystorhinostomy. Med. ibera *1:*545–547, April 27, '29

BATALIN, A. K.: Correction of entropion in trachoma by modified Chronis method. Sovet. vestnik oftal. *3:*398–399, '33

BATE, J. T.: Instrument for subcutaneous removal of fascia lata strips for suture purposes. Ann. Surg. *95:*313–314, Feb '32

BATE, J. T.: Method of treating nerve ends in amputations. Am. J. Surg. *64:*373–374, June '44

BATE, J. T.: Operations for correction of locking of proximal interphalangeal joint in hyperextension. J. Bone and Joint Surg. *27:*142–144, Jan '45

BATEMAN, G. H. (see DAGGETT, W. I.) March '34

BATEMAN, J. E.: Universal splint for deformities of hand. J. Bone and Joint Surg. *28:*169–173, Jan '46

BATSELAERE, R. (see MUYLE, G.) July '36

BATSON, O. V.: Use of gelatin prosthesis in restoration of face. Tr. Am. Acad. Ophth. *40:*317-326, '35

BATTISTA, A.: Basocellular epithelioma of ear treated surgically. Rinasc. med. *6:*31–34, Jan 15, '29

BATTISTA, A.: Hypertrichosis following burns. Folia med. *16:*1420–1431, Oct 30, '30

BATTISTA, A.: Rigid fixation of jaws due to forward luxation; arthroplasty. Riforma med. *46:*1122–1127, July 14, '30

BATTISTA, A.: Surgical cure of elephantiasis. Urol. and Cutan. Rev. *34:*431–436, July '30

BATTY-SMITH, C. G.: Operation for increasing range of independent extension of ring finger for pianists. Brit. J. Surg. *29:*397–400, April '42

BAU, R. G. (see GURDIN, M. M. *et al*) March '44

BAUDET, G.: Ulcerated radiodermatitis of hand cured by perihumeral sympathectomy; case. Bull. et mem. Soc. nat. de chir. *61:*991-994, July 20, '35

BAUDOLINO, M.: Significance of specific immunity of organs during growth of homoplastic grafts. Gior. di batteriol. e immunol. *2:*381-389, June '27

BAUDOUIN, A. *et al:* Action of slow continuous injections of epinephrine in shock. Compt. rend. Soc. de biol. *119:*474-476, '35

BAUER, G.: Transplantation of nerves in facial palsy. Acta chir. Scandinav. *81:*130-138, '38

BAUER, I.: Venesection and blood transfusion as methods of treating extensive burns in infants. Deutsche med. Wchnschr. *64:*1064-1066, July 22, '38

BAUER, K. H.: Homeotransplants in uniovular twins. Beitr. z. klin. Chir. *141:*442-447, '27

BAUM, H. L.: Plastic surgery of nose; with special reference to correction of "saddle nose" deformities. Colorado Med. *22:*140-144, April '25

BAUM, G.: Operation for pendulous breasts. Med. Welt *3:*684, May 11, '29

BAUMANN, A. (see MONTANT, R.) Jan '38

BAUMANN, E.: Tendon suture after injuries. Zentralbl. f. Chir. *53:*3037-3038, Nov 27, '26

BAUMANN, E.: Treatment of surgical and traumatic shock. Schweiz. med. Wchnschr. *57:*1045-1047, Oct 29, '27

BAUMANN, R.: Treatment of finger injuries; plastic replacement of parts of thumb in industrial accident. Schweiz. med. Wchnschr. *58:*918-925, Sept 15, '28

BAUMGARTNER, C. J.: Branchial cysts and fistulas in children. Also: thyroglossal duct cysts and fistulas. Surg., Gynec. and Obst. *56:*948-955, May '33

BAUMGARTNER, C. J. AND STEINDEL, S.: Differential diagnosis between thymic duct fistulas and branchial cleft fistulas; case of bilateral aural fistulas and bilateral thymic duct fistulas. Am. J. Surg. *59:*99-103, Jan '43

BAUMRUCK, K. O. (see SITTIG, O.) April '38

BAUZÁ, J. A. (see BONABA, J.) Dec '28

BAUZÁ, J. A.: Partial biphallism (double penis) associated with exstrophy of bladder and multiple abnormalities of hands and feet; case. Arch. de pediat. d. Uruguay *3:*353-355, Aug '32

BAXTER, H. (see ELVIDGE, A.) Dec '44

BAXTER, H. (see SWEEZEY, E. *et al*) Jan '44

BAXTER, H.: Congenital fistulas of lower lip; case. Am. J. Orthodontics *25:*1002-1007, Oct '39

BAXTER, H.: New method of elongating short palates. Canad. M. A. J. *46:*322-325, April '42

BAXTER, H.: New method of treatment of depressed fracture of zygomatic bone (splint). Canad. M. A. J. *44:*5-9, Jan '41

BAXTER, H.: Plastic correction of protruding ears in children. Canad. M. A. J. *45:*217-220, Sept '41

BAXTER, H.: Plastic repair of congenital harelip. McGill M. J. *13:*151-156, April '44

BAXTER, H.: Tantalum in plastic surgery. McGill M. J. *12:*287-291, Dec '43

BAXTER, H. *et al:* Effect of different agents on rate of epithelial regeneration; use of dermatone donor area in obtaining clinical data. Canad. M. A. J. *50:*411-415, May '44

BAY, R. P. AND DORSEY, B. M.: Fractures of lower jaw. Am. J. Surg. *42:*532-535, Dec '38

BAYLEY DE CASTRO, A.: Accessory mouth. Indian M. Gaz. *58:*162-163, April '23 (illus.)

BAYMA, F.: Giant hemangiofibroma of nose; case. Ann. paulist. de med. e cir. *18:*1-10, Jan '27

BAYR, G.: Rare muscular contractures of hand following poisoning with carbon monoxide, phosphorus and ethyl gasoline. Deut. Militararzt *8:*623, Nov '43

BAZALA, W.: Plastic methods of construction of vagina; 10 cases. Ztschr. f. Geburtsh. u. Gynak. *100:*85-114, '31

BEACH, W. V.: Urgent surgery for hand. J. Roy. Nav. M. Serv. *27:*258-267, July '41

BEADNELL, C. M.: Congenital malformation of hands. Lancet *2:*800, Oct 18, '24

BEALL, L. L.: Treatment of facial wounds. Mississippi Doctor *19:*370-372, April '42

BEARD, J. W. (see BLALOCK, A. *et al*) Dec '31

BEARD, J. W. (see COOPER, G. R. *et al*) June '43

BEARD, J. W. AND BLALOCK, A.: Experimental shock; composition of fluid that escapes from blood stream after burns. Arch. Surg. *22:*617-625, April '31

BEARDSLEY, J. M. AND ZECCHINO, V.: Reconstruction of thumb. Am. J. Surg. *71:*825-827, June '46

BEARSE, C.: Ganglions of tendon sheaths; method of treatment. J.A.M.A. *109:*1626, Nov 13, '37

BEARSE, C.: Necrosis of terminal phalanx of finger; method of treatment. Boston M. and S. J. *197:*1083-1086, Dec 8, '27

BEATON, L. E. (see MASON, M. L. *et al*) Jan '40

BEATTIE, D. A.: Case of severe sepsis with hand infection; with some note on general treatment of such conditions. St. Barth. Hosp. J. *39:*147-152, May '32

BEATTY, H. G.: Care of cleft palate patients. Tr. Am. Laryng., Rhin. and Otol. Soc. *41:*165-

187, '35 also: Laryngoscope *46:*203–226, March '36

BEATTY, H. G.: Cleft palate. Ann. Otol. Rhin. and Laryng. *55:*572–579, Sept '46

BEATTY, H. G.: Etiology of cleft palate and harelip. J. Speech Disorders, pp. 13–20, March '36

BEATTY, H. G.: Harelip and cleft palate. West Virginia M. J. *32:*501–516, Nov '36

BEATTY, H. G.: Retractor for use in neck surgery. Arch. Otolaryng. *35:*651–652, April '42

BEATTY, S. R.: Roentgen therapy of Dupuytren's contracture. Radiology *30:*610–612, May '38

BEAUJON, O.: Recidivating symblepharon in leper treated with conjunctival transplant; case. Arch. venezol. Soc. de oto-rino-laring., oftal., neurol. *2:*23–27, March '41

Beaumetz Operation: See Dujardin-Beaumetz Operation

BEAUX, A. R.: Correction of protruding ears; Malbec technic. Prensa med. argent. *32:*2314–2320, Nov 23, '45

BEAUX, A. R.: Postage stamp grafts; technic and results. Bol. y trab., Soc. argent. de cirujanos *7:*355–362, '46 also: Rev. Asoc. med. argent. *60:*587–589, July 15, '46

BEAUX, A. R.: Spring finger due to partial hernia of flexor tendon. Prensa med. argent. *29:*1694–1698, Oct 21, '42

BEAVIS, J. O.: Problems associated with reconstructive procedures for cleft lip and palate. Ohio State M. J. *34:*1115–1117, Oct '38

BECART, A: Importance of rhythmic injection of blood or its substitutes (preserved blood, human plasma and Bayliss, Normet or physiologic serum) in acute hemorrhage and shock. Presse med. *47:*1681–1682, Dec 27–30, '39

BECART, A.: Traumatic shock and its therapy, with special reference to blood transfusion; importance of rhythmic injection. Monde med., Paris *49:*859–862, Dec '39

BECCARI, C.: Tannic acid in burns. Policlinico (sez. prat.) *44:*1637–1643, Aug 30, '37

BECHET, A. (see FOLLIASSON, A.) July '32

BECK, C. (see SMITH, S. *et al*) Oct '39

BECK, C.: Hand infections and fingers. Am. J. Surg. *8:*301–304, Feb '30

BECK, C.: *A Monograph on the Various Types of Deformities of the Hand and Arm*. J. B. Lippincott Co., Phila., 1925

BECK, C. AND BECK, W. C.: Plastic correction of pendulous breast. S. Clin. North America *14:*769–773, Aug '34

BECK, C. AND BECK, W. C.: Plastic reconstruction of fingers by transplantation of toes. S. Clin. North America *14:*763–767, Aug '34

BECK, C. K.: Nasal fractures. Kentucky M. J. *27:*387–390, Sept '29

BECK, C. S.: Burns. Kentucky M. J. *42:*68–72, March '44

BECK, C. S. AND POWERS, J. H.: Burns treated by tannic acid. Ann. Surg. *84:*19–36, July '26

BECK, E. G.: Carcinoma of external ear; combined surgical and radium treatment. Internat. Clinics *1:*29, '21

BECK, E. G.: Epithelioma of lower lip; combined surgical and radium treatment. Internat. Clinics *1:*31, '21

BECK, H.: Formation of artificial vagina. Orvosi hetil. *80:*207–209, March 7, '36

BECK, H.: Mechanism of temporomaxillary fractures. Ztschr. f. Stomatol. *38:*201–221, March 22, '40

BECK, J. C.: Anatomy, psychology, diagnosis and treatment of congenital malformation and absence of ear. Laryngoscope *35:*813–831, Nov '25

BECK, J. C.: Conclusive remarks from personal experience in plastic surgery. Ann. Otol., Rhin. and Laryng. *44:*90–93, March '35

BECK, J. C.: Personal and practical experiences with neoplasms about head and neck, with special reference to ear, nose and throat. Pennsylvania M. J. *34:*467–469, April '31

BECK, J. C.: Plastic and reconstructive surgery about face and head—then and now. Illinois M. J. *76:*237–242, Sept '39

BECK, J. C.: Plastic surgery about face, head and neck. J. Indiana M. A. *18:*167–184, May '25

BECK, J. C.: Principles in plastic surgery about head and neck (and nose). Illinois M. J. *48:*194–202, Sept '25

BECK, J. C.: Review of 25 years' observation in plastic surgery, with special reference to rhinoplasty. Laryngoscope *31:*487, July '21

BECK, J. C. AND GUTTMAN, M. R.: Plastic repair of defect following operative treatment of carcinoma of antrum and upper jaw. S. Clin. North America *14:*775–782, Aug '34

BECK, J. C. AND GUTTMAN, M. R.: Present day status of irradiation and surgery of cancer of neck. South. M. J. *29:*606–609, June '36

BECK, K.: Method of treating atresia of pharynx. Chirurg *8:*957–958, Dec 15, '36

BECK, O.: Causes of facial asymmetry in muscular wry-neck and jaw dislocations. Ztschr. f. orthop. Chir. *49:*424–449, May 18, '28

Beck Operation

Postoperative lymphedema of arm (in breast cancer); (Beck operation). GUTHRIE, D. AND GAGNON, G. Ann. Surg. *123:*925–936, May '46

Beck-Von Hacker Operation

Treatment of anterior balanic and penile hypospadias with Beck-von Hacker operation. MADIER, J. J. de chir. *18:*234-242, Sept '21 (illus.) J.A.M.A. *78:*688, March 4, '22 (abstr.)

BECK, W.: Congenital contracture of thumb. Arch. f. orthop. u. Unfall-Chir. *40:*318-325, '40
BECK, W. C. (see BECK, C.) Aug. '34
BECK, W. C.: Branchiogenic cysts in infancy. Surgery *1:*792-799, May '37
BECK, W. C.: Chemical burns of face. S. Clin. North America *18:*13-20, Feb '38
BECKER, E.: Suppurative inflammation of milkers' hands. Chirurg *2:*708-711, Aug 1, '30
BECKER, F. T.: Congenital auricular fistula. Arch. Dermat. and Syph. *48:*520-522, Nov '43
BECKER, J.: Branchial fistulas of neck. Beitr. z. klin. Chir. *134:*470-472, '25
BECKER, J.: Etiology and therapy of contracture of fingers. Zentralbl. f. Chir. *68:*2070-2072, Nov 1, '41
BECKER, J.: Myogenic traumatic ankylosis of jaws; case. Med. Welt *2:*681, May 5, '28
BECKER, O. J.: Aids in rhinoplastic procedures. Ann. Otol., Rhin. and Laryng. *55:*562-571, Sept '46
BECKER, O. J.: Surgical correction of protruding ears. Eye, Ear, Nose and Throat Monthly *24:*177-181, April '45
BECKER, S. W.: Melanoma of skin. Am. J. Cancer *22:*17-40, Sept '34
BECKER, S. W. AND BRUNSCHWIG, A.: Sinus preauricularis (fistula preauricularis congenita). Am. J. Surg. *24:*174-177, April '34
BECKERMAN, L. S.: Thermic burns and their therapy. Sovet. vrach. zhur. *43:*1163-1174, Dec 30, '39
BECUWE (see PIQUET, J.) May '37
BEDER, O. E.: Cleft palate children. Hygeia *24:*834-835, Nov '46
BEDER, O. E.: Obturators for palate; review. J. Oral Surg. *2:*356-368, Oct '44
BEDER, O. E.: Use of stents in skin grafting in mouth. J. Oral Surg. *2:*32-38, Jan '44
BEDER, O. E. AND SAPORITO, L. A.: Orofacial cripple. Am. J. Orthodontics (Oral Surg. Sect.) *32:*351-358, June '46
BEDER, O. E. *et al:* Correction of cleft palate using stress-breaker type partial appliance with obturator attached. Am. J. Orthodontics (Oral Surg. Sect.) *31:*377-380, June '45
BEECHER, H. K. AND MCCARRELL, J. D.: Reduction of fluid loss from damaged tissues (burns) by a barbiturate (pentobarbital sodium). J. Pharmacol. and Exper. Therap. *78:*39-48, May '43
BEEK, C. H.: Question of relationship between nevus and carcinoma. Nederl. tijdschr. v. geneesk. *82:*1199-1203, March 12, '38
BEEKMAN, F.: Grafts and transplants. Am. J. Surg. *26:*528-532, Dec '34
BEEKMAN, F.: Tannic acid in burns; end-results in 114 cases compared with 320 treated by other methods. Arch. Surg. *18:*803-806, March '29
BEEKMAN, F.: Use of pedicle graft for chronic osteomyelitis. S. Clin. North America *17:*185-190, Feb '37
BEEKMAN, F. AND O'CONNELL, R. J. JR.: Healing of surface wounds for prevention of deformities. Ann. Surg. *98:*394-407, Sept '33
BEER, E.: Exstrophy of bladder. S. Clin. North America *12:*283-285, April '32
BEER, H.: Treatment of traumatic hematoma of fingernails. Munchen. med. Wchnschr. *76:*1635, Sept 27, '29
BEGG, C. L. (see LOWSLEY, O. S.) Feb '38
BEGG, J. D.: Electric shock with extensive injuries requiring immediate amputation of left arm and right leg; case. M. J. Australia *2:*263-264, Aug 14, '37
BEGG, R. C.: Perineal hypospadias; case, treatment by tunnelling and skin graft. New Zealand M. J. *34:*378-383, Dec '35

Behcet Syndrome

Recurrent aphthous ulceration of oral mucous membrane and genitals associated with recurrent hypopyon iritis (Behcet syndrome); 3 cases. KATZENELLENBOGEN, I. Brit. J. Dermat. *58:*161-172, Jul-Aug '46

BEHDJET, H.: Diathermic treatment of rhinophyma; 2 cases. Dermat. Wchnschr. *88:*129-130, Jan 26, '29
BEHNCKE: Practical bandage for finger. Deutsche med. Wchnschr. *63:*558-559, April 2, '37
BEHREND, M.: Contractures due to burns of face, neck and body. S. Clin. N. America *6:*237-243, Feb '26
BEHREND, M.: Rhinoplasty to replace nose bitten off by a rat. J.A.M.A. *76:*1752, June 18, '21
BEHRENS, B.: Injuries to finger tips caused by stamping press. Med. Welt *12:*1706-1710, Nov 26, '38
BEHRMAN, W.: Nasal perforation; free transplantation; experiments with fascia lata. Acta oto-laryng. *34:*78-81, '46
BEHRMAN, W.: Ways of treating most anterior portions during submucous resection. Acta oto-laryng. *21:*248-255, '34
BEINFIELD, H. H.: Common errors in plastic

surgery and how to avoid them. Eye, Ear, Nose and Throat Monthly *25:*491–495, Oct '46

BEKKER, E. K. S.: Ultraviolet rays in burn therapy. Eksper. med. (no. 3) *8:*53–60, '41

BELCHOR, G.: Modern burn therapy. Rev. san. mil., Buenos Aires *42:*420–424, June '43 also: Prensa med. argent. *30:*1093–1096, June 16, '43

BELCHOR, G.: Prevention of infection in burns. Semana med. *2:*714–717, Sept 23, '43

BELFORT MATTOS, W.: Conjunctival palpebral autoplasty. Arq. brasil. de oftal. *8:*103–109, '45

BELISARIO, J. C.: Treatment of early carcinoma of lip, with special reference to use of low kilovoltage x-rays. M. J. Australia *1:*91–95, Jan 16, '37

BELK, W. P. Branchiogenic tumors of neck. S. Clin. N. Amer. *7:*453–468, April '27

BELL, B. T.: Principles of orthopedic treatment of rheumatoid arthritis. Pennsylvania M. J. *44:*1304–1305, July '41

BELL, J.: New pedigrees of hereditary disease; polydactylism and syndactylism. Ann. Eugenics *4:*41–48, April '29

BELL, J. G. Y.: Epithelioma following burns. Clin. J. *57:*525–527, Oct 31, '28

BELL, L. P.: Surgical treatment of imperforate anus; with report of case. Am. J. Obst. and Gynec. *14:*603–608, Nov '27

BELL, P. S.: Treatment of granulating areas in burns. Tr. Roy. Soc. Trop. Med. and Hyg. *27:*511–516, March '34

BELLELLI, F.: Esthetic surgery of saddle nose. Riforma med. *49:*442–448, March 25, '33

BELLELLI, F.: Problem of abnormal thumbs and thumbs with 3 phalanges. Riforma med. *53:*320, Feb 27, '37

BELLELLI, F.: Pseudo-atrophy of fingers or Ledderhose-Secrétan syndrome. Riforma med. *46:*257–258, Feb 17, '30

BELLINGER, D. H. (see WEAVER, D. F.) Oct '46

BELLINGER, D. H.: Blood and lymph vessel tumors involving mouth. J. Oral Surg. *2:*141–151, April '44

BELLINGER, D. H.: Fractures and dislocations of jaws and wounds of face. Am. J. Surg. *46:*535-541, Dec '39

BELLINGER, D. H.: Temporomandibular ankylosis and its surgical correction. J. Am. Dent. A. *27:*1563–1568, Oct '40

BELLINGER, D. H.; HENNY, F. A. AND PETERSON, L. W.: Fractures of mandibular condyle. J. Oral Surg. *1:*48–58, Jan '43

BELLO, E.: Infections of fingers and hands. Rev. med. peruana *9:*169–178, April '37

BELLO, E.: Modern therapy of burns. Cron. med., Lima *55:*173–177, June '38

BELLOCQ, PHILIPPE B.: *Anatomie medico-chirurgicale, Fascicles 2 and 3, La Face.* Masson et Cie, Paris, 1926

BELLONE, A.: Osteo-aponeurotic cavities of palm of hand in infections; roentgen study to determine mode of propagation of suppurative processes. Arch. di radiol. *15:*491–495, July–Oct '39

BELLONE, G.: Therapy of serous cysts of neck. Riv. san. siciliana *23:*1717–1724, Dec 1, '35

BELLOSO, R. A. AND GOLDIE, J. C.: Juvenile gigantomastia; surgical therapy of case. Arch. urug. de med., cir. y especialid. *17:*35–52, July '40

Belloste, Augustin

Augustin Belloste and treatment for avulsion of scalp; old history of operation in head surgery. STRAYER, L. M. New England J. Med. *220:*901–905, June 1, '39

BELLOT, A. (see DEGRAIS, P.) 1927

BELLOT, A. (see DEGRAIS, P.) March '32

Bell's Palsy: See Facial Paralysis

Surgical treatment of Bell's palsy. MORRIS, W. M. Lancet *1:*429–431, Feb 19 '38

BELOSOR, I.: Result of transplantations of blood vessels in Filatov cutaneous pedicle; experiments. Arch. f. klin. Chir. *168:*199–208, '31

BELOT, F.: Therapy of recent wounds of hands and fingers in miners. Scalpel *86:*1272–1276, Dec 2, '33

BELOT, J.: Physiotherapy of keloids. Bull. Soc. franc. de dermat. et syph. (Reunion dermat., Strasbourg) *38:*965–976, July '31

BELOT, J.: Therapy of keloids. J. de med. et chir. prat. *103:*77–87, Feb 10, '32

BELOT, J. AND BUHLER, Y. E.: Treatment of surface cancers of face with scraping and roentgen therapy; value in relation to other methods. Rev. d'actinol. *6:*91–107, March–April '30

BELOT, J. AND LEPENNETIER, F.: Epithelioma of face treated by grattage and radiotherapy. Bull. et mem. Soc. de radiol. med. de France *16:*227, Nov '28

BELOT, J. AND MÉNÉGAUX, G.: Parotid gland cancer, surgical therapy, recurrence and cure by radiotherapy. J. de radiol. et d'electrol. *15:*90–91, Feb '31

BELOU, PEDRO: *La revisión de la morfología arterial en las regiones anatómicas que atañen a la oto-rino-laringología.* La Sociedad Argentina de Oto-rino-laringología, Buenos Aires, 1939

BELOUSOVA, N. M. (see KOTELNIKOV, F. S.) 1941

BELSKAYA, V. M.: Alcohol block in delayed consolidation of maxillary fractures. Khirurgiya, no. 7, pp. 46-49, '44
BELTRAMI, G.: Therapy of maxillary fractures. Marseille-med. *1:*32-37, Jan 15, '40
BELYAEVA, V. I. AND POSTNIKOV, B. N.: Open method of burn therapy. Vestnik khir. *34:*93-106, '34
BEN, F.: Hemiatrophy of face and scleroderma. Dermat. Wchnschr. *83:*1366-1371, Sept 11, '26
BENATTI, D. (see ROSSELLO, H.) May '26
BENAVENTE, O. (see BERGARA, R. A. *et al*) Oct '34
BENDER, E.: Sincipital hydro-encephalocele with deformity of nose. Arch. f. klin. Chir. *161:*625-632, '30
BENEDEK, L. AND KULCSÁR, F.: Facial hemiatrophy; case. Gyogyaszat *73:*356-357, June 4, '33
BENEDETTI-VALENTINI, F.: New method of arthroplasty in bilateral ankylosis of jaw caused by trauma. Policlinico (sez. chir) *37:*201-215, May '30
BENEDICT, E. B. AND MEIGS, J. V.: Study of 225 cases of parotid tumors with complete end-results in 80 cases. Surg., Gynec. and Obst. *51:*626-647, Nov '30
BENEDICT, W. L.: Treatment of eyelid spasm. (blepharospasm) Tr. Am. Ophth. Soc. *39:*227-241, '41
BENEDICT, W. L. AND ASBURY, M. K.: Treatment of cancer of eyelids. New York State J. Med. *29:*675-677, June 1, '29
BENESI, O.: Role of nervous system in causation of congenital malformations of external and middle ear. Handb. d. Neurol. d. Ohres (Teil 1) *2:*89-112, '28
BENGOLEA, A. J.: Exstrophy of bladder treated by transfixion suture of ureters into large intestine (Coffey operation) in new-born infant. Bol. y trab. de la Soc. de cir. de Buenos Aires *17:*894-896, Sept 13, '33
BENJAMIN, B. (see TARLOV, I. M.) March '42
BENJAMIN, B. (see TARLOV, I. M.) March '43
BENJAMINS, C. E.: Congenital epithelial ducts and cysts of bridge of nose. Nederl. tijdschr. v. geneesk. *80:*1886-1890, May 2, '36 also: Acta oto-laryng. *24:*284-297, '36
BENJAMINS, C. E. AND STIBBE, F. H.: Congenital anomaly of external nose. Nederl. Tijdschr. v. Geneesk. *2:*2543-2549, Dec 4, '26
BENJAMINS, C. E. AND STIBBE, F. H.: Congenital deformity of nasal bones. Acta oto-laryng. *11:*274-284, '27
BENJAMINS, C. E. AND VAN ROMUNDE, L. H.: Plastic operation on lacrimal canal. Nederlandsch Tijdschr. v. Geneesk. *2:*33-35, July 1, '22 (illus.)
BENNETT, A. B.: Cure of mastoid fistula with fat graft; case. M. Ann. District of Columbia *2:*117-118, May '33

Bennett Fracture

Bennett fracture of thumb. WHEELER W. I. DE C., J. Bone and Joint Surg. *19:*520-521, April '37

BENNETT, I. B. AND CHILTON, N. W.: Traumatic cysts of mandible; case. J. Am. Dent. A. *32:*51-59, Jan 1, '45
BENNETT, L. C.: Radical operation with plastic closure, for cure of ingrowing nails. Mil. Surgeon *94:*361-364, June '44
BENON, R.: Jaw fracture with chronic asthenia. J. de med. et chir. prat. *99:*208-214, March 25, '28
BENSON, R. E. (see DIXON, C. F.) Sept '45
BENSON, R. E. (see MALCOLM, R. B.) Feb '40
BENTHIN, W.: Construction of artificial vagina. Zentralbl. f. Gynak. *45:*1330, Sept 17, '21
BENTLEY, F. H. AND HILL, M.: Nerve grafting. Brit. J. Surg. *24:*368-387, Oct '36
BENTLEY, F. H. AND HILL, M.: Possibilities of nerve transplantation. Brit. M. J. *2:*352-353, Sept 14, '40
BENTLEY, J. P. (see MORLEY, G. H.) Jan '43
BENVENUTO, E.: Bifid uvula in school children; statistical study. Valsalva *15:*492-494, Nov '39
BÉRARD; SARGNON AND EVRARD: Medial cervical fistula probably of thyroglossal origin; recovery after surgical intervention. Lyon med. *151:*611-613, May 14, '33
BÉRARD, L. AND CREYSSEL, J.: Treatment of large epitheliomas after failure of radiotherapy. (on face) Paris med. *1:*237-243, March 15, '30
BÉRARD, L. AND DUNET: Spreading epitheliomas, recurring after radium therapy; cure by surgical treatment. (face) Lyon chir. *26:*562-565, Aug-Sept '29
BÉRARD, L.; COLSON, C. R. AND DARGENT, M.: Indications for and limits of surgical therapy in extensive cancers of buccofacial region; 3 cases. Lyon chir. *35:*318-327, May-June '38
BERARD, M. (see SANTY, P.) Jan-Feb '36
BERARIU, A.: Etiologic study of multiple congenital malformations, with report of case of acrocephalosyndactylia. Rev. pediat. si puericult. *1:*314-318, May-Aug '37
BERCEANU, D.: Burn therapy. Rev. de chir., Bucuresti *41:*297-310, March-April '38
BERCHER: Cooperation between maxillofacial surgeon and other surgeons in treatment of soldiers with multiple wounds. Rev. de stomatol. *41:*759-769, '40

BERCHER, J.: Fracture of condylar region of maxilla; 6 cases. Rev. de chir. *61:*200-218, '23 (illus.)

BERCHER, J.: Fractures of jaws. Arch. de med. et pharm. mil. *76:*268-282, March '22 (illus.)

BERCHER, J.: Malignant tumors of jaws. Paris med. *11:*205, Sept 3, '21 abstr: J.A.M.A. *77:*1289, Oct 15, '21

BERCHER, J.: Question of need for resecting basculated condyle in subcondylar fractures. (jaw) Rev. de stomatol. *41:*196-197, March '39

BERCHER, J.: Treatment of war wounds of face and jaws. Mil. Surgeon *58:*130-132, Feb '26

BERCHER, J. AND FRIEZ, P.: Classification of anterior luxations of temporomaxillary joint. Presse med. *41:*644-646, April 22, '33

BERCHER, J. AND GINESTET, G.: Osteosynthesis by external fixation apparatus in fractures of lower jaw; technic and description of apparatus. Rev. de stomatol. *36:*294-300, May '34

BERCHER, J. AND LEPROUST: Unicondylar hypertrophy; late result after jaw resection; case. Rev. de stomatol. *41:*257-262, April '39

BERCHER, J.; PUIG, J. AND FLEURY: Continual dislocation of jaw at temporomaxillary articulation. Rev. d'hyg. *49:*605-607, Oct '27

BERCOWWITSCH, G. G.: Restoration of face. Dental Cosmos *70:*167-170, Feb '28

BERDICHEVSKIY, G. A.: Plastic surgery (grafts) in pathology and in clinical conditions. Novy khir. arkhiv *28:*79-87, '33

BERDICHEVSKIY, G. A.: Skin as plastic material for closure of large abdominal hernias. Novy khir. arkhiv. *45:*225-229, '40

BERENDES, J.: Nose and sinus injuries; necessity of early surgical intervention. Deut. Militararzt *7:*579-581, Sept '42

BERENS, C.: Canaliculus dilator in eye. Am. J. Ophth. *25:*725-726, June '42

BERENS, C.: Double-edged knife for removing mucous membrane and skin grafts. Tr. Sect. Ophth., A.M.A., p. 291, '40

BERENS, C. AND LOUTFALLAH, M.: Resection of left inferior oblique muscle at its scleral attachment for postoperative left hypotropia and left pseudoptosis. Am. J. Ophth. *26:*528-533, May '43

BERESOW, E. L.: Removal of submaxillary salivary glands and lymph glands in operations for carcinoma of lower lip. Deutsche Ztschr. f. Chir. *213:*391-415, '29

BERESOW, E. L.: Removal of submaxillary salivary glands in operations for carcinoma of lower lip; responses to questionnaire. Arch. f. klin. Chir. *151:*767-784, '28

BERESOW, S. L.: Insulin-dextrose treatment of surgical shock. Zentralbl. f. Chir. *53:*3214-3217, Dec 18, '26

Beresowski Operation

Beresowski method in surgical treatment of ankylosis of lower jaw. SOKOLOW, N. N. Deutsche Ztschr. f. Chir. *231:*294-298, '31

BERETTA, A.: Treatment of fractures of maxillary bones. Gior. di med. mil. *81:*952-956, Nov '33

BEREZINSKAYA, D. I.: Chemical burns to eyes. Sovet. vestnik oftal. *8:*319-332, '36

BEREZINSKAYA, D. I.: Role of paracentesis in therapy of chemical burns to eyes. Vestnik oftal. *13:*361-367, '38

BEREZKIN, N. F.: Autoplastic skin grafts for covering defects on extremities. Vestnik khir. *58:*196-204, Sept '39

BEREZKIN, N. F.: Visor-like method of cutaneous grafts in open wounds of bones and joints. Ortop. i travmatol. (no. 2) *13:*38-41, '39

BEREZOV, Y. E.: Antireticular cytotoxic serum in therapy of ulcerating cicatrix. Med. zhur. *13:*101-103, '44

BERG, A.: Complete harelip and cleft palate on left side, with absence of left half of intermaxillary bone, of philtrum and of cartilaginous portion of nasal septum. Arch. f. klin. Chir. *140:*168-171, '26

BERG, A.: Results of surgical therapy of carcinoma and sarcoma of lower jaw, some in advanced stage, over last 20 years. Ztschr. f. Stomatol. *35:*933-947, July 23, '37

BERG, R. (see COTTON, F. J.) Nov '29

BERGAGLIO, E. O.: Correction of flattened nose without graft, according to Gonzalez Loza procedure; author's experience. Rev. otorrinolaring. d. litoral *1:*373-377, March '42

BERGARA, C. (see BERGARA, R. A.) 1932

BERGARA, C. (see BERGARA, R. A.) Jan '33

BERGARA, C. (see BERGARA, R. A.) Jan '34

BERGARA, C. (see BERGARA, R. A. *et al*) Oct '34

BERGARA, R. A. AND BERGARA, C.: Bilateral congenital preauricular fistula, with report of case in congenital syphilitic. Rev. Asoc. med. argent. *48:*44-50, Jan '34

BERGARA, R. A. AND BERGARA, C.: Congenital auriculo-hyoid fistula; medical therapy; case. An. de oto-rino-laring. d. Uruguay *2:*117-130, '32

BERGARA, R. A. AND BERGARA, C.: Thyroglossal fistula; medical therapy, case. Rev. Asoc. med. argent. *47:*1983-1986, Jan '33

BERGARA, R. A.; BERGARA, C. AND BENAVENTE, O.: Modifying liquids in therapy of congenital fistulas of lateral region of neck; new case with recovery. Rev. Asoc. med. argent. *48:*1212-1215, Oct '34

Berge, C. A.: Septic branchial cyst eradicated by electrical cauterization; case. J. Michigan M. Soc. *40:*189-191, March '41

Bergel, D.: Question of Dupuytren's contracture as industrial injury meriting compensation. Med. Welt *10:*16-18, Jan 4, '36

Bergenfeldt, E.: Exstrophy of bladder with hydronephrosis and hydroureter on one side; surgical therapy by Coffey-Mayo operation. Ztschr. f. urol. Chir. *41:*515-521; '36

Bergenfeldt, E.: Prosthetic treatment of defects of mandible following unilateral exarticulation of mandible for adamantinoma; case. Acta chir. Scandinav. *64:*473-492, '29

Bergenhem Operation

Exstrophy of bladder, operation by Bergenhem method. Disque, T. L. Pennsylvania M. J. *33:*546, May '30

Remote sequelae of rectal implantation of ureters for exstrophy; findings at necropsy 14 years after Bergenhem operation. Richey, DeW. G. Arch. Surg. *11:*408-416, Sept '25

Berger, A.: Correction of case of cicatricial oral atresia. J. Am. Dent. A. *32:*1427-1430, Nov 1-Dec 1, '45

Berger, A.: Extra-articular bony ankylosis of temporomandibular joint. Bull. Hosp. Joint Dis. *2:*27-33, Jan '41

Berger, A.: Fractures of mandibular condyle. J. Am. Dent. A. *30:*819-833, June 1, '43

Berger, A.: *Principles and Technique of Oral Surgery*. Dental Items of Interest Publishing Co., Brooklyn, 1923

Berger, A.: Symposium on reparative surgery; osteomyelitis of jaws. S. Clin. North America *24:*392-403, April '44

Berger, R. A. (see Hodges, F. M. *et al*) May '39

Bergeret, A. and Martin, J.: Esthetic breast surgery; various technics. Gynec. et obst. *29:*55-70, Jan '34

Bergeret, P.M. (see Pacaud, H. E. L.) Oct '30

Bergeron, G. A. (see Green, H. D.) March '45

Berggren, S. and Froste, N.: Combined plastic surgery on facial and facial-hypoglossal nerves for facial paralysis. Acta oto-laryng. *30:*325-327, '42

Bergk, W.: Perforated duodenal ulcer and ileus following burn; case. Chirurg *10:*548-552, Aug 1, '38

Bergman, H. C. (see Prinzmetal, M. *et al*) Dec '44

Bergman, H. C. (see Hechter, O. *et al*) April '45

Bergman, H. C. (see Prinzmetal, M.) May-June '45

Bergman, H. C. (see Prinzmetal, M.) Dec '45

Bergman, H. C. and Printzmetal, M.: Antishock action of certain drugs in burned mice. J. Lab. and Clin. Med. *31:*663-671, June '46

Bergman, H. C. and Prinzmetal, M.: Antishock action of ethanol (ethyl alcohol) in burned mice; effect of edema formation and capillary atony. J. Lab. and Clin. Med. *31:*654-662, June '46

Bergman, H. C. and Prinzmetal, M.: Influence of environmental temperature on shock in burns. Arch. Surg. *50:*201-206, April '45

Bergman, H. C.; Hechter, O. and Prinzmetal, M.: Effect of short-term nutritional stress upon resistance to scald shock. Am. Heart J. *29:*513-515, April '45

Bergman, H. C. *et al:* Ineffectiveness of adrenocortical hormones, thiamine, ascorbic acid, nupercaine and post-traumatic serum in shock due to scalding burns. Am. Heart J. *29:*506-512, April '45

Bergmann, E.: Principles of cineplastic operations. J. Internat. Coll. Surgeons *9:*99-103, Jan-Feb '46

Bering, F.: Elastic prosthesis for defects of nose and ear. Munchen. med. Wchnschr. *86:*253-254, Feb 17, '39 (Comment on Siemens' article).

Berke, R. N.: Resection of levator palpebrae in ptosis (eye), with anatomic studies. Tr. Am. Ophth. Soc. *42:*411-435, '44; also: Arch. Ophth. *33:*269-280, April '45

Berkley, W. L.: Treatment of cicatricial entropion. U. S. Nav. M. Bull. *41:*729-736, May '43

Berkove, A. B.: Hypertelorism. Arch. Otolaryng. *38:*587-589, Dec '43

Berkovich, E. M.: Intracisternal injection of potassium phosphate according to Shtern method in therapy of traumatic shock at the front. Khirurgiya, no. 7, pp. 8-12, '44

Berkow, S. G.: Burns incident to war (treatment). Clinics *2:*1265-1294, Feb '44

Berkow, S. G.: Ectropion of lower eyelids following burns and scalds; new early pathognomonic sign. J.A.M.A. *90:*1708-1709, May 26, '28

Berkow, S. G.: Program for emergency treatment of extensive burns. U. S. Nav. M. Bull. *41:*946-952, July '43

Berkow, S. G.: Tape method of skin grafting. U. S. Nav. M. Bull. *45:*1-13, July '45

Berkow, S. G.: Value of surface-area proportions in prognosis of cutaneous burns and scalds. Am. J. Surg. *11:*315-317, Feb '31

BERLIEN, I. C. AND DAVIS, J.R.: Cod-liver oil and vaseline in burns. Ohio State M. J. *35:*267-269, March '39

BERLINER, M. L.: Unilateral microphthalmia with congenital anterior synechiae and syndactyly. Arch. Ophth. *26:*653-660, Oct '41

BERMAN, H. L.: Nasal fractures. M. Rec. *140:*17, July 4, '34

BERMAN, H. L.: Submucous resection. Laryngoscope *45:*184-187, March '35

BERMAN, J. K.; PETERSON, L. AND BUTLER, J.: Treatment of burn shock with continuous hypodermoclysis of physiologic saline solution into burned area; experimental study. Surg., Gynec. and Obst. *78:*337-345, April '44

BERMAN, J. K.; PIERCE, G. S.; AND BEST, M. M.: Burn shock; Treatment with continuous hypodermoclysis of isotonic solution of sodium chloride into burned areas; clinical studies in 2 cases. Arch. Surg. *53:*577-587, Nov '46

BERMUDEZ, E.: Therapy of burns in last war. Gac. med. Lima *2:*275-281, March '46

BERNALDEZ SARMIENTO, P.: Surgical therapy of elephantiasis of extremities; review apropos of case. Rev. espan. cir., traumatol. y ortop. *3:*146-156, Sept '45

BERNARD, E.: Tannin in burns. Bull. et mem. Soc. d. chirurgiens de Paris *27:*583-586, Dec 6, '35

BERNARD, G. T. (see GREENBLATT, R. B. *et al*) Feb '36

BERNARD, MME. I. (see CLAOUE, C.) Oct '36

BERNARD, R.: Management of facial teguments in extensive exeresis for cancers of inferior maxilla, of floor of mouth, of tonsils and of pharynx. Presse med. *41:*748-751, May 10, '33

BERNARDI, R. (see GRIMALDI, F. E.) Sept '41

BERNARDI, R. (see GRIMALDI, F.E.) Sept-Oct '41

BERNDORFER, A.: Esthetics of plastic surgery (face). Gyogyaszat *78:*638-641, Oct 30, '38

BERNDORFER, A.: Harelip and cleft palate. Gyogyaszat *76:*499, Aug 30-Sept 6, '36; 527, Sept 13, '36

BERNDORFER, A.: Psychology of plastic surgery of ear. Gyogyaszat *79:*349-351, June 4, '39

BERNDORFER, A.: Surgical and phonetic problems of harelip and cleft palate. Gyogyaszat 277:433, July 18-25; 452, Aug 1-8, '37

BERNE, L. P.: Rhinoplastic surgeon versus rhinologist. Tr. Sect. Laryng., Otol. and Rhin., A.M.A., pp. 118-121, '23

BERNE, L. P.: Rhinoplasty from an artist's standpoint. J. M. Soc. New Jersey *21:*121-123, April '24

BERNFELD, K.: Congenital functional defect of soft palate and uvula with other malformations of first and second branchial arches in unshortened palate. Monatschr. f. Ohren., *66:*916-921, Aug '32

BERNHEIMER, L. B.: Ivory implant in atrophic rhinitis. Illinois M. J. *55:*420-422, June '29

BERNIER, J. L. AND CANBY, C. P.: Histologic studies on reaction of alveolar bone to vitallium implants (preliminary report). J. Am. Dent. A. *30:*188-197, Feb 1, '43

BERNSTEIN, E.: Hemiatrophia alternans facialis progressiva with hemilateral alopecia; pigment displacement and atrophy of skin; case. Dermat. Wchnschr. *90:*235-237, Feb 15, '30

BERNSTEIN, M. A.: Clinical aspect of tendon transposition. Surg., Gynec. and Obst., *34:*84-90, Jan '22 (illus.)

BERNSTEIN, P.: Gastroschisis, rare teratologic condition in new-born; case. Arch. Pediat. *57:*505-513, '40

BERNSTIEN, J.: Treatment (with ivory implants) of atrophic rhinitis. J. Laryng. and Otol. *48:*603-607, Sept '33

BERNTSEN, A.: BIlateral congenital manus vara without defects of bones of forearm; 3 cases. Acta chir. Scandinav. *67:*61-67, '30

BERNUCCI, F.: Possibility of transmission of biologic properties of skin from animal to animal by means of transplantation. Gior. ital. di dermat. e sif. *73:*1373-1379, Aug '32

BERNUCCI, F.: Tardy result of burn from toxic gas. Gior. ital. di dermat. e sifil. *66:*1349-1357, Oct '25

BERRI, C. (see CORA ELISEHT, F.) April '39

BERROCAL URIBE, E. (see ISELIN, M.) Feb '32

BERRY, G.: Branchial cyst; 2 instructive cases. Ann. Otol. Rhin. and Laryng., *43:*287-293, March '34

BERRY, H. C.: Care of military and civilian injuries; implantation method of setting fractured mandibles. Am. J. Orthodontics (Oral Surg. Sect) *28:*292-306, May '42

BERRY, H. C.: New departure from orthodox methods of setting fractured edentulous mandibles. J. Am. Dent. A. *28:*388-392, March '41

BERRY, H. C.: Simple skeletal fixation method for quick repair in war surgery. (Jaws) J. Am. Dent. A. *30:*1377-1378, Sept 1, '43

BERRY, J.: Operation for cleft palate. Brit. J. Surg. *8:*364, Jan '21

BERRY, M. F.: Correction of cleft-palate speech by phonetic instruction. Quart. J. Speech Educ. *14:*523-529, Nov '28

BERRY, T. B. (see BEYERS, C. F.) Dec '25

BERRY, T. B. AND KRITZINGER, F. J.: Surgical and dental treatment of cleft palate. South African M. J. *15:*497-498, Dec 27, '41

BERSHON, A. L. (see CHOLLETT, B. G.) March '31

BERSON, M. I.: Complete reconstruction of auricle. Am. J. Surg. *60:*101–104, April '43

BERSON, M. I.: Construction of ideal nose with aid of masks and measurements. M. Rec. *149:*80–82, Feb 1, '39

BERSON, M. I.: Derma-fat-fascia transplants used in building up breasts. Surgery *15:*451–456, March '44

BERSON, M. I.: Important considerations in rhinoplastic procedures. Eye, Ear, Nose and Throat Monthly *22:*424–430, Nov '43

BERSON, M. I.: Mammaplasty for pendulous hypertrophied breasts. M. Rec. *153:*89–92, Feb 4, '41

BERSON, M. I.: Monocaine hydrochloride; clinical experiences and technic of administration in rhinoplasty. Anesth. and Analg. *23:*189–195, Sept–Oct '44

BERSON, M. I.: New rhinometer. Am. J. Surg. *63:*148–149, Jan '44

BERSON, M. I.: Plastic repair for protruding ears. Eye, Ear, Nose and Throat Monthly *24:*423–426, Sept '45

BERSON, M. I.: Prevention of nasal deformity in corrective rhinoplasty (description of rhinometer.) Laryngoscope *53:*276–287, April '43

BERSON, M. I.: Rebuilding bony depressions of face and skull. J. Internat. Coll. Surgeons *9:*243–247, Mar–Apr '46

BERSON, M. I.: Relation of deflections of nasal septum to rhinoplasty. M. Rec. *158:*734–736, Dec '45

BERSON, M. I.: Surgical removal of hemangioma of face with grafting. Am. J. Surg. *51:*362–365, Feb '41

BERTANZI, R.: Basocellular epithelioma of face with clinical syndrome simulating scleroderma. Gior. ital. di dermat. e sifil. *70:*1344–1348, Oct '29

BERTEIN: Fracture of 3 orbital walls with suppurative ethmoiditis; case. Lyon med. *142:*79, July 15, '28

BERTEIN, P. (see SARGNON, A.) Sept '29

BERTEIN, P.: Physiologic troubles in patients with old wounds and injuries of face. Bull. med., Paris *44:*947–949, Dec 27, '30

BERTI, A. (see ARAUJO, D. G.) 1940

BERTINI, G.: Vascularization of autoplastic bone implants. Arch. ital. di chir. *16:*105–121, '26

BERTOCCHI, A.: Periarterial decortication as aid to skin grafting. Gior. d. r. Accad. di med. di Torino *33:*129–134, March '27

BERTOCCHI, A.: Periarterial decortication by Leriche method and autoplastic and homoplastic grafts. Arch. ital. di chir. *29:*1–36, '31

BERTOCCHI, A.: Osteoplastic amputation with graft of fixed heteroplastic bone. Arch. ital. di chir. *50:*315–321, '38

BERTOCCHI, A.: Skin grafts. Arch. ital. di chir. *11:*445–482, '25 abstr: J.A.M.A. *85:*1095, Oct 3, '25

BERTOCCHI, A.: Transplantation of fat tissue previously treated with fixation fluid. Arch. ital. di chir. *12:*621–652, '25

BERTOCCHI, A. AND BIANCHETTI, C. F.: Experimental researches on homoplastic transplantation of striated muscle preserved in vitro. Arch. per le sc. med. *51:*347–363, '27

BERTOCCHI, A. AND BIANCHETTI, C. F.: Experimental researches on homoplastic transplantation of striated muscle preserved in vitro. Gior. d. r. Accad. di med. di Torino *90:*434–438, Aug '27

BERTOCCHI, A. AND BIANCHETTI, C. F.: Tendon and fascia autografts drawn through channel in bone or joint. Chir. d. org. di movimento *7:*225–243, June '23 (illus.) abstr: J.A.M.A. *81:*964, Sept 15, '23

BERTOLA, V. J.: Cervicofacial arc, apparatus for isolating surgical field. Prensa med. argent. *27:*997–998, May 8, '40

BERTOLA, V. J.: Compass for symmetrical measured tracing in plastic surgery of breast. Semana med. *2:*197–198, July 16, '36

BERTOLA, V. J.: New periosteotome for hard palate. Prensa med. argent. *26:*1853–1854, Sept 20, '39

BERTOLA, V. J.: Procedure for treating habitual or recidivating luxation of temporomaxillary joint. Prensa med. argent. *29:*536–542, April 1, '42

BERTOLA, V. J.: Resection of lower jaw by oral route. Prensa med. argent. *28:*323–327, Feb 5, '41

BERTOLA, V. J. AND MOREYRA BERNAN, L.: Maxillofacial prognathism; surgical therapy of case. Bol. y trab., Soc. de cir. de Cordoba *6:*59–75, '45

BERTOLA, V. J.; SALA, F. AND ORTIZ, C.: Fracture of penis; surgical therapy of case. Prensa med. argent. *32:*703–707, April 20, '45

BERTOLA, V. J.; YADAROLA, D. AND SALA, F.: Resection of superior cervical ganglion (Leriche operation) in therapy of peripheral facial paralysis; 3 cases. Prensa med. argent. *23:*2414–2427, Oct 21, '36

BERTOLINO, P.: Burn therapy. Profilassi *7:*201–219, June '34

BERTOTTO, E. V.: Buccal mucosal grafts in therapy of total symblepharon. Rev. med. de Rosario *35:*317–322, April '45

BERTRAND, P. AND FREIDEL, C.: Craniofacial disjunction; case. Lyon chir. *30:*632–634, Sept–Oct '32

BERTRAND, P. AND FREIDEL, C.: Treatment of fracture of lower jaw without loss of sub-

stance. Bull. med. Paris *45:*585–587, Aug 22, '31
Bertreux, H. (see Pauchet, V. *et al*) Dec '33
Bertwistle, A. P.: Harelip treatment; suggestion. Clin. J. *71:*71–72, March–April '42
Bertwistle, A. P.: Results of operations on thyroglossal tract and a note on thyroid secretions. Canad. M. A. J. *15:*400–401, April '25
Bertwistle, A. P.: Skin grafting in general practice. Practitioner *113:*440–441, Dec '24
Bertwistle, A. P.: Treatment of facial paralysis due to exposure. Brit. M. J. *2:*494, Sept 17, '27
Bertwistle, A. P.: "Tulip fingers." Brit. M. J. *2:*255, Aug 10, '35
Bertwistle, A. P. and Frazer, J. E.: Study of thyroglossal tract. Brit. J. Surg. *12:*561–578, Jan '25
Beselin, O. (see Kafemann, A. W.) Dec '26
Beselin, O.: Etiology and operation of congenital dermoid on dorsum of nose. Arch. f. Ohren-, Nasen-u. Kehlkopfh. *129:*47–49, June 6, '31
Besser, E. L.: Role of adrenal glands in shock; value of desoxycorticosterone acetate (adrenal preparation) in prevention of operative shock. Arch. Surg. *43:*249–256, Aug '41
Besser, E. L.: Stored dextrose-citrate plasma in treatment of operative shock. Arch. Surg. *43:*451–457, Sept '41
Best, C. H. and Solandt, D. Y.: Concentrated serum in treatment of traumatic shock in experimental animals. Brit. M. J. *1:*799–802, May 18, '40
Best, M. M. (see Berman, J. K. *et al*) Nov '46
Best, R. R.: Anatomical and clinical study of hand infections. Ann. Surg. *89:*359–378, March '29
Bett, W. R.: Traumatic cleft palate; Micrococcus catarrhalis meningitis; recovery. Brit. M. J. *1:*494–495, March 21, '31
Bettazzi, G.: Lesions of hand and face caused by colored copying pencil. Policlinico (sez. chir.) *35:*501–505, Oct '28
Bettman, A. G.: Back as source for pedicled grafts. Northwest Med. *32:*453–456, Nov '33
Bettman, A. G.: Burns; treatment of shock and toxemia; healing wound; reconstruction. Am. J. Surg. *20:*33–37, April '33
Bettman, A. G.: Homogenous Thiersch grafting as life saving measure in burns. Am. J. Surg. *39:*156–162, Jan '38
Bettman, A. G.: New Thiersch graft razor. J.A.M.A. *89:*451, Aug 6, '27
Bettman, A. G.: Pedicled skin grafts. Northwest Med. *27:*78–86, Feb '28
Bettman, A. G.: Plastic surgery about eyes. Ann. Surg. *88:*994–1006, Dec '28
Bettman, A. G.: Plastic surgery of nose. M. J. and Rec. *123:*417–421, April 7; 499–501, April 21, '26
Bettman, A. G.: Plastic surgery; psychology of appearances. Northwest Med. *28:*182–185, April '29
Bettman, A. G.: Rationale of tannic acid-silver nitrate treatment of burns. J.A.M.A. *108:*1490–1494, May 1, '37
Bettman, A. G.: Simpler technic for promoting epithelization and protecting skin grafts (oxyquinoline sulphate scarlet R ointment). J.A.M.A. *97:*1879–1881, Dec 19, '31
Bettman, A. G.: Syndactylizing fingers preliminary to skin grafting. Northwest Med. *31:*70–71, Feb '32
Bettman, A. G.: Tannic acid and silver nitrate in burns. Am. J. Nursing *37:*1333–1339, Dec '37
Bettman, A. G.: Tannic acid and silver nitrate in burns. Surg., Gynec. and Obst. *62:*458–463, Feb (no. 2A) '36
Bettman, A. G.: Tannic acid-silver nitrate in burns; method of minimizing shock and toxemia and shortening convalescence. Northwest Med. *34:*46–51, Feb '35
Bettman, A. G.: Total reconstruction of ear; original technic. Rev. de chir. plastique, pp. 3–13, May '34
Bettman, E. Jr.: Traumatic hard edema of hand. Arch. f. orthop. u. Unfall-Chir. *32:*570–575, '33
Bettmann, E. H. (see Stein, H. C.) Nov '40
Betts, L. O.: Injuries of flexor tendons of hand. M. J. Australia *2:*457–460, Nov 9, '40
Bevan, A. D.: X-ray burns. S. Clin. N. Amer. *1:*935, Aug '21
Bevilacqua, E.: Wounds of fingers during work. Gazz. d. osp. *59:*506–510, May 15, '38
Beyer, A. R.: Volkmann's contracture. J. Florida M. A. *15:*599–600, June '29
Beyers, C. F. and Berry, T. B.: Case of facial deformity (jaw also). M. J. S. Africa *21:*127–131, Dec '25
Beynes, E.: Congenital choanal imperforation; operation. Arch. internat. de laryng. *34:*179–183, Feb '28
Béyoul, A.: Dupuytren's contracture; clinical study. Rev. de chir., Paris *73:*351–357, May '35
Beyul, A. P. and Kogan, A. V.: False Dupuytren's contracture. Khirurgiya, no. 3, pp. 98–102, '37
Bezerra, M.: Free grafts of whole skin. Arq. brasil. de cir. e ortop. *(12):*165–174, '44
Bezza, P.: Possibility of repairing loss of bony substance of cranium by means of graft of bladder mucosa. Arch. ital. di chir. *55:*405–429, '39

BHADRA, A. C.: Treatment of burns. Indian M. J. *39:*174–175, June '45
BHANDARI, S. L.: Hypospadias, case with double channel urethra. Indian M. Gaz. *66:*444, Aug '31
BHAVE, Y. M.: Method of removing tight ring from finger. Indian M. Gaz. *75:*354, June '40
BIAILLE DE LANGIBAUDIERE, M.: Technic of Italian graft in hand injuries. Bull. Soc. med.-chir. de l'Indochine *13:*387–396, May '35
BIANCALANA, L.: Ombredanne operation in hypospadias; case. Boll. e mem. Soc. piemontese di chir. *6:*18–25, '36
BIANCALANA, L.: Posterior hypospadias cured by Ombredanne operation; case. Boll. e mem. Soc. piemontese di chir. *7:*325–327, '37
BIANCALANI, A.: Evaluation of pluridigital lesions (injuries). Rassegna d. previd. sociale *26:*40–44, Sept '39
BIANCHERI, A.: Right osseous temporomaxillary ankylosis; surgical therapy; case. Arch. ital. di chir. *50:*396–403, '38
BIANCHETTI, C. F. (see BERTOCCHI, A.) June '23
BIANCHETTI, C. F. (see BERTOCCHI, A.) 1927
BIANCHETTI, C. F. (see BERTOCCHI, A.) Aug '27
BIANCHI, A. E. AND PAVLOVSKY, A.: Branchiogenous cysts and cystadenolymphomas. An. Inst. modelo de clin. med. *21:*436–452, '40
BIANCHI, G.: Alcohol and insulin in severe burns; preliminary report. Riforma med. *51:*1179–1180, Aug 3, '35
BIANCHI, R. G.: Graft of cadaver skin; preliminary report. Dia med. *17:*1168, Oct 8, '45 also: Prensa med. argent. *32:*1997, Oct 12, '45
BIANCHINI, A.: Syndactylia with acrocephaly; case. Radiol. med. *14:*1–12, Jan '27
BIANCULLI, H.: Plastic surgery of nose. Semana med. *1:*741–748, March 28, '29
BIANCULLI, H.: Plastic surgery of nose. Semana med. *1:*292–297, Jan 29, '31
BICHLMAYR, A.: First aid in facial injuries. Munchen. med. Wchnschr. *85:*1267–1275, Aug 19, '38
BICHLMAYR, A.: Therapy of complicated fractures of lower jaw. Med. Welt *9:*158–160, Feb 2, '35
BICK, M. AND DREVERMANN, E. B.: Use of pooled human serum for treatment of hemorrhage and shock. M. J. Australia *1:*750–754, June 21, '41
BICKEL, W. H.; MEYERDING, H. W. AND BRODERS, A. C.: Melanoepithelioma (melanosarcoma, melanocarcinoma, malignant melanoma) of extremities. Surg., Gynec. and Obst. *76:*570–576, May '43
BIDART MALBRÁN, J. C.: Thyroglossal fistula, four times recurrent; case. Bol. y trab. de la Soc. de cir. de Buenos Aires *12:*491–498, Sept 5, '28

Bidder Operation: See Landerer-Bidder Operation

BIDDLE, A. G.: Improved breast lifting operation. Am. J. Surg. *67:*488–494, March '45
BIDDLE, A. G.: Improved technic for restoration of pendulous breast. Am. J. Surg. *23:*191–193, Jan '34
BIDGOOD, C. Y.: Treatment of hypospadias; analysis of 28 cases. Virginia M. Monthly *51:*634–642, Jan '25
BIEDERMANN, H.: Reconstruction of palate after injury. Beitr. z. klin. Chir. *125:*444–450, '22 (illus.) abstr: J.A.M.A. *79:*84, July 1, '22
BIESENBERGER, H.: Care, preservation and repair of female breasts; review of Erna Glaesmer's "Die Formfehler und die plastischen Operationen de weiblichen Brust," and H. Biesenberger's "Deformitaten und Operationen de weiblichen Brust." SELLHEIM, H. Deutsche med. Wchnschr. *58:*1414–1417, Sept 2, '32
BIESENBERGER, H.: Cosmetic corrections of the legs. Wien. med. Wchnschr. *82:*735–738, June 4, '32
BIESENBERGER, H.: *Deformitäten und kosmetische Operationen der weiblichen Brust.* Wilhelm Maudrich, Vienna, 1931
BIESENBERGER, H.: New method of mammaplasty. Zentralbl. f. Chir. *55:*2382–2387, Sept 22, '28
BIESENBERGER, H.: New methods of treatment of hypertrophy of breast by plastic surgery. Zentralbl. f. Chir. *57:*2971–2975, Nov 29, '30 (Addendum)
BIESENBERGER, H.: Plastic operation on protruding ears (Gersuny). Zentralbl. f. Chir. *51:*1126–1127, May 24, '24
BIESENBERGER, H.: Surgical correction of breast. Wien. med. Wchnschr. *82:*734–735, June 4, '32
BIESENBERGER, H.: Unilateral surgical correction of asymmetric breasts. Wien. med. Wchnschr. *82:*732–733, June 4, '32
BIETTI, G.: Surgical technic in congenital eyelid ptosis (modifications and additions to existing procedure of substituting frontal muscle). Boll. d'ocul. *21:*721–727, Nov-Dec '42
BIGELOW, H. M.: Facial restorations. J. Am. Dent. A. *30:*509–512, April 1, '43
BIGELOW, H. M.: Treatment of fractures of mandible with vitallium screws. M. Bull. Vet. Admin. *17:*54–56, July '40
BIGELOW, H. M.: Vitallium bone screws and appliances for fracture of mandible. J. Oral Surg. *1:*131–137, April '43

BIGGER, I. A. (see EVANS, E. I.) Oct '45
BIGGER, I. A.: Hypertonic sodium chloride solution intravenously in treatment of extensive superficial burns. South. M. J. *19:*302-306, April '26
BIGGS, A. D. (see LLEWELLYN, J. S.) March '43
BIGGS, T. J.: Lymphedema of leg. M. J. Australia *1:*623-624, May 18, '35
BILLET, H.: Present status of traumatic shock and hemorrhage. Arch. de med. et pharm. mil. *74:*473-486, May '21
BILLICH, H. U.: "Carpenter's hand." Mitt. a. d. Grenzgeb. d. Med. u. Chir. *40:*638-647, '28
BILLIG, H. E. JR. AND VAN HARREVELD, A.: New aspect of muscle reinnervation; preliminary report. U. S. Nav. M. Bull. *41:*410-414, March '43
BILLINGTON, R. W.: Tendon transplantation for musculospiral (radial) nerve injury. J. Bone and Joint Surg. *4:*538-547, July '22 (illus.)
BILLINGTON, W.: Two-stage operation for cleft palate. Brit. M. J. *1:*15, Jan 1, '27
BILLINGTON, W. AND ROUND, H.: Bone-grafting of mandible, with report of 7 cases. Brit. J. Surg. *13:*497-505, Jan '26
BILLINGTON, W. AND ROUND, H.: Bone grafting the mandible. Am. Dent. Surgeon *50:*185-188, May '30
BILLINGTON, W. AND ROUND, H.: Bone-grafting the mandible. Proc. Roy. Soc. Med (sect. Odont.) *23:*7-13, March '30
BILLINGTON, W. AND ROUND, H.: Two-stage operation for cleft palate. Proc. Roy. Soc. Med. (sect. Odont.) *23:*13-20, March '30
BINET, L. AND STRUMZA, M. V.: Intravenous injections of diluted blood; experimental study in shock. Bull. Acad. de med., Paris *123:*592-595, Aug 6-27, '40
BINET, L. AND STRUMZA, M. V.: Study of shock and therapeutic deductions. Presse med. *48:*825-828, Oct 16-19, '40
BINGEL, K.: Local metabolism and tissue reaction; effect of transplantation into heterogenic tissue and of application of salt solution and of organ extract on growth of transplanted cartilage. Beitr. z. path. Anat. u. z. allg. Path. *99:*205-223, '37
BINGHAM, D. L. C. AND JACK, E. A.: "Buttonholed" extensor expansion of finger. Brit. M. J. *2:*701-702, Oct 9, '37
BINGHAM, R.: Nonadherent surgical dressings (especially nylon surgical gauze). Arch. Surg. *52:*610-618, May '46
BINHOLD: Homoplastic transplantations of human skin, with special consideration of blood characteristics. Deutsche Ztschr. f. Chir. *252:*183-195, '39
BINTCLIFFE, E. W. (see KELIKIAN, H.) Dec '46
BIOLATO, D.: Bilateral plastic surgery of second phalanx of thumbs almost severed in industrial accident; functional and anatomic recovery of case. Boll. e mem. Soc. piemontese di chir. *6:*277-285, '36

Bipp Operation

"Bipp" method of treatment of bone cavities and bone grafts. MORISON, R. Surg., Gynec. and Obst., *34:*642-666, May '22 (illus.)

BIRAM, J. H.: Minor and medium burns; treatment with sulfathiazole (sulfanilamide derivative). Indust. Med. *11:*462-463, Oct '42
BIRCKEL, A.: Phalangization of stumps of forearm amputations (Putti-Krukenberg operation); 13 cases. Strasbourg-med. (pt. 2) *85:*437-447, Dec '20, '27
BIRD, C. E. (see BROHM, C. G.) March '35
BIRDSALL, S. E.: Hematoma, abscess and necrosis of septum (especially following injury). St. Barth. Hosp. J. *47:*68-70, Feb '43
BIRILLO, I. A.: Intra-arterial blood transfusion in shock therapy. Khirurgiya, no. 8, pp. 3-17, '39
BIRKE, L.: Birth injuries to nose of new-born. Monatschr. f. Geburtsh. u. Gynak. *98:*144-152, Nov '34
BIRKENFELD, W.: Congenital pendulous hypertrophic breasts in female twins; case. Arch. f. klin. Chir. *168:*568-576, '32
BIRKENFELD, W.: Hereditary nature of harelip and cleft palate. Arch. f. klin. Chir. *141:*729-753, '26
BIRKENFELD, W.: Operative treatment of hypospadias in man. Arch. f. klin. Chir. *145:*445-454, '27
BIRKENFELD, W.: Study of twins with cleft lip, jaw, and palate from standpoint of pathologic heredity. Beitr. z. klin. Chir. *141:*257-267, '27
BIRKETT, G. E.: Principles of and results in radium treatment of buccal carcinoma. Canad. M. A. J. *23:*780-784, Dec '30
BIRKHOLZ: Depth of action of percaine solution by application to mucous membrane of nose in surgical anesthesia. Klin. Wchnschr. *9:*72, Jan 11, '30
BIRNBAUM, I. R.: Thiocresol in wound healing and in skin grafting. Ann. Surg. *96:*467-470, Sept '32
BIRNBAUM, W. AND CALLANDER, C. L.: Acute suppurative gonococcic tenosynovitis. J.A.M.A. *105:*1025-1028, Sept 28, '35
BIRO, E.: Hereditary character of eyelid ptosis. Arch. d'opht. *53:*685-693, Sept '36
BIRT, E.: Combined operations for elephantiasis of leg. Deutsche Ztschr. f. Chir. *184:*110-114, '24

BIRT, E.: Terminology and therapy of elephantiasis. Tung-Chi Med. Monatschr. *14:*205-214, June '39

BIRT, E.: Therapy of elephantiasis of leg. Tung-chi, Med. Monatschr. *2:*108-113, Dec '26

BISHOP, G. H.: Regeneration of skin after experimental removal in man. Am. J. Anat. *76:*153-181, March '45

BISI, R. H. (see MARFORT, A.) Feb '39

BISI, R. H. (see MARFORT, A. *et al*) Feb '39

BISI, R. H. AND EMILIANI, C. M.: Amygdaloid branchial cyst of neck; embryologic considerations. Rev. Asoc. med. argent. *52:*935-937, Sept 15, '38

Bisi Operation

External agenesis of ear treated surgically by Humberto and Ricardo Bisi. IVANISSEVICH, O. Bol. y trab., Acad. argent. de cir. *29:*666-668, Aug 1, '45

BISNOFF, H. L.: Care of military and civilian injuries; external traction appliance for jaw fractures. Am. J. Orthodontics (Oral Surg. Sect) *29:*96-101, Feb '43

BISSON, C.: Dislocations of fingers in children and fractures. Ann. med.-chir. de l'Hop. Sainte-Justine, Montreal *3:*36-43, May '39

BISSON, C. AND ROYER, A.: Burns and shock in children; Mentana Street disaster in Montreal, September 1945. Ann. med.-chir. de l'Hop. Sainte-Justine, Montreal *5:*5-19, '46

Bite, Human

Human bite infections of hand. WELCH, C. E. New England J. Med. *215:*901-908, Nov 12, '36

BITTENCOURT, J.: Construction of artificial vagina in case of congenital absence. Rev. med. de Pernambuco *12:*315-325, Dec '42

BITTNER, W.: Etiology and therapy of ischemic paralysis of forearm (Volkmann contracture); 4 cases. Beitr. z. klin. Chir. *152:*510-513, '31

BIVINGS, L.: Discussion of angiomata and pigmented nevi. South. M. J. *38:*241-244, April '45

BIVINGS, L.: Simple instrument for inverted or retracted nipples. J. M. A. Georgia *17:*120-121, March '28

BIZARD, G.; RAZEMON, AND DEBURGE: Pathologic rupture of tendon of extensor pollicis longus. Echo med. du nord. *36:*368-369, July 30, '32

BIZE, P. R. (see TIXIER, L.) April '27

BJELOSOR, I. (see POLISSADOWA, X.) 1929

BJERRUM, O.: Fracture-dislocation of mandible. Acta chir. Scandinav. *79:*209-218, '37

BJÖRKENHEIM, G. A.: Plastic surgery for pendulous breast. Finska lak.-sallsk. handl. *76:*57-77, Jan '34

BLACK, B. W.: Paraffin treatment preferred for burns of all types. Mod. Hosp. *61:*108, Dec '43

BLACK, C. E.: Plastic surgery in Mississippi Valley; David Prince. Tr. West. S. A. (1937) *47:*287-309, '38

BLACK, D. A. K.: Treatment of burn shock with plasma and serum. Brit. M. J. *2:*693-697, Nov 23, '40

BLACK, J. I. M.: Nasal fractures. Newcastle M. J. *20:*74-80, July-Oct '40

BLACK, J. I. M.: Nasal injury. Clin. J. *70:*177-183, July '41

BLACK, J. R. (see MEYERDING, H. W. *et al*) March '41

BLACK, J. R. AND MACEY, H. B.: Plastic operation (skin grafting); case. (tendon grafting). Proc. Staff Meet., Mayo Clin. *12:*497-500, Aug 11, '37

BLACKBURN, J. D.: Arthroplasty of temporomandibular joint; case. J. M. A. Georgia *21:*314-315, Aug '32

BLACKBURNE, G.: Successful operative procedure for reshaping lower limbs. J. M. Soc. New Jersey *31:*214-215, April '34

BLACKFIELD, H. M.: Burn contractures of hand. Surg., Gynec. and Obst. *68:*1066-1073, June '39

BLACKFIELD, H. M.: Burn therapy. California and West. Med. *61:*187-190, Oct '44

BLACKFIELD, H. M.: Treatment of Dupuytren's contracture by means of radical excision of palmar fascia. Brunn, Med.-Surg. Tributes, pp. 59-72, '42

BLACKFIELD, H. M. AND GOLDMAN, L.: Burns in children. J.A.M.A. *112:*2235-2240, June 3, '39

BLACKWELL, H. B.: Clinical observations on correction of external deformities of nose by intranasal route, with lantern demonstration. Laryngoscope *33:*21-26, Jan '23 (illus.)

Bladder

Case of plastic operation including urethra, bladder and vagina. JORGE, J. M. Semana med. *2:*499-502, Sept 13, '23 (illus)

Artificial vagina from bladder. SCHMID, H. H. Monatschr. f. Geburtsh. u. Gynak. *72:*330-336, March '26

Formation of artificial vagina and bladder from sigmoid. RUDOLF, A. Beitr. z. klin. Chir. *153:*103-109, '31

Abnormalities and plastic surgery of lower urogenital tract (Roman Guiteras lecture). YOUNG, H. H., J. Urol. *35:*417-480, April '36

Free autoplastic graft of gastric mucosa to replace urinary bladder tissue loss. STE-

Bladder—Cont.
FANINI, P. Arch. ed atti d. Soc. ital. di chir. *43:*951-967, '37

Bladder, Exstrophy

Ectopia vesicae successfully treated by transplantation of trigone into the sigmoid. BROWN, H. H. Brit. M. J. *1:*15, Jan 1, '21
Exstrophy of bladder in female. BURKE, J. Ann. Surg. *73:*100, Jan '21
Exstrophy of urinary bladder with carcinoma. LOWER, W. E. Ann. Surg. *73:*354, March '21
Operation for treatment of ectopia vesicae. ROBERTS, C. Lancet *1:*1125, May 28, '21
Remote results of Maydl's operation for exstrophy of bladder. MUGNIÉRY, E. Lyon chir. *18:*481, July-Aug '21 abstr: J.A.M.A. *77:*1606, Nov 12, '21
Extroversion of bladder. LENDON, A. A. AND NEWLAND, H. S. Brit. M. J. *2:*38, July 9, '21 also: M. J. Australia *2:*103, Aug 6, '21
Formation of cloaca in treatment of exstrophy of bladder. MAYO, C. H., S. Clin. N. Amer. *1:*1257, Oct '21
Results of operative treatment of exstrophy of bladder. DEMEL, R. Mitt. a. d. Grenzgeb. d. Med. u. Chir. *33:*533, '21 abstr: J.A.M.A. *77:*1294, Oct 15, '21
Successful treatment of exstrophy of bladder. PFLAUMER, E. Beitr. z. klin. Chir. *122:*346, '21
Extroversion of bladder treated by vesico-colostomy. MACEWEN, J. A. C. Lancet *1:*531, March 18, '22
Potential malignancy in exstrophy of bladder. SCHOLL, A. J. JR. Ann. Surg. *75:*365-371, March '22 (illus.)
Exstrophy of bladder. GRANT, W. W. Southern M. J. *15:*297-302, April '22 (illus.)
Cancer in exstrophy of bladder. DUPONT, R. J. d'urol. *13:*433-444, June '22 (illus.) abstr: J.A.M.A. *79:*855, Sept 2, '22
Treatment of exstrophy of bladder. DRACHTER, R. Arch. f. klin. Chir. *120:*291-297, '22 (illus.) abstr: J.A.M.A. *79:*1370, Oct 14, '22
Case operated according to method of Maydl-Borelius (exstrophy of bladder). BRATTSTRÖM, E. Acta chir. Scandinav. *55:*33-37, '22 (illus.; in English) abstr: J.A.M.A. *79:*1562, Oct 28, '22
Modified operation for ectopia vesicae. ZAAIJER, J. H. Zentralbl. f. Chir. *50:*114-115, Jan 27, '23 (illus.)
Maydl-Borelius operation for exstrophy of bladder. BRATTSTRÖM, E. Beitr. z. klin. Chir. *127:*419-421, '22 Abstr: J.A.M.A. *80:*364, Feb 3, '23
Embryologic study of case of exstrophy of bladder with umbilical hernia and aplasia of anus and rectum. GARCIA, C. L. Semana med. *1:*347-355, Feb 22, '23 (illus.)
Treatment of exstrophy of bladder. CAMERA, U. Arch. ital. di chir. *6:*421-432, Dec '22 (illus.) abstr: J.A.M.A. *80:*806, March 17, '23
Case of exstrophy of bladder. CÚNEO, N. L. Semana med. *1:*490-491, March 15, '23 (illus.)
Exstrophy of bladder with successful transplantation of ureters into rectum, report of 2 cases. HUTCHINS, E. H. AND HUTCHINS, A. F. Surg., Gynec. and Obst. *36:*731-741, June '23 (illus.)
Correction of exstrophy of bladder. LOTSCH, F. Ztschr. f. Urolog. *17:*385-396, '23 abstr: J.A.M.A. *81:*967, Sept 15, '23
Case of exstrophy of bladder in woman aged 39. BARDON, J., J. d'urol. *16:*384-389, Nov '23
Treatment of exstrophy of bladder by Makkas-Lengemann technic. GAZA, W. V. Arch. f. klin. Chir. *126:*515-522, '23
Etiology of exstrophy of bladder. VON GELDERN, C. E. Arch. Surg. *8:*61-99, (pt. 1) Jan '24
Transplantation of ureters into rectum, end-results in 35 cases of exstrophy of bladder. MAYO, C. H. AND WALTERS, W., J.A.M.A. *82:*624-626, Feb 23, '24
New operation for exstrophy of bladder; preliminary report. BURNS, J. E., J.A.M.A. *82:*1587-1590, May 17, '24
Makkas operation in case of exstrophy of bladder. WALLER, J. B. Zentralbl. f. Chir. *51:*1841-1842, Aug 23, '24
Unusual example of exstrophy of bladder with marked separation of pubic bones. SAGE, E. C. Am. J. Obst. and Gynec. *8:*497-500, Oct '24
Operation for exstrophy of bladder. ROLOFF. Zentralbl. f. Chir. *51:*2432-2433, Nov 1, '24
Exstrophy of bladder. VALERIO, A. Brazil-med. *2:*295-298, Nov 22, '24
Surgical treatment of exstrophy of bladder, with report of a case. DAVIS, L. Boston M. and S. J. *191:*1201-1206, Dec 25, '24
Ectopia of urinary bladder in an infant. EPSTEIN, J., M. F. and Rec. *121:*151-152, Feb 4, '25
Case of exstrophy of bladder. CAMERON, D. A., M. J. Australia *1:*509-510, May 16, '25
Remote sequelae of rectal implantation of ureters for exstrophy; findings at necropsy 14 years after Bergenhem operation. RICHEY, DEW. G. Arch. Surg. *11:*408-416, Sept '25

Bladder, Exstrophy—Cont.
Interesting case of exstrophic bladder with neoplastic implant. McCarthy, J. F. and Klemperer, P., J. Urology *14:*419–427, Oct '25
Exstrophy of bladder (day in Dr. Charles M. Mayo's clinic). Hendricks, W. A. Internat. Clin. *1:*182–184, March '26
Interesting case of ectopia vesicae. David, M. D. Indian M. Gaz. *61:*290, June '26
Extroversion of bladder treated by transplantation of ureters. Levin, J. J., M. J. S. Africa *21:*336–339, July '26
Exstrophy of bladder. Mayo, C. H. and Hendricks, W. A. Surg., Gynec. and Obst. *43:*129–134, Aug '26
Exstrophy of bladder; junction of ureters with upper part of rectum; results 24 years after operation. Estor, E., J. d'urol. *22:*242–243, Sept '26
Complete exstrophy of bladder with split pelvis; Peter's operation in 1912 with subsequent complication of pregnancy; caesarean section and recovery in 1926. Green-Armytage, V. B., J. Obst. and Gynec. Brit. Emp. *33:*436–438, '26
Late results after operation for exstrophy of bladder. Robinson, T. A. and Foulds, G. S. Brit. J. Surg. *14:*529–539, Jan '27
Exstrophy of bladder; case. Colby, F. H. Boston M. and S. J. *196:*1033–1036, June 23, '27
Formation of artificial bladder in exstrophy; 3 cases. Garmsen, B. M. Zentralbl. f. Chir. *54:*1736–1741, July 9, '27
Operative treatment of exstrophy of bladder. Mayer, A. Zentralbl. f. Gynak. *51:*1887–1898, July 23, '27
Morphological genesis of cleft of abdomen and bladder (ectopia vesicae). Sternberg, H. Urol. and Cutan. Rev. *31:*475–479, Aug '27
Exstrophy of bladder, treatment by Heitz-Boyer-Hovelacque operation; 9 cases. Rivarola, R. A. Semana med. *2:*1023–1027, Oct 20, '27
Late result in ectopia vesicae. Starr, F. N. G. Brit. J. Surg. *15:*328, Oct '27
Formation of artificial bladder in exstrophy of bladder. Isserson, M. Vestnik Khir. *10:*245–248, '27
Demonstration of value of urea tolerance test as indication of functional condition of kidney in patient with total exstrophy of bladder; case. Köhler, H. Zentralbl. f. Chir. *55:*1412–1417, June 9, '28
Pathogenesis of exstrophy of bladder; embryological study; case. Vicente Carcellar, M. Clin. y lab. *12:*115–122, Aug '28
Pregnancy terminated by caesarean section after ureteral transplantation into sigmoid for exstrophy of bladder. Eberbach, C. W. and Pierce, J. M. Surg., Gynec. and Obst. *47:*540-542, Oct '28
Exstrophy of bladder. Mayo, C. H. Proc. Staff Meet., Mayo Clin. *3:*289, Oct 3, '28
Repair of epispadias and exstrophy of bladder. Rockey, E. W., S. Clin. N. Amer. *8:*1503–1509, Dec '28
Ectopia vesicae. Roux, C. Beitr. z. klin. Chir. *142:*482–489, '28
Ureteral transplantation in exstrophy of bladder. Dixon, C. F. Proc. Staff. Meet., Mayo Clin. *4:*33, Jan 30, '29
Exstrophy of bladder, case. Lorthior, P. Bruxelles-med. *9:*778–780, May 5, '29
Exstrophy of bladder, case with abnormalities of genitals. Pavlovsky, A. J. and Savage, R. Bol. Soc. de obst. y ginec. *8:*64–74, June 5, '29 also: Semana med. *2:*615–620, Aug 29, '29
Cancer of sigmoid flexure 10 years after ureteral implantation for exstrophy of bladder. Hammer, E., J. d'urol. *28:*260–263, Sept '29
Exstrophy of bladder, case with operations. Fuller, E. B., J. M. A. South Africa *3:*525–526, Sept 28, '29
Fate of patient in whom exstrophy of bladder was cured by Trendelenburg operation (synchondroseotomy). Heinsius, F. Zentralbl. f. Gynak. *55:*322–332, Feb 7, '31 abstr.: Ztschr. f. Geburtsh. u. Gynak. *99:*187–191, '30
Ureteral transplantation for exstrophy of bladder. Mayo, C. H. and Dixon, C. F., S. Clin. N. Amer. *10:*1–6, Feb '30
Exstrophy of bladder, operation by Bergenhem method. Disque, T. L. Pennsylvania M. J. *33:*546, May '30
Unusual anomaly of pelvis with exstrophy of bladder. Dugan, W. M. and Upson, W. O. J. Michigan M. Soc. *29:*512–515, July '30
Exstrophy of bladder. Robertson, T. S. Illinois M. J. *58:*66–69, July '30
Remote results of Maydl's operation for exstrophy. Roloff, F. Zentralbl. f. Chir. *57:*1977–1979, Aug 9, '30
Exstrophy of bladder; operation by Borelius-Maydl method. Müller, S. Hospitalstid. (Dansk kir. selsk. forh.) *73:*23, Aug 14, '30
Exstrophy of bladder; case. Pizzagalli, L. Boll. d. spec. med.-chir. *4:*321–328, '30
Exstrophy of bladder with abnormal symphysis pubis. Nuri, M. K., J. de radiol. et d'electrol. *15:*254, May '31
Transplantation of ureters into sigmoid in exstrophy. Donovan, E. J., S. Clin. North

Bladder, Exstrophy – Cont.
America *11:*511-512, June '31
Ectopy of bladder, remains of cloacal duct, perineal hernia of caudal gut and aparent doubling of external genitals. GRUBER, G. B. Beitr. z. path. Anat. u. z. allg. Path. *87:*455-465, June 27, '31
Transplantation of ureters into sigmoid in exstrophy; 3 operations on 2 cases. PRICE, P. B. China M. J. *45:*634-643, July '31
Ureterosigmoidal transplantation and plastic operations on penis in exstrophy of bladder. WALTERS, W. *et al.* S. Clin. North America *11:*823-828, Aug '31
Transplantation of ureters into rectum in exstrophy. HIGGINS, C. C. Ohio State M. J. *27:*705-708, Sept '31
Exstrophy of bladder, case. MCEACHERN, J. S. Canad. M. A. J. *25:*324, Sept '31
Treatment of exstrophy by ureteral transplantations. CABOT, H. New England J. Med. *205:*706-711, Oct 8, '31
Ectopia vesicae. MADHOK, G. D. Indian M. Gaz. *66:*633, Nov '31
Transplantation of ureters into rectosigmoid portion of intestines in exstrophy, with extirpation of bladder; 76 cases. WALTERS, W. Arch. f. klin. Chir. *167:*589-600, '31
Transplantation of ureters to rectosigmoid and cystectomy in exstrophy; 76 cases. WALTERS, W. Am. J. Surg. *15:*15-22, Jan '32
Treatment of total ectopy in adults. VON JASCHKE, R. T. Zentralbl. f. Gynak. *56:*322-326, Feb 6, '32
Late results of Peters operation for exstrophy. FOULDS, G. S. AND ROBINSON, T. A. Brit. J. Urol. *4:*20-26, March '32
Transplantation of ureters in exstrophy; case. WISE, B. T., J. M. A. Georgia *21:*100-103, March '32
Exstrophy of bladder. BEER, E., S. Clin. North America *12:*283-285, April '32
Exstrophy of bladder complicated by other congenital anomalies. BRAKELEY, E. Am. J. Dis. Child. *43:*931-935, April '32
Combined congenital exstrophy of female bladder and cloaca. KERNWEIN, G. A. Arch. Path. *13:*926-930, June '32 also: Tr. Chicago Path. Soc. *14:*4-9, June 1, '32
Implantation of ureters for inoperable vesicovaginal fistula and ectopia vesicae; new technic. GREEN-ARMYTAGE, V. B. Brit. J. Surg. *20:*130-138, July '32 also: Indian M. Gaz. *67:*631-636, Nov '32
Partial biphallism (double penis) associated with exstrophy of bladder and multiple abnormalities of hands and feet; case. BAUZA, J. A. Arch. de pediat. d. Uruguay *3:*353-

Bladder, Exstrophy – Cont.
355, Aug '32
Transplantation of ureters into sigmoid colon for exstrophy of bladder incontinence (unilateral versus simultaneous bilateral transplantation). WALTERS, W. Proc. Staff Meet., Mayo Clin. *7:*470-472, Aug 10, '32
Makkas operation for exstrophy of bladder in child; case. TAVERNIER. Lyon chir. *29:*587-591, Sept-Oct '32
Transplantation of ureters into large intestine by submucous implantation; clinical application of technic 3 in exstrophy of bladder. COFFEY, R. C., J.A.M.A. *99:*1320-1323, Oct 15, '32
Ectopia vesicae; surgical treatment of 3 cases. LINDSTRÖM, E. Acta chir. Scandinav. *72:*134-145, '32
Further studies and experiences with transfixion suture technic (technic 3) for transplantation of ureters into large intestine. COFFEY, R. C. Northwest Med. *32:*31-34, Jan '33
Ectopia vesicae; full report of case treated by transplantation of ureters into recto-sigmoid and complete cystectomy. EL-KATIB, A., J. Egyptian M. A. *16:*3-16, Jan '33
Transplantation of ureters into sigmoid in exstrophy of bladder. NORTHROP, H. L., J. Am. Inst. Homeop. *26:*33-34, Jan '33
Transplantation of ureters to sigmoid colon for exstrophy of bladder and other ureteral abnormalities with urinary incontinence. WALTERS, W. Minnesota Med. *16:*416-419, June '33
Aseptic uretero-intestinal anastomosis in exstrophy. HIGGINS, C. C. Surg., Gynec. and Obst. *57:*359-361, Sept '33 also: Am. J. Surg. *22:*207-209, Nov '33
Exstrophy of bladder treated by transfixion suture of ureters into large intestine (Coffey operation) in new-born infant. BENGOLEA, A. J. Bol. y trab. de la Soc. de cir. de Buenos Aires *17:*894-896, Sept 13, '33
Historical data on ureteral transplantation in exstrophy; Peters operation. FOULDS, G. S. Am. J. Surg. *22:*217-219, Nov '33
Operation for exstrophy without involving intestine. JANSSEN, P. Zentralbl. f. Chir. *60:*2658-2662, Nov 11, '33
Drainage after uretero-intestinal anastomosis for exstrophy of bladder. MOORHEAD, S. W. Am. J. Surg. *22:*215-216, Nov '33
Congenital ectopia vesicae with recovery after operation. SUZUKI, T. Okayama-Igakkai-Zasshi *45:*2615, Nov '33
Exstrophy of bladder associated with pregnancy and labor. DAWSON, J. B., J. Obst. and Gyaec. Brit. Emp. *40:*1214-1219, Dec

Bladder, Exstrophy–Cont.
'33
Ureterorectomneostomy by transfixion suture method in exstrophy of bladder, Coffey's technic 3. HELPER, A. B., S. Clin. North America *13:*1387-1391, Dec '33
Exstrophy of bladder; surgery and later complications; case. FORSHELL, Y. P. Acta path. et microbiol. Scandinav., supp. 16, pp. 350–357, '33
Ureterosigmoidal transplantation for exstrophy of bladder. MAYO, C. H. Sovet. khir. (nos. 1–3) *5:*308–313, '33
Treatment of ectopy of bladder. NUBOER, J. F. Deutsche Ztschr. f. Chir. *240:*390–393, '33
Implantation of both ureters into rectum; prolongation of life 24 years. Exstrophy of bladder. ESTES, W. L. Ann. Surg. *99:*223–226, Jan '34
Exstrophy of bladder (persistent cloaca) associated with intestinal fistulas, with brief analysis of 36 cases of anal and rectal anomalies from records of Charity Hospital in New Orleans. VEAL, J. R. AND MCFETRIDGE, E. M., J. Pediat. *4:*95–103, Jan '34
Ureteral transplantation to rectosigmoid for exstrophy of bladder, complete epispadias and other urethral abnormalities with total urinary incontinence; 85 cases operated. WALTERS, W. AND BRAASCH, W. F. Am. J. Surg. *23:*255–270, Feb '34
Surgical therapy of exstrophy of bladder in young children. MONNIER, E. Schweiz. med. Wchnschr. *64:*202–203, March 10, '34
Construction of continent urethra in female; application in exstrophy. MARION, G., J. d'urol. *37:*393-402, May '34
Pregnancy and parturition following bilateral ureteral transplantation for congenital exstrophy of bladder. RANDALL, L. M. AND HARDWICK, R. S. Surg., Gynec. and Obst. *58:*1018–1020, June '34
Ureterosigmoidal transplantation for exstrophy and complete epispadias with absent urinary sphincters. WALTERS, W. Am. J. Surg. *24:*776–792, June '34
Complete inversion of bladder; case. WERHATZKY, N. P. Zentralbl. f. Gynak. *58:*1543–1546, June 30, '34
Late results of Segond operation for exstrophy of bladder. DOTTI, E. Gior. veneto di sc. med. *8:*730–739, July '34
Problems of surgical therapy of exstrophy of bladder. JUARISTI, V. Arch. espan. de pediat. *18:*385–390, July '34
Transplantation of solitary ureter to sigmoid colon for exstrophy of bladder; case. WALTERS, W. Proc. Staff Meet., Mayo Clin. *9:*485–486, Aug 15, '34
Surgical treatment of exstrophy of bladder. MULLER, G. P., S. Clin. North America *15:*275–283, Feb '35
Small exstrophy of bladder in women; case in girl 4½ years old; surgical therapy with use maintained for 5 years. GAUTIER, J. Bull. et mem. Soc. nat. de chir. *61:*708–713, June 1, '35
Pelvic prerectal transposition in surgical therapy of exstrophy of bladder. GODARD, H. Bull. Soc. de pediat. de Paris *33:*408–415, June '35 also: Bull. Soc. franc. d'urol., pp. 291–298, July 9, '35
Exstrophy of bladder; case. TAYLOR, R. C. Memphis M. J. *10:*43–44, July '35
Ureteral transplantation for exstrophy of bladder and carcinoma. HIGGINS, C. C. Cleveland Clin. Quart. *2:*32–42, Oct '35
Exstrophy of bladder; case. ISMAIL, M., J. Egyptian M. A. *18:*704–715, Oct '35
Exstrophy of bladder, cure by Marion-Heitz-Boyer method (transplantation of ureters into rectum) in man 20 years old. NANDROT. Bull. et mem. Soc. nat. de chir. *61:*1103–1105, Nov 2, '35
Exstrophy of bladder, surgical therapy by Coffey operation; 2 cases. DERMAN, I. A. Ztschr. f. Urol., *29:*856–859, '35
Makkas operation in exstrophy of bladder. GORODINSKIY, D. M. Novy khir. arkhiv *33:*290–294, '35
Transplantation of ureter to rectum in exstrophy of bladder. COLOMBINO, S. Boll. e mem. Soc. piemontese di chir. *5:*333–341, '35
Ectopia vesicae, imperforate rectum and anus, true hermaphroditism and other anomalies. POTTER, A. H. Am. J. Surg. *31:*172–178, Jan '36
Exstrophy of bladder, uretero-intestinal anastomosis. BAGGETT, L. G. South. Surgeon *5:*31–41, Feb '36
Successful restoration in exstrophy of bladder resulting in continence and enabling urination by natural channels. GODARD, H. Bull. Soc. franc. d'urol., pp. 157–160, March 16, '36
Exstrophy of bladder, ureteral transplantation. HANSSEN, S. A. Hospitalstid *79:*285–292, March 24, '36
Rare case of exstrophy of bladder. SARAZIN, A. Bull. et mem. Soc. de radiol. med. de France *24:*324–327, April '36
Ureteral transplantations in exstrophy of bladder. FOSTER, G. V. Pennsylvania M. J. *39:*874–877, Aug '36

Bladder, Exstrophy—Cont.

Total inversion of bladder; case. HEIDLER, H. Wien. med. Wchnschr. *86:*1007–1009, Sept 5, '36

Exstrophy of bladder with genital malformations; case in new-born infant. TALAMO, P. Clin. ostet. *38:*516–520, Oct '36

Late results of Maydl operation for congenital ectopy of bladder. GRAUBNER, E. Zentralbl. f. Chir. *63:*2657–2658, Nov 7, '36

Exstrophy of bladder with hydronephrosis and hydroureter on one side; surgical therapy of Coffey-Mayo operation. BERGENFELDT, E. Ztschr. f. urol. Chir. *41:*515–521, '36

Incontinence due to severe hypospadias of female urethra with simultaneous ectopy of ureteral orifice; case. DE GIRONCOLI, F. Ztschr. f. urol. Chir. u. Gynak. *42:*152–156, '36

Exstrophy of bladder, transplantation of ureters into intestine (Coffey operation). HELLSTRÖM, J. Ztschr. f. urol. Chir. *41:*522–528, '36

Therapy of ectopic bladder. MAKKAS, M. Beitr. z. klin. Chir. *163:*554–570, '36

Ureteral transplantation in very young (infant 4 months old) with exstrophy of bladder; case. LOWER, W. E. Cleveland Clin. Quart. *4:*23–25, Jan '37

Congenital ectopy of bladder cured by operation 15 years previously. SZEKELY, L. Zentralbl. f. Chir. *64:*464–467, Feb 20, '37

Technic of Mayo-Walters operation in exstrophy of bladder. KRABBEL, M. Zentralbl. f. Chir. *64:*693–696, March 20, '37

Ectopia vesicae, surgically treated 15 years ago; case. SZEKELY, L. Budapesti orvosi ujsag *35:*221–223, March 4, '37

Exstrophy of bladder (treated by ureterosigmoidostomy). LADD, W. E. AND LANMAN, T. H. New England J. Med. *216:*637–645, April 15, '37

Ectopia vesicae; case. LAIDLEY, J. W. S. Australian and New Zealand J. Surg. *6:*398–399, April '37

Transplantation of ureters into sigmoid in therapy of urinary incontinence due to grave congenital malformation; case. (exstrophy of bladder). BUFALINI, M. Policlinico (sez. prat.) *44:*880–883, May 3, '37

Extroversion of bladder with control of micturition. THOMPSON, A. R. Brit. M. J. *2:*3–5, July 3, '37

Extroversion of bladder; case. KEARNS, W. M. Wisconsin M. J. *36:*820–824, Oct '37

Exstrophy of bladder; case. TANER, F., J. d'urol. *44:*340–342, Oct '37

Surgical therapy of exstrophy of bladder. LUHMANN, K. Beitr. z. klin. Chir. *165:* 221–242, '37

Clinical anatomy of cases of epispadias and extroversion of bladder. THOMPSON, A. R. Brit. J. Child. Dis. *35:*36–43, Jan–March '38

Transplantation of ureters into rectosigmoid in young children and infants with exstrophy of bladder; preliminary report. LOWER, W. E., J. Mt. Sinai Hosp. *4:*650–653, March–April '38

Partial exstrophy of bladder; embryologic considerations; case. GAUDIN, H. J. AND CABOT, H. Proc. Staff Meet., Mayo Clin. *13:*216–220, April 6, '38

Progress in plastic operations performed during childhood (for exstrophy of bladder and harelip, cleft palate). MONNIER, E. Schweiz. med. Wchnschr. *68:*613–614, May 21, '38

Case of ureteral transplantation (Peters' operation) for exstrophy of bladder surviving 22 years. FISHER, J. H. Brit. J. Urol. *10:*241–244, Sept '38

Coffey operation for exstrophy of bladder; cases. FEVRE, M. Mem. Acad. de chir. *64:*1114–1123, Oct 26, '38

Exstrophy of bladder complicated by carcinoma. JUDD, E. S. AND THOMPSON, H. L. Arch. Surg. *17:*641–657, Oct '28

Exstrophy of bladder; with report of case in adult. DE GRISOGONO, A. Clin. ostet. *40:*560–569, Nov '38

Surgical therapy of exstrophy of bladder; case. HENRY, G., J. belge d'urol. *11:*538–545, Dec '38

Exstrophy of bladder and masculine epispadias; treatment by prerectal pelvic transposition of bladder. GODARD, H., J. d'urol. *47:*97–109, Feb '39

Exstrophy of bladder, case presenting many unusual features. RUSSELL, K. F. Brit. J. Urol. *11:*31–47, March '39

Coffey operation in exstrophy of bladder; case. YOVTCHITCH, J. Mem. Acad. de chir. *65:*368–369, March 8, '39

Transplantation of ureters in infants with exstrophy of bladder. HIGGINS, C. C., J. Urol. *41:*464–472, April '39

Modification of Makkas operation in therapy of exstrophy of bladder. MATOLAY, G. Zentralbl. f. Chir. *66:*1130–1133, May 20, '39

Creation of new bladder with aid of loop of small intestine in case of exstrophy. ETIENNE, *et al.* Arch. Soc. d. sc. med. et biol. de Montpellier *20:*285–291, June '39

Transplantation of ureters into rectum by Mirotvortzeff's method in exstrophy of

Bladder, Exstrophy—Cont.
bladder. SHILOVTZEFF, S. P. Lancet *2:*412-415, Aug 19, '39
Exstrophy of bladder, association with congenital prolapse of uterus; case. ISMAIL, M. J. Egyptian M. A. *22:*587-589, Oct '39
Exstrophy of bladder, Coffey-Mayo operations and their results. MATTOS, S. O. Rev. de obst. e ginec. de Sao Paulo *4:*107-126, Oct-Dec '39
Transplantation of ureters into sigmoid and cystectomy in radical therapy of exstrophy; late results in case. AREZZI, G. Arch. ital. di urol. *16:*384-405, Dec '39
Coffey operation in exstrophy of bladder. GÜRSEL, A. E. Turk tib cem. mec. *5:*90-91, '39
Exstrophy of bladder; treatment by uretero-intestinal anastomosis. HAMM, F. C. Brooklyn Hosp. J. *2:*14-24, Jan '40
Exstrophy of bladder and epispadias (surgical technic). LADD, W. E. AND LANMAN, T. H. New England J. Med. *222:*130-134, Jan 25, '40
Maydl operation in child 1½ years old for exstrophy. HEYN, W. Zentralbl. f. Gynak. *64:*194-198, Feb 3, '40
Carcinoma of bladder in exstrophy. MCCOWN, P. E., J. Urol. *43:*533-542, April '40
Extroversion of primitive hind gut. MORISON, J. E. Arch. Dis. Childhood *15:*105-114, June '40
Experimental and clinical study of cases of exstrophy (technic of Lyman-Farrell operation). KIMBALL, G. H. AND DRUMMOND, N. R., J. Oklahoma M. A. *33:*2-8, Aug '40
Therapy of congenital bladder ectopia. OBERNIEDERMAYR, A. Med. Klin. *36:*971-973, Aug 30, '40
Ectopy of bladder and nephrolithiasis; case. KOVALEVA, T. F. Novy khir. arkhiv *45:*253-255, '40
Clinical study of therapy of exstrophy of bladder. IADEVAIA, F. Clinica *7:*33-46, Jan '41
Plastic operations for exstrophy of bladder. YOUNG, H. H. Proc. Interst. Postgrad. M. A. North America (1941) pp. 241-244, '42
Ectopia vesicae. DAVIES, D. V. Brit. J. Urol. *14:*1-10, March '42
First case of exstrophy of bladder in which normal bladder and urinary control have been obtained by plastic operation. YOUNG, H. H. Surg., Gynec. and Obst. *74:*729-737, March '42
Pregnancy in woman 25 years old after Maydl operation in childhood for exstrophy of bladder and cleft pelvis; review of clini-

Bladder, Exstrophy—Cont.
cal aspects of exstrophy. SCHUMANN, H. Geburtsh. u. Frauenh. *4:*318-333, Aug '42
Ureterointestinal anastomosis by Reimer method; preliminary results in case of exstrophy in boy. HART, A. Zentralbl. f. Chir. *69:*1485-1495, Sept 12, '42
Surgical therapy of exstrophy of bladder with intestinal transplantation of ureters. ORTH, O. Ztschr. f. Urol. *36:*214-216, '42
Coffey method of ureteral implantation in exstrophy of bladder. HAGENBACH, E. Helvet. med. acta *10:*321-324, June '43
Exstrophy of bladder in pseudohermaphrodite; case. LOEWEN, S. L. AND RUPE, L. O. J. Kansas M. Soc. *44:*186-189, June '43
Case of exstrophy of bladder. COURI, A. A. An. brasil de ginec. *16:*335-347, Nov '43
Transplantation of ureters into rectosigmoid in infants with exstrophy of bladder; review of 19 cases. HIGGINS, C. C., J. Urol. *50:*657-666, Dec '43
Surgical therapy of exstrophy of bladder, with special reference to Maydl and Coffey operations. TILK, G. U. Deutsche Ztschr. f. Chir. *257:*287, '43
Exstrophy of bladder in twins. HIGGINS, C. C. Cleveland Clin. Quart. *11:*25, Jan '44
Exstrophy of bladder and its therapy. ADAMS, F. Arch. f. klin. Chir. *205:*695, '44
Intestinal hernia with eversion and exstrophic bladder. SINCLAIR, J. G., J. Pediat. *26:*78-81, Jan '45
Case of exstrophy of bladder with procidentia. CLAYTON, S. G., J. Obst. and Gynaec. Brit. Emp. *52:*177-179, April '45
Report of 2 patients with exstrophy of bladder operated upon at 2 months of age. SCHAEFER, A. A. AND SAKAGUCHI, S., J. Pediat. *26:*492-500, May '45

Bladder, Exstrophy—Cancer

Exstrophy with cancer of bladder and absence of umbilicus; report of case. MURPHY, D. P., J.A.M.A. *82:*784-785, March 8, '24
Interesting case of exstrophic bladder with neoplastic implant. MCCARTHY, J. F., AND KLEMPERER, P. J. Urology. *14:*419-427, Oct '25

BLAESEN, C.: Congenital median and lateral fistulas in neck. Deutsche Ztschr. f. Chir. *167:*60-64, '21
BLAINE, E. S.: X-ray burn of third degree followed by rapid healing. Am. J. Roentgenol. *8:*183, April '21
BLAINE, G.: Use of plastic materials in plastic

surgery. M. Press *216:*223–224, Sept 25, '46 also: Lancet *2:*525–528, Oct 12, '46

Blaine, G.; Dollar, J. M. and Sorsby, A.: Use of plastic materials for scleral wounds. Tr. Ophth. Soc. U. Kingdom (1944) *64:*187–194, '45

Blair, E. G.: Surgical treatment of X-ray burns. J. Radiol. *5:*149–152, May '24

Blair, V. P.: Delayed transfer of long pedicle flaps in plastic surgery (face). Surg., Gynec. and Obst. *33:*261, Sept '21

Blair, V. P.: Repair of major defects of face. Texas State J. Med. *17:*301, Oct '21

Blair, V. P.: Rhinoplasty, with special reference to saddle nose. J.A.M.A. *77:*1479, Nov 5, '21

Blair, V. P.: Reconstruction surgery of face. Surg., Gynec. and Obst. *34:*701–716, June '22 (illus.)

Blair, V. P. (with Robert H. Ivy and, in the second and third editions, J. B. Brown): *Essentials of Oral Surgery*. C. V. Mosby Co., St. Louis, 1923. Second Edition, 1936. Third Edition, 1944.

Blair, V. P.: Restoration of burnt child. Southern M. J. *16:*522–527, July '23 (illus.)

Blair, V. P.: Congenital facial clefts. Surg., Gynec. and Obst. *37:*530–533, Oct '23

Blair, V. P.: Radical operation for extrinsic carcinoma of larynx. Ann. Otol., Rhin. and Laryng. *33:*373–378, June '24

Blair, V. P.: Full thickness skin graft. Ann. Surg. *80:*298–324, Sept '24

Blair, V. P.: Restoration of function of mouth. Ann. Clin. Med. *3:*242–244, Sept '24

Blair, V. P.: Influence of mechanical pressure on wound healing. Illinois M. J. *46:*249–252, Oct '24

Blair, V. P.: Nasal deformities associated with congenital cleft of lip. J.A.M.A. *84:*185–187, Jan 17, '25

Blair, V. P.: Surgical restoration of lining of mouth. Surg., Gynec. and Obst. *40:*165–174, Feb '25

Blair, V. P. and Brown, J. B.: Course and treatment of simple osteomyelitis of jaws. S. Clin. N. America *5:*1413–1436, Oct '25

Blair, V. P.: Total and subtotal restoration of nose. J.A.M.A. *85:*1931–1935, Dec 19, '25

Blair, V. P.: Problem of bringing forward retracted upper lip and nose in harelip. Surg., Gynec. and Obst. *42:*128–132, Jan '26

Blair, V. P.: Operative correction of facial paralysis. South. M. J. *19:*116–120, Feb '26

Blair, V. P.: Repair of defects caused by surgery and radium in cancer of hand, mouth and cheek. Am. J. Roentgenol. *17:*99–100, Jan '27

Blair, V. P. and Brown, J. B.: Septic osteomyelitis of bones of skull and face; plea for conservative treatment. Ann. Surg. *85:*1–26, Jan '27

Blair, V. P.: Plastic surgery of face, neck and chest skin losses. Tr. Am. S. A. *45:*190–199, '27

Blair, V. P.: Consideration of contour as well as function in operations for organic ankylosis of lower jaw. Surg., Gynec. and Obst. *46:*167–179, Feb '28

Blair, V. P.: Why and how of harelip correction. Ann. Otol., Rhin. and Laryng. *37:*196–205, March '28

Blair, V. P.; Brown, J. B. and Womack, N. A.: Cancer in and about mouth; 211 cases. Ann. Surg. *88:*705–724, Oct '28

Blair, V. P.: Plastic surgery of nose; patient's viewpoint. Tr. Am. Acad. Ophth. *33:*436–444, '28

Blair, V. P.: Nasal deformities. Tr. Am. Laryng. A. *50:*36–40, '28

Blair, V. P.; Brown, J. B. and Womack, N. A.: Cancer in and about mouth; 211 cases. Tr. Am. S. A. *46:*414, '28

Blair, V. P. and Brown, J. B.: Use and uses of large split-skin grafts of intermediate thickness. Tr. South. S. A. *41:*409–424, '28 also: Surg., Gynec. and Obst. *49:*82–97, July '29

Blair, V. P: Why and how of harelip correction. Internat. J. Orthodontia *15:*1112–1119, Nov '29

Blair, V. P.: Consideration of contour as well as function in operations for organic ankylosis of mandible. Internat. J. Orthodontia *16:*62–80, Jan '30

Blair, V. P.; Brown, J. B. and Womack, N. A.: Cancer in and about mouth; 211 cases. Internat. J. Orthodontia *16:*188–209, Feb '30

Blair, V. P.; Brown, J. B. and Moore, S.: Osteomyelitis of jaws. J. Missouri M. A. *27:*173–176, April '30

Blair, V. P. and Brown, J. B.: Mirault operation for single harelip. Surg., Gynec. and Obst. *51:*81–98, July '30

Blair, V. P.: Further observation upon compensatory use of live tendon strips in facial paralysis. Ann. Surg. *92:*694–703, Oct '30

Blair, V. P.: Compensatory use of live tendon strips; further observations in facial paralysis. Tr. Am. S. A. *48:*369–378, '30

Blair, V. P.: Hypospadias and epispadias, indications for and technique of their operative correction. Tr. South. S. A. (1929) *42:*163–165, '30

Blair, V. P.: Plea for better average harelip repairs. Dallas M. J. *17:*4–9, Jan '31

Blair, V. P.; Brown, J. B. and Moore, S.:

Osteomyelitis of jaws. Internat. J. Orthodontia *17:*169-175, Feb '31

Blair, V. P.: Facial abnormalities, fancied and real; reaction of patient; attempted correction. (including nose). Proc. Inst. Med., Chicago *8:*217-223, April 15, '31

Blair, V. P. and Brown, J. B.: Mirault operation for single harelip. Internat. J. Orthodontia *17:*370-396, April '31

Blair, V. P. and Brown, J. B.: Plea for better average harelip repairs. Internat. J. Orthodontia *17:*472-483, May '31

Blair, V. P. and Brown, J. B.: Early and late repair of extensive burns. Dallas M. J. *17:*59-70, May '31

Blair, V. P.: Promotion of early healing in burns and correction and prevention of late complications. J. Oklahoma M.A. *24:*271-272, Aug '31

Blair, V. P.: Congenital atresia or obstruction of air passages. Ann. Otol., Rhin. and Laryng. *40:*1021-1035, Dec '31 also: Tr. Am. Laryng. A. *53:*229-246, '31 also: Internat. J. Orthodontia *18:*516-526, May '32

Blair, V. P. and Brown, J. B.: Defects of nose—fancied and real; reaction of patient; attempted correction. Surg., Gynec. and Obst. *53:*797-819, Dec '31

Blair, V. P. and Brown, J. B.: Nasal abnormalities, fancied and real; reaction of patient; attempted correction. Internat. J. Orthodontia *18:*363-401, April '32

Blair, V. P.; Brown, J. B. and Hamm, W. G.: Early care and repair of defects in burns. J.A.M.A. *98:*1355-1359, April 16, '32

Blair, V. P.: Correction of losses and deformities of external nose, including those associated with harelip. California and West. Med. *36:*308-313, May '32

Blair, V. P.; Brown, J. B. and Hamm, W. G.: Correction of epicanthus. eyelid ptosis. Arch. Ophth. *7:*831-846, June '32

Blair, V. P.; Brown, J. B. and Hamm, W. G.: Surgery of inner canthus and related structures. Am. J. Ophth. *15:*498-507, June '32

Blair, V. P.: Types of contour repair in plastic surgery. South. Surgeon *1:*162-166, July '32

Blair, V. P.: Repairs and adjustments of eyelids. J.A.M.A. *99:*2171-2176, Dec 24, '32

Blair, V. P.; Brown, J. B. and Hamm, W. G.: Surgical therapy of post-radiation keratosis. Radiology *19:*337-344, Dec '32

Blair, V. P.: Repairs and adjustments of eyelids. Tr. Sect. Ophth., A.M.A., pp. 328-341, '32

Blair, V. P.; Brown, J. B. and Hamm, W. G.: Release of axillary and brachial scar fixation. Tr. South. S. A. *45:*258-274, '32

Blair, V. P.; Brown, J. B. and Hamm, W. G.: Types of reconstructive surgery of orbital region. South. Surgeon *1:*293-300, Jan '33

Blair, V. P.: Summary of 65 "cures" of cancer about mouth. Surg., Gynec. and Obst. *56:*469, Feb (No. 2A) '33

Blair, V. P.; Brown, J. B. and Hamm, W. G.: Radical treatment of cancer of lips. Am. J. Roentgenol. *29:*229-233, Feb '33

Blair, V. P. (see Brown, J. B. *et al*) April '33

Blair, V. P. and Brown, J. B.: Treatment of cancerous or potentially cancerous cervical lymph-nodes (as result of cancers of mouth). Ann. Surg. *98:*650-661, Oct '33

Blair, V. P.; Brown, J. B. and Hamm, W. G.: Correction of epispadias and scrotal hypospadias. Surg., Gynec. and Obst. *57:*646-653, Nov '33

Blair, V. P. and Brown, J. B.: Dieffenbach-Warren operation for closure of congenitally cleft palate. Surg., Gynec. and Obst. *59:*309-320, Sept '34

Blair, V. P. (see Brown, J. B.) Feb '35

Blair, V. P. (see Brown, J. B. *et al*) May, June '35

Blair, V. P.; Brown, J. B. and Byars, L. T.: Cancer of cheek and neighboring bone. Am. J. Surg. *30:*250-253, Nov '35

Blair, V. P.: Plastic surgery of head, face and neck; psychic reactions. J. Am. Dent. A. *23:*236-240, Feb '36

Blair, V. P.; Brown, J. B. and Byars, L. T.: Cancer of cheek and neighboring bone. Internat. J. Orthodontia *22:*183-188, Feb '36

Blair, V. P. and Brown, J. B.: Dieffenbach-Warren operation for closure of congenitally cleft palate. Internat. J. Orthodontia *2:*853-868, Aug '36

Blair, V. P. (see Brown, J. B. *et al*) Sept '36

Blair, V. P.; Brown, J. B. and Byars, L. T.: Plantar warts, flaps and grafts. J.A.M.A. *108:*24-27, Jan 2, '37

Blair, V. P.; Brown, J. B. and Byars, L. T.: Early local care of facial wounds. Surg., Gynec. and Obst. *64:*358-371, Feb (no. 2A) '37 also: Internat. J. Orthodontia *23:*515-533, May '37

Blair, V. P.; Brown, J. B. and Byars, L. T.: Treatment of fracture of upper jaw. Surgery *1:*748-760, May '37

Blair, V. P.; Brown, J. B. and Byars, L. T.: Observations on sinus abnormalities in congenital total and hemi-absence of nose. Ann. Otol., Rhin and Laryng. *46:*592-599, Sept '37

Blair, V. P.; Brown, J. B. and Byars, L. T.: Our responsibility toward oral cancer. Ann. Surg. *106:*568-576, Oct '37

Blair, V. P. Cleft palate surgery. J. Speech Disorders *2:*195-198, Dec '37

Blair, V. P.: Sinus abnormalities in congenital

total and hemiabsence of nose. Tr. Am. Laryng. A. *59:*223-229, '37

BLAIR, V. P. AND BYARS, L. T.: Treatment of wounds resulting from deep burns. J.A.M.A. *110:*1802-1804, May 28, '38

BLAIR, V. P.; BROWN, J. B. AND BYARS, L. T. Treatment of cancer of tongue. S. Clin. North America *18:*1255-1274, Oct '38

BLAIR, V. P.; BROWN, J. B. AND BYARS, L. T.: Prevention and correction of disfigurement in facial fractures. Am. J. Surg. *42:*536-541, Dec '38

BLAIR, V. P. AND BYARS, L. T.: Hypospadias and epispadias (surgical correction). J. Urol. *40:*814-825, Dec '38

BLAIR, V. P. (see BROWN, J. B. *et al*) Feb '39

BLAIR, V. P.: Distortions accompanying congenital single lip cleft. Nebraska M. J. *24:*41-43, Feb '39

BLAIR, V. P. AND BYARS, L. T.: Paralysis of lower eyelid and scleral scars and grafts. Surg., Gynec. and Obst. *70:*426-437, Feb (no. 2A) '40

BLAIR, V. P. AND BYARS, L. T.: Cancer of face. Mississippi Valley M. J. *62:*90-93, May '40

BLAIR, V. P. AND BYARS, L. T.: Toe to finger transplant. Ann. Surg. *112:*287-290, Aug '40

BLAIR, V. P. AND BYARS, L. T.: Current treatment of cancer of lip (and involved lymph nodes); clinical speculation. Surgery *8:*340-352, Aug '40

BLAIR, V. P., MOORE, S., AND BYARS, L. T.: *Cancer of the Face and Mouth*. C. V. Mosby Co., St. Louis, 1941

BLAIR, V. P.: Role of plastic surgeon in care of war injuries. Ann. Surg. *113:*697-704, May '41

BLAIR, V. P. AND BYARS, L. T.: Desirability of early proper treatment of facial fractures. Texas State J. Med. *38:*533-537, Jan '43

BLAIR, V. P. AND BYARS, L. T.: Cancer of mouth (and face). Texas State J. Med. *38:*641-645, March '43

BLAIR, V. P.: Relation of early care to final outcome of major wounds of face in war surgery. Mil. Surgeon *92:*12-17, Jan '43 also: Cincinnati J. Med. *24:*121-127, May '43

BLAIR, V. P.: Uses of transplanted pedicle flaps for restoration or correction of nose. Tr. Am. Soc. Plastic and Reconstructive Surg. *12:*23-24, '43

BLAIR, V. P.: Symposium on plastic surgery; treatment of battle casualities and street or industrial wounds. (face) Surgery *15:*16-21, Jan '44

BLAIR, V. P. AND BYARS, L. T.: "Hits, strikes and outs" in use of pedicle flaps for restoration or correction of nose. Surg. Gynec. and Obst. *82:*367-385, April '46

Blair Operation (See also Brown-Blair Operation)

Vilray P. Blair's modification of Mirault operation for cleft lip. BROWN, R. G., M. J. Australia *1:*499-503, April 11, '36

Blair-Brown Operation

Blair-Brown modification of Mirault method of treating unilateral harelip; results in cases. CHIATELLINO, A. Gior. med. d. Alto Adige *11:*131-145, March '39

BLAIRE, G. (see PERIN, L.) Dec '37

BLAISDELL, F. E. (see POLLOCK, W. E. *et al*) Feb '29

BLAISDELL, J. H.: Vascular nevi and their treatment. New England J. Med. *215:*485-488, Sept 10, '36

BLALOCK, A. (see BEARD, J. W.) April '31

BLALOCK, A. (see JOHNSON, G. S.) April '31

BLALOCK, A. (see CRESSMAN, R. D.) Dec '39

BLALOCK, A. (see WOOD, G. O. *et al*) Aug '40

BLALOCK, A. (see MINOT, A. S.) Oct '40

BLALOCK, A. (see DUNCAN, G. W.) Aug '42

BLALOCK, A.: Causes of shock associated with injury to tissues. Internat. Clin. *1:*144-161, March '33

BLALOCK, A.: Comparison of effects of local application of heat and of cold in prevention and treatment of experimental traumatic shock. Surgery *11:*356-359, March '42

BLALOCK, A.: Experimental shock; importance of local loss of fluid in production of low blood pressure after burns. Arch. Surg. *22:*610-616, April '31

BLALOCK, A.: Gordon Wilson lecture; shock or peripheral circulatory failure. Tr. Am. Clin. and Climatol. A. (1941) *57:*2-11, '42

BLALOCK, A.: Mechanism of production and treatment of shock. J.M.A. Alabama *1:*94-99, Sept '31

BLALOCK, A.: Present status of problem; "problem on shocks," Surgery *14:*487-508, Oct '43

BLALOCK, A.: Prevention and treatment of shock in military medicine. Dia med. *14:*1063-1066, Oct 12, '42

BLALOCK, A: Prevention and treatment of shock; symposium on military surgery. S. Clin. North America *21:*1663-1683, Dec '41

BLALOCK, A.: Shock treatment, with particular reference to use of blood plasma. J. Tennessee M. A. *34:*254-257, July '41

BLALOCK, A.: Trauma; occupational diseases and hazards; shock and hemorrhage. Bull. New York Acad. Med. *12:*610-622, Nov '36

BLALOCK, A.: Traumatic shock and hemorrhage. South. M. J. *27:*126-130, Feb '34

BLALOCK, A.: Treatment of shock or peripheral circulatory failure. South. Surgeon *7:*150-156, April '38

BLALOCK, A. AND CRESSMAN, R. D.: Experimental traumatic shock; further studies with particular reference to role of nervous system. Surg., Gynec. and Obst. *68:*278-287, Feb (no. 2A) '39

BLALOCK, A. AND DUNCAN, G. W.: Traumatic shock—consideration of several types of injuries (Donald C. Balfour lecture). Surg., Gynec. and Obst. *75:*401-409, Oct '42

BLALOCK, A. AND MASON, M. F.: Blood and blood substitutes in treatment and prevention of shock, with particular reference to their uses in warfare. Ann. Surg. *113:*657-676, May '41

BLALOCK, A. AND MASON, M. F.: Comparison of effects of heat and cold in shock therapy. Arch. Surg. *42:*1054-1059, June '41

BLALOCK, A. AND Price, P. B.: Panel discussions; traumatic shock; early signs, prevention and treatment. Bull. Am. Coll. Surgeons *27:*102-105, April '42

BLALOCK, A.; BEARD, J. W. AND JOHNSON, G. S.: Experimental shock; production and treatment. Tr. Sect. Surg., Gen. and Abd., A.M.A. pp. 294-303, '31

BLALOCK, A.; BEARD, J. W. AND JOHNSON, G. S.: Therapy in experimental shock. J.A.M.A. *97:*1794-1797, Dec 12, '31

BLANC, H.: Section of 2 extensor tendons of fingers; delayed suture; case. Bull. et mem. Soc. de chir. de Paris *21:*42, Jan 4, '29

BLANC FORTACÍN, J.: Bone grafting into infected field. Siglo med. *82:*117-120, Aug 11, '28

BLANC FORTACÍN, J.: Surgical grafts. Rev. ibero-am. de cien. med. *7:*193-204, Dec '32 Also: Siglo med. *90:*641-645, Dec 17, '32

BLANCHARD, H. E.: Corrective rhinoplasty. Rhode Island M. J. *9:*161-165, Oct '26

BLANCHARD, J. (see DECOURT, J. *et al*) March-April '41

BLANCO, T.: Two new methods of plastic surgery of eyelids. Arch. de oftal. hispano-am. *31:*79-84, Feb '31

BLANKSTEIN, W. G.: Cysts of bursa mucosa of subhyoid region of neck. Acta oto-laryng. *24:*379-385, '36

BLASI, R.: Roentgenotherapy of rhinophyma. Gior. ital. di mal. esot. e trop. *7:*16-22, Jan 31, '34

BLASKOVICS (see also DE BLASKOVICS, AND VON BLASKOVICS)

BLASKOVICS, L.: Total blepharoplasty. Orvosi hetil. *81:*1050-1055, Oct 16, '37

Blaskovics Operation

Blaskovics operation for eyelid ptosis. LINDNER, K. Klin. Monatsbl. f. Augenh. *93:*1-12, July '34

Blaskovics operation for eyelid ptosis. SHCHEKINA, A. N. Sovet. vestnik oftal. *8:*551-558, '36

Blaskovics operation for eyelid ptosis. GOLDFEDER, A. E. AND BUSHMICH, D. G. Vestnik oftal. *11:*824-829, '37

Blaskovics operation for eyelid ptosis. DIACICOV, M. Rev. san. mil., Bucuresti *36:*730-735, Aug '37

Bilateral eyelid ptosis operation; Blaskovics method. REA, R. L. Proc. Roy. Soc. Med. *31:*667-669, April '38

Blaskovics operation for eyelid ptosis. VON GERNET, R. Klin. Monatsbl. f. Augenh. *101:*422-423, Sept '38

Blaskovics operation for eyelid ptosis on basis of statistics of Moscow Ophthalmologic Hospital. KLYKOVA, A. L. AND TOKAREVA, B. A. Vestnik oftal. *12:*495-498, '38

BLASKOVICS operation: Modified Blaskovics operation for ptosis of eyelids, Bull. Pract. Ophth. *12:*7-9, Jan '42

BLATT, N.: Operation for eyelid ptosis. Wien. klin. Wchnschr. *34:*134, March 24, '21

BLAUSTEN, S.: Modified maxillary fracture splint for jaw. Bull. U. S. Army M. Dept. (no. 84) pp. 119-121, Jan '45

BLAVET DI BRIGA, C.: Successful experimental substitution of cartilage fixed in alcohol for loss of cranial substance. Arch. per. le sc. med. *54:*63-70, Jan '30

BLAVET DI BRIGA, C.: Experimental transplantation of cartilage fixed in bone. Arch. ital. de biol. *83:*26-33, July 30, '30

BLEDSOE, N. C.: Burn therapy. Southwest Med. *16:*313-317, Aug '32

BLEGVAD, N. R.: Cosmetic operations of nose; paraffin injections. Ugesk. f. Laeger *89:*1141-1144, Dec 8, '27

BLEGVAD, N. R.: Cosmetic operations on nose and paraffin injections; 6 cases. Ugesk. f. Laeger *90:*286-290, March 29, '28

BLENCKE, A.: Transplantation of skin in amputations of foot. Zentralbl. f. Chir. *56:*2050-2054, Aug 17, '29

BLENCKE, B.: Therapy of open injuries of fingers. Ztschr. f. arztl. Fortbild. *29:*301-302, May 15, '32

Blepharoplasty

One-stage plastic reconstruction of upper eyelid together with muscle fibers and eye-

Blephoroplasty—Cont.
lashes. KAZ, R. Zentralbl. f. Chir. *48:*1239, Aug 27, '21
Plastic surgery of eyelids and orbit. WALDRON, C. W. Minnesota Med. *4:*504, Aug '21
Plastic repair of eyelids by pedunculated skin grafts. CROSS, G. H. J.A.M.A. *77:*1233, Oct 15, '21
Plastic surgery in and about eyelids. NUTTING, R. J. California State J. Med. *20:*15-16, Jan '22
Reconstruction of lower eyelid. JIMÉNEZ LÓPEZ, C. AND RIBÓN, V. Semana med. *2:*832, Oct 19, '22 (illus.)
Reconstruction of eyelids. JOSEPH, H. Beitr. z. klin. Chir. *131:*52-65, '24
Autoplastic skin implant in blepharoplasty. D'ALESSANDRO, A. Semana med. *2:*1531-1534, Dec 17, '25
Plastic operations on face, in region of eye. VARIOUS AUTHORS. Proc. Roy. Soc. Med. (sect. Ophth.) *19:*14-38, June '26
Plastic repair of eyelid after excision of tumor. Bull. Soc. d'opht. de Paris, pp. 411, Oct '26
Etude des Blepharoplasties, by PIERRE BOUCHAUD. Arnette, Paris, 1927
Ophthalmic plastic surgery; clinical procedure in certain cases. PARKER, W. R. Am. J. Ophth. *10:*109-113, Feb '27
Formation of new upper eyelid from auricle. ROCHAT, G. F. Nederl. Tijdschr. v. Geneesk. *2:*709, Aug 6, '27
Lidplastik und plastische Operationen anderer Weichteile des Gesichts, By JOSEF IMRE. Studium, Budapest, 1928
Operation for pouches under eyes (Bourguet's operative technic). BOURGUET. Arch. franco-belges de chir. *31:*133-137, Feb '28
Operative treatment for sunken upper lid following enucleation. LÖWENSTEIN, A. Klin. Monatsbl. f. Augenh. *80:*233-236, Feb 24, '28
Plastic repair of right lower eyelid. MCKEE, S. H. Canad. M.A.J. *18:*307-308, March '28
Hungarian method of forming lower eyelid. SZOKOLIK, E. Klin. Monatsbl. f. Augenh. *80:*652-655, May 25, '28
Treatment of eyelid abnormalities by plastic surgery. BOURGUET, J. Monde med., Paris *39:*725-731, July 1, '29
Plastic surgery of eyelid. MENESTRINA, G. Boll. d'ocul. *8:*667-685, July '29
Cancer of upper eyelid; plastic operation; case. FROTHINGHAM, G. E., J. Michigan M. Soc. *28:*632-633, Sept '29
Machine for shaping skinflaps in anaplasty

Blepharoplasty—Cont.
of eyelids. LÉNÁRD, E. Klin. Monatsbl. f. Augenh. *83:*526-530, Oct-Nov '29
Two new methods of plastic surgery of eyelids. BLANCO, T. Arch. de oftal. hispano-am. *31:*79-84, Feb '31
Epithelioma of face secondary to extensive epithelioma of eyelids; three-stage operation; removal of tumor, skin graft and restoration of eyelids. TIXIER, L. AND BONNET, P. Lyon chir. *28:*719-722, Nov-Dec '31
New eyelid clamp. CRUICKSHANK, M. M. Indian M. Gaz. *67:*82-83, Feb '32 also: Am. J. Ophth. *15:*349, April '32
Pedicled flap in plastic surgery of eyelids. SPAETH, E. B. Pennsylvania M. J. *35:*560-562, May '32
Biological principles which underlie plastic surgery of eyelids. SPAETH, E. B. Am. J. Ophth. *15:*589-603, July '32
Repairs and adjustments of eyelids. BLAIR, V. P., J.A.M.A. *99:*2171-2176, Dec 24, '32
Argumosa blepharoplastic methods. MARQUEZ, M. Arch. de oftal. hispano-am. *33:*1-8, Jan '33
Surgery and plastic replacement of eyelids. BÜCKLERS, M. Chirurg *5:*460-472, June 15, '33
Plastic operations for restoration of lower eyelid. EL-TOGBY, A. F. Bull. Ophth. Soc. Egypt *26:*1-7, '33
Plastic surgery of eyelids. GLEZEROV, S. Y. Sovet. vestnik oftal. *3:*305-307, '33
Therapy of cancer of eyelid by evisceration followed by plastic surgery; case. AGUILAR, H. AND ZAVALETA, D. Hosp. argent. *4:*506-512, Jan 15, '34
Correction of ocular disfigurements. WIENER, M. Surg., Gynec. and Obst. *58:*390-394, Feb (no 2A) '34
Principles of plastic surgery of eyelids, with special reference to Hungarian school. KATZ, D. Arch. Ophth. *12:*220-227, Aug '34
Plastic repair of congenital and acquired deformities of palpebral margin by means of cartilage from auricle. LÖWENSTEIN, A. Klin. Monatsbl. f. Augenh. *93:*320-323, Sept '34
Closure of defects of lower eyelid on side nearest to nose by means of skin grafts from nose. KRAUPA, E. Ztschr. f. Augenh. *84:*216-217, Oct '34
Biologic flap to form 2 eyelids at same time; case. ESSER, J. F. S. Rev. espan. de cir. *17:*1-3, Jan-Feb '35
Operations on eyelids in Foville syndrome; case. COPPEZ, J. H. J. belge de neurol. et de psychiat. *35:*206-208, April '35

Blepharoplasty – Cont.
External canthal ligament in surgery of lower eyelid. HILDRETH, H. R. Am. J. Ophth. *18:*437–439, May '35
Plastic operations for restoration of upper eyelid. EL TOBGY, A. F. Bull. Ophth. Soc. Egypt *28:*21–25, '35
Plastic surgery of eyelids. GILLIES, H. D. Tr. Ophth. Soc. U. Kingdom *55:*357–373, '35
Comparative evaluation of marginoplastic operations of eyelids. LUZHINSKIY, G. F. Sovet. vestnik oftal. *7:*137–142, '35
Indications and comparative evaluation of Hungarian method of blepharoplasty. KOPP, I. F. Sovet. vestnik oftal. *7:*603–609, '35
Euroblepharon; case. WEVE, H. Nederl. tijdschr. v. geneesk. *80:*1213–1217, March 21, '36
Total blepharoplasty. BLASKOVICS, L. Orvosi hetil. *81:*1050–1055, Oct 16, '37
Sources of grafts for plastic surgery about eyes. WHEELER, J. M. New York State J. Med. *36:*1372–1376, Oct 1, '36
Instruments for eyelid treatment. HEATH, P. Tr. Sect. Ophth., A.M.A., pp. 272–283, '36 also: Arch. Ophth. *17:*894–895, May '37
Marginal cutaneous blepharopexy in plastic surgery. DUPUY-DUTEMPS, L. Ann. d'ocul. *174:*312–317, May '37
Plastic repair of eyelid hernia with fascia lata. SAKLER, B. R. Am. J. Ophth. *20:*936–938, Sept '37
Technic of blepharoplasty. KALT, E. Bull. Soc. d'opht. de Paris *49:*723–725, Dec '37
Technic of median nonmutilating blephorrhaphy. KLEEFELD, G. Bull. Soc. belge d'opht., no. 74, pp. 16–21, '37
Autoplasty of eyelids. LEONARDI, Bull. et mem. Soc. franc. d'opht. *50:*20–24, '37
Blepharoplasty by means of free transplants of skin. LEVITSKIY, M. A. Vestnik oftal. *11:*798–802, '37
Plastic surgery of eyelids; use of pedicled flaps with handle VON SEEMEN, H. Deutsche Ztschr. f. Chir. *248:*411–419, '37
Pedicled dermomuscular blepharoplasty; 12 cases. CHARAMIS, J. S. Arch. d'opht. *2:*206–218, March '38
Plastic and esthetic reparative surgery of eyelid. MAZZI, L. Chir. plast., *4:*138–141, July–Sept '38
Plastic surgery of eyelids. KREIBIG, W. Ztschr. f. Augenh. *95:*269–275, Aug '38
Advantages of use of coagulants, especially in plastic operations on eyes. BUSACCA, A. Arch. Ophth. *20:*406–409, Sept '38
Review of some modern methods for plastic surgery of eyes. SPAETH, E. B. Am. J. Surg. *42:*89–100, Oct '38

Blepharoplasty – Cont.
Use of orbicularis palpebrarum muscle in eyelid surgery. WHEELER, J. M. Am. J. Surg. *42:*7–9, Oct '38
Eyelid surgery; about sliding-flap, known also as Hungarian plastic. CZUKRASZ, I. Tr. Ophth. Soc. U. Kingdom (pt. 2) *58:*561–575, '38
Technic of Millingen-Sapezhko operation (eyelid). MITSKEVICH, L. D. Vestnik oftal. *13:*848–849, '38
Results of reconstruction of eyelids following loss of substance due to grave trauma. NICOLATO, A. Ann. di ottal. e clin. ocul. *67:*81–92, Feb '39
Hughes procedure for rebuilding lower eyelid. GIFFORD, S. R. Arch. Ophth. *21:*447–452, March '39
Plastic surgery of eyelid following removal of epithelioma caused by irradiation. LAUBER, H. Ophthalmologica *97:*312–316, July '39
Discussion on plastic surgery of eyelids. KILNER, T. P. AND IMRE, J. Proc. Roy. Soc. Med. *32:*1247–1260, Aug '39
Operation in patient with large eyelids and maintained levator function. FAZAKAS, A. Klin. Monatsbl. f. Augenh. *103:*621–624, Dec '39
Blepharoplasty with free skin flap from auricle BULACH, K. Vestnik oftal. (no. 6) *14:*46–48, '39
Correction of massive defects of both eyelids. SPAETH, E. B. Pennsylvania M. J. *43:*663–668, Feb '40
Plastic surgery of eyelids. SHANKS, J. M. Rec. *152:*408, Dec 4, '40
Plastic reconstruction of upper eyelid. McLEAN, J. M. Am. J. Ophth. *24:*46–48, Jan '41
Plastic operations of total defect of eyelids and symblephara orbitalia. INOUE, S. Far East. Sc. Bull. *1:*3, April '41 (abstract)
Plastic repair of deformities of eyelids. MORGAN, A. L. Canad. M.A.J. *44:*560–562, June '41
Some phases of plastic surgery about eye. McLEAN, J. M. Mississippi Doctor *19:*335–339, Dec '41
Hughes operation for total loss of lower eyelid. DELLEPIANE RAWSON, R. Arq. de cir. clin. e exper. *6:*235–251, April–June '42
Hughes operation for total loss of lower eyelid. DELLEPIANE RAWSON, R. Dia med. *14:*461, May 25, '42
Plastic repair of baggy eyelids. ZENO, L. Bol. Soc. de cir. de Rosario *9:*131–133, June '42
Plastic surgery of eyelids. AJO, A. Nord. med. *15:*2437–2440, Sept 5, '42
Cure of depression of lower eyelid following

Blepharoplasty – Cont.

reinsertion of inferior rectus muscle; case. INCIARDI, J. A. Arch. Ophth. *28:*464-466, Sept '42

Recent advances in eyelid surgery. HAGUE, E. B. Dis. Eye, Ear, Nose and Throat *2:*353-359, Dec '42

"Pocket-flap" as method for total restoration of eyelid; preliminary report. KURLOV, I. N. Vestnik oftal. (nos. 1-2) *20:*12-19, '42

Plastic reconstruction of lower and upper eyelids. RAPIN, M. Ophthalmologica *105:*233-239, May '43

Argumosa's 2 methods of blepharoplasty for tumors usually attributed to other authors (especially Dieffenbach). MARQUEZ, M. J. Internat. Coll. Surgeons *7:*63-67, Jan-Feb '44

Tarsoconjunctival sliding-graft technics for reconstruction of eyelids. SUGAR, H. S. Am. J. Ophth. *27:*109-123, Feb '44

Reconstruction of ablated lower eyelid. WHALMAN, H. F. Arch. Ophth. *32:*66-67, July '44

Reconstruction of lower eyelid by Hughes method. FOSTER, J. Brit. J. Ophth. *28:*515-519, Oct '44

Minor surgery of eyelids. ALVIN, B. Y. Tr. Indiana Acad. Ophth. and Otolaryng. *28:*78-93, '44

Reconstructive surgery of eyelids; case. CASTROVIEJO, R. Arch. Asoc. para evit. ceguera Mexico *2:*189-194, '44

Surgical reconstruction of upper eyelid. HAGUE, E. B. Am. J. Ophth. *28:*886-889, Aug '45

Total reconstruction of upper lid (blepharopoiesis). HUGHES, W. L. Am. J. Ophth. *28:*980-992, Sept '45

Reconstruction of eyelids. HUGHES, W. L. Am. J. Ophth. *28:*1203-1211, Nov '45

Plastic procedures of eyelids. PUNTENNEY, I. Illinois M. J. *88:*238-242, Nov '45

Conjunctival palpebral autoplasty. BELFORT MATTOS, W. Arq. brasil. de oftal. *8:*103-109, '45

Methods of repair and reconstruction. (eyelids). FOX, S. A. Am. J. Ophth. *29:*452-458, Apr '46

Surgery of eyelids. LODGE, W. O. J. Internat. Coll. Surgeons *9:*383-388, May-June '46

Plastic restoration of upper lid and socket. LUC, J. Brit. J. Ophth. *30:*665-668, Nov '46

Blepharoplasty, Cosmetic

New principles in plastic operations of eyelids and face. IMRE, J. JR. J.A.M.A. *76:*1293, May 7, '21

Blepharoplasty, Cosmetic – Cont.

Operation for pouches under eyes (Bourguet's operative technic). BOURGUET. Arch. franco-belges de chir. *31:*133-137, Feb '28

Plastic surgery in removal of excessive cutaneous tissues obstructing vision. KAHN, K. New York State J. Med. *34:*781-783, Sept 1, '34

Operation for senile ectropion. IMRE, J. Klin. Monatsbl. f. Augenh. *95:*303-305, Sept '35

Esthetic surgery of eyelids. DANTRELLE, A. J. de med. de Paris. *55:*997-1004, Nov 14, '35

Surgery for trachomatous ectropion. KITAEVA, A. Sovet. vestnik oftal. *7:*387-388, '35

Cosmetic correction of ptosis of lower eyelid. EITNER, E. Wien. med. Wchnschr. *87:*423-424, April 10, '37

Plastic repair of eyelid hernia with fascia lata. SAKLER, B. R. Am. J. Ophth. *20:*936-938, Sept '37

Plastic and esthetic reparative surgery of eyelid. MAZZI, L. Chir. plast. *4:*138-141, July-Sept '38

Plastic operation of eyelids. IMRE, J. Tr. Ophth. Soc. U. Kingdom (pt. 2, 1937) *57:*494-508, '38

Plastic repair of baggy eyelids. ZENO, L. Bol. Soc. de cir. de Rosario, *9:*131-133, June '42

Blepharoplasty for Ectropion

So-called lacrymal or senile ectropion of lower eyelid, and its treatment. AUBARET. Medecine *7:*261-262, Jan '26

Technic of total ectropion operation. VERNON, E. L. Am. J. Ophth. *9:*598-600, Aug '26

Surgical treatment of senile ectropion. DE ROSA, G. Arch. di ottal. *34:*15-19, Jan '27

Easy and successful operation for over-eversion of eyelids. BAKRY, M. Bull. Ophth. Soc. Egypt *2:*20-23, '29

Resection of orbicular muscle in ectropion paralysis. HOLLOS, L. Orvosi hetil. *74:*1094-1095, Oct 25, '30 also: Ztschr. f. Augenh. *73:*27-31, Dec '30

New method of blepharoplastic operation for cicatricial ectropion using free transplant from ear flap. GOLDFEDER, A. E. Sovet. vestnik. oftal. *6:*173-177, '35

Cicatricial ectropion as result of mucocele of frontal sinus; plastic repair. MCLEOD, J. AND LUX, P. Arch. Ophth. *15:*994-997, June '36

Operation for correction of eversion of inferior lacrimal point. TIKHOMIROV, P. E. Vestnik oftal. *11:*216-217, '37

New technic in therapy of eversion of lacri-

Blepharoplasty for Ectropion – Cont.

mal point and ectropion of lower lid; preliminary report. POKHISOV, N. Vestnik oftal. *11:*218–222, '37

Free full-thickness grafts of skin to eyelids; cases. ZENO, L. Bol. Soc. de cir. de Rosario *7:*127–135, May '40 also: An. de cir. *6:*156–164, June '40

Ectropion and its therapy. COVARRUBIAS ZENTENO, R. Rev. med. de Chile *68:*1187–1190, Sept '40

Therapy of cicatricial ectropion. BURMISTROVA, E. Vestnik oftal. *18:*89, '41

Principles of plastic surgery in cicatricial ectropion of lower eyelid. GLEZEROV, S. Y. Vestnik oftal. *18:*397–400, '41

Subcutaneous splitting of eyelid in operative treatment of senile ectropion. LYTTON, H. Brit. J. Ophth. *29:*378–380, July '45

Blepharoplasty for Entropion

Entropion following influenza with new surgical procedure. CLAPP, C. A. Am. J. Ophth. *5:*542–544, July '22 (illus.)

Autoplastic operation on lower margin of tarsus for ingrown eyelash. SHIMKIN, N. Klin. Monatsbl. f. Augenh. *77:*538–546, Oct 30, '26

Operative procedure in trachomatous entropion of upper lid. OLÁH, E. Klin. Monatsbl. f. Augenh. *79:*388, Sept 30, '27

Transplantation of cartilage from auricle into eyelid in trachomatous cicatricial entropion. GOLDFEDER, A. E. Klin. Monatsbl. f. Augenh. *82:*809–813, June 21, '29

New method in correction of cicatricial entropion. SALVATI, G. Ann. d'ocul. *167:*311–314, April '30

Marginoplasty by means of cartilage of auricle without skin in partial trichiasis of eyelid. GOLDFEDER, A. E. Klin. Monatsbl. f. Augenh. *86:*218–225, Feb '31

New marginoplastic method of operation in trichiasis of eyelids. POCHISSOFF, N. Klin. Monatsbl. f. Augenh. *86:*213–218, Feb '31

Surgical therapy of entropion and trichiasis. LAUTERSTEIN, M. Ztschr. f. Augenh. *75:*183, Sept '31

Removal of cartilage in trachomatous entropion. WARSCHAWSKI, J. Klin. Monatsbl. f. Augenh. *87:*378–382, Sept '31

Surgical therapy of trichiasis and entropion of upper eyelid. CHRONIS, P. Cong. internat. de med. trop. et d'hyg., Compt. rend. (1928) *3:*755–757, '31

New surgical technic in entropion musculare and trichiasis of lower eyelid. CHRONIS, P. Cong. internat. de med. trop. et d'hyg., Compt. rend. (1928) *3:*759, '31

Blepharoplasty for Entropion – Cont.

Low tarsotomy and horizontal suture in trachomatous entropion of upper eyelid. JUNÈS, E. Ann. d'ocul. *169:*704–717, Sept '32

Radical operation in therapy of trichiasis and entropion of upper eyelid. CHRONIS, P. Folia ophth. orient. *1:*187–190, Feb '33

New technic of operation in case of hypertrophy of tarsal plate, with trichiasis as complication. TSHERNOFF, L. Hebrew Physician *2:*55, '33

Therapy of trachomatous entropion. MEDVEDEV, N. I. Sovet. vestnik oftal. *3:*36–42, '33

Resection of orbicularis oculi in therapy of spasmodic entropion. DUSSELDORP, M. Rev. Asoc. med. argent. *48:*296–298, March-April '34 also: Rev. oto-neuro-oftal. *9:*207–209, June '34

Internal plastic surgery of tarsus in posttrachomatous entropion and trichiasis. WORONYTSCH, N. Ztschr. f. Augenh. *84:*58–72, Aug '34

Entropion in newborn and its treatment. CHOW, K. V. Chinese M. J. *48:*830–832, Sept '34

External tarsorrhaphy in therapy of spontaneous entropion of lower eyelid. HAMBRESIN, L. Bull. Soc. belge d'opht., no. 68, pp. 68–71, '34

Late results of Snellen and Millingen-Sapezhko operations for correction of trachomatous entropion. ZAKHAROV, A. P. Sovet. vestnik oftal. *4:*491–497, '34

Surgical therapy of entropion of external angular origin. POULARD, A. Ann. d'ocul. *172:*97–105, Feb '35

Correction of trachomatous entropion of upper eyelid. BALDINO, S. Rassegna ital. d'ottal. *4:*212–217, March-April '35

Correction of trichiasis of eyelids by transplantation of cartilage from auricle. CHEPURIN, N. S. Sovet. vestnik oftal. *7:*368–373, '35

Operation for spastic entropion. POKHISOV, N. Y. Sovet. vestnik oftal. *6:*131–135, '35

Removal of tarsal section of orbicular muscle of upper eyelid in therapy of entropion and trichiasis and for prevention of recurrence of trachomatous processes. BUSACCA, A. Ztschr. f. Augenh. *88:*100–106, Jan '36

Surgical therapy of entropion and trichiasis in trachoma patients. IFY, I. Budapesti orvosi ujsag *34:*774–776, Sept 17, '36

Satisfactory operation for entropion of upper eyelid. GODDARD, F. W. Chinese M. J. *50:*1505, Oct '36

Method for correction of entropion in trachomatous patients, with particular atten-

Blepharoplasty for Entropion – Cont.

tion to esthetic results. BUSACCA, A. Arch. Ophth. *16:*822–828, Nov '36

Linear incision for entropion or trichiasis due to trachoma. LÜTFÜ, Ö. AND BASTUG, K. Ö. Deutsche med. Wchnschr. *62:*2014–2015, Dec 4, '36

Surgical therapy of cicatricial trachoma. ABDULAEV, G. G. Sovet. vestnik oftal. *8:*712–715, '36

Operation for cicatricial entropion of lower eyelid. KIPARISOV, N. M. Vestnik oftal. *11:*223–225, '37

Vertical section and flat incisions of cartilage of eyelids in therapy of trachomatous entropion. SHEVELEV, M. M. Vestnik oftal. *11:*383–386, '37

Surgical treatment of trachoma (complicated by entropion). RAMBO, V. C. Am. J. Ophth. *21:*277–285, March '38

Simple surgical method in post-trachomatous entropion and trichiasis. MIRIC, B. Klin. Monatsbl. f. Augenh. *101:*381–386, Sept '38

Surgical therapy of cicatricial entropion of lower eyelid. PARADOKSOV, L. F. Vestnik oftal. *13:*550–551, '38

Simplified taroplastic in cicatricial entropion. KREIKER, A. Ophthalmologica *97:*69–78, May '39

Spastic entropion correction by orbicularis transplantation. WHEELER, J. M. Am. J. Ophth. *22:*477–483, May '39

Barg operation (eyelids) according to data of Trachoma Institute in Turkmenistan. VASILEVA, N. A. Vestnik oftal (no. 2) *15:*46–48, '39

Inversion of tarsus as surgical procedure in correction of granulous entropion. NIZETIC, Z. Ann. d'ocul. *177:*211–217, June '40

Operation for spastic entropion. MEEK, R. E. Arch. Ophth. *24:*547–551, Sept '40

Technic of operation for correction of trachomatous entropion. NIZETIC, Z. Klin. Monatsbl. f. Augenh. *105:*641–647, Dec '40

Treatment of spastic entropion. ROBBINS, A. R. Arch. Ophth. *25:*475–476, March '41

Spasmodic entropion; new surgical technic in therapy. TORRES ESTRADA, A. Bol. d. Hosp. oftal. de Ntra. Sra. de la Luz *1:*265–272, Nov–Dec '41

New surgical technic for treating spasmodic entropion. TORRES ESTRADA, A. Cir. y cirujanos *9:*559–569, Dec 31, '41

Best operation against spastic entropion. HABACHI, S. Bull. Ophth. Soc. Egypt. *34:*57–63, '41

Paganelli's modification of operation for entropion. PAGANELLI, T. R. Dis. Eye, Ear, Nose and Throat *2:*347–349, Nov '42

Operations for trachomatous eversion of eyelids and trichiasis. MAKHLIN, I. M. Sovet. med. (nos. 1–2) *6:*22–23, '42

Modified Ewing operation for cicatricial entropion. SMITH, J. E. AND SINISCAL, A. A. Am. J. Ophth. *26:*382–389, April '43

Treatment of cicatricial entropion. BERKLEY, W. L., U. S. Nav. M. Bull. *41:*729–736, May '43

Operation for entropion of trachoma. COCKBURN, C. Brit. J. Ophth. *27:*308–310, July '43

New treatment of entropion. MACDONALD, A. E. Tr. Am. Ophth. Soc. *43:*372, '45

Blepharoptosis

Operation for eyelid ptosis. BLATT, N. Wien. klin. Wchnschr. *34:*134, March 24, '21

Blepharochalasis with ptosis; report of case. HECKEL, E. B. Am. J. Ophth. *4:*273, April '21

Motais operation for eyelid ptosis, report of 6 cases. O'CONNOR, R. California State J. Med. *19:*409, Oct '21

Use of living sutures in treatment of eyelid ptosis. WRIGHT, W. W. Arch. Ophth. *51:*99–102, March '22 (illus.)

On permanence of results of Motais' operation for eyelid ptosis. BRUNS, H. D. Am. J. Ophth. *5:*269–270, April '22 (illus.)

Operative treatment of ptosis of eyelid. CAMPOS, E. Brazil-med. *2:*345–349, Dec 2, '22 (illus.) abstr: J.A.M.A. *80:*514, Feb 17, '23

New operation for eyelid ptosis with shortening of levator and tarsus. DE BLASKOVICS, L. Arch. Ophth. *52:*563–573, Nov '23 (illus.)

Hereditary ptosis of eyelids. KILLIAN, H. Klin. Wchnschr. *2:*2286, Dec 10, '23

Operation for blepharoptosis with formation of a fold in eyelid. REESE, R. G. Arch. Ophth. *53:*26–30, Jan '24

Unilateral congenital eyelid ptosis corrected by Hunt-Tansley operation. LOEB, C. Am. J. Ophth. *7:*216–217, March '24

An operation for congenital eyelid ptosis. YOUNG, G. Brit. J. Ophth. *8:*272–275, June '24

Congenital ptosis of upper lid. LEAL, J. Brazil-med. *2:*179–180, Sept 20, '24 abstr: J.A.M.A. *83:*1626, Nov 15, '24

Automatic pseudocorrection in ocular ptosis and strabismus. PAULIAN, E. D. Encephale *19:*506–508, Sept–Oct '24 abstr: J.A.M.A. *83:*1623, Nov 15, '24

Operation for ptosis of eyelids. BRAUNSTEIN, E. P. Arch. f. Ophth. *116:*452–456, '26

Bilateral eyelid ptosis cured by Hunt-Tansley operation. LOEB, C. Am. J. Ophth. *10:*191–192, March '27

Blepharoptosis – Cont.

Post-traumatic ptosis and atrophic myopathies of eyelid. MOLIN DE TEYSSIEU, AND PONS. Rev. d'oto-neuro-ocul. *5:*284-287, April '27

Treatment of blepharoptosis. ESTEBAN ARANJUEZ, M. Arch. de med., cir. y espec. *26:*696-700, June 4, '27

Methods of surgical treatment of congenital ptosis; case. VERDERAME, F. Rev. gen. d'opht. *41:*277-288, July '27

Young's operation for eyelid ptosis; case. BUTLER, T. H. Tr. Ophth. Soc. U. Kingdom *47:*387, '27

Case of myasthenia gravis operated on for eyelid ptosis by Hess's method. HARDIE, D. Brit. J. Ophth. *12:*31-33, Jan '28

Correction of eyelid ptosis by fascia lata hammock. DERBY, G. S. Am. J. Ophth. *11:*352-354, May '28

Modified Motais operation for eyelid ptosis. KIRBY, D. B. Arch. Ophth. *57:*327-331, July '28

Operation according to Shoemaker method for ptosis. SCARLETT, H. W. Am. J. Ophth. *11:*779-780, Oct '28

Technique of Motais operation for ptosis. WEEKS, W. W. Am. J. Ophth. *11:*879-883, Nov '28

Congenital eyelid ptosis with Gunn's phenomenon; case. DUPUY-DUTEMPS, L. Bull. Soc. d'opht. de Paris, pp. 136-140, March '29

New technic of operation for eyelid ptosis. BARDELLI, L. Boll. d'ocul. *8:*289-301, April '29

Treatment of eyelid ptosis. MORTON, H. M. Eye, Ear, Nose and Throat Monthly *8:*155-158, May '29

Operative treatment of eyelid ptosis; case. RENEDO. Arch. de med., cir. y espec. *30:*628-631, May 25, '29

Treatment of ptosis; formation of fold in eyelid and resection of levator and tarsus. VON BLASKOVICS, L. Arch. Ophth. *1:*672-680, June '29

Ptosis of eyelid; case operated by new method. NIDA, M. Ann. d'ocul. *166:*639-645, Aug '29

Palliative operation for eyelid ptosis. SCHNEIDER, R. Ber. u. d. Versamml. d. deutsch. ophth. Gesellsch. (1928) *47:*274-277, '29

Formation of folding lid in ptosis operation. VON BLASKOVICS, L. Ber. u. d. Versamml. d. deutsch. ophth. Gesellsch. (1928) *47:*277-283, '29

Hereditary eyelid ptosis with epicanthus;

Blepharoptosis – Cont.

case with pedigree extending over 4 generations. MCILROY, J. H. Proc. Roy. Soc. Med. (sect. Ophth.), *23:*17-20, Jan '30

Balance ptosis of eyelids; case. CARAMAZZA, F. Riv. oto-neuro-oft. *7:*165-177, March-April '30

Family of 18th century with eyelid ptosis; hereditary aspect. VAN SETERS, W. H. Nederl. tijdschr. v. geneesk. *74:*1775-1779, April 5, '30

Treatment of congenital ptosis of eyelids. BOURGUET. Bull. et mem. Soc. de chir. de Paris *22:*313-319, May 2, '30

Surgical technic in therapy of eyelid ptosis. NOCITO, J. P. Semana med. *2:*496-497, Aug 14, '30

Operative treatment of eyelid ptosis. BAER, A. J., J. Kansas M. Soc. *32:*262-265, Aug '31

Congenital epicanthus and ptosis of eyelid transmitted through 4 generations. ROSS, N. Brit. M. J. *1:*378-379, Feb 27, '32

Correction of epicanthus and eyelid ptosis. BLAIR, V. P., BROWN, J. B., AND HAMM, W. G. Arch. Ophth. *7:*831-946, June '32

Machek operation in eyelid ptosis. GIFFORD, S. R. Arch. Ophth. *8:*495-502, Oct '32

Plastic surgery of eyelid ptosis. BOURGUET, J. Monde med. Paris *42:*962-971, Nov 15, '32

Use of prisms in bilateral eyelid ptosis; case. OLSHO, S. L. Am. J. Ophth. *16:*141-142, Feb '33

Acrocephalosyndactylia, microcephaly, ptosis of eyelids and infantillism; addition of acute spasmodic paraplegia. EUZIÈRE, J.; *et al.* Arch. Soc. d. sc. med. et biol. de Montpellier *14:*110-119, March '33

Eyelid ptosis. VEIL, P. Rev. gen. de clin. et de therap. *47:*310-311, May 13, '33

Cosmetic therapy of mild forms of eyelid ptosis. MÁRQUEZ, M. Arch de oftal. hispano-am. *33:*363-366, June '33

Partial cryptophthalmos with epicanthus and congenital ptosis of upper eyelid; author's technic for surgical correction; 2 cases. SATANOWSKY, P. Semana med. *1:*1953-1958, June 15, '33 abstr: Rev. Asoc. med. argent. *47:*2718-2724, June '33

Operation for relief of congenital eyelid ptosis. GREEVES, R. A. Proc. Roy. Soc. Med. *26:*1478-1482, Sept '33

Partial cryptophthalmos with epicanthus and congenital ptosis of upper eyelid; author's technic for surgical correction; 2 cases. SATANOWSKY, P. Arch. de oftal. hispano-am. *33:*643-652, Nov '33

Operation for relief of congenital ptosis of

Blepharoptosis – Cont.
eyelids. GREEVES, R. A. Brit. J. Ophth. *17:*741–745, Dec '33
Heredofamilial eyelid ptosis. LYUBARSKŜYA, T. E. Sovet. nevropat., psikhiat. i psikhogig. (no. 3) *2:*103–104, '33
Modification of Motais' operation for ptosis of eyelid. TAGGART, H. J. Tr. Ophth. Soc. U. Kingdom *53:*417–421, '33
Relative ptosis of eyelids. WOLFF, E. Tr. Ophth. Soc. U. Kingdom *53:*317–319, '33
Supporting suture in ptosis operations. FROST, A. D. Am. J. Ophth. *17:*633, July '34
Blaskovics operation for eyelid ptosis. LINDNER, K. Klin. Monatsbl. f. Augenh. *93:*1–12, July '34
Progress with tarsal graft of Müller's muscle in pseudoptosis due to enophthalmos. GALLENGA, R. Rassegna ital. d'ottal. *3:*626–636, July–Aug '34
Bilateral congenital epicanthus inversus and ptosis; case. LUO, T. H. Chinese M. J. *48:*814–818, Sept '34
Temporary and permanent eyelid ptosis in trachoma. BUSACCA, A. Rev. internat. du trachome *11:*204–213, Oct '34
Tarsectomy in incomplete eyelid ptosis. ALEXANDER, C. S. Texas State J. Med. *30:*511–514, Dec '34
Surgical therapy of eyelid ptosis. JAENSCH, P. A. Klin. Monatsbl. f. Augenh. *94:*183–189, Feb '35
Surgical treatment of eyelid ptosis. KISKADDEN, W. S. Am. J. Surg. *27:*499–501, March '35
Hereditary congenital eyelid ptosis; report of pedigree and review of literature. RODIN, F. H. AND BARKAN, H. Am. J. Ophth. *18:*213–225, March '35
Congenital eyelid ptosis; cases. TIRELLI, G. Rassegna ital. d'ottal. *4:*224–236, March–April '35
Operation for congenital eyelid ptosis; case. ADAMS, W. M. Memphis M. J. *10:*16, April '35
Congenital eyelid ptosis associated with ocular abnormalities; 3 cases. PERGOLA, A. Rassegna ital. d'ottal. *4:*371–384, May–June '35
Improved eyelid crutch for ptosis. DODGE, W. M. JR. Arch. Ophth. *14:*989–990, Dec '35
Simple procedure of advancement of levator combined with tarsectomy in trachomatous as well as in congenital ptosis. FEIGENBAUM, A. Folia ophth. orient. *2:*50–58, '35
Treatment of trachomatous eyelid ptosis. KAGAN, Y. A. Sovet. vestnik oftal. *6:*416, '35
Eyelid ptosis operation. TRAINOR, M. E. Tr. Sect. Ophth., A.M.A., pp. 93-97, '35
Pedigree of four generations of hereditary congenital ptosis affecting only one eye and pedigree of one generation of congenital ptosis with epicanthus. RODIN, F. H. Am. J. Ophth. *19:*597–599, July '36
Eyelid ptosis, superior-rectus fascia-lata sling in correction. DICKEY, C. A. Am. J. Ophth. *19:*660–664, Aug '36
Correction by 2 strips of fascia lata, eyelid ptosis. MAGNUS, J. A. Brit. J. Ophth. *20:*460–464, Aug '36
Hereditary character of eyelid ptosis. BIRO, E. Arch. d'opht. *53:*685–693, Sept '36
Necessity for examination of corneal sensitivity before operating for congenital eyelid ptosis. FAYN, I. E. Sovet. vestnik oftal. *9:*905, '36
Blaskovic's operation for eyelid ptosis. SHCHEKINA, A. N. Sovet. vestnik oftal. *8:*551–558, '36
Plastic surgery of ptosis of upper left eyelid; case in child. MALBEC, E. F. Semana med. *1:*521–525, Feb 18, '37
Cosmetic correction of ptosis of lower eyelid. EITNER, E. Wien. med. Wchnschr. *87:*423–424, April 10, '37
Ox-fascia-transplant operation in eyelid ptosis. HILDRETH, H. R. South. M. J. *30:*471–473, May '37
Blaskovics operation for eyelid ptosis. DIACICOV, M. Rev. san. mil., Bucuresti *36:*730–735, Aug '37
Surgical management of eyelid ptosis, with special reference to use of superior rectus muscle. JAMESON, P. C. Arch. Ophth. *18:*547–557, Oct '37
Eyelid ptosis. PICKERILL, H. P. New Zealand M. J. *36:*308–309, Oct '37
Surgical treatment of eyelid ptosis. RUEDEMANN, A. D. S. Clin. North America *17:*1503–1509, Oct '37
Eyelid ptosis and its surgical correction. SPAETH, E. B. J.A.M.A. *109:*1889–1894, Dec 4, '37
Eyelid ptosis and its surgical correction. SPAETH, E. B. Tr. Sect. Ophth., A.M.A., pp. 66–89, '37
New modification of operation for eyelid ptosis. LAZAREV, E. G. Vestnik oftal. *11:*76–80, '37
Correction of eyelid ptosis by transplantation of fascia lata. TSITOVSKIY, M. L. Vestnik oftal. *11:*373–377, '37
Blaskovics operation for eyelid ptosis. GOLDFEDER, A. E. AND BUSHMICH, D. G. Vestnik oftal. *11:*824–829, '37
Congenital unilateral partial blepharoptosis;

Blepharoptosis – Cont.

case. Tupinamba, J. Rev. de oftal. de Sao Paulo, *6:*29–32, Jan–Mar '38

Modification of Motais operation for eyelid ptosis. de Saint-Martin, R. Bull. Soc. d'opht. de Paris *50:*100–102, Feb '38

Bilateral eyelid ptosis operation; Blaskovics method. Rea, R. L. Proc. Roy. Soc. Med. *31:*667–669, April '38

Surgical correction of eyelid ptosis. Fazakas, S. Orvosi hetil. *82:*492–494, May 21, '38

Congenital eyelid ptosis with rhinomalacia (lack of ossification of nasal bones); case. Rebelo Neto, J. Rev. Assoc. paulista de med. *12:*455–464, May '38

Modified Motais operation for eyelid ptosis. de Saint-Martin, R. Ann. d'ocul. *175:*589–596, Aug '38

Blaskovics operation for eyelid ptosis. von Gernet, R. Klin. Monatsbl. f. Augenh. *101:*422–423, Sept '38

Blaskovics operation for eyelid ptosis on basis of statistics of Moscow Ophthalmologic Hospital. Klykova, A. L. and Tokareva, B. A. Vestnik oftal. *12:*495–498, '38

Familial bilateral eyelid ptosis. Wängler, K. Arch. f. Kinderh. *114:*102–107, '38

Correction of eyelid ptosis by attachment of strips of orbicularis muscle to superior rectus muscle. Wheeler, J. M. Tr. Sect. Ophth., A.M.A., pp 130–137, '38 Also: Arch. Ophth. *21:*1–7, Jan '39

Surgical therapy of eyelid ptosis with special reference to Nida technic; results in cases. Valerio, M. Rassegna ital. d'ottal. *8:*62–83, Jan–Feb 8, '39

Ptosis of eyelids. Zeeman, W. P. C. Nederl. tijdschr. v. geneesk. *83:*2714–2720, June 10, '39

Plastic surgery for Hutchinson's facies and various accompanying ptoses. Bourguet, J. Monde med., Paris *49:*659–667, June 15, '39

Nida method of correcting ptosis of upper eyelid. Bardanzellu, T. Rassegna ital. d'ottal. *8:*449–453, July–Aug '39

Miotic ptosis; case of Fuchs' progressive muscular dystrophy in man. Ferreira, F. Brasil-med. *53:*1087–1088, Dec 2, '39

Correction of eyelid ptosis by means of buried sutures. Askalonova, T. M. and Zakharov, A. P. Vestnik oftal. (no. 6) *14:*64–66, '39

Lexer operation in eyelid ptosis. Butler, R. D. W. Tr. Ophth. Soc. U. Kingdom (pt. 2), *59:*579–585, '39

Eyelid ptosis; cases. Ferreira, F. Rev. med. Bahia *8:*9–13, Jan '40

Blepharoptosis – Cont.

Fascia lata transplant in eyelid ptosis. Rosenburg, S. Am. J. Surg. *47:*142–148, Jan '40

Blepharoptosis; technic of surgical correction. Kirby, D. B. Surg., Gynec. and Obst. *70:*438–449, Feb (no. 2A) '40

Surgical management of eyelid ptosis. Fink, W. H. Journal-Lancet *60:*245–246, May '40

Paradoxic monocular ptosis. Yanes, T. R. Arch. Ophth. *23:*1169–1172, June '40

Eyelid ptosis operation. Glezerov, S. Vestnik oftal. *17:*132–134, '40

Surgical treatment of eyelid ptosis. Chang, S. K. Nat. M. J. China *27:*239, April '41

Eyelid ptosis operations. Sun, K. S. Nat. M. J. China *27:*245–246, April '41

Hess operation: new bandage substitute (eyelid ptosis). Pereira, R. F. Arch. de oftal. de Buenos Aires, *16:*241–242, May '41

Eyelid ptosis; insertions of levator palpebrae muscle. Hildreth, H. R. Am. J. Ophth. *24:*749–758, July '41

Ptosis; applied anatomy of eye; relation to ophthalmic surgery. Meek, R. E. Arch. Ophth. *26:*494–513, Sept '41

Surgical correction of eyelid ptosis. Malbran, J. Semana med. *2:*1456–1462, Dec 18, '41

Lexer operation for ptosis of eyelids. Armstrong, T. M. Tr. Ophth. Soc. Australia (1940) *2:*84–85, '41

Modified Blaskovics operation for ptosis of eyelids. Bull. Pract. Ophth. *12:*7–9, Jan '42

Resection of levator palpebrae muscle by conjunctival route; simplified technic. Agatston, S. A. Arch. Ophth. *27:*994–996, May '42

Modification of Dickey operation in eyelid ptosis. Gifford, S. R. and Putenney, I. Arch. Ophth. *28:*814–820, Nov '42

Surgical technic in congenital eyelid ptosis (modifications and additions to existing procedure of substituting frontal muscle). Bietti, G. Boll. d'ocul. *21:*721–727, Nov–Dec '42

Ptosis of eyelids; combined operation. Ellis, O. H. Tr. Pacific Coast Oto-Ophth. Soc. *27:*159–166, '42

Congenital blepharoptosis – classification; principles of surgical correction. Spaeth, E. B. Tr. Am. Acad. Ophth. (1942) *47:*285–301, March–April '43

Resection of left inferior oblique muscle at its scleral attachment for postoperative left hypotropia and left pseudoptosis. Berens, C. and Loutfallah, M. Am. J. Ophth. *26:*528–533, May '43

Blepharoptosis – Cont.

Ptosis of eyelids. SATHAYE, V. D. Indian J. Ophth. *4:*54–55, July '43

Combined operation for ptosis of eyelids. ELLIS, O. H. Am. J. Ophth. *26:*1048–1053, Oct '43

Congenital eyelid ptosis; simple useful corrective operation; case. ZENO, L. Bol. y trab., Acad. argent. de cir. *27:*930–935, Oct 6, '43 also: An. de chir. *10:*38–42, March–June '44

Dickey operation for eyelid ptosis; results in 21 patients and 30 lids. CORDES, F. C. AND FRITSCHI, U. Tr. A. Acad. Ophth. (1943) *48:*266–279, March–April '44 also: Arch. Ophth. *31:*461–468, June '44

Bilateral congenital ptosis of eyelids treated by Traynor operation. DURAN RODRIGUEZ, C. Vida nueva *53:*245–249, May '44

Bilateral ptosis and atypical slant eyes associated with unilateral syndactylia, adactylia and brachyphalangia. GIRI, D. V. Proc. Roy. Soc. Med. *37:*360–361, May '44

Congenital ectropion associated with bilateral ptosis – case. GORDON, S. AND CRAGG, B. H. Brit. J. Ophth. *28:*520–521, Oct '44

Operations for correction of ptosis of eyelids. ALVIS, B. Y. Tr. Indiana Acad. Ophth. and Otolaryng. *28:*97–115, '44

Resection of levator palpebrae in ptosis (eye), with anatomic studies. BERKE, R. N. Tr. Am. Ophth. Soc. *42:*411–435, '44 also: Arch. Ophth. *33:*269–280, April '45

Modified sling operation for correction of ptosis (eye). LAVAL, J. Arch. Ophth. *33:*482–483, June '45

Prosthetic device for support of eyelids. KOHOUT, J. J. Bull. U. S. Army M. Dept. *4:*117–118, July '45

Blepharospasm

Surgery of blepharospasm. SACHS, M. Wien. klin. Wchnschr. *38:*215, Feb 19, '25 abstr: J.A.M.A. *84:*1161, April 11, '25

Causes and treatment of eyelid spasms and tics. CANTONNET, A. AND VINCENT, C. Rev. gen. de clin. et de therap. *40:*787, Nov 20; 805, Nov 27, '26

Senile blepharospasm. MADAN, K. E. Brit. J. Ophth. *11:*385–386, Aug '27

Surgical treatment of intractable cases of eyelid spasm. GURDJIAN, E. S. AND WILLIAMS, H. W. J.A.M.A. *91:*2053–2056, Dec 29, '28

Peripheral neurectomy in blepharospasm. FRIEDE, R. Ztschr. f. Augenh. *72:*299–303, Oct '30

Surgical treatment of eyelid spasm. FRAZIER, C. H. Ann. Surg. *93:*1121–1125, June '31

Blepharospasm – Cont.

Encephalitic blepharospasm and its therapy. ZLATOVEROV, A. I. Nevropat. i. psikhiat. (nos. 1–2) *9:*160–163, '40

Treatment of eyelid spasm (blepharospasm). BENEDICT, W. L. Tr. Am. Ophth. Soc. *39:*227–241, '41

BLESSING, G. AND ROST, F.: Resection of lower jaw in acromegaly. Zentralbl. f. Chir. *52:*855–857, April 18, '25

BLOCH, J. C. AND BONNET, P.: Injuries of tendons of hand; surgical repair. J. de chir. *34:*456–474, Oct '29

BLOCH, J. C. AND TAILHEFER, A.: Plastic operations on tendon flexors of fingers; technic. Gaz. d. hop. *102:*5, Jan 2, '29

BLOCH, J. C. AND ZAGDOUN, J.: Therapy of digital wounds of flexor tendons; St. Bünnell operation using tendon graft; technic and results; 14 cases. J. de chir. *47:*376–391, March '36

BLOCH, J. J. AND BONNET, P.: Evolution and treatment of wounds of tendons of hand. Gaz. d. hop. *102:*1581, Nov 6, '29

BLOCK, F. B.: Artificial vagina. Am. J. M. Sc. *198:*567–576, Oct '39

BLOCK, L. S. AND HARRIS, E.: Approach to rational study and treatment of temporomandibular joint problems. J. Am. Dent. A. *29:*349–358, March '42

BLOCK, W.: Plastic surgery of face following injury due to strong current. Chirurg *9:*510–514, July 1, '37

BLOCKER, T. G. JR: Plastic construction of artificial vagina. Texas State J. Med. *37:*345–348, Sept '41

BLOCKER, T. G. JR.: Free full-thickness skin graft for relief of burn contracture of neck. South. Surgeon *10:*849–857, Dec '41

BLOCKER, T. G. JR. AND WEISS, L. R.: Maxillofacial injuries. J. Indiana M. A. *39:*60–63, Feb '46

BLOCKER, T. G. JR. AND WEISS, L. R.: Use of cancellous bone in repair of defects about jaws. Ann. Surg. *123:*622–638, April '46

BLOCKER, T. G. JR. AND WEISS, L. R.: Use of cancellous bone in repair of defects of jaw. Tr. South. S. A. (1945) *57:*153–169, '46

BLOKHIN, N. N.: Skin plastic procedures in war injuries. Am. Rev. Soviet. Med. *2:*104–107, Dec '44

BLOKHIN, V. N.: Therapy of nonhealing wounds, ulcers and contractures by transplantation of chemically treated tissues according to Krauze. Khirurgiya No. 6, pp. 3–10, '45

BLOND, K. Hypertrophy of mammary gland. Med. Klin. *17:*497, April 24, '21

Blond, K.: Experiences with decapitation finger cap. Zentralbl. f. Gynak. *50:*2907–2909, Nov 6, '26

Blondin-Walther, J. (see Thalheimer, M.) April '31

Bloodgood, J. C.: Method of operative attack for central lesions of lower jaw. New York State J. Med. *24:*379–385, March 21, '24

Bloodgood, J. C.: Moles, pigmented and nonpigmented, and other skin defects in precancerous stage. Northwest Med. *28:*543–547, Dec '29

Bloom, A. R.: Hereditary multiple ankylosing arthopathy (congenital stiffness of finger joints). Radiology *29:*166–171, Aug '37

Bloom, H.: "Cellophane" dressing for second degree burns. Lancet *2:*559, Nov 3, '45

Bloom, J. D.: Macrodactylism. New Orleans M. and S. J. *90:*29–30, July '37

Blotevogel, H.: Vitamin B_1 and dextrose in burns. Arch. f. orthop. u. Unfall-Chir. *40:*280–282, '39

Blount, W. P.: Late rupture of extensor pollicus longus tendon following Colles' fracture. Wisconsin M. J. *37:*912–916, Oct '38

Blum, G.: Experimental observations of use of absorbable and nonabsorbable plastics. Proc. Roy. Soc. Med. *38:*169–171, Feb '45

Blum, L.: Partial myotomy in treatment of divided flexor tendons in hand; 2 cases. Ann. Surg. *113:*460–463, March '41

Blum, L.: Use of myotomy in repair of divided flexor tendons. Ann. Surg. *116:*461–469, Sept '42

Blum, L.: Myotomy in repair of divided flexor tendons. U. S. Nav. M. Bull. *42:*1317–1322, June '44

Blum, L. L.: Hematogenic shock; recent advances in early recognition and treatment. Urol. and Cutan. Rev. *47:*401–409, July '43

Blum, V.: Plastic restoration of penis; case. J. Mt. Sinai Hosp. *4:*506–511, March–April '38

Blume, and Scholz: Simple method for raising corner of mouth in facial paralysis. Deutsche med. Wchnschr. *55:*272, Feb 15, '29

Blumenfeld, L.: Rhinocanalicular anastomosis with reconstruction of lacrimal sac. Arch. Ophth. *31:*248–249, March '44

Bobbio, A.: Craniofacial disjunction; case. Boll. e mem. Soc. piemontese di chir. *8:*515–520, '38

Bockenheimer: Treatment of ankylosis of jaw. Deutsche med. Wchnschr. *48:*729–730, June 2, '22

Bockenheimer, P.: Surgical treatment of furunculosis of axilla. Zentralbl. f. Chir. *48:*1317, Sept 10, '21

Bockstein, F.: New operative method in anterior nasal atresia. Ztschr. f. Hals-, Nasen-u. Ohrenh. *17:*180–187, Jan 31, '27

Bodart, M. (see Hamant, A.) Sept '28

Bodart (see Hamant, A. *et al*) Jan '33

Bodenham, D. C.: Penicillin; value for infected burns. Lancet *2:*725–728, Dec 11, '43

Bodenham, D. C.: Problem of fractures with associated burn injuries; principles of treatment. Proc. Roy. Soc. Med. *36:*657–662, Oct '43

Bodenham, D. C.: Restoration of function in burnt hand. Lancet *1:*298–300, March 6, '43

Bodenham, D. C.: Splint for control of ulnar deviation of fingers in rheumatoid arthritis. Lancet *2:*354–355, Sept 18, '43

Bodenheimer, M. and Goldman, M. L.: Case of genital aplasia; artificial vagina successfully constructed by Baldwin operation. J. Mt. Sinai Hosp. *7:*310–315, Jan–Feb '41

Bodian, D.: Repair of traumatic gaps in peripheral nerves. J.A.M.A. *121:*662–664, Feb 27, '43

Bodine, R. L.: Maxillofacial prosthesis. Internat. J. Orthodontia *14:*998, Nov; 1076, Dec '28; *15:*42, Jan; 163, Feb; 254, March; 371, April '29

Bodkin, L. G.: Rectal stricture (method for surgical relief). Am. J. Surg. *61:*277–279, Aug '43

Bøe, H. W.: Facial hemiatrophia progressiva treated with expansion prosthesis in mouth; case. Acta psychiat. et neurol. *9:*1–27, '34

Bøe, H. W.: Modern therapy of collum fractures of lower jaw. Med. rev., Bergen *55:*627–639, Dec '38

Bøe, H. W.: Progressive facial hemiatrophy treated by means of expansion prosthesis of oral cavity; case. Med. rev., Bergen *50:*212–225, May '33

Boecker, P.: New splint with surface for supporting injured fingers. Zentralbl. f. Chir. *64:*2134–2137, Sept 11, '37

Boecker, W.: Fascia implant to correct respiratory sinking in of nasal wings. Zentralbl. f. Chir. *48:*1796–1797, Dec 10, '21

Boehs, C. J.: Precaution against hemorrhage and infections following intranasal operations. Texas State J. Med. *32:*824–827, April '37

Boeminghaus, H.: Surgical treatment of epispadias of second degree. Chirurg *2:*11–14, Jan 1, '30

Bogart, D. W. (see Hughes, W. L. *et al*) Sept '41

Bogoljuboff, W. L.: Various uses of transplanted twisted skin in surgery. Arch. f. klin. Chir. *149:*412–414, '28

Bogomolets, O.: Why homotransplantation fails. Med. zhur. *5:*137–141, '35

Bogoraz, N.: Plastic construction of penis capable of accomplishing coitus; case. Zentralbl. f. Chir. *63:*1271–1276, May 30, '36

BOGORAZ, N. A.: Plastic restoration of penis. Sovet. khir., no. 8, pp. 303–309, '36

BOGORODIZKY, W. A.: Rhinoplasty over silver frame. Zentralbl. f. Chir. *52:*2830–2835, Dec 12, '25

Böhler Operation

Fractures of lower jaw; therapy by Böhler method. MONA, C. Policlinico (sez. prat.) *48:*659–666, April 14, '41

Böhler's Splint

Value of Böhler's wire-finger splint in treatment of severe injuries of fingers. FELSENREICH, F. Wien. klin. Wchnschr. *42:*1046–1048, Aug 8, '29

BÖHM, J.: Congenital cysts and fistulas of neck. Hals-, Nasen-u. Ohrenarzt (Teil 1) *30:*130–138, March '39

BÖHMER, L.: Therapy of keloids. Med. Welt *4:*1472–1474, Oct 11, '30

BÖHMIG, R.: Discussion of problem of bone transplantation on basis of histologic examination of Albee's transplant. Beitr. z. klin. Chir. *149:*663–676, '30

BOIDE AND RENAUD, MME. A.: Accidents due to heat; prevention and therapy in army. Rev. med. franc. *19:*387–400, May '38

BOIES, L. R.: Compound dislocation fracture of distal phalanx of finger; report of case. Minnesota Med. *10:*773–775, Dec '27

BOIES, L. R. *et al:* Osteogenic sarcoma of maxilla; case. J. Oral Surg. *4:*56–60, Jan '46; correction *4:*126, Apr '46

BOILER. W. F.: Nasal septum trephine. Laryngoscope *40:*438–439, June '40

BOISSERIE-LACROIX, J.: Congenital hemiatrophy of face with facial paralysis and microphthalmus; case. J. de med. de Bordeaux *113:*419–420, May 30, '36

BOISSON, R.: Clinical cases in stomatology (including fractures). Rev. de stomatol. *38:*625–662, Sept '36

BOIVIN, J. (see DUBECQ, X. J.) Jan '40

BOIX POU, M. (see Zorraquín, G.) Dec '31

BOIX POU, M. (see Zorraquín, G.) April '34

BÓKAY, J.: Cases of diphallus. Orvosi hetil. *73:*1138–1141, Nov 16, '29 also: Jahrb. f. Kinderh. *127:*127–136, April '30

BOLAÑOS, J. M. (see BANET, V.) April '33

BOLINTINEANU, G. AND BĂJEU, G.: Cystic lymphangioma of neck. Spitalul *52:*26–27, Jan '32

BOLK, L.: Lips and teeth and cyclopia and harelips. Ztschr. f. d. ges. Anat. (Abt. 1) *85:*762–783, May 21, '28

BOLLA, I. (see ARENAS, N.) April '40

BOLMAN, R. M.: Bilateral branchial cleft cysts. Am. J. Surg. *71:*96–99, Jan '46

BOLOT, F. AND DAUSSET: Shock; resuscitation in surgery. Afrique franc. chir. *2:*39–43, Jan–March '44

BOLOTOW, N. A.: Surgical treatment of nasal obstruction; indications for plastic approach to septal deformity; details of plastic procedures. Arch. Otolaryng. *40:*198–202, Sept '44

BOLTE, R.: Use of first metacarpus in plastic restoration of thumb; case. J. de l'Hotel-Dieu de Montreal *7:*359–365, Nov–Dec '38

BOM, G. S.: Comparative evaluation of bone autotransplants and heterotransplants in correction of bone defects. Ortop. i travmatol. (no. 4) *10:*107–113, '36

BOMBELLI, U.: Surgical diathermy in cicatricial stenosis of larynx. Oto-rhino-laryng. internat. *22:*16–24, Jan '38

BONÀ, T.: Cancer of lips. Cluj. med. *10:*652–656, Dec 1, '29

BONÀ, T. Reconstruction of extensive urethral defects by transplantation of pedicled flap. Rev. de chir., Bucuresti *41:*347–352, May–June '38

BONÀ, T.: Traumatic wounds of tendons. Cluj. med. *10:*435–439, Sept 1, '29

BONABA, J. AND BAUZÁ, J. A.: Acrocephalosyndactylia; case. Rev. de med., Rosario *3:*419–424, Dec '28

BONACCORSI, A.: Experiments with skin grafts in plastic surgery of tendons. Clin. chir. *36:*839–853, July–Aug '33

BONAFOS, (see LAFFONT,) Nov '34

BONAMOUR, (see BONNET, P. *et al*) March '34

BONAR, B. E. AND OWENS, R. W.: Bilateral congenital facial paralysis; review of literature and classification. Am. J. Dis. Child. *38:*1256–1272, Dec '29

BOND, B. J.: Small type skeletal traction apparatus (fingers). U. S. Nav. M. Bull. *46:*124–126, Jan '46

BOND, D. D. AND WRIGHT, D. G.: Treatment of hemorrhage and traumatic shock by intravenous use of lyophile serum. Ann. Surg. *107:*500–510, April '38

BONDURANT, C. P.: Epithelioma of lip and face. J. Oklahoma M. A. *20:*252–256, Sept '27

BONDY, G.: Plastic surgery of ear. Monatschr. f. Ohrenh. *62:*1227, Oct '28

Bone

Atrophy of bone (Sudeck) following burns. DUBS, J. Munchen. med. Wchnschr. *68:*1141, Sept 9, '21

Bone—Cont.
Skin grafting upon dry bone. BABCOCK, W. W., S. Clin. N. Amer. *8:*773–775, Aug '28
Comparative evaluation of bone autotransplants and heterotransplants in correction of bone defects. BOM, G. S. Ortop. i travmatol. (no. 4) *10:*107–113, '36
Bone drilling in resistant chronic ulcers; new principle. ALBEE, F. H. Am. J. Surg. *54:*605–608, Dec '41
Use of skin flaps in repair of scarred defects over bone and tendons. PADGETT, E. C. AND GASKINS, J. H. Surgery *18:*287–298, Sept '45
Acrylic resin (methyl methacrylate) for closure of defects; preliminary report. SMALL, J. M. AND GRAHAM, M. P. Brit. J. Surg. *33:*106–113, Oct '45
Early nerve and bone repair in war wounds. SCHWARTZ, H. G. AND PARKER, J. M., J. Neurosurg. *2:*510–515, Nov '45
Deep burns involving bones. McDOWELL, F. J. Indiana M.A. *39:*108–109, Mar '46
Use of pedicled flaps in surgical treatment of chronic osteomyelitis resulting from compound fractures. STARK, W. J., J. Bone and Joint Surg. *28:*343–350, April '46
Fixation of tendons, ligaments and bone by Bunnell's pull-out wire suture. KEY, J. A. Tr. South. S. A. (1945) *57:*187–194, '46

Bone Derivatives, Grafting

Study of experimental transplantation of bone, with special reference to effect of "decalcification." GHORMLEY, R. K. AND STUCK, W. G. Proc. Staff Meet. Mayo Clin. *8:*253–254, April 26, '33
Experimental bone transplantation, with special reference to effect of "decalcification." GHORMLEY, R. K. AND STUCK, W. G. Arch. Surg. *28:*742–770, April '34
Interposition of os purum in osteosynthesis after osteotomy, resections of bones and joints, etc. (interposition-osteosynthesis). ORELL, S. Surg., Gynec. and Obst. *59:*638–643, Oct '34
Bone implantation and new growth; implantation of "os purum" and transplantation of "os novum." ORELL, S. Acta chir. Scandinav. (supp. 31) *74:*1–274, '34
Graft of osseous tissue using bouillon and paste of living bone. BAILLEUL, AND REGNER. Bull. et mem. Soc. d. chirurgiens de Paris *27:*414–418, July 5, '35
Surgical implantation of pure bone, new bone and boiled bone. ORELL, S. Mem. Acad. de chir. *61:*1376–1378, Dec 21, '35
Flexible bone transplants. VON ERTL, J. Zentralbl. f. Chir. *64:*362–371, Feb 6, '37

Bone Derivatives, Grafting—Cont.
Surgical grafting with "os purum," "os novum" and "boiled bone." ORELL, S. J. Bone and Joint Surg. *19:*873–885, Oct '37 also: J. de chir. *49:*857–870, June '37
Use of os purum in implantations (bone). ORELL, S. Surg., Gynec. and Obst. *66:*23–36, Jan '38
Os purum as biologic element of internal prosthesis. DE ROMANA, J. Dia med. (Ed. espec.), no. 2, pp. 19–20, April '39
Ability of bone tissue (including "os novum") to survive in pedicled grafts. HELLSTADIUS, A. Acta chir. Scandinav. *86:*85–109, '42

Bone Formation by Grafts of Bladder Mucosa

Possibility of repairing loss of bony substance of cranium by means of graft of bladder mucosa. BEZZA, P. Arch. ital. di chir. *55:*405–429, '39

Bone Grafts

Auto-bone implants. GOUVÉA, J. Brazil-med. *35:*61, Jan 29, '21
Study of series of bone graft cases operated in U. S. Army Hospitals. WALKER, J. B. Ann. Surg. *73:*1, Jan '21
Bone implants. CHRISTOPHE, L. Presse med. *29:*204, March 12, '21
Bone-periosteum transplants. DELAGÉNIÈRE, H., J. de chir. *17:*305, April '21 abstr: J.A.M.A. *76:*1372, May 14, '21
Present status of bone transplantation. DURAND, M. Lyon med. *130:*473, June 10, '21
Autogenous bone transplantation. HENDERSON, M. S., J.A.M.A. *77:*165, July 16, '21
Certain fundamental laws underlying surgical use of bone graft. ALBEE, F. H. Ann. Surg. *74:*196, Aug '21
Reconstruction, bone implants for reconstruction of jaw. CAVINA, C. Chir. d. org. di movimento *5:*417, Aug '21 abstr: J.A.M.A. *77:*1374, Oct 22, '21
Grafts of long bones and joints. FIESCHI, D. Chir. d. org. di movimento *5:*359, Aug '21 abstr: J.A.M.A. *77:*1373, Oct 22, '21
Repair of loss of bone substance and reconstruction of bones by osteo-periosteal grafts taken from tibia, (with 118 new personal cases). DELAGÉNIÈRE, H. Am. J. Surg. *35:*281, Sept '21
Function in relation to transplantation of bone. HAAS, S. L. Arch. Surg. *3:*425, Sept '21
Values of various methods of bone graftings judged by 1,390 reported cases. McWILLIAMS, C. A. Ann. Surg. *74:*286, Sept '21

Bone Grafts—Cont.

Surgiology and survival of bone grafts. REGARD, G. L. Paris med. *11:*292, Oct 8, '21 abstr: J.A.M.A. *77:*1847, Dec 3, '21

Biology of bone development in its relation to bone transplantation. NATHAN, P. W. New York M. J. *114:*454, Oct 19, '21

Study of some methods of bone-grafting. FORRESTER-BROWN, M. F. Brit. J. Surg. *9:*179, Oct '21

Bone graft. MAMOURIAN, M. Brit. M. J. *2:*934, Dec 3, '21

Autogenous bone inlay; its indications and advantages. HANNETT, J. W. Southwestern Med. *5:*1, Dec '21

Bone grafting and its clinical application. KURLANDER, J. J. Ohio State M. J. *17:*816, Dec '21

"Dovetail" bone graft. MOREAU, J. Arch. franco-belges de chir. *25:*256-267, Dec '21 (illus.) abstr: J.A.M.A. *78:*618, Feb 25, '22

Fate of bone graft. JONAS, A. F. Wisconsin M. J. *20:*407-410, Jan '22

Bone grafts. POATE, H. R. G., M. J. Australia *1:*209-215, Feb 25, '22 (illus.)

Spontaneous healing inherent in transplanted bone. HAAS, S. L., J. Bone and Joint Surg. *4:*209-214, April '22 (illus.)

Some observations on bone-grafting; with special reference to bridge-grafts. PAGE, C. M. AND PERKINS, G. Brit. J. Surg. *9:*540-552, April '22 (illus.)

Results of osteoperiosteal bone grafts. DELAGÉNIÈRE, H. Arch. franco-belges de chir. *25:*673-718, May '22 (illus.)

"Bipp" method of treatment of bone cavities and bone grafts. MORISON, R. Surg., Gynec. and Obst. *34:*642-666, May '22 (illus.)

Notes on use of bone graft with illustrated cases. WELCHMAN, W. M., J. South Africa *17:*224-228, June '22

Experimental growth of bone and cartilage. POLETTINI, B. Arch. ital. di chir. *6:*179-191, Nov '22 (illus.) abstr: J.A.M.A. *80:*360, Feb 3, '23

Osteoperiosteal bone grafts. DELAGÉNIÈRE, H. Bull. Acad. de med., Par. *88:*396-416, Dec 5, '22 abstr: J.A.M.A. *80:*434, Feb 10, '23

Grafts of bone tissue. SIMON, R. Rev. de chir. *60:*207-286, '22 (illus.) abstr: J.A.M.A. *79:*1276, Oct 7; 2122, Dec 16, '22

Bone grafting. ADAMS, W. R. Surg., Gynec. and Obst. *36:*97-98, Jan '23 (illus.)

Association of surgeon and radiologist in bone grafting. BUXTON, ST. J. D. Arch. Radiol. and Electroth. *27:*289-304, March '23 (illus.)

Bone Grafts—Cont.

Bone grafts. MONACO, U. Policlinico (sez. chir.) *30:*203-220, April '23 abstr: J.A.M.A. *81:*341, July 28, '23

Principles of bone graft surgery. MORISON, A. E. Tr. Medico-Chir. Soc., Edinburgh, pp. 65-80, '22-'23; in Edinburgh M. J., April '23

Principles for bone transplanting. ALBEE, F. H. Nederlandsch Tijdschr. v. Geneesk. *1:*2230-2233, May 26, '23

Bone implants in treatment of Pott's disease (Albee method). GONZALEZ LIZCANO, J. Siglo med. *71:*624-629, June 30, '23; *72:*652-656, July 7; 680-682, July 14; 701-705, July 21; 726-729, July 28; 752-754, Aug 4, '23

Fractures in transplanted bone. HAAS, S. L. Surg., Gynec. and Obst. *36:*749-762, June '23 (illus.)

Ideal bone graft as determined by experimental investigations. HAAS, S. L. S. Clin. N. America *3:*761-763, June '23

Evolution of bone implants. SATTA, F. Chir. d. org. di movimento *7:*345-366, June '23 (illus.)

Nonunion in fractures; massive bone graft. HENDERSON, M. S. J.A.M.A. *81:*463-468, Aug 11, '23 (illus.)

Bone grafting. TROELL, A. Acta chir. Scandinav. *56:*59-72, '23 (illus., in English) abstr: J.A.M.A. *81:*1062, Sept 22, '23

Bone grafts. IMBERT, L. Bull. Acad. de med., Par. *90:*174-182, Oct 16, '23 abstr: J.A.M.A. *82:*163, Jan 12, '24 also: Bull. Acad. de med., Par. *91:*371-375, March 18, '24

Fundamentals in bone transplantation, experiences in 3,000 bone graft operations. ALBEE, F. H. J.A.M.A. *81:*1429-1432, Oct 27, '23

Fate of bone transplants. LEXER, E. Acta chir. Scandinav. *56:*164-180, '23 (illus., in German)

Greffes et Transplants Osseux chez l'Homme, by A. D. RADULESCO. Romaneasca, Bucharest, 1924

Bone transplants and failure to heal. LEXER, E. Zentralbl. f. Chir. *51:*258-259, Feb 16, '24

Importance of periosteum and endosteum in repair of transplanted bone. HAAS, S. L. Arch. Surg. *8:*535-556, March '24

Remote result of a periosteal bone implant. CAPRIOLI, N. Pediatria *32:*418-421, April 1, '24

Treatment of ununited fractures and other bone defects by bone grafts and bone comminution. STEVENSON, G. H. Glasgow M. J. *101:*274-286, May '24

Bone Grafts—Cont.

Experiments on transplants of fresh and preserved bone. TRAVERSA GAUDIOSO, E. Policlinico (sez. prat.) *31:*735-740, June 9, '24 abstr: J.A.M.A. *83:*227, July 19, '24

End results of 158 consecutive autogenous bone grafts for non-union in long bone (A) in simple fractures; (B) in atrophic bone following war wounds and chronic suppurative osteitis (osteomyelitis). KIRK, N. T. J. Bone and Joint Surg. *6:*760-799, Oct '24

Fragment method in bone grafts. IMBERT, L. Bull. Acad. de med., Par. *92:*1285-1290, Dec 2, '24

Bone graft; reconstructive surgery. ALBEE, F. H. Internat. clinics *2:*225-236, June '25

Autoplastic bone transplantation from viewpoint of biology and architectonic. HOFFMANN, V. Arch. f. klin. Chir. *135:*413-485, '25

Transplants of living bones. LAZZARINI, L. Arch. ital. di chir. *11:*109-138, '25 abstr: J.A.M.A. *85:*155, July 11, '25

Fate of bone transplants. WERESCHINSKI, A. Arch. f. klin. Chir. *136:*545-567, '25

Research on bone graft; heterotopic autografts. IMBERT, L. Bull. Acad. de med., Paris *95:*538-542, May 25, '26

Experimental research on bone grafting. IMBERT, L., J. de chir. *27:*710-724, June '26

Importance of spongiosa in bone transplantation. BÁRON, A. Zentralbl. f. Chir. *53:*2332-2341, Sept 11, '26

Biologic processes in bone transplantation. DOLJANSKY, J. Zentralbl. f. Chir. *53:*2523-2526, Oct 2, '26

Vascularization of autoplastic bone implants. BERTINI, G. Arch. ital. di chir. *16:*105-121, '26

Autoplastic bone transplants in man. SERAFINI, G. AND ANTONIOLI, G. M. Arch. ital. di chir. *16:*273-293, '26

Bone transplantation. SCHWARTZ, A. Bull. et mem. Soc. nat. de chir. *53:*767-775, June 4, '27

Bone transplantation. GREEF, J. H. H. J.M.A.S. Africa *1:*474-475, Sept 24, '27

Transplantation and growth of bones. KORNEFF, P. Vestnik khir. (no. 34) *12:*10-61, '27

Action of periosteum and connective tissue of host in grafts of bone without periosteum. LAZZARINI, L. Arch. di ortop. *43:*65-72, '27

Grafts and bony implants for repairing large deficiencies in epiphysis and diaphysis; concealed internal prosthesis. MAUCLAIRE. Bull. et mem. Soc. nat. de chir. *53:*1363-1373, Dec 17, '27

Bone Grafts—Cont.

Formation of radius congenitally absent; condition 7 years after implantation of bone graft. ALBEE, F. H. Ann. Surg. *87:*105-110, Jan '28

Comparison of various forms of bone transplantation. LAZZARINI, L. Gazz. d. osp. *49:*97-100, Jan 29, '28

Bone transplantation. RANKIN, J. O., W. Virginia M. J. *24:*18-24, Jan '28

Experimental researches on autotransplantation of bones. DE JOSSELIN DE JONG, R. AND EYKMAN VAN DER KEMP, P. H. Beitr. z. path. Anat. u. z. allg. Path. *79:*268-332, Feb 15, '28

Bone transplantation. STEIN, G. Ztschr. f. Stomatol. *26:*284-309, March '28

Role of periosteum in bone grafts. TRÈVES, A. Arch. franco-belges de chir. *31:*213-219, March '28

Use of cortical inlay bone-graft in non-union; importance and technic by avoiding encircling bone sutures; clinical and experimental study. McWHORTER, G. L., S. Clin. N. Amer. *8:*555-560, June '28

Role of periosteum in osseous grafts. TRÈVES, A. Bull. et mem. Soc. de chir. de Paris *20:*550, June 15, '28

Bone grafting into infected field. BLANC FORTACÍN, J. Siglo med. *82:*117-120, Aug 11, '28

Sixteen years maintenance of autoplastic bone graft; case. ANNOVAZZI, G. Clin. chir. *31:*1051-1081, Oct '28

Necessity for transplantation of living bone and cartilage; cases. PINEDA, J. C. Rev. de med. y cir. de la Habana *33:*862, Dec 31, '28

Utilization of autoplastic bone grafts in orthopedic and plastic surgery. RIGNEY, P. Southwestern Med. *12:*564-565, Dec '28

Data on autoplastic bone grafting and cartilage. GORBOUNOFF, V. P. Vestnik khir. (nos. 37-38) *13:*71-85, '28

Bone autoplasty; 3 cases. POGGI, J. Folha med. *10:*13-17, Jan 15, '29

Viability of bone grafts; experimental study. POLLOCK, W. E. *et al.* Arch. Surg. *18:*607-623, Feb '29

Anatomical survival, growth and physiological function of epiphyseal bone transplant. STRAUB, G. F. Surg., Gynec. and Obst. *48:*687-690, May '29

Osteotomy and transplantation of substantia spongiosa. MATTI, H. Schweiz. med. Wchnschr. *59:*1254-1258, Dec 7, '29

Appearance of bone autotransplant of 2 month's duration; case. KALIMA, T. Acta chir. Scandinav. *65:*196-208, '29

Bone Grafts – Cont.
Growth of bone transplants; experimental study. KORNEW, P. G. Arch. f. klin. Chir. *154:*499-564, '29
Autogenous bone graft. HILL, H. G. Memphis M. J. *7:*21-25, Feb '30
Late results of bone grafts; microscopic study. IMBERT, L. Ann. d'anat. path. *7:*291-315, March '30
Various uses of bone transplants. ALBEE, F. H. Proc. Roy. Soc. Med. (Sect. Orthop.) *23:*31-36, April '30
Hinged bone-graft. HENRY, A. K. Brit. M. J. *1:*737-738, April 19, '30
Histologic examination of bone transplant after 15 years. MATWEJEW, D. N. Monatschr. f. Ohrenh. *64:*417-422, April '30
Experimental transplantation of cartilage fixed in bone. BLAVET DI BRIGA, C. Arch. ital. de biol. *83:*26-33, July 30, '30
Osteoperiosteal bone grafts. DORRANCE, G. M. Ann. Surg. *92:*161-168, Aug '30
Discussion of problem of bone transplantation on basis of histologic examination of Albee's transplant. BÖHMIG, R. Beitr. z. klin. Chir. *149:*663-676, '30
Sequels and role of bone transplants. KARTASHEFF, Z. I. Vestnik khir. (nos. 58-60) *20:*282-296, '30
Free autoplastic bone transplantation; especially of small bone fragments. KARTASCHEW, S. I. Arch. f. klin. Chir. *156:*758-805, '30
Fate of cortical bone graft. DAVISON, C. AND KRAFT, A. Arch. Surg. *22:*94-97, Jan '31
Bone transplantation. GALLIE, W. E. Brit. M. J. *2:*840-844, Nov 7, '31
Free transplantation of substantia spongiosa (bone). MATTI, H. Arch. f. klin. Chir. *168:*236-258, '31
Experimental studies and application of bone transplantation in practical surgery; preliminary report. ORELL, S. Deutsche Ztschr. f. Chir. *232:*701-713, '31
Late results of cranioplasty by hinging method of bone grafts. MAYET. Bull. et mem. Soc. d. chirurgiens de Paris *24:*138-140, Feb 19, '32
Fundamental principles of bone transplantation. HART, V. L. J. Michigan M. Soc. *31:*184-187, March '32
Massive bone grafts; cases. MILLER, O. L. South M. J. *25:*211-218, March '32
Use of periosteal flap with skin graft in radical mastoid surgery. ZIEGELMAN, E. F. Laryngoscope *42:*170-176, March '32
Vascularization of long bones by autotransplantation. RUBASCHEWA, A. AND PRIWES, M. G. Beitr. z. klin. Chir. *156:*299-312, '32

Bone Grafts – Cont.
Effect of periarterial sympathectomy on autoplastic grafts (including bone); experimental study. SANTI, E. Arch. ital. di chir. *31:*209-227, '32
Operation to make posterior bone block at ankle to limit foot-drop. GILL, A. B. J. Bone and Joint Surg. *15:*166-170, Jan '33
Alternating life of tissues; importance in bone transplantation. IMBERT, R. Paris med. *1:*267-270, March 25, '33
Results of 11 cases of bone grafts. LE FUR, R. Bull. et mem. Soc. d. chirurgiens de Paris *25:*187-192, March 17, '33
Influence of periosteum on survival of bone grafts. HALDEMAN, K. O. J. Bone and Joint Surg. *15:*302-319, April '33
Massive graft in repair of defects in long bones. COMPERE, E. L. S. Clin. North America *13:*1261-1273, Oct '33
New methods of free bone autotransplantation. KRASIN, P. M. AND OSIPOVSKIY, V. M. Novy khir. arkhiv *28:*231-235, '33
Twenty-five year old bone transplant. PETROW, N. Arch. f. klin. Chir. *175:*176-180, '33
Practical significance and uses of bone grafts. VON MATOLCSY, T. Arch. f. klin. Chir. *176:* 319-334, '33
Reparation of bone loss by Ollier osteoperiostic grafts, segmentary bone grafts, bone implantations and hidden internal prostheses. MAUCLAIRE. Rev. med. franc. *15:*263-273, March '34
Dovetail joint simplified for bone graft purposes. WATKINS, A. B. K. M. J. Australia *1:*430-431, March 31, '34
Small bone grafts. KEITH, W. S. J. Bone and Joint Surg. *16:*314-330, April '34
Behavior of transplanted bone; clinical consideration. HARBIN, M. AND LIBER, K. E. Surg., Gynec. and Obst. *59:*149-160, Aug '34
Role of bone marrow and endosteum in regeneration; experimental study of bone marrow and endosteal transplants. McGAW, W. H. AND HARBIN, M. J. Bone and Joint Surg. *16:*816-821, Oct '34
Experimental bone regeneration using lime salts and autogenous grafts as source of available calcium. STEWART, W. J. Surg., Gynec. and Obst. *59:*867-871, Dec '34
Bone transplantation. ORELL, S. Acta chir. Scandinav. *74:*424-425, '34
Formation of new bone in transplantation. LEVANDER, G. Acta chir. Scandinav. *74:*425-426, '34
Nature of bone transplants. CAMITZ, H. *et al.* Acta chir. Scandinav. *75:*1-67, '34

Bone Grafts—Cont.
Present status of bone transplantation. KNOBLOCH, J. Rozhl. v chir. a gynaek. (cast chir.) *13:*191-199, '34
Vascularization of entire reimplanted radii in dog; relation to regeneration of bone and marrow, to growth and to joint cartilage. MAY, H. Beitr. z. klin. Chir. *160:*30-74, '34
Clinical evolution of bone grafts. INCLAN, A. Cir. ortop. y traumatol. *3:*161-173, July-Sept '35
Immediate transplantation of bone, cartilage and soft tissues in accident cases. CARTER, W. W. Laryngoscope *45:*730-738, Sept '35
Bone transplantation. MACAULEY, H. F. Irish J. M. Sc., pp. 669-675, Dec '35
Free transplantation of bone. EPSTEIN, I. Bucuresti med. *7:*138-146, '35
Massive onlay bone grafts. (arm fractures). WEST, W. K., J. Oklahoma M. A. *29:*39-45, Feb '36
Fate of transplanted cow's horn in treatment of bone fractures. SIEGLING, J. A. AND FAHEY, J. J., J. Bone and Joint Surg. *18:*439-444, April '36
Massive bone graft in fracture. HENDERSON, M. S., J.A.M.A. *107:*1104-1107, Oct 3, '36
Comparative evaluation of bone autotransplants and heterotransplants in correction of bone defects. BOM, G. S. Ortop. i travmatol. (no. 4) *10:*107-113, '36
Fate of bone transplanted into soft tissue; experimental study. POKOTILO, V. L. AND KOZDOBA, A. Z. Sovet. khir., no. 1, pp. 73-82, '36
Fate of bone explants grafted into soft tissue; experimental studies. POKOTILO, W. L. AND KOZDOBA, A. Z. Mitt. a. d. Grenzgeb. d. Med. u. Chir. *44:*390-400, '36
Regeneration of bone transplants. MAY, H. Ann. Surg. *106:*441-453, Sept '37
Results of autoplastic transplantation of spongy bone; experimental studies. BAHLS, G. AND KALAMBOKAS, A. Beitr. z. klin. Chir. *166:*647-655, '37
Fate of osseous tissue in autoplastic transplantation. BAHLS, G. Beitr. z. klin. Chir. *166:*535-583, '37
Transformation of osseous tissue used for filling bone defects. NIKITIN, A. A. Ortop. i travmatol. (no. 6) *11:*64-65, '37
Method of grafting long bones. STAMM, T. T. Proc. Roy. Soc. Med. *31:*461-464, March '38
Use of hyoid bone as graft in laryngeal stenosis. LOOPER, E. A. Arch. Otolaryng. *28:*106-111, July '38
Regenerative-reconstructive operations and

Bone Grafts—Cont.
late results of bone and tissue transplantations. ERTL, J. Budapesti orvosi ujsag *36:*949-953, Nov 3, '38
Orell method of bone transplantation; cases. RISINGER, W. Acta orthop. Scandinav. *9:*152-180, '38
Bone transplantation. MASMONTEIL, F. Bull. et mem. Soc. de med. de Paris *143:*376-379, June 9, '39
Autogenous bone graft. CAMPBELL, W. C. J. Bone and Joint Surg. *21:*694-700, July '39
Action on general ossification with bone transplantation. ENSELME, J. AND TRINTIGNAC, P. Lyon chir. *36:*434-436, July-Aug '39
Behavior of bone transplants; clinical and anatomicopathologic study. FRANCESCHELLI, N. Arch. di orthop. *55:*297-320, Sept 30, '39
Bone Graft Surgery in Disease, Injury, and Deformity, by FRED H. ALBEE AND ALEXANDER KUSHNER. Appleton-Century Co., New York, 1940
New technic of bone transplantation. CHESTER, J. B. Surg., Gynec. and Obst. *70:*819-825, April '40
Evaluation of Wolff's law of bone formation as related to transplantation. KUSHNER, A., J. Bone and Joint Surg. *22:*589-596, July '40
Value of periosteum in grafting operation. POLLOCK, G. A. AND HENDERSON, M. S. Proc. Staff Meet., Mayo Clin. *15:*443-448, July 10, '40
Experimental studies on influences of previous fractures on behavior of transplants of bone. YUHARA, K. Tr. Soc. path. jap. *30:*738-741, '40
Surgical bone transplantation; review. ORELL, S. Zentralbl. f. Chir. *68:*1398-1403, July 26, '41
Sources of regeneration of transplanted bone; experimental study. NOVACHENKO, N. P. Ortop. i travmatol. (no. 1) *15:*5-13, '41
Formation of blood cells in devitalized bone transplants. RÖHLICH, K. Ztschr. f. mikr.-anat. Forsch. *49:*616-625, '41
Bone tissue as filling material in loss of substances. ORTIZ TIRADO, A. Cir. y cirujanos *10:*65-70, Feb 28, '42
Choice of graft methods in bone and joint surgery. GHORMLEY, R. K. Ann. Surg. *115:*427-434, March '42
Bone transplantation with report of cases. ZENO, L. An. de cir. *8:*216-232, Sept '42
Internal prosthesis with autotransplant of

Bone Grafts—Cont.

bone or cartilage. JORGE, J. M. AND MEALLA, E. S. Arq. de cir. clin. e exper. *6:*539-540, April-June '42

Effect of sulfanilamide crystals, used topically, on fate of transplanted bone; experimental and clinical observations. HORWITZ, T. Surgery *11:*690-697, May '42

Regeneration of joint transplants and intracapsular fragments. MAY, H. Ann. Surg. *116:*297-310, Aug '42

Application of Wolff's law to bone transplants. PUYO VILLAFANE, E. Semana med. *2:*840-843, Oct 8, '42

Transplantation of skin together with implanted bone to cover defects of soft tissues and bones. KLEINSCHMIDT, O. Chirurg *14:*737-742, Dec 15, '42

Use of cancellous bone grafts in orthopedic surgery. ABBOTT, L. C. AND GILL, G. G. Brunn, Med.-Surg. Tributes, pp. 1-11, '42

Small bone grafts of extremities. MURRAY, G. Canad. M. A. J. *48:*137-139, Feb '43

Treatment of bone cavities (including use of molds for grafts). QUICK, B. Australian and New Zealand J. Surg. *13:*3-10, July '43

Recovery of function with autoplastic bone graft and tubular skin flaps. JENTZER, A. Schweiz. med. Wchnschr. *73:*1023, Aug 21, '43

Repair of fractures by bone transplantation. PHEMISTER, D. B. Proc. Interst. Postgrad. M. A. North America (1942) pp. 105-108, '43

Use of delayed bone grafts in ununited fractures. DONOHUE, E. S. J. Iowa M. Soc. *35:*8-10, Jan '45

Surgical obliteration of cavities following traumatic osteomyelitis (by bone and skin transplantation). KNIGHT, M. P. AND WOOD, G. O. J. Bone and Joint Surg. *27:*547-556, Oct '45

Molded bone graft. BARSKY, A. J. Surgery *18:*755-763, Dec '45

Traumatic osteomyelitis; use of grafts; subsequent treatment. KELLY, R. P. *et al.* Ann. Surg. *123:*688-697, April '46

Use of penicillin therapy in conjunction with free bone grafting in infected areas. ABBOTT, L. C. AND OTHERS. Surg. Gynec. and Obst. *83:*101-106, July '46

Cancellous grafts for infected bone defects; single stage procedure. COLEMAN, H. M.; *et al.* Surg. Gynec. and Obst. *83:*392-398, Sept '46

Traumatic osteomyelitis; use of grafts; subsequent treatment. KELLY, R. P.; *et al.* Tr. South. S. A. (1945) *57:*219-228, '46

Bone Grafts, Pedicled

Pedunculated bone grafts. GAZZOTTI, L. G. Policlinico (sez. chir.) *28:*548-555, Dec '21 (illus.) abstr: J.A.M.A. *78:*691, March 4, '22

Indications and advantages of pedunculated bone grafts. CURTILLET, J. AND TILLIER, R. Lyon chir. *22:*789-804, Nov-Dec '25 abstr: J.A.M.A. *86:*1487, May 8, '26

Repair of skull defects by new pedicle bone-graft operation. JONES, R. W. Brit. M. J. *1:*780-781, May 6, '33

Late results of pedicle bone-graft for fractured mandible; 3 cases. COLE, P. Proc. Roy. Soc. Med. *31:*1131-1134, July '38

Pathologic fracture of mandible; nonunion treated with pedicled bone graft. COLE, P. P. Lancet *1:*1044-1045, June 8, '40

Ability of bone tissue (including "os novum") to survive in pedicled grafts. HELLSTADIUS, A. Acta chir. Scandinav. *86:*85-109, '42

Bone Grafts, Preserved

Disadvantages of dead bone implants in pseudoarthrosis or fracture of femur. GIRODE, C. Rev. de chir. *60:*60-80, '22 (illus.) abstr: J.A.M.A. *79:*507, Aug 5, '22

Grafts of bones kept in alcohol and bone regeneration. CHRISTOPHE, L. Arch. franco-belges de chir. *26:*13-56, Jan '23 (illus.) abstr: J.A.M.A. *80:*1180, April 21, '23

Bone transplantation with devitalized grafts. IMBERT, L. Bull. Acad. de med., Par. *93:*204-214, Feb 24, '25 abstr: J.A.M.A. *84:*1240, April 18, '25

Bone graft with dead bone. TAVERNIER. Lyon chir. *27:*233-236, March-April '30

Dead bone grafts to repair skull defects. PANKRATIEV, B. E. Ann. Surg. *97:*321-326, March '33

Formation of new bone substance in devitalized bone transplants. RÖHLICH, K. Ztschr. f. mikr. -anat. Forsch. *50:*132-145, '41

Use of preserved bone graft in orthopedic surgery. INCLAN, A. J. Bone and Joint Surg. *24:*81-96, Jan '42

Bone Grafts to Face

Preoperative and postoperative prosthesis in application of skin, cutaneomucosal, cartilage and bone grafts and in improvement of cicatrix of face. DARCISSAC, M. Bull. et mem. Soc. d. chirurgiens de Paris *28:*424-433, June 19, '36

Skin, cartilage and bone grafts to face. NEW, G. B. Proc. Staff Meet., Mayo Clin. *11:*791-794, Dec 9, '36

Use of iliac bone in facial and cranial repair.

Bone Grafts to Face—Cont.

SHEEHAN, J. E. Am. J. Surg. *52:*55-61, April '41

Palatine fistula, plastic closure by means of turbinate bone. DE MARTINI, R. Boll. d. mal. d. orecchio, d. gola, d. naso *59:*172-177, May '41

Bone grafts in pseudarthrosis and loss of substance of upper jaw. GINESTET AND CHEMIN. Rev. de stomatol. *47:*137-139, May-June '46

Bone Grafts to Hand

Transplantation of bone in hand. MICHON, L. J. de chir. *20:*260-273, Sept '22 (illus.) abstr: J.A.M.A. *79:*1884, Nov 25, '22

Case showing anatomical and functional reproduction of metacarpal by bone-graft. FOWLER, A. Brit. J. Surg. *14:*675-676, April '27

Restoration of thumb from carpal bone. SHIPOV, A. K. Sovet. khir., no. 8, p. 163, '35

Reconstruction of left thumb by skin and osteoperiosteal grafts; case. DESPLAS, B. Mem. Acad. de chir. *62:*1292-1296, Nov 25, '36

Restoration of thumb by transposition of second metacarpal; indications and technic; 2 cases. ISELIN, M. AND MURAT, J. Presse med. *45:*1099-1102, July 28, '37

Restoration of thumb using bone and skin grafts. HUARD, P. AND LONG, M. Bull. Soc. med. -chir. de l'Indochine *15:*855-860, Aug-Sept '37

Use of first metacarpus in plastic restoration of thumb; case. BOLTE, R. J. de l'Hotel-Dieu de Montreal *7:*359-365, Nov-Dec '38

Phalangization of first metacarpal bone in plastic restoration of thumb; anatomic basis of author's method. SHIROKOV, B. A. Khirurgiya, no. 7, pp. 115-122, '39

Finger tip reconstruction; new operation (using bone and skin grafts). LAUTEN, W. F. Indust. Med. *8:*99-100, March '39

Successful substitution of second metacarpal bone for missing thumb; case. WITTEK, A. Chirurg *13:*577-581, Oct 1, '41

Simultaneous osteocutaneous graft in reconstruction of thumb. LABOK, D. M. Khirurgiya, no. 2, pp. 73-75, '44

Conservation of metacarpus by skin and bone grafting in 3 patients. MORONEY, P. B. Brit. J. Surg. *32:*464-466, April '45

Bone Grafts to Mandible

Plastic surgery, 40 cases of bone-grafted mandibles. CHUBB, G. Lancet *1:*640, March 26, '21

Bone Grafts to Mandible—Cont.

Traumatic fracture of mandible, preoperative preparation; type of bone-graft; adaption of bone-graft. WOOLSEY, J. H. S. Clin. N. America *2:*333-340, April '22 (illus.)

Treatment of nonunion of fractures of mandible by free autogenous bone-grafts. RISDON, F. J.A.M.A. *79:*297-299, July 22, '22

Bone grafting in pseudoarthrosis of lower jaw. ROUVILLOIS, H. Paris med. *2:*237-245, Sept 26, '25 abstr: J.A.M.A. *85:*1422, Oct 31, '25

Bone-grafting of mandible, with report of 7 cases. BILLINGTON, W. AND ROUND, H. Brit. J. Surg. *13:*497-505, Jan '26

Osteoperiosteal bone graft; experimental and clinical data concerning its application for repair of bone defect and extra-articular ankylosis. DORRANCE, G. M. AND WAGONER, G. W., J.A.M.A. *87:*1433-1435, Oct 30, '26

Bone grafting for defects of mandible. IVY, R. H. AND EPES, B.M. Mil. Surgeon *60:*286-293, March '27

Successful treatment of jaw fractures by reduction, retention and grafts. CAVINA, C. Rev. de stomatol. *29:*815-842, Nov '27

Bone transplantation from crest of ilium for reconstruction of ascending ramus and two-thirds of body of lower jaw-bone. NEW, G. B., S. Clin. N. America *7:*1483-1486, Dec '27

Free transplantation of bone with periosteum in jaw surgery; 2 cases of excision of tumors. AXHAUSEN, G. Chirurg *1:*23-30, Nov 1, '28

Operative technic of osseous transplantation on lower jaw. CAVINA, C. Arch. ed atti d. Soc. ital. di chir. (1927) *34:*672-675, '28

Bone graft to jaw. MOOREHEAD, F. B., S. Clin. N. Amer. *9:*321-323, April '29

Bone-grafting the mandible. BILLINGTON, W. AND ROUND, H. Proc. Roy. Soc. Med. (sect. Odont.) *23:*7-13, March '30

Bone grafting the mandible. BILLINGTON, W. AND ROUND, H. Am. Dent. Surgeon *50:*185-188, May '30

Implantation of bone into lower jaw. AXHAUSEN, G. Deutsche Ztschr. f. Chir. *227:*368-385, '30

Bone transplantation by Axhausen's method in case of pseudoarthrosis of lower jaw resulting from defective healing. NISSEN, R. Deutsche Ztschr. f. Chir. *229:*140-142, '30

Operative treatment of tumors of jaw by Axhausen method of bone transplantation. KLEINSCHMIDT, O. Arch. f. klin. Chir. *164:*205-212, '31

Bone Grafts to Mandible – Cont.

Transplantation of bone and tissues in reconstruction of lower jaw. WEISSENFELS, G. Deutsche Zahnh., Hft. 79, pp. 1-30, '31

Reconstruction of lower jaw with tibial grafts. ROCHER, H. L. Bordeaux chir. *3:*272-277, July '32

Osteoplastic repair of congenital and acquired defects of lower jaw. GÖBELL, R. Arch. di chir. inf. *1:*111-125, Jan '34

Autoplastic osseous and cutaneous grafts in destruction of lower jaw. DUFOURMENTEL, L. Bull. et mem. Soc. d chirurgiens de Paris *27:*82-85, Feb 1, '35

Methods of transplanting bone into lower jaw. WASSMUND, M. Deutsche Ztschr. f. Chir. *244:*704-705, '35

Hemiresection of lower jaw with immediate osteoperiosteal graft in multilocular cancer; technical study. PRUDENTE, A. Rev. de cir. de Sao Paulo *3:*245-258, Aug '37

Bone graft of mandible with prosthetic objective. MARTINEZ SUAREZ, M., J. Internat. Coll. Surgeons *3:*260-261, June '40

Therapy of loss of substance of lower jaw by autoplastic bone graft. SANCHEZ GALINDO, J. Med. espan. *4:*35-45, July '40

Bone transplantation in major resections of lower jaw; case of osteofibroma. AXHAUSEN, G. Chirurg *12:*442-444, Aug 1, '40

Technic of bone transplantation in traumatic defects of lower jaw; author's experiences. GANZER, H. Plast. chir. *1:*113-154, '40

Implantation of bone in chin in severe case of mandibular retraction; case. LUSSIER, E. F. AND DAVIS, A. D. Am. J. Orthodontics *27:*267-274, May '41

Cosmetic and functional aspects of bone grafting in mandibular fractures. MACKENZIE, C. M. AND SHARPLESS, D. H. Northwest Med. *40:*372-374, Oct '41

Use of bone grafts in reconstructing mandible. FALLIS, R. J. Mil. Surgeon *9:*535-545, May '42

Primary bone grafting in resected tumor of mandible. STROMBECK, J. P. Acta chir. Scandinav. *86:*554-560, '42

Bone grafts to mandible. NEW, G. B. AND ERICH, J. B. Am. J. Surg. *63:*153-167, Feb '44

Hemiresection of lower jaw; immediate prosthesis with later iliac bone graft. FINOCHIETTO, R.; *et al.* Semana med. (tomo cincuent., fasc. 1) pp. 65-71, '44

Screw-pin for use in connection with mandibular fractures and grafts. WALKER, F. A. Brit. Dent. J. *78:*266-267, May 4, '45

Spindle cell sarcoma of mandible with excision and subsequent bone graft; case. DINGMAN, R. O. J. Oral Surg. *3:*235-240, July '45

Haynes splint in case of bone graft of lower jaw. INCLAN, A. JR. Cir. ortop. y traumatol. Habana *12:*132-137, July-Sept '45

Use of cancellous bone in repair of defects about jaws. BLOCKER, T. G. and WEISS, L. R. Ann. Surg. *123:*622-638, April '46

Role of cancellous bone in plastic surgery. GORDON, S. Surgery *20:*202-203, Aug '46

Reconstruction of bony defects, with special reference to cancellous iliac bone. MACOMBER, D. W. Surg. Gynec. and Obst. *83:*761-766, Dec '46

Use of cancellous bone in repair of defects of jaw. BLOCKER, T. G. J. AND WEISS, L. R. Tr. South. S. A. (1945) *57:*153-169, '46

Bone Grafts to Nose

Value and ultimate fate of bone and cartilage transplants in correction of nasal deformities. CARTER, W. W. Laryngoscope *33:*196-202, March '23 (illus.)

Depressed nasal deformities, comparison, of prosthetic values of paraffin, bone, cartilage and celluloid, with report of cases corrected with celluloid implants by author's method. LEWIS, J. D. Ann. Otol., Rhin. and Laryng. *32:*321-365, June '23 (illus.)

Rib implant for depressed bridge of nose. EADIE, C. M. M. J. Australia *2:*137-139, Aug 1, '25

How soon should nasal deformities, due to abscess of septum be corrected by transplantation of bone. CARTER, W. W. M. J. and Rec. *122:*247-248, Sept 2, '25

Case of developmental deformity of nose corrected by bone and cartilage transplants. CARTER, W. W. Laryngoscope *36:*664-666, Sept '26

Correction of pronounced types of saddle nose with mixed implants of bone and cartilage. COHEN, L. Ann. Otol. Rhin. and Laryng. *36:*639-647, Sept '27

Correction of pronounced types of saddle nose with mixed implants of bone and cartilage. COHEN, L. Tr. Am. Laryng., Rhin. and Otol. Soc. *33:*233-242, '27

Plastic surgery of nose with bone graft and paraffin. CHÉRIDJIAN, Z. Rev. med. de la Suisse Rom. *49:*751-753, Oct 25, '29

Cartilaginous and osteo-cartilaginous rib grafts in correction of nasal deformities. METZ, W. R. New Orleans M. and S. J. *82:*831-840, June '30

Surgical therapy of ozena by transplantation

Bone Grafts to Nose—Cont.
of bone into septum. OLIVARES, M. G. An. Soc. mex. de oftal. y oto-rino-laring. *9:*28-32, July-Sept '31
Ultimate fate of bone when transplanted into nose for purpose of correcting deformity. CARTER, W. W. Arch. Otolaryng. *15:*563-573, April '32
Correction of nasal deformities by plastic methods and by transplantation of bone and cartilage (from rib). CARTER, W. W. Internat. J. Orthodontia *19:*1012-1016, Oct '33
Value of bone and cartilage grafts in rhinoplasty. CARTER, W. W. Laryngoscope *43:*905-910, Nov '33
Correction of posttraumatic saddle nose by costal graft. PERI. Rev. de chir. plastique, pp. 334-338, Jan '34
Correction of depressed deformities of external nose with rib graft. COHEN, L. South. M. J. *30:*680-685, July '37
Endonasal free graft in therapy of old fractures of nose. SARGNON, A. Rev. de chir. structive, pp. 185-204, Oct '37
Use and behavior of iliac bone grafts in restoration of nasal contour; clinical and radiographic observations. MOWLEM, R. Rev. de chir. structive *8:*23-29, May '38
Advantage of mixed bone and cartilage grafts in correction of saddle nose and other depressed deformities of dorsum. COHEN, L. Ann. Otol., Rhin. and Laryng. *49:*410-417, June '40
Advantage of mixed bone and cartilage grafts in correction of saddle nose and other depressed deformities of dorsum. COHEN, L. Tr. Am. Laryng., Rhin. and Otol. Soc. *46:*370-376, '40
Osseous autotransplantations in partial rhinoplasties. MALBEC, E. F. Semana med. *2:*350-354, Aug 7, '41
Bone (iliac) and cartilage transplants to ear and nose; use and behavior. MOWLEM, R. Brit. J. Surg. *29:*182-193, Oct '41
Bone autografts in partial rhinoplasties. MALBEC, E. F. Arq. de cir. clin. e exper. *6:*163-171, April-June '42
Elevation of bridge line of nose (use of iliac bone). MACCOLLUM, D. W. Surgery *12:*97-108, July '42
Osteocartilaginous homogenous grafts in partial rhinoplasties. MALBEC, E. F. Dia med. *15:*644-645, June 21, '43
Cancellous bone transplants for correction of saddle nose. FOMON, S. *et al.* Ann. Otol. Rhin. and Laryng. *54:*518-533, Sept '45

Bone Grafts to Skull
Method of cranioplasty using as a graft one-half the thickness of bone part of rib. BALLIN, M. Surg., Gynec. and Obst. *33:*79, July '21
Costo-chondral graft for the repair of skull defects. HANSON, A. M. Minnesota Med. *7:*610-612, Sept '24
Case of successful grafting of ribs into skull for cranial defect. LEVIN, J. J., M. J. South Africa *20:*61-63, Oct '24
Separate tangentially cut bone-periosteum flaps from tibia to close gap in skull. BUFALINI, M. Arch. ital. di chir. *12:*529-554, '25
Bone grafting for cranial defect; cases. LEVIN, J. J., M. J. S. Africa *21:*283-284, May '26
Skull defects repaired by tibial grafts. HADLEY, F. A., J. Coll. Surgeons, Australasia *1:*208-213, Nov '28
Cranioplasty with osseous grafts for large loss of substance of frontal bone; case. TILLIER, R. Bull. et mem. Soc. nat. de chir. *56:*1277-1282, Nov 29, '30
Use of portion of scapula to fill bony defects of cranium. ILLYIN, G. A. Vestnik khir. (nos. 68-69) *23:*84-94, '31
Osteoplastic restoration of skull. MONEY, R. A., M. J. Australia *2:*269-270, Aug 27, '32
Autoplastic covering of cranial defects by transplants from iliac crest. LEXER, E. W. Deutsche Ztschr. f. Chir. *239:*743-749, '33
Cranioplasty by sterilized grafts from human cadaver. DAMBRIN, L. AND DAMBRIN, P. Bordeaux chir. *7:*279-286, July '36
Cranioplasty using parallel split costal grafts (protective grille). FAGARASANU, I. Tech. chir. *29:*57-64, May-June '37
Plastic use of crest of ilium in repair of loss of substance of cranium. KLAGES, F. Zentralbl. f. Chir. *66:*1580-1587, July 15, '39
Repair of cranial defects by cast chip-bone grafts; preliminary report. CONVERSE, J. M.; *et al.* J. Lab. and Clin. Med. *29:*546-559, May '44
Repair of defects, with special reference to use of cancellous bone in cranium. CARMODY, J. T. B. New England J. Med. *234:*393-399, March 21, '46
Repair of defects by bone grafting (especially from ilium) in cranium. MONEY, R. A. Surgery *19:*627-650, May '46

Bone Heterografts
Autoplastic and heteroplastic bone grafts. TROELL, A. Hygiea *85:*79-92, Feb 15, '23

Bone Heterografts – Cont.

(illus.) abstr: J.A.M.A. *80:*1112, April 14, '23

Free homoplastic and heteroplastic grafts of periosteum and of bone in sensitized animals. GAGLIO, V. Ann. ital. di chir. *11:*2017-2030, Oct '32

Use of spongy tissue of young calf as bone mortar. CALVE, J. Rev. med. franc. *16:*797-806, Dec '35 abstr: Bull. et mem. Soc. nat. de chir. *61:*1170-1174, Nov 16, '35

Late result of grafts of heterogenous bone tissue. LERICHE, R. Mem. Acad. de chir. *61:*1341-1343, Dec 14, '35

Autoplastic and heteroplastic bone grafts in osteosynthesis. DANIS, R. Bull. Acad. roy. de med. de Belgique *1:*88-94, '36 also: J. de med. de Paris *56:*631-633, July 30, '36

Autoplastic and heteroplastic bone grafts. AMBROS, Z. Chir. narz. ruchu *10:*345-356, '37

Osteoplastic amputation with graft of fixed heteroplastic bone. BERTOCCHI, A. Arch. ital. di chir. *50:*315-321, '38

Heterogenous bone grafts. LOPEZ ESNAURRIZAR, M., J. Internat. Coll. Surgeons *3:*151-155, April '40

Segmental regeneration of bone due to heteroplastic grafts; experimental study. LIBERTI, V. Ann. ital. di chir. *19:*389-430, May-June '40

Heterogenous bone grafts. LOPEZ ESNAURRIZAR, M. Medicina, Mexico *20:*384-392, July 25, '40

Use of bone from cattle in restoration of saddle nose. GONZALEZ ULLOA, M. Rev. mex. de cir., ginec. y cancer *9:*321-329, Aug '41

Use of bone from cattle in restoration of saddle nose. GONZALEZ ULLOA, M. Arq. de cir. clin. e exper. *6:*535-538, April-June '42

Transplantation of dead heterologous bone in surgery; present status of problem; preparation of Orell's os purum. CASANUEVA DEL C. M. AND VELASCO S., A. Rev. med. de Chile *70:*424-428, June '42

Bone Homografts

Grafts of bones of embryos. SIMON, R. AND ARON, M. Arch. franco-belges de chir. *25:*869-883, July '22 (illus.) abstr: J.A.M.A. *80:*65, Jan 6, '23

Homoplastic bone graft in tibia. VANDER ELST. Arch. franco-belges de chir. *26:*181-183, Feb '23 (illus.)

Successful 15 1/2 year old homeoplastic bone graft in man. ELLMER, G. AND SCHMINCKE, A. Zentralbl. f. Chir. *52:*562-565, March 14, '25 abstr: J.A.M.A. *84:*1463, May 9, '25

Experimental bone grafts; homogenous grafts. IMBERT, L. Bull. Acad. de med., Paris *94:*1086-1090, Dec 1, '25

Autotransplantation and homoiotransplantation of cartilage and bone in rat. LOEB, L. Am. J. Path. *2:*315-333, July '26

Comparative study of bony new growth in auto- and homoplastic grafts of periosteum and young bones. POLACCO, E. Arch. per le sc. med. *53:*476-480, Aug '29 also: Gior. d. r. Accad. di med. di Torino *92:*153-157, April-June '29

Survival of bone marrow and bone in homoplastic grafting. VILLATA, G. Gior. d. r. Accad. di med. di Torino *93:*167-174, July-Sept '30

Auto- and homotransplantation of bone and cartilage. GORBUNOFF, W. P. Arch. f. klin. Chir. *161:*651-670, '30

Free homoplastic and heteroplastic grafts of periosteum and of bone in sensitized animals. GAGLIO, V. Ann. ital. di chir. *11:*2017-2030, Oct 31, '32

Method of homoplastic bone grafts. ASTRAKHANSKIY, V. A. Sovet. khir. *4:*202-209, '33

Behavior of homoplastic transplants of bone prophylactically treated with blood serum of host; preliminary report. GRISANTI, S. Riv. san. siciliana *22:*3-18, Jan 1, '34

Bone graft from mother to child. MASSART, R. Bull. et mem. Soc. d. Chirurgiens de Paris *27:*142-144, March 1, '35

Cranioplasty by sterilized grafts from human cadaver. DAMBRIN, L. AND DAMBRIN, P. Bordeaux chir. *7:*279-286, July '36

Postoperative parathyroid tetany treated by autoplastic and homoplastic bone graft. IACOBOVICI, I. Rev. de chir., Bucuresti *42:*567-570, July-Aug '39

Bone Infections

End results of 158 consecutive autogenous bone grafts for non-union in long bone (A) in simple fractures; (B) in atrophic bone following war wounds and chronic suppurative osteitis (osteomyelitis). KIRK, N. T. J. Bone and Joint Surg. *6:*760-799, Oct '24

Method of dealing with chronic osteomyelitis by saucerization followed by skin grafting. ARMSTRONG, B. AND JARMAN, T. F. J. Bone and Joint Surg. *18:*387-396, April '36

Osteomyelitis of hands. KOCH, S. L. Surg., Gynec. and Obst. *64:*1-8, Jan '37

Use of pedicle graft for chronic osteomyelitis. BEEKMAN, F. S. Clin. North America *17:*185-190, Feb '37

Bone Infections – Cont.
Correction of acquired asymmetry caused by osteomyelitis of lower jaw. AXHAUSEN, G. Deutsche Ztschr. f. Chir. *248:*533–551, '37
Fistulized tuberculous trochanteritis with extensive bone loss; immediate transplantation of pedicled cutaneous flap into residual cavity; case with recovery. INGIANNI, G. Arch. ed atti d. Soc. ital. di chir. *44:*873–875, '38
Dermo-epidermal grafts and pedicled tubular grafts in surgical therapy of osteomyelitis. INGIANNI, G. Arch. ed atti d. Soc. ital. di chir. *45:*724–730, '39
Technical results of grafting skin into cavity of bone after surgical therapy of osteomyelitis. INGIANNI, G. Accad. med., Genova *54:*25–33, Jan '39
Double incisions in therapy of phlegmon of sheath and empyema of joints. KLAPP, R. Zentralbl. f. Chir. *66:*753–758, April 1, '39
Filling of osteomyelitis cavities by means of fat transplants. LEONTE, C. Rev. de chir., Bucuresti *43:*801–805, Nov–Dec '40
Use of muscular flap to fill bone cavities in osteomyelitis due to gunshot wounds. STOTZ, W. Zentralbl. f. Chir. *69:*427, March 14, '42
Sequestrectomy and autoplasty with skin flaps in therapy of subacute and chronic nonspecific osteomyelitis. PARODI, L. Ann. ital. di chir. *21:*307–314, May '42
Surgical obliteration of cavities following traumatic osteomyelitis (by bone and skin transplantation). KNIGHT, M. P. AND WOOD, G. O. J. Bone and Joint Surg. *27:*547–556, Oct '45
Osteomyelitis treated by radical saucerization and early grafting. (skin) McCLINTOCK, J. A. J. Indiana M. A. *39:*9–14, Jan '46
Traumatic osteomyelitis; use of grafts; subsequent treatment. KELLY, R. P. Ann. Surg. *123:*688–697, April '46
Reconstructive surgery following treatment of osteomyelitis by saucerization and early grafting. McCLINTOCK, J. A. J. Indiana M. A. *39:*436–439, Sept '46
Skin grafting in treatment of osteomyelitic war wounds. KELLY, R. P. J. Bone and Joint Surg. *28:*681–691, Oct '46
Traumatic osteomyelitis; use of grafts; subsequent treatment. KELLY, R. P.; *et al.* Tr. South. S. A. (1945) *57:*219–228, '46

BONHAM, W. L.: Congenital choanal occlusion. South. M. J. *35:*252–257, March '42
BONHAM, W. L. Postoperative results in 2 cases of congenital choanal occlusion. Eye, Ear, Nose and Throat Monthly *25:*387–393, Aug '46
BÖNHEIM, E: Peripheral facial paralysis and progressive facial hemiatrophy as sequels of teeth extraction. Deutsche Monatschr. f. Zahnh. *45:*353–366, Avil 15, '27
BONIKOWSKY, H.: Tendon suture; location of proximal end of tendon. Arch. f. klin. Chir. *145:*598, '27
BONNARD, R. (see LAIGNEL-LAVASTINE *et al*) Dec '34
BONNE: Prevention and treatment of bed-sores. Med. Klinik *20:*784–785, June 8, '24
BONNEAU, R.: Forward dislocations of phalangeal joints. Rev. gen. de clin. et de therap. *40:*824, Dec 4, '26
BONNET: Surgical treatment of acute hand infections. Arch. de med. et pharm. mil. *97:*1–23, July '32
BONNET, L.: Familial syndactylia. Bull. et med. Soc. de chir. de Paris *20:*677–681, Oct 19, '28
BONNET, P. (see BLOCH, J. C.) Oct '29
BONNET, P. (see BLOCH, J. J.) Nov '29
BONNET, P. (see TIXIER, L.) Nov–Dec '31
BONNET, P.: Fractures involving frontal sin; 2 cases. Bull. Soc. d'opht. de Paris *51:*83–84, Jan '39
BONNET, P.: Fracture of orbit and superior maxilla followed by subcutaneous and deep emphysema from secondary infection. Lyon chir. *28:*718–819, Nov–Dec '31
BONNET, P.: Prognosis of fractures of frontal sinus. Bull. Soc. d'opht. de Paris, pp. 327–328, May '32
BONNET, P. AND CARCASSONNE, F.: Anatomic restoration of injured thumb by graft of mutilated and useless index finger. Lyon chir. *28:*247–248, March–April '31
BONNET, P. AND CARCASSONNE, F.: Anatomic restoration of thumb by graft of functionally useless index finger; case. Lyon chir. *28:*529–540, Sept–Oct '31
BONNETT, P. AND CARCASSONNE, F.: Phalangization of first metacarpal bone; technic, indications and results. Rev. de chir., Paris *50:*341–355, May '31
BONNETT, P. AND DELAYE: Results of suture of flexor tendon of thumb after healing of wound; case. Lyon chir. *28:*189–190, March–April '31
BONNET, P. AND MICHON, L.: Wound of flexor tendon of thumb; perfect functional cure. Lyon chir. *26:*849–852, Nov–Dec '29
BONNET, P.; PAUFIQUE, AND BONAMOUR: Congenital bilateral coloboma of upper eyelid. Bull. Soc. d'opht. de Paris, pp. 229–232, March '34

BONNET-ROY, F.: Cancer of upper maxilla and lip; operation; recovery. Odontologie *66:*39, Jan '28

BONNEY, V. AND MCINDOE, A. H.: Unique constructive operation in artificial vagina. J. Obst. and Gynaec. Brit. Emp. *51:*24–29, Feb '44

BONNIOT, (see MARTIN, L.) June '32

BONOLA, A.: Tendon transplantation in therapy of inveterate radial paralysis; physiologic aims, technic and results. Chir. d. org. di movimento *22:*239–254, Aug '36

BONOLI, U.: Intra-arterial medication of deep diffuse hand phlegmon. Policlinico (sez. prat.) *36:*851–853, June 17, '29 Comment by CINQUEMANI, P. Policlinico (sez. prat.) *36:*1395–1396, Sept 30, '29

BONOLI, U.: Intra-arterial medication with colloidal silver in treatment of deep phlegmon of hand. (Reply to Scollo). Policlinico (sez. prat.) *37:*949–950, June 30, '30

Bonoli, U.

Therapy of deep phlegmon of hand by intra-arterial injection of colloidal silver. (Comment on Bonoli's article). SCOLLO, G. Policlinico (sez. prat.) *37:*546–548, April 14, '30

Reply to article by Bonoli on hand infections. SCOLLO, G. Policlinico (sez. prat.) *37:*1103, July 28, '30

BONZON: Congenital absence of right thumb; attempt at functional restoration. Scalpel *86:*799–801, May 27, '33

BOOKHALTER, S. (see MURRAY, J. J.) Sept '38

Books (Alphabetically by first authors)

Bone Graft Surgery in Disease, Injury, and Deformity. ALBEE, FRED H., AND KUSHNER, ALEXANDER. Appleton-Century-Crofts Co., New York, 1940

Inheritance of Harelip and Cleft Palate. ANDERSEN, POUL FOGH. Nyt Nordisk Forlag Arnold Busck, Copenhagen, 1942

Chirurgie de la face et de la région maxillo-faciale. AUBRY, MAURICE AND FREIDEL, CHARLES. Masson et Cie, Paris, 1942

Technique de la parotidectomie totale avec conservation integrale du nerf facial. AUDOUIN, J., AND NEVEU, J. Maloine, Paris, 1941

Technik und Ergebnisse der Gaumenplastik. AXHAUSEN, GEORG. Georg Thieme, Stuttgart, 1936

Technik und Ergebnisse der Lippenplastik. AXHAUSEN, GEORG. Georg Thieme, Leipzig, 1941

Moderne Kosmetik unter besonderer Berücksichtigung der chirurgischen Kosmetik.

Books—Cont.

BAB, MARTIN. Karger, Basel, 1929

Die frühindische Plastik. BACHHOFER, LUDWIG. K. Wolff, Munich, 1929

Plastic Surgery. BANKOFF, GEORGE. Medical Publications, London, 1944

Surgical Anatomy of the Head and Neck. BARNHILL, JOHN F. Wm. Wood and Co., New York, 1937. Second Edition (with William J. Mellinger), 1940

Plastic Surgery. BARSKY, ARTHUR J. W. B. Saunders Co., Phila., 1938

A Monograph of the Various Types of Deformity of the Hand and Arm. BECK, CARL. J. B. Lippincott Co., Phila., 1925

Anatomie medico-chirurgicale, Fascicles 2 and 3, La Face. BELLOCQ, PHILIPPE B. Masson et Cie, Paris, 1926

La revisión de la morfología arterial en las regiones anatómicas que atañen a la oto-rino-laringología. BELOU, PEDRO. La Sociedad Argentina de Oto-rino-laringología, Buenos Aires, 1939

The Principles and Technique of Oral Surgery. BERGER, ADOLPH. Dental Items of Interest Publishing Co., Brooklyn, 1923

Deformitäten und kosmetische Operationen der weiblichen Brüst. BIESENBERGER, HERMANN. Wilhelm Maudrich, Vienna, 1931

Essentials of Oral Surgery. BLAIR, VILRAY P., AND IVY, ROBERT H. C. V. Mosby Co., St. Louis, 1923. (With Brown, James Barrett), Second Edition 1936, Third Edition 1944

Etude des Blepharoplasties. BOUCHAUD, PIERRE. Arnette, Paris, 1927

La véritable chirurgie esthétique du visage. BOURGUET, JULIEN. Librairie Plon, Paris, 1936

Theory and Treatment of Fractures of the Jaws in Peace and War. BOYLE, HORACE H. Henry Kimpton, London, 1940

Treatment of Hand and Forearm Infections. BRICKEL, A. C. J. C. V. Mosby Co., St. Louis, 1939

Cleft Lip and Palate. BROPHY, TRUMAN W. Blakiston Co., Phila., 1923

Modern Plastic Surgical Prosthetics. BROWN, ADOLPH M. Grune and Stratton Co., New York, 1947

The Surgery of Oral and Facial Diseases and Malformations. BROWN, GEORGE V. I. Lea and Febiger, Phila., 1938

Skin Grafting of Burns. BROWN, J. BARRETT AND MCDOWELL, FRANK. J. B. Lippincott Co., Phila., 1943

Facial Prosthesis. BULBULIAN, ARTHUR H. W. B. Saunders Co., Phila., 1945

Books—Cont.

Surgery of the Hand. BUNNELL, STERLING. J. B. Lippincott Co., Phila., 1944

Tratamiento quirúrgico del promentonismo-mandibulo-megalia y otras deformidades mandibulares. Tesis. CARREA, RAUL M. E. University Press, Buenos Aires, 1943

La pratique stomatologique. Tome VIII: Restauration et prothèse maxillofaciales. CHOMPRET, Editor. Masson et Cie, Paris, 1935

Technique and Results of Grafting Skin. CHRISTIE, H. KENRICK. H. K. Lewis and Co., London, 1930

Chirurgie plastique abdominale; cure chirurgicale de ptose cutanée abdominale, ventre en tablier. CLAOUÉ, CHARLES. Maloiné, Paris, 1940

Propos sur la chirurgie esthétique. CLAOUÉ, CHARLES. Maloine, Paris, 1932

Plastique mammaire. CLAOUÉ, CHARLES AND BERNARD, IRENE. Maloine, Paris, 1936

Facial and Body Prosthesis. CLARKE, CARL D. C. V. Mosby Co., St. Louis, 1945

Technik und Ergebnisse der Lippenplastik, by Georg Thieme, Leipzig, 1941

Surgery of the Hand. COUCH, JOHN H. Univ. Toronto Press, Toronto, 1939

Making of a Beautiful Face, or Face-Lifting Unveiled. CRUM, J. HOWARD. Walton Book Co., New York, 1931

The Hand; Its Disabilities and Diseases. CUTLER, CONDICT W., JR. W. B. Saunders Co., Phila., 1942

Chirurgie réparatrice: Plastique et esthétique de la poitrine, des seins, et de l'abdomen. DARTIGUES, L. Lépine, Paris, 1936

The Operative Story of Cleft Palate. DORRANCE, GEORGE. W. B. Saunders Co., Phila., 1933

Chirurgie de l'articulation temporomaxillaire. DUFOURMENTEL, LÉON. Masson et Cie, Paris, 1928

Chirurgie correctrice du nez. DUFOURMENTEL, LÉON. University Press of France, Paris, 1929

Diagnostic, Traitement, et Expertise des Sequelles des Accidents des Regions Maxillofaciales. DUFOURMENTEL, LÉON, AND FRISON, LÉON. J. B. Baillière et fils, Paris, 1922

Plastic Surgery of the Nose. EASTMAN, J. EASTMAN. Paul Hoeber Co., New York, 1925. Second Edition, 1927 (Macmillan Co., New York)

Kosmetische Operationen. EITNER, ERNST. Springer-Verlag, Berlin, 1932

Traumatic Injuries of Facial Bones. ERICH, JOHN B., AND AUSTIN, Louie T. W. B. Saunders Co., Phila., 1944

Books—Cont.

Harelip and Cleft Palate. FEDERSPIEL, MATTHEW. C. V. Mosby Co., St. Louis, 1927

Infections of the Hand. FIFIELD, LIONEL R. H. K. Lewis and Co., London, 1926. Second Edition, 1939

The Surgery of Injury and Plastic Repair. FOMON, SAMUEL. Wm. Wood and Co., New York, 1939

Les luxations habituelles sans blocage de l'articulation temporo-maxillaire. FRIEZ, PIERRE. Le François, Paris, 1933

Korrektiv-kosmetische Chirurgie der Nase, der Ohren, und des Gesichts. FRÜHWALD, VICTOR. Wilhelm Maudrich, Vienna, 1932. (Also English edition, translated by Geoffrey Morey)

Die Formfehler und die plastischen Operationen der weiblichen Brust. GLÄSMER, ERNA. F. Enke, Stuttgart, 1930

Manual of Diagnosis and Management of Peripheral Nerve Injuries. GROFF, ROBERT A., AND HOUTZ, SARA. J. J. B. Lippincott Co., Phila., 1945

Surgery of the Hand. HANDFIELD-JONES, R. M. E. and S. Livingstone Ltd., Edinburgh, 1946

Treatment of Burns. HARKINS, HENRY. C C Thomas Co., Springfield, Ill., 1942

Anatomy of the Head and Neck. HILL, ROBERT T. Lea and Febiger Co., Phila., 1946

Plastic Surgery of the Head, Face, and Neck. HUNT, H. LYONS. Lea and Febiger Co., Phila., 1926

Lidplastik und plastische Operationen anderer Weichteile des Gesichts. IMRE, JOSEF. Studium, Budapest, 1928

Chirurgie de la main, livre du chirurgien: Chirurgie réparatrice des tramatismes de la main. ISELIN, MARC. Masson et Cie, Paris, 1945

Plaies et maladies infectieuses des mains. ISELIN, MARC. Masson et Cie, Paris, 1928. Second Edition, 1932. Third Edition, 1938

Fractures of the Jaws. IVY, ROBERT H., AND CURTIS, LAWRENCE. Lea and Febiger, Phila., 1931, Second Edition, 1938, Third Edition, 1945

Injuries of the Jaws and Face. JAMES, W. WARWICK, AND FICKLING, B. W. Bale, London, 1940

The Principles of Anatomy as Seen in the Hand. JONES, FREDERIC W. Baillière, Tindall and Cox, London, 1942

Eine Nasenplastik, ausgeführt in Lokalanesthesie. Kinegrammata medica. JOSEPH, JACQUES. (In German, English, French, Italian, Russian, and Spanish text) Pp. 14. G. Stilke, Berlin, 1927

Nasenplastik und sonstige Gesichtsplastik.

Books—Cont.
Nebst einem Anhang über Mammaplastik. JOSEPH, JACQUES. C. Kabitsch, Leipzig, 1928
Nasenplastik und sonstige Gesichtsplastik. Nebst einem Anhang über Mammaplastik und . . . Korperplastik. JOSEPH, JACQUES. C. Kabitsch, Leipzig, 1931
Infections of the Hand. KANAVEL, ALLEN B. Sixth Edition. Lea and Febiger, Phila., 1933. Seventh Edition, 1939
Allgemeine und spezielle chirurgische Operationslehre. Band III, Die Eingriffe an der Brüst and Brüsthöhle. KIRSCHNER, MARTIN (Editor). von Otto Kleinschmidt. Springer-Verlag, Berlin, 1940
Die Chirurgie: . . . Band II, Pp. 393–602, Die plastischen Operationen der Haut. KIRSCHNER, M., AND NORDMANN, O. (Editors). by K. Tiesenhausen. Urban, Berlin, 1927
Die verletzte Hand. KRÖMER, KARL. Wilhelm Maudrich, Vienna, 1938
Introduction à la chirurgie réparatrice. LAUWERS, E. E. Masson et Cie, Paris, 1934
Il viso. Igiene cutanea, terapia estetica, chirurgia plastica. LIBERA, DONATO. Hoepli, Milan, 1938
Fractures of the Jaws and Other Facial Bones. MAJOR, GLENN. C. V. Mosby Co., St. Louis, 1943
Sculpture in the Living. MALINIAK, JACQUES W. Lancet Press, New York, 1934
Evolution of Plastic Surgery. MALTZ, MAXWELL. Froben Press, New York, 1946
New Faces—New Futures; Rebuilding Character with Plastic Surgery. MALTZ, MAXWELL. Richard R. Smith, New York, 1936
Living Canvas: A Romance of Aesthetic Surgery. MARGETSON, ELISABETH. Methuen, London, 1936
Surgery of Repair, Injuries, and Burns. MATTHEWS, DAVID N. C C Thomas Co., Springfield, Ill., 1946
Chirurgie maxillofaciale. MAUREL, G. Maloine, Paris, 1931. Second Edition, 1940, Le François, Paris
Surgery of Head and Neck. MCQUILLAN, ARTHUR S. Oxford Press, London, 1942
Oral Surgery. MEAD, STERLING V. C. V. Mosby Co., St. Louis, 1933. Second Edition, 1940. Third Edition, 1946
Cannula Implants and Review of Implantation Technics in Esthetic Surgery. MILLER, CHARLES C. Oak Printing and Pub. Co., Chicago, 1926
Cosmetic Surgery: The Correction of Featural Imperfections. MILLER, CHARLES C. F. A. Davis Co., Phila., 1924

Books—Cont.
Chirurgie plastique des seins. MONTANT, C., AND DUBOIS, F. Maloine, Paris, 1933
Cleft Palate and Speech. MORLEY, MURIEL E. E. and S. Livingstone Ltd., Edinburgh, 1945
Frühe Plastik in Griechenland und Vorderasien. MULLER, VALENTIN. (rund 3000 bis 600 v. Christ). B. Filser, Augsburg, 1929
La chirurgie esthétique, son role social. NOËL, A. Masson et Cie, Paris, 1926. (German translation by A. Hardt published by Barth, Leipzig, 1932)
Speech Training for Cases of Cleft Palate. OLDFIELD, MICHAEL C. H. K. Lewis and Co., London, 1938
Les hermaphrodites et la chirurgie. OMBREDANNE, L. Masson et Cie, Paris, 1923
Fascial Grafting in Principle and Practice. ORRIN, H. C. Oliver and Boyd, Ltd., London, 1928
Tumors of the Hands and Feet. PACK, GEORGE T. (Editor). C. V. Mosby Co., St. Louis, 1939
Skin Grafting from a Personal and Experimental Viewpoint. PADGETT, EARL C. C C Thomas Co., Springfield, Ill., 1942
Surgical Diseases of the Mouth and Jaws. PADGETT, EARL C. W. B. Saunders Co., Phila., 1938
Cirugía estética. PALACIO POSSE, RAMÓN. El Ateñeo Press, Buenos Aires, 1946
Reconstruction of the Fingers. PARIN, B. V. U.S.S.R. "Medgiz" Press, Moscow, 1944
Synopsis of Traumatic Injuries of the Face and Jaws. PARKER, DOUGLAS B. C. V. Mosby Co., St. Louis, 1942
Chirurgie esthétique pure. PASSOT, RAYMOND. Gaston Doin et Cie, Paris, 1930
Brenthurst Papers. PENN, JACK (Editor). Witwatersrand Univ. Press, Johannesburg, 1944
The Human Face. PICARD, MAX. (translated from the German by G. Endore). Cassell and Co., London, 1931
Facial Surgery. PICKERILL, H. P. Wm. Wood and Co., New York, 1924
Speech Training for Cleft Palate Patients. PICKERILL, H. P. Whitcombe and Tombs, Ltd., London, 1937
Chirurgische und konservative Kosmetik der Gesichtes. POHL, LEANDER (Editor). Urban and Schwarzenberg, München, 1931
Greffes et Transplants Osseux chez l'Homme. RADULESCO, A. D. Romaneasca, Bucharest, 1924
Corrective Rhinoplastic Surgery. SAFIAN, JOSEPH. Paul Hoeber Co., New York, 1935
Chirurgia plastica del naso. SANVENERO-

Books—Cont.

ROSSELLI, GUSTAVO. Luigi Pozzi, Rome, 1931

Considerations sur les fractures du maxillaire inferieur. SCHIESS, EMILE. Hans Huber, Berne, 1932

As Others See You: The Story of Plastic Surgery. SCHIRESON, HENRY J. Macauley, New York, 1938

Correction chirurgicale des difformités congenitales et acquises de la pyramide nasale. SEBILEAU, PIERRE, AND DUFOURMENTEL, LÉON. Arnette, Paris, 1927

General and Plastic Surgery with Emphasis on War Injuries. SHEEHAN, J. EASTMAN. Paul Hoeber Co., New York, 1945

Manual of Reparative Plastic Surgery. SHEEHAN, J. EASTMAN. Paul Hoeber Co., New York, 1938

Plastic Surgery of the Orbit. SHEEHAN, J. EASTMAN. Macmillan Co., New York, 1927

Principles and Practice of Oral Surgery. SILVERMAN, S. L. Blakiston Co., Phila., 1926

Newer Methods of Ophthalmic Plastic Surgery. SPAETH, EDMUND B. Blakiston Co., Phila., 1925

Les techniques et les résultats actuals de la réparation des tendons de la main et des doigts. TAILHEFER, ANDRÉ. Arnette, Paris, 1928

Traumatic Surgery of the Jaws, Including First-Aid Treatment. THOMA, KURT H. C. V. Mosby Co., St. Louis, 1942

Plastic Surgery of the Breast and Abdominal Wall. THOREK, MAX. C C Thomas Co., Springfield, Ill. 1942

De la prosthèse immédiate des maxillaires. TULASNE, R. LeGrand, Paris, 1928

Cleft Palate Speech. VAN THAL, J. H. George Allen and Unwin, Ltd., London, 1934

Congenital Cleft Lip, Cleft Palate, and Associated Nasal Deformities. VAUGHN, HAROLD S. Lea and Febiger Co., Phila., 1940

Division palatine, anatomie, chirurgie, phonetique. VEAU, VICTOR, AND BOREL, S. Masson et Cie, Paris, 1931

Bec-de-lièvre. VEAU, VICTOR, AND RÉCAMIER, JACQUES. Masson et Cie, Paris, 1938

Epithelioma du Maxillaire Superieur. VERGER. Doin, Paris, 1925

Chirurgie esthétique; le sein. VIRENQUE, M. Maloine, Paris, 1928

Chirurgie réparatrice maxillo-faciale. VIRENQUE, M. Maloine, Paris, 1940

The Treatment of Burns. WALLACE, A. B. Oxford Press, London, 1941

Maxillo-Facial Injuries, Report of Army Standing Ctte. WAR OFFICE, GREAT BRITAIN. H. M. Stationery Office, London, 1935

Books—Cont.

Operative Oral Surgery. WINTER, LEO. C. V. Mosby Co., St. Louis, 1941

Overcoming Cleft Palate Speech. YOUNG, EDNA H. Hill-Young School, Minneapolis, 1928

Cirugía plástica. ZENO, LELIO. El Ateñeo Press, Buenos Aires, 1943

BOORSTEIN, S. W.: Cleft hand; case. J. Bone and Joint Surg. *12:*172–176, Jan '30

BOOTH, F. A.: Cosmetic surgery of face, neck and breast. Northwest Med. *21:*170–172, June '22 (illus.)

BOPPE: Use of silk in musculotendinous and ligamentary reparative surgery. Mem. Acad. de chir. *68:*452–456, Dec 9–16, '42

BOPPE, M. AND FAUGERON, P.: Treatment of syndactylias by total free skin grafts. Paris med. *1:*522–527, June 17, '39

BOR, H. A.: Jaw fractures. Geneesk. tijdschr. v. Nederl.-Indie *75:*1530–1536, Sept 3, '35

BORCHERS, E.: Epidermal grafts in correction of severe forms of hypospadias; further study. Chirurg *11:*713–722, Oct 15, '39

BORCHERS, E.: Operative treatment of severe forms of hypospadias in male. Ztschr. f. Urol. *22:*808–822, '28

Borchers Operation: See Nove-Josserand-Borchers Operation

BORDEIANU, I.: Skin grafts for great loss of skin. Bucuresti med. *4:*1–2, '32

BORDEN, C. R. C.: Pulmonary complications following nose and throat operations. Laryngoscope *31:*851, Nov '21

BORDIER, H.: Cancer of hand in radiologist, cured by diathermo-coagulation; case. Cancer, Bruxelles *4:*328–330, '27

BORDIER, H.: Effective use of electric coagulation in rhinophyma. Presse med. *38:*538–539, April 19, '30

BORDIER, H.: Technic of diathermic epilation. Am. J. Phys. Therapy *8:*273–274, Jan '32 also: Monde med., Paris *42:*78–81, Feb 1, '32

BORDONI, L.: Double phalanx in thumb of acromegalic subject. Radiol. med. *14:*775–781, Sept '27

BOREL, (see VEAU, V.) July '28

BOREL, S. (see VEAU, V.) June '29

BOREL, S. (see VEAU, V.) 1931

BOREL, S. (with VICTOR VEAU): *Division palatine, anatomie, chirurgie, phonetique.* Masson et Cie, Paris, 1931

BOREL-MAISONNY, MME. (see VEAU, V.) Nov '33

BOREL-MAISONNY, MME. (see VEAU, V.) July '36

BOREL-MAISONNY, MME. (see VEAU, V. *et al*) May '37

BOREL-MAISONNY, MME.: Phonetic results obtained after cleft palate therapy. Rev. de stomatol. *39:*733–754, Oct '37

Borelius Operation (See also Maydl Operation)

Exstrophy of bladder; operation by Borelius-Maydl method. MÜLLER, S. Hospitalstid. (Dansk kir. selsk. forh.) *73:*23, Aug 14, '30

BORELLI, E.: Dislocation of fingers. Policlinico (sez. prat.) *28:*115, Jan 24, '21 abstr: J.A.M.A. *76:*826, March 19, '21

BORGES DE SOUZA, A.: Surgical therapy of incoercible senile spasmodic entropion. Lisboa med. *13:*169–177, March '36

BORGHESAN, E.: Technic of surgical therapy of osseous choanal diaphragm. Valsalva *14:*73–75, Feb '38

BORGHI, M.: Experimental researches on grafting cartilage on to tendons. Arch. per. le sc. med. *50:*437–465, '27

BORISOV, M. V.: Transplantation of toes for fingers. Sovet. khir., no. 10, pp. 136–140, '35

BORKOWSKI, J.: Retro-auricular salivary fistula; therapy. Warszawskie czasop. lek. *9:*653, July 14, '32

BORLAND, V. G. (see ANDERSON, J. K.) July '36

BORN, R.: Unusual urethral calculus containing hair; use of scrotal skin in restoration of hypospadias as probable cause; case. Ztschr. f. Urol. *31:*552–554, '37

BORNEMEIER, W. C. AND PARSONS, L.: Report of 155 cases of burn treatment. Surg. Gynec. and Obst. *82:*311–318, Mar '46

BOROVSKAYA, V. M.: Shock following war wounds; changes of blood in. Byull. eksper. biol. i med. (nos. 1–2) *19:*33–36, '45

BOROVSKIY, M. L. Peripheral nerve injuries; therapy. Khirurgiya, no. 5, pp. 50–52, '45

BORRAS, J. A.: Practical efficacious procedure in burns. Med. clin. Barcelona *4:*235–239, March '45

BORRAS, P. E.: Creation of artificial vagina in congenital absence. Bol. Soc. de cir. de Rosario *4:*24–34, '37

BORRI, N.: Absence of ulnar derivations of hand; case. Sett. med. *27:*450–455, April 13, '39

BORS, E.: New instrument for use in skin grafting. Zentralbl. f. Chir. *54:*2890–2891, Nov 12, '27

BORST, J. G. G. AND VEENING, H. P.: Task of internist in treatment of war injuries; post-traumatic (secondary) shock. Nederl. tijdschr. v. geneesk. *84:*914–922, March 9, '40

BOSCH OLIVES, V.: Clubhand due to partial absence of ulna; case. Cir. d. ap. locom. *2:*284–287, July '45

BOSDEVEIX, G. L.: Lateral branchial cysts of neck. Ann. d. mal. de l'oreille, du larynx *48:*826–842, Aug '29

BOSE, P.: Accessory external ear. Indian M. Gaz. *57:*139–140, April '22

BOSERUP, O. AND KRAGH, J.: Operation to correct crooked nose. Ugesk. f. Laeger *85:*808, Nov 15; 830, Nov 22, '23

BOST, C.: Progressive facial hemiatrophy; case in child. Arch. Pediat. *44:*497–501, Aug '27

BOSTOCK, J.: Acrocephaly with associated syndactylism. M. J. Australia *1:*572–574, May 12, '28

BOSVIEL, J.: Aspiration of ala nasi and its operative treatment. J. de med. de Paris, *46:*417, May 26, '27

BOSVIEL, J.: Outline of methods of nasal plastic surgery. J. de med. de Paris *46:*87, Jan 31, '27

BOTASHEFF, V. A.: Treatment of burns of first and second degree. Vrach. gaz. *34:*1748–1750, Dec 15, '30

BOTERO JARAMILLO, L. E.: Traumatic tearing off of fifth finger and of corresponding flexor tendon; case. Colombia med. *2:*82–85, March–April '40

BOTHMAN, L. (see WALSH, T. E.) Sept '37

BOTTO MICCA, A.: Cavernous angiomas of tendons of hands. Riv. san. siciliana *22:*568–577, April 15, '34

BOTTURA, G.: Rare case of congenital malformation of external ear. Ann. di laring., Otol. *29:*323–328, Nov '28

BOUCHAUD, PIERRE: *Etude des Blepharoplasties*. Arnette, Paris, 1927

BOUCHER, R.: Macrocheilia. Union med. du Canada *75:*461–462, April '46

BOUDREAUX, J.: Clawhand following violent compression of long flexor muscles of forearm; study of case. Mem. Acad. de chir. *68:*124–126, Feb 11–March 4, '42

BOULOGNE: Dupuytren's contracture; etiologic conception based on 2 similar cases. Rev. neurol. *63:*991–992, June '35

BOURDON, E. (see AUBRY, M.) Oct–Dec '45

BOURGEOIS, P.; FEIL, AND LOIREAU: Ectrodactylia with syndactylia; case. Bull. et mem. Soc. med. d. hop. de Paris *49:*320–322, March 13, '33

BOURGOYNE, J. R.: Extraoral splinting of mandible. J. Am. Dent. A. *30:*1390–1392, Sept 1, '43

BOURGOYNE, J. R.: Fixation of pathologic fractures of mandible. Am. J. Orthodontics (Oral Surg. Sect.) *31:*492–500, Aug '45

BOURGOYNE, J. R.: Open reduction vs. skeletal fixation in jaw fractures. Am. J. Orthodontics (Oral Surg. Sect.) *31:*519–532, Aug '45

BOURGUET (see DUPUY-DUTEMPS, L.) Oct '30

BOURGUET: Esthetic surgery of face. Arch. franco-belges de chir. *28:*293–297, April '25

BOURGUET: Operation for pouches under eyes (Bourguet's operative technic.). Arch. franco-belges de chir. *31:*133–137, Feb '28

BOURGUET: Treatment of congenital ptosis of eyelids. Bull. et mem. Soc. de chir. de Paris *22:*313–319, May 2, '30

BOURGUET; PONROY, AND CABROL: Bicondyloid resection in deviations of lower jaw and prognathism. Rev. de stomatol. *33:*715, Dec '31

BOURGUET, J.: Curative and plastic surgery in different deformities of temporomaxillary joint. Monde med., Paris *40:*109–114, Feb 15, '30

BOURGUET, J.: Esthetic surgery (face). Bull. et mem. Soc. d. chirurgiens de Paris *25:*282–288, May 5, '33

BOURGUET, J.: Esthetic surgery in correction of abnormally protruding pinna. Clinique, Paris *28:*318–320, Oct (B) '33

BOURGUET, J.: Esthetic surgery in lower jaw prognathism. Monde med., Paris *46:*81–88, Feb 1, '36

BOURGUET, J.: Exophthalmos, treatment by plastic surgery. Monde med., Paris *42:*104–113, Feb 15, '32

BOURGUET, J.: *La véritable chirurgie esthétique du visage*. Librairie Plon, Paris, 1936

BOURGUET, J.: Plastic surgery for Hutchinson's facies and various accompanying ptoses. Monde med., Paris *49:*659–667, June 15, '39

BOURGUET, J.: Plastic surgery in abnormalities of direction, convolution and flexion of external ear. Monde med., Paris *41:*483–492, April 1, '31

BOURGUET, J.: Plastic surgery of different parts of face. Cong. internat. de med. trop. et d'hyg., Compt. rend (1928)

BOURGUET, J.: Plastic surgery of eyelid ptosis. Monde med., Paris *42:*962–971, Nov 15, '32

BOURGUET, J.: Special technic for surgical correction of hypertrophy of breast. Bull. et mem. Soc. de med. de Paris *140:*411–417, June 27, '36

BOURGUET, J.: Surgical correction of deformities of external ear; 3 cases. Bull. et mem. Soc. de med. de Paris *137:*656–659, Dec 8, '33

BOURGUET, J.: Surgical therapy of abnormalities of external ear. Bull. Acad. de med., Paris *109:*602–604, April 25, '33

BOURGUET, J.: Surgical therapy of prognathism; bicondyloid resection and section of ascending branch of lower jaw; cases. Rev. de stomatol. *37:*152–169, March '35

BOURGUET, J.: Treatment of eyelid abnormalities by plastic surgery. Monde med., Paris *39:*725–731, July 1, '29

BOURGUET, J.: Treatment of facial wrinkles; 17 photographs. Monde med., Paris *38:*41–51, Jan 15, '28

BOURGUET, M.: Surgical therapy of prognathism; Jaboulay method of bicondyloid resection; Lane method in section of ascending branch of lower jaw. Rev. de stomatol. *35:*61–79, Feb '33

Bourguet Operation

- Dupuy-Dutemps and Bourguet's plastic dacryocystorhinostomy in chronic dacryocystitis. HUSSON, A. AND JEANDELIZE, P. Medecine *5:*256–259, Jan '24
- Surgical relief of chronic dacryocystitis and epiphora; Dupuy-Dutemps et Bourguet technique; direct anastomosis of tear sac with nasal mucous membrane. CORBETT, J. J. M. J. and Rec. *128:*158–160, Aug 15, '28 also: New England J. Med. *199:* 459–461, Sept 6, '28 also: Am. J. Ophth. *11:*774–778, Oct '28
- Dupuy-Dutemps and Bourguet technic in dacryocystotomy. BARBEROUSSE. Bull. Soc. d'opht. de Paris, p. 226, March '31
- Dacryocystorhinostomy according to plastic procedure of Bourguet-Dupuy-Dutemps. VANCEA, P. Rev. san. mil., Bucuresti *35:*393–395, April '36

BOURGUIGNON (see DUJARIER, C.) April '27

BOURGUIGNON, G. (see CROUZON, O. *et al*) June '32

BOURGUIGNON, G.: Iontophoresis in treatment of deforming or adherent scars. Paris med. *2:*515–520, Dec 20, '24 abstr: J.A.M.A. *84:*404, Jan 31, '25

BOURGUIGNON, G.: Late result of hypoglossofacial anastomosis: inadaptation of centers. Rev. neurol. *73:*601–603, Nov–Dec '41

BOUROULLEC, (see FRANCAIS) March '38

BOUTAREAU (see HUARD, P.) Dec '35

BOUTROUX (see PONROY, *et al*) Nov '27

BOUTROUX (see PONROY, *et al*) Sept '28

BOUYSSET (see LAROYENNE) Feb '27

BOUYSSOU (see CADENAT *et al*) Oct–Dec '45

BOVE, C.: Shock. M. Rec. *155:*463–466, Oct '42

BOVE, C.: Suturing of flexor tendons (transfixation) in hand. M. Rec. *153:*94, Feb 5, '41

BOVE, C.: War burns. New York State J. Med. *42:*1366–1370, July 15, '42

BOVENSIEPEN, F. G.: Surgical therapy of furunculosis. Zentralbl. f. Chir. *68:*909–912, May 17, '41

BOWEN, A.: Development and surgical applications of absorbable tubular membrane; preliminary report. Am. J. Surg. *34:*122–124, Oct '36

Bowen, F. H.: Branchial fistulae, 2 cases. J. Florida M. A. *27:*500–502, April '41
Bowen, W. W.: Epithelioma of face. J. Iowa M. Soc. *14:*154–157, April '24
Bower, R. L.: Maxillofacial injuries. J. Missouri M. A. *34:*448–449, Dec '37
Bowers, V. H. (see Gordon, R. A.) Oct '42
Bowers, W. F.: Nature and treatment of shock. Mil. Surgeon *89:*41–48, July '41
Bowler, R. G. (see Crooke, A. C. *et al*) Nov '44
Boyce, F. F.: Hepatic (hepatorenal) factor in burns. Arch. Surg. *44:*799–818, May '42
Boyce, F. F.: Human bites of hand; analysis of 90 (chiefly delayed and late) cases from Charity Hospital of Louisiana at New Orleans. South. M. J. *35:*631–638, July '42
Boyce, W. A.: Splint for unusual break of face. Laryngoscope *36:*266–269, April '26
Boyd, G. L. (see Robertson, B.) Feb '23
Boyd, G. L. (see Robertson, B.) Oct '23
Boyd, H. M. E.: Congenital atresia of posterior nares; descriptions of technics used in meeting operative difficulties and report of case. Arch. Otolaryng. *41:*261–271, April '45
Boyd, J. E.: Cancer of lip, resulting deformity, plastic repair. J. Florida M. A. *12:*27–29, Aug '25
Boyd, W.: Tumors and cysts of neck. Tr. West. S. A. (1938) *48:*172–182, '39
Boyd, W. C. (see Malkiel, S.) Aug '46
Boyden, R. C. (see Ebert, E. C.) Oct '38
Boyer, B. E. (see Good, R. W.) Feb '32
Boyer, B. E.: Reconstruction of lip after cancer. J. Med. *20:*543–544, Feb '40

Boyer Operation: See Heitz-Boyer-Hovelacque Operation
Boyer Operation: See Marion-Heitz-Boyer Operation

Boyes, J. H. (see Bunnell, S.) April '39
Boykin, I. M.: Lymphangioma of axilla and upper lip. S. Clin. N. Amer. *9:*1229–1230, Oct '29
Boyle, H. E. G.: Combined gag and tongue retractor. Lancet *2:*1130, Nov 25, '22 (illus.)
Boyle, Horace H.: *Theory and Treatment of Fractures of the Jaws in Peace and War.* Henry Kimpton, London, 1940. C. V. Mosby Co., St. Louis, 1941
Boyne, H. N.: Correcting deformities of velum and mesopharynx to insure better speech following cleft palate surgery. Nebraska M. J. *19:*407–409, Nov '34
Boyne, H. N.: Early care of facial injuries. Nebraska M. J. *28:*111–113, April '43
Bozzini, M.: Extirpation of small sebaceous cysts. Rev. med. del Rosario *25:*800–805, July '35
Braasch, W. F. (see Walters, W.) Feb '34
Bracco, J. A. and d'Albo, E. A.: Amygdaloid cysts; clinical, surgical and histologic study. (neck) Prensa med. argent. *30:*2058–2067, Oct 27, '43
Brachetto-Brian, D. (see Rodríguez Villegas, R.) Oct '30
Brachetto-Brian, D.: Amygdaloid cysts and tumors; origin, structure and classification of vestigial formations in neck. Prensa med. argent. *18:*1177–1187, Feb 10, '32
Bradbeer, W. H.: Skin grafting in operations of the frontal sinus. J. Laryng. and Otol. *59:*36–37, Jan '44
Bradburn, M.: Tendon reconstruction. S. Clin. N. America *2:*1363–1365, Oct '22 (illus.)
Bradford, C. H. (see Cotton, F. J. *et al*) July '38
Bradford, F. K. and Livingston, K. E.: Failure in early secondary repair of cranial defects with tantalum. J. Neurosurg. *3:*318–328, July '46
Bradley, J. L. (see Christiansen, G. W.) May '45
Bradley, J. L. (see Christiansen, G. W.) July '45
Bradley, R. A. and Snoke, P. O.: Treatment of advanced carcinoma of skin of face with radium. S. Clin. N. Amer. *7:*165–168, Feb '27
Bradley, R. M.: Aneurysm of palmar arteries; case. Mil. Surgeon *97:*486–489, Dec '45
Bradshaw, T. L.: Compound, comminuted fracture of both maxillae and mandible. Internat. J. Orthodontia *21:*260–262, March '35
Brady, L.: Methods of constructing vagina. Ann. Surg. *121:*518–519, April '45
Brady, L.: Methods of construction of artificial vagina. Tr. South. S. A. (1944) *56:*134–145, '45
Braendstrup, P.: Fractures in zygomatic region. Nord. med. (Hospitalstid.) *7:*1527–1534, Sept 14, '40
Bragagnolo, J. (see Marottoli, O. R.) July '44
Bragman, L. J.: Progressive facial hemiatrophy; early case. Arch. Pediat. *52:*686–688, Oct '35
Braimbridge, C. V.: Cyst of neck; case. East Africa M. J. *14:*393–395, March '38
Braimbridge, C. V.: Fracture of terminal phalanx of finger. Brit. M. J. *1:*838, May 27, '22
Braimbridge, C. V.: Surgical notes on burn therapy. East African M. J. *20:*93–95, March '43
Braine, J.: Case of total phlegmon of left hand flexors; antibrachiopalmar incision; recovery with remarkable functional restitution. Bull. et mem. Soc. nat. de chir. *54:*524–529, April 7, '28

BRAITHWAITE, J. V. C.: Case of hypertelorism described, relation of hypertelorism to mongolism. Arch. Dis. Childhood *1:*369-372, Dec '26

BRAITHWAITE, L. R.: Unusual case of congenital naevus of forefinger and thumb. Brit. J. Surg. *14:*538-540, Jan '27

BRAKE, B. S.: Artificial penis. West Virginia M. J. *41:*45-47, Feb '45

BRAKELEY, E.: Exstrophy of bladder complicated by other congenital anomalies. Am. J. Dis. Child. *43:*931-935, April '32

BRAMBILLA, A. (see VES LOSADA, C.) April '37

BRANCH, C. D.; WILKINS, G. F. AND ROSS, F. P.: Coagulum contact method (Sano) of skin grafting. Surgery *19:*460-466, April '46

BRANCH, H. E.: Extensive burns; treatment with silver nitrate and methyl rosaniline. Arch. Surg. *35:*478-485, Sept '37

BRANCH, J. L.: Hand infections. J.M.A. Alabama *5:*1-3, July '35

Branchial Cysts and Fistulas (See also: Lateral Cervical Fistula)

- Branchial fistulae; with report of surgical case. MILLER, L. I. Colorado Med. *18:*110, May '21
- Branchial cysts and fistulas. GILMAN, P. K. J.A.M.A. *77:*26, July 2, '21
- Clinical aspects of branchial cysts. BAILEY, H. Brit. J. Surg. *10:*565-572, April '23 (illus.)
- Branchial fistulas of neck. BECKER, J. Beitr. z. klin. Chir. *134:*470-472, '25
- Branchial cysts. CROW, I. N. J. Iowa M. Soc. *15:*524-528, Oct '25
- Cysts and fistulas of lateral branchial canal. REINECKE, R. Arch. f. klin. Chir. *136:*99-108, '25
- Congenital complete branchiogenetic cyst and duct. MEYER, H. W. Am. J. Surg. *40:*121, May '26
- Branchial fistula; its clinical relation to irritation of vagus. CARP, L. Surg., Gynec. and Obst. *42:*772-777, June '26
- Congenital lymphoid cysts in lateral portion of neck. SOUBEIRAN, M. Arch. franco-belges de chir. *29:*514-521, June '26
- Branchial cyst. SEED, L. S. Clin. N. Amer. *6:*1029-1031, Aug '26
- Branchial cysts and fistulae; report of 5 cases. JOHNSON, J. A. Minnesota Med. *9:*514-517, Sept '26
- Deep branchiogenous cysts in right side of neck. ANARDI, T. Tumori *12:*217-225, '26
- Branchial cyst; case. THOMSON, J. W. Lancet *1:*76, Jan 8, '27
- Branchiogenic tumors of neck. BELK, W. P. S. Clin. N. Amer. *7:*453-468, April '27

Branchial Cysts and Fistulas – Cont.

- Branchial fistula. BAILEY, H. Clin. J. *56:*619, Dec 28, '27
- Pedigree of anomalies in first and second branchial cleft, inherited according to laws of Mendel, and contribution to technique of extirpation of congenital lateral fistulae coli. PŘECECHTĚL, A. Acta oto-laryng. *11:*23-30, '27
- Anomalies and neoplasms of branchial apparatus; 32 cases with follow-up results. CARP, L. AND STOUT, A. P. Ann. Surg. *87:*186-209, Feb '28
- Hereditary transmission of branchial fistulas; case. STARKENSTEIN, E. Med. Klin. *24:*701, May 4, '28
- Diagnosis of branchial cyst, with note upon its removal. BAILEY, H. Brit. M. J. *1:*940-941, June 2, '28
- Nasopharyngeal cyst of branchial origin; case. GIUSSANI, M. Ann. di laring., otol. *29:*213-226, July '28
- Branchial cysts and fistulae. FAGGE, C. H. Clin. J. *57:*421-423, Sept 5, '28
- Lateral and internal cysts and fistula of neck. TOMILOFF, N. L. Vestnik khir. (nos. 43-44) *14:*234-237, '28
- Clinical manifestations of branchial cysts. WAKELEY, C. P. G. Clin. J. *58:*109-111, March 6, '29
- Complete congenital branchial fistula. BARAJAS Y DE VILCHES, J. M. Siglo med. *84:*85-86, July 27, '29
- Branchial cysts of parotid gland. CUNNINGHAM, W. F. Ann. Surg. *90:*114-117, July '29
- Simple method of dealing with congenital branchial fistulae. LOVE, R. J. M. Lancet *2:*122, July 20, '29
- Lateral branchial cysts of neck. BOSDEVEIX, G. L. Ann. d. mal. de l'oreille, du larynx *48:*826-842, Aug '29
- Embryologic origin and pathologic changes to which the branchial apparatus gives rise, with presentation of familial group of fistulas. HYNDMAN, O. R. AND LIGHT, G. Arch. Surg. *19:*410-452, Sept '29
- Branchiogenetic cyst of larynx removed by thyrotomy. IMPERATORI, C. J. Laryngoscope *39:*679-683, Oct '29
- Congenital branchial fistula; cases. DEBEYRE, A. AND SALEZ. Echo m. du nord *33:*541-544, Nov 16, '29
- Branchial anomalies. SWEET, P. W. Tr. A. Resid. and ex-Resid. Physicians, Mayo Clin. (1928) *9:*94-103, '29
- Pathologic changes, with presentation of familial group of branchial fistulas. HYND-

Branchial Cysts and Fistulas—Cont.

MAN, O. R. AND LIGHT, G. J. Iowa M. Soc. *20:*260–262, June '30
Patent branchial cleft. JOHNS, A. H. G. Brit. M. J. *1:*1047, June 7, '30
Operative technic in congenital branchial fistulas. ESTELLA, J. AND MORALES, L. Arch. de med., cir. y espec. *33:*73–84, July 26, '30
Successful surgical treatment of large suppurative cyst of second branchial cleft; case. BÁRÁNY, R. Acta oto-laryng. *14:*556–559, '30
Branchiogenic anomalies (cysts and fistulas) associated with larynx. ROSENAUER, F. Deutsche Ztschr. f. Chir. *226:*304–307, '30
Branchial cysts. VASSILIEFF, A. I. Vestnik khir. (nos. 58–60) *20:*181–187, '30
Branchiogenous cyst with postoperative recurrence; recovery after iodine injection; case. SCHWERS, H. Liege med. (supp.) *24:*1–4, Feb 8, '31
Differentiation of branchial from other cervical cysts by x-ray examination. WANGENSTEEN, O. H. Ann. Surg. *93:*790–792, March '31
Double branchial cysts complicated by carcinoma of larynx. HERMAN, A. L. Minnesota Med. *14:*555–557, June '31
Ambulant treatment of branchial fistulas. KLEINSCHMIDT, O. Deutsche med. Wchnschr. *57:*1549–1551, Sept 4, '31
Similarity of certain tuberculous cervical abscesses and branchial cysts. BAILEY, H. Brit. J. Tuberc. *25:*167–170, Oct '31
Developmental abnormalities of second branchial slit. PŘECECHTĚL, A. Otolaryng. slavica *3:*437–449, Oct '31
Cysts and fistulae (branchial). SHEDDEN, W. M. New England J. Med. *205:*800–811, Oct 22, '31
Branchial cyst. SCHWARTZ, L. JR. New York State J. Med. *31:*1376–1377, Nov. 15, '31
Plastic reconstruction of intestinal branchial apparatus and its derivatives in human embryos. BRUNI, A. C. Monitore zool. ital. (supp.) *41:*196–199, 1930–1931
Tumors of hyo-thyro-pharyngeal region; laryngocele and branchial cyst. VAN DEN WILDENBERG, L. Scalpel *85:*265–271, Feb 27, '32
Cervicofacial branchiomas. SOUBEIRAN, M. Arch. franco-belges de chir. *33:*542–554, June '32
Origin of cysts, fistulas and tumors of lateral region of neck. ROSSANO, I. Rev. de path. comparee *32:*951, Sept; 1127, Oct '32
Clinical and pathologic aspects of branchiogenic cysts. RUTTIN, E. Monatschr. f. Ohrenh. *66:*1111–1114, Sept '32

Branchial Cysts and Fistulas—Cont.

Branchial fistulas in children. KETELBANT. Scalpel *85:*1433–1435, Nov 26, '32
Occurrence of branchial cysts in neck; case. KOCH, F. Monatschr. f. Ohrenh. *66:*1331–1334, Nov '32
Origin of cysts, fistulas and tumors of lateral region of neck. ROSSANO, I. Rev. de path. comparee *32:*1269–1307, Nov '32
Cysts and fistulas of lateral region of neck. KOLKMAN, D. Nederl. tijdschr. v. geneesk. *77:*862–865, Feb 25, '33
Branchial cyst with dermic steatonecrosis; case. BANET, V. AND BOLAÑOS, J. M. Bol. Liga contra el cancer *8:*97–104, April '33
Branchial cysts and fistulas in children. also: thyroglossal duct cysts and fistulas. BAUMGARTNER, C. J. Surg., Gynec. and Obst. *56:*948–955, May '33
Fistulized preauricular branchial fibrochondroma; case. JACOD, M. Lyon med. *151:*613–615, May 14, '33
Lateral cyst of neck; surgical removal followed by development of malignant branchioma; clinical and pathologic study. PAGLIANI, F. Bull. d. sc. med., Bologna *105:*405–428, Sept-Oct '33
Clinical aspects of branchial fistula. BAILEY, H. Brit. J. Surg. *21:*173–182, Oct '33
Branchial fistula. KLEINERT, M. N. Arch. Otolaryng. *18:*510–515, Oct '33
Cystic tumors of neck; branchial and thyroglossal cysts. MCNEALY, R. W. S. Clin. North America *13:*1083–1100, Oct '33
Branchial fistulas; treatment with sclerosing fluids; case presentation and report. ROBITSHEK, E. C. Minnesota Med. *16:*760–762, Dec '33
Branchial cyst; 2 instructive cases. BERRY, G. Ann. Otol., Rhin. and Laryng. *43:*287–293, March '34
Cervical branchioma; 3 cases. TRUFFERT, P. Bull. et mem. Soc. nat. de chir. *60:*602–611, May 5, '34
Branchiogenic tumors; surgical therapy. MOLLÁ, V. M. Cron. med., Valencia *38:*501–509, July 15, '34
Branchiogenic cysts of neck; 2 cases. NISHIMURA, I. Okayama-Igakkai-Zasshi *47:*235, Jan '35
Branchiogenetic or branchial fistulae. MACGUIRE, D. P. Am. Med. *41:*324–327, June '35
Branchial and thyroglossal duct cysts and fistulas. BROWN, J. M. Ann. Otol., Rhin. and Laryng. *44:*644–652, Sept '35
Branchial fistula; case. PARISEAU, L. J. de l'Hotel-Dieu de Montreal *4:*276–283, Nov '35

Branchial Cysts and Fistulas – Cont.

Fistulas of first branchial arch. JOSA, L. Zentralbl. f. Chir. *63:*1760–1763, July 25, '36
Fistulas of first branchial arch. JOSA, L. Orvosi hetil. *80:*973–974, Oct 10, '36
Branchial cysts. OCHSNER, C. G. Minnesota Med. *20:*31–33, Jan '37
Relation of tonsil to branchiogenetic cysts. MEEKER, L. H. Laryngoscope *47:*164–183, March '37
Branchiogenic cysts in infancy. BECK, W. C. Surgery *1:*792–799, May '37
Branchiogenetic cysts. LARSON, E. California and West. Med. *47:*244–248, Oct '37
True branchiogenic cyst and fistula of neck. MEYER, H. W. Arch. Surg. *35:*766–771, Oct '37
Congenital branchiogenic anomalies; 82 cases. LADD, W. E. AND GROSS, R. E. Am. J. Surg. *39:*234–248, Feb '38
Congenital branchial cyst of floor of mouth; case. CHAVES, D. A. Rev. med.-cir. do Brasil *46:*620–626, May '38
Branchial cyst; case. MASI, C. AND MARINI, J. Semana med. *1:*1061–1062, May 12, '38
Therapy of congenital branchial fistulas. NYLANDER, P. E. A. Zentralbl. f. Chir. *65:*1095–1097, May 7, '38
Lateral or branchial cysts of neck; 13 cases. JACKSON, A. S. Wisconsin M. J. *37:*641–646, Aug '38
Amygdaloid branchial cyst of neck; embryologic considerations. BISI, R. H. AND EMILIANI, C. M. Rev. Assoc. med. argent. *52:*935–937, Sept 15, '38
Problems of congenital origin of lateral fistulas and cysts of neck. MARX, J. Beitr. z. klin. Chir. *168:*435–447, '38 also: Orvosi hetil. *82:*891–895, Sept 10, '38
Congenital cyst of right lateral cervical region developed from lateral vestiges of "cervical sinus." BARGE, P. Ann. d'anat. path. *15:*1025–1031, Dec '38
Bilateral congenital branchial fistulas; case. DUMALLE, G. AND HOUOT, A. Ann. Fac. franc. de med. et de pharm. de Beyrouth *7:*129–133, '38
Branchial cyst; case. KASARCOGLU. Turk tib cem. mec. *4:*182–183, '38
Congenital lateral neck cyst; case. TAKAHARA, T. AND WATANABE, D. Oto-rhino-laryng. *12:*44–45, Jan '39
Branchial cysts; with report of 2 cases of cyst of cervical sinus. MALCOLM, R. B. AND BENSON, R. E. Surgery *7:*187–203, Feb '40
Branchiogenous cysts and cystadenolymphomas. BIANCHI, A. E. AND PAVLOVSKY, A. An. Inst. modelo de clin. med. *21:*436–452, '40

Branchial Cysts and Fistulas – Cont.

Septic branchial cyst eradicated by electrical cauterization; case. BERGE, C. A. J. Michigan M. Soc. *40:*189–191, March '41
Branchial fistulae, 2 cases. BOWEN, F. H. J. Florida M. A. *27:*500–502, April '41
Branchial cysts and sinuses. LAHEY, F. H. AND NELSON, H. F. Ann. Surg. *113:*508–512, April '41
Clinical conditions arising from anomalies or maldevelopments of branchial arches and clefts. HOOVER, W. B. Ann. Otol., Rhin. and Laryng. *50:*834–849, Sept '41
Branchial cysts; 2 cases. PONTES, A. Brasil-med. *55:*610–614, Sept 6, '41
Branchial fistula; case. ARTHUR, H. R. Brit. J. Surg. *29:*440–441, April '42
Bilocular branchiogenic cyst of neck; case. FERNICOLA, C. Bol. Soc. de cir. de Rosario *9:*511–519, Sept '42
Clinical aspects of branchial fistulas, with case report of bilateral complete fistulas. ANDERSON, E. R. Minnesota Med. *25:*789–795, Oct '42
Relation of precervical sinus and branchial clefts. CORDIER, G. AND DELMAS, A. Bull. Acad. de med., Paris *126:*485–486, Oct 27–Nov 10, '42
Cystic tumors; branchial and thyroglossal cysts. MCNEALY, R. W. J. Am. Dent. A. *29:*1808–1818, Oct 1, '42
Cervicolaryngeal cyst of branchial orgin; case. MARTIN CALDERIN, A. Semana med. espan. *6:*91, Jan 23, '43
Lymphoepithelial papilliferous cystomas of branchial, thyroglossal and thyropharyngeal origin. LUPPI, J. E. Rev. med. de Rosario *33:*608–623, July '43
Complications in diabetic; nodular thyroid and branchial cleft fistulas. WARTHEN, H. J. AND JORDAN, W. R. South. M. J. *36:*536–537, July '43
Cervical lesions of branchial origin. SOMMER, G. N. J. JR.; *et al*. Am. J. Surg. *61:*266–270, Aug '43
Branchial dermoepidermic cysts, with report of cases. PUENTE DUANY, N. Arch. cubanos cancerol. *3:*133–156, April–June '44
Branchiogenic malformations of neck region. LADEWIG, P. AND SERT, D. Schweiz. Ztschr. f. Path. u. Bakt. *7:*1–12, '44
Bilateral branchial cleft cysts. BOLMAN, R. M. Am. J. Surg. *71:*96–99, Jan '46
Branchial cysts of lateral cervical region. VAN CANEGHEM, D. Belg. tijdschr. geneesk. *2:*236–246, May '46
Treatment of branchial cleft cysts by aspiration and injection of pure carbolic acid

Branchial Cysts and Fistulas – Cont.

(phenol). JARMAN, T. F. Brit. M. J. *1:*953-954, June 22, '46

Branchiogenic cyst of right carotid region; case of difficult diagnosis. CABALLERO, A. AND TORTI, D. D. Rev. med.-quir. de pat. fem. *25:*283-291, July '46

BRANCHINI, C.: Mandibular fracture; symptomatology, evolution and outcome in case involving teeth. Arch. ital. di chir. *50:*595-600, '38

BRANDENBURG, E.: Avulsion fracture of flexor side of terminal phalanx of left little finger. Zentralbl. f. Chir. *58:*1065-1067, April 25, '31

BRANDES, W. W.; WHITE, W. C. AND SUTTON, J. B.: Accidental transplantation of cancer (in skin of donor site) in operation room, with case report. Dia med. *18:*153-154, Feb 25, '46 also: Surg. Gynec. and Obst. *82:*212-214, Feb '46

BRANDI, B.: Treatment of fractures, ischemic contractures, cicatricial contractures and nerve injuries to fingers. Chirurg *3:*263-269, March 15, '31

BRANDSON, B. J. AND HILLSMAN, J. A.: Use of fluids in burns and shock. Canad. M. A. J. *26:*689-698, June '32

BRANDT: Application to study of human constitution, of biological laws discovered by transplantation of extremities. Verhandl. d. anat. Gesellsch. *37:*38-41, '28

BRANDT, G.: New operation for epispadias. Arch. f. klin. Chir. *183:*607-610, '35

BRANSFIELD, J. W. (see DORRANCE, G. M.) Feb '22

BRANSFIELD, J. W. (see DORRANCE, G. M.) April '23

BRANSFIELD, J. W. (see DORRANCE, G. M.) Oct '23

BRANSFIELD, J. W. (see DORRANCE, G. M.) Nov '42

BRANSFIELD, J. W. (see DORRANCE, G. M.) Jan '43

BRANSFIELD, J. W.: Surgical reconstruction of nose. Atlantic M. J. *27:*637-640, July '24

BRANTIGAN, O. C. AND HEBB, D.: Compression treatment of burns. Bull. School Med. Univ. Maryland *28:*12-20, July '43

BRATTSTRÖM, E.: Case operated according to method of Maydl-Borelius (exstrophy of bladder). Acta chir. Scandinav. *55:*33-37, '22 (illus.; in English) abstr: J.A.M.A. *79:*1562, Oct 28, '22

BRATTSTRÖM, E.: Maydl-Borelius operation for exstrophy of bladder. Beitr. z. klin. Chir. *127:*419-421, '22 Abstr: J.A.M.A. *80:*364, Feb 3, '23

BRATU, I. (see CONSTANTINESCO, M.) Sept-Oct '40

BRAUN, A. A. AND ORLOVA, G. N.: Experiments on heterotopic transplantation of skin. Compt. rend. Acad. d. sc. URSS *47:*138-139, April 20, '45

BRAUN, K.: Typical combination of congenital abnormalities of hand and foot. Ztschr. f. menschl. Vererb.-u. Konstitutionslehre *23:*510-515, '39

BRAUN, W.: Skin grafts. Med. Klin. *17:*398, April 3, '21

BRAUN, W.: Ultimate outcome of skin grafts. Med. Klinik *20:*1383-1385, Oct 5, '24 abstr: J.A.M.A. *83:*1628, Nov 15, '24

Braun's Operation

Braun's skin grafting after amputations. LIHOTZKY. Med. Klin. *22:*1757-1758, Nov 12, '26

Operation for ptosis of eyelids. BRAUNSTEIN, E.P. Arch. f. Ophth. *116:*452-456, '26

Therapy of acute infections of hand and forearm. BRAVO GARCÍA, R. Med. latina *6:*375-394, Aug '33

BREA, C. A. AND CASTRO O'CONNOR, R.: Vaginal aplasia (complete absence); formation of new vagina by McIndoe technic. Bol. y trab., Acad. argent. de cir. *30:*313-326, June 19, '46

BREA, M. M.: Diagnosis and treatment of hand infections. Dia med. *3:*357, Nov 24, '30

Breasts (See also: Gynecomastia; Mammaplasty, Various Divisions)

Abdominal flap to cover defect after mammectomy. SOUPAULT, R. Presse med. *31:*177-178, Feb 24, '23 (illus.)

Congenital absence of pectoralis muscles and of right mammary gland. SZCZAWINSKA, W. Nourrisson *11:*187-190, May '23 (illus.)

Abdominal skin flap after amputation of breast. HEIDENHAIN, L. Zentralbl. f. Gynak. *48:*2649-2650, Nov 29, '24

Plastic covering of large defects following breast amputation. GRUCA, A. Zentralbl. f. Chir. *54:*1293-1297, May 21, '27

Plastic covering of defects following breast amputation. KRAFT, R. Deutsche Ztschr. f. Chir. *207:*171-183, '27

Indications and advantages of areolar incision in breast surgery. DUFOURMENTEL, L. Bull. et mem. Soc. de chir. de Paris *20:*9-14, Jan 6, '28

Atypical epithelial proliferation of transplanted mammary tissue. POLISSADOWA, X. AND BJELOSOR, I. Virchows Arch. f. path. Anat. *272:*759-762, '29

Breasts–Cont.

Technic of complete operation on breast. BARTLETT, E. I. Surg., Gynec. and Obst. *52:*71–78, Jan '31

Total mastoneoplasty following amputation of breast. REINHARD, W. Deutsche Ztschr. f. Chir. *236:*309–317, '32

Plastic removal of skin from breast as aid in treating scars on breast and neck resulting from burns; case. BREITFUSS, F. F. Zentralbl. f. Chir. *61:*436–437, Feb 24, '34

Routes of access in reparative surgery of breast. CLAOUE. Bull. et mem. Soc. de med. de Paris *139:*205–212, March 23, '35

Cicatrix in reparative surgery of breast. CLAOUE, C. AND BERNARD, MME. I. J. de med. de Bordeaux *113:*695–697, Oct 10, '36

Late results after transplantation of mammary gland in closure of facial defect. IGNATEV, S. S. Vestnik khir. *47:*103, '36

Pedicle breast flap for amputation-stump; structive surgery applied to amputation stump at knee. ESSER, J. F. S. Ann. Surg. *105:*469–472, March '37

Use of skin of female breast in plastic surgery. ESSER, J. F. S. Brit. M. J. *2:*1256–1257, Dec 17, '38

Arteries of mammary gland; importance in esthetic surgery; anatomic and roentgenographic study. SALMON, M. Ann. d'anat. path. *16:*477–500, April '39

Method for closure of operative wound in cancer of breast; skin grafting. KOROLEV, B. A. Novy khir. arkhiv. *46:*48–51, '40

Latex prosthesis for cosmetic restoration of amputated breast. BROWN, A. M. South. Surgeon *11:*181–188, March '42

Attempted plastic surgery in extirpation of breast cancer. ROFFO, A. E. Bol. Inst. de med. exper. para el estud. y trat. d. cancer *21:*163–179, April '44

Prosthetic restorations of breast; technic using sponge rubber. BROWN, A. M. Arch. Surg. *48:*388–394, May '44

Breast tissue as new source for heterogenous implants; preliminary report. LA ROE, E. K. Am. J. Surg. *66:*58–67, Oct '44

Free transplant of areola preliminary to amputation of breast for benign tumor; free fat graft; case. ZENO, L. An. de cir. *10:*190–194, Sept-Dec '44

Skin transposition in incisional defects; modification of Z plastic for primary skin closure following extensive breast surgery. SINAIKO, E. S. Surgery *18:*650–652, Nov '45

Partial or total mammectomy by simple or enlarged areolar route. CABANIE, G. Paris med. *2:*373–375, Aug 24, '46; abstr: Mem. Acad. de chir. *72:*68, Feb 6–20, '46

Breasts–Cont.

Darier's fibrosarcoma on scar of human bite on male breast; case. SYLVESTRE BEGNIS, C. AND PICENA, J. P. Rev. med. de Rosario *36:*233–239, May '46

Breasts, Atrophy

Postpartum traumatic gynatresia, 2 cases. GARCIA BIRD, J. Bol. Asoc. med. de Puerto Rico *37:*205–207, June '45

Breasts, Augmentation: See Mammaplasty, Augmentation

Breasts, Cancer

Accidental autogenous transplantation of mammary carcinoma to thigh during skin graft operation; case. SPIES, J. W.; *et al.* Am. J. Cancer *20:*606–609, March '34

Unusual metastatic manifestations of breast cancer: metastasis to mandible, with report of 5 cases. ADAIR, F. E. AND HERRMANN, J. B. Surg. Gynec. and Obst. *83:*289–295, Sept '46

Breasts, Deformity

Unilateral symbrachydactylia with defect of thoracic wall and amastia; case. STÖHR, F. J. Ztschr. f. Morphol. u. Anthrop. *26:*384–390, '27

Anisomastia (unilateral hyperplasia) of breast. DE ANGELIS, E. AND ALTSCHUL, R. Deutsche Ztschr. f. Nervenh. *112:*165–176, '30

Unilateral surgical correction of asymmetric breasts. BIESENBERGER, H. Wien. med. Wchnschr. *82:*732–733, June 4, '32

Unilateral amastia; case. FABRE, M. Bull. Soc. franc. de dermat. et syph. (Reunion dermat., Lyon) *40:*1072–1074, July '33

Monolateral amastia; case. PUTZU DONEDDU, F. Arch. di ostet. e ginec. *41:*1–13, Jan '34

Asymmetrical deformities of breast. MALINIAK, J. W. Ann. Surg. *99:*743–752, May '34

Plastic surgical therapy of dystrophy of breast. MONTANT. Tech. chir. *27:*155–164, Oct '35

Surgical therapy of breast abnormalities. DARTIGUES, L. Bull. et mem. Soc. de med. de Paris *139:*575–569, Nov 7, '35

Breast deformities; anatomic and physiologic considerations in plastic repair. MALINIAC, J. W. Am. J. Surg. *39:*54–61, Jan '38

Breast malformations and suggestions for treatment. KAPP, J. F. M. Rec. *147:*252–253, March 16, '38

Malformations of mammary glands and their

Breasts, Deformity—Cont.

surgical correction. HEIJL, C. Hygiea (Festband) *100:*118-127, '38

Breasts, Hypertrophy

Hypertrophy of mammary gland. BLOND, K. Med. Klin. *17:*497, April 24, '21
Bilateral hypertrophy of breasts. MARQUES, A. Brazil-med. *35:*129, Sept. 17, '21
Massive hypertrophy of breast. KEYSER, L. D. Surg., Gynec. and Obst. *33:*607, Dec '21
Puberal mammary hypertrophy. GREIG, D. M. Edinburgh M. J. *28:*153-167, April '22 (illus.)
Hyperplasia of breast. NITTER, H. Norsk Mag. f. Laegevidensk. *83:*673-677, Sept '22 (illus.) abstr: J.A.M.A. *79:*1730, Nov 11, '22
Diffuse hypertrophy of mamma at puberty. HEYN, A. Zentralbl. f. Gynak. *47:*263-265, Feb 17, '23 (illus.)
Hypertrophy of breasts at puberty. TOURNEUX, J. P. Rev. franc. de gynec. et d'obstet. *18:*454-459, July 10-25, '23
Brachial hypotony and hypertrophy of mamma. CALLIGARIS, G. Rev. neurol. *2:*365-377, Oct '23 (illus.)
Case of diffuse hypertrophy of breast. GHOSH, N. Indian M. Gaz. *61:*395-396, Aug '26
Massive hypertrophy of breasts. PLUMMER, S. C. AND BUMP, W. S. Ann. Surg. *85:*61-66, Jan '27
Massive hypertrophy of breast; 2 cases. BROHEE, G. Arch. franco-belges de chir. *31:*451-468, June '28
Diffuse hypertrophy of breast during pregnancy; case. RAMÍREZ OLIVELLA, J. Rev. med. cubana *41:*131-137, Feb '30
Macromastia in girl of 17; case. MELO, N. L. Rev. med. veracruzana *11:*238-240, Feb 1, '31
Diffuse hypertrophy of breasts in girl aged 17. WAKELEY, C. P. G. Tr. M. Soc. London *54:*146-148, '31
Massive breast enlargement. GREENWOOD, H. H. Lancet *1:*232-234, Jan 30, '32
Bilateral hypertrophy of breasts treated by x-rays. LAIRD, A. H. Brit. J. Radiol. *5:*249, March '32
Diffuse breast hypertrophy; preliminary case report. BURNELL, M. J. Michigan M. Soc. *31:*324-325, May '32
Breast hypertrophies and hypoplasias. KAPP, J. F. Fortschr. d. Med. *50:*652-654, Aug 5, '32
Congenital pendulous hypertrophic breasts in female twins; case. BIRKENFELD, W. Arch. f. klin. Chir. *168:*568-576, '32
Massive hypertrophy of breast in puerperium. FERRO, A. Riv. d'ostet. e ginec. prat. *15:*198-203, May '33
Massive diffuse breast hypertrophy in girls; 4 cases. WAKELEY, C. P. G. Practitioner *132:*608-613, May '34
Mastitis gargantuan; unusual case of puberty hypertrophy. GOODMAN, B. A. J.A.M.A. *103:*335-336, Aug 4, '34
Massive puberty hypertrophy of breast. GAINES, J. A. Am. J. Obst. and Gynec. *34:*130-136, July '37
Hypertrophy of breasts. GESCHICKTER, C. F. Surgery *3:*916-949, June '38
Giant breast; case. KARUBE, R. AND KOJIMA, K. J. Orient. Med. (Abst. Sect) *30:*272, June '39
Supernumerary nipples. Congenital hemihypertrophy and congenital hemiatrophy of breast. LANDAUER, W. Human Biol. *11:*447-472, Dec '39
Massive hypertrophy breast (approximate weight 35 pounds) in adolescence; notable case. FISHER, G. A.; *et al.* West. J. Surg. *51:*349-355, Sept '43

Breasts, Hypoplasia

Breast hypertrophies and hypoplasias. KAPP, J. F. Fortschr. d. Med. *50:*652-654, Aug 5, '32

Breasts, Nipple Operations

Simple instrument for inverted or retracted nipples. BIVINGS, L. J.M.A. Georgia *17:*120-121, March '28
Therapy of inverted nipples. PÖPPELMANN, W. Med. Welt *6:*1317, Sept 10, '32
Noël technic in plastic surgery of nipple. VENETIANER, P. Gyogyaszat *73:*553-555, Sept 3, '33
Polymastia. MASON, L. W. Colorado Med. *31:*141-142, April '34
Plastic reconstruction of nipples. MICHALEK-GRODZKI, S. Bull. et mem. Soc. d. chirurgiens de Paris *28:*387-399, June 19, '36
Plastic reconstruction in deformities of nipples. MICHALEK-GRODSKY, Rev. de chir. structive, pp. 126-136, June '37
Operation to correct crater nipple; contribution to problem of necrosis of nipple and areola. KAST, H. Chirurg. *14:*181-184, March 15, '42

Breasts, Pendulous (See also: Mammaplasty, Mastopexy)

Appliance for pendulous breasts. GLASS, E. Deutsche med. Wchnschr. *51:*660, April 17, '25 abstr: J.A.M.A. *84:*1881, June 13, '25

Breasts, Pendulous—Cont.

Congenital pendulous hypertrophic breasts in female twins; case. BIRKENFELD, W. Arch. f. klin. Chir. *168:*568–576, '32

Breasts, Reconstruction

Late results of fat transplantation in breast surgery. WREDE, L. Deutsche Ztschr. f. Chir. *203-204:*672–685, '27

Reconstruction of atrophic mammary gland by means of autotransplantation of fat. PASSOT, R. Presse med. *38:*627–628, May 7, '30

Artificial breasts formed by union of 3 flaps following mammectomy for adenofibroma; case. ZORRAQUÍN, G. AND BOIX POU, M. Rev. de cir. de Buenos Aires *13:*244–248, April '34

Technic of reconstruction of breast. CLAOUE, C. Bull. et mem. Soc. de med. de Paris *140:*33–36, Jan 9, '36

Reparative surgery; distribution of skin on neoformed breast. CLAOUE. Bull. et mem. Soc. de med. de Paris *140:*418–423, June 27, '36

Plastic surgery of hypoplasia of breast. HAGENBACH, E. Helvet. med. acta *3:*811–812, Dec '36

Arterial supply of breast; revised anatomic data relating to reconstructive surgery. MALINIAC, J. W. Arch. Surg. *47:*329–343, Oct '43

Reconstruction of breast deformities. (atrophy) (pendulous) MAY, H. Surg., Gynec. and Obst. *77:*523–529, Nov '43

Derma-fat-fascia transplants used in building up breasts. BERSON, M. I. Surgery *15:*451–456, March '44

Free transplant of areola preliminary to amputation of breast for benign tumor; free fat graft; case. ZENO, L. An. de cir. *10:*190–194, Sept-Dec '44

Operative replacement of mammary prominence. GILLIES, H. Brit. J. Surg. *32:*477–479, April '45

Breasts, Reduction: See Mammaplasty, Reduction

Breasts, Supernumerary

Supernumerary nipples. Congenital hemihypertrophy and congenital hemiatrophy of breast. LANDAUER, W. Human Biol. *11:*447–472, Dec '39

Supernumerary breasts, with special reference to pseudomamma type (case of large breast in inguinal region). WEINSHEL, L. R. AND DEMAKOPOULOS, N. Am. J. Surg. *60:*76–80, April '43

Supernumerary breasts; surgical therapy of case. DE MORAES, A. Obst. y ginec. latino-am. *4:*1–6, Jan '46

Breasts, Suspension: See Mammaplasty, Mastopexy

BRECHET, J.: Cyst of ductus thymopharyngeus; case. Zentralbl. f. alig. Path. u. path. Anat. *69:*353–357, March 30, '38

BRECHOT, AND LEBOURG, L.: Fractures at symphysis and below both condyles of jaw. Odontologie *67:*144–148, March 30, '29

BRECKWOLDT, H.: Teeth in cyclopia and congenital cleft of face. Beitr. z. path. Anat. u. z. allg. Path. *98:*115–135, '36

BREHANT, J.: Therapy of recidivating luxation of jaws by pre-articular osseous abutment; cases. Mem. Acad. de chir. *65:*893–897, June 21, '39

BREIDENBACH, L.: Burn therapy. S. Clin. North America *23:*575–588, April '43

BREITFUSS, F. F.: Plastic removal of skin from breast as aid in treating scars on breast and neck resulting from burns; case. Zentralbl. f. Chir. *61:*436–437, Feb 24, '34

BREITINGER, E.: Healed fractures of lower jaw, from early Bronze Age. Arch. f. Gesch. d. Med. *32:*103–110, '39

BREITKOPF, E.: Operative treatment of tumors of lower jaw. Beitr. z. klin. Chir. *142:*738–741, '28

BREITMAN, M. Y.: Abortive burn treatment with alcohol. Sovet. vrach. gaz. p. 248, Feb 29, '32

BREITNER, B.: Surgical organotherapy by grafts. Wien. klin. Wchnschr. (Sonderbeil. 32) *40:*4–5, '27

BREMER, J. L.: Hypospadias and epispadias; philological note. New England J. Med. *207:*537–539, Sept 22, '32

BRENIZER, A. G.: Skin and fascia grafting. Am. J. Surg. *47:*265–279, Feb '40

BRENIZER, A. G.: Use of fascia and ribbon catgut in harelip and cleft palate repair. Ann. Surg. *107:*692–700, May '38

BRENNER, C.: Peripheral nerve injuries; review of recent literature. War Med. *5:*21–35, Jan '44

BRENNER, F.: Low grade burns as cause of pathologic changes in internal organs (liver, heart, gallbladder, kidney), Zentralbl. f. allg. Path. u. path. Anat. *65:*97–101, May 30, '36

BRENNER, M.: Artificial vagina. Monatschr. f.

Geburtsh. u. Gynak. *54:*112, Feb '21 abstr: J.A.M.A. *76:*1436, May 21, '21
BRENTA, Mme.: (see COPPEZ, J. H.) 1936
BRESSOT, E.: Use of Normet's citrated solution in shock. Cron. med. mex. *30:*207–209, May '31
BRETECHE; MILLANT, AND NOËL, A.: Regional anesthesia of breast with procaine hydrochloride in plastic surgery. Bull. med., Paris *49:*685–686, Oct. 5, '35
BREUER, F.: Congenital fistula of external ear; case. Deutsche Ztschr. f. Chir. *202:*278–282, '27
BREWER, G. E.: Carcinoma of lip and cheek; general principles involved in operation and results obtained at Presbyterian, Memorial, and Roosevelt Hospitals. Surg., Gynec. and Obst. *36:*169–184, Feb '23
BREWER, J. H.: (see CURTIS, R. M.) Feb '44
BREYTFUS, F. F.: Technic of resection of lower lip in cancer; cases. Khirurgiya, no. 5, pp. 61–62, '37
BREZIN, D.: Sulfathiazole (sulfonamide)-cod liver oil ointment in postoperative care of septic hand. Am. J. Surg. *68:*232–233, May '45
BREZINA, P. S. (see LAWRENCE, E. A.) Aug '45
BRICAGE, R. (see FEVRE, M.) March '36
BRICKEL, A. C. J.: *Treatment of Hand and Forearm Infections.* C. V. Mosby Co., St. Louis, 1939.
BRIGGS, R. AND JUND, L.: Successful grafting of frozen and thawed mouse skin. Anat. Rec. *89:*75–85, May '44
BRINDEAU, A.: Formation of artificial vagina with membrane from fetus at term; case. Gynec. et obst. *29:*385–392, May '34
BRINITZER, W.: Dactylomegaly; case. Indian M. Gaz. *76:*286–287, May '41
BRINITZER, W.: Spontaneous entropion. Med. Klin. *24:*1310, Aug 24, '28
BRINKMAN, H.: Burn therapy. J. Maine M. A. *34:*1, Jan '43
BRISOTTO, P.: Cases of cheiloplasty; description of apparatus for feeding infants with harelip and cleft palate. Also: rhinoplasty. Boll. d. mal. d. oreccio, d. gola, d. naso *56:*89–99, March '38
BRISTOW, W. R. (see PLATT, H.) Jan '24
BRITES, G.: Syndactylia and hypophalangism of spoon-shaped hand; case. Folia anat. univ. conimb. (nos. 7-8) *5:*1–5, '30
BRITTO, R.: Neck lesions; therapy. Imprensa med., Rio de Janeiro *19:*59–70, Sept '43
BRITTON, H. A.: Treatment for acute traumatic hematoma of external ear. J.A.M.A. *89:*111–112, July 9, '27
BROCA, A.: Results of operative treatment for cleft palate. Paris med. *12:*58–63, July 15, '22 abstr: J.A.M.A. *79:*1003, Sept 16, '22
BROCHIER, A. (see VORON) Jan '28
BROCK, R.C.: Simple instrument for finger extension. Lancet *1:*382, Feb 16, '35
BRÖCKER, W.: Treatment of injuries with rays of long wave length. Strahlentherapie *42:*551–570, '31
BRÖDEL, M.: Case of Reverdin skin grafting exhibited in Dr. Halsted's clinic on wound healing. Bull. Johns Hopkins Hosp. *36:*60, Jan '25
BRODERICK, R. A.: Life-masks in conjunction with models of mouth in cleft palate. Proc. Roy. Soc. Med. *28:*1667–1672, Oct '35
BRODERS, A. C. (see BICKEL, W. H. *et al*) May '43
BRODERS, A. C. (see MEYERDING, H. W. *et al*) March '41
BRODERS, A. C. (see NEW, G. B. *et al*) Feb '32
BRODERS, A. C.: A study of 63 cases of epithelioma of ear. S. Clin. N. Amer. *1:*1401, Oct '21
BRODERS, A. C.: Squamous-cell epithelioma of skin. Ann. Surg. *73:*141, Feb '21
BRODIN, P. AND SAINT-GIRONS, F.: Transfusion of plasma instead of whole blood in massive hemorrhages; use in war. Bull. et mem. Soc. d. hop. de Paris *55:*1224–1226, Nov 10, '39
BRODY, H.: Fracture and necrosis of mandible; case. Dental Cosmos *69:*242–247, March '27
BROEKMAN, R. W.: Hapsburg family type of prognathism. Tijdschr. v. tandheelk. *35:*174–186, March 15, '28
BROEMAN, C. J.: Carcinoma of lip. W. Virginia M. J. *20:*27–31, Jan '25
BROEMAN, C. J.: Cosmetic facial surgery. Urol. and Cutan. Rev. *34:*319–323, May '30
BROESAMLE, K. M.: Fracture of mandible. U. S. Nav. M. Bull. *42:*47–55, Jan '44
BROFELDT, S. A.: Leukoplakia of lip, and its relations to cancer. Arb. a. d. path. Inst. *5:*34–109, '27
BROGGI, M. (see PONS-TORTELLA, E.) Oct '45
BROGGI, M. AND DOMENECH-ALSINA, F.: Emergency therapy of gunshot wounds of face with fracture of lower jaw. Med. espan. *9:*70–74, Jan '43
BROHEE, G.: Baldwin operation in congenital absence of vagina; result after 11 years. J. de chir. et ann. Soc. belge de chir. (32-30):13–16, Jan '33
BROHEE, G.: Baldwin operation in congenital absence of vagina; result after 11 years. Scalpel (86):825–829, June 3, '33
BROHEE, G.: Massive hypertrophy of breast; 2 cases. Arch. franco-belges de chir. *31:*451–468, June '28

BROHM, C. G. AND BIRD, C. E.: Primary repair of severed parotid duct; method of fixation of inlying dowel. J.A.M.A. *104:*733–734, March 2, '35

BROHOVICI, H.: Cheiloplasty of lower lip; case. Rev. de chir. structive, pp. 210–213, Oct '37

BRONAUGH, W.: Ambulatory method of grafting small areas of skin by use of elastic adhesive. West Virginia M. J. *32:*180–181, April '36

Bronchial Fistula

Treatment of persistent bronchial fistula by use of pedicled muscle flap. GARLOCK, J. H. S. Clin. North America *14:*307–313, April '34

Pedicled muscle flap in treatment of bronchial fistulas; 16 cases. CRAFOORD, C. AND LINTON, P. J. Thoracic Surg. *9:*606–611, Aug '40

BRONNER, H.: Zygoma fractures; diagnosis and treatment. Chirurg *2:*606–611, July 1, '30

BROOKE, C. R.: Fractures of finger with infections. Physical Therap. *47:*91–94, Jan 26, '29

BROOKE, E. M.: Burn therapy among Emergency Medical Service hospital in-patients. Brit. M. J. *1:*259–260, Feb. 24, '45

BROOKE, R.: Facial paralysis treated by fascial grafts; case. Brit. J. Surg. *20:*523–526, Jan '33

BROOKE, R.: Wire extension in treatment of mandibular fractures. Brit. M. J. *2:*498–499, Sept. 14, '35

BROOKE, R. AND ROOKE, C. J.: Grease-gun finger; 2 cases. Brit. M. J. *2:*1186, Dec. 16, '39

BROOKES, H. S. JR. (see PROBSTEIN, J. G.) Sept '24

BROOKES, W. L.: Case of complete avulsion of scalp. Indian M. Gaz. *61:*128, March '26

BROOKS, B.: Case of spontaneous aneurysm of first portion of axillary artery associated with unilateral clubbing of fingers and Dupuytren's contracture. S. Clin. North America *10:*741–755, Aug '30

BROPHY, T. W.: *Cleft Lip and Palate*. Blakiston Co., Phila., 1923.

BROPHY, T. W.: Cleft lip and palate. J. Am. Dent. A. *14:*1108–1115, June '27

BROPHY, T. W.: Cleft palate and harelip procedures. Minnesota Med. *4:*283, May '21

BROPHY, T. W.: Cleft palate extraordinary. Surg., Gynec. and Obst. *32:*182, Feb '21

BROPHY, T. W.: Cleft palate in young infants. New York J. Med. *24:*483–488, April 4, '24

BROPHY, T. W.: Fundamental principles and recent conclusions in surgery of congenital cleft palate. Minnesota Med. *7:*327–336, May '24

BROSCH, F.: Possibility and practical value of universal method in therapy of mandibular fractures. Ztschr. f. Stomatol. *39:*123–144, Feb 28, '41 comment by Reichenbach *39:*144–147, Feb 28, '41

BROSSMANN, H.: Operative formation of vagina. Zentralbl. f. Gynak. *45:*789, June 4, '21

BROVER, B. I.: Transplantation of conserved skin according to Filatov method in therapy of chronic crural ulcers; preliminary report. Vrach. delo *21:*105–110, '39

BROWDER, J.: Encephaloma or so-called nasal glioma. Ann. Otol. Rhin. and Laryng. *38:*395–403, June '29

BROWN, A.: Facial nerve anastomosis for relief of paralysis. Illinois M. J. *59:*130, Feb '31

BROWN, A.: Results of hypoglossofacial anastomosis for facial paralysis in 2 cases. Surg., Gynec. and Obst. *42:*608–613, May '26

BROWN, A. AND HARPER, R. A. K.: Craniofacial dysostosis; significance of ocular hypertelorism Quart. J. Med. *15:*171–181, July '46

BROWN, A. L.: Lime burns to eyes; use of rabbit peritoneum to prevent severe delayed effects; experimental studies and report of cases. Arch. Ophth. *26:*754–769, Nov '41

BROWN, A. L.: (Cincinnati) Lime burns to eye; use of rabbit peritoneum to prevent severe delayed effects; experimental studies and report of cases. Tr. Sect. Ophth., A.M.A., pp. 40–57, '41

BROWN, A. L.: Endocutaneous (Eloesser) flap; application in various types of intrathoracic lesions. Brunn, Med. -Surg. Tributes, pp. 73–79, '42

BROWN, A. M. (see DAVIDSON, J. B.) July '40

BROWN, A. M.: Correction of facial defects with latex prostheses; technic. Arch. Otolaryng. *35:*720–731, May '42

BROWN, A. M.: Extensive mutilating defect of face; cosmetic correction with latex mask. Surgery *12:*957–961, Dec '42

BROWN, A. M.: Latex prosthesis for cosmetic restoration of amputated breast. South. Surgeon *11:*181–188, March '42

BROWN, A. M.: *Modern Plastic Surgical Prosthetics*. Grune and Stratton Co., New York, 1947

BROWN, A. M.: Plastic operations for hump nose; notes on artistic anatomy. Arch. Otolaryng. *31:*827–837, May '40

BROWN, A. M.: Prostheses for eye and orbit. Arch. Ophth. *32:*208–212, Sept '44

BROWN, A. M.: Prosthetic restorations of breast; technic using sponge rubber. Arch. Surg. *48:*388–394, May '44

BROWN, A. M.: Sculpturally molded synthetic implants (methyl methacrylate) in plastic surgery of face. Arch. Otolaryng. *39:*179–183, Feb '44

BROWN, C. E. AND CRANE, G. L.: Bilateral cortical necrosis of kidneys following severe burns. J.A.M.A. *122:*871–873, July 24, '43

BROWN, C. F.: Imperforate anus. China M. J. *43:*274–277, March '29

BROWN, C. P.: Three cases of skin grafting. Surg. J. *34:*20, Sept-Oct '27

BROWN, D.: Mangled forearm; treatment in skeleton splint with fixed skeletal traction. Brit. M. J. *2:*425–426, Oct 10, '42

BROWN, D. AND LUMSDEN, R.: (Plastic) surgery heals scars of war. Hygeia *22:*26, Jan '44

BROWN, D. O.: Repair of limb wounds by use of direct skin flaps. Brit. J. Surg. *30:*307–314, April '43

BROWN, E.: Treatment of alar collapse of nose. J. Laryng. and Otol. *46:*545–546, Aug '31

BROWN, G. V. I.: Nasal relation of harelip operations. J.A.M.A. *77:*1954, Dec 17, '21

BROWN, G. V. I.: Principles of plastic surgery of importance to general practitioners (for face.) Proc. Internat. Assemb. Inter-State Post-Grad. M. A., North America (1928), pp. 542–547, '29

BROWN, G. V. I.: Recent advances in plastic surgery. Wisconsin M. J. *22:*427–428, Feb '24

BROWN, G. V. I.: Reconstruction in times of war and peace. Proc. Interst. Postgrad. M. A. North America (1942) pp. 63–66, '43

BROWN, G. V. I.: Surgical treatment of cleft palate; new method which is primarily reconstructive application of parts of many old operative procedures revised to form what is in effect a new operation. J.A.M.A. *87:*1379–1384, Oct. 23, '26

BROWN, G. V. I.: *The Surgery of Oral and Facial Diseases and Malformations*. Lea and Febiger, Phila., 1938.

BROWN, H. H.: Ectopia vesicae successfully treated by transplantation of trigone into the sigmoid. Brit. M. J. *1:*15, Jan 1, '21

BROWN, J. B.: (see BLAIR, V. P.) Oct '25

BROWN, J. B.: (see BLAIR, V. P.) Jan '27

BROWN, J. B.: (see BLAIR, V. P.) 1928

BROWN, J. B.: (see BLAIR, V. P. *et al*) 1928

BROWN, J. B.: (see BLAIR, V. P. *et al*) Oct '28

BROWN, J. B.: (see BLAIR, V. P. *et al*) Feb '30

BROWN, J. B.: (see BLAIR, V. P. *et al*) April '30

BROWN, J. B.: (see BLAIR, V. P.) July '30

BROWN, J. B.: (see BLAIR, V. P. *et al*) Feb '31

BROWN, J. B.: (see BLAIR, V. P.) April '31

BROWN, J. B.: (see BLAIR, V. P.) May '31

BROWN, J. B.: (see BLAIR, V. P.) Dec '31

BROWN, J. B.: (see BLAIR, V. P. *et al*) 1932

BROWN, J. B.: (see BLAIR, V. P.) April '32

BROWN, J. B.: (see BLAIR, V. P. *et al*) April '32

BROWN, J. B.: (see BLAIR, V. P. *et al*) June '32

BROWN, J. B.: (see BLAIR, V. P. *et al*) Dec '32

BROWN, J. B.: (see BLAIR, V. P. *et al*) Jan '33

BROWN, J. B.: (see BLAIR, V. P. *et al*) Feb '33

BROWN, J. B.: (see BLAIR, V. P.) Oct '33

BROWN, J. B.: (see BLAIR, V. P. *et al*) Nov '33

BROWN, J. B.: (see BLAIR, V. P.) Sept '34

BROWN, J. B.: (see BLAIR, V. P. *et al*) Nov '35

BROWN, J. B.: (see BLAIR, V. P. *et al*) Feb '36

BROWN, J. B.: (see BLAIR, V. P.) Aug '36

BROWN, J. B.: (see BLAIR, V. P. *et al*) Jan '37

BROWN, J. B.: (see BLAIR, V. P. *et al*) Feb '37

BROWN, J. B.: (see BLAIR, V. P. *et al*) May '37

BROWN, J. B.: (see BLAIR, V. P. *et al*) Sept '37

BROWN, J. B.: (see BLAIR, V. P. *et al*) Oct '37

BROWN, J. B.: (see BLAIR, V. P. *et al*) Oct '38

BROWN, J. B.: (see BLAIR, V. P. *et al*) Dec '38

BROWN, J. B.: (see MCDOWELL, F.) Dec '40

BROWN, J. B.: (see MCDOWELL, F.) March '44

BROWN, J. B.: Care of compound injuries of face. South. M. J. *32:*136–144, Feb '39 also: New Orleans M. and S. J. *91:*474–480, March '39

BROWN, J. B.: Cancer of mouth. South. Surgeon *3:*47–52, March '34

BROWN, J. B.: Double elongations of partially cleft palates and elongations of palates with complete clefts. Am. J. Orthodontics *26:*910–915, Sept '40

BROWN, J. B.: Double elongations of partially cleft palates and elongations of palates with complete clefts. Surg., Gynec. and Obst. *70:*815–818, April '40

BROWN, J. B.: Deep block anesthesia of second and third divisions of fifth nerve. Internat. J. Orthodontia *18:*193–199, Feb '32

BROWN, J. B.: Deep block anesthesia of second and third divisions of fifth nerve. Surg., Gynec. and Obst. *53:*832–835, Dec '31

BROWN, J. B.: Elongation of partially cleft palate. Am. J. Orthodontics *24:*878–883, Sept '38

BROWN, J. B.: Elongation of partially cleft palate. Surg., Gynec. and Obst. *63:*768–771, Dec '36

BROWN, J. B.: Facial bone fractures. Surg., Gynec. and Obst. *68:*564–573, Feb. (no. 2A) '39 also: Am. J. Orthodontics *25:*432–446, May '39

BROWN, J. B.: Feeding of liquid diet in jaw fractures. Internat. J. Orthodontia *18:*614–617, June '32

BROWN, J. B.: Homografting, with report of success in identical twins. Surgery *1:*558–563, April '37

BROWN, J. B.: New type of tissue forceps. Am. J. Surg. *49:*397, Aug '40

BROWN, J. B.: Plastic surgery of burns. Delaware State M. J. *16:*35–38, March '44

BROWN, J. B.: Panel discussions; treatment of injuries to face. Bull. Am. Coll. Surgeons *27:*132–134, April '42

BROWN, J. B.: Preserved and fresh cartilage homotransplants. Surg., Gynec. and Obst. *70:*1079–1082, June '40

BROWN, J. B.: Plastic surgery of face. Internat. Abstr. Surg., pp. 297–311, Oct '33

BROWN, J. B.: Repair of surface defects of hand. Ann. Surg. *107:*952–971, June '38

BROWN, J. B.: Restoration of entire skin of penis. Surg., Gynec. and Obst. *65:*362–365, Sept '37

BROWN, J. B.: Surface repair of compound injuries of extremities. J. Bone and Joint Surg. *26:*448–454, July '44

BROWN, J. B.: Surface defects of hand. Am. J. Surg. *46:*690–699, Dec '39

BROWN, J. B.: Skin graft covering of raw surfaces. Internat. Abstr. Surg. *67:*105–116, '38; in Surg., Gynec. and Obst. Aug '38

BROWN, J. B.: Switching of vermilion-bordered lip flaps. Surg., Gynec. and Obst. *46:*701–704, May '28

BROWN, J. B.: Types of chronic infection about mouth. Internat. J. Orthodontia *18:*1311, Dec '32; *19:*59, Jan '33

BROWN, J. B.: Utilization of temporal muscle and fascia in facial paralysis. Am. J. Orthodontics *26:*80–87, Jan '40

BROWN, J. B.: Utilization of temporal muscle and fascia for facial paralysis. Ann. Surg. *109:*1016–1023, June '39

BROWN, J. B.: (with VILRAY P. BLAIR AND ROBERT H. IVY): *Essentials of Oral Surgery*. C. V. Mosby Co., St. Louis.

BROWN, J. B. AND BLAIR, V. P.: Repair of defects resulting from full thickness loss of skin from burns. Surg., Gynec. and Obst. *60:*379–389, Feb. (no. 2A) '35

BROWN, J. B.; BLAIR, V. P. AND BYARS, L. T.: Repair of surface defects, from burns and other causes, with thick split skin grafts. South M. J. *28:*408, May; 529, June '35

BROWN, J. B.; BLAIR, V. P. AND BYARS, L. T.: Ulceration of lower extremities and grafts. Am. J. Surg. *43:*452–457, Feb '39

BROWN, J. B.; BLAIR, V. P. AND HAMM, W. G.: Release of axillary and brachial scar fixation. Surg., Gynec. and Obst. *56:*791–798, April '33

BROWN, J. B. AND BYARS, L. T.: Interstitial radiation treatment of hemangiomata. Am. J. Surg. *39:*452–457, Feb '38

BROWN, J. B. AND BYARS, L. T.: Malignant melanomas, with report of 4 and 7 year cures. Surg., Gynec. and Obst. *71:*409–415, Oct '40

BROWN, J. B. AND BYARS, L. T.: Spontaneous and surgical covering (grafts) of raw surfaces. Journal-Lancet *60:*503–512, Nov '40

BROWN, J. B. AND BYARS, L. T.: Malignant melanomas with report of 4- and 7-year cures. Am. J. Orthodontics (Oral Surg. Sect) *27:*90–100, Feb '41

BROWN, J. B.; BYARS, L. T. AND BLAIR, V. P.: Repair of ulcerations of lower extremity with thick split skin grafts. Surg., Gynec. and Obst. *63:*331–340, Sept '36

BROWN, J. B.; BYARS, L. T. AND MCDOWELL, F.: Preoperative and postoperative care in reconstructive surgery. Arch. Surg. *40:*1192–1210, June '40

BROWN, J. B. AND CANNON, B.: Plastic surgery and its association with orthopedic surgery. Am. Acad. Orthop. Surgeons, Lect. pp. 212–216, '44

BROWN, J. B. AND CANNON, B.: Repair of surface defects of foot. Tr. Am. S. A. *62:*417–430, '44

BROWN, J. B. AND CANNON, B.: Repair of surface defects of foot. Ann. Surg. *120:*417–430, Oct '44

BROWN, J. B. AND CANNON, B.: Full-thickness skin grafts from neck for function and color in eyelid. Tr. South. S. A. (1944) *56:*255–259, '45

BROWN, J. B. AND CANNON, B.: Full-thickness skin grafts from neck for function and color in eyelid. Ann. Surg. *121:*639–643, May '45

BROWN, J. B. AND CANNON, B.: Composite free grafts of skin and cartilage from ear. Surg. Gynec. and Obst. *82:*253–255, Mar '46

BROWN, J. B. AND HAFFNER, H.: Lesions of tongue; collective review. Am. J. Orthodontics *25:*1213–1223, Dec '39

BROWN, J. B. AND HAMM, W. G.: Diagnosis and treatment of lesions preventing normal opening of mouth; 6 illustrative cases. Internat. J. Orthodontia *18:*353–362, April '32

BROWN, J. B. AND MCDOWELL, F.: Syndactylism with absence of pectoralis major. Surgery *7:*599–601, April '40

BROWN, J. B. AND MCDOWELL, F.: Care of severe injuries of face and jaws. Jounral-Lancet *60:*260–267, June '40

BROWN, J. B., AND MCDOWELL, F.: Review of reconstructive surgery of the face, 1938–1940. Laryng., *50:*1117, Dec. '40

BROWN, J. B. AND MCDOWELL, F.: Persistence of function of skin grafts through long periods of growth. Surg., Gynec. and Obst. *72:*848–853, May '41

BROWN, J. B. AND MCDOWELL, F.: Secondary repair of cleft lips and their nasal deformities. Ann. Surg. *114:*101–117, July '41

BROWN, J. B. AND MCDOWELL, F.: Persistence of function of grafts through long periods of growth. J. Iowa M. Soc. *31:*457–462, Oct '41

BROWN, J. B. AND MCDOWELL, F.: Secondary

repair of cleft lips and their nasal deformities. Am. J. Orthodontics (Oral Surg. Sect) *27:*712–727, Dec '41

BROWN, J. B. AND MCDOWELL, F.: Internal wire fixation of jaw fractures; preliminary report. Surg., Gynec. and Obst. *74:*227–230, Feb '42

BROWN, J. B. AND MCDOWELL, F.: Massive repairs with thick split-skin grafts; emergency "dressing" with homografts in burns. Ann. Surg. *115:*658–674, April '42

BROWN, J. B. AND MCDOWELL, F.: Plastic repair with free skin grafts in burns. Clinics *1:*25–36, June '42

BROWN, J. B. AND MCDOWELL, F.: Review of reconstructive surgery of face—1940-1942. Laryngoscope *52:*489–504, June '42

BROWN, J. B. AND MCDOWELL, F.: "Field-fire" and invasive basal cell carcinoma—basal-squamous type. Surg., Gynec. and Obst. *74:*1128–1132, June '42

BROWN, J. B. AND MCDOWELL, F.: Epithelial healing and transplantation. Ann. Surg. *115:*1166–1181, June '42

BROWN, J. B. AND MCDOWELL, F.: Internal wire fixation, with note on external bar fixation. Surg., Gynec. and Obst. *75:*361–368, Sept '42

BROWN, J. B. AND MCDOWELL, F.: Care of military and civilian injuries; internal wire fixation of jaw fractures; preliminary report. Am. J. Orthodontics (Oral Surg. Sect.) *29:*86–91, Feb '43

BROWN, J. B. AND MCDOWELL, F.: *Skin Grafting of Burns.* J. B. Lippincott Co., Phila., 1943

BROWN, J. B. AND MCDOWELL, F.: Treatment of metastatic carcinoma of neck. Tr. South. S. A. (1943) *55:*254–266, '44

BROWN, J. B. AND MCDOWELL, F.: Treatment of metastatic carcinoma of neck. Ann. Surg. *119:*543–555, April '44

BROWN, J. B. AND MCDOWELL, F.: Neck dissections for metastatic carcinoma. Surg., Gynec. and Obst. *79:*115–124, Aug '44

BROWN, J. B. AND MCDOWELL, F.: Simplified design for repair of single cleft lips. Surg., Gynec. and Obst. *80:*12–26, Jan '45

BROWN, J. B. AND PETERSON, L. W.: Ankylosis and trismus resulting from war wounds involving coronoid region of mandible; 3 cases J. Oral Surg. *4:*258–266, July '46

BROWN, J. B. AND TUNG, P. C.: Osteomyelitis of jaws. South. Surgeon *4:*12–26, March '35

BROWN, J. B. AND TUNG, P. C.: Osteomyelitis of jaws. Internat. J. Orthodontia *22:*69–80, Jan '36

BROWN, J. B. *et al*: Direct flap repair of defects of arm and hand; preparation of gunshot wounds for repair of nerves, bones and tendons. Ann. Surg. *122:*706–715, Oct '45

BROWN, J. L.: Observation on series of 15 fractures of mandible. U. S. Nav. M. Bull. *18:*245–248, Feb '23

BROWN, J. L. (see CARSON, L. D.) April '34

BROWN, J. M.: Branchial and thyroglossal duct cysts and fistulas. Ann. Otol., Rhin. and Laryng. *44:*644–652, Sept '35

BROWN, K. T.: Submucous resection of nasal septum. J. Indiana M. A. *14:*339, Oct '21

BROWN, O. F.: Notes on maxillofacial centers, Warwick, October, 1642. Brit. Dent. J. *77:*195–197, Oct 6, '44

BROWN, R. C.: Cranioplasty by split rib method. J. Coll. Surgeons, Australasia *1:*238–246, Nov '28

BROWN, R. G.: Modification of Davis Boyle gag. Lancet *2:*756, Oct 11, '24

BROWN, R. G.: Cancer of lips; treatment by radium needles. M. J. Australia *1:*421–423, March 30, '29

BROWN, R. G.: Vilray P. Blair's modification of Mirault operation for cleft lip. M. J. Australia *1:*499–503, April 11, '36

BROWN, R. K. AND DZIOB, J. M.: Fractures of hand. New York State J. Med. *42:*1824–1832, Oct 1, '42

BROWN, W. L.: (see DAVIS, A. H.) March '38

Brown-Blair Operation

Complete unilateral harelip; immediate result of operation by Brown-Blair method. DELLEPIANE RAWSON, R. Dia med. *15:*146–147, Feb 22, '43

Brown Operation (See also Blair-Brown Operation

Cleft palate therapy; Brown operation. MARINO, H. Arq. de cir. clin. e exper. *6:*333–336, April-June '42

BROWNE, D.: Cleft palate operation. Brit. J. Surg. *20:*7–25, July '32

BROWNE, D.: Congenital deformities of mouth (including cleft lip and palate). Practitioner *132:*658–670, June '34

BROWNE, D.: Orthopedic operation in cleft palate. Brit. M. J. *2:*1093–1095, Dec 7, '35

BROWNE, D.: Hypospadias operation. Lancet *1:*141–143, Jan. 18, '36

BROWNE, H. S.: Nasal septal perforation. J. Oklahoma M. A. *25:*382–383, Sept '32

BROWNE, J. S. L. (see ROSE, B. *et al)* May '41

BROWNE, J. S. L. (see WEIL, P. G. *et al)* July '40

BROWNE, W. E.: Necessity for use of splints at certain stages in treatment of hand infections, with demonstration of some of the newer types. New England J. Med. *215:*743-749, Oct 22, '36

BROWNE, W. E.: Diagnosis and primary surgical treatment of injuries of hand. Rhode Island M. J. *28:*875, Dec '45 also: J. Maine M. A. *37:*21, Feb '46

BROWNELL, D. H.: Congenital atresia of posterior choana of nose. Univ. Bull. Ann Arbor *5:*68, Sept '39

BROWNLEE, J. J.: Burn therapy. New Zealand M. J. *41:*192-197, Oct '42

BROWNSON, H. N.: Handy bandage for jaw fractures. J. Oral Surg. *1:*271, July '43

BRUCH, H.: (see MERRITT, K. K. *et al*) March '37

BRÜCKNER, S. AND OBSTÄNDER, E.: So-called facial hemiatrophy; case. Psychiat.-neurol. Wchnschr. *34:*448-451, Sept 10, '32

BRÜDA, B. E. AND KREINER, W.: Homeoplasty and reticulo-endothelial system; effect of injuries of reticulo-endothelial system on rapidity with which transplanted tissue heals. Deutsche Ztschr. f. Chir. *222:*285-301, '30

BRUGGER, Congenital ankylosis of finger joints. Munchen. med. Wchnschr. *70:*874-875, July 6, '23 (illus.)

BRUHN, C.: Surgical-orthopedical removal of deformations of jaws. Internat. J. Orthodontia *13:*65-79, '27

BRUHN, C.: Surgical-orthopedical removal of deformations of jaws. Internat. Orthodont. Cong. *1:*245-259, '27

BRUHN, C.: Fracture of lower jaw; essentials of treatment. Tung-chi, Med. Monatschr. *2:*144-150, Jan '27

BRUHN, C.: Surgico-orthopedic treatment of congenital and acquired jaw defects. Stomatol. *27:*905-926, Nov '29

Bruhn Operation: See Darcissac-Bruhn-Petroff Operation

DE BRUIN, J.: Acrocephalosyndactylia. Nederl. Tijdschr. v. Geneesk. *2:*2380-2393, Nov 28, '25 also: Acta Paediat. *5:*280-293, '26 abstr: J.A.M.A. *86:*456, Feb 6, '26

DE BRUIN, T. R.: Plastic surgery (modified Ombredanne operation) in therapy of epispadias with urinary incontinence; case. Nederl. Tijdschr. v. Geneesk. *90:*1127-1129, Sept 7, '46

BRUN, J. (see FROMENT, J. *et al)* Oct '36

BRUN, M. (see LAROYENNE, L.) Jan '33

BRUNEL. (see RONNEAUX, G.) Nov '33

BRUNEMEIER, E. H.: Imperforate anus; report of case. China M. J. *37:*748-749, Sept '23

BRUNER, E.: Treatment of roentgen ulcerations of skin. Strahlentherapie *36:*373-384, '30

BRUNER, J. M.: Hand; treatment of war injuries in U. S. Army. J. Iowa M. Soc. *36:*509-511, Dec '46

BRUNER, M. A.: Hand hazards. Hygeia *20:*424, June '42

BRUNET, P.: Congenital deformities of hands. Arch. d'anat., d'histol. et d'embryol. *13:*1-31, '31

BRUNETTI, F.: Absence of several fingers and fibroma of middle finger of right hand in new-born infant. Rinasc. med., *9:*7-8, Jan 1, '32

BRUNI, A.: Clinical aspects and treatment of skeletal injuries of hand in industry. Rassegna d. previd. soc. *15:*27-41, Dec '28

BRUNI, A.: Neuritis of median nerve due to compression by luxated semilunar bone; case in workman. Rassegna d. previd. sociale *24:*42-43, Nov-Dec '37

BRUNI, A. C.: Plastic reconstruction of intestinal branchial apparatus and its derivatives in human embryos. Monitore zool. ital. (supp.) *41:*196-199, 1930-1931

BRUNINGS: New restorative operation following partial extirpation for cancer. Ztschr. f. Krebsforsch. *49:*278-286, '39

BRUNNER, H.: Surgical treatment of facial paralysis. Ztschr. f. Hals-, Nasen-u. Ohrenh. *15:*379-382, Oct 6, '26

BRUNNER, H.: Plastic operations for paralysis of facial nerve. Arch. f. klin. Chir. *140:*85-100, '26

BRUNNER, H.: Endoral plastic correction of results of paralysis of facial nerve. Wien. klin. Wchnschr. *41:*876-877, June 21, '28

BRUNS, H. D.: On permanence of results of Motais' operation for eyelid ptosis. Am. J. Ophth., *5:*269-270, Apr '22 (illus.)

BRUNSCHWIG, A.: Tumors of synovia, tendons and joint capsules (hand). Surgery *5:*101-111, Jan '39

BRUNSCHWIG, A. (see BECKER, S. W.) April '34

BRUNSTING, L. A. AND GHORMLEY, R. K.: Treatment of extensive gasoline burns of legs (due to explosion) with correction of deformity; case. Proc. Staff Meet., Mayo Clin. *11:*129-131, Feb 26, '36

BRUNZEL, H. F.: Surgical treatment of intractable furunculosis of axilla. Zentralbl. f. Chir. *48:*991, July 16, '21

BRUSCHI, F.: Fracture of lower jaw in girl 10 years old; results of therapy. Stomatol. *35:*17-33, Jan '37

BRUSKIN, J.: Construction of vagina from intestine. Zentralbl. f. Gynak. *48:*1597-1599, July 19, '24

BRUSOTTI, A.: Nasal deformities plastic repair; cases. Stomatol. *25:*161-181, March '27

BRUSOTTI, A.: Bucco-facial prosthesis in case of grave mutilation. Stomatol. *25:*649-658, Aug '27

BRUZZONE, C.: Ear injury due to electric discharge; case. Ann. di laring., otol. *34:*147-150, '34

BRUZZONE, I. A.: (see FERRARI, R. A.) Dec '33

BRYAN, W. A.: Correction of cleft palate. Southern M. J. *16:*117-121, Feb '23 (illus.)

BRYANT, B. L.: Endonasal tear sac operation. California and West. Med. *51:*376-378, Dec '39

BRZHOZOVSKIY, A. A.: Value of primary skin grafts in fresh cutaneous wounds. Sovet. khir., no. 7, pp. 72-73, '35

BUBB, C. H. (see COLE, P. P. *et al*) May '30

BUBNOV, M. A.: Therapy of traumatic shock according to experimental data. Khirurgiya, no. 9, pp. 38-45, '37

BUCCI, P.: Intravenous injections of salt-gum solutions in shock from hemorrhage. Boll. d. Soc. ital. di biol. Sper. *2:*965-972, Nov '27

BUCHANAN, A. R.: Concepts of anatomy of head and neck. Am. J. Orthodontics *28:*152-166, March '42

BUCHANAN, J. M.: Technic of plastic repair in wounds of vagina. Australian and New Zealand J. Surg. *8:*300-307, Jan '39

BUCHANAN, J. S.: Hand infections. Tr. Roy. Med.-Chir. Soc. Glasgow, pp. 117-128; 129-130, '34-'35 in Glasgow M. J. Sept., Oct '35

BUCHHOLZ, R. R. (see DOUGLAS, B.) May '43

BÜCKLERS, M.: Surgery and plastic replacement of eyelids. Chirurg *5:*460-472, June 15, '33

Bucknall Operation

Modification of operation of Bucknall for hypospadias. HARVEY, S. C. Ann. Surg. *77:*572-579, May '23 (illus.)

Bucknall Operation Complication

Ball of hair in urethra; late complication of Bucknall operation for hypospadias. VERMOOTEN, V. New England J. Med. *202:*658-660, April 3, '30

BUCKY, G.: Cure of epithelioma of nose with Bucky's border rays (grenz rays). Arch. f. Dermat. u. Syph. *155:*109-111, '28

BUDDE, W.: Surgical therapy of hypospadias. Zentralbl. f. Chir. *69:*1080, June 27, '42

BUDETTI, J. A.: Unilateral exophthalmos; case report of unusual result Ann. Otol. Rhin. and Laryng. *55:*434-439, June '46

BUDINA, R. Y.: Pathogenesis of facial hemiatrophy and heterochromia of iris. Sovrem. psikhonevrol. *11:*316-323, '30

BÜDINGER, K.: Mummifying gangrene following phlegmons on finger and hand. Wien. klin. Wchnschr. *45:*1093, Sept 2, '32

Buediner-Diffenbach Operation

Buediner's modification of Diffenbach's operation for early epithelioma of lower lid. WRIGHT, R. E. Brit. J. Ophth. *8:*58-61, Feb '24

BUENO PLEMONT, I.: Aplasia of vagina. Rev. med.-cir. do Brasil *50:*899-906, Sept '42

BUENO DOS REIS, J. D. (see FERRAZ ALVIM, J. *et al*) Feb '34

BUENO RODRIGO, L.: Artificial vagina in case of total absence of uterus and vagina. Siglo med. *91:*549-550, May 27, '33

BUFALINI, M.: Separate tangentially cut bone-periosteum flaps from tibia to close gap in skull. Arch. ital. di chir. *12:*529-554, '25

BUFALINI, M.: Transplantation of ureters into sigmoid in therapy of urinary incontinence due to grave congenital malformation; case. (exstrophy of bladder). Policlinico (sez. prat.) *44:*880-883, May 3, '37

BUFFINGTON, C. B.: Finger injuries. West Virginia M. J. *37:*499-502, Nov '41

BUHLER, Y. E. (see BELOT, J.) March-April '30

BÜHR, R.: Dangers of permitting anyone except rhinologist to operate on nose. Deutsche med. Wchnschr. *55:*1554, Sept 13, '29

BUIRGE, R. E.: Secondary carcinoma of mandible; analysis of 71 cases. Surgery *15:*553-564, April '44

BUIZARD, C.: Transmission for several generations of double pure cubital club-hand. Bull. et mem. Soc. de chir. de Paris *20:*711-714, Nov 2, '28

BULACH, K.: Transplantation of hyaline cartilage. Sovet. vestnick oftal. *9:*329-331, '36

BULACH, K.: Blepharoplasty with free skin flap from auricle. Vestnik oftal. (no. 6) *14:*46-48, '39

BULBULIAN, A. H.: Simple and practical technic for making facial casts. J. Am. Dent. A. *26:*347-354, March '39

BULBULIAN, A. H.: Improved technic for prosthetic restoration of defects of face by use of latex compound. Proc. Staff Meet., Mayo Clin. *14:*433-439, July 12, '39

BULBULIAN, A. H.: Prosthetic restorations of defects of face by use of latex compound; further detailed description of technic used. Proc. Staff Meet., Mayo Clin. *14:*721-727, Nov 15, '39

BULBULIAN, A. H.: Artificial ear. and nose. Hygeia *18:*980-982, Nov '40

BULBULIAN, A. H.: Repair of facial defects with prosthesis using latex compound. J. Am. Dent. A. *28:*559-571, April '41 abstr., Mil. Surgeon *88:*179-182, Feb '41

BULBULIAN, A. H.: Prosthetic reconstruction of

nose and ear with latex compound. J.A.M.A. *116:*1504–1506, April 5, '41

Bulbulian, A. H.: Congenital and postoperative loss of ear; reconstruction by prosthetic method. J. Am. Dent. A. *29:*1161–1168, July 1, '42

Bulbulian, A. H.: *Facial Prosthesis.* W. B. Saunders Co., Phila., 1945

Bulfaro, J. A. (see Delrio, J. M. A.) 1945

Bulfaro, J. A. H.: Dermoepidermal grafts in grave traumas of upper extremity; case. Bol. y trab. Soc. argent. de cirujanos *7:*340–343, '46 also: Rev. Asoc. med. argent. *60:*605–606, July 15 '46

Bullo, J.: Facial progressive hemiatrophy; facioabdominocrural hemidystrophic form; case. Dia med. *17:*444–445, 448, May 14, '45

Bullock, H.: Plastic operation on face and lips. M. J. Australia *2:*220, Sept. 17, '21

Bullowa, J. G. M. and Fox, C. L. Jr. Newer conceptions in burn therapy. Hebrew M. J. *1:*192, '43

Bullowa, J. G. M. (see Rothman, M. *et al*) Nov '42

Bulmer, J. W.: Plasma and its clinical use in shock. M. Times, New York *70:*3–8, Jan '42

Bulmer, J. W.: Present day treatment of burns. New York State J. Med. *43:*2192–2195, Nov 15, '43

v. Bülow, W. (see Kurtzahn, H.) 1926

Bulson, A. E. and Bulson, E. L.: Cerebrospinal rhinorrhea following nasal surgery. J. A. M. A. *93:*1969–1970, Dec 21, '29

Bulson, A. E. Jr.: A new local anesthetic for nose and throat work. Ann. Otol. Rhinol. and Laryngol. *31:*131–136, March '22

Bulson, E. L. (see Bulson, A. E.) Dec '29

Bumba, J. and Lucksch, F.: Case of bulldog nose. Virchow's Arch. f. path. Anat. *264:*554–562, '27

Bumin, H.: Hypertrophy of breast corrected by plastic surgery according to Nissen. Turk tib cem. mec. *5:*173–183, '39

Bumm, E.: Duplication of upper jaw. Arch. f. klin. Chir. *135:*506–519, '25

Bump, W. S. (see Plummer, S. C.) Jan '27

Bunnell, S.: Repair of tendons in fingers. Surg. Gynec. and Obst., *35:*88–97, July '22 (illus.)

Bunnell, S.: Reconstructive surgery of hand. Surg., Gynec. and Obst. *39:*259–274, Sept '24

Bunnell, S.: Surgery of nerves of hand. Surg., Gynec. and Obst. *44:*145–152, Feb '27

Bunnell, S.: Suture of facial nerve within temporal bone, with report of first successful case. Surg., Gynec. and Obst. *45:*7–12, July '27

Bunnell, S.: Cleft palate repair; cause of failure in infants and its prevention. Surg., Gynec. and Obst. *45:*530–533, Oct '27

Bunnell, S.: Repair of nerves and tendons of hand and grafting. J. Bone and Joint Surg. *10:*1–26, Jan '28 abstr: Arch. franco-belges de chir. *30:*93–97, Feb '27

Bunnell, S.: Treatment of hand injuries. California and West. Med. **30:**1–5, Jan '29

Bunnell, S.: Physiological reconstruction of thumb after total loss. Surg., Gynec. and Obst. *52:*245–248, Feb '31

Bunnell, S.: Vertical skin-grafts for reconstruction of eyebrows. Surg., Gynec. and Obst. *53:*239–240, Aug '31

Bunnell, S.: Contractures of hand from infections. J. Bone and Joint Surg. *14:*27–46, Jan '32

Bunnell, S.: Surgical repair in facial paralysis. Arch. Otolaryng. *25:*235–259, March '37

Bunnell, S.: Reconstruction of injured hand. Rocky Mountain M. J. *35:*194–200, March '38

Bunnell, S.: Opposition of thumb. J. Bone and Joint Surg. *20:*269–284, April '38

Bunnell, S.: Surgery for opposition of thumb. J. Bone and Joint Surg. *20:*1072, Oct '38

Bunnell, S.: Primary repair of severed tendons; use of stainless steel wire. Am. J. Surg. *47:*502–516, Feb '40

Bunnell, S.: Treatment of tendons in compound injuries to hand. J. Bone and Joint Surg. *23:*240–250, April '41

Bunnell, S.: Surgery of intrinsic muscles other than those producing opposition of thumb. J. Bone and Joint Surg. *24:*1–31, Jan '42

Bunnell, S.: Suturing tendons. Am. Acad. Orthop. Surgeons, Lect., pp. 1–5, '43

Bunnell, S.: Primary and secondary repair of flexor tendons. Tr. Am. Soc. Plastic and Reconstructive Surg. *12:*65–67, '43

Bunnell, S.: Muscle transplants; opposition of thumb. Am. Acad. Orthop. Surgeons, Lect., pp. 283–288, '44

Bunnell, Sterling: *Surgery of the Hand.* J. B. Lippincott Co., Phila., 1944

Bunnell, S.: Suggestions to improve early treatment of hand injuries. Bull. U.S. Army M. Dept. (no. 88) pp. 78–82, May '45

Bunnell, S.: Suggestions to improve early treatment of hand injuries. Arch. Phys. Med. *26:*693–697, Nov '45

Bunnell, S. Knuckle bender splint. Bull. U.S. Army M. Dept. *5:*230–231, Feb '46

Bunnell, S.: Active splinting of hand J. Bone and Joint Surg. *28:*732–736, Oct. '46

Bunnell, S.: Reconstructive surgery of hand Guy's Hosp. Gaz. *60:*293–296, Oct 26, '46

Bunnell, S. and Boyes, J. H.: Nerve grafts.

Am. J. Surg. *44:*64-75, April '39

Bunnell Operation

Surgical therapy of otogenic facial paralysis according to Ballance-Duel and Bunnell: 35 cases. KETTEL, K. Nord. med. (Hospitalstid.) *24:*1783-1795, Oct 6, '44

Therapy of digital wounds of flexor tendons; St. Bunnell operation using tendon graft; technic and results; 14 cases. BLOCH, J. C. AND ZAGDOUN, J., J. de Chir. *47:*376-391, March '36

Bunnell operation to repair loss of grasping power of thumb (paralysis of opponens pollicis) after infantile paralysis; case. (transplantation of tendon). INCLAN, A. AND RODRIGUEZ, R. Cir. ortop. y traumatol., Habana, *6:*140-145, July-Sept '38

Restoration of flexion of fingers by Sterling Bunnel's method. DZHANELIDZE, U. U. Vestnik khir. (nos. 56-57) *19:*39-53, '30

Fixation of tendons, ligaments and bone by Bunnell's pull-out wire suture. KEY, J. A. Tr. South. S. A. (1945) *57:*187-194, '46

Significance of early resumption of function following plastic repair of tendons according to Bunnell. NIKOLAEV, G. F. Novy khir. arkhiv. *45:*327-331, '40

Experimental data on plastic surgery of tendons according to Bunnell. NIKOLAEV, G. F. Ortop. i travmatol. (no. 6) *11:*3-11, '37

Instruments for restoration of severed flexor tendons of fingers according to Bunnell method. Rozov, V. I. Sovet. khir. (nos. 3-4) *6:*458-461, '34

Tendoplasty according to Bunnell method. KRINITISKIY, Y. M. Ortop. i travmatol. (no. 5) *11:*149-151, '37

Bunnell Suture

Fixation of ligaments by Bunnell's pull-out wire suture. KEY, J. A. Ann. Surg. *123:* 656-663, April '46

BUNTEN, W. A.: Neurolysis of facial nerve after 10 years inclusion within scar tissue; operation, with returning function. Nebraska M. J. *16:*169-173, May '31

BUNYAN, J.: Envelope method of burn therapy. Proc. Roy. Soc. Med. *34:*65-70, Nov '40

BUNYAN, J.: Burn therapy with envelope method (using electrolytic sodium hypochlorite solution). Brit. M. J. *2:*1-7, July 5, '41 also: M. Press *206:*103-109, July 30, '41

BUNYAN, J.: Envelope method of burn therapy (using electrolytic sodium hypochlorite solution). Gen. Practitioner *14:*190-193, Nov 15, '43

BURCH, J. C. AND FISHER, H. C.: The problem of tumors of the parotid gland. S. Clin. North America *26:*489-494, April '46

BURCH, J. C. (see BURCH, L. E.) June '37

BURCH, J. E.: Simple pliable finger splint. J. A. M. A. *108:*2036-2037, June 12, '37

BURDESHAW, H. B.: Blood and blood substitutes in hemorrhage and shock. J. M. A. Alabama *12:*79-81, Sept '42

BURDICK, C. G.: Harelip and cleft palate; analysis of 184 cases. Ann. Surg. *92:*35-50, July '30

BURFORD, W. N. AND ACKERMAN, L. V.: Carcinoma of buccal mucosa. Am. J. Orthodontics (Oral Surg. Sect) *31:*547-551, Sept '45

BURFORD, W. N. AND ACKERMAN, L. V.: Hemangioma of lip. Am. J. Orthodontics (Oral Surg. Sect.), *31:*559-560, Sept '45

BURFORD, W. N. AND ACKERMAN, L. V.: Lesions of lower lip. Am. J. Orthodontics (Oral Surg. Sect.) *31:*560-574, Sept '45

BURFORD, W. N.; ACKERMAN, L. V. AND ROBINSON, H. B. G.: Symposium on 20 cases of benign and malignant lesions of oral cavity, from Ellis Fischel State Cancer Hospital, Columbia, Missouri. Am. J. Orthodontics (Oral Surg. Sect.) *30:*353-398, July '44

BURGDORF, K.: Necrosis of septum after correction in latent syphilis; 2 cases. Arch. f. Ohren-, Nasen-u. Kehlhopfh. *129:*175-180, July 21, '31

BURGER, CHARLES (KAROLY) See: BURGER, K.

BURGER, H.: Fatalities after operations on nose. Nederlandsch Tijdschr. v. Geneesk. *1:*2356-2366, June 2, '23 abstr: J.A.M.A. *81:* 1061, Sept. 22, '23

BURGER, H.: Nasal speech and cleft palate. Nederl. Tijdschr. v. Geneesk. *1:*1563-1571, March 31, '28

BURGER, K.: New method of construction of artificial vagina. Orvosi hetil. *81:*788-790, July 31, '37

BURGER, K.: Use of fetal membranes in formation of artificial vagina. Zentralbl. f. Gynak. *61:*2437-2440, Oct 16, '37

BURGER, K.: Use of fetal membranes in vaginal reconstruction. Geburtsh. u. Frauenh. *1:*183-187, March '39

BURGER, K.: Biologic significance of fetal membranes (including use as grafts); Joseph Price oration (Artificial vagina). Am. J. Obst. and Gynec. *37:*572-584, April '39

BURGESS, F. (see ALLEN, J. W. *et al*) April '44

BURGESS, N.: Epithelioma developing on site of recurrent herpes simplex of lips. Brit. M. J. *2:*249, Aug. 16, '30

BURIAN, F.: Plastic surgery of breast. Casop. lek. cesk. *73:*373, April 6; 397, April 13, '34

BURIAN, F.: Reconstruction of hard palate. Rev. de chir. *59:*49, '21

BURIAN, F.: Correction of deformity from facial paralysis. Rev. de chir. *59:*52, '21

BURIAN, F.: Physiology and technic of free skin transplant. Casop. lek. cesk. *70:*667, May 8; 714, May 15, '31

BURIAN, F.: Tubular skin transplants. Casop. lek. cesk. *70:*741–743, May 22, '31

BURIAN, F.: Plastic surgery of nose by Italian method using tubular grafts. Presse med. *39:*1418–1420, Sept. 26, '31

BURIAN, F.: Present status of therapy of cleft lip and palate. Casop. lek. cesk. *72:*420, April 7; 454, April 14; 491, April 21, '33

BURIAN, F.: Cartilage autograft. Rev. de chir. plastique, pp. 15–19, May '34

BURIAN, F.: Plastic surgery of crippled hand and injured hand. Rozhl. v chir. a gynaek. (cast chir.) *13:*252–270, '34

BURIAN, F.: Plastic surgery of facial defects. Casop. lek. cesk. *74:*261–263, March 8, '35

BURIAN, F.: Technic of increasing tone of skin and removing wrinkles. Med. Welt *10:*930–931, June 27, '36

BURIAN, F.: Pathology and embryogenesis of deformities of nose and lip. Casop. lek. cesk. *76:*101, Jan 29, '37; 138, Feb 5, '37

BURIAN, F.: Experiences of Prague Institute for Plastic Surgery with free whole thickness grafts. Rev. de chir. structive, pp. 264–266, Dec '37

BURIAN, F.: Experience with mammaplasties. Rev. de chir. structive *8:*35–37, May '38

BURKE, G. R.: Results in Porto Rico of Kondoleon operations for elephantiasis of extremities. Surg., Gynec. and Obst. *47:*843–847, Dec '28

BURKE, H. D.; MURPHY, D. L. AND MCNICHOLS, W. A.: Skeletal fixation of mandibular fractures; 5 cases with 9 fractures. Arch. Surg. *51:*279–282, Nov-Dec '45

BURKE, J.: Exstrophy of bladder in female. Ann. Surg. *73:*100, Jan '21

BURKET, L. W.: Congenital bony temporomandibular ankylosis and facial hemiatrophy; review of literature and report of case. J. A. M. A. *106:*1719–1722, May 16, '36

BURKHARDT, C. F.: Modification of present radical operation for deflection of nasal septum. Illinois M. J. *56:*353–355, Nov '29

BURKHARDT, L.: Histology of fat transplantation. Deutsche Ztschr. f. Chir. *254:*372–378, '41

BÜRKLE-de la CAMP, H.: Plastic reconstruction of osseous defects of cranium; surgical therapy of early traumatic epilepsy. Zentralbl. f. Chir. *65:*2578–2584, Nov. 19, '38

BURMAN, C. E. L.: Two cases of keloid formation, with comments. Brit. J. Surg. *21:*527–529, Jan '34

BURMAN, M.: Kinetic disabilities of hand and their classification; study in balance and imbalance of hand muscles. Am. J. Surg. *61:*167–214, Aug '43

BURMAN, M.: Nylon fabric arthroplasty of carpometacarpal joint of thumb. Bull. Hosp. Joint Dis. *4:*74–78, Oct '43

BURMAN, M. AND ABRAHAMSON, R. H.: Use of plastics in reconstructive surgery; lucite in arthroplasty; tissue tolerance for lucite, its use as interposition mold in arthroplasty of phalangeal joints; 3 cases. Mil. Surgeon *93:*405–414, Nov '43

BURMAN, M. S.: Spastic hand. J. Bone and Joint Surg. *20:*133–145, Jan '38

BURMAN, M. S.: Vitallium cap arthroplasty of metacarpophalangeal and interphalangeal joints of fingers. Bull. Hosp. Joint Dis. *1:*79–89, Oct '40

BURMAN, M. S.: Use of nylon sheath in secondary repair of torn finger flexor tendons. Bull. Hosp. Joint Dis. *5:*122–133, Oct '44

BURMISTROVA, E.: Therapy of cicatricial ectropion. Vestnik oftal. *18:*89, '41

BURNELL, G. H.: Closure of defect in hard palate by pedicled tube graft. M. J. Australia *2:*484, Oct 7, '33

BURNELL, M.: Diffuse breast hypertrophy; preliminary case report. J. Michigan M. Soc. *31:*324–325, May '32

BURNETT, J. H.: Gas bacillus infections, burns and tetanus. Am. J. Orthodontics (Oral Surg. Sect.) *27:*698–700, Dec '41

BURNHAM, C.: Fracture of terminal phalanx of finger with rupture of common extensor tendon. Brit. M. J. 141, Jan 28, '22

BURNHAM, DeW. K. (see HOSMER, M. N. *et al*) Oct '40

BURNIER, (see GOUGEROT, H.) Nov '29

Burns

Burns, a case report. WHELCHEL, H. C., J. M. A. Georgia *10:*239, Jan '21

Blood concentration changes in extensive superficial burns, and their significance for systemic treatment. UNDERHILL, F. P. *et al*. Arch. Int. Med. *32:*31–49, July '23

Notes on group of burn cases. JONES, J. F. X. AND KEEGAN, A. P., M. J. and Record *119:*86–87, Jan 16, '24

Extensive superficial burns. SHEPARD, G. W. U.S. Nav. M. Bull. *20:*697-701, June '24

Gastrointestinal ulceration following cutaneous burns; with report of case. NOVAK, E. Am. J. M. Sc. *169:*119–125, Jan '25

Burns and scalds. SOUTTAR, H. S. Lancet *1:*142–143, Jan 17, '25

Cause of death in burns. MLLS, H. P. Southwestern Med. *9:*111, March '25

Burns—Cont.

Burns. SCHREINER, P. K. Med. Klinik *21:*1187–1189, Aug 7; 1231–1233, Aug 14, '25

Extensive burns. PARAVICINI. Schweiz. med. Wchnschr. *57:*22, Jan. 1, '27

Study of burns, their classification and treatment. GOLDBLATT, D. Ann. Surg. *85:*490–501, April '27

Burns in children. FRASER, J. Brit. M. J. *1:*1089–1092, June 18,'27

Superficial burns. RAVDIN, I. S. Atlantic M. J. *30:*679–683, Aug '27

Burns in children. McCULLOUGH, J. W. S. Canad. M. A. J. *17:*1176–1177, Oct '27

Burns of larynx. FLURIN, H. AND MAGDELEINE, J. Ann. d. mal. de l'oreille, du larynx *46:*1207–1221, Dec '27

Changes in blood concentration with special reference to treatment of extensive superficial burns. UNDERHILL, F. P. Ann. Surg. *86:*840–849, Dec '27

Extensive burn of body with recovery. LEIGH, A. M. Kentucky M. J. *26:*477–478, Sept '28

Crush-burns of hand. MACLURE, F. J. Coll. Surgeons, Australasia *1:*233–235, Nov '28

Burns in children. WAKELEY, C. P. G., M. Press *128:*32, July 10, '29

Burns of scalp in women. FINDLAY, R. T. Am. J. Surg. *8:*389–396, Feb '30

Cutaneous burns. MORTON, A. M., M. Times, New York. *58:*73, March '30

Cutaneous burns. BANCROFT, F. W. New England J. Med. *202:*811–822, April 24, '30

Hypertrichosis following burns. BATTISTA, A. Folia med. *16:*1420–1431, Oct. 30, '30

Value of surface-area proportions in prognosis of cutaneous burns and scalds. BERKOW, S. G. Am. J. Surg. *11:*315–317, Feb '31

Prognosis, therapy and complications in burns. RIEHL, G. JR. Arch. f. Dermat. u. Syph. *164:*409–471, '31

Unusual cicatrix following burns. SOLCARD, AND MORVAN, Ann. d'anat. path. *8:*530, May '31

Severe burns. TRUEBLOOD, D. V. West. J. Surg. *39:*543–546, July '31

Cutaneous burns. LITTLE, W. D., J. Indiana M. A. *24:*415–417, Aug '31

Burns of oral cavity. NADOLECZNY, M. Arch. f. Ohren-, Nasen-u. Kehlkopfh. *133:*283–287, '32

Extensive burn of arms. THOMPSON, C. F. J. Indiana M. A. *25:*301–302, July '32

Studies of scalding. SAITO, R. Mitt. d. med. Gesellsch. zu Tokio *46:*2137–2138, Dec '32

Management of cutaneous burns in children. DAVIDSON, E. C. Kentucky M. J. *31:*46–50, Jan '33

Burns—Cont.

Peripheral burns. MYERS, B. L., J. Missouri M. A. *30:*25–29, Jan '33

Symposium on acute burns; biochemical studies. OSTERBERG, A. E. Proc. Staff Meet., Mayo Clin. *8:*121–123, Feb. 22, '33

Presence of toxic substances in artificial fluid circulating through burned area. LORETO, C. Arch. ed atti d. Soc. ital. di chir. *39* 1058–1067, '33

Extensive cutaneous burns. Mc IVER, M. A. Ann. Surg. *97:*670–682, May '33

Burns in very young children. RIEHL, G. JR. Wien. klin. Wchnschr. *46:*1147–1150, Sept 22, '33

Extensive cutaneous burns. CAMP, J. H. Texas State J. Med. *29:*639–642, Feb '34

Extensive burns. STANLEY-BROWN, M. M. Clin. North America *17:*1393–1405, March '34

Pharyngolaryngeal burns and scalds; prognosis, complications and therapy. AGUERRE, J. A. JR. Arch. de pediat. d. Uruguay *5:*181–190, May '34

Clinical note on burns. OMAR BEY, T., J. Egyptian M. A. *17:*653, July '34

Tar burns; case. DRACKLE, W. Deutsche med. Wchnschr. *60:*1961–1962, Dec. 21, '34

Review of burn cases treated in Glasgow Royal Infirmary during past hundred years (1833–1933), with some observations on present-day treatment. DUNBAR, J. Glasgow M. J. *122:*239–255, Dec '34

Cause of death of badly burned persons; case of grave icterus. MASSABUAU, *et al.* Arch. Soc. d. sc. med. et biol. de Montpellier *16:*213–218, April '35

Extensive burns. STANLEY-BROWN, M. S. Clin. North America *15:*375–385, April '35

Causes of early death from scalding. ISHIZAWA, G. Tohoku J. Exper. Med. *26:*527–545, July 31, '35

Extensive burns and scalds. WILSON, W. C. Tr. Med.-Chir. Soc. Edinburgh, pp. 177–192, '34–'35; in Edinburgh M. J. Oct '35

Review of modern burn problem. PFOHL, A. C. J. Iowa M. Soc. *26:*100–103, Feb '36

Treatment of extensive gasoline burns of legs (due to explosion) with correction of deformity; case. BRUNSTING, L. A. AND GHORMLEY, R. K. Proc. Staff Meet., Mayo Clin. *11:*129–131, Feb 26, '36

Extensive burns. DUFOUR, A. Hopital, *24:*187–190, March (B) '36

Epidemolysis bullosa dystrophica; etiopathogenic study of case following burn in tuberculous child. CIACCIO, I. Arch. ital. di dermat., sif. *12:*326–344, May '36

Burns—Cont.

Time changes in relative mortality from accidental burns among children in different geographic regions of United States, 1925–32; studies on fatal accidents of childhood. GAFAFER, W. M. Pub. Health Rep. *51:*1308–1316, Sept 18, '36

Statistical study of 1206 burn cases. WILLEMS, J. D. AND KUHN, L. P. Am. J. Surg. *34:*254–258, Nov. '36

Severe burns complicated by appendicitis. ROSE, H. W. Northwest Med. *36:*113–114, April '37

Two case reports of extensive burns in children; both recovered; one with Curling ulcer. SHERRILL, W. P. Southwestern Med. *21:*135–138, April '37

Humorotissular syndrome in extensive burns; pathogenesis and therapy. LAMBRET, O. AND DRIESSENS, J. Rev. de chir., Paris, *75:*319–354, May '37

Peripheral radial paralysis following burns. BAHLS, G. Med. Welt *11:*857–858, June 19, '37

Pathogenesis of death due to burns; role of acidosis. PELAGATTI, V. Ateneo parmense *9:*209–227, July-Aug '37

Experiences with "Hindenburg" patients and review of cutaneous burns. HOLTERS, O. R. J. M. Soc. New Jersey *34:*545–548, Sept '37

Scalds of pharynx in small children. IDEMITSU, K. Oto-rhino-laryng. *10:*1047, Nov '37

Industrial burn. WITTMER, J. J. New York State J. Med. *37:*1931–1937, Nov. 15, '37

Recent extensive cutaneous burns. MOURGUE-MOLINES, E. Montpellier med., *12:* 201–212, Dec '37

Burns in children. HARRENSTEIN, R. J. Maandschr. v. kindergeneesk. *7:*179–191, Feb '38

Recent advances in study of burns. HARKINS, H. N. Surgery *3:*430–465, March '38

Mast cells as system of local and general defense in burns of mammals. SCEVOLA, P. Arch. ital. di otol. *50:*169–199, April '38

Clinical course and pathology of burns and scalds under modern methods of treatment. WILSON, W. C.; *et al.* Brit. J. Surg. *25:*826–865, April '38

Cutaneous burns. LAZYNSKA, W. Pediatria polska, *18:* 340–343, June '38

Burns in childhood. YONIS, Z. Harefuah *15:*ii–iii, July-Aug '38

Burns. TYNICKI, M. Polska gaz. lek., *17:*653–657, Aug. 7, '38; 679–682, Aug 21, '38

Plaster casts in simple and complicated burns. ZENO, L. Bol. y trab. de la Soc. de cir. de Buenos Aires *22:*712–722, Sept 28, '38

Burns—Cont.

Severe burns. PEDOTTI, F. Helvet. med. acta *5:*914–915, Dec '38

Hyperthermic epidermal destruction. NAGLE, P. S., J. Oklahoma M. A. *32:*7–14, Jan '39

Clinic study of burn therapy, with special reference to metabolic disturbances. CAVALCANTI, H. Rev. med. -cir. do Brasil, *47:*65–181, Feb '39

Burns in childhood. CLARK, A. M., M. Press *201:*182–185, Feb 15, '39

Burns. SEEGER, S. J., J. Michigan M. Soc. *38:*133–138, Feb '39 also: Wisconsin M. J., *38:*279–282, April '39

Clinical study of burns. ZAVALETA, D. E. Dia med., *11:*162–168, Feb 27, 39

Burns, unsolved problem. COHN, I. New Orleans M. and S. J. *91:*465–474, March '39

Wounds of larynx due to burns during childhood. RIECKE, H. G. Hals-, Nasen-u. Ohrenarzt (Teil 1) *30:*111–118, March '39

Cutaneous burns. JOHNSON, G. N., J. Maine M. A. *30:*91–93, May '39

Changes in blood chemistry after burning injuries; with reference to treatment by desoxycorticosterone acetate (suprarenal preparation). WILSON, W. C. AND STEWART. C. P. Tr. Med.-Chir. Soc. Edinburgh, pp. 153–173, '38–'39; in Edinburgh M. J., Nov '39

Severe burns. MCCLURE, R. D., J.A.M.A. *113:*1808–1812, Nov. 11, '39

Burns and scalds in children. DENNISON, W. M. Lancet *2:*1107–1110, Nov. 25, '39

Bacterial flora of content of vesicles produced by burns. KANEKEVICH, M. I. Ortop. i travmatol. (no. 3) *13:*77–81, '39

Third-degree burns. KNAPPER, C. Nederl. tijdschr. v. geneesk. *84:*382–387, Feb. 3, '40

Syndrome due to serious burns. COURTY, L. Rev. gen. de clin. et de therap. *54:*73–77, Feb, 17, '40

Grave burns. BARMAK, M. AND CONCILIO, L. Rev. Assoc. paulista de med. *16:*306–315, May '40

Burns and frostbite. MICHAËL, P. R. Geneesk. gids *18:*476, May 31, '40; 494, June 7, '40

Emergency care of burns and injuries to skin. CHORMLEY, R. K. Proc. Staff Meet., Mayo Clin. *15:*741, Nov. 20, '40

Injuries to face (soft tissues) (with burns). ECKHOFF, N. L. Guy's Hosp. Gaz. *54:*345–350, Nov. 30, '40

Cause and treatment of lethal factors in burns (Honyman Gillespie lecture). WILSON, W. C. Edinburgh M. J. *48:*85–93, Feb '41

Burns—Cont.

Grave burns during pregnancy; case. PERRUELO, N. N. Semana med. *1:*452-456, Feb. 20, '41

Serious burns. MONTEIRO, O. Hospital, Rio de Janeiro *19:*929-935, June '41

Extensive cutaneous burns. TENERY, R. M. Surg., Gynec. and Obst. *72:*1018-1027, June '41

Burns. DESJARDINS, E. Union med. du Canada *70:*770-771, July '41

Clinical and physiopathologic study of burns. FERNANDES, J. F. JR. Rev. med. Brasil. *11:*117-133, Aug '41

Burns and scalds in infants and children. FINCKE, B. Monatschr. f. Kinderh. *86:*73-95, '41

Cutaneous burns. TENERY, R. M. Am. J. M. Sc. *203:*293-300, Feb '42

Burns. NOYA BENITEZ, J. Bol. Asoc. med. de Puerto Rico *34:*90-95, March '42

Extensive burns. TODD, M. C. Illinois M. J. *81:*329-331, April '42

Severe burns. ALLEN, H. S. AND KOCH, S. L. Surg., Gynec. and Obst. *74:*914-924, May '42

Burns and scalds; etiology and prognosis. HOFFMAN, J. M. Am. J. Surg. *56:*463-468, May '42

General considerations of burn problem. RAVDIN, I. S. Clinics *1:*1-5, June '42

Plan for grave burns. SANTAS, A. A. *et al.* Bol. d. Inst. clin. quir. *18:*549-553, Aug '42

Burns of skin due to molten magnesium. WILSON, J. A. AND EGEBERG, B. Indust. Med., *11:*436-437, Sept '42

Modern theories on burns. DA ROCHA AZEVEDO, L. G. An. paulist, de med. e cir., *44:*277-297, Oct '42

Recent developments in severe third degree burns. WOLFF, W. A. *et al.* Nebraska M. J. *27:*369-374, Nov '42

Cocoanut Grove disaster in Boston; preliminary account. FAXON, N. W. AND CHURCHILL, E. D., J.A.M.A., *120:*1385-1388, Dec. 26, '42

Burns and scalds. KERR, W. G. East African M. J. *19:*274-288, Dec '42

Clinical aspect of severe burns. DE NICOLA, C. P. AND VILAFANE, A. R. An. Cong. brasil. e am. cir., *3:*364-374, '42

Burns and explosions in anesthesia. EHLERS, G. Deutsche Ztschr. f. Chir. *255:*485-522, '42

Cutaneous burns. RIVEROS, M. An. Cong. Brasil. e am. cir. *3:*174-278, '42

Skin Grafting of Burns, by J. B. Brown and Frank McDowell, J. B. Lippincott Co., Phila., 1943

Burns—Cont.

Burn progress. MACOMBER, D. W. Rocky Mountain M. J. *40:*34-36, Jan '43

Burn problem. RAVDIN, I. S. Am. J. Surg. *59:*330-340, Feb '43

Early mortality as influenced by rapid tanning and by transfusions in burns. ELMAN, R. Ann. Surg. *117:*327-331, March '43

Medical report on St. John's conflagration. FARMER, A. W.; *et al.* Canad. M. A. J. *48:*191-195, March '43

Thermal burns. GORDON, S. D. AND GORDON, R. A. Canad. M. A. J. *48:*302-309, April '43

Burns. SCHAFF, R. A., J. M. Soc. New Jersey *40:*128-133, April '43

Symposium on management of Cocoanut Grove burns at Massachusetts General Hospital; foreword. COPE, O. Ann. Surg. *117:*801-802, June '43

Symposium on management of Cocoanut Grove burns at Massachusetts General Hospital; treatment of surface burns. COPE, O. Ann. Surg. *117:*885-893, June '43

Trend in burns. SILER, V. E. Cincinnati J. Med. *24:*163-167, June '43

Care of victims of Cocoanut Grove fire at Massachusetts General hospital. COPE, O. New England J. Med., *229:*138-147, July 22, '43

Mangle burn injuries. LYLE, F. M. Am. J. Surg. *61:*148-149, July '43

Magnesium burns. JARZYNKA, F. J. Indust. Med. *12:*427-431, July '43

Statistical study of minor industrial burns. MCCLURE, R. D. AND LAM, C. R., J.A.M.A. *122:*909-911, July 31, '43

Burn review. Quemaduras. Semana med., *2:*33-37, July 1, '43

Basic principles in thermal burns. WHIPPLE, A. O. Ann. Surg. *118:*187-192, Aug '43

Major and minor burns. ALDRICH, R. H. M. Clin. North America *27:*1229-1246, Sept '43

Clinical test for differentiating second from third degree burns. DINGWALL, J. A. III Ann. Surg., *118:*427-429, Sept '43

Extensive (60 percent) burn; case. DONOVAN, S. J. AND CARR, F. J. JR. U.S. Nav. M. Bull. *41:*1410-1412, Sept '43

Burns. LUND, C. C. Rhode Island M. J. *26:*197-200, Oct '43

Studies on destruction of red blood cells; mechanism and complications of hemoglobinuria in patients with thermal burns; spherocytosis and increased osmotic fragility of red blood cells. SHEN, S. C. AND HAM, T. H. New England J. Med. *229:*701-713, Nov. 4, '43

Burns—Cont.

Burns. Richards, R. T. Rocky Mountain M. J. *40:*810-815, Dec '43

Burns. Beck, C. S. Kentucky M. J. *42:*68-72, March '44

Carbohydrate metabolism after burning. Clark, E. J. and Rossiter, R. J. Quart. J. Exper. Physiol. *32:*279-300, March '44

Changes in blood following thermal burns. Gordon, S. D. and Gordon, R. A. J. Canad. M. Serv. *1:*312-320, May '44

Problem of thermal burns: 1944. Harkins, H. N., J.A.M.A. *125:*533-536, June 24, '44

Physiologic analysis of burns. Glenn, W. W. L. Ann. Surg. *119:*801-814, June '44

Diagnosis of depth of skin destruction in burns and its bearing on treatment. Patey, D. H. and Scarff, R. W. Brit. J. Surg. *32:*32-35, July '44

The burned patient. Sampson, W. C. J. Nat. M. A. *36:*143-151, Sept '44

Pantocrine in thermal and chemical burns. Pavlenko, S. M. Khirurgiya, no. 5, pp. 19-22, '44

Treatment of burns complicated by fractures of extremities. Warthen, H. J. Jr. Ann. Surg. *119:*526-532, April '44

Treatment of burns complicated by fractures of extremities. Warthen, H. J. Jr. Tr. South. S. A. (1943) *55:*237-243, '44

Burns with partial skin destruction; illustrative case. Patey, D. H. and Scarff, R. W. Lancet *1:*146, Feb 3, '45

Statistical analysis of study of prevention of infection in burns, with special reference to sulfonamides. Meleney, F. L. and Whipple, A. O. Surg. Gynec. and Obst., *80:*263-296, March '45

Thermal burns in diabetes mellitus. Root, H. F. New England J. Med. *232:*279, March 8, '45

Significance of blood changes in treatment of patient with burns. Gordon, R. A. Anesth. and Analg., *24:*78-84, March-April '45

Physiology and metabolism of severe burn. Sturgis, S. H. Mil. Surgeon *97:*215-224, Sept '45

Extensive second and third degree burns. Maguire, D. L. Jr. J. South Carolina M. A. *41:*246-248, Oct '45

The critically burned patient. Urkov, J. C. Am. J. Surg. *71:*242-252, Feb '46

Collective review of burns. Lund, C. C.; *et al* Internat. Abst. Surg. *82:*443-478, '46, in Surg. Gynec. and Obst. June '46

Burns, Anesthesia for

Anesthetization in burns. Laqueur, B. Therap. d. Gegenw. *73:*144, March '32

Burns, Anesthesia for—Cont.

Intravenous novocain (procaine hydrochloride) for analgesia in burns; preliminary report. Gordon, R. A. Canad. M. A. J. *49:*478-481, Dec '43

Influence of ether, morphine and nembutal (Pentobarbital) on mortality in experimental burns. Elman, R. Ann. Surg. *120:*211-213, Aug '44

Local anesthesia in burn therapy. Rivas Diez, B. and Delrio, J. M. A. Bol. y trab., Acad. argent. de cir. *28:*1182-1192, Nov 22, '44

Anesthesia for patient in burn therapy. Papper, E. M. Surgery *17:*116-121, Jan '45

Burns, Bones, and Fractures with

Burns and compound fractures; review of their closed treatment. Alexander, H. H. Jr. Indust. Med. *12:*434-436, July '43

Problem of fractures with associated burn injuries; principles of treatment. Bodenham, D. C. Proc. Roy. Soc. Med., *36:*657-662, Oct '43

Treatment of burns complicated by fractures of extremities. Warthen, H. J. Jr. Ann. Surg. *119:*526-532, April '44

Treatment of burns complicated by fractures of extremities. Warthen, H. J. Jr. Tr. South. S. A. (1943) *55:*237-243, '44

Fracture of mandible associated with burns of head. Karnes, T. W. J. Oral Surg. *3:*83-86, Jan '45

Deep burns involving bones. Mc Dowell, F. J. Indiana M. A. *39:*108-109, Mar '46

Burns, Cancer in

Development of carcinoma in scar tissue following burns. Johnson, F. M. Ann. Surg. *83:*165-169, Feb '26

Epithelioma of forearm developed upon scar of ancient burn. Roussy, *et al.* Bull. de l'Assoc. franc. p. l'etude du cancer *16:*504-509, June '27

Epithelioma following burns. Bell, J. G. Y. Clin. J. *57:*525-527, Oct 31, '28

Professional epithelioma of lower eyelid following burn by hot tar; case. Milian, G. and Garnier, G. Bull. Soc. franc. de dermat. et syph. *35:*793, Nov '28

Cancer forming in inflamed tissue following burns; case. Stauffer, H. Ztschr. f. Krebsforsch. *28:*418-430, '29

Acute, spinocellular epithelioma developed after burn with flaming asphalt; case. Gunsett, A. Bull. Assoc. franc. p. l'etude du cancer *19:*459-462, June '30

Traumatic burns in etiology of cancer. Genkin, I. I. Vrach. delo *15:*496-499, '32

Burns, Cancer in – Cont.

Carcinoma developing on extensive scars; inefficiency of pinch grafts as prophylactic measure. DANZIS, M; *et al.* Am. J. Surg. *41:*304-306, Aug '38

Rare case of horny epithelioma on burn cicatrix; surgical extirpation and plastic repair of residual defect by free skin graft of Davis type. HALLEY MIRALLES, G. Bol. Liga. contra el cancer *18:*41-46, Feb '43

Fibrosarcoma protuberans arising on old burn scar. NEIDELMAN, M. L. Ann. Surg. *123:*311-314, Feb '46

Burns, Chemical

Treatment of acid and alkali burns. SMITH, A. K. Mod. Med. *3:*232, April '21

Treatment of lime burn of eye. BARKAN, O. AND BARKAN, H. J.A.M.A. *83:*1567-1569, Nov 15, '24

Phenol burns of left eyelids, eyeball, upper face and temporal area. SHEEHAN, J. E. Laryngoscope *35:*55, Jan '25

Tardy result of burn from toxic gas. BERNUCCI, F. Gior. ital. di dermat. e sifil. *66:*1349-1357, Oct '25

Treatment of lime burns of cornea by 10 per cent neutral ammonium tartrate. WOLFF, E. Brit. J. Ophth. *10:*196-197, April '26

Treatment of acid and alkali burns; experimental study. DAVIDSON, E. C. Ann. Surg. *85:*481-489, April '27

Favorable results of iridectomy in case of ammonia burn of eyes. THIES, O. Klin. Monatsbl. f. Augenh. *79:*534-536, Oct 28, '27

Acid and alkali burns of eyes; experimental study. COSGROVE, K. W. AND HUBBARD, W. B. Ann. Surg. *87:*89-94, Jan '28

Burns of larynx from swallowing sodium hydroxide; 2 cases. FOTIADE, V. Arch. internat. de laryng. *34:*22-30, Jan '28

Ammonia burns of eyes. THIES, O. Zentralbl. f. Gewerbehyg. *5:*83-88, March '28

Davidson's method in acid burns. KORNMAN, I. E. AND SMERETCHINSKY, T. M. Odessky M. J. *4:*13-16, '29

Roentgen treatment of thermal and chemical burns of skin. TAMIYA, C. AND KOYAMA, M. Strahlentherapie *34:*808-812, '29

Early plastic operation (transplantation of oral mucosa) in caustic injuries of eye. THIES, O. Arch. f. Ophth. *123:*165-170, '29

Chemical injuries (burns). KARSTED, A. Am. J. Surg. *8:*360-361, Feb '30

Burns from chlorosulphonic acid in industrial plant. ARTZ, L. Dermat. Wchnschr. *97:*995-997, July 8, '33

Burns due to sulfur dioxide of eyes; 2 cases.

Burns, Chemical – Cont.

DETROY, Echo med. du Nord *4:*742bis-743, Oct 27, '35

Treatment of chemical burns in industry. KASHKAROV, S. E. Sovet. khir., no. 8, pp. 3-8, '35

First aid in chemical burns. RAKHMANOV, V. A. Sovet. khir., no. 8, pp. 10-15, '35

Plastic surgery for deformity and contractures after nitric acid burns to face (case). MONEY, R. A., M. J. Australia *2:*848-853, Dec 19, '36

Chemical burns to eyes. MOSS, O. W. New Orleans M. and S. J. *89:*302-306, Dec '36

Chemical burns to eyes. BEREZINSKAYA, D. I. Sovet. vestnik oftal. *8:*319-332, '36

Burns to eyes with sulfuric acid. COPPEZ, J. H. AND BRENTA, MME. Bull. Soc. belge d'opht., no. 72, pp. 88-100, '36

Alkali burns to eyes; experimental study. VINOGOROV, D. R. AND KOPIT, R. Z. Sovet. vestnik oftal. *8:*333-347, '36

Chemical burns of mouth. DELPH, J. F. S. Clin. North America *17:*585-592, April '37

Chemical burns. RUDANOVSKAYA, V. A. AND STRUCHKOV, V. I. Novy khir. arkhiv., *38:*471-475, '37

Chemical burns of face. BECK, W. C., S. Clin. North America *18:*13-20, Feb '38

Caustic burns of eyes. HUBBARD, W. B. Arch. Ophth. *19:*968-975, June '38

Vinethene (vinyl ether) burn of face. LYONS, S. S., J.A.M.A. *111:*1284-1285, Oct 1, '38

Ammonia gas burns; account of 6 cases. SLOT, G. M. J. Lancet *2:*1356-1357, Dec 10, '38

Role of paracentesis in therapy of chemical burns to eyes. BEREZINSKAYA, D. I. Vestnik oftal. *13:*361-367, '38

Cement burn; etiology, pathology and treatment. MEHERIN, J. M. AND SCHOMAKER, T. P., J.A.M.A., *112:*1322-1326, April 8, '39

Phenol burns of both eyes and their general sequels; therapy of chemical burns. WINKLER, A. Klin. Monatsbl. f. Augenh. *102:*810-815, June '39

First aid in case of burns of eye due to lime. KAPLAN, Y. D. Vestnik oftal. (nos. 2-3) *14:*114-118, '39

Skin injuries from incendiary bombs and war chemicals. FUHS, H. Wien. klin. Wchnschr. *53:*40-44, Jan 12, '40

Rational therapy of chemical burns to eyes. BURSUK, G. G. AND SHULTS, V. A. Vestnik oftal. *17:*55-56, '40

Surgical therapy of chemical burns to eyes. DASHEVSKIY, A. I. AND MARMORSHTEYN, F. F. Vestnik oftal. *16:*415-420, '40

Chemical burns to eyes. RAMEEV, R. S. Vestnik oftal., *16:*381-383, '40

Burns, Chemical — Cont.

Chemical burns. SEYEWETZ, A. Avenir med., *37*:27, Jan '40

Severe chemical burns to eyes. THIES. O. Klin. Monatsbl. f. Augenh., *106*:47–56, Jan '41

Burn of eyes caused by brilliant green. KRÜCKELS, H. Klin. Monatsbl. f. Augenh. *106*:571–574, May '41

Conjunctival burn due to ammonia treated by Denig method (excision of tissue and graft of buccal mucosa); case. VON GROLMAN, G. Prensa med. argent. *28*:839–840, April 16, '41

Lime burns to eyes; use of rabbit peritoneum to prevent severe delayed effects; experimental studies and reports of cases. BROWN, A. L. Arch. Ophth., *26*:754–769, Nov '41

Lime burns to eye; use of rabbit peritoneum to prevent severe delayed effects; experimental studies and report of cases. BROWN, A. L. Tr. Sec. Ophth., A. M. A., pp. 40–57, '41

Therapy of chemical burns. WAKELEY, C. P. G. M. Press *208*:360–363, Dec 2, '42

Creosote burns. JONAS, A. D., J. Indust. Hyg. and Toxicol. *25*:418–420, Nov '43

Phosphates in therapy of chemical burns. POSER, E. AND HAAS, E., J.A.M.A. *123*:630–631, Nov 6, '43

Early transplantation of buccal mucosa and conjunctiva in chemical burns of eyes. PAVISIC, Z. Ophthalmologica *108*:297–304, Dec '44

Pantocrine in thermal and chemical burns. PAVLENKO, S. M. Khirurgiya, no. 5, pp. 19–22, '44

Methyl bromide burns. BUTLER, E. C. B.; *et al.* Brit. J. Indust. Med. *2*:30–31, Jan '45

Improved treatment for chemical burns of eye. OAKS, L. W. Am. J. Ophth. *28*:370–373, April '45

Chemical burn of penis. HOOPES, B. F., U.S. Nav. M. Bull. *44*:846–847, April '45

Burns, Complications

Atrophy of bone (Sudeck) following burns. DUBS, J. Munchen. med. Wchnschr. *68*:1141, Sept 9, '21

Tetanus after burn from high power current. FÖRSTER, W. Munchen. med. Wchnschr. *68*:1655, Dec 23, '21

Cause of death from burns. VACCAREZZA, R. A. Rev. Asoc. med. argent. *35*:48–53, Jan–April '22 abstr: J.A.M.A. *79*:859, Sept 2, '22

Burns, Complications — Cont.

Toxemia of severe superficial burns in children. ROBERTSON, B. AND BOYD, G. L. Am. J. Dis. Child. *25*:163–167, Feb '23

Toxemia of severe superficial burns. ROBERTSON, B. AND BOYD. G. L., J. Lab. and Clin. Med. *9*:1–14, Oct '23

Unusual deformity sequential to a burn of hand. PACK, G. T. AND PARSONS, J. L. Am. J. Surg. *38*:159, June '24

Duodenal ulcers in case of grave burns. RONCHESE, F. Riforma med. *40*:753–755, Aug 11, '24 abstr.: J.A.M.A., *83*:1038, Sept 27, '24

Gastrointestinal ulceration following cutaneous burns; with report of case. NOVAK, E. Am. J. M. Sc. *169*:119–125, Jan '25

Pathogenesis of death from burns and its relation to anaphylaxis. GIAMPAOLO, R. Policlinico (sez. prat.) *32*:207–208, Feb 9, '25

Poisoning from use of picric acid in burn therapy. ACHARD, C. Rev. gen. de clin. et de therap. *41*:65–68, Jan 29, '27

Note of caution on use of picric acid solution as burn dressing. COLQUHOUN, K. G., M. J. Australia *2*:652, Nov 24, '28

Duodenal ulcers following burns, with report of 2 cases. LEVIN, J. J. Brit. J. Surg. *17*:110–113, July '29

Tetanus after burns. SCHREINER, K. AND STOCKER, H. Wien. med. Wchnschr. *79*:1020–1022, Aug 3, '29

Extrabuccal scarlet fever after burns; cases. BYTCHKOFF, V. S. AND ALEXEEFF, O. A. Mosk. med. j. (no. 1) *9*:23–30, '29

Gastrostaxis following burns. D'EWART, J. Brit. M. J. *1*:242, Feb 8, '30

Haemorrhage into suprarenal capsule and haemorrhage from duodenal ulcer in burns; case. HARRIS, R. I. Clin. J. *59*:150–152, March 26, '30

Curling's ulcer; duodenal ulcer following superficial burns. MAES, U. Ann. Surg. *91*:527–532, April '30

Use of insulin in second-degree burn developing hyperglycemia and glycosuria. TEOPACO, R. L., J. Philippine Islands M. A. *10*:162–165, April '30

Curling's ulcer in burns; with report of 2 cases. MAES, U. M. Rec. and Ann. *24*:564–568, June '30

Delirium tremens excited by infected burns. DAMAYE, H. AND POIRIER, B. Progres med., p. 1340, Aug 2, '30

Epidemiology and prophylaxis of scarlet fever after burns. MINKEWITSCH, I. Med. Welt *4*:1397, Sept 27, '30

Burns, Complications – Cont.

Peptic ulcer following burns of skin; 5 cases. RIEHL, G. JR. Acta dermat.-venereol. *11:*277–294, Sept '30

"Curling's ulcer" in burns, with report of case. LAIRD, W. R. AND WILKERSON, W. V. West Virginia M. J. *27:*128–130, March '31

Determination of fatal cases in burns of skin. KERNBACH, M. AND GIURGIU, V. Cluj. med. *12:*406–408, July 1, '31

Burns causing death; review of past and recent literature. RIEHL, G. JR. Zentralbl. f. Haut-u. Geschlechtskr. *38:*289–296, Sept 5, '31

Course of infectious process in burns. SMORODINTZEFF, A. A. AND TOGUNOVA, E. F. Microbiol. j. *13:*27–35, '31

Curling ulcer in burns. MILLER, T. AND RUBENSTEIN, B. DALLAS M. J., *18:*8–9, Jan '32

Unusual case of burn complication (development of Curling ulcer; recovery). MILLER, T. AND RUBENSTEIN, B. Texas State J. Med. *27:*873, April '32

Mistakes, dangers and unforeseen complications in burn therapy. FILATOV, A. Chirurg, *4:*568–576, July 15, '32

Duodenal ulcer following skin burns; 2 cases with recovery. FITZGIBBON, J. H. Northwest Med., *31:*427–430, Sept '32

Curling ulcer in burns; study of intestinal ulceration associated with suprarenal damage. MCLAUGHLIN, C. W. Arch. Surg. *27:*490–505, Sept '33

Fat embolism after injury from blunt force and after burns; 130 cases. STRASSMANN, G. Deutsche Ztschr. f. d. ges. gerichtl. Med., *22:*272–298, '33

Mechanism of production of Curling's ulcer in burns. KAPSINOW, R. South. M. J. *27:*500–503, June '34

Changes in Golgi apparatus of kidney, liver and suprarenal cells produced by burning. HIROTA, K. Nagasaki Igakkai Zassi *12:*1143–1144, Aug 25, '34

Complications associated with treatment of burns. PENBERTHY, G. C. AND WELLER, C. N. Am. J. Surg. *26:*124–132, Oct '34

Prophylaxis of tetanus following burns. FASAL, P. Wien. klin. Wchnschr. *48:*181–182, Feb 8, '35

Megacolon, with report of traumatic case (anal stricture due to burn), treated by left lumbar sympathectomy. FOWLER, L. H. AND HANSON, W. A. Minnesota Med., *18:*646–655, Oct '35

Cause of death of badly burned persons; case of grave icterus. MASSABUAU, *et al.* Arch. Soc. d. sc. med. et biol. de Montpellier *16:*213–218, April '35

Bacterial infection in burns. CRUICKSHANK, R. Tr. Roy. Med.-Chir. Soc. Glasgow, pp. 79–82, '34–'35; in Glasgow M. J., July '35, also: J. Path. and Bact. *41:*367–369, Sept '35

Causes of early death from scalding. ISHIZAWA, G. Tohoku J. Exper. Med. *26:*527–545, July 31, '35

Low grade burns as cause of pathologic changes in internal organs (liver, heart, gallbladder, kidney). BRENNER, F. Centralbl. f. allg. Path. u. path. Anat. *65:*97–101, May 30, '36

Anuria after burn with hypertensive crisis and bradycardia treated successfully by sodium bicarbonate and transfusions of noncitrated blood; case. FROMENT, J.; *et al.* Lyon med. *158:*412–415, Oct 11, '36

Generalized edema following extensive burns; pathogenesis of edema; role of serum protein equilibrium. CLAVELIN, C. AND HUGONOT. Bull. et mem. Soc. med. d. hop. de Paris *52:*1444–1449, Nov 16, '36

Duodenal ulcer following burns; medicolegal importance with report of case following industrial accident. TORCHIANA, L. Policlinico (sez. prat.) *43:*2105–2112, Nov 23, '36

Infections and burns. MCELROY, T. J. Oklahoma M. A. *29:*443–446, Dec '36

Rare case of tetanus following burn. MUKHIN, M. V. Sovet. vrach. zhur., pp. 1820–1821, Dec 15, '36

Tetanus after burns. KUDRINSKIY, A. A. Sovet. khir., no. 9, pp. 522–524, '36

Clinically atypical, but histologically typical lupus immediately following burn; case. GOUGEROT, H. AND MEYER, J. Bull Soc. franc. de dermat. et syph. *44:*269–270, Feb '37

Immediate application of tannic acid for extensive burns; death in 7 days due to anuria and progressive azotemia; case. LERICHE, R. Rev. de chir., Paris, *75:*143–144, Feb '37

Severe burns complicated by appendicitis. ROSE, H. W. Northwest Med. *36:*113–114, April '37

Two case reports of extensive burns in children; both recovered; one with Curling ulcer. SHERRILL, W. P. Southwestern Med., *21:*135–138, April '37

Tetanus after burn by high tension electric current; 2 cases in workmen. CHAVANNAZ, J. Ann. de med. leg. *17:*800–801, July '37

Burns, Complications—Cont.

Pathogenesis of death due to burns; role of acidosis. PELAGATTI, V. Ateneo parmense *9:*209-227, July-Aug '37

Fatal tetanus following burns; case. MAZZINI, O. F. Bol. y trab. de la Soc. de cir. de Buenos Aires *21:*651-654, Aug 25, '37

Fatal tetanus in burn; case. MAZZINI, O. F. Prensa med. argent. *25:*554-556, March 16, '38

Acute ulcer of duodenum (Curling's ulcer) as complication of burns; relation to sepsis; report of case with study of 107 cases collected from literature, 94 with necropsy, 13 with recovery; experimental studies. HARKINS, H. N. Surgery *3:*608-641, April '38

Peculiar case of purpura developing after burns. DE HAAN, H. R. M. Nederl. tijdschr. v. geneesk. *82:*2556-2557, May 21, '38

New conception of mechanism of death from burns. CHRISTOPHE, L. Presse med. *46:*1054-1055, July 2, '38

Perforated duodenal ulcer and ileus following burn; case. BERGK, W. Chirurg *10:*548-552, Aug 1, '38

Rapid death due to extensive burns. DUVAL, P. Dia med. *10:*877-880, Aug 29, '38

Immunologic connection with burn sepsis. HUGHES, W. H. Lancet *2:*670-672, Sept 17, '38

Otitis media and cerebellar abscess developing after burns. ROSTA, G. Budapesti orvosi ujsag *36:*902-904, Oct 20, '38

Mechanism of death following burns. RUDLER, J. C. Bull. med., Paris *52:*765-767, Oct 22, '38

Tetanus after burns. MAURER, G. Zentralbl. f. Chir. *65:*2771-2772, Dec 10, '38

Collapse following burns. EWIG, W. Verhandl. d. deutsch. Gesellsch. f. Kreislaufforsch., pp. 148-157, '38

Systemic disturbances in severe burns and their treatment. ELKINTON, J. R. Bull. Ayer Clin. Lab., Pennsylvania Hosp. *3:*279-292, Dec '39

Treatment (especially tannic acid) of infected burns. MURLESS, B. C. Brit. M. J. *1:*51-53, Jan 13, '40

Problems in treatment of burns; liver necrosis as lethal factor. MC CLURE, R. D. AND LAM, C. R. South. Surgeon *9:*223-234, April '40

Gas bacillus infections, burns and tetanus. BURNETT, J. H. Am. J. Orthodontics (Oral Surg. Sect.) *27:*698-700, Dec '41

Relation of tannic acid to liver necrosis in burns. WELLS, D. B.; *et al.* New England J. Med. *226:*629-636, April 16, '42

Experimental investigation of gastrointestinal secretions and motility following burns and their relation to ulcer. NECHELES, H. AND OLSON, W. H. Surgery *11:*751-765, May '42

Hemorrhage complicating cutaneous burn (zinc peroxide therapy). ALTEMEIER, W. A. Cincinnati J. Med. *23:*176-178, June '42

Infected burns with hemorrhage. ALTEMEIER, W. A. AND CARTER, B. N. Ann. Surg. *115:*1118-1124, June '42

Toxic blood-level of sulfanilamide from local application in burns. GORDON, R. A. AND BOWERS, V. H. Lancet, *2:*484, Oct 24, '42

Severe burns associated with duodenal ulceration. WHIGHAM, J. R. M. Brit. J. Surg., *30:*178-179, Oct '42

Complications of burns. DA SILVA, CANDIDO. Amatus *1:*781-798, Nov '42

Infected burns in naval personnel. HEGGIE, R. M. AND HEGGIE, J. F. Lancet *2:*664-667, Dec 5, '42

Grave burn in girl 6 years old; death on fifty-second day due to progressive emaciation; role of adrenal insufficiency. HOUOT, A. Union med. du Canada *72:*25-27, Jan '43

Pathologic picture as revealed at autopsy in series of 61 fatal burn cases treated (with and without tannic acid) at Hospital for Sick Children, Toronto, Canada. ERB, I. H.; *et al.* Ann. Surg. *117:*234-255, Feb '43

Perforated esophagus with burns. ROBSON, L. C. Brit. M. J. *1:*414, April 3, '43

Symposium on management of Cocoanut Grove burns at Massachusetts General Hospital; note on thrombophlebitis encountered. MOORE, F. D. Ann. Surg. *117:*931-936, June '43

Bilateral cortical necrosis of kidneys following severe burns. BROWN, C. E. AND CRANE, G. L., J.A.M.A. *122:*871-873, July 24, '43

Tannic acid toxicity in burn therapy. BARNES, J. M. AND ROSSITER, R. J. Lancet *2:*218-222, Aug 21, '43

Liver necrosis in burns. HARTMAN, F. W. AND ROMENCE, H. L. Ann. Surg. *118:*402-416, Sept '43

Wound infection; preliminary note on combined clinical and bacteriologic investigation of 708 wounds. (and burn) DE WAAL, H. L. Edinburgh M. J. *50:*577-588, Oct '43

Chemotherapy in prevention and treatment of infection in burns; panel discussion; introduction. MELENEY, F. L. Am. Acad. Orthop. Surgeons, Lect., pp. 314-316, '43

Tannic acid in burn therapy; liver necrosis following therapy. JACKSON, A. V., M. J. Australia *2:*352-354, Sept 30, '44

Burns, Complications–Cont.

Tannic acids in burns; useful and dangerous fixative. SAINT-ONGE, G. J. de l'Hotel-Dieu de Montreal *13:*270–282, Sept–Oct '44

Phlebitis and burns (role of pressure bandages). MEYER, O. Indust. Med. *14:*440, May '45

Extensive infected burns. MARINO, H. Gac. med., Lima *1:*177–178, June '45 also: Rev. san. de policia *5:*185–196, July–Aug '45

Anemia of thermal burns. MOORE, F. D.; *et al.* Ann. Surg. *124:*811–839, Nov '46

Burns, Contractures

Surgical treatment of burn scars. PIERCE, G. W. S. Clin. N. America *3:*841–855, June '23 (illus.)

Correction of burn scar deformity by Z-plastic method. MCCURDY, S. L., J. Bone and Joint Surg. *6:*683–688, July '24

Exercise after burns. SCHWARTZ, A. Paris med., *2:*175–176, Aug 30, '24

Contractures due to burns of face, neck and body. BEHREND, M., S. Clin. N. America, *6:*237–243, Feb '26

Treatment of contracture deformities secondary to burns. MILLER, O. L. Southern M. J., *17:*522–526, July '24

Surgical treatment of large contraction scars of burns according to Morestin's plastic operations. STEGEMANN, H. Zentralbl. f. Chir. *53:*1880–1884, July 24, '26

Contracture from burn with extensive ulcer in popliteal space; excision and full-thickness skin graft. JONES, H. T., S. Clin. N. America *7:*1447–1449, Dec '27

Contracture of axilla from burns; 3 cases. JONES, H. T. Minnesota Med. *11:*210–214, April '28

Wry-neck following burns, relieved by skin flaps; case report. MILLER, O. R. Kentucky M. J. *26:*190–192, April '28

Ectropion of lower eyelids following burns and scalds; new early pathognomonic sign. BERKOW, S. G., J.A.M.A. *90:*1708–1709, May 26, '28

Contractures due to burns; treatment with free full thickness grafts and pedunculated flaps. KOCH, S. L. AND KANAVEL, A. B. Tr. Sect. Surg, General and Abd., A. M. A., pp. 208–227, '28

Contracture due to burns; treatment with free full thickness grafts and pedunculated flaps. KOCH, S. L. AND KANAVEL, A. B. J.A.M.A. *92:*277–281, Jan 26, '29

Whirlpool baths and posterior splinting to overcome contractures in burns. HILBERT, J. W., J.A.M.A. *95:*1021, Oct 4, '30

Hypertension of hand and fingers from burn;

Burns, Contractures–Cont.

correction by single pedicled skin and fascial flap from anterior abdominal wall. JACKSON, C. AND BABCOCK, W. W., S. Clin. North America *10:*1285–1286, Dec '30

Morestin operation in dermatogenous contractures after burns. PRISELKOFF, P. V. Vestnik khir. (no. 64) *22:*111–114, '30

Plastic operation for cicatricial ectropion of eyelids resulting from burn. WEINGOTT, L. Arch. d'opht. *48:*505–507, July '31

Plastic surgery in cicatrices of eyelid caused by burn; case. ROY, J. N. Bull. med. de Quebec *32:*322–328, Oct '31

Plastic surgery of face and neck to remove cicatricial adhesions caused by burns; case. VASCONCELLOS ALVARENGA, E. Rev. brasil. de med. e pharm. *7:*334–337, '31

Release of axillary and brachial scar fixation. BLAIR, V. P.; *et al.* Tr. South. S. A. *45:*258–274, '32

Contractures of neck following burns (treatment by use of tubular skin graft). MIXTER, C. G. New England J. Med. *208:*190–196, Jan 26, '33

Burn therapy to prevent contractures. BURTON, J. F., J. Oklahoma M. A. *26:*36–38, Feb '33

Cicatricial contraction of neck. NEW, G. B. S. Clin. North America *13:*868–869, Aug '33

Reconstructive surgery and old facial burns. UPDEGRAFF, H. L., J.A.M.A. *101:*1138–1140, Oct 7, '33

Palmar contracture of hand as sequel of burn received in infancy; therapy with Gillies tubular graft at age 17 years. LLUESMA URANGA, E. Cron. med., Valencia *38:*11–14, Jan 15, '34

Plastic removal of skin from breast as aid in treating scars on breast and neck resulting from burns; case. BREITFUSS, F. F. Zentralbl. f. Chir. *61:*436–437, Feb 24, '34

Z plastic or web splitting operation for relief of scar contractures of extremities. JONES, H. T. Surg. Gynec. and Obst., *58:*178–182, Feb '34

Burn contractures of axilla. KOCH, S. L. S. Clin. North America *14:*751–761, Aug '34

Radium as adjuvant to operation in case of deformity of eyelids from burn with keloid scars. HUDSON, A. C. Proc. Roy. Soc. Med. *27:*1611, Oct '34

Plastic surgery of contracture after burns. GRZYWA, N. Geneesk. tijdschr. v. Nederl.-Indie *74:*1539–1540, Nov 6, '34

Treatment (with skin grafts) of deformities from burns. MILLER, O. L. AND ROBERTS, W. M. South. Surgeon *4:*52–62, March '35

Scarring of face and neck with keloid from

Burns, Contractures—Cont.

burn treated with radium and plastic operation; case. New, G. B. Proc. Staff Meet., Mayo Clin. *10:*283-285, May 1, '35

Surgical restoration by means of grafts in severe burns of face with cicatrix. Sanvenero-Rosselli, G. Bull. et mem. Soc. d. chirurgiens de Paris *27:*391-403, July 5, '35

Plastic repair of talipes calcaneovalgus due to cicatricial adhesions following burns; case. Pascau. I. Cir. ortop. y traumatol. *3:*185-189, July-Sept '35

Malocclusion produced by formation of scar tissue (from burn). Howes, A. E. Internat. J. Orthodontia *21:*1141-1143, Dec '35

Tourniquet method in retractile cicatrices caused by burns in articular regions. Michel, L. J. de med. de Bordeaux *113:*184-185, March 10, '36

Repair of contractures resulting from burns. (grafts). Kazanjian, V. H. New England J. Med. *215:*1104-1120, Dec 10, '36

Symphysis of both thighs due to burn cicatrix; surgical therapy of case. Gutiérrez, A. Rev. de cir. de Buenos Aires *16:*13-21, Jan '37

Burns, discussion on their treatment, both immediate and remote, with special emphasis on prevention of scars and contractures. Coakley, W. A. Am. J. Surg. *36:*50-53, April '37

Choice method in plastic restoration of face following extensive burns causing cicatricial disfigurement. Dantrelle, M. Rev. de chir. structive, pp. 108-109, June '37

Extensive cicatrices of legs and feet due to burns; cicatricial pes talus; autoplasty and disarticulation of Chopart's joint of left foot; case. Rocher, H. L. Rev. de chir. structive, pp. 111-114, June '37

Tubular graft in autoplastic therapy of burn cicatrix; case. Tecqmenne, C. Liege med. *30:*818-820, July 11, '37

Cicatricial ectropion of upper eyelid and contracture of lower lip following burn; blepharoplasty and labioplasty; case. Roy, J. N. Rev. de chir. structive *8:*85-90, Aug '38

Therapy of cicatrical contracture of hand and fingers after burns. Bakushinskiy, R. N. Ortop. i travmatol. (no. 2) *12:*76-83, '38

Surgical therapy of cicatricial contracture of neck after burns. Mikhelson, N. M. Ortop. i travmatol. (no. 1) *12:*74-82, '38

Reconstruction of 4 eyelids for ectropion resulting from cicatrix of severe facial burn, by means of free cutaneous grafts; case. de Lieto Vollaro, A. Arch. ital. di chir. *51:*588-595, '38

Contractures due to burns. Coughlin, W. T.

Burns, Contractures—Cont.

Surg., Gynec. and Obst. *68:*352-361, Feb (no. 2A) '39

Whole-thickness grafts in correction of contractures due to burn scars; 3 cases. Conway, H. Ann. Surg. *109:*286-290, Feb '39

Fibrous contracture of head and neck after extensive burns. Gjankovic, H. Lijecn. vjes. *61:*279-284, May '39

Burn contractures of hand. Blackfield, H. M. Surg., Gynec. and Obst. *68:*1066-1073, June '39

Management of old contractures of hand resulting from third degree burns. Jones, R. Jr. Surgery *7:*264-275, Feb '40 also: North Carolina M. J. *1:*148-152, March '40

Therapy for deformities of extremities due to burn cicatrices. Rebaudi, F. and Musso, A. Gior. di med. mil. *88:*46-55, Jan '40

Esthetic results of grafts of Anglo-Russian type in facial burn; case. Codazzi Aguirre, J. A. Semana med., *1:*651-655, March 14, '40

Labiomentothoracic synechia due to burn; plastic repair of case. Johow, A. and Urzua, R. Rev. med. de Chile *68:*1482-1487, Nov '40

Plastic reconstruction of scars after burns, with report of 6 cases. Pickerill, H. P. New Zealand M. J. *39:*327-329, Dec '40

Management of old contractures of upper extremity resulting from third degree burns. Jones, R. R., Jr. South. M. J. *34:*789-797, Aug '41

Relief of contractures of knee following extensive burns. Hamm, W. G. and Kite, J. H. South. Surgeon *10:*795-801, Nov '41

Hand and finger contracture due to burns. Hohmann, G. Chirurg. *14:*289, May 15, '42

Prevention of contracture deformities following burns by use of Padgett dermatome. Thompson, H. A. South. Med. and Surg. *105:*51-55, Feb '43

Thoracofacial synechia following burn; case. Covarrubias Zenteno, R. Rev. med. de Chile *71:*899-901, Sept '43

Tubed pedicle graft in therapy of burn cicatrix; resulting keloids. Pedemonte, P. V. Bol Soc. cir. d. Uruguay *14:*106-108, '43 also: Arch. urug. de med., cir. y especialid. *23:*296-298, Sept '43

Deep burns and contractures. Kite, J. H. J. M. A. Georgia *33:*139-143, May '44

Late plastic care of burn scars and deformities (contractures). Davis, J. S., J.A.M.A. *125:*621-628, July 1, '44

Esthetic repair of face (after burn) by free grafts of skin; case. Rocher, H. L. Bordeaux chir. *3-4:*98-100, July-Oct '44

Burns, Contractures – Cont.

Treatment of deformity from burns. KAZANJIAN, V. H. Connecticut M. J. *8:*661-670, Oct '44

Plastic repair of extensor hand contractures following healed deep second degree burns. GREELEY, P. W. Surgery *15:*173-177, Jan '44

Plastic considerations of burn scars and contractures of hand and forearm. MACOMBER, W. B. Am. Acad. Orthop. Surgeons, Lect., pp. 174-179, '44

Autoplastic grafts in cicatrical deformities due to burns. PASSALACQUA, L. A. Bol. Asoc. med. de Puerto Rico *37:*285-295, Aug '45

Correction of cicatricial contractures of axilla, elbow joint and knee. MAY, H., S. Clin. North America, *25:*1229-1241, Oct. '45

Burns, Debridement

Value of debridement in treatment of burns. WILLIS, A. M., J.A.M.A. *84:*655-658, Feb. 28, '25

Excision as method of treatment of third degree burns. GORBUNOV, V. P. Sovet. vrach. gaz., pp. 637-639, April 30, '34

Enzymatic debridement (with papain-cysteine-salicylate solution) in local treatment of burns; preliminary report. COOPER, G. R.; *et al.* Am. J. Dis. Child. *65:*909-911, June '43

Burns, Electrical

Pathology of electric current "burns". JELLINEK, S. Wien. klin. Wchnschr. *34:*239, May 19, '21

Tetanus after burn from high power current. FÖRSTER, W. Munchen. med. Wchnschr. *68:*1655, Dec 23, '21

Injury of skin from electric current. JELLINEK, S. Wien. klin. Wchnschr. *36:*157-158, March 1, '23

Electric burns of skin. MIEREMET, C. W. G. Klin. Wchnschr. *2:*1362-1364, July 16, '23

Live-wire injuries of skin. RIEHL, G. Munchen. med. Wchnschr. *70:*1119-1120, Aug 31, '23

Character of skin changes from electric burns. JELLINEK, S. Arch. f. Dermat. u. Syph. *148:*433-440, '25

Electrical burns and electrical shock. GABY, R. E. Canad. M. A. J. *17:*1343-1345, Nov '27

Ear injury by electric current; 2 cases. CALICETI, P. Ann. di laring., otol. *29:*16-21, Jan '28

Treatment of electric burns by immediate

Burns, Electrical – Cont.

resection and skin graft. WELLS, D. B. Ann. Surg. *90:*1069-1078, Dec '29

Cases of burns of high voltage electricity. KAPLAN, A. D. Profess. pat. i gig., no. 6, pp. 91-118, '29

Injuries of ear by electricity. PETZAL, E. Internat. Zentralbl. f. Ohrenh. *34:*65-76, July '31

Plastic surgery for extensive loss of bony substance of cranium after passage of electric current; case. LEOTTA, Arch. ed atti d. Soc. ital. di chir. *37:*633-639, '31

Ear injuries due to electricity. NAGER, F. R. AND RÜEDI, L. Rassegna ital. di oto-rino-laring. *5:*129-140, Jan-Dec '31

Massive electrical burns with destruction of part of larynx and trachea. BABCOCK, W. W., S. Clin. North America *12:*1415-1417, Dec '32

Ear injury due to electric discharge; case. BRUZZONE, C. Ann. di laring., otol. *34:*147-150, '34

Injuries to ear due to electric current. HAARMANN, H. Hals-, Nasen-u. Ohrenarzt (Teil 1) *28:*49-58, Feb '37

Plastic surgery of face following injury due to strong current. BLOCK, W. Chirurg *9:*510-514, July 1, '37

Tetanus after burn by high tension electric current; 2 cases in workmen. CHAVANNAZ, J. Ann. de med. leg. *17:*800-801, July '37

Electric shock with extensive injuries requiring immediate amputation of left arm and right leg; case. BEGG, J. D., M. J. Australia *2:*263-264, Aug 14, '37

Late gangrene of finger after electrical injuries; case. SCHNETZ, H. Ztschr. f. klin. Med. *132:*120-127, '37

Facial burns from electric current in small children and use of plastic surgery in therapy; 4 cases. LEMPKE, H. Deutsche Ztschr. f. Chir. *251:*331-342, '38

Mechanism and therapy of electric injuries. VIGLIANI, E. C. Rassegna di med. indust. *10:*143-158, March '39

Electrical injuries of oral cavity. OPPIKOFER, E. Schweiz. med. Wchnschr. *69:*1197-1198, Nov 25, '39

Injuries of external and middle ear in lightning stroke clinical study of case. CRESPI REGHIZZI, A. Arch. ital. di otol. *52:*49-60, Feb '40

Accidents with electricity; burns of mouth. MORHARDT, P. E. Presse med. *48:*480, May 8-11, '40

Burn of cranium due to electric current; rare case. MUNOZ ARENOS, J. M. Semana med. espan. *3:*1070-1073, Aug 31, '40

Burns, Electrical – Cont.

Electric injury to ear. MIKHLIN, E. G. Sovet. med. (no. 23) *4:*29-30, '40

Injuries of region of oral cavity by strong electric current. LINDEMANN, AND LEMPKE, H. Med. Klin. *37:*155-160, Feb 14, '41

Electric shock, electric burns and their treatment. GORDIN, A. E. Indust. Med. *10:*87-91, March '41

Electric accidents to eyes; shock, burns and glare injuries. FISHER, H. E. Arch. Phys. Therapy *22:*611-617, Oct '41

Electrical burns and their treatment. WAKELEY, C. P. G., M. Press *206:*482-484, Dec 31, '41

Case of delayed death following lightning burns. SJÖVALL, H. Acta chir. Scandinav. *85:*455-472, '41

Symposium on medical aspects of chemical warfare; treatment of burns (including thermal and electric). HERRLIN, J. O. JR. AND GLASSER, S. T. Bull. New York M. Coll., Flower and Fifth Ave. Hosps. *5:*79-84, June-Oct '42

Burns, Experimental Work

Experiments with adrenalin in burn therapy. VIOLATO, A. Umbria med. *7:*1237-1239, May '27

Reaction of reticulo-endothelial system in severe burns. SCHREINER, K. AND WENDLBERGER, J. Wien. med. Wchnschr. *83:*891-894, Aug 5, '33

Lymphatic pathology in relation to "toxin" of burns. FENDER, F. A. Surg., Gynec. and Obst. *57:*612-620, Nov '33

Experimental research on cutaneous burns; trials of serotherapy; preliminary report. SCHÜTZ, F. Boll. d. Ist. sieroterap. milanese. *13:*253-262, April '34

Depressor action of extracts of burned skin. HARKINS, H. N.; *et al.* Proc. Soc. Exper. Biol. and Med. *32:*913-914, March '35

Low grade burns as cause of pathologic changes in internal organs (liver, heart, gallbladder, kidney). BRENNER, F. Centralbl. f. allg. Path. u. path. Anat. *65:*97-101, May 30, '36

Correlation of clinical treatment of burns with recent experimental studies. HARKINS, H. N. Illinois M. J. *70:*332-338, Oct '36

Relation between burns and development of anaphylaxis; experimental study. GILIBERTI, P. Gior. di batteriol. e immunol. *20:*19-35, Jan '38

Therapy of severe burns with cortical suprarenal hormone and vitamin C; animal experiments. EINHAUSER, M. Klin. Wchnschr. *17:*127-134, Jan 22, '38

Burns, Experimental Work – Cont.

Circulatory histopathology following burns. ZINCK, K. H. Verhandl. d. deutsch. Gesellsch. f. Kreislaufforsch., pp. 263-275, '38

Immunobiologic state of patients immediately after burns. KANEKEVICH, M. I. Eksper. med., no. 2, pp. 17-22, '39

Hepatic (hepatorenal) factor in burns. BOYCE, F. F. Arch. Surg. *44:*799-818, May '42

Flow of lymph from burned tissue, with particular reference to effects of fibrin formation upon lymph drainage and composition. GLENN, W. W. L.; *et al.* Surgery *12:*685-693, Nov '42

Biology of burn lesions. GREUER, W. Ztschr. f. d. ges. exper. Med. *111:*120-144, '42

Gelatin-glucose-salts solution; influence on hemoconcentration of experimental burns. ELY, J. O. AND ANGULO, A. W., J. Franklin Inst. *235:*197-204, Feb '43

Reduction of fluid loss from damaged tissues (burns) by a barbiturate (pentobarbital sodium). BEECHER, H. K. AND MCCARRELL, J. D., J. Pharmacol. and Exper. Therap. *78:*39-48, May '43

Experimental burns; effect of elastic pressure applied to burned area (effect on hemoconcentration and mortality). LISCHER, C. E. AND ELMAN, R. War Med. *3:*482-483, May '43

Abnormal nitrogen metabolism in patients with thermal burns. TAYLOR, F. H. L.; *et al.* New England J. Med. *229:*855-859, Dec 2, '43

Experimental burns; changes in plasma albumin and globulin. LISCHER, C.; *et al.* War Med. *5:*43-45, Jan '44

Problem of nutrition in presence of excessive nitrogen requirement in seriously ill patients, with particular reference to thermal burns. TAYLOR, F. H. L.; *et al.* Connecticut M. J. *8:*141-148, March '44

Case of severe burn; abnormal nitrogen metabolism. DEAVER, J. M.; *et al.* U. S. Nav. M. Bull. *42:*1162-1163, May '44

Significance of nitrogen loss in exudate from surface burns. HIRSHFELD, J. W. *et al.* Surgery *15:*766-773, May '44

Nitrogen requirement of patients with thermal burns. TAYLOR, F. H. L. J. Indust. Hyg. and Toxicol. *26:*152-155, May '44

Untoward effects of various substances recommended in burn therapy; experimental tests on rats. BAKER, R. D. Arch. Surg. *48:*300-304, April '44

Nutritional care of cases of extensive burns; with special reference to oral use of amino

Burns, Experimental Work – Cont.

acids (amigen, hydrolyzed casein) in 3 cases. Co TUI *et al.* Ann. Surg. *119:*815-823, June '44

Interrelationship of salt solutions, serum and defibrinated blood in treatment of severely scalded, anesthetized dogs. MOYER, C. A., *et al.* Ann. Surg. *120:*367-376, Sept '44

Effects of applying pressure to experimental thermal burns. CAMERON, G. R. *et al.* J. Path. and Bact. *57:*37-46, Jan '45

Experimental human burns; partial report. ASHE, W. F. JR. AND ROBERTS, L. B. War Med. *7:*82-83, Feb '45

Effect of methionine upon nitrogen losses in urine following severe burns. CROFT, P. B. AND PETERS, R. A. Nature, London *155:*175-176, Feb 10, '45

Alterations following thermal burns; effect of variations in food intake on nitrogen balance of burned patients. HIRSHFELD, J. W. *et al.* Arch. Surg. *50:*194-200, April '45

Quantitative evaluation of certain treatments in healing of experimental third degree burns. RHODE, C. M.; *et al.* J. Clin. Investigation *24:*372-379, May '45

Acceleration of healing by pressure application to experimental thermal burns. CAMERON, G. R.; *et al.* J. Path. and Bact. *58:*1-9, Jan '46

Effect of local temperature (application of cold) on fluid loss in thermal burns. COURTICE, F. C., J. Physiol. *104:*321-345, Jan 15, '46

Burns, Eyes and Eyelids

Case after operation for extensive burn of left lids, eyeball, upper face and temporal area. SHEEHAN, J. E., M. J. and Rec. *121:*291-292, March 4, '25

Transplantation of oral mucosa in diseases of cornea and burns of eyes. DENIG, R. Arch. f. Ophth. *118:*729-737, '27

Destruction of capsule of crystalline lens by fire. KRAUPA, E. Klin. Monatsbl. f. Augenh. *87:*397, Sept '31

Plastic surgery in cicatrices of eyelid caused by burn; case. ROY, J. N. Bull. med. de Quebec *32:*322-328, Oct '31

Early grafting of mucous membrane in burns of eye. O'CONNOR, G. B. Arch. Ophth. *9:*48-51, Jan '33

Radium as adjuvant to operation in case of deformity of eyelids from burn with keloid scars. HUDSON, A. C. Proc. Roy. Soc. Med. *27:*1611, Oct '34

Application of grafts early in burns of eye. O'CONNOR, G. B. Rev. de chir. structive, pp. 273-277, June '36

Burns, Eyes and Eyelids – Cont.

Immediate treatment of eye injuries including burns. RUEDEMANN, A. D., S. Clin. North America *16:*979-989, Aug '36

Denig operation for burns of eyes. AVIZONIS, V. Medicina, Kaunas *19:*309-315, April '38

Management of burns of cornea. CULLER, A. M. Ohio State M. J. *34:*873-878, Aug '38

Reasons for early operation in cases of severe burns of eyes. THIES, O. Arch. f. Ophth. *138:*686-692, '38

Therapy of ocular burns by transplantation of conjunctiva from cadaver. ZENKINA, L. V. Vestnik oftal. (no. 2) *15:*28-29, '39

Mucosal graft in therapy of corneoconjunctival burns. VON GROLMAN, G. Arch. de oftal. de Buenos Aires *15:*429-434, Sept '40 also: Rev. med. y cien. afines *2:*629-632, Sept 30, '40

Bilateral burns to eyes; case. FINK, M. V. Vestnik oftal. *16:*509-510, '40

Discussion on burns of eyelids and conjunctiva. WAKELEY, C. P. G. *et al.* Proc. Roy. Soc. Med. *37:*29-33, Nov '43

Buccal mucous membrane grafts in treatment of burns of eye. SIEGEL, R. Arch. Ophth. *32:*104-108, Aug '44

Burn of cornea and conjunctiva; how to prevent symblepharon. PAVIA, J. L. Rev. otoneuro-oftal. *19:*159-171, Nov-Dec '44 also: Semana med. *2:*1117-1122, Dec 7, '44

Transplantation of mucous membrane (Denig operation) in severe burns of eyes. MITERSTEIN, B. AND KORNBLUETH, W. Harefuah *29:*152, Oct 1, '45

Burns, History

History of burns in connection with Fabricius Hildanus' book published in 1610. RUBASHEV, S. M. Vestnik khir. *56:*876-880, Dec '38

Treatment of Burns, by HENRY HARKINS. CC Thomas Co., Springfield, Ill., 1942

Ambroise Paré's onion treatment of burns. SIGERIST, H. E. Bull. Hist. Med. *15:*143-149, Feb '44

Burns, Radiation: See Radiation Injuries

Burns, Scars (See also: Burns, Contractures; Burns, Skin Grafting)

Cicatricial contracture of buttocks nearly occluding anus; plastic operation on buttocks. ASHHURST, A. P. C., S. Clin. N. America *2:*77-79, Feb '22 (illus.)

Surgical treatment of burn scars. PIERCE, G. W., S. Clin. N. America *3:*841-855, June '23 (illus.)

Plastic surgery of cicatrical contractures of

Burns, Scars – Cont.

underarm. VIDEMAN, G. K. Vestnik khir. (nos. 56–57) *19:*323–328, '30

Unusual cicatrix following burn. SOLCARD, AND MORVAN. Ann. d'anat. path. *8:*530, May '31

Contracted dense scar of neck despite use of many Thiersch grafts. BABCOCK, W. W., S. Clin. North America *12:*1405–1407, Dec '32

Plastic removal of skin from breast as aid in treating scars on breast and neck resulting from burns; case. BREITFUSS, F. F. Zentralbl. f. Chir. *61:*436–437, Feb 24, '34

Possible uses of Reverdin skin flap for plastic surgery, primarily for covering skin defects, and secondarily for scar contractures. EHALT, W. Munchen. med. Wchnschr. *82:*669–671, April 25, '35

Malocclusion produced by formation of scar tissue (from burn). HOWES, A. E. Internat. J. Orthodontia *21:*1141–1143, Dec '35

Tourniquet method in retractile cicatrices caused by burns in articular regions. MICHEL, L., J. de med. de Bordeaux *113:*184–185, March 10, '36

Delay of cicatrization in burns; use of cod liver oil dressings in therapy. CABANAC, Arch. Soc. d. sc. med. et biol. de Montpellier *18:*38–40, Feb '37

Burns, discussion on their treatment, both immediate and remote, with special emphasis on prevention of scars and contractures. COAKLEY, W. A. Am. J. Surg. *36:*50–53, April '37

Choice method in plastic restoration of face following extensive burns causing cicatricial disfigurement. DANTRELLE, M. Rev. de chir. structive, pp. 108–109, June '37

Extensive cicatrices of legs and feet due to burns; cicatricial pes talus; autoplasty and disarticulation of Chopart's joint of left foot; case. ROCHER, H. L. Rev. de chir. structive, pp. 111–114, June '37

Cutaneous full thickness graft in therapy of cicatrix due to burn of elbow fold; case. COELST, Rev. de chir. structive *8:*124–126, Aug '38

Therapy of deformities of extremities due to burn cicatrices. REBAUDI, F. AND MUSSO, A. Gior. di med. mil. *88:*46–55, Jan '40

Good effects of vitamin A on burn cicatrization. COMBEMALE, P. Echo med. du Nord *11:*53–57, March '40

Plastic reconstruction of scars after burns, with report of 6 cases. PICKERILL, H. P. New Zealand M. J. *39:*327–329, Dec '40

Skin grafting and "three quarter" thickness skin graft for prevention and correction of cicatricial formation. PADGETT, E. C. Ann.

Burns, Scars – Cont.

Surg. *113:*1034–1049, June '41

Late plastic care of burn scars and deformities (contractures). DAVIS, J. S., J.A.M.A. *125:*621–628, July 1, '44

Plastic considerations of burn scars and contractures of hand and forearm. MACOMBER, W. B. Am. Acad. Orthop. Surgeons, Lect., pp. 174–179, '44

Correction of cicatrical contractures of axilla, elbow joint and knee. MAY, H., S. Clin. North America *25:*1229–1241, Oct '45

Burns, Shock

Blood transfusion in severe burns in infants and young children. ROBERTSON, B. Canad. M. A. J. *11:*744, Oct '21

Treatment of severe burns by blood transfusion. RIEHL, G. Wien. klin. Wchnschr. *38:*833–834, July 23, '25 abstr: J.A.M.A. *85:*860, Sept 12, '25

Hypertonic sodium chloride solution intravenously in treatment of extensive superficial burns. BIGGER, I. A. South. M. J. *19:*302–306, April '26

Twenty-eight cases of grave burns treated by blood transfusion. RIEHL, G. JR. Arch. f. Dermat. u. Syph. *153:*41–65, '27

Experimental shock; composition of fluid that escapes from blood stream after burns. BEARD, J. W. AND BLALOCK, A. Arch. Surg. *22:*617–625, April '31

Experimental shock; importance of local loss of fluid in production of low blood pressure after burns. BLALOCK, A. Arch. Surg. *22:*610–616, April '31

Use of fluids in burns and shock. BRANDSON, B. J. AND HILLSMAN, J. A. Canad. M. A. J. *26:*689–698, June '32

Burns; treatment of shock and toxemia; healing wound; reconstruction. BETTMAN, A. G. Am. J. Surg. *20:*33–37, April '33

Bleeding volume in severe burns. HARKINS, H. N. Ann. Surg. *102:*444–454, Sept '35

Surgical shock from burns, freezing and similar traumatic agents. HARKINS, H. N. Colorado Med. *33:*871–876, Dec '36

Therapy of primary shock due to burns; 2 cases. WANDERLEY FILHO, E. AND GALVAO, H. Arq. brasil. de cir. e ortop. *5:*308–318, March '38

Traumatic shock and burns. HILLSMAN, J. A. AND GUNN, J. A. Manitoba M. A. Rev. *18:*65–68, April '38

Venesection and blood transfusion as methods of treating extensive burns in infants. BAUER, I. Deutsche med. Wchnschr. *64:*1064–1066, July 22, '38

Attempts at therapy after extensive burns;

Burns, Shock – Cont.

consideration of blood volume. HELDERWEIRT, G.; *et al.* Arch. internat. de pharmacodyn. et de therap. *60:*462–465, Dec 31, '38

Shock in burns. STAJANO, C. An. Fac. de med. de Montevideo *23:*923–941, '38

Theories of shock and their relation to burns. DEVINE, J. B., M. J. Australia *1:*14–17, Jan 7, '39

Burn shock; question of water intoxication as complicating factor; blood chemical studies and report of extensive burn treated by repeated transfusions of blood and blood plasma. TRUSLER, H. M.; *et al.* J.A.M.A. *113:*2207–2213, Dec 16, '39

Pathology of collapse following burns. GÜNTHER, G. W. Arch. f. klin. Chir. *194:*539–557, '39

Blood transfusion in extensive burns. STRUCHKOV, V. I. Khirurgiya, no. 6, pp. 53–57, '39

Pathology of shock in man; visceral effects of burns.- trauma, hemorrhage and surgical operat. DAVIS, H. A. Arch. Surg. *41:*123–146, July '40

Plasma transfusion in treatment of fluid shift in severe burns. ELKINTON, J. R.; *et al.* Ann. Surg. *112:*150–157, July '40

Death due to shock after scalding of pharynx and larynx. TANAKA, H. Oto-rhino-laryng. (Abstr. Sect.) *13:*45–46, Oct '40

Treatment of burn shock with plasma and serum. BLACK, D. A. K. Brit. M. J. *2:*693–697, Nov 23, '40

Calcedral (suprarenal preparation) in severe burns. DOSKAROVA, V. Ceska dermat. *19:*141–145, '40

Therapeutic significance of plasma protein replacement in severe burns. ELMAN, R. J.A.M.A. *116:*213–216, Jan 18, '41

Management of shock and toxemia in severe burns. LEE, W. E.; *et al.* Pennsylvania M. J. *44:*1114–1117, June '41

Use of adrenal cortical extract in treatment of traumatic shock of burns. RHOADS, J. E.; *et al.* Ann. Surg. *113:*955–968, June '41

Symposium on military medicine, and shock burn therapy. STRUMIA, M. M.; *et al.* M. Clin. North America *25:*1813–1827, Nov '41

Military symposium; blood and blood substitutes in burn treatment. MUDD, S. AND FLOSDORF, E. W. New England J. Med. *225:*868–870, Nov 27, '41

Blood plasma in therapy of burn case with severe shock. ST-ONGE, G. J. de l'Hotel-Dieu de Montreal *10:*396–408, Nov–Dec '41

Burn shock; consideration of its mechanism and management. WILSON, H. Memphis M. J. *17:*3–5, Jan '42

Use of plasma in hospital ship for burns. WOLFE, H. R. I. AND CLEGG, H. W. Lancet *1:*191–193, Feb 14, '42

Nervous factor in etiology of shock in burns. KABAT, H. AND HEDIN, R. F. Surgery *11:*766–776, May '42 also: Proc. Soc. Exper. Biol. and Med. *49:*114–116, Feb '42 (abstract)

Shock due to extensive superficial burns; case. LABRECQUE, R. Ann. med.-chir. de l'Hop. Sainte-Justine, Montreal *4:*131–140, May '42

Use of plasma in treatment of burn shock. RHOADS, J. E.; *et al.* Clinics *1:*37–42, June '42

Treatment of shock of burns. DAVISON, G. Newcastle M. J. *21:*78–82, July '42

Shock, without or with hemorrhage, and burns. FENNEL, E. A. Hawaii M. J. *1:*385–389, July '42

Burns of thermal origin. (with shock) HULL, H. C. Arch. Surg. *45:*235–252, Aug '42

Plasma in severe burns. HARKINS, H. N.; *et al.* Surg., Gynec. and Obst. *75:*410–420, Oct '42

Acute protein deficiency (hypoproteinemia) in shock due to severe hemorrhage and in burns, intestinal obstruction and general peritonitis, with special reference to use of plasma and hydrolized protein (amigen). ELMAN, R., J.A.M.A. *120:*1176–1180, Dec 12, '42

Experimental chemotherapy of burns; effects of local therapy upon mortality from shock. ROSENTHAL, S. M. Pub. Health Rep. *57:*1923–1935, Dec 18, '42

Controlled fluid therapy in burns; case report illustrating severe hemoconcentration, electrolyte changes and futility of formulas in replacement therapy. SCUDDER, J. AND ELLIOTT, R. H. E. JR. South. Med. and Surg. *104:*651–658, Dec '42

Grave burn in infant; case with recovery after therapy with cortin (adrenal preparation) associated with tannic acid and silver nitrate (Bettmann). HOUOT, A. Union med. du Canada *72:*169–171, Feb '43

Experimental chemotherapy of burns and shock; effects of systemic therapy on early mortality. ROSENTHAL, S. M. Pub. Health Rep. *58:*513–522, March 26, '43

Symposium on management of Cocoanut Grove burns at Massachusetts General Hospital; problem of burn shock complicated by pulmonary damage. COPE, O. AND RHINELANDER, F. W. Ann. Surg. *117:*915–928, June '43

Burns, Shock—Cont.

Albuminotherapy, plasma therapy and blood transfusion in burns. MACIEL, H. Rev. brasil. de cir. *12:*375-384, June '43 also: Bol. Col. brasil. de cirurgioes *18:*195-204, July '43

Occurrence of vasoconstrictor substance in blood during shock induced by trauma, hemorrhage and burns. PAGE, I. H. Am. J. Physiol. *139:*386-398, July '43

Principle from liver effective against shock due to burns; preliminary report. PRINZMETAL, M.; *et al.* J.A.M.A. *122:*720-723, July 10, '43

Intensive human serum treatment of burn shock; modified formula for calculating amount of infusion. PRESSMAN, D. L. *et al.* J.A.M.A. *122:*924-928, July 31, '43

Sternal transfusions in burns. LIEBERMAN, S. L., J.A.M.A. *123:*721, Nov 13, '43

Failure of plasma and serum tranfusion prolonged during 8 days in extensive burns. LOMBARD, P. Afrique franc. chir. *1:*375-378, Nov-Dec '43

Treatment of burn shock. COONEY, E. A. Bull. New England M. Center *5:*248-256, Dec '43

Adrenal cortical extract in burn shock; further experiences. RHOADS, J. E.; *et al.* Ann. Surg. *118:*982-987, Dec '43

Plasma loss in burns (review of literature, prepared on behalf of Burns Sub-Committee, M.R.C. War Wounds Committee). ROSSITER, R. J. Bull. War Med. *4:*181-189, Dec '43

Biologic properties of blood and spinal fluid in traumatic shock complicated by burns. GROMAKOVSKAYA, M. M. AND KAPLAN, L. E. Byull. eksper. biol. i med. (no. 6) *15:*12-16, '43

Blood transfusion in burn therapy. FEDOROVICH, D. P. Sovet. med. (no. 9) *7:*28, '43

Treatment of burns (including shock). PENBERTHY, G. C. AND WELLER, C. N. Am. Acad. Orthop. Surgeons, Lect., pp. 188-198, '43

Therapy of traumatic shock complicated by burns. SHTERN, L. S. *et al.* Byull. eksper. biol. i med (no. 6) *15:*6-9, '43

Oral sodium lactate in burn shock. FOX, C. L. JR. J.A.M.A. *124:*207-212, Jan 22, '44

Another failure of transfusion in severe burns; case. LOMBARD, P. Afrique franc. chir. *2:*77-79, Jan-March '44

Treatment of burn shock with continuous hypodermoclysis of physiologic saline solution into burned area; experimental study. BERMAN, J. K.; *et al.* Surg., Gynec. and Obst. *78:*337-345, April '44

Plasma therapy in burns. ROMERO ALVAREZ, A. M. Semana med. *1:*1117-1129, June 1, '44

Plasma and blood in treatment of shock in burns. LUNDY, J. S.; *et al.* S. Clin. North America *24:*798-807, Aug '44

Closed plaster method of burn therapy in prevention of shock. SELLERS, E. A. AND GORANSON, E. S. Canad. M. A. J. *51:*111-114, Aug '44

Principle from liver effective against shock due to burns. PRINZMETAL, M.; *et al.* J. Clin. Investigation *23:*795-806, Sept '44

Shock associated with deep muscle burns. ANTOS, R. J.; *et al.* Proc. Soc. Exper. Biol. and Med. *57:*11-13, Oct '44

Demonstration of 2 types of shock in burns. PRINZMETAL, M.; *et al.* Surgery *16:*906-913, Dec '44

Cortin (adrenal preparation) in burn therapy. HOUOT, A. Union med. du Canada *74:*289-296, March '45

Influence of environmental temperature on shock in burns. BERGMAN, H. C. AND PRINZMETAL, M. Arch. Surg. *50:*201-206, April '45

Comparison of therapeutic effectiveness of serum and sodium chloride in scald shock. HECHTER, O.; *et al.* Am. Heart J. *29:*484-492, April '45

Role of renal pressor system in shock of burns. HECHTER, O.; *et al.* Am. Heart J. *29:*493-498, April '45

Liver principle which is effective against burn shock; further studies. HECHTER, O. *et al.* Am. Heart J. *29:*499-505, April '45

Ineffectiveness of adrenocortical hormones, thiamine, ascorbic acid, nupercaine and post-traumatic serum in shock due to scalding burns. BERGMAN, H. C.; *et al.* Am. Heart J. *29:*506-512, April '45

Effect of short-term nutritional stress upon resistance to scald shock. BERGMAN, H. C.; *et al.* Am. Heart J *29:*513-515, April '45

Early massive plasma therapy in burns of children; preliminary report. ROMERO ALVAREZ, A. M. Dia med. *17:*309-313, April 9, '45

Closed plaster method in prevention of shock after burns. SELLERS, E. A. AND GORANSON, E. S. J., Canad. M. Serv. *2:*431-437, May '45

Metabolic alterations following thermal burns; effect of treatment with whole blood and electrolyte (salt) solution or with plasma following experimental burn. ABBOTT, W. E.; *et al.* Surgery *17:*794-804, June '45

Mechanism of shock from burns and trauma traced with radiosodium. FOX, C. L. JR.

Burns, Shock – Cont.

AND KESTON, A. S. Surg., Gynec. and Obst. *80:*561-567, June '45

Metabolic alterations following thermal burns; use of whole blood and electrolyte solution (salt) in treatment of burned patients. ABBOTT, W. E. *et al.* Ann. Surg. *122:*678-692, Oct '45

Rationale of whole blood therapy in severe burns; clinical study. EVANS, E. I. AND BIGGER, I. A. Ann. Surg. *122:*693-705, Oct '45

Metabolic changes in shock after burns. HARKINS, H. N. AND LONG, C. N. H. Am. J. Physiol. *144:*661-668, Oct '45

Electrolyte changes and chemotherapy in experimental burn and traumatic shock and hemorrhage (use of isotonic sodium chloride solution). ROSENTHAL, S. M. AND TABOR, H. Arch. Surg. *51:*244-252, Nov-Dec, '45

Nature of circulatory changes in burn shock. PRINZMETAL, M. AND BERGMAN, H. C. Clin. Sc. *5:*205-227, Dec '45

Extent and cause of blood volume reduction in traumatic, hemorrhagic and burn shock. NOBLE, R. P. AND GREGERSEN, M. I. J. Clin. Investigation *25:*172-183, Mar '46

Present policies in treatment of severely burned patient; outline of treatment including use of whole blood transfusions. LANGE, H. J.; *et al.* J. Michigan M. Soc. *45:*619-633, May '46

Antishock action of ethanol (ethyl alcohol) in burned mice; effect of edema formation and capillary atony. BERGMAN, H. C. AND PRINZMETAL, M. J. Lab. and Clin. Med. *31:*654-662, June '46

Antishock action of certain drugs in burned mice. BERGMAN, H. C. AND PRINZMETAL, M. J. Lab. and Clin. Med. *31:*663-671, June '46

Blood changes in shock following burns. GORDIENKO, A. N. Bull. War Med. *6:*473, July '46 (abstract)

Importance of whole blood transfusions in management of severe burns. McDONALD, J. J.; *et al.* Ann. Surg. *124:*332-353, Aug '46

Burns and shock in children; Mentana Street disaster in Montreal, September 1945. BISSON, C. AND ROYER, A. Ann. med.-chir. de l'Hop. Sainte-Justine, Montreal *5:*5-19, '46

Burn shock; Treatment with continuous hypodermoclysis of isotonic solution of sodium chloride into burned areas; clinical studies in 2 cases. BERMAN, J. K.; *et al.* Arch. Surg. *53:*577-587, Nov '46

Burns, Skin Grafting

Restoration of the burnt child. BLAIR, V. P. Southern M. J. *16:*522-527, July '23 (illus.)

Burns, Skin Grafting – Cont.

Immobilizing cage in burn therapy and skin grafts. HOSMER, A. J. Am. J. Surg. *3:*23-30, July '27

Burns on both forearms and back of hand; treatment by graft from thigh. MIRIZZI, P. L. Bull. et mem. Soc. nat. de chir. *55:*780-785, June 8, '29

Buried skin grafts of burned children; new use of old method of grafting. HENSON, E. B. West Virginia M. J. *26:*557-559, Sept '30

Early and late repair of extensive burns. BLAIR, V. P. AND BROWN, J. B. Dallas M. J. *17:*59-70, May '31

Reconstruction of burned hand. (grafts) VON WEDEL, C., J. Oklahoma M. A. *24:*164-165, May '31

Promotion of early healing in burns and correction and prevention of late complications. BLAIR, V. P. J. Oklahoma M. A. *24:*271-272, Aug '31

Treatment of extensive granulating areas, with special reference to use of physical therapy measures in burns and skin grafts. POTTER, E. B. AND PECK, W. S. Am. J. Surg. *14:*472-476, Nov '31

Early care and repair of defects in burns. BLAIR, V. P.; *et al.* J.A.M.A. *98:*1355-1359, April 16, '32

Skin grafting with reference to extensive burns. SUTTON, H. T. Ohio State M. J. *27:*943-949, Dec '31

Treatment of old unhealed burns. (grafts).DAVIS, J. S. AND KITLOWSKI, E. A. Ann. Surg. *97:*648-669, May '33

Early and late treatment of burns. PADGETT, E. C., J. Kansas M. Soc. *34:*184-188, May '33

Modified technic of application of Davis grafts in extensive burns. DANTLO, R. Rev. de chir. plastique, pp. 219-237, Oct '33

Autoplasty using digital flap in therapy of stubborn ulcers resulting from burns received in childhood. CHAUVENET, A. Bordeaux chir. *6:*18-25, Jan '35

Repair of defects resulting from full thickness loss of skin from burns. BROWN, J. B. AND BLAIR, V. P. Surg., Gynec. and Obst. *60:*379-389, Feb (no. 2A) '35

Repair of surface defects, from burns and other causes, with thick split skin grafts. BROWN, J. B.; *et al.* South M. J. *28:*408, May; 529, June '35

Thermal burns. GUNN, J. AND HILLSMAN, J. A. Ann. Surg. *102:*429-443, Sept '35

Burn therapy. (skin grafts). RITTER, H. H. Am. J. Surg. *31:*48-55, Jan '36

Dermo-epidermal grafts in delayed healing of burn wounds; 2 cases. CLEMENTE, D. Policlinico (sez. prat.) *43:*1861-1863, Oct 19, '36

Burns, Skin Grafting–Cont.

Care of severely burned, with special reference to skin grafting. PADGETT, E. C. Arch. Surg. *35:*64–86, July '37

Replacement of almost entire skin of upper extremity by skin graft; case. REYNBERG, G. A. Khirurgiya, no. 12, pp. 144–145, '37

Plaster of paris bandage in therapy of burns of extremities. ZENO, L. AND BARENBOYM, S. Novy khir. arkhiv *38:*435, '37

Homogenous Thiersch grafting as life saving measure in burns. BETTMAN, A. G. Am. J. Surg. *39:*156–162, Jan '38

Treatment of wounds resulting from deep burns. BLAIR, V. P. AND BYARS, L. T. J.A.M.A. *110:*1802–1804, May 28, '38

Cutaneous full thickness graft in therapy of cicatrix due to burn of elbow fold; case. COELST. Rev. de chir. structive *8:*124–126, Aug '38

Free graft in reparation of extensive axillary wound after burns. ALICH, S. Turk tib cem. mec *4:*183–187, '38

Skin grafting in severe burns. PADGETT, E. C. Am. J. Surg. *43:*626–636, Feb '39

Burns in children. BLACKFIELD, H. M. AND GOLDMAN, L., J.A.M.A. *112:*2235–2240, June 3, '39

Autoplastic skin grafts for covering defects on extremities. BEREZKIN, N. F. Vestnik khir., *58:*196–204, Sept '39

Dermo-epidermoid graft in third degree burns. CANIZARES, RAUL AND CANIZARES, RAFAEL. Vida nueva *45:*113–118, Feb '40

Early skin grafts in burns. KRIKENT, R. K. Ortop. i. travmatol. (no. 2) *14:*26–28, '40

Treatment of superficial injuries and burns of hand. ALLEN, H. S., J.A.M.A. *116:*1370–1373, March 29, '41

Burns of hand. MACCOLLUM, D. W. J.A.M.A. *116:*2371–2377, May 24, '41

Use of abdominal skin to correct cervical defect due to burn. GABARRO, P. Rev. Fac. de med., Bogota *10:*339–342, Oct '41

New skin for burns. MILLER, L. M. Hygeia *19:*884–885, Nov '41

Biologic orientation in burn therapy in plastic surgery. ZENO, L. Bol. y trab., Soc. argent. de cirujanos *2:*904–961, '41

Burns and reconstructive surgery. LEVEN, N. L. Proc. Interest. Postgrad. M. A. North America (1941) pp. 267–269, '42

Implant skin grafting; case in burns. HORTON, W. S. S. Am. J. Surg. *55:*597–599, March '42

Massive repairs with thick split-skin grafts; emergency "dressing" with homografts in burns. BROWN, J. B. AND MCDOWELL, F. Ann. Surg. *115:*658–674, April '42

Burns, Skin Grafting–Cont.

Plastic surgery of burns. GILLIES, H. Rev. Assoc. med. argent. *56:*196–198, April 15–30, '42

Epithelial healing and the transplantation of skin. BROWN, J. B., AND MCDOWELL, F. Ann. Surg., *115:*1166, June '42

Plastic repair with free skin grafts in burns. BROWN, J. B. AND MCDOWELL, F. Clinics *1:*25–36, June '42

Preservation of function in burnt hand (including description of steering wheel apparatus). AINSWORTH-DAVIS, J. C. Brit. M. J. *1:*724, June 13, '42

Immediate skin grafting in burns; preliminary report. YOUNG, F. Ann. Surg. *116:*445–451, Sept '42

Skin Grafting of Burns. BROWN, J. B., AND MCDOWELL, F., J. B. Lippincott Co., Phila., 1943

Burn therapy. BURTON, J. F., J. Oklahoma M. A. *36:*4–5, Jan '43

Burn experience at Hospital for Sick Children. FARMER, A. W. Am. J. Surg. *59:*195–209, Feb '43

Restoration of function in burnt hand. BODENHAM, D. C. Lancet *1:*298–300, March 6, '43

Burn therapy. (hands). BARNES, J. M. Brit. M. J. *1:*408–410, April 3, '43

Plastic surgery; early repair of skin defects caused by severe burns. EVANS, E. I. Bull. Am. Coll. Surgeons *28:*142–143, June '43

Plastic procedures in burn therapy. KIRKHAM, H. L. D. Bull. Am. Coll. Surgeons *28:*144–145, June '43

Burn therapy. LEVEN, N. L. Minnesota Med. *26:*534–537, June '43

Dermatome pattern graft and its use in reconstruction (after burns) KANTHAK, F. F. Surg., Gynec. and Obst. *77:*610–614, Dec '43

Plastic repair of extensor hand contractures following healed deep second degree burns. GREELEY, P. W. Tr. Am. Soc. Plastic and Reconstructive Surg. *12:*79–82, '43

Plastic procedures in burn therapy. KIRKHAM, H. L. D. Am. Acad. Orthop. Surgeons, Lect., pp. 202–208, '43

Rehabilitation following severe burns; experience with victims of Boston night club (Cocoanut Grove) fire. CANNON, B. Surgery *15:*178–185, Jan '44

The burned hand. MCINDOE, A. H., M. Press *211:*57–61, Jan 26, '44

Repair of burned hand. PIERCE, G. W.; *et al.* Surgery *15:*153–172, Jan '44

Plastic surgery of burns. BROWN, J. B. Delaware State M. J. *16:*35–38, March '44

Burns, Skin Grafting—Cont.

Surgical repair of burns. McDowell, F. and Brown, J. B. Wisconsin M. J. *43:*310–315, March '44

Surgical reconstruction following serious burns. Siler, V. E. South. M. J. *37:*187–195, April '44

Modified technic in skin grafting of extensive deep burns. Saltonstall, H. and Lee, W. E. Ann. Surg. *119:*690–693, May '44

Plastic surgery of severe burns. Evans, E. I. and Alm, T. J. Virginia M. Monthly *71:*342–350, July '44

Finger exerciser for burned hands. Oldfield, M. C. and King, C. J. Lancet *2:*109, July 22, '44

Burn therapy. Matthews, D. N. Practitioner *153:*86–93, Aug '44

Penicillin and skin grafting in burns. Hirshfeld, J. W.; *et al.* J.A.M.A. *125:*1017–1019, Aug 12, '44

Burn therapy. Blackfield, H. M. California and West. Med. *61:*187–190, Oct '44

Penicillin as adjunct in skin grafting of severe burns. Lam, C. R. and McClure, R. D. Proc. Am. Federation Clin. Research *1:*56, '44

Principles and indications of burn therapy. Marino, H. Bol. y trab., Soc. de cir. de Cordoba *5:*361–375, '44

Selection of time for grafting of skin to extensive defects resulting from deep thermal burns. McCorkle, H. J. and Silvani, H. Ann. Surg. *121:*285–290, March '45

Case of serious burns; problem of reconstructive surgery. Smith, P. E. Mississippi Doctor *22:*258–262, March '45

Dermoplasty of healed burned dorsum of hand. Pick, J. F., J. Internat. Coll. Surgeons *8:*217–223, May–June '45

Resurfacing of dorsum of hand following burns. Farmer, A. W. and Woolhouse, F. M., Ann. Surg. *122:*39–47, July '45

Therapy of thermal burns. Gordon, S. D. Bull. Vancouver M. A. *21:*283–286, Aug '45

Routine for early skin grafting of deep burns. Rawles, B. W. Jr. Surgery *18:*696–706, Dec '45

Surgical impressions from England; burns and plastic surgery. ten Kate, J. Geneesk. gids. *24:*25, Jan 31, '46; 52, Feb 28, '46

Burns and their sequels; therapy with free skin grafts. Pavlowsky, A. J.; *et al.* Rev. Assoc. med. Argent. *60:*78–83, Feb. 15–28, '46

Management and surgical resurfacing of serious burns. Clarkson, P. and Lawrie, R. S., Brit. J. Surg. *33:*311–323, Apr '46

Burns, Skin Grafting—Cont.

Problem of skin grafts in severe burns. Del-Rio, J. M. A. Bol. y trab. Acad. argent. de cir. *30:*363–376, Jun 26, '46

Free graft in form of cutaneous "bandage"; use in severe burns. Marino, H. Bol. y trab. Acad. argent. de cir. *30:*451–459, July 17, '46

Skin grafting burned dorsum of hand. Webster, G. V. and Rowland, W. D. Ann. Surg. *124:*449–462, Aug '46

Burns, Topical Therapy

Dichloramine T treatment of burns. Horan, F. P. Illinois M. J. *40:*123, Aug '21

Burns from splashing of molten metal; advantages of picric acid treatment. van Gelderen, D. N. Nederlandsch Tijdschr. v. Geneesk. *2:*2793–2794, Dec 3, '21

Burns, with special reference to acetic acid treatment. Dorrance, G. M. and Bransfield, J. W., S. Clin. N. America *2:*299–307, Feb '22

Modern treatment of burns (paraffin). de Moraes, A. Brasil-med. *1:*242–244, May 13, '22 abstr: J.A.M.A. *79:*858, Sept 2, '22

Hot air mineral oil treatment of extensive burns. Steel, W. A. New York M. J. *116:*418–419, Oct 4, '22

Paraffin spray in burns. Rebaudi, L. Munchen. med. Wchnschr. *70:*179, Feb 9, '23

Hydrogen dioxide in treatment of burns. de Groot, A. Nederlandsch Tijdschr. v. Geneesk. *2:*354, July 28, '23

Linimentum calcis chlorinatae in treatment of burns. Tomb, J. W. Brit. M. J. *1:*711, April 19, '24

Treatment of burns and ulcers with Veroform and Epithelan. Linden. Deutsche med. Wchnschr. *50:*719–720, May 30, '24

Tannic acid in treatment of burns. Davidson, E. C. Surg., Gynec. and Obst. *41:*202–221, Aug '25

Burns; chemotherapy of local suppuration, acriflavine and boric acid compared. Graham, J. G. Brit. M. J. *2:*826, Nov 7, '25

Prevention of toxemia of burns; treatment by tannic acid solution. Davidson, E. C. Am. J. Surg. *40:*114–116, May '26

Local treatment of burns with use of dusting powders and exposure to air. Mandanas, A. Y. J. Philippine Islands M. A. *6:*161–162, May '26

Paraffin treatment for burns and denuded areas. Trueblood, D. V. Northwest Med. *25:*255–258, May '26

Treatment of burns by actinotherapy. Kes-

Burns, Topical Therapy—Cont.

SLER, E. B. Arch. Physical Therapy *7:*347–354, June '26

Burns treated by tannic acid. BECK, C. S. AND POWERS, J. H. Ann. Surg. *84:*19–36, July '26

Treatment of burns and scalds by sterilized cocoanut oil. GOPALAN, N. Indian M. Gaz. *61:*549, Nov '26

Tannic acid treatment of burns; case report. LINDSAY, J. C. Canad. J. Med. and Surg. *61:*9, '27 also: Canad. M.A.J. *17:*86, Jan '27

Tea in treatment of burns. SHEN, J. K. China M. J. *41:*150–153, Feb '27

Beerwort in burn therapy. CAPPELLETTI, A. Semana med. *1:*815–817, March 31, '27

Dressing for burns. FIST, H. S., J.A.M.A. *88:*1483, May 7, '27 addendum, 1922

Tannic acid in burns. REBHORN, E. H. Bull. Moses Taylor Hosp. *1:*21–23, May '27

Desitin salve in burns. JACOB, F. J. Med. Klin. *23:*1032, July 8, '27

Tannic acid in burns. FLORESCO, A. Gaz. d. hop. *100:*1281–1285, Sept 28, '27

Severe and extensive burn treated with solution of tannic acid. HUNTER, J. Canad. M. A.J. *17:*1357–1358, Nov '27

Tannic acid in burns. SEEGER, S. J. Wisconsin M. J. *27:*1–6, Jan '28

Chlorinated carron oil for burns. TOMB, J. W. M. Press *125:*99, Feb 1, '28

Burn therapy with tannic acid. GORDON, R. M. Lancet *1:*336–337, Feb 18, '28

Local and general use of melted paraffin at 54°–60° C. in burns. VAN DER HOEVEN, L. Geneesk. Gids *6:*176–182, Feb 24, '28

Tannic acid in burns. BARLING, S. Birmingham M. Rev. *3:*58–61, March '28 also: Clin. J. *57:*277–281, June 13, '28

Tannic acid in burns. HARROLD, T. JR. J. M. A. Georgia *17:*286–288, July '28

Treatment of burns and scalds by tannic acid. WILSON, W. C. Brit. M. J. *2:*91–94, July 21, '28

Note of caution on use of picric acid solution as burn dressing. COLQUHOUN, K. G., M. J. Australia *2:*652, Nov 24, '28

Naphthalene ointment in burns. GILLERSON, A. B. AND EPSTEIN. Vrach. gaz. *32:*1645, Dec 15, '28

Treatment of ulcers of thigh and burns with polysan (magnesium hydroxide preparation). JANOUŠEK, B. Ceska dermat. *9:*154–159, '28

Treatment of burns and scalds by tannic acid. HERZFELD, G. Practitioner *122:*106–111, Feb '29

Tannic acid treatment of burns in children.

Burns, Topical Therapy—Cont.

MONTGOMERY, A. H. Surg., Gynec. and Obst. *48:*277–280, Feb '29

Tannic acid in burns; end-results in 114 cases compared with 320 treated by other methods. BEEKMAN, F. Arch. Surg. *18:*803–806, March '29

Rational treatment of burns (including tannic acid). DUNN, E. P. Am. J. Surg. *6:*519–521, April '29

Local burn therapy. MAKAI, E. Munchen. med. Wchnschr. *76:*574–575, April 5, '29

Local actinotherapy in burns. LEMARIÉE, P. Rev. d'actinol. *5:*371–390, May–June '29

Tannic acid treatment in burns. BALTZELL, N. A., J. Florida M. A. *15:*597–599, June '29

Tannic acid in burns. PACKARD, G. B. JR. Colorado Med. *26:*173–176, June '29

Tannic acid in burn therapy. HUTTON, A. J. Glasgow M. J. *112:*1–8, July '29

Local burn therapy. KENDIG, E. L. Virginia M. Monthly *56:*219–222, July '29

Ultra-violet light for burns, with special reference to technique used by C. B. Heald, M. D., M. R. C. P. PEAKE, J., Brit. J. Actinotherapy *4:*96–97, Aug '29

Ionized silver in burns. SHILLITO, L. Brit. M. J. *2:*668, Oct 12, '29

Tannic acid for burns. KERNODLE, S. E., J. Oklahoma M. A. *22:*384–387, Nov '29

Roentgen treatment of thermal and chemical burns of skin. TAMIYA, C. AND KOYAMA, M. Strahlentherapie *34:*808–812, '29

Early treatment of severe, extensive burns, without dressing. PATEL, M. AND PONTHUS, P. Progres med., pp. 497–501, March 22, '30

Silver foil in burn therapy. PFAB, B. Munchen. med. Wchnschr. *77:*857–858, May 16, '30

Tannic acid in burns. WOLLESEN, J. M. Ugesk. f. laeger *92:*487–491, May 22, '30

Modern methods of burn therapy, especially tannic acid. PEREZ DUEÑO, F. Arch. de med., cir. y espec. *32:*593–597, June 7, '30

First-aid treatment of burns with tannic acid. CHRISTOPHER, F. Internat. J. Med. and Surg. *43:*363–367, July '30 also: Journal-Lancet *50:*317–321, July 15, '30

Actinotherapy in burns. LEMARIÉE, P. Paris med. *2:*161–164, Aug 23, '30

Tannic acid treatment of cutaneous burns. ROBITSHEK, E. C. Journal-Lancet *50:*470–472, Oct 1, '30

Paraffin-wax treatment of burns. COOK, C. K. Wisconsin M. J. *29:*609–613, Nov '30

Use of tannic acid in children with burns.

Burns, Topical Therapy—Cont.
Davidson, E. C. Minnesota Med. *13:*775-783, Nov '30
Treatment of burns in children with tannic acid. Davidson, E. C. and Penberthy, G. C. Proc. Internat. Assemb. Inter-State Post-Grad. M. A., North America (1929) *5:*265-268, '30
Treatment of burns of face without dressings; 2 cases. Sassard, P. Lyon med. *147:*43, Jan 11, '31
Tannic acid in burns. Mourgue-Molines, E. Montpellier med. *53:*45, Feb 1; 79, Feb 15, '31
Freshly prepared tannic acid solution in burns. van der Spek Jszn., J. Nederl. tijdschr. v. geneesk. *75:*873-877, Feb 21, '31
Tannin solution and other means for treatment of extensive burns. Klug, W. Ztschr. f. arztl. Fortbild. *28:*278-281, May 1, '31
Localized light therapy in burns. Lemariée, P. Arch. d'electric. med. *39:*269, July '31
Aqueous solution of tannic acid in burns. Patrignani, F. Riv. osp. *21:*257-264, Aug '31
Extensive burns treated by exposure to air. Patel. Lyon chir. *28:*617-618, Sept-Oct '31
Abortive burn therapy with alcohol. Iokhelson, S. A. Vrach. gaz. *35:*1449-1451, Oct 15, '31
Topography of burns of normal man who catches on fire; therapy with gutta-percha. Zorraquín, G. and Boix Pou, M. Prensa med. argent. *18:*995-999, Dec 30, '31
Ichtoxyl (sulphoichthyolate preparation) in burns. Ramiš, V. Ceska dermat. (supp.) *12:*517-522, '31
Paraffin in burns. Steiger-Kazal, P. Orvosi hetil. (mell.) *76:*2-3, Jan 9, '32
Tannic acid in burns. Saegesser, M. Schweiz. med. Wchnschr. *62:*117-118, Jan 30, '32
Burn therapy without bandaging; continuous exposure to hot air and electric light. Riche, V. *et al.* Arch. Soc. d. sc. med. et biol. de Montpellier *13:*36-45, Jan '32
Abortive burn treatment with alcohol. Breitman, M. Y. Sovet. vrach. gaz. p. 248, Feb 29, '32
Six years of tannic acid treatment in burns. Glover, D. M. Surg., Gynec. and Obst. *54:*798-805, May '32
Modern treatment (tannic acid) of burns and scalds. Wilson, W. C. Practitioner *129:* 183-193, July '32
Burn therapy in out-patients with reinforced tannic acid dressings. Hunt, J. H. and Scott, P. G. Lancet *2:*774-776, Oct 8, '32
Hydrogen-ion concentration value of tannic acid solutions in burn therapy. Seeger, S. J. Surg., Gynec. and Obst. *55:*455-463, Oct '32
Burn therapy with paraffin and paraffin mixture, with special regard to local effect of paraffinoderm bandage. Cholnoky, L. Gyogyaszat *72:*673-675, Oct 30, '32
Granugenol in burns. Muller, H. Deutsche med. Wchnschr. *58:*1759-1760, Nov 4, '32
Tannic acid in burns. Gymnich, W. Med. Welt *6:*1646, Nov 12, '32
Burn therapy with report of 278 cases (tannic acid in 158 cases). Seeger, S. J. Wisconsin M. J. *31:*755-759, Nov '32
Burn treatment (use of rubber sponge bandage). Luxenberg, L. Pennsylvania M. J. *36:*334-335, Feb '33
Role of infection in burns. Rx-gentian violet. Aldrich, R. H. New England J. Med. *208:*299-309, Feb 9, '33
Burn treatment (use of tannic acid). Madler, N. A. Colorado Med. *30:*46-49, Feb '33
Treatment of burns and scalds, with especial reference to use of tannic acid (Hunterian lecture). Mitchiner, P. H. Lancet *1:*233-239, Feb 4, '33 also: Brit. M. J. *1:*447-452, March 18, '33
Burn therapy with especial reference to use of gentian violet. Penick, R. M. Jr. Internat. Clin. *1:*31-42, March '33
Tannic acid therapy of burns; case. Leriche, R. and Jung, A. Lyon chir. *30:*177-179, March-April '33
Tannic acid treatment of burns. Martin, J. D. Jr. South M. J. *26:*321-325, April '33
Gentian violent in burns; preliminary report. Connell, J. H.; *et al.* J.A.M.A. *100:*1219-1220, April 22, '33
Evaluation of tannic acid treatment of burns. Mason, J. B. Ann. Surg. *97:*641-647, May '33
Tannic acid treatment of fresh burns; erroneous methods of application. Seifert, E. Zentralbl. f. Chir. *60:*1051-1055, May 6, '33
Results of tannic acid therapy in children (in burns). Langer, M. Wien. klin. Wchnschr. *46:*689-690, June 2, '33
Treatment of burns and scalds (with special reference to use of tannic acid). Mitchiner, P. H. St. Thomas's Hosp. Gaz. *34:*71-78, June '33
Paraffin therapy of burns produced by heat and cold and for cicatrices. Jouan, S.; *et al.* Rev. med. latino-am. *18:*1424-1427, Sept '33
Aseptic tannic acid treatment of diffuse superficial burns. Wells, D. B., J.A.M.A. *101:*1136-1138, Oct 7, '33

Burns, Topical Therapy—Cont.
Tannin ointment in burns. WIENECKE, H. Med. Welt 7:1643–1644, Nov 18, '33
Ultraviolet rays in burn therapy. LARIN, N. AND GOLONZKO, L. Y. Sovet. khir. *4:*44–50, '33
New technic (application of hot air immediately after spraying with tannic acid) of burn therapy. EL DIWANY, M. A. M., J. Egyptian M. A. *17:*112–114, Jan '34
Brilliant green in burns. KORYTKIN-NOVIKOV, L. E. Sovet. vrach. gaz., pp. 21–23, Jan 15, '34 also: Zentralbl. f. Chir. *61:*253–256, Feb 3, '34
First aid treatment of burns with tannic acid. MALMSTONE, F. A. Internat. J. Med. and Surg. *47:*72–77, Feb '34
Treatment of granulating areas in burns. BELL, P. S. Tr. Roy. Soc. Trop. Med. and Hyg. *27:*511–516, March '34
Cod liver oil therapy of extensive burns of first, second and third degrees. LÖHR, W. Chirurg *6:*263–276, April 1, '34
Tannin in burns. MITTELSTAEDT. Kinderarztl. Praxis *5:*152–153, April '34
Practical hints on use of tannic acid for burns and scalds. MITCHINER, P. H. Clin. J. *63:*221–224, June '34
Trypaflavine (acridine dye) compresses in burns. SOSODORO-DJATIKOESOEMO, R. Geneesk. tijdschr. v. Nederl.-Indie *74:*759–760, June 5, '34
Tannic acid in burns. HEMPEL-JØRGENSEN, E. Ugesk. f. laeger *96:*625–626, June 14, '34
Cod liver oil salve treatment of burns with and without use of plaster of paris cast. LÖHR, W. Zentralbl. f. Chir. *61:*1686–1695, July 21, '34
Modern burn therapy, with special reference to use of tannin. LEIBOVICI, R., J. de med. de Paris *54:*765–766, Sept 6, '34
Davidson method of burn therapy. SZÁNTÓ, M. Gyogyaszat *74:*555–556, Sept 23, '34
Tannic acid in burns. DESJARDINS, E., J. de l'Hotel-Dieu de Montreal *3:*410–416, Nov–Dec '34
Open method of burn therapy. BELYAEVA, V. I. AND POSTNIKOV, B. N. Vestnik khir. *34:*93–106, '34
Application of cultures of Bacillus bulgaricus in treatment of purulent wounds after burns. POLISADOVA, K. I. AND SINITSKIY, A. A. Sovet. khir. (no. 6) *6:*786–794, '34
Tannic acid in burns. PENBERTHY, G. C., J. Michigan M. Soc. *34:*1–4, Jan '35
Tannic acid in burns. HANSEN, P. Ugesk. f. laeger *97:*1–6, Jan 3, '35
Tannic acid-silver nitrate in burns; method of

Burns, Topical Therapy—Cont.
minimizing shock and toxemia and shortening convalescence. BETTMAN, A. G. Northwest Med. *34:*46–51, Feb '35
Tannic acid in burns; principles, advantages, method and results of application. MASMONTEIL, F. Bull. et mem. Soc. d. chirurgiens de Paris *27:*91–96, Feb 1, '35
Ultraviolet therapy of burns. BACH, H. Med. Welt *9:*235–237, Feb 16, '35
Extensive cutaneous burns; ultraviolet light as adjunct to the repair of defects. TRUSLER, H. M., J. Indiana M. A. *28:*113–118, March '35
Davidson tannic acid treatment of burns; 10 year results. MCCLURE, R. D. AND ALLEN, C. I. Am. J. Surg. *28:*370–388, May '35
Burn therapy with special reference to use of tannic acid (Davidson method). NOGUERA, A. M. Gac. med. de Caracas *42:*223–224, July 31, '35
Alcohol and insulin in severe burns; preliminary report. BIANCHI, G. Riforma med. *51:*1179–1180, Aug 3, '35
Cod liver oil in burns. STEEL, J. P. Lancet *2:*290–292, Aug 10, '35
Burn therapy, with special reference to use of tannic acid (Davidson method). NOGUERA, A. M. Gac. med. de Caracas *42:*226–240, Aug 15, '35
Use of ambrine (paraffin dressing) in burns. BALTODANO BRICENO, E. Med. de los ninos *36:*300–304, Oct '35
Vitamins A and D and camphorated oil in burns; preliminary report. FRANZETTI, C. O. Semana med. *2:*998, Oct 3, '35
Ferric chloride coagulation in burns, with resume of tannic acid treatment. COAN, G. L. Surg., Gynec. and Obst. *61:*687–692, Nov '35
Cleansing and painting extensive burns with mercurochrome; therapy without use of bandages. SORREL, E. *et al.* Bull. Soc. de pediat. de Paris *33:*564–568, Nov '35
Contribution to treatment of burns (use of mercurochrome). TURNER, A. C. Brit. M. J. *2:*995–996, Nov 23, '35
Tannin in burns. BERNARD, E. Bull. et mem. Soc. d. chirurgiens de Paris *27:*583–586, Dec 6, '35
Tannic acid-silver nitrate in burns. COTTER, A. P. AND KIMBELL, N. K. B. New Zealand M. J. *34:*384–388, Dec '35
Radiant energy from artificial light in burns. MAZEL, Z. A. *et al.* Vrach. delo *18:*913–916, '35
Drying of burns by means of heliotherapy. SHIMANKO, I. I. Sovet. khir., no. 6, pp. 226–230, '35

Burns, Topical Therapy–Cont.
Tannin in burns. SNELLMAN, A. Duodecim *51:*579-603, '35
Burn in children and their therapy with powdered chalk dressings. TERNOVSKIY, S. D. Vestnik khir. *39:*3-8, '35
Gentian violet in burns. DEHART, R. M. Virginia M. Monthly *62:*594-595, Jan '36
Camphorated oil in treatment of minor industrial wounds (burns). MCINTURFF, D. N. JR. U. S. Nav. M. Bull. *34:*70-72, Jan '36
Tannic acid and silver nitrate in burns. BETTMAN, A. G. Surg., Gynec. and Obst. *62:*458-463, Feb (no. 2A) '36
Painting burns with methylthionine chloride; case. VIOLET, H. Lyon med. *157:*308-310, March 15, '36
Brilliant green in burn therapy. KORYTKIN-NOVIKOV, L. E. Sovet. vrach. zhur., pp. 421-422, March 30, '36 also: Zentralbl. f. Chir. *63:*2427-2430, Oct 10, '36
Misuse of tannic acid in burns. TAYLOR, F. J.A.M.A. *106:*1144-1146, April 4, '36
Tannic acid in burns. BARRET, M. Clinique, Paris *31:*135-138, May (A) '36
Initial cold water treatment of burns. ROSE, H. W. Northwest Med. *35:*267-270, July '36
Tannic acid in burns. RACZ, B. Orvosi hetil. *80:*756-757, Aug 8, '36
Burn wounds and their therapy. WOLFER, J. A. Northwest Med. *35:*339-342, Sept '36
Tannic acid in burns. WOLLESEN, J. M. Chirurg *8:*732-740, Sept 15, '36
Therapy of first and second degree burns with taktocut, substance used in tanning. JÄGER, R. AND JÄGER, F. Munchen. med. Wchnschr. *83:*1597-1598, Sept 25, '36
Lapis ointment (silver nitrate) in burns. KISSMEYER, A. Ugesk. f. laeger *98:*1032-1033, Oct 22, '36
Treatment of burns and scalds with silver nitrate ointment. KISSMEYER, A. Lancet *2:*985, Oct 24, '36
Small burns, with special reference to use of amertam (tannic acid preparation). DE FARIA, J. Rev. brasil. de cir. *5:*503-516, Nov '36
Question of local vitamin deficiency; therapy of burns with vitaderm (carotene preparation). BALAKHOVSKIY, S. D. *et al.* Novy khir. arkhiv. *36:*49-64, '36
Activate charcoal in therapy of slowly healing ulcers after burns. LYAKER, B. Sovet. khir., no. 12, pp. 911-913, '36
Compound of aniline dyes (acriviolet and brilliant green) in burns. ALDRICH, R. H. Maine M. J. *28:*5-7, Jan '37

Burns, Topical Therapy–Cont.
Case report of severe burn, with special reference to tannic acid treatment. WEYER, S. M. Nebraska M. J. *22:*23-25, Jan '37
Applications of vitamin A in burns; 5 cases. CHEVALLIER, A. *et al.* Progres med., pp. 89-90, Jan 16, '37
Delay of cicatrization in burns; use of cod liver oil dressings in therapy. CABANAC. Arch. Soc. d. sc. med. et biol. de Montpellier *18:*38-40, Feb '37
Evaluation of tannic acid; clinical study of 556 burns so treated over period of 11 years. GLOVER, D. M. Ohio State M. J. *33:*146-151, Feb '37
External use of cod liver oil in burns; review. HOLMES, A. D. Indust. Med. *6:*77-83, Feb '37
Treatment of minor burns by amyl salicylate and other salicyl esters. STEWART, R. L. Brit. M. J. *1:*380-383, Feb 20, '37
Tannic acid-silver nitrate burn treatment in children. LOW, M. B. New England J. Med. *216:*553-556, April 1, '37
Brilliant green in burns. NARAT, J. K. Am. J. Surg. *36:*54-56, April '37
Tannic acid and silver nitrate in burns. WOLLESEN, J. M. Ugesk. f. laeger. *99:*405-409, April 15, '37
Rationale of tannic acid-silver nitrate treatment of burns. BETTMAN, A. G., J.A.M.A. *108:*1490-1494, May 1, '37
Tannic acid in burns. GHEESLING, G. Indust. Med. *6:*306, May '37
Silver nitrate ointment in burns. KISSMEYER, M. Bull. med., Paris *51:*323, May 15, '37
Mercurochrome in burns. GUNN, W. D., J. Roy. Nav. M. Serv. *23:*260-261, July '37
Compound solution of tannic acid in burn therapy. FANTUS, B. AND DYNIEWICZ, H. A. J.A.M.A. *109:*200-203, July 17, '37
Tannic acid in burns. BECCARI, C. Policlinico (sez. prat.) *44:*1637-1643, Aug 30, '37
Extensive burns; treatment with silver nitrate and methyl rosaniline. BRANCH, H. E. Arch. Surg. *35:*478-485, Sept '37
Biologic therapy of burns; rest and immobilization with plaster of paris bandaging. ZENO, L. An. de cir. *3:*228-232, Sept '37
Tannic acid in therapy of burns in children. SEVERIN, E. Nord. med. tidskr. *14:*1787-1789, Oct 30, '37
Pro-vitamin A ointment in burns. BAKER, W. B. AND VONACHEN, H. A. Indust. Med. *6:*584-589, Nov '37
Burn therapy with compound of aniline dyes (acrioviolet and brilliant green). ALDRICH, R. H. New England J. Med. *217:*911-914, Dec 2, '37

Burns, Topical Therapy—Cont.

Tannic acid and silver nitrate in burns. BETTMAN, A. G. Am. J. Nursing. *37:*1333-1339, Dec '37

Treatment of burns (tannic acid and silver nitrate). MONTGOMERY, A. H. Indust. Med. *6:*639-642, Dec '37

Use of tea in burn therapy. PEIRIS, M. V. P. Indian M. Gaz. *72:*718-720, Dec '37

Comparative value of closed and open methods of burn therapy. KOMISSAROV, M. K. Novy khir. arkhiv. *38:*464-468, '37

Burn therapy; fumigation with iodine vapors. MUSHKATIN, V. I. Novy khir. arkhiv *39:*485-503, '37

Chalk dressing in ambulant burn therapy. POSTNIKOV, B. N. Khirurgiya, no. 1, pp. 28-33, '37

Burn therapy, open method as practiced at Traumatologic Clinic of Sklifasovskiy Institute. SAMSONOVA, Z. P. Novy khir. arkhiv *38:*476-479, '37

Plaster of paris bandage in therapy of burns of extremities. ZENO, L. AND BARENBOYM, S. Novy khir. arkhiv *38:*485, '37

Plaster of paris bandages in treatment of burns of extremities. ZENO, L. AND KAPLAN, A. V. Vestnik khir. *51:*16-18, '37

Clinical studies in burn therapy (tannic acid). MARTIN, J. D. JR. J. M. A. Georgia *27:*39-46, Feb '38

Burn therapy with special reference to tannin. LEIBOVICI, R., J. de med. de Paris *58:*177-178, March 3, '38

Vitamin oils in burns; experimental study. PUESTOW, C. B.; *et al.* Surg., Gynec. and Obst. *66:*622-627, March '38

Combined burn therapy with rivanol (acridine dye) and cod liver oil. TAMAI, T. Bull. Nav. M. A., Japan (Abstr. Sect.) *27:*15, March 15, '38

Burn management and therapy, with special reference to use of tannin. FASAL, P. Chirurg *10:*454-462, July 1, '38

Therapy of burns of extremities with plaster of paris bandages. GORBAN, I. A. Vestnik khir. *56:*100, July '38

Burn therapy in home (tannic acid). HARRIS, M. H. Virginia M. Monthly *65:*403-404, July '38

Tannic acid in burns; results from Maria Hospital and description of simplified quick method. RÖDEN, S. H. Nord. med. tidskr. *16:*1188-1191, July 23, '38

Continuous bath medicated with tannin in burns. JEANNENEY, G. AND SOUBIRAN. J. de med. de Bordeaux *115:*153-157, Aug 20-27, '38

Burns, Topical Therapy—Cont.

Plaster casts in simple and complicated burns. ZENO, L. Bol. y trab. de la Soc. de cir. de Buenos Aires *22:*712-722, Sept 28, '38

Biologic therapy in burns; rest and immobilization in plaster cast. ZENO, L. Arq. brasil. de cir. e ortop. *6:*295-300, Sept-Dec '38

Comparative study of foille with tannic acid and tannic acid preparations. TERRELL, T. C. Texas State J. Med. *34:*409-415, Oct '38

Therapy of first, second and third degree burns with biologic pomade; case. DE SOUSA DIAS, A. Hospital, Rio de Janeiro *14:*1415-1417, Dec '38

Tannic acid in burns. MARTIN, J. D. JR. Internat. Clin. *4:*148-153, Dec '38

Burns (fundamentals of tannic acid therapy). PICKELL, F. W., J. M. A. Alabama *8:*203-208, Dec '38

Bettman therapy in burns; results in 5 cases. ZARAZAGA, J. Dia med. *10:*1316-1317, Dec 19, '38

Clinical study and pathology of burns of second and third degree (with criticism of tannin therapy). LÖHR, W. AND ZACHER, K. Zentralbl. f. Chir. *66:*5-24, Jan 7, '39

Rapid epithelization (following use of scarlet red ointment); case, without skin grafting in extensive third degree burns. HERZ, L. F., M. Rec. *149:*43-44, Jan 18, '39

Results of new therapies for serious recent burns, with special reference to tannin. HOUOT, A.; *et al.* Ann. Fac. franc. de med. et de pharm. de Beyrouth *8:*32-54, Jan-Feb '39

Cod-liver oil and vaseline in burns. BERLIEN, I. C. AND DAVIS, J. R. Ohio State M. J. *35:*267-269, March '39

Therapy of simple and complicated burns by means of plaster casts. ZENO, L. Arch. urug. de med., cir. y especialid. *14:*322-324, March '39

Unguentolan (cod liver oil ointment) and plaster casts in industrial burns. WICHMANN, F. W. Zentralbl. f. Chir. *66:*655-662, March 25, '39

Burn therapy; with special reference to use of solutions of silver nitrate, aniline dyes (especially gentian violet) and their combination. CHEN, C. Y. Chinese M. J. *55:*407-426, May '39

Paraffin film treatment of burns of eyelids. SHUMAN, G. H. Pennsylvania M. J. *42:*907-909, May '39

Three-dye treatment of burns. DEVINE, J. B. M. J. Australia *1:*924-928, June 24, '39

Antiseptic compounds (especially trinitro-

Burns, Topical Therapy – Cont.
phenolate of ethyl aminobenzoate) in burns. MEREDITH, D. T. AND LEE, C. O., J. Am. Pharm. A. *28:*369-373, June '39
Treatment of extensive burns and scalds (with special reference to Unna's paste, zinc oxide preparation). OCHSNER, E. H. New Zealand M. J. *38:*180-187, June '39 also: M. Rec. *150:*193-196, Sept 20, '39
Use of foille in burns. GALT, S. Dallas M. J. *25:*81-86, July '39
Results of exposure to air and use of tannic acid in burns. PATEL. Lyon chir. *36:*474-476, July-Aug '39
Aloes in treatment of burns and scalds. CREWE, J. E. Minnesota Med. *22:*538-539, Aug '39
Industrial burns and their therapy by tannic acid or silver nitrate. FERNANDEZ DEL VALLE, A. Rev. d. trab. *4:*203-207, Aug '39
Burn therapy; with special reference to tannin salve. HERTZBERG, G. Kinderarztl. Praxis *10:*364-370, Aug '39
Treatment and management of burn cases (with special reference to bath procedure). LAVENDER, H. J. Am. J. Surg. *45:*534-538, Sept '39
Frekasan (tannin preparation) in burns. MAJER, E. Munchen. med. Wchnschr. *86:*1433-1435, Sept 22, '39
Therapy of cutaneous burns according to Davidson method. FELDSTEINAS, L. Medicina, Kaunas *20:*875-881, Oct-Nov '39
New treatment for burns (use of hydrogen peroxide and electric lamp attachment); cases. HENRY, H. B., M. Bull. Vet. Admin. *16:*143-145, Oct '39
Warm moist air therapy in burns. SMITH, S. *et al.* Arch. Surg. *39:*686-690, Oct '39
Studies on hexyl-chloro-m-cresol and other carbocyclic antiseptics (for use with tannic acid) in burns. HARTMAN, F. W. AND SCHELLING, V. Am. J. Surg. *46:*460-467, Dec '39
Histologic study of effect of local application of certain medicaments in third degree burns. ANAGNOSTIDIS, N. Deutsche Ztschr. f. Chir. *252:*248-256, '39
Critical study of usual methods of burn therapy; cod liver oil, with special reference to third degree burns. KRIEG, W. Arch. f. klin. Chir. *195:*203-249, '39
Leukoplast for bandaging burns. SMIRNOV, V. I. Khirurgiya, no. 1, pp. 54-59, '39
Use of antiseptic anesthetic agent locally in extensive burn. NAGLE, P. J. Oklahoma M. A. *33:*14-16, Jan '40
Cod liver oil in burns. HARDIN, P. C. North Carolina M. J. *1:*82-91, Feb '40

Burns, Topical Therapy – Cont.
Modern trends, with special reference to tannic acid and cod liver oil. Burns. LAMBOMBARDA, G. Clinica *6:*59-76, Feb '40
Tannin; practical application in burns. JOLY, P. AND DE VADDER, A. Presse med. *48:*171-172, Feb 7-10, '40
Good effects of vitamin A on burn cicatrization. COMBEMALE, P. Echo med. du Nord *11:*53-57, March '40
Coagulant medications in burns. RUATA, G. Rassegna di med. indust. *11:*213-220, April '40
Sulfanilamide in burns. GRIGSBY, B. C. Virginia M. Monthly *67:*306-307, May '40
Comparative evaluation of Bettmann-Davidson method in burns. NORENBERG, A. E. Vestnik khir. *60:*9-17, July-Aug '40
Tannin and gentian violet in burn therapy. MORHARDT, P. E. Presse med. *48:*660, Aug 14-17, '40
Antiseptic analgesic tannic acid jelly in burns. HEGGIE, J. F. AND HEGGIE, R. M. Lancet *2:*391, Sept 28, '40
Envelope method of burn therapy. BUNYAN, J. Proc. Roy. Soc. Med. *34:*65-70, Nov '40
Silver nitrate, tannic acid and gentian violet in burn therapy. ROSS, J. A. AND HULBERT, K. F. Brit. M. J. *2:*702-703, Nov 23, '40
Tannic acid versus saline in burns. COHEN, S. M. Brit. M. J. *2:*754-755, Nov 30, '40
Therapy of extensive burns, with special reference to use of tannic acid. PAOLUCCI, R. Ann. di med. nav. e colon. *46:*501-504, Nov-Dec '40
Methyl violet in burns. RAPOPORT, D. M. Sovet. vrach. zhur. *44:*843-846, Dec '40
Burn treatment (with paraffin dressing). ZEISS, C. R. Illinois M. J. *78:*540-544, Dec '40
Ammargen (silver-ammonia compound) in burn therapy. KOVANOV, V. V. Sovet. med. (no. 3) *4:*21-22, '40
Methyl violet in burns. RAPOPORT, D. M. Sovet. med. (nos. 13-14) *4:*15-16, '40
Local application of cod liver oil in therapy of burns of eyes. TIKHOVA, V. A. Vestnik oftal. *17:*396-397, '40
Atomizer for burn therapy with vitaderm (carotene preparation). TITOV, E. S. Ortop. i. travmatol. (no. 2) *14:*24-25, '40
Burn therapy with vitaderm (carotene preparation). USPENSKIY, A. A. Ortop. i travmatol. (no. 2) *14:*12-23, '40
Dressing of open wounds and burns with tulle gras. MATTHEWS, D. N. Lancet *1:*43-44, Jan 11, '41
Author's application of Lohr method using cod liver oil in burns. GOMEZ OLIVEROS, L. Rev. clin. espan. *2:*170-173, Feb 1, '41

Burns, Topical Therapy—Cont.
Bag bandage for hand burns. STRECKFUSS, H. Chirurg *13:*96, Feb 1, '41
Criticism of ointments and skin-forming preparations, especially in relation to third degree burns. HAASE, W. Zentralbl. f. Chir. *68:*350–353, Feb 22, '41
Fifteen years of tannic acid method in burns. GLOVER, D. M. AND SYDOW, A. F. Am. J. Surg. *51:*601–619, March '41
Powdered tannin in burns. POPESCU, A. AND VLAD, V. Romania med. *19:*73–74, March 15, '41
Perforated oiled silk in burns. STOPFORD-TAYLOR, R. Brit. M. J. *1:*403–404, March 15, '41
Physical chemistry of oils in burn treatment. THOMSON, D.; *et al.* Lancet *1:*341–343, March 15, '41
Glycerin-sulfonamide paste (euglamide, acetylsulfanilamide preparation) in burns. ROBSON, J. M. AND WALLACE, A. B. Brit. M. J. *1:*469–472, March 29, '41
Absorption of sulfanilamide from burned surfaces. HOOKER, D. H. AND LAM, C. R. Surgery *9:*534–537, April '41
Question of cod liver oil or tannin; comparative study in burns. GEY, R. Deut. Militararzt *6:*287–288, May '41
Cod liver oil in burns. HARDIN, P. C. South. Surgeon *10:*301–338, May '41
Crude vegetable oil (Calophyllum oil) for local burn treatment. SANYAL, S. N. Calcutta M. J. *38:*255–258, May '41
Treatment of fresh burns with scarlet red bandage and moist sulfanilamide dressings. GOWER, W. E., J. Iowa M. Soc. *31:*234–237, June '41
Burn therapy with envelope method (using electrolytic sodium hypochlorite solution). BUNYAN, J. Brit. M. J. *2:*1–7, July 5, '41 also: M. Press *206:*103–109, July 30, '41
Burn therapy by coated silk fabric (including envelopes); report upon conclusion drawn from treatment of 82 cases (by irrigation with electrolytic sodium hypochlorite solution). HUDSON, R. V. Brit. M. J. *2:*7–12, July 5, '41
Burn therapy with envelope irrigation (with electrolytic sodium hypochlorite solution). HANNAY, J. W. Brit. M. J. *2:*46–48, July 12, '41
Local treatment of burns (using tulle gras with sulfanilamide powder or envelope irrigation with electrolytic sodium hypochlorite solution). PEARSON, R. S. R.; *et al.* Brit. M. J. *2:*41–45, July 12, '41
Burn therapy with foille not acceptable for N. R. CARBISULPHOIL COMPANY. J.A. M.A. *117:*363–365, Aug 2, '41

Burns, Topical Therapy—Cont.
Treatment of superficial granulating surface (burns). EDMUNDS, A. Lancet *2:*130, Aug 2, '41
New burn treatment (spraying solution of sulfadiazine, sulfanilamide derivative); preliminary report. PICKRELL, K. L. Bull. Johns Hopkins Hosp. *69:*217–221, Aug '41
Sulfhydryl solution (hydrosulphosol) in burns; preliminary report. PIERCE, W. F. Am. J. Surg. *53:*434–439, Sept '41
Modern burn treatment with special reference to new dressing, "foille." HAMILTON, J. E., Indust. Med. *10:*427–432, Oct '41
Acetylsulfanilamide ointment in local therapy of burns. HRAD, O. Deutsche med. Wchnschr. *67:*1147–1150, Oct 17, '41
Biochemical investigation of tannic acid and sulfanilamide in burns. DE VIDAS, J. AND McEACHERN, A. C., M. J. Australia *2:*470–474, Oct 25, '41
Closed-plaster burn treatment. ROULSTON, T. J. Brit. M. J. *2:*611–613, Nov 1, '41
Ultraviolet rays in burn therapy. BEKKER, E. K. S. Eksper. med. (no. 3) *8:*53–60, '41
Local burn treatment with special reference to sulfadiazine (sulfanilamide derivative). ADAMS, W. M. Memphis M. J. *17:*5–8, Jan '42
New sulfhydryl solution (hydrosulphosol) in burns. MELLON, R. R. Indust. Med. *11:*14–18, Jan '42
Tannin therapy of burns of all degrees. BALTIN, W. Monatschr. f. Unfallh. *49:*65–80, March '42
Treatment of burns of eyes and face with sulfhydryl solution (hydrosulphosol). CRUTHIRDS, A. E. Indust. Med. *11:*109–112, March '42
Superficial granulating areas treated with antiseptic emulsions in burns. HEGGIE, R. M.; *et al.* Lancet *1:*347–350, March 21, '42
Chemical coagulants in burn therapy. MEDAWAR, P. B. Lancet *1:*350–352, March 21, '42
Color film of treatment by cod liver oil and sulfanilamide in burns. CLARK, A. M. Tr. Roy. Med.-Chir. Soc. Glasgow, pp. 17–18, '41–42; in Glasgow M. J. April '42
Sulfadiazine (sulfanilamide derivative) spray in burns; case. KEITER, W. E. North Carolina M. J. *3:*190–192, April '42
Phototherapy of burns. LEONENKO, P. M. Am. Rev. Soviet Med. *1:*340–343, April '44 also: Khirurgiya, no. 7, pp. 42–46, '42
Relation of tannic acid to liver necrosis in burns. WELLS, D. B.; *et al.* New England J. Med. *226:*629–636, April 16, '42

Burns, Topical Therapy—Cont.
Sulfadiazine (sulfanilamide derivative) in burns. ADAMS, W. M. AND CRAWFORD, J. K. South. Surgeon *11:*324–340, May '42
Sulfathiazole (sulfanilamide preparation) ointment in burns. ALLEN, J. G.; *et al.* Arch. Surg. *44:*819–828, May '42
Plaster casts in local burn therapy. BALESDENT, E. Hospital, Rio de Janeiro *21:*753–768, May '42
Triple dye treatment of burns and scalds. DREOSTI, A. E. South African M. J. *16:*181, May 9, '42
Local treatment of burns. HAMILTON, J. E. Kentucky M. J. *40:*207–211, June '42
Local treatment of burns. HARKINS, H. N. Clinics *1:*6–24, June '42
Clinical and experimental studies with Koch method in heat burns. SILER, V. E. AND REID, M.R. Ann. Surg. *115:*1106–1117, June '42
Sulfathiazole (sulfanilamide derivative) emulsion; further experience in burns. ACKMAN, D. AND WILSON, G. Canad. M. A. J. *47:*1–7, July '42
Burn wounds; their treatment. WEAVER, D. D. California and West Med. *57:*9–12, July '42
Boric-butyn-petrolatum gauze treatment in burns. HUGHES, G. K., J. Michigan M. Soc. *41:*653–656, Aug '42
Primary cleansing, compression and rest in burn treatment. SILER, V. E. Surg., Gynec. and Obst. *75:*161–164, Aug '42 also: Am. J. Nursing *42:*994–1000, Sept '42
Local burn treatment (with sulfathiazole, sulfanilamide derivative, and cod liver oil ointment) in the Army. THIESSEN, N. W. AND STEINREICH, O. S. Mil. Surgeon *91:*208–211, Aug '42
Value of local chemotherapy (with sulfanilamide and its derivative, sulfathiazole); Hunterian lecture, abridged. (Burns) MATTHEWS, D. N. Lancet *2:*271–275, Sept 5, '42
Minor and medium burns; treatment with sulfathiazole (sulfanilamide derivative). BIRAM, J. H. Indust. Med. *11:*462–463, Oct '42
Comparison of certain drugs (tannic acid and gentian violet) used as local applications. (Burns) DOWNS, T. M., U. S. Nav. M. Bull. *40:*936–938, Oct '42
Sulfanilamide and its derivatives in burns. DUBE, E. Union med. du Canada *71:*1062–1066, Oct '42
Immediate treatment of burn patient (coagulation regime). GLOVER, D. M. Australian and New Zealand J. Surg. *12:*91–102, Oct '42

Burns, Topical Therapy—Cont.
Cod liver oil in burns. HARDIN, P. C. South. Surgeon *11:*691–728, Oct '42
Therapy of burns (coagulation therapy; saline regime; skin grafting). RANK, B. K. Australian and New Zealand J. Surg. *12:*103–110, Oct '42
Sulfonamides (sulfanilamide and its derivatives) in local treatment of burns. RHOADS, J. E.; *et al.* Pennsylvania M. J. *46:*13–16, Oct '42
Microcrystalline sulfathiazole (sulfanilamide derivative) in superficial burns. SHAAR, C. M.; *et al.* U. S. Nav. M. Bull. *40:*954–957, Oct '42
Paper tissue-cod liver oil ointment dressings after surgical cleansing of burns. CALLAHAN, G. B. Illinois M. J. *82:*368–373, Nov '42
Practical concept for major and minor burns (including use of sulfathiazole, sulfanilamide derivative, emulsion and "sulfamesh" dressing); importance of timing therein. GURD, F. B.; *et al.* Ann. Surg. *116:*641–657, Nov '42
Burn therapy with 2.5 per cent sulfadiazine (sulfanilamide derivative) in 8 per cent triethanolamine solution. ROTHMAN, M.; *et al.* J.A.M.A. *120:*803–805, Nov 14, '42
Local burn treatment with sulfadiazine (sulfanilamide derivative) spray. COLOVIRAS, G. J. JR.; *et al.* Canad. M. A. J. *47:*505–514, Dec '42
Better local application for first and second degree burns (picric acid in flexible collodion). GUILD, W. A., J. Am. Inst. Homeop. *35:*532–533, Dec '42
Comparative study of local burn treatments. HAMILTON, J. E. Am. J. Surg. *58:*350–364, Dec '42
Intrasternal administration of plasma in burns; sulfadiazine (sulfonamide) complications. MUIRHEAD, E. E. AND HILL, J. M. Dallas M. J. *28:*156–161, Dec '42
Burn therapy with special reference to use of casts. ZENO, L. An. de cir. *8:*265–280, Dec '42
Burn therapy; chemotherapeutic membranes (containing sulfanilamide, sulfonamide, with and without azochloramid, hypochlorite derivative. ANDRUS, W. DEW.; *et al.* Arch. Surg. *46:*1–8, Jan '43
Treatment of acute stage of burns (with alcohol compresses). COMPTON, W. C. Cincinnati J. Med. *23:*540–547, Jan '43
Hexenol in burns of limited areas. LEVINE, B. Am. J. M. Sc. *205:*125–130, Jan '43
Human red cell concentrate for surgical dressings for burns. MOORHEAD, J. J. AND

Burns, Topical Therapy—Cont.
UNGER, L. J. Am. J. Surg. *59:*104–105, Jan '43
Burn therapy with special reference to use of sulfadiazine (sulfonamide). RENNIE, J. G. Virginia M. Monthly *70:*24–30, Jan '43
Local burn treatment. THIESSEN, N. W. South. Med. and Surg. *105:*1–3, Jan '43
Plastic film (containing sulfonamides) in treatment of experimental burns. SKINNER, H. G. AND WAUD, R. A. Canad. M. A. J. *48:*13–18, Jan '43
Triple dyes in burn therapy. TRABUE, C. C. J. Tennessee M. A. *36:*13–19, Jan '43
Propamidine for burns at an E. M. S. hospital. KOHN, F.; *et al.*Lancet *1:*140–141, Jan 30, '43
Propamidine in burns. MORLEY, G. H. AND BENTLEY, J. P. Lancet *1:*138–139, Jan 30, '43
Burn therapy with A and D vitaminized oil; case. GARCIA-SALA, J. Rev. clin. espan. *8:*201–202, Feb 15, '43
Diffusion of sulfonamides (sulfathiazole and sulfanilamide) out of certain bases in burn therapy. WAUD, R. A. AND RAMSAY, A. Canad. M. A. J. *48:*121–123, Feb '43
Tannic acid jelly (tanaburn); use in experimental burns. MATSON, D. D. Surgery *13:*394–400, March '43
Detergents; use in cleansing and local treatment of burns. ROSENBERG, N. Surgery *13:*385–393, March '43
Burn therapy; cod liver oil ointment-paper tissue dressing, peace-time dressing brought to war. CALLAHAN, G. B. Mil. Surgeon *92:*439–442, April '43
Local and general therapy of grave burns; authors' experience. RUA, L. AND VENTURINO, H. Dia med. *15:*356–363, April 19, '43
Local therapy for industrial burns; series of 96 cases ($1^1/_2$ per cent sulfadiazine in ethanolamines with methyl cellulose as treatment of choice). COLLINGS, G. H. JR. Indust. Med. *12:*301–303, May '43
Local therapy of burns with author's formula containing prontosil (sulfonamide) and tannic acid; preliminary report. GIULIANO, A. Rev. Asoc. med. argent. *57:*254–257, May 15-30, '43 also: Semana med. *1:*1434–1438, June 24, '43
Sulfadiazine (sulfonamide) treatment of burns; comparative study (bismuth tribromophenate pressure dressings.) MEYER, K. A. AND GRADMAN, R. Surg., Gynec. and Obst. *76:*584–586, May '43
Sulfonamide (sulfacetimide) ointment; local treatment of burns. HRAD, O. Bull. War Med. *3:*542–543, June '43 (abstract)

Burns, Topical Therapy—Cont.
Paraffin wax open air treatment of burns. PENDLETON, R. C., J.A.M.A. *122:*414–417, June 12, '43
Sulfonamides in burn therapy. ROA, R. L. Dia med. *15:*608, June 14, '43
Compression treatment of burns. BRANTIGAN, O. C. AND HEBB, D. Bull. School Med. Univ. Maryland *28:*12–20, July '43
Burns of ear, nose, mouth and adjacent tissues (with special reference to therapy with hydrosulphosol, sulfhydryl solution). CRUTHIRDS, A. E. Laryngoscope *53:*478–494, July '43
Sulfonamides in war wounds and burns. FOX, C. L. Spec. Libraries *34:*244–247, July–Aug '43
Closed-plaster method of burn therapy, with certain physiologic considerations implicit in success of this technic. GLENN, W. W. L.; *et al.* J. Clin. Investigation *22:*609–625, July '43
Tannic acid toxicity in burns; experimental investigation. CAMERON, G. R.; *et al.* Lancet *2:*179–186, Aug 14, '43
Sulfonamides; local use in burns. BARRABIA VARALLA, A. Semana med. *2:*568–569, Sept 2, '43
Triple-dye-soap mixture in burn therapy. ROBINSON, C. N. Lancet *2:*351–353, Sept 18, '43
Sulfanilamide (sulfonamide); absorption from burned surfaces. WELBORN, M. B., J. Indiana M. A. *36:*447–448, Sept '43
Burn therapy with tanning by means of sulfonamides. DELRIO, J. M. A. Rev. Asoc. med. argent. *57:*866–873, Oct 30, '43
Treatment of burns of external genitalia. DRUMMOND, A. C., J. Urol. *50:*497–502, Oct '43
Sulfanilamide (sulfonamide) ointment treatment of severe burns. EVANS, E. I. AND HOOVER, M. J. Surg., Gynec. and Obst. *77:*367–375, Oct '43
Treatment of hand burns with close fitting plaster of paris casts. LEVENSON, S. M. AND LUND, C. C., J.A.M.A. *123:*272–277, Oct 2, '43
Bio-dyne ointment in burns. HIRSHFELD, J. W.; *et al.* J.A.M.A. *123:*476, Oct 23, '43
Treatment of burns with tanning agents, with special reference to tannic acid. LEONI IPARRAGUIRRE, C. A. Rev. Asoc. med. argent. *57:*862–866, Oct 30, '43
Human fibrin as burn dressing. MACFARLANE, R. G. Brit. M. J. *2:*541–543, Oct 30, '43
Pressure dressings in burns. OWENS, N., S. Clin. North America *23:*1354–1366, Oct '43

Burns, Topical Therapy—Cont.
Viacutan (silver dianphthylmethane disulfonate) in burn therapy (hand). PICK, F. AND BARTON, D. Lancet *2:*408–410, Oct 2, '43
Neoprontosil (sulfonamide); local therapy of second degree burn. VISCONTI, C. Semana med. *2:*1017, Oct 28, '43
Biologic fundamentals of immobilization and exposure to air. (burns) ZENO, L. Rev. Asoc. med. argent. *57:*854–862, Oct 30, '43
Envelope method of burn therapy (using electrolytic sodium hypochlorite solution). BUNYAN, J. Gen. Practitioner *14:*190–193, Nov 15, '43
Local burn treatment. CHRISMAN, R. B. JR. J. Tennessee M. A. *36:*413–415, Nov '43
Surface treatment of burns; comparison of results of tannic acid, silver nitrate, triple dye, and vaseline or boric ointment as surface treatments in 150 cases. CLOWES, G. H. A. JR.; *et al.* Ann. Surg. *118:*761–779, Nov '43
Pressure ointment method of burn therapy. MEYER, O. Indust. Med. *12:*727–728, Nov '43
Paraffin treatment preferred for burns of all types. BLACK, B. W. Mod. Hosp. *61:*108, Dec '43
Effect of plaster bandages and local cooling on hemoconcentration and mortality rate in burns. SELLERS, E. A. AND WILLARD, J. W. Canad. M. A. J. *49:*461–464, Dec '43
Burns of ear, nose, mouth and adjacent tissues (including use of hydrosulphosol, sulfhydryl solution). CRUTHIRDS, A. E. Tr. Am. Laryng., Rhin. and Otol. Soc., pp. 219–235, '43
Paraffin wax open air treatment of burns. PENDLETON, R. C. Am. Acad. Orthop. Surgeons, Lect., pp. 198–202, '43
Topical use of medicated (with sulfanilamide, sulfonamide) human plasma in burns. ABBOTT, M. D. AND GEPFERT, J. R. U. S. Nav. M. Bull. *42:*193–194, Jan '44
Therapy of burns with special emphasis on transparent jacket system. DOUGLAS, B. Surgery *15:*96–143, Jan '44
Sulfamide therapy in burns due to occupational accidents. FILIPATO, A. J. J. Prensa med. argent. *31:*119–121, Jan 12, '44
Local treatment of burns. HARKINS, H. N. Dia med. *16:*30–34, Jan 10, '44
Prevention of infection in wounds, fractures and burns (report of 1500 cases, especially evaluation of sulfonamides). MELENEY, F. L. Bull. U. S. Army M. Dept. (no. 72) pp. 41–46, Jan '44

Burns, Topical Therapy—Cont.
Controlled external pressure and edema formation in burns. ROSSITER, R. J. and PETERS, R. A. Lancet *1:*9–11, Jan 1, '44
Report on management of burns with sulfathiazole emulsion, using occlusive compression dressing. ACKMAN, D.; *et al.* Ann. Surg. *119:*161–177, Feb '44
Casein in local treatment of burns. CURTIS, R. M. AND BREWER, J. H. Arch. Surg. *48:*130–136, Feb '44
Ambroise Pare's onion treatment of burns. SIGERIST, H. E. Bull. Hist. Med. *15:*143–149, Feb '44
Extensive burns treated in open irrigation chamber (with sodium hypochlorite solution). GOLDBERG, H. M. Lancet *1:*371–372, March 18, '44
Modified nonadherent gauze pressure treatment of burns. MARSHALL, W. AND GREENFIELD, E. Am. J. Surg. *63:*324–328, March '44
Emergency dressing for burns of extermities. McGRAW, A. B. Hosp. Corps Quart. (no. 2) *17:*40–44, March '44
Liver function after burns in childhood; changes in levulose tolerance (especially in relation to tannic acid therapy). RAE, S. L. AND WILKINSON, A. W. Lancet *1:*332–334, March 11, '44
Toxic effects of propamidine therapy in burns. ALLEN, J. W.; *et al.* J. Path. and Bact. *56:*217–223, April '44
Prontosil (sulfonamide); indications for use in burns. PAZ, J. C. Dia med. *16:*354–357, April 10, '44
Topical application of horse serum in extensive burns. RABINOWITZ, H. M. AND PELNER, L. Am. J. Surg. *64:*55–63, April '44
Cod liver oil, sulfanilamide-sulfathiazole (sulfonamides) powder dressing in burns. FLAX, H. J., Bol. Asoc. med. de Puerto Rico *36:*208–214, May '44
General principles underlying primary local treatment of burns; review. LEVENSON, S. M., J. Indust. Hyg. and Toxicol. *26:*156–161, May '44
Local treatment of burns. NELSON, O. G., J. Tennessee M. A. *37:*159–161, May '44
Dried plasma sheets in burn therapy; preliminary reports. POLLOCK, B., U. S. Nav. M. Bull. *42:*1171–1173, May '44
Value of sulfonated oils (for cleansing) in treatment of burns and other denuded surfaces. ROGERS, W. L.; *et al.* U. S. Nav. M. Bull. *42:*1125–1128, May '44
Effect of plaster confinement applied at varying intervals after burning. ALRICH, E. M.

Burns, Topical Therapy – Cont.

AND LEHMAN, E. P. Surgery *15:*899-907, June '44

"Cellophane" (medicated with sulfanilamide, sulfonamide) treatment of burns. FARR, J. Brit. M. J. *1:*749-750, June 3, '44

Paraffin wax open air treatment of burns. PENDLETON, R. Semana med. *1:*1344-1346, June 29, '44

Local treatment of surface burns. PRIOLEAU, W. H. South. Med. and Surg. *106:*201-202, June '44

Early plastic care of deep burns (including use of pressure dressing with sulfathiazole, sulfonamide). GURD, F. B. AND GERRIE, J. W., J.A.M.A. *125:*616-621, July 1, '44

Fibrinogen and thrombin in surface treatment of burns. HAWN, C. V. *et al.* J. Clin. Investigation *23:*580-585, July '44

Surgical cleanliness, compression, and rest as primary surgical principles in burn therapy. KOCH, S. L., J.A.M.A. *125:*612-616, July 1, '44

Tannic acid method of burn therapy; present status. LEE, W. E. AND RHOADS, J. E. J.A.M.A. *125:*610-612, July 1, '44

Treatment of burns and wounds with skin loss by envelope method (using electrolytic sodium hypochlorite solution.) OSBORNE, R. P. Brit. J. Surg. *32:*24-32, July '44

Proflavine (acridine dye) powder in burn wounds. RAVEN, R. W. Lancet *2:*73-75, July 15, '44

Sulfanilamide (sulfonamide) ointment in local therapy of burns (in Hebrew). SEIDMAN, M. Harefuah *27:*6-8, July 2, '44

Analysis of modern treatment (especially with closed plaster) of severe burns. DRINKER, C. K., J. Oklahoma M. A. *37:*339-346, Aug '44

Open air, immobilization and protection in burn therapy. BAHAMONDE Q., A. Arch. Soc. cirujanos hosp. *14:*476-483, Sept '44

Healing of deep thermal burns; preliminary report (on local application of acids, expecially pyruvic acid). CONNOR, G. J. AND HARVEY, S. C. Ann. Surg. *120:*362-366, Sept '44

Comparison of various types of local treatment in burns (especially results with sulfonamide-impregnated plastic film) in controlled series of experimental burns in human volunteers. DINGWALL, J. A. III AND ANDRUS, W. DEW. Ann. Surg. *120:*377-386, Sept '44

Tannic acid in burn therapy; liver necrosis following therapy. JACKSON, A. V., M. J. Australia *2:*352-354, Sept 30, '44

Burns, Topical Therapy – Cont.

Tannic acid in burn therapy; an obsequy. McCLURE, R. D. *et al.* Ann. Surg. *120:*387-398, Sept '44

Hemostatic globulin and plasma clot dressing in local treatment of burns. MISCALL, L. AND JOYNER, A. Surgery *16:*419-421, Sept '44

Tannic acid in burns; useful and dangerous fixative. SAINT-ONGE, G., J. de l'Hotel-Dieu de Montreal *13:*270-282, Sept-Oct '44

Prontosil (sulfonamide) in burns; cases. HASENBALG, A. Semana med. *2:*755-756, Oct 12, '44

Tannic acid in burn therapy; experimental study with particular reference to its effect on local fluid loss and healing. HAM, A. W. Ann. Surg. *120:*698-706, Nov '44

Comparative experimental study including medicated (with potassium iodide and sulfathiazole, sulfonamide) pliable gelatin film (sulfagel) in burns; effect of firm dressings on rate of healing. ROBACK, R. A. AND IVY, A. C. Surg., Gynec. and Obst. *79:*469-477, Nov '44

Prontosil (sulfonamide) in burn therapy. GINI LACORTE, F. D. AND GEFFNER, S. Dia med. *16:*1492-1493, Dec 4, '44

Healing of deep thermal burns; preliminary report (on local application of acids, especially pyruvic acid). CONNOR, G. J. AND HARVEY, S. C. Tr. Am. S. A. *62:*362-366, '44

Comparison of various types of local treatment (especially results with sulfonamide-impregnated plastic film) in controlled series of experimental burns in human volunteers. DINGWALL, J. A., III AND ANDRUS, W. DEW. Tr. Am. S. A. *62:*377-386, '44

Sulfonamides in treatment of war burns. FOX, C. L. JR. Smithsonian Inst. Annual Rep. (1943) pp. 569-574, '44

Tannic acid in burns; an obsequy. McCLURE, R. D.; *et al.* Tr. Am. S. A. *62:*387-405, '44

Sulfathiazole (sulfonamide) ointment; further studies on preparation and use. (in burns) JENKINS, H. P. *et al.* Surg., Gynec. and Obst. *80:*85-96, Jan '45

Treatment of patient (burns), with reference to proflavine (acridine dye) powder technic. RAVEN, R. W. Brit. M. J. *1:*261-262, Feb 24, '45

Sulfonamides (in ointment base); absorption from burn surface. EVANS, E. I.; *et al.* Surg., Gynec. and Obst. *80:*297-302, March '45

"Cellophane" (medicated with sulfanilamide,

Burns, Topical Therapy—Cont.

sulfonamide) treatment of burns. FARR, J. D. Rev. san. mil. Buenos Aires *44:*313–317, March '45

Local treatment of burns with pressure dressings and films containing sulfonamide. REESE, E. C. Am. J. Surg. *67:*524–529, March '45

Local therapy including facial, interdigital and perineal burns; preliminary report. ZORRAQUIN, G. AND ZORRAQUIN, G. F. Dia med. *17:*329–331, April 16, '45

Results of sulfonamides and penicillin in serious burns. MALAQUIAS, G. Folha med. *26:*79–80, May 25, '45

Boric acid ointment in burn therapy; study of possible intoxication. PFEIFFER, C. C. J.A.M.A. *128:*266–274, May 26, '45

Pyruvic acid method of burn slough removal; experimental investigation. LAM, C. R. AND PUPPENDAHL, M. Ann. Surg. *121:*866–871, June '45

Preliminary report of new gelatin product used in burns (containing sulfadiazine, sulfonamide)-sulfagel. FLACK, H. L.; *et al.* J. Am. Pharm. A. (Scient. Ed.) *34:*187–190, July '45

Cod liver oil ointment in surgery of burns; topical application. DAUGHTRY, DEW. C. Surgery *18:*510–515, Oct '45 also: Alexander Blain Hosp. Bull. (no. 3) *4:*2–6, Nov '45

New dressing for burns (medicated ointment in perforated cellophane envelope). KING, G. S. Indust. Med. *14:*796–797, Oct '45

"Cellophane" dressing for second degree burns. BLOOM, H. Lancet *2:*559, Nov 3, '45

Local treatment of thermal burns. GREEN, F. H. K. Prensa med. argent. *33:*94–102, Jan 11, '46

Plaster casts in burns. DE MORAES LEME, J. Rev. paulista de Med. *28:*109–125, Feb '46

Plaster bandages in burns. FAURA, C. Actas dermo-sif. *37:*705–707, Feb '46

Merbromin (mercury compound) in local therapy of second degree burns. GROB, M. Helvet. paediat. acta *1:*267–275, Feb '46

Use of saline solution, glycerin, and acetic acid in care of burns; odorless method of treating burns. LUDWIG, F. E. Surgery *19:*486–491, Apr '46

Burn dressing (cellophane). KING, G. S. New York State J. Med. *46:*1567, July 15, '46

Treatment (with picric acid) of minor burns acquired in laboratory and at home. MALKIEL, S. AND BOYD, W. C., J. Missouri M. A. *43:*538–539, Aug '46

Hydrophilic acid ointments for debridement

Burns, Topical Therapy—Cont.

of burns. MATTOCKS, A.M. AND LAZIER, W.A., J. Am. Pharm. A. (Scient. Ed.) *35:*275–279, Sept '46

Pyruvic acid method in deep clinical burns. CONNOR, G. J. AND HARVEY, S. C. Ann. Surg. *124:*799–810, Nov '46

Treatment of burns under plexiglass covers. ERUSALIMSKIY, A. L. Vrach. delo (nos. 7–8) *26:*549–552, '46

Burns, Treatment

Treatment of burns. WORKMAN, J. B., J. S. Carolina M. A. *17:*176, July '21

Treatment of burns. FLÖRCKEN, H. Therap. Halbmonatsh. *35:*460, Aug 1, '21

Burns and their treatment. HARTTUNG, H. Therap. Halbmonatsh. *35:*464, Aug 1, '21

Successful treatment of a case of scalding. DEY, P. K. Indian M. Gaz. *56:*338, Sept '21

Burns. PEASE, H. E., J. Missouri M. A. *18:*323, Sept '21

Burn treatment. TUNGER. Deutsche med. Wchnschr. *48:*95, Jan 19, '22

Newer method in treatment of burns with report of cases. MICKLETHWAITE, G. R. Ohio State M. J. *18:*198–200, March '22

Burn therapy. KOTZAREFF, A. Rev. de chir. *60:*5–29, '22 abstr: J.A.M.A. *79:*507, Aug 5, '22

Epinephrin in treatment of burns. ARSENIO PLAZA. Siglo med. *70:*560–562, Dec 9, '22 abstr: J.A.M.A. *80:*438, Feb 10, '23

Burns and their treatment. GOSS, E. L. Journal-Lancet *44:*510–515, Oct 15, '24

Treatment of burns with epinephrin. DOUGLAS, B. Compt. rend. Soc. de biol. *92:*267–268, Feb 6, '25

Treatment of burns. HOGAN, M., J. Kansas M. Soc. *25:*35–37, Feb '25

Early treatment of superficial burns. RAVDIN, I. S. AND FERGUSON, L. K. Ann. Surg. *81:*439–456, Feb '25

Burn therapy. PAGENSTECHER, G. A. J.A.M.A. *84:*1917, June 20, '25

Management and treatment of burns. RING, H. J. California and West. Med. *23:*1296–1297, Oct '25

Treatment of burns. SAYRE, B. E. Illinois M. J. *48:*325–327, Oct '25

Treatment of superficial burns. RAVDIN, I. S. S. Clin. N. America *5:*1579–1583, Dec '25

Rational treatment of burns. FRATTIN, G. Zentralbl. f. Chir. *53:*201–203, Jan 23, '26

Burn therapy. COLGIN, I. E. Texas State J. Med. *21:*668–670, March '26

Treatment of cutaneous burns. BANCROFT, F. W. AND ROGERS, C. S. Ann. Surg. *84:*1–18, July '26

Burns, Treatment—Cont.
Detoxication in treatment of burns. WILSON, W. R. Brit. M. J. *1:*54-55, Jan 8, '27
Parasan and pituitrin in burns. McDOUGALL, C. Ugesk. f. Laeger *89:*59, Jan 20, '27
Treatment of burns. MACKENZIE, D. Brit. M. J. *1:*421-422, March 5, '27
Burn therapy. SOKOVNINA, R. Vrach. Gaz. *31:*524, April 15, '27
Treatment of extensive burns. DAVIS, M. B. J. Tennessee M. A. *20:*6-9, May '27
Surgical treatment of burns. LEE, W. E. Internat. J. Med. and Surg. *40:*189-194, May '27
Burn therapy. BARMONDIERE. Prat. med. franc. *6:*258-260, June (B) '27
Burn therapy. MACLENNAN, A. Brit. M. J. *2:*590-591, Oct 1, '27
Late treatment of burns. BANCROFT, F. W. AND ROGERS, C. S. Tr. South. S. A. *40:*73-81, '27
Tschmarke's antiseptic treatment of burns. RESCHKE, K. Arch. f. klin. Chir. *146:*763-776, '27
Late burn treatment. BANCROFT, F. W. AND ROGERS, C. S. Arch. Surg. *16:*979-999, May '28
Burn therapy. ROSTOCK, P. Fortschr. d. Therap. *4:*386-388, June 25, '28
Radium treatment of burns. SORET. Paris med. *1:*534, June 9, '28
Present status of burn therapy. CHRISTOPHER, F. Am. J. Surg. *5:*61-65, July '28
Simple treatment of extensive burns. SCOTT, J. F. Northwest Med. *27:*347-348, July '28
Burn therapy. THELEN, W. P. Surg. J. *34:*146-149, July-Aug '28
Burn therapy. CUTTING, R. A. New Orleans M. and S. J. *81:*112-120, Aug '28
Surgical treatment of burns. LEE, W. E., S. Clin. N. Amer. *8:*901-909, Aug '28
Burn therapy in Presbyterian Hospital of Philadelphia. GRIFFITH, G. C. Internat. Clin. *4:*129-131, Dec '28
Normal horse serum in burns; cases. MONTEITH, S. R. AND CLOCK, R. O. J.A.M.A. *92:*1173-1177, April 6, '29
Horse serum in burns; cases. MONTEITH, S. R. Gazz. d. osp. *50:*550-554, April 28, '29
Burn therapy. AYYAR, T. G. R., J. Ayurveda *5:*413, May '29
Prevention of deaths from burns by treatment with medicaments, particularly vasano (scopolamine preparation). SCHREINER, K. Med. Klin. *25:*706-708, May 3, '29
Surgical treatment of burns. HEATLEY, T. F. Internat. J. Med. and Surg. *42:*360, July '29

Burns, Treatment—Cont.
Burn therapy. HAYWARD. Med. Klin. *25:*1510-1511, Sept 27, '29
Burn therapy. KREIBICH, C. Med. Klin. *25:*1656-1657, Oct 25, '29
Burn therapy. SCHMIDT, E. R. Am. J. Surg. *8:*274-276, Feb '30
Use of insulin in second-degree burn developing hyperglycemia and glycosuria. TEOPACO, R. L., J. Philippine Islands M. A. *10:*162-165, April '30
Immediate treatment of severely injured (including burn). WEST, C. O., J. Kansas M. Soc. *31:*129-131, April '30
Burn therapy. SCHREINER, K. Wien. klin. Wchnschr. *43:*871-876, July 10, '30
Prevention of pain and treatment of burns. NOVAK, M. Munchen. med. Wchnschr. *77:*1669-1670, Sept 26, '30
Modern methods of burn therapy. PEREZ DUEÑO, F. Cron. med. mex. *29:*511-516, Nov 1, '30
Treatment of burns of first and second degree. BOTASHEFF, V. A. Vrach. gaz. *34:*1748-1750, Dec 15, '30
Detoxification treatment in burns. LUTTERLOH, P. W. AND STROUD, H. A. Internat. J. Med. and Surg. *44:*16-18, Jan '31
Burns and their treatment. LAVENDER, H. J. J. med. *11:*635-643, Feb '31
Tschmarke method of burn therapy. RESCHKE, K. Med. Welt *5:*444, March 28, '31
Therapy of burns. GREEN, J. L. JR. Southwestern Med. *15:*194-198, May '31
Application of physical therapy measures in burns. PECK, W. S. Arch. Phys. Therapy *12:*327-333, June '31 abstr: Brit. J. Phys. Med. *6:*175, Nov '31
Burns and scalds. LLOYD, E. I. Brit. M. J. *2:*177-179, Aug 1, '31
Modern treatment of burns. MASON, E. C., J. Oklahoma M. A. *24:*273-274, Aug '31
Burn therapy. KLEINSCHMIDT, O. Deutsche med. Wchnschr. *57:*1546-1548, Sept 4, '31
Immediate treatment of extensive superficial burns. CUTTING, R. A. Am. J. Surg. *14:*705-724, Dec '31
Present status of burn therapy. ROBINSON, C. C., J. Indiana M. A. *24:*652-656, Dec '31
Theories on therapy of extended burns. KABELÍK. Ceska dermat. *12:*313-316, '31
Methods of burn therapy. MECCA, G. Prat. pediat. *10:*61-65, Feb '32
Burns and their treatment; review of 352 cases. STRAUSS, A. Ohio State M. J. *28:*101-106, Feb '32
Burn therapy. CIPOLLETTA, B. Gazz. internaz. med.-chir. *40:*244-247, April 30, '32

Burns, Treatment—Cont.

Are we up to date in our treatment of burns? CLEMENTS, H. J. Northwest Med. *31:*209-215, May '32

Ozone in burns; preliminary report. SIMONETTI, G. Osp. maggiore *20:*287-290, May '32

Convalescent serum in treatment of grave burns of children; 2 cases. AMADO, C. F. Semana med. *1:*1696-1698, June 2, '32

Modern burn treatment. MASON, R. F., J. Tennessee M. A. *25:*267-271, July '32

Burn therapy. BLEDSOE, N. C. Southwest Med. *16:*313-317, Aug '32

Burn therapy. POENARU-CAPLESCU. Romania med. *10:*239-242, Oct 15, '32

Burn therapy. SATULLO, B. Policlinico (sez. prat.) *39:*1947-1950, Dec 12, '32

Philonin (irradiated cholesterol preparation) in burns. LUTTENBERGER, A. Wien. med. Wchnschr. *83:*88-89, Jan 14, '33

Symposium on acute burns; medical care. BANNICK, E. G. Proc. Staff. Meet., Mayo Clin. *8:*123-126, Feb 22, '33

Burn therapy to prevent contractures. BURTON, J. F., J. Oklahoma M. A. *26:*36-38, Feb '33

Symposium on acute burns; surgical care. GHORMLEY, R. K. Proc. Staff Meet., Mayo Clin. *8:*126-127, Feb 22, '33

Burns; treatment of shock and toxemia; healing wound; reconstruction. BETTMAN, A. G. Am. J. Surg. *20:*33-37, April '33

Burn therapy. HILGENFELDT, O. Med. Klin. *29:*490-492, April 7, '33

Recent advances in burn therapy. WARTHEN, H. J. JR. Virginia M. Monthly *60:*30-36, April '33

Burn therapy. LOCK, N. Clin. J. *62:*200-203, May '33

Extensive burns on both forearms and back of hand; remote results of resection of retractile scar and pedicled graft from thigh. MIRIZZI, P. L. Bull. et mem. Soc. nat. de chir. *59:*694-695, May 6, '33

Early and late treatment of burns. PADGETT, E. C., J. Kansas M. Soc. *34:*184-188, May '33

Prognosis and therapy of severe burns. MOURGUE-MOLINES, E. Gaz. d. hop. *106:*1013, July 8, '33; 1045, July 15, '33

New apparatus for wire skeletal traction used in therapy of fractures, burns and traumas. ROVIRALTA, E. But. Soc. catalana de pediat. *6:*233-237, July-Aug '33

Burns and their treatment. MUNGER, I. C. JR. Nebraska M. J. *18:*300-306, Aug '33

Pathology and therapy of burns. RIEHL, G. JR. Wien. klin. Wchnschr. *46:*1041-1043, Aug 25, '33

Burns, Treatment—Cont.

Story of burns, treatment of burns. ALDRICH, R. H. Am. J. Nursing *33:*851-855, Sept '33

Review of modern burn treatment. BARNES, J. P. Arch. Surg. *27:*527-544, Sept '33

Fomentobiol (vaccine broth) in burns; 5 cases. ABASCAL, H. Cron. med.-quir. de la Habana *59:*411-413, Oct '33

Surgical therapy of severe burns. NEXULA, R. Casop. lek. cesk. *72:*1487-1491, Nov 24, '33

Burn therapy. BARON, C. Kentucky M. J. *31:*579, Dec '33

Therapy of general manifestations of burns; experimental study; preliminary report. LORETO, C. Arch. ed atti d. Soc. ital. di chir. *39:*1068-1072, '33

Burn therapy. RAMIRO MORENO, A. Rev. mex. de cir., ginec. y cancer *2:*28-45, Jan '34

Management of burns. KIRKHAM, H. L. D. Texas State J. Med. *29:*636-638, Feb '34

Burn therapy. BERTOLINO, P. Profilassi *7:*201-219, June '34

Burn therapy. MORROW, J. Minnesota Med. *17:*330-332, June '34

Burns and their treatment. PRIMLANI, C. H. Sind M. J. *7:*1-7, June '34

Practical therapy of burns. GOMOIU, V. Spitalul *54:*302-305, July-Aug '34

Mendez biologic method of burn therapy. TORVISO, R. E. Semana med. *2:*732-734, Sept 6, '34

Burn therapy. WHITEHILL, N. M., J. Iowa M. Soc. *24:*481-482, Sept '34

Burn therapy. WEAVER, D. California and West. Med. *41:*222-226, Oct '34

Burn therapy of Cook County Hospital. FANTUS, B., J.A.M.A. *103:*1446-1447, Nov 10, '34

Burn therapy. SEEGER, S. J. AND SCHAEFER, A. A. Physiotherapy Rev. *14:*174-176, Nov-Dec '34

Urgent therapy of grave burns. GOTTLIEB, F. M. Bucuresti med. *6:*109-110, '34

Burn therapy. CLARK, A. M. AND CRUICKSHANK, R. Lancet *1:*201-204, Jan 26, '35

Burn therapy. HOLMGREN, B. Nord. med. tidskr. *9:*413-420, March 16, '35

Thermal burns and their treatment. LOWELL, H. M., J. Med. *16:*28-30, March '35

Burn therapy. ROBB, J. J. Brit. M. J. *1:*466-467, March 9, '35

Modern burn therapy; 2 cases. GUBERN-SALISACHS, L. Rev. de cir. de Barcelona *9:*325-348, April '35

Burn therapy. PUSITZ, M. E., J. Kansas M. Soc. *36:*148, April '35

Methods of burn therapy. ARZT, L. Wien. klin. Wchnschr. *48:*644-647, May 18, '35

Burns, Treatment—Cont.

Modern therapy of superficial burns in medical practice. RUDLER, J. C. Bull. med., Paris *49:*343-347, May 18, '35

Therapy of burns. GÓMEZ, O. Bol. y trab. de la Soc. de cir. de Buenos Aires *19:*484-491, July 17, '35

Burn therapy. SNEDECOR, S. T., J. M. Soc. New Jersey *32:*535-537, Sept '35

Treatment of severe cutaneous burns. WALSH, J. N., J. South Carolina M. A. *31:*189-194, Oct '35

Burn therapy. MARRE, P. Avenir med. *32:*266-269, Nov '35

Burn therapy. SEEGER, S. J. Texas State J. Med. *31:*488-494, Dec '35

Burns and their therapy. GORINEVSKAYA, V. V. AND SAMSONOVA, Z. P. Sovet. khir., no. 6, pp. 216-224, '35

Disturbance in acid-base equilibrium due to burns and its treatment with thiosulfate. GRINCHAR, F. N. Sovet. khir., no. 6, pp. 232-244, '35

Burn therapy. KATSNELSON, Z. N. Sovet. khir., no. 8, pp. 16-20, '35

Treatment of extensive gasoline burns of legs (due to explosion) with correction of deformity; case. BRUNSTING, L. A. AND GHORMLEY, R. K. Proc. Staff Meet., Mayo Clin. *11:*129-131, Feb 26, '36

Burn therapy. PENBERTHY, G. C. New England J. Med. *214:*306-310, Feb 13, '36

Modern burn therapy. CONNELL, J. H. New Orleans M. and S. J. *88:*575-578, March '36

Clinical aspects of burns. TIMOFEEV, S. L. Sovet. vrach. zhur., pp. 416-420, March 30, '36

Modern methods of burn therapy. WILSON, W. C. Practitioner *136:*394-403, April '36

Burn therapy. CRILE, G. JR. M. Clin. North America *19:*1941-1947, May '36

Significance of loss of serum protein in therapy of severe burns. WEINER, D. O.; *et al.* Proc. Soc. Exper. Biol. and Med. *34:*484-486, May '36

Practical therapy of burns. DE BIL. Avenir med. *33:*180-183, June '36

Burn therapy. SUNDARANADANAM, B. M. Indian M. Rec. *56:*129-131, June '36

Early operation for severe burns. LÄWEN, A. Zentralbl. f. Chir. *63:*1576-1581, July 4, '36

Burn therapy. VOHWINKEL, K. H. Therap. d. Gegenw. *77:*313-315, July '36

New method of burn treatment. NAKONOVA, E. I. Sovet. vrach. zhur., pp. 1262-1263, Aug 30, '36

Analysis of 235 cases burn therapy. POYNER, H. Texas State J. Med. *32:*274-279, Aug '36

Burns, Treatment—Cont.

Surgical therapy of localized third degree burns. GEKTIN, F. L. Vestnik khir. *46:*205-208, '36

Burn therapy. HILGENFELDT, O. Ergebn. d. Chir. u. Orthop. *29:*102-210, '36

Burn therapy. LEBEDEVA, M. P. Med. zhur. *6:*535-538, '36

Present status of problem of burn therapy. FASAL, P. Klin. Wchnschr. *16:*697, May 15, '37; 729, May 22, '37

Burn therapy. CZIRER, L. Orvosi hetil. *81:*591-594, June 5, '37

Detoxin (glutathione preparation) in therapy of toxinemia in children following burns. JELINEK, K. Dermat. Wchnschr. *104:*692-695, June 5, '37

Repair of loss of substance of throat due to extensive burns. PRUDENTE, A. Rev. Assoc. paulista de med. *11:*43-51, July '37

Burn therapy. FRAMPTON, W. H. Indust. Med. *6:*501-503, Sept '37

Burn therapy. McSWAIN, G. H., J. Florida M. A. *24:*165-167, Sept '37

Pathologic physiology and therapy of recent extensive cutaneous burns. DUVAL, P. AND MOURGUE-MOLINES, E., J. de chir. *50:*471-488, Oct '37

Burn therapy. WRIGHT, W. A. Journal-Lancet *57:*449-450, Oct '37

Physiopathology and therapy of recent cutaneous burns. GISMONDI, A. Prat. pediat. *15:*195-197, Nov '37

Burn therapy. LOOS, J. W. Nederl. tijdschr. v. geneesk. *81:*5674-5675, Nov 27, '37

Modern treatment of severe burns. DUFOUR, A. Hopital *25:*643-647, Dec (A) '37

Burn therapy. CHARUGIN, A. I. Novy khir. arkhiv *38:*447-452, '37

Burns and their treatment; 400 cases. GORBAN, I. A. Novy khir. arkhiv *38:*479-482, '37

Surgical methods in burn therapy. ISHCHENKO, I. N. AND LEBEDEVA, M. P. Novy khir. arkhiv *38:*452-456, '37

Burn therapy. NALIVKIN, P. A. Novy khir. arkhiv *38:*436-447, '37

Combined open method of burn therapy. PARAMONOV, V. A. Khirurgiya, no. 10, pp. 37-39, '37

Primary treatment of burns. VASILKOVAN, V. Y. Novy khir. arkhiv *38:*456-464, '37

Primary burn treatment. VASILKOVAN, V. Y. Khirurgiya, no. 10, pp. 29-36, '37

Burn therapy. McGANDY, R. F. Minnesota Med. *21:*17-23, Jan '38

Burns and scalds; therapy. MITCHINER, P. H. Brit. M. J. *1:*27-30, Jan 1, '38

Burns, Treatment—Cont.

Burn therapy. JENNINGS, W. K., S. Clin. North America *18:*145-159, Feb '38

Early and late burn treatment in children. MACCOLLUM, D. W. Am. J. Surg. *39:*275-311, Feb '38

Burn therapy. BERCEANU, D. Rev. de chir., Bucuresti *41:*297-310, March-April '38

Burn therapy, review of literature. GUISO, L. Ann. di med. nav. e colon *44:*149-156, March-April '38

Burn therapy by practitioner. ARRIVAT. Rev. gen. de clin. et de therap. *52:*293-296, April 30, '38

Immediate and subsequent treatment of burns. HEDIN, R. F. Minnesota Med. *21:*229-236, April '38

Newer burn treatment. JOPLIN, R. O. Kentucky M. J. *36:*134-136, April '38

Burn therapy. MOCHALOV, S. P. Vestnik khir. *55:*531-536, May '38

Modern therapy of burns. BELLO, E. Cron. med., Lima *55:*173-177, June '38

Action of infra-red irradiation on humorotissular syndrome in extensive burns. LAMBRET, O.; *et al.* Rev. de chir., Paris *76:*478-502, July '38

First aid in cases of severe burns. LE PICARD. Gaz. med. de France *45:*733-734, July 1-15, '38

Burns. GIOIA, T. Semana med. *2:*543-549, Sept 8, '38

Zeno method of burn therapy by immobilization in plaster cast. AFONSO, J. Arq. brasil. de cir. e ortop. *6:*302-309, Sept-Dec '38

Burn therapy. MCKEE, T. K. Virginia M. Monthly *65:*522-523, Sept '38

Modern burn treatment; evaluation of various methods used in 968 cases in Cook County Hospital. MEYER, K. A. AND WILKEY, J. L. Minnesota Med. *21:*644-649, Sept '38

Burn therapy. GEBHARD, U. E. Indust. Med. *7:*622-623, Oct '38

Treatment of industrial burns, with report of 350 cases. POYNER, H. Am. J. Surg. *42:*744-749, Dec '38

Burns. TRAUB, E. F. Hygeia *16:*1064, Dec '38

Burn therapy. PEDOTTI, F. Arch. ital. di chir. *53:*499-500, '38

Modern concepts and theories of burn therapy. TAUBER, E. B. Arch. de med. int. *4:*210-219, '38

Infra-red light in burns. GAUTIER, J. Arch. med. d'Angers *43:*65-68, April '39 also: Presse med. *47:*139-141, Jan 28, '39

Burns by running water; physiopathologic mechanism. GONALONS, G. P. Prensa med. argent. *26:*1117-1119, June 7, '39

Burns, Treatment—Cont.

Results of therapy of extensive burns in children. GUILLEMINET. Lyon chir. *36:*476-479, July-Aug '39

Modern burn therapy. LÖHR, W. Ztschr. f. arztl. Fortbild. *36:*449-452, Aug 1, '39

Burn therapy. PATTON, C. L. Illinois M. J. *76:*141-144, Aug '39

Burn therapy. COGSWELL, H. D. AND SHIRLEY, C. Am. J. Surg. *45:*539-545, Sept '39

Burn therapy. GOLDHAHN, R. Deutsche med. Wchnschr. *65:*1472-1474, Sept 22, '39

Burn therapy. MARTIN, J. D. JR. Indust. Med. *8:*384-386, Sept '39

Burn therapy. MCCLURE, R. D., J. Connecticut M. Soc. *3:*479-483, Sept '39

Internal treatment of extensive second degree burns. MELCHER, K. Orvosi hetil. *83:*878-879, Sept 9, '39

General accidents and treatment (burns). RUDLER, J. C. Presse med. *47:*1366-1368, Sept 27, '39

Infra-red light in burns. TOPA, P. Rev. de chir., Bucuresti *42:*718-721, Sept-Oct '39

Burn therapy. MORISON, J. H. S., M. Bull. Vet. Admin. *16:*146-148, Oct '39

Surgical and medical therapy of third degree burns. PAUTIENIS, K. Medicina, Kaunas *20:*869-874, Oct-Nov '39

Physiologic and pharmacologic aspects of burn therapy. ALLEN, A. M. Indust. Med. *8:*480-482, Nov '39

Thermic burns and their therapy. BEKERMAN, L. S. Sovet. vrach. zhur. *43:*1163-1174, Dec 30, '39

Systemic disturbances in severe burns and their treatment. ELKINTON, J. R. Bull. Ayer Clin. Lab., Pennsylvania Hosp. *3:*279-292, Dec '39

Modern therapy of burns. FAVREAU, J. C. Union med. du Canada *68:*1329-1330, Dec '39

Present status of treatment of burn patient. OWEN, H. R. AND NORTH, J. P., S. Clin. North America *19:*1489-1511, Dec '39

Burn therapy. PENBERTHY, G. C. AND WELLER, C. N. Am. J. Surg. *46:*468-476, Dec '39

Vitamin B_1 and dextrose in burns. BLOTEVOGEL, H. Arch. f. orthop. u. Unfall-Chir. *40:*280-282, '39

Rational treatment of burns. KALMANOVSKIY, S. M. Khirurgiya, no. 1, pp. 63-72, '39

Burn therapy. VILLANUEVA, A. Arch. am. de med. *15:*43-44, '39

Burn therapy. GOLDHAHN, R. Med. Welt *14:*107-109, Feb 3, '40

Burn therapy. LAFAYETTE PINTO, I. Rev. med. brasil. *8:*211-236, Feb '40

Burns, Treatment—Cont.
Rational treatment of burns. ORSOS, J. I. Gyogyaszat *79:*613, Nov 26; 626, Dec 3, '39 also: Munchen. med. Wchnschr. *87:*297–299, March 15, '40
Therapy of thermal burns. SCHAEFER, A. A. Marquette M. Rev. *4:*101–106, March '40
Burn therapy. HANSEN, T. L. Indust. Med. *9:*251–254, May '40
Burn therapy. McCLURE, R. D. AND LAM, C. R. Am. J. Nursing *40:*498–501, May '40
Burn therapy. POULSEN, V. Ugesk. f. laeger *102:*578–579, May 30, '40
Burn therapy with infra-red light. BART, C.; *et al*. Rev. stiint. med. *29:*490–495, June '40
Early care of severe thermal injuries. McCORKLE, H. California and West. Med. *53:*72–74, Aug '40
Modern therapy of extensive burns. SIMON, H. Therap. d. Gegenw. *81:*295–298, Aug '40
Modern therapy of burns. COURTY, L. Dia med. *12:*829–830, Sept 9, '40
Burn therapy. WALLACE, A. B. Practitioner *145:*180–187, Sept '40
Insulin in burn therapy. FLYNN, S. E., U. S. Nav. M. Bull. *38:*538–540, Oct '40
Burn therapy. WILSON, W. C., J. Roy. Nav. M. Serv. *26:*352–361, Oct '40
Burn therapy. ATKINS, H. J. B. Guy's Hosp. Gaz. *54:*320–324, Nov 2, '40
Emergency care of burns and injuries to skin. GHORMLEY, R. K. Proc. Staff Meet., Mayo Clin. *15:*741, Nov 20, '40
Cortical adrenal extract in severe burns. IVORY, H. S. Mil. Surgeon *87:*423–429, Nov '40
Accidental skin transplantation in Tschmarke brushing therapy of severe burns. MATYAS, M. Zentralbl. f. Chir. *67:*2245–2246, Nov 30, '40
More recent ideas on burn therapy. NOLAND, L. AND WILSON, C. H., J.M.A. Alabama *10:*157–162, Nov '40
Burn therapy. WAKELEY, C. P. G. *et al*. Proc. Roy. Soc. Med. *34:*43–72, Nov '40
Burn therapy. SAEGESSER, M. Chirurg *12:*708–711, Dec 1, '40
Treatment of burns with blood and serum of convalescents. SEGAL, G. I. AND UZDIN, Z. M. Sovet. vrach. zhur. *44:*835–840, Dec '40
Therapy of second degree burns. BABIN, V. V. Sovet. med. (no. 1) *4:*45–46, '40
Burn therapy with high frequency currents; preliminary report. MAZEL, Z. A. Vrach. delo *22:*269–274, '40
Burn therapy at surgical clinic in Munich. PÖHLMANN, G. Arch. f. klin. Chir. *197:*666–722, '40

Burns, Treatment—Cont.
The Treatment of Burns, by A. B. WALLACE. Oxford Press, London, 1941
Severe burn therapy. SHAWVER, J. R., M. Bull. Vet. Admin. *17:*319–321, Jan '41
Burn therapy. HARTTUNG, H. Med. Klin. *37:*129–132, Feb 7, '41
Burn therapy. MOWLEM, R. Proc. Roy. Soc. Med. *34:*221–224, Feb '41
Therapy of extensive burns. PRIMA, C. Zentralbl. f. Chir. *68:*243–245, Feb 8, '41
Persistence of function of skin grafts through long periods of growth. J. B. BROWN AND F. McDOWELL. Surg., Gynec. and Obst., *72:*848, May 1941. Also in J. Iowa State Med. Soc., *31:*457, Oct 1941
Massage in burn therapy. LEROY, R. Presse med. *49:*535–536, May 14–17, '41
Burn therapy. Wisconsin M. J. *40:*391–393, May '41
Burn therapy. HEWITT, W. R., J. Missouri M. A. *38:*191–195, June '41
Burn therapy. RICHARDS, R. T. Rocky Mountain M. J. *38:*521–525, July '41
Burn therapy. OGILVIE, W. H. East Africa M. J. *18:*131–139, Aug '41
Heat tent for patients having severe burns of trunk and extremities. BURNS, M. E. Am. J. Nursing *41:*1057–1058, Sept '41
Burn therapy. GASCO PASCUAL, J. Med. espan. *6:*242–251, Sept '41
Infra-red irradiation as therapy in serious burns of children; cases. PELLINI, M. Pediatria *49:*507–516, Sept '41
Burn therapy. (and physiopathology) GASCO PASCUAL, J. Med. espan. *6:*324–337, Oct '41
Emergency treatment of burns. TENERY, W. C. AND TENERY, J. H. South. Surgeon *10:*759–764, Oct '41
Surgical treatment of burns. SILER, V. E. Cincinnati J. Med. *22:*451–456, Dec '41
Immediate treatment of burns. GLOVER, D. M. Proc. Interst. Postgrad. M. A. North America (1940) pp. 98–102, '41
Treatment of Burns, by HENRY HARKINS. C C Thomas Co., Springfield, Ill., 1942
Burn management in children; analytic study of 250 cases. LAVENDER, H. J. J.A.M.A. *118:*344–349, Jan 31, '42
Burns and their therapy. MARQUARDT, P. Fortschr. d. Therap. *18:*27–34, Jan '42
Burn therapy. WILSON, T. E., M. J. Australia *1:*131–133, Jan 31, '42
Critical survey of burn therapy. ALDRICH, R. H., J. Maine M. A. *33:*21–30, Feb '42
Emergency care of burns and other injuries. BANCROFT, F. W. New York State J. Med. *42:*361–368, Feb 15, '42
Burn therapy. PENBERTHY, G. C. AND

Burns, Treatment–Cont.
WELLER, C. N. Surg., Gynec. and Obst. *74:*428-432, Feb (no. 2A) '42
Practical treatment of extensive burns, with report of case. MORRIS, S. L. JR. South. Surgeon *11:*210-217, March '42
Medical therapy of burns. ROBERT, P. Union med. du Canada *71:*262-268, March '42
Emergency care of burns. KITLOWSKI, E. A. South. Med. and Surg. *104:*189-190, April '42
Burn therapy. KOCH, S. L. Quart. Bull., Northwestern Univ. M. School *16:*191-196, '42 also: Bull. Am. Coll. Surgeons *27:*106-108, April '42
Panel discussions on burn therapy. LAM, C. R. AND HARKINS, H. N. Bull. Am. Coll. Surgeons *27:*109-110, April '42
Burn therapy. ORIENTE, L. AND DE ALMEIDA MOURA, J. C. Arq. de cir. clin e exper. (supp.) *6:*1-56, April-June '42
Reorientation in burn therapy. PICKERILL, H. P. New Zealand M. J. *41:*70-78, April '42
Burn therapy based on etiopathogenesis. STILMAN, I. Semana med. *1:*882-883, April 30, '42
Surgical therapy in burns. LARICHELLIERE, R. Union med. du Canada *71:*491-494, May '42
Burn therapy. MARTIN, J. D. JR. South. M. J. *35:*513-518, May '42
Present-day therapy of burns. SEDAM, M. S. M. Woman's J. *49:*129-133, May '42
Physiologic treatment of burns. WEBB, A. JR. North Carolina M. J. *3:*220-223, May '42
Epithelial healing and the transplantation of skin. J. B. BROWN AND F. MCDOWELL. Ann. Surg., *115:*1166, June 1942. Also in Trans. American Surg. Assn., *60:*1166, June 1942. Also in Digest of Treatment, *6:*481, Jan 1943. Also in Anales de Cirugia (Span.), pp. 272, 1942
The plastic repair of burns with free skin grafts. J. B. BROWN AND F. MCDOWELL. Clinics, *1:*25, June '42
Burn therapy. GRISWOLD, R. A. Kentucky M. J. *40:*203-207, June '42
Local treatment of thermal burns. HARKINS, H. N. Ann. Surg. *115:*1140-1151, June '42
Recent trends in burn therapy. LEE, W. E.; *et al.* Ann. Surg. *115:*1131-1139, June '42
Burn therapy. PENBERTHY, G. C. Indust. Med. *11:*277-280, June '42
Management of burned patient. GEIST, D. C. Am. J. Surg. *57:*20-25, July '42
Burn therapy. HAILES, W. A. Australian and New Zealand J. Surg. *12:*30-33, July '42
Emergency treatment of burns. KIMBROUGH,

Burns, Treatment–Cont.
J. W., U. S. Nav. M. Bull. *40:*723, July '42
Burn therapy. WELBORN, M. B., J. Indiana M. A. *35:*363-364, July '42
Care and treatment of burns. COAKLEY, W. A., M. Times, New York *70:*267-273, Aug '42
Burn therapy. FARMER, W. A. Bull. Vancouver M. A. *18:*333-336, Aug '42
Burn therapy. HOWARD, N. J. Stanford M. Bull. *1:*34-36, Aug '42
Practical outline for burn therapy. MACCOLLUM, D. W. New England J. Med. *227:*331-336, Aug 27, '42
Symposium on industrial surgery; burn therapy. PENBERTHY, G. C.; *et al.* S. Clin. North America *22:*1215-1233, Aug '42
Plan for grave burns. SANTAS, A.; *et al.* Semana med. *2:*424-426, Aug 20, '42
Trends in burn therapy. PENBERTHY, G. C. Surgery *12:*345-348, Sept '42
Burn therapy. WELLS, D. B. Connecticut M. J. *6:*704-708, Sept '42
Modern burn treatment. AINSLIE, J. P., M. J. Australia *2:*339-340, Oct 10, '42
Burn therapy. BROWNLEE, J. J. New Zealand M. J. *41:*192-197, Oct '42
Principles of burn therapy. COPE, O., J. Missouri M. A. *39:*310-314, Oct '42
Burn therapy. GAMARRA ANTEZANA, J. Prensa med., La Paz *2:*221-225, Oct '42
Symposium on emergency treatment of burns. KITLOWSKI, E. A., S. Clin. North America *22:*1501-1519, Oct '42
Burn therapy. PETTAVEL, C. A. Rev. med. de la Suisse Rom. *62:*769-798, Oct 25, '42
Modern burn treatment (with special reference to physiologic changes). RICHARDSON, F. M., M. J. Australia *2:*337-339, Oct 10, '42
Modern burn therapy. SMITH, A. D., M. J. Australia *2:*335-337, Oct 10, '42
Burn therapy. KAISER, G. Zentralbl. f. Gewerbehyg. *19:*201-204, Nov '42
Modern concepts of burn therapy. PEARMAN, R. O. AND THOMPSON, F. G. JR. Missouri M. A. *39:*342-346, Nov '42
Modern treatment of burns. CHAKRAVARTI, D. C. Indian M. Rec. *62:*359-382, Dec '42
Authors' technic of burn therapy, especially in children. GONI MORENO, I. AND GIGLIO, H. An. Cong. brasil. e am. cir. *3:*375-383, '42
Burn therapy. ROCHA AZEVEDO, L. An. Cong. brasil. e am. cir. *3:*384-395, '42
New apparatus (heat tent) in burn therapy. ROGACHEVSKIY, S. L. Klin. med. (no. 7) *20:*91-92, '42
Burn therapy. BALABAN, M. Dia med. *15:*24-25; 33-35, Jan 11, '43

Burns, Treatment—Cont.
Burn therapy. BRINKMAN, H., J. Maine M. A. *34:*1, Jan '43
Burn therapy; Cocoanut Grove disaster in Boston; preliminary account. FAXON, N. W. AND CHURCHILL, E. D. Hospitals *17:*13-18, Jan '43
Burn management. REEVE, B. B. Illinois M. J. *83:*26-31, Jan '43
Burn therapy. KING, M. K. Virginia M. Monthly *70:*106-109, Feb '43
Surgical notes on burn therapy. BRAIMBRIDGE, C. V. East African M. J. *20:*93-95, March '43
Burn therapy. CURRY, D. E., M. Rec. and Ann. *37:*528-531, March '43
Rehabilitation of burns. WAKELEY, C. P. G. M. Press *209:*173-175, March 17, '43
Burn therapy. BREIDENBACH, L., S. Clin. North America *23:*575-588, April '43
Problem of burn therapy. DOSTROVSKY, A. AND SAGHER, F. Harefuah *24:*114, April 1, '43
Burn therapy. ELLIS RIBEIRO, F. Rev. med.-cir. do Brasil *51:*255-286, April-June '43
Treatment of phosphorus burns (with note on acute phosphorus poisoning). RABINOWITCH, I. M. Canad. M. A. J. *48:*291-296, April '43
Reduced temperature in burn therapy. ALLEN, F. M.; *et al.* New York State J. Med. *43:*951-952, May 15, '43
Penicillin and propamidine; elimination of hemolytic streptococci and staphylococci (in burns). CLARK, A. M. *et al.* Lancet *1:*605-609, May 15, '43
Practical outline for burn therapy. MACCOLLUM, D. W. Am. J. Orthodontics (Oral Surg. Sect.) *29:*247-254, May '43
Burn therapy. PENBERTHY, G. C.; *et al.* Dia med. *15:*518-522, May 24, '43
Modern burn therapy. BELCHOR, G. Rev. san. mil., Buenos Aires *42:*420-424, June '43 also: Prensa med. argent. *30:*1093-1096, June 16, '43
Symposium on management of Cocoanut Grove burns at Massachusetts General Hospital; procedures in rehabilitation of severely burned. CANNON, B. Ann. Surg. *117:*903-910, June '43
Burn therapy. CASTELLANOS FONSECA, E. Rev. med.-quir. de Oriente *4:*87-95, June '43
Symposium on management of Cocoanut Grove burns at Massachusetts General Hospital; metabolic observations. COPE, O.; *et al.* Ann. Surg. *117:*937-958, June '43
Surgical operations (on burns) with the Navy

Burns, Treatment—Cont.
Medical Corps in South Pacific. JOHNSTON, W. M. Am. J. Surg. *60:*313-318, June '43
Symposium on management of Cocoanut Grove burns at Massachusetts General Hospital; problems of infection and chemotherapy (especially with penicillin and sulfadiazide sulfonamide). LYONS, C. Ann. Surg. *117:*894-902, June '43
Modern burn treatment; review. SMYTH, C. M. JR. Clinics *2:*201-217, June '43
Symposium on management of Cocoanut Grove burns at Massachusetts General Hospital; note on physical therapy (hands). WATKINS, A. L. Ann. Surg. *117:*911-914, June '43
Symposium on management of Cocoanut Grove burns at Massachusetts General Hospital. VARIOUS AUTHORS. Ann. Surg. *117:*801-975, June '43
Program for emergency treatment of extensive burns. BERKOW, S. G., U. S. Nav. Bull. *41:*946-952, July '43
Burns. ECKHOFF, N. L. Guy's Hosp. Gaz. *57:*156-162, July 24, '43
Summary of present burn treatment. HAYDEN, R. New York State J. Med. *43:*1213-1219, July 1, '43
Treatment of severely burned patient, with special reference to controlled protein therapy. MAHONEY, E. B. AND HOWLAND, J. W. New York State J. Med. *43:*1307-1315, July 15, '43
Present status of burn therapy. MARTINEZ CORDOBA, F.; *et al.* Semana med. *2:*488-493, Aug 26, '43
Tissue reactions to medications used in local treatment of burns. MAUN, M. E.; *et al.* Surgery *14:*229-238, Aug '43
Prevention of infection in contaminated accidental wounds, compound fractures and burns (report on 1500 cases, especially evaluation of sulfonamides). MELENEY, F. L. Ann. Surg. *118:*171-186, Aug '43
Modern burn treatment. SCHAEFER, A. A. Marquette M. Rev. *8:*93-97, Aug '43
Problems of protein nutrition in burn patients. TAYLOR, F. H. L. *et al.* Ann. Surg. *118:*215-224, Aug '43
Burn therapy founded on cellular stimulation. WALSH, T. F. P. AND NUTINI, L. G. South. Med. and Surg. *105:*341-350, Aug '43
Prevention of infection in burns. BELCHOR, G. Semana med. *2:*714-717, Sept 23, '43
Burn therapy. HARKINS, H. N. Illinois M. J. *84:*103-106, Aug '43 (abstract) also: S. Clin. North America *23:*1233-1258, Oct '43

Burns, Treatment—Cont.
Prevention of infection in burns. BELCHOR, G. Semana med. *2:*714-717, Sept 23, '43
Biologic (plasma) and chemical therapy of burns. SANTAS, A. A. Rev. Asoc. med. argent. *57:*850-854, Oct 30, '43 also: Bol. d. Inst. clin. quir. *19:*690-697, Dec '43
Burn therapy. SCHAEFER, A. A. Wisconsin M. J. *42:*1052-1054, Oct '43
Present day treatment of burns. BULMER, J. W. New York State J. Med. *43:*2192-2195, Nov 15, '43
Medical progress; treatment of thermal burns; general outline. NATIONAL RESEARCH COUNCIL. New England J. Med. *229:*817-823, Nov 25, '43
Grave burns; physiopathology and therapy. TEJERINA FOTHERINGHAM, W. Dia med. *15:*1255-1259, Nov 15, '43
Penicillin; value for infected burns. BODENHAM, D. C. Lancet *2:*725-728, Dec 11, '43
Early treatment of thermal burns. CARLISLE, J. M., J. M. Soc. New Jersey *40:*459-461, Dec '43
Treatment of third degree burns. KLUMPP, J. S. West Virginia M. J. *39:*406-414, Dec '43
Medical progress; treatment of thermal burns; recent developments. LUND, C. C. New England J. Med. *229:*868-873, Dec 2, '43
Severe burns treated by blood transfusion, adrenal cortical hormone and ascorbic acid. OVNBOL, A. Ugesk. f. laeger *105:*1331, Dec 30, '43
Burns. REGGI, J. P. Dia med. *15:*1424-1427, Dec 20, '43
Newer conceptions in burn therapy. BULLOWA, J. G. M. AND FOX, C. L. JR. Hebrew M. J. *1:*192, '43
Burn therapy. HARKINS, H. N. Proc. Interst. Postgrad. M. A. North America (1942) pp. 245-246, '43
Physiologic aspects of burn therapy. HARKINS, H. N. Am. Acad. Orthop. Surgeons, Lect., pp. 186-188, '43
Treatment of burns. KRYAZHEVA, V. I. Sovet. med. (nos. 7-8) *7:*24-25, '43
Burn therapy with report of cases. RIVEROS, M. An. Fac. de cien. med., Asuncion (no. 18) *11:*7-68, '43
Burn therapy. SEABRA, D. DOS S. Bahia med. *14:*45-53, '43
Physiopathology of extensive burns and their therapy in light of endocrinology. DE MESQUITA SAMPAIO, J. A. AND DA ROCHA AZEVEDO, L. G. Sao Paulo med. *1:*25-55, Jan '44
General care and treatment of burns. HOGG, B. M. Air Surgeon's Bull. (no. 1) *1:*19-21, Jan '44
Burn therapy. MAY, H. Am. J. Surg. *63:*34-46, Jan '44
Burn therapy. MOUROT, A. J. Virginia M. Monthly *71:*25-28, Jan '44
Burn therapy in infants. DA ROCHA AZEVEDO, L. G. Rev. paulista de med. *24:*87-91, Feb '44
Burn therapy in general practice. MUKERJI, A., J. Indian M. A. *13:*146-148, Feb '44
Management of heat burns. SILER, V. E. J.A.M.A. *124:*486-487, Feb 19, '44
Early treatment of burns. FARMER, A. W. Surgery *15:*144-152, Jan '44 also: Am. J. Orthodontics (Oral Surg. Sect.) *30:*146-153, March '44
Principles of burn therapy. FRANKLIN, R. H. Practitioner *152:*167-173, March '44
Treatment of burns. FUHS, H. Wien. klin. Wchnschr. *57:*120, March 10, '44
Burn after-treatment. HULLSTRUNG, H. Med. Klin. *40:*164, March 17, '44
Management of severe burns. KING, W. E. West Virginia M. J. *40:*83-85, March '44
Surgical repair of burns. F. MCDOWELL AND J. B. BROWN. Wisconsin Med. J., *43:*310, March '44
Trophoanesthetic treatment of burns; preliminary report. RIVAS DIEZ, B. AND DELRIO, J. M. A. Dia med. *16:*209, March 6, '44
Treatment of burns. WOLFRAM, S. Wien. klin. Wchnschr. *57:*142, March 24, '44
Trial of method of management of severe burns, with reports of cases and commentary. BURT, L. I., M. J. Australia *1:*342-343, April 15, '44
First aid treatment of burns and scalds. COLEBROOK, L.; *et al.* Brit. J. Indust. Med. *1:*99-105, April '44
Carbon tetrachloride; new and important applications in medical therapy of burns. FASTING, G. F. New Orleans M. and S. J. *96:*439-445, April '44
Perspective review of burn therapy. KUMMER, W. M. AND LEGG, G. E. Hahneman. Monthly *79:*175, April; 221, May '44
Burns and their therapy. NEUMANN, H. Med. Klin. *40:*245, April 28, '44
New methods of burn therapy. PORRITT, A. E. Mil. Surgeon *94:*227-228, April '44
Brief survey of burn therapy, with account of new method adopted by author. RAJASINGHAM, A. S., J. Ceylon Br., Brit. M. A. *40:*136-146, April '44
Burn management. WALTON, F. E. Surgery *15:*547-552, April '44

Burns, Treatment—Cont.
Present treatment of burns. HAYDEN, R. J. Internat. Coll. Surgeons *7:*179-190, May-June '44
Burn therapy critique. LIMOGES, J. E. Ann. med.-chir. de l'Hop. Sainte-Justine, Montreal *4:*69-72, May '44
Burns and their treatment. VANCE, C. L., U. S. Nav. M. Bull. *42:*1129-1133, May '44
General care of burn patient. LAM, C. R. J.A.M.A. *125:*543-546, June 24, '44
Burn therapy. LAROCHELLE, J. L. Laval med. *9:*413-419, June '44
Burn therapy in industry. MORANI, A. D. Am. J. Surg. *64:*361-372, June '44
Evolution of burn treatment. NOVELLA MONLEON, F. Med. clin., Barcelona *2:*505-509, June '44
Burn therapy. CAULFIELD, P. A., M. Ann. District of Columbia *13:*251, July '44
Chemical aspects of burn therapy. COPE, O. J.A.M.A. *125:*731, July 8, '44
Burn therapy. PAGE. M. Bull. Bombay *12:*261-264, July 8, '44
Grave burns, with special reference to hypoproteinemia. AGUILAR, H. D. Prensa med. argent. *31:*1446-1449, Aug 2, '44
Burn therapy. ALVES, E. Hora med., Rio de Janeiro *2:*45-51, Aug '44
Symptomatology and general therapy of extensive burns. MEDINA AGUILAR, R. Medicina, Mexico *24:*323-340, Aug 25, '44
Modern concepts of burn therapy. BAHR, S. J. Arch. Soc. cirujanos hosp. *14:*467-475, Sept '44
New acquisitions in burn therapy. DA ROCHA AZEVEDO, L. G. Rev. paulista de med. *25:*227-232, Oct '44
Physiologic management of burns. WILLIAMS, V. T., J. Missouri M. A. *41:*205-206, Oct '44
Modern methods of burn therapy. PORRIT, A. E. AND BARBIERI, P. Rev. san. mil., Buenos Aires *43:*1366-1368, Oct '44
Penicillin and deep burns. COPE, O. Bull. New England M. Center *6:*255, Dec '44
Rational treatment of burns. SEWELL, S. A. M. J. Australia *2:*590-592, Dec 2, '44
Cheap method of burn therapy. ALTUKHOV, P. P. Sovet. med. (no. 6) *8:*27-28, '44
Burn therapy. GURD, F. B. Proc. Interst. Postgrad. M. A. North America (1943) pp. 141-146, '44
Symposium on industrial medicine in wartime—or widening field of industrial medicine; treatment of burns. ROONEY, J. C. California and West. Med. *62:*23-24, Jan '45

Burns, Treatment—Cont.
Burn therapy. CONKLIN, F. L. Mil. Surgeon *96:*139-142, Feb '45
Refrigeration in burns. CROSSMAN, L. W. AND SAFFORD, F. K. JR. Mod. Hosp. *64:*90, Feb '45
Burn therapy. HARKINS, H. N., J. South Carolina M. A. *41:*27-30, Feb '45
Practical efficacious procedure in burns. BORRAS, J. A. Med. clin., Barcelona *4:*235-239, March '45
Modern aspects of burn therapy. CARBONELL ANTOLI, C. Rev. espan. cir., traumatol. y ortop. *2:*187-202, March '45
Burn therapy. FERGUSON, L. K. Bull. New York Acad. Med. *21:*127-144, March '45
Recent advances in burn therapy. LEE, W. E.; *et al.* Pennsylvania M. J. *48:*563-565, March '45
Treatment of extensive burns, with report of case. CRADDOCK, F. H. JR. J.M.A. Alabama *14:*236-239, April '45
Newer aspects of burn therapy. RHODES, J. E. Clinics *3:*1618-1622, April '45
General care of burn patient. HARKINS, H. N. Nebraska M. J. *30:*175-176, May '45
Nutrition of patients with thermal burns. LEVENSON, S. M.; *et al.* Surg., Gynec. and Obst. *80:*449-469, May '45
Treatment of burns. BHADRA, A. C. Indian M. J. *39:*174-175, June '45
Fluid and nutritional therapy in burns. HARKINS, H. N. *et al.* J.A.M.A. *128:*475-479, June 16, '45
Therapy of thermal burns. RENNIE, S. W. Delaware State M. J. *17:*111-113, June '45
Physiologic analysis of nature and treatment of burns. GLENN, W. W. L. Prensa med. argent. *32:*1298-1300, July 6, '45
Recent advances in burn therapy. LAM, C. R. Indust. Med. *14:*610, July '45
Adequate nutrition gains emphasis as vital factor in burn surgery. MACOMBER, M. H. Hospitals (no. 7) *19:*73-74, July '45
Recent advances in burn therapy. MERRY, C. R., J. Nat. M. A. *37:*117-120, July '45
Practical treatment of burns. GUERIN, J. Presse med. *53:*424, Aug 4, '45
Present status of burn treatment; review of literature. IMPERATI, L. Gior. ital. chir. (no. 2) *1:*51-53, Aug '45
Plea for simplicity in burn treatment. FLEMMING, C. W. Brit. M. J. *2:*314-316, Sept 8, '45
Treatment of burns. MISRA, B. Antiseptic *42:*488-491, Sept '45
Practical aspects of burn therapy. SIEGEL, S. A.; *et al.* Surgery *18:*298-305, Sept '45

Burns, Treatment–Cont.
Recent progress in burn treatment. GOSSET, J. Presse med. *53:*539, Oct 6, '45
Treatment of severely burned patient; outline of present policies. LANGE, H. J. AND CAMPBELL, K. N. Univ. Hosp. Bull., Ann Arbor *11:*90-96, Nov '45
Severe burns; case. HOLMES, H. B., M. J. Australia *2:*465-466, Dec 22, '45
Practical method of burn treatment; preliminary report. RIBEIRO, E. B. Bol. San. Sao Lucas *7:*93-95, Dec '45
Modern therapy of burns. WALLENTIN Y SPRINGER, R. Rev. med. y cien. afines. Mexico *4:*409-444, Jan '46
Burns and treatment of third degree. SARKAR, K. D. Antiseptic *43:*126-130, Feb '46
Report of 155 cases of burn treatment. BORNEMEIER, W. C. AND PARSONS, L. Surg., Gynec. and Obst. *82:*311-318, Mar '46
Modern treatment of burns. VALONE, J. A. Mississippi Doctor *23:*610-614, Apr '46
Present status of burn therapy in United States. MONASTERIO ODENA, R. Dia med. (supp) *3:*1-12, April 15, '46
Modern therapy of burns; review of literature. PIGNATELLI, G. Progr. med. Napoli *2:*307-310, May 15, '46
Modern methods of burn therapy. OSBORNE, R. P., J. Roy. Inst. Pub. Health and Hyg. *9:*169-177, June '46
Burn physiology applied to modern surgery; symposium; fluid therapy. GUISS, J. M. Northwest Med. *45:*488-491, July '46
Therapy outline for severe burns. LEVENSON, S. M.; *et al.*New England J. Med. *235:*76-79, July 18, '46
Severe burns; clinical findings with simplified plan of early treatment. ELMAN, R.; *et al.* Surg., Gynec. and Obst. *83:*187-199, Aug '46

Burns, War
War lesions due to toxic gases and incendiary projectiles. (burns). TROTOT, R. Tunisie med. *29:*293-304, July-Aug '35
Burn therapy in army medical department. CLAVELIN, C. AND CARILLON, R. J. Rev. serv. de san. mil. *106:*571-596, April '37
Burns due to explosion. ANDERSON, C. B. C. AND DOUGLAS, J. P., J. Roy. Army M. Corps *70:*168-177, March '38
Accidents due to heat; prevention and therapy in army. BOIDE, AND RENAUD, MME. A. Rev. med. franc. *19:*387-400, May '38
Incendiary air raids; incendiary bombs, extinction of fires and treatment of burns. SIMON, L. Strasbourg med. *98:*175-179, May 15, '38

Burns, War–Cont.
Death resulting from burns on military field. LEYVA PEREIRA, L. Rev. Fac. de med., Bogota *7:*149-154, Oct '38
Burn therapy under war conditions. MITCHINER, P. H., M. Press *202:*26-31, July 12, '39
First aid in burns, with special consideration of conditions prevailing in air raids. FICK. Ztschr. f. arztl. Fortbild. *36:*584-592, Oct 1, '39
Burn therapy in sanitary services of army. MASINI, P. Hopital *27:*517, Nov.; 544, Dec '39
First aid for thermal war injuries. HOCHE, O. Med. Klin. *35:*1532, Dec 1; 1563, Dec 8, '39; *36:*39, Jan 12; 67, Jan 19; 94, Jan 26; 154, Feb 9; 239, March 1; 265, March 8; 291, March 15, '40
Skin injuries from incendiary bombs and war chemicals. FUHS, H. Wien. klin. Wchnschr. *53:*40-44, Jan 12, '40
War burns. FLÖRCKEN, H. Chirurg *12:*89-92, Feb 15, '40
Treatment of air raid burn casualties at base hospital; experiences in Chinese war. REIMERS, C. Chirurg *12:*145-152, March 15, '40
Local first aid treatment of burns during naval combat. GUISO, L. Ann. di med. nav. e colon *46:*151-154, March-April '40
Experience in treatment of war burns. COHEN, S. M. Brit. M. J. *2:*251-254, Aug 24, '40
Combination of burns and wounds; treatment. FLEMMING, C. Proc. Roy. Soc. Med. *34:*53, Nov '40
War burns. KENDALL, A. W., M. Press *205:*42-45, Jan 15, '41
War burns. WAKELEY, C. P. G., J. Roy. Nav. M. Serv. *27:*20-34, Jan '41 also: Surgery *10:*207-232, Aug '41
War burns and their treatment. WAKELEY, C. P. G. Practitioner *146:*27-37, Jan '41
First aid in burns. WAKELEY, C. P. G., M. Press *205:*93-96, Jan 29, '41
Burn therapy in peacetime and war. HENSCHEN, C. Helvet. med. acta *8:*77-148, April '41
Treatment of 100 war wounds and burns. ROSS, J. A. AND HULBERT, K. F. Brit. M. J. *1:*618-621, April 26, '41
Suggestions for first aid of burns at front. WESTERMANN, H. H. Deut. Militararzt *6:*209-211, April '41
Injuries due to burns from point of view of naval surgery. KOCH, F. Svenska lak.-tidning. *38:*1351-1356, June 13, '41
Burn therapy in wartime. DENNISON, W. M. AND DIVINE, D., J. Roy. Army M. Corps *77:*14-18, July '41

Burns, War—Cont.
Burn therapy in wartime. OLDFIELD, M. C., J. Roy. Army M. Corps. *77:*1-13, July '41
First aid treatment in burns. WALLACE, A. B. Practitioner *147:*513-517, Aug '41
First aid in burns. MCINDOE, A. H. Lancet *2:*377-378, Sept 27, '41
Management of war burns. HALFORD, F. J. Hawaii M. J. *1:*191-192, Jan '42
War burns; survey of treatment and results in 100 cases. MAITLAND, A. I. L., J. Roy. Nav. M. Serv. *28:*3-17, Jan '42
Treatment of burns. E. M. S. Memorandum. M. J. Australia *1:*356, March 21, '42
Care of military and civilian injuries (burns). HICKEY, M. J. Am. J. Orthodontics (Oral Surg. Sect.) *28:*177-182, April '42
Wartime burns. PASSALACQUA, L. A. Bol. Asoc. med. de Puerto Rico *34:*140-146, April '42
Burn casualties at Pearl Harbor. RAVDIN, I. S. AND LONG, P. H., U. S. Nav. M. Bull. *40:*353-358, April '42
Late end-results of war burns. WAKELEY, C. P. G. Lancet *1:*410-412, April 4, '42
Burn therapy in wartime. (Ernest Edward Irons lecture) HARKINS, H. N., J.A.M.A. *119:*385-390, May 30, '42
War surgery; management of burns. ATKINS, H. J. B., Brit. M. J. *1:*704, June 6, '42: 729, June 13, '42
Symposium on medical aspects of chemical warfare; treatment of burns (including thermal and electric). HERRLIN, J. O. JR. AND GLASSER, S. T. Bull. New York M. Coll., Flower and Fifth Ave. Hosps. *5:*79-84, June-Oct '42
War burns. LINDSAY, H. C. L. Urol. and Cutan. Rev. *46:*386-390, June '42
War Burns. BOVE, C. New York State J. Med. *42:*1366-1370, July 15, '42
"Solace" (hospital ship) in action (burns). ECKERT, G. A. AND MADER, J. W., U. S. Nav. M. Bull. *40:*552-557, July '42
Newer concepts, with suggestions for management of wartime thermal injuries. FOX, T. A., U. S. Nav. M. Bull. *40:*557-570, July '42
Burns en masse (at Pearl Harbor). SAXL, N. T., U. S. Nav. M. Bull. *40:*570-576, July '42
Military burns; analysis of 308 cases. KNOEPP, L. F. Am. J. Surg. *57:*226-230, Aug '42
War burns. PALMER, E. P. AND PALMER, E. P. JR. Southwestern Med. *26:*251-255, Aug '42
Burn therapy. GAY, E. C. Mil. Surgeon *91:*298-305, Sept '42

Burns, War—Cont.
Plan for larger numbers of burns. SPANGLER, P. C. Hawaii M. J. *2:*40-41, Sept-Oct '42
Early management of burn cases in mass quantity. CAVENY, E. L., U. S. Nav. M. Bull. *40:*824-828, Oct '42
War burns; varieties according to method of production. DE ARAGON, E. R. Rev. med.-social san. y benef. mumic. *2:*309-314, Oct-Dec '42
War burns and their treatment. RAU, U. M. Antiseptic *39:*655-665, Oct '42
Burns, various types; treatment and prognosis from military as well as civilian viewpoint. WIDMEYER, R. S., J. Florida M. A. *29:*165-168, Oct '42
Human albumin in military medicine; clinical evaluation (burns). WOODRUFF, L. M. AND GIBSON, S. T., U. S. Nav. M. Bull. *40:*791-796, Oct '42
Burn therapy for medical defense unit, with reference to early and late therapy. MARCKS, K. M. Am. J. Surg. *58:*174-180, Nov '42
War burns. GONCALVES BOGADO, L. Rev. med.-cir. do Brasil *50:*1087-1098, Dec '42
Gunpowder burns in munitions factory. GRONEMANN. Zentralbl. f. Gewerbehyg. *19:* 217, Dec '42
Newer concepts, with suggestions for management of wartime thermal injuries. FOX, T. A., J. Lab. and Clin. Med. *28:*474-484, Jan '43
Preparation of jelly in the field for burn therapy. KEENAN, H. J. Hosp. Corps. Quart. *16:*49-50, Jan '43
Burn therapy in war. YEMM, W. A. Physiotherapy Rev. *23:*13-16, Jan-Feb '43
Forum on therapy of wartime injuries (burns). HOUCK, J. S. New York State J. Med. *43:*226-228, Feb 1, '43
Clinical observations on patients (sailors) with scalding burns. MIYATA, S. AND KAYASHIMA, K. Far East. Sc. Bull. *3:*12, March '43 (abstract)
Most recent advances in burn therapy; question of therapy used in present war. PETIT ODDO. Publ. med., Sao Paulo *14:*43-56, March-April '43
Burn therapy; activities of Naval Hospital at Pearl Harbor following Japanese air raid of December 7, 1941; comments on care of battle casualties. HAYDEN, R. Am. J. Surg. *60:*161-181, May '43
Burn therapy at Tobruk. LOGIE, N. J. Lancet *1:*609-611, May 15, '43
Burn cases off the U.S.S. Wasp. JACOBS, R. G., J. Oklahoma M. A. *36:*235-236, June '43

Burns, War—Cont.
Local therapy of war burns. DESJARDINS, E. Union med. du Canada *72:*790-792, July '43
Experiences with burns at Naval Hospital, Pearl Harbor during and after Japanese air raid of December 7, 1941. HAYDEN, R. J. Internat. Coll. Surgeons *6:*259-268, July-Aug '43
Burn therapy with human serum albumin concentrated; clinical indications and dosage. KENDRICK, D. B. JR.; *et al.* Army M. Bull. (no. 68) pp. 107-112, July '43
Burn therapy in warfare. MACEY, H. B. Proc. Staff Meet., Mayo Clin. *18:*241-246, July 28, '43
Burn therapy in the field. STEIN, J. J. Hosp. Corps Quart. *16:*113-115, July '43
Late treatment of flash burns. STRANGE, W. W. AND MOUROT, A. J., U. S. Nav. M. Bull. *41:*953-960, July '43
War burns and their therapy. COUTINHO, A. Rev. med. de Pernambuco *13:*175-190, Aug '43
War burns; traumatologic study on action of flame throwers and explosives. PARANAGUA, C. Imprensa med., Rio de Janeiro *19:*57-72, Aug '43
Ophthalmic injuries (including burns) of war. MATTHEWS, J. L. War Med. *4:*247-261, Sept '43
Burns treated as war wounds. SHEEHAN, J. E. Am. J. Surg. *61:*331-338, Sept '43
Discussion of burns based on experience with 360 cases seen on board a U. S. hospital ship. KERN, R. A.; *et al.* U. S. Nav. M. Bull. *41:*1654-1678, Nov '43
Therapy of war burns. MARQUES PORTO, E. Rev. med.-cir. do Brasil *51:*585-608, Nov '43
Burn therapy at an Army Air Forces advanced flying school. WEINSHEL, L. R. Mil. Surgeon *93:*389-399, Nov '43
Therapy of war burns. HAMILTON, J. E. AND BARNETT, L. A., S. Clin. North America *23:*1575-1588, Dec '43
Symposium on war surgery; rehabilitation of burned hand. MEHERIN, J. M. AND GREELEY, P. W., S. Clin. North America *23:*1651-1665, Dec '43
Discussion based on experience with 360 burn cases seen on board a U. S. hospital ship. KERN, R. A. *et al.* U. S. Nav. M. Bull. *42:*59-81, Jan '44
Burns incident to war (treatment). BERKOW, S. G. Clinics *2:*1265-1294, Feb '44
Therapy of war burns. RANKIN, F. W. *et al.* Clinics *2:*1194-1218, Feb '44

Burns, War—Cont.
Treatment of burns incident to war; Wellcome prize essay. RODDIS, L. H. Mil. Surgeon *94:*65-75, Feb '44
Burn therapy at sea. CZWALINSKI, P. F., U. S. Nav. M. Bull. *42:*838-840, April '44
Burn therapy experience from South Pacific area. YANDELL, H. R., U. S. Nav. M. Bull. *42:*829-837, April '44
Burn therapy in forward areas. JOHNSTON, C. C. Bull. U. S. Army M. Dept. (no. 75) pp. 109-113, May '44
Local treatment of war burns. STOCKTON, A. B. Stanford M. Bull. *2:*71-73, May '44
Burn therapy in warfare. LOGIE, N. J. Lancet *2:*138-140, July 29, '44
How they treat burn cases aboard U.S.S. Solace. SHAW, C. E. W. Mod. Hosp. *63:*72-75, Nov '44
Review of burn cases treated in overseas general hospital. RAWLES, B. W. JR. AND MASSIE, J. R. JR. Virginia M. Monthly *71:*605-609, Dec '44
Therapy at the front for burns. SHEYNKMAN, S. S. Khirurgiya, no. 12, pp. 41-46, '44
Burn therapy among Emergency Medical Service hospital in-patients. BROOKE, E. M. Brit. M. J. *1:*259-260, Feb 24, '45
Plastic surgery in burns among naval personnel; current experiences. GREELEY, P. W. Am. J. Surg. *67:*401-411, Feb '45
Organization for treatment of burns; important aspect of preparedness. ROSENQVIST, H. Nord. med. *25:*419-423, March 9, '45
Care of burn casualty. WANAMAKER, F. H. U. S. Nav. M. Bull. *44:*1239-1244, June '45
Eighty-three percent body surface burn with recovery. JOHNSON, J. R., U. S. Nav. M. Bull. *45:*163-165, July '45
Dermoepidermal grafts in early treatment of severe war burns. HUBER, J. P. Semaine d. hop. Paris *21:*741-747, July 21, '45 also: Bull. internat. serv. san. *18:*197-209, Aug '45
Flashburn protection. COREY, E. L. Hosp. Corps Quart. (no. 10) *18:*27-30, Oct '45
Late end-results of war burns. WAKELEY, C. P. G.; *et al.* Tr. M. Soc. London (1940-1943) *63:*129-142, '45
Major burns in naval warfare. MCLAUGHLIN, C. W. JR. Nebraska M. J. *31:*11-19, Jan '46
Short review of treatment of service burns during the war. HILL. M. Bull. Bombay *14:*13-15, Jan 28, '46
Therapy of burns in last war. BERMUDEZ, E. Gac. med. Lima *2:*275-281, March '46
Modern therapy of burns in war. DRIESSEN, H. E. Nederl. tijdschr. v. geneesk. *90:*497-500, May 18, '46

BURNS, J. E.: New operation for exstrophy of bladder; preliminary report. J.A.M.A. *82:*1587-1590, May 17, '24
BURNS, M. E.: Heat tent for patients having severe burns of trunk and extremities. Am. J. Nursing *41:*1057-1058, Sept '41
BURNS, S. R. (see MCCARTHY, W. D.) Oct '76
BURROWS, H.: Restoration of sunken nose. Brit. M. J. *2:*688-689, Oct 14, '22 (illus.)
BURSTEIN, T.: Plastic repair of leg ulcers (skin grafting). M. Rec. *150:*207-308, Nov 1, '39
BURSUK, G. G.: Modification of operation for trachomatous entropion (trichiasis) by means of free transplant. Sovet. vestnik oftal. *2:*251-252, '33
BURSUK, G. G.: Canthoplasty. Vestnik oftal. *16:*243-245, '40
BURSUK, G. G. AND SHULTS, V. A.: Rational therapy of chemical burns to eyes. Vestnik oftal. *17:*55-56, '40
BURT, L. I.: Trial of method of management of severe burns, with reports of cases and commentary. M. J. Australia *1:*342-343, April 15, '44
BURT, L. I.: Treatment of suppurative tenosynovitis in fingers. M. J. Australia *1:*399, Mar 23, '46
BURTON, J. F.: Burn therapy to prevent contractures. J. Oklahoma M. A. *26:*36-38, Feb '33
BURTON, J. F.: Skin grafts. J. Oklahoma M. A. *27:*363-367, Oct '34
BURTON, J. F.: Role of plastic surgery in treatment of malignancies about face. South. M. J. *32:*67-68, Jan '39
BURTON, J. F.: Brachiothoracic adhesions. Surg., Gynec. and Obst. *70:*938-944, May '40
BURTON, J. F.: Burn therapy. J. Oklahoma M. A. *36:*4-5, Jan '43
BURTY: Autoplasty by flap; cases. Bull. et mem. Soc. de chir. de Paris *20:*848-850, '28
BURTY: Result of graft of extensor tendon of left index finger in repair of flexor tendon of same finger. Bull. et mem. Soc. d. chirurgiens de Paris *26:*659-660, Dec 7, '34
BUSACCA, A.: Transplantation of preserved tendons; comment on Weidenreich's article. Virchows Arch. f. path. Anat. *258:*238-245, '25
BUSACCA, A.: Temporary and permanent eyelid ptosis in trachoma. Rev. internat. du trachome *11:*204-213, Oct '34
BUSACCA, A.: Removal of tarsal section of orbicular muscle of upper eyelid in therapy of entropion and trichiasis and for prevention of recurrence of trachomatous processes. Ztschr. f. Augenh. *88:*100-106, Jan '36
BUSACCA, A.: Method for correction of entropion in trachomatous patients, with particular attention to esthetic results. Arch. Ophth. *16:*822-828, Nov '36
BUSACCA, A.: Advantages of use of coagulants, especially in plastic operations on eyes. Arch. Ophth. *20:*406-409, Sept '38
BUSH, L. F. (see FERGUSON, L. K. *et al*) Jan '41
BUSHMICH, D. G. (see GOLDFEDER, A. E.) 1937
BUSTAMANTE, S.: Therapy of microstomia; case. Ann. Casa de Salud Valdecilla *4:*281-282, '33
BUSULENGA, A.: Rare variety of congenital syndactylia. Cluj. med. *8:*219-222, June '27
BUSSE GRAWITZ, P.: Method of fractional implantation and other systematic implantation experiments. Ztschr. d. d. ges. exper. Med. *111:*1-9, '42 (Reply to Hora)
BUSSE-GRAWITZ, P.: Reactions in tissues of mummies following implantation. Arch. f. exper. Zellforsch. *24:*320-358, '42

Busse-Grawitz Experiments

Question of "cellular tissue decomposition" or wandering of leukocytes; testing of Busse-Grawitz experiments. HEINEMANN, K. Beitr. z. path. Anat. u. z. allg. Path. *106:*525-534, '42

BÜSSEMAKER, J.: Shock and circulatory collapse. Jahresk. f. arztl. Fortbild. *30:*20-27, Feb '39
BUSSOLA, E.: Acrocephalosyndactylia with postneurotic atrophy of optic nerves. Riv. otoneuro-oft. *5:*503-520, Nov-Dec '28
BUTCHER, E. O.: Fate and activity of autografts and homografts in white rats. Arch. Dermat. and Syph. *36:*53-56, July '37
BUTCHER, E. O.: Hair growth in skin transplanted under skin and into peritoneal cavity in rat. Anat. Rec. *96:*101-109, Oct '46
BUTLER, C.: Treatment of cancer and precancer of lip; clinical and therapeutic study of 191 cases. An. de Fac. de med., Montevideo *10:*985-998, Dec '25 abstr: J.A.M.A. *87:*447, Aug 7, '26
BUTLER, E.: Indications for infusion of blood substitutes and transfusion of blood in cases of traumatic hemorrhage and shock. California State J. Med. *19:*145, April '21
BUTLER, E.: Facial injuries. Am. J. Surg. *8:*336-337, Feb '30
BUTLER, E.: Photographic records in plastic surgery, with special reference to textual aspects of facial portrayal. M. Press *209:*109-112, Feb 17, '43
BUTLER, E. C. B.; PERRY, K. M. A. AND WILLIAMS, J. R. F.: Methyl bromide burns. Brit. J. Indust. Med. *2:*30-31, Jan '45

BUTLER, J. (see BERMAN, J. K. *et al*) April '44
BUTLER, R. D. W.: Lexer operation in eyelid ptosis. Tr. Ophth. Soc. U. Kingdom (pt. 2) *59:*579–585, '39
BUTLER, T. H.: Young's operation for eyelid ptosis; case. Tr. Ophth. Soc. U. Kingdom *47:*387, '27
BUTOIANU, S. AND STOIAN, C.: Maxillofacial surgery. Rev. san. mil., Bucuresti *28:*344–355, Sept '29
BUTTERWORTH, T. AND KLAUDER, J. V.: Malignant melanomas arising in moles; report of 50 cases. J.A.M.A. *102:*739–745, March 10, '34
BÜTTNER, G.: Therapy of slowly-healing crural ulcers by "circumcision," i.e. by transplantation of active epithelium. Zentralbl. f. Chir. *59:*2530–2531, Oct 15, '32
BÜTTNER, G.: Therapy of slowly-healing crural ulcers by "circumcision," i.e., by transplantation of active epithelium. Zentralbl. f. Chir. *59:*3092, Dec 29, '32 (Addendum)

Buttocks

Regeneration technic in plastic surgery of buttocks, using blood as "nutritive bed"; illustrative case. PRUDENTE, A. Arq. de cir. clin. e exper. *6:*270–272, April–June '42

BUXTON, ST. J. D.: Association of surgeon and radiologist in bone grafting. Arch. Radiol. and Electroth. *27:*289–304, March '23 (illus.)
BUXTON, ST. J. D.: Common injuries to joints of fingers and wrist. Clin. J. *63:*270–274, July '34
BUZELLO, A.: Plastic transposition of index finger to replace entire thumb. Zentralbl. f. Chir. *63:*2945–2952, Dec 12, '36
BUZOIANU, G. (see JIANU, I.) March '27
BUZOIANU, G. (see JIANU, J.) Nov–Dec '27
BUZOIANU, G. (see JIANU, J.) Jan–Feb '28
BUZOIANU, G. V. (see POPESCU, S.) March '29
BUZZARD, E. F.: Treatment of traumatic facial paralysis. Proc. Roy. Soc. Med. (Sect. Otol.) *20:*35–39, May '27
BUZZARD, E. F.: Treatment of traumatic facial paralysis. J. Laryng. and Otol. *42:*437–439, July '27
BUZZI, A.: Technic of immediate treatment of jaw fractures. Rev. de cir. *7:*215, May '28 also: Prensa med. argent. *15:*235–236, July 20, '28
BUZZI, A. AND CORNEJO SARAVIA, E.: Plastic operation of penis; case. Bol. y trab. de la Soc. de cir. de Buenos Aires *13:*143, May 22, '29
BUZZI, A.; COSTA, A. J. AND DERQUI, M. N.: Injuries to fingers caused by aniline pencils; surgical treatment. Semana med. *2:*1064–1068, Oct 10, '29
BYARS, L. T.: Free full thickness grafts; principles involved and technic of application. Surg., Gynec. and Obst. *75:*8–20, July '42
BYARS, L. T.: Avulsion of scrotum and skin of penis; technic of delayed and immediate repair (using skin grafts). Surg., Gynec. and Obst. *77:*326–329, Sept '43
BYARS, L. T.: Tattooing of free grafts and pedicle flaps. Tr. South. S. A. (1944) *56:*260–264, '45
BYARS, L. T.: Tattooing of free grafts and pedicle flaps. Ann. Surg. *121:*644–648, May '45
BYARS, L. T. AND KAUNE, M. M.: Plastic surgery; possibilities and limitations. Am. J. Nursing *44:*334–342, April '44
BYARS, L. T. AND SARNAT, B. G.: Surgery of mandible; ameloblastoma. Surg., Gynec. and Obst. *81:*575–584, Nov '45
BYARS, L. T. AND SARNAT, B. G.: Surgery of mandible; ameloblastoma. Am. J. Orthodontics (Oral Surg. Sect.) *32:*34–46, Jan '46
BYARS, L. T. (see BLAIR, V. P.) May '38
BYARS, L. T. (see BLAIR, V. P.) Dec '38
BYARS, L. T. (see BLAIR, V. P.) Feb '40
BYARS, L. T. (see BLAIR, V. P.) May '40
BYARS, L. T. (see BLAIR, V. P.) Aug '40
BYARS, L. T. (see BLAIR, V. P.) 1941
BYARS, L. T. (see BLAIR, V. P.) Jan '43
BYARS, L. T. (see BLAIR, V. P.) March '43
BYARS, L. T. (see BLAIR, V. P.) April '46
BYARS, L. T. (see BLAIR, V. P. *et al*) Nov '35
BYARS, L. T. (see BLAIR, V. P. *et al*) Feb '36
BYARS, L. T. (see BLAIR, V. P. *et al*) Jan '37
BYARS, L. T. (see BLAIR, V. P. *et al*) Feb '37
BYARS, L. T. (see BLAIR, V. P. *et al*) May '37
BYARS, L. T. (see BLAIR, V. P. *et al*) Sept '37
BYARS, L. T. (see BLAIR, V. P. *et al*) Oct '37
BYARS, L. T. (see BLAIR, V. P. *et al*) Oct '38
BYARS, L. T. (see BLAIR, V. P. *et al*) Dec '38
BYARS, L. T. (see BROWN, J. B.) Feb '38
BYARS, L. T. (see BROWN, J. B.) Oct '40
BYARS, L. T. (see BROWN, J. B.) Nov '40
BYARS, L. T. (see BROWN, J. B.) Feb '41
BYARS, L. T. (see BROWN, J. B. *et al*) May, June '35
BYARS, L. T. (see BROWN, J. B. *et al*) Sept '36
BYARS, L. T. (see BROWN, J. B. *et al*) Feb '39
BYARS, L. T., BROWN, J. B., AND MCDOWELL, F.: Preoperative and postoperative care in reconstructive surgery. Arch. Surg., *40:*1192, June '40
BYARS, L. T. *et al*: Color matching of skin grafts and flaps with permanent pigment injection. Surg. Gynec. and Obst. *79:*624, Dec '44
BYARS, L. T., BROWN, J. B., AND MCDOWELL, F.: Fundamental principles of skin grafting. The Interne, *12:*558, Sept '46
BYFORD, W. H.: Pathogenesis of Dupuytren's

contracture of palmar fascia. Med. Rec. *100:*487, Sept 17, '21
BYRNE, J. J.: Grease gun injuries to fingers. J.A.M.A. *125:*405–407, June 10, '44
BYRNES, C. M. JR.: Trophic lesions in multiple sclerosis (decubitus). J. Nerv. and Ment. Dis. *82:*373–380, Oct '35
BYTCHKOFF, V. S. AND ALEXEEFF, O. A.: Extrabuccal scarlet fever after burns; cases. Mosk. med. j. (no. 1) *9:*23–30, '29

C

DEC. M. SAUNDERS, J. B. (see SAUNDERS)
CABALLERO, A. AND TORTI, D. D.: Branchiogenic cyst of right carotid region; case of difficult diagnosis. Rev. med.-quir. de pat. fem. *25:*283-291, July '46
CABALLOL Y DE VERA, F.: Fracture of both condyles of lower jaw; case. Rev. san. mil., Habana *4:*63–65, Jan–March '40
CABANA, E. (see COMTOIS, A. *et al*) May '41
CABANAC: Delay of cicatrization in burns; use of cod liver oil dressings in therapy. Arch. Soc. d. sc. med. et biol. de Montpellier *18:*38–40, Feb '37
CABANAC (see LAPEYRIE) Jan '34
CABANES, E. AND XICLUNA, R.: Baldwin operation in case of pseudohermaphroditism and vulviform hypospadias. Algerie med. *43:*333–336, July '39
CABANIE, G.: Sectional urethrectomy in therapy of fistulas of perineobulbar portion of urethra. J. d'urol. *50:*124-126, March-April '42
CABANIE, G.: Technic and indications for sectional urethrectomy in urethroperineal fistula. J. d'urol. *52:*66–73, May–June '44
CABANIE, G.: Partial or total mammectomy by simple or enlarged areolar route. Paris med. *2:*373–375, Aug 24, '46; abst. Mem. Acad. de chir. *72:*68, Feb 6–20, '46
CABITZA, A.: Congenital cystic lymphangioma cured by subcutaneous anastomosis (marsupialization); case in infant. Riv. di clin. pediat. *38:*681-684, Nov '40
CABOT, C. M. (see NEW, G. B.) Nov '34
CABOT, C. M. (see NEW, G. B.) 1935
CABOT, C. M. (see NEW, G. B.) May '35
CABOT, H.: Plastic operations for epispadias and hypospadias. Proc. Staff Meet., Mayo Clin. *5:*315, Nov 5, '30
CABOT, H.: Treatment of exstrophy by ureteral transplantations. New England J. Med. *205:*706–711, Oct 8, '31
CABOT, H.; WALTERS, W. AND COUNSELLER, V. S.: Principles of treatment of hypospadias. J. Urol. *33:*400–407, April '35
CABOT, H.: Improved operation for hypospadias. Proc. Staff. Meet., Mayo Clin. *10:*796–798, Dec 11, '35
CABOT, H.: Hypospadias treatment in theory and practice. New England J. Med. *214:*871–876, April 30, '36
CABOT, H.: Epispadias; treatment in male. Proc. Staff Meet., Mayo Clin. *12:*793–795, Dec 15, '37
CABOT, H. (see GAUDIN, H. J.) April '38
CABRAL JUNIOR, A.: Wharton operation in case of partial aplasia of vagina. An. brasil. de ginec. *20:*87–107, Aug '45
CABROL: Plastic surgery after bicondyloid resection of mandible; case. Rev. de stomatol. *33:*720–722, Dec '31
CABROL: Technic for taking imprint for construction of cleft palate prosthesis. Rev. de stomatol. *47:*157–159, May–June '46
CABROL (see BOURGUET, *et al*) Dec '31
CABROL (see PONROY) Feb '33
CACCIALANZA, P.: Tubular skin flaps. Boll. Soc. med.-chir. Modena *42:*455–460, '41–'42
CACCIALANZA, P.: Tubular grafts. Boll. Soc. ital. biol. sper. *17:*94, Feb '42

Cadaver

Reactions in tissues of mummies following implantation. BUSSE-GRAWITZ, P. Arch. f. exper. Zellforsch. *24:*320–358, '42
Study of surgical technic in cadaver; hemiresection of lower jaw. MARISCAL, E. Prensa med. mex. *9:*59–61, '44

CADENAT, E.: Embryo with harelip. Compt. rend. Soc. de biol. *90:*181–183, Feb 1, '24
CADENAT, E.: Abnormalities along median line of face. Bruxelles-med. *7:*1151–1153, July 10, '27
CADENAT, E.: Origin of harelip. Presse med. *38:*270–271, Feb 22, '30
CADENAT, F. M.: Tendon sheath abscess; diagnosis; treatment. Hopital *15:*106–108, Feb (B) '27
CADENAT, F. M.: Cuts and punctures of fingers; treatment. Semaine d. hop. de Paris *4:*395–408, July 15, '28
CADENAT, F. M.: Operative treatment in inflammation of digital tendon sheaths. Bull. et mem. Soc. nat. de chir. *57:*522, April 25, '31
CADENAT, F. M.: Method for correcting paralysis of lower part of face due to nerve injury in extirpation of benign parotid tumors. Mem. Acad. de chir. *62:*961-962, June 17, '36
CADENAT, F. M.: Extirpation of benign parotid tumors; use of digastric muscle as guide during operation and in correction of facial paralysis. J. de chir. *48:*625–629, Nov '36

CADENAT, M. E.: Muscles and nerves in total bilateral harelip. Ann. d'anat. path. *8:*353–358, April '31

CADENAT; BOUYSSOU AND LAURENS: Surgical therapy of mandibular fracture by Kirschner nails; case. Rev. de stomatol. *46:*130–133, Oct–Dec '45

Cadenat Operation

Malignant tumor of parotid gland treated by Duval operation, with transplantation of digastric muscle to relieve resulting paralysis (Cadenat operation); case. MIRIZZI, P. L. AND URRUTIA, J. M. Bol. y trab., Soc. de cir. de Cordoba (no. 4) *1:*52–55, '40

CADÉRAS, J. (see RICHE, V. *et al*) Jan '32

CADMAN, E. F. (see MCDONALD, J. J. *et al*) Aug '46

CAEIRO, J. A.: Remote results of suture of ulnar and median nerves. Semana med. *2:*495–497, Aug 27, '25

CAEIRO, J. A.: Periarterial sympathectomy in Volkmann's contracture. Semana med. *1:*1185–1190, May 17, '28

CAEIRO, J. A.: Arthroplasty of interphalangeal joint for correction of "hammer finger." Semana med. *2:*1346–1347, Nov 7, '29

CAEIRO, J. A.: Results of stellectomy in facial paralysis due to section of nerve involved in parotid tumor; case. Bol. y trab. de la Soc. de cir. de Buenos Aires *19:*392–403, June 26, '35

CAEIRO, J. A.: Results of stellectomy in facial paralysis due to section of facial nerve involved in parotid tumor; case. Semana med. *1:*572–579, Feb 20, '36

CAFFIER, P.: Artificial vagina construction using transplanted amniotic membrane as lining. Zentralbl. f. Gynak. *62:*1186–1192, May 28, '38

CAFORIO, L.: New method of skin grafting, "à godet." Rinasc. med. *9:*84–86, Feb 15, '32

CAFORIO, L.: Technic of autoplastic operation to restore whole nose. Rinasc. med. *9:*467–469, Oct 15, '32

CAFORIO, L.: Skin grafting in therapy of paraffinomas due to self-mutilation during World War. Riforma med. *52:*1414–1417, Oct 17, '36

CAGNOLI, H.: Rupture of tendon of extensor pollicis longus as sequel of fracture of lower end of radius; case. Arch. urug. de med., cir. y especialid. *19:*598–603, Dec '41

CAHALL, W. L.: Treatment of facial paralysis. Arch. Physical Therapy *11:*78–81, Feb '30

CAHILL, J. A. JR. AND CAULFIELD, P. A.: Complete avulsion of scalp and loss of right ear; reconstruction by pedunculated tube grafts and costal cartilage. Surg., Gynec. and Obst. *66:*459–465, Feb (no. 2A) '38

CAHN, L. R.: Surgery of labial frenum. Am. J. Surg. *38:*254–255, Oct '24

CAHN, L. R. AND LEVY, J.: Case of facial fistula due to submaxillary sialolithiasis. Am. J. Surg. *36:*11, Jan '22 (illus.)

CAIN, H.: Inhibition of coagulation necrosis of implants by means of oxalate and enzyme poisons. Frankfurt. Ztschr. f. Path. *58:*171, '43

CAIRNS, H. (see CALVERT, C. A.) Oct '42

CAL, G. AND CAMBIAGGI, J. E.: Compound fracture of mandible due to gunshot wound. Rev. san. mil., Buenos Aires *43:*873–875, June '44

CALABRO, N.: Therapy of maxillofacial war lesions in territorial hospitals. Stomatol. ital. *2:*297–302, April '40

CALDERIN, A. M. (see MARTIN CALDERIN, A.)

Caldwell-Luc Operation

After-examination of 131 patients who had been operated on according to Caldwell-Luc procedure. HAASE, E. B. Acta oto-laryng. *34:*23–30, '46

Unusual complication of radical antrum operation (hemiatrophy of face following Caldwell-Luc operation). FULLER, T. E. South. M. J. *31:*1094–1095, Oct '38

CALICETI, (see CITELLI) Aug '21

CALICETI, P.: Ear injury by electric current; 2 cases. Ann. di laring., otol. *29:*16–21, Jan '28

CALISSANO, G.: Experiences with interposition of fixed cartilage grafts between bone stumps to induce nearthrosis. Arch. ital. di chir. *22:*206–217, '28

CALLAHAN, A.: Removal of adjacent nevi of eyelids. Am. J. Ophth. *29:*563–565, May '46

CALLAHAN, G. B.: Paper tissue-cod liver oil ointment dressings after surgical cleansing of burns. Illinois M. J. *82:*368–373, Nov '42

CALLAHAN, G. B.: Burn therapy; cod liver oil ointment-paper tissue dressing, peace-time dressing brought to war. Mil. Surgeon *92:*439–442, April '43

CALLANDER, C. L. (see PLAYER, L. P.) March '27

CALLANDER, C. L. (see BIRNBAUM, W.) Sept '35

CALLEWAERT, H.: Learning to write again after mutilation or amputation of right hand. Arch. serv. san. Parmeé belge *99:*71–77, Mar–Apr '46

CALLIGARIS, G.: Brachial hypotony and hypertrophy of mamma. Rev. neurol. *2:*365–377, Oct '23 (illus.)

CALLILAR, N.: Complications of malignant furuncle of upper lip and their prevention. Turk tip cem mec *12:*44–50, '46

CALLISTER, A. C.: Hypoplasia of mandible (micrognathy) with cleft palate; treatment in early infancy by skeletal traction. Am. J. Dis. Child. *53:*1057–1059, April '37

CALLISTER, A. C.: Practical problems in surgical correction of harelip and nose, palate defects. Rocky Mountain M. J. *35:*698–701, Sept '38

CALLISTER, A. C.: Hygroma colli cysticum. Rocky Mountain M. J. *38:*562–564, July '41

CALLISTER, A. C.: Hypertelorism with facies bovinia. Rocky Mountain M. J. *40:*36–40, Jan '43

CALLUM, E. N.: Congenital deformities of hands and feet (case). Brit. M. J. *2:*991, Nov 12, '38

CALVE, J.: Use of spongy tissue of young calf as bone mortar. Rev. med. franc. *16:*797–806, Dec '35 abstr: Bull. et mem. Soc. nat. de chir. *61:*1170–1174, Nov 16, '35

CALVER, G. W.: Problem of surgical shock. U. S. Nav. M. Bull. *42:*358–380, Feb '44

CALVERT, C. A. AND CAIRNS, H.: Discussion on injuries of frontal and ethmoidal sinuses. Proc. Roy. Soc. Med. *35:*805–810, Oct '42 also: J. Laryng. and Otol. *57:*499–508, Nov '42

CALZETTA, J. C. (see CEBALLOS, A.) Jan '45

CAMEIAGGI, J. E. (see CAL, G.) June '44

CAMERON, D. A.: Case of exstrophy of bladder. M. J. Australia *1:*509–510, May 16, '25

CAMERON, D. M. (see GHORMLEY, R. K.) Aug '40

CAMERON, G. R.; MILTON, R. F. AND ALLEN, J. W.: Tannic acid toxicity in burns; experimental investigation. Lancet *2:*179–186, Aug 14, '43

CAMERON, G. R. *et al*: Effects of applying pressure to experimental thermal burns. J. Path. and Bact. *57:*37–46, Jan '45

CAMERON, G. R. *et al*: Acceleration of healing by pressure application to experimental thermal burns. J. Path. and Bact. *58:*1–9, Jan '46

CAMERON, G. R. (see ALLEN, J. W. *et al*) April '44

CAMERON, J. E. (see ELKINS, C. W.) May '46

CAMERA, U.: New treatment of hypospadias. Arch. ital. di chir. *6:*277–296, Nov '22 (illus.) abstr: J.A.M.A. *80:*436, Feb 10, '23

CAMERA, U.: Treatment of exstrophy of bladder. Arch. ital. di chir. *6:*421–432, Dec '22 (illus.) abstr: J.A.M.A. *80:*806, March 17, '23

CAMERER, C. B.: Treatment of a "saddle nose" by costal cartilage graft. U. S. Nav. M. Bull. *15:*397, April '21

CAMERER, C. B.: Plastic repair of "saddle nose" deformity by autogenous cartilaginous graft. U. S. Nav. M. Bull. *22:*186, Feb '25

CAMERER, J. W. AND SCHLEICHER, R.: Etiology of "snapping finger"; simultaneous appearance in uniovular twins. Med. Klin. *31:*245–246, Feb 22, '35

CAMES, O. AND MAROTTOLI, O. R.: Recidivating temporomaxillary luxation; author's experience with therapy. An. de cir. *3:*274–279, Sept '37

CAMES, O. AND MAROTTOLI, O. R.: Therapy of recidivating luxation of jaw; authors' experience. Bol. y trab. de la Soc. de cir. de Buenos Aires *21:*756–763, Sept 8, '37

CAMINITI MANGANARO, E.: New technical procedure for preparation of tubular cutaneous graft for plastic surgery; experimental study. Rinasc. med. *16:*11–12, Jan 15, '39

CAMITZ, H.; HOLMGREN, H. AND JOHANSSON, H.: Nature of bone transplants. Acta chir. Scandinav. *75:*1–67, '34

CAMMERMEYER, J.: Extensive cerebral changes in case of "sudden" death following plastic transfer of skin on neck under local anesthesia. Acta path. et microbiol. Scandinav. *15:*307–329, '38

CAMP, J. D. AND ALLEN, E. P.: Microtia and congenital atresia of external auditory canal; demonstration of external auditory canal by means of tomography. Am. J. Roentgenol. *43:*201–203, Feb '40

CAMP, J. H.: Extensive cutaneous burns. Texas State J. Med. *29:*639–642, Feb '34

CAMP, M. N. (see TERHUNE, S. R.) Sept '42

CAMPBELL, A.: Closure of congenital clefts of hard palate. Brit. J. Surg. *13:*715–719, April '26

CAMPBELL, C. A.: New perichondrium elevator for resection of nasal septum. Laryngoscope *31:*973, Dec '21 (illus.)

CAMPBELL, C.A.: Nasal suturing instrument. Arch. Otolaryng. *11:*95–96, Jan '30

CAMPBELL, D.: Thumb with 3 phalanges; case. Fortschr. a. d. Geb. d. Rontgenstrahlen *39:*479–481, March '29

CAMPBELL, D.: Hemiatrophy of face. Fortschr. a. d. Geb. d. Rontgenstrahlen *47:*198–202, Feb '33

CAMPBELL, E. H. JR.: Peripheral nerves; missile injuries. M. Bull. Mediterranean Theat. Op. *3:*246–251, June '45

CAMPBELL, H. H.: Plastic surgery in orthopedics. Tr. Roy. Med.-Chir. Soc. Glasgow, pp. 7–12, '42–'43; in Glasgow M. J. Dec '42

CAMPBELL, K.: Absence of vagina; successful treatment without operation. M. J. Australia *2:*650, Dec 6, '41

CAMPBELL, K. N. (see LANGE, H. J.) Nov '45

CAMPBELL, K. N. (see LANGE, H. J. *et al*) May '46

CAMPBELL, M. D.: Repair of lacerations of lacrimal canaliculus. Air Surgeon's Bull. (no. 12) *1:*18, Dec '44
CAMPBELL, W. C.: Mobilization of ankylosed jaw. J. Am. Dent. A. *19:*1222–1229, July '32
CAMPBELL, W. C.: Surgery of arthritis. South. Surgeon *4:*353–371, Oct '35
CAMPBELL, W. C.: Autogenous bone graft. J. Bone and Joint Surg. *21:*694–700, July '39
DEL CAMPO, R. M. AND SELLERA CASTRO, R.: Fractures of lower jaw in children. Rev. ortop. y traumatol. *1:*357–371, Jan '32
CAMPORA, G. (see CANESTRO, C.) Jan–Feb '27
DE CAMPOS, A.: Local supracutaneous serotherapy used in skin diseases and surgery for esthetic results. Rev. paulista de med. *20:*12–19, Jan '42
CAMPOS, E.: Operative treatment of ptosis of eyelid. Brazil-med. *2:*345–349, Dec 2, '22 (illus.) abstr: J.A.M.A. *80:*514, Feb 17, '23
CAMPOS, E.: Case of spastic entropion. Brazil-med. *1:*309, May 31, '24
CAMPOS, E.: Case of diffuse angioma of eyelid cured by electrolysis. Brazil-med. *2:*233, Oct 18, '24
CAMPOS, F.: Plastic surgery, human aspects. Arq. de cir. clin. e exper. *6:*280–286, April–June '42
CAMPOS, F.: Bilateral gynecomastia and its surgical therapy; case. Arq. de cir. clin. e exper. *6:*703–705, April–June '42
CAMPOS, J.: Old and new methods of palate surgery. Ars med. *5:*229–238, July '29
CAMPOS MARTIN, R.; USUA MARINE, J. AND ALVAREZ-ZAMORA, R.: Skin grafts in therapy of late reactions to roentgen or radium therapy; cases. Actas dermo-sif. *34:*564–575, April '43
CAMPOS MARTIN, R. AND USUA MARINE, J.: Giant epithelioma of lower extremity; roentgenotherapy and Reverdin grafts; case. Actas dermo-sif. *34:*747–750, June '43
CAMPOS, R.: Combined use of surgery and radium in treatment of rhinophyma. Ars med., Barcelona *12:*85–91, Feb '36
CANALE, A.: Improvised emergency apparatus for fractured jaw. Semana med. *2:*1189–1193, Dec 7, '22 (illus.)
CANALE, A.: Therapy of fracture of ascending branch of lower jaw. Semana med. *2:*381–386, Aug 6, '36
CANALE, A. (see FINOCHIETTO, R. *et al*) 1944
CANALS MAYNER, R.: Temporomaxillary ankylosis; case. Rev. med. de Barcelona *15:*3–21, Jan '31
CANAVERO, G.: Skin grafts derived from scrotum. Policlinico (sez. chir.) *36:*61–69, Feb '29
CANBY, C. P. (see BERNIER, J. L.) Feb '43

Cancer

Relationship of cellular differentiation, fibrosis, hyalinization, and lymphocytic infiltration to postoperative longevity of patients with squamous-cell epithelioma of skin and lip. POWELL, L. D. J. Cancer Research *7:*371–378, Oct '22 (illus.)
Multiple malignant skin epitheliomas in the young. PICCARDI, G. Gior. ital. d. mal. ven. *65:*338–343, April '24
Destructive and constructive surgery of malignancy. RITCHIE, H. P. Minnesota Med. *8:*4–7, Jan '25
Suggestion for relief of pain from carcinoma of mouth and cheek. GRANT, F. C. Ann. Surg. *81:*494–498, Feb '25
Surgical relief of pain in deep carcinoma of face and neck. FAY, T. Am. J. Roentgenol. *14:*1–5, July '25
Surgical removal and pathological study of massive squamous cell epithelioma associated with angioma of scalp. PULFORD, D. S. AND ADSON, A. W. Surg., Gynec. and Obst. *42:*846–848, June '26
Cancer of lip, breast and cervix; end result study. WAINWRIGHT, J. M. Bull. Moses Taylor Hosp. *1:*9–14, May '27
Plastic correction of defects remaining after original operation. MANASSE, P. Deutsche med. Wchnschr., *53:*1790, Oct 14, '27
Epithelioma following burns. BELL, J. G. Y. Clin. J. *57:*525–527, Oct 31, '28
Statistics on 1,323 operations on mouth, pharynx and esophagus for cancer. SIMEONI, V. Valsalva *5:*86–89, Feb '29
Reconstructive surgery in relation to cancer defects. SHEEHAN, J. E. Internat. J. Med. and Surg. *42:*177–180, April '29
Construction of gluteal anus in treatment of recurring rectal prolapse following amputation in case of adenocarcinoma. BREITNER, B. Wien. klin. Wchnschr. *42:*638–639, May 9, '29
Relief of pain with cancer of face. GRANT, F. C. Pennsylvania M. J. *32:*548–551, May '29
Epithelioma of cheek from drop of carbon disulphide; case. GOUGEROT, H. AND BURNIER. Bull. Soc. franc. de dermat. et syph. *36:*1041, Nov '29
Plastic surgery of lip, chin and cheek in man after resection for cancer. CAVINA, C. Arch. ed atti d. Soc. ital. di chir. *35:*526–541, '29
Epithelioma developing on site of recurrent

Cancer—Cont.
herpes simplex of lips. BURGESS, N. Brit. M. J. *2:*249, Aug 16, '30
Naso-orbital epitheliomas; 10 cases. ABOULKER, H. AND GOZLAN, A. Ann. d'oto-laryng., pp. 381–398, April '31
Production of malignant tumors by transplantation of embryonal tissues. KLEE-RAWIDOWWICZ, E. Deutsche med. Wchnschr. *58:*1439–1440, Sept 9, '32
Review of cases of squamous cell carcinoma at New Haven Hospital from January 1, 1920, to November 1, 1931. ROBERTS, F. W. Yale J. Biol. and Med. *4:*187–198, Dec '31
Five year cures in cancer of mouth, lip, nose, etc. SMITH, F. Surg., Gynec. and Obst. *56:*470–471, Feb (no. 2A) '33
Therapy of cancer by means of transplantation of normal organs; review. NYKA, W. AND LAVEDAN, J. Paris med. *1:*229–240, March 18, '33
Five year cures of cancer of larynx and mouth and pharynx. NEW, G. B. AND FIGI, F. A. Surg., Gynec. and Obst. *60:*483–484, Feb (no. 2A) '35
Deep epitheliomas of benign evolution; 6 cases. DUFOURMENTEL, L. Bull. et mem. Soc. d. chirurgiens de Paris *27:*586–596, Dec 6, '35
Epitheliomata; clinical notes. MONTGOMERY, D. W. California and West. Med. *45:*134–137, Aug '36
Metastasis of tumor of rectum to mandible (case). IVY, R. H. AND CURTIS, L. Ann. Dent. *3:*133–137, Sept '36
Epitheliomas and their therapy. NUYTTEN, J. Echo med. du Nord. *6:*544–563, Sept 27, '36
Restorative surgery following surgical or pathologic loss of substance in cancer and leprosy. PRUDENTE, A. Rev. de chir. structive, pp. 148–154, June '37
Plastic surgery as allied with treatment of cancer (grafts). OWENS, N. New Orleans M. and S. J. *90:*417–424, Jan '38
Skin grafts in protection of exposed area after extirpation of cancer. PRUDENTE, A. Arch. urug. de med., cir. y especialid. *12:*196–209, Feb '38
Salivary gland cancer. MACFEE, W. F. Ann. Surg. *109:*534–550, April '39
Cancer of head and neck; management of lesions with borderline operability and curability. KIME, E. N. Arch. Phys. Therapy *20:*282–287, May '39
New restorative operation following partial extirpation for cancer. BRÜNINGS. Ztschr. f. Krebsforsch. *49:*278–286, '39

Cancer—Cont.
Reconstruction of scalp following excision for malignancy. STEISS, C. F. Am. J. Surg. *52:*378–380, May '41
Use of cold air blast on precancerous skin lesions and hemangiomas. POPPE, J. K. Surgery *11:*460–465, March '42
Keysser's work and plastic surgery of cancer. PRUDENTE, A. Arq. de cir. clin. e exper. *6:*316–320, April–June '42
Skin graft restoration after excision for malignant disease. PICKERILL, H. P. Australian and New Zeland J. Surg. *13:*147–154, Jan '44
Attempted plastic surgery in extirpation of breast cancer. ROFFO, A. E. Bol. Inst. de med. exper. para el estud. y trat. d. cancer *21:*163–179, April '44
Surgical treatment of pain; malignant lesions of face, nose and mouth. ROBERTSON, J. S. Tr. Roy. Med.-Chir. Soc. Glasgow, pp. 29–31, '43–'44; in Glasgow M. J. May '44
Cancer of skin, lip and tongue. MARTIN, H. Bull. Am. Soc. Control Cancer *26:*82–83, July '44
Plastic repair after electrothermal operations (cancer). VIANNA, J. B. Med. cir. farm., pp. 598–606, Nov '44
Therapy of anorectal cancers exteriorized to perineum by diathermocoagulation; subsequent plastic operation. MOULONGUET, P. Mem. Acad. de chir. *71:*298–300, June 13–20, '45
Recidivation of vulvar cancer in arm, due to graft to prevent local recurrence; case. PIULACHS, P. AND PLANAS-GUASCH, J. Med. clin., Barcelona *6:*334–336, May '46
Darier's fibrosarcoma on scar of human bite on male breast; case. SYLVESTRE BEGNIS, C. AND PICENA, J. P. Rev. med. de Rosario *36:*233–239, May '46
Unusual metastatic manifestations of breast cancer: metastasis to mandible, with report of 5 cases. ADAIR, F. E. AND HERRMANN, J. B. Surg., Gynec. and Obst. *83:*289–295, Sept '46

Cancer, Antrum

Lymphosarcoma of antrum treated 12 years ago; no recurrence. NEW, G. B. Proc. Staff Meet., Mayo Clin. *7:*317–318, June 1, '32
Plastic repair of defect following operative treatment of carcinoma of antrum and upper jaw. BECK, J. C. AND GUTMAN, M. R. S. Clin. North America *14:*775–782, Aug '34
Curability of malignant tumors of upper jaw and antrum. NEW, G. B. AND CABOT, C. M.

Cancer, Antrum–Cont.

Tr. Am. Laryng., Rhin. and Otol. Soc. *41:*584–590, '35

Transplantation of parotid (Stensen's) duct in cancer of antrum. FIGI, F. A. Proc. Staff Meet., Mayo Clin. *11:*241–243, April 15, '36

Cancer in Artificial Vagina

Primary carcinoma of vagina following Baldwin reconstruction operation for congenital absence of vagina. RITCHIE, R. N. Am. J. Obst. and Gynec. *18:*794–799, Dec '29

Late cancer of artificial vagina formed from rectum (Schubert operation); case. LAVAND'HOMME, P. Bruxelles-med. *19:*14–15, Nov 6, '38

Cancer, Basal Cell

Surgical treatment of extensive basal cell carcinoma. HORSLEY, J. S., J.A.M.A. *78:*412–416, Feb 11, '22 (illus.)

Basal-cell carcinoma of skin. HORSLEY, J. S. S. Clin. N. America *2:*1247–1257, Oct '22

Transplantation of distant skin flaps for cure of intractable basal-cell carcinoma. HORSLEY, J. S. Ann. Surg. *82:*14–29, July '25

Basal-cell carcinoma of face. SCHAMBERG, J. F. S. Clin. N. Amer. *7:*113–115, Feb '27

Treatment of baso-cellular epithelioma of face. MARIN, A. Union med. du Canada *56:*489–500, Sept '27

Basocellular epithelioma of face with clinical syndrome simulating scleroderma. BERTANZI, R. Gior. ital. di dermat. e sifil. *70:*1344–1348, Oct '29

Coexistence of basal celled epithelioma of temporal region and spinocellular epithelioma of lip; case. MARIN, A. Union med. du Canada *61:*770–772, June '32

Neglected and recurrent basal cell epitheliomas of face. MEYER, H. W. Surg., Gynec. and Obst. *64:*675–683, March '37

Treatment of persistent recurrent basal cell carcinoma. YOUNG, F. Surg., Gynec. and Obst. *73:*152–162, Aug '41

Metastasizing basal cell carcinoma of face. DE NAVASQUEZ, S., J. Path. and Bact. *53:*437–439, Nov '41

"Field-fire" and invasive basal cell carcinoma–basal-squamous type. BROWN, J. B. AND McDOWELL, F. Surg., Gynec. and Obst. *74:*1128–1132, June '42

Free grafts and pedicle flaps in treatment of recurring basal cell epitheliomas; cases. WEAVER, D. F. Laryngoscope *53:*336–342, May '43

Basal cell lesions of nose, cheek and lips. DAVIS, W. B. Ann. Surg. *119:*944–948, June '44

Cancer, Basal-Squamous

Field-fire and invasive basal cell carcinoma; basal-squamous carcinoma. J. B. BROWN AND F. McDOWELL. Surg., Gynec. and Obst. *74:*1128, June '42

Cancer, Burn Scars: See Burns, Cancer in

Cancer, Cheek (See also Cancer, Mouth)

Carcinoma of cheek, case report. SHERRILL, J. G. Kentucky M. J. *20:*284–285, April '22

Carcinoma of lip and cheek; general principles involved in operation and results obtained at Presbyterian, Memorial, and Roosevelt Hospitals. BREWER, G. E. Surg., Gynec. and Obst. *36:*169–184, Feb '23

Case report of plastic repair of mutilating operations of lip and cheek following radical removal of carcinoma. COPP, F. A., J. Florida M. A. *12:*29–35, Aug '25

Radio-active substances; their therapeutic uses and applications; radiation of cancer of cheek. MUIR, J. Radiology *7:*131–136, Aug '26

New method of treating carcinoma of cheek. PATTERSON, N. Lancet *2:*703, Oct 1, '27

Electrocoagulation of cancer of cheek. CLAIRMONT, P. AND SCHÜRCH, O. Deutsche Ztschr. f. Chir. *227:*115–125, '30

Plastic operations on cheeks and nose for cancer. WOLF, H. Arch. f. klin. Chir. *160:*105–117, '30

Cancer of cheek, with special reference to results of surgical therapy. THEODORESCO, D. AND HOFER, O. Presse med. *42:*2040–2043, Dec 19, '34

Cancer of cheek and neighboring bone. BLAIR, V. P.; BROWN, J. B., AND BYARS, L. T. Am. J. Surg. *30:*250–253, Nov '35

Cancer of cheek and neighboring bone. BLAIR, V. P.; BROWN, J. B., AND BYARS, L. T. Internat. J. Orthodontia *22:*183–188, Feb '36

Carcinoma of cheek; original method of treatment, with reports on 10 cases. PATTERSON, N. Brit. J. Surg. *25:*330–336, Oct '37

Treatment of epitheliomas of nasolabial fold. MELAND, O. N. Am. J. Roentgenol. *38:*730–739, Nov '37

Ulcerating epithelioma of cheek; case treated with 500,000 volt therapy. MERSHON, H. F. South. Surgeon *7:*262, June '38

Cancer of lips and cheeks. FIGI, F. A. Proc. Staff Meet., Mayo Clin. *16:*280–282, April 30, '41

Plastic reconstruction of cheek after exten-

Cancer, Cheek—Cont.

sive epithelioma. FLYNN, R., M. J. Australia *1:*555–556, May 9, '42

Full thickness defects of cheek (cancer) involving angle of mouth; method of repair. MACFEE, W. F. Surg., Gynec. and Obst. *76:*100–105, Jan '43

Large carcinoma of cheek. NATHANSON, I. T. Am. J. Orthodontics (Oral Surg. Sect.) *31:*284–286, April '45

Cancer, Ear

A study of 63 cases of epithelioma of ear. BRODERS, A. C., S. Clin. N. Amer. *1:*1401, Oct '21

Carcinoma of external ear; combined surgical and radium treatment. BECK, E. G. Internat. Clinics *1:*29, '21

Epithelioma of face and ear. YOUNG, W. J. Kentucky M. J. *20:*367–368, May '22

Epithelioma of auricle. MONTGOMERY, D. W. AND CULVER, G. D. Arch. Dermat. and Syph. *7:*472–478, April '23

Prosthesis after removal of auricle for carcinoma. FENTON, R. A. AND LUPTON, I. M. Northwest Med. *22:*212, June '23 (illus.)

Radium treatment of epithelioma of ear. KENNEDY, W. H. Radiology *7:*249–252, Sept '26

Results of surgical and diathermic-surgical treatment of cancer of concha of ear. GIESE, A. Ztschr. f. Laryng., Rhin. *19:*414–423, July '30

Epithelioma of auricle and its therapy. DESAIVE, P. Cancer, Bruxelles *12:*273–286, '35

Epithelioma of pinna. DUGOUJON, F. Rev. de laryng. *57:*439–501, April '36

Cancer in Exstrophied Bladders

Exstrophy of urinary bladder with carcinoma. LOWER, W. E. Ann. Surg. *73:*354, March '21

Cancer in exstrophy of bladder. DUPONT, R. J. d'urol. *13:*433–444, June '22 (illus.) abstr: J.A.M.A. *79:*855, Sept 2, '22

Exstrophy with cancer of bladder and absence of umbilicus; report of case. MURPHY, D. P. J.A.M.A. *82:*784–785, March 8, '24

Interesting case of exstrophic bladder with neoplastic implant. McCARTHY, J. F. AND KLEMPERER, P. J. Urology *14:*419–427, Oct '25

Exstrophy of bladder complicated by carcinoma. JUDD, E. S. AND THOMPSON, H. L. Arch. Surg. *17:*641–657, Oct '28

Cancer of sigmoid flexure 10 years after ureteral implantation for exstrophy of bladder. HAMMER, E. J. d'urol. *28:*260–263, Sept '29

Cancer in Exstrophied Bladders—Cont.

Carcinoma of bladder in exstrophy. McCOWN, P. E., J. Urol. *43:*533–542, April '40

Cancer, Eyelid

Carcinoma of eyelids treated with radium. WITHERS, S. Am. J. Ophth. *4:*8, Jan '21

Case of epithelioma of outer canthus of eye. MEYER, H. W., S. Clin. N. Amer. *1:*1643, Dec '21

Transplantation flap repair of lower eyelid following removal of epithelioma. MINCHEW, B. H., J.M.A. Georgia *11:*110–111, March '22

Buediner's modification of Dieffenbach's operation for early epithelioma of lower lid. WRIGHT, R. E. Brit. J. Ophth. *8:*58–61, Feb '24

Case of sarcoma of eyelids. FISHER, J. A. Am. J. Ophth. *7:*619–620, Aug '24

Sarcoma of eyelid. SATANOWSKY, P. Semana med. *2:*169–177, July 23, '25 abstr: J.A.M.A. *85:*1264, Oct 17, '25

Treatment of epithelioma of face and eyelid. SIMPSON, C. A. Virginia M. Monthly *52:*337–340, Sept '25

Skin grafting in 2 cases of epithelioma of eyelids. MORAX, V. Ann. d'ocul. *164:*6–15, Jan '27

Superiority of radium to surgery in cancer of eyelids; cures without risk of recurrence, mutilation or pain. DEGRAIS, P. AND BELLOT, A. Bull. Soc. d'opht. de Paris, no. 9, pp. 536–544, '27 also: Clinique, Paris *22:*397–403, Oct (B) '27

Cancer of eyelid; radium therapy; case. CAPIZZANO, N. Bol. Inst. de med. exper. para el estud. y trat. del cancer *4:*139, April '28

Treatment of cancer of eyelids. BENEDICT, W. L. AND ASBURY, M. K. New York State J. Med. *29:*675–677, June 1, '29

Cancer of upper eyelid; plastic operation; case. FROTHINGHAM, G. E., J. Michigan M. Soc. *28:*632–633, Sept '29

Epithelioma of eyelids; indications for radium treatment and surgical intervention. VILLARD, H. Medecine *11:*19–23, Jan '30

Radium treatment of epitheliomas of eyelids. APPELMANS, M. Rev. belge sc. med. *2:*829–840, Dec '30

Epithelioma of eyelid; case. CORBETT, J. J. New England J. Med. *204:*774–776, April 9, '31

Recurrence after roentgenotherapy and then after excision of epithelioma of internal angle and of upper right eyelid; case. COSTE, J. Bull. Soc. franc. de dermat. et syph. (Reunion dermat., Lyon) *38:*501–504, April '31

Cancer, Eyelid–Cont.
Epithelioma of eyelid; excision. CASTROVIEJO, R. JR. Am. J. Ophth. *14:*634-635, July '31
Epithelioma of eyelid. LEHMANN, C. F. Texas State J. Med. *27:*422-426, Oct '31
Radiotherapy of epithelioma of eyelids; aesthetic results. ARCELIN, F. Lyon med. *149:*289-292, March 6, '32
Therapy of cancer of eyelid by evisceration followed by plastic surgery; case. AGUILAR, H. AND ZAVALETA, D. Hosp. argent. *4:*506-512, Jan 15, '34
Pigmented basocellular epithelioma of palpebral skin. SEDAN, J. Bull. Soc. d'opht. de Paris, pp. 341-348, April '36
Excision of cancer of eyelids and autoplastic surgery according to Imre technic. DE SAINT-MARTIN. Bull. Soc. d'opht. de Paris *49:*36-40, Jan '37
Symptomatology and therapy of cancer of eyelids. DOLLFUS, M. A. Bull. med., Paris *51:*375-380, May 29, '37
Successfully operated basalioma of eyelid; case. LOTIN, A. V. Vestnik oftal. *10:*891-892, '37
Partial resection of eyelid and plastic repair for epithelioma involving margin of lid. REESE, A. B. Arch. Ophth. *32:*173-178, Sept '44

Cancer, Face
Treatment of basal epithelioma of face. YOUNG, W. J. Kentucky M. J. *19:*154, April '21
Extensive epitheliomatous ulcer of side of face. MCKILLOP, L. M., M. J. Australia *2:*456, Nov 19, '21
Radiotherapy in treatment of superficial malignant disease of face. JOSSELYN, R. B., J. Maine M. A. *13:*279-284, June '23 (illus.)
Epithelioma of face. BOWEN, W. W., J. Iowa M. Soc. *14:*154-157, April '24
Treatment of malignant growths about the face. WITHERS, S. AND RANSON, J. R. Colorado Med. *21:*92-97, April '24
Radium treatment of epithelioma of face. KENNEDY, W. H., J. Radiol. *6:*52-55, Feb '25
Radium treatment of cancer of face. TRUEHART, M., J. Kansas M. Soc. *25:*70-73, March '25
Relief for pain in carcinoma of face. GRANT, F. C., J.A.M.A. *86:*173-176, Jan 16, '26
Treatment of advanced carcinoma of skin of face with radium. BRADLEY, R. A. AND SNOKE, P. O., S. Clin. N. Amer. *7:*165-168, Feb '27

Cancer, Face–Cont.
Radium treatment in 13 cases of cancer of face. FRUCHAUD, H. AND MARY, A. Gazettes med., Paris, pp. 465-471, Aug 15, '27
X-ray treatment of epithelioma of face. MARTIN, J. M. Proc. Inter-State Post-Grad. M. Assemb., North America (1927) *3:*303-305, '28
Relief of pain of facial cancer. MIXTER, W. J. AND GRANT, F. C. Tr. Am. S. A. *45:*473-482, '27 also: Ann. Surg. *87:*179-185, Feb '28
Multiple epitheliomata of face developed from keratoma senile. WIENER, E. Nederl. Tijdschr. v. Geneesk. *1:*614-616, Feb 4, '28
Treatment of facial cancer by irradiation. KAPLAN, I. I. Am. J. Roentgenol. *19:*437-439, May '28
Cancer of face. MEYER, H. W. Am. J. Surg. *5:*352-357, Oct '28
Epithelioma of face treated by grattage and radiotherapy. BELOT, J. AND LEPENNETIER, F. Bull. et mem. Soc. de radiol. med. de France *16:*227, Nov '28
Multiple dermal cancer in face and on neck; case. ODQVIST, H. Acta radiol. *9:*302-304, '28
Roentgentherapy in inoperable epithelioma of face. SCADUTO, G. Urol. and Cutan. Rev. *33:*28-35, Jan '29
Neglected treatment of cancer of face; case. HEILBRONN, S. Munchen. med. Wchnschr. *76:*374, March 1, '29
Primary double epithelioma of face; case. ABERNETHY, D. A. Brit. J. Surg. *16:*687-689, April '29
Diagnosis of cutaneous cancer of face. RAMOND, L. Presse med. *37:*951-952, July 20, '29
Spreading epitheliomas, recurring after radium therapy; cure by surgical treatment (face). BÉRARD, L. AND DUNET. Lyon chir. *26:*562-565, Aug-Sept '29
Biologic aspects of cancer of face in view of results of treatment. VON DOELINGER DA GRACA. Folha med. *10:*384-386, Nov 5, '29
Value of radium in treatment of cancer of face. LARKIN, A. J. Am. J. Surg. *8:*164-165, Jan '30
Use of small amounts of radium at distance in treatment of cancer of face. PETTIT, R. T. Radiology *14:*55-59, Jan '30
Etiology of cancer of face; prevention. DARIER, J. Monde med., Paris *40:*65-73, Feb 1, '30
Recurring epithelioma of face. FIGI, F. A., S. Clin. N. Amer. *10:*105-107, Feb '30
Treatment of large epitheliomas after failure of radiotherapy (on face). BÉRARD, L. AND

Cancer, Face—Cont.

CREYSSEL, J. Paris med. *1:*237–243, March 15, '30

Unusual case of cancer of face. WILLIS, R. A. J. Coll. Surgeons, Australasia *2:*417–421, March '30

Epithelioma of face; treatment and subsequent surgical reconstruction. NEW, G. B. AND HAVENS, F. Z., J.A.M.A. *97:*687–690, Sept 5, '31

Epithelioma of face; treatment and subsequent surgical reconstruction. NEW, G. B. AND HAVENS, F. Z. Tr. Sect. Surg., Gen. and Abd., A.M.A., pp. 166–176, '31

Surgery for cancer of face and lip. TRUEBLOOD, D. V. West. J. Surg. *40:*401–404, Aug '32

Squamous cell epitheliomata of face; 26 cases. TRAUB, E. F. AND TOLMACH, J. A. New York State J. Med. *33:*875–881, July 15, '33

Terebrant cancers of face. IMBERT, R. Rev. de chir., Paris *74:*331–373, May '36

Thermocauterization in therapy of facial cancer. MERIC, A. J. L. Rev. de laryng. *57:*768–802, July–Aug '36

Plastic repair of defects resulting from radical extirpation of facial cancer. OWENS, N. South. M. J. *29:*654–664, July '36

Cancer of face, especially in region of eye; method of treatment. ALBRIGHT, H. L. Am. J. Surg. *33:*176–179, Aug '36

Reconstruction following ablation of cancer of face. PRUDENTE, A. Bull. et mem. Soc. d. chirurgiens de Paris *28:*485–496, Nov 6, '36

Results of roentgen rays, radium, diathermocoagulation and surgery in therapy of cutaneous epithelioma (face); 14 cases. MARTIN, J. Arch. d'electric. med. *44:*444–460, Dec '36

Indications for and limits of surgical therapy in extensive cancers of buccofacial region; 3 cases. BÉRARD, L.; COLSON, E. R., AND DARGENT, M. Lyon chir. *35:*318–327, May–June '38

Experiences in reconstruction in surgical treatment of malignant diseases of face with skin grafts. KILNER. Rev. de chir. structive *8:*170–180, '38

Role of plastic surgery in treatment of malignancies about face. BURTON, J. F. South. M. J. *32:*67–68, Jan '39

Plastic reconstruction after therapy for facial cancer. SCHÜRCH, O. Plast. chir. *1:*60–70, '39

Cancer of face. BLAIR, V. P. AND BYARS, L. T. Mississippi Valley M. J. *62:*90–93, May '40

Cancer of the Face and Mouth. BLAIR, V. P., MOORE, S., AND BYARS, L. T., C. V. Mosby Co., St. Louis, 1941

Cancer of face. NEW, G. B. Proc. Staff Meet., Mayo Clin. *16:*71–72, Jan 29, '41

Treatment of cancer of face, including reconstructive surgery. NEW, G. B., S. Clin. North America *21:*969–978, Aug '41

Principles of plastic surgery in treatment of malignant tumors of face. CONWAY, H. Surg., Gynec. and Obst. *74:*449–457, Feb (no. 2A) '42

Field-fire and invasive basal cell carcinoma; basal-squamous carcinoma. J. B. BROWN AND F. MCDOWELL. Surg., Gynec. and Obst. *74:*1128, June '42

Clinical and statistical study of 1062 cases facial cancer. DE CHOLNOKY, T. Ann. Surg. *122:*88–101, July '45

Cancer, Hand

Epithelioma of hand, with tendency to spontaneous cure. CORLETTE, C. E. AND INGLIS, K., M. J. Australia *1:*250, March 26, '21

Surgical treatment of epithelioma of hand. MANNA, A. Policlinico (sez. prat.) *29:*753–755, June 5, '22 (illus.) abstr: J.A.M.A. *79:*776, Aug 26, '22

Epithelioma of back of hand. MONTGOMERY, D. W. AND CULVER, G. D. New York M. J. *118:*674–676, Dec 5, '23 (illus.)

Cancer of back of hand. TOURNEUX, J. P. Progres med., pp. 149–158, Jan 24, '31

Epitheliomas of hand; types and treatment. ADAIR, F. E., S. Clin. North America *13:*423–430, April '33

Chondrosarcoma of fingers; case. ALLENDE, G. Rev. ortop. y tramatol. *6:*71–81, July '36

Recurrent epithelioma of arm; method of covering defect after radical excision illustrating 2 useful types of skin transplantation. GARLOCK, J. H., J. Mt. Sinai Hosp. *5:*75–78, July–Aug '38

Giant epithelioma of lower extremity; roentgenotherapy and Reverdin grafts; case. CAMPOS MARTIN, R. AND USUA MARINE, J. Actas dermo-sif. *34:*747–750, June '43

Cancer, Jaws

Malignant disease of superior maxillary bone; continued report. DABNEY, S. G. Kentucky M. J. *19:*125, March '21

Malignancy of face and jaws. FORT, F. T. Kentucky M. J. *19:*456, Aug '21

Malignant tumors of jaws. BERCHER, J. Paris med. *11:*205, Sept 3, '21 abstr. J.A.M.A. *77:*1289, Oct 15, '21

Treatment of cancer of jaws; observations

Cancer, Jaws – Cont.

continued since 1918, covering 26 additional cases. OCHSNER, A. J. Ann. Surg. *76:*328-332, Sept '22

Atypical operations on jaws for malignant growths. MCARTHUR, L. L., J.A.M.A. *79:*1484-1487, Oct 28, '22

Certain difficult problems in treatment of carcinoma of lower jaw. JOHNSON, F. M. Radiology *5:*280-285, Oct '25

Surgery associated with radium in treatment of epitheliomas of upper jaw. HAUTANT, A. *et al*. J. de chir. *28:*257-274, Sept '26

Treatment of epithelioma of lower jaw. SIMON, J. Marseille med. *1:*629, May 15, '27

Statistical postoperative prognosis of malignant tumors of upper jaw. OLAISON, F. Hygiea *89:*705-710, Sept 30, '27

Osteoplastic partial resection of lower jaw by Krassin's method for removal of lingual cancer; 5 cases. NASAROW, N. N. AND KUSCHEWA, M. N. Deutsche Ztschr. f. Chir. *215:*145-146, '29

Late results of operations on maxillary bone in cancer of oral cavity; 5 cases. DEBERNARDI, L. Boll. e mem. Soc. piemontese di chir. *2:*1114-1148, '32

Cancer of maxilla and ethmoid; survey of 50 cases. DAVIS, E. D. D. Brit. M. J. *1:*53-55, Jan 13, '34

Curability of malignant tumors of upper jaw and antrum. NEW, G. B. AND CABOT, C. M. Proc. Staff Meet., Mayo Clin. *9:*684-685, Nov 7, '34

Curability of malignant tumors of upper jaw and antrum. NEW, G. B. AND CABOT, C. M. Surg., Gynec. and Obst. *60:*971-977, May '35

Therapy of mandibular epithelial cancers by electrocoagulation followed by curietherapy. GERNEZ, L.; *et al*. Bol. Liga contra el cancer *10:*293-308, Oct '35

Surgical therapy of cancer of jaws. ALTERI. Morgagni *77:*1199-1201, Nov 10, '35

Malignant tumors of upper jaw. PORTMANN, G. AND DESPONS, J. Rev. de laryng. *57:*1-44, Jan '36

Results of surgical therapy of carcinoma and sarcoma of lower jaw, some in advanced stage, over last 20 years. BERG, A. Ztschr. f. Stomatol. *35:*933-947, July 23, '37

Malignant tumors of jaw and their differential diagnosis. HAMMER, H. Med. Welt *12:*261-264, Feb 19, '38

Jaw cancer; electrosurgery; segmental bone resection without interruption of continuity. KROEFF, M. Hospital, Rio de Janeiro *14:*337, Aug; 595, Sept; 1007, Oct '38

Cancer, Jaws – Cont.

Cancer of mandible. THOMA, K. H. Am. J. Orthodontics *24:*995-999, Oct '38

Plastic and prosthetic therapy after resection of upper jaw for cancer; cases. FRENCKNER, P. AND SUNDBERG, S. Acta oto-laryng. *27:*147-158, '39

Adenocarcinoma of maxilla. THOMA, K. H. Am. J. Orthodontics (Oral Surg. Sect.) *28:*65-85, Feb '42

Benign and malignant tumors of palate. MARTIN, H. E. Arch. Surg. *44:*599-635, April '42

Malignant tumors of upper jaw; Skinner lecture, 1943. WINDEYER, B. W. Brit. J. Radiol. *16:*362, Dec '43; *17:*18, Jan '44

Cancer of chin; extirpation in case. FERNANDEZ, L. L. Prensa med. argent. *31:*291-292, Feb 9, '44

Secondary carcinoma of mandible; analysis of 71 cases. BUIRGE, R. E. Surgery *15:*553-564, April '44

Recent advances in treatment of carcinoma of jaw. SOMERVELL, T. H. Brit. J. Surg. *32:*35-43, July '44

Malignant tumors of upper jaw. ORSI, J. L. Rev. med. de Rosario *34:*983-1011, Oct '44

Spindle cell sarcoma of mandible with excision and subsequent bone graft; case. DINGMAN, R. O., J. Oral Surg. *3:*235-240, July '45

Cancer, Larynx

Statistics and technique in treatment of malignant neoplasms of larynx. QUICK, D. A. AND JOHNSON, F. M. Am. J. Roentgenol. *9:*599-606, Sept '22

Surgical treatment of laryngeal cancer with an analysis of 70 cases. MACKENTY, J. E. New York State J. Med. *22:*456-462, Oct '22

Radical operation for extrinsic carcinoma of larynx. BLAIR, V. P. Ann. Otol., Rhin. and Laryng. *33:*373-378, June '24

Carcinoma of larynx. NEW, G. B. Minnesota Med. *9:*365-368, July '26

Carcinoma of larynx and laryngopharynx treated with radium; analysis of 30 cases. IMPERATORI, C. J. Arch. Otolaryng. *4:*151-159, Aug '26

Ten years' experience with radium therapy of cancer of larynx. SARGNON, A., J. de radiol. et d'electrol. *10:*553-555, Dec '26

Intrinsic cancer operated on by laryngo-fissure; immediate and ultimate results. THOMSON, ST. C. Eye, Ear, Nose and Throat Monthly *7:*266-270, June '28 also: Arch. Otolaryng. *8:*377-385, Oct '28

Cancer, Larynx – Cont.

Extrinsic epithelioma of larynx. NEW, G. B. S. Clin. N. Amer. *9:*84–87, Feb '29

Cancer of larynx in young. FIGI, F. A. AND NEW, G. B. Arch. Otolaryng. *9:*386–391, April '29

Intrinsic laryngeal cancer; lasting cure in 76 per cent of cases by laryngo-fissure. THOMSON, ST. C. Canad. M. A. J. *21:*4–8, July '29

Carcinoma of larynx in young. FIGI, F. A. AND NEW, G. B. Tr. Am. Laryng., Rhin. and Otol. Soc. *35:*350–357, '29

Intrinsic laryngeal cancer; lasting recovery in 76 per cent of cases of laryngofissure. THOMSON, ST. C. Ann. d. mal. de l'oreille, du larynx *48:*1079–1088, Nov '29 also: Union med. du Canada *59:*5–16, Jan '30

Results of radium therapy in cancer of larynx; 150 cases. ESCAT, *et al.* Cancer, Bruxelles *7:*121–126, '30

Double branchial cysts complicated by carcinoma of larynx. HERMAN, A. L. Minnesota Med. *14:*555–557, June '31

Laryngectomy for cancer. JACKSON, C. AND BABCOCK, W. W., S. Clin. North America *11:*1207–1227, Dec '31

Status of thyrotomy in cancer of larynx. NEW, G. B. Tr. Am. Laryng., Rhin. and Otol. Soc. *37:*241–247, '31

Late results of fractional roentgenotherapy of intrinsic cancer of larynx; results of 5 years' experience. GUNSETT, A. Gaz. med. de France (supp. radiol.), pp. 173–177, May 1, '32

Treatment of laryngeal cancer by laryngofissure. JACKSON, C. South. Surgeon *1:*223–229, Oct '32

Selection of treatment for cancer of larynx. NEW, G. B. AND FLETCHER, E. J.A.M.A. *99:*1754–1758, Nov 19, '32

Selection of treatment of cancer of larynx. NEW, G. B. AND FLETCHER, E., J.A.M.A. Laryng., Otol. and Rhin., A.M.A., pp. 27–42, '32

Statistical report on 5 year cures of cancer of larynx. LEWIS, F. O. Surg., Gynec. and Obst. *56:*466–467, Feb (No. 2A) '33

Radium therapy of cancer of larynx; results in 150 cases. CAPIZZANO, N. Bol. Inst. de med. exper. para el estud. y trat. del cancer *10:*575–579, Oct '33

Laryngectomy for cancer of larynx; results in 140 cases. CETRÁ, C. M. Bol. Inst. de med. exper. para el estud. y trat. del cancer *10:*564–573, Oct '33

Curability of cancer of larynx by laryngofissure. JACKSON, C. Surg., Gynec. and Obst. *58:*431–432, Feb (no. 2A) '34

Cancer, Larynx – Cont.

Curability of cancer of larynx. NEW, G. B. AND WAUGH, J. M. Surg., Gynec. and Obst. *58:*841–844, May '34

Analysis of 58 cases of cancer of larynx treated with laryngofissure. CLERF, L. H. Arch. Otolaryng. *19:*653–659, June '34

Observations in 200 consecutive cases of cancer of larynx. TUCKER, G. Arch. Otolaryng. *21:*1–8, Jan '35

Laryngectomy for carcinoma in aged patient; case. NEW, G. B. Proc. Staff Meet., Mayo Clin. *10:*186–187, March 20, '35

Statistics on results of 393 surgically treated cases of laryngeal cancer from May 1919 to July 1934 inclusive. HAJEK, M. AND HEINDL, A. Monatschr. f. Ohrenh. *69:*385, April; 583, May '35

Study of 133 cases of laryngeal cancer. MULLIN, W. V. AND DARSIE, L. L., S. Clin. North America *15:*851–858, Aug '35

Cancer of larynx and its therapy. DE SANSON, R. D. Rev. oto-laring. de Sao Paulo *3:*197–214, May–June '35 also: Rev. de laryng. *56:*964–985, Sept–Oct '35

Treatment of laryngeal cancer by laryngofissure and laryngectomy. JACKSON, C. AND JACKSON, C. L. Am. J. Surg. *30:*3–17, Oct '35

Study of 202 cases of laryngeal cancer with end results. GARFIN, S. W. New England J. Med. *213:*1109–1123, Dec 5, '35

Treatment of carcinoma of larynx. NEW, G. B. AND FIGI, F. A. Surg., Gynec. and Obst. *62:*420–423, Feb (no. 2A) '36

Diagnosis and surgical cure of cancer of larynx. TUCKER, G. Delaware State M. J. *8:*80–82, May '36

Surgical therapy of cancer of larynx; 200 cases. CETRÁ, M. C. Bol. Inst. de med. exper. para el estud. y trat. d. cancer, *14:*169–188, April '37

Results of roentgenotherapy of cancer of larynx after 5 and 10 years of control. COUTARD, H., J. de radiol. et d'electrol. *21:*402–409, Sept '37

Cancer of larynx. JACKSON, C. AND JACKSON, C. L., S. Clin. North America *17:*1791–1795, Dec '37

Surgical treatment of cancer of larynx. LOOPER, E. A. South. M. J. *31:*367–374, April '38

Surgical treatment of cancer of larynx. NEW, G. B. Surg., Gynec. and Obst. *68:*462–466, Feb (no. 2A) '39

Surgical treatment of cancer of larynx; results. ORTON, H. B. Mississippi Doctor *17:*128–135, Aug '39

Therapy of cancer of larynx. ALONSO, J. M.

Cancer, Larynx – Cont.

An. de oto-rino-laring. d. Uruguay *9:*215-232, '39

Surgical treatment of laryngeal cancer. McCREADY, J. H. Radiology *34:*146-148, Feb '40

Diagnosis and surgical treatment of cancer of larynx. LOOPER, E. A. South. Surgeon *9:*513-521, July '40

Results of treatment of malignant tumors of larynx and hypopharynx. WOODWARD, F. D. AND ARCHER, V. W. Virginia M. Monthly *67:*751-755, Dec '40

Surgical solution to carcinoma of larynx. CETRÁ, M. Rev. otorrinolaring. d. litoral *3:*99-117, Jan-June '44

Cancer, Lip

Epithelioma of lip. NASSAU, C. F., S. Clin. N. Amer. *1:*197, Feb '21

Results of surgical treatment of epithelioma of lip. SISTRUNK, W. E. Ann. Surg., *73:*521, May '21

Radium in treatment of epithelioma of lip. QUICK, D., J. Radiol. *2:*1, Dec '21

Epithelioma of lower lip, combined surgical and radium treatment. BECK, E. G. Internat. Clinics *1:*31, '21

Radium treatment of cancer of lip. DUBOIS-ROQUEBERT. Paris med. *12:*110-112, Feb 4, '22

Epithelioma of lip. TWYMAN, E. D., J.A.M.A. *78:*348-349, Feb 4, '22

Precancer lesion of lip. ANZILOTTI, G. Riforma med., *38:*411-413, May 1, '22

Modern treatment of cancer of lip. PANCOAST, H. K. Surg., Gynec. and Obst. *34:*589-593, May '22

Cancer of lip treated by radiation or combined with electro-coagulation and surgical procedures. PFAHLER, G. E., J. Radiol. *3:*213-218, June '22 (illus.)

Squamous-cell epithelioma of lip, its surgical indications. SHEPHARD, J. H. Surg., Gynec. and Obst. *35:*107-109, July '22 (illus.)

Cancer of lip. HAMILTON, C. M., J. Tennessee M. A. *15:*190-192, Aug '22

Treatment of cancer of lip by radiation. LAIN, E. S. Tr. Sect. Dermat. and Syphilol., A. M. A. pp. 220-233, '22 (illus.) also: Arch. Dermat. and Syph. *6:*434-447, Oct '22

Cancer of lip treated by electrocoagulation and radiation. PFAHLER, G. E. Arch. Dermat. and Syph., *6:*428-433, Oct '22 also: Tr. Sect. Dermat. and Syphilol., A.M.A., pp. 213-219, '22

Squamous epithelioma of lower lip. MILIANI, A. Arch. ital. di chir. *6:*105-124, Nov '22 (illus.) abstr: J.A.M.A. *80:*360, Feb 3, '23

Cancer, Lip – Cont.

Results of operations for cancer of lip at Massachusetts General Hospital from 1909 to 1919. SIMMONS, C. C. AND DALAND, E. M. Surg., Gynec. and Obst. *35:*766-771, Dec '22

Cancer of lip, its treatment by radium and surgery combined. WALL, C. K., J.M.A. Georgia *12:*67-69, Feb '23

Cancer of lip. RODRIGUEZ VILLEGAS, R. Semana med. *1:*398-403, March 1, '23 abstr: J.A.M.A. *81:*169, July 14, '23

Surgical treatment of carcinoma of lower lip. LEIGHTON, W. E., J. Missouri M. A. *20:*90-95, March '23 (illus.)

Radium treatment of carcinoma of lip. TAUSSIG, L. R., M. Clin. N. America *6:*1579-1586, May '23 (illus.)

Cancer of lips. PRAT, D. An. de Fac. de med., Montevideo *8:*865-883, Sept '23

Local treatment of cancer of lip. PEÑA NOVO, P. Siglo med. *73:*371-372, April 12, '24

Model of carcinoma of lip reconstructed from serial section. WARWICK, M., J.A.M.A. *82:*1119-1120, April 5, '24

Treatment of cancer of lower lip. NORSWORTHY, O. L. Texas State J. Med. *20:*184-188, July '24

Contribution to treatment of cancer of lip by irradiation; report on 136 cases. SCHREINER, B. F. AND KRESS, L. C. J. Cancer Research *8:*221-223, July '24

Carcinoma of lower lip. MASON, J. T., S. Clin. N. America *4:*1095-1104, Oct '24

Epithelioma of lip treated with radium. MONTGOMERY, D. W. AND CULVER, G. D. California and West. Med. *22:*628-631, Dec '24

Carcinoma of lip. BROEMAN, C. J., W. Virginia M. J. *20:*27-31, Jan '25

Epithelioma of lip, observations on 150 cases. KENNEDY, W. H. Radiology *4:*319-324, April '25

Cancer of lip, resulting deformity, plastic repair. BOYD, J. E., J. Florida M. A. *12:*27-29, Aug '25

Cancer of lower lip. MCGUFFIN, W. H. Canad. M. A. J. *15:*1046-1049, Oct '25

Epithelioma of lip treated by radiation. JACOBS, A. W., M. J. and Rec. *123:*803, June 16, '26

Radio-active substances; their therapeutic uses and applications; radium treatment of carcinoma of lower lip. MUIR, J. Radiology, *7:*51-58, July '26

Treatment of cancer and precancer of lip; clinical and therapeutic study of 191 cases. BUTLER, C. An. de Fac. de med., Monte-

Cancer, Lip—Cont.
video *10:*985-998, Dec '25 abstr: J.A.M.A. *87:*447, Aug 7, '26
Treatment of cancer of lip. WASSINK, W. F. Nederl. Tijdschr. v. Geneesk. *2:*1059-1069, Sept 4, '26 abstr: J.A.M.A. *87:*1524, Oct 30, '26
Cancer of lip; report of 25 cases treated with radium. TRUEHEART, M., J. Kansas M. Soc. *26:*311-313, Oct '26
Epidermoid carcinoma (epithelioma) of lip; diagnosis, pathology, and discussion of treatment by non-surgical measures. PENDERGRASS, E. P., S. Clin. N. Amer. *7:*117-163, Feb '27
Results of surgical treatment of epithelioma of lip from Massachusetts General Hospital and Cancer Commission of Harvard University. SHEDDEN, W. M. Boston M. and S. J. *196:*262-270, Feb 17, '27
Spontaneous cure of cancer of lip. AVRAMOVICI, A. Lyon chir. *24:*257-268, May-June '27
Squamous cell carcinoma of lower lip; case. LANDHAM, J. W. Piedmont Hosp. Bull. *4:*32-35, July-Aug '27
Plastic operation for ulcerative epithelioma of upper lip and cheek. ZAGNI, L. Stomatol. *25:*591-594, July '27
Epithelioma of lip and face. BONDURANT, C. P., J. Oklahoma M. A. *20:*252-256, Sept '27
Deductions from 191 cases of cancer of lips. FONTS, E. Bol. de la Liga contra el cancer *3:*4-9, Jan 1, '28
Cancer of lips. MCKILLOP, L. M., M. J. Australia *1:*260-263, March 3, '28
Radium and radon in treatment of epithelioma of lips. SIMPSON, F. E. AND FLESHER, R. E. Arch. Physical Therapy *9:*207-208, May '28
Epithelioma of lip; case from Postgraduate Hospital, New York City. ANDERSON, N. P. Physical Therap. *46:*350-352, July '28
Radium and radon in treatment of epithelioma of lips. SIMPSON, F. E. AND FLESHER, R. E. Illinois M. J. *54:*48-50, July '28
Cancer of lower lip; operative technic in plastic repair. FAIRCHILD, F. R. Arch. Surg. *17:*630-640, Oct '28
Cutaneous epithelioma developing rapidly on upper lip after diathermic treatment of supposed verruca carnea; case. HECHT, H. Dermat. Wchnschr. *88:*501-502, April 6, '29
Cancer of lips; treatment by radium needles. BROWN, R. G., M. J. Australia *1:*421-423, March 30, '29
Epithelioma of lips; radium therapy. LENTH, V. Radiol. Rev. and Chicago M. Rec. *51:*132-135, March '29

Cancer, Lip—Cont.
Treatment of cancer of lips. QUICK, D. Am. J. Roentgenol. *21:*322-327, April '29
End-results of irradiation of cancer of lips; based on study of 173 cases, January 1914 to January 1924. SCHREINER, B. F. AND SIMPSON, B. T. Radiol. Rev. and Chicago M. Rec. *51:*235-245, June '29
Results of radium treatment of epithelioma of lips; statistics. LACASSAGNE, A. Arch. d'electric. med. *39:*358-366, Oct '29
Cancer of lips. BONÀ, T. Cluj. med. *10:*652-656, Dec 1, '29
Electrothermic surgery of cancer of lips. STEVENS, J. T. Am. J. Surg. *7:*831-835, Dec '29
Rational therapy for cancer of lower lip. FISCHEL, E. Tr. South. S. A. (1929) *42:*306-321, '30
Cancer of lips. JAMES, W. D. Am. J. Surg. *8:*593-597, March '30
Epithelioma of lip with visceral metastases. WRIGHT-SMITH, R. J., J. Coll. Surgeons, Australasia *2:*421-424, March '30
Early diagnosis and treatment of cancer of lips and mouth. FIGI, F. A. Minnesota Med. *13:*788-792, Nov '30
Radium treatment of early epithelioma of lips. HAILEY, H. South. M. J. *23:*1121-1125, Dec '30
X-ray therapy as conservative method in cancer of lower lip. MARTIN, J. M. Proc. Internat. Assemb. Inter-State Post-Grad. M. A., North America (1930) *6:*399-403, '31
Treatment of bulky lesions of lips by combination of external and interstitial irradiation. DUFFY, J. J. Am. J. Cancer *15:*246-254, Jan '31
Treatment of uncomplicated primary carcinoma of lips. HAAGENSEN, C. D. Am. J. Cancer *15:*239-245, Jan '31
Bulky carcinoma of lip treated by irradiation, wide surgical excision and plastic closure. MARTIN, H. E. Am. J. Cancer *15:*261-266, Jan '31
Differential diagnosis of cancer of lip. NELSON, P. A. Am. J. Cancer *15:*230-238, Jan '31
Special clinic on epithelioma of lips. QUICK, D. Am. J. Cancer *15:*229-270, Jan '31
Treatment of cancer of lips. FISCHEL, E. Colorado Med. *28:*57-61, Feb '31
Etiology of cancer of lips. FRIEDRICH, R. Wien. klin. Wchnschr. *44:*177-179, Feb 6, '31
Epithelioma of lip. FINNERUD, C.W., M. Clin. North America *14:*1148-1150, March '31
Malignancy of lower lip complicated by mouth infections. WILSON, S. J. South. M. J. *24:*359-363, April '31

Cancer, Lip – Cont.
Treatment of cancer of lips. MONTGOMERY, D. W. AND CULVER, G. D., M. J. and Rec. *133:*573-575, June 17, '31
Rational therapy for lower lip cancer. FISCHEL, E. Am. J. Cancer *15:*1321-1337, July '31
Squamous-celled epithelioma of lower lip; radium therapy. HAILEY, H., J. M. A. Georgia *20:*386-388, Oct '31
Report of 88 cases of cancer of lips from Steiner Clinic. STEWART, C. B. Surg., Gynec. and Obst. *53:*533-535, Oct '31
Radium treatment of cancer of lips. VAN STUDDIFORD, M. T. New Orleans M. and S. J. *84:*252-259, Oct '31
Plastic reconstruction of lower lip in cancer. DALAND, E. M. New England J. Med. *205:*1131-1142, Dec 10, '31
Epithelioma of mucous membrane of lower lip; recovery after radium therapy complicated by partial necrosis of inferior maxilla; case. HOCHE, L. AND ROY. Bull. Assoc. franc. p. l'etude du cancer, *21:*381-384, May '32
Cheiloplasty for advanced carcinoma. MARTIN, H. E. Surg., Gynec. and Obst. *54:*914-922, June '32
Diagnosis of cancer of lips. WHITEHILL, N. M. J. Iowa M. Soc. *22:*533-534, Nov '32
Therapy of cancer of lower lip. RUBINROT, S. Nowotwory *7:*240-244, '32
Analysis of 137 cases of cancer of lips treated in services of department of laryngology of Instituto del Cancer in Havana. GROS, J. C. Bol. Liga contra el cancer *8:*8-11, Jan '33
Radical treatment of cancer of lips. BLAIR, V. P.; BROWN, J. B., AND HAMM, W. G. Am. J. Roentgenol. *29:*229-233, Feb '33
Surgical and radiotherapy of cancer of lips. HARRISON, R. S. Strahlentherapie *46:*401-434, '33 abstr: Schweiz. med. Wchnschr. *63:*159-162, Feb 18, '33
Surgical management of cancer of lips. SMITH, F. Surg., Gynec. and Obst. *56:*782-785, April '33
Idiopathic (glandular and exfoliative) cheilitis; relation to epithelioma of lower lip; case. GAY PRIETO, J. AND CAZORLA ROMERO, J. Actas dermo-sif. *25:*700-706, May '33
Radium therapy of cancer of lips, with especial consideration of permanent results. ARTZ, L. AND FUHS, H. Wien. klin. Wchnschr. *46:*706-708, June 9, '33
Cancer of lower lip in child 9 years old. ABDANSKI, A. Rev. de chir., Paris *52:*557-559, July '33

Cancer, Lip – Cont.
Report of results of treatment at Collis P. Huntington Memorial Hospital from 1918-1926, cancer of lip. LUND, C. C. AND HOLTON, H. M. Am. J. Roentgenol. *30:*59-66, July '33
Five-year end-results obtained by radiation treatment of cancer of lips. SCHREINER, B. F. AND MATTICK, W. L. Am. J. Roentgenol. *30:*67-74, July '33
Treatment and results of cancer of lips; 130 cases. WANGENSTEEN, O. H. AND RANDALL, O. S. Am. J. Roentgenol. *30:*75-81, July '33
Operation for epithelioma of lips. WEBSTER, J. P. Am. J. Roentgenol. *30:*82-88, July '33
Clinicopathologic analysis of 77 cases of cancer of lips and suggestion for rational plan of treatment. HYNDMAN, O. R. Arch. Surg. *27:*250-266, Aug '33
Curability of cancer of lips. JUDD, E. S. AND PHILLIPS, J. R. Proc. Staff Meet., Mayo Clin. *8:*637-640, Oct 18, '33
Cancer of lower lip; efficient treatment by radiation. MUIR, J. Internat. J. Med. and Surg. *46:*590-591, Dec '33
Surgical therapy of cancer of lips. WIEDHOPF, O. Deutsche Ztschr. f. Chir. *238:*741-744, '33
Early diagnosis of cancer of lips. CURRY, W. A. Canad. M. A. J. *30:*50-53, Jan '34
Abrasive cheilitis; clinical and histologic study of precancerous lesions. MANGANOTTI, G. Arch. ital. di dermat., sif. *10:*25-67, Jan '34
Results of treatment of cancer of lips by electrocoagulation and irradiation. PFAHLER, G. E. AND VASTINE, J. H. Pennsylvania M. J. *37:*385-389, Feb '34
Glandular cheilitis, precancerous state of lower lip. TOURAINE, A. AND SOLENTE. Presse med. *42:*191-194, Feb 3, '34
Epitheliomas of lips; survey of 100 cases. DELREZ, L. AND DESAIVE, P. Liege med. *27:*2057-2085, Oct 7, '34
Epithelioma of lower lip; results of treatment. FIGI, F. A. Surg., Gynec. and Obst. *59:*810-819, Nov '34
Standard methods of treatment of cancer of lips by surgery and radiation. FISCHEL, E. Surg., Gynec. and Obst. *60:*505-512, Feb (no. 2A) '35
Epithelioma of lips; 385 cases. IACOBOVICI, I. AND ONACA. Rev. de chir., Bucuresti *38:*1-16, March-April '35
Cancer of lip and intra-oral mucous membrane. FRANK, L. W. South. Surgeon *4:*444-456, Dec '35
Surgical therapy of cancer of lips. NARBUTOVSKIY, S. D. Novy khir. arkhiv. *33:*3-14, '35

Cancer, Lip—Cont.
Treatment of carcinoma of lip. HOLLANDER, L. Arch. Phys. Therapy *17:*17–24, Jan '36
Diagnosis and treatment of cancer of lip, mouth and throat. CHRISTIE, A. C. Fortschr. a. d. Geb. d. Rontgenstrahlen *53:*529–534, March '36
General considerations, pathology, clinical picture and diagnosis of cancer of lips. PADGETT, E. C. Internat. J. Orthodontia *22:*387–394, April '36
Cheiloplasty in cancer of lips. PADGETT, E. C. Internat. J. Orthodontia *22:*939–947, Sept '36
Late results of operation for carcinoma of lower lip. KOGON, A. I. Novy khir. arkhiv *37:*227–240, '36
Treatment of early carcinoma of lip, with special reference to use of low kilovoltage x-rays. BELISARIO, J. C., M. J. Australia *1:*91–95, Jan 16, '37
Results of therapy in four hundred and twenty-five cases of cancer of lips followed from one to ten years. WILE, U. J. AND HAND, E. A., J.A.M.A. *108:*374–382, Jan 30, '37
Malignancy and potential malignancy of lower lip. KENNEDY, R. H., S. Clin. North America *17:*297–301, Feb '37
Cancer of lower lip; technic of surgical therapy. MARINO, H. Rev. de cir. de Buenos Aires *16:*53–62, Feb '37
Diagnosis and treatment of cancer of lips. JORSTAD, L. H. Radiol. Rev. and Mississippi Valley M. J. *59:*63–64, March '37
Radiation therapy of cancer of lips. KAPLAN, I. I. Radiology *28:*533–543, May '37
Treatment of epithelioma of lip by electrodesiccation technic and preliminary report of results during past 5 years. MORROW, H. *et al.* Arch. Dermat. and Syph. *35:*821–830, May '37
Cancer of lip and oral cavity and skin. HOLLANDER, L. Pennsylvania M. J. *40:*749–750, June '37
Interstitial radium treatment of cancer of lips; review of 71 cases. DE MONCHAUX, C. M. J. Australia *2:*221–225, Aug 7, '37
Life expectancy and incidence; carcinoma of lip and oral cavity. WELCH, C. E. AND NATHANSON, I. T. Am. J. Cancer *31:*238–252, Oct '37
Technic of resection of lower lip in cancer; cases. BREYTFUS, F. F. Khirurgiya, no. 5, pp. 61–62, '37
Radical inferior cheiloplasty for advanced carcinoma of lower lip; 2 cases. WIRTH, J. E. Northwest Med. *37:*109–112, April '38

Cancer, Lip—Cont.
Malignant tumors of upper and lower lip treated at Oncologic Institute of Leningrad in past 10 years. SHANIN, A. P. Vestnik khir. *57:*43–62, Jan '39
Treatment of cancer of lips. PADGETT, E. C. J. Missouri M. A. *36:*154–157, April '39
Clinical and pathologic study of 390 cases lip cancer, with report of 5 year cures. NEWELL, E. T., JR. Arch. Surg. *38:*1014–1029, June '39
Repair of large defects of lips after removal for cancer. DALAND, E. M. Surg., Gynec. and Obst. *69:*347–357, Sept '39
Superficial cancer of lip. TRUEHEART, M., J. Kansas M. Soc. *40:*419, Oct '39
Treatment of cancer of lips. SHARP, G. S. AND SMITH, H. D. West. J. Surg. *47:*695–705, Dec '39
Reconstruction of lip after cancer. BOYER, B. E., J. Med. *20:*543–544, Feb '40
Prophylaxis, diagnosis and treatment of cancer of lips. HUNT, H. B. Nebraska M. J. *25:*133, April; 187, May '40
Management of cancer of lips. WILSON, H. Memphis M. J. *15:*80–82, May '40
Method of therapy of cancer of lower lip. GEXTIN, F. L. Novy khir. arkhiv *46:*52–59, '40
Carcinoma of lower lip; interval statistical survey of end-results in all cases treated at Brooklyn Cancer Institute, 1930 to 1939 inclusive. HOWES, W. E. AND LA ROSA, F. J. Am. J. Roentgenol. *47:*39–49, Jan '42
Epidermoid carcinoma of lower lip; case with recovery and survival for 14 years after surgical therapy. MONTEIRO, A. Acta med., Rio de Janeiro *9:*51–58, Feb '42
Cancer of lips. DUNNE, R. E. Connecticut M. J. *6:*175–176, March '42
Results of irradiation treatment for cancer of lips; analysis of 636 cases from 1926–1936. SCHREINER, B. F. AND CHRISTY, C. J. Radiology *39:*293–297, Sept '42
Repair of extensive loss of substance of lower lip (due to cancer). VIANNA, J. B. Hospital, Rio de Janeiro *23:*69–79, Jan '43
Clinical study of 778 cases of cancer of lips with particular regard to predisposing factors and radium therapy. EBENIUS, B. Acta radiol., supp. 48, pp. 1–232, '43
Study of 56 5-year cases of cancer of lips. WHITCOMB, C. A. Am. J. Surg. *63:*304–315, March '44
Cancer of lips. CAZAP, S. Bol. Inst. de med. exper. para el estud. y trat. d. cancer *21:*215–188, April '44
Treatment of epithelioma of lips. LINDBERG, L. Arizona Med. *1:*128–130, May–June '44

Cancer, Lip – Cont.

Cancer of lips. DOUGLAS, S. J. Brit. J. Radiol. *17:*185-189, June '44

Cancer of lips. GARLAND, J. G. AND DAVIES, J. A. Marquette M. Rev. *9:*113-118, June '44

Lip carcinoma. ECKERT, C. T. AND PETRY, J. L., S. Clin. North America *24:*1064-1076, Oct '44

Cancer of lips. FREEMAN, D. B. Illinois M. J. *87:*94-96, Feb '45

Acute epithelioma of lip; case. MERCADAL PEYRI, J. AND PEDRAGOSA, R. Actas dermosif. *36:*521-526, Feb '45

Cancer, Lupus

Spinocellular epithelioma of cheek in patient with old lupus. VIGNE, P. Marseille med. *2:*369-371, Dec 15, '30

Extensive lupus erythematosus with subsequent carcinoma of lower lip (case). GRAHAM-LITTLE, E. Proc. Roy. Soc. Med. *25:*1741, Oct '32

Cancer, Lymph Nodes: See Neck Dissections

Cancer, Metastases: See Neck Dissections

Cancer, Mouth (See also Cancer, Cheek)

Surgery in cancer of mouth and throat. HEIDRICH, L. Beitr. z. klin. Chir. *128:*310-347, '23 abstr: J.A.M.A. *80:*1348, May 5, '23

Carcinoma of floor of mouth. QUICK, D. Am. J. Roentgenol. *10:*461-470, June '23 (illus.)

Cancer of mouth. GRANT, W. W. Colorado Med. *20:*248-251, Sept '23 (illus.)

Treatment of precancerous and cancerous lesions in mouth. SCHMIDT, W. H. New York M. J. *118:*732-737, Dec 19, '23 (illus.)

Malignancies of oral cavity. PETTIT, J. A. Northwest Med. *23:*153-157, April '24

Radium emanation in treatment of intra-oral cancer; with report of 141 cases. SIMPSON, F. E. AND FLESHER, R. E. Tr. Sect. Dermat. and Syphil., A.M.A., pp. 120-129, '25

Epithelioma of face and buccal cavity. WETZEL, J. O. New York State J. Med. *26:*634-639, July 15, '26

Cancer of skin and mouth. KING, J. M., J. Tennessee M. A. *19:*115-121, Sept '26

Technique of operations for carcinoma of buccal mucous membranes. PÓLYA, E. Surg., Gynec. and Obst. *43:*343-354, Sept '26

Cancer of mouth; results of treatment by operation and radiation; 376 cases observed at Massachusetts General and Collis P. Huntington Memorial Hospitals in three-year period, 1918-1920. SIMMONS, C. C. Surg., Gynec. and Obst. *43:*377-382, Sept '26

Precancerous lesions of oral cavity and their treatment. BASS, H. H. Internat. J. Med. and Surg. *40:*321-323, Aug '27

Surgery of cancer of mouth. JUDD, E. S. AND NEW, G. B. Radiology *9:*380-383, Nov '27

Treatment of cancer of mucosa of cheek. HÜNERMANN, T. Deutsche Ztschr. f. Chir. *203-204:*332-336, '27

Carcinoma of mucosa of cheek treated surgically; 10 cases. SERAFINI, G. AND ANTONIOLI, G. M. Gior. d. r. Accad. di med. di Torino *91:*51-56, Jan-March '28 also: Minerva med. (pt. 2) *8:*599-610, Sept 15, '28

Cancer in and about mouth; 211 cases. BLAIR, V. P.; BROWN, J. B., AND WOMACK, N. A. Ann. Surg. *88:*705-724, Oct '28

Cancer in and about mouth; study of 211 cases. BLAIR, V. P.; BROWN, J. B., AND WOMACK, N. A. Tr. Am. S. A. *46:*395-414, '28

Management of intra-oral cancers at Radium Institute of University of Paris. PACK, G. T. Ann. Surg. *90:*15-25, July '29

Five year end-results of radiation treatment of cancer of oral cavity, nasopharynx and pharynx, based on study of 309 cases, 1912-1923. SCHREINER, B. F. AND SIMPSON, B. T. Radiol. Rev. and Chicago M. Rec. *51:*327-332, Aug '29

Carcinoma of mouth and lip. LELAND, G. A. New England J. Med. *201:*1196-1199, Dec 12, '29

Plastic surgery of floor of mouth after excision of malignant tumors. GAIDUKOFF, M. F. Odessky M. J. *4:*332-334, '29

Cancer in and about mouth; study of 211 cases. BLAIR, V. P.; *et al.* Internat. J. Orthodontia *16:*188-209, Feb '30

Necessity of early diagnosis and early treatment of cancer of mouth for effective therapy; 202 cases treated in hospitals of Eastern Switzerland from 1919-1928. SCHÜRCH, O. Schweiz. med. Wchnschr. *60:*96-101, Feb 1, '30

Treatment of malignant tumors of mouth and throat. FIGI, F. A. Am. J. Roentgenol. *23:*648-653, June '30

Intraoral cancer and its treatment. SOILAND, A. AND MELAND, O. N. California and West. Med. *33:*559-562, Aug '30

Principles of and results in radium treatment of buccal carcinoma. BIRKETT, G. E. Canad. M. A. J. *23:*780-784, Dec '30

Results of treatment of cancer of mouth in 82 cases. SEGALE, G. C. Arch. ed atti d. Soc. ital. di chir. *36:*770, '30

Position of surgery and radium in treatment

Cancer, Mouth – Cont.

of cancer of mouth. PADGETT, E. C., J. Kansas M. Soc. *32:*167–172, May '31

Radiation therapy of cancer of lips and mouth. MARTIN, J. M. Radiology *16:*881–892, June '31

Analysis of cases at Pondville Hospital; cancer of lip and mouth. TAYLOR, G. W. Am. J. Cancer (supp.) *15:*2380–2385, July '31

Cancer in and about mouth, treated with irradiation by European method. MARTIN, C. L. AND MARTIN, J. M. Texas State J. Med. *27:*286–291, Aug '31

Malignant and other growths about mouth. LYONS, C. J., J. Am. Dent. A. *20:*3–16, Jan '33

Summary of 65 "cures" of cancer about mouth. BLAIR, V. P. Surg., Gynec. and Obst. *56:*469, Feb (no. 2A) '33

Carcinoma of buccal mucosa; end results 1918–1926. LUND, C. C. AND HOLTON, H. M. New England J. Med. *208:*775–780, April 13, '33

Carcinoma of mucosa of cheek treated by irradiation only; patient living and free of disease 5 years, 3 months. MARTIN, H. E. S. Clin. North America, *13:*442–443, April '33

Carcinoma of mouth and its treatment. STACY, H. S., M. J. Australia *1:*549–550, May 6, '33

Carcinoma of lip and mouth. MARTIN, C. L. Radiology *22:*136–146, Feb '34

Cancer of mouth. BROWN, J. B. South. Surgeon *3:*47–52, March '34

Carcinoma of buccal mucosa; analysis of cases observed at Massachusetts General Hospital in 3 year period 1924–1926. TAYLOR, G. W. Surg., Gynec. and Obst. *58:*914–916, May '34

Role of surgery in carcinoma of buccal cavity. STACY, H. S., M. J. Australia *1:*712–717, June 2, '34

Cancer of mouth. FIGI, F. A., S. Clin. North America *15:*1233–1240, Oct '35

Malignant disease of mouth and accessory structures. NEW, G. B. Am. J. Surg. *30:*46–52, Oct '35

Cancer of mouth. FIGI, F. A., J. Am. Dent. A. *23:*216–224, Feb '36

Epidermoid carcinoma of mouth; general considerations and etiologic factors. PADGETT, E. C. Internat. J. Orthodontia *22:*283–293, March '36

Pathology, clinical features and diagnosis of cancer of mouth. PADGETT, E. C. Internat. J. Orthodontia *22:*504–515, May '36

Results and prognosis of cancer in and about oral cavity. PADGETT, E. C. Internat. J. Orthodontia *22:*1255–1267, Dec '36

Early diagnosis and therapy of cancer of mouth. LINDEMANN, A. Ztschr. f. Stomatol. *35:*145–171, Jan 22, '37

Management of cancer in and about oral cavity. PADGETT, E. C. Internat. J. Orthodontia *23:*73–82, Jan '37

Diagnosis and treatment of malignancy of mouth. FITZGERALD, L. M., J. Am. Dent. A. *24:*763–770, May '37

Our responsibility toward oral cancer. BLAIR, V. P.; BROWN, J. B., AND BYARS, L. T. Ann. Surg. *106:*568–576, Oct '37

Cancer of lip and mouth. HAY, A. W. S. Manitoba M. A. Rev. *18:*231–234, Dec '38

Cancer of the Face and Mouth. BLAIR, V. P., MOORE, S., AND BYARS, L. T., C. V. Mosby Co., St. Louis, 1941

Cancer of mouth (and face). BLAIR, V. P. AND BYARS, L. T. Texas State J. Med. *38:*641–645, March '43

Cancer of floor of mouth. KAPLAN, I. I., J. Am. Dent. A. *30:*737–740, May 1 '43

Cancer of mouth and jaws (with emphasis on therapy). SOMERVELL, T. H. Indian J. Surg. (no. 2) *5:*5–28, June '43

Therapy of malignant tumors of mouth at Bern. RUEDI, J. AND MINDER, W. Pract. oto-rhino-laryng. *6:*113–114, '44

Carcinoma of oral cavity; 10 year survey in general hospital. LAWRENCE, E. A. AND BREZINA, P. S., J.A.M.A. *128:*1012–1016, Aug 4, '45

Carcinoma of buccal mucosa. BURFORD, W. N. AND ACKERMAN, L. V. Am. J. Orthodontics (Oral Surg. Sect.) *31:*547–551, Sept '45

Present day treatment of cancer of mouth. MAYNE, W. Am. J. M. Sc. *210:*548–554, Oct '45

Cancer of oral mucosa and circumoral areas. MASUDA, B. J. Am. J. Orthodontics (Oral Surg. Sect.) *31:*730–740, Dec '45

Cancer, Neck: See Neck Dissections

Cancer, Nevi

Moles, pigmented and nonpigmented, and other skin defects in precancerous stage. BLOODGOOD, J. C. Northwest Med. *28:*543–547, Dec '29

Cutaneous epithelioma developed on pigmented nevi. HALKIN, H. Cancer, Bruxelles *9:*241–247, '32

Use of cobra venom in generalized nevocarcinoma; case. PRUD'HOMME, E., J. de l'Hotel-Dieu de Montreal *4:*372–378, Dec '35

Cancer, Nevi – Cont.

Diathermocoagulation as only therapy for nevocarcinoma. JOLY, M. Bull. et mem. Soc. de med. de Paris *140:*70–71, Jan 25, '36

Epitheliomas developing on pigmented nevi and pigmented epitheliomas; cases. HALKIN, H. Paris med. *1:*242–249, March 30, '37

Nevocarcinoma of eyelids and conjunctiva. VEIL, P. Bull. med., Paris *51:*371–375, May 29, '37

Nevocarcinoma of cheek in child 3 years old. PERIN, L. AND BLAIRE, G. Rev. franc. de dermat. et de venereol. *13:*491–499, Dec '37

Question of relationship between nevus and carcinoma. BEEK, C. H. Nederl. tijdschr. v. geneesk. *82:*1199–1203, March 12, '38

Giant nevus with malignant degeneration; case. PINHEIRO, J. AND BARRETO NETO, M. Arq. Serv. nac. doen. ment., pte. 1, pp. 173–205, '43

Cancer, Nose

Clinical study of carcinoma of nose. SUTTON, R. L., J.A.M.A. *77:*1561, Nov 12, '21

Basocellular epithelioma of nose. GATÉ, J. AND MASSIA, G. Bull. Soc. franc. de dermat. et syph. *33:*668–673, Nov '26

Therapy of epitheliomas of septum of nose. GROS, J. C. Bol. Liga contra el cancer *12:*148–154, May '37

Epithelioma of nose in girl of 15. FOLLMANN, E. Dermat. Wchnschr. *85:*940–943, July 2, '27

Cancer of nose and mouth, with special reference to treatment by irradiation. EWING, J. Radiology *9:*359–365, Nov '27

Payment epithelial cancer of nasal cavity cured by roentgen treatment; case. MAYER, O. Wien. med. Wchnschr. *78:*587, April 28, '28

Infiltrating cancer of nose; acute evolution; treatment by radium; case. MARTÍNEZ, E. AND PUENTE DUANY, N. Bol. de la Liga contra el cancer *3:*145–149, July 1, '28

Cure of epithelioma of nose with Bucky's border rays (grenz rays). BUCKY, G. Arch. f. Dermat. u. Syph. *155:*109–111, '28

One stage plastic surgery after removal of epithelioma of nose and contiguous areas. KURTZAHN, H. Beitr. z. klin. Chir. *144:*50–57, '28

Operative treatment of radium resistant epitheliomata; cases. (of nose.) HAUTANT, A. AND MONOD, O. Ann. d. mal. de l'oreille, du larynx *49:*394–410, April '30

Surgical diathermy of cancer of nose. HESSE, W. Deutsche med. Wchnschr. *56:*1479–1481, Aug 29, '30

Cancer, Nose – Cont.

Rhinophyma with carcinomatous degeneration; case. NOVY, F. G. JR. Arch. Dermat. and Syph. *22:*270–273, Aug '30

Radium therapy of cancer of nose. MORAN, H. M., M. J. Australia *2:*814–817, Dec 20, '30

Operation followed by radium therapy in epithelioma of nasal septum; 2 cases. SAKON, H. Ann. d'oto-laryng., pp. 55–60, Jan '31

Epithelioma on bridge of nose; case. DERR, J. S. Radiology *16:*955–956, June '31

Destruction of nose and part of face by squamous-celled carcinoma of rodent ulcer type. RIDOUT, C. A. S. Proc. Roy. Soc. Med. *25:*1767, Oct '32

Curability of carcinoma of skin of nose. ERICKSEN, L. G., J. Iowa M. Soc. *25:*309–311, June '35

Reparation of loss of substance due to electrosurgical therapy of nasofacial cancer. PRUDENTE, A. Rev. oto-laring. de Sao Paulo (no. 5, bis) *4:*749–810, Sept–Oct '36

Treatment of cancer of nose. KING, E. Ohio State M. J. *36:*627–628, June '40

Early diagnosis and therapy of cancer of nose. GROS, J. C. Bol. Liga contra el cancer *15:*305–311, Nov '40

Plastic surgery in exeresis of epitheliomas of dorsum of nose. SILVEIRA, L. M. Arq. de cir. clin. e exper. *6:*573–577, April–June '42

Epithelioma of nose; free graft of whole skin; case. MALBEC, E. F. Prensa med. argent. *29:*1763–1765, Nov 4, '42

Free full thickness skin graft in nasal cancer; case. MALBEC, E. F. Semana med. *2:*1489–1491, Dec 17, '42

Restoration of ala nasi following its excision for cancer. AUBRY, M. AND DUCOURTIOUX, M. pp. 89–92, July–Sept '44

Cancer, Parotid

Operation on two cases of secondary carcinoma and on one case of primary cystadenoma of parotid gland; relation of lobes of parotid to facial nerve. MC WHORTER, G. L. S. Clin. N. Amer. *7:*489–505, June '27

Parotid gland cancer, surgical therapy, recurrence and cure by radiotherapy. BELOT, J. AND MÉNÉGAUX, G., J. de radiol. et d'electrol. *15:*90–91, Feb '31

Cancer of parotid gland, indications and technic for total removal; 2 cases. SANTOS, M. Bol. do coll. brasil. de cir. *3:*10–20, April–July '32

Questions of malignancy of parotid tumors, diagnosis and therapy. FRENYÓ, L. Deutsche Ztschr. f. Chir. *235:*130–139, '32

Cancer, Parotid – Cont.
Cancer of parotid in new-born. MC KNIGHT, H. A. Am. J. Surg. *45:*128–130, July '39

Cancer, Pharynx
Treatment of malignant tumors of pharynx and nasopharynx. NEW, G. B. Surg., Gynec. and Obst. *40:*177–182, Feb '25
Repair of defects after operation on pharynx for removal of malignant tumours. COLLEDGE, L. Proc. Roy. Soc. Med. (sect. Laryng.) *24:*14–17, Feb '31 also: J. Laryng. and Otol. *46:*409–413, June '31
Highly malignant tumors of pharynx and nasopharynx. NEW, G. B. Tr. Am. Acad. Ophth. *36:*39–44, '31
Highly malignant tumors of pharynx and base of tongue; identification and treatment. NEW, G. B. *et al.* Surg., Gynec. and Obst. *54:*164–174, Feb '32
Selection of treatment of cancer of pharynx. FIGI, F. A. Radiol. Rev. and Mississippi Valley M. J. *58:*13–19, Jan '36
Diagnosis and therapy of malignant tumors of nasopharynx. GERLINGS, P. G. AND DEN HOED, D. Nederl. tijdschr. v. geneesk. *81:*581–589, Feb 6, '37
Cancer of pharynx, treatment and its results. COLLEDGE, L. Brit. M. J. *2:*167–168, July 23, '38
Surgical therapy of laryngopharyngeal cancer. AUBRY, M. Ann. d'oto-laryng., pp. 905–908, Nov–Dec '39
Malignant tumors of nasopharynx; anatomicopathologic study. VILLATA, I. Oto-rinolaring. ital. *10:*106–151, March '40
Surgical therapy of cancer of hypopharynx. ALONSO, J. M. An. Fac. de med. de Montevideo *28:*81–818, '43
Total pharynogoplasty in cancer. MARINO, H. Prensa med. argent. *31:*1509–1516, Aug 9, '44

Cancer, Radiation Dermatitis
Electrocoagulation of desiccation in treatment of keratoses and malignant degeneration which follow radiodermatitis. PFAHLER, G. E. Am. J. Roentgenol. *13:*41–48, Jan '25
Cancer of hand in radiologist, cured by diathermo-coagulation; case. BORDIER, H. Cancer, Bruxelles *4:*328–330, '27
Symposium on cancer: radiation damage to tissue and its repair. DALAND, E. M. Surg., Gynec. and Obst. *72:*372–383, Feb (no. 2A) '41
Skin grafts in extirpation of cancer due to roentgen irradiation. PEYRI, J. Actas dermo-sif. *32:*736–738, May '41
Subtotal replacement of skin of face for acti-

Cancer, Radiation Dermatitis – Cont.
nodermatitis due to roentgenotherapy with multiple areas of squamous cell carcinoma. JENKINS, H. P. Ann. Surg. *122:*1042–1048, Dec '45

Cancer, Skin (See also Cancer, Basal Cell; Skin, Cancer)
Squamous-cell epithelioma of skin. BRODERS, A. C. Ann. Surg. *73:*141, Feb '21
Caustic treatment of superficial cancer of ear, nose. CITELLI AND CALICETI. Tumori *8:*165, Aug '21 abstr: J.A.M.A. *77:*1139, Oct 1, '21
Unusual types of skin cancer with remarks on its genesis. ELIASSOW, A. Dermat. Wchnschr. *78:*365–370, March 29, '24
Precancerous eruptions of skin. KNOWLES, F. C., J. Iowa M. Soc. *14:*403–407, Sept '24
Cancerous and precancerous conditions of the skin. MACCORMAC, H. Brit. M. J. *2:*457–460, Sept 13, '24
Cancerous and precancerous conditions of the skin. SAVATARD, L. Brit. M. J. *2:*460–463, Sept 13, '24
Treatment of skin cancer. PFAHLER, G. E. New York M. J. *116:*553–555, Nov 15, '22
Precancerous dermatoses, report of case. FUKAMACHI, T. Arch. Dermat. and Syph. *10:*714–721, Dec '24
Superficial epitheliomas of skin. MARTINOTTI, L. Arch. ital. di chir. *10:*471–556, '24
Electrocoagulation and desiccation of surface malignancies. PLANK T. H. Physical Therap. *44:*363–367, July '26
Cancer of skin of face and neck. LOUNSBERRY, C. R. California and West. Med. *26:*800–801, June '27
Treatment of surface cancers of face with scraping and roentgen therapy; value in relation to other methods. BELOT, J. AND BUHLER, Y. E. Rev. d'actinol. *6:*91–107, March–April '30
Old and new facts about Chaoul method of close exposure (plesioroentgenotherapy) for cancer of skin and lip; 42 cases. LIEBMANN, G. Dermat. Wchnschr. *104:*293–300, March 6, '37
Recurrent epithelioma of arm; method of covering defect after radical excision illustrating 2 useful types of skin transplantation. GARLOCK, J. H., J. Mt. Sinai Hosp. *5:*75–78, July–Aug '38
Therapy of external cancer by extirpation and Padgett grafts. FERRARI, R. C. AND VIACAVA, E. P. Bol. y trab., Acad. argent. de cir. *28:*959–970, Oct 18, '44
Closure of defects of skin after surgery for cancer. MAY, H. Clinics *4:*53–62, June '45

Cancer, Skin—Cont.
Common precanceroses of skin. DUNCAN, C. S. West Virginia M. J. *42:*299-301, Dec '46

Cancer, Tongue

Carcinoma of tongue; general principles involved in operations and results obtained at Mayo Clinic. JUDD, E. S. AND NEW, G. B. Surg., Gynec. and Obst. *36:*163-169, Feb '23 (illus.)
Radium therapy of cancer of tongue; 143 cases. CAPIZZANO, N. Rev. med. latino-am. *13:*464-470, Dec '27
Cancer of tongue and floor of mouth. DORRANCE, G. M. AND MC SHANE, J. K. Ann. Surg. *88:*1007-1021, Dec '28
Analysis of 138 cases of cancer of tongue treated at Instituto del Cancer in Havana. MARTÍNEZ, E. Bol. Liga contra el cancer *8:*12-21, Jan '33
Cancer of tongue and lower jaw. NEW, G. B. Tr. Am. Laryng., Rhin. and Otol. Soc. *41:*610-613, '35
Five year end-results in treatment of cancer of tongue, lip and cheek. MARTIN, H. E. Surg., Gynec. and Obst. *65:*793-797, Dec '37
Analysis of 73 consecutive cases of tongue cancer; preliminary report. TURNER, J. W. AND RIFE, C. S. Univ. Hosp. Bull., Ann Arbor *4:*33-35, May '38
Treatment of cancer of tongue. BLAIR, V. P.; BROWN, J. B., AND BYARS, L. T., S. Clin. North America *18:*1255-1274, Oct '38
Epithelioid giant cell tumor of tongue, locally malignant; report of case. DINGMAN, R. O. J. Oral Surg. *2:*77-80, Jan '44

Cancer, Transplantation of by Skin Grafting

Cases of cancer after skin transplantation. KORKHOV, V. Vestnik khir. (no. 41) *14:*137-142, '28
Factors of resistance and receptivity in skin transplanted in epitheliomatous regions. PERAZZO, G. Gior. ital. di dermat. e sif. *7:*573-584, Dec '31
Transplantation of skin cancer by use of superficial grafts of epidermis covering epithelioma. CROSTI, A. Gior. ital. di dermat. e sif. *79:*1091-1108, Dec '38
Autogenous transplantation of fibrosarcoma during application of full-thickness skin graft. HARRELL, G. T. AND FALK, A. DET. Ann. Surg. *111:*285-291, Feb '40
Accidental transplantation of cancer (in skin of donor site) in operation room, with case report. BRANDES, W. W. *et al.* Dia. med. *18:*153-154, Feb 25, '46 also: Surg. Gynec. and Obst. *82:*212-214, Feb '46

CANESTRO, C. AND CAMPORA, G.: Hypoglossal-facial nerve anastomosis. Riv. oto-neuro-oftal. *4:*81-90, Jan-Feb '27
CANFIELD, N.: Injuries to nose, paranasal sinuses, mouth and ears. Connecticut M. J. *6:*796-798, Oct '42
CANFIELD, N.: Nose and sinuses; primary war injuries. Proc. Roy. Soc. Med. *38:*627-628, Sept '45
CANFIELD, N.: Primary war injuries involving nose and sinuses. J. Laryng. and Otol. *60:*458-460, Nov '45
CANGE, A.: Surgical treatment of entropion by method of Panas. Medecine *4:*261-262, Jan '23 abstr: J.A.M.A. *80:*1183, April 21, '35
CANGE, A. AND DUBOUCHER, H.: Lacrimal fistula. Arch. d'opht. *48:*161-185, March '31
CANIZARES, RAFAEL (see CANIZARES, RAUL) Feb '40
CANIZARES, RAUL AND CANIZARES, RAFAEL: Dermo-epidermoid graft in third degree burns. Vida nueva *45:*113-118, Feb '40
CANNADAY, J. E.: Use of cutis graft in repair of certain types of incisional herniae and other conditions. Ann. Surg. *115:*775-781, May '42
CANNADAY, J. E.: Skin transplantation; uses in surgery. Am. J. Surg. *59:*409-419, Feb '43
CANNADAY, J. E.: Skin grafts in general surgery, orthopedic surgery and gynecology. West Virginia M. J. *40:*277-282, Sept '44
CANNADAY, J. E.: Review of results in skin grafting; additional cases. Tr. South. S. A. (1944) *56:*372-386, '45
CANNADAY, J. E.: Additional report on uses of cutis graft material in reparative surgery. Am. J. Surg. *67:*382-390, Feb '45
CANNADAY, J. E.: Cutis graft in surgery; review of results obtained, with comments on indications and technic and report of cases. Arch. Surg. *52:*286-303, March '46
CANNON, A. B. (see MC LEAN, S.) Sept '25
CANNON, A. B.: Pigmented growths of skin; their significance and treatment. New York State J. Med. *29:*857-864, July 15, '29
CANNON, A. B.: Treatment of x-ray burns and other superficial disfigurements of skin (and keloids). New York State J. Med. *40:*391-399, March 15, '40
CANNON, A. B.: Treatment of common disfigurements of skin. New York State J. Med. *40:*1567-1572, Nov 1, '40
CANNON, B.: Split vermilion bordered lip flap in cleft lip. Surg., Gynec. and Obst. *73:*95-97, July '41
CANNON, B.: Use of vermilion bordered flaps in surgery about mouth. Surg., Gynec. and Obst. *74:*458-462, Feb. (no. 2A) '42

CANNON, B.: Use of vermilion bordered flaps in surgery about mouth. Am. J. Orthodontics (Oral Surg. Sect.) *28:*423–430, July '42

CANNON, B.: Care of military and civilian injuries; use of remote flaps in regarding defects of face and mouth. Am. J. Orthodontics (Oral Surg. Sect.) *29:*77–85, Feb '43

CANNON, B.: Symposium on management of Cocoanut Grove burns at Massachusetts General Hospital; procedures in rehabilitation of severely burned. Ann. Surg. *117:*903–910, June '43

CANNON, B.: Rehabilitation following severe burns; experience with victims of Boston night club (Cocoanut Grove) fire. Surgery *15:*178–185, Jan '44

CANNON, B. AND COPE, O.: Rate of epithelial regeneration; clinical method of measurement, and effect of various agents recommended in treatment.

CANNON, B. AND GRAHAM, W. C.: Plastic and reconstructive surgery of hand. Mil. Surgeon *97:*137–139, Aug '45

CANNON, B. (see BROWN, J. B.) 1944

CANNON, B. (see BROWN, J. B.) Oct '44

CANNON, B. (see BROWN, J. B.) 1945

CANNON, B. (see BROWN, J. B.) May '45

CANNON, B. (see BROWN, J. B.) (St. Louis) Mar '46

CANNON, W. B.: Studies in experimental traumatic shock; evidence of toxic factor in wound shock. Arch. Surg. *4:*1–22, Jan '22

CANNON, W. B.: Recent evidence as to nature of wound shock. Northwest Med. *21:*351–355, Sept '22

CANNON, W. B.: Traumatic shock. Sovet. khir., no. 1, pp. 3–9, '36

CANNON, W. B. AND CATTELL, McK.: Studies in experimental traumatic shock; critical level in a falling blood pressure. Arch. Surg. *4:*300–323, March '22 (illus.)

CANOSA, F.: Shock treatment in war medicine. Rev. med.-social san. y benef. munic. *2:*282–290, Oct–Dec '42

CANTONNET, A. AND VINCENT, C.: Causes and treatment of eyelid spasms and tics. Rev. gen. de clin. et de therap. *40:*787, Nov 20; 805, Nov 27, '26

CANTOR, B. B.: Prosthesis for palate; treatment of case with hollow-ball obturator. Am. J. Orthodontics (Oral Surg. Sect.) *31:*740–743, Dec '45

CAPELLI, E.: Multiple skeletal malformations and Dupuytren syndrome in congenital syphilis; case. Dermosifilografo *17:*19–32, Jan '42

CAPIZZANO, N.: Radium therapy of cancer of tongue; 143 cases. Rev. med. latino-am. *13:*464–470, Dec '27

CAPIZZANO, N.: Cancer of eyelid; radium therapy; case. Bol. Inst. de med. exper. para el estud. y trat. del cancer *4:*139, April '28

CAPIZZANO, N.: Radium therapy of cancer of larynx; results in 150 cases. Bol. Inst. de med. exper. para el estud. y trat. del cancer *10:*575–579, Oct '33

CAPONNETTO, A.: Abnormalities of nerves in palmar region of man. Monitore zool. ital. *41:*180–183, '30

CAPPA, O.: Bilateral ankylosis of mandible; case of traumatic origin; surgical therapy. Policlinico (sez. prat.) *42:*59–62, Jan 14, '35

CAPPELLETTI, A.: Beerwort in burn therapy. Semana med. *1:*815–817, March 31, '27

CAPRIO, G.: Hermaphroditisim pseudo- and true; surgical possibilities. An. d. atenecolin. quir. *7:*414–429, Aug '41

CAPRIOLI, N.: Remote result of a periosteal bone implant. Pediatria *32:*418–421, April 1, '24

CAPRIOLI, N.: Operative treatment in case of gigantic rhinophyma. Rinasc. med. *7:*144, March 15, '30

CARAMAZZA, F.: Balance ptosis of eyelids; case. Riv. oto-neuro-oft. *7:*165–177, March–April '30

CARAMAZZA, F.: Large angiomas of upper eyelid treated with surgical diathermy. Boll. d'ocul. *13:*742–753, June '34

CARANDO, V.; GALANTE, E. AND ROBBIO CAMPOS, J.: Complications of submucosal resection (Killian operation). Semana med. *1:*225–227, Jan 21, '37

CARBISULPHOIL COMPANY: Burn therapy with foille not acceptable for N. N. R., J.A.M.A. *117:*363–365, Aug 2, '41

Carbon Dioxide Freezing

Treatment of angiomas with carbon dioxide snow and electrolysis. TRIER, K. Hospitalstid. *68:*117–118, Feb 5, '25

Carbon dioxide snow in treatment of keloids. RAMIREZ, V. Gac. med. de Mexico *57:*318–320, May–June '26

Carbon dioxide snow in treatment of angiomas. VENTURELLI, G. Riforma med. *42:*1039–1041, Nov 1, '26

Carbon dioxide snow in injuries of skin due to x-ray. EISNER. Zentralbl. f. Haut-u. Geschlechtskr. *24:*580, Oct 5, '27

Therapy of cutaneous angiomas with sclerosing injections of quinine and urea hydrochloride associated with cryotherapy with carbon dioxide snow. SÉZARY, A. *et al.* Presse med. *41:*260, Feb 15, '33

Therapy of small cutaneous angiomas by systematic association of cryotherapy with carbon dioxide snow and diathermy. DUR-

Carbon Dioxide Freezing – Cont.
AND. Bull. Soc. franc. de dermat. et syph. (Reunion dermat.) *41:*587-589, April '34
Treatment of angiomas with carbon dioxide snow pencil. SEMON, H. C. Lancet *1:*1167-1169, June 2, '34
Treatment of hemangiomas of skin in children by carbon dioxide snow. WRONG, N. M., Canad. M. A. J. *41:*571-572, Dec '39
Carbon dioxide snow in therapy of hemangioma. CREMER, G. Nederl. tijdschr. v. geneesk. *84:*520-524, Feb 10, '40
Therapy of "Knuckle pads" with carbon dioxide snow. ASBECK, F. Dermat. Wchnschr. *110:*457-461, June 1, '40
Failure with cryotherapy (using carbon dioxide slush) in treatment of acne scars. FRIEDLANDER, H. M. Arch. Dermat. and Syph. *46:*734-736, Nov '42

CARBONELL ANTOLI, C.: Modern aspects of burn therapy. Rev. espan. cir., traumatol. y ortop. *2:*187-202, March '45
CARCASSONNE: Syndactylia; cases. Lyon med. *143:*778, June 23, '29
CARCASSONNE, F. AND DARGENT: Sprains of fingers. Lyon med. *152:*5-8, July 2, '33
CARCASSONNE, F. AND LĒNA, A.: Value of amputation after trauma of fingers and hand. Marseille-med. *2:*643-651, Nov 25, '34
CARCASSONNE, F. (see BONNET, P.) March-April '31
CARCASSONNE, F. (see BONNET, P.) May '31
CARCASSONNE, F. (see BONNET, P.) Sept-Oct '31
CARCASSONNE, F. (see WERTHEIMER, P.) Sept-Oct '31
CARCASSONNE, F. (see TIXIER, L. *et al*) Nov-Dec '31
CARCASSONNE, F. (see DE ROUGEMONT, J.) Feb '33
CARCASSONNE, F. (see CHEVALLIER, A. *et al*) Jan '37
CARDELLE PENICHET, G. AND GARCIA LOPEZ, A.: Cystic hygroma (lymphangioma); 3 cases. Arch. de med. inf. *10:*104-117, April-June '41
CARDI, G.: Congenital malformation of hand with syndactylia and hypoplasia of fourth metacarpal bone; case. Arch. di ortop. *52:*427-434, Sept 30, '36
CARDIA, A. AND LIGAS, A.: Effects of moist-heat medication on free autoplastic skin transplants. Riv. di pat. sper. *12:*475-484, '34
CARDIN, M.: Closure of orifices of tracheotomy; Aubry procedure (graft). Ann. d'oto-laryng. *12:*305-314, April-June '45
CARDINALE, J. R. (see LIMA, E. J. *et al*) May '38
CARDWELL, E. P.: Cutaneous femoris lateralis nerve, direct implantation of free nerve grafts between facial musculature and facial trunk; first case to be reported. Arch. Otolaryng. *27:*469-471, April '38
CARILLON, R. J. (see CLAVELIN, C.) April '37
CARLING, E. R.: Construction of artificial vagina from loop of sigmoid. Brit. M. J. *1:*373-376, March 3, '34
CARLISLE, J. M.: Early treatment of thermal burns. J. M. Soc. New Jersey *40:*459-461, Dec '43
CARLSON, A. C.: Volkmann's contracture; presentation of case with moving pictures. Southwestern Med. *14:*367-368, Aug '30
CARLTON, C. H.: Factors in foot reconstruction. Lancet *2:*605-606, Sept 21, '29
CARLTON, C. H.: Case of fractured mandible complicated by infection with Streptothrix. Tr. M. Soc., London *55:*51-53, '32
CARLU, L.: Ionization of magnesium chloride in therapy of keloids and keloid cicatrices. Ann. de dermat. et syph. *5:*162-169, Feb '34 abstr: Bull. et mem. Soc. de med. de Paris *137:*478-481, June 24, '33
CARMAN, G. A. (see Schapiro, I. E. *et al*) Sept '45
CARMICHAEL, E. B. (see SEARCY, H. B. *et al*) March '44
CARMICHAEL, J. L.: Skin transplantation with especial reference to split thickness graft. J.M.A. Alabama *14:*11-13, July '44
CARMODY, J. T. B.: Repair of defects, with special reference to use of cancellous bone in cranium. New England J. Med. *234:*393-399, March 21, '46
CARMONA, L.: Autoplastic, homoplastic and heteroplastic skin grafts. Ann. ital. di chir. *6:*1234-1256, Dec '27
CARMONA, L.: Effect of thyroid injection and skin grafts in sensitized animals. Arch. ital. di chir. *21:*436-456, '28
CARNEVALE-RICCI, F.: Lateral congenital fistula of neck. Arch. ital. di otol. *45:*473-482, July '34
CARNEY, H. J.: Facial prosthesis. Am. J. Orthodontics (Oral Surg. Sect.) *27:*689-697, Dec '41
CARONES, C.: Dupuytren's contracture due to work; case. Rev. med. leg. y jurisp. med. *4:*244-247, Oct-Dec '40
CAROTHERS, J. C.: Comparison of 2 methods of skin grafting (in ulcers). East African M. J. *13:*345, Feb '37
CARP, L.: Branchial fistula; its clinical relation to irritation of vagus. Surg., Gynec. and Obst. *42:*772-777, June '26
CARP, L.: Distal anterior closed space infections of fingers. Surg., Gynec. and Obst. *46:*484-495, April '28
CARP, L. AND STOUT, A. P.: Anomalies and

neoplasms of branchial apparatus; 32 cases with follow-up results. Ann. Surg. *87:*186-209, Feb '28

Carpenter, A. R.: End-result study of 458 tendon transplantations. J. Bone and Joint Surg. *21:*921-932, Oct '39

Carpue, J. C.: Joseph Constantine Carpue and revival of rhinoplasty. Internat. Abstract Surg., pp. 275-280, Oct '30

Carr, F. J. Jr. (see Donovan, S. J.) Sept '43

Carr, M. W.: Significant developments that have contributed to advancement of oral and maxillofacial surgery. Ann. Dent. *5:*206-212, Dec '38

Carr, R. W.: Caliper for reduction of phalangeal and metacarpal fractures by skeletal traction. South. M. J. *32:*543-546, May '39

Carr, W. P.: End-results of operations for bony ankylosis of jaw. Ann. Surg. *73:*314, March '21

Carrari, G.: Plastic operations in laryngostomy; 2 cases. Arch. ital. di otol. *44:*731-737, Dec '33

Carrea, Raul M. E.: *Tratamiento quirurgico del promentonismo mandibulo-megalia y otras deformidades mandibulares.* (Tesis) University Press, Buenos Aires, 1943

Carriere, G. and Paris, J.: Clinical forms of ulnar paralysis. Gaz. d. hop. *113:*5, Jan 3-6; 21, Jan 10-13, '40

Carrington, G. L.: Molded plaster splints in treatment of hand fractures. North Carolina M. J. *3:*195-196, April '42

Carroll, W. (see Davis, L. *et al*) 1945

Carroll, W. (see Davis, L. *et al*) May '45

Carroll, W. W.: Venous surgery (skin transplantation for stasis ulcers). Quart. Bull. Northwestern Univ. M. School *20:*373-379, '46

Carruthers, F. W.: Care and treatment of harelip and cleft palate. J. Arkansas M. Soc. *25:*93-97, Oct '28

Carscadden, W. G.: Hand infections. St. Michael's Hosp. M. Bull. *4:*11-26, June '30

Carson, L. D. and Brown, J. L.: Hematoma auris. U. S. Nav. M. Bull. *32:*204-205, April '34

Cartelli, N. and Albornoz, I.: Impassable stricture of urethra; resection of 8 cm with plastic repair; case (graft). Rev. argent. de urol. *6:*242-249, May-June '37

Carter, B. N. (see Altemeier, W. A.) June '42

Carter, D. M.: Hand infections. Internat. J. Med. and Surg. *48:*187-189, May-June '35

Carter, D. M.: Minor injuries to fingers. Guy's Hosp. Gaz. *54:*142-144, May 18, '40

Carter, R. M.: Treatment of finger infections. Wisconsin M. J. *24:*312-315, Nov '25

Carter, W. W.: Recent fractures of nose; how to diagnose and treat them. Med. Rec. *101:*237-239, Feb 11, '22

Carter, W. W.: Bone surgery of nose. Surg., Gynec. and Obst. *34:*800-803, June '22 (illus.)

Carter, W. W.: Transplantation for correction of depressed deformities of nose. New York M. J. *117:*59-60, Jan 3, '23

Carter, W. W.: Value and ultimate fate of bone and cartilage transplants in correction of nasal deformities. Laryngoscope *33:*196-202, March '23 (illus.)

Carter, W. W.: Abscesses of nasal septum, their etiology and treatment with reference to resulting deformities. M. J. and Rec. *119:*11-13, Feb 6, '24

Carter, W. W.: How soon should nasal deformities, due to abscess of septum, be corrected by transplantation of bone. M. J. and Rec. *122:*247-248, Sept 2, '25

Carter, W. W.: Use of gold-wire splints in intranasal plastic surgery. Laryngoscope *35:*942-943, Dec '25

Carter, W. W.: Correction of nasal deformities. New York State J. Med. *25:*1070-1073, Dec 1, '25

Carter, W. W.: Case of developmental deformity of nose corrected by bone and cartilage transplants. Laryngoscope *36:*664-666, Sept '26

Carter, W. W.: Relation of minor injuries of nose during childhood to subsequent deformities of organ. Ann. Otol., Rhin. and Laryng. *35:*825-833, Sept '26

Carter, W. W.: Use of autogenous transplants vs. foreign bodies in correction of nasal deformities. Am. Med. *23:*363-366, May '28

Carter, W. W.: Prevention of nasal deformity following submucous resection. Arch. Otolaryng. *8:*555-563, Nov '28

Carter, W. W.: Importance of early treatment of recent nasal fractures. Am. J. Surg. *6:*51-55, Jan '29

Carter, W. W.: Prevention of deformities following submucous resection. Tr. Am. Laryng., Rhin. and Otol. Soc. *34:*123-131, '28 also: Laryngoscope *39:*52-57, Jan '29

Carter, W. W.: Relief of obstruction in children without subsequent deformity of nose. Laryngoscope *40:*55-58, Jan '30

Carter, W. W.: Relief of obstruction of nose in children due to deviation of septum. Ann. Otol., Rhin. and Laryng. *39:*199-203, March '30

Carter, W. W.: Treatment of split fingernails. M. J. and Rec. *131:*599-600, June 18, '30

Carter, W. W.: Importance of plastic surgery of nose. Laryngoscope *40:*502-506, July '30

Carter, W. W.: Transposition of section from

auricle for correction of nasal defect; case. Arch. Otolaryng. *12:*178-183, Aug '30

CARTER, W. W.: Prevention of nasal deformities (fractures). Ann. Otol., Rhin. and Laryng. *39:*696-700, Sept '30

CARTER, W. W.: Development of nose; dynamic relation to traumatic injuries and to submucous resection. Laryngoscope *42:*189-194, March '32

CARTER, W. W.: Ultimate fate of bone when transplanted into nose for purpose of correcting deformity. Arch. Otolaryng. *15:*563-573, April '32

CARTER, W. W.: Treatment of automobile accidents in cases where nose and face are involved. Ann. Otol., Rhin. and Laryng. *41:*571-575, June '32

CARTER, W. W.: Abscess (traumatic) of nasal septum in children; importance of early diagnosis and treatment. Eye, Ear, Nose and Throat Monthly *11:*352-354, Oct '32

CARTER, W. W.: Injuries to nose in automobile accidents; importance of early treatment. Eye, Ear, Nose and Throat Monthly *12:*150-152, May '33

CARTER, W. W.: Nasal obstruction in children due to septal abnormalities; what shall we do for them? Laryngoscope *43:*377-382, May '33

CARTER, W. W.: Correction of nasal deformities by plastic methods and by transplantation of bone and cartilage (from rib). Internat. J. Orthodontia *19:*1012-1016, Oct '33

CARTER, W. W.: Value of bone and cartilage grafts in rhinoplasty. Laryngoscope *43:*905-910, Nov '33

CARTER, W. W.: Treatment of traumatic injuries to nose in automobile accidents. Arch. Otolaryng. *20:*513-517, Oct '34

CARTER, W. W.: Importance of correct technic in primary treatment of nasal injuries. M. Rec. *140:*465-466, Nov 7, '34

CARTER, W. W.: Ideals in rhinoplastic surgery. Am. J. Surg. *26:*524-527, Dec '34

CARTER, W. W.: Clinical observations on influence of septum on development of nose and palatal arch. Laryngoscope *45:*355-365, May '35

CARTER, W. W.: Tattooing of nose and face following automobile injuries. New York State J. Med. *35:*573-585, June 1, '35

CARTER, W. W.: Immediate transplantation of bone, cartilage and soft tissues in accident cases. Laryngoscope *45:*730-738, Sept '35

Cartilage Grafts

Treatment of a "saddle nose" by costal cartilage graft. CAMERER, C. B., U. S. Nav. M. Bull. *15:*397, April '21

Cartilage transplantation. COUGHLIN, W. T.

Cartilage Grafts—Cont.

Southern M. J. *14:*311, April '21

Costochondral graft for repair of skull defects. HANSON, A. M. *et al.* Mil. Surgeon *48:*691, June '21

Cranioplasty with cartilage. COUGHLIN, W. T., S. Clin. N. America *2:*1627-1636, Dec '22 (illus.)

Value and ultimate fate of bone and cartilage transplants in correction of nasal deformities. CARTER, W. W. Laryngoscope *33:*196-202, March '23 (illus.)

Depressed nasal deformities, comparison of prosthetic values of paraffin, bone, cartilage and celluloid, with report of cases corrected with celluloid implants by author's method. LEWIS, J. D. Ann. Otol., Rhin. and Laryng. *32:*321-365, June '23 (illus.)

Operation of cartilage-cranioplasty. MUNROE, A. R. Canad. M. A. J. *14:*47-49, Jan '24

Costo-chondral graft for the repair of skull defects. HANSON, A. M. Minnesota Med. *7:*610-612, Sept '24

Free cartilage grafts. (nasal deformities.) RUEF, H. Med. Klinik *20:*1428-1429, Oct 12, '24 abstr: J.A.M.A. *83:*1722, Nov 22, '24

Plastic repair of "saddle nose" deformity by autogenous cartilaginous graft. CAMERER, C. B., U. S. Nav. M. Bull. *22:*186, Feb '25

Method of nasal plastic repair by cartilage graft. WATSON-WILLIAMS, E. Brit. M. J. *2:*987-988, Nov 28, '25

Case of developmental deformity of nose corrected by bone and cartilage transplants. CARTER, W. W. Laryngoscope *36:*664-666, Sept '26

Free autoplastic cartilage transplantation. MANNHEIM, A. AND ZYPKIN, B. Arch. f. klin. Chir. *141:*668-672, '26 abstr: J.A.M.A. *87:*2132, Dec 18, '26

Reconstruction of nasal bridge by means of autogenous rib cartilage grafts. GARRETSON, W. T., J. Michigan M. Soc. *26:*36-41, Jan '27

New method of obtaining costal cartilage for plastic and reconstructive surgery. KELLY, J. D. Surg., Gynec. and Obst. *44:*687-689, May '27

Rhinoplasty by cartilaginous grafts. LECLERC, G. Bull. et mem. Soc. nat. de chir. *53:*671-678, May 21, '27

Correction of pronounced types of saddle nose with mixed implants of bone and cartilage. COHEN, L. Ann. Otol., Rhin. and Laryng. *36:*639-647, Sept '27

Closure of cranial openings by cartilaginous autotransplantation. PASCALIS, G. Gaz. d. hop. *100:*1314-1316, Oct 5, '27

Cartilage Grafts – Cont.

Cartilage and ivory in plastic surgery of nose. SALINGER, S. Arch. Otolaryng. *6:*552–558, Dec '27

Autoplastic cartilage transplantation. BABSKY, A. A. AND LISIANSKAIA, V. S. Vestnik Khir. (no. 26–27) *9:*240–243, '27

Correction of pronounced types of saddle nose with mixed implants of bone and cartilage. COHEN, L. Tr. Am. Laryng., Rhin. and Otol. Soc. *33:*233–242, '27

Enucleation of eye-ball and cartilage transplantation as basis for prosthesis. FABER, A. Beitr. z. klin. Chir. *141:*524–527, '27

Late results of cartilage transplantation. MANNHEIM, A. AND ZYPKIN, B. Arch. f. klin. Chir. *149:*31–39, '27

Resector for removing shaped piece of rib cartilage for nasal transplant. FORNELL, C. H. Laryngoscope *38:*733–734, Nov '28

Orbital grafting of cartilage from nasal ala; technic. DANTRELLE, AND SHEEHAN. Ann. d'ocul. *165:*902–909, Dec '28

Necessity for transplantation of living bone and cartilage; cases. PINEDA, J. C. Rev. de med. y cir. de la Habana *33:*862, Dec 31, '28

Repair of roof of orbit by means of cartilaginous graft. RHÉAUME, P. Z. AND BABEAUX, F. Presse med. *36:*1604, Dec 15, '28

Data on autoplastic bone grafting and cartilage. GORBOUNOFF, V. P. Vestnik khir. (nos. 37–38) *13:*71–85, '28

Cartilage graft to malar bone. MOOREHEAD, F. B., S. Clin. N. Amer. *9:*331–332, April '29

Cartilage graft to nose. MOOREHEAD, F. B., S. Clin. N. Amer. *9:*327–328, April '29

Plastic operation with costal cartilage in concave nose; cases. ROY, J. N. Union med. du Canada *58:*408–414, July '29

Bridging of osseous defects of forehead, using metal models as guides for shaping cartilage transplants. RUSH, L. V. *et al.* Am. J. Surg. *7:*805–807, Dec '29

Transplantation of cartilage; experiments. FOHL, T. Arch. f. klin. Chir. *155:*232–243, '29

Transplantation of pedicled cartilaginous symphysis. RESCHKE, K. Beitr. z. klin Chir. *146:*713–720, '29

Autogenous free cartilage transplanted into joints; experimental study. HARBIN, M. AND MORITZ, A. R. Arch. Surg. *20:*885–896, June '30

Cartilaginous and osteo-cartilaginous rib grafts in correction of nasal deformities. METZ, W. R. New Orleans M. and S. J. *82:*831–840, June '30

Narrowing of wide alae of nose by reimplantation of cartilage from tip of nose. ÉRCZY, N. Ztschr. f. Hals-, Nasen-u. Ohrenh. *26:*194–197, July 3, '30

Problem of cartilage implant (face). UPDEGRAFF, H. L. Am. J. Surg. *14:*492–498, Nov '31

Lesions of jaw, nose and cheek; cleft lip and palate; cartilage transplant; tube graft. MOOREHEAD, F. B., S. Clin. North America *12:*57–66, Feb '32

Traumatic scarring and depressed fracture of right malar bone and orbital border; cartilage implant. FIGI, F. A., S. Clin. North America *12:*949–951, Aug '32

Syphilitic origin of perforation of palate and destruction of nose; uranoplasty; reconstruction of nose by tubular grafts with cartilaginous support of costal origin. ROCHER, H. L. Bull. et mem. Soc. de chir. de Bordeaux et du Sud-Ouest, pp. 150–152, '32

Cartilage and ivory; indications and contraindications for their use as nasal support. MALINIAK, J. W. Arch. Otolaryng. *17:*649–657, May '33

Restoration of shape of nose by cartilaginous autograft after old fracture. DANTLO, R. Strasbourg med. *93:*485–487, July 15, '33

New instruments for use of rib cartilage grafts in rhinoplasty. MALINIAK, J. W. Arch. Otolaryng. *18:*79–82, July '33

Correction of nasal deformities by plastic methods and by transplantation of bone and cartilage (from rib). CARTER, W. W. Internat. J. Orthodontia *19:*1012–1016, Oct '33

Value of bone and cartilage grafts in rhinoplasty. CARTER, W. W. Laryngoscope *43:*905–910, Nov '33

Cartilage autograft. BURIAN, F. Rev. de chir. plastique. pp. 15–19, May '34

Restoration of depressed nose by grafting of cartilage; 6 cases. MCINDOE, A. H. Proc. Roy. Soc. Med. *27:*1278–1284, July '34

Combined nasal plastic and chin plastic; correction of microgenia by osteocartilaginous transplant from large hump nose. AUFRICHT, G. Am. J. Surg. *25:*292–296, Aug '34

Correction of saddle nose by autograft from costal cartilage. TETU, I. AND DUMITRESCU, J. Spitalul *55:*65–66, Feb '35

Immediate transplantation of bone, cartilage and soft tissues in accident cases. CARTER, W. W. Laryngoscope, *45:*730–738, Sept '35

Two instruments for modelling transplanted cartilage in closure of laryngeal and tracheal defects. MAYER, F. J. Monatschr. f. Ohrenh. *69:*1193–1196, Oct '35

Cartilage Grafts – Cont.

Influence of parathyroid extract on calcification of tissues studied by observation of free transplants (including cartilage). LERICHE, R. *et al.* Ann. d'anat. path. *13:*551-555, May '36

Cartilage transplants in facial surgery. BAMES, H. O. Rev. de chir. structive, pp. 281-285, June '36

Preoperative and postoperative prosthesis in application of skin, cutaneomucosal, cartilage and bone grafts and in improvement of cicatrix of face. DARCISSAC, M. Bull. et mem. Soc. d. chirurgiens de Paris *28:*424-433, June 19, '36

Correction of saddle nose with ozena by endonasal inclusions of costal grafts; case. PERI, M. Rev. de chir. structive, pp. 299-302, June '36

Costal graft and ivory inclusions in reconstruction of saddle nose by transsupraciliary route. ALVES, O. Rev. oto-laring. de Sao Paulo (no. 5, bis) *4:*843-863, Sept-Oct '36

Skin, cartilage and bone grafts to face. NEW, G. B. Proc. Staff Meet., Mayo Clin. *11:*791-794, Dec 9, '36

Transplantation of hyaline cartilage. BULACH, K. Sovet. vestnik oftal. *9:*329-331, '36

Chondral autoplasty in correction of saddle nose. PRISANT, M. Folia oto-laryng. orient. *3:*205-211, '36

Repair of depressed disfiguring scars by means of rib cartilage implant. TRUSLER, H. M., J. Indiana M. A. *30:*194-196, April '37

Use of costal cartilage in restorative surgery of saddle nose; 3 cases. PERI, M. Rev. de chir. structive, pp. 103-107, June '37

Saddle nose; ivory and cartilage implants. SALINGER, S. Illinois M. J. *72:*412-417, Nov '37

Free transplantation of cartilage in rhinoplasty. DUJARDIN, E. Ugesk. f. laeger *99:*1292, Dec 2, '37

Complete avulsion of scalp and loss of right ear; reconstruction by pedunculated tube grafts and costal cartilage. CAHILL, J. A. JR. AND CAULFIELD, P. A. Surg., Gynec. and Obst. *66:*459-465, Feb (no. 2A) '38

Implantation of costal cartilage for correction of nasal deformities. GILL, E. G. Virginia M. Monthly *65:*279-281, May '38

Intolerance of cartilage grafts. THEVENIN, J. Rev. de chir. structive *8:*7-12, May '38

Principle to be considered in transplanting costal cartilage for repairing deficiencies of nasal skeleton. YOUNG, F. Ann. Surg. *108:*1113-1117, Dec '38

Laryngotracheal reconstruction with free autoplastic cartilaginous grafts. GIUSSANI, M. Arch. ital. di chir. *52:*472-483, '38

Cartilage autograft in therapy of saddle nose; case. MOERS Bull. Soc. belge d'otol., rhinol., laryng., pp. 23-24, '38

Fate of living and dead cartilage transplanted in humans. PEER, L. A. Surg., Gynec. and Obst. *68:*602-610, March '39

Plastic repair with cartilagoperiosteal bridge in drooping (or dog) ear. RIGG, J. P. AND WALDAPFEL, R., J.A.M.A. *113:*125-126, July 8, '39

Correction of saddleback deformities of nose by specially cut cartilage from ear. HARBERT, F. Arch. Otolaryng. *31:*339-341, Feb '40

Plastic surgery with cartilage for saddle nose. REHN, E. Zentralbl. f. Chir. *67:*548-550, March 30, '40

Advantage of mixed bone and cartilage grafts in correction of saddle nose and other depressed deformities of dorsum. COHEN, L. Ann. Otol., Rhin. and Laryng. *49:*410-417, June '40

Graft of costal cartilage in therapy of saddle nose; case. PEDEMONTE, P. V. Arch. urug. de med., cir. y especialid. *17:*65-67, July '40

Sulfathiazole (sulfanilamide derivative) used with cartilage implants for repair of facial defects. CHILDREY, J. H. Ann. Otol., Rhin. and Laryng. *49:*709-712, Sept '40

Prevention and correction of dorsal depressions by septal implants (nose). GOLDMAN, I. B. Arch. Otolaryng. *32:*524-529, Sept '40

Advantage of mixed bone and cartilage grafts in correction of saddle nose and other depressed deformities of dorsum. COHEN, L. Tr. Am. Laryng., Rhin. and Otol. Soc. *46:*370-376, '40

Method to prevent fresh costal cartilage grafts from warping. NEW, G. B. AND ERICH, J. B. Proc. Staff Meet., Mayo Clin. *16:*199-200, March 26, '41

Autogenous cartilage grafts; experimental study. YOUNG, F. Surgery *10:*7-20, July '41

Reconstructive otoplasty (by transplantation of cartilage). GREELEY, P. W. Surgery *10:*457-461, Sept '41

Bone (iliac) and cartilage transplants to ear and nose; use and behavior. MOWLEM, R. Brit. J. Surg. *29:*182-193, Oct '41

Fate of autogenous cartilage after transplantation in human tissues. PEER, L. A. Arch. Otolaryng. *34:*696-709, Oct '41

Cartilage Grafts – Cont.

Method to prevent fresh cartilage grafts from warping (facial surgery). New, G. B. and Erich, J. B. Am. J. Surg. *54:*435–438, Nov '41

Cartilage graft restoration of jaw ankylosis; new operation. Pickerill, H. P. Australian and New Zealand J. Surg. *11:*197–206, Jan '42

Use of meniscus of knee in plastic surgery (ear). Dellepiane Rawson, R. Prensa med. argent. *29:*654–658, April 22, '42

Internal prosthesis with autotransplant of bone or cartilage. Jorge, J. M. and Mealla, E. S. Arq. de cir. clin. e exper. *6:*539–540, April–June '42

Diced cartilage grafts; new method for repair of skull defects. Peer, L. A. Arch. Otolaryng. *38:*156–165, Aug. '43

Cartilage transplantation. Peer, L. A., S. Clin. North America *24:*404–419, April '44

Cast and precast cartilage grafts; use in restoration of contour of face. Young, F. Surgery *15:*735–748, May '44

Cartilage implants in therapy of ozena; first cases in Venezuela. Celis Perez, A. Gac. med. de Caracas *54:*14–16, Jan–Mar '45

Boiled cartilage implants. Firestone, C. Am. J. Surg. *72:*153–160, Aug '46

Cartilage Grafts, Cadaver: See Cartilage Grafts, Preserved

Cartilage Grafts, Ear

Transplantation of cartilage from auricle into eyelid in trachomatous cicatricial entropion. Goldfeder, A. E. Klin. Monatsbl. f. Augenh. *82:*809–813, June 21, '29

Marginoplasty by means of cartilage of auricle without skin in partial trichiasis of eyelid. Goldfeder, A. E. Klin. Monatsbl. f. Augenh. *86:*218–225, Feb '31

Plastic repair of congenital and acquired deformities of palpebral margin by means of cartilage from auricle. Löwenstein, A. Klin. Monatsbl. f. Augenh. *93:*320–323, Sept '34

Correction of trichiasis of eyelids by transplantation of cartilage from auricle. Chepurin, N. S. Sovet. vestnik oftal. *7:*368–373, '35

Histopathologic changes in freely transplanted tissue from human auricle. Kyandskiy, A. A. Sovet. khir., no. 9, pp. 66–69, '35

Rhinoplasty with free transplantation from auricle. Limberg, A. A. Sovet. khir., no. 9, pp. 70–90, '35

Cartilage Grafts, Ear – Cont.

Experimental studies on transplantation of cartilage (ear) to cover tracheal defect. Mori, S. Okayama-Igakkai-Zasshi *48:*516, March '36

Transplantation of cartilage (ear) in surgical therapy of strabismus. Dubinov, O. A. Sovet. vestnik oftal. *8:*250–255, '36

Transplanted conchae auriculae as new method of correcting spastic entropion of upper eyelid following total tarsectomy. Shimkin, N. I. Rev. internat. du trachome *15:*15–20, Jan '38 also: Brit. J. Ophth. *22:*282–287, May '38

Use of tubular flap for transplantation of cartilage (ear) in surgical restoration of alae nasi. Novoshinova, E. N. Zhur. ush., nos. i gorl. bolez. *15:*164–168, '38

Technical modifications in operation for strabismus by transplanting auricular cartilage. Ivanov, A. I. Vestnik oftal. (no. 2) *15:*43–45, '39

Rare complication following peritomy and transplantation of auricular cartilage in therapy of pannus. Mitskevich, L. D. Vestnik oftal. (no. 1) *14:*118–119, '39

Correcting spastic entropion of upper lid following total tarsectomy, by transplanting a shaving from concha auriculae. Anand, H. L. Indian J. Ophth. *1:*20–23, Jan '40

New free graft (of skin and ear cartilage) applied to reconstruction of nostril. Gillies, H. Brit. J. Surg. *30:*305–307, April '43

Cartilage Grafts, Experimental

Experimental growth of bone and cartilage. Polettini, B. Arch. ital. di chir. *6:*179–191, Nov '22 (illus.) abstr: J.A.M.A. *80:*360, Feb 3, '23

Experimental transplantation of cartilage and skin for repair of concha. Gussio, S. Valsalva *3:*58–77, Feb '27

Experimental implantation of cartilage into kidney and transplantation of cartilage into bone defects. Nigrisoli, P. Arch. per. le sc. med. *49:*689–703, Dec '27

Experimental researches on grafting cartilage on to tendons. Borghi, M. Arch. per. le sc. med. *50:*437–465, '27

Experiences with interposition of fixed cartilage grafts between bone stumps to induce nearthrosis. Calissano, G. Arch. ital. di chir. *22:*206–217, '28

Cranioplasty with autografts of elastic cartilage; experiments. Mairano, M. and Virano, G. Clin. chir. *32:*1687–1705, Dec '29

Transplantation of cartilage; experiments. Fohl, T. Arch. F. klin. Chir. *155:*232–243, '29

Cartilage Grafts, Experrimental – Cont.

Experimental transplantation of cartilage fixed in bone. BLAVET DI BRIGA, C. Arch. ital. de biol. *83:*26-33, July 30, '30

Further observation on transplantation of epiphyseal cartilage plate. HAAS, S. L. Surg., Gynec. and Obst. *52:*958-963, May '31

Influence of parathyroid extract on calcification of tissues studied by observation of free transplants (including cartilage). LERICHE, R. *et al.* Ann. d'anat. path. *13:*551-555, May '36

Fate of living and dead cartilage transplanted in humans. PEER, L. A. Surg., Gynec. and Obst. *68:*603-610, March '39

Actual growth of young cartilage transplants in rabbits; experimental studies. DUPERTUIS, S. M. Arch. Surg. *43:*32-63, July '41

Transplantation of epiphysial cartilage. WENGER, H. L. Arch. Surg. *50:*148-151, March '45

Experimental observations on growth of human cartilage grafts. PEER, L. A. Arch. Otolaryng. *42:*384-396, Nov-Dec '45

Experimental observations on growth of young human cartilage grafts. PEER, L. A. Plast. and Reconstruct. Surg. *1:*108-112, July '46

Cartilage Grafts, Preserved

Experiences with interposition of fixed cartilage grafts between bone stumps to induce nearthrosis. CALISSANO, G. Arch. ital. di chir. *22:*206-217, '28

Successful experimental substitution of cartilage fixed in alcohol for loss of cranial substance. BLAVET DI BRIGA, C. Arch. per. le sc. med. *54:*63-70, Jan '30

Cartilage transplanted beneath skin of chest in man; experimental studies with sections of cartilage preserved in alcohol and buried from 7 days to 14 months. PEER, L. A. Arch. Otolaryng. *27:*42-58, Jan '38

Refrigerated cartilage isografts in facial surgery. O'CONNOR, G. B. AND PIERCE, G. W. Surg., Gynec. and Obst. *67:*796-798, Dec '38

Merthiolate (mercury compound): tissue preservative and antiseptic (for "refrigerated cartilage isografts"). O'CONNOR, G. B. Am. J. Surg. *45:*563-565, Sept '39

Cadaver cartilage as material for free transplantation. MIKHELSON, N. M. Khirurgiya, no. 10, pp. 29-34, '39

Refrigerated cartilage isografts; source, storage and use. O'CONNOR, G. B. California and West. Med. *52:*21-23, Jan '40

Cartilage Grafts, Preserved – Cont.

Use of preserved cartilage in ear reconstruction. KIRKHAM, H. L. D. Ann. Surg. *111:*896-902, May '40

Preserved and fresh cartilage homotransplants. BROWN, J. B. Surg., Gynec. and Obst. *70:*1079-1082, June '40

Grafts of preserved cartilage in restorations of facial contour. STRAITH, C. L. AND SLAUGHTER, W. B., J.A.M.A. *116:*2008-2013, May 3, '41

Preserved human cartilage in reconstructive surgery of face. IGLAUER, S. Ann. Otol., Rhin. and Laryng. *50:*1072-1078, Dec '41

Transplantation of cartilage from cadaver according to Mikhelson method in correction of nasal deformities. LITINSKIY, A. M. Novy khir. arkhiv. *48:*211-214, '41

New method for formation of stump after enucleation by transplantation of cadaver's cartilage into Tenon's capsule of eye. SVERDLOV, D. G. Vestnik oftal. (nos. 5-6) *19:*45-50, '41

Refrigerated cartilage for use in plastic surgery. ADLER, D. Arq. de cir. clin. e exper. *6:*608-611, April-June '42

Reconstructive plastic surgery of absent ear with necrocartilage; original method. LAMONT, E. S. Arch. Surg. *48:*53-72, Jan '44

Cadaver cartilage banks. NUNN, L. L. Bull. U. S. Army M. Dept. (no. 74) pp. 99-101, March '44

Utilization of cadaver cartilage in surgery. GONZALEZ ULLOA, M. Medicina, Mexico *25:*495-503, Dec 10, '45

Use of cadaver cartilage in surgery. GONZALEZ ULLOA, M. Rev. brasil. de cir. *14:*663-670, Dec '45 also: Prensa med. argent. *33:*705-709, April 5, '46

Receded chin; correction with preserved cartilage. WOLF, G. D. Am. J. Surg. *72:*74-77, July '46

Cartilage Heterografts

Heterotransplantation of cartilage and fat tissue and reaction against heterotransplants in general. LOEB, L. AND HARTER, J. S. Am. J. Path. *2:*521-537, Nov '26

Entropion spasticum after tarsectomia totalis of upper eyelid cured by hemoplastica tarsi; 3 cases. SHIMKIN, N. Cong. internat. de med. trop. et d'hyg., Compt. rend. (1928) *3:*743-751, '31

Alloplastic and heteroplastic grafts in reconstruction of facial defects; use of ivory and cartilage. SPANIER, F. Rev. de chir. structive, pp. 391-401, Dec '36

Local metabolism and tissue reaction; effect

Cartilage Heterografts—Cont.
of transplantation into heterogenic tissue and of application of salt solution and of organ extract on growth of transplanted cartilage. BINGEL, K. Beitr. z. path. Anat. u. z. allg. Path. *99:*205-223, '37
Human cartilage heterografts in plastic surgery. GUTTERIDGE, E., M. J. Australia *1:*9-10, Jan 6, '45

Cartilage Homografts (See also Cartilage Grafts, Preserved; Homografts)

Autotransplantation and homoiotransplantation of cartilage in guinea-pig. LOEB, L. Am. J. Path. *2:*111-122, March '26
Autotransplantation and homoiotransplantation of cartilage and bone in rat. LOEB, L. Am. J. Path. *2:*315-333, July '26
Auto- and homotransplantation of bone and cartilage. GORBUNOFF, W. P. Arch. f. klin. Chir. *161:*651-670, '30
Cartilage homografts. DUFOURMENTEL, L. Oto-rhino-laryng. internat. *21:*461-462, Aug '37
Reconstruction of external ear with special reference to use of maternal ear cartilage as supporting structure (cases). GILLIES, H. Rev. de chir. structive, pp. 169-179, Oct '37
Osteocartilaginous homogenous grafts in partial rhinoplasties. MALBEC, E. P. Dia med. *15:*644-645, June 21, '43
Homogenous cartilage grafts; experimental study. YOUNG, F. Surgery *17:*616-621, April '45
Device for cutting cartilage isografts. STAGMAN, J. Arch. Otolaryng. *42:*284, Oct '45

CARTWRIGHT, F. S.: Orthodontic treatment of jaw fractures and cleft palate. Internat. J. Orthodontia *23:*159-163, Feb '37
CARTY, T. J. A.: Decubitus ulcer, treatment with elastic adhesive plaster. Brit. M. J. *1:*105-106, Jan 19, '35
DE CARVALHO FRANCO, D.: Two cases of keloid therapy. Ann. paulist. de med. e cir. *26:*375-384, Nov '33
CARVALHO LUZ, F.: Crushing of extremities with resulting shock. Brasil-med. *56:*35-41, Jan 17, '42
CASADESÚS CASTELLS, F.: Indications for dacryocystorhinostomy. Med. ibera *2:*229, Sept 25; 249, Oct 2, '26
CASANUEVA DEL C., M.: Hand wounds; medicosocial problem. Arch. Soc. cirujanos hosp., num. espec., pp. 39-50, Dec '41
CASANUEVA DEL C., M. AND CROQUEVIELLE G., A.: Buttonhole rupture-luxation of extensor tendon of fingers. Rev. med. de Chile *70:*57-63, Jan '42
CASANUEVA DEL C., M. AND FLUHMANN D., G.: Wounds of hand tendons; analysis of 168 cases. Rev. med. de Chile *72:*1044-1048, Dec '44
CASANUEVA DEL C., M. AND VELASCO S., A.: Transplantation of dead heterologus bone in surgery; present status of problem; preparation of Orell's os purum. Rev. med. de Chile *70:*424-428, June '42
CASANUEVA DEL C., M. AND VILLARROEL, E.: Thyroglossal fistula, with report of case. Arch. Soc. cirujanos hosp. *12:*79-84, May-Aug '42
CASCO, C. M.: Therapy of cicatrices of fingers by "pocketbook" graft. Dia med. *18:*788-789, June 24, '46
CASE, C. S.: Mechanical correction of cleft palate. Dominion Dent. J. *40:*69-72, March '28
CASELLA, E.: Cleft palate and harelip. Rev. med. latino-am. *19:*119-159, Nov '33
CASH, J. R. (see YOUNG, H. H.) May '21
CASHMAN, C. J.: Early treatment of war wounds of face. Rev. san. mil., Buenos Aires *42:*291-298, May '43
CASHMAN, C. J.: Delayed union of mandibular fractures. J. Oral Surg. *4:*166-171, April '46
CASKEY, C. R.: Therapy of birthmarks. California and West. Med. *41:*385-388, Dec '34
CASSEGRAIN, O. C.: Small deep graft (skin); experiences and results of last 3 years. Surg., Gynec. and Obst. *38:*557-559, April '24
CASSELS, W. H. (see HELFRICH, L. S. *et al*) Feb '42
CASSIDY, W. A.: Intratemporal repair of facial nerve for facial paralysis (Ballance-Duel operation). Nebraska M. J. *25:*47-50, Feb '40
CASSIRER, R. AND UNGER, E.: Nerve transplants to bridge nerve defects. Deutsche med. Wchnschr. *47:*586, May 26, '21
CASTAY: Rare congenital malformation of right portion of lower and upper jaw (unilateral micrognathia); case. Bull. et mem. Soc. de radiol. med. de France *25:*125-126, Feb '37
CASTELLANO, J. L. AND GIGANTI, I. J.: Plastic and esthetic surgery; cases. Semana med. *1:*1337-1343, June 8, '39
CASTELLANO, J. L. AND GIGANTI, I. J.: Therapy of palatine fissure by combined Veau and Axhausen technics. Semana med. *2:*887-889, Oct 14, '43
CASTELLANOS FONSECA, E.: Burn therapy. Rev. med.-quir. de Oriente *4:*87-95, June '43
CASTELNAU, M.: Tracheotomy for grave subcutaneous emphysema following cervicofacial trauma; cases. Oto-rhino-Laryng. internat. *22:*195-196, April '38

CASTERÁN, E.: Heterotopy of pinna of ear and congenital facial paralysis; case. Rev. de especialid. *4:*1035–1038, Sept '29

CASTERÁN, E. (see ZAMBRINI, A. R.) Aug '32

CASTIGLIONI, G.: New experiments with homoplastic transplantation of organs. Atti d. Soc. di sc. med. e biol. *16:*34–49, Jan–Feb '27

CASTILLO ODENA, I. (see FINOCHIETTO, E. *et al*) July '40

CASTILLO ODENA, I.: Anatomy and physiology in relation to tendon transplantation. Dia med. *13:*246–249, April 7, '41

CASTILLO ODENA, I.: Technic of muscular evaluation; examination of flexor and extensor muscles of toes. Prensa med. argent. *33:*980–982, May 10, '46

DE CASTRO, A.: Oxycephalosyndactylia; case. Rev. neurol. *1:*359–367, March '34

CASTRO O'CONNOR, R.: Fractures of middle third of face in civil and military practice according to British experience. Dia med. *16:*361–367, April 17, '44

CASTRO O'CONNOR, R.: Facial traumatisms in war surgery. Bol. d. Inst. clin. quir. *21:*95–98, Feb '45

CASTRO O'CONNOR, R. (see BREA, C. A.) June '46

CASTROVIEJO, R.: Reconstructive surgery of eyelids; case. Arch. Asoc. para evit. ceguera Mexico *2:*189–194, '44

CASTROVIEJO, R. JR.: Epithelioma of eyelid; excision. Am. J. Ophth. *14:*634–635, July '31

CASU, C.: Technics of formation of artificial vagina; case. Rassegna d'ostet. e ginec. *44:*208–228, April 30, '35

CATALANO, F. E.: Polydactylia and syndactylia; case. Prensa med. argent. *27:*1081–1082, May 22, '40

CATALANO, F. E. AND SIBILLA, C. E.: Mixed tumors of parotid, with report of cases. Rev. Asoc. med. argent. *59:*507–510, May 15, '45

CATALANO, F. E. (see SIBILLA, C. E.) 1945

CATALAO, P. V. B.: Valle operation (lacrimal), Brazilian contribution. Brasil-med. *57:*213, May 1–15, '43

CATANIA, V.: Two wounds resulting from firearms, with multiple lesions of jaw bones. Stomatol. *31:*179–200, Feb '33

CATES, B. B.: A knife for harelip and cleft palate operations. Am. J. Surg. *36:*70, March '22

CATES, B. B. Plea for early cleft palate operations. Am. J. Surg. *36:*221–222, Sept '22 (illus.)

CATES, B. B.: Few points in technic of cleft palate operations. Am. J. Surg. *37:*231–232, Sept '23

CATES, B. B.: Technique of cleft palate operations. Boston M. and S. J. *191:*1166–1168, Dec 18, '24

CATES, B. B.: Special periostetomes for cleft palate work. Boston M. and S. J. *193:*728–729, Oct 15,'25

CATES, B. B.: Harelip and cleft palate operations. Internat. J. Med. and Surg. *41:*8–11, Jan '28

CATEULA, J.: New type of forceps used as accessory element in depilation by diathermocoagulation. Semana med. *2:*628, Sept 14, '39

CATO, E.: Plastic repair of patulous anus by means of fascia lata strips. Australian and New Zealand J. Surg. *4:*315–317, Jan '35

CATTANI, P.: Treatment of deformities of lips. Schweiz. med. Wchnschr. *53:*85–88, Jan 25, '23 (illus.)

CATTELL, McK.: Studies in experimental traumatic shock; action of ether on circulation in traumatic shock. Arch. Surg. *6:*41–84, (pt. 1), Jan '23

CATTELL, McK.: Studies in experimental traumatic shock; influence of morphine on blood pressure and alkali reserve in traumatic shock. Arch. Surg. *7:*96–110, July '23 (illus.)

CATTELL, McK. (see CANNON, W. B.) March '22

CAUHEPE, J.: Maxillary deformities and their orthopedic therapy. Medecine *18:*657–658, Aug '37

CAULDWELL, E. W. (see MCCORMACK, L. J. *et al*) Jan '45

CAULFIELD, P. A.: Cut tendon. M. Ann. District of Columbia *7:*207–211, July '38

CAULFIELD, P. A.: Burn therapy. M. Ann. District of Columbia *13:*251, July '44

CAULFIELD, P. A. (see CAHILL, J. A.) Feb '38

CAUSSADE, L. AND NICHOLAS: Acrocephalosyndactylia; 2 cases. Paris med. *2:*399–402, Nov 2, '29

CAUSSADE, L.; DOUZAIN, AND ROUSSEL, J. M.: Agenesis of abdominal wall in infant. Rev. med. de Nancy *66:*262–265, March 15, '38

CAUSSADE, L.; GOEPFERT, AND MEIGNANT: Acrocephalosyndactylia; evolution of case. Rev. med. de Nancy *65:*576–586, July 1, '37

CAVALCANTI, H.: Clinic study of burn therapy, with special reference to metabolic disturbances. Rev. med.-cir. do Brasil *47:*65–181, Feb '39

CAVALCANTI, J.: Fractures of phalanges of fingers, with report of cases. Arq. brasil. de cir. e ortop. *7:*326–337, Dec '39

CAVALLI, M.: Behavior of lymphatic vessels in autoplastic skin grafts. Sperimentale, Arch. di biol. *89:*504–508, '35

CAVANAGH, J. R. (see YATER, W. M.) Sept '32

CAVAZZUTTI, A. M.: Osteomyelitis of superior maxilla in infant; surgical treatment. Semana med. *1:*95–96, Jan 10, '29

CAVENY, E. L.: Early management of burn cases in mass quantity. U. S. Nav. M. Bull. *40:*824–828, Oct '42

CAVINA, C.: Reconstruction, bone implants for reconstruction of jaw. Chir. d. org. di movimento *5:*417, Aug '21 abstr: J.A.M.A. *77:*1374, Oct 22, '21

CAVINA, C.: Plastic operation to reconstruct syphilitic defect in palate. Gior. ital. di dermat. e sifil. *66:*678–679, April '25

CAVINA, C.: Successful treatment of jaw fractures by reduction, retention and grafts. Rev. de stomatol. *29:*815–842, Nov '27

CAVINA, C.: Operative technic of osseous transplantation on lower jaw. Arch. ed atti d. Soc. ital. di chir. (1927) *34:*672–675, '28

CAVINA, C.: Treatment of jaw fractures. Stomatol. *26:*657-678, July '28

CAVINA, C.: Plastic surgery of lip, chin and cheek in man after resection for cancer. Arch. ed atti d. Soc. ital. di chir. *35:*526–541, '29

CAVINA, C.: Therapy of fractures of mandible due to firearms. Gior. di med. mil. *83:*713–722, Aug '35

CAVINA, C.: Therapy of extensive fractures of mandible due to firearms. Gior. di med. mil. *83:*809, Sept; 923, Oct '35

CAVINA, C. (see CHIAROLANZA, R.) 1928

CAWLEY, J. J. JR. (see ROBERTSON, R. C. *et al*) Jan '46

CAWTHORNE, T.: Nerve transplantation in facial paralysis. Tr. M. Soc. London *60:*171–177, '37

CAZAP, S.: Cancer of lips. Bol. Inst. de med. exper. para el estud. y trat. d. cancer *21:*188–215, April '44

CAZIN, M.: Evolution and treatment in wounds of tendons of hands and fingers. Paris chir. *21:*179–190, Sept–Oct '29

CAZORLA ROMERO, J. (see GAY PRIETO, J.) May '33

CEBALLOS, A. AND CALZETTA, J. C.: Conservative treatment in grave trauma of arm and forearm. Prensa med. argent. *32:*31–34, Jan 5 '45

CEBALLOS, A. AND GIOIA, T.: Volkmann's contracture, treatment by humeral sympathectomy. Bol. y trab. de la Soc. de cir. *11:*147–153, May 11, '27

CEBALLOS, A. AND GIOIA, T.: Volkmann's syndrome; case; periarterial sympathectomy; permanent recovery. Bol. y trab. de la. Soc. de cir. de Buenos Aires *12:*185–191, June 6, '28

CECCARELLI, G.: Skin grafts and conditions which favor their vitality and attachment; experimental research. Arch. ital. di chir. *15:*353–412, '26 abstr: J.A.M.A. *87:*284, July 24, '26

CECIL, A. B.: Treatment of case of male hypospadias. S. Clin. N. Amer. *8:*1343–1350, Dec '28

CECIL, A. B.: Treatment of case of male epispadias. S. Clin. N. Amer. *8:*1351–1356, Dec '28

CECIL, A. B.: Surgery of hypospadias and epispadias in male. Tr. Am. A. Genito-Urin. Surgeons *24:*253–302, '31 also: J. Urol. *27:*507–537, May '32

CECIL, A. B.: Surgery of hypospadias and epispadias in male. West. J. Surg. *40:*297–315, June '32

CECIL, A. B.: Cure of epispadias; further report. J. Urol. *34:*278–283, Sept '35

CECIL, A. B.: Repair of hypospadias and fistula. J. Urol. *56:*237–242, Aug '46

CELIS PEREZ, A.: Cartilage implants in therapy of ozena; first cases in Venezuela. Gac. med. de Caracas *54:*14–16, Jan–Mar '46

CERDEIRO, A. M. (see GAREISO, A. *et al*) Aug '38

Cerebral Fungus, Skin Grafting

Hernia cerebri treated by Thiersch grafts. WRIGHT, A. D. Proc. Roy. Soc. Med. *32:*213–214, Jan '39

Treatment of major cranial wounds; cerebral fungus; skin grafting. HYNDMAN, O. R. Surgery *11:*466–471, March '42

CERESETO, P. L.: Therapy of hand phlegmons; cases. Dia med. *10:*64–68, Jan 24, '38

CERNEA AND LAMBERT: Hemiatrophy of face. Rev. de stomatol. *43:*185–187, Nov–Dec '42

DE CERQUEIRA FALCAO, E.: Vascular tumors of face; 2 cases. Rev. oto-laring. de Sao Paulo *3:*533–538, Nov–Dec '35 also: Brasil-med. *50:*134–139, Feb 15, '36

DE CERQUEIRA FALCAO, E.: Therapy of postoperative hematoma of nasal septum by means of laminaria. Rev. oto-laring. de Sao Paulo *6:*471–477, Nov–Dec '38 also: Brasil-med. (no. 5) *53:*143–145, '39

CERVENANSKY, J.: Fistulography with lipiodol (iodized oil) as new therapy of congenital cervical fistula. Wien. med. Wchnschr. *91:*886–890, Nov 1, '41

CESARI, M.: Operation for pendulous breasts. Bull. d. sc. med. *5:*373–379, Sept–Oct '27

CETRÁ, C. M.: Laryngectomy for cancer of larynx; results in 140 cases. Bol. Inst. de med. exper. para el estud. y trat. del cancer *10:*564–573, Oct '33

CETRÁ, M.: Surgical solution to carcinoma of larynx. Rev. otorrinolaring. d. litoral *3:*99–117, Jan–June '44

CETRÁ, M. C.: Surgical therapy of cancer of

larynx; 200 cases. Bol. Inst. de med. exper. para el estud. y trat. del. cancer *14:*169-188, April '37
CEVARIO, L.: Serous cysts of neck. Gazz. d. osp. *42:*200, Feb 27, '21
CHAKRAVARTI, D. C.: Modern treatment of burns. Indian M. Rec. *62:*359-382, Dec '42
CHALNOT, (see HAMANT, A. *et al*) Jan '33
CHAMBERLIN, W. B.: Prevention of hematoma after submucous resection. Tr. Am. Laryng. A. *61:*21-28, '39
CHAMBERS, J. V.: Plastic reconstruction following gunshot wound of lip; case. U. S. Nav. M. Bull. *46:*588-590, April '46
CHAN, L. F.: Occupational injury of hand (palmar tendon injury of agricultural workers). Caribbean M. J. (no. 5) *6:*341-342, '44
CHANDLER, P. A.: Dacryocystorhinostomy. Tr. Am. Ophth. Soc. *34:*240-263, '36
CHANG, S. K.: Surgical treatment of eyelid ptosis. Nat. M. J. China *27:*239, April '41
CHANG CHI: Skin grafts. Nat. M. J., China *15:*20-27, Feb '29
CHAPIN, W. C.: Congenital harelip and cleft palate; case I, (unfinished case). Internat. Orthodont. Cong. *1:*485-492, '27
CHARAMIS, J.: Surgical therapy of congenital coloboma of eyelids. Ann. d'ocul. *173:*810-819, Oct '36
CHARAMIS, J. S.: Pedicled dermomuscular blepharoplasty; 12 cases. Arch. d'opht. *2:*206-218, March '38
CHARBONNEAU, L. O.: Improved finger splint. Hosp. Corps Quart. (no. 12) *18:*57, Dec '45
CHARBONNEL: Reconstruction of muscles and tendons. J. de med. de Bordeaux *92:*437, Aug 10, '21 abstr: J.A.M.A. *77:*1210, Oct 8, '21
CHARBONNEL AND BARROUX, R.: Tendon transplant for complete radial paralysis; case. Bordeaux chir. *1-2:*55, Jan-Apr '44
CHARBONNEL, AND MASSE: Dislocation of thumb; surgical treatment. Arch. franco-belges de chir. *32:*229-230, March '30
CHARNOCK, D. A. AND KISKADDEN, W. S.: Hypospadias. J. Urol. *49:*444-449, March '43
CHARRIER, J. (see GOSSET, A.) Jan '22
CHARRY, R.: Arthroplastic reconstruction in joints. Rev. d'orthop. *31:*186-194, Sept-Dec '45
CHARSCHAK, M. J.: Surgical treatment of chronic stenosis of larynx; 148 cases. Monatschr. f. Ohrenh. *65:*57-80, Jan '31
CHARUGIN, A. I.: Hand infections in surgeons. Novy khir. arkhiv *31:*414-417, '34
CHARUGIN, A. I.: Burn therapy. Novy khir. arkhiv *38:*447-452, '37
CHASANOW, M.: Etiology of facial hemiatrophy. Ztschr. f. d. ges. Neurol. u. Psychiat. *140:*473-485, '32
CHASE, I. C.: Hand infections. Texas State J. Med. *27:*31-34, May '31
CHATAGNON, C. (see CHATAGNON, P. *et al*) July '38
CHATAGNON, P.; SOULAIRAC, A. AND CHATAGNON, C.: Dupuytren's contracture in patient with melancholia; biochemical and clinical study. Ann. med.-psychol. (pt. 2) *96:*238-245, July '38
CHATON, M.: Treatment of section of tendons of fingers. Rev. gen. de clin. et de therap. *43:*289-296, May 4, '29
CHATTERTON, C. C. (see PHALEN, G. S.) Nov '42
CHATZKELSON, B.: Extra-oral emergency bandage in fractures of lower jaw. Munchen. med. Wchnschr. *78:*98, Jan 16, '31
CHAUMERLIAC, J. (see HANNS, *et al*) Dec '28
CHAUNCEY, L. R. (see GRAY, H. K.) Jan '39
CHAUVENET, A.: Autoplasty using digital flap in therapy of stubborn ulcers resulting from burns received in childhood. Bordeaux chir. *6:*18-25, Jan '33
CHAVANNAZ, G.: Tumor of cheek and problem of surgical restoration. J. de med. de Bordeaux *110:*7-9, Jan 10, '35
CHAVANNAZ, J.: Tetanus after burn by high tension electric current; 2 cases in workmen. Ann. de med. leg. *17:*800-801, July '37
CHAVANY, J. A.: Orbitotemporal osteoma with exorbitism in syphilitics, with report of cases. Presse med. *53:*702, Dec 22, '45
CHAVANY, J. A. (see ZIMMERN, A.) June '30
CHAVES, D. A.: Congenital branchial cyst of floor of mouth; case. Rev. med.-cir. do Brasil *46:*620-626, May '38
CHAVES, D. A.: Surgical therapy of cleft palate and harelip. Rev. med. munic. *3:*259-270, March '42
CHAVEZ, E. JR.: Technical study of accidents to longshoremen of Minatitlan (including hand injuries). Rev. d. trab. *2:*167-172, May '38
CHAVEZ TRUJILLO, A.: Clinical evolution of traumatic and surgical shock. Medicina, Mexico *25:*54-56, Feb 25, '45
CHAWLA, G. S.: Case of abnormal salivary fistula. Indian M. Gaz. *61:*233, May '26

Cheiloplasty

Cheiloplasty; using upper lip to make new lower lip. PÓLYA, E. Zentralbl. f. Chir. *48:*262, Feb 26, '21
Plastic operation on lips. KÖNIG, F. Beitr. z. klin. Chir. *122:*288, '21 abstr: J.A.M.A. *77:*656, Aug 20, '21
Plastic operation on face and lips. BULLOCK, H., M. J. Australia *2:*220, Sept 17, '21

Cheiloplasty – Cont.
Reconstruction of lower lip. TZAÏCO, A. Presse med. *29:*723, Sept 10, '21 abstr: J.A.M.A. *77:*1606, Nov 12, '21
Plastic surgery of lip. KAZANJIAN, V. H. J.A.M.A. *77:*1959, Dec 17, '21
Reconstruction of upper lip. DUFOURMENTEL, L. Presse med. *30:*344–346, April 22, '22 (illus.) abstr: J.A.M.A. *78:*1851, June 10, '22
Reconstruction to insure function after plastic operation on lower lip. PICHLER, H. Zentralbl. f. Chir. *49:*1363–1365, Sept 16, '22 (illus.)
Case of "hypospadias perinealis." CHELLIAH, S. Internat. A. M. Museums Bull., pp. 162–164, Dec '22
Plastic operations on corner of mouth. FESSLER, J. Deutsche Ztschr. f. Chir. *172:*427–429, '22 (illus.)
Modification of Estlander's operation for lip defect. TWYMAN, E. D. Surg., Gynec. and Obst. *38:*824–825, June '24
Operative correction of paralysis of lower lip. SCHMERZ, H. Arch. f. klin. Chir. *131:*353–360, '24 abstr: J.A.M.A. *83:*1464, Nov 1, '24
Reconstruction of lower lip. HOFMANN, M. Arch. f. klin. Chir. *131:*338–342, '24
Cancer of lip, resulting deformity, plastic repair. BOYD, J. E., J. Florida M. A. *12:*27–29, Aug '25
Reconstruction of lower lip according to round pedicle method. WOLOSCHINOW, W. Arch. f. klin. Chir. *135:*770–775, '25
Plastic reconstruction of upper and lower lips. DEMEL, R. Deutsche Ztschr. f. Chir. *196:*210–214, '26
Plastic surgery of lower lip. EHLER, F. Casop. lek. cesk. *66:*141–144, Jan 21, '27
Excision and restoration of upper lip. PICKERILL, H. P. Brit. J. Surg. *14:*536–538, Jan '27
Certain fundamental principles of esthetic surgery; with method of plastic reconstruction of lower lip for cicatricial deformity. GIANTURCO, G. Rinasc. med. *4:*507, Nov 1, '27
Why and how of harelip correction. BLAIR, V. P. Ann. Otol. Rhin. and Laryng. *37:*196–205, March '28
Cancer of lower lip; operative technic in plastic repair. FAIRCHILD, F. R. Arch. Surg. *17:*630–640, Oct '28
Restoration of upper lip. AXT, E. F. Dental Cosmos *70:*1158–1160, Dec '28
Plastic surgery of lower lip for noma. KOLDAEFF, S. M. Vrach. gaz. *32:*1177–1181, '28
Reconstruction of upper lip and portion of

Cheiloplasty – Cont.
nose. NEW, G. B., S. Clin. N. Amer. *9:*75–78, Feb '29
Plastic reconstruction of lower lip. FREEMAN, L. Colorado Med. *26:*160–162, June '29
Use of double skin flap in restoration of lip defects. VON CZEYDA-POMMERSHEIM, F. Zentralbl. f. Chir. *56:*2381–2382, Sept 21, '29
Cheiloplastic methods. HAGENTORN, A. Zentralbl. f. Chir. *56:*3031–3032, Nov 30, '29
Cheiloplasty of upper lip. KURTZAHN. Deutsche Ztschr. f. Chir. *218:*378–383, '29
Restoration of lower lip by means of Filatov's tubular skin flap. KARTASCHEW, S. Deutsche Ztschr. f. Chir. *229:*395–400, '30
Surgical treatment of double lips. MEYER, H. Deutsche Ztschr. f. Chir. *222:*305–309, '30
Bulky carcinoma of lip treated by irradiation, wide surgical excision and plastic closure. MARTIN, H. E. Am. J. Cancer *15:*261–266, Jan '31
Aesthetic correction of lips. DE ASÍS, R. Siglo med. *87:*269–270, March 14, '31
Plastic reconstruction of lower lip in cancer. DALAND, E. M. New England J. Med. *205:*1131–1142, Dec 10, '31
Partial cheiloplasty by transplantation from one person to another. DUJARDIN, E. Ugesk. f. laeger *94:*382–383, April 14, '32
Method for cheiloplasty of lower lip. SANCHÍS PERPIÑÁ, V. Actas Soc. de cir. de Madrid *1:*329–352, April–June '32
Plastic replacement of upper lip in case of epitheliomatous ulcer resulting from x-ray treatment of sycosis barbae. HUTTON, A. J. Glasgow M. J. *117:*225–230, May '32
Cheiloplasty for advanced carcinoma. MARTIN, H. E. Surg., Gynec. and Obst. *54:*914–922, June '32
Recurring epithelioma of lower lip and chin; diathermy and cautery excision; reconstruction of lower lip. FIGI, F. A., S. Clin. North America *12:*951–954, Aug '32
Technic of plastic surgery for correction of microstomia resulting from Estlander cheiloplasty. TUOMIKOSKI, V. Duodecim *48:*691–698, '32
Surgery of upper lip to correct loss of tissue due to actinomycosis. DESELAERS, H. Ars med., Barcelona *9:*143–144, April '33
Method for cheiloplasty of lower lip. SANCHÍS PERPIÑÁ, V. Arch. de med., cir. y especialid. *36:*449–458, April 22, '33
Restoration of vermilion border in certain operation. BALDWIN, J. F. Am. J. Surg. *22:*232, Nov '33
Therapy of microstomia; case. BUSTAMANTE,

Cheiloplasty – Cont.
S. Ann. Casa de Salud Valdecilla *4:*281-282, '33
Author's cheiloplastic method of surgery of lower lip. SANCHÍS PERPIÑÁ, V. Beitr. z. klin. Chir. *158:*367-380, '33
Plastic method of correcting microstomia, particularly of type following Estlander cheiloplastic operation. TUOMIKOSKI, V. Acta chir. Scandinav. *70:*353-362, '33
Surgical therapy of cancer of lips. WIEDHOPF, O. Deutsche Ztschr. f. Chir. *238:*741-744, '33
Preservation of innervation and circulation supply in plastic restoration of upper lip. ESSER, J. F. S. Ann. Surg. *99:*101-111, Jan '34
Frontal flaps of lips; special practice of biological- or artery flaps. ESSER, J. F. S. Rev. de chir. plastique, pp. 288-294, Jan '34
New method of reconstruction of lips. PIERCE, G. W. AND O'CONNOR, G. B. Arch. Surg. *28:*317-334, Feb '34
Cheiloplasty by Estlander technic. ALFREDO, J. Rev. med. de Pernambuco *5:*233-237, June '35
Cheiloplasty in plastic repair of harelip; author's technic. CODAZZI AGUIRRE, J. A. Rev. med. del Rosario *25:*953-965, Aug '35
Surgical therapy of cancer of lips. NARBUTOVSKIY, S. D. Novy khir. arkhiv. *33:*3-14, '35
Esthetic surgery of lips. DANTRELLE, A., J. de med. de Paris *56:*57-62, Jan 23, '36
Repair of postoperative defects involving lips and cheeks secondary to removal of malignant tumors. NEW, G. B. AND FIGI, F. A. Surg., Gynec. and Obst. *62:*182-190, Feb '36
New method of muscular transplantation applied to cheiloplasty; case. REBELO NETO, J., Rev. de chir. structive, pp. 199-209, March '36
Cheiloplasty in cancer of lips. PADGETT, E. C. Internat. J. Orthodontia *22:*939-947, Sept '36
Double lip; surgical therapy of case. RODRIGUEZ VILLEGAS, R. AND TAULLARD, J. C. Bol. y trab. de la Soc. de cir. de Buenos Aires *21:*45-48, April 14, '37
Cheiloplasty of lower lip; case. BROHOVICI, H. Rev. de chir. structive, pp. 210-213, Oct '37
Cheilorthocaliplasty (esthetic surgery of mouth). CODAZZI AGUIRRE, J. A. Rev. med. del Rosario *27:*1111-1131, Nov '37
Technic of resection of lower lip in cancer; cases. BREYTFUS, F. F. Khirurgiya, no. 5, pp. 61-62, '37

Cheiloplasty – Cont.
Plastic surgery of double lip. ZENO, L. An. de cir. *4:*11-13, March '38
Radical inferior cheiloplasty for advanced carcinoma of lower lip; 2 cases. WIRTH, J. E. Northwest Med. *37:*109-112, April '38
Switching of vermilion-bordered lip flaps. BROWN, J. B. Surg., Gynec. and Obst. *46:*701-704, May '28
Improved method of lip fixation in harelip. EBERT, E. C. AND BOYDEN, R. C., U. S. Nav. M. Bull. *36:*501, Oct '38
Plastic correction of lips. EITNER, E. Wien. med. Wchnschr. *89:*89-90, Jan 28, '39
Repair of postoperative defects of lips. NEW, G. B. AND ERICH, J. B. Am. J. Surg. *43:*237-248, Feb '39
Cheiloplasty for extensive loss of substance of lower lip; 2 cases. LOMBARD, P. Presse med. *47:*525-526, April 8, '39
Plastic correction after unsatisfactory healing following operation for harelip. AXHAUSEN, G. Chirurg *11:*321-334, May 1, '39
Repair of large defects of lips after removal for cancer. DALAND, E. M. Surg., Gynec. and Obst. *69:*347-357, Sept '39
Surgical and anatomic aspects of case of double lower lip. MASON, M. L. *et al.* Surg., Gynec. and Obst. *70:*12-17, Jan '40
Reconstruction of lip after cancer. BOYER, B. E., J. Med. *20:*543-544, Feb '40
New Cupid's-bow operation (in harelip). HARDY, E. A. Lancet *1:*361, Feb 24, '40
Reconstruction of lower lip. CUNNINGHAM, A. F. Northwest Med. *39:*336-337, Sept '40
Extensive plastic repair for restoration of lower lip; report of procedure in case in which lower lip was entirely removed for eradication of epithelioma. FEDERSPIEL, M. N. Am. J. Orthodontics (Oral Surg. Sect) *28:*163-166, March '42
Restoration of subseptum and lower lip by process of tubular autoplasty; case. DA SILVA, G. Arq. de cir. clin. e exper. *6:*287-299, April-June '42
Hypermotility of upper lip, surgery of. DORRANCE, G. M. AND LOUDENSLAGER, P. E. Surg., Gynec. and Obst. *75:*790-791, Dec '42
Repair of extensive loss of substance of lower lip (due to cancer). VIANNA, J. B. Hospital, Rio de Janeiro *23:*69-79, Jan '43
Plastic surgery of upper lip with skin flaps from chin. FREY, S. Zentralbl. f. Chir. *70:*539, April 10, '43
Plastic reconstruction of lower lip (French method). IVANISSEVICH, O. *et al.* Bol. y trab., Acad. argent. de cir. *27:*353-362, June 23, '43

Cheiloplasty – Cont.

Simplified method of rotating skin and mucous membrane flaps for complete reconstruction of lower lip. OWENS, N. Surgery *15:*196–206, Jan '44

Plastic operation for lengthening congenitally short upper lip; preliminary report. FORD, J. F., J. Oral Surg. *2:*260–265, July '44

Cheiloplasties. COVARRUBIAS ZENTENO, R. Rev. med. de Chile *72:*696–698, Aug '44

New technic for correction of macrostomia. HARRIS, H. I., J. Oral Surg. *3:*156–163, April '45

Orotracheal anesthesia for cheiloplasty. SLOCUM, H. C. AND ALLEN, C. R. Anesthesiology *6:*355–358, July '45

Macrocheilia. BOUCHER, R. Union med. du Canada *75:*461–462, April '46

Cosmetic reduction of full, everted lower lip. FIRESTONE, C. Northwest Med. *45:*499–501, July '46

Chemical Peeling

Truth and fallacies of face peeling and face lifting. BAMES, H. O., M. J. and Rec. *126:*86–87, July 20, '27

Surgical treatment of lupus of face (use of tubular cranial flaps and application of Filhos' caustic for destruction of minor facial lesions of lupus). MOURE, P. French M. Rev. *2:*415–419, Oct '32

Skin peeling and scarification in treatment of pitted scars, pigmentations and certain facial blemishes. ELLER, J. J. AND WOLFE, S. J.A.M.A. *116:*2208, May 10, '41

Skin peeling. GOODMAN, H. Hygeia *20:*514, July '42

CHEMIN (see GINESTET) May–June '46

CHEN, C. Y.: Burn therapy; with special reference to use of solutions of silver nitrate, aniline dyes (especially gentian violet) and their combination. Chinese M. J. *55:*407–426, May '39

CHEN, C. Y. (see SZUTU, C.) June '40

CHEN, C. Y. (see WHITACRE, F. E.) June '45

CHEN, H. I. (see TUNG, P. C.) Feb '35

CHENET, H.: Maxillofacial prosthesis. Odontologie *67:*831–850, Dec '29

CHENET, H.: Preparation and adjustment of prosthesis in loss of auricular substance. Odontologie *68:*861–870, Dec '30 also: Ann. d'oto-laryng., pp. 1–9, Jan '31

CHENUT, A.: Results of suture of radial nerve in therapy of fracture of radius. Bull. et mem. Soc. de chir. de Bordeaux et du Sud-Ouest, pp. 254–257, '32

CHENUT, A.: Results of suture of median and radial nerves in therapy of fracture of left radius. Bordeaux chir. *3:*136–138, April '32

CHEPURIN, N. S.: Correction of trichiasis of eyelids by transplantation of cartilage from auricle. Sovet. vestnik oftal. *7:*368–373, '35

CHÉRIDJIAN, Z.: Plastic surgery of nose with bone graft and paraffin. Rev. med. de la Suisse Rom. *49:*751–753, Oct 25, '29

CHERKASSOV, F. M. (see BALAKHOVSKIY, S. D. *et al)* 1936

CHERNIGOVSKY, N. N.: Artificial vagina formation by transplantation of piece of ileum. J. akush. i zhensk. boliez. *39:*329–332, '28

Chest

Combined satchel handle or tubed pedicle and large delayed whole skin pedicle flaps in case of plastic surgery of face, neck and chest. ALDEN, B. F. Surg., Gynec. and Obst. *41:*493–496, Oct '25

Treatment of funnel-shaped chest. ZAHRADNIČEK, J. Cas. lek. cesk. *64:*1814–1817, Dec 12, '25 abstr: J.A.M.A. *86:*456, Feb 6, '26

Plastic operation on chest. SHIPLEY, A. M. Ann. Surg. *84:*246–250, Aug '26

Cystic lymphangioma of chest wall. SAILER, K. Orvosi hetil. *71:*811–813, July 17, '27

Plastic surgery of face, neck, and chest skin losses. BLAIR, V. P. Tr. Am. S. A. *45:*190–199, '27

Unilateral symbrachydactylia with defect of thoracic wall and amastia; case. STÖHR, F. J. Ztschr. f. Morphol. u. Anthrop. *26:*384–390, '27

Median cleft of lower lip and mandible, cleft sternum and absence of basihyoid (inferior gnathoschisis); case. MORTON, C. B. AND JORDAN, H. E. Arch. Surg. *30:*647–656, April '35

Surgery of funnel chest. KRAUSS, H. Deutsche Ztschr. f. Chir. *250:*715–826, '38

Funnel chest; successfully operated case. HÄBERLIN, F. Schweiz. med. Wchnschr. *72:*126–128, Jan 31, '42

Pectus excavatum; 2 cases successfully operated upon. SWEET, R. H. Ann. Surg. *119:*922–934, June '44

Funnel chest; case successfully treated by chondrosternal resection. PHILLIPS, J. R. Dis. of Chest. *10:*422–426, Sept–Oct '44

CHESTER, J. B.: New technic of bone transplantation. Surg., Gynec. and Obst. *70:*819–825, April '40

CHEVALLIER, A.; CARCASSONNE, F. AND LUCCIONI: Applications of vitamin A in burns; 5 cases. Progres med., pp. 89–90, Jan 16, '37

CHIANELLO, C.: Treatment of old extensive destruction of tendons (hand). Cultura med. mod. *6:*104–106, March 1, '27

CHIARIELLO, A.: Absence of hand; 3 cases. Rev. d'orthop. *15:*242–251, May '28

CHIARIELLO, A. G.: Plastic surgery of tendons and nerves of hand. Policlinico (sez. prat.) *39:*520–525, April 4, '32

CHIARIELLO, A. G.: Therapy of lymphangiomas of neck. Folia med. *20:*590–594, May 30, '34

CHIAROLANZA, R. AND CAVINA, C.: Technic of facial surgery. Arch. ed atti d. Soc. ital. di chir. (1927) *34:*cxvi, '28

CHIAROLANZA, R.: Avoiding postoperative recurrence of thyroglossal fistula in surgical therapy; necessity of resection of hyoid bone. Arch. ital. di chir. *51:*331–336, '38

CHIAROLANZA, R.: Plastic surgery of face; cases. Chir. plast. *4:*114–123, July–Sept '38

CHIAROLANZA, R.: Surgical therapy of simple harelip; technic and results. Rinasc. med. *17:*128–131, March 15, '40

CHIASSERINI, A.: Free grafts of nerves. Policlinico (sez. chir.) *30:*489–497, Oct '23 (illus.)

CHIATELLINO, A.: Blair-Brown modification of Mirault method of treating unilateral harelip; results in cases. Gior. med. d. Alto Adige *11:*131–145, March '39

CHIBUKMAKHER, N. B.: Peripheral nerves; reconstructive surgery following gunshot wounds. Khirurgiya, no. 5, pp. 45–50, '45

CHIBUKMAKHER, N. B.: Restorative operations in reflex disorders caused by nerve trauma. Vrach. delo (nos. 7–8) *26:*435–440, '46

CHICHE, P.: Traumatic shock; recent physiopathologic data. Presse med. *53:*407–409, July 28, '45

CHILD, C. G., III: Traumatic shock; prevention and treatment. S. Clin. North America *23:*321–332, April '43

CHILDREY, J. H.: Atresia of choana of nose; case. Laryngoscope *48:*51–53, Jan '38

CHILDREY, J. H.: Simplified intranasal suture. Arch. Otolaryng. *27:*618, May '38

CHILDREY, J. H.: Sulfathiazole (sulfanilamide derivative) used with cartilage implants for repair of facial defects. Ann. Otol., Rhin. and Laryng. *49:*709–712, Sept '40

CHILDREY, J. H.: Fractures of malar bone; cases. Laryngoscope *52:*473–479, June '42

CHILDREY, J. H. (see NEW, G. B. *et al)* Feb '32

CHILTON, N. W. (see BENNETT, I. B.) Jan '45

Chin

Reconstruction of jaw and chin. EISELSBERG, A. AND PICHLER, H. Arch. f. klin. Chir. *122:*337–369, '22 (illus.) abstr: J.A.M.A. *80:*732, March 10, '23

Chin – Cont.

Repair of defects about chin, from standpoint of general surgeon. COUGHLIN, W. T. J.A.M.A. *83:*989–993, Sept 27, '24

Skin flap transplantation for lupus of neck and chin. SALOMON, A. Deutsche med. Wchnschr. *52:*1821, Oct 22, '26

Plastic surgery of chin and mouth mucosa; case. SMITAL, W. Zentralbl. f. Chir. *55:*142–145, Jan 21, '28

Use of visor flaps from chest in plastic operations upon neck, chin and lip. FREEMAN, L. Ann. Surg. *87:*364–368, March '28

Rhinophyma, case with unusual involvement of chin. SAMS, W. M. Arch. Dermat. and Syph. *26:*834–837, Nov '32

Combined nasal plastic and chin plastic; correction of microgenia by osteocartilaginous transplant from large hump nose. AUFRICHT, G. Am. J. Surg. *25:*292–296, Aug '34

Plastic surgery of soft parts of chin, with report of case treated by scalp graft. FINOCHIETTO, R. AND MARINO, H. Prensa med. argent. *21:*1672–1685, Sept 5, '34

Median cleft of lower lip and mandible, cleft sternum and absence of basihyoid (inferior gnathoschisis); case. MORTON, C. B. AND JORDAN, H. E. Arch. Surg. *30:*647–656, April '35

Congenital median cleft of chin. STEWART, W. J. Arch. Surg. *31:*813–815, Nov '35

Reconstruction of deformed chin in its relationship to rhinoplasty; dermal graft – procedure of choice. MALINIAC, J. W. Am. J. Surg. *40:*583–587, June '38

Receding chin; plastic reconstruction. SAFIAN, J. New York State J. Med. *38:*1331–1335, Oct 15, '38

Retruded chins; correction by plastic operation. NEW, G. B. AND ERICH, J. B. J.A.M.A. *115:*186–191, July 20, '40

Correction of asymmetric chins. ZENO, L. Semana med. *1:*674–679, March 20, '41

One stage operation for closure of large defects of lower lip and chin. MAY, H. Surg., Gynec. and Obst. *73:*236–239, Aug '41

Use of osteocartilaginous hump of nose for correction of underdeveloped chin. PALACIO POSSE, R. Arq. de cir. clin. e exper. *6:*299–301, April–June '42

Deformed chin and lower jaw. SCHER, S. L. Ann. Surg. *115:*869–879, May '42

Use of biologic flaps and Esser inlay to form chin and lip. PENHALE, K. W. AND ESSER, J. F. S., J. Am. Dent. A. *29:*1417–1420, Aug 1, '42

Plastic surgery of upper lip with skin flaps from chin. FREY, S. Zentralbl. f. Chir. *70:*539, April 10, '43

Chin—Cont.

Cancer of chin; extirpation in case. FERNANDEZ, L. L. Prensa med. argent. *31:*291-292, Feb 9, '44

Surgical correction of chin malformations. EISENSTODT, L. W. Am. J. Surg. *71:*491-501, Apr '46

Rhinoplasty; importance of microgenia of jaw. MARINO, H. Prensa med. argent. *33:*1500-1503, July 19, '46

Receded chin; correction with preserved cartilage. WOLF, G. D. Am. J. Surg. *72:*74-77, July '46

CHIODIN, L.: Embryology, clinical aspects and treatment of harelip. Rev. med. del Rosario, *20:*70-84, Feb '30

CHIODIN, L.: Vulviform hypospadias; case. Bol. Soc. de cir. de Rosario *5:*151-160, June '38

CHISTYAKOV, N. L.: Ganglions and their therapy (of tendon sheath). Khirurgiya, no. 5, pp. 84-95, '39

CHISTYAKOV, N. L.: Use of cellophane in treatment of wounds. Am. Rev. Soviet Med. *3:*490-493, Aug '46

CHISTYAKOV, P. I.: Morax operation in correction of symblepharon orbitale. Vestnik oftal. *11:*795-797, '37

CHOISSER, R. M. AND RAMSEY, E. M.: Use of ascitic fluid in primary shock. Proc. Soc. Exper. Biol. and Med. *38:*651-652, June '38

CHOLLETT, B. G. AND BERSHON, A. L.: Surgery in certain types of arthritis. Ohio State M. J. *27:*205-209, March '31

CHOLMELEY, J. A.: Plastic splint for opponens pollicis paralysis. Brit. M. J. *1:*357, March 9, '46

CHOLNOKY, L.: Burn therapy with paraffin and paraffin mixture, with special regard to local effect of paraffinoderm bandage. Gyogyaszat *72:*673-675, Oct 30, '32

DE CHOLNOKY, T.: Malignant melanoma; clinical study of 117 cases. Ann. Surg. *113:*392-410, March '41

DE CHOLNOKY, T.: Clinical and statistical study of 1062 cases of facial cancer. Ann. Surg., *122:*88-101, July '45

CHOMPRET (Editor): *La pratique stomatologique. Tome VIII: Restauration et prosthese maxillofaciales*. Masson et Cie, Paris, 1935

CHOTZEN, F.: Unusual familial developmental disturbance of face (acrocephalosyndactylia, craniofacial dysostosis and hypertelorism). Monatschr. f. Kinderh. *55:*97-122, '32

CHOW, K. V.: Entropion in newborn and its treatment. Chinese M. J. *48:*830-832, Sept '34

CHRISMAN, R. B. JR.: Local burn treatment. J. Tennessee M. A. *36:*413-415, Nov '43

CHRIST, H. G.: Jaw injuries; work and therapeutic aims of front line specialized unit; results in the Army on Eastern Front IV. Munchen. med. Wchnschr. *89:*832, Sept 25, '42

CHRISTIANSEN, G. W.: Penicillin in oral and maxillofacial surgery. Mil. Surgeon *96:*51-54, Jan '45

CHRISTIANSEN, G. W.: Maxillofacial injuries. M. Ann. District of Columbia *14:*76-77, Feb '45

CHRISTIANSEN, G. W.: Open operation and tantalum plate insertion for fracture of mandible. J. Oral Surg. *3:*194-204, July '45

CHRISTIANSEN, G. W. AND BRADLEY, J. L.: Palatal flap in cleft palate. U. S. Nav. M. Bull. *44:*1018-1022, May '45

CHRISTIANSEN, G. W. AND BRADLEY, J. L.: Treatment of depressed fracture of zygomatic arch by Gillies method. U. S. Nav. M. Bull. *44:*1066-1068, May '45

CHRISTIANSEN, G. W. AND BRADLEY, J. L.: Bilateral depressed zygomatic fractures. U. S. Nav. M. Bull. *45:*153-155, July '45

CHRISTIANSEN, G. W. (see HARRIS, L. W.) July '45

CHRISTIANSEN, T.: Acrocephalosyndactylia in brother and sister. Hospitalstid. *72:*178-184, Feb 14, '29

CHRISTIE, A. C.: Diagnosis and treatment of cancer of lip, mouth and throat. Fortschr. a. d. Geb. d. Roentgenstrahlen *53:*529-534, March '36

CHRISTIE, H. KENRICK: *Technique and Results of Grafting Skin*. H. K. Lewis and Co., London, 1930

CHRISTMANN, F. E.: Surgical shock. Dia med. *12:*1175-1180, Dec 23, '40

CHRISTOFFERSEN, A. K.: Modification of extension treatment in fractures of fingers. Ugesk. f. laeger *95:*1239-1240, Nov 16, '33

CHRISTOPHE, J. (see CROUZON, O. *et al)* June '32

CHRISTOPHE, L.: Bone implants. Presse med. *29:*204, March 12, '21

CHRISTOPHE, L.: Grafts of bones kept in alcohol and bone regeneration. Arch. franco-belges de chir. *26:*13-56, Jan '23 (illus.) abstr: J.A.M.A. *80:*1180, April 21, '23

CHRISTOPHE, L.: Restorative surgery of peripheral nerves. J. de chir. et ann. Soc. belge de chir., Seances extraord., pp. 122-154, June 25-26, '38

CHRISTOPHE, L.: New conception of mechanism of death from burns. Presse med. *46:*1054-1055, July 2, '38

CHRISTOPHER, F.: Present status of burn therapy. Am. J. Surg. *5:*61-65, July '28

CHRISTOPHER, F.: Lateral cervical fistula; paraffin injection as aid to excision. S. Clin. N. Amer. *10:*351-353, April '30
CHRISTOPHER, F.: First-aid treatment of burns with tannic acid. Internat. J. Med. and Surg. *43:*363-367, July '30 also: Journal-Lancet *50:*317-321, July 15, '30
CHRISTY, C. J. (see SCHREINER, B. F.) Sept '42
CHRONIS, P.: Surgical therapy of trichiasis and entropion of upper eyelid. Cong. internat. de med. trop. et d'hyg., Compt. rend. (1928) *3:*755-757, '31
CHRONIS, P.: New surgical technic in entropion musculare and trichiasis of lower eyelid. Cong. internat. de med. trop. et d'hyg., Compt. rend. (1928) *3:*759, '31
CHRONIS, P.: Radical operation in therapy of trichiasis and entropion of upper eyelid. Folia ophth. orient. *1:*187-190, Feb '33

Chronis Operation

Correction of entropion in trachoma by modified Chronis method. BATALIN, A. K. Sovet. vestnik oftal. *3:*398-399, '33

CHRYSSICOS, J. AND LAMBADARIDIS, A.: Results of surgical therapy and radiotherapy of epitheliomas of mouth, tongue and larynx. Ztschr. f. Hals-, Nasen-u. Ohrenh. *40:*410-413, '37
CHUBB, G.: Plastic surgery, 40 cases of bone-grafted mandibles. Lancet *1:*640, March 26, '21
CHULIA, V.: Surgical therapy of very extensive symblepharon. Arch. soc. oftal. hispano-am. *4:*1070-1071, Nov-Dec '44
CHURCHILL, E. D. (see FAXON, N. W.) Dec '42
CHURCHILL, E. D. (see FAXON, N. W.) Jan '43
CIACCIA, S.: Treatment of contracture of fingers. Chir. d. org. di movimento *6:*666-684, Nov '22 (illus.) abstr: J.A.M.A. *80:*513, Feb 17, '23
CIACCIO, I.: Epidermolysis bullosa dystrophica; etiopathogenic study of case following burn in tuberculous child. Arch. ital. di dermat., sif. *12:*326-344, May '36
DI CIANNI, E.: Cystic lymphangioma of neck; case. Rinasc. med. *9:*128-129, March 15, '32
CICCHETTI, N. J. (see RONCORONI, E. J.) May '45
CID, J. M. (see SALOJ, C. D.) June '35
CIERI, G.: Grafts of fixed fat tissues. Rassegna di terap. e pat. clin. *4:*587-597, Oct '32
CIESLAK, A. K. AND STOUT, A. P.: Traumatic and amputation neuromas. Arch. Surg. *53:*646-651, Dec '46
CIEZA RODRÍGUEZ, M.: Fistula in center of neck; recidivation because of inflammation of Boyer's bursa; case. Semana med. *1:*552-554, Feb 26, '31
CILLERUELO: Dacryocystorhinostomy. Informacion med. *7:*179-189, Aug '30
CINELLI, A. A.: Crooked nose. Laryngoscope *48:*760-764, Oct '38
CINELLI, A. A. AND CINELLI, J. A.: Saddle nose. New York State J. Med. *38:*977-981, July 1, '38
CINELLI, A. A.: Nasal atresia; surgical critique. Ann. Otol., Rhin. and Laryng. *49:*912-923, Dec '40
CINELLI, A. A.: Collapse of nares. Arch. Otolaryng. *33:*683-693, May '41
CINELLI, A. A.: Secondary nasal deformities following correction of cleft lip. Laryngoscope *51:*1053-1058, Nov '41
CINELLI, A. A.: Ideal nose. New York State J. Med. *42:*64-66, Jan 1, '42
CINELLI, A. A.: High cartilaginous septal trauma. Dis. Eye, Ear, Nose and Throat *2:*6-9, Jan '42
CINELLI, J. A.: Correction of nasal deformities. New York State J. Med. *37:*1018-1024, June 1, '37
CINELLI, J. A.: Rhinophyma. New York State J. Med. *40:*1672-1674, Nov 15, '40
CINELLI, J. A.: New instruments for use in rhinoplastic surgery. Arch. Otolaryng. *32:*1102-1106, Dec '40
CINELLI, J. A. (see CINELLI, A. A.) July '38
CINQUEMANI, F.: Intra-arterial medication of deep diffuse phlegmon of hand (comment on Bonoli's article.) Policlinico (sez. prat.) *36:*1395-1396, Sept 30, '29
ČÍPEK, J.: Familial syndactylia. Casop. lek. cesk. *71:*806-811, June 24, '32
CIPOLLARO, A. C.: Electrolysis for hair removal; discussion of equipment, method of operation, indications, contraindications and warnings concerning its use. J.A.M.A. *111:*2488-2491, Dec 31, '38
CIPOLLARO, A. C.: Hair removal; electrolysis; surgical procedure. New York State J. Med. *39:*1475-1480, Aug 1, '39
CIPOLLETTA, B.: Burn therapy. Gazz. internaz. med.-chir. *40:*244-247, April 30, '32
CISNEROS, R.: Lateral congenital fistula of neck; case. Bol. y trab., Acad. argent. de cir. *29:*247-259, May 9, '45
CITELLI, AND CALICETI: Caustic treatment of superficial cancer of ear, nose. Tumori *8:*165, Aug '21 abstr: J.A.M.A. *77:*1139, Oct 1, '21
CITELLI, S.: Plastic method to correct occlusions of meatus and auditory canal. Oto-rino-laring. ital. *12:*300-305, '42
CITOLER SESÉ, R.: Fractures of lower jaw; pros-

thetic therapy. Clin. y lab. *25:*129–132, Aug '34
CLAFLIN, R. S.: Construction of nose by prosthesis (case). Am. J. Orthodontics *25:*92–93, Jan '39
CLAIBORN, L. N.: Injuries to soft tissues of face. Connecticut M. J. *6:*793–795, Oct '42
CLAIRMONT, P.: Free skin grafts. Rev. de chir. structive, p. 268, Dec '37
CLAIRMONT, P. AND SCHÜRCH, O.: Electrocoagulation of cancer of cheek. Deutsche Ztschr. f. Chir. *227:*115–125, '30
CLAOUÉ, CHARLES: *Propos sur la Chirurgie Esthetique*. Maloine, Paris, 1932
CLAOUÉ, C.: Technic of surgical restoration of aged face. Bull. Acad. de med., Paris *109:*257–265, Feb 28, '33
CLAOUÉ: Marks of alignment in plastic surgery of breast. Bull. et mem. Soc. de med. de Paris *139:*130–134, Feb 23, '35
CLAOUÉ: Routes of access in reparative surgery of breast. Bull. et mem. Soc. de med. de Paris *139:*205–212, March 23, '35
CLAOUÉ, C.: Technic of plastic reduction of breast volume. Bull. et mem. Soc. de med. de Paris *139:*454–458, June 29, '35
CLAOUÉ, CHARLES AND BERNARD, IRENE: *Plastique Mammaire*. Maloine, Paris, 1936
CLAOUÉ, C.: Technic of reconstruction of breast. Bull. et mem. Soc. de med. de Paris *140:*33–36, Jan 9, '36
CLAOUÉ: Rhinoplasty using cutaneous flap from abdomen via forearm. Bull. et mem. Soc. de med. de Paris *140:*208–209, March 28, '36
CLAOUÉ: Reparative surgery; distribution of skin on neoformed breast. Bull. et mem. Soc. de med. de Paris *140:*418–423, June 27, '36
CLAOUÉ, C.: Technic of rhinoplasty by tubular grafts. J. de med. de Bordeaux *113:*633–635, Sept 10–30, '36
CLAOUÉ, C. AND BERNARD, MME. I.: Cicatrix in reparative surgery of breast. J. de med. de Bordeaux *113:*695–697, Oct 10, '36
CLAOUÉ, C.: Restorative surgery of breast in hypertrophy; author's technic. Bull. et mem. Soc. med. et chir. de Bordeaux, pp. 168–182, '36
CLAOUÉ: Rhinoplasty using cutaneous flap from abdomen via forearm. Bull. et mem. Soc. de med. de Paris *141:*278–280, April 24, '37
CLAOUÉ: Plastic surgery of breast; presentation of colored motion picture. Arch. f. klin. Chir. *189:*538–547, '37
CLAOUÉ: Plastic surgery of nose; technic and instruments. Ztschr. f. Hals-, Nasen-u. Ohrenh. *40:*660–662, '37
CLAOUÉ, C.: Alignment points in plastic surgery of breast. Chir. plast. *4:*26–28, Jan–April '38
CLAOUÉ, C.: "Les brides," vestibulo-alveolare; destruction for the plastic reconstruction of the gingivo-jugo-labial groove. Bull. et mem. Soc. de med. de Paris, *142:*523–528, June 25, '38
CLAOUÉ, C.: Vestibulo-alveolar adhesions; destruction by plastic reconstruction of gingivo-jugo-labial groove. Oto-rhino-laryng. internat. *24:*41–45, Feb '40 also: Rev. gen. de clin. et de therap. *54:*95–96, Feb 24, '40
CLAOUÉ: Tubular flaps transferred by dermal inclusion (leech method). Monde med., Paris *50:*149–152, May '40
CLAOUÉ, CHARLES: *Chirurgie plastique abdominale; cure chirurgicale de ptose cutanée abdominale, ventre en tablier*. Maloine, Paris, 1940
CLAPP, C. A.: Entropion following influenza, with new surgical procedure. Am. J. Ophth., *5:*542–544, July '22 (illus.)

Clapp's Operation

Plastic operation of mandibular region by Clapp's method; case. TSUNODA, E. Mitt. a. d. med. Akad. zu Kioto *8:*131–132, '33

CLARK, A.: Surgical shock. Glasgow M. J. *123:*1–7, Jan '35
CLARK, A. M.: Burns in childhood. M. Press *201:*182–185, Feb 15, '39
CLARK, A. M.: Color film of treatment by cod liver oil and sulfanilamide in burns. Tr. Roy. Med.-Chir. Soc. Glasgow, pp. 17–18, '41–'42; in Glasgow M. J. April '42
CLARK, A. M. *et al.* Penicillin and propamidine; elimination of hemolytic streptococci and staphylococci (in burns). Lancet *1:*605–609, May 15, '43
CLARK, A. M. AND CRUICKSHANK, R.: Burn therapy. Lancet *1:*201–204, Jan '35
CLARK, A. M.; MILNE, G. R. AND TODD, J. P.: Fixation of grafts with human plasma and thrombin. Lancet *1:*498–499, April 21, '45
CLARK, C. M.: Harelip and cleft palate. Ohio State M. J. *18:*417–423, June '22 (illus.)
CLARK, C. M.: Angiomas of face and mouth. Ohio State M. J. *30:*438–441, July '34
CLARK, C. P.: Laceration of eyelids. J. Indiana M. A. *36:*245–247, May '43
CLARK, E. J. AND ROSSITER, R. J.: Carbohydrate metabolism after burning. Quart. J. Exper. Physiol. *32:*279–300, March '44
CLARK, H. B. JR.: Fractures of upper jaw; 150 cases in overseas maxillofacial center. J. Oral Surg. *3:*286–303, Oct '45

CLARK, W. G.; STRAKOSCH, E. A. AND LEVEN, L. N.: "Prefabricated eschar" or bandage, containing sulfonamide. Journal-Lancet *62:*455-456, Dec '42

CLARK, W. L.: Electrodesiccation and electrocoagulation in neoplastic and allied diseases of oral cavity and adjacent parts; clinical, physical, historical and photographic studies based upon 20 years' experience. Am. J. Surg. *6:*257-275, March '29

CLARKE, C. D.: Moulage prosthesis for face. J. Lab. and Clin. Med. *26:*901-912, Feb '41 also: Am. J. Orthodontics (Oral Surg. Sect) *27:*214-225, April '41

CLARKE, C. D.: Application and wearing of facial prostheses. J. Lab. and Clin. Med. *27:*123-126, Oct '41

CLARKE, C. D.: Coloring and applying prosthesis to face. J. Lab. and Clin. Med. *28:*1517-1534, Sept '43

CLARKE, C. D.: Prosthesis in relation to war wounds of face. M. Bull. North African Theat. Op. (no. 1) *1:*17-24, Jan '44 also: J. Lab. and Clin. Med. *29:*667-672, June '44

CLARKE, CARL D.: *Facial and Body Prosthesis*. C. V. Mosby Co., St. Louis, 1945

CLARKE, C. D. (see CONVERSE, J. M. *et al*) May '44

CLARKE, D. A. (see FLACK, H. L. *et al*) July '45

CLARKE, L. T.: Economy in use of cocaine, by Moffett method of postural instillation. J. Roy. Army M. Corps. *82:*135-137, March '44

CLARKSON, P.: Plastic surgery tour of United States centers. Guy's Hosp. Gaz. *60:*141, May 25, '46; 165, June 22, '46

CLARKSON, P. AND LAWRIE, R. S.: Management and surgical resurfacing of serious burns. Brit. J. Surg. *33:*311-323, Apr '46

CLARKSON, P. AND SCHORSTEIN, J.: Treatment of denuded external table of skull. Brit. M. J. *2:*422-423, Sept 29, '45

CLARKSON, P. AND WILSON, T. H. H.: Recommendations for treatment of maxillofacial cases in forward areas. Brit. Dent. J. *77:*229-234, Oct 20, '44

CLARKSON, P.; WILSON, T. H. H. AND LAWRIE, R. S.: Treatment of 1,000 fractures (in British army) of jaw. Ann. Surg. *123:*190-208, Feb '46 also: Brit. Dent. J. *80:*69, Feb 1, '46; 107, Feb 15, '46

CLAUS, G.: Complications following resections of submucous septum. Ztschr. f. Hals-, Nasen-u. Ohrenh. *23:*444-449, Sept 10, '29

CLAUS, G.: Plastic surgery with bridge flap for correction of retroauricular defects. Deutsche med. Wchnschr. *57:*1779-1780, Oct 16, '31

CLAUS, G.: Correction of saddle nose, with special reference to implantation of ivory. Ztschr. f. Hals-, Nasen-u. Ohrenh. *35:*198-211, '34

CLAUS, H.: Easy method of dacryocystorhinostomy. Beitr. z. Anat., Physiol., Path. u. Therap. d. Ohres *26:*121-124, Nov '27

CLAVELIN, C. AND CARILLON, R. J.: Burn therapy in army medical department. Rev. serv. de san. mil. *106:*571-596, April '37

CLAVELIN, C. AND HUGONOT: Generalized edema following extensive burns; pathogenesis of edema; role of serum protein equilibrium. Bull. et mem. Soc. med. d. hop. de Paris *52:*1444-1449, Nov 16, '36

Clawhand

Clawhand. JANSEN, M. Ztschr. f. orthop. Chir. *58:*193-199, '32

Tenoplasty of flexor muscles of fingers for clawhand (pseudo-Volkmann contracture); results in case. DIAMANT-BERGER, L. Bull. et mem. Soc. d. chirurgiens de Paris *27:*541-545, Nov 22, '35

Clawhand; Morestin plastic surgery with free full-thickness skin graft. ZENO, L. Bol. Soc. de cir. de Rosario *7:*308-315, Aug '40 also: An. de cir. *6:*315-321, Sept '40

Clawhand following violent compression of long flexor muscles of forearm; study of case. BOUDREAUX, J. Mem. Acad. de chir. *68:*124-126, Feb 11-March 4, '42

Clawhand resulting from mechanical constriction of forearm in plaster casts. LEVEUF, J. Rev. de chir., Paris *80:*79-106, April-Dec '42

Clawhand; capsulotomies. NUNZIATA, A. Prensa med. argent. *31:*2169-2171, Oct 25, '44

Adaption of structure of hand to disturbed function following deep burns (clawhand). HUDACK, S. S. Am. Acad. Orthop. Surgeons, Lect., pp. 208-211, '44

Splint to correct deformity (clawhand) resulting from injury to ulnar nerve. PRUCE, A. M., J. Bone and Joint Surg. *28:*397, Apr '46

CLAY, G. E. AND BAIRD, J. M.: Restoration of orbit and repair of conjunctival defects, with grafts from prepuce and labia minora. Tr. Sect. Ophth., A.M.A., pp. 252-259, '36

CLAY, G. E. AND BAIRD, J. M.: Restoration of orbit and repair of conjunctival defects, with grafts from prepuce and labia minora. J.A.M.A. *107:*1122-1125, Oct 3, '36

CLAY, R. C.: Fibroma of palmar fascia. Ann. Surg. *120:*224-231, Aug '44

CLAY, R. C. (see PICKRELL, K. L.) April '44

CLAYTON, S. G.: Case of exstrophy of bladder with procidentia. J. Obst. and Gynaec. Brit. Emp. *52:*177-179, April '45

CLAYTON, S. G.: Melanoma of vulva with pregnancy. Proc. Roy. Soc. Med. *39:*578–579, July '46

CLAYTON, W. (see THOMSON, D. *et al*) March '41

Cleft Hand

Plastic reconstruction of fingers with particular regard to formation of cleft hand. ZOLLINGER, A. Deutsche Ztschr. f. Chir. *196:*271–287, '26

Cleft hand; case. BOORSTEIN, S. W., J. Bone and Joint Surg. *12:*172–176, Jan '30

Cleft hand; 2 cases. MIKI, Y. Okayama-Igakkai-Zasshi *44:*2295–2296, Aug '32

Cleft hands and cleft feet with oligodactylia. KELLNER, A. W. Klin. Wchnschr. *13:*1507–1509, Oct 20, '34

Syndrome of "forked hands and feet" and oligophrenia; 2 cases. MUYLE, G. AND BATSELAERE, R., J. belge de neurol. et de psychiat. *36:*441–455, July '36

Split-hand deformity. POPENOE, P., J. Hered. *28:*174–176, May '37

Acrocephalosyndactylia with cleft hand in one of a pair of uniovular twins. GOLL, H. AND KAHLICH-KOENNER, D. M. Ztschr. f. menschl. Vererb.-u. Konstitutionslehre *24:*516–535, '40

Study of anatomy and heredity of cleft foot and hand deformities in siblings. KLAGES, F. AND JACOB, R. Ztschr. f. Orthop. *70:*265–281, '40

Cleft Lip

Repair of harelip and cleft palate deformity. RITCHIE, H. P. Minnesota Med. *4:*15, Jan '21

Correction of unilateral harelip. VEAU, V. AND RUPPE, C. Presse med. *29:*321, April 23, '21 abstr: J.A.M.A. *76:*1712, June 11, '21

Cleft palate and harelip procedures. BROPHY, T. W. Minnesota Med. *4:*283, May '21

Cleft palate and harelip. SHEARER, W. L. Minnesota Med. *4:*293, May '21

Hare-lip and cleft palate; a war influence. AYMARD, J. L. Brit. M. J. *2:*405, Sept 10, '21

Certain non-technical considerations in treatment of harelip and cleft palate. COE, H. E. Arch. Pediat. *38:*658, Oct '21

Substitute for adhesive plaster bandage in hare-lip operations. FRÜND, H. Zentralbl. f. Chir. *48:*1426, Oct 1, '21

Hare-lip surgery; a suggestion. SAMUELS, L. Lancet *2:*860, Oct 22, '21

Simplification of technique in operations for hare-lip and cleft palate. THOMPSON, J. F. Ann. Surg. *74:*394, Oct '21

Harelip and cleft palate. VON WEDEL, C. Southwest J. Med. and Surg. *29:*148–149, Nov '21 (illus.)

Nasal relation of harelip operations. BROWN, G. V. I., J.A.M.A. *77:*1954, Dec 17, '21

Correction of congenital cleft palate and harelip, surgical principles involved. MOOREHEAD, F. B., J.A.M.A. *77:*1951, Dec 17, '21

Operation for harelip and cleft palate. MILNER, R. Zentralbl. f. Chir. *49:*80–81, Jan 21, '22 (illus.)

Harelip and cleft palate. DAVIS, W. B., S. Clin. N. America *2:*199–223, Feb '22 (illus.)

Correction of nose deformities at operations for harelip. MEYER, H. Zentralbl. f. Chir. *49:*220, Feb 18, '22 (illus.)

A knife for harelip and cleft palate operations. CATES, B. B. Am. J. Surg. *36:*70, March '22

Harelip and cleft palate. MCCURDY, S. L. Pennsylvania M. J. *25:*560–564, May '22 (illus.)

Harelip and cleft palate. CLARK, C. M. Ohio State M. J. *18:*417–423, June '22 (illus.)

Harelip and cleft palate deformities, some types and their operative treatment. DAVIS, W. B. Ann. Surg. *76:*133–142, Aug '22 (illus.)

Classification of congenital clefts of lip and palate, with suggestions for recording these cases. DAVIS, J. S. AND RITCHIE, H. P., J.A.M.A. *79:*1323–1327, Oct 14, '22 (illus.)

Harelip and cleft palate operation. EDBERG, E. Acta chir. Scandinav. *55:*1–26, '22 (in English) abstr: J.A.M.A. *79:*1562, Oct 28, '22

Operation for complex harelip. RAMSTEDT, C. Zentralbl. f. Chir. *49:*1556–1558, Oct 21, '22

Atypical plastic operations for congenital fissures of lip and palate. THOMPSON, J. E., S. Clin. N. America *2:*1387–1401, Oct '22 (illus.)

Tripartite cleft palate and double harelip in identical twins. DAVIS, A. D. Surg., Gynec. and Obst. *35:*586–592, Nov '22 (illus.)

Harelip and cleft palate. FEDERSPIEL, M. N. Laryngoscope *32:*909–928, Dec '22 (illus.)

Treatment of harelip. OMBREDANNE, L. Medecine *4:*21–27, Oct '22 abstr: J.A.M.A. *79:*1962, Dec 2, '22

Rhino-laryngologic phases of harelip and cleft palate work. DAVIS, W. B. Internat. Clinics *2:*258–266, '22 (illus.)

Cleft Lip—Cont.

Cleft Lip and Palate, by TRUMAN W. BROPHY. Blakiston Co., Phila., 1923

Treatment of harelip. LADD, W. E. Boston M. and S. J. *188:*270–272, March 1, '23 (illus.)

Correction of nasal deformities associated with harelip and cleft palate. DAVIS, W. B. J. M. Soc. New Jersey *20:*113–119, April '23 (illus.)

Bandaging after harelip operation. RANFT, G. Zentralbl. f. Chir. *50:*598–600, April 14, '23 (illus.)

Reasons for operations in early infancy on cleft-lip and cleft palate. SILVERMAN, S. L. J. M. A. Georgia *12:*143–147, April '23 (illus.)

Spontaneous correction of harelip. AUSEMS, A. W. Nederlandsch Tijdschr. v. Geneesk. *2:*1942, Nov 10, '23

Cleft palate and harelip. SUDLER, M. T., J. Kansas M. Soc. *24:*18–20, Jan '24

Embryo with harelip. CADENAT, E. Compt. rend. Soc. de biol. *90:*181–183, Feb 1, '24

Cleft palate and cleft lip cases. SHEARER, W. L. Nebraska M. J. *9:*160–164, May '24

Heredity of malformations, especially harelip and polydactylism. LÜCKER, F. C. Monatschr. f. Geburtsh. u. Gynak. *66:*327–336, July '24 abstr: J.A.M.A. *83:*882, Sept 13, '24

Congenital clefts of lip and palate, incidence of. DAVIS, J. S. Ann. Surg. *80:*363–374, Sept '24

Fissure of lip; a simple and efficient method of treatment. MICHELSON, H. E. Arch. Dermat. and Syph. *10:*332, Sept '24

Treatment of unilateral harelip with special reference to associated deformity of nose. COLEMAN, C. C. Virginia M. Monthly *51:*393–399, Oct '24

Treatment of cleft lip and palate. BAIRD, J. P. J. Tennessee M. A. *17:*257–264, Dec '24

Treatment of congenital cleft lip and palate. FARR, R. E. Minnesota Med. *8:*149–153, March '25

Treatment of congenital cleft of lip and palate. KAHN, L. Am. J. Surg. *39:*142–144, June '25 also: Kentucky M. J. *23:*491–493, Oct '25

Treatment of hare-lip. MACAULEY, H. F. Brit. M. J. *2:*253–254, Aug 8, '25

Treatment of congenital cleft lip. MULLEN, T. F., M. J. and Rec. (supp.) *122:*402–407, Oct 7, '25

Treatment of harelip. MEYER, H. Beitr. z. klin. Chir. *135:*136–149, '25

Problem of bringing forward retracted upper lip and nose in harelip. BLAIR, V. P. Surg., Gynec. and Obst. *42:*128–132, June '26

Cleft Lip—Cont.

Four generations of harelip. MASON, R., J. Hered. *17:*52, Feb '26

Role of median nasal process in development of face; study of hare-lip. VEAU, V. Ann. d'anat. path. *3:*305–348, April '26 abstr: J.A.M.A. *87:*1160, Oct 2, '26

Types of harelip and cleft-palate deformities and operative results. DAVIS, W. B. Surg., Gynec. and Obst. *42:*704–709, May '26

Harelip and cleft palate. LADD, W. E. Boston M. and S. J. *194:*1016–1025, June 3, '26

Rare congenital malformations of nose; case histories, and treatment: (1) fibrolipoma of septum, harelip; (2) bull-dog nose, fibrolipoma of dorsum of nose. FEYGIN, N. Zentralbl. f. Chir. *53:*1686, July 3, '26

Congenital cleft lip and palate; muscle theory repair of cleft lip. RITCHIE, H. P. Ann. Surg. *84:*211–222, Aug '26

Important factors in treatment of cleft lip and palate. VAUGHAN, H. S. Ann. Surg. *84:*223–232, Aug '26

Operation for cleft palate and hare-lip. HOHMEIER, F. Deutsche med. Wchnschr. *52:*1604–1606, Sept 17, '26

Surgery of mouth and face with special reference to cleft palate and cleft lip. LOGAN, W. H. G. Kentucky M. J. *24:*498–505, Oct '26

Prosthetic treatment of harelip and cleft palate complication. RUPPE, L. AND RUPPE, C. Odontologie *64:*831–845, Dec 30, '26

Hare-lip and other developmental lesions of face. RANKIN, W. Glasgow M. J. *106:*350–358, Dec '26

Congenital cleft lip and palate; series of congenital clefts. RITCHIE, H. P. Minnesota Med. *9:*664–666, Dec '26

Management of cleft-lip and palate cases. SPRAGUE, E. W., S. Clin. N. Amer. *6:*1481–1496, Dec '26

Complete harelip and cleft palate on left side, with absence of left half of intermaxillary bone, of philtrum and of cartilaginous portion of nasal septum. BERG, A. Arch. f. klin. Chir. *140:*168–171, '26

Hereditary nature of harelip and cleft palate. BIRKENFELD, W. Arch. f. klin. Chir. *141:*729–753, '26

Harelip with cleft palate; 2 cases. PIETRANTONI, L. Sperimentale Arch. di biol. *80:*651–664, Jan 25, '27

Shortcomings in surgery of cleft lip and palate, with suggestions for meeting them. FARR, R. E. Minnesota Med. *10:*70–76, Feb '27

Harelip and cleft palate. HORSLEY, J. S. JR. Virginia M. Monthly *53:*782–787, March '27

Cleft Lip – Cont.
Congenital cleft lip and palate. WOOLSEY, J. H. California and West. Med. *26:*633–636, May '27
Cleft lip and palate. BROPHY, T. W., J. Am. Dent. A. *14:*1108–1115, June '27
Operative procedure in cleft palate and harelip. LYONS, C. J., J. Am. Dent. A. *14:*1080–1094, June '27
Congenital cleft lip and palate; some personal observations. MOOREHEAD, F. B., J. Am. Dent. A. *14:*1098–1107, June '27
Operative treatment of harelip and cleft palate. HELBING, C. Allg. deutsche Hebam.-Ztg. *42:*193, July 1, '27
Orthodontia and its uses in preliminary treatment of extreme cases of harelip and cleft palate. MILLARD, J., J. Internat. Orthodont. Cong. *1:*493–496, '27 also: Internat. J. Orthodontia *13:*621–624, July '27
Cleft lip and palate. FREW, A. L. Texas State J. Med. *23:*333–335, Sept '27
Importance of pediatric care in operative treatment of harelip and cleft palate. HENSKE, J. A., J.A.M.A. *89:*1666–1670, Nov. 12, '27
Surgical correction of cleft lip and palate. JOBSON, G. B. Arch. Otolaryng. *6:*434–445, Nov '27
Harelip operation by Orlovsky method. MASLOV, I. Vestnik khir. (no. 33) *11:*146–150, Nov. 22, '27
Harelip, SHANK, R. A., J. Med. *8:*434–437, Nov '27
Cleft palate and harelip; familial manifestations. LEVEN. Arch. f. Rassen-u. Gesellsch.-Biol. *20:*71, Dec. 20, '27
Study of twins with cleft lip, jaw, and palate from standpoint of pathologic heredity. BIRKENFELD, W. Beitr. z. klin. Chir. *141:*257–267, '27
Congenital harelip and cleft palate; case I (unfinished case). CHAPIN, W. C. Internat. Orthodont. Cong. *1:*485–492, '27
Transplantation of strip of cheek and naris in harelip therapy. EHRENFELD, H. Arch. f. klin. Chir. *144:*486–488, '27
Congenital cleft lip and palate; embryology of upper jaw interpreted in terms of surgical repair of process and palate of clefts. RITCHIE, H. P. Tr. Am. S. A. *45:*170–178, '27
Harelip and Cleft Palate, by MATTHEW FEDERSPIEL. C. V. Mosby Co., St. Louis, 1927
Harelip and cleft palate operations. CATES, B. B. Internat. J. Med. and Surg. *41:*8–11, Jan '28
Problem of child with harelip and cleft palate. MCEACHERN, J. D. Canad. M. A. J. *18:*170–174, Feb '28

Cleft Lip – Cont.
Harelip operation. HAGENTORN, A. Zentralbl. f. Chir. *55:*528–533, March 3, '28
End-results after harelip operations. HORSLEY, J. S. JR. Virginia M. Monthly *54:*753–757, March '28
Harelip and cleft palate; study of 425 consecutive cases. DAVIS, W. B. Ann. Surg. *87:*536–554, April '28
Surgical treatment of clefts of palate and lip. PARKER, D. B. Am. J. Surg. *4:*385–389, April '28
Lips and teeth and cyclopia and harelips. BOLK, L. Ztschr. f. d. ges. Anat. (Abt. 1) *85:*762–783, May 21, '28
Plastic surgery of face and harelip and nose and cleft palate. JOBSON, G. B. Atlantic M. J. *31:*716–723, July '28
Harelip in univitelline twins; case. LÉVY, G. Bull. Soc. d'obst. et de gynec. *17:*661, July '28
Clinical aspects and treatment of harelip. ESTELLA Y BERMÚDEZ DE CASTRO, J. Clin. y lab. *12:*177–199, Sept '28
Care and treatment of harelip and cleft palate. CARRUTHERS, F. W., J. Arkansas M. Soc. *25:*93–97, Oct '28
Discussion on treatment of harelip. VEAU, V. *et al.* Proc. Roy. Soc. Med. (sect. Surg.) *21:*100–120, Oct '28
Treatment of harelip and cleft palate. RISDON, F., J. Am. Dent. A. *15:*2017–2020, Nov '28
Technic of operation for harelip. HAGENTORN, A. Deutsche Ztschr. f. Chir. *212:*391–398, '28
Unilateral harelip; fundamental principles of operation. HÄRTEL, F. Beitr. z. klin. Chir. *144:*313–319, '28
Surgery of labio-maxillo-palatine fissure. LASAGNA, F. Arch. ital. di chir. *20:*661–679, '28
Surgical therapy of harelip by Orlowsky's method. MASSLOFF, I. D. Arch. f. klin. Chir. *150:*322–327, '28
Why and how of harelip correction. BLAIR, V. P. Ann. Otol. Rhin. and Laryng. *37:*196–205, March '28
Anatomy of total, unilateral harelip. VEAU, V. Ann. d'anat. path., *5:*601–632, June '28
Surgical treatment of harelip. LÓPEZ VILLORIA, L. Gac. med. de Caracas *36:*85–88, March 31, '29
Surgical treatment under regional anesthesia for harelip. GINESTET, G. AND GINESTET, F. Rev. de stomatol. *31:*212, April '29
Repair of harelip and accompanying nasal deformity. PADGETT, E. C., J. Kansas M. Soc. *30:*143–147, May '29

Cleft Lip – Cont.
Why and how of harelip correction. BLAIR, V. P. Internat. J. Orthodontia *15:*1112–1119, Nov '29
Operation of harelip. HAGENTORNAS, A. Medicina, Kaunas *10:*917–918, Dec '29
Origin of harelip. CADENAT, E. Presse med. *38:*270–271, Feb 22, '30
Embryology, clinical aspects and treatment of harelip. CHIODÍN, L. Rev. med. del Rosario *20:*70–84, Feb '30
Hare-lip and its treatment. WARBURTON, G. B. Brit. M. J. *1:*732–734, April 19, '30
Etiology of cleft palate and lip; fundamental principles in operative procedure. LYONS, C. J., J. Am. Dent. A. *17:*827–843, May '30
Mirault operation for single harelip. BLAIR, V. P. AND BROWN, J. B. Surg. Gynec. and Obst. *51:*81–98, July '30
Harelip and cleft palate; analysis of 184 cases. BURDICK, C. G. Ann. Surg. *92:*35–50, July '30
Dental cyst in patient operated for harelip; case. ARELLANO, E. R. Cron. med. mex. *29:*337–342, Aug '30
Opportune time and method for cosmetic and functional repair of congenital cleft palate and harelip. HOFER, O. Wien. klin. Wchnschr. *43:*1184, Sept 18, '30
Pathology and therapy of cleft palate and harelip. ROSENTHAL, W. Fortschr. d. Zahnh. *6:*953–972, Nov '30
Treatment of harelip and other facial fissures. HÄRTEL, F. F. Chirurg *2:*1057–1061, Dec 1, '30
Plea for better average harelip repairs. BLAIR, V. P. Dallas M. J. *17:*4–9, Jan '31
Mirault operation for single harelip. BLAIR, V. P. AND BROWN, J. B. Internat. J. Orthodontia *17:*370–396, April '31
Surgical correction of cleft lip and palate. DAVIS, A. D. Surg., Gynec. and Obst. *52:*875–883, April '31
Freezing of facial nerve in treatment of harelip. GOETZE, O. Zentralbl. f. Chir. *58:*927–930, April 11, '31
Cleft palate and harelip treated by mobilization of 2 triangular osseous segments from cleft palate. BASTIANELLI, P. Boll. d. mal. d. orecchio, d. gola. e d. naso *29:*137–153, May '31
Plea for better average harelip repairs. BLAIR, V. P. AND BROWN, J. B. Internat. J. Orthodontia *17:*472–483, May '31
Dimensions and growth of palate in infant with gross maldevelopment of upper lip and palate; quantitative study. PEYTON, W. T. Arch. Surg. *22:*704–737, May '31

Cleft Lip – Cont.
Hereditary aspect of harelip and cleft palate. COENEN, H. Chirurg *3:*501–505, June 1, '31
Operative methods in unilateral harelip. VEAU, V. AND PLESSIER, P. Bull. et mem. Soc. nat. de chir. *57:*861–863, June 13, '31
Treatment of harelip. MOURE, P. Bull. et mem. Soc. nat. de chir. *57:*899–901, June 27, '31
Role of orthodontia following cleft lip and palate surgery. DAVIS, A. D. Pacific Dent. Gaz. *39:*571–580, Aug '31
Harelip and cleft palate. NEW, G. B., S. Clin. North America. *11:*761–765, Aug '31
Plastic surgery of cleft lip. EHRENFELD, H. Gyogyaszat *71:*607, Sept. 27, '31
Surgical correction of harelip and cleft palate. DAVIS, A. D. California and West. Med. *35:*357–361, Nov '31
Surgical treatment of harelip and cleft palate. in children. RISDON, F. Canad. M. A. J. *25:*563–565, Nov '31
Hereditary aspect of cleft lip and palate. SCHRÖDER, C. H. Arch. f. Rassen-u. Gesellsch.-Biol. *25:*369–394, Nov. 25, '31
Cleft lip and cleft palate. ARMBRECHT, E. C. West Virginia M. J. *28:*59–64, Feb '32
Lesions of jaw, nose and cheek; cleft lip and palate; cartilage transplant; tube graft. MOOREHEAD, F. B., S. Clin. North America *12:*57–66, Feb '32
Cleft lip and palate; surgical correction. DAVIS, A. D. Internat. J. Orthodontia *18:*282–290, March '32
Surgical therapy of cleft lip and palate. WASSMUND, M. Deutsche med. Wchnschr. *58:*445–448, March 18, '32
Cradle suspended from ceiling for quieting infants after surgical therapy for harelip. FREUDENBERG, E. Kinderarztl. Praxis *3:*213–214, May '32
Preoperative and postoperative care of congenital clefts of lip and palate. KITLOWSKI, E. A. Ann. Surg. *95:*659–666, May '32
Similarity of reasons for operative failures in congenital harelip and traumatic tear of lip. RENDU, A. Gaz. med. de France, pp. 351–353, May 15, '32
Therapy of harelip and cleft palate. EDBERG, E. Hygiea *94:*529–558, July 31, '32
Method of placing dressing in order to relieve tension of suture after operation for harelip. PORZELT, W. Zentralbl. f. Chir. *59:*2165–2167, Sept. 3, '32
Surgery of fetal clefts (harelip, cleft palate, etc.); review of literature. ROSENTHAL, W. Zentralbl. f. Chir. *59:*2345–2379, Sept. 24, '32

Cleft Lip – Cont.
Cosmetic surgery of incomplete (operated) harelip and nasal deformities combined with harelip. ÉRCZY, M. Gyogyaszat *72:*719–721, Nov. 20, '32
Surgical therapy of harelip in children. HARRENSTEIN, R. J. Nederl. tijdschr. v. geneesk. *76:*5557–5566, Dec. 3, '32
Congenital clefts of face and jaw; survey of 350 operated cases. RITCHIE, H. P. Tr. West. S. A. *42:*37–98, '32
Surgical treatment of harelip and cleft palate. SKINNER, M., J. M. A. Alabama *2:*253–259, Jan '33
Present status of therapy of cleft lip and palate. BURIAN, F. Casop. lek. cesk. *72:*420, April 7; 454, April 14; 491, April 21, '33
Harelip. FOUCAR, H. O. Canad. M. A. J. *28:*373–376, April '33
Principles to be observed in treatment of congenital harelip and cleft palate. HYSLOP V. B. Wisconsin M. J. *32:*246–248, April '33
Cleft palate and harelip. CASELLA, E. Rev. med. latino-am. *19:*119–159, Nov '33
Anatomic examination of human hemicephalic fetus 10 months old with harelip, cleft palate, hyperdactylia, syndactylia, etc. IKEDA, Y. Arb. a. d. anat. Inst. d. kaiserlich-japan. Univ. zu Sendai. Hft. 15, pp. 61–212, '33
Operations on congenital harelip and cleft of both hard and soft palates. PICHLER, H. Wien. klin. Wchnschr. *47:*70–72, Jan. 19, '34
Cleft lip and palate surgery. FREW, A. L., J. Am. Dent. A. *21:*251–255, Feb '34
Surgical therapy of harelip and cleft palate; possibilities of results. ERNST, F. Kinderarztl. Praxis *5:*120–128, March '34
Cleft lip repair under bilateral infra-orbital nerve block at infra-orbital foramina. NYI, P. C. Chinese M. J. *48:*373–374, April '34
Congenital clefts of face and jaws; 350 cases in which operation was performed. RITCHIE, H. P. Arch. Surg. *28:*617–658, April '34
Congenital deformities of mouth (including cleft lip and palate). BROWNE, D. Practitioner *132:*658–670, June '34
Dimensions and growth of palate in infants with gross maldevelopment of upper lip and palate; further investigations (including cleft lip and palate). PEYTON, W. T. Am. J. Dis. Child. *47:*1265–1268, June '34
Cleft palate and harelip; adolescent case treated orthodontically in conjunction with lip-stretching device and skin grafting of labial sulcus. HARDY, E. A. Internat. J. Orthodontia *20:*750–758, Aug '34

Cleft Lip – Cont.
Cleft palate and cleft lip. SHEARER, W. L., J. Am. Dent. A. *21:*1446–1454, Aug '34
Inheritance of harelip and cleft palate. SANDERS, J. Genetica *15:*433–510, '34
Surgical repair of facial injuries and harelip and cleft palate deformities. RISDON, E. F. Canad. M. A. J. *32:*51–54, Jan '35
Skeletal malformations in total unilateral and bilateral harelip. VEAU, V. Ann. d'anat. path. *11:*873–904, Dec '34 abstr.: Schweiz. med. Wchnschr. *65:*99–101, Jan. 26, '35
Hypothesis on initial malformation in harelip; role of skeleton and muscles. VEAU, V. Ann. d'anat. path. *12:*389–424, April '35
Initial malformation in harelip. VEAU, V. Bull. et mem. Soc. nat. de chir. *61:*496–502, April 6, '35
Technic of surgical correction of harelip. FUSS, H. Chirurg *7:*372–375, June 1, '35
Cheiloplasty in plastic repair of harelip; author's technic. CODAZZI AGUIRRE, J. A. Rev. med. del Rosario *25:*953–965, Aug '35
Inheritance of harelip and cleft palate in man. DROOGLEEVER FORTUYN, A. B. Genetica *17:*349–366, '35
Surgical therapy of harelip. FUSS, H. Arch. f. klin. Chir. *182:*253–272, '35
Studies on heredity of harelip, and cleft palate with particular regard to mode of transmission. SCHRÖDER, C. H. Arch. f. klin. Chir. *182:*299–330, '35
Clinical forms of unilateral harelip. VEAU, V. Deutsche Ztschr. f. Chir. *244:*595–610, '35
Correction of cleft lip. and palate. FREW, A. L. J. Am. Dent. A. *23:*29–34, Jan '36
Present day conception of cleft lip and palate surgery. KIRKHAM, H. L. D. Texas State J. Med. *31:*571–574, Jan '36
Basic trends in surgical therapy of harelip. VEAU, V. Chirurg *8:*1–12, Jan. 1, '36
Harelip. STEPHENS, H. D. Brit. M. J. *1:*5–8, Jan. 4, '36 also: M. J. Australia *1:*494–498, April 11, '36
Etiology of cleft palate and harelip. BEATTY, H. G., J. Speech Disorders, pp. 13–20, March '36
Normal and anomalous formation of primary palate; embryology of harelip. VEAU, V. AND POLITZER, G. Ann. d'anat. path. *13:*275–326, March '36
Vilray P. Blair's modification of Mirault operation for cleft lip. BROWN, R. G., M. J. Australia *1:*499–503, April 11, '36
Harelip. FAGGE, C. H. Australian and New Zealand J. Surg. *5:*359–365, April '36
Harelip and cleft palate. BERNDORFER, A.

Cleft Lip – Cont.
Gyogyaszat *76:*499, Aug. 30-Sept. 6, '36; 527, Sept. 13, '36
Therapy of cleft lip, jaw and palate with protruding intermaxillary bone. TOMOFF, W. Zentralbl. f. Chir. *63:*2535–2538, Oct. 24, '36
Harelip and cleft palate. BEATTY, H. G. West Virginia M. J. *32:*501–516, Nov '36
Quantitative studies on congenital clefts. PEYTON, W. T. AND RITCHIE, H. P. Arch. Surg. *33:*1046–1053, Dec '36
Teeth in cyclopia and congenital cleft of face. BRECKWOLDT, H. Beitr. z. path. Anat. u. z. allg. Path. *98:*115–135, '36
Development of harelip and cleft palate in embryo 22 mm. in length. MAURER, H. Ztschr. f. Anat. u. Entwcklngsgesch. *105:*359–373, '36
Origin of facial cleft, harelip and cleft palate. POLITZER, G. Monatschr. f. Ohrenh. *71:*63–73, Jan '37
Thoracopagus, one with harelip and cleft palate. SANGVICHIEN, S. Anat. Rec. *67:*157–158, Jan. 25, '37
Cleft lips and cleft palate. CUNNINGHAM, A. F. Am. J. Nursing *37:*339–341, April '37
New approach in plastic operations of cleft palate and harelip. HERLYN, K. E. Zentralbl. f. Chir. *64:*815–818, April 3, '37
Anesthesia (endotracheal oxygen-ether vapor) for harelip and cleft palate operations on babies. AYRE, P. Brit. J. Surg. *25:*131–132, July '37
Harelip and cleft palate. ERNST, F. Med. Welt *11:*1061–1064, July 31, '37
Surgical and phonetic problems of harelip and cleft palate. BERNDORFER, A. Gyogyaszat *77:*433, July 18–25; 452, Aug. 1–8, '37
Aids in surgery of harelip. DOUGLAS, B. Ann. Surg. *106:*293–296, Aug '37
Review of recent literature on cleft lip and palate surgery. IVY, R. H. Internat. J. Orthodontia *23:*844–849, Aug '37
Surgical therapy of harelip and cleft palate. OBERNIEDERMAYR, A. Chirurg *9:*641–645, Sept. 1, '37
Problems of unilateral harelip repair. YOUNG, F. Surg., Gynec. and Obst. *65:*348–354, Sept. '37
Atypical cartilage in nose, upper lip and palate in cheilognathopalatoschisis. STUPKA, W. Monatschr. f. Ohrenh. *71:*1333–1344, Nov '37
Cleft lip and palate repair technic. KILNER, T. P. St. Thomas's Hosp. Rep. *2:*127–140, '37
Healing process in harelip and cleft palate in

Cleft Lip – Cont.
embryo 23.3 mm. in length. MAURER, H. Ztschr. f. Anat. u. Entwcklngsgesch. *107:*203–211, '37
Optimal age for operations in cases of cleft palate and harelip. SOIVIO, A. Duodecim *53:*335–344, '37
Bec-de-lièvre, by VICTOR VEAU AND JACQUES RÉCAMIER. Masson et Cie, Paris, 1938
Surgery of cleft lip, jaw and palate. AXHAUSEN, G. Chirurg *10:*1–10, Jan. 1, '38
Cases of cheiloplasty; description of apparatus for feeding infants with harelip and cleft palate also: rhinoplasty. BRISOTTO, P. Boll. d. mal. d. oreccio, d. gola, d. naso *56:*89–99, March '38
Harelip cleft palate; congenital deformities of mouth and face. KIMBALL, G. H., J. Oklahoma M. A. *31:*85–89, March '38
Use of fascia and ribbon catgut in harelip and cleft palate repair. BRENIZER, A. G. Ann. Surg. *107:*692–700, May '38
Progress in plastic operations performed during childhood (for exstrophy of bladder and harelip) cleft palate. MONNIER, E. Schweiz. med. Wchnschr. *68:*613–614, May 21, '38
Harelip treatment (and cleft palate). PENN, J. South African M. J. *12:*425–429, June 25, '38
Harelip; and cleft palate age at operation and results in therapy. LUHMANN, K. Therap. d. Gegenw. *79:*300–303, July '38
Use of celluloid to cover operations for harelip. COELST. Rev. de chir. structive *8:*99–101, Aug '38
Harelip and cleft palate in relation to eugenic sterilization, according to German law. MARTINY. Ztschr. f. Stomatol. *36:*947, Aug 26; 1004, Sept 9, '38
Cleft-lip correction (and palate). STUMPF F. W., J. Am. Dent. A. *25:*1196–1201, Aug '38
Practical problems in surgical correction of harelip and nose, palate defects CALLISTER, A. C. Rocky Mountain M. J., *35:*698–701, Sept '38
Harelip repair (cleft palate). OWENS, N. South. M. J. *31:*959–968, Sept '38
Problems associated with reconstructive procedures for cleft lip and palate. BEAVIS, J. O. Ohio State M. J. *34:*1115–1117, Oct '38
Improved method of lip fixation in harelip. EBERT, E. C. AND BOYDEN, R. C., U. S. Nav. M. Bull. *36:*501, Oct '38
Embryology of face in relation to harelip. VEAU, V. Bull. Acad. de med., Paris *120:*227–233, Oct 18, '38
Congenital clefts of lip and palate. DOOLIN, W. Irish J. M. Sc., pp. 708–720, Nov '38

Cleft Lip—Cont.

Harelip in embryo. HOEPKE, H. AND MAURER, H. Ztschr. f. Anat. u. Entwcklngsgesch. *108:*768–774, '38 (Comment on Fleischmann's and Veau's articles).

Fissures of face, apropos of case of unusual labiogenal malformation. PREVOT, M. Rev. de chir. structive *8:*196–198, '38

Harelip and cleft palate from eugenic point of view. UEBERMUTH, H. Arch. f. klin. Chir. *193:*224–229, '38

Harelip in relation to embryology of face. VEAU, V. Arch. ital. di chir. *54:*824–845, '38

Harelip of human embryo 21–23 mm. long. VEAU, V. Ztschr. f. Anat. u. Entwcklngsgesch. *108:*459–493, '38

Experiences in treatment of children with harelip and cleft palate. EDBERG, E. Nord. med. *1:*89–92, Jan 14, '39

Distortions accompanying congenital single lip cleft. BLAIR, V. P. Nebraska M. J. *24:*41–43, Feb '39

Blair-Brown modification of Mirault method of treating unilateral harelip; results in cases. CHIATELLINO, A. Gior. med. d. Alto Adige *11:*131–145, March '39

Surgical therapy of harelip. GUILLEMINET, AND GUILLET. Lyon chir. *36:*197–201, March-April '39

Plastic correction after unsatisfactory healing following operation for harelip. AXHAUSEN, G. Chirurg *11:*321–334, May 1, '39

Question of age for operating on simple or complicated harelip. FORERO, A. Rev. argent. de oto-rino-laring. *8:*191–206, May-June '39

Factor of heredity in harelip. LITTLE, J. L. Canad. M. A. J. *40:*482–483, May '39

Most favorable age for harelip operation in infants. TAVERNIER, L. Lyon chir. *36:*345–346, May–June '39

Harelip problem and cleft palate. KELLY, C. C., J. Connecticut M. Soc. *3:*490–491, Sept '39

Skeletal anomalies associated with cleft palate and harelip. LYONS, D. C. Am. J. Orthodontics *25:*895–897, Sept '39

Surgical therapy of harelip and cleft palate in Denmark. ANDERSEN, P. F. Ugesk. f. Laeger *101:*1187–1193, Oct 12, '39

Harelip and cleft palate in uniovular twins. SCHRÖDER, C. H. Zentralbl. f. Chir. *66:*2299–2308, Oct 21, '39

Veau operation for correction of harelip. TJIONG NJAN HAN. Geneesk. tijdschr. v. Nederl.-Indie *79:*3034–3045, Nov 28, '39

Harelip and cleft palate. SOIVIO, A. Nord. med. (Duodecim) *4:*3705–3709, Dec 23, '39

Surgical therapy of harelip in Denmark; results of 4 years of using Veau method. ANDERSEN, V. F. Plast. chir. *1:*35–38, '39

Cleft Lip—Cont.

Importance of immobilization in plastic surgery of harelip. APOLO, E. An. de oto-rino-laring. d. Uruguay *9:*207–214, '39

Therapy of harelip and of velopalatine fissures. APOLO, E. AND ALVAREZ GRAU, J. An. de oto-rino-laring. d. Uruguay *9:*102–109, '39

Hereditary transmission of harelip. FLORIS, M. Boll. d. Soc. eustachiana *37:*25–32, '39

Plastic surgery of face (including harelip and cleft palate). HAGENTORN, A. Arch. f. klin. Chir. *195:*455–488, '39

Harelip with cleft jaw and palate in relation to law on prevention of hereditary defects. LEHMANN, W. AND RITTER, R. Ztschr. f. menschl. Vererb.-u. Konstitutionslehre *23:*1–16, '39

Studies on family groups with harelip and clefts of jaw and palate. MENGELE, J. Ztschr. f. menschl. Vererb.-u. Konstitutionslehre *23:*17–42, '39

Congenital cardiac defects and harelip with clefts of jaw and palate in twins. RABL, R. AND SCHULZ, F. Virchows Arch. f. path. Anat. *305:*505–520, '39

Hereditary relations between harelip and cleft palate and other malformations, especially of spine. SCHRÖDER, C. H. Beitr. z. klin. Chir. *169:*402–413, '39

Effect of certain experimental conditions on development of hereditary harelip in mice. STEINIGER, F. Ztschr. f. menschl. Vererb.-u. Konstitutionslehre *24:*1–12, '39

Harelip in human embryo of 18 mm. STRÖER, W. F. H. Ztschr. f. Anat. u. Entwckingsgesch. *109:*339–343, '39

Surgical therapy of harelip. VEAU, V. Plast. chir. *1:*29–33, '39

Harelip and its therapy at surgical clinic of children's hospital during 14 years. VENGEROVSKIY, I. S. Novy khir. arkhiv *44:*302–305, '39

Congenital Cleft Lip, Cleft Palate, and Associated Nasal Deformities, by HAROLD S. VAUGHAN. Lea & Febiger Co., Phila., 1940

New Cupid's-bow operation (in harelip). HARDY, E. A. Lancet *1:*361, Feb 24, '40

Surgical therapy of simple harelip; technic and results. CHIAROLANZA, R. Rinasc. med. *17:*128–131, March 15, '40

Harelip and cleft palate. FRASER, K. B., M. J. Australia *1:*361–381, March 16, '40

Methods preferred in cleft lip and cleft palate repair. DAVIS, W. B., J. Internat. Coll. Surgeons. *3:*116–124, April '40

Complete harelip; correction of large unilat-

Cleft Lip – Cont.
eral fissures of adult. MARINO, H. AND CRAVIOTTO, M. Semana med. *1:*1003-1008, April 25, '40
Therapy of harelip and cleft palate. ROY, F. Laval med. *5:*197-201, May '40
Operation for harelip. WADE, R. Australia and New Zealand J. Surg. *10:*75-76, July '40
Harelip and cleft palate. MILLER, S. J. C. Univ. West. Ontario M. J. *11:*14-19, Nov '40
Surgical therapy of harelip should be at birth. REBELO NETO, J. Rev. brasil. de otorino-laring. *8:*601-608, Nov-Dec '40
Harelip inheritance in man. MATHER, K. AND PHILIP, U. Ann. Eugenics *10:*403-416, Dec '40
Heredopathology of fissures of lips, jaws and palate; report on unselected series of 41 pairs of twins. IDELBERGER, A. AND IDELBERGER, K. Ztschr. f. menschl. Vererb.-u.-Konstitutionslehre *24:*417-479, '40
Rare congenital malformation of face; median harelip with dissociation without deformation of 2 halves of nose (double nose); case. STEFANI, F. Plast. chir. *1:*162-166, '40
Interrelation of dentistry and surgery in treatment of harelip. KAZANJIAN, V. H. Am. J. Orthodontics (Oral Surg. Sect) *27:*10-30, Jan '41
Plastic surgery of simple harelip. FLORES, A. Rev. med. peruana *13:*55-58, Feb '41
Anesthesia for harelip surgery during infancy. SPAID, J. D., J. Indiana M. A. *34:*143-145, March '41
Harelip with special reference to therapy. DUBE, E. Ann. med.-chir. de l'Hop. Sainte-Justine, Montreal *3:*89-93, May 41
Heredity of congenital fossette of lip in conjunction with clefts of upper jaw. TRAUNER, R. Wien. klin. Wchnschr. *54:*427-429, May 16, '41 addendum: *54:*454, May 23, '41
Secondary repair of cleft lips and their nasal deformities. BROWN, J. B. AND McDOWELL, F. Ann. Surg. *114:*101-117, July '41
Orthodontics in treatment of harelip and cleft palate. LIFTON, J. C. Am. J. Orthodontics *27:*423-453, Aug '41
Treatment of cleft lip and palate. ABRAMSON, P. D. Tri-State M. J. *14:*2559, Nov '41
Secondary nasal deformities following correction of cleft lip. CINELLI, A. A. Laryngoscope *51:*1053-1058, Nov '41
Incidence of supernumerary and congenitally missing lateral incisor teeth in 81 cases of harelip and cleft palate. MILLHON, J. A. AND STAFNE, E. C. Am. J. Orthodontics

Cleft Lip – Cont.
(Oral Surg. Sect) *27:*599-604, Nov '41
Congenital clefts of face and jaws; report of operations used and discussion of results. RITCHIE, H. P. Surg., Gynec. and Obst. *73:*654-670, Nov '41
Embryologic study of harelip cysts. STEINIGER, F. Ztschr. f. menschl. Vererb.-u. Konstitutionslehre *25:*1-27, '41
Inheritance of Harelip and Cleft Palate, by POUL FOGH ANDERSEN. Nyt Forlag Arnold Busck, Copenhagen, 1942
Harelip treatment; suggestion. BERTWISTLE, A. P. Clin. J. *71:*71-72, March-April '42
Surgical therapy of cleft palate and harelip. CHAVES, D. A. Rev. med. munic. *3:*259-270, March '42
Nasal deformity in harelip; anatomic study. APOLO, E. Arq. de cir. clin. e exper. *6:*339-343, April-June '42
Nasal deformity in harelip; surgical problem. APOLO, E. Arq. de cir. clin. e exper. *6:*645-651, April-June '42
Uncomplicated unilateral harelip; general review. DE MORAIS LEME, J. B. Arq. de cir. clin. e exper. *6:*359-457, April-June '42
Harelip and cleft palate; results of plastic surgery. DE SANSON, R. D. Arq. de cir. clin. e exper. *6:*336-339, April-June '42
Paraffinoma, harelip, cicatrices, auricular prosthesis in plastic surgery. GONCALVES, G. Arq. de cir. clin. e exper. *6:*307-316, April-June '42
Harelip and cleft palate; 70 consecutive cases. PICKERILL, C. M. New Zealand M. J. *41:*121-129, June '42
Technical devices in surgical therapy of harelip and velopalatine fissures, with report of cases. REBELO NETO, J. Arq. de cir. clin. e exper. *6:*343-358, April-June '42
Rehabilitation of children with cleft palate, harelip or both. PERKINS, H. W. AND SILVER, E. I. Am. J. Orthodontics *28:*567-575, Sept '42
Histology of harelip. FINOCHIETTO, R.; *et al* Bol. Acad. nac. de med. de Buenos Aires, pp. 627-636, Nov '42
Significance of occult spina bifida in heredity of harelip and cleft palate. SCHRODER, C. H. AND HILLENBRAND, H. J. Arch. f. klin. Chir. *203:*328-342, '42
"Heteropenetration" and twin discordance in hereditary harelip and cleft palate. STEINIGER, F. AND VEIT, G. Ztschr. f. menschl. Vererb-. u. Konstitutionslehre *26:*75-92, '42
Complete unilateral harelip; immediate result of operation by Brown-Blair method. DELLEPIANE RAWSON, R. Dia med. *15:*146-

Cleft Lip – Cont.
147, Feb 22, '43
Labiovelopalatine fissure; surgical therapy with report of cases. DE SANSON, R. D. AND AMARANTE, R. C. L. Rev. brasil. de cir. *12:*215–246, March '43
Harelip and cleft palate. ANDERSEN, P. FOGH. Nord. med. *19:*1597–1598, Sept. 25, '43
Case showing partial deficient fusion of maxillary process with lateral nasal process on one side. DODDS, G. E. Brit. J. Ophth. *27:*414–415, Sept '43
Three generations of mucous cysts occurring with harelip and cleft palate. STRAITH, C. L. AND PATTON, H. S., J.A.M.A. *123:*693–694, Nov. 13, '43
Postoperative immobilization and holding of sutured flaps in harelips. ZENO, L. Bol. y trab., Soc. argent. de cirujanos *4:*648–653, '43 also: An. de cir. *9:*236–241, Sept–Dec '43 also: Rev. Asoc. med. argent. *57:*945–947, Nov. 15, '43
Multiple cleft formations of maxillofacial region and their combination with other malformations. GERKE, J. Munchen. med. Wchnschr. *90:*712, Dec 17, '43
Frequency of occurrence of cleft palates and harelips. GRACE, L. G., J. Dent. Research *22:*495–497, Dec '43
Surgical therapy of simple and complicated harelip. PASSALACQUA, L. A. Bol. Asoc. med. de Puerto Rico *36:*56–61, Feb '44
Plastic repair of congenital harelip. BAXTER, H. McGill M. J. *13:*151–156, April '44
Restoration of facial contour in surgery of secondary cleft lip and palate. DAVIS, A. D. AND SELLECK, G. A. Am. J. Surg. *64:*104–114, April '44
Postoperative immobilization and holding of sutured flaps in harelip. ZENO, L. Pediat. Americas *2:*238–240, April 15, '44
Complicated harelip; surgical therapy of case. LOZOYA SOLIS, J. Bol. med. d. Hosp. inf., Mexico *1:*58–67, July–Aug '44
Care of cleft lip and palate in babies. SCHULTZ, L. W. Illinois M. J. *86:*138–159, Sept '44
Simplified design for repair of single cleft lips. BROWN, J. B. AND McDOWELL, F. Surg., Gynec. and Obst. *80:*12–26, Jan '45
Congenital cleft palate and harelip in infants; mode of nutrition in preoperative period. TAYLOR, H. P. Brit. Dent. J. *78:*1–7, Jan 5, '45
Surgical repair of harelip. PETERSEN, N. South African M. J. *19:*132–134, April 28, '45
Plastic surgery of harelip. Science and art of plastic surgery; present and future status. SANVENERO-ROSSELLI, G. Salud y belleza *1:*8–9, April–May '45
Cleft palate and cleft lip. SHEARER, W. L. Nebraska M. J. *30:*125–126, April '45
Surgical therapy of harelip. VEAU, V. Salud y belleza *1:*10–11; 42, April–May '45
Harelip and cleft palate; plan of management. PRIOLEAU, W. H., J. South Carolina M. A. *41:*129–130, June '45
Surgical therapy of harelip. TORRES POSSE, A. Bol. Soc. de cir. de Rosario *12:*88–107, June '45
Surgical therapy of harelip; technic and results. DETCHESSARRY, R. Arch. argent. de pediat. *24:*197–204, Sept '45
Management of cleft lip. OVENS, J. M. Arizona Med. *2:*298–303, Sept '45
Surgical correction of harelip; 26 cases. REBAUDI, F. AND JANNUZZI, V. Boll. Soc. ital. di med. e ig. trop. (nos. 5–6) *5:*253–264, '45
Surgical treatment of harelip and cleft palate. WODAK, E. M. Acta oto-larying. orient. *1:*13–17, '45
Surgical treatment of harelip and cleft palate. WODAK, E. M. Acta oto-larying. orient. *1:*42–45, '45
Harelip and cleft palate. KAUFMAN, I. Am. J. Orthodontics (Oral Surg. Sect.) *32:*47–51, Jan '46
Harelip – urgent maxillofacial surgery. SCHULTZ, L. W. M. Times, New York *74:*33, Feb.; 63, Mar '46
Vinesthene (vinyl ether) anesthesia for repair of harelip and cleft palate. DAPLYN, P. F. L. Brit. M. J. *2:*117–119, July 27, '46
Treatment of secondary deformity of harelip. RAGNELL, A., M. Press. *216:*281–286, Oct 16, '46
Surgical treatment of vicious cicatrices involving cheek, lip and alveolar process in cleft lip and palate cases. IVY, R. H. Am. J. Orthodontics (Oral Surg. Sect.) *32:*673–674, Nov '46
Harelip and cleft palate; 1,000 patients submitted to operation. ANDERSEN, P. FOGH. Acta chir. Scandinav. *94:*213–242, '46

Cleft Lip, Bilateral

Case of bilateral harelip. MERTENS, G. Zentralbl. f. Chir. *48:*1794–1795, Dec 10, '21
Treatment of complex bilateral harelip. VEAU, V. AND LASCOMBE, J., J. de chir. *19:*113–136, Feb '22 (illus.) abstr: J. A. M. A. *78:*1168, April 15, '22
Operative treatment of complete double harelip. VEAU, V. Ann. Surg. *76:*143–156, Aug '22 (illus.)

Cleft Lip, Bilateral – Cont.

Operation for double cleft palate and harelip. PICHLER, H. Deutsche Ztschr. f. Chir. *195:*104–107, '26

Harelip operation by Orlovsky method. MASLOV, I. Vestnik khir. (no. 33) *11:*146–150, Nov 22, '27

Reich-Matti operation for double harelip. FRÜND, H. Munchen. med. Wchnschr. *75:*1067–1070, June 22, '28

Surgical therapy of harelip by Orlowsky's method. MASSLOFF, I.D. Arch. f. klin. Chir. *150:*322–327, '28

Value of Orloff's method in double harelip. MASSLOFF, I. D. Vestnik khir. (no. 51) *17:*69–73, '29

Orlowski's method in double harelip. MASSLOFF, I. D. Chirurg *2:*220, March 1, '30

Muscles and nerves in total bilateral harelip. CADENAT, M. E. Ann. d'anat. path. *8:*353–358, April '31

Double harelip and cleft palate showing importance of proper surgical and orthodontic treatment of premaxillary lobe or process. KELSEY, H. E. Internat. J. Orthodontia *18:*145–147, Feb '32

Surgical therapy of bilateral harelip and total cleft palate; case. VIGNARD. Avenir med. *29:*41, Feb '32

Double harelip. HORSLEY, J. S. JR. South. Med. and Surg. *94:*197–201, April '32

Repair of bilateral harelip. LYERLY, J. G. Virginia M. Monthly *59:*85–88, May '32

Surgery of double harelip. HAGENTORNAS, A. Zentralbl. f. Chir. *59:*1460–1463, June 11, '32

Operation for total bilateral harelip; technic and results. VEAU, V. AND PLESSIER, P., J. de chir. *40:*321–357, Sept '32 abstr: Bull. et mem. Soc. nat. de chir. *56:*1079–1082, July 16, '32

Postoperative double harelip deformity. NEW, G. B., S. Clin. North America *13:* 867–868, Aug '33

Causes and prevention of failures in surgical therapy for bilateral harelip. KALLIUS, H. U. Chirurg *5:*704–712, Sept 15, '33

Treatment of prominent intermaxillary bone in therapy of harelip and cleft palate. HAGENBACH, E. Schweiz. med. Wchnschr. *63:*949–950, Sept 23, '33

Complete double harelip complicated by protrusion of premaxillae. KAHN, K., M. Times and Long Island M. J. *62:*176–178, June '34

Underlying principles in repair of double harelip. LEE, F. C., J. M. A. Georgia *23:*383–389, Oct '34

Skeletal malformations in total unilateral and bilateral harelip. VEAU, V. Ann. d'anat. path. *11:*873–904, Dec '34 abstr.: Schweiz. med. Wchnschr. *65:*99–101, Jan 26, '35

Complications of unilateral harelip. SCARCELLA PERINO, G. Stomatol. *33:*56–62, Jan '35

Fundamentals in treatment of protruding intermaxillary bone in bilateral harelip. FELDMANN, E. Zentralbl. f. Chir. *62:*434–437, Feb. 23, '35

Structural plan of jaw and question of treating projections of intermaxillary bone in harelip and cleft palate. KULENKAMPFF, D. Zentralbl. f. Chir. *62:*1394–1396, June 15, '35

Therapy of cleft lip, jaw and palate with protruding intermaxillary bone. TOMOFF, W. Zentralbl. f. Chir. *63:*2535–2538, Oct. 24, '36

Hyperpyrexia following harelip operation. IRISH, H. E. AND STEPAN, C. E. Am. J. Dis. Child. *58:*320–331, Aug. '39

Bilateral cleft lip reconstruction. SCHULTZ, L. W., J. Am. Dent. A. *29:*248–250, Feb '42

Management of bilateral cleft lip. DAVIS, W. B. Tr. Am. Soc. Plastic and Reconstructive Surg. *12:*99–116, '43

Bilateral complicated harelip with bilateral palpebral coloboma and left iridic coloboma; total ectromelia of right upper extremity. ROCHER, H. L. AND PESME. J. de med. de Bordeaux *121–122:*493–494, Oct '45

Orbicularis oris muscle in double harelip. LEE, F. C. Arch. Surg. *53:*407–413, Oct '46

Cleft Lip, Median

Median upper hare-lip. VEAU, V. AND RUPPE, C. Arch. de med. d. enf. *24:*241, April '21

Median cleft of upper lip; case. DICK, B. M. Edinburgh M. J. *34:*45–47, Jan '27

Congenital median fistula, with report of case. DE GAETANO, L. Riforma med. *53:*523–526, April 10, '37

Median harelip and bifid nose; case. LAGOS GARCIA, A. Semana med. *2:*237–241, Aug. 3, '44

Median harelip, cleft palate and glossal agenesis. SINCLAIR, J. G. AND MCKAY, J. Anat. Rec. *91:*155–160, Feb '45

Bifid nose associated with midline cleft of upper lip. WEAVER, D. F. AND BELLINGER, D. H. Arch. Otolaryng. *44:*480–482, Oct '46

Cleft Lip; Secondary Deformity

Reconstruction of nostril in simple hare-lip. OMBRÉDANNE, L. Presse med. *29:*703, Sept. 3, '21

Cleft Lip; Secondary Deformity–Cont.
Nasal relation of harelip operations. BROWN, G. V. I., J. A. M. A. *77:*1954, Dec. 17, '21
Correction of nose deformities at operations for harelip. MEYER, H. Zentralbl. f. Chir. *49:*220, Feb. 18, '22 (illus.)
Correction of nasal deformities associated with harelip and cleft palate. DAVIS, W. B. J. M. Soc. New Jersey *20:*113–119, April '23 (illus.)
Recommended procedure for relief of ala deformity in certain cases in adult associated with harelip and its mechanical counterpart. SHEEHAN, J. E., M. J. and Rec. *120:*72–73, July 16, '24
Treatment of unilateral harelip with special reference to associated deformity of nose. COLEMAN, C. C. Virginia M. Monthly *51:*393–399, Oct '24
Nasal deformities associated with congenital cleft of lip. BLAIR, V. P., J. A. M. A. *84:* 185–187, Jan. 17, '25
Cleft lip and palate; correction of late deformities resulting from neglect or improper treatment. FARR, R. E. Minnesota Med. *8:*561–568, Sept '25
Problem of bringing forward retracted upper lip and nose in harelip. BLAIR, V. P. Surg., Gynec. and Obst. *42:*128–132, Jan '26
Role of median nasal process in development of face; study of hare-lip. VEAU, V. Ann. d'anat. path. *3:*305–348, April '26 abstr: J. A. M. A. *87:*1160, Oct. 2, '26
Surgery of mouth and face with special reference to cleft plate and cleft lip. LOGAN, W. H. G. Kentucky M. J. *24:*498–505, Oct '26
Transplantation of strip of cheek and naris in harelip therapy. EHRENFELD, H. Arch. f. klin. Chir. *144:*486–488, '27
Flat nose, consequent to harelip operations; operative treatment. OMBRÉDANNE, L. AND OMBRÉDANNE, M. Ann. d. mal. de l'oreille, du larynx *47:*1090–1111, Dec '28
Orthodontic treatment and result of case of malocclusion of teeth brought by conditions associated with congenital cleft palate and harelip; case. HELLMAN, M. Internat. J. Orthodontia *15:*135–138, Feb '29
Repair of harelip and accompanying nasal deformity. PADGETT, E. C., J. Kansas M. Soc. *30:*143–147, May '29
Treatment of secondary deformity in cases of harelip (nose). NEW, G. B. AND FIGI, F. A. Minnesota Med. *14:*514–516, June '31
Primary and secondary repair of cleft lip. KISKADDEN, W. S. AND THOLEN, E. F. Internat. J. Orthodontia *18:*863–873, Aug '32 also: West. J. Surg. *40:*18–27, Jan '32
Correction of losses and deformities of external nose, including those associated with harelip. BLAIR, V. P. California and West. Med. *36:*308–313, May '32
Cosmetic surgery of incomplete (operated) harelip and nasal deformities combined with harelip. ÉRCZY, M. Gyogyaszat *72:*719–721, Nov. 20, '32
Operations for correction of secondary deformities of cleft lip. GILLIES, H. AND KILNER, T. P. Lancet *2:*1369–1375, Dec. 24, '32
Plastic correction of nasal deformities after operation for harelip. EITNER, E. Deutsche Ztschr. f. Chir. *238:*644–646, '33
Atypical cartilage in nose, upper lip and palate in cheilognathopalatoschisis. STUPKA, W. Monatschr. f. Ohrenh. *71:*1333–1344, Nov '37
Correction of alar deformity in cleft lip. McINDOE, A. H. Lancet *1:*607–609, March 12, '38
Nostril in secondary harelip. HUMBY, G. Lancet *1:*1275, June 4, '38
Practical problems in surgical correction of harelip and nose, palate defects. CALLISTER, A. C. Rocky Mountain M. J. *35:*698–701, Sept '38
Embryology of face in relation to harelip. VEAU, V. Bull. Acad. de med., Paris, *120:*227–233, Oct. 18, '38
Nasal deformities in harelip; surgical therapy. MICHALEK-GRODZKI. Rev. de chir. structive *8:*205–210, '38
Harelip in relation to embryology of face. VEAU, V. Arch. ital. di chir. *54:*824–845, '38
Distortions accompanying congenital single lip cleft. BLAIR, V. P. Nebraska M. J. *24:*41–43, Feb '39
Nasal deformity in harelip; technic of plastic correction. ZENO, L. Bol. Soc. de cir. de Rosario *7:*408–414, Oct '40 also: An. de cir. *6:*388–394, Dec '40
Secondary repair of cleft lips and their nasal deformities. BROWN, J. B. AND McDOWELL, F. Ann. Surg. *114:*101–117, July '41
Split vermilion bordered lip flap in cleft lip. CANNON, B. Surg., Gynec. and Obst. *73:*95–97, July '41
Secondary nasal deformities following correction of cleft lip. CINELLI, A. A. Laryngoscope *51:*1053–1058, Nov '41
Secondary repair of cleft lips and their nasal deformities. J. B. BROWN AND F. McDOWELL. Am. J. Orthodontics and Oral Surg., *27:*712, Dec. 1941
Nasal deformity in harelip; anatomic study. APOLO, E. Arq. de cir. clin. e exper. *6:*339–343, April-June '42
Nasal deformity in harelip; surgical problem.

Cleft Lip; Secondary Deformity—Cont.
APOLO, E. Arq. de cir. clin. e exper. *6:*645-651, April-June '42
Wide nostril in unilateral cleft lip. VAUGHAN, H. S. Tr. Am. Soc. Plastic and Reconstructive Surg. *12:*117-123, '43
Restoration of facial contour in surgery of secondary cleft lip and palate. DAVIS, A. D. AND SELLECK, G. A. Am. J. Surg. *64:*104-114, April '44
Treatment of secondary deformity of harelip RAGNELL, A., M. Press. *216:*281-286, Oct. 16, '46
Surgical treatment of vicious cicatrices involving cheek, lip and alveolar process in cleft lip and palate cases. IVY, R. H. Am. J. Orthodontics (Oral Surg. Sect.) *32:*673-674, Nov '46

Cleft Palate
Operation for cleft palate. BERRY, J. Brit. J. Surg. *8:*364, Jan '21
Repair of harelip and cleft palate deformity. RITCHIE, H. P. Minnesota Med. *4:*15, Jan '21
Cleft palate extraordinary. BROPHY, T. W. Surg., Gynec. and Obst. *32:*182, Feb '21
A new principle in surgical treatment of "congenital cleft palate," and its mechanical counterpart. GILLIES, H. D. AND FRY, W. K. Brit. M. J. *1:*335, March 5, '21
Cleft palate and harelip procedures. BROPHY, T. W. Minnesota Med. *4:*283, May '21
Cleft palate and harelip. SHEARER, W. L. Minnesota Med. *4:*293, May '21
Hare-lip and cleft palate; a war influence. AYMARD, J. L. Brit. M. J. *2:*405, Sept. 10, '21
Certain non-technical considerations in treatment of harelip and cleft palate. COE, H. E. Arch. Pediat. *38:*658, Oct '21
Advantages of two-stage operation for cleft palate. KELLOCK, T. H. Brit. J. Surg. *9:*290, Oct '21
Cleft palate operations. MONNIER, E. Schweiz. med. Wchnschr. *51:*970, Oct. 20, '21
Simplification of technique in operations for hare-lip and cleft palate. THOMPSON, J. F. Ann. Surg. *74:*394, Oct '21
Harelip and cleft palate. VON WEDEL, C. Southwest J. Med. and Surg. *29:*148-149, Nov '21 (illus.)
Correction of congenital cleft palate and harelip, surgical principles involved. MOOREHEAD, F. B., J. A. M. A. *77:*1951, Dec. 17, '21
Reconstruction of hard palate. BURIAN, F. Rev. de chir. *59:*49, '21
Operation for harelip and cleft palate. MILNER, R. Zentralbl. f. Chir. *49:*80-81, Jan. 21, '22 (illus.)

Cleft Palate—Cont.
Harelip and cleft palate. DAVIS, W. B., S. Clin. N. America *2:*199-223, Feb '22 (illus.)
Some consideration of cleft palate surgical technic. PETTIT, J. A. Northwest Med. *21:*52-55, Feb '22 (illus.)
A knife for harelip and cleft palate operations. CATES, B. B. Am. J. Surg. *36:*70, March '22
Harelip and cleft palate. MCCURDY, S. L. Pennsylvania M. J. *25:*560-564, May '22 (illus.)
Harelip and cleft palate. CLARK, C. M. Ohio State M. J. *18:*417-423, June '22 (illus.)
Results of treatment of cleft palate. VEAU, V. AND RUPPE, C. Rev. de chir. *60:*81-99, '22 (illus.) abstr: J. A. M. A. *78:*1998, June 24, '22
Results of operative treatment for cleft palate. BROCA, A. Paris med. *12:*58-63, July 15, '22 abstr: J. A. M. A. *79:*1003, Sept. 16, '22
Harelip and cleft palate deformities, some types and their operative treatment. DAVIS, W. B. Ann. Surg. *76:*133-142, Aug '22 (illus.)
Correction of cleft palate. VEAU, V. AND RUPPE, C. J. de chir. *20:*113-144, Aug. '22 (illus.) abstr: J. A. M. A. *79:*1179, Sept. 30, '22
Plea for early cleft palate operations. CATES, B. B. Am. J. Surg. *36:*221-222, Sept '22 (illus.)
Classification of congenital clefts of lip and palate, with suggestion for recording these cases. DAVIS, J. S. AND RITCHIE, H. P. J. A. M. A. *79:*1323-1327, Oct. 14, '22 (illus.)
Harelip and cleft palate operation. EDBERG, E. Acta chir. Scandinav. *55:*1-26, '22 (in English) abstr: J. A. M. A. *79:*1562, Oct. 28, '22
Atypical plastic operations for congenital fissures of lip and palate. THOMPSON, J. E., S. Clin. N. America *2:*1387-1401, Oct. '22 (illus.)
Harelip and cleft palate. FEDERSPIEL, M. N. Laryngoscope *32:*909-928, Dec '22 (illus.)
Cleft Lip and Palate, by TRUMAN W. BROPHY. Blakiston Co., Phila., 1923
Correction of cleft palate. BRYAN, W. A. Southern M. J. *16:*117-121, Feb '23 (illus.)
Congenital perforate soft palate and double uvula, with repair of perforation. TRINDER, J. H. J. A. M. A. *80:*914, March 31, '23 (illus.)
Correction of nasal deformities associated with hare-lip and cleft palate. DAVIS, W. B., J. M. Soc. New Jersey *20:*113-119, April '23 (illus.)
Reasons for operations in early infancy on

Cleft Palate—Cont.

cleft-lip and cleft palate. SILVERMAN, S. L. J. M. A. Georgia *12:*143-147, April '23 (illus.)

Ultimate results of Langenbeck's operation for cleft palate. STAHL, O. Arch. f. klin. Chir. *123:*271-316, '23 (illus.) abstr: J. A. M. A. *80:*1421, May 12 '23

Few points in technic of cleft palate operations. CATES, B. B. Am. J. Surg. *37:*231-232, Sept '23

Staphylorrhapy. VEAU, V. Medecine *5:*21-25, Oct '23

A new method of operation for congenital cleft palate. NAEGELI, T. Schweiz. med. Wchnschr. *54:*62-63, Jan. 10, '24

Cleft palate and harelip. SUDLER, M. T., J. Kansas M. Soc. *24:*18-20, Jan '24

Some factors in cleft palate work. KIRKHAM, H. L. D. Texas State J. Med. *19:*577-579, Feb '24

Cleft palate in young infants. BROPHY, T. W. New York J. Med. *24:*483-488, April 4, '24

Fundamental principles and recent conclusions in surgery of congenital cleft palate. BROPHY, T. W. Minnesota Med. *7:*327-336, May '24

Cleft palate and cleft lip cases. SHEARER, W. L. Nebraska M. J. *9:*160-164, May '24

Plastic operations on hard palate. ROSENTHAL, W. Zentralbl. f. Chir. *51:*1621-1627, July 26, '24

Plea for preservation of premaxillary bones in congenital cleft palate. DAVIS, A. D. Lancet *2:*749-751, Oct. 11, '24

Two problems in treatment of cleft palate. GOYDER, F. W. Brit. M. J. *2:*615, Oct. 4, '24

Treatment of cleft palate. FRY, W. K. Lancet *2:*1081-1082, Nov. 22, '24

Treatment of cleft lip and palate. BAIRD, J. P. J. Tennessee M. A. *17:*257-264, Dec '24

Technique of cleft palate operations. CATES, B. B. Boston M. and S. J. *191:*1166-1168, Dec. 18, '24

Remote results of cleft palate operations. MONNIER, E. Jahrb. f. Kinderh. *105:*200-211, '24

Harelip operation in 1808. VAN DER HOEVEN, J. Nederl. Tidjschr. v. Geneesk. *1:*44-51, Jan. 3, '25

Plastic operations on hard palate; comment on Rosenthal's article. ERNST, F. Zentralbl. f. Chir. *52:*464-470, Feb. 28, '25

Surgical treatment of cleft palate. DOWD, C. N. Ann. Surg. *81:*573-584, March '25

Treatment of congenital cleft lip and palate. FARR, R. E. Minnesota Med. *8:*149-153, March '25

Cleft-palate, some pitfalls in operation. ADDISON, O. L. Lancet *1:*818-819, April 18, '25

Cleft Palate—Cont.

Operative treatment of cleft-palate, record of results in 125 consecutive cases. RAYNER, H. H. Lancet *1:*816-817, April 18, '25

Treatment of congenital cleft of lip and palate. KAHN, L. Am. J. Surg. *39:*142-144, June '25 also: Kentucky M. J. *23:*491-493, Oct '25

Repair of inoperable cleft of soft palate by utilizing faucial tonsils. SHEEHAN, J. E. M. J. and Rec. *122:*185-188, Aug. 19, '25

Special periostetomes for cleft palate work. CATES, B. B. Boston M. and S. J. *193:*728-729, Oct. 15, '25

Surgical treatment of cleft palate. KIRSCHNER, M. Arch. f. klin. Chir. *138:*515-533, '25

Closure of congenital clefts of hard palate. CAMPBELL, A. Brit. J. Surg. *13:*715-719, April '26

Types of harelip and cleft-palate deformities and operative results. DAVIS, W. B. Surg., Gynec. and Obst. *42:*704-709, May '26

Harelip and cleft palate. LADD, W. E. Boston M. and S. J. *194:*1016-1025, June 3, '26

Plea for co-operation in congenital cleft palate treatment. MOORE, J. R. A., S. African M. Record *24:*335-338, Aug. 14, '26

Congenital cleft lip and palate; muscle theory repair of cleft lip. RITCHIE, H. P. Ann. Surg. *84:*211-222, Aug '26

Important factors in treatment of cleft lip and palate. VAUGHAN, H. S. Ann. Surg. *84:*223-232, Aug '26

Operation for cleft palate and hare-lip, HOHMEIER, F. Deutsche med. Wchnschr. *52:*1604-1606, Sept. 17, '26

Surgical treatment of cleft palate; new method which is primarily reconstructive application of parts of many old operative procedures revised to form what is in effect a new operation. BROWN, G. V. I., J. A. M. A. *87:*1379-1384, Oct. 23, '26

Surgery of mouth and face with special reference to cleft palate and cleft lip. LOGAN, W. H. G. Kentucky M. J. *24:*498-505, Oct '26

Use of septal flap in closure of unilateral clefts of palate. THOMPSON, J. E., J. A. M. A. *87:*1384-1388, Oct. 23, '26

Congenital cleft lip and palate; series of congenital clefts. RITCHIE, H. P. Minnesota Med. *9:*664-666, Dec '26

Cleft palate. SHEARER, W. L. Nebraska M. J. *11:*462-468, Dec '26

Management of cleft-lip and palate cases. SPRAGUE, E. W., S. Clin. N. Amer. *6:*1481-1496, Dec '26

Complete harelip and cleft palate on left side, with absence of left half of intermaxillary bone, of philtrum and of cartilaginous por-

Cleft Palate—Cont.
tion of nasal septum. BERG, A. Arch. f. klin. Chir. *140:*168-171, '26
Free fat transplantation in therapy of cleft palate. v. GAZA, W. Arch. f. klin. Chir. *142:*590-599, '26
Harelip and Cleft Palate, by MATTHEW FEDERSPIEL. C. V. Mosby Co., St. Louis, 1927
Two-stage operation for cleft palate. BILLINGTON, W. Brit. M. J. *1:*15, Jan. 1, '27
Cleft palate; clinical study of method for its treatment. FORBES, A. M. Canad. M. A. J. *17:*76-78, Jan '27
Technic of uranostaphylorrhaphy. PIZZAGALLI, L. Boll. d. spec. med.-chir. *1:*7-16, Jan-March '27
Harelip with cleft palate; 2 cases. PIETRANTONI, L. Sperimentale Arch. di biol. *80:*651-664, Jan. 25, '27
Shortcomings in surgery of cleft lip and palate, with suggestions for meeting them. FARR, R. E. Minnesota Med. *10:*70-76, Feb '27
Preliminary paper on improvement of speech in cleft palate cases. KIRKHAM, H. L. D. Surg., Gynec. and Obst. *44:*244-246, Feb '27
Cleft palate. PADGETT, E. C., J. Kansas M. Soc. *27:*50-51, Feb '27
Harelip and cleft palate. HORSLEY, J. S. JR. Virginia M. Monthly *53:*782-787, March '27
Closure of defects of palate by flaps of mucosa from nasal septum. PERWITZSCHKY, R. Arch. f. Ohren-, Nasen-u. Kehlkopfh. *116:*196-203, March '27
Cleft palate. HOLLAND, C. L., W. Virginia M. J. *23:*262-263, May '27
Congenital cleft lip and palate. WOOLSEY, J. H. California and West. Med. *26:*633-636, May '27
Cleft lip and palate. BROPHY, T. W., J. Am. Dent. A. *14:*1108-1115, June '27
Operative procedure in cleft palate and harelip. LYONS, C. J., J. Am. Dent. A. *14:*1080-1094, June '27
Congenital cleft lip and palate; some personal observations. MOOREHEAD, F. B., J. Am. Dent. A. *14:*1098-1107, June '27
Operative treatment of harelip and cleft palate. HELBING, C. Allg. deutsche Hebam.-Ztg. *42:*193, July 1, '27
Innovations in operative methods for cleft palate. LIMBERG, A. Zentralbl. f. Chir. *54:*1745-1750, July 9, '27
Cleft lip and palate. FREW, A. L. Texas State J. Med. *23:*333-335, Sept '27
Cleft palate repair; cause of failure in infants and its prevention. BUNNELL, S. Surg., Gynec. and Obst. *45:*530-533, Oct '27

Cleft Palate—Cont.
Treatment of cleft palate. FREW, A. L., J. Am. Dent. A. *14:*1857-1859, Oct '27
Discussion on treatment of cleft palate by operation. VARIOUS AUTHORS. Proc. Roy. Soc. Med. (Sect. Surg.) *20:*127-185, Oct '27
Surgical correction of cleft lip and palate. JOBSON, G. B. Arch. Otolaryng. *6:*434-445, Nov '27
Treatment of congenital cleft palate. BAGGER, H. Acta oto-larying. *10:*361-370, '27
Congenital harelip and cleft palate; case I, (unfinished case). CHAPIN, W. C. Internat. Orthodont. Cong. *1:*485-492, '27
Treatment of perforations and fissures of palate and soft palate. CRESPI, R. A. Semana med. *1:*666; 710; 755, '27
Surgical treatment of cleft palate. DEUBNER, W. Arch. f. klin. Chir. *146:*430-461, '27
Operative treatment of cleft palate in older children and adults. DEUBNER, W. Deutsche Ztschr. f. Chir. 201:117-121, '27
Various methods of treatment of cleft palate. LEXER, E. Deutsche Ztschr. f. Chir. *200:*109-128, '27
Operative treatment of cleft palate. TSCHMARKE, G. Arch. f. klin. Chir. *144:*697-722, '27
Harelip and cleft palate operations. CATES, B. B. Internat. J. Med. and Surg. *41:*8-11, Jan '28
Cleft palate. DORRANCE, G. M. Atlantic M. J. *31:*351-355, Feb '28
Problem of child with harelip and cleft palate. MCEACHERN, J. D. Canad. M. A. J. *18:*170-174, Feb '28
Nasal speech and cleft palate. BURGER, H. Nederl. Tijdschr. v. Geneesk. *1:*1563-1571, March 31, '28
Harelip and cleft palate; study of 425 consecutive cases. DAVIS, W. B. Ann. Surg. *87:*536-554, April '28
Surgical treatment of clefts of palate and lip. PARKER, D. B. Am. J. Surg. *4:*385-389, April '28
Facial paralysis, palatal repair and some other plastic operations. PICKERILL, P., M. J. Australia *1:*543-548, May 5, '28
Plastic surgery of face and harelip and nose and cleft palate. JOBSON, Q. B. Atlantic M. J. *31:*716-723, July '28
Cleft palate. WARDILL, W. E. M. Brit. J. Surg. *16:*127-148, July '28
Removal of blood from mouth by suction during operations (staphylorrhaphy). VULLIET, M. Zentralbl. f. Chir. *55:*1996-1997, Aug. 11, '28
Treatment and diagnostic considerations in cleft palate. SAMENGO, L. AND ERRECART, P. L. Semana med. *2:*913-914, Oct. 4, '28

Cleft Palate—Cont.
Cleft palate. FORBES, A. M. Surg., Gynec. and Obst. *47:*707-709, Nov '28
Treatment of harelip and cleft palate. RISDON, F., J. Am. Dent. A. *15:*2017-2020, Nov '28
Relations of osseous fragments in total cleft palates. RUPPE, C. Rev. de stomatol. *30:*670-681, Nov '28
Cleft palate. SHEARER, W. L. J. Am. Dent. A. *15:*2135-2140, Nov '28
Surgical and phonetic results of late cleft palate operations. HALLE. Med. Klin. *24:*1976-1979, Dec. 21, '28
Cleft palate operation with multiple mobilization. EICHHOFF, E. AND HELLMANN, K. Beitr. z. klin. Chir. *143:*290-319, '28
Surgery of labio-maxillo-palatine fissure. LASAGNA, F. Arch. ital. di chir. *20:*661-679, '28
Cleft palate; cases. LEMBERK, B. E. Odont. i stomatol. (no. 12) *6:*16-22, '28
Treatment of cleft palate. MITCHELL, V. E. Dental Cosmos *71:*230-235, March '29
Cleft palate repair after unsuccessful operations, with special reference to cases with extensive loss of palatal tissue. PADGETT, E. C. Tr. Sect. Surg. General and Abd., A. M. A., pp. 336-358, '29 also: Arch. Surg. *20:*453-472, March '30
When and how should cleft palate be treated? FENNER, E. D. New Orleans M. and S. J. *81:*718-722, April '29
Technic of cleft palate operation. MONNIER, E. Schweiz. med. Wchnschr. *59:*595, June 8, '29
Cleft palate treatment in children. OMBRÉDANNE. Rev. odont. *50:*230-237, June '29
Suture technic of palate. SCHOEMAKER, J. Chirurg *1:*1012, Oct. 1, '29
Operative treatment of cleft palate; new method. MACKENTY, J. E. Arch. Otolaryng. *10:*491-512, Nov '29
Pathology and therapy of cleft palate. ROSENTHAL, W. Fortschr. d. Zahnheilk. *5:*1044-1054, Nov '29
Technic of staphylorrhaphy in simple division of palate. VEAU, V., J. de chir. *35:*1-21, Jan '30
Two-stage operation for cleft palate. BILLINGTON, W. AND ROUND, H. Proc. Roy. Soc. Med. (sect. Odont.) *23:*13-20, March '30
Gillies tubed pedicle flap in cleft palate. QUICK, B., J. Coll. Surgeons; Australasia *2:*395-400, March '30
Treatment of cleft palate. DEBENHAM, L. S. AND BADCOCK, C. E. Brit. Dent. J. *51:*347-353, April 1, '30
Operative method in cleft palate. DE MELLO, C. Beitr. z. Anat., Physiol., Path. u. Therap. d. Ohres *28:*120-123, May '30
Etiology of cleft palate and lip; fundamental principles in operative procedure. LYONS, C. J., J. Am. Dent. A. *17:*827-843, May '30
Harelip and cleft palate; analysis of 184 cases. BURDICK, C. G. Ann. Surg. *92:*35-50, July '30
Cleft palate. FRASER, J. Practitioner *125:*203-218, July '30
Surgical therapy of cleft palate. WALDHEIM C., E. Salubridad *1:*538, July-Sept '30
Uranostaphylorrhaphy. GATTI, G. Surg., Gynec. and Obst. *51:*224-226, Aug '30
Opportune time and method for cosmetic and functional repair of congenital cleft palate and harelip. HOFER, O. Wien. klin. Wchnschr. *43:*1184, Sept. 18, '30
Treatment of cleft palate with sutures; case. BARBARO. Bull. et mem. Soc. nat. de chir. *56:*1186-1195, Nov. 15, '30
Pathology and therapy of cleft palate and harelip. ROSENTHAL, W. Fortschr. d. Zahnh. *6:*953-972, Nov '30
Surgical technic in cleft palate. JORGE, J. M. Bol. y trab. de la Soc. de cir. de Buenos Aires *14:*1019-1025, Dec. 3, '30
Division palatine, anatomie chirurgie, phonetique, by VICTOR VEAU AND S. BOREL. Masson et Cie, Paris, 1931
Surgical correction of cleft lip and palate. DAVIS, A. D. Surg., Gynec. and Obst. *52:*875-883, April '31
Cleft palate and harelip treated by mobilization of 2 triangular osseous segments from cleft palate. BASTIANELLI, P. Boll. d. mal. d. orecchio, d. gola. e d. naso *49:*137-153, May '31
Uranoplasty at several sittings. EICHHOFF, E. Chirurg *3:*595-599, July 1, '31
Harelip and cleft palate. NEW, G. B., S. Clin. North America. *11:*761-765, Aug '31
Veau operation for cleft palate. RUPPE, C. Ann. D'oto-laryng., pp. 1029-1043, Oct '31
Surgical therapy of cleft palate. LIEBERMANN, T. Orvosi hetil. *75:*1065, Oct. 31, '31
Surgical correction of harelip and cleft palate. DAVIS, A. D. California and West. Med. *35:*357-361, Nov '31
Surgical treatment of harelip and cleft palate in children. Canad. M. A. J. *25:*563-565, Nov '31
Pathology and therapy of cleft palates. ROSENTHAL, W. Fortschr. d. Zahnh. *7:*989-1016, Nov '31
Surgical therapy of cleft palate; 150 cases. MONNIER, E. Schweiz. med. Wchnschr. *61:*1207, Dec. 12, '31

Cleft Palate—Cont.
Cleft palate operations. KINZEL, H. Beitr. z. klin. Chir. *152:*618-624, '31
Surgical therapy of congenital cleft palate. PIZZAGALLI, L. Boll. d. spec. med.-chir. *5:*129-266, '31
Simple plastic method of covering palatal defects. SPANIER, F. Deutsche Ztschr. f. Chir. *231:*284-293, '31
Cleft palate. TURNER, G. G. Proc. Internat. Assemb. Inter-State Post-Grad. M.A., North America (1930) *6:*255-260, '31
Cleft lip and cleft palate. ARMBRECHT, E. C. West Virginia M. J. *28:*59-64, Feb '32
Double harelip and cleft palate showing importance of proper surgical and orthodontic treatment of premaxillary lobe or process. KELSEY, H. E. Internat. J. Orthodontia *18:*145-147, Feb '32
Cleft palate. SHEARER, W. L. Nebraska M. J. *17:*66-70, Feb '32
Cleft lip and palate; surgical correction. DAVIS, A. D. Internat. J. Orthodontia *18:*282-290, March '32
Cleft palate. HUNTER, J. B. Guy's Hosp. Gaz. *46:*102-109, March 19, '32
Surgical therapy of cleft lip and palate. WASSMUND, M. Deutsche med. Wchnschr. *58:*445-448, March 18, '32
Preoperative and postoperative care of congenital clefts of lip and palate. KITLOWSKI, E. A. Ann. Surg. *95:*659-666, May '32
Uranostaphylorrhaphy according to method of Victor Veau. French M. Rev. *2:*259-275, May '32
Simple surgical therapy of cleft palate. Gac. med. de Mexico *63:*327-332, June '32
Cleft palate operation. BROWNE, D. Brit. J. Surg. *20:*7-25, July '32
Therapy of harelip and cleft palate. EDBERG, E. Hygiea *94:*529-558, July 31, '32
Surgery of fetal clefts (harelip, cleft palate, etc.); review of literature. ROSENTHAL, W. Zentralbl. f. Chir. *59:*2345-2379, Sept. 24, '32
Cleft palate repair, with notes on administration of anesthetics. MITCHELL, A. and MACKENZIE, J. R. Brit. J. Surg. *20:*214-219, Oct '32
Late anatomic and functional results of cleft palate operation; 150 cases. PAGNAMENTA, E. Deutsche Ztschr. f. Chir. *235:*214-233, '32
Congenital clefts of face and jaw; survey of 350 operated cases. RITCHIE, H. P. Tr. West. S. A. *42:*37-98, '32
Modern therapy of cleft palate. ROSENTHAL, W. Ztschr. f. Stomatol. *30:*530-540. '32
Surgical therapy of cleft palate. VON LIEBER-

Cleft Palate—Cont.
MANN, T. Ztschr. f. Hals-, Nasen-u. Ohrenh. *30:*556-559, '32
The Operative Story of Cleft Palate, by GEORGE M. DORRANCE. W. B. Saunders Co., Phila., 1933
Surgical treatment of harelip and cleft palate. SKINNER, M., J. M. A. Alabama *2:*253-259, Jan '33
Cleft palate procedures; experiences and observations. VOORHEES, I. W. Arch. Pediat. *50:*73-80, Feb '33
Extreme cleft of hard and soft palate closed with use of author's tension plates. FEDERSPIEL, M. N. Wisconsin M. J. *32:*172-177, March '33
Advance in surgery of cleft palate. LEVI, D. Lancet *1:*515-518, March 11, '33
Present status of therapy of cleft lip and palate. BURIAN, F. Casop. lek. cesk. *72:*420, April 7; 454, April 14; 491, April 21, '33
Principles to be observed in treatment of congenital harelip and cleft palate. HYSLOP, V. B. Wisconsin M. J. *32:*246-248, April '33
Surgery of cleft palate. VAUGHAN, H. S. Am. Med. *39:*149-154, April '33 abstr: Eye, Ear, Nose and Throat Monthly *12:*25-27, Feb '33
Lateral expansion of upper jaw in case of marked atresia in patient 30 years old; amelioration of nasal permeability. DARCISSAC, M. Bull. et mem. Soc. d. chirurgiens de Paris *25:*296-300, May 5, '33
Securing successful results in surgical therapy of cleft palate. HALLE. Rev. de chir. plastique, pp. 17-21, May '33
Treatment of prominent intermaxillary bone in therapy of harelip and cleft palate. Schweiz. med. Wchnschr., *63:*949-950, Sept. 23, '33
Hunterian lecture; cleft palate. WARDILL, W. E. M. Brit. J. Surg. *21:*347-369, Oct '33
Cleft palate and harelip. CASELLA, E. Rev. med. latino-am. *19:*119-159, Nov '33
Functional results of 200 staphylorrhaphies. VEAU, V. AND BOREL-MOISONNY, MME. Bull. et mem. Soc. nat. de chir. *59:*1372-1382, Nov. 25, '33
Results of surgical therapy in cleft palate. WARDILL, W. E. M. Arch. f. klin. Chir. *177:*504-509, '33
Operations on congenital harelip and cleft of both hard and soft palates. PICHLER, H. Wien. klin. Wchnschr. *47:*70-72, Jan. 19, '34
Cleft lip and palate surgery. FREW, A. L., J. Am. Dent. A. *21:*251-255, Feb '34
Surgical therapy of harelip and cleft palate; possibilities of results. ERNST, F. Kinderarztl. Praxis *5:*120-128, March '34

Cleft Palate – Cont.
Cleft palate associated with congenital and hypo-alimentary debility and pulmonary tuberculosis; case. PÉREZ MORENO, B. Siglo med. *93:*325–328, March 24, '34
Congenital clefts of face and jaws; 350 cases in which operation was performed. RITCHIE, H. P. Arch. Surg. *28:*617–658, April '34
Plastic surgery of traumatic cleft of hard palate in adult; case. PESSANO, J. E. AND GOÑI MORENO, I. Semana med. *1:*1678–1679, May 31, '34
Congenital deformities of mouth (including cleft lip and palate). BROWNE, D. Practitioner *132:*658–670, June '34
New mouth gag for cleft palate operation. NEWKIRK, H. D. Laryngoscope *44:*587, July '34
Cleft palate and cleft lip. SHEARER, W. L., J. Am. Dent. A. *21:*1446–1454, Aug '34
Dieffenbach-Warren operation for closure of congenitally cleft palate. BLAIR, V. P. AND BROWN, J. B. Surg., Gynec. and Obst. *59:*309–320, Sept '34
Cleft palate procedures in surgery; experiences with Veau and Dorrance technic. IVY, R. H. AND CURTIS, L. Ann. Surg. *100:*502–511, Sept '34
Correcting deformities of velum and mesopharynx to insure better speech following cleft palate surgery. BOYNE, H. N. Nebraska M. J. *19:*407–409, Nov '34
Treatment of cleft palate. FALTIN, R. Finska lak. -sallsk. handl. *76:*961–984, Nov '34
Surgical repair of facial injuries and harelip and cleft palate deformities. RISDON, E. F. Canad. M. A. J. *32:*51–54, Jan '35
Velopalatine fissure; result of staphylorrhaphy in case. ROUDIL, G. AND ASSALI, J. Marseille-med. *1:*37–38, Jan. 5, '35
Cleft palate. TUNG, P. C. Chinese M. J. *49:*22–41, Jan '35
New surgical technics; Limberg pterygoid displacement in cleft palate. DUFOURMENTEL, L. Bull. et mem. Soc. d. chirurgiens de Paris *27:*130–135, March 1, '35 also: Prat. med. franc. *17:*339–345, June (A–B) '36
Structural plan of jaw and question of treating projections of intermaxillary bone in harelip and cleft palate. KULENKAMPFF, D. Zentralbl. f. Chir. *62:*1394–1396, June 15, '35
Cleft palate. WARDILL, W. E. M. Lancet *1:*1435–1437, June 22, '35
Cleft palate operations. RIEMKE, V. Hospitalstid. *78:*741, July 9; 753, July 16, '35
Operative repair of cleft palate. LEMESURIER, A. B. Canad. M. A. J. *33:*150–157, Aug. '35

Cleft Palate – Cont.
Technic and results of plastic surgery of the palate. AXHAUSEN, G. Zentralbl. f. Chir. *62:*2211–2215, Sept. 14, '35
Life-masks in conjunction with models of mouth in cleft palate. BRODERICK, R. A. Proc. Roy. Soc. Med. *28:*1667–1672, Oct '35
Value of speech training in cleft palate. SCHARFE, E. E. Arch. Oto-laryng. *22:*585–596, Nov '35 also: Canad. M. A. J. *33:*641–647, Dec '35
Orthopedic operation in cleft palate. BROWNE, D. Brit. M. J. *2:*1093–1095, Dec. 7, '35
Treatment of protruding intermaxillary bone in case of cleft palate. LUHMANN, K. Beitr. z. klin. Chir. *161:*539–547, '35
Surgical therapy of cleft palate. MICHAËL, P. R. Beitr. z. klin. Chir. *161:*468–475, '35
Technik und Ergebnisse der Gaumenplastik, by GEORG AXHAUSEN. Georg Thieme, Stuttgart, 1936
Correction of cleft lip and palate. FREW, A. L. J. Am. Dent. A. *23:*29–34, Jan '36
Present day conception of cleft lip and palate surgery. KIRKHAM, H. L. D. Texas State J. Med. *31:*571–574, Jan '36
Care of cleft palate patients. BEATTY, H. G. Tr. Am. Laryng., Rhin & Otol. Soc. *41:*165–187, '35 also: Laryngoscope *46:*203–226, March '36
Radical uranoplasty (Limberg): new opertion. (for closure of cleft palate). SCHULTZ, L., J. Am. Dent. A. *23:*407–415, March '36
Technic of plastic surgery of cleft palate. AXHAUSEN, G. Chirurg *8:*299–313, April 15, '36
Surgical therapy of cleft palate by Veau technic. DE SANSON, R. D. Rev. oto-laring. de Sao Paulo *4:*349–364, July–Aug. '36
Therapy of cleft palate by uranoplasty. KAMIMURA, S. Oto-rhino-laryng. *9:*608, July '36
Effect of suture of cleft palate on phonation. VEAU, V. AND BOREL-MAISONNY, S. Monatschr. f. Ohrenh. *70:*858–864, July '36
Harelip and cleft palate. BERNDORFER, A. Gyogyaszat *76:*499, Aug. 30–Sept. 6, '36; 527, Sept. 13, '36
Dieffenbach-Warren operation for closure of congenitally cleft palate. BLAIR, V. P. AND BROWN, J. B. Internat. J. Orthodontia *22:*853–868, Aug '36
Oblique-angled knife for resetting lower end of dislocated septal cartilage and operations on harelip and cleft palate. METZENBAUM, M. Arch. Otolaryng. *24:*199, Aug '36
Cleft palate. VIGNARD. Avenir med. *33:*240–241, Sept–Oct '36
Therapy of cleft lip, jaw and palate with pro-

Cleft Palate – Cont.
truding intermaxillary bone. TOMOFF, W. Zentralbl. f. Chir. *63:*2535–2538, Oct. 24, '36
Principles of plastic operation for cleft palate (Langenbeck-Axhausen). VEAU, V. Deutsche Ztschr. f. Chir. *247:*300–316, '36 also: J. de chir. *48:*465–481, Oct '36 (comment on Axhausen's book).
Harelip and cleft palate. BEATTY, H. G. West Virginia M. J. *32:*501–516, Nov '36
Surgical therapy of congenital cleft palate. SANVENERO-ROSELLI, G. Rev. de chir. structive, pp. 413–418, Dec '36
Surgical technic in cleft palate. SOIVIO, A. Duodecim *52:*723–735, '36
Principles of plastic operation (Langenbeck-Axhausen) of cleft palate. (Reply to Veau). AXHAUSEN, G., J. de chir. *49:*47–53, Jan '37
Cleft lips and cleft palate. CUNNINGHAM, A. F. Am. J. Nursing *37:*339–341, April '37
New approach in plastic operations of cleft palate and harelip. HERLYN, K. E. Zentralbl. f. Chir. *64:*815–818, April 3, '37
Pharyngo-staphylo-uranoplasty, operation in older children and adults. TROELL, A. Svenska lak. -tidning. *34:*521–524, April 9, '37
Mechanism of speech in cleft palates. WARDILL, W. E. M. Monatschr. f. Ohrenh. *71:*424–429, April '37
Harelip and cleft palate. ERNST, F. Med. Welt *11:*1061–1064, July 31, '37
Cleft palate repair technic affording better speech results. HYSLOP, V. B. Wisconsin M. J. *36:*540–543, July '37
Plastic operation of cleft palate according to Ernst method. STANČIUS, P. Medicina, Kaunas *18:*558–562, July '37
Technic of operation for cleft palate. WARDILL, W. E. M. Brit. J. Surg. *25:*117–130, July '37
Surgical and phonetic problems of harelip and cleft palate. BERNDORFER, A. Gyogyaszat *77:*433, July 18–25; 452, Aug. 1–8, '37
Review of recent literature on cleft lip and palate surgery. IVY, R. H. Internat. J. Orthodontia *23:*844–849, Aug '37
Surgical therapy of harelip and cleft palate. OBERNIEDERMAYR, A. Chirurg *9:*641–645, Sept. 1, '37
Surgical therapy of fissures of palate inoperable by classic methods. COELST, M. Bull. Soc. belge d'otol., rhinol., laryng., pp. 377–380, '37
Technic of suture of cleft palate. HERLYN, K. E. Beitr. z. klin. Chir. *165:*276–277, '37
Results of bridge plastic (Axhausen) operation for cleft palate in 45 cases. IMMENKAMP, A. Deutsche Ztschr. f. Chir. *249:*326–336, '37

Cleft Palate – Cont.
Cleft lip and palate repair technic. KILNER, T. P. St. Thomas's Hosp. Rep. *2:*127–140, '37
New methods of plastic surgery in cleft palate. LINDEMANN, A. Deutsche Ztschr. f. Chir. *249:*68–78, '37
Present status of surgical therapy of cleft palate. PHILIPPIDES, D. Ergebn. d. Chir. u. Orthop. *30:*316–371, '37
The Surgery of Oral and Facial Diseases and Malformations, by GEORGE V. I. BROWN. Lea and Febiger, Phila., 1938
Surgery of cleft lip, jaw and palate. AXHAUSEN, G. Chirurg *10:*1–10, Jan. 1, '38
Harelip, cleft palate; congenital deformities of mouth and face. KIMBALL, G. H. J. Oklahoma M. A. *31:*85–89, March '38
Suggested aid in treatment of cleft palate in older children or adults. FLYNN, R. Australian and New Zealand J. Surg. *8:*82–84, July '38
Causes of surgical failure in cleft palate repair. VOORHEES, I. W. Am. J. Surg. *40:*588–595, June '38
Harelip treatment (and cleft palate). PENN, J. South African M. J. *12:*425–429, June 25, '38
Use of fascia and ribbon catgut in harelip and cleft palate repair. BRENIZER, A. G. Ann. Surg. *107:*692–700, May '38
Harelip and cleft palate; age at operation and results in therapy. LUHMANN, K. Therap. d. Gegenw. *79:*300–303, July '38
Cleft-lip correction (and palate). STUMPF, F. W., J. Am. Dent. A. *25:*1196–1201, Aug '38
Practical problems in surgical correction of harelip and nose, palate defects. CALLISTER, A. C. Rocky Mountain M. J. *35:*698–701, Sept '38
Harelip repair (cleft palate). OWENS, N. South. M. J. *31:*959–968, Sept '38
Problems associated with reconstructive procedures for cleft lip and palate. BEAVIS, J. O. Ohio State M.J. *34:*1115–1117, Oct '38
Cooperation necessary in treatment of cleft palate. FITZ-GIBBON, J. J. Ann. Dent. *5:*143–153, Sept '38
Care and treatment of harelip. and cleft palate. CARRUTHERS, F. W., J. Arkansas M. Soc. *25:*93–97, Oct '38
Correction of cleft-palate speech by phonetic instruction. BERRY, M. F. Quart. J. Speech Educ. *14:*523–529, Nov '28
Congenital clefts of lip and palate. DOOLIN, W. Irish J. M. Sc., pp. 708–720, Nov '38
Rubber plate as support for mouth following cleft palate operation. JANTZEN, J. Deutsche Ztschr. f. Chir. *249:*651–656, '38

Cleft Palate – Cont.
Operative treatment of cleft palate. LE MESURIER, A. B. Am. J. Surg. *39:*458–469, Feb '38
Uranostaphylorrhaphy with Donati suture. SCHOEMAKER, J. Arch. ital. di chir. *54:*513–515, '38
Experiences in treatment of children with harelip and cleft palate. EDBERG, E. Nord. med. *1:*89–92, Jan. 14, '39
New data on surgical therapy of cleft palate. THEODORESCO, D. Rev. de chir., Bucuresti *42:*126–134, Jan–Feb '39
New mouth gag for surgery of cleft palate. LUHMANN, K. Zentralbl. f. Chir. *66:*243–244, Feb. 4, '39
Plastic surgery by Axhausen method in cleft palate; case. MARFORT, A. AND BISI, R. H. Rev. Asoc. med. argent. *53:*93–94, Feb. 15–28, '39
Cleft palate surgery. SCHULTZ, L. W. Illinois M. J., *75:*127–131, Feb. '39
Surgical therapy of unilateral cleft palate. WASSMUND, M. Zentralbl. f. Chir. *66:*994–999, April 29, '39
New mouth gag for operation of cleft palate. LUHMANN, K. Therap. d. Gegenw. *80:*284–285, June '39
Surgery of cleft palate. SMITH, A. E. AND JOHNSON, J. B. Am. J. Surg. *45:*93–103, July '39
Harelip problem and cleft palate. KELLY, C. C., J. Connecticut M. Soc. *3:*490–491, Sept '39
Orthopedic correction of congenital fissures of jaws. PETRIK, L. Ztschr. f. Stomatol. *37:*1235–1252, Sept '39
Surgical therapy of harelip and cleft palate in Denmark. ANDERSEN, P. F. Ugesk. f. Laeger *101:*1187–1193, Oct. 12, '39
Value of osteoplastic flaps in cleft palate repair. DAVIS, W. B. Pennsylvania M. J. *43:*153–158, Nov '39
New surgical procedure for repair of cleft palate. JAKABHAZY, I. Gyogyaszat *79:*651–652, Dec. 17, '39
Harelip and cleft palate. SOIVIO, A. Nord. med. (Duodecim) *4:*3705–3709, Dec. 23, '39
Therapy of harelip and of velopalatine fissures. APOLO, E. and ALVAREZ GRAU, J. An. de oto-rino-laring. d. Uruguay *9:*102–109, '39
Plastic surgery of face (including harelip and cleft palate). HAGENTORN, A. Arch. f. klin. Chir. *195:*455–488, '39
Results of cleft palate operation. HERLYN, K. E. Beitr. z. klin. Chir. *169:*397–401, '39
Experiences in surgical therapy of cleft palate. PERMAN, E. Acta chir. Scandinav.

Cleft Palate – Cont.
*83:*83–89, '39
Congenital cardiac defects and harelip with clefts of jaw and palate in twins. RABL, R. AND SCHULZ, F. Virchows Arch. f. path. Anat. *305:*505–520, '39
Cleft palate. SOIVIO, A. Duodecim *55:*607–620, '39
Cleft palate therapy in Finland. SOIVIO, A. Acta Soc. med. fenn. duodecim (Ser. B, Fasc. 1–2, art. 25) *27:*1–8, '39
Congenital Cleft Lip, Cleft Palate, and Associated Nasal Deformities, by HAROLD S. VAUGHAN. Lea and Febiger Co., Phila., 1940
Harelip and cleft palate. FRASER, K. B., M. J. Australia *1:*361–381, March 16, '40
Care of cleft palate. CONWAY, H. S. Clin. North America *20:*593–602, April '40
Methods preferred in cleft lip and cleft palate repair. DAVIS, W. B., J. Internat. Coll. Surgeons *3:*116–124, April '40
Therapy of harelip and cleft palate. ROY, F. Laval med. *5:*197–201, May '40
Experiences in surgery of cleft palate. IVY, R. H. Ann. Surg. *112:*775–782, Oct '40
Harelip and cleft palate. MILLER, S. J. C. Univ. West. Ontario M. J. *11:*14–19, Nov '40
Congenital defect of lower jaw associated with cleft palate (case). SACKS, S. South African M. J. *15:*34, Jan. 25, '41
Functional surgical therapy of cleft palate. SEGRE, R. Rev. Asoc. med. argent. *55:*89–91, Feb. 15–28, '41
Congenital velopalatine fissure, with special reference to therapy. JEREZ TABLADA, G. Rev. mex. de cir. ginec. y cancer *9:*273–279, July '41
Surgical therapy of cleft palate. VAN DER HOFF, H. L. M. Chirurg *13:*396–403, July 1, '41
Extensive cleft of hard palate; case. MORIKAWA, G. Oto-rhino-laryng. *14:*574, Aug '41
Treatment of cleft lip and palate. ABRAMSON, P. D. Tri-State M. J. *14:*2559, Nov '41
Incidence of supernumerary and congenitally missing lateral incisor teeth in 81 cases of harelip and cleft palate. MILLHON, J. A. AND STAFNE, E. C. Am. J. Orthodontics (Oral Surg. Sect) *27:*599–604, Nov '41
Congenital clefts of face and jaws; report of operations used and discussion of results. RITCHIE, H. P. Surg., Gynec. and Obst. *73:*654–670, Nov '41
Surgical and dental treatment of cleft palate. BERRY, T. B. AND KRITZINGER, F. J. South African M. J. *15:*497–498, Dec. 27, '41

Cleft Palate—Cont.
Inheritance of Harelip and Cleft Palate, by POUL FOGH ANDERSEN. Nyt Nordisk Forlag Arnold Busck, Copenhagen, 1942
Surgical therapy of cleft palate and harelip. CHAVES, D. A. Rev. med. munic. *3:*259-270, March '42
Light aspirator in surgery of palatine fissure and in general surgery. MARINO, H. Prensa med. argent. *29:*481-483, March 18, '42
Cleft palate therapy; Brown operation. MARINO, H. Arq. de cir. clin. e exper. *6:*333-336, April-June '42
Harelip and cleft palate; results of plastic surgery. DE SANSON, R. D. Arq. de cir. clin. e exper. *6:*336-339, April-June '42
Maxillary osteotomy in extensive palatine fissures of adult. MARINO, H. Arq. de cir. clin. e exper. *6:*615-620, April-June '42
Technical devices in surgical therapy of harelip and velopalatine fissures, with report of cases. REBELO NETO, J. Arq. de cir. clin. e exper. *6:*343-358, April-June '42
Harelip and cleft palate; 70 consecutive cases. PICKERILL, C. M. New Zealand M. J. *41:*121-129, June '42
Method of keeping palatal mucoperiosteum against bony structures following surgery. GROSS, P. P. Am. J. Orthodontics (Oral Surg. Sect) *28:*522-524, Sept. '42
Rehabilitation of children with cleft palate, harelip or both. PERKINS, H. W. AND SILVER, E. I. Am. J. Orthodontics *28:*567-575, Sept '42
Cleft palate. DORRANCE, G. M. AND BRANSFIELD, J. W. Ann. Surg. *117:*1-27, Jan '43
Labiovelopalatine fissure; surgical therapy with report of cases. DE SANSON, R. D. AND AMARANTE, R. C. L. Rev. brasil. de cir. *12:*215-246, March '43
Harelip and cleft palate. ANDERSEN, P. FOGH. Nord. med. *19:*1597-1598, Sept. 25, '43
Therapy of palatine fissure by combined Veau and Axhausen technics. CASTELLANO, J. L. AND GIGANTI, I. J. Semana med. *2:*887-889, Oct. 14, '43
Plastic surgery of cleft palate. MARINO, H. Prensa med. argent. *30:*2350-2352, Dec. 8, '43
Frequency of occurrence of cleft palates and harelips. GRACE, L. G., J. Dent. Research *22:*495-497, Dec '43
Functional surgical therapy of cleft palate. GARCIA CASTELLANOS, J. A. AND MAURETTE, R. Bol. y trab., Soc. de cir. de Cordoba *4:*141-148, '43
Review of recent literature on technic of surgical therapy of cleft palate. TRAUNER, R. Beitz. z. klin. Chir. *174:*599, '43
Surgical correction of congenital cleft palate. VAUGHAN, H. S., S. Clin. North America *24:*370-380, April '44
Cleft palate. KEMPER, J. W., J. Oral Surg. *2:*227-238, July '44
Preliminary graft of buccal mucosa in closure of extensive perforations of hard palate. REBELO NETO, J. Rev. brasil. de oto-rino-laring. *12:*297-301, July-Oct '44
Care of cleft lip and palate in babies. SCHULTZ, L. W. Illinois M. J. *86:*138-159, Sept '44
Procedure for closing cleft palate (uranoplasty for uranoschisis). MENDIZABAL, P. Cir. y cirujanos *12:*432-435, Oct-Nov '44
Schema of surgical technic in congenital fissures (palate). REBELO NETO, J. Rev. brasil. de oto-rino-laring. *12:*393-400, Nov-Dec '44
Congenital cleft palate and harelip in infants; mode of nutrition in preoperative period. TAYLOR, H. P. Brit. Dent. J. *78:*1-7, Jan. 5, '45
Cleft palate and cleft lip. SHEARER, W. L. Nebraska M. J. *30:*125-126, April '45
Palatal flap in cleft palate. CHRISTIANSEN, G. W. AND BRADLEY, J. L., U. S. Nav. M. Bull. *44:*1018-1022, May '45
Harelip and cleft palate; plan of management. PRIOLEAU, W. H., J. South Carolina M. A. *41:*129-130, June '45
Surgical treatment of harelip and cleft palate. WODAK, E. M. Acta oto-laryng. orient. *1:*13-17, '45
Surgical treatment of harelip and cleft palate. WODAK, E. M. Acta oto-laryng. orient. *1:*42-45, '45
Harelip and cleft palate. KAUFMAN, I. Am. J. Orthodontics (Oral Surg. Sect.) *32:*47-51, Jan '46
Cleft palate. BEATTY, H. G. Ann. Otol. Rhin. and Laryng. *55:*572-579, Sept '46
Responsibility of orthodontist in cleft palate problem. COOPER, H. K. Am. J. Orthodontics (Oral Surg. Sect.) *32:*675-683, Nov. '46
Present status of surgical treatment of cleft hard palate. DAVIS, W. B. Am. J. Orthodontics (Oral Surg. Sect.) *32:*671-672, Nov '46
Surgical treatment of vicious cicatrices involving cheek, lip and alveolar process in cleft lip and palate cases. IVY, R. H. Am. J. Orthodontics (Oral Surg. Sect.) *32:*673-674, Nov '46
Responsibility of surgeon in treating palatal and related defects. KEMPER, J. W. Am. J.

Cleft Palate—Cont.
Orthodontics (Oral Surg. Sect.) *32:*667-670, Nov '46
Harelip and cleft palate; 1,000 patients submitted to operation. ANDERSEN, P. FOGH. Acta chir. Scandinav. *94:*213-242, '46

Cleft Palate, Age for Operation

Age for surgery of cleft palate. HAGENBACH. Schweiz. med. Wchnschr. *55:*487-488, May 28, '25
Surgical therapy of cleft palate must be performed before child begins to talk. ROVIRALTA, E. Ars med., Barcelona, *7:*395-398, Dec '31
Most favorable time for surgical correction of cleft palate. EICHHOFF, E. Chirurg *5:*263-265, April 1, '33
Optimal age for operations in cases of cleft palate and harelip. SOIVIO, A. Duodecim *53:*335-344, '37
At what age should cleft palate operation be performed? KUBANYI, E. Zentralbl. f. Chir. *65:*1798-1799, Aug. 13, '38
Optimum age for operation of cleft palate, with special reference to normal speech development. SPANIER, F., J. Internat. Coll. Surgeons *4:*338-343, Aug '41

Cleft Palate, Associated Anomalies

Developmental anomalies of face and neck and their surgical significance (also cleft palate). SINGLETON, A. O. Texas State J. Med. *25:*659-663, Feb '30
Facial coloboma with complete, unilateral, velopalatine fissure; case. ROCHER, H. L. AND PESME, P., J. de med. de Bordeaux *107:*763, Oct. 10, '30
Late syphilis with destructive gummatous manifestations in nasal bones and first cervical vertebrae; cleft palate; case. RADAELI, A. Gior. ital. di dermat. e sif. *73:*531, Feb '32
Cleft palate and bilateral lack of development of upper extremities; case. RYLL-NARDZEWSKA, J. Ginek. polska *11:*678-683, July-Sept '32
Anatomic examination of human hemicephalic fetus 10 months old with harelip, cleft palate, hyperdactylia, syndactylia, etc. IKEDA, Y. Arb. a d. anat. Inst. d. kaiserlich-japan. Univ. zu Sendai, Hft. 15, pp. 61-212, '33
Teeth in cyclopia and congenital cleft of face. BRECKWOLDT, H. Beitr. z. path. Anat. u. z. allg. Path. *98:*115-135, '36
Thoracopagus, one with harelip and cleft palate. SANGVICHIEN, S. Anat. Rec. *67:*157-158, Jan. 25, '37

Cleft Palate, Associated Anomalies—Cont.
Hypoplasia of mandible (micrognathy) with cleft palate; treatment in early infancy by skeletal traction. CALLISTER, A. C. Am. J. Dis. Child. *53:*1057-1059, April '37
Congenital median fistula, with report of case. DE GAETANO, L. Riforma med. *53:*523-526, April 10, '37
Atypical cartilage in nose, upper lip and palate in cheilognathopalatoschisis. STUPKA, W. Monatschr. f. Ohrenh. *71:*1333-1344, Nov '37
Encephalocele associated with hypertelorism and cleft palate. OLDFIELD, M. C. Brit. J. Surg. *25:*757-764, April '38
Progress in plastic operations performed during childhood (for exstrophy of bladder and harelip) (cleft palate). MONNIER, E. Schweiz. med. Wchnschr. *68:*613-614, May 21, '38
Enlarged thymus (especially in relation to cleft palate operations and roentgenotherapy). TYLER, A. F. AND HOLMES, W. E. Nebraska M. J. *24:*121-125, April '39
Skeletal anomalies associated with cleft palate and harelip. LYONS, D. C. Am. J. Orthodontics *25:*895-897, Sept '39
Hereditary relations between harelip and cleft palate and other malformations, especially of spine. SCHRÖDER, C. H. Beitr. z. klin. Chir. *169:*402-413, '39
Ocular hypertelorism with cleft palate and giant-cell tumor. POSNER, I. AND PIATT, A. D. Radiology *35:*79-81, July '40
Congenital bilateral anophthalmos vera with unilateral polydactyly and cleft palate; case. APPLEBAUM, A. AND MARMELSTEIN, M. Arch. Ophth. *29:*258-265, Feb '43
Spina bifida and cranium bifidum; unusual nasopharyngeal encephalocele (with cleft palate). INGRAHAM F. D. AND MATSON, D. D. New England J. Med. *228:*815-820, June 24, '43
Three generations of mucous cysts occurring with harelip and cleft palate. STRAITH, C. L. AND PATTON, H. S., J.A.M.A. *123:* 693-694, Nov. 13, '43
Median harelip, cleft palate and glossal agenesis. SINCLAIR, J. G. AND MCKAY, J. Anat. Rec. *91:*155-160, Feb '45
Palatal flap in cleft palate. CHRISTIANSEN, G. W. AND BRADLEY, J. L., U. S. Nav. M. Bull. *44:*1018-1022, May '45

Cleft Palate, Bilateral (See also Cleft Palate)

Operation for double cleft palate and harelip. PICHLER, H. Deutsche Ztschr. f. Chir. *195:*104-107, '26

Cleft Palate, Bilateral—Cont.

Complete bilateral cleft palate: case. LAL, R. B. Indian M. Gaz. *66:*268, May '31

Double harelip and cleft palate showing importance of proper surgical and orthodontic treatment of premaxillary lobe or process. KELSEY, H. E. Internat. J. Orthodontia *18:*145–147, Feb. '32

Surgical therapy of bilateral harelip and total cleft palate; case. VIGNARD. Avenir med. *29:*41, Feb '32

Cleft Palate, Complications

Treatment of complications arising from cleft palate. URBAN, W. G. Am. J. Orthodontics *24:*87–89, Jan '38

Frequent occurrence of scarlet fever following cleft palate operations. SCHEPPOKAT. Deutsche Ztschr. f. Chir. *218:*383–386, '29

Cleft Palate, Ear Problems

Rhino-laryngologic phases of harelip and cleft palate work. DAVIS, W. B. Internat. Clinics *2:*258–266, '22 (illus.)

Cleft palate and rhinopharyngeal functions; case. SEGRÈ, R. Arch. ital. di otol. *40:*633–643, Oct '29

Oral surgical problems of interest to rhinologists (including cleft palate). DORRANCE, G. M. New York State J. Med. *32:*1226–1228, Nov. 1, '32

Tubal (Eustachian) function in cleft palate. SEGRE, R. Valsalva, *9:*856–875, Nov '33

Diseases of ear in patients with cleft palate. MEISSNER, K. Hals-, Nasen-u. Ohrenarzt (Teil 1) *30:*6–20, Jan '39

Cleft Palate, Elongation of

Lengthening soft palate in cleft palate operations. DORRANCE, G. M. Ann. Surg. *82:*208–211, Aug '25

Prolongation of palate by retrotransposition of pterygoid processes in cleft palate. PŘECECHTĚL, A. Casop. lek. cesk. *66:*541–543, March 28, '27

Operation for lengthening palate. LVOFF, P. P. Vestnik khir (nos. 37–38) *13:*212–221, '28

Congenital insufficiency of cleft palate. DORRANCE, G. M. Arch. Surg. *21:*185–248, Aug '30

Cleft palate repair; palatine insertion of superior constrictor muscle of pharynx and its significance in cleft palate, with remarks on "push-back operation." DORRANCE, G. M. Ann. Surg. *95:*641–658, May '32

"Push-back operation" of palate. DORRANCE, G. M. Ann. Surg. *101:*445–459, Jan '35

Role of push-back operation in surgery of cleft palate. DORRANCE, G. M. AND SHIRAZY, E., J. Am. Dent. A. *22:*1108–1117, July '35

Cleft Palate, Elongation of—Cont.

Cleft palate—surgical repair; with special reference to lengthening soft palate. VAUGHAN, H. S. Am. J. Surg. *31:*5–9, Jan '36

Elongation of partially cleft palate. BROWN, J. B. Surg., Gynec. and Obst. *63:*768–771, Dec '36

Elongation of partially cleft palate. BROWN, J. B. Am. J. Orthodontics *24:*878–883, Sept '38

Double elongations of partially cleft palates and elongations of palates with complete clefts. BROWN, J. B. Surg., Gynec. and Obst. *70:*815–818, April '40

Double elongations of partially cleft palates and elongations of palates with complete clefts. BROWN, J. B. Am. J. Orthodontics *26:*910–915, Sept '40

Cleft Palate, Etiology

Hare-lip and cleft palate; a war influence. AYMARD, J. L. Brit. M. J. *2:*405, Sept. 10, '21

Tripartite cleft palate and double harelip in identical twins. DAVIS, A. D. Surg., Gynec. and Obst. *35:*586–592, Nov '22 (illus.)

Hereditary nature of harelip and cleft palate. BIRKENFELD, W. Arch. f. klin. Chir. *141:*729–753, '26

Cleft palate and harelip; familial manifestations. LEVEN. Arch. f. Rassen-u. Gesellsch.-Biol. *20:*71, Dec. 20, '27

Study of twins with cleft lip, jaw, and palate from standpoint of pathologic heredity. BIRKENFELD, W. Beitr. z. klin. Chir. *141:*257–267, '27

Cause and treatment of cleft palate. SAMENGO, L. AND ERRECART, P. L. Rev. de especialid. *3:*658–662, Nov '28

Hereditary aspect of harelip and cleft palate. COENEN, H. Chirurg *3:*501–505, June 1, '31

Hereditary aspect of cleft lip and palate. SCHRÖDER, C. H. Arch. f. Rassen-u. Gesellsch.-Biol. *25:*369–394, Nov. 25, '31

Cleft palate found in only one of identical twins. WRIGHT, H. B. Internat. J. Orthodontia *20:*649–657, July '34

Inheritance of harelip and cleft palate. SANDERS, J. Genetica *15:*433–510, '34

Inheritance of harelip and cleft palate in man. DROOGLEEVER FORTUYN, A. B. Genetica *17:*349–366, '35

Heredity of submucous cleft of palate. MAHLSTEDT, H. Ztschr. f. Laryng., Rhin., Otol. *26:*347–352, '35.

Cleft Palate, Etiology—Cont.

Studies on heredity of harelip, and cleft palate, with particular regard to mode of transmission. SCHRÖDER, C. H. Arch. f. klin. Chir. *182:*299–330, '35

Etiology of cleft palate and harelip. BEATTY, H. G., J. Speech Disorders, pp. 13–20, March '36

Development of harelip and cleft palate in embryo 22 mm. in length. MAURER, H. Ztschr. f. Anat. u. Entwcklngsgesch. *105:*359–373, '36

Origin of facial cleft, harelip and cleft palate. POLITZER, G. Monatschr. f. Ohrenh. *71:*63–73, Jan '37

Healing process in harelip and cleft palate in embryo 23.3 mm. in length. MAURER, H. Ztschr. f. Anat. u. Entwcklngsgesch. *107:*203–211, '37

Harelip and cleft palate in relation to eugenic sterilization, according to German law. MARTINY. Ztschr. f. Stomatol. *36:*947, Aug. 26; 1004, Sept. 9, '38

Harelip and cleft palate from eugenic point of view. UEBERMUTH, H. Arch. f. klin. Chir. *193:*224–229, '38

Hairy polyus of soft palate as cause of cleft formation; case. NASE, H. Zentralbl. f. Chir. *66:*29–32, Jan. 7, '39

Harelip and cleft palate in uniovular twins. SCHRÖDER, C. H. Zentralbl. f. Chir. *66:*2299–2308, Oct. 21, '39

Harelip with cleft jaw and palate in relation to law on prevention of hereditary defects. LEHMANN, W. AND RITTER, R. Ztschr. f. menschl. Vererb.-u. Konstitutionslehre, *23:*1–16, '39

Studies on family groups with harelip and clefts of jaw and palate. MENGELE, J. Ztschr. f. menschl. Vererb.-u. Konstitutionslehre *23:*17–42, '39

Hereditary relations between harelip and cleft palate and other malformations, especially of spine. SCHRÖDER, C. H. Beitr. z. klin. Chir. *169:*402–413, '39

Heredopathology of fissures of lips, jaws and palate; report on unselected series of 41 pairs of twins. IDELBERGER, A. AND IDELBERGER, K. Ztschr. f. menschl. Vererb.-u. Konstitutionslehre *24:*417–479, '40

The Inheritance of Harelip and Cleft Palate. POUL FOGH-ANDERSEN. Nyt Nordisk Forlag, Arnold Busch, Copenhagen, 1942

Significance of occult spina bifida in heredity of harelip and cleft palate. SCHRODER, C. H. AND HILLENBRAND, H. J. Arch. f. klin. Chir. *203:*328–342, '42

"Heteropenetration" and twin discordance in hereditary harelip and cleft palate. STEINIGER, F. AND VEIT, G. Ztschr. f. menschl.

Cleft Palate, Etiology—Cont.

Vererb-. u. Konstitutionslehre *26:*75–92, '42

Eugenic aspect of cleft palate and other facial deformities. OLINGER, N. A., J. Am. Dent. A. *31:*1431–1434, Nov. 1, '44

Cleft Palate, Extra-Oral Flaps for

Gillies tubed pedicle flap in cleft palate. QUICK, B., J. Coll. Surgeons, Australasia *2:*395–400, March '30

Pedicled grafts in therapy of defects of hard palate. PUTSCHKOWSKY, A. Ztschr. f. Laryng., Rhin., Otol. *22:*98–102, '31

Lesions of jaw, nose and cheek; cleft lip and palate; cartilage transplant; tube graft. MOOREHEAD, F. B., S. Clin. North America *12:*57–66, Feb '32

Plastic closure of palate defects by means of tube-pedicle flap. SMYRNOFF, S. A. Am. Med. *39:*115, March '33

Closure of defect in hard palate by pedicled tube graft. BURNELL, G. H., M. J. Australia *2:*484, Oct. 7, '33

Plastic closure of defective hard palate by means of round pedicled flap (Filatov). FRANKENBERG, B. E. Sovet. khir. *4:*591–595, '33

Palatoplasty using extra-oral tissues. DAVIS, A. D. Ann. Surg. *99:*94–100, Jan '34

Two cases illustrating elastic traction in plastic surgery; pedicle flap to close large opening in hard palate. MOOREHEAD, F. B., S. Clin. North America *14:*745–749, Aug '34

Cleft Palate Growth (See also Cleft Palate)

Dimensions and growth of palate in infant with gross maldevelopment of upper lip and palate; quantitative study. PEYTON, W. T. Arch. Surg. *22:*704–737, May '31

Dimensions and growth of palate in infants with gross maldevelopment of upper lip and palate; further investigations. (including cleft lip and palate). PEYTON, W. T. Am. J. Dis. Child. *47:*1265–1268, June '34

Cleft Palate Incidence

Quantitative studies on congenital clefts. PEYTON, W. T. AND RITCHIE, H. P. Arch. Surg. *33:*1046–1053, Dec '36

Congenital clefts of lip and palate, incidence of. DAVIS, J. S. Ann. Surg. *80:*363–374, Sept '24

The Inheritance of Harelip and Cleft Palate. POUL FOGH-ANDERSEN. NYT Nordisk Forlag, Arnold Busch, Copenhagen, 1942

Frequency of occurrence of cleft palates and harelips. GRACE, L. G., J. Dent. Research *22:*495–497, Dec '43

Cleft Palate Obturators

Artificial velum for congenital cleft palate. PAYNE, J. L. Proc. Roy. Soc. Med. (Sect. Odontology) *14:*36, Feb '21

Dental aspect of treatment of congenital cleft palates. FRY, W. K. Proc. Roy. Soc. Med. (Sect. Odontology), *14:*57, Oct '21

Prosthetic treatment of harelip and cleft palate complications. RUPPE, L. AND RUPPE, C. Odontologie *64:*831-845, Dec. 30, '26

Aids to palatal sufficiency after cleft palate operations. WOODS, R. Brit. M. J. *1:*371-372, Feb. 26, '27

Prosthesis for cleft palate. RUPPE, L. AND RUPPE, C. Odontologie *65:*276-302, April '27

Mechanical correction of cleft palate. CASE, C. S. Dominion Dent. J. *40:*69-72, March '28

Form of new obturator (meatus obturator) for preventing nasal speech in cleft palate. FRÖSCHELS, E. Ztschr. f. Stomatol. *26:*882-888, Sept '28

New obturator (meatus obturator) for preventing nasal speech in cleft palate. SCHALIT, A. Ztschr. f. Stomatol. *26:*888-898, Sept '28

Fasting of protective celluloid plates in uranoplasty. LIMBERG, A. A. Odont. i stomatol. (no. 11) *6:*5-8, '28

Principles of prosthetic treatment in cleft palate. FISCHER, A. Ugesk. f. Laeger *91:*108-110, Feb 7, '29

Phonetic results of 100 staphylorrhaphies. VEAU, V. AND BOREL, S. Bull. et mem. Soc. nat. de chir. *55:*894-909, June 29, '29

New obturator to combat nasalization in patients with cleft of hard palate. FRÖSCHELS, E. AND SCHALIT, A. Wien. klin. Wchnschr. *42:*1442-1444, Nov. 7, '29

Prosthetic treatment of congenital gnathopalatoschisis; case. BAGGER, H. Ugesk. f. laeger *92:*66-69, Jan. 16, '30

Correction of congenital cleft-palate speech by appliances. FITZ-GIBBON, J., J. Dental Cosmos *72:*231-238, March '30

Correction of nasal speech from congenital defects of palate by obturators. REICHENBACH, E. Vrtljsschr. f. Zahnh. *46:*418-434, '30

Fitz-Gibbon's prosthesis for correcting phonetic troubles in congenital cleft palate. FITZ-GIBBON, J., J. Odontologie *69:*760-767, Nov '31

Experiences with new obturator in cleft palate. MELA, B. AND SEGRE, R. Stomatol. *30:*854-869, Sept '32

New obturator for use in case of unsuccessful uranoplasty, with reference to surgical and prosthetic therapeutic methods in palatine defects. KAHN, W. Ztschr. f. Stomatol. *32:*18-27, Jan. 12, '34

Cleft Palate Obturators – Cont.

Protective prosthesis for plastic operation on palate. HOTTA, H. Ztschr. d. japan, chirurg. Gesellsch. *36:*100-101, '35

Prosthetic therapy for cleft palate. SEGRE, R. Monatschr. f. Ohrenh. *70:*865-884, July '36

Claims of various obturators, from standpoint of correction of speech defects in cleft palate. REICHENBACH, E. Hals-, Nasen-. u. Ohrenarzt. (Teil 1) *28:*29-33, Feb '37

Prosthetic treatment of cleft palate. BAGGER, H. Nord. med. tidskr., *13:*685-689, May 1, '37

Cleft palate operation supplemented by obturator in treatment. FITZGERALD, R. R. Brit. J. Surg. *25:*816-825, April '38

Prosthetic therapy of acquired palatal defects. EHRICKE, A. Med. Welt *12:*775-776, May 28, '38

Construction of simple obturator in cleft palate. GEMMELL, J. A. M. Brit. Dent. J. *76:*69-70, Feb. 4, '44

Obturators for palate; review. BEDER, O. E. J. Oral Surg. *2:*356-368, Oct '44

Cleft palate prosthesis. SCHOLE, M. L. AND KATZ, T. Bull. U. S. Army M. Dept. (no. 84) pp. 90-93, Jan '45

Correction of cleft palate using stress-breaker type partial appliance with obturator attached. BEDER, O. E. *et al.* Am. J. Orthodontics (Oral Surg. Sect.) *31:*377-380, June '45

Technic for taking imprint for construction of prosthesis for cleft palate. CABROL. Rev. de stomatol. *47:*157-159, May-June '46

Prosthetic restoration of congenital cleft palate. OLINGER, N. A. Am. J. Orthodontics (Oral Surg. Sect.) *32:*456-468, July '46

Responsibility of prosthodontist in treatment of cleft palate. HARKINS, C. S. Am. J. Orthodontics (Oral Surg. Sect.) *32:*684-687, Nov '46

Obturator of choice for congenital cleft palate. SCHALIT, A. Am. J. Orthodontics (Oral Surg. Sect.), *32:*688-713, Nov '46

Cleft Palate Operations, Anesthesia for

Endotracheal anesthesia supplementing avertin (tribrom-ethanol) in cleft palate operations. LEIGH, M. D. AND FITZGERALD, R. R. Canad. M. A. J. *35:*427-428, Oct '36

Anesthesia (endotracheal oxygen-ether vapor) for harelip and cleft palate operations on babies. AYRE, P. Brit. J. Surg. *25:*131-132, July '37

Endotracheal anesthesia for babies with cleft palate. AYRE, P. Anesth. & Analg. *16:*330-333, Nov-Dec '37

Cleft Palate Operations, Anesthesia for—Cont.

Protection of surgeon against anesthetic gases while performing plastic surgery on cleft palate. REBELO NETO, J. Arq. de cir. clin. e exper. *6:*641-645, April-June '42

Vinesthene (vinyl ether) anesthesia for repair of harelip and cleft palate. DAPLYN, P. F. L. Brit. M. J. *2:*117-119, July 27, '46

Anesthesia during surgical therapy of cleft palate. LOMBARD, P. Presse med. *54:*566, Aug. 31, '46

Cleft Palate Orthodontia

Surgical correction of maxillary and palatal defects in cooperation with orthodontist and prosthodontist. VAUGHAN, H. S. Dental Cosmos *69:*63-67, Jan '27

Orthodontia and its uses in preliminary treatment of extreme cases of harelip and cleft palate. MILLARD, J., J. Internat. Orthodont. Cong. *1:*493-496, '27 also: Internat. J. Orthodontia *13:*621-624, July '27

Congenital cleft lip and palate; embryology of upper jaw interpreted in terms of surgical repair of process and palate of clefts. RITCHIE, H. P. Tr. Am. S. A. *45:*170-178, '27

Orthodontic treatment and result of case of malocclusion of teeth brought by conditions associated with congenital cleft palate and harelip; case. HELLMAN, M. Internat. J. Orthodontia *15:*135-138, Feb '29

Combined orthodontic and prosthetic treatment of cleft palate. LIFTON, J. C. Dental Items Interest *52:*503-513, July '30

Immediate dental treatment of cleft palate babies. WEARN, W. J. Australia J. Dent. *34:*423-435, Dec '30

Role of orthodontia following cleft lip and palate surgery. DAVIS, A. D. Pacific Dent. Gaz. *39:*571-580, Aug '31

Cleft palate and harelip; adolescent case treated orthodontically in conjunction with lip-stretching device and skin grafting of labial sulcus. HARDY, E. A. Internat. J. Orthodontia *20:*750-758, Aug '34

Orthodontic treatment of jaw fractures and cleft palate. CARTWRIGHT, F. S. Internat. J. Orthodontia *23:*159-163, Feb '37

Orthodontics as aid in repairing congenital cleft palate. ABELSON, J. M. Am. J. Orthodontics *25:*154-158, Feb '39

Orthopedic correction of congenital fissures of jaws. PETRIK, L. Ztschr. f. Stomatol. *37:*1235-1252, Sept '39

Orthodontics in treatment of harelip and cleft palate. LIFTON, J. C. Am. J. Orthodontics *27:*423-453, Aug '41

Malnutrition in infants with cleft palate,

Cleft Palate, Pediatric Care

with description of new external obturator. FOOTE, J. A. Am. J. Dis. Child. *30:*343-346, Sept '25

Importance of pediatric care in operative treatment of harelip and cleft palate. HENSKE, J. A. J.A.M.A. *89:*1666-1670, Nov. 12, '27

Cases of cheiloplasty; description of apparatus for feeding infants with harelip and cleft palate. also: rhinoplasty. BRISOTTO, P. Boll. d. mal. d. oreccio, d. gola, d. naso *56:*89-99, March '38

Feeding infant with cleft palate with aid of dental plate; 5 cases. SILLMAN, J. H. Am. J. Dis. Child. *56:*1055-1058, Nov '38

Obturator (acrylic) for newborn infant with cleft palate. SCHAPIRO, I. E.; *et al*. J. Pediat. *27:*288-290, Sept '45

Incidence of supernumerary and congenitally missing lateral incisor teeth in 81 cases of harelip and cleft palate. MILLHON, J. A. AND STAFNE, E. C. Am. J. Orthodontics (Oral Surg. Sect) *27:*599-604, Nov '41

Cleft Palate, Pharyngeal Flap

Schönborn-Rosenthal operation for cleft palate. FRÜND, H. Zentralbl. f. Chir. *54:*3206-3210, Dec. 10, '27

Staphylopharyngoplasty by Rosenthal's method. HARBITZ, H. F. Norsk. Mag. f. Laegevidensk. *90:*13-16, Jan '29

Cleft Palate Pushback: See Cleft Palate Elongation

Cleft Palate, Secondary Operations

Cleft lip and palate; correction of late deformities resulting from neglect or improper treatment. FARR, R. E. Minnesota Med. *8:*561-568, Sept '25

Correction of secondary palate defects. MOOREHEAD, F. B., J.A.M.A. *90:*1614-1615, May 19, '28

Repair of cleft palates after unsuccessful operations, with special reference to cases with extensive loss of palatal tissue. PADGETT, E. C. Internat. J. Orthodontia *16:*1299-1316, Dec '30

Repair of palates primarily unsuccessfully operated upon. PADGETT, E. C. Surg., Gynec. & Obst. *63:*483-496, Oct '36

Secondary deformities in cleft palate patients. KAZANJIAN, V. H. Ann. Surg. *109:*442-467, March '39

Restoration of facial contour in surgery of secondary cleft lip and palate. DAVIS, A. D. AND SELLECK, G. A. Am. J. Surg. *64:*104-114, April '44

Cleft Palate, Social Problems

Surgical therapy of cleft palate from social-medical point of view. PERMAN, E. Svenska lak.-tidning. *35:*2025–2029, Dec. 9, '38

Cleft palate children. BEDER, O. E. Hygeia *24:*834–835, Nov '46

Responsibility of public health agencies in cleft palate. DODDS, P. Am. J. Orthodontics (Oral Surg. Sect.) *32:*665–666, Nov '46

Cleft Palate, Speech

Training the speech after operations for cleft palate. SEEMANN, M. Cas. lek. cesk. *61:*811–815, Sept. 2, '22

Training of speech in children with cleft palate. RUPPE, L. AND RUPPE, C. Arch. de med. d. enf. *26:*19–35, Jan '23 (illus.)

Peripheric expressive or articular speech defects; cleft palate. VAN BAGGEN, N. Y. P. M. J. & Rec. *125:*535–537, April 20, '27

Overcoming Cleft Palate Speech, by Edna H. Young. Hill-Young School, Minneapolis, 1928

Cleft palate and re-education of speech. WARD, W. K. Brit. J. Dent. Sc. *72:*1–4, Jan '28

Phonetic result of surgical treatment of cleft palate; case. VEAU, V. AND BOREL. Bull. et mem. Soc. nat. de chir. *54:*1017, July 14, '28

Re-educating cleft palate speech. WARD, W. K. Practitioner *123:*147–152, Aug '29

Surgical and phonetic results of late operations for cleft palate. HALLE, M. Verhandl. d. Berl. med. Gesellsch. (1928) *59:*267–276, '29

Speech training of children with cleft palate. SCHLEUSS, W. Eos *21:*29–38, '29

Speech training without obturator in children with cleft palate who have not had operations. HELWIG, K. Ztschr. f. Kinderforsch. *36:*178–194, Jan. 18, '30

Speech exercises after cleft palate operation. GUTZMANN, H. Chirurg *2:*1019–1027, Nov. 15, '30

Cleft palate speech. GLASSBURG, J. A. Arch. Otolaryng. *12:*820–821, Dec '30

Surgical therapy of cleft palate must be performed before child begins to talk. ROVIRALTA, E. Ars med., Barcelona *7:*395–398, Dec '31

Phonation after operations for palatal division. VEAU, V. AND BOREL, S. Rev. franc. de pediat. *7:*333–342, '31

Handicap of cleft-palate speech. WOLDSTAD, D. M. Ment. Hyg. *16:*281–288, April '32

Nasal lisping and speech in palatoschisis; palatographic study. GUMPERTZ, F. Wien. med. Wchnschr. *82:*901–903, July 9, '32

Cleft Palate, Speech – Cont.

Perfect phonetic results of uranostaphylorrhaphy (Langenbeck-Trelat method). ROCHER. J. de med. de Bordeaux *109:*402–403, May 20, '32

Study of improvement of speech after operation for cleft hard palate; case. LAMBECK, A. Ztschr. f. Kinderforsch. *42:*369–384, '33

Cleft Palate Speech, by J. H. Van Thal. George Allen & Unwin, Ltd., London, 1934

Phonetic education of patients with palatal fissures. FIORINI, J. M. Semana med. *1:*1985–1997, June 21, '34

Phonetic results in 200 cases of staphylorrhaphy. VEAU, V. Helvet. med. acta *1:*99–103, June '34

Speech training for cleft palate patients. PARSONS, F. Proc. Roy. Soc. Med. *27:*1301–1303, July '34

Palatographic researchers on phonation in cleft palate. RICHERI, S. Arch. ital. di otol. *45:*487–509, July '34

Comment on phonetic education in palatal fissures in article by Fiorini. FIKH, E. Semana med. *2:*735–738, Sept. 6, '34

Value of speech training in cleft palate. SCHARFE, E. E. Tr. Sect. Laryng. Otol. & Rhin., A.M.A., pp. 116–128, '35

Phonation and staphylorraphy. VEAU, V. AND BOREL-MAISONNY, S. Rev. franc. de phoniatrie *4:*133–141, July '36

Speech Training for Cleft Palate Patients, by H. P. Pickerill. Whitcombe & Tombs, Ltd., London, 1937

Treatment of cleft-palate speech. WARD, W. K. South African M. J. *11:*433–435, June 26, '37

Correlation of anatomic and functional results following operation for cleft palate. RITCHIE, W. P. Arch. Surg. *35:*548–570, Sept '37

Phonetic results obtained after cleft palate therapy. BOREL-MAISONNY, Mme. Rev. de stomatol. *39:*733–754, Oct '37

Cleft palate surgery. BLAIR, V. P. J. Speech Disorders *2:*195–198, Dec '37

Speech Training for Cases of Cleft Palate, by Michael C. Oldfield. H. K. Lewis & Co., London, 1938

Pedogogic therapy of speech disturbances in congenital palatoschisis. LIISBERG, H. B. Valsalva *14:*346–351, July '38

Phonetic reeducation for velopalatine division; conditions necessary for improving speech. FROMENT, AND FEYEUX, A. Lyon chir. *36:*201–207, March-April '39

Cleft Palate, Speech—Cont.
Physiopathology of phonetic formation and education of cleft palate patients treated surgically. LIMA, J. Rev. med. Bahia *9:*74-85, March '41
Cleft palate and mechanism of speech. (Arris and Gale lecture). OLDFIELD, M. C. Brit. J. Surg. *29:*197-227, Oct '41
Correction of phonetic disorders in cleft palate lacking timely surgical therapy. ROVIRALTA, E. Rev. clin. espan. *4:*48-49, Jan. 15, '42
Speech re-education following palatal reconstruction. HUBER, M. Canad. M.A.J., *46:*325-326, April '42
Speech function following 300 palate operations. AXHAUSEN, G. Zentralbl. f. Chir. *69:*770, May 9, '42
Speech reeducation in cleft palate. RUMSEY, H. ST. J. Guy's Hosp. Gaz. *58:*6-8, Jan. 8, '44
Cleft Palate and Speech, by Muriel E. Morley. E. & S. Livingstone Ltd., Edinburgh, 1945
Speech training center for cleft palate children. WELLS, C. G. Quart. J. Speech *31:*68-73, Feb '45
Improving speech of cleft palate child. WELLS, C. G. J. Speech Disorders *10:*162-168, June '45
Responsibility of speech correctionist in treatment of patient who has received surgical or prosthetic treatment. KOEPP-BAKER, H. Am. J. Orthodontics (Oral Surg. Sect.) *32:*714-717, Nov '46

Cleft Palate, Submucous
Submucous fissure of palate. SEEMANN, M. Cas. lek. cesk. *62:*641-646, June 16, '23 (illus.) abstr: J.A.M.A. *81:*1734, Nov 17, '23
Submucous bone defect of palate. MÓSCISKER, E. Wien. med. Wchnschr. *78:*961, July 14, '28
Submucous cleft of palate; case. KLESTADT, W. Ztschr. f. Laryng., Rhin. *19:*279-287, May '30
Submucous cleft palate with impairment of hearing; case. SEELER, E. Beitr. z. Anat., Physiol., Path. u. Therap. d. Ohres *28:*427-430, Jan '31
Submucous clefts of palate. SEGRE, R. Monatschr. f. Ohrenh. *67:*649-670, June '33
Submucosal palatoschisis. SEGRE, R. Valsalva *14:*356-363, July '38
Bifid uvula in school children; statistical study. BENVENUTO, E. Valsalva *15:*492-494, Nov '39
Submucous cleft of palate. HAYASHI, Y. Otorhino-laryng. (Abstr. Sect.) *13:*60, Nov '40
Unusual case of submucosal cleft palate in conjunction with deformity of soft palate and nasal speech. ARNOLD, G. E. Arch. f. Ohren-, Nasen-u. Kehlkopfh. *147:*173-176, '40
Submucous cleft palate; traumatic perforation by denture. GINGRASS, R. P. Am. J. Orthodontics (Oral Surg. Sect.) *28:*113-114, Feb '42

Cleft Palate, Traumatic
Traumatic cleft palate; Micrococcus catarrhalis meningitis; recovery. BETT, W. R. Brit. M. J. *1:*494-495, March 21, '31
Question of traumatic cleft palate. AXHAUSEN, G. Deutsche Zahn-, Mund-u. Kieferh. *1:*340-342, '34

Cleft Palate, X-Ray Studies
Functional results of plastic surgery of cleft palate as shown in roentgenograms. VEAU, V. *et al.* Ztschr. f. Stomatol. *35:*597-606, May 14, '37
Roentgenologic studies of closure of oropharynx against nasopharynx and position of tongue during blowing up of cheeks in persons with cleft palate; function tests of soft palate. SEIFERTH, L. B. Klin. Wchnschr. *14:*897-899, June 22, '35

CLEGG, H. W. (see WOLFE, H. R. I.) Feb '42
CLEGG, J. W. AND DIBLE, J. H.: Preparation and use of human serum for blood transfusion. Lancet *2:*294-296, Sept 7, '40
CLEMENT, F. W.: Shock and some associated factors. Anesth. & Analg. *16:*271-274, Sept-Oct '37
CLÉMENT, R. (see LESNÉ, E. *et al*) Dec '28
CLEMENTE, D.: Dermo-epidermal grafts in delayed healing of burn wounds; 2 cases. Policlinico (sez. prat.) *43:*1861-1863, Oct 19, '36
CLEMENTS, H. J.: Are we up to date in our treatment of burns? Northwest. Med. *31:*209-215, May '32
CLEMETSEN, N.: Late rupture of tendon of extensor pollicus longus after fracture of radius; case. Norsk mag. f. laegevidensk. *99:*1322-1328, Dec '38
CLERC, J. P.: Acute postoperative decubitus following gynecologic and obstetric interventions. Monatschr. f. Geburtsh. u. Gynak. *115:*128-137, '43
CLERF, L. H.: Analysis of 58 cases cancer of larynx treated with laryngofissure. Arch. Otolaryng. *19:*653-659, June '34
CLERY, A. B.: Rhinoplastic surgery through ages. Irish J. M. Sc., pp. 170-176, April '32
CLEVELAND, D.: Facial paralysis treatment; collective review from 1932 to 1938. Internat. Abstr. Surg. *69:*545-555, '39; in Surg., Gynec.

& Obst. Dec '39
CLEVELAND, D. (see DAVIS, L.) June '36
CLEVELAND, D. A. (see DAVIS, L.) Feb '34
CLEVELAND, H. E.: Repair of tendons of hand. Journal-Lancet *59:*524-525, Dec '39
CLEVELAND, M.: Suppurative tenosynovitis of flexor muscles of hand. Arch. Surg. *7:*661-686, Nov '23 (illus.)
CLEVELAND, M.: Restoration of digital portion of flexor tendon and sheath. J. Bone & Joint Surg. *15:*762-765, July '33
CLEVELAND, M.: Medical progress; saving injured hand. New York Med. (no. 17) *2:*19-22, Sept 5, '46
CLEWER, D.: Injuries to jaws and face; outline of treatment. J. Roy. Army M. Corps *48:*286-295, April '27
CLIMO, S.: Plasma, nutrient dusting powder used to nullify rubber cement used in connection with Padgett dermatome. U. S. Nav. M. Bull. *46:*1291-1296, Aug '46
CLOCK, R. O. (see MONTEITH, S. R.)

Cloquet Operation

Cleft-thumb operated on by Cloquet's method. VAN NECK, M. Arch. franco-belges de chir. *28:*607-608, July '25
Surface treatment of burns; comparison of results of tannic acid, silver nitrate, triple dye, and vaseline or boric ointment as surface treatments in 150 cases. CLOWES, G. H. A. JR.; LUND, C. C. AND LEVENSON, S. M. Ann. Surg., *118:*761-779, Nov '43

Club Hand

A case of clubhand. MOURAD, A. Lancet *2:*1222, Dec 9, '22 (illus.)
Rare type of congenital club hand. JONES, H. W. AND ROBERTS, R. E. J. Anat. *60:*146-147, Jan '26
Case of club-hand associated with congenital syphilis. SCHWARZ, E. G. South. M. J. *19:*105-106, Feb '26
Congenital club hand with subluxation of phalanges; case. GRUCA, A. Rev. d'orthop. *14:*407-412, Sept '27
Congenital bilateral club hand with absence of thumbs; case. PETRIDIS, P. A. Rev. d'orthop., *14:*419-421, Sept '27
Friedreich's disease with club-hand in hereditary syphilitic; case. ROGER, H. *et al.* Gaz. d. hop. *101:*501-504, April 4, '28
Talipomanus (congenital club hand). ELTERICH, T. O. Atlantic M. J. *31:*953-954, Sept '28
Transmission for several generations of double pure cubital club-hand. BUIZARD, C. Bull. et mem. Soc. de chir. de Paris *20:*711-714, Nov 2, '28

Club Hand—Cont.

Club hands; case. MUKHERJI, M. Brit. J. Radiol *4:*507-508, Oct '31
Congenital absence of radius and club hand; case. GRANT, D. N. W. Mil. Surgeon *69:*518-521, Nov '31
Surgical treatment of acquired club-hand. RESCHKE, K. Deutsche Ztschr. f. Chir. *232:*458-462, '31
Deformed fetus complicating clubhands and microtia. FUKE, T. Jap. J. Obst. & Gynec. *15:*255-258, June '32
Congenital bilateral clubhand; roentgen study of case. GRIZAUD, H. J. de radiol. et d'electrol. *16:*515-516, Oct '32
Bilateral congenital radial clubhand complicated in one case by luxation of elbow, in other by luxation of shoulder. ROCHER, H. L. AND ROCHER, C., J. de med. de Bordeaux *112:*880-882, Nov 30, '35
Syndrome characterized by bilateral clubfoot and clubhand associated with special type of amyotrophy of upper and lower extremities, dating from birth; case. THOMAS, A. AND HUC, G. Rev. neurol. *64:*918-925, Dec '35
Clubhand resulting from congenital absence of radius; 3 cases. DRINNENBERG, A. Ztschr. f. orthop. Chir., *63:*297-307, '35
Case of congenital clubhand (and absence of radius) with review of etiology of condition. FORBES, G. Anat. Rec. *71:*181-199, June 25, '38
Surgical therapy of clubhand due to spastic paralysis of cerebral origin; cases. SATANOWSKY, S. Rev. ortop. y traumatol. *9:*19-25, July '39
Congenital club-hand deformity associated with absence of radius; surgical correction; case. DAVIDSON, A. J. AND HORWITZ, M. T. J. Bone & Joint Surg. *21:*462-463, April '39
Question of physical deformities, especially clubhand; special case of amniotic stricture. ROSGEN AND MAMIER. Ztschr. f. Orthop. *74:*45-52, '42
Clubhand due to partial absence of ulna; case. BOSCH OLIVES, V. Cir. d. ap. locom. *2:*284-287, July '45

CLUTE, H. M.: Kondoleon operation for elephantiasis. S. Clin. N. Amer. *8:*119-122. Feb '28
CLUTE, H. M. (see LEECH, J. V. *et al*) Sept '28
COAKLEY, W. A.: Burns, discussion on their treatment, both immediate and remote, with special emphasis on prevention of scars and contractures. Am. J. Surg. *36:*50-53, April '37
COAKLEY, W. A.: Care and treatment of burns. M. Times, New York *70:*267-273, Aug '42

Coakley, W. A. and Baker, J. M.: Analysis of 212 cases of fractured jaw. Am. J. Surg. *65:*244-247, Aug '44

Coakley, W. A. and White, M. F.: Report of 72 consecutive cases of zygoma fractures. Surg., Gynec. & Obst. *77:*360-366, Oct '43

Coan, G. L.: Ferric chloride coagulation in burns, with resume of tannic acid treatment. Surg., Gynec. & Obst. *61:*687-692, Nov '35

Coate, J. D.: Congenital gigantism of hand. Radiog. & Clin. Photog. *11:*16-17, April '35

Coates, G. M.: Problem of rhinoplastic surgery. Tr. Am. Acad. Ophth. *51:*11-17, Sep-Oct '46

Cobb, S. A.: Traumatic surgery of hand. Maine M. J. *26:*33-36, March '35

Cobey, M. C.; Hansen, H. C. and Morris, M. H.: Use of skeletal traction in hand fractures. Army M. Bull. (no. 68) pp. 135-141, July '43

Cobey, M. C.; Hansen, H. C. and Morris, M. H.: Use of skeletal traction in hand. South. M. J. *37:*309-313, June '44

Cockayne, E. A.: Hypertelorism. Brit. J. Child. Dis. *22:*265-274, Oct-Dec '25

Cockayne, E. A.: Unusual form of brachyphalangy and syndactylia, with double proximal phalanx in middle fingers. J. Anat. *67:*165-167, Oct '32

Cockburn, C.: Operation for entropian of trachoma. Brit. J. Ophth. *27:*308-310, July '43

Codazzi Aguirre, J. A.: Esthetic surgery and its development. Semana med. *1:*1245-1248, April 25, '35

Codazzi Aguirre, J. A.: Cheiloplasty in plastic repair of harelip; author's technic. Rev. med. del Rosario *25:*953-965, Aug '35

Codazzi Aguirre, J. A.: Use of medicated gauze dressing (tulle gras) in plastic and esthetic surgery. Rev. med. del Rosario *25:*441-446, April '35

Codazzi Aguirre, J. A.: Progress of plastic and esthetic surgery in Buenos Aires. Semana med. *1:*464-467, Feb 6, '36

Codazzi Aguirre, J. A.: Extreme hypertrophy of nasal pyramid (exclusively osseous); plastic surgery of case. Rev. med. del Rosario *26:*654-660, July '36

Codazzi Aguirre, J. A.: Importance of plastic surgery for relieving mental condition of deformed individuals (psychocosmeticopathy). Semana med. *1:*675-680, March 4, '37

Codazzi Aguirre, J. A.: Cheilorthocaliplasty (esthetic surgery of mouth). Rev. med. del Rosario *27:*1111-1131, Nov '37

Codazzi Aguirre, J. A.: Tubular graft (Gillies-Filatov Anglo-Russian graft) in repair of facial defects; cases. Rev. med. de Rosario *30:*208-218, Feb '40

Codazzi Aguirre, J. A.: Esthetic results of grafts of Anglo-Russian type in facial burn; case. Semana med. *1:*651-655, March 14, '40

Codazzi Aguirre, J. A.: Harmful effects of malformed ears in school; plastic surgery of protruding ears. Semana med. *1:*456-462, Feb 20, '41

Codazzi Aguirre, J. A.: Mastortocaliplasty in hypertrophic ptosis of breasts. Rev. med. de Rosario *31:*564-572, June '41

Codazzi Aguirre, J. A.: Esthetic surgery for hypertrophy of breast. Rev. Med. de Rosario *32:*163-167, March '42

Codazzi Aguirre, J. A.: References to esthetic surgery in work of Hippocrates. Arq. de cir. clin. e exper. *6:*137-144, April-June '42

Codazzi Aguirre, J. A.: Nasal defects in students; psychologic aspects and plastic correction. Arq. de cir. clin. e exper. *6:*194-197, April-June '42

Codazzi Aguirre, J. A.: Esthetic breast surgery. Arq. de cir. clin. e exper., *6:*595-597, April-June '42

Codazzi Aguirre, J. A.: Nasal deformities in students; psychologic aspects and plastic correction. Semana med. *1:*981-988, May 14, '42

Codazzi Aguirre, J. A.: References to nasal and auricular esthetic surgery in work of Hippocrates. Semana med. *1:*445-449, Feb 25, '43

Coe, H. E.: Certain non-technical considerations in treatment of harelip and cleft palate. Arch. Pediat., *38:*658, Oct '21

Coe, H. E.: Congenital deformities of ear. Northwest Med. *38:*135-136, April '39

Coe, H. E.: Use of stainless steel wire in operation for hypospadias. Urol. & Cutan. Rev. *45:*297-298, May '41

Coe, H. E.: Correction of lop ears. Northwest Med. *41:*126, April '42

Coelst, M.: Cosmetic surgery of pendulous humped nose. Brux.-med. *7:*530-532, Feb 20, '27

Coelst, M.: Plastic surgery of nasal fractures. Rev. de chir. plastique, pp. 54-68, April '32

Coelst, M.: Possibility of reconstructing whole face by full thickness, free cutaneous grafts, using several flaps. Rev. de chir. structive, pp. 105-125, Dec '35

Coelst, M.: Further application of author's method of outlay on celluloid frame. (facial surgery). Rev. de chir. structive, pp. 195-198, March '36

Coelst, M.: Surgical therapy of fissures of palate inoperable by classic methods. Bull. Soc. belge d'otol., rhinol., laryng., pp. 377-380, '37

Coelst, M.: Method of free whole thickness skin graft. Rev. de chir. structive, pp. 253-

258, Dec '37

COELST, M.: Use of celluloid in facial surgery. Rev. de chir. structive. *8:*161–162, '38

COELST, M.: Use of full thickness free grafts in surgical therapy of microtia; case. Rev. de chir. structive. *8:*155–159, '38

COELST, M.: Fractures of nose and their otorhinolaryngologic complications. Bull. Soc. belge d'oto., rhinol., laryng., pp. 69–71, '38

COELST, M.: Use of celluloid to cover operations for harelip. Rev. de chir. structive *8:*99–101, Aug '38

COELST, M.: Plastic surgery in complete loss of lobules and subpartition of nose; case. Rev. de chir. structive. *8:*103–105, Aug '38

COELST, M.: Plastic surgery in therapy of postoperative facial paralysis; case. Rev. de chir. structive. *8:*107–109, Aug '38

COELST, M.: Free full thickness graft in restoration of loss of substance of auricle; case. Rev. de chir. structive *8:*111–112, Aug '38

COELST, M.: Repair of permanent cavity behind left ear, following petromastoid evident; excision of concha of ear; case. Rev. de chir. structive. *8:*113–115, Aug '38

COELST, M.: Construction of the amputated shoulder in order to fit a prosthesis with a mechanical arm. Rev. de chir. structive. *8:*117–122, Aug '38

COELST, M.: Cutaneous full thickness graft in therapy of cicatrix due to burn of elbow fold; case. Rev. de chir. structive. *8:*124–126, Aug '38

COELST, M.: Permanent fistula of floor of mouth; case. Rev. de chir. structive. *8:*128–130, Aug '38

COELST, M.: Nasal surgery in women. Bull. Soc. belge d'otol., rhinol., laryng., pp. 316–318, '39

COELST, M.: Use of medicated paper dressing in facial surgery. Bull. Soc. belge d'otol., rhinol. laryng., pp. 319–320, '39

COELST, M.: Modern surgical therapy of total loss of nose. Bull. Soc. belge d'otol., rhinol., laryng., pp. 103–106, '40

COENEN, H.: Cause of rupture of extensor pollicis longus tendon in typical fracture of radius. Arch. f. Orthop. *28:*193–206, May 6, '30

COENEN, H.: Use of silk in plastic construction of tendons of fingers. Deutsche Ztschr. f. Chir. *234:*699–709, '31

COENEN, H.: Hereditary aspect of harelip and cleft palate. Chirurg, *3:*501–505, June 1, '31

COENEN, H.: Dupuytren's contracture of finger. Med. Klin. *31:*1657–1661, Dec 20, '35

COFFEY, R. C.: Transplantation of ureters into large intestine by submucous implantation; clinical application of technic 3 in exstrophy of bladder. J.A.M.A. *99:*1320–1323, Oct 15, '32

COFFEY, R. C.: Further studies and experiences with transfixion suture technic (technic 3) for transplantation of ureters into large intestine. Northwest Med. *32:*31–34, Jan '33

Coffey's Operation

- Ureterorectomneostomy by transfixion suture method in exstrophy of bladder, Coffey's technic 3. HELPER, A. B., S. Clin. North America *13:*1387–1391, Dec '33
- Exstrophy of bladder treated by transfixion suture of ureters into large intestine (Coffey operation) in new-born infant. BENGOLEA, A. J. Bol. y trab. de la Soc. de cir. de Buenos Aires *17:*894–896, Sept 13, '33
- Exstrophy of bladder, surgical therapy by Coffey operation; 2 cases. DERMAN, I. A. Ztschr. f. Urol. *29:*856–859, '35
- Exstrophy of bladder with hydronephrosis and hydroureter on one side; surgical therapy by Coffey-Mayo operation. BERGENFELDT, E. Ztschr. f. urol. Chir. *41:*515–521, '36
- Exstrophy of bladder, transplantation of ureters into intestine (Coffey operation). HELLSTRÖM, J. Ztschr. f. urol. Chir. *41:*522–528, '36
- Coffey operation for exstrophy of bladder; cases. FEVRE, M. Mem. Acad. de chir. *64:*1114–1123, Oct 26, '38
- Coffey operation in exstrophy of bladder; case. YOVTCHITCH, J. Mem. Acad. de chir. *65:*368–369, March 8, '39
- Exstrophy of bladder, Coffey-Mayo operations and their results. MATTOS, S. O. Rev. de obst. e ginec. de Sao Paulo *4:*107–126, Oct–Dec '39
- Coffey operation in exstrophy of bladder. GÜRSEL, A. E. Turk tib cem. mec. *5:*90–91, '39
- Coffey method of ureteral implantation in exstrophy of bladder. HAGENBACH, E. Helvet. med. acta *10:*321–324, June '43
- Surgical therapy of exstrophy of bladder, with special reference to Maydl and Coffey operations. TILK, G. U. Deutsche Ztschr. f. Chir. *257:*287, '43

COFFIN, F.: Use of acrylic resin for prostheses of face. Brit. Dent. J. *77:*36–39, July 21, '44

COGNIAUX, P.: Extensive resection and graft in therapy of recidivating radioresistant tumors. J. de chir. et ann. Soc. belge de chir. *37–35:*270–275, Oct '38

COGNIAUX, P.: Parotidectomy with conservation of superior facial nerve (Duval operation); 2 cases. J. de chir. et ann. Soc. belge de chir. *38-36:*370-372, Dec '39

COGNIAUX, P. AND MARIQUE, P.: Conservative therapy in crushing of thumb and index finger; late result. Scalpel (86):995-996, July 1, '33

COGNIAUX, P. AND SIMON, S.: Modern trends in therapy of parotid tumors. J. de chir. et ann. Soc. belge de chir. (no. 4) *36-34:*152-163, May '37

COGSWELL, H. D. AND SHIRLEY, C.: Burn therapy. Am. J. Surg. *45:*539-545, Sept '39

COGSWELL, H. D. AND TRUSLER, H. M.: Modified Agnew operation for syndactylism. Surg., Gynec. & Obst. *64:*793, April '37

COGSWELL, H. D. (see TRUSLER, H. M.) June '35

COGSWELL, W. W.: Problems involving mandibular nerve (paresthesia of lip). J. Am. Dent. A. *29:*964-969, June 1, '42

COHEN, H. H.: Adjustable volar-flexion splint. J. Bone & Joint Surg. *24:*189-192, Jan '42

COHEN, L.: Management of recent fractures of nose. Ann. Otol. Rhinol. & Laryng. *30:*690, Sept '21

COHEN, L.: Corrective rhinoplasty, some anatomicosurgical considerations. Surg., Gynec. & Obst. *34:*794-799, June '22 (illus.)

COHEN, L.: Corrective rhinoplasty, some reasons for faulty results. Tr. Sect. Laryng., Otol. & Rhin., A.M.A., pp. 122-133, '23 (illus.)

COHEN, L.: Immediate and late treatment of nasal fractures. Laryngoscope *33:*847-853, Nov '23 (illus.)

COHEN, L.: Corrective rhinoplasty; some reasons for faulty results. Ann. Otol. Rhin. & Laryng. *33:*342-350, June '24

COHEN, L.: Correction of pronounced types of saddle nose with mixed implants of bone and cartilage. Tr. Am. Laryng., Rhin. & Otol. Soc. *33:*233-242, '27

COHEN, L.: Correction of pronounced types of saddle nose with mixed implants of bone and cartilage. Ann. Otol. Rhin. & Laryng. *36:*639-647, Sept '27

COHEN, L.: Results obtained in corrective rhinoplasty. M. J. & Rec. *127:*354-357, April 4, '28

COHEN, L.: Recent results in rhinoplasty. Virginia M. Monthly *55:*781-788, Feb '29

COHEN, L.: External nasal deformities corrected and removal of existing intranasal obstruction advantageously accomplished at same operation. Ann. Otol., Rhin. & Laryng. *44:*233-241, March '35

COHEN, L.: Correction of depressed deformities of external nose with rib graft. South. M. J. *30:*680-685, July '37

COHEN, L.: Advantage of mixed bone and cartilage grafts in correction of saddle nose and other depressed deformities of dorsum. Tr. Am. Laryng., Rhin. & Otol. Soc. *46:*370-376, '40

COHEN, L.: Advantage of mixed bone and cartilage grafts in correction of saddle nose and other depressed deformities of dorsum. Ann. Otol., Rhin. & Laryng. *49:*410-417, June '40

COHEN, L. AND FOX, S. L.: Atresia of auditory canal. Arch. Otolaryng. *38:*338-346, Oct '43

COHEN, M. A. AND FELDMAN, L.: Rational treatment of Bell's palsy. Am. J. Phys. Therapy *4:*59-61, May '27

COHEN, M. M.: Fissural cysts of median palatine suture. Am. J. Orthodontics (Oral Surg. Sect.) *29:*442-451, Aug '43

COHEN, S.: Lower nasal deflection; new operation for its correction. Arch. Otolaryng. *8:*399-404, Oct '28

COHEN, S.: Plastic surgery of nose. Pennsylvania M. J. *33:*50-52, Nov '29

COHEN, S.: Plastic surgery of nose. Eye, Ear, Nose & Throat Monthly *10:*493-498, Jan '32

COHEN, S.: Plastic surgery of nasal deformities. M. Rec. *140:*536-539, Nov 21, '34

COHEN, S.: Correction of displaced nasal cartilage, especially in children. Pennsylvania M. J. *40:*925-930, Aug '37

COHEN, S.: New approach for nasal implants. Ann. Otol., Rhin. & Laryng. *47:*1101-1106, Dec '38

COHEN, S.: Role of septum in surgery of nasal contour. Arch. Otolaryng. *30:*12-20, July '39

COHEN, S.: Plastic surgery of nose. Laryngoscope *51:*363-377, April '41

COHEN, S.: Complications of plastic surgery of nasal septum. Dis. Eye, Ear, Nose & Throat *2:*235-243, Aug '42

COHEN, S.: Planning rhinoplasty. Arch. Otolaryng. *43:*283-922, Mar '46

COHEN, S. M.: Experience in treatment of war burns. Brit. M. J. *2:*251-254, Aug. 24, '40

COHEN, S. M.: Tannic acid versus saline in burns. Brit. M. J. *2:*754-755, Nov 30, '40

COHEN, T. M. (see ROGERS, W. L. *et al*) May '44

COHN, I.: Plastic surgery in industry. (industrial surgery) New Orleans M. & S. J. *83:*623-631, March '31

COHN, I.: Incised wound of palm; severance of median nerve; immediate nerve suture. Internat. Clin. *2:*104-106, June '31

COHN, I.: Burns, unsolved problem. New Orleans M. & S. J. *91:*465-474, March '39

COHN, M.: Late results of tendon transplantation. Deutsche Ztschr. f. Chir. *230:*220-238, '31

COHN, R.: Hand infections following human

bites. Surgery *7:*546–554, April '40
COHN, R. D.: Few notes on Halle's Clinic; with special reference to his endonasal surgery. California State J. Med. *22:*6–8, Jan '24
COIMBRA, A.: Tenosynovitis; cases. Arq. de cir. e ortop. *2:*159–168, Dec '34
COKKALIS, P.: Dupuytren's contracture of palmar and plantar aponeurosis. Deutsche Ztschr. f. Chir. *194:*256–258, '26
COLBY, F. AND BARR, H. B.: Vincent's disease following bite of hand. Texas State J. Med. *28:*467–470, Nov '32
COLBY, F. H.: Exstrophy of bladder; case. Boston M. & S. J. *196:*1033–1036, June 23, '27
COLDREY, R. S.: Treatment of rhinophyma. Brit. M. J. *2:*518, Sept. 27, '30
COLDWATER, K. B. (see CONWAY, H.) April '46
COLE, H. N. AND SROUB, W. E.: Glomus tumor: arterial angioneuromyoma of Masson. J.A.M.A. *107:*428–429, Aug. 8, '36
COLE, P.: Late results of pedicle bone-graft for fractured mandible; 3 cases. Proc. Roy. Soc. Med. *31:*1131–1134, July '38
COLE, P. P.: Extended use of whole thickness skin graft. Practitioner *116:*311–313, April '26
COLE, P. P.: Circumferential wiring in fractures of mandible. Lancet *1:*749–750, April 8, '33
COLE, P. P.: Pathologic fracture of mandible; nonunion treated with pedicled bone graft. Lancet *1:*1044–1045, June 8, '40
COLE, P. P.: War injuries of jaws and face. Post-Grad. M. J. *16:*233–244, July '40
COLE, P. P.: Reparative surgery of upper limb (in contractures of hands or arms). Brit. J. Surg. *28:*585–607, April '41
COLE, P. P.; BUBB, C. H. AND ROWBOTHAM, S. E.: Fractures of mandible. Practitioner *124:*489–505, May '30
COLE, P. P. AND LEDERMAN, M.: Glycerin-gelatin base for irradiation dermatitis and burns. Lancet *2:*329, Sept. 13, '41
COLE, T. C.: Tendon repair. U. S. Nav. M. Bull. *43:*241–244, Aug '44
COLE, W. H.: Hand injuries and wrist. Minnesota Med. *20:*727–730, Nov '37
COLE, W. H.: Clinical considerations of surgical shock. Illinois M. J. *83:*162–165, March '43
COLE, W. H. AND GREELEY, P. W.: Utilization of pedicle skin grafts in correction of cicatrical stenosis of anus. Surgery *12:*349–354, Sept '42
COLE, W. H. (see HELFRICH, L. S. *et al*) Feb '42
COLEBROOK, L.; GIBSON, T. AND TODD, J. P.: First aid treatment of burns and scalds. Brit. J. Indust. Med. *1:*99–105, April '44
COLEMAN, C. C.: Surgical treatment of facial paralysis. Virginia M. Monthly *49:*180–188, July '22 (illus.)
COLEMAN, C. C.: Correction of facial defects with special reference to nutrition of skin flaps and planning of repair. Virginia M. Monthly *49:*301–306, Sept '22 (illus.)
COLEMAN, C. C.: Treatment of unilateral harelip with special reference to associated deformity of nose. Virginia M. Monthly *51:*393–399, Oct '24
COLEMAN, C. C.: Fracture of skull involving paranasal sinuses and mastoids. Tr. Sect. Laryng., Otol. & Rhin., A. M. A., pp. 58–67, '37
COLEMAN, C. C.: Surgical treatment of facial spasm. Ann. Surg. *105:*647–657, May '37
COLEMAN, C. C.: Fracture of skull involving paranasal sinuses. J.A.M.A. *109:*1613–1616, Nov. 13, '37
COLEMAN, C. C.: Results of facio-hypoglossal anastomosis in treatment of facial paralysis. Ann. Surg. *111:*958–970, June '40
COLEMAN, C. C.: Surgical lesions of facial nerve, with comments on anatomy. Tr. South SA (1943) *55:*318–332, '44
COLEMAN, C. C.: Peripheral nerve injuries; surgical treatment. Surg., Gynec. & Obst. *78:*113–124, Feb '44 abstr: Tr. Am. Neurol. A. *69:*51–55, '43
COLEMAN, C. C.: Surgical lesions of facial nerve, with comments on anatomy. Ann. Surg. *119:*641–655, May '44
COLEMAN, E. P.: Method of repair of scalp defects (grafts). Illinois M. J. *49:*40–43, Jan '26
COLEMAN, F.: Fractures of mandible; sign of and method of treatment. Proc. Roy. Soc. Med. *34:*212–214, Feb '41
COLEMAN, H. A.: Coexistence of congenital amputations and syndactylism. J.A.M.A. *83:*1164–1165, Oct. 11, '24
COLEMAN, H. M. *et al:* Cancellous grafts for infected bone defects; single stage procedure. Surg. Gynec. & Obst. *83:*392–398, Sept. '46
COLETTI, C. J. (see LAPIDUS, P. W. *et al*) Aug '43
COLGIN, I. E.: Burn therapy. Texas State J. Med. *21:*668–670, March '26
COLIN, (see DELORD, E. *et al*) Dec '34
COLL, J. J. (see WELLS, D. B.) April '42
COLLEDGE, L.: Unusual complication (suppuration of sternoclavicular joint) following laryngectomy. J. Laryng. & Otol. *43:*661–663, Sept '28
COLLEDGE, L.: Repair of defects after operation on pharynx for removal of malignant tumours. Proc. Roy. Soc. Med. (Sect. Laryng.) *24:*14–17, Feb '31
COLLEDGE, L.: Cancer of pharynx, treatment and its results. Brit. M. J. *2:*167–168, July 23, '38
COLLEDGE, L. (see BALLANCE, C. *et al*) Jan '26

COLLER, F. A.: Use of paraffin as primary dressing for skin grafts. Surg., Gynec. & Obst. *41:*221-225, Aug '25

COLLER, F. A. AND YGLESIAS, L.: Infections of lip and face. Surg., Gynec. & Obst. *60:*277-290, Feb. (no. 2A) '35

COLLER, F. A. (see LANGE, H. J. *et al*) May '46

COLLIER, D. J. *et al:* Discussion on limitations of operative treatment in traumatic facial paralysis. Proc. Roy. Soc. Med. *34:*575-584, July '41 also: J. Laryng. & Otol. *56:*207-222, June '41

COLLIER, J.: Facial paralysis and its operative treatment (Hunterian lecture abridged). Lancet *2:*91-94, July 27, '40

COLLINGS, G. H. Jr.: Local therapy for industrial burns; series of 96 cases ($1^1/_2$ per cent sulfadiazine in ethanolamines with methyl cellulose as treatment of choice). Indust. Med. *12:*301-303, May '43

COLLIN, E.: Radium therapy of cancer of lips, with study of metastasis into regional lymph nodes. Acta radiol. *13:*232-237, '32

COLLINS, C. G.: Cotton sutures in vaginal plastic operations about bladder and urethra. S. Clin. North America *26:*1221-1229, Oct. '46

COLLINS, E. G.: Ear wounds and injuries among battle casualties of Western Desert. J. Laryng. & Otol. *59:*1-15, Jan '44

COLLINS, J. (see MILLER, N. F. *et al*) Dec '45

COLLINS, J. L. (see WHITE, C. S. *et al*) Jan '41

COLLINS, J. L. (see WHITE, C. S. *et al*) May '41

COLLINS, J. L. (see WHITE, C. S. *et al*) Dec '41

COLMEIRO LAFORET, C.: Vaginal aplasia; modern trends in therapy. Rev. med. cubana *50:*423-427, May '39

COLOMBINO, C. AND SANVENERO ROSSELLI, G.: Construction of artificial vagina by Kirschner-Wagner operation. Atti Soc. ital. di ostet. e ginec., *35:*460-464, Sept-Oct '39

COLOMBINO, S.: Transplantation of ureter to rectum in exstrophy of bladder. Boll. e mem. Soc. piemontese di chir. *5:*333-341, '35

COLONNA, P. C.: Tendon sheath infections. Am. J. Surg. *50:*509-511, Dec '40

COLONNA, P. C.: Role of surgery in chronic arthritic patient (Nathan Lewis Hatfield lecture). Clinics *2:*955-965, Dec '43

COLONNA, P. C.: Method for fusion of wrist. South. M. J. *37:*195-199, April '44

COLOVIRAS, G. J. Jr.; WEST, W. T. AND ARMOUR, J. C.: Local burn treatment with sulfadiazine (sulfanilamide derivative) spray. Canad. M. A. J. *47:*505-514, Dec '42

COLP, R.: Use of pedicle grafts in traumatic surgery. Internat. Clin. *1:*189-206, March '28

COLP, R. (see KLINGENSTEIN, P.) Dec '25

COLQUHOUN, K. G.: Note of caution on use of picric acid solution as burn dressing. M. J. Australia *2:*652, Nov. 24, '28

COLRAT, A.: Congenital fistula of lacrimal sac. Bull. Soc. d'opht. de Paris. pp. 60-62, Jan '33

COLSON, C. R. (see BERARD, L. *et al*) May-June '38

COLT, G. H.: Surgical treatment of "de-gloved" hand. Brit. J. Surg. *14:*560-568, April '27

COLVER, B. N.: Congenital choanal atresia; 2 cases of complete bilateral obstruction. Ann. Otol., Rhin., and Laryng. *46:*358-375, June '37

COLYER, S.: Chronic deep infection of jaws. Lancet *1:*175-176, Jan. 28, '22

COMBAULT, A.: Tendon transplantation for radial paralysis. Clinique, Paris *21:*315-320, Nov '26

COMBECHER, W.: Septal hematomas and their complications. Ztschr. f. Laryng., Rhin., Otol. *26:*156-171, '35

COMBEMALE, P.: Good effects of vitamin A on burn cicatrization. Echo med. du Nord *11:*53-57, March '40

COMBIER, V. AND MURARD, J.: Habitual jaw dislocation cured by excision of meniscus; case. Bull. et mem. Soc. nat. de chir. *53:*1271, Nov. 26, '27

COMBY, J.: Hypertelorism. Arch. de med. d. enf. *28:*570-573, Sept '25

COMEL, M.: Eudermic grafts in plastic surgery. Plast. chir. *1:*78-88, '39

COMER, M. C.: Persistent or patent thymic duct. Southwestern Med. *11:*308-309, July '27

COMOLLI, A.: Neurotization of muscular tissues transplanted into striated muscles. Arch. ed atti d. Soc. ital. di chir. *36:*967, '30

COMOLLI, A.: Attachment of autoplastic grafts of striated muscles in relation to their nervous connections. Chir. d. org. di movimento *16:*51-180, June '31

COMORA, H. C.: Rhinoplasty. Laryngoscope *49:*484-488, June '39

COMPERE, E. L.: Bilateral snapping thumbs. Ann. Surg. *97:*773-777, May '33

COMPERE, E. L.: Massive graft in repair of defects in long bones. S. Clin. North America *13:*1261-1273, Oct '33

COMPERE, E. L.: Tendon transplantation. Physiotherapy Rev. *20:*131-133, May-June '40

Composite Flaps

Transplantation of pedicled cartilaginous symphysis. RESCHKE, K. Beitr. z. klin. Chir. *146:*713-720, '29

Plastic closure of laryngostomic fistulas and enlargement of lumen of trachea or larynx by implantation of chondrocutaneous flap.

Composite Flaps – Cont.

BABCOCK, W. W. Arch. Otolaryng. *19:*585–589, May '34

New free graft (of skin and ear cartilage) applied to reconstruction of nostril. GILLIES, H. Brit. J. Surg. *30:*305–307, April '43

Tarsoconjunctival sliding-graft technics for reconstruction of eyelids. SUGAR, H. S. Am. J. Ophth. *27:*109–123, Feb '44

Simultaneous osteocutaneous graft in reconstruction of thumb. LABOK, D. M. Khirurgiya, no. 2, pp. 73–75, '44

Composite Grafts

One-stage plastic reconstruction of upper eyelid together with muscle fibers and eyelashes. KAZ, R. Zentralbl. f. Chir. *48:*1239, Aug 27, '21

Formation of new upper eyelid from auricle. ROCHAT, G. F. Nederl. Tijdschr. v. Geneesk. *2:*709, Aug 6, '27

Restoration of completely destroyed eyelid by cutaneous and tarso-conjunctival grafts from other lid; 3 cases. DUPUY-DUTEMPS, L. Ann. d'ocul. *164:*915–926, Dec '27

Transplantation of fleshy tip of toe to tip of nose. KURTZAHN, H. Deutsche Ztschr. f. Chir. *209:*401–402, '28

Margino-tarsal graft in treatment of trichiasis and cicatricial entropion of both eyelids. VITALE, F. Gior. di ocul. *9:*61–65, June '28

Repair of entirely destroyed eyelid by cutaneous and tarso-conjunctival graft taken from other eyelid. DUPUY-DUTEMPS, L. Bull. med., Paris *43:*935–938, Aug 31, '29

Marginotarsal graft in correction of cicatricial entropion of lower eyelid. VITALE, F. Cultura med. mod. *9:*588–592, July 31, '30

Transposition of section from auricle for correction of nasal defect; case. CARTER, W. W. Arch. Otolaryng. *12:*178–183, Aug '30

Autoplastic graft of conjunctiva and of eyelid; 2 cases. DÉJEAN, C. Arch. Soc. d. sc. med. et biol. de Montpellier *12:*23–25, Jan '31

Rhinoplasty with free transplantation from auricle. LIMBERG, A. A. Soviet. khir., no. 9, pp. 70–90, '35

Restoration of partial defect of auricle by free transplantation, ERCZY, M. Gyogyaszat *79:*319–320, May 21, '39

Blepharoplasty with free skin flap from auricle. BULACH, K. Vestnik oftal. (no. 6) *14:*46–48, '39

Use of osteocartilaginous hump of nose for correction of underdeveloped chin. PALACIO POSSE, R. Arq. de cir. clin. e exper. *6:*299–301, April–June '42

Composite Grafts – Cont.

Total graft of nail and of matrix; case. IVANISSEVICH, O. AND RIVAS, C. I. Bol. d. Inst. clin. quir. *18:*640–642, Sept '42

Free transplantation of nipples and areolae in breast hypertrophy. ADAMS, W. M. Surgery *15:*186–195, Jan '44

Twenty-five years' experience with plastic reconstruction of breast and transplantation of nipple. THOREK, M. Am. J. Surg. *67:*445–466, March '45

Composite free grafts of skin and cartilage from ear. BROWN, J. B. AND CANNON, B. Surg. Gynec. and Obst. *82:*253–255, Mar '46

Plastic reconstruction of breast and free transplantation of nipple (author's one-stage operation; microscopic proof of survival of transplanted nipple.) THOREK, M. J. Internat. Coll. Surgeons *9:*194–224, Mar–Apr '46

COMPTON, W. C.: Treatment of acute stage of burns (with alcohol compressed). Cincinnati J. Med. *23:*540–547, Jan '43

COMTOIS, A.; CABANA, E. AND GAUTHIER, F.: Hemangioma of upper lip; case. Ann. med.-chir. de l'Hop. Sainte-Justine, Montreal *3:*80–88, May '41

CONCILIO, L. (see BARMAK, M.) May '40

CONDOLEON, E.: Therapy of elephantiasis. Arch. ital. di chir. *51:*464–469, '38

CONEJO MIR, J.: Plastic induration of penis and Dupuytren's disease with negative Frei reaction; case. Actas dermo-sif. *32:*834–836, June '41

CONGDON, E. D.; ROWHANAVONGSE, S. AND VARAMISARA, P.: Human congenital auricular and juxta-auricular fossae, sinuses and scars (including so-called aural and auricular fistulae) and bearing of their anatomy upon theories of their genesis. Am. J. Anat. *51:*439–463, Nov '32

CONGER, K. B. New method for repair of small defects left following urethroplasty. J. Urol. *47:*689–691, May '42

CONKLIN, F. L.: Burn therapy. Mil. Surgeon *96:*139–142, Feb '45

CONLEY, J. J.: Atresia of external auditory canal occurring in military service; correction of this condition in 10 cases. Arch. Otolaryng. *43:*613–622, June '46

CONLEY, J. J. (see SOMMER, G. N. J. JR. *et al*) Aug '43

CONLEY, J. J. (see STEWART, M. B.) Oct '46

CONN, H. R.: Tenosynovitis. Ohio State M. J. *27:*713–716, Sept '31

CONNELL, J. E. A.: Severe hand infections. Colorado Med. *30:*17–19, Jan '33

CONNELL, J. H.: Modern burn therapy. New Orleans M. and S. J. *88:*575–578, March '36

CONNELL, J. H. *et al:* Gentian violet in burns; preliminary report. J.A.M.A. *100:*1219–1220, April 22, '33

CONNELL, J. H. (see MCFARLAND, O. W.) Jan '41

CONNELLY, J. H. (see MACK, C. H.) Jan '34

CONNER, P. K. (see HEYMAN, J. A.) April '31

CONNER, T.: Osteomyelitis of mandible. J. Am. Dent. A. *22:*1190–1193, July '35

CONNER, W. H.: Osteomyelitis of jaws; cases successfully treated by early radical operation. M. Bull. Vet. Admin. *9:*184–186, Oct '32

CONNOLLY, E. A.: Skin grafting by implantation. Nebraska M. J. *15:*323–324, Aug '30

CONNOR, W. H.: Osteomyelitis of jaws; cases successfully treated by early radical operation. M. Bull. Vet. Admin., *9:*184–186, Oct. '32

CONNOLLY, E. A.: Skin grafting by implantation. Nebraska M. J. *15:*323–324, Aug '30

CONNOLLY, E. A. AND JENSEN, W. P.: Skin defects repaired with grafts. Nebraska M. J. *24:*253–256, July '39

CONNOR, G. J. AND HARVEY, S. C.: Healing of deep thermal burns; preliminary report (on local application of acids, especially pyruvic acid). Tr. Am. S. A. *62:*362–366, '44

CONNOR, G. J. AND HARVEY, S. C.: Healing of deep thermal burns; preliminary report (on local application of acids, especially pyruvic acid). Ann. Surg. *120:*362–366, Sept '44

CONNOR, G. J. AND HARVEY, S. C.: Pyruvic acid method in deep clinical burns. Ann. Surg. *124:*799–810, Nov. '76

CONROY, C. F.: Shock therapy. Wisconsin M. J. *42:*498–500. May '43

CONSTANTINESCO, M. M.; TUCHEL, V. AND BRATU, I.: Single kidney and congenital absence of uterus and vagina; vaginoplasty. Rev. de chir., Bucuresti *43:*713–714, Sept–Oct '40

CONSTANTINESCU, M. AND COVALI, N.: Artificial vagina; plastic surgery according to Baldwin-Mori. Rev. de chir., Bucuresti *43:*296–298, March–April '40

CONSTANTINESCU, M.; TUCHEL, V. AND CORACIU, G.: Congenital bilateral contracture (Dupuytren's); case. Zentralbl. f. Chir. *65:*191–194, Jan. 22, '38

Constantini Operation

Formation of artificial vagina by Baldwin method with Constantini's modification. TICHONOVICH, A. J. Akush. i Zhensk. Boliez. *38:*301–305, May–June '27

CONTIADES, X. J.: Old luxation of fifth finger with double pseudarthrosis. Ann. d'anat. path. *7:*1011–1013, Nov '30

CONTIADES, X. J.: Habitual temporomaxillary luxation; cure of 3 years duration after meniscopexy; case. Mem. Acad. de chir. *62:*18–21, Jan. 15, '36

Contracture

Webbing of left arm. MANSON, J. S. Lancet *1:*1182, June 4, '21

Cicatricial contracture of buttocks nearly occluding anus; plastic operation on buttocks. ASHHURST, A. P. C., S. Clin. N. America *2:*77–79, Feb '22 (illus.)

Treatment of contracture of fingers. CIACCIA, S. Chir. d. org. di movimento *6:*666–684, Nov '22 (illus.) abstr: J.A.M.A. *80:*513, Feb 17, '23

Resection of bone to remedy finger contracture. ECKSTEIN, H. Zentralbl. f. Chir. *49:*547–548, April 22, '22 abstr: J.A.M.A. *79:*598, Aug 12, '22

Plastic operation on contracted finger. RAHM, H. Beitr. z. klin. Chir. *127:*214–217, '22 (illus.) abstr: J.A.M.A. *79:*1726, Nov 11, '22

Cicatricial contractures. VAN NECK, M. Arch. franco-belges de chir. *26:*245–257, March '23 (illus.) abstr: J.A.M.A. *80:*1813, June 16, '23

Operation for relief of flexion-contracture in forearm. PAGE, C. M., J. Bone and Joint Surg. *5:*233–234, April '23

Treatment of weblike dermatogenic contractures of large joints. LOEFFLER, F. Zentralbl. f. Chir. *51:*681–683, March 29, '24

Contractures of thumbs in children. HAUCK, G. Med. Klinik *20:*1465–1466, Oct. 19, '24

Case of contracture of mouth. NARASIMHAN, N. S. Indian M. Gaz. *60:*72, Feb '25

Congenital familial finger contracture and associated familial knee-joint subluxation. MURPHY, D. P., J.A.M.A. *86:*395–397, Feb 6, '26

Flexion contracture of fingers. REICH, W. Zentralbl. f. Chir. *53:*1503–1504, June 12, '26

Flexion contracture of fingers. SEBENING, W. Zentralbl. f. Chir. *53:*2526–2527, Oct. 2, '26

Ischemic contracture; experimental study. JEPSON, P. N. Ann. Surg. *84:*785–795, Dec '26

Contractures in peripheral facial paralysis. LESCHTSCHENKO, G. D. Ztschr. f. d. ges. Neurol. u. Psychiat. *104:*586–595, '26

New plastic operation for chronic cases of contracture of jaws. ROSENTHAL, W.

Contracture – Cont.
Vrtljschr. f. Zahnh. *42:*499-507, '26
Role of capsule in joint contractures; with especial reference to subperiosteal separation. SILVER, D., J. Bone and Joint Surg. *9:*96-105, Jan '27
Orthopedic treatment of hand and finger contractures. Ztschr. f. orthop. Chir. *48:*21-31, Feb. 11, '27
Details in repair of cicatricial contractures of neck. DOWD, C. N. Surg., Gynec. and Obst. *44:*396-399, March '27
Splint for overcoming contractures of fingers. MONTGOMERY, A. H. Surg., Gynec. and Obst. *44:*404-405, March '27
Prevention of contractures following infections of hand. KOCH, S. L., J.A.M.A. *88:*1214-1217, April 16, '27
Therapy of contractures with aid of free full thickness skin-grafts and pedunculated flaps. KOCH, S. L., S. Clin. North America *7:*611-626, June '27
Scar contracture of flexor sublimis digitorum. KOVACS, R. Physical Therap. *45:*383-384, Aug '27
Eyelid surgery for partial contraction of socket. GREEVES, R. A. Tr. Ophth. Soc. U. Kingdom *47:*101-106, '27
Plastic operation for web-like dermatogenous contractures of large joints. ARNOLDS, A. Zentralbl. f. Chir. *55:*838-840, April 7, '28
Surgical treatment of spastic adductor contraction of thumb by dorsal suspension of metacarpus of thumb by fascial sling. HENSCHEN, C. Schweiz. med. Wchnschr. *58:*621-625, June 23, '28
Congenital contractures of fingers and clinodactyly; 4 cases. TOMESKU, I. Arch. f. Orthop. *26:*126-137, '28
Orthopedic treatment of contracture of temporomaxillary joint. KNORR, H. Zentralbl. f. Chir. *56:*1229-1232, May 18, '29
Contracture of right hand treated by full-thickness skin grafts. JONES, H. T., S. Clin. N. Amer. *9:*939-940, Aug '29
Slow screw extension in contractures of fingers. WOLF, J. Monatschr. f. Unfallh. *36:*447-451, Oct '29
Familial symmetrical finger contracture (camptodactylia). HEERUP, L. Ugesk. f. laeger *91:*1072-1075, Nov. 28, '29
Treatment of flexion contracture of knee by means of fascioplasty (fascia lata). CAMITZ, H. Acta chir. Scandinav. *65:*267-282, '29
Treatment of ischemic contracture of wrist. RESCHKE, K. Beitr. z. klin. Chir. *147:*302-307, '29
Surgical and physical therapy of contractures. SAXL, A. Wien. klin. Wchnschr.

Contracture – Cont.
*42:*1266-1267, Sept. 26, '29
Low voltage currents in contractures of hand. GRIES, L. Arch. Physical Therapy *11:*10-13, Jan '30
Surgical treatment and physiotherapy of contractures. SAXL, A. Wien. med. Wchnschr. *80:*203-207, Feb 1, '30
Splint to prevent contracture in surgery of hand. GAGE, E. L., J.A.M.A. *94:*1063-1064, April 5, '30
Acquired contractures of hand. KOCH, S. L. Am. J. Surg. *9:*413-423, Sept '30
Method of reconstruction of axilla for contracture. GARLOCK, J. H. Surg., Gynec. and Obst. *51:*705-710, Nov '30
Contracture of fingers (ischemic myositis). OEHLECKER, F. Beitr. z. klin. Chir. *149:*333-364, '30
Plastic surgery of cicatricial contractures of underarm. VIDEMAN, G. K. Vestnik khir. (nos. 56-57) *19:*323-328, '30
Thumb contractures in children. STRACKER, O. Wien. klin. Wchnschr. *44:*197-199, Feb 6, '31
Treatment of fractures, ischemic contractures, cicatricial contractures and nerve injuries to fingers. BRANDI, B. Chirurg *3:*263-269, March 15, '31
Contractures of hand from infections. BUNNELL, S. J. Bone and Joint Surg. *14:*27-46, Jan '32
New treatment of palatopharyngeal synechiae of traumatic origin. LEMOINE, J. Ann. d'oto-laryng., pp. 404-410, April '32
Therapy of contracture of underarm. (Comment on Kappis' article.) ODELBERG, A. Zentralbl. f. Chir. *59:*2915-2918, Dec 3, '32
Contracture of underarm; therapy. KAPPIS, M. Zentralbl. f. Chir. *59:*2209-2215, Sept 10, '32
Successful therapy of severe contractures of fingers and hand by cotton redressments. ŠPIŠIĆ, B. Ztschr. f. orthop. Chir. *57:*195-202, '32
Complicated contractures of hand; their treatment by freeing fibrosed tendons and replacing destroyed tendons with grafts. KOCH, S. L. Ann. Surg. *98:*546-580, Oct '33
Cicatricial adhesive contracture of thumb with surface of hand; surgical therapy. SITTERLI, A. Ztschr. f. orthop. Chir. *59:*142-144, '33
Z plastic or web splitting operation for relief of scar contractures of extremities. JONES, H. T. Surg., Gynec. and Obst. *58:*178-182, Feb '34
Tubed pedicle flap for scar contracture. NASSAU, C. F., S. Clin. North America *14:*13-

Contracture – Cont.
18, Feb '34
Correction appliance for contracture of fingers and wrist. HOWITT, F. Lancet *2:*1394–1395, Dec 22, '34
Functional therapy of finger contractures. ORBACH, E. Arch. f. orthop. u. Unfall-Chir. *34:*572–579, '34
Snapping finger (intermittent reflex contraction) in electric welders. VEGER, A. M. Novy khir. arkhiv *30:*321–325, '34
Distribution of palmar aponeurosis in relation to contracture of thumb. HARPER, W. F., J. Anat. *69:*193–195, Jan '35
Surgery of muscles and tendons for contracture. GILL, A. B., S. Clin. North America *15:*203–212, Feb '35
Retraction of palmar aponeurosis with syringomyelic dissociation of sensitivity; 2 cases. URECHIA, C. I. AND DRAGOMIR, L. Paris med. *2:*274–276, Oct 5, '35
Contracture of fingers due to cicatrices on back of hand. NAPALKOV, N. Ortop. i. travmatol. (no. 6) *9:*43–47, '35
Prevention of decubitus ulcers during therapy of contracture by Mommsen cast method. VERESHCHAKOVSKIY, I. I. Ortop. i travmatol. (no. 1) *9:*100, '35
Spring fingers and flexion contracture due to blockage of digital tendons. FEVRE, M. Rev. d'orthop. *23:*137–142, March '36
Plastic surgery of elbow after transplantation of skin in ankylosis with cicatricial contracture; case. VON SEEMEN, H. Zentralbl. f. Chir. *63:*946–950, April 18, '36
Contracture of hands with arthropathies in postencephalitic parkinsonism; clinical and anatomicopathologic study of cases. PENNACCHIETTI, M. Minerva med. *1:*423–431, May 5, '36
Necrosis of finger tips following use of local anesthetic in operation for contracture; study of epinephrine toxicity. HANKE, H. Chirurg *8:*684–687, Sept 1, '36
Orthopedic treatment of contraction of fingers. HOHMANN, G. Munchen. med. Wchnschr. *83:*2088–2089, Dec 18, '36
Surgical treatment of congenital webbed skin across joints. MATOLCSY, T. Orvosi hetil. *80:*1159–1161, Dec 5, '36
Surgical therapy of congenital webbed skin. MATOLCSY, T. Arch. f. klin. Chir. *185:*675–681, '36
Splint for correction of finger contracture. OPPENHEIMER, E. D., J. Bone and Joint Surg. *19:*247–248, Jan '37
Concomitance of muscular torticollis and contracture of fingers. DECKNER, K. Zentralbl. f. Chir. *65:*1192–1195, May 21, '38

Contracture – Cont.
Contracture of middle fingers as new occupational deformation in milkers; case. ALKIEWICZ, J. Dermat. Wchnschr. *107:*1233–1234, Oct 15, '38
Skin grafts in surgical correction of defective cicatrix of hand causing contracture; 2 cases. BARBERIS, J. C. Bol. Soc. de cir. de Rosario *5:*469–477, Nov '38
Flexion contracture of thumb in small children, typical phenomenon. RUSCHENBERG, E. Ztschr. f. Orthop. *68:*172–178, '38
Diagnosis and treatment of contractures of fingers. THOMSEN, W. Arch. f. orthop. u. Unfall-Chir. *39:*201–205, '38
New banjo splint (for extension of contractures of metacarpophalangeal and interphalangeal joints). COZEN, L. Mil. Surgeon *85:*67–68, July '39
Free full thickness skin grafts in hand contracted by cicatrix; technical problems in case. ZENO, L. Rev. ortop. y traumatol. *9:*73–77, July '39
Technic of free graft of whole skin for cicatricial contracture of hand. ZENO, L. Bol. y trab., Soc. de cir. de Buenos Aires *23:*525–531, July 26, '39
Pathology and operative correction of finger deformities due to contractures of extensor digitorum tendon. KAPLAN, E. B. Surgery *6:*451, Sept '39
Technic of full thickness free grafts for cicatricial contracture of hand. ZENO, L. Semana med. *2:*829–831, Oct 12, '39
Reconstruction of axillary space in cases of cicatricial contracture of shoulder. TARTAKOVSKIY, B. S. Novy khir. arkhiv *44:*201–204, '39
Congenital contracture of thumb. BECK, W. Arch. f. orthop. u. Unfall-Chir. *40:*318–325, '40
Reparative surgery of upper limb (in contractures of hands or arms). COLE, P. P. Brit. J. Surg. *28:*585–607, April '41
Symposium on sequelae to war wounds; scarring and contracture. MOWLEM, R. M. Press *205:*384–387, May 7, '41
Flexor contracture of little finger, typical late tertiary symptom of tropical frambesia. PRONK, K. J. Geneesk. tijdschr. v. Nederl.-Indie *81:*1403–1407, July 1, '41
Management of old contractures of upper extremity resulting from third degree burns. JONES, R. R., JR. South. M. J. *34:*789–797, Aug '41
Contracture therapy, extension treatment of shoulder joint. JORDE, A. AND MAGNUSSON, R. Nord. med. (Hygiea) *11:*2471–2474, Aug 30, '41

Contracture – Cont.

Synechia of frenum linguae. MAEKAWA, S. AND HASHIMOTO, T. Oto-rhino-laryng. *14:*666, Sept '41

Etiology and therapy of contracture of fingers. BECKER, J. Zentralbl. f. Chir. *68:*2070–2072, Nov 1 '41

Relief of contractures of knee following extensive burns. HAMM, W. G. AND KITE, J. H. South. Surgeon *10:*795–801, Nov '41

Abrasions and accidental tattoos, scars, keloids and scar contractures and nasal deformities. GREELEY, P. W., S. Clin. North America *22:*253–276, Feb '42

Correction of disabling flexion contracture of thumb. KAPLAN, E. B. Bull. Hosp. Joint Dis. *3:*51–54, April '42

Relation between sympathetic phenomena and contracture in facial paralysis; therapeutic conclusions. PONTHUS, P.; *et al.* Presse med. *50:*308–309, April 20, '42

Therapy of flexion contracture of leg stumps. CORSI, G. Arch. ortop. *57:*320–340, Jul-Aug '42

Contractures of fingers and toes after war wounds. SQUIRE, C. M. Proc. Roy. Soc. Med. *36:*665–666, Oct '43

Rare muscular contractures of hand following poisoning with carbon monoxide, phosphorus and ethyl gasoline. BAYR, G. Deut. Militararzt *8:*623, Nov '43

Plastic repair of scar contractures. GREELEY, P. W. Surgery *15:*224–241, Feb '44

Contractures following gunshot wounds; prophylaxis and therapy. MARKS, V. O. Khirurgiya, no. 11, pp. 9–18, '44

Contracture of fingers and hand following gunshot wounds. FRIDLAND, M. O. Khirurgiya, no. 8, pp. 56–61, '44

Splint for correction of extension contractures of metacarpophalangeal joints. NACHLAS, I. W., J. Bone and Joint Surg. *27:*507–512, July '45

Operation for irreducible contractures of fingers. ZATSEPIN, T. S. Khirurgiya, No. 5, pp. 81–83, '45

Therapy of nonhealing wounds, ulcers and contractures by transplantation of chemically treated tissues according to Krauze. BLOKHIN, V. N. Khirurgiya, No. 6, pp. 3–10, '45

Post traumatic contractures. SPERANSKI, A. D. Am. Rev. Soviet Med. *4:*22–24, Oct '46

Contracture, Burn (See also Burns, Contractures)

Arm-chest adhesions; brachio-thoracic adhesions; axillary webs. DAVIS, J. S. J. Bone and Joint Surg. *6:*167–187, Jan '24 also:

Contracture, Burn – Cont.

Arch. Surg. *8:*1–23 (pt. 1), Jan '24

Treatment of contracture deformities secondary to burns. MILLER, O. L. Southern M. J. *17:*522–526, July '24

Contractures due to burns of face, neck and body. BEHREND, M., S. Clin. N. America *6:*237–243, Feb '26

Surgical treatment of large contraction scars of burns according to Morestin's plastic operations. STEGEMANN, H. Zentralbl. f. Chir. *53:*1880–1884, July '24, '26

Contracture of axilla from burns; 3 cases. JONES, H. T. Minnesota Med. *11:*210–214, April '28

Contractures due to burns; treatment with free full thickness grafts and pedunculated flaps. KOCH, S. L. AND KANAVEL, A. B. Tr. Sect. Surg, General and Abd., A.M.A., pp. 208–227, '28

Contracture due to burns; treatment with free full thickness grafts and pedunculated flaps. KOCH, S. L. AND KANAVEL, A. B. J.A.M.A. *92:*277–281, Jan 26, '29

Whirlpool baths and posterior splinting to overcome contractures in burns. HILBERT, J. W., J.A.M.A. *95:*1021, Oct 4, '30

Morestin operation in dermatogenous contractures after burns. PRISELKOFF, P. V. Vestnik khir. (no. 64) *22:*111–114, '30

Plastic surgery of face and neck to remove cicatricial adhesions caused by burns; case. VASCONCELLOS ALVARENGA, E. Rev. brasil. de med. e pharm. *7:*334–337, '31

Plastic surgery of cicatricial contractures of skin. KARFÍK, V. Casop. lek. cesk. *71:*1289–1292, Oct 7, '32

Contractures of neck following burns (treatment by use of tubular skin graft). MIXTER, C. G. New England J. Med. *208:*190–196, Jan 26, '33

Arm-chest adhesions and their plastic reconstruction by tube flap method. KULOWSKI, J. Ann. Surg. *97:*683–692, May '33

Extensive burns on both forearms and back of hand; remote results of resection of retractile scar and pedicled graft from thigh. MIRIZZI, P. L. Bull. et mem. Soc. nat. de chir. *59:*694–695, May 6, '33

Cicatricial contraction of neck. NEW, G. B., S. Clin. North America *13:*868–869, Aug '33

Palmar contracture of hand as sequel of burn received in infancy; therapy with Gillies tubular graft at age 17 years. LLUESMA URANGA, E. Cron. med., Valencia *38:*11–14, Jan 15, '34

Burn contractures of axilla. KOCH, S. L., S. Clin. North America *14:*751–761, Aug '34

Plastic surgery of contracture after burns.

Contracture, Burn – Cont.
GRZYWA, N. Geneesk. tijdschr. v. Nederl.-Indie *74:*1539–1540, Nov 6, '34
Possible uses of Reverdin skin flap for plastic surgery, primarily for covering skin defects, and secondarily for scar contractures. EHALT, W. Munchen. med. Wchnschr. *82:*669–671, April 25, '35
Tubular skin graft in therapy of extensive contracture of neck. KARTASHEV, Z. I. Sovet. khir., no. 11, pp. 22–30, '35
Plastic repair of talipes calcaneovalgus due to cicatricial adhesions following burns; case. PASCAU, I. Cir. ortop. y traumatol. *3:*185–189, July–Sept '35
Repair of contractures resulting from burns (grafts). KAZANJIAN, V. H. New England J. Med. *215:*1104–1120, Dec 10, '36
Plastic surgery for deformity and contractures after nitric acid burns to face (case). MONEY, R. A., M. J. Australia *2:*848–853, Dec 19, '36
Burns, discussion on their treatment, both immediate and remote, with special emphasis on prevention of scars and contractures. COAKLEY, W. A. Am. J. Surg. *36:*50–53, April '37
Surgical therapy of cicatricial contracture of neck after burns. MIKHELSON, N. M. Ortop. i travmatol. (no. 1) *12:*74–82, '38
Therapy of cicatricial contracture of hand and fingers after burns. BAKUSHINSKIY, R. N. Ortop. i travmatol. (no. 2) *12:*76–83, '38
Whole-thickness grafts in correction of contractures due to burn scars; 3 cases. CONWAY, H. Ann. Surg. *109:*286–290, Feb '39
Contractures due to burns. COUGHLIN, W. T. Surg., Gynec. and Obst. *68:*352–361, Feb (no. 2A) '39
Fibrous contracture of head and neck after extensive burns. GJANKOVIC, H. Lijecn. vjes. *61:*279–284, May '39
Burn contractures of hand. BLACKFIELD, H. M. Surg., Gynec. and Obst. *68:*1066–1073, June '39
Epithelial inlay for scars in neck dragging lower jaw downwards. ESSER, J. F. S. Am. J. Surg. *45:*148–149, July '39
Management of old contractures of hand resulting from third degree burns. JONES, R. JR. Surgery *7:*264–275, Feb '40 also: North Carolina M. J. *1:*148–152, March '40
Brachiothoracic adhesions. BURTON, J. F. Surg., Gynec. and Obst. *70:*938–944, May '40
Technic of pedicled flaps in plastic surgery of skin; use in treating cicatricial contracture of hand. ZENO, L. Semana med. *2:*1058–1061, Nov 7, '40 also: Bol. y trab., Acad. argent. de cir. *24:*886–890, Sept 18, '40
Labiomentothoracic synechia due to burn; plastic repair of case. JOHOW, A. AND URZUA, R. Rev. med. de Chile *68:*1482–1487, Nov '40
Free full-thickness skin graft for relief of burn contracture of neck. BLOCKER, T. G., JR. South. Surgeon *10:*849–857, Dec '41
Hand and finger contracture due to burns. HOHMANN, G. Chirurg. *14:*289, May 15, '42
Prevention of contracture deformities following burns by use of Padgett dermatome. THOMPSON, H. A. South. Med. and Surg. *105:*51–55, Feb '43
Thoracofacial synechia following burn; case. COVARRUBIAS ZENTENO, R. Rev. med. de Chile *71:*899–901, Sept '43
Plastic repair of extensor hand contractures following healed deep second degree burns. GREELEY, P. W. Tr. Am. Soc. Plastic and Reconstructive Surg. *12:*79–82, '43
Plastic repair of extensor hand contractures following healed deep second degree burns. GREELEY, P. W. Surgery *15:*173–177, Jan '44
Deep burns and contractures. KITE, J. H. J.M.A. Georgia *33:*139–143, May '44
Late plastic care of burn scars and deformities (contractures). DAVIS, J. S. J.A.M.A. *125:*621–628, July 1, '44
Plastic considerations of burn scars and contractures of hand and forearm. MACOMBER, W. B. Am. Acad. Orthop. Surgeons, Lect., pp. 174–179, '44
Correction of cicatricial contractures of axilla, elbow joint and knee. MAY, H. S. Clin. North America *25:*1229–1241, Oct '45

Contracture, Dupuytren's

Induratio penis plastica and Dupuytren's contracture. MARTENSTEIN, H. Med. Klin. *17:*44, Jan. 9, '21
Pathogenesis of Dupuytren's contracture of palmer fascia. BYFORD, W. H. Med. Rec. *100:*487, Sept 17, '21
Pathogenesis of Dupuytren's contracture. KROGIUS, A. Acta chir. Scandinav. *54:*33, '21
Contracture of aponeurosis of palms and soles plus neuralgia treated with X-ray. SPECKLIN, P. AND STOEBER, R. Presse med. *30:*743–745, Aug 30, '22 abstr: J.A.M.A. *79:*1368, Oct 14, '22
Dupuytren's contraction of palmar fascia and some other deformities. TUBBY, A. H. Practitioner *110:*214–220, March '23

Contracture, Dupuytren's – Cont.
Dupuytren's contracture. VAN BRAAM HOUCKGEEST, A. Q. Nederlandsch Tijdschr. v. Geneesk. *2:*1032–1034, Sept 8, '23
Heredity in Dupuytren's contracture. LOWI, J. Zentralbl. f. inn. Med. *44:*51–52, Jan 27, '23 abstr: J.A.M.A. *80:*1279, April 28, '23
Etiology of Dupuytren's contracture. SCHUBERT, A. Deutsche Ztschr. f. Chir. *177:*362–377, '23
Dupuytren's contracture. SILVA, F. Brazil-med. *2:*269–272, Nov. 8, '24 abstr: J.A.M.A. *84:*557, Feb 14, '25
Four cases of contraction of palmar fascia in lead-poisoning. MICHAUX, J.; *et al.* Bull. et mem. Soc. med. d. hop. de Par. *49:*782–786, May 22, '25 abstr: J.A.M.A. *85:*308, July 25, '25
Hereditary contracture of palmar fascia; efficiency of radium emanation. APERT, E. Bull. et mem. Soc. med. d. hop. de Paris *49:*1502–1505, Nov. 27, '25 abstr: J.A.M.A. *86:*380, Jan 30, '26
Dupuytren's disease from traumatic cause; medicolegal testimony in case. MASCIOTRA, A. A. Semana med. *2:*1615–1617, Dec 24, '25
Problem of heredity of Dupuytren's contracture. SPROGIS, G. Compt. rend. Soc. de biol. *94:*631–632, March 12, '26 abstr: J.A.M.A. *87:*131, July 10, '26
Dupuytren's contraction. ELY, L. W., S. Clin. N. Amer. *6:*421–424, April '26
Dupuytren's contracture. WAINWRIGHT, L. Practitioner *117:*263–265, Oct '26
Dupuytren's contracture of palmar and plantar aponeurosis. COKKALIS, P. Deutsche Ztschr. f. Chir. *194:*256–258, '26
Theory of heredity of Dupuytren's contracture. SPROGIS, G. Deutsche Ztschr. f. Chir. *194:*259–263, '26
Family tree of hereditary transmission of Dupuytren's contracture. KARTSCHIKJAN, S. I. Ztschr. f. orthop. Chir. *48:*36–38, Feb 11, '27
Dupuytren's contraction. PICARD, J. Vie med. *8:*225–228, Feb 4, '27
Trauma and Dupuytren's contracture. SCHUBERT, A. Med. Klin. *23:*549–551, April 15, '27
Association of scleroderma and Dupuytren's disease in syphilitic. LECHELLE, P. *et al.* Bull. et mem. Soc. med. d. hop. de Paris *51:*622–629, May 19, '27
Traumatic origin of Dupuytren's contracture. NIEHUES. Aerztl. Sachverst.-Ztg. *33:*250–255, Sept 15, '27

Contracture, Dupuytren's – Cont.
Dupuytren's contracture treated with humanol injections. STAHNKE, E. Zentralbl. f. Chir. *54:*2438–2442, Sept 24, '27
Clinical and histological study of Dupuytren's contracture. ANTONIOLI, G. M. Ann. ital. di chir. *6:*1011–1037, Oct '27
Dupuytren's contracture, cases. DUTTO, U. Gazz. med. di Roma *54:*198, Oct '28
Dupuytren's contracture; case. MASSAROTTI, G. Gior. di med. mil. *76:*600–602, Nov '28
Histology and pathogenesis of Dupuytren's contracture. IKLÉ, C. Deutsche Ztschr. f. Chir. *212:*106–118, '28
Dupuytren's contracture among Polynesians of Truk. MATSUNAGA, T. Acta dermat. *13:*101, Jan '29
Description of palmar fascia, review of literature, and report of 29 surgically treated cases of Dupuytren's contracture. KANAVEL, A. B.; *et al.* Surg., Gynec. and Obst. *48:*145–190, Feb '29
Dupuytren's contracture; review of literature and report of new technique in surgical treatment; preliminary statement. ABBOTT, A. C. Canad. M. A. J. *20:*250–253, March '29
Dupuytren's contracture not occupational accident; case. OLLIER, A. Ars med. *5:*96–98, March '29
Dupuytren's contracture as result of industrial accident. OLLER, A. Arch. de med., cir. y espec. *30:*333–335, March 16, '29
Dupuytren's contracture, industrial accident or disease? DECREF, J. Siglo med. *83:*569–570, April 13, '29
Supposed pathogenesis; case of polyneuritis with retraction of palmar aponeurosis. DE VILLAVERDE, J. M. Med. ibera *2:*213–222, Aug 31, '29
Dupuytren's contracture, clinical case. UNGUREÀNU, V. Cluj. med. *10:*522–524, Nov 1, '29
Familial predisposition to Dupuytren's contracture. CSÖRSZ, K. Budapesti orvosi ujsag *28:*59–61, Jan 16, '30
Dupuytren's contracture with congenital dislocations of hip joint. CSÖRSZ, K. Budapesti orvosi ujsag *28:*61–63, Jan 16, '30
Tobiášek's method of operation for Dupuytren's disease. TOBIÁŠEK. Casop. lek. cesk. *69:*421, March 14; 459, March 21, '30
Gangrene of fingers after operation for Dupuytren's contracture. ROEDELIUS, E. Zentralbl. f. Chir. *57:*936–939, April 12, '30
Dupuytren's contracture. SICARD, A. Ann. d'anat. path. *7:*745–746, June '30
Case of spontaneous aneurysm of first por-

Contracture, Dupuytren's—Cont.
tion of axillary artery associated with unilateral clubbing of fingers and Dupuytren's contracture. BROOKS, B. S. Clin. North America *10:*741–755, Aug '30
Retraction of superficial palmar aponeurosis; case. RODRÍGUEZ VILLEGAS, R. AND BRACHETTO-BRIAN, D. Bol. y trab. de la Soc. de cir. de Buenos Aires *14:*809–821, Oct 29, '30
Dupuytren's contracture localized to 2 last fingers of left hand and accompanied by Bernard-Horner ocular sympathetic syndrome of same side, observed 15 years after lesion of cubital nerve of opposite side. ALAJOUANINE, T. *et al*. Rev. neurol. *2:*679–683, Dec '30
Relation of retraction of palmar aponeurosis to hypocalcemia and parathyroid insufficiency. LERICHE, R. AND JUNG, A. Presse med. *38:*1641–1642, Dec 3, '30
Surgical treatment of Dupuytren's contracture. RITTER, C. Deutsche Ztschr. f. Chir. *227:*544–546, '30
Dupuytren's contracture; etiology, especially in young adults. SCHOLLE, W. Deutsche Ztschr. f. Chir. *223:*328–339, '30
Continued improvement of Dupuytren's contracture after injections of patient's own blood mixed with testicular extract. FILDERMAN. Bull. et mem. Soc. de med. de Paris, no. 4, pp. 115–117, Feb 28, '31
Contracture of hand. KOCH, S. L. Surg., Gynec. and Obst. *52:*367–370, Feb (No. 2A) '31
Etiology of Dupuytren's contracture. POMMÉ, B. *et al*. Rev. neurol. *1:*633–638, May '31
Heredity and Dupuytren's contracture. MANSON, J. S. Brit. M. J. *2:*11, July 4, '31
Dupuytren's contracture; case. TRUMPER, W. A. Lancet *2:*17, July 4, '31
Dupuytren's contracture and the unconscious; preliminary statement of problem. JELLIFFE, S. E. Internat. Clin. *3:*184–199, Sept '31
Surgical treatment of Dupuytren's contracture. HAYWARD. Med. Klin. *27:*1721–1722, Nov 20, '31
New light on cause and possibility of physiotherapy (Dupuytren's contracture). POWERS, H. Am. J. Phys. Therapy *8:*239–241, Dec '31
Retraction of palmar aponeurosis; therapy; case. ROUTIER. Bull. et mem. Soc. nat. de chir. *57:*1467, Dec 5, '31
Etiology of finger contracture (Dupuytren's). REICHEL. Deutsche Ztschr. f. Chir. *230:*291–295, '31
Pathogenesis of Dupuytren's contracture.

Contracture, Dupuytren's—Cont.
NOICA, I. AND PÂRVULESCU, N. Rev. san. mil., Bucuresti *31:*3–9, Jan–Feb '32
Surgical therapy of Dupuytren's contracture. DESPLAS, AND MEILLÈRE, J. Bull. et mem. Soc. nat. de chir. *58:*424–429, March 12, '32
Surgical therapy of Dupuytren's contracture. FREDET, P. Bull. et mem. Soc. nat. de chir. *58:*440–444, March 19, '32
Review of 31 cases of Dupuytren's contracture, with assessment of comparative value of different methods of therapy. DAVIS, A. A. Brit. J. Surg. *19:*539–547, April '32
Nervous etiology of Dupuytren's contracture. NOICA, D. AND PARVULESCO. Rev. neurol. *1:*703–708, April '32
Serrated plastic surgery; one of several beneficial methods of treating syndactylia and Dupuytren's. PALMÉN, A. J. Zentralbl. f. Chir. *59:*1377–1379, May 28, '32
Dupuytren's contracture, with note on incidence of contracture in diabetes. DAVIS, J. S. AND FINESILVER, E. M. Arch. Surg. *24:*933–989, June '32
Division of palmar fascia in therapy of Dupuytren's contracture. ORBACH, E. Med. Welt *6:*955–956, July 2, '32
Dupuytren's contracture, development favored by existence of diabetes mellitus; case. SCHLOSSER. Munchen. med. Wchnschr. *79:*1238, July 29, '32
Surgical therapy of Dupuytren's contracture. DESPLAS, B. AND MEILLIÈRE, J. Monde med., Paris *42:*795–802, Aug 1–15, '32
Dupuytren's contracture; etiology, with report of case. SAJDOVÁ, V. Rev. v neurol. a psychiat. *29:*188–194, Sept '32
Contracture of palmar aponeurosis. PARDO-CASTELLO, V. Acta dermat.-venereol. *13:*649–654, Dec '32
Surgical therapy of Dupuytren's contracture. WAGNER, W. Beitr. z. klin. Chir. *155:*271–274, '32
Cure of Dupuytren's contracture associated with diabetes by roentgen irradiation of hypophysis; case. BARISON, F. Gior. di psichiat. e di neuropat. *60:*45–64, '32
Dupuytren's contracture; relation to occupation. NIEDERLAND, W. Arch. f. Gewerbepath. u. Gewerbehyg. *3:*23–43, '32
Dupuytren's contracture; relation to occupation. NIEDERLAND, W. Med. Welt *7:*126–127, Jan 28, '33
Dupuytren's contracture; case, probably of medullary origin complicating sensory disturbances of syringomyelic type. TOLOSA,

Contracture, Dupuytren's – Cont.

A. Bol. Soc. de med. e cir. de Sao Paulo *16:*158–162, Jan '33

Dupuytren's contracture. Koch, S. L. J.A.M.A. *100:*878–880, March 25, '33

Dupuytren's contracture and nervous disturbances. Richon, *et al.* Rev. med. de l'est *61:*231–237, March 15, '33

Contracture (Dupuytren's) of fingers as result of injury; case. Niederland, W. Med. Klin. *29:*614–615, April 28, '33

Nervous etiology of Dupuytren's contracture; cases. Gubern-Salisachs, L. Rev. de cir. de Barcelona *6:*81–115, Sept '33

Retraction of palmar aponeurotic fascia. Palmer, R. G. Gaz. d. hop. *106:*1369–1375, Sept 23, '33

True and false Dupuytren contracture in relation to traumatic etiogenesis of condition; interest from medicolegal viewpoint. Macaggi, D. Policlinico (sez. chir.) *40:*743–759, Dec '33

Association of retraction of palmar aponeurosis and scleroderma; relation to diseases of endocrine glands and of sympathetic nervous system. Weill, J. and Maire, R. Paris med. *1:*263–268, March 24, '34

Heredity of Dupuytren's contracture. Schröder, C. H. Zentralbl. f. Chir. *61:*1056–1059, May 5, '34

Three cases of Dupuytren's contracture. Mazzoni, E. Gazz. d. osp. *55:*1323–1329, Oct 28, '34

Retraction of palmar aponeuroses and scleroderma. Norsa, G. Gazz. d. osp. *55:*1285–1287, Oct. 21, '34

One hundred years after Dupuytren; interpretation. Powers, H. J. Nerv. & Ment. Dis. *80:*386–409, Oct '34

Traumatic Claude Bernard-Horner syndrome associated with Dupuytren's contracture and paroxysmal anxiety (precordial pain) caused by aerophagy; case. Laignel-Lavastine, *et al.* Rev. neurol. *2:*784–787, Dec '34

Genealogical table showing appearance of Dupuytren's contracture in siblings. Debrunner, H. Ztschr. f. orthop. Chir. *62:*321–323, '34

Failure of parathyroid extract in Dupuytren's contracture; 4 cases. Previtera, A. Arch. ed atti d. Soc. ital. di chir. *40:*578–583, '34

Dupuytren's contracture and its relation to trauma and occupation. Schröder, C. H. Deutsche Ztschr. f. Chir. *244:*140–149, '34 abstr.: Arch. f. orthop. u. Unfall-Chir. *35:*125–127, '34

Contracture, Dupuytren's – Cont.

Attempt to culture tissue from Dupuytren's contracture in adults. Tůma, V. Arch. f. exper. Zellforsch. *15:*173–178, '34

Hemithoracic pain following zona, with disturbances of cutaneous pigmentation; bilateral contracture of palmer aponeuroses; case. Poinso, R. *et al.* Marseille-med. 1:20–29, Jan 5, '35

Radium therapy of Dupuytren's contracture. Tománek, F. Casop. lek. cesk. *74:*46–47, Jan 11, '35

Distribution of palmar aponeurosis in relation to contracture of thumb. Harper, W. F. J. Anat. *69:*193–195, Jan '35

Unusual case of contracture of palmar fascia of both hands. Koster, S. Nederl. tijdschr. v. geneesk. *79:*674–678, Feb 16, '35 also: Rev. neurol. *63:*281–285, Feb '35

Significance of occupational and sport injuries in etiology of Dupuytren's contracture. Schnitzler, O. Munchen. med. Wchnschr. *82:*248–249, Feb 14, '35

Dupuytren's contracture; clinical study. Béyoul, A. Rev. de chir., Paris *73:*351–357, May '35

Dupuytren's contracture; etiologic conception based on 2 similar cases. Boulogne, Rev. neurol. *63:*991–992, June '35

Traumatic development of Dupuytren's contracture. Kohlmayer, H. Zentralbl. f. Chir. *62:*1928–1931, Aug 17, '35

Dupuytren's contracture. Meyerding, H. W. Proc. Staff Meet., Mayo Clin. *10:*694–696, Oct 30, '35

Dupuytren's contracture. Niederland, W. Zentralbl. f. Chir. *62:*2238–2243, Sept 21, '35

Etiology of Dupuytren's contracture; relation to occupation and trauma. Gerritzen, P. Monatschr. f. Unfallh. *42:*545–551, Nov '35

Dupuytren's contracture of finger. Coenen, H. Med. Klin. *31:*1657–1661, Dec 20, '35

Bilateral Dupuytren's contracture. Meyerding, H. W. & Overton, L. M. Proc. Staff Meet., Mayo Clin. *10:*801–803, Dec 18, '35

Traumatic etiology of Dupuytren's contracture. David, V. Rozhl. v chir. a gynaek. (cast chir.) *14:*126–129, '35

Surgical and bloodless therapy of Dupuytren's contracture. Krinke, J. Rozhl. v chir. a gynaek. (cast chir.) *14:*129–133, '35

Question of Dupuytren's contracture as industrial injury meriting compensation. Bergel, D. Med. Welt 10:16–18, Jan 4, '36

Dupuytren's contracture of finger. Moser, E. Zentralbl. f. Chir. *63:*149–151, Jan 18, '36

Contracture, Dupuytren's – Cont.
Dupuytren's contracture. MEYERDING, H. W. Arch. Surg. *32:*320–333, Feb '36
Spring finger and Dupuytren's contracture; case in woman. RUIZ MORENO, A. Semana med. 1:939–946, March 19, '36
Physical therapy for Dupuytren's contracture. Physiotherapy Rev. *16:*42–45, March–April '36
Familial appearance of Dupuytren's contracture; case. IMBER, I. Note e riv. di psichiat. *65:*209–222, April–June '36
New data on pathogenesis of Dupuytren's contracture. NOICA, D. *et al.* Rev. san. mil., Bucuresti *35:*513–518, May '36
Pathogenic study of case of Dupuytren's contracture. DUSATTI, C. Minerva med. *2:*79–80, July 28, '36
Importance of predisposition, chronic trauma and accident in genesis of Dupuytren's contracture. SCHAEFER, V. Zentralbl. f. Chir. *63:*1712–1716, July 18, '36
Radium therapy in Dupuytren's contracture. FEURSTEIN, J. G. Wien. klin. Wchnschr. *49:*1090–1092, Sept 4, '36
Dupuytren's contracture as industrial injury. NIEDERLAND, W. Jahresk. f. arztl. Fortbild. *27:*60–65, Sept '36
Dupuytren's contracture of palmer fascia and its treatment. MAURER, G. Deutsche Ztschr. f. Chir. *246:*685–692, '36
Dupuytren's contracture, two cases. PILON, A., J. de l'Hotel-Dieu de Montreal *5:*75–81, '36
Pathogenesis and etiology of Dupuytren's contracture. VERMEL, S. S. Novy khir. arkhiv *36:*249–252, '36
Operation for Dupuytren's contracture. VON SEEMEN, H. Deutsche Ztschr. f. Chir. *246:*693–696, '36
Surgical therapy of Dupuytren's contracture. YOVANOVICH, B. Y. Voj.-san. glasnik *7:*331–347, '36
Successful surgical therapy of Dupuytren's contracture, 2 cases. FERNANDEZ, J. C. Semana med. 1:260–262, Jan 28, '37
Dupuytren's contracture, covering palmer defects with skin from little finger. FRANKENTHAL, L. Zentralbl. f. Chir. *64:*211–214, Jan 23, '37
Plastic induration of penis with retraction of palmar aponeurosis; case. POLICARO, R. D. Gior. med. d. Alto Adige *9:*13–16, Jan '37
Dupuytren's contracture and industrial accident; case. WETTE, W. Monatschr. f. Unfallh. *44:*195–197, April '37
Surgical therapy of Dupuytren's contracture. REICHL, E. Zentralbl. f. Chir. *64:*1570–1573, July 3, '37

Contracture, Dupuytren's – Cont.
Bilateral Dupuytren's contracture due to injury of cubital nerve in lower third of forearm. NOICA, D. *et al.* Romania med. *15:*261–262, Oct 15, '37
False Dupuytren's contracture. BEYUL, A. P. & KOGAN, A. V. Khirurgiya, no. 3, pp. 98–102, '37
Congenital bilateral contracture (Dupuytren's); case. CONSTANTINESCU, M. *et al.* Zentralbl. f. Chir. *65:*191–194, Jan 22, '38
Dupuytren's contracture. GILL, A. B. Ann. Surg. *107:*122–127, Jan '38
Note on Dupuytren's contracture, camptodactylia and knuckle-pads. WEBER, F. P. Brit. J. Dermat. *50:*26–31, Jan '38
Roentgen therapy of Dupuytren's contracture. BEATTY, S. R. Radiology *30:*610–612, May '38
Retraction of palmer aponeurosis or Dupuytren's disease due to industrial trauma; medicolegal expertise in case. MASCIOTRA, A. A. Semana med. *1:*1063–1066, May 12, '38
Dupuytren's contracture in patient with melancholia; biochemical and clinical study. CHATAGNON, P. *et al.* Ann. med.-psychol. (pt. 2) *96:*238–245, July '38
Identical Dupuytren's contracture in identical twins. COUCH, H. Canad. M. A. J. *39:*225–226, Sept '38
Dupuytren's contracture in connection with palmer fascia. KAPLAN, E. B. Surgery *4:*415–422, Sept '38
Dupuytren's contracture and retraction of connective tissue fibers. VALCARCEL, A. G. Zentralbl. f. Chir. *65:*2506–2508, Nov 5, '38
Dupuytren's contracture; importance of morbid processes of cervical spine in pathogenesis. PACIFICO, A. Rassegna di neurol. veget. *1:*34–80, '38
Technic for surgical therapy of Dupuytren's contracture. SAUERBRUCH, F. AND VON DANCKELMAN, A. Arch. ital. di chir. *54:*502–507, '38
Diagnosis and treatment of contractures of fingers. THOMSEN, W. Arch. f. orthop. u. Unfall-Chir. *39:*201–205, '38
Report of 30 cases of Dupuytren's contracture observed in 1932–1938. RIEDL, L. Zentralbl. f. Chir. *66:*1093–1096, May 13, '39
Pathologic anatomy and etiopathogenesis of Dupuytren's contracture; review. FERRARINI, M. Gior. d. r. Accad. di med. di Torino (parte seconda) *102:*40–51, Jan–March '39
Dupuytren's contracture; nature and therapy. DECKNER, K. Therap. d. Gegenw. *80:*69–72, Feb '39

Contracture, Dupuytren's – Cont.

Dupuytren's contracture; plastic surgery of hands. (grafts) MASON, M. L., S. Clin. North America *19:*227–248, Feb '39

Dupuytren's contracture; etiology. REICHL, E. Wien. klin. Wchnschr. *52:*315–316, March 31, '39

Dupuytren's contracture among upholsterers. SMITH, K. D. AND MASTERS, W. E. J. Indust. Hyg. & Toxicol. *21:*97–100, March '39

Dupuytren's contracture. DUDLEY, H. D. Northwest Med. *38:*138–139, April '39

Report of 30 cases of Dupuytren's contracture observed in 1932–1938. RIEDL, L. Zentralbl. f. Chir. *66:*1093–1096, May 13, '39

Dupuytren's contracture of palmer and plantar fascias. GREENBERG, L., J. Bone & Joint Surg. *21:*785–788, July '39

Dupuytren's contracture; operation based on anatomy of palmer fascia. KAPLAN, E. B. Bull. Russian M. Soc. New York, pp. 78–83, Sept '39

Dupuytren's contracture as occupational disease. TELEKY, L. J. Indust. Hyg. & Toxicol. *21:*233–235, Sept '39

Permanent retraction of fingers, produced by affection of palmer fascia. DUPUYTREN, G. M. Classics *4:*142–150, Oct '39 (Reprint). also: M. Classics *4:*127–141, Oct '39 (Reprint; in French)

Iontophoresis in treatment of Dupuytren's contracture and keloids. NIJKERK, M. Nederl. tijdschr. v. geneesk. *83:*5135–5140, Oct 28, '39

Bilateral Dupuytren's contracture in three children of one family; case. RIEDL, L. Casop. lek. cesk. *78:*1114–1115, Oct 6, '39

Dupuytren's contracture. MARIN GATICA, J. Rev. med. de Chile *67:*1221–1232, Nov '39

Dupuytren's contracture as example for concurrent action of hereditary and environmental factors for development of variable characteristics. DECKNER, K. Ztschr. f. menschl. Vererb.-u. Konstitutionslehre *22:*734–790, '39

Dupuytren's contracture; pathologic anatomy and etiopathogenesis; review of literature and report of cases. FERRARINI, M. Arch. ital. di chir. *57:*1–110, '39

Dupuytren's contracture and its therapy. MELESHKO, E. R. Khirurgiya, no. 12, pp. 78–85, '39

Dupuytren's contracture; concordant occurrence in fingers of 3 sets of twins. THEN BERGH, H. Allg. Ztschr. f. Psychiat. *112:*327–336, '39

Dupuytren's contracture can be considered as occupational disease. FERRARINI, M. Rassegna di med. indust. *11:*70–97, Feb '40

Dupuytren's contracture. KÖNIG, E. Med. Klin. *36:*568–571, May 24, '40

Dupuytren's contracture. HANCOCK, J. D. Kentucky M. J. *38:*290–293, July '40

Aberrant manifestations; retraction of palmer aponeurosis. FINOCHIETTO, E. *et al.* Prensa med. argent. *27:*1421–1424, July 10, '40

Treatment of Dupuytren's contracture. MEYERDING, H. W. Am. J. Surg. *49:*94–103, July '40

Dupuytren's contracture due to work; case. CARONES, C. Rev. med. leg. y jurisp. med. *4:*244–247, Oct–Dec '40

So-called retraction of palmer aponeurosis; case. COUCEIRO, A. Neurobiologia *3:*396–403, Dec '40

Dupuytren's contracture. ADAMS, H. D. Lahey Clin. Bull. *2:*75–78, Jan '41

Etiology and pathology of Dupuytren's contracture. MEYERDING, H. W. *et al.* Surg., Gynec. & Obst. *72:*582–590, March '41

Plastic induration of penis and Dupuytren's disease with negative Frei reaction; case. CONEJO MIR, J. Actas dermo-sif. *32:*834–836, June '41

Dupuytren's contracture. JONES, A. R., M. Press *206:*14–16, July 2, '41

Operative correction of Dupuytren's contracture by use of tunnel skin graft. SKINNER, H. L. Surgery *10:*313–317, Aug '41

New operative procedure for Dupuytren's contracture. STERN, E. L. Am. J. Surg. *54:*711–715, Dec '41

Dupuytren's contracture, relation to plastic induration of penis. VOLAVSEK, W. Ztschr. f. Urol. *35:*173–178, '41

Dupuytren's contracture in both hands and both feet. HOHMANN, G. Ztschr. f. Orthop. *73:*45, '41

Clinical connection between Dupuytren's contracture, fibroma plantae, periarthrosis humeri, helodermia, induratio penis plastica and epilepsy, with attempt at pathogenetic valuation. LUND, M. Acta psychiat. et neurol. *16:*465–492, '41

Multiple skeletal malformations and Dupuytren syndrome in congenital syphilis; case CAPELLI, E. Dermosifilografo *17:*19–32, Jan '42

Dupuytren's contracture; consideration of anatomy of fibrous structures of hand in relation to this condition, with interpretation of histology. HORWITZ, T. Arch. Surg. *44:*687–706, April '42

Contracture, Dupuytren's – Cont.

Plastic induration of penis and Dupuytren's contracture; cases. LANA MARTINEZ, F. AND LANA SALARRULLANA, F. Med. espan. *7:*450–456, May '42

Dupuytren's contracture. ADAMS, H. D., S. Clin. North America *22:*899–906, June '42

Dupuytren's contracture; with report of case. PAOLINI LANDA, J. AND FARINA, R. C. Semana med. *2:*1607–1612, Dec 31, '42

Treatment of Dupuytren's contracture by means of radical excision of palmar fascia. BLACKFIELD, H. M. Brunn, Med.-Surg. Tributes, pp. 59–72, '42

Orientation in etiology of permanent retraction of fingers. MAY, J. An. Fac. de med. de Montevideo *28:*675–685, '43

Plastic surgery of hand; fingers in flexion contracture; semeiologic and therapeutic study. PEDEMONTE, P. V. Arch. urug. de med., cir. y especialid. *24:*249–274, Mar '44

Dupuytren's contracture. CORLETTE, C. E., M. J. Australia *2:* 177–182, Aug. 19, '44

FERRE, R. L. Dia med. *16:*487–490, May 15, '44

Dupuytren's contracture. CORLETTE, C. E. M. J. Australia *2:*177–182, Aug. 19, '44

Fibroma of palmar fascia. CLAY, R. C. Ann. Surg. *120:*224–231, Aug '44

Bilateral symmetric contractures of hand and phalanges; case. SPISIC, B. Ztschr. f. Orthop. *75:*33, '44

Neuroma of palmer fascia simulating Dupuytren's contracture. GRIFFITHS, D. L. AND CRAWFORD, T. J. Roy. Army M. Corps *84:*130–131, March '45

Bridge operation for Dupuytren's contracture. PALMER, L. A. AND SOUTHWORTH, J. L. Am. J. Surg. *68:*351–354, June '45

Study apropos of 150 cases Dupuytren's contracture. DESPLAS, B. AND TOSTIVINT, R. Mem. Acad. de chir. *71:*373–379, Oct 17–31, '45

Report of 64 cases Dupuytren's contracture among Veterans Guard of Canada. AYRE, W. B., J. Canad. M. Serv. *3:*57–61, Nov '45 also: Canad. M. A. J. *54:*158–160, Feb '46

Clinical and etiopathogenetic study of 2 rare cases of Dupuytren's contracture. FERRARI, A. (Adolfo) Minerva med. *2:*230–235, Dec 1 '45

New method of treatment (vitamin E) of Dupuytren's contracture, form of fibrositis. STEINBERG, C. L. M. Clin. North America *30:*221–231, Jan '46

Treatment of Dupuytren's contracture. EINARSSON, F. Acta chir. Scandinav. *93:*1–22, '46

Contracture, Volkmann's

Volkmann's ischemic contracture. JEANNE. Bull. Acad. de med., Par. *92:*1266–1270, Nov 25, '24 abstr: J.A.M.A. *84:*235, Jan 17, '25

Volkmann's ischemic contracture. PEREMANS, G. Arch. franco-belges de chir. *27:*1076–1086, Dec '24

Volkmann's ischemic contracture. JORGE, J. M. Semana med. *1:*833–842, May 3, '23

Volkmann's ischemic paralysis. JENSEN, E. Ugesk. f. Laeger *87:*729–734, Aug 20, '25

Volkmann's ischemic paralysis. JENSEN, E. Ugesk. f. Laeger *87:*756–759, Aug 27, '25

Pathogenic and therapeutic considerations of Volkmann's contracture. SÉNÈQUE, J. Presse med. *34:*133–135, Jan 30, '26

Volkmann's disease. MOUCHET, A., J. de med. et chir. prat. *98:*229–238, April 10, '27

Volkmann's contracture, treatment by humeral sympathectomy. CEBALLOS, A. AND GIOIA, T. Bol. y trab. de la Soc. de cir. *11:*147–153, May 11, '27

Treatment of posttraumatic Volkmann contracture by sympathectomy and shortening of bones of forearm. DE GAETANO, L. Ann. ital. di chir. *6:* 447–479, May '27

Volkmann's contracture, case. JORGE. Boll. y trab. de la Soc. de cir. *11:*204, June 1, '27

Volkmann's contracture. LUGONES, C. Rev. med. latino-amer. *13:*39–69, Oct '27

Volkmann's syndrome: treatment by ramisection. JUARISTI, V. Rev. de chir. *6:*760–765, Dec '27

Volkmann contracture; case with surgical treatment; good results. DEFINE, D. Ann. de Fac. de med. de Sao Paulo *2:*533–551, '27

Mommsen's bloodless treatment of Volkmann's contracture. TANCREDI, G. Arch. di ortop. *43:*362–377, '27

Etiology, pathogenesis, semeiology, surgical and nonsurgical treatment of Volkmann's contracture. OLIVARES, L. Med. ibera *1:*313–319, March 24, '28

Periarterial sympathectomy in Volkmann's contracture. CAEIRO, J. A. Semana med. *1:*1185–1190, May 17, '28

Volkmann's syndrome; case; periarterial sympathectomy; permanent recovery. CEBALLOS, A. AND GIOIA, T. Bol. y trab. de la. Soc. de cir. de Buenos Aires *12:*185–191, June 6, '28

Ischemic contracture, treatment by transplantation of internal epicondyle. BAILEY, H. Brit. J. Surg. *16:*335–337, Oct '28

Volkmann's contracture, with special reference to treatment. JONES, R. Brit. M. J. *2:*639–642, Oct 13, '28

Contracture, Volkmann's – Cont.
Prognosis and treatment of Volkmann's ischemic paralysis. RANCKEN, D. Finska lak.-sallsk. handl. *71:*22–28, Jan '29
Treatment of Volkmann's ischemic paralysis; case. ALBANESE, A. Rinasc. med. *6:*181–183, April 15, '29
Volkmann's disease and syndromes of arterial obliteration in extremities. NARIO, C. V. An. de Fac. de med., Montevideo *14:*422–589, May–June '29
Volkmann's contracture. BEYER, A. R., J. Florida M. A. *15:*599–600, June '29
Volkmann's contracture. DICKSON, F. D. New Orleans M. & S. J. *82:*119–126, Sept '29
Treatment of Volkmann's contracture by transplantation of internal epicondyle. HODGSON, N. Brit. J. Surg. *17:*317–318, Oct '29
Volkmann's ischaemic contracture treated by transplantation of internal condyle. MEADE, H. S. Clin. J. *59:*8, Jan 1, '30
Volkmann's ischemic contracture. MEYERDING, H. W., S. Clin. N. Amer. *10:*49–52, Feb '30
Volkmann's contracture; case. GODOY MOREIRA, F. E. Chir. d. org. di movimento *14:*573–582, March '30
Volkmann's ischemic contracture. MEYERDING, H. W., J.A.M.A. *94:*394–400, Feb 8, '30 abstr: Gazz. d. osp. *51:*338–343, March 16, '30
Volkmann syndrome in obstetric fractures of humerus. ROCHER, H. L. Arch. franco-belges de chir. *32:*625–627, July '30
Volkmann's contracture; presentation of case with moving pictures. CARLSON, A. C. Southwestern Med. *14:*367–368, Aug '30
Volkmann's contracture. DRIVER, S. South. M. J. *23:*953–956, Oct '30
Volkmann's retraction; surgical treatment; case. DURANTE, L. Arch. ital. di chir. *25:*429–439, '30
Surgical treatment of Volkmann's contracture. HAYWARD, Med. Klin. *27:*473–474, March 27, '31
Volkmann's contracture with report of case. SHIH, H. E. Nat. M. J., China *17:*315–322, June '31
Therapy of Volkmann's contracture. HABERLER, G. Zentralbl. f. Chir. *58:*1774–1781, July 11, '31
Impending Volkmann's ischaemic contracture treated by incision of deep fascia; case. FLEMMING, C. W. Lancet *2:*293, Aug 8, '31
Pathogenesis and treatment of Volkmann contracture; ESPERABÉ Y GONZÁLEZ, J. M. Med. ibera *2:*285–294, Sept 5, '31

Contracture, Volkmann's – Cont.
Volkmann contracture. MASSABUAU, G. Rev. gen. de clin. et de therap. (no. 42, bis) *45:*691–695, Oct 21, '31
Etiology and therapy of ischemic paralysis of forearm (Volkmann contracture); 4 cases. BITTNER, W. Beitr. z. klin. Chir. *152:*510–513, '31
Volkmann's contracture. MEYERDING, H. W. Physiotherapy Rev. *12:*96–97, March–April '32
Volkmann contracture of hand; therapy by Henle operation; case. SÁNCHEZ TOLEDO, P. Cir. ortop. y traumatol. *1:*113–118, April '33
Volkmann contracture; 6 cases in children. DE ARAUJO, A. Rev. brasil. de cir. *2:*377–399, Sept '33
Ischemic Volkmann contracture. JOVČIĆ, M. Chir. narz. ruchu *6:*249–265, Sept '33
Partial resection of wrist for Volkmann contracture; case. POUZET, F. Lyon chir. *30:*581–584, Sept–Oct '33
Volkmann contracture; causes and treatment. GOLDBERG, H. Kentucky M. J. *31:*531–533, Nov '33
Therapy of Volkmann syndrome. ARNAUD, M. Marseille-med. *1:*229–232, Feb 15, '34
Volkmann contracture; clinical and pathogenetic study. ROGER, H. Marseille-med. *1:*213–228, Feb. 15, '34
Volkmann contracture. TERHUNE, S. R. J.M.A. Alabama *4:*116–117, Sept '34
Volkmann contracture. KOCH, S. L. Tr. West. S. A. *44:*222–235, '34
Volkmann syndrome; therapeutic measures; 4 cases in children. THOMAS, A. *et al.* Rev. neurol *63:*505–528, April '35
Volkmann syndrome; new technic of resection of bones of forearm (chevron osteotomy). SORREL, E. Paris med. *1:*569–573, June 15, '35
Volkmann contracture. JONES, S. G., J. Bone & Joint Surg. *17:*649–655, July '35
Volkmann's ischemic contracture associated with supracondylar fracture of humerus. MEYERDING, H. W., J.A.M.A. *106:*1139–1144, April 4, '36
Volkmann syndrome. SENEQUE, J. Prat. med. franc. *17:*427–435, Oct (A-B) '36
Muscular infarct and necrotic lesions of nerves in Volkmann syndrome; biopsy study. TAVERNIER, L. *et al.* J. de med. de Lyon *17:*815–826, Dec 20, '36
Advantages and method of surgical therapy in Volkmann contracture; case. MONTEMARTINI, G. Policlinico (sez. chir.) *44:*12–19, Jan '37
Initial lesions in Volkmann paralysis; 2

Contracture, Volkmann's – Cont.
cases. Tavernier, L. and Dechaume, J. Lyon chir. *34:*117-122, Jan-Feb '37
Volkmann contracture; case. Guilleminet, M. Lyon chir. *34:*183-187, March-April '37
Volkmann paralysis; appearance of lesions 70 hours after beginning circulatory disturbances; case. Pouzet, F. and Leclerc, G. Lyon chir. *34:*187-190, March-April '37
Volkmann syndrome limited to 2 fingers following accidental trauma; case. Corret, P. Rev. med. de Nancy *66:*184-187, Feb 15, '38
Straightening apparatus for Volkmann contracture. Corret, P. Presse med. *46:*748, May 7, '38
Elective traumatism of extensor digitorum and flexor digitorum profundus in injury to forearm; reflex inhibition of extension; infiltration of stellate ganglion; Volkmann contracture; tendinous transmutation. Froment, J. and Mallet-Guy, P. Lyon chir. *35:*623-629, Sept-Oct '38
Pathogenesis of Volkmann contracture. de Leo, F. Chir. d. org. di movimento *30:*90-105, Jan-Mar '46

Contreras, M. V. and Rocca, E. D.: Plastic aspects of neurosurgery, with special reference to use of tantalum. Arch. Soc. cirujanos hosp. *16:*353-358, Mar '46
Converse, J. M.: Corrective surgery of nasal tip. Ann. Otol., Rhin. & Laryng. *49:*895-911, Dec '40
Converse, J. M.: Orthopedic aspects of plastic surgery; early replacement of skin losses in war injuries to extremities. Proc. Roy. Soc. Med. *34:*791-799, Oct '41
Converse, J. M.: Early skin grafting in war wounds of extremities. Ann. Surg. *115:*321-335, March '42
Converse, J. M.: Face injuries in war. Tr. Am. Acad. Ophth. (1941) *46:*250-255, May-June '42
Converse, J. M.: New forehead flap for nasal reconstruction. Proc. Roy. Soc. Med. *35:*811-812, Oct '42 also: J. Larying. & Otol. *57:*508-509, Nov '42
Converse, J. M.: External skeletal fixation of mandibles. J. Oral Surg. *1:*210-214, July '43
Converse, J. M.: Emergency plastic surgery in war injuries of face. Ann. Otol., Rhin. & Laryng. *52:*637-654, Sept '43
Converse, J. M: Two plastic operations for repair of orbit following severe trauma and extensive comminuted fracture. Arch. Ophth. *31:*323 325, April '44
Converse, J. M.: Appliances for external fixation of mandible and cranial fixation of maxilla. Am. J. Orthodontics (Oral Surg. Sect.) *31:*111-112, Feb '45
Converse, J. M.: Skin graft of dorsum of hand; use of large size dermatome to obtain one-piece pattern. Ann. Surg. *121:*172-174, Feb '45
Converse, J. M.: Jaws, early and late treatment of gunshot wounds in French battle casualties in North Africa and Italy. J. Oral. Surg. *3:*112-137, April '45
Converse, J. M.; Clarke, C. D. and Guidi, H.: Repair of cranial defects by cast chip-bone grafts; preliminary report. J. Lab. & Clin. Med. *29:*546-559, May '44
Converse, J. M. and Robb-Smith, A. H. T.: Healing of surface cutaneous wounds (donor areas); analogy with healing of superficial burns. Ann. Surg. *120:*873-885, Dec '44
Converse, J. M. and Waknitz, F. W.: External skeletal fixation in fractures of mandibular angle. J. Bone & Joint Surg. *24:*154-160, Jan '42
Conway, H.: Whole-thickness grafts in correction of contractures due to burn scars; 3 cases. Ann. Surg. *109:*286-290, Feb '39
Conway, H.: Bathing trunk nevus. Surgery *6:*585-597, Oct '39
Conway, H.: Sweating function of transplanted skin. Surg., Gynec. & Obst. *69:*756-761, Dec '39
Conway, H.: Care of cleft palate. S. Clin. North America *20:*593-602, April '40
Conway, H.: Surgical management of postradiation scars and ulcers. Surgery *10:*64-84, July '41
Conway, H.: Principles of plastic surgery in treatment of malignant tumors of face. Surg., Gynec. & Obst. *74:*449-457, Feb (no. 2A) '42
Conway, H. and Coldwater, K. B. Principles in reparative plastic surgery; experiences in general hospital in tropics. Surgery *19:*437-459, April '46
Conway, J. H.: Technical details of skin grafting. Surg., Gynec. & Obst. *63:*369-371, Sept '36
Cook, C. K.: Paraffin-wax treatment of burns. Wisconsin M. J. *29:*609-613, Nov '30
Cook, J.: Treatment of parotid fistula. Lancet *1:*1239, May 30, '36
Cook, J. A. L.: Congenital atresia of posterior choanae. South African M. J. *15:*498-499, Dec 27, '41
Cook, T. J.; Royster, H. P. and Kirby, C. K.: Treatment of gunshot fractures of mandible J. Oral Surg. *3:*326-335, Oct '45
Cook, W. C (see Moore, A. T.) April '44

COONEY, E. A.: Treatment of burn shock. Bull. New England M. Center *5:*248–256, Dec '43

COONSE, G. K. *et al*: Traumatic and hemorrhagic shock; experimental and clinical study. New England J. Med. *212:*647–663, April 11, '35

COOPER, G. R.; HODGE, G. B. AND BEARD, J. W.: Enzymatic debridement (with papain-cysteine-salicylate solution) in local treatment of burns; preliminary report. Am. J. Dis. Child. *65:*909–911, June '43

COOPER, H. K.: Responsibility of orthodontist in cleft palate problem. Am. J. Orthodontics (Oral Surg. Sect.) *32:*675–683, Nov '46

COOPER, R. N.: Shock therapy. Indian Physician *1:*305–314, July '42

COPE, O.: Principles of burn therapy. J. Missouri M. A. *39:*310–314, Oct '42

COPE, O.: Symposium on management of Cocoanut Grove burns at Massachusetts General Hospital; foreword. Ann. Surg. *117:*801–802, June '43

COPE, O.: Symposium on management of Cocoanut Grove burns at Massachusetts General Hospital; treatment of surface burns. Ann. Surg. *117:*885–893, June '43

COPE, O.: Care of victims of Cocoanut Grove fire at Massachusetts General Hospital. New England J. Med. *229:*138–147, July 22, '43

COPE, O: Chemical aspects of burn therapy. J.A.M.A. *125:*731, July 8, '44

COPE, O.: Penicillin and deep burns. Bull. New England M. Center *6:*255, Dec '44

COPE, O. *et al*: Symposium on management of Cocoanut Grove burns at Massachusetts General Hospital; metabolic observations. Ann. Surg. *117:*937–958, June '43

COPE, O. AND RHINELANDER, F. W.: Symposium on management of Cocoanut Grove burns at Massachusetts General Hospital; problem of burn shock complicated by pulmonary damage. Ann. Surg. *117:*915–928, June '43

COPE, O. (see CANNON, B.) Jan '43

COPE, V. Z.: Prevention and treatment of bedsores. Brit. M. J. *1:*737–738, April 8, '39

COPEMAN, R. (see SWEEZEY, E. *et al*) Jan '44

COPP, F. A.: Case report of plastic repair of mutilating operations of lip and cheek following radical removal of carcinoma. J. Florida M. A. *12:*29–35, Aug '25

COPPEZ, J. H.: Operations on eyelids in Foville syndrome; case. J. belge de neurol. et de psychiat. *35:*206–208, April '35

COPPEZ, J. H. AND BRENTA, MME: Burns to eyes with sulfuric acid. Bull. Soc. belge d'opht., no. 72, pp. 88–100, '36

CORA ELISEHT, F.: Rhinoplasty. Rev. argent. de oto-rino-laring. *7:*301–341, Sept–Oct '38

CORA ELISEHT, F.: Rhinocele; case. Rev. Asoc. med. argent. *53:*18–19, Jan. 15–30, '39

CORA ELISEHT, F.: Cutaneous cicatrix. Prensa med. argent. *29:*1648–1654, Oct 14, '42

CORA ELISEHT, F.: Deficient respiration due to malformation of lobe of nose; surgical therapy of case. Prensa med. argent. *30:*175–179, Jan 27, '43

CORA ELISEHT, F. AND AUBONE, J.: Deformation of auricular pavilion and its surgical corrections. Rev. argent. de oto-rino-laring. *7:*411–421, Nov–Dec '38

CORA ELISEHT, F. AND BERRI, C.: Gonzalez Loza operation for removing tip of nose. Rev. Asoc. med. argent. *53:*214–215, April 15, '39

CORA ELISEHT, F.; MONTERO, J. AND CORREAS MOYA, I.: Microtia; therapeutic problem. Prensa med. argent. *31:*1671–1673, Aug 23, '44

CORA ELISEHT, F. (see GALLINO, J. A.) Dec '45

CORACHAN, M.: Basal skin grafts. Bull. et mem. Soc. nat. de chir. *59:*1185–1192, July 22, '33

CORACHAN, M.: Use of movable tubular skin graft; 2 cases. Rev. de cir. de Barcelona *10:*36–41, July–Aug '35

CORACIU, G. (see CONSTANTINESCU, M. *et al*) Jan '38

CORBET, G. G.: Infected hand followed by loss of power in extensors of fingers and thumb. Canad. M. A. J. *16:*1502, Dec '26

CORBET, G. G.: Minor injuries resulting in death (including hand). Canad. M. A. J. *20:*40–41, Jan '29

CORBETT, J. J.: Surgical relief of chronic dacryocystitis and epiphora; Dupuy-Dutemps et Bourguet technique; direct anastomosis of tear sac with nasal mucous membrane. M. J. & Rec. *128:*158–160, Aug 15, '28 also: New *England J. Med. 199:*459–461, Sept 6, '28 also: Am. J. Ophth. *11:*774–778, Oct '28

CORBETT, J. J.: Epithelioma of eyelid; case. New England J. Med. *204:*774–776, April 9, '31

CORBIN, F. R.: Fractures of malar zygoma. Mil. Surgeon *89:*750–754, Nov '41

CORDEIRO LOBATO, J.: Cicatricial atresia of nasal fossa; 5 cases. Lisboa med. *9:*155–163, Feb '32

CORDES, F. C. AND FRITSCHI, U.: Dickey operation for eyelid ptosis; results in 21 patients and 30 lids. Tr. A. Acad. Ophth. (1943) *48:*266–279, March–April '44 also: Arch. Ophth. *31:*461–468, June '44

CORDES, F. C. (see Horner, W. D.) Dec '29

CORDIER, G. AND DELMAS, A.: Relation of precervical sinus and branchial clefts. Bull. Acad. de med., Paris *126:*485–486, Oct 27–Nov 10, '42

CORDIER, P. AND COULOUMA, P.: Anatomy of hand and surgery of phlegmons of palm; new data on cellular spaces. Echo med. du nord *1:*513, April 8; April 15, '34

CORDIER, P. AND COULOUMA, P.: Anatomy of hand and surgery of phlegmons of palm; new data on cellular spaces. Echo med. du nord *1:*661–674, May 6, '34

CORDIER, P. AND COULOUMA, P.: New data on cellular space of palm; roentgen study; importance in infections. Rev. de chir., Paris *53:*563–588, Oct '34

CORDONNIER, J. J.: Fistula of penile urethra; method of repair utilizing stainless steel "pull-out" sutures. J. Urol. *55:*278–286, Mar '46

COREY, E. L.: Flashburn protection. Hosp. Corps Quart. (no. 10) *18:*27–30, Oct '45

CORLETTE. C. E.: Dupuytren's contracture. M. J. Australia *2:*177–182, Aug 19, '44

CORLETTE, C. E. AND INGLIS, K.: Epithelioma of hand, with tendency to spontaneous cure. M. J. Australia *1:*250, March 26, '21

CORNEJO SARAVIA, E.: Plastic surgery of penis; case and scrotum. Rev. de cir. *6:*662–670, Dec '27

CORNEJO SARAVIA, E.: Lateral congenital neck fistula; 2 cases. Bol. y trab. de la Soc. de cir. de Buenos Aires *17:*1224–1237 Nov. 22, '33

CORNEJO SARAVIA, E. (see BUZZI, A.) May '29

CORNELL, C. (see SMITH, B. *et al*) Oct '45

CORNET, E.: Dacryocystorhinectomy in stenoses of lacrimal sac; new technic. Rev. med. franc. d'Extreme-Orient *16:*551–554, May '38

CORNET, E.: Dacryocystorhinectomy; new technic. Ann. d'ocul. *175:*842–845, Nov '38

CORNET, J.: Recovery after late suture of flexor tendon of index finger. Scalpel *85:*1296–1297, Oct 22, '32

CORNILLON, A. AND ROJO, J. J.: Importance of good technic in therapy of fractures of lower jaw; technic proposed by authors. Gac. med. de Mexico *72:*591–597, Dec 31, '42

CORNILLOT, M. (see LAMBRET, O. *et al*) July '38

CORRADO, P. C.: Adrenal cortical hormone (preoperative administration in prevention of shock). M. Times, New York *69:*155–162, April '41

CORREA CASTILLO, H. (see VARGAS MOLINARE, R.) June '45

CORREA ITURRASPE, M.: Melanoma of skin. Dia med. *17:*1449–1454, Dec 10, '45

CORRÊA NETTO, A. AND ETZEL, E.: Acacia therapy in surgical shock. Rev. Assoc. paulista de med. *3:*244–264, Nov '33

CORREAS MOYA, I. (see CORA Eliseht, F. *et al*) Aug '44

CORREIA NETO, A. AND MONTEIRO, J.: Shock; treatment in 32nd Field Hospital, Nov. 22, 1944 to March 22, 1945, Brazilian Expeditionary Forces, North American Fifth Army. Rev. med.-cir. do Brasil (nos. 9–10) *53:*349–357, Sept–Oct, '45

CORREIA NETTO, A. AND ETZEL, E.: Shock and its therapy by gum acacia. Rev. de cir. de Sao Paulo *2:*137–148, Dec '35

CORRET, P.: Volkmann syndrome limited to 2 fingers following accidental trauma; case. Rev. med. de Nancy *66:*184–187, Feb. 15, '38

CORRET, P.: Straightening apparatus for Volkmann contracture. Presse med. *46:*748, May 7, '38

CORRET, P.: Subcutaneous rupture of long extensor tendon of thumb; case. Rev. med. de Nancy *66:*867–870, Oct 15, '38

CORSARO, J. F. (see GOODMAN, J. I.) Oct '41

CORSI, G.: Therapy of flexion contracture of leg stumps. Arch. ortop. *57:*320–340, Jul–Aug '42

CORTE, P. (see ALESSANDRINI, I. *et al*) Dec '31

COSGROVE, K. W. AND HUBBARD, W. B.: Acid and alkali burns of eyes; experimental study. Ann. Surg. *87:*89–94, Jan '28

Cosmetics

Concealment of scars (with covermark). TAMERIN, J. A. Am. J. Surg. *36:*91–92, April '37

Medicamentous cosmetics for plastic covering of grave cicatrices left by various diseases. DAUBRESSE-MORELLE, E. Rev. Franc. de dermat. et de venereol. *14:*355–362, Sept–Oct '38

COSMETTATOS, G. F.: Pathogenesis of congenital fistulas of lacrimal sac. Ann. d'ocul. *170:*594–599, July '33

COSSIO, P.: Shock and syncope in postoperative period. Dia med. *13:*1309–1313, Dec. 15, '41

COSTA, A. J.: Tumor of neuro-myo-arterial glomus in left index finger; anatomicopathologic and histologic study. Bol. y trab. de la Soc. de cir. de Buenos Aires *16:*1514–1524, Nov 30, '32

COSTA, A. J. (see BUZZI, A. *et al*) Oct '29

COSTA, O. G.: Case of keloids of unusual size. Arch. Dermat. and Syph. *48:*411–412, Oct '43

COSTE, F.; FORESTIER, J. AND MANDE, R.: Dangers of surgical interventions on joints in course of evolute period of chronic polyarthritis. Presse med. *45:*729–730, May 15, '37

COSTE, J.: Recurrence after roentgenotherapy and then after excision of epithelioma of internal angle and of upper right eyelid; case. Bull. Soc. franc. de dermat. et syph. (Reunion dernat., Lyon) *38:*501 504, April '31

COSTELLO, M. J.: How to remove superfluous hair. Hygeia *18:*584–586, July '40
COSTELLO, M. J.: Keloids and their treatment. M. Record *154:*205–207, Sept. 17, '41
COSTELLO, M. J.: Microaerophilic hemolytic streptococcus infection causing destruction of nose. J. A. M. A. *121:*36–38, Jan. 2, '43
COSTELLO, M. J. AND SHEPARD, J. H.: Supernumerary ears. Arch. Otolaryng. *29:*695–698, April '39
DE COSTER: New method of morphologic analysis in dentofacial orthopedics. Rev. de stomatol. *32*:552–564, June '30
DE COSTER, L.: Orthopedic therapy of fractures of lower jaw; new apparatuses. Rev. de stomatol. *41*:933–947, '40
COSTANTINI, AND FERRARI: Colpoplasty by modified Baldwin technic for congenital absence of vagina; case. Mem. Acad. de chir. *62*:1213–1215, Oct 28, '36
COSTANTINI, H.: Modified technic for artificial vagina. Presse med. *32*:798, Oct. 4, '24 abstr: J.A.M.A. *83*:1543, Nov 8, '24
COSTANTINI, H.: Antethoracic esophagoplasty using loop of small intestine and tubal skin graft in cicatricial inflammatory stenosis of esophagus; case. Bull. et mem. Soc. nat. de chir. *61*:1312–1315, Dec 7, '35
COSTANTINI, H.: New methods of treatment of parotid fistula; cauterization and silence cure. Afrique franc. chir., nos. 3-4, pp. 65–68, May–Aug '45
COSTANTINI, H. AND CURTILLET: É. Loss of substance of sole of foot; treatment by autoplastic grafts from ischiatic region. Rev. de chir., Paris *67*:515–539, '29
COSTANTINI, H. AND CURTILLET, É.: Bilateral spinofacial anastomosis and resection of superior cervical ganglion for bilateral facial paralysis; case. Lyon chir. *32*:291–305, May-June '35
COSTANTINI, H. AND CURTILLET, É.: Spinofacial anastomosis for bilateral traumatic facial paralysis; late results. Lyon chir. *36*:50–53, Jan-Feb '39
COSTESCU, P. AND TURAI, I.: Temporomaxillary ankylosis; resection of mandibular condyle and neck followed by recovery; 2 cases. Rev. de chir., Bucuresti *43*:405–410, May-June '40
COSTESCU, P. (see STOIAN, C.) Jan '36
CO TUI *et al:* Nutritional care of cases of extensive burns; with special reference to oral use of amino acids (amigen, hydrolyzed casein) in 3 cases. Ann. Surg. *119*:815–823, June '44
COTSAFTIS, G. G. (see: AUGÉ, A.) Feb '28
COTTALORDA, J. (see: IMBERT, L.) June '22
COTTE, G. Schubert operation for artificial vagina; case. Mem. Acad. de chir. *64;*1365–1374, Dec 14, '38
COTTE, G. AND BARDONNET: Pregnancy following surgical intervention in gynandroid with closed scrotum. Gynec. et obst. *44*:12, '44
COTTENOT, P.: Treatment of vascular nevi in children with roentgen and radium therapy. Med. inf. *37*:72–83, March '30 also: J. de med. de Paris *50*:376–378, May 1, '30
COTTER, A. P. AND KIMBELL, N. K. B.: Tannic acid-silver nitrate in burns. New Zealand M. J. *34*:384–388, Dec '35
COTTINI, G. F.: Surgical correction of facial paralysis; results in cases. Bol. y trab., Soc. argent. de cirujanos *6*:443–448, '45
COTTLE, G. F.: Avulsion of scrotum, left testicle and sheath of penis. U. S. Nav. M. Bull. *20*:457–460, April '24
COTTLE, G. F.: Diathermy in shock; case. U. S. Nav. M. Bull. *25*:340–343, April '27
COTTLE, M. H.: Nasal septal surgery in children. Illinois M. J. *75*:161–163, Feb '39
COTTLE, M. H. AND LORING, R. M.: Corrective surgery of external pyramid and septum for restoration of normal physiology. Illinois M. J. *90*:119–131, Aug '46
COTTON, F. J.: Scar excision; two-stage flap-graft. S. Clin. N. Amer. *1*:904, June '21
COTTON, F. J.: Technic of fat grafts. New England J. Med. *211*:1051–1053, Dec 6, '34
COTTON, F. J.: AND BERG, R. Two-stage pedicle graft to replace unsatisfactory scar. New England J. Med. *201*:981–982, Nov 14, '29
COTTON, F. J.; MORRISON, G. M. AND BRADFORD, C. H.: De Quervain's disease; radial styloid tendovaginitis. New England J. Med. *219*:120–123, July 28, '38
COTTON, F. J. AND SAWYER, E. J.: Stiff fingers. Boston M. and S. J. *186*:183–185, Feb 9, '22 (illus.)
COUCEIRO, A.: So-called retraction of palmar aponeurosis; case. Neurobiologia *3*:396–403, Dec '40
COUCH, H.: Identical Dupuytren's contracture in identical twins. Canad. M. A. J. *39*:225–226, Sept '38
COUCH, JOHN H.: *Surgery of the Hand.* Univ. Toronto Press, Toronto, 1939
COUCH, J. H.: Principles of tendon suture. Canad. M. A. J. *41*:27–30, July '39
COUDANE, R. AND FABRE, A.: Complete thyroglossal fistula; 2 cases. Ann. d'oto-laryng, pp. 93–99, July–Sept '44
COUGHLIN, W. T.: Cartilage transplantation. Southern M. J. *14*:311, April '21
COUGHLIN, W. T.: Injuries to face and jaws. Southwestern Med. *6*:356–359, Oct '22

COUGHLIN, W. T.: Ununited fracture of mandible. S. Clin. N. America *2*:1609–1626, Dec '22 (illus.)

COUGHLIN, W. T.: Cranioplasty with cartilage. S. Clin. N. America *2*:1627–1636, Dec '22 (illus.)

COUGHLIN, W. T.: Repair of defects about chin, from standpoint of general surgeon. J.A.M.A. *83*:989–993, Sept 27, '24

COUGHLIN, W. T.: New procedure for relief of facies scaphoidea-dish face. Surg., Gynec. and Obst. *40*:109–111, Jan '25

COUGHLIN, W. T.: New treatment for undeveloped lower jaw. J.A.M.A. *84*:419–421, Feb 7, '25

COUGHLIN, W. T.: Sarcoma of nasal bones; subtotal removal of nose and its reconstruction. Arch. Otolaryng. *7*:588–600, June '28

COUGHLIN, W. T.: Jaw fractures. J. Missouri M. A. *25*:292–296, July '28

COUGHLIN, W. T.: Contractures due to burns. Surg., Gynec. and Obst. *68*:352–361, Feb (no. 2A) '39

COULANCE, (see ROGER, H. *et al*) April '28

COULLAUD.: "Godets" method of dermo-epidermic graft. Bull. et mem. Soc. nat. de chir. *53*:389–405, March 19, '27

COULOUMA, P. (see CORDIER, P.) April '34

COULOUMA, P. (see CORDIER, P.) May '34

COULOUMA, P. (see CORDIER, P.) Oct '34

COUNSELLER, V. S.: Congenital anomalies with particular reference to cryptorchidism, hypospadias and congenital absence of vagina (surgical treatment). J. Michigan M. Soc. *37*:689–697, Aug '38

COUNSELLER, V. S.: Congenital absence and traumatic obliteration of vagina and its treatment with inlaying Thiersch grafts. Am. J. Obst. and Gynec. *36*:632–638, Oct '38

COUNSELLER, V. S.: New surgical treatment for congenital absence and traumatic obliteration of vagina (skin grafting). S. Clin. North America *19*:1047–1052, Aug '39

COUNSELLER, V. S. AND PALMER, B. M.: Avulsion of skin of penis and scrotum. S. Clin. N. Amer. *9*:993–996, Aug '29

COUNSELLER, V. S. AND SLUDER, F. S.: Artificial vagina in treatment for congenital absence. S. Clin. North America *24*:938–942, Aug '44

COUNSELLER, V. S.: (see CABOT, H. *et al*) April '35

COUREAUD.: Accident from compressed air; hand shattered with bony lesions and open fracture of forearm; conservative treatment. Bull. et mem. Soc. nat. de chir. *55*:1374–1377, Dec 21, '29

COURI, A. A.: Case of exstrophy of bladder. An. brasil. de ginec. *16*:335–347, Nov 43

COURNAND, A. *et al:* Clinic use of concentrated human serum albumin; comparison with whole blood and with rapid saline infusion. J. Clin. Investigation *23*:491–505, July '44

COURTICE, F. C.: Effect of local temperature (application of cold) on fluid loss in thermal burns. J. Physiol. *104*:321–345, Jan 15, '46

COURTIS, B. (see ARGANARAZ, R. *et al*) 1938

COURTNEY, J. E.: Management of acute hand infections. Nebraska M. J. *25*:299–301, Aug '40

COURTY, L.: Syndrome due to serious burns. Rev. gen. de clin. et de therap. *54*:73–77, Feb 17, '40

COURTY, L.: Modern therapy of burns. Dia med. *12*:829–830, Sept 9, '40

COUTARD, H.: Results of roentgenotherapy of cancer of larynx after 5 and 10 years of control. J. de radiol. et d'electrol. *21*:402–409, Sept '37

COUTINHO, A.: Ankylosis of jaws, correction by bilateral resection; case. Rev. brasil. de cir. *2*:469–479, Nov '33

COUTINHO, A.: Unilateral hyperplasia of breast in virgin; study apropos of case treated with plastic surgery. An. brasil. de ginec. *16*:20–27, July '43

COUTINHO, A.: War burns and their therapy. Rev. med. de Pernambuco *13*:175–190, Aug '43

COUTO, DEOLINDO: Ascending neuropathy due to injury of hand; predominance and unusual nature of trophic phenomena. Cultura med. *3*:355–370, Feb '42

COVALI, N. AND TROOMAIER, C.: Multiple open fractures of cranial and facial bones; 2 cases with recovery after operation. Rev. de chir., Bucuresti *41*:284–287, March-April '38

COVALI, N.: (see CONSTANTINESCU, M.) March–April '40

COVARRUBIAS ZENTENO, R.: Guillies-Filatov tubal graft used to replace loss of substance of thigh; case. Rev. med. de Chile *67*:903–907, Aug '39

COVARRUBIAS ZENTENO, R.: Year's work in plastic surgery. Rev. med. de Chile *68*:227–237, March '40

COVARRUBIAS ZENTENO, R.: Ectropion and its therapy. Rev. med. de Chile *68*:1187–1190, Sept '40

COVARRUBIAS ZENTENO, R.: Rhinoplasties by Italian and Hindu methods. Rev. med. de Chile *68*:1331–1346, Oct '40

COVARRUBIAS ZENTENO, R.: Grafts using Padgett dermatome. Rev. med. de Chile *71*:729–741, Aug '43

COVARRUBIAS ZENTENO, R.: Scalping treated

with free skin grafts. Arch. Soc. cirujanos hosp. *13*:115–118, Sept '43

Covarrubias Zenteno, R.: Thoracofacial synechia following burn; case. Rev. med. de Chile *71*:899–901, Sept '43

Covarrubias Zenteno, R.: Reparative surgery in the war. Arch. Soc. cirujanos hosp. *14*:49–56, March '44

Covarrubias Zenteno, R.: Large skin grafts in surgery. Arch. Soc. cirujanos hosp. *14*:303–305, March '44

Covarrubias Zenteno, R.: Cheiloplasties. Rev. med. de Chile *72*:696–698, Aug '44

Cowell, E.: Pathology and treatment of traumatic (wound) shock. Proc. Roy. Soc. Med. (War Sect.) *21*:39–46, July '28 also: J. Roy. Army M. Corps *51*:81–102, Aug '28

Cowell, E. M.: Prevention and treatment of shock. Brit. M. J. *1*:883–885, April 29, '39

Cowell, E. M. (see Mitchiner, P. H.) Jan '39

Cowell, E. M. (see Mitchiner, P. H.) March '39

Cowen, S. B.: Dacryocystorhinoplasty, Mosher's modification of Toti method. Ohio State M. J. *21*:902–905, Dec '25

Cowles, A. G.: Agenesis of vagina (surgical treatment). Texas State J. Med. *35*:685–688, Feb '40

Cowley Campodonico, R.: Tannic acid therapy of decubitus ulcers. Rev. de med. y cir. de la Habana *40*:555–557, Oct 31, '35

Cox, F. J.; Parnell, H. S. and Sobatier, J. A.: New type of hand dressing to improve function. M. Bull. Mediterranean Theat. Op. *2*:168–169, Dec '44

Cox, G. H.: Treatment of nasal fractures. M. Times and Long Island M. J. *62*:171–175, June '34

Cox, G. H.: Correction of recent and old nasal fractures. Laryngoscope *45*:188–197, March '35

Cox, G. H.: Treatment of facial bone fractures. New York State J. Med. *37*:52–58, Jan. 1, '37

Cox, G. H.: Deformities of ear and nose treated by plastic surgery. New York State J. Med. *39*:1956–1961, Oct 15, '39

Cox, G. H.: Surgery of auricle, including total reconstruction and protuberant ears. Laryngoscope *51*:791–797, Aug '41

Cox, L. B. and Maclure, A. F.: Facial hemiatrophy, with description of 3 cases. Australian and New Zealand J. Surg. *5*:68–76, July '35

Cozen, L.: New banjo splint (for extension of contractures of metacarpophalangeal and interphalangeal joints). Mil. Surgeon *85*:67–68, July '39

Crabtree, W. C.: Rhinophyma. California and West. Med. *45*:485–487, Dec '36

Craddock, F. H. and Whetstone, G.: Diathermy in treatment of shock. South. M. J. *19*:812–813, Nov '26

Craddock, F. H. Jr.: Treatment of extensive burns, with report of case. J.M.A.Alabama *14*:236–239, April '45

Crafoord, C. and Linton, P.: Pedicled muscle flap in treatment of bronchial fistulas; 16 cases. J. Thoracic Surg. *9*:606–611, Aug '40

Cragg, B. H. (see Gordon, S.) Oct '44

Craig, W. M.: War wounds of peripheral nerves. U. S. Nav. M. Bull. *41*:613–624, May '43

Craig, W. M.: Surgical shock. J. Internat. Coll. Surgeons *7*:103–106, March-April '44

Craig, W. M. (see Steenrod, E. J. *et al*) May '37

Cramer, F. E. K.: Technical difficulties and complications of dacryocystorhinostomy by external route. Semana med. *2*:604–610, Sept 9, '43

Cramer, F. E. K. and Balza, J.: New drills for dacryocystorhinostomy. Semana med. *1*:294–295, Jan 30, '41

Cramer, F. J. (see Woodhall, B.) Nov '45

Cran, B. S.: Unsuspected chronic bronchiectasis from inhalation of fragment of bone—unusual sequel to comminuted fracture of nasal bones. J. Laryng and Otol. *48*:821–823, Dec '33

Crane, G. L. (see Brown, C. E.) July '43

Craniofacial Deformity (See also Apert's Syndrome; Crouzon's Syndrome; Hypertelorism)

Scaphocephaly, oxycephaly and hypertelorism, with reports of cases. Ogilvie, A. G. and Posel, M. M. Arch. Dis. Childhood *2*:146–154, June '27

Acrocephalic dysostosis; study of cranium of patient with acrocephalosyndactylia. Apert, and Regnault, F. Bull. et mem. Soc. med. d. hop. de Paris *53*:832–835, July 1, '29

Sincipital hydro-encephalocele with deformity of nose. Bender, E. Arch. f. klin. Chir. *161*:625–632, '30

Anatomic examination of human hemicephalic fetus 10 months old with harelip, cleft palate, hyperdactylia, syndactylia, etc. Ikeda, Y. Arb. a. d. anat. Inst. d. kaiserlich-japan. Univ. zu Sendai, Hft. 15, pp. 61–212, '33

Arhinencephalia with incomplete development of nose; case. Henze, K. Beitr. z. prakt. u. theoret. Hals-, Nasen-u. Ohrenh. *31*:241–247, '34

Craniofacial Deformity – Cont.

Cranial deformities due to premature synosteoses of sutures with particular reference to Crouzon's disease (craniofacial dysostoses) and Apert syndrome (acrocephaly and syndactylia). MASTROMARINO, A. Arch. di ortop. *51*:233–304, June 30, '35

Craniofacial hemihypertrophy; case. LEREBOULLET, P. AND ECTORS, MME. M. L. Arch. de med. d. enf. *39*:37–39, Jan '36

Spina bifida and cranium bifidium; unusual nasopharyngeal encephalocele (with cleft palate). INGRAHAM F. D. AND MATSON, D. D. New England J. Med. *228*:815–820, June 24, '43

Atypical craniofacial dysostosis associated with atrophy of optic nerve. MORONE, G. Arch. ottal. *50*:45–74, Mar–Apr '46

Premature synostosis in children. EXPOSITO, L. Rev. cubana pediat. *18*:497–508, Aug '46

Craniofacial Injuries

Complete separation of facial bones from base of skull. ASPINALL, A., M. J. Australia *1*:292–294, March 17 '23 (illus.)

Craniofacial disjunction; case. BERTRAND, P. AND FREIDEL, C. Lyon chir. *30*:632–634, Sept–Oct '32

Nasal fractures in connection with fracture of facial cranium. CSILLAG, S. Monatschr. f. Ohrenh. *68*:663–669, June '34 also: Orvosi hetil. *78*:586–588, June 30, '34

Therapy of scalping wounds. (head) SOLOVEV, A. G. Sovet. khir. (no. 6) *6*:805–813, '34

Traumatic craniofacial disjunctions; clinical study. FREIDEL, C. *et al*. J. de chir. *51*:27–43, July '37

Fracture of skull involving paranasal sinuses. COLEMAN, C. C. J.A.M.A. *109*:1613–1616, Nov 13, '37

Fracture of skull involving paranasal sinuses and mastoids. COLEMAN, C. C. Tr. Sect. Laryng., Otol. and Rhin., A. M. A., pp. 58–67, '37

Therapy of fractures of cranial base involving nasal sinuses. NATHANSON, G. Acta otolaryng. *25*:430–439, '37

Multiple open fractures of cranial and facial bones; 2 cases with recovery after operation. COVALI, N. AND TROCMAIER, C. Rev. de chir., Bucuresti *41*:284–287, March–April '38

Craniofacial disjunction; case. BOBBIO, A. Boll. e mem. Soc. piemontese di chir. *8*:515–520, '38

Fracture of upper maxilla associated with

Craniofacial Injuries – Cont.

extensive trauma of left half of forehead, injury to right optic canal and blindness of right eye; case. SVERDLOV, D. G. AND GOLDIN, L. B. Vestnik oftal. *12*:515–516, '38

Burn of cranium due to electric current; rare case. MUNOZ ARENOS, J. M. Semana med. espan. *3*:1070–1073, Aug 31, '40

Multiple fractures of skull complicated by fractures of jaws. GARFIN, S. W. Am. J. Surg. *52*:460–465, June '41

Total craniofacial disjunction; case. DUFOURMENTEL, L. Bull. et mem. Soc. d. chirurgiens de Paris *32*:69–71, '41

Reduction of faciocranial fractures. SMITH, G. C., J. Missouri M. A. *39*:178–180, June '42

Plastic surgery in case of severe wound of cranium and face. DE VASCONCELOS MARQUES, A. Amatus *1*:612–615, July '42

Immediate covering of denuded area of skull. DORRANCE, G. M. AND BRANSFIELD, J. W. Am. J. Surg. *58*:236–239, Nov '42

Proposal to prevent necrosis of tabula externa of skull denuded of periosteum (scalping). ENGEL, D. Brit. M. J. *1*:185, Feb 5, '44

Management of jaw fractures complicated by intracranial injuries. KINGSBURY, B. C., U. S. Nav. M. Bull. *42*:915–920, April '44

Treatment of denuded external table of skull. CLARKSON, P. AND SCHORSTEIN, J. Brit. M. J. *2*:422–423, Sept 29, '45

Management of orbitocranial wounds. WEBSTER, J. E. *et al*. J. Neurosurg. *3*:329–336, July '46

Cranioplasty (*See also Bone Grafts to Skull*)

Comparison of various methods of repair of gaps in skull. MAUCLAIRE, P. Maris med. *11*:153, Feb. 19, '21 abstr: J.A.M.A. *76*:1049, April 9, '21

Costochondral graft for repair of skull defects. HANSON, A. M. *et al*. Mil. Surgeon *48*:691, June '21

Method of cranioplasty using as a graft one-half the thickness of bony part of rib. BALLIN, M. Surg., Gynec. and Obst. *33*:79, July '21

Repair of bony defects of cranium. SHUTTLEWORTH, C. B. Canad. M. A. J. *11*:562, Aug '21

Cranioplasty with cartilage. COUGHLIN, W. T., S. Clin. N. America *2*:1627–1636, Dec '22 (illus.)

Operation of cartilage-cranioplasty. MUNROE, A. R. Canad. M. A. J. *14*:47–49, Jan '24

Cranioplasty – Cont.
Costo-chondral graft for the repair of skull defects. HANSON, A. M. Minnesota Med. *7*:610–612, Sept '24
Case of successful grafting of ribs into skull for cranial defect. LEVIN, J. J., M. J. South Africa *20*:61–63, Oct '24
Separate tangentially cut bone-periosteum flaps from tibia to close gap in skull. BUFALINI, M. Arch. ital. di chir. *12*:529–554, '25
Bone grafting for cranial defect; cases. LEVIN, J. J., M. J. S. Africa *21*:283–284, May '26
Closure of cranial openings by cartilaginous autotransplantation. PASCALIS, G. Gaz. d. hop. *100*:1314–1316, Oct 5, '27
Technic of temporary craniectomy and of plastics in cranium defects. SOKOLOV, V. Vestnik khir. (no. 32) *11*:115–116, Nov 5, '27
Cranioplasty by split rib method. BROWN, R. C., J. Coll. Surgeons, Australasia *1*:238–246, Nov '28
Skull defects repaired by tibial grafts. HADLEY, F. A., J. Coll. Surgeons, Australasia *1*:208–213, Nov '28
Cranioplasty with autografts of elastic cartilage; experiments. MAIRANO, M. AND VIRANO, G. Clin. chir. *32*:1687–1705, Dec '29
Successful experimental substitution of cartilage fixed in alcohol for loss of cranial substance. BLAVET DI BRIGA, C. Arch. per. le sc. med. *54*:63–70, Jan '30
Cranioplasty with osseous grafts for large loss of substance of frontal bone; case. TILLIER, R. Bull. et mem. Soc. nat. de chir. *56*:1277–1282, Nov 29, '30
Use of portion of scapula to fill bony defects of cranium. ILLYIN, G. A. Vestnik khir. (nos. 68-69) *23*:84–94, '31
Plastic surgery for extensive loss of bony substance of cranium after passage of electric current; case. LEOTTA. Arch. ed atti d. Soc. ital. di chir. *37*:633–639, '31
Plastic method of repairing defects in soft coverings of cranium due to trauma. FLICK, K. AND TRAUM, E. Zentralbl. f. Chir. *59*:908–909, April 2, '32
Late results of cranioplasty by hinging method of bone grafts. MAYET. Bull. et mem. Soc. d. chirurgiens de Paris *24*:138–140, Feb 19, '32
Osteoplastic restoration of skull. M. J. Australia *2*:269–270, Aug 27, '32
Dead bone grafts to repair skull defects. PANKRATIEV, B. E. Ann. Surg. *97*:321–326, March '33
Repair of skull defects by new pedicle bone-

Cranioplasty – Cont.
graft operation. JONES, R. W. Brit. M. J. *1*:780–781, May 6, '33
Technic of plastic repair of cranium. SOBOL, I. Rev. oto-neuro-oftal. *8*:351–355, Oct '33
Autoplastic covering of cranial defects by transplants from iliac crest. LEXER, E. W. Deutsche Ztschr. f. Chir. *239*:743–749, '33
Cranioplasty by sterilized grafts from human cadaver. DAMBRIN, L. AND DAMBRIN, P. Bordeaux chir. *7*:279–286, July '36
Cranial prosthesis and restoration of nose in fractures of nose and frontal part of cranium. PONT, A. Rev. de chir. structive, pp. 34–37, March '37
Cranioplasty using parallel split costal grafts (protective grille). FAGARASANU, I. Tech. chir. *29*:57–64, May–June '37
Treatment of acquired defects of skull (especially use of celluloid plates). PRINGLE, J. H. Brit. M. J. *2*:1105–1107, Dec 4, '37
Plastic surgery in loss of bone substance of cranium. ZENO, L. An. de cir. *4*:16–18, March '38
Buried grafts used to repair depressions in brow, eye socket, skull and nose. PEER, L. A., J. M. Soc. New Jersey *35*:601–605, Oct '38
Plastic reconstruction of osseous defects of cranium; surgical therapy of early traumatic epilepsy. BÜRKLE-DE LA CAMP, H. Zentralbl. f. Chir. *65*:2578–2584, Nov 19, '38
Repair of cranial defects with celluloid. NEY, K. W. Am. J. Surg. *44*:394–399, May '39
Plastic use of crest of ilium in repair of loss of substance of cranium. KLAGES, F. Zentralbl. f. Chir. *66*:1580–1587, July 15, '39
Possibility of repairing loss of bony substance of cranium by means of graft of bladder mucosa. BEZZA, P. Arch. ital. di chir. *55*:405–429, '39
Types of buried grafts used to repair deep depressions of cranium. PEER, L. A. J.A.M.A. *115*:357–360, Aug 3, '40
Use of iliac bone in facial and cranial repair. SHEEHAN, J. E. Am. J. Surg. *52*:55–61, April '41
Cranial depressions; plastic surgery, with report of cases. BABBINI, R. J. *et al.* Bol. Soc. de cir. de Rosario *8*:299–339, Oct '41 also: Rev. argent. de neurol. y psiquiat. *6*:221–250, Dec '41
Diced cartilage grafts; new method for repair of skull defects. PEER, L. A. Arch. Otolaryng. *38*:156–165, Aug '43
Repair of cranial defects by cast chip-bone grafts; preliminary report. CONVERSE, J. M.; *et al.* J. Lab. and Clin. Med. *29*:546–559, May '44

Cranioplasty—Cont.

Plastic closure of defect of cranium; case report illustrating use of tantalum plate and pedicle-tube graft. HARRIS, M. H. AND WOODHALL, B. Surgery *17*:422–428, March '45

Management of extensive defects in craniocerebral injuries. BALKIN, S. G. *et al.* J.A.M.A. *128*:70–72, May 12, '45

Cranioplasty with tantalum, case. MOUNT, L. A. Rev. argent. de neurol. y psiquiat. *10*:127–131, June '45

Extradural pneumatocele following tantalum cranioplasty. WOODHALL, B. AND CRAMER, F. J., J. Neurosurg. *2*:524–529, Nov '45

Tantalum cranioplasty. BAKODY, J. T. Ohio State M. J. *42*:29–33, Jan '46

Cranioplasty; metallic inserts.WOOLF, J. I. AND WALKER, A. E. Rev. oto-neuro-oftal. *21*:16–18 Jan–Feb '46

Repair of defects with special reference to use of tantalum in cranium. VORIS, H. C., S. Clin. North America *26*:33–55, Feb '46

Rebuilding bony depressions of face and skull. BERSON, M. I., J. Internat. Coll. Surgeons *9*:243–247, Mar–Apr '46

Repair of defects, with special reference to use of cancellous bone in cranium. CARMODY, J. T. B. New England J. Med. *234*:393–399, March 21, '46

Use of tantalum for repair of defects in infected cases in cranium. GARDNER, W. J. Cleveland Clin. Quart. *13*:72–87, Apr '46

Cranioplasty with acrylic plates. ELKINS, C. W. AND CAMERON, J. E., J. Neurosurg. *3*:199–205, May '46

Repair of defects by bone grafting (especially from ilium) in cranium. MONEY, R. A. Surgery *19*:627–650, May '46

Tantalum cranioplasty. TURNER, O. A. Ohio State M. J. *42*:604–607, June '46

Failure in early secondary repair of cranial defects with tantalum. BRADFORD, F. K. AND LIVINGSTON, K. E., J. Neurosurg. *3*:318–328, July '46

Experimental observations on use of stainless steel for cranioplasty; comparison with tantalum. SCOTT, M. AND WYCIS, H. T., J. Neurosurg. *3*:310–317, July '46

Cranioplasty with tantalum plate in postwar period. BAKER, G. S., S. Clinics North America *26*:841–845, Aug '46

Problems in late management of craniocerebra injuries, with special reference to repair of defects with tantalum plate; analysis of 170 cases SPIEGEL, I. J. Am. J. Surg. *72*:448–467, Sept '46

Use of tantalum for cranioplasties; further studies. FULCHER, O. H. U. S. Nav. M. Bull *46*:1493–1498 Oct '46

Simplified technic for fabrication of tantalum plates in cranial surgery. GERRY, R. G., U. S. Nav. M. Bull *46*:1499–1505, Oct '46

Cranium, Osteomyelitis of

Septic osteomyelitis of bones of skull and face; plea for conservative treatment. BLAIR, V. P. AND BROWN, J. B. Ann. Surg. *85*:1–26, Jan '27

Cranium, Tumors of

Cirsoid craniofacial angiomas; cases. DUFOURMENTEL, L. Bull. et mem. Soc. d. chirurgiens de Paris *28*:103–109, March 6, '36

Orbitotemporal osteoma with exorbitism in syphilitics, with report of cases. CHAVANY, J. A. Presse med. *53*:702, Dec 22, '45

CRAVIOTTO, M. (see MARINO, H.) April '40

CRAVIOTTO, M. (see MARINO, H.) Sept '46

CRAWFORD, J. K. (see ADAMS, W. M.) May '42

CRAWFORD, M. J.: Applicances and attachments for treatment of upper jaw fractures. U. S. Nav. M. Bull. *41*:1151–1157, July '43

CRAWFORD, T. (see GRIFFITHS, D. L.) March '45

CREEVY, C. D.: Operative treatment of hypospadias, with report of 13 cases. Surgery *3*:719–731, May '38

CREEVY, C. D.: Straightening hypospadiac penis. Surgery *8*:777–780, Nov '40

CREMER, G.: Carbon dioxide snow in therapy of hemangioma. Nederl. tijdschr. v. geneesk. *84*:520–524, Feb. 10, '40

CREMER, H. D.: Chemical research on traumatic shock. Deut. Militararzt 7:79, Feb '42 also: Bull. War Med. *3:*150–151, Nov. '42 (abstract)

CRESCENZI, G.: Urethral fistulas in women. Policlinico (sez. chir.) *30*:497–502, Oct '23

CRESPI, R. A.: Treatment of perforations and fissures in hard and soft palates. Semana med. *1*:666–683, April 1, '26; *1*:710–723, April 8; *1*:755–776, April 15, '26

CRESPI, R. A.: Treatment of perforations and fissures of palate and soft palate. Semana med. *1*:666; 710; 755, '27

CRESPI REGHIZZI, A.: Injuries of external and middle ear in lightning stroke, clinical study of case. Arch. ital. di otol. *52*:49–60, Feb '40

CRESSMAN, R. D. AND BLALOCK, A.: Prevention and treatment of surgical shock. Am. J. Surg. *46*:417–425, Dec '39

CRESSMAN, R. D. (see BLALOCK, A.) Feb '39

CREWE, J. E.: Aloes in treatment of burns and scalds. Minnesota Med. *22*:538–539, Aug '39

CREYSSEL, J. AND SAUTOT, J.: Fibrous tumor developing on laparotomy cicatrix; case. Lyon chir. *41*:67–68, Jan–Feb '46

CREYSSEL, J. AND SUIRE, P.: Traumatic shock of war wounded. J. de med. de Lyon *21*:83–96, March 5, '40

CREYSSEL, J. AND SUIRE, P.: Traumatic shock of war wounded; bilateral procaine hydrochloride infiltration of carotid sinus; case. Mem. Acad. de chir. *66*:762–765, Nov 6–20, '40

CREYSSEL, J. AND SUIRE, P.: Bilateral procaine hydrochloride infiltration of carotid sinus region in therapy of traumatic shock. Lyon chir. *37*:101–104, '41–'42

CREYSSEL, J. (see: BÉRARD, L.) March '30

CRICH, W. A.: Double fracture of mandible predisposed by impacted third molar. Canad. M. A. J. *19*:207–210, Aug '28

CRIGLER, C. M.: Urologic complications following operation for imperforate hymen (use of bladder to form artificial vagina). J. Urol. *56*:211–222, Aug '46

CRILE, G.: Energy background of genesis of gallstones and of prevention of immediate postoperative shock. Surg., Gynec. and Obst. *60*:818–825, April '35

Crile, G.

- Ideas of Dr. Crile on operative shock and their clinical application. DE NECKER, J. Arch. franco-belges de chir. *27*:411–421, May '24
- Shockless surgery; Crile's contribution to humanity and to the medical profession; with simple and dependable method of preparation of patient for same; and remarks. SMYTHE, F. D., J. Tennessee M. A. *16:*313–317, Jan '24

CRILE, G. JR.: Burn therapy. M. Clin. North America *19*:1941–1947, May '36

CRILE, G. W.: Carcinoma of jaws, tongue, cheek, and lips; general principles involved in operations and results obtained at Cleveland Clinic. Surg., Gynec. and Obst. *36*:159–162, Feb '23 (illus.)

CRIMMINS, M. L.: Treatment of shock in rattlesnake bites. Texas State J. Med. *26*:449–450, Oct '30

CRIMMINS, M. L.: Therapy of shock in rattlesnake bites. Mil. Surgeon *69*:42–44, July '31

CRISP, N. W.: Toxemia producing shock after operation; report of case. Proc. Staff Meet., Mayo Clin. *5:*128, May 7, '30

CRISTODULO (see THEODORESCO, D.) July–Aug '38

CRITCHLEY, M. AND GILLIES, H.: Treatment of facial paralysis. Tr. M. Soc. London *60:*166–171, '37

CROCE, E. J.; SCHULLINGER, R. N., AND SHEARER, T. P.: Operative treatment of decubitus ulcer. Ann. Surg. *123:*53–69, Jan '46

CROCQUEFER: Use of cranial supports in reduction of fractures of mandibular angle. Rev. de stomatol *34:*347–351, June '32

CROCQUEFER: Fissural cyst of cheek; case. Rev. de stomatol. *37:*513–518, Aug '35

CROFT, P. B. AND PETERS, R. A.: Effect of methionine upon nitrogen losses in urine following severe burns. Nature, London *155:*175–176, Feb 10, '45

CRON, R. S. (see DAVIS, C. H.) Feb '28

CRONIN, T. D.: Plastic surgery field. M. Rec. and Ann. *36:*260–264, March '42

CRONIN, T. D.: Syndactylism; correction. Tri-State M. J. *15:*2869, Jan '43

CRONK, F. Y.: Injuries to small bones of hand and wrist. J. Oklahoma M. A. *19:*64–66, March '26

CRONKITE, E. P.; LOZNER, E. L. AND DEAVER, J. M.: Use of thrombin and fibrinogen in skin grafting; preliminary report. J.A.M.A. *124:*976–978, April 1, '44

CRONKITE, E. P. (see DEAVER, J. M. *et al*) May '44

CROOKE, A. C.; MORRIS, C. J. O. R. AND BOWLER, R. G.: General anesthesia in shock. Brit. M. J. *2:*683–686, Nov 25, '44

CROQUEVIELLE G., A. (see CASANUEVA DEL C., M.) Jan '42

CROSBY, E. H. AND GALASINSKI, R. E.: New arthroplasty for small joints. Connecticut M. J. *9:*926–928, Dec '45

CROSS, C. D. (see KOHN, F. *et al*) Jan '43

CROSS, G. H.: Plastic repair of eyelids by pedunculated skin grafts. J.A.M.A. *77:*1233, Oct 15, '21

CROSSMAN, L. W. AND SAFFORD, F. K. JR.: Refrigeration in burns. Mod. Hosp. *64:*90, Feb '45

CROSSMAN, L. W. (see ALLEN, F. M. *et al*) May '43

CROSTI, A.: Transplantation of skin cancer by use of superficial grafts of epidermis covering epithelioma. Gior. ital. di dermat. e sif. *79:*1091–1108, Dec '38

CROUZON, O.: Hereditary craniofacial dysostosis and its relations with acrocephalosyndactylia. Bull. et mem. Soc. med. d. hop. de Paris *48:*1568–1574, Dec 12, '32

CROUZON, O.; BOURGUIGNON, G. AND CHRISTOPHE, J.: Subcutaneous rupture of extensor pollicis longus simulating partial radial paralysis; case. Bull. et mem. Soc. med. d. hop. de Paris *48:*1043–1046, June 27, '32

CROUZON, O. (see REGNAULT, F.) May '30

Crouzon's Syndrome

Craniofacial dysostosis and multiple malformations. MACERA, J. M. AND FEIGUES, I. Semana med. *2:*793–800, Sept. 12, '29

Isolated case of craniofacial dysostosis (Crouzon's disease) with ectrodactylia. GARCIN, R.; *et al*. Bull. et mem. Soc. med. d. hop. de Paris *48:*1458–1466, Nov 28, '32

Hereditary craniofacial dysostosis and its relations with acrocephalosyndactylia. CROUZON, O. Bull. et mem. Soc. med. d. hop. de Paris *48:*1568–1574, Dec 12, '32

Craniofacial dysostosis (dyscephaly, Crouzon's disease) associated with syndactylia of 4 extremities (dyscephalodactylia). VOGT, A. Klin. Monatsbl. f. Augenh. *90:*441–454, April '33

Isolated case of craniofacial dysostosis (Crouzon's disease) with ectrodactylia. GARCIN, R.; *et al*. Arch. de med. d. enf. *36:*359–365, June '33

Cranial deformities due to premature synostoses of sutures with particular reference to Crouzon's disease (craniofacial dysostoses) and Apert syndrome (acrocephaly and syndactylia). MASTROMARINO, A. Arch. di ortop. *51:*233–304, June 30, '35

Craniofacial dysostosis with hypertelorism in congenital syphilis; case. TOURAINE, A.; *et al*. Bull. Soc. franc. de dermat. et syph. *43:*612–618, March '36

Craniofacial dysostosis and congenital malformation of hands; case. KOSTEČKA, F. Ztschr. f. Stomatol. *35:*113–120, Jan 9, '37

Pneumatization of bones of face in Crouzon's disease, Apert's syndrome and oxycephaly; 13 cases. DE GUNTEN, P. Schweiz. med. Wchnschr. *68:*268–270, March 12, '38

Crouzon's disease (craniofacial dysostosis); case. OSORIO, L. A. An. Fac. de med. de Porto Alegre (fasc. 2) *5:*98–99, July–Dec '44

Craniofacial dysostosis; significance of ocular hypertelorism. BROWN, A. AND HARPER, R. A. K. Quart. J. Med. *15:*171–181, July '46

CROW, I. N.: Branchial cysts. J. Iowa M. Soc. *15:*524–528, Oct '25

CRUICKSHANK, J. N.: Persistent cloaca with imperforate anus as a cause of foetal ascites. Brit. M. J. *2:*980, Dec 10, '21

CRUICKSHANK, M. M.: New eyelid clamp. Indian M. Gaz. *67:*82–83, Feb '32 also: Am. J. Ophth. *15:*349, April '32

CRUICKSHANK, R.: Bacterial infection in burns. Tr. Roy. Med.-Chir. Soc. Glasgow, pp. 79–82, '34–'35; in Glasgow, M. J., July '35 also: J. Path. and Bact. *41:*367–369, Sept '35

CRUICKSHANK, R. (see CLARK, A. M.) Jan '35

CRUM, J. HOWARD: *Making of a Beautiful Face, or Face-Lifting Unveiled*. Walton Book Co., New York, 1931

CRUTHIRDS, A. E.: Treatment of burns of eyes and face with sulfhydryl solution (hydrosulphosol). Indust. Med. *11:*109–112, March '42

CRUTHIRDS, A. E.: Burns of ear, nose, mouth and adjacent tissues (including use of hydrosulphosol, sulfhydryl solution). Tr. Am. Laryng., Rhin. and Otol. Soc., pp. 219–235, '43

CRUTHIRDS, A. E.: Burns of ear, nose, mouth and adjacent tissues (with special reference to therapy with hydrosulphosol, sulfhydryl solution). Laryngoscope *53:*478–494, July '43

CRUZ, A. (see SANTOS, H. A. *et al*) Nov '40

CRYMBLE, P. T.: Two cases of ankylosis of left temporo-mandibular joint. Brit. M. J. *1:*996–997, June 7, '24

Cryotherapy

Results of cryotherapy in angiomas of face in nurslings and in angiomas of eyelids. LORTAT-JACOB, L. Bull. et mem. Soc. med. d. hop. de Paris *52:*527–528, March 29, '28

Therapy of cutaneous angiomas with sclerosing injections of quinine and urea hydrochloride associated with cryotherapy with carbon dioxide snow. SÉZARY, A.; *et al*. Presse med. *41:*260, Feb 15, '33

Is cryotherapy treatment of choice for angiomas? LORTAT-JACOB, E. Monde med., Paris *44:*781–782, July 1, '34

Surface angioma of face treated with cryotherapy and radium. MARIN, A. Union med. du Canada *65:*446–449, May '36

Cryotherapy of cutaneous tuberous angioma and injections of sclerosing substances in subcutaneous forms. Gaz. med. de France *45:*1061–1062, Dec 1, '38

Cryotherapy (with mixture containing carbon dioxide snow) for acne and its scars. KARP, F. L.; *et al*. Arch. Dermat. and Syph. *39:*995–998, June '39

Evaluation of cryotherapy of post-acne scars. HOLLANDER, L. AND SHELTON, J. M. Pennsylvania M. J. *45:*226–228, Dec '41

Use of cold air blast on precancerous skin lesions and hemangiomas. POPPE, J. K. Surgery *11:*460–465, March '42

Formula for cryotherapy (with carbon dioxide slush) for acne and postacne scarring. ZUGERMAN, I. Arch. Dermat. and Syph. *54:*209–210 Aug '46

CSAPODY, I.: Plastic surgery of orbit. Gyogyaszat *72:*65–67, Jan 31, '32

CSAPODY, I.: Fixation of artificial eye in conjunctival sac made of skin graft. Budapesti orvosi ujsag *33:*337–343, April 11, '35

CSAPODY, I.: Plastic construction of artificial conjunctival sac using skin flaps. Orvosi hetil. *81:*1217–1219, Dec 4, '37

CSERNYEI, G.: Prosthetic nose and face. Schweiz. med. Wchnschr. *62:*116, Jan 30, '32

CSERNYEI, J. See: CSERNYEI, G.

CSILLAG, S.: Nasal fractures in connection with fracture of facial cranium. Monatschr. f. Ohrenh. *68:*663–669, June '34 also: Orvosi hetil. *78:*586–588, June 30, '34

CSILLAG, S.: Accidental severing of ear and its suturing; case. Budapesti orvosi ujsag *38:*268–269, June 6, '40

CSÖRSZ, K.: Familial predisposition to Dupuytren's contracture. Budapesti orvosi ujsag *28:*59–61, Jan 16, '30

CSÖRSZ, K.: Dupuytren's contracture with congenital dislocations of hip joint. Budapesti orvosi ujsag *28:*61–63, Jan 16, '30

CUCCO, A.: Plastic or esthetic surgery of face. Ann. di ottal. e clin. ocul. *59:*253–271, March '31

CUCCO, A.: Lesions of eye with permanent disfigurement of face; medicolegal study of case. Riv. san. siciliana *24:*137–141, Feb 1, '36

Cuénod-Saunders Operation

Cuénod and Nataf modification of Saunders' operation for trichiasis and entropion. CUNNINGHAM, E. R. Chinese M. J. *48:*819–829, Sept '34

CUFF, C. H.: Application of fascia lata in plastic surgery. Brit. M. J. *1:*599–600, April 15, '22

CULLA, E.: Error in diagnosis and treatment of nevus; case. Bol. d. Inst. clin. quir. *18:*643–645, Sept '42

CULLEN, S. C.: Adjuvant secondary therapy in shock. West. J. Surg. *50:*392–395, Aug '42

CULLEN, S. C.: Anesthesia in otorhinolaryngology. Tr. Am. Acad. Ophth. (1943) *48:*240–247, March–April '44

CULLER, A. M.: Management of burns of cornea. Ohio State M. J. *34:*873–878, Aug '38

CULVER, G. D. (see MONTGOMERY, D. W.) April '23

CULVER, G. D. (see MONTGOMERY, D. W.) Dec '23

CULVER, G. D. (see MONTGOMERY, D. W.) Dec '24

CULVER, G. D. (see MONTGOMERY, D. W.) June '31

CUMMINS, H.: Spontaneous amputation of human supernumerary digits; pedunculated postminimi. Am. J. Anat. *51:*381–416, Nov '32

CUMMINS, R. C.: "Dead hand"; lesion produced by rapid vibration. Irish J. M. Sc., pp. 171–175, April '40

CUMSTON, C. G.: Ankylosis of lower jaw, surgical treatment. Internat. Clinics. *1:*65, '21

CÚNEO, N. L.: Case of exstrophy of bladder. Semana med. *1:*490–491, March 15, '23 (illus.)

CUNNING, D. S.: End-results in 20 cases of primary skin grafts in radical mastoidectomies. Laryngoscope *41:*484–486, July '31

CUNNING, D. S.: Series of cases of radical mastoidectomy with skin graft. Laryngoscope *45:*776–781, Oct '35

CUNNINGHAM, A. F.: Cleft lips and cleft palate. Am. J. Nursing *37:*339–341, April '37

CUNNINGHAM, A. F.: Reconstruction of lower lip. Northwest Med. *39:*336–337, Sept '40

CUNNINGHAM, E. R: Cuénod and Nataf modification of Saunders' operation for trichiasis and entropion. Chinese M. J. *48:*819–829, Sept '34

CUNNINGHAM, W. F.: Branchial cysts of parotid gland. Ann. Surg. *90:*114–117, July '29

COPAR, I.: Surgical therapy of cysts of jaws. Ztschr. f. Stomatol. *35:*1339–1346, Oct 22, '37

CUPAR, I.: Facial and maxillary injuries in war. Voj.-san. glasnik *11:*457–471, '40

Curling's Ulcer

Duodenal ulcers in case of grave burns. RONCHESE, F. Riforma med. *40:*753–755, Aug 11, '24 abstr: J.A.M.A. *83:*1038, Sept 27, '24

Duodenal ulcers following burns, with report of 2 cases. LEVIN, J. J. Brit. J. Surg. *17:*110–113, July '29

Haemorrhage into suprarenal capsule and haemorrhage from duodenal ulcer in burns; case. HARRIS, R. I. Clin. J. *59:*150–152, March 26, '30

Curling's ulcer; duodenal ulcer following superficial burns. MAES, U. Ann. Surg. *91:*527–532, April '30

Curling's ulcer in burns; with report of 2 cases. MAES, U., M. Rec. and Ann. *24:*564–568, June '30

Peptic ulcer following burns of skin; 5 cases. RIEHL, G. JR. Acta dermat.-venereol. *11:*277–294, Sept '30

"Curling's ulcer" in burns, with report of case. LAIRD, W. R. AND WILKERSON, W. V. West Virginia M. J. *27:*128–130, March '31

Curling ulcer in burns. MILLER, T. AND RUBENSTEIN, B. Dallas M. J. *18:*8–9, Jan '32

Unusual case of burn complication (development of Curling ulcer; recovery). MILLER, T. AND RUBENSTEIN, B. Texas State J. Med. *27:*873, April '32

Duodenal ulcer following skin burns; 2 cases with recovery. FITZGIBBON, J. H. Northwest Med. *31:*427–430, Sept '32

Curling's Ulcer—Cont.
Mechanism of production of Curling's ulcer in burns. KAPSINOW, R. South. M. J. *27:*500–503, June '34
Two case reports of extensive burns in children; both recovered; one with Curling ulcer. SHERRILL, W. P. Southwestern Med. *21:*135–138, April '37
Acute ulcer of duodenum (Curling's ulcer) as complication of burns; relation to sepsis; report of case with study of 107 cases collected from literature, 94 with necropsy, 13 with recovery; experimental studies. HARKINS, H. N. Surgery *3:*608–641, April '38
Perforated duodenal ulcer and ileus following burn; case. BERGK, W. Chirurg *10:*548–552, Aug. 1, '38
Experimental investigation of gastrointestinal secretions and motility following burns and their relation to ulcer. NECHELES, H. AND OLSON, W. H. Surgery *11:*751–765, May '42
Severe burns associated with duodenal ulceration. WHIGHAM, J. R. M. Brit. J. Surg. *30:*178–179, Oct '42

CURNOCK, J. E.: Spontaneous fracture of mandible; case. Proc. Roy. Soc. Med. *25:*885, April '32
CURR, J. F.: Salivary gland tumor of upper lip. Brit. M. J. *2:*605, Nov. 3, '45
CURRAN, J. A.: Partial or pseudoankylosis of jaws. China M. J. *43:*241–244, March '29
CURRAN, M.: Case of undiagnosed cavernous sinus thrombophlebitis; untreated fracture of mandible. J. Oral Surg. *2:*7–12, Jan '44
CURRY, D. E.: Burn therapy. M. Rec. and Ann. *37:*528–531, March '43
CURRY, G. J.: Treatment of simple and compound finger fractures; finger amputations. Am. J. Surg. *71:*80–83, Jan. '46
CURRY, G. J.: Finger amputations. Amer. J. Surg. *72:*40–42, July '46
CURRY, W. A.: Early diagnosis of cancer of lips. Canad. M. A. J. *30:*50–53, Jan '34
CURTILLET, A. (see GOINARD, P.) July '34
CURTILLET, E.: Shock; treatment during Tunisian campaign of 1942–1943. Afrique franc. chir. *1:*297–303, Sept–Oct '43
CURTILLET, E.: Specialized surgery (plastic surgery). Afrique franc. chir., nos. 5–6, pp. 201–213, Sept–Dec '45
CURTILLET, É. (see COSTANTINI, H.) 1929
CURTILLET, E. (see COSTANTINI, H.) May–June '35
CURTILLET, E. (see COSTANTINI, H.) Jan–Feb '39
CURTILLET, J. AND TILLER, R.: Indications and advantages of pedunculated bone grafts. Lyon chir. *22:*789–804, Nov–Dec '25 abstr: J.A.M.A. *86:*1487, May 8, '26
CURTIN, L. J.: Limitations of septum operation. J. Laryng. and Otol. *44:*24–26, Jan '29
CURTIS, G. M. AND KREDEL, F. E.: Imperforate anus. Ohio State M. J. *29:*183–184, March '33
CURTIS, J. F.: Infections of tendon sheaths. Univ. Toronto M. J. *7:*16–22, Nov '29
CURTIS, LAWRENCE (with ROBERT H. IVY): *Fractures of the Jaws*. Lea and Febiger, Phila., 1931. Second Edition, 1938. Third Edition, 1945
CURTIS, L.: Jaw fractures. Mil. Surgeon *89:*648–652, Oct '41
CURTIS, L. (see IVY, R. H.) Oct '28
CURTIS, L. (see IVY, R. H.) April '29
CURTIS, L. (see IVY, R. H.) Dec '30
CURTIS, L. (see IVY, R. H.) April '31
CURTIS, L. (see IVY, R. H.) Sept '31
CURTIS, L. (see IVY, R. H.) Dec '32
CURTIS, L. (see IVY, R. H.) Sept '34
CURTIS, L. (see IVY, R. H.) Jan '36
CURTIS, L. (see IVY, R. H.) April '36
CURTIS, L. (see IVY, R. H.) Sept '36
CURTIS, L. (see IVY, R. H.) Jan '37
CURTIS, L. (see IVY, R. H.) Nov '37
CURTIS, L. (see IVY, R. H.) Sept '42
CURTIS, L. (see IVY, R. H.) Oct '43
CURTIS, L. (see IVY, R. H.) Nov '45
CURTIS, R. M. AND BREWER, J. H.: Casein in local treatment of burns. Arch. Surg. *48:*130–136, Feb '44
CUTHBERT, J. B.: Comminuted fractures of mandible; 25 consecutive cases from plastic and jaw unit, Emergency Medical Service. Lancet *1:*748–750, June 10, '44
CUTHBERT, J. B.: Comminuted fractures of mandible; 25 consecutive cases from plastic and jaw unit, Emergency Medical Service. Dia med. *16:*1395–1397, Nov 13, '44
CUTHBERT, J. B.: Late treatment of dorsal injuries associated with loss of skin in hand. Brit. J. Surg. *33:*66–71, July '45
CUTHBERTSON, D. P.: Postshock metabolic response (Arris and Gale lecture). Lancet *1:*433–436, April 11, '42
CUTLER, C. W. Jr.: Acute osteomyelitis of lower jaw. S. Clin. North America *15:*483–494, April '35
CUTLER, C. W. Jr.: Injuries to hands by puncture wounds and foreign bodies, S. Clin. North America *21:*485–493, April '41
CUTLER, CONDICT W. Jr.: *The Hand: Its Disabilities and Diseases*. W. B. Saunders Co., Phila., 1942
CUTLER, C. W. Jr.: Early and late repair of extensor tendons. Tr. Am. Soc. Plastic and Reconstructive Surg. *12:*69–77, '43
CUTLER, C. W. Jr.: Early management of hand

wounds. Bull. U. S. Army M. Dept. (no. 85) pp. 92–98, Feb '45

CUTLER, G. D. AND ROCK, J. C.: Congenital tumors of maxilla; report of case with operation. Boston M. and S. J. *192:*1001–1002, May 21, '25

CUTLER, N. L.: Fascia lata transplant for rectrotarsal atrophy of upper lid following enucleation. Am. J. Ophth. *29:*176–179, Feb '46

CUTTING, C. C.: Hand fractures. California and West. Med. *62:*21–22, Jan '45 also: Indust. Med. *14:*242, March '45

CUTTING, R. A.: Burn therapy. New Orleans M. and S. J. *81:*112–120, Aug '28

CUTTING, R. A.: Immediate treatment of extensive superficial burns. Am. J. Surg. *14:*705–724, Dec '31

CYRIAX, E.: Minor displacements of phalanges. Brit. J. Phys. Med. *2:*21–22, Jan '39

Cystic Hygroma (See also Lymphangioma)

Serous cysts of neck. CEVARIO, L. Gass. d. osp. *42:*200, Feb 27, '21

Hygroma cystica treated with radium. NEW, G. B., S. Clin. N. America *4:*527–528, April '24

Multilocular serous cyst in neck, probably of congenital origin. MENESES, J. G. J. Arch. espan. de pediat. *9:*91–95, Feb '25

Lymphatic cysts of neck with report of case. WAFFLE, E. B., AND FOWLER, F. E. Northwest Med. *25:*142–144, March '26

Congenital serous cyst of neck; case. MASSABUAU *et al.* Bull. Soc. d. sc. med. et biol. de Montpellier *8:*354–358, Aug '27

Radium in treatment of multilocular lymph cysts (cystic hygromas) of neck in children. FIGI, F. A. Am. J. Roentgenol. *21:*473–480, May '29

Cystic hygroma of neck. NEW, G. B., S. Clin. North America *11:*771–773, Aug '31

Cystic hygroma; 2 cases. (neck). MASON, J. T. AND BAKER, J. W., S. Clin. North America *11:*1091–1095, Oct '31

Pseudo-unilocular serous cyst of neck in infant; case. TERCERO, M. Arch. espan. de pediat. *16:*306–309, July '32

Hygroma cysticum colli; case report with review of literature. HYATT, C. N., J. Iowa M. Sco. *22:*406–408, Aug '32

Treatment of cystic hygroma by sodium morrhuate. HARROWER, J. G. Brit. M. J. *2:*148, July 22, '33

Cystic hygroma of neck; report of case and review of literature. VAUGHN, A. M. Am. J. Dis. Child. *48:*149–158, July '34

Cystic hygroma of neck. MACGUIRE, D. P. Arch. Surg. *31:*301–307, Aug '35

Cystic lymphangioma associated with grave congenital malformations; study of cervical hygromas. QUADRI, S. Clin. pediat. *17:*755–777, Oct '35

Cystic Hygroma—Cont.

Therapy of serous cysts of neck. BELLONE, G. Riv. san siciliana *23:*1717–1724, Dec 1, '35

Cystic hygroma of neck; 2 cases in Bulu children. MCCRACKIN, R. H. Am. J. Dis. Child. *51:*349–352, Feb '36

Tendovaginitis and tendon nodules, ganglion, hygroma and bursitis. STORCK, H. Med. Welt *10:*522–525, April 11, '36

New developments in study of hygroma. DUFFY, J. J., J. Iowa M. Soc. *27:*205–208, May '37

Cystic hygroma. BAILEY, H. Clin. J. *66:*242–244, June '37

Hygroma colli cysticum and hygroma axillare; pathologic and clinical study and report of 12 cases. GOETSCH, E. Arch. Surg. *36:*394–479, March '38

Cystic hygroma of neck. FLEMING, B. L. J.A.M.A. *110:*1899–1900, June 4, '38

Cystic hygroma (of neck). BAILEY, H. J. Internat. Coll. Surgeons *2:*31–33, Jan–April '39

Cystic hygroma of neck; 27 cases. GROSS, R. E. AND GOERINGER, C. F. Surg., Gynec. and Obst. *69:*48–60, July '39

Cystic hygroma (lymphangioma); 3 cases. CARDELLE PENICHET, G. AND GARCIA LOPEZ, A. Arch. de med. inf. *10:*104–117, April–June '41

Hygroma colli cysticum. CALLISTER, A. C. Rocky Mountain M. J. *38:*562–564, July '41

Cervicomediastinal lymphangioma (cystic hygroma); 2 cases in infants. ARNHEIM, E. E. J. Mt. Sinai Hosp. *10:*404–410, Sept–Oct '43

Congenital lymphangiomatous macroglossia with cystic hygroma of neck. LIERLE, D. M. Ann. Otol., Rhin. and Laryng. *53:*574–757, Sept '44

Congenital lymphangiomatous macroglossia with cystic hygroma. LIERLE, D. M. Tr. Am. Laryng. A. *66:*194–196, '44

Cystic hygroma; 3 cases. PORTMANN, U. V. Cleveland Clin. Quart. *12:*98–104, July '45

Cysts and Fistulas

Midline congenital cervical fistula of tracheal origin. SEELIG, M. G. Arch. Surg. *2:*338, March '21

Congenital fistula of neck. DETZEL, L. Munchen. med. Wchnschr. *68:*1227, Sept 23, '21

Congenital cysts and fistulas in neck. DEGAETANO, L. Arch. ital. di chir. *4:*265–324, Nov '21, (illus.) abstr: J.A.M.A. *78:*250, Jan 21, '22

Congenital median and lateral fistulas in

Cysts and Fistulas – Cont.
neck. BLAESEN, C. Deutsche Ztschr. f. Chir. *167:*60–64, '21
Complete median fistula of neck. TAKEDA. Deutsche med. Wchnschr. *48:*1649–1650, Dec 8, '22
Congenital cysts in neck. GOBBI, L. Policlinico (sez. chir.) *30:*372–388, July '23 (illus.)
Case of symmetrical bilateral multiple small cysts in neck. MARTINOTTI, L. Gior. ital. d. ma. ven. *65:*19–25, Feb '24
Fistulae and cysts of neck. LIPSHUTZ, B. Ann. Surg. *79:*499–505, April '24
Congenital cysts and fistulas in neck. BACCARINI, L. Arch. ital. di chir. *9:*279–335, '24 abstr: J.A.M.A. *83:*73, July 5, '24
Fistulae and congenital cysts of lateral region of neck; 3 personal cases. SIMON, R. *et al*. Arch. franco-belges de chir. *28:*203–258, March '25
Two cases of congenital complete lateral pharyngo-cervico-sternal fistulas of neck and their extirpation. DE GAETANO, L. Riforma med. *41:*889–896, Sept 21, '25
Congenital salivary fistula of neck. SMITH, R. R. AND TORGERSON, W. R. Surg., Gynec. and Obst. *41:*318–319, Sept '25
Case of lateral fistulas in neck. MÜLLER, S. Deutsche Ztschr. f. Chir. *193:*401–408, '25
Congenital lymphoid cysts in lateral portion of neck. SOUBEIRAN, M. Arch. franco-belges de chir. *29:*514–521, June '26
Operation for complete fistula of neck. GROSS, W. Zentralbl. f. Chir. *53:*2076–2080, Aug 14, '26
Dermoid cyst of neck. SEED, L. S. Clin. N. Amer. *6:*1033–1035, Aug '26
Cystic tumors of neck; struma papillomatosa cystica lateralis. RÜHL, A. Deutsche Ztschr. f. Chir. *198:*90-98, '26
Congenital cysts of neck in children. PAYNE, R. L. Am. J. Surg. *3:*1–5, July '27
Congenital serous cyst of neck; case. MASSABUAU, *et al*. Bull. Soc. d. sc. med. et biol. de Montpellier *8:*354–358, Aug '27
Bilateral complete cervical fistulae. WOODEN, W. AND HUTCHENS, D. K. Am. J. Surg. *3:*377–378, Oct '27
Venous cyst of neck. LUSENA, G. Arch. ital. di chir. *19:*93–108, '27
Congenital cervical fistulae and cysts. NYLANDER, P. E. A. Arb. a. d. path. Inst. *5:*114–231, '27
So-called congenital fistulae of neck. NIENHUIS, J. H. Geneesk. Gids *6:*625–633, July 6, '28
Amygdaloid cyst of neck; case. REBATTU, J. AND PARTHIOT. Rev. de laryng. *49:*771–773, Dec 31, '28

Cysts and Fistulas – Cont.
Cysts and fistulae of median cervical line. MAGLIULO, A. Sperimentale, Arch. di biol. *82:*455–504, '28
Congenital median fistula of neck. DE MARCHI, E. Arch. ital. di chir. *22:*91–100, '28
Lateral and internal cysts and fistula of neck. TOMILOFF, N. L. Vestnik khir. (nos. 43–44) *14:*234–237, '28
Lateral cyst of neck of thyroid origin. ZAMPA, G. Policlinico (sez. chir.) *36:*51–60, Jan '29
Screw curet; use in curettage and in excision of fistulous tracts. YOUNG, H. H. J. A. M. A. *93:*110–113, July 13, '29
Treatment of congenital fistula of neck with diathermy (electrocoagulation). HOFER, G. Arch. f. klin. Chir. *156:*274–283, '29
Parathyroidal cyst of neck; case. NYLANDER, P. E. A. Acta chir. Scandinav. *64:*539–547, '29
Treatment of congenital fistula of neck. FRANGENHEIM, P. Zentralbl. f. Chir. *57:*259–260, Feb 1, '30
Developmental anomalies of face and neck and their surgical significance. (also cleft palate). SINGLETON, A. O. Texas State J. Med. *25:*659–664, Feb '30
Congenital anomalies of the neck. PAGENSTECHER, G. A. Texas State J. Med. *25:*786–789, April '30
Formation of medial cysts of neck. KORKHOFF, U. Vrach. gaz. *34:*779–781, May 31, '30
Rare neck cyst. FRASER, I. Brit. J. Surg. *18:*338–339, Oct '30
Plastic reconstruction of intestinal branchial apparatus and its derivatives in human embryos. BRUNI, A. C. Monitore zool. ital. (supp.) *41:*196–199, 1930–1931
Anatomy, pathogenesis and clinical aspects of congenital fistulas of neck. MOATTI, L. Rev. med. franc. *12:*39–57, Jan '31
Pathogenesis of lateral fistulae and cysts of neck. MOATTI, L. Ann. d'oto-laryng., pp. 11–41, Jan '31
Fistula in center of neck; recidivation because of inflammation of Boyer's bursa; case. CIEZA RODRÍGUEZ, M. Semana med. *1:*552–554, Feb 26, '31
Differentiation of branchial from other cervical cysts by x-ray examination. WANGENSTEEN, O. H. Ann. Surg. *93:*790–792, March '31
Treatment of wide fecal fistula of sacral region in case with rectal prolapse. NUSSBAUM, J. Zentralbl. f. Chir. *58:*2024–2027, Aug 8, '31
Similarity of certain tuberculous cervical ab-

Cysts and Fistulas – Cont.
scesses and branchial cysts. BAILEY, H. Brit. J. Tuberc. *25:*167–170, Oct '31
Congenital cysts of neck. SÀFTA, E. Cluj. med. *12:*595–598, Nov 1, '31
Congenital cartilaginous remains in neck; relation to lateral cervical fistulas. NIEDEN, H. AND ASBECK, C. Beitr. z. klin. Chir. *153:*47–59, '31
Fate of free transplants of epidermis into deep-lying tissues; relation to epithelial cysts. ZIMCHES, J. L. Frankfurt, Ztschr. f. Path. *42:*203–227, '31
Amygdaloid cysts and tumors; origin, structure and classification of vestigial formations in neck. BRACHETTO-BRIAN, D. Prensa med. argent. *18:*1177–1187, Feb 10, '32
Congenital cysts and fistulas of neck. MEYER, H. W. Ann. Surg. *95:*1, Jan; 226, Feb '32
Hemorrhagic cyst on side of neck. IWATÔ, Y. Okayama-Igakkai-Zasshi *44:*1727–1728, June '32
Cervicofacial branchiomas. SOUBEIRAN, M. Arch. franco-belges de chir. *33:*542–554, June '32
Technic of closure of esophageal fistula; significance in surgical treatment of laryngo-esophageal cancer. PORTMANN, G. AND DESPONS, J. Bordeaux chir. *3:*252–261, July '32
Origin of cysts, fistulas and tumors of lateral region of neck. ROSSANO, I. Rev. de path. comparee *32:*951, Sept; 1127, Oct; 1269, Nov '32
Congenital auriculo-hyoid fistula; medical therapy; case. BERGARA, R. AND BERGARA, C. An. de oto-rino-laring. d. Uruguay *2:*117–130, '32
Erroneous diagnoses in cases of aural and cervical fistulas and cysts. ZÖLLNER, F. Ztschr. f. Hals-, Nasen-u. Ohrenh. *32:*54–61, '32
Cysts and fistulas of lateral region of neck. KOLKMAN, D. Nederl. tijdschr. v. geneesk. *77:*862–865, Feb 25, '33
Congenital fistula of neck. KANAI, T. Taiwan Igakkai Zasshi (Abstr. Sect.) *32:*125, Sept '33
Lateral cyst of neck; surgical removal followed by development of malignant branchioma; clinical and pathologic study. PAGLIANI, F. Bull. d. sc. med., Bologna *105:*405–428, Sept–Oct '33
Cystic tumors of neck; branchial and thyroglossal cysts. MCNEALY, R. W. S. Clin. North America *13:*1083–1100, Oct '33
Cervical cysts and fistulae; 3 cases. PASCHOUD, H. Rev. med. de la Suisse Rom. *54:*300–319, March 25, '34
Congenital fistulas of neck. FALENI, R. A. Prensa med. argent. *21:*882, May 9; 932, May 16; 980, May 23, '34
Lateral congenital fistula of neck. CARNEVALE-RICCI, R. Arch ital. di otol. *45:*473–482, July '34
Congenital median fistula of neck; pathogenesis and histology. ŚWIATLOWSKI, B. Monatschr. f. Ohrenh. *68:*1096–1106, Sept '34
Modifying liquids in therapy of congenital fistulas of lateral region of neck; new case with recovery. BERGARA, R. A., *et al.* Rev. Asoc. med. argent. *48:*1212–1215, Oct '34
Cysts and fistulae of neck. RUSSELL, R. D. Ann. Otol., Rhin. and Laryng. *44:*532–543, June '35
Lympho-epithelial cysts of neck; cases. SALOJ, C. D., AND CID, J. M. An. de cir. *1:*48–60, June '35
Fissural cyst of cheek; case. CROCQUEFER. Rev. de stomatol. *37:*513–518, Aug '35
Congenital median cysts and fistulae of neck. IONESCU, N. V. Rev. san. mil., Bucuresti *35:*71–80, Jan '36
Roentgenographic examination of midcervical fistula. RUCKENSTEINER, E. Fortschr. a. d. Geb. d. Rontgenstrahlen *54:*321–325, Sept '36
Suppurative cyst of neck; case. DIEULAFE, R. Bordeaux chir. *7:*452–453, Oct '36
Cysts and sinuses of neck. GASTON, E. A. Cleveland Clin. Quart. *3:*311–322, Oct '36
Cysts of neck, nine cases. GILL, E. G. Virginia M. Monthly *63:*482–487, Nov '36
Cysts of bursa mucosa of subhyoid region of neck. BLANKSTEIN, W. G. Acta oto-Laryng. *24:*379–385, '36
Pathologic and clinical study of lamellar cysts of neck. LANG, C. Arch. f. klin. Chir. *185:*527–536, '36
Unguentolan (cod liver oil ointment) in therapy of decubitus and postoperative fistula and wound infection; 15 cases. WEBER, H. Wien. med. Wchnschr. *87:*219–221, Feb 20, '37
Congenital median fistula, with report of case. DE GAETANO, L. Riforma med. *53:*523–526, April 10, '37
Fistulas and cysts of neck. SUERMONDT, W. F. Nederl. tijdschr. v. geneesk. *81:*1528–1535, April 10, '37
Dermoid cysts of neck and head. NEW, G. B. AND ERICH, J. B. Surg., Gynec. and Obst. *65:*48–55, July '37
Congenital cysts and fistulas of neck. DE

Cysts and Fistulas – Cont.
GAETANO, L. Arch. di ortop. *53:*455–479, Sept 30, '37
Low lateral congenital fistulas of neck. JANKOVSKY, P. Ann. d'oto-laryng., pp. 1133–1146, Dec '37
Results of electrocoagulation therapy of congenital fistulas of neck. SPITZY, M. Zentralbl. f. Chir. *65:*114–117, Jan 15, '38
Cyst of neck; case. BRAIMBRIDGE, C. V. East Africa M. J. *14:*393–395, March '38
Laryngotracheoplasty by Mangoldt technic in therapy of laryngotracheal fistula. LASKIEWICZ, A. Rev. de laryng. *59:*463–471, May '38
Tumors of neck; diagnosis and treatment, cervical cysts and fistulas. HICKEN, N. F. AND POPMA, A. M. Nebraska M. J. *23:*209–212, June '38
Therapy of inoperable cysts of neck. MURESANU, J. Zentralbl. f. Chir. *65:*1453–1455, June 25, '38
Permanent fistula of floor of mouth; case. COELST. Rev. de chir. structive *8:*128–130, Aug '38
Retromaxillary tonsillar cysts; removal by predigastric incision; case. LERICHE, R. Lyon chir. *35:*574–575, Sept–Oct '38
Congenital cyst of right lateral cervical region developed from lateral vestiges of "cervical sinus." BARGE, P. Ann. d'anat. path. *15:*1025–1031, Dec '38
Medial cervical fistula due to persistence of thryoglossal tract; case. RASTELLI, E. Gior. med. d. Alto Adige *11:*3–14, Jan '39
Congenital lateral neck cyst; case. TAKAHARA, T. AND WATANABE, D. Oto-rhino-laryng. *12:*44–45, Jan '39
Congenital cysts and fistulas of neck. BÖHM, J. Hals-, Nasen-u. Ohrenarzt (Teil 1) *30:*130–138, March '39
Congenital fistula of neck; case. GONZALEZ, N. B. Rev. mex. de cir., ginec. y cancer *7:*471–477, Oct '39
Tumors and cysts of neck. BOYD, W. Tr. West. S. A. (1938) *48:*172–182, '39
Cysts and fistulas of neck. GOROKHOV, A. V. Zhur. ush. nos. i gorl. bolez. *16:*444–447, '39
Anomalies and complex abnormalities of region of first pharyngeal arch. GÜNTHER, H. Ztschr. f. menschl. Vererb. -u. Konstitutionslehre *23:*43–52, '39
Branchial cysts; with report of 2 cases of cyst of cervical sinus. MALCOLM, R. B. AND BENSON, R. E. Surgery *7:*187–203, Feb '40
Congenital fistula of neck communicating with middle ear (with aural malformations). DRUSS, J. G. AND ALLEN, B. Arch. Otolaryng. *31:*437–443, March '40
Congenital fistulas and cysts of neck, with

Cysts and Fistulas – Cont.
report of 17 cases. MAGGIOROTTI, U. Valsalva *16:*337–365, Sept '40
Congenital cysts of neck, with report of cases. VELASCO, L. R. Rev. otorrinolaring. *1:*27–30, Sept '41
Fistulography with lipiodol (iodized oil) as new therapy of congenital cervical fistula. CERVENANSKY, J. Wien. med. Wchnschr. *91:*886–890, Nov 1, '41
Embryologic study of harelip cysts. STEINIGER, F. Ztschr. f. menschl. Vererb. -u. Konstitutionslehre *25:*1–27, '41
Lymphoepithelial papilliferous cystomas of branchial, thyroglossal and thyropharyngeal origin. LUPPI, J. E. Rev. med. de Rosario *33:*608–623, July '43
Method of treating cystic tumors of neck. LYLE, F. M. Am. J. Surg. *61:*443–444; Sept '43
Amygdaloid cysts; clinical, surgical and histologic study. (neck) BRACCO, J. A. AND D'ALBO, E. A. Prensa med. agent. *30:*2058–2067, Oct. 27, '43
Grafts of pedicled soft tissue flaps in therapy of osseous fistulas following gunshot fractures. HUNDEMER, W. Munchen. med. Wchnschr. *91:*154, March 24, '44
Blood cysts of neck. OSTENFELD, J. Nord. med. (Hospitalstid.) *22:*758–759, April 21, '44
Cysts and sinuses of neck. DOSTER, J. T. JR. Mississippi Doctor *22:*205–210, Jan '45
Simple method of therapy of congenital cervical fistulas. LENGGENHAGER, K. Schweiz. med. Wchnschr. *76:*607–609, July 6, '46

Cysts and Fistulas, Branchial

Congenital lateral cervical fistula. LEVINGER. Munchen. med. Wchnschr. *68:*304, March 11, '21
Congenital lateral fistulas of neck. GRIESSMANN, B. Munchen. med. Wchnschr. *68:*460, April 15, '21
Branchial fistulae; with report of surgical case. MILLER, L. I. Colorado Med. *18:*110, May '21
Branchial cysts and fistulas. GILMAN, P. K. J.A.M.A. *77:*26, July 2, '21
Clinical aspects of branchial cysts. BAILEY, H. Brit. J. Surg. *10:*565–572, April '23 (illus.)
Fistulae and congenital cysts of lateral regions of neck; 3 personal cases. SIMON, R. *et al.* Arch. franco-belges de chir. *28:*203–258, March '25
Branchial cysts. BROW, I. N., J. Iowa M. Soc. *15:*524–528, Oct '25
Branchial fistulas of neck. BECKER, J. Beitr. z. klin. Chir. *134:*470–472, '25

Cysts and Fistulas, Branchial—Cont.
Case of lateral fistulas in neck. MÜLLER, S. Deutsche Ztschr. f. Chir. *193:*401–408, '25
Cysts and fistulas of lateral branchial canal. REINECKE, R. Arch. f. klin. Chir. *136:*99–108, '25
Congenital complete branchiogenetic cyst and duct. MEYER, H. W. Am. J. Surg. *40:*121, May '26
Branchial fistula; its clinical relation to irritation of vagus. CARP, L. Surg., Gynec. and Obst. *42:*772–777, June '26
Congenital lymphoid cysts in lateral portion of neck. SOUBEIRAN, M. Arch. franco-belges de chir. *29:*514–521, June '26
Lateral cervical fistulae. KRAMER, R. Laryngoscope *36:*517–522, July '26
Branchial cyst. SEED, L., S. Clin N. Amer. *6:*1029–1031, Aug '26
Branchial cysts and fistulae; report of 5 cases. JOHNSON, J. A. Minnesota Med. *9:*514–517, Sept '26
Case of lateral fistula of neck. HUIZINGA, E. Nederl. Tijdschr. v. Geneesk. *2:*1775–1777, Oct 16, '26
Deep branchiogenous cysts in right side of neck. ANARDI, T. Tumori *12:*217–225, '26
Branchial cyst; case. THOMSON, J. W. Lancet *1:*76, Jan 8, '27
Branchiogenic tumors of neck. BELK, W. P. S. Clin. N. Amer. *7:*453–468, April '27
Branchial fistula. BAILEY, H. Clin. J. *56:*619, Dec 28, '27
Lateral cervical fistula; case. HUIZINGA, E. Laryngoscope *37:*878–879, Dec '27
Pedigree of anomalies in first and second branchial cleft, inherited according to laws of Mendel, and contribution to technique of extirpation of congenital lateral fistulae coli. PŘECECHTĚL, A. Acta oto-laryng. *11:*23–30, '27
Anomalies and neoplasms of branchial apparatus; 32 cases with follow-up results. CARP, L. AND STOUT, A. P. Ann. Surg. *87:*186–209, Feb '28
Hereditary transmission of branchial fistulas; case. STARKENSTEIN, E. Med. Klin. *24:*701, May 4, '28
Diagnosis of branchial cyst, with note upon its removal. BAILEY H. Brit. M. J. *1:*940–941, June 2, '28
Nasopharyngeal cyst of branchial origin; case. GIUSSANI, M. Ann. di laring., otol. *29:*213–226, July '28
Branchial cysts and fistulae. FAGGE, C. H. Clin. J. *57:*421–423, Sept 5, '28
Lateral, congenital, cervical fistula; clinical aspects, histogenesis, operative technic; case. SANTORO, E. Ann. ital. di chir. *8:*59–71, Jan '29

Cysts and Fistulas, Branchial—Cont.
Clinical manifestations of branchial cysts. WAKELEY, C. P. G. Clin. J. *58:*109–111. March 6, '29
Complete congenital branchial fistula. BARAJAS Y DE VILCHES, J. M. Siglo med. *84:*85–86, July 27, '29
Branchial cysts of parotid gland. CUNNINGHAM, W. F. Ann. Surg. *90:*114–117, July '29
Simple method of dealing with congenital branchial fistulae. LOVE, R. J. M. Lancet *2:*122, July 20, '29
Lateral branchial cysts of neck. BOSDEVEIX, G. L. Ann. d. mal. de l'oreille, du larynx *48:*826–842, Aug '29
Embryologic origin and pathologic changes to which the branchial apparatus gives rise, with presentation of familial group of fistulas. HYNDMAN, O. R., AND LIGHT, G. Arch. Surg. *19:*410–452, Sept '29
Branchiogenetic cyst of larynx removed by thyrotomy. IMPERATORI, C. J. Laryngoscope *39:*679–683, Oct '29
Congenital branchial fistula; cases. DEBEYRE, A. AND SALEZ. Echo m. du nord *33:*541–544, Nov 16, '29
Genesis of congenital lateral cervical fistulas and cysts. NYLANDER, P. E. A. Deutsche Ztschr. f. Chir. *215:*139–145, '29
Branchial anomalies. SWEET, P. W. Tr. A. Resid. and ex-Resid. Physicians, Mayo Clin. (1928) *9:*94–103, '29
Lateral cervical fistula; paraffin injection as aid to excision. CHRISTOPHER, F., S. Clin. N. Amer. *10:*351–353, April '30
Pathologic changes, with presentation of familial group of branchial fistulas. HYNDMAN, O. R., AND LIGHT, G. J. Iowa M. Soc. *20:*260–252, June '30
Patent branchial cleft. JOHNS, A. H. G. Brit. M. J. *1:*1047, June 7, '30
Operative technic in congenital branchial fistulas. ESTELLA, J. AND MORALES, L. Arch. de med., cir. y espec. *33:*73–84, July 26, '30
Successful surgical treatment of large suppurative cyst of second branchial cleft; case. BÁRÁNY, R. Acta oto-laryng. *14:*556–559, '30
Branchiogenic anomalies (cysts and fistulas) associated with larynx. ROSENAUER, F. Deutsche Ztschr. f. Chir. *226:*304–307, '30
Branchial cysts. VASSILIEFF, A. I. Vestnik khir. (nos. 58-60) *20:*181–187, '30
Pathogenesis of lateral fistulae and cysts of neck. MOATTI, L. Ann. d'oto-laryng., pp. 11–41, Jan '31
Branchiogenous cyst with postoperative recurrence; recovery after iodine injection;

Cysts and Fistulas, Branchial – Cont.
case. SCHWERS, H. Liege med. (supp.) *24:*1-4, Feb 8, '31
Differentiation of branchial from other cervical cysts by x-ray examination. WANGENSTEEN, O. H. Ann. Surg. *93:*790-792, March '31
Ambulant treatment of branchial fistulas. KLEINSCHMIDT, O. Deutsche med. Wchnschr. *57:*1549-1551, Sept 4, '31
Similarity of certain tuberculous cervical abscesses and branchial cysts. BAILEY, H. Brit. J. Tuberc. *25:*167-170, Oct '31
Developmental abnormalities of second branchila slit. PŘECECHTĚL, A. Otolaryng. slavica *3:*437-449, Oct '31
Cysts and fistulae (branchial). SHEDDEN, W. M. New England J. Med. *205:*800-811, Oct 22, '31
Branchial cyst. SCHWARTZ, L. JR. New York State J. Med. *31:*1376-1377, Nov 15, '31
Congenital cartilaginous remains in neck; relation to lateral cervical fistulas. NIEDEN, H. AND ASBECK, C. Beitr. z. klin. Chir. *153:*47-59, '31
Tumors of hyo-thyro-pharyngeal region; laryngocele and branchial cyst. VAN DEN WILDENBERG, L. Scalpel *85:*265-271, Feb 27, '32
Cervicofacial branchiomas. SOUBEIRAN, M. Arch. franco-belges de chir. *33:*542-554, June '32
Clinical and pathologic aspects of branchiogenic cysts. RUTTIN, E. Monatschr. f. Ohrenh. *66:*1111-1114, Sept '32
Origin of cysts, fistulas and tumors of lateral region of neck. ROSSANO, I. Rev. de path. comparee *32:*951, Sept; 1127, Oct '32
Branchial fistulas in children. KETELBANT. Scalpel *85:*1433-1435, Nov 26, '32
Occurrence of branchial cysts in neck; case. KOCH, F. Monatschr. f. Ohrenh. *66:*1331-1334, Nov '32
Origin of cysts, fistulas and tumors of lateral region of neck. ROSSANO, I. Rev. de path. comparee *32:*1269-1307, Nov '32
Cysts and fistulas of lateral region of neck. KOLKMAN, D. Nederl. tijdschr. v. geneesk. *77:*862-865, Feb 25, '33
Branchial cyst with dermic steatonecrosis; case. BANET, V. AND BOLAÑOS, J. M. Bol. Liga contra el cancer *8:*97-104, April '33
Branchial cysts and fistulas in children. also: thyroglossal duct cysts and fistulas. BAUMGARTNER, C. J. Surg., Gynec. and Obst. *56:*948-955, May '33
Fistulized preauricular branchial fibrochondroma; case. JACOD, M. Lyon med. *151:*613-615, May 14, '33

Cysts and Fistulas, Branchial – Cont.
Congenital fistula of lateral region of neck. JACQUES, P. AND GRIMAUD. Oto-rhino-laryng. internat. *17:*437-439, June '33
Lateral cyst of neck; surgical removal followed by development of malignant branchioma; clinical and pathologic study. PAGLIANI, F. Bull. d. sc. med., Bologna *105:*405-428, Sept-Oct '33
Clinical aspects of branchial fistula. BAILEY, H. Brit. J. Surg. *21:*173-182, Oct '33
Branchial fistula. KLEINERT, M. N. Arch. Otolaryng. *18:*510-515, Oct '33
Lateral congenital neck fistula; 2 cases. CORNEJO SARAVIA, E. Bol. y trab. de la Soc. de cir. de Buenos Aires *17:*1224-1237 Nov 22, '33
Branchial fistulas; treatment with sclerosing fluids; case presentation and report. ROBITSHEK, E. C. Minnesota Med. *16:*760-762, Dec '33
Branchial cyst; 2 instructive cases. BERRY, G. Ann. Otol., Rhin. and Laryng. *43:*287-293, March '34
Cervical branchioma; 3 cases. TRUFFERT, P. Bull. et mem. Soc. nat. de chir. *60:*602-611, May 5, '34
Lateral congenital fistula of neck. CARNEVALE-RICCI, F. Arch. ital. di otol. *(45):*473-482, July '34
Branchiogenic tumors: surgical therapy. MOLLÁ, V. M. Cron. med., Valencia *38:*501-509, July 15, '34
Modifying liquids in therapy of congenital fistulas of lateral region of neck; new case with recovery. BERGARA, R. A. *et al.* Rev. Asoc. med. argent. *48:*1212-1215, Oct '34
Branchiogenic cysts of neck; 2 cases. NISHIMURA, I. Okayama-Igakkai-Zasshi *47:*235, Jan '35
Branchiogenetic or branchial fistulae. MACGUIRE, D. P. Am. Med. *41:*324-327, June '35
Branchial and thyroglossal duct cysts and fistulas. BROWN, J. M. Ann. Otol., Rhin. and Laryng. *44:*644-652, Sept '35
Branchial fistula; case. PARISEAU, L. J. de l'Hotel-Dieu de Montreal *4:*276-283, Nov '35
Fistulas of first branchial arch. JOSA, L. Zentralbl. f. Chir. *63:*1760-1763, July 25, '36
Fistulas of first branchial arch. JOSA, L. Orvosi hetil. *80:*973-974, Oct 10, '36
Branchial cysts. OCHSNER, C. G. Minnesota Med. *20:*31-33, Jan '37
Relation of tonsil to branchiogenetic cysts. MEEKER, L. H. Laryngoscope *47:*164-183, March '37

Cysts and Fistulas, Branchial – Cont.
Branchiogenic cysts in infancy. BECK, W. C. Surgery *1:*792–799, May '37
Branchiogenetic cysts. LARSON, E. California & West. Med. *47:*244–248, Oct '37
True branchiogenic cyst and fistula of neck. MEYER, H. W. Arch. Surg. *35:*766–771, Oct '37
Low lateral congenital fistulas of neck. JANKOVSKY, P. Ann. d'oto-laryng., pp. 1133–1146, Dec '37
Congenital branchiogenic anomalies; 82 cases. LADD, W. E. AND GROSS, R. E. Am. J. Surg. *39:*234–248, Feb '38
Congenital branchial cyst of floor of mouth; case. CHAVES, D. A. Rev. med.-cir. do Brasil *46:*620–626, May '38
Branchial cyst; case. MASI, C. AND MARINI, J. Semana med. *1:*1061–1062, May 12, '38
Therapy of congenital branchial fistulas. NYLANDER, P. E. A. Zentralbl. f. Chir. *65:*1095–1097, May 7, '38
Lateral or branchial cysts of neck; 13 cases. JACKSON, A. S. Wisconsin M. J. *37:*641–646, Aug '38
Amygdaloid branchial cyst of neck; embryologic considerations. BISI, R. H. AND EMILIANI, C. M. Rev. Assoc. med. argent. *52:*935–937, Sept. 15, '38
Problems of congenital origin of lateral fistulas and cysts of neck. MARX, J. Beitr. z. klin. Chir. *168:*435–447, '38 also: Orvosi hetil. *82:*891–895, Sept. 10, '38
Congenital cyst of right lateral cervical region developed from lateral vestiges of "cervical sinus." BARGE, P. Ann. d'anat. path. *15:*1025–1031, Dec '38
Bilateral congenital branchial fistulas; case. DUMALLE, G. AND HOUOT, A. Ann. Fac. franc. de med, et de pharm. de Beyrouth *7:*129–133, '38
Branchial cyst; case. KASARCOGLU. Turk tib cem. mec. *4:*182–183, '38
Congenital lateral neck cyst; case. TAKAHARA, T. AND WATANABE, D. Oto-rhino-laryng. *12:*44–45, Jan '39
Branchial cysts; with report of 2 cases of cyst of cervical sinus. MALCOLM, R. B. AND BENSON, R. E. Surgery *7:*187–203, Feb '40
Branchiogenous cysts and cystadenolymphomas. BIANCHI, A. E. AND PAVLOVSKY, A. An. Inst. modelo de clin. med. *21:*436–452, '40
Septic branchial cyst eradicated by electrical cauterization; case. BERGE, C. A. J. Michigan M. Soc. *40:*189–191, March '41
Brachial fistulae, 2 cases. BOWEN, F. H., J. Florida M. A. *27:*500–502, April '41

Cysts and Fistulas, Branchial – Cont.
Branchial cysts and sinuses. LAHEY, F. H. AND NELSON, H. F. Ann. Surg. *113:*508–512, April '41
Clinical conditions arising from anomalies or maldevelopments of branchial arches and clefts. HOOVER, W. B. Ann. Otol., Rhin. and Laryng. *50:*834–849, Sept '41
Branchial cysts; 2 cases. PONTES, A. Brasil-med. *55:*610–614, Sept. 6, '41
Branchial fistula; case. ARTHUR, H. R. Brit. J. Surg. *29:*440–441, April '42
Bilocular branchiogenic cyst of neck; case. FERNICOLA, C. *et al.* Bol. Soc. de cir. de Rosario *9:*511–519, Sept '42
Clinical aspects of branchial fistulas, with case report of bilateral complete fistulas. ANDERSON, E. R. Minnesota Med. *25:*789–795, Oct '42
Relation of precervical sinus and branchial clefts. CORDIER, G. AND DELMAS, A. Bull. Acad. de med., Paris *126:*485–486, Oct. 27–Nov. 10, '42
Cystic tumors; branchial and thyroglossal cysts. McNealy, R. W., J. Am. Dent. A. *29:*1808–1818, Oct. 1, '42
Cervicolaryngeal cyst of branchial origin; case. MARTIN CALDERIN, A. Semana med. espan. *6:*91, Jan. 23, '43
Complications in diabetic; nodular thyroid and branchial cleft fistulas. WARTHEN, H. J. AND JORDAN, W. R. South. M. J. *36:*536–537, July '43
Cervical lesions of branchial origin. SOMMER, G. N. J. JR. *et al.* Am. J. Surg. *61:*266–270, Aug '43
Branchial dermoepidermic cysts, with report of cases. PUENTE DUANY, N. Arch. cubanos cancerol. *3:*133–156, April–June '44
Dermoepidermal branchial cysts. PUENTE DUANY, N. Rev. med. cubana *55:*398, May; 449, June '44
Branchiogenic malformations of neck region. LADEWIG, P. AND SERT, D. Schweiz. Ztschr. f. Path. u. Bakt. *7:*1–12, '44
Lateral congenital fistula of neck; case. CISNEROS, R. Bol. y trab., Acad. argent. de cir. *29:*247–259, May 9, '45
Lateral cervical (branchial) cysts and fistulas; clinical and pathologic study. NEEL, H. B. AND PEMBERTON, J. DEJ. Surgery *18:*267–286, Sept '45
Bilateral branchial cleft cysts. BOLMAN, R. M. Am. J. Surg. *71:*96–99, Jan '46
Treatment of sebaceous cysts by electrosurgical marsupialization. DANNA, J. A. Ann. Surg. *123:*952–956, May '46
Branchial cysts of lateral cervical region.

Cysts and Fistulas, Branchial—Cont.
VAN CANEGHEM, D. Belg. tijdschr. geneesk. *2:*236–246, May '46
Treatment of branchial cleft cysts by aspiration and injection of pure carbolic acid (phenol) JARMAN, T. F. Brit. M. J. *1:*953–954, June 22, '46
Branchiogenic cyst of right carotid region; case of difficult diagnosis. CABALLERO, A. AND TORTI, D. D. Rev. med.-quir. de pat. fem. *25:*283–291, July '46

Cysts and Fistulas, Thyroglossal (See also Cysts and Fistulas)
Cysts and fistulae of thyroglossal duct. GILMAN, P. K. Surg., Gynec. and Obst. *32:*141, Feb '21
Cysts of thyroglossal tract. SISTRUNK, W. E. S. Clin. N. Amer. *1:*1509, Oct '21
Thyroglossal cyst and fistula. GESSNER, H. B. Southern M. J. *17:*428–430, June '24
Thyroglossal cysts and fistulae. BAILEY, H. Brit. J. Surg. *12:*579–589, Jan '25
Case of true congenital thyroglossal fistula. BAILEY, H. Proc. Roy. Soc. Med. (Clin. Sect.) *18:*6–7, Jan '25
Study of thryoglossal tract. BERTWISTLE, A. P. AND FRAZER, J. E. Brit. J. Surg. *12:*561–578, Jan '25
Results of operations on thyroglossal tract and a note on thyroid secretions. BERTWISTLE, A. P. Canad. M. A. J. *15:*400–401, April '25
Congenital cysts and fistulae of neck; review of 42 thyroglossal cysts and fistulae. KLINGENSTEIN, P. AND COLP, R. Ann. Surg. *82:*854–864, Dec '25
Median cervical fistulae. HLAVÁČEK, V. Casop. lek. Cesk. *66:*511–514, March 28, '27
Persistent or patent thymic duct. COMER, M. C. Southwestern Med. *11:*308–309, July '27
Thyroglossal fistula, four times recurrent; case. BIDART MALBRÁN, J. C. Bol. y trab. de la Soc. de cir. de Buenos Aires *12:*491–498, Sept. 5, '28
Cysts and fistulae; thyroglossal; with notes of case. ARMSTRONG, H. G. St. Michael's Hosp. M. Bull. *3:*90–93, Dec '28
Congenital median fistula of neck. DE MARCHI, E. Arch. ital. di chir. *22:*91–100, '28
Thyroglossal fistula; classification, clinical aspects, surgical treatment; cases. EGÜES, A. Bol. Inst. de clin. quir. *4:*313–367, '28
Cysts and fistulae of median cervical line. MAGLIULO, A. Sperimentale, Arch. di biol *82:*455–504, '28
Formation of medial cysts of neck. KORKHOFF, U. Vrach. gaz. *34:*779–781, May 31, '30

Cysts and Fistulas, Thyroglossal—Cont.
Fistula in center of neck; recidivation because of inflamation of Boyer's bursa; case. CIEZA RODRÍGUEZ, M. Semana med. *1:*552–554, Feb. 26, '31
Thyroglossal cysts and fistulae. JARVIS, H. G. New England J. Med. *205:*987–991, Nov. 19, '31
Thyroglossal fistula; medical therapy; case. BERGARA, R. AND BERGARA, C. Rev. Asoc. med. argent. *47:*1983–1986, Jan '33
Thyroglossal fistula with submental opening (case). PARSONS, W. B. JR. Ann. Surg. *97:*143, Jan '33
Thyroglossal fistula in children; surgical therapy; 2 cases. NOGUEIRA, P. Rev. Assoc. paulista de med. *2:*206–212, April '33
Medial cervical fistula probably of thyroglossal origin; recovery after surgical intervention. BÉRARD *et al.* Lyon med. *151:*611–613, May 14, '33
Congenital median fistula of neck; pathogenesis and histology. ŚWIATLOWSKI, B. Monatschr. f. Ohrenh. *68:*1096–1106, Sept '34
Thyroglossal fistulae. BASTOS, E. Rev. otolaring. de Sao Paulo *3:*227–238, May–June '35
Branchial and thyroglossal duct cysts and fistulas. BROWN, J. M. Ann. Otol., Rhin. and Laryng. *44:*644–652, Sept '35
Congenital median cysts and fistulae of neck. IONESCU, N. V. Rev. san. mil., Bucuresti *35:*71–80, Jan '36
Management of cysts and fistulas (thyroglossal). HENDRICK, J. W. Texas State J. Med. *32:*34–36, May '36
Complete thyroglossal fistula; case. PASQUALINO, G. Riv. san. siciliana *25:*586–593, May 15, '37
Persistence of thyroglossal duct; median cervical fistula; 2 cases. SORU, S. *et al.* Rev. de chir., Bucuresti *41:*48–56, Jan–Feb '38 also: Ann. d'oto-laryng., pp. 318–324, April '38
Cyst of ductus thymopharyngeus; case. BRECHET, J. Zentralbl. f. alig. Path. u. path. Anat. *69:*353–357, March 30, '38
Avoiding postoperative recurrence of thyroglossal fistula in surgical therapy; necessity of resection of hyoid bone. CHIAROLANZA, R. Arch. ital. di chir. *51:*331–336, '38
Medial cervical fistula due to persistance of thryoglossal tract; case. RASTELLI, E. Gior. med. d. Alto Adige *11:*3–14, Jan '39
Complete thyroglossal fistulas. KINSELLA, V. J. Brit. J. Surg. *26:*714–720, April '39
Injection treatment of chronic sinuses; case of infected thyroglossal duct cured by copper

Cysts and Fistulas, Thyroglossal—Cont.

sulfate injections. HUGHES, R. P. AND SMITH, L. M. Southwestern Med. *23:*187, June '39

Thyroglossal fistulas and cysts. OTTOBRINI COSTA, M. AND LABATE, F. Pediatria prat., Sao Paulo *10:*287–300, July-Aug '39

Technic for extirpation of thyroglossal fistulas. FINOCHIETTO, R. AND VEPPO, A. A. Prensa med. argent. *26:*1920–1926, Oct. 4, '39

Extirpation of hyoid bone in therapy of thyroglossal cyst; 3 cases. SUMERMAN, S. Turk tib cem. mec. *5:*265–271, '39

Thyroglossal cysts, sinuses and fistulae; results in 293 surgical cases. PEMBERTON, J. DE J. AND STALKER, L. K. Ann. Surg. *111:*950–957, June '40

Thyroglossal fistula due to persistence of thyroglossal tract; cases. ALTAVISTA, A. E. Rev. otorrinolaring. d. litoral *1:*232–241, March '42

Thyroglossal fistula, with report of case. CASANUEVA DEL C., M. AND VILLARROEL, E. Arch. Soc. cirujanos hosp. *12:*79–84, May-Aug '42

Cystic tumors; branchial and thyroglossal cysts. MCNEALY, R. W., J. Am. Dent. A. *29:*1808–1818, Oct. 1, '42

Complete thyroglossal fistula; 2 cases. COUDANE, R. AND FABRE, A. Ann. d'oto-laryng., pp. 93–99, July-Sept '44

Thyroglossal cysts and fistulas; 8 cases. SIBILIA, C. E. Rev. Asoc. med. argent. *58:*888–891, Oct. 15, '44

Thyroglossal cysts and fistulas; 8 cases. SIBILLA, C. E. Bol. y trab., Soc. argent. de cirujanos *5:*543–553, '44

Salivary fistula of submaxillary gland following excision of thyroglossal cyst. JENKINS, H. B. Am. J. Surg. *70:*118–120, Oct '45

Cysts, Implantation

Post-traumatic epidermoid cysts of hands and fingers. KING, E. S. J. Brit. J. Surg. *21:*29–43, July '33

Mechanism of development of epithelial cysts; behavior of autogenous skin particle implanted subcutaneously. ŌKUMA, M. Nagasaki Igakkai Zasshi *14:*94–96, Jan. 25, '36

Traumatic implantation of epithelial cyst in phalanx. YACHNIN, S. C. AND SUMMERILL, F., J.A.M.A. *116:*1215–1218, March 22, '41

Cysts, Sebaceous (See also Cysts and Fistulas; Dermoid Cysts

Bygone operations in surgery; removal of sebaceous cyst from King George IV. POWER, D'A. Brit. J. Surg. *20:*361–365, Jan '33

Cysts; sebaceous, mucous, dermoid and epidermoid. ERICH, J. B. Am. J. Surg. *50:*672–677, Dec '40

Sebaceous cysts of face; extirpation. FINOCHIETTO, R. Prensa med. argent. *30:*1876–1877, Sept. 29, '43

Cysts, Thymic

Congenital cyst of thymic origin in neck. PEZCOLLER, A. Clin. chir. *32:*272–284, March '29

Thymic cyst; case. HYDE, T. L. *et al.* Texas, State J. Med. *39:*539–540, Feb '44

CZIRER, L.: Burn therapy. Orvosi hetil. *81:*591–594, June 5, '37

CZUKRASZ, I.: Eyelid surgery; about sliding-flap, known also as Hungarian plastic. Tr. Ophth. Soc. U. Kingdom (pt. 2) *58:*561–575, '38

CZUKRASZ, I.: Epithelial inlay with Kerr-material to form eye socket. Brit. J. Ophth. *23:*343–347, May '39

CZWALINSKI, P. F.: Burn therapy at sea. U.S. Nav. M. Bull. *42:*838–840, April '44

D

DABNEY, S. G.: Malignant disease of superior maxillary bone; continued report. Kentucky M. J. *19:*125, March '21

DABNEY, S. G.: Salivary fistula; case report. Kentucky M. J. *20:*589, Sept '22

D'ABREU, A. R.: Congenital bilateral absence of radius and thumb. Indian M. Gaz. *65:*505–507, Sept '30

D'ABREU, A. R.: Bilateral absence of radius and thumb. Indian M. Gaz. *67:*266–267, May '32

Dacryocystorhinostomy

Mosher-Toti operation on lacrimal sac. MOSHER, H. P. Laryngoscope *31:*284, May '21

Plastic operation on lacrimal canal. BENJAMINS, C. E. AND VAN ROMUNDE, L. H. Nederlandsch Tijdschr. v. Geneesk. *2:*33–35, July 1, '22 (illus.)

Indications, contraindications and preparation for dacrycystorhinostomy. FENTON, R. A. Ann. Otol., Rhin. and Laryng. *32:*67–83, March '23 (illus.)

Dacryocystorhinostomy; combined methods. SAUER, W. E. Ann. Otol., Rhin. and Laryng. *32:*25–43, March '23 (illus.)

Dacryocystorhinostomy – Cont.

Dupuy-Dutemps and Bourguet's plastic dacryocystorhinostomy in chronic dacryocystitis. HUSSON, A. AND JEANDELIZE, P. Medecine *5:*256–259, Jan '24

Dacryocystorhinostomy. GILLUM J. R., J. Indiana M. A. *17:*113–116, April '24

Plastic operations for obtaining nasolacrimal passages. KRUSIUS, F. F. Deutsche med. Wchnschr. *50:*954–955, July 11, '24

Treatment of lacrimal fistula following dacryocystectomy. HANDS, S. G., J. Iowa M. Soc. *15:*598–600, Nov '25

Dacryocystorhinoplasty, Mosher's modification of Toti method. COWEN, S. B. Ohio State M. J. *21:*902–905, Dec '25

Toti-Mosher operation; dacryocystorhinostomy; combined endonasal and external technic. SIBBALD, D. AND O'FARRELL, G. Rev. Soc. argent. de Oftal. *1:*79–82, '25

Indications for dacryocystorhinostomy. CASADESÚS CASTELLS, F. Med. ibera *2:*229, Sept. 25; 249, Oct. 2, '26

Historical observation on improvement of Toti's operation (dacryocystorhinostomy). OHM, J. Klin. Monatsbl. f. Augenh. *77:*825–832, Dec '26

Toti-Mosher operation; dacryocystorhinostomy. SIBBALD, AND O'FARRELL. Rev. de especialid. *1:*568–573, '26

Toti's dacryocystorhinostomy. WISSELINK, G. W. Klin. Monatsbl. f. Augenh. *78:*550, April '27

Indications for dacryocystorhinostomy. URBANEK, J. Wien. med. Wchnschr. *77:*1109, Aug. 20, '27

Easy method of dacryocystorhinostomy. CLAUS, H. Beitr. z. Anat., Physiol., Path. u. Thereap. d. Ohres *26:*121–124, Nov '27

Dacryocystorhinostomy; 2 cases. POLYACK, G. D. Ann. d'ocul. *164:*942–951, Dec '27

Dacryocystorhinostomy; radical cure for lacrimation. MANES, A. J. Semana med. *1:*1020–1027, April 26, '28

Dacryocystorhinostomy. LARSSON, S. Acta ophth. *6:*193–215, '28

Technic and indications of dacryocystorhinostomy. RUBBRECHT, R. Technic and indications of dacryocystorhinostomy. Bull. Soc. belge d'opht., no. 57, pp. 94–106, '28

End-results in dacryocystorhinostomy. BASZERRA, J. Med. ibera *1:*545–547, April 27, '29

Reconstruction of destroyed lacrimal excretory apparatus. ASCHER, K. W. Med. Klin. *25:*749–750, May 10, '29

Simplified dacryocystorhinostomy, modification of Toti's method. DE LIETO VOLLARO, A. Boll. d'ocul. *8:*561–574, June '29

Dacryocystorhinostomy – Cont.

Dacryocystorhinostomy by method of Dupuy-Dutemps and Bourguet. POTIQUET, H. Ann. d'ocul. *166:*470–487, June '29

Modification of Toti's dacryocystorhinostomy. POLJAK, G. D. Klin. Monatsbl. f. Augenh. *83:*510–515, Oct–Nov '29

Technical points suggesting dacryocystorhinostomy. ANDINA, M. Rev. cubana de oft. *1:*424–426, Nov '29

New instruments for Toti operation (dacryocystorhinostomy). GUTZEIT, R. Klin. Monatsbl. f. Augenh. *84:*92, Jan '30

Hemo-aspiration and trephining with aid of electric apparatus in dacryocystorhinostomy. SUBILEAU, J. M. Ann. d'ocul. *167:*301–306, April '30

Dacryocystorhinostomy. CILLERUELO. Informacion med. *7:*179–189, Aug '30

Mosher-Toti dacryocystorhinostomy. SPAETH, E. B. Arch. Ophth. *4:*487–496, Oct '30

External dacryocystorhinostomy. LOPES DE ANDRADE. Med. contemp. *49:*21–29, Jan. 18, '31

West's dacryocystorhinostomy in 300 cases. ALCAINO, A. AND RODRÍGUEZ, D. M. Arch. de oftal. hispano-am. *31:*65–79, Feb '31

Technic in dacryocystorhinostomy. GÓMEZ-MÁRQUEZ. Arch. de oftal. hispano-am. *31:*147–176, March '31

Dacryocystorhinostomies; 517 cases. GÓMEZ-MÁRQUEZ. Klin. Monatsbl. f. Augenh. *86:*620–629, May '31

Dacryocystorhinostomy, Dupuy-Dutemps method; 25 cases. GONZÁLEZ LLANOS, N. Rev. de especialid. *6:*237, May '31

Grave hemorrhage as late complication of dacryocystorhinostomy; 2 cases. MARÍN AMAT, M. Siglo med. *87:*673–675, June 20, '31 also: Arch. d'opht. *48:*632–638, Sept '31

Technic in external dacryocystorhinostomy. TORRES ESTRADA, A. Gac. med. de Mexico *62:*339–360, Aug '31

Operations on lacrimal ducts. SATTLER, C. H. Ztschr. f. Augenh. *75:*237–239, Oct '31

Severe hemorrhage as late complication of dacryocystorhinostomy. MARÍN-AMAT, M. Bull. et mem. Soc. franc. d'opht. *44:*269–278, '31 also: Arch. de oftal. hispano-am. *31:*629–636, Nov '31

Formation of new lacrimonasal canal after excision of lacrimal sac. MATHEWSON, G. H. Am. J. Ophth. *14:*1252, Dec '31

New instrument for detachment of sac in dacryocystectomy. NEUSCHULER, I. Arch. d'opht. *48:*829–831, Dec '31

Dacryocystorhinostomy; indications and

Dacryocystorhinostomy – Cont.
technic; case. GRAUE Y GLENIE, E. An. Soc. mex. de oftal. y oto-rino-laring. *9:*114–116, Jan–March '32
Technic of dacryocystorhinostomy. WEEKS, W. W. Arch. Ophth. *7:*443–447, March '32
Technic of external dacryocystorhinostomy. TORRES ESTRADA, A. An. Soc. mex. de oftal. y oto-rino-laring. *9:*131–157, April–June '32
Statistics on 1000 plastic dacryocystotomies. DUPUY-DUTEMPS, L. Bull. Soc. d'opht. de Paris, pp. 392–399, June '32
External dacryocystorhinostomy according to Gutzeit method. DIAZ-CANEJA, E. Ann. d'ocul. *170:*384–414, May '33 also: An. Casa de Salud Valdecilla *3:*292–313, '32
Observations on 1000 plastic dacryocystotomies. DUPUY-DUTEMPS, L. Ann. d'ocul. *170:*361–384, May '33
Results of intranasal dacryocystorhinostomy (West operation). HENRY, L. M. J. Brit. J. Ophth. *17:*550–552, Sept '33
Toti-Mosher operation (lacrimal ducts) and its end results. MARTIN, R. C. Tr. Pacific Coast Oto-Ophth. Soc. *21:*50–58, '33
Dacryocystorhinostomy by modified Gutzeit method. MATA, P. Arch. de oftal. hispano-am. *34:*141–147, March '34
External dacryocystorhinostomy. PREOBRAZHENSKIY, V. V. Sovet. vrach. gaz., pp. 388–390, March 15, '34
Result of surgical therapy of suppuration of lacrimal sac after implantation of lower end of lacrimal sac into nose; modified Toti operation. STOCK, W. Klin. Monatsbl. f. Augenh. *92:*433–435, April '34
Dacryocystorhinostomy. WODON. Arch. med. belges *87:*95–97, June '34
New knife for dacryocystorhinostomy. MEURMAN, Y. Acta otolaryng. *21:*343–345, '34
Dacryocystorhinostomy and its clinical results. MOREU, A. Arch. de oftal. hispano-am. *35:*127–139, March '35
External dacryocystorhinostomy. DE ALMEIDA, A. Rev. brasil. de cir. *4:*181–188, April '35
Dacryocystorhinostomy; easy and sure method. WEEKERS, L. Arch. d'opht. *52:*241–246, April '35
Technic of extranasal dacryocystorhinostomy. BASTERRA, J. Cron. med., Valencia *39:*354–363, May 15, '35
Technic of endonasal dacryocystorhinostomy. (Halle operation); cases. JUST TISCORNIA, B. AND MERCANDINO, C. P. Rev. med. latino-am. *20:*1118–1136, July '35
Plastic dacryocystorhinostomy in 1200 cases.

Dacryocystorhinostomy – Cont.
AVERBAKH, M. AND IVANOVA, MME. Ann. d'ocul. *172:*913–936, Nov '35
Dacryocystorhinostomy by nasal route. PETTERINO PATRIARCA, A. AND DUC, C. Rassegna ital. d'ottal. *5:*205–224, March–April '36
Technic of extranasal dacryocystorhinostomy. BASTERRA, J. Arch. de oftal. hispano-am. *36:*208–216, April '36
Dacryocystorhinostomy according to plastic procedure of Bourguet-Dupuy-Dutemps. VANCEA, P. Rev. san. mil., Bucuresti *35:*393–395, April '36
Cause of failure of dacryocystorhinostomy. ESTEBAN, M. Rev. cubana de oto-neuro-oftal. *5:*99–100, May–June '36
Plastic dacryocystorhinostomy. FILHO, A. P. Rev. oto-laring. de Sao Paulo (no. 5, bis) *4:*731–747, Sept–Oct '36
Progress in dacryocystorhinostomy. FRIEBERG, T. Nord. med. tidskr. *12:*1686–1687, Oct. 10, '36
Dacryocystorhinostomy. AMSLER, M. Schweiz. med. Wchnschr. *66:*1268–1270, Dec. 12, '36
Dacryocystorhinostomy (Mosher-Toti operation). HOOVER, W. B., S. Clin. North America *16:*1695–1699, Dec '36
Dacryocystorhinostomy. CHANDLER, P. A. Tr. Am. Ophth. Soc. *34:*240–263, '36
Surgical therapy of flow of tears after removal of lacrimal sac. TOWBIN, B. G. Arch. f. Ophth. *135:*579–580, '36
Artificial restoration of nasolacrimal duct. GERKE, J. Ztschr. f. Augenh. *91:*50–52, Jan '37
Technic of dacryocystostomy. ZARZYCKI, P. Bull. Soc. d'opht. de Paris *49:*9–12, Jan '37
Simplified modification of external dacryocystorhinostomy. KALEFF, Ztschr. f. Augenh. *91:*140–157, Feb '37
Dacryocystorhinostomy; technic and results. WEVE, H. J. M. AND KENTGENS, S. K. Klin. Monatsbl. f. Augenh. *98:*195–205, Feb '37
Simplification of classic technic of external dacryocystorhinostomy. TORRES ESTRADA, A. Cir. y cirujanos *5:*219–250, May–June '37
Dacryocystorhinostomy. WRIGHT, R. E. Lancet *2:*250–251, July 31, '37
Results of intranasal dacryocystorhinostomy. WALSH, T. E. AND BOTHMAN, L. Am. J. Ophth. *20:*939–941, Sept '37
Dacryocystorhinectomy in stenoses of lacrimal sac; new technic. CORNET, E. Rev. med. franc. d'Extreme-Orient (16):551–554, May '38

Dracryocystorhinostomy—Cont.

Modified Brigg's retractor for dacryocystorhinostomy. Stallard, H. B. Brit. J. Ophth. *22:*361, June '38

Turbinotome for "ab externo" dacryocystorhinostomy. Rassegna ital. d'ottal. *7:*499–503, July–Aug '38

Congenital stenosis of nasolacrimal duct; complications and treatment. Granström, K. O. Nord. med. tidskr. *16:*1280–1283, Aug. 13, '38

Dacryocystorhinostomy by external route; technic. Venco, L. Rassegna ital. d'ottal. *7:*593–612, Sept–Oct '38

Chisel for dacryocystorhinostomy. Haas, E. Bull. Soc. d'opht. de Paris *50:*468–469, Oct '38

Dacryocystorhinostomy; new technic. Cornet, E. Ann. d'ocul. *175:*842–845, Nov '38

Dacryocystorhinostomy; critieria of operability, indications, complications and results. Venco, L. Riv. oto-neuro-oftal. *15:*510–531, Nov–Dec '38

Simple dacryocystorhinostomy. Guy, L. Arch. Ophth. *20:*954–957, Dec '38

Dacryocystorhinostomy by nasal route (West operation) and its results. Arganaraz, R. *et al.* Cong. argent. de oftal. (1936) *2:*491–496, '38

Treatment of congenital atresia of nasolacrimal duct. Larsson, S. Acta ophth. *16:*271–278, '38

Treatment of epiphora, with special reference to some cases treated by dacryocystorhinostomy. Morgan, O. G. Tr. Ophth. Soc. U. Kingdom (pt. 1) *58:*163–172, '38

Late results of external dacryocystorhinostomy. Tomkevich, A. I. Vestnik oftal. *13:*388–396, '38

Construction of lacrimal passages. Nizetic, Z. Klin. Monatsbl. f. Augenh. *102:*67–71, Jan '39

Two-stage dacryocystorhinostomy. Nizetic, Z. Klin. Monatsbl. f. Augenh. *102:*71–76, Jan '39

Dacryocystostomy by nasal route. Matsui, T. Oto-rhino-laryng. *12:*238–241, March '39 (in Japanese).

Surgical technic for construction of pituitary conjunctival canal (artificial lacrimal canal). da Silva Costa, A. Bull. Soc. d'opht. de Paris *5:*385–388, June '39

Transplantation (implantation) of lacrimal sac in chronic dacryocystitis. Stokes, W. H. Arch. Ophth. *22:*193–210, Aug '39

External dacryocystorhinostomy by Torres Estrada technic. Gurria Urgell, D. Gac. med. de Mexico *69:*336–340, Oct. 30, '39

Importance of suture of lacrimal sac and nasal mucosa in dacryocystorhinostomy. Balacco, F. Boll. d'ocul. *18:*876–880, Nov '39

Dacryocystorhinostomy by way of pyriform aperture. Kofler, K. Monatschr. f. Ohrenh. *74:*299–306, June '40

New Technic for dacryocystorhinostomy. Vaquero, L. Rev. med. d. Hosp. gen. *3:*244–253, Dec. 15, '40

Dacryocystorhinostomy; author's experience. Pereira, R. F. Arch. de oftal. de Buenos Aires *15:*603–613, Dec '40

New drills for dacryocystorhinostomy. Cramer, F. E. K. and Balza, J. Semana med. *1:*294–295, Jan. 30, '41

Dacryocystorhinostomy; interesting points on operation. Yanes, T. R. Arch. Ophth. *26:*12–20, July '41

Dacryocystorhinostomy. Ayuyao, C. D. and Yambao, C. V., J. Philippine M. A. *21:* 391–393, Aug '41

Dacryocystorhinostomy. Hughes, W. L. *et al.* Surg., Gynec. and Obst. *73:*375–380, Sept '41

Question of external or internal dacryocystorhinostomy. Hausmann, R. Arch. f. Ohren-, Nasen-u. Kehlkopfh. *149:*309–316, '41

Dacryocystorhinostomy in Venezuela. Rhode, J. Arch. venezol. Soc. de oto-rino-laring., oftal., neurol. *3:*1–56, March '42

Dacryocystorhinostomy versus dacryocystectomy. Yanes, T. R. Vida nueva *49:*132–136, April '42

Plastic dacryocystorhinostomy; technic. Lathrop, F. D., S. Clin. North America *22:*675–679, June '42

Instruments to facilitate mucosal suture in dacryocystorhinostomy. Bangerter, A. Ophthalmologica *104:*171–174, Sept '42

Simple method for preparing dacryocystorhinostomy needles. Balod, K. Klin. Monatsbl. f. Augenh. *108:*626, Sept–Oct '42

Dacryocystotomy and canaliculorhinostomy. Valle, D. Arq. brasil. de oftal. *5:*236–251, Oct '42

Construction of lacrimal passage. Guy, L. P. Arch. Ophth. *29:*575–577, April '43

Intranasal approach to lacrimal sac (transparent dacryocystotomy). Matis, E. T. Laryngoscope *53:*357–365, May '43

Dacryocystorhinostomy; logical treatment of occlusion of lacrimal sac. Hallum, A. V., J. M. A. Georgia *32:*186–189, June '43

Technical difficulties and complications of dacryocystorhinostomy by external route. Cramer, F. E. K. Semana med. *2:*604–610, Sept. 9, '43

Dacryocystorhinostomy – Cont.
Dacryocystorhinostomy in Venezuela. RHODE, J. Gac. med. de Caracas *50:*231, Nov. 30, '43; 241, Dec. 15, '43; 251, Dec. 31, '43 *51:*261, Jan. 15, '44 comment by Lopez Villoria *51:*264, Jan. 15, '44; 11, Jan. 31 '44
Dacryocystorhinostomy for obstruction. AMSLER, M. Ophthalmologica *107:*50–51, Jan-Feb '44
Simplified technic for dacryocystorhinostomy. TORRES ESTRADA, A., J. Internat. Coll. Surgeons *7:*147–158, March-April '44
Rhinocanalicular anastomosis. WALDAPFEL, R. Arch. Ophth. *31:*432–433, May '44
Simplified external dacryocystorhinostomy. WILLIAMS, J. L. D. AND HILL, B. G. Brit. J. Ophth. *28:*407–410, Aug '44
Twenty-five years of dacryorhinostomy (1919–1944). SURLA. Arch. Soc. oftal. hispano-am. *4:*807–812, Sept-Oct '44
Autoplastic dacryorhinostomy; new process for reconstructing lacrimal organs by means of labial mucosal graft. NIEMEYER, W. Arq. brasil. de oftal. *8:*181–185, Dec '45
New instruments for dacryocystorhinostomy. SANCHEZ BULNES, L. AND SILVA, D. Arch. Asoc. para evit. ceguera Mexico *3:*249–255, '45
West operation (endonasal dacryocystostomy). MCARTHUR, G. A. D., M. J. Austalia *1:*508–510, April 13, '46
Operation for chronic dacryocystitis (plastic dacryocystorhinostomy). HAMILTON, R. G. Pennsylvania M. J. *49:*1327–1330, Sept '46

D'AGATA, G.: Rhinoplasty by rotation of flaps from cheek. Policlinico (sez. prat.) *34:*168, Jan 31, '26
DAGGETT, W. I. AND BATEMAN, G. H.: Secondary Thiersch grafting of radical mastoid cavity through meatus. J. Laryng. and Otol. *49:*169–174, March '34
DAHL, G. M.: Experiences in therapy of maxillary injuries during Russian-Finnish war. Acta odont. Scandinav. *2:*1–18, June '40
DAHLBERG, A. A.: Treatment of lip and cheek in cases of facial paralysis (by plastic lip cradle). J.A.M.A. *124:*503–504, Feb 19, '44
DAHMANN, H.: Cork as plastic material for correction of saddle noses. Ztschr. f. Laryng., Rhin. *20:*451–457, March '31
DAINELLI, M.: Surgical technic employed in therapy of extremely short stumps in amputations of thigh; preliminary report. Policlinico (sez. prat.) *49:*377–383, Mar 16, '42
DAITÔ, T.: Rhinolalia clausa palatina functionalis. Fukuoka-Ikwadaigaku-Zasshi *24:*87–90, Sept '31
DALAND, E. M.: Plastic reconstruction of lower lip in cancer. New England J. Med. *205:*1131–1142, Dec 10, '31
DALAND, E. M.: Repair of large defects of lips after removal for cancer. Surg., Gynec. and Obst. *69:*347–357, Sept '39
DALAND, E. M.: Symposium on cancer: radiation damage to tissue and its repair. Surg., Gynec. and Obst. *72:*372–383, Feb (no. 2A) '41
DALAND, E. M. (see SIMMONS, C. C.) Dec '22
D'ALBO, E. A. (see BRACCO, J. A.) Oct '43
DALE, H. (see HOLT, R. L. *et al*)
DALE, H. W. L.: Regional anesthesia of nose. Lancet *1:*562–563, April 29, '44
D'ALESSANDRO, A.: Autoplastic skin implant in blepharoplasty. Semana med. *2:*1531–1534, Dec 17, '25
DALEPPA, K.: Lipoma of cheek and neck. Indian M. Gaz. *62:*385–386, July '27
DALEY, J.: Retaining correct septolabial angle in rhinoplasty. Arch. Otolaryng. *39:*348–349, April '44
DALEY, J.: Introduction of artistic point of view in regard to rhinoplastic diagnosis. Arch. Otolaryng. *42:*33–41, July '45
DALGER, J.: Action of periarterial sympathectomy on skin grafts. Lyon chir. *23:*451–452, July-Aug '26
DAL LAGO: (see LAGO)
DALLING, E. J.: Notes from maxillofacial centers; intraoral methods of immobilizing mandibular fractures. Bull. War Med. *3:*555, June '43 (abstract)
DALLING, E. J.: Maxillofacial surgical unit mobile dental laboratory. Brit. Dent. J. *78:*10–12, Jan 5, '45
DALSGAARD, S.: Treatment of disrupted extensor tendon from terminal phalanx of finger by means of simple splint. Ugesk. f. laeger *96:*273–274, March 8, '34 abstr: Acta chir.Scandinav. *74:*429, '34
DALTON, S. E.: Self-retaining illuminating palate retractor. Tr. A. Acad. Ophth. (1941) *46:*151, Jan-Feb '42
DALY, R. F.: Prophylactic and therapeutic use of adrenal cortical substances in shock; preliminary report. Rev. M. Progr., pp. 33–35, '41
DAMAYE, H. AND POIRIER, B.: Delirium tremens excited by infected burns. Progres med., p. 1340, Aug 2, '30
DAMBRIN, L.: Macrodactylia. Rev. D'orthop. *3:*215–229, May '36
DAMBRIN, L. AND DAMBRIN, P.: Cranioplasty by sterilized grafts from human cadaver. Bordeaux chir. *7:*279–286, July '36
DAMBRIN, P. (see DAMBRIN, L.) July '36
DAMEL, C. S.: Reconstruction of conjunctival culdesac and eyelid in patients after enuclea-

tion of eye; technic. Rev. Asoc. med. argent. *47:*2733–2738, June '33

DANCHAKOFF, V. AND DANCHAKOFF, V. E.: Age factor in transplantation. Contrib. Embryol. (no. 124) *21:*125–140, June '30

DANCHAKOFF, V. E. (see DANCHAKOFF, V.) June '30

DANDY, W. E.: Method of restoring nerves requiring resection (by removing neuroma, shortening bone and suturing nerve). J.A.M.A. *122:*35–36, May 1, '43

DANDY, W. E. (see HANRAHAN, E. M.) April '44

DANE, P. G.: Results of 98 cases of nerve suture. Brit. M. J. *1:*885, June 18, '21

DANELIUS, B.: Example of Joseph nose improvement. Acta oto-laryng. *9:*49–52, '26 (in English).

DANIEL, C.: Artificial vagina made from intestine; 13 cases. Rev. Franc. de gynec. et d'obst. *19:*305–321, May 25, '24

DANIEL, G. H.: Hereditary anarthrosis of index finger, with associated abnormalities in proportions of fingers; case. Ann. Eugenics *7:*281–297, Nov '36

DANIEL, R. A. JR.: Treatment of facial fractures. J. Tennessee M.A. *33:*419–426, Nov'40

DANIELS, J. (see RUBENSTEIN, A. D. *et al*) Nov '45

DANIS, R.: Autoplastic and heteroplastic bone grafts in osteosynthesis. Bull. Acad. roy. de med. de Belgique *1:*88–94, '36 also: J. de med. de Paris *56:*631–633, July 30, '36

DANNA, J. A.: Treatment of sebaceous cysts by electrosurgical marsupialization. Ann. Surg. *123:*952–956, May '46

DANNREUTHER, W. T.: Frank-Geist operation for congenital absence of vagina (skin graft). Am. J. Obst. and Gynec. *35:*452–468, March '38

DANNREUTHER, W. T.: Partial congenital aplasia of vagina (transplantation of fetal membranes for artificial vagina in one case). Am. J. Obst. and Gynec. *44:*1063–1073, Dec '42 also: Tr. Am. Gynec. Soc. (1942) *67:*35–45, '43

DANTLO, R.: Restoration of shape of nose by cartilaginous autograft after old fracture. Strasbourg med. *93:*485–487, July 15, '33

DANTLO, R.: Modified technic of application of Davis grafts in extensive burns. Rev. de chir. plastique, pp. 219–237, Oct '33

DANTRELLE: Free skin grafts. Rev. de chir. plastique, pp. 3–15, April '32

DANTRELLE: Technic of transplanting mucosa. Rev. de chir. plastique, pp. 274–287, Oct '32

DANTRELLE: Technic of incisions and sutures in plastic surgery (face). Rev. de chir. plastique, pp. 75–108, Aug '33

DANTRELLE: Cicatrization and scars. Rev. de chir. plastique, pp. 301–319, Jan '34

DANTRELLE AND SHEEHAN: Orbital grafting of cartilage from nasal ala; technic. Ann. d'ocul. *165:*902–909, Dec '28

DANTRELLE, A.: Esthetic surgery of nose. J. de med. de Paris *55:*865–870, Oct. 3, '35

DANTRELLE, A.: Esthetic surgery of eyelids. J. de med. de Paris *55:*997–1004, Nov 14, '35

DANTRELLE, A.: Injuries and plastic surgery of face from medicolegal point of view. Rev. de chir. structive, pp. 133–147, Dec '35

DANTRELLE, A.: Esthetic surgery of lips. J. de med. de Paris *56:*57–62, Jan. 23, '36

DANTRELLE, M.: Choice method in plastic restoration of face following extensive burns causing cicatricial disfigurement. Rev. de chir. structive, pp. 108–109, June '37

DANZIGER, F.: Epispadias; operation. Ztschr. f. urol. Chir. *25:*21–24, '28

DANZIS, M.; FRIEDMAN, M. AND LEVINSON, L. J.: Carcinoma developing on extensive scars; inefficiency of pinch grafts as prophylactic measure. Am. J. Surg. *41:*304–306, Aug '38

DAPLYN, P. F. L.: Vinesthene (vinyl ether) anesthesia for repair of harelip and cleft palate Brit. M. J. *2:*117–119, July 27, '46

DARCISSAC, M.: Correction of ankylosis of jaws. Paris med. *12:*227–229, Sept 2, '22 (illus.) abstr: J.A.M.A. *79:*1884, Nov 25, '22

DARCISSAC, M.: Temporomaxillary ankylosis; surgical and prosthetic treatment. J. de med. et chir. prat. *99:*581–590, Aug 25, '28

DARCISSAC, M.: Plastic surgery in loss of substance of alveolar border of incisive region of upper jaw; case. Bull. et mem. Soc. d. chirurgiens de Paris *23:*507–511, July 3, '31

DARCISSAC, M.: Lateral expansion of upper jaw in case of marked atresia in patient 30 years old; amelioration of nasal permeability. Bull. et mem. Soc. d. chirurgiens de Paris *25:*296–300, May 5, '33

DARCISSAC, M.: Mandibular automobilizer; use in therapy of postoperative temporomaxillary ankylosis. Bull. et mem. Soc. d. chirurgiens de Paris *26:*561–568, Oct 19, '34

DARCISSAC, M.: Preoperative and postoperative prosthesis in application of skin, cutaneomucosal, cartilage and bone grafts and in improvement of cicatrix of face. Bull. et mem. Soc. d. chirurgiens de Paris *28:*424–433, June 19, '36

DARCISSAC, M.: Prosthesis in restorative surgery of face. Rev. de chir. structive, pp. 420–424, Dec '36

DARCISSAC, M.: Therapy of acute invading form of osteomyelitis of lower jaw; author's technic. J. de med. de Bordeaux *114:*387–408, Oct 30, '37

DARCISSAC, M.: Bilateral temporomaxillary luxation of 5 months' duration, considered irreducible, but reduced under local anesthesia by elastic traction on transangular metallic loops. Rev. de stomatol. *43:*5-13, Jan-Feb '42
DARCISSAC, M. (see DUFOURMENTEL, L.) Nov '28
DARCISSAC, M. (see DUFOURMENTEL, L.) June '32
DARCISSAC, M. (see DUFOURMENTEL, L. *et al*) Dec '32
DARCISSAC, M. (see DUFOURMENTEL, L.) May '33
DARCISSAC, M. (see DUFOURMENTEL, L. *et al*) June '33
DARCISSAC, M. (see DUFOURMENTEL, L.) Oct '33
DARCISSAC, M. (see DUFOURMENTEL, L.) May '34
DARCISSAC, M. (see DUFOURMENTEL, L.) July '34
DARCISSAC, M. (see DUFOURMENTEL, L.) March '35
DARCISSAC, M. (see DUFOURMENTEL, L.) 1939

Darcissac-Bruhn-Petroff Operation

Extension treatment of fractures of mandible by combined method (Darcissac-Bruhn-Petroff). TOMIRDIARO, O. Deutsche Monatschr. f. Zahnh. *49:*1112-1116, Nov 15, '31

DARGENT, M. (see CARCASSONNE, F.) July, '33
DARGENT, M. AND DUROUX, P. E.: Anatomic findings concerning morphology and relations of intraparotid facial nerve. Presse med. *54:*523-524, Aug 10, '46
DARGENT, M. (see BERARD, L. *et al*) May-June '38
DARGENT, M. (see PONTHUS, P. *et al*) April '42
DARGENT, M. (see SANTY, P.) April-May, '46
DARIER, J.: Etiology of cancer of face; prevention. Monde med., Paris *40:*65-73, Feb 1, '30
D'ARMAN, S.: Articular lesions due to crushing of fingers. Gior. veneto di sc. med. *8:*597-603, June '34
DARNALL, W. L.: Use of modified Baker anchorage in naval dental service for fractured jaw. U. S. Nav. M. Bull. *19:*42-45, July '23 (illus.)
DARNER, L. D.: Injuries to carpal bones. Internat. J. Med. and Surg. *45:*541-546, Dec '32
DARSIE, L. L. (see MULLIN, W. V.) Aug '35
DARTIGUES, L.: Surgical correction of pendulous breasts. Arch. franco-belges de chir. *28:*313-328, April '25
DARTIGUES, L.: Breast surgery with graft of areolar region; 2 cases. Monde med., Paris *38:*75-85, Feb 1, '28
DARTIGUES, L.: New operative technic of animal grafts in women. Rev. espan. de med. y cir. *11:*271-275, May '28
DARTIGUES, L.: Total mammectomy; free autograft of nipple and areola; bilateral aesthetic amputation. Bull. et mem. Soc. de chir. de Paris *20:*739-744, Nov 2, '28
DARTIGUES, L.: Apparatus for localization of transplanted areolae of breast in plastic surgery. Bull. et mem. Soc. de chir. de Paris *21:*43, Jan 4, '29
DARTIGUES, L.: Excision of breast combined with autoplastic areolomammary graft. Paris chir. *21:*11-19, Jan-Feb '29
DARTIGUES, L.: Description of new circular incision for breast plastic surgery. Bull. et mem. Soc. de chir. de Paris *21:*263, March 15, '29
DARTIGUES, L.: French law and aesthetic surgery. Vie med. *10:*289-298, March 25, '29
DARTIGUES, L.: Transpectoral costal mastopexy by peri-areolar route. Bull. et mem. Soc. de chir. de Paris *21:*287-289, April 19, '29
DARTIGUES, L.: Total bilateral mammectomy with free graft of nipple and areola. Bull. et mem. Soc. d. chirurgiens de Paris *25:*289-291, May 5, '33
DARTIGUES, L.: Present status of plastic surgery of breast. Clin. y lab. *23:*737-741, Sept '33
DARTIGUES, L.: Alignment points of nipples in relation to thorax in plastic surgery of breast. Clin. y lab. *28:*27-37, Jan '36 abstr: Bull. et mem. Soc. de med. de Paris *139:*494-499, Oct 10, '35
DARTIGUES, L.: Surgical therapy of breast abnormalities. Bull. et mem. Soc. de med. de Paris *139:*569-575, Nov 7, '35
DARTIGUES, L.: Method of examination of pendulous breasts before reconstructive surgery. Bull. et mem. Soc. de med. de Paris *140:*151-160, Feb 29, '36
DARTIGUES, L.: Alignment points of breast in relation to thorax in plastic surgery. Spitalul *56:*57-59, Feb '36 also: Rev. de chir. structive, pp. 287-291, June '36
DARTIGUES, L.: Medical responsibility in plastic surgery; possible precautions for protection of practitioner; how much should patient know of risks. Vie med. *17:*893-899, Dec 10, '36
DARTIGUES, L.: *Chirurgie réparatrice: Plastique et esthétique de la poitrine, des seins, et de l'abdomen.* Lépine, Paris, 1936
DAS, S. C.: Bilateral dislocation of mandible; case. Indian M. Gaz. *62:*86, Feb '27
DASHEVSKIY, A. I. AND MARMORSHTEYN, F. F.: Surgical therapy of chemical burns to eyes. Vestnik oftal. *16:*415-420, '40

DAUBRESSE-MORELLE, E.: Nasal prosthesis in lupus treated with ultraviolet rays. Ann. de l'Inst. chir. de Bruxelles *29:* 161–165, Nov 15, '28

DAUBRESSE-MORELLE, E.: Medicamentous cosmetics for plastic covering of grave cicatrices left by various diseases. Rev. Franc. de dermat. et de venereol. *14:*355–362, Sept-Oct '38

DAUGHTRY, DEW. C.: Cod liver oil ointment in surgery of burns; topical application. Surgery *18:*510–515, Oct '45 also: Alexander Blain Hosp. Bull (no. 3) *4:*2–6, Nov '45

DAUSSET, (see BOLOT, F.) Jan-March '44

DAVID, M. D.: Interesting case of ectopia vesicae. Indian M. Gaz. *61:*290, June '26

DAVIDOFF, R. B.: New traction finger splint for fractures. New England J. Med. *198:*79–80, March 1, '28

DAVIDSON, A. J. AND HORWITZ, M. T.: Congenital club-hand deformity associated with absence of radius; surgical correction; case. J. Bone and Joint Surg. *21:*462–463, April '39

DAVEY, H. W. (see LISCHER, C. *et al)* Jan '44

DAVIDSON, C. S. AND LEVENSON, S. M.: Skin graft in hemophilia with preparation of thrombin and sulfanilamide (sulfonamide). J.A.M.A. *128:*656–657, June 30, '45

DAVIDSON, C. S. (see TAYLOR, F. H. L. *et al)* March '44

DAVIDSON, E. C.: Tannic acid in treatment of burns. Surg., Gynec. and Obst. *41:*202–221, Aug '25

DAVIDSON, E. C.: Prevention of toxemia of burns; treatment by tannic acid solution. Am. J. Surg. *40:*114–116, May '26

DAVIDSON, E. C.: Treatment of acid and alkali burns; experimental study. Ann. Surg. *85:*481–489, April '27

DAVIDSON, E. C.: Use of tannic acid in children with burns. Minnesota Med. *13:*775–783, Nov '30

DAVIDSON, E. C.: Management of cutaneous burns in children. Kentucky M. J. *31:*46–50, Jan '33

DAVIDSON, E. C. AND PENBERTHY, G. C.: Treatment of burns in children with tannic acid. Proc. Internat. Assemb. Inter-State Post-Grad. M. A., North America (1929) *5:*265–268, '30

DAVIDSON, J. B. AND BROWN, A. M.: Management of fractures of maxilla. Mil. Surgeon *87:*26–42, July '40

DAVIES, D. V.: Ectopia vesicae. Brit. J. Urol. *14:*1–10, March '42

DAVIES, J. A. (see GARLAND, J. G.) June '44

DAVIS, A. A.: Review of 31 cases of Dupuytren's contracture, with assessment of comparative value of different methods of therapy. Brit. J. Surg. *19:*539–547, April '32

DAVIS, A. D.: Surgical principles of mouth. Nebraska M. J. *7:*27–29, Jan '22

DAVIS, A. D.: Tripartite cleft palate and double harelip in identical twins. Surg., Gynec. and Obst. *35:*586–592, Nov '22 (illus.)

DAVIS, A. D.: Plea for preservation of premaxillary bones in congenital cleft palate. Lancet *2:*749–751, Oct 11, '24

DAVIS, A. D.: Plastic surgery of nose, ear, face. Arch. Otolaryng. *10:*575–584, Dec '29

DAVIS, A. D.: Surgical correction of cleft lip and palate. Surg., Gynec. and Obst. *52:*875–883, April '31

DAVIS, A.D.: Role of orthodontia following cleft lip and palate surgery. Pacific Dent. Gaz. *39:*571–580, Aug '31

DAVIS, A. D.: Surgical correction of harelip and cleft palate. California and West. Med. *35:*357–361, Nov '31

DAVIS, A. D.: Cleft lip and palate; surgical correction. Internat. J. Orthodontia *18:*282–290, March '32

DAVIS, A. D.: Role of plastic surgery in relation to orthodontia. Internat. J. Orthodontia *19:*1214–1222, Dec '33

DAVIS, A. D.: Palatoplasty using extra-oral tissues. Ann. Surg. *99:*94–100, Jan '34

DAVIS, A. D.: Role of plastic surgery in general practice. Urol. and Cutaneous Rev. *42:*40–45, Jan '38

DAVIS, A.D.: Value and limitations of plastic surgical procedures. M. Times., New York *67:*158–163, April '39

DAVIS, A. D. AND DUNN, R.: Micrognathia; suggested treatment for correction in early infancy. Am. J. Dis. Child. *45:*799–806, April '33

DAVIS, A. D. AND SELLECK, G. A.: Restoration of facial contour in surgery of secondary cleft lip and palate. Am. J. Surg. *64:*104–114, April '44

DAVIS, A. D. (see HOSMER, M. N. *et al)* Oct '40

DAVIS, A. D. (see LUSSIER, E. F.) May '41

DAVIS, A. G.: Reconstructive surgery of extremities today; introduction. J. Bone and Joint Surg. *26:*435–436, July '44

DAVIS, A. H. AND BROWN, W. L.: Radium treatment of keloids. Radiol. Rev. and Mississippi Valley M. J. *60:*67–69, March '38

DAVIS, C. H. AND CRON, R. S.: Two cases of absence of vagina treated by plastic operations. Am. J. Obst. and Gynec. *15:*196–201, Feb '28

DAVIS, D. M.: Epispadias in females; surgical treatment. Surg., Gynec. and Obst. *47:*680–696, Nov '28 abstr: J. Urol. *20:*673–678, Dec '28

DAVIS, D. M.: Surgical treatment of genital

elephantiasis in male. Ann. Surg. *92:*400–404, Sept '30
DAVIS, D. M.: Pedicle tube-graft in surgical treatment of hypospadias in male, with new method of closing small fistulas. Surg., Gynec. and Obst. *71:*790–796, Dec '40
DAVIS, D. M.: New operation for midscrotal hypospadias. J. Urol. *52:*340–345, Oct '44
DAVIS, D. M.: New operation for midscrotal hypospadias. Tr. Am. A. Genito-Urin. Surgeons (1944) *37:*27–33, '45
DAVIS, E. D. D.: Cancer of maxilla and ethmoid; survey of 50 cases. Brit. M. J. *1:*53–55, Jan 13, '34
DAVIS, E. D. D.: Treatment and primary suture of facial wounds. Brit. M. J. *1:*381–383, March 9, '40
DAVIS, E. D. D.: Minor nasal surgery. Practitioner *148:*244–249, April '42
DAVIS, E. D. D. (see HOWARTH, W.) Aug '39
DAVIS, E. W. (see LIVINGSTON, K. E. *et al*) May '46
DAVIS, G. G.: Ball splint for hand fractures. Internat. Clin. *1:*182–183, March '28
DAVIS, G. G. AND HUEY, W. B.: Operation for elevation of depressed zygomatic fractures. Indust. Med. *4:*404–408, Aug '35
DAVIS, H. A.: Physiologic availability of fluids in secondary shock. Arch. Surg. *35:*461–477, Sept '37
DAVIS, H. A.: Factors in treatment of shock; experimental study (Davidson lecture abstract). M. Ann. District of Columbia *6:*344–349, Dec '37
DAVIS, H. A.: Pathology of shock in man; visceral effects of burns.-trauma, hemorrhage and surgical operat. Arch. Surg. *41:*123–146, July '40
DAVIS, H. A.: Physiologic effects of high concentrations of oxygen in experimental secondary shock. Arch. Surg. *43:*1–13, July '41
DAVIS, H. A. AND EATON, A. G.: Intravenous administration of bovine serum albumin as blood substitute in experimental secondary shock. Proc. Soc. Exper. Biol. and Med. *49:*20–22, Jan '42
DAVIS, H. A. AND EATON, A. G.: Comparative effects of horse serum, horse serum albumin and horse serum globulin in experimental shock. Proc. Soc. Exper. Biol. and Med. *49:*359–361, March '42
DAVIS, H. A. AND WHITE, C. S.: Human ascitic fluid as blood substitute in secondary shock. Proc. Soc. Exper. Biol. and Med. *38:*462–465, May '38
DAVIS, J. R. (see BERLIEN, I. C.) March '39
DAVIS, J. S.: General plastic surgery. Ann. Surg. *77:*257–262, March '23
DAVIS, J. S.: Arm-chest adhesions; brachio-thoracic adhesions; axillary webs. J. Bone and Joint Surg. *6:*167–187, Jan '24 also: Arch. Surg. *8:*1–23 (pt. 1), Jan '24
DAVIS, J. S.: Congenital clefts of lip and palate, incidence of. Ann. Surg. *80:*363–374, Sept '24
DAVIS, J. S.: Treatment of deep roentgen-ray burns by excision and tissue shifting. J.A.M.A. *86:*1432–1435, May 8, '26
DAVIS, J. S.: Art and science of plastic surgery. Ann. Surg. *84:*203–210, Aug '26
DAVIS, J. S.: Transplantation of skin. Surg., Gynec. and Obst. *44:*181–189, Feb '27
DAVIS, J. S.: Small deep graft; development; relationship to true Reverdin graft; technic. Tr. South. S. A. *41:*395–408, '28
DAVIS, J. S.: Small deep graft; relationship to true Reverdin graft. Ann. Surg. *89:*902–916, June '29
DAVIS, J. S.: Removal of wide scars and large disfigurements of skin by gradual partial excision with closure. Ann. Surg. *90:*645–653, Oct '29
DAVIS, J. S.: Small deep skin graft. Ann. Surg. *91:*633–635, April '30
DAVIS, J. S.: Deep x-ray burns. Tr. South. S. A. *44:*227–236, '31
DAVIS, J. S.: Relaxation of scar contractures by means of Z-, or reversed Z-type incision; stressing use of scar infiltrated tissues. Tr. Am. S. A. *49:*381–394, '31
DAVIS, J. S.: Relaxation of scar contractures by means of Z-, or reversed Z-type incision; stressing use of scar infiltrated tissues. Ann. Surg. *94:*871–884, Nov '31
DAVIS, J. S.: Deep roentgen-ray burns. Am. J. Roentgenol. *26:*890–893, Dec '31
DAVIS, J. S.: Division of plastic surgery; its needs; its field of usefulness. Tr. West. S. A. *42:*209–225, '32
DAVIS, J. S.: Division of plastic surgery; organization, needs and field of usefulness. South. Surgeon *2:*136–142, June '33
DAVIS, J. S.: On-end or vertical mattress suture. Ann. Surg. *98:*941–951, Nov '33
DAVIS, J. S.: Decubitus ulcers; operative treatment of scars following bedsores. Surgery *3:*1–7, Jan '38
DAVIS, J. S.: Use of relaxation incision in treatment of scars. Pennsylvania M. J. *41:*565–572, April '38
DAVIS, J. S.: Use of small deep grafts in repair of surface defects. Am. J. Surg. *47:*280–298, Feb '40
DAVIS, J. S.: Address of president; story of plastic surgery. Ann. Surg. *113:*641–656, May '41
DAVIS, J. S.: History of plastic surgery. Bol. d. Inst. clin. quir. *18:*34–48, Jan-April '42

Davis, J. S.: Late plastic care of burn scars and deformities (contractures). J.A.M.A. *125:*621-628, July 1, '44

Davis, J. S.: Plastic surgery in World War I and in World War II. Tr. South. S. A. (1945) *57:*141-152, '46

Davis, J. S.: Plastic surgery in World War I and in World War II. Ann. Surg. *123:*610-621, April '46

Davis, J. S.: Present evaluation of merits of Z-plastic operation (for scar contractures) Plast. and Reconstruct. Surg. *1:*26-38, July '46

Davis, J. S. and Finesilver, E. M.: Dupuytren's contracture, with note on incidence of contracture in diabetes. Arch. Surg. *24:*933-989, June '32

Davis, J. S. and German, W. J.: Syndactylism. Arch. Surg. *21:*32-75, July '30

Davis, J. S. and Kitlowski, E. A.: Immediate skin graft contraction and its cause. Arch. Surg. *23:*954-965, Dec '31

Davis, J. S. and Kitlowski, E. A.: Treatment of old unhealed burns. (grafts) Ann. Surg. *97:*648-669, May '33

Davis, J. S. and Kitlowski, E. A.: Regeneration of nerves in grafts and flaps. Am. J. Surg. *24:*501-545, May '34

Davis, J. S. and Kitlowski, E. A.: General sensations in pedunculated skin flaps. Arch. Surg. *29:*982-1000, Dec '34

Davis, J. S. and Kitlowski, E. A.: Method of tubed flap formation. South. M. J. *29:*1169-1174, Dec '36

Davis, J. S. and Kitlowski, E. A.: Abnormal prominence of ear; method of readjustment. Surgery *2:*835-848, Dec '37

Davis, J. S. and Kitlowski, E. A.: Theory and practical use of Z-incision for relief of contractures. Ann. Surg. *109:*1001-1015, June '39

Davis, J. S. and Ritchie, H. P.: Classification of congenital clefts of lip and palate, with suggestion for recording these cases. J.A.M.A. *79:*1323-1327, Oct 14, '22 (illus.)

Davis, J. S. and Traut, H. F.: Origin and development of blood supply of whole-thickness skin grafts; experimental study. Ann. Surg. *82:*871-879, Dec '25

Davis, J. S. and Traut, H. F.: Method of obtaining greater relaxation with whole thickness skin grafts. Surg., Gynec. and Obst. *42:* 710-711, May '26

Davis, J. S. and Wilgis, H. E.: Treatment of hemangiomata by excision. South. M. J. *27:*283-290, April '34

Davis, J. S. (see German, W. *et al*) Jan '33

Davis, J. W.: Hand infections complicating injuries. Indust. Med. *6:*309-310, May '37

Davis, J. W.: Hand injuries. South. M. J. *31:*251-254, March '38

Davis, J. W.: Hand injuries. Indust. Med. *9:*565-567, Nov '40

Davis, J. W.: Hand injuries. South. Med. and Surg. *103:*258-259, May '41

Davis, L.: Surgical treatment of exstrophy of bladder, with report of a case. Boston M. and S. J. *191:*1201-1206, Dec 25, '24

Davis, L.: Return of sensation to transplanted skin. Surg., Gynec. and Obst. *59:*533-543, Sept '34

Davis, L. and Aries, L. J.: Experimental study upon prevention of adhesions about repaired nerves and tendons (especially by use of allantoic and amniotic membranes). Surgery *2:*877-888, Dec '37

Davis, L. and Cleveland, D. A.: Experimental studies in nerve transplantation. Ann. Surg. *99:*271-283, Feb '34

Davis, L. and Cleveland, D.: Surgical treatment of facial paralysis. West. J. Surg. *44:*313-317, June '36

Davis, L. and Hiller, F.: Nerve regeneration in end to end sutures, grafts and gunshot nerve injuries. Tr. Am. Neurol. A. *70:*178-179, '44

Davis, L.; Perret, G. and Carroll, W.: Surgical principles underlying use of peripheral nerve grafts in repair of injuries. Tr. West. S. A. (1944) *52:*526-537, '45

Davis, L.; Perret, G. and Carroll, W. Peripheral nerve injuries; surgical principles underlying use of grafts in repair. Tr. South. S. A. (1944) *56*:302-315, '45

Davis, L.; Perret, G. and Carroll, W. Peripheral nerve injuries; surgical principles underlying use of grafts in repair. Ann. Surg. *121:*686-699, May '45

Davis, L. *et al*: Peripheral nerve injuries; experimental study of recovery of function following repair by end to end sutures and nerve grafts. Surg., Gynec. and Obst. *80:*35-59, Jan '45

Davis, L. (see Pollock, L. J.) June '32

Davis, L. (see Pollock, L. J.) Aug '32

Davis, L. (see Pollock, L. J.) Dec '32

Davis, M. B.: Treatment of extensive burns. J. Tennessee M. A. *20:* 6-9, May '27

Davis, V.: Traumatic etiology of Dupuytren's contracture. Rozhl. v chir. a gynaek. (cast chir.) *14:*126-129, '35

Davis, W. B.: Rhino-laryngologic phases of harelip and cleft palate work. Internat. Clinics *2:*258-266, '22 (illus.)

Davis, W. B.: Harelip and cleft palate. S. Clin. N. America *2:*199-223, Feb '22 (illus.)

Davis, W. B.: Harelip and cleft palate deformities, some types and their operative treatment. Ann. Surg. *76:*133–142, Aug '22 (illus.)

DAVIS, W. B.: Correction of nasal deformities associated with harelip and cleft palate. J. M. Soc. New Jersey *20:*113–119, April '23 (illus.)

DAVIS, W. B.: Types of harelip and cleft-palate deformities and operative results. Surg., Gynec. and Obst. *42:*704–709, May '26

DAVIS, W. B.: Harelip and cleft palate; study of 425 consecutive cases. Ann. Surg. *87:*536–554, April '28

DAVIS, W. B.: Congenital facial deformities; types found in series of 1,000 cases. Surg., Gynec. and Obst. *61:*201–209, Aug '35

DAVIS, W. B.: Value of delayed single pedicle skin flaps in plastic repair of scalp. Surg., Gynec. and Obst. *66:*899–901, May '38

DAVIS, W. B.: Value of osteoplastic flaps in cleft palate repair. Pennsylvania M. J. *43:*153–158, Nov '39

DAVIS, W. B.: Methods preferred in cleft lip and cleft palate repair. J. Internat. Coll. Surgeons *3:*116–124, April '40

DAVIS, W. B.: External nasal deformities and methods used in their repair. Tr. A. Laryng. A. *64:*80–90, '42

DAVIS, W. B.: External deformities of nose and methods used in their repair. Arch. Otolaryng. *36:*619–628, Nov '42

DAVIS, W. B.: Management of bilateral cleft lip. Tr. Am. Soc. Plastic & Reconstructive Surg. *12:*99–116, '43

DAVIS, W. B.: Deformities of face and their correction. Surgery *15:*43–55, Jan '44

DAVIS, W. B.: Basal cell lesions of nose, cheek and lips. Ann. Surg. *119:*944–948, June '44

DAVIS, W. B.: Present status of surgical treatment of cleft hard palate. Am. J. Orthodontics (Oral Surg. Sect.) *32:*671–672, Nov '46

DAVISON, C.: Hypospadias. Internat. Clinics *2:*10–16, '22 (illus.)

DAVISON, C. AND KRAFT, A.: Fate of cortical bone graft. Arch. Surg. *22:*94–97, Jan '31

DAVISON, G.: Treatment of shock of burns. Newcastle M. J. *21:*78–82, July '42

DAVISON, T. C.: Observation on nature and treatment of surgical shock. J. M. A. Georgia *10:*779, Nov '21

DAVISON, T. C.: Use of prepuce to epithelialize tract in treatment of imperforate anus. South. Surgeon *7:*68–70, Feb '38

DAWSON, J. B.: Exstrophy of bladder associated with pregnancy and labor. J. Obst. & Gynaec. Brit. Emp. *40:*1214–1219, Dec '33

DAWSON, J. B.: Pregnancy and labor complicated by ascending myelitis and bedsore of unusual size. J. Obst. & Gynaec. Brit. Emp. *50:*63, Feb '43

DAWSON, J. B.: Formation of artificial vagina without operation. New Zealand M. J. *44:*132–133, June '45

DAY, H. F.: Reconstruction of ears. Boston M. & S. J. *185:*146, Aug 4, '21

DAY, H. F.: Immediate flap grafts following trauma (of fingers). New England J. Med. *218:*758–759, May 5, '38

DE AJURIAGUERRA (see THOMAS, A.) Nov–Dec '42

DE ALMEIDA, A.: External dacryocystorhinostomy. Rev. brasil. de cir. *4:*181–188, April '35

DE ALMEIDA MOURA, J. C. (see ORIENTE, L.) April–June '42

DEAN, H. T.: Fractures of mandible; analysis of 50 cases. J. Am. Dent. A. *17:*1074–1085, June '30

DEAN, S. R.: Dermigraft. Surg., Gynec. & Obst. *68:*930–931, May '39

DE ANDRADE, M. A.: Temporomandibular ankylosis; surgical therapy in cases. Med. cir. pharm., pp. 45–58, Jan '44

DE ANDRADE, P. C.: Surgical therapy of facial paralysis with free aponeurotic graft. Bol. coll. brasil. de cirurgioes *5:*39–40, June–July '34

DE ANDRADE MEDICIS, J.: Wounds of neck and lesions of larynx, trachea and esophagus in war surgery. Arq. brasil. de cir. e ortop. *10:*155–179, '42

DE ANGELIS, H.: Plastic surgery of sebaceous cysts. Semana med. *1:*1176–1177, April 9, '36

DE ANGELIS, E. AND ALTSCHUL, R.: Anisomastia (unilateral hyperplasia) of breast. Deutsche Ztschr. f. Nervenh. *112:*165–176, '30

DE ARAGON, E. R.: Local anesthesia in plastic surgery of vagina. Vida nueva *39:*272–275, April 15, '37

DE ARAGON, E. R.: War burns; varieties according to method of production. Rev. med.-social san. y benef. mumic. *2:*309–314, Oct–Dec '42

DE ARAUJO, A.: Volkmann contracture; 6 cases in children. Rev. brasil. de cir. *2:*377–399, Sept '33

DE ARAUJO, A.: Megalodactylia and megalosyndactylia. Rev. brasil. de orthop. e traumatol. *1:*341–368, May–June '40

DE ARAUJO, A.: Post-traumatic dorsal torsion of hand; late results of surgical therapy; case. Rev. brasil. de orthop. e traumatol. *2:*339–355, May–June '41

DE ASÍS, R.: Aesthetic correction of lips. Siglo med. *87:*269–270, March 14, '31

DEAVER, C. G.: Athletic injuries to tendons. S. Clin. North America *16:*753–761, June '36

DEAVER, J. M.; CRONKITE, E. P. AND PHILLIPS, R. B.: Case of severe burn; abnormal nitrogen metabolism. U. S. Nav. M. Bull. *42:*1162–1163, May '44

DEAVER, J. M. (see CRONKITE, E. P. *et al*) April '44
DE AZEVEDO, M.: Plasma therapy in shock; importance. Rev. clin. de Sao Paulo *13:*6–16, Jan '43
DE BAKEY, M. (see LERICHE, R. *et al*) May '36
DE BAKEY, M. (see BAKEY, M.)
DEBELUT, J.: Transplantation of tendons in therapy of paralytic clubfoot. Semaine d. hop. de Paris *14:*353–354, July 15, '38
DEBENHAM, L. S. AND BADCOCK, C. E.: Treatment of cleft palate. Brit. Dent. J. *51:*347–353, April 1, '30
DEBENHAM, M.: Primary repair of tendons; end-results in 207 cases. California & West. Med. *54:*273–276, May '41
deBERNARDI, L.: Late results of operations on maxillary bone in cancer of oral cavity; 5 cases. Boll. e mem. Soc. piemontese di chir. *2:*1114–1148, '32
DEBEYRE, A.: Gunshot injuries of nerves during war; general considerations, regeneration and transplants. Echo med. du Nord *7:*769–783, June 13, '37
DEBEYRE, A. AND SALEZ: Congenital branchial fistula; cases. Echo m. du nord *33:*541–544, Nov 16, '29
DE BIL: Practical therapy of burns. Avenir med. *33:*180–183, June '36
DE BLASKOVICS, L.: New operation for eyelid ptosis with shortening of levator and tarsus. Arch. Ophth. *52:*563–573, Nov '23 (illus.)
DE BLOIS, E. (see WEILLE, F. L.) Jan '44
DEBRUNNER, H.: Genealogical table showing appearance of Dupuytren's contracture in siblings. Ztschr. f. orthop. Chir. *62:*321–323, '34
DEBURGE, (see BIZARD, G. *et al*) July '32
DEBUSMANN: Familial combination of deformities in region of first visceral arch. Arch. f. Kinderh. *120:*133–139, '40
DEC. M. SAUNDERS, J. B. (see SAUNDERS)
DECHAUME: Chronic osteomyelitis of jaws; cases. Rev. de stomatol. *32:*148–156, March '30
DECHAUME, J. (see TAVERNIER, L. *et al*) Dec '36
DECHAUME, J. (see TAVERNIER, L.) Jan–Feb '37
DECHAUME, M.: Parahyoid cellulitis following fracture of lower jaw. Rev. de stomatol. *38:*457–458, June '36
DECHAUME, M.: Therapy of osteomyelitis of jaws. Presse med. *46:*265–266, Feb 16, '38
DECHAUME, M.: Role of sympathetic in maxillary fractures. Presse med. *46:*714–715, May 4, '38
DECHAUME, M.: Incomplete fractures of upper maxilla and their sinusal complications. Presse med. *48:*627–628, July 31-Aug 3, '40
DECHAUME, M. (see PONROY *et al*) July '34
DECKNER, K.: Concomitance of muscular torticollis and contracture of fingers. Zentralbl. f. Chir. *65:*1192–1195, May 21, '38
DECKNER, K.: Dupuytren's contracture; nature and therapy. Therap. d. Gegenw. *80:*69–72, Feb '39
DECKNER, K.: Dupuytren's contracture as example for concurrent action of hereditary and environmental factors for development of variable characteristics. Ztschr. f. menschl. Vererb. -u. Konstitutionslehre *22:*734–790, '39
DECOURT, J.; AUDRY, M. AND BLANCHARD, J.: Associated facial, lingual and velopalatine hemiatrophy and Basedow's disease; case. Rev. neurol. *73:*135–140, March–April '41
DECREF, J.: Dupuytren's contracture, industrial accident or disease? Siglo med. *83:*569–570, April 13, '29
DEDONCKER *et al*: Emergency treatment and primary apparatus for war fractures of jaw (reports of various countries). Internat. Cong. Mil. Med. & Pharm. *2:*206–218 '39
DEENETZ, B. J.: Complete absence of vagina in two sisters and operation of artificial formation by fasciae method. Vrach. Gaz. *31:*362–365, March 15, '27
DEES, J. E.: Epispadias with incontinence in male. Surgery *12:*621–630, Oct '42
DEFINE, D.: Volkmann contracture; case with surgical treatment; good results. Ann. de Fac. de med. de Sao Paulo *2:*533–551, '27

Deformities (See also Anatomical Area and Plastic Surgery)

Congenital abnormalities (with surgical therapy of prominent ear). FOUCAR, H. O. Canad. M. A. J. *43:*26–27, July '40
Congenital anomalies in otorhinolaryngology. VAN DEN WILDENBERG. Bull. Soc. belge d'otol., rhinol., laryng., pp. 282–292, '37
Mental and psychic condition of certain malformed individuals; value of plastic surgery. MALBEC, E. F. Semana med. *1:*716–722, March 30, '39

DEGA, W.: Plastic surgery of thumb. Rev. d' orthop. *13:*497–501, Nov '26
DEGAUDENZI, C.: Oral and genital aphthae of mutilating character; case. Dermosifilografo *17:*520–526, Sept '42
DEGRAIS, P. AND BELLOT, A.: Superiority of radium to surgery in cancer of eyelids; cures without risk of recurrence, mutilation or

pain. Bull. Soc. d'opht. de Paris, no. 9, pp. 536–544, '27 also: Clinique, Paris *22:*397–403, Oct (B) '27

DEGRAIS, P. AND BELLOT, A.: Radium in therapy of cicatrices & keloids. Bull. med., Paris *46:*196–198, March 12, '32

DEICKE, H.: Suppurative tenosynovitis; treatment and ultimate outcome. Beitr. z. klin. Chir. *158:*461–480, '33

DÉJEAN, C.: Autoplastic graft of conjunctiva and of eyelid; 2 cases. Arch. Soc. d. sc. med. et biol. de Montpellier *12:*23–25, Jan '31

DÉJEAN, C. (see ETIENNE, E.) Feb '32

DÉJEAN, C. (see DELORD, E. *et al*) Dec '34

DELAGÉNIÈRE, H.: Bone-periosteum transplants. J. de chir. *17:*305, April '21 abstr: J.A.M.A. *76:*1372, May 14, '21

DELAGENIÈRE, H.: Repair of loss of bony substance and reconstruction of bones by osteoperiosteal grafts taken from tibia, (with 118 new personal cases). Am. J. Surg. *35:*281, Sept '21

DELAGENIÈRE, H.: Results of osteoperiosteal bone grafts. Arch. franco-belges de chir. *25:*673–718, May '22 (illus.)

DELAGENIÈRE, H.: Osteoperiosteal bone grafts. Bull. Acad. de med., Par. *88:*396–416, Dec 5, '22 abstr: J.A.M.A. *80:*434, Feb 10, '23

DELANEY, W. E. JR.: High traumatic amputation of thigh and treatment of shock. Indust. Med. *9:*28–29, Jan '40

DELANY, H. B. JR.: Fracture of mandible. J. Nat. M. A. *29:*80–82, May '37

DELARUE, J. (see MILIAN, G.) March '27

DELARUE, J. (see BABONNEIX, L. *et al*) March '28

DELAYE. (see BONNET, P.) March–April '31

DELBET, P.: Phlegmon of flexor tendon of thumb; vaccinotherapy; case. Bull. et mem. Soc. nat. de chir. *54:*666–672, May 12, '28

DELBET, P.: Use of rubber in plastic operations on tendons and nerves, in repairing defects in abdominal wall, in hernia and in fractures with loss of substance. Rev. de chir. *66:*181–213, '28

DELCHEF, J.: Tendon transplantation; case. Scalpel (86):1099–1100, July 15, '33

DELITALA, F.: Surgical therapy of ankylosis of jaw; case. Gior. veneto di sc. med. *13:*236–237, April '39

DELLA-MANO, N.: Cystic lymphangioma of neck; case. Gazz. d. osp. *51:*43–53, Jan 12, '30

DELLEPIANE RAWSON, R.: Primary tumors of facial bones. Semana med. *1:*652–654, March 19, '25

DELLEPIANE RAWSON, R.: Sheehan's method of plastic surgery of nose. Rev. med. latino-am. *15:*1055–1090, May '30

DELLEPIANE RAWSON, R.: Nasal spine as stenosing factor; surgical therapy. Rev. otoneuro-oftal. *11:*343–344, Dec '36

DELLEPIANE RAWSON, R.: Hughes operation for total loss of lower eyelid. Arq. de cir. clin. e exper. *6:*235–251, April–June '42

DELLEPIANE RAWSON, R.: Use of meniscus of knee in plastic surgery (ear). Prensa med. argent. *29:*654–658, April 22, '42

DELLEPIANE RAWSON, R.: Hughes operation for total loss of lower eyelid. Dia med. *14:*461, May 25, '42

DELLEPIANE RAWSON, R.: Plastic surgery of face. Dia med. *14:*1052–1055, Oct 12, '42

DELLEPIANE RAWSON, R.: Free grafts in plastic surgery. Prensa med. argent. *29:*1643–1648, Oct 14, '42

DELLEPIANE RAWSON, R.: Complete unilateral harelip; immediate result of operation by Brown-Blair method. Dia med. *15:*146–147, Feb 22, '43

DELLEPIANE RAWSON, R.: Plastic surgery of face; synthesis. Dia med. *15:*638–640, June 21, '43

DELLEPIANE RAWSON, R.: Grafts of refrigerated skin; Filatov graft. Dia med. *15:*1150–1151, Oct 4, '43

DELLEPIANE RAWSON, R. AND VIVOLI, D.: Fibroglioma of nose; case. Rev. med. latino-am. *14:*860–868, May '29

DELLEPIANE RAWSON, R. AND GONZÁLEZ AVILA, E.: Congenital ocular hypertelorism; case. Rev. de especialid. *5:*1090–1096, Aug '30 also: Semana med. *2:*1206–1209, Oct 16, '30

DELLEPIANE RAWSON, R. AND GONZÁLEZ AVILA, E.: Nasal surgery. Semana med. *2:*1351–1357, Oct 30, '30

DELLEPIANE RAWSON, R. AND JAROLAVSKY, N. N.: Angled bistoury with retrograde uniform cutting edge for use in plastic surgery of nose. Dia med. *14:*1280, Dec 7, '42

DELLEPIANE RAWSON, R. AND PEREZ FERNANDEZ, M.: Nasal deformity of syphilitic type due to injury; loss of mucosa and of supporting bone and cartilage; modified Gillies operation in therapy of case. Arq. de cir. clin. e exper. *6:*492–503, April–June '42

DELMAS, A. (see CORDIER, G.) Oct-Nov, '42

DELORD, E.; COLIN, AND DEJEAN, C.: Truc operation in ectropion; technic and review of cases. Arch. d'opht. *51:*763–774, Dec '34

Delorme-Juvara Operation

Delorme-Juvara operation in rectal prolapse; 3 cases. ALPEROVICH, A. Bol. y trab. de la Soc. de cir. de Buenos Aires *22:*6–11, April 6, '38

Delorme-Juvara Operation—Cont.

Modification of Delorme-Juvara operation in therapy of total rectal prolapse in adults. STAMATIU, C. Rev. san. mil., Bucuresti *36:*421–432, May '37

Rectal prolapse with special reference to Delorme-Juvara method of therapy. ALPEROVICH, A. Semana med. *1:*1365–1374, June 16, '38

DELPH, J. F.: Chemical burns of mouth. S. Clin. North America *17:*585–592, April '37

DELPRAT, G. D.: Traumatic avulsion of entire penis (both corpora cavernosa and urethra). J.A.M.A. *125:*274–275, May 27, '44

DELREZ, L. AND DESAIVE, P.: Epitheliomas of lips; survey of 100 cases. Liege med. *27:*2057–2085, Oct 7, '34

DELRIO, J. M. A.: Nonsurgical therapy of dermoid cysts, with report of cases. Bol. y trab., Soc. argent. de cirujanos *4:*284–290, '43 also: Rev. Asoc. med. argent. *57:*490–492, July 30, '43

DELRIO, J. M. A.: Burn therapy with tanning by means of sulfonamides. Rev. Asoc. med. argent. *57:*866–873, Oct 30, '43

DELRIO, J. M. A.: Problem of skin grafts in severe burns. Bol. y trab. Acad. argent. de cir. *30:*363–376, Jun 26, '46

•DELRIO, J. M. A. AND BULFARO, J. A.: Instruments for dermoepidermal grafts. Bol. y trab., Soc. argent. de cirujanos *6:*745–748, '45 also: Rev. Asoc. med. argent. *59:*1328–1329, Nov 30, '45

DELRIO, J. M. A. (see RIVAS DIEZ, B.) March '44

DELRIO, J. M. A. (see RIVAS DIEZ, B.) Nov '44

DEMAKOPOULOS, N. (see WEINSHELL, L. R.) April '43

DEMEL, R.: Results of operative treatment of exstrophy of bladder. Mitt. a. d. Grenzgeb. d. Med. u. Chir. *33:*533, '21 abstr: J.A.M.A. *77:*1294, Oct 15, '21

DEMEL, R.: Plastic reconstruction of upper and lower lips. Deutsche Ztschr. f. Chir. *196:*210–214, '26

DEMEL, R.: Plastic use of fascia in treatment of facial paralysis. Zentralbl. f. Chir. *61:*1445–1448, June 23, '34

DEMEL, R.: Results of treatment of protruding ears. Wien. klin. Wchnschr. *48:*1185, Sept 27, '35

DEMEL, R.: Reparative surgery. Arch. f. klin. Chir. *188:*207–214, '37

DEMEL, R. AND FEIGL, E.: Surgical correction of protruding ears. Deutsche Ztschr. f. Chir. *233:*453–459, '31

DEMING, C. L.: Epispadias in female, transplantation of gracilis muscle for incontinence. J.A.M.A. *86:*822–825, March 20, '26

DENEHY, W. J. AND AMIES, A.: Treatment of adherent and deficient palates following injury. M. J. Australia *1:*150–154, Feb 4, '33

DENIG, R.: Transplantation of oral mucosa in diseases of cornea and burns of eyes. Arch. f. Ophth. *118:*729–737, '27

DENIG, R.: Circumcorneal transplantation of oral mucosa as curative measure in diseases of eye. Arch. Ophth. *1:*351–357, March '29

Denig Operation

Histologic changes in membrane transplanted from lip to trachomatous eye (Denig's method). TOWBIN, B. G. Arch. f. Ophth. *125:*643–651, '31

Denig operation in trachomatous pannus (grafting). DERKAČ, V. Klin. Monatsbl. f. Augenh. *85:*409–411, Sept 26, '30

Transplantation of mucous membrane (Denig operation) in severe burns of eyes. MITERSTEIN, B. AND KORNBLUETH, W. Harefuah *29:*152, Oct 1, '45

Transplantation of lip mucosa by Denig method in treatment of trachoma. KAMINSKI, D. S. Klin. Monatsbl. f. Augenh. *87:*60–70, July '31

Denig operation for burns of eyes. AVIZONIS, V. Medicina, Kaunas *19:*309–315, April '38

Unsatisfactory results of Denig operation (in pannus). KARBOWSKI, M. Klin. Monatsbl. f. Augenh. *85:*411–414, Sept 26, '30

Denker Operation: See Rouge-Denker Operation

DENNISON, W. M.: Burns and scalds in children. Lancet *2:*1107–1110, Nov 25, '39

DENNISON, W. M. AND DIVINE, D.: Burn therapy in wartime. J. Roy. Army M. Corps *77:*14–18, July '41

DEPLAEN, P.: Roentgen and radium treatment in prevention and therapy of keloids. Rev. de chir. structive, pp. 99–102, June '37

DEPP, M. E. (see LINDENBAUM, I. S.) 1936

De Quervain's Syndrome

Stenosing tendovaginitis on styloid process of radius (styloidalgia). WINTERSTEIN, O. Munchen. med. Wchnschr. *74:*12–15, Jan 7, '27

Stenosing tendovaginitis of long abductor and of short extensor of thumb. LAROYENNE, AND BOUYSSET. Arch. franco-belges de chir. *30:*98–104, Feb '27 also: Lyon med. *140:*573–575, Nov 27, '27

Styloidalgia radii and some other cases of tendovaginitis stensans. JAGERINK, T. A. Nederl. Tijdschr. v. Geneesk. *1:*3227, June 30, '28

De Quervain's Syndrome—Cont.
Stenosing fibrous tendovaginitis over radial styloid (de Quervain). SCHNEIDER, C. C. Surg., Gynec. & Obst. *46:*846–850, June '28
Stenosis of tendon sheath of wrist. WINTERSTEIN, O. Schweiz. med. Wchnschr. *58:*746–748, July 28, '28
Stenosing tendovaginitis of first portion of styloid process of radius; its nature and treatment. LASSEN, E. Ugesk. f. laeger *91:*837–840, Oct 3, '29
Stenosing tendovaginitis of DeQuervain; case. WATKINS, J. T. AND PITKIN, H. C. California & West Med. *32:*101–102, Feb '30
Stenosing tendovaginitis at radial styloid process. FINKELSTEIN, H., J. Bone & Joint Surg. *12:*509–540, July '30
Stenosing tendovaginitis at radial styloid process. HOFFMANN, P., J. Bone & Joint Surg. *13:*89–90, Jan '31
Snapping hand. HINRICHSMEYER, C. Zentralbl. f. Chir. *58:*834–837, April 4, '31
Diagnosis of deQuervain's chronic stenosing inflammation of tendons. WEISSENBACH, R. J. AND FRANCON, F. Bull. med., Paris *45:*378–382, May 30, '31
De Quervain's chronic stenosing tendovaginitis; 3 cases. LAMY, L. Bull. et mem. Soc. d. chirurgiens de Paris *24:*373–377, June 3, '32
De Quervain's stenosing tendovaginitis (Winterstein's styloidalgia radii); 8 cases. SCHETTINO, M. Riforma med. *48:*1142–1145, July 23, '32
Acute forms of de Quervain's stenosing tendovaginitis; 2 cases. LAROYENNE, L. AND BRUN, M. Lyon med. *151:*3–9, Jan 1, '33
De Quervain's disease; stenosing tendovaginitis at radial styloid. PATTERSON, D. C. New England J. Med. *214:*101–103, Jan 16, '36
Tendovaginitis stenosans of extensor pollicis longus sinister. POHL, H. Med. Klin. *32:*1596–1597, Nov 20, '36
Stenosing tendovaginitis at radial styloid process (de Quervain's disease). KEYES, H. B. Ann. Surg. *107:*602–606, April '38
De Quervain's disease; radial styloid tendovaginitis. COTTON, F. J. *et al.* New England J. Med. *219:*120–123, July 28, '38
Stenosing tendovaginitis at radial styloid process (de Quervain's disease). McDONALD, J. E. AND STUART, F. A., J. Bone & Joint Surg. *21:*1035, Oct '39
De Quervain's disease; frequently missed diagnosis. DIACK, A. W. AND TROMMALD, J. P. West. J. Surg. *47:*629–633, Nov '39
Stenosing tendovaginitis at radial styloid process (de Quervain's disease). WOOD, C. F. South. Surgeon *10:*105–110, Feb '41
Chronic stenosing tenosynovitis (de Quervain's disease); symptoms, diagnosis and therapy. WEISSENBACH, R. J. AND FRANCON, F. Rev. argent. de reumatol. *5:*299–305, March '41
De Quervain's tendovaginitis as sequel to hand injury. WIBERG, G. Nord. med. (Hygiea) *10:*1929–1933, June 21, '41

DER BRUCKE, M. G.: Simple surgical method for esthetic correction of pendulous breasts. Am. J. Surg. *11:*324–327, Feb '31
DERBY, G. S.: Correction of eyelid ptosis by fascia lata hammock. Am. J. Ophth. *11:*352–354, May '28
DEREUX, J.: Case of hyperostosis of one-half of face. Bull. et mem. Soc. med. d. hop. de Paris *50:*307–311, Feb 26, '26 abstr: J.A.M.A. *86:*1486, May 8, '26
DERKAČ, V.: Plastic correction of coloboma of eyelid. Klin. Monatsbl. f. Augenh. *96:*102–104, Jan '36

Dermal Grafts
Uses of dermal graft and delayed flap. RITCHIE, H. P., S. Clin. N. America *3:*1371–1387, Oct '23 (illus.)
Use of dermal graft in repair of small saddle defects. (nose) STRAATSMA, C. R. Arch. Otolaryng. *16:*506–509, Oct '32
Cysts; fate of buried skin grafts in man. PEER, L. A. Arch. Surg. *39:*131–144, July '39
Closure of large hernial apertures by means of skin grafts. JUNGHANNS, H. AND JUZBASIC, D. M. Chirurg *12:*742–746, Dec 15, '40
Skin as plastic material for closure of large abdominal hernias. BERDICHEVSKIY, G. A. Novy khir. arkhiv. *45:*225–229, '40
Use of cutis graft in repair of certain types of incisional herniae and other conditions. CANNADAY, J. E. Ann. Surg. *115:*775–781, May '42
Additional report on uses of cutis graft material in reparative surgery. CANNADAY, J. E. Am. J. Surg. *67:*382–390, Feb '45
Cutis grafts. Clinical and experimental studies on use as reinforcing patch in repair of large ventral and incisional hernias. HARKINS, H. N. Ann. Surg. *122:*996–1015, Dec '45
Skin transplantation in treatment of recidivating hernias. JUNQUEIRA, A. Hospital, Rio de Janeiro *29:*11–16, Jan '46

Dermal Grafts–Cont.

Cutis graft in surgery; review of results obtained, with comments on indications and technic and report of cases. CANNADAY, J. E. Arch. Surg. *52:*286–303, March '46

Derman, I. A.: Exstrophy of bladder, surgical therapy by Coffey operation; 2 cases. Ztschr. f. Urol. *29:*856–859, '35

Dermoid Cysts

Dermoid cysts of dorsum of nose. MARCHINI, F. Policlinico (sez. prat.) *30:*1422, Oct 29, '23

Unusual dermoid cyst of eyelid. GRADLE, H. S. AND STEIN, J. C. Arch. Ophth. *53:*254–257, May '24

Dermoid cyst of neck. SEED, L., S. Clin. N. Amer. *6:*1033–1035, Aug '26

Dermoid cyst of dorsum of nose; citation of case. HART, V. K. Laryngoscope *37:*760–763, Oct '27

Dermoid cysts of palm. JAUREGUI, P. Bol. y trab. de la Soc. de cir. de Buenos Aires *13:*233–239, June 12, '29

Dermoid cyst of nose; case. TRAMPNAU. Ztschr. f. Hals-, Nasen-u. Ohrenh. *28:*163–165, March 3, '31

Etiology and operation of congenital dermoid on dorsum of nose. BESELIN, O. Arch. f. Ohren-, Nasen-u. Kehlkopfh. *129:*47–49, June 6, '31

Dermoid cysts of dorsum of nose; 3 cases. HACQUEBORD, P. Geneesk. gids *9:*721–728, July 31, '31

Dermoid cyst of nasal dorsum. POWELL, L. S. Arch. Otolaryng. *19:*67–68, Jan '34

Cysts of skin graft into rectovaginal septum; case. ROSSI, D. Clin. ostet. *38:*464–470, Sept '36

Dermoid cysts of neck & head. NEW, G. B. AND ERICH, J. B. Surg., Gynec. & Obst. *65:*48–55, July '37

Cysts; sebaceous, mucous, dermoid and epidermoid. ERICH, J. B. Am. J. Surg. *50:*672–677, Dec '40

Sacrococcygeal dermoid cysts; Lahey plastic repair using bipedicled flap. BAILA, A. E. Bol. y trab., Soc. argent. de cirujanos *4:*292–293, '43 also: Rev. Asoc. med. argent. *57:*495, July 30, '43

Nonsurgical therapy of dermoid cysts, with report of cases. DELRIO, J. M. A. Bol. y trab., Soc. argent. de cirujanos *4:*284–290, '43 also: Rev. Asoc. med. argent. *57:*490–492, July 30, '43

Dermoid cyst in floor of mouth. MASUDA, B. J. Am. J. Orthodontics (Oral Surg. Sect.) *32:*252–256, Apr '46

DEROW, D.: Short wave epilation. Arch. Phys. Therapy *20:*101–102, Feb '39

DERQUI, M. N. (see BUZZI, A. *et al*) Oct '29

DERR, J. S.: Epithelioma on bridge of nose; case. Radiology *16:*955–956, June '31

DERRA, E. AND RUBERG, G.: Late results of surgical therapy in injuries to tendons of hand. Monatschr. f. Unfallh. *45:*305–315, June '38

DESAIVE, P.: Epithelioma of auricle and its therapy. Cancer, Bruxelles *12:*273–286, '35

DESAIVE, P. (see DELREZ, L.) Oct '34

DESAULNIERS, L. AND DUGAL, L. P.: Influence of pH on cicatrization. Rev. canad. de biol. *4:*325–333, '45

DESELAERS: Inversion of ala nasi. Rev. espan. de med. y cir. *15:*9–10, Jan '32

DESELAERS: Plastic and esthetic surgery in hemangioma. (face). Rev. de chir. plastique, pp. 70–73, April '32

DESELAERS, H.: Plastic surgery cases. Rev. espan. de med. y cir. *13:*2–11, Jan '30

DESELAERS, H.: Plastic surgery in therapy of trichiasis & free skin graft for hemangioma. Rev. espan. de med. y cir. *15:*353–355, July '32

DESELAERS, H.: Plastic surgery in therapy of maxillotemporal ankylosis; case. Rev. espan. de med. y cir. *16:*114–116, March '33

DESELAERS, H.: Surgery of upper lip to correct loss of tissue due to actinomycosis. Ars med., Barcelona *9:*143–144, April '33

DESFOSSES, P. (see MOUCHET, A.) July '28

DESGOUTTES, L.: Resection of maxillary angle in temporomaxillary ankylosis. Tech. chir. *25:*97–102, June '33

DESGOUTTES, L.: Technic of surgical therapy of rhinophyma. Tech. chir. *25:*117–188, Oct '33

DESJACQUES, R.: Crushing of right hand and wrist; conservation of useful "grip" formed from thumb and small portion of index finger. Rev. d'orthop. *20:*315–318, July–Aug '33

DESJACQUES, R.: Probability of existence of diabetes in patients with panaris or phlegmons of hand. Presse med. *42:*1431–1432, Sept 12, '34

DESJACQUES, R. AND MILLET: Loss of cutaneous substance in ulceration of thigh cured by Davies graft. Lyon med. *152:*222–223, Aug 27, '33

DESJARDINS, E.: Hyperplastic angioma of fingers; 7 cases. J. de l'Hotel-Dieu de Montreal *2:*99–114, March–April '33

DESJARDINS, E.: Tannic acid in burns. J. de l'Hotel-Dieu de Montreal *3:*410–416, Nov–Dec '34

DESJARDINS, E.: Burns. Union med. du Canada *70:*770–771, July '41

DESJARDINS, E.: Benign tumors of hand and fingers. Union med. du Canada *70:*999–1001, Sept '41

DESJARDINS, E.: Phlegmons of hand. Union med. du Canada *70:*1329–1331, Dec '41

DESJARDINS, E.: Local therapy of war burns. Union med. du Canada *72:*790–792, July '43

DESMAREST, E. AND EBRARD, D.: Treatment of imperforate anus. Arch. de med. d. enf. *29:*96–101, Feb '26

DESOILLE, H. (see OLIVER, E. *et al*) Oct '37

D'Espine Operation

Prolapse of rectum in children; D'Espine method of. ALEXANDER, E. G. Ann. Surg. *76:*496–499, Oct '22

DESPLAS, B.: Ephedrine and its compounds in treatment of shock in spinal anesthesia. Rev. crit. de path. et de therap. *2:*669–674, Sept '31

DESPLAS, B.: Ephedrine and its compounds in treatment of shock in spinal anesthesia. Bull. et mem. Soc. nat. de chir. *58:*158–162, Feb 6, '32

DESPLAS, B.: Reconstruction of left thumb by skin and osteoperiosteal grafts; case. Mem. Acad. de chir. *62:*1292–1296, Nov 25, '36

DESPLAS, B.: Septic puncture of fingers in industry. Arch. d. mal. profess. *6:*231–232, '44–'45

DESPLAS, B. AND MEILLIÈRE, J.: Surgical therapy of Dupuytren's contracture. Bull. et mem. Soc. nat. de chir. *58:*424–429, March 12, '32

DESPLAS, B. AND MEILLIÈRE, J.: Surgical therapy of Dupuytren's contracture. Monde med., Paris *42:*795–802. Aug 1–15, '32

DESPLAS, B. AND TOSTIVINT, R.: Study apropos of 150 cases Dupuytren's contracture. Mem. Acad. de chir. *71:*373–379, Oct 17–31, '45

DESPONS, J. (see PORTMANN, G.) July '32

DESPONS, J. (see PORTMANN, G.) Jan '36

DESVERNINE, C. M.: Syndrome characterized by fracture of radius, hematoma of forearm, dyskinesia of flexor muscles of fingers, with fingers in permanent extension; surgical therapy of case. Cron. med.-quir. de la Habana *62:*343–349, Aug '36

DETCHESSARRY, R.: Surgical therapy of harelip; technic and results. Arch. argent. de pediat. *24:*197–204, Sept '45

DETROY, L.: Burns due to sulfur dioxide of eyes; 2 cases. Echo med. du Nord *4:*742bis–743, Oct 27, '35

DETROY, L. (see PIQUET, J.) June '38

DETWILER, R. H.: Digital injury in infant from silk wool blanket. Arch. Pediat. *54:*625–626, Oct '37

DETZEL, L.: Congenital fistula of neck. Munchen. med. Wchnschr. *68:*1227, Sept 23, '21

DEUBNER, W.: Operative treatment of cleft palate in older children and adults. Deutsche Ztschr. f. chir. *201:*117–121, '27

DEUBNER, W.: Surgical treatment of cleft palate. Arch. f. klin. Chir. *146:*430–461, '27

DEUCHER, W. G. AND OCHSNER, A. E. W.: Free homeoplastic skin grafting. Arch. f. klin. Chir. *132:*470–479, '24. Comment by Ascher, K. W., Arch. f. klin. Chir., *137:*198, '25

DEVENISH, E. A.: Infections of hand; 3 years' experience in clinic for study of whitlow. Arch. Surg. *37:*726–734, Nov '38

DEVENISH, E. A.: Hematoma of flexor tendon sheaths following penetrating wounds (hand). Lancet *1:*447–448, Feb 25, '39

DEVENISH, E. A. AND JESSOP, W. H. G.: Nature and cause of swelling of upper limb after radical mastectomy. Brit. J. Surg. *28:*222–238, Oct '40

DEVINE, H.: Review of acute postoperative circulatory disturbances. Australian and New Zealand J. Surg. *8:*145–155, Oct '38

DEVINE, H.: Shock. M. J. Australia *2:*19–26, July 11, '42

DEVINE, J. B.: Theories of shock and their relation to burns. M. J. Australia *1:*14–17, Jan 7, '39

DEVINE, J. B.: Three-dye treatment of burns. M. J. Australia *1:*924–928, June 24, '39

DEVINE, K. D. (see NEW, G. B.) Aug '46

D'EWART, J.: Gastrostaxis following burns. Brit. M. J. *1:*242, Feb. 8, '30

DEWEL, B. F.: Dentofacial musculature. Am. J. Orthodontics *27:*469–488, Sept '41

DEXELMANN, J.: Denudation of penis and scrotum; case. Zentralbl. f. Chir. *59:*2760–2761, Nov 12, '32

DEY, P. K.: Successful treatment of a case of scalding. Indian M. Gaz. *56:*338, Sept '21

DHALLUIN, A.: Congenital non-existence of vagina and its treatment; 2 cases. Arch. franco-belges de chir. *25:*808–816, June '22 (illus.) abstr: J.A.M.A. *79:*2039, Dec 9, '22

DHALLUIN, A.: Rare malformation of hands, polydactylia, syndactylia and thumb with 3 phalanges. Arch. franco-belges de chir. *25:*931–933, July '22 (illus.)

DHALLUIN, M.: Radium treatment of angioma of external ear in infant. Gaz. med. de France (supp. radiol.) no. 6, pp. 136–138, Oct 1, '31

DIACICOV, M.: Blaskovics operation for eyelid ptosis. Rev. san. mil., Bucuresti *36:*730–735, Aug '37

DIACK, A. W. AND TROMMALD, J. P.: De Quervain's disease; frequently missed diagnosis. West. J. Surg. *47:*629–633, Nov '39

DIAL, D. E.: Hand injury due to injection of oil at high pressures. J.A.M.A. *110:*1747, May 21, '38

DIAL, D. E.: Reconstruction of thumb after traumatic amputation. J. Bone and Joint Surg. *21:*98–100, Jan '39

DIAMANT-BERGER, L.: Tenoplasty of flexor muscles of fingers for clawhand (pseudo-Volkmann contracture); results in case. Bull. et mem. Soc. d. chirurgiens de Paris *27:*541–545, Nov 22, '35

DIAZ-CANEJA, E.: External dacryocystorhinostomy according to Gutzeit method. Ann. d'ocul. *170:*384–414, May '33 also: An. Casa de Salud Valdecilla *3:*292–313, '32

DIAZ Y GOMEZ, E.: Technic of surgical therapy in diffuse phlegmons of hand and forearm. Med. ibera *1:*436–442, March 16, '35

DIAZ INFANTE, A.: Avulsion of scalp, treated by large free skin flaps by "grate" or "sieve" method; case. Medicina, Mexico *17:*107–114, March 10, '37

DIBAN, P. AND DIENERMANN, J.: Plastic with round pedicle. Deutsche Ztschr. f. Chir. *191:*164–169, '25

DIBLE, J. H. (see CLEGG, J. W.) Sept '40

DICK, A.: Free grafts. M. Ann. District of Columbia, *15:*262, June '46

DICK, B. M.: Median cleft of upper lip; case. Edinburgh M. J. *34:*45–47, Jan '27

DICK, W.: Lymph vessels of human omentum; contribution to treatment of elephantiasis. Beitr. z. klin. Chir. *162:*296–314, '35

DICKEY, C. A.: Eyelid ptosis, superior-rectus fascia-lata sling in correction. Am. J. Ophth. *19:*660–664, Aug '36

Dickey Operation

Modification of Dickey operation in eyelid ptosis. GIFFORD, S. R. AND PUNTENNEY, I. Arch. Ophth. *28:*814–820, Nov '42

Dickey operation for eyelid ptosis; results in 21 patients and 30 lids. CORDES, F. C. AND FRITSCHI, U. Tr. A. Acad. Ophth. (1943) *48:*266-279, March-April '44 also: Arch. Ophth. *31:*461–468, June '44

DICKMANN, G. H. (see FINOCHIETTO, R.) Nov '35

DICKSON, D. D. (see MEYERDING, H. W.) April '39

DICKSON, F. D.: Volkmann's contracture. New Orleans M. and S. J. *82:*119–126, Sept '29

DICKSON, F. D.: Surgical therapy of arthritis. Ann. Surg. *113:*869-876, May '41

DICKSON, J. A.: Treatment of webbed fingers; syndactylism; case. Cleveland Clin. Quart. *6:*72–74, Jan '39

Didot's Operation

Congenital web fingers; addition to Didot's operation for syndactylism. JONES, H. T. S. Clin. N. Amer. *7:*1450–1452, Dec '27

DIECKMANN, F.: Rhinophyma; representations in art and literature. Dermat. Ztschr. *62:* 20–31, Sept '31

Dieffenbach-Warren Operation

Dieffenbach-Warren operation for closure of congenitally cleft palate. BLAIR, V. P. AND BROWN, J. B. Surg., Gynec. and Obst. *59:*309–320, Sept '34

Dieffenbach-Warren operation for closure of congenitally cleft palate. BLAIR, V. P. AND BROWN, J. B. Internat. J. Orthodontia *22:*853–868, Aug '36

Argumosa's 2 methods of blepharoplasty for tumors usually attributed to other authors (especially Dieffenbach). MARQUEZ, M. J. Internat. Coll. Surgeons *7:*63–67, Jan–Feb '44

DIENERMANN, J. (see DIBAN, P.) 1925

DIETERICH: Ultimate outcome of suture of nerves. Med. Klinik *19:*237–238, Feb. 25, '23 abstr: J.A.M.A. *80:*1742, June 9, '23

DIEULAFÉ, L.: Lymphangioma of lower lip; case. Rev. de stomatol. *29:*193–195, April '27

DIEULAFÉ, L.: Angioma of upper lip; case. Rev. de stomatol. *29:*390–392, July '27

DIEULAFÉ, L.: Treatment of fractures of lower jaw by bone suture with silver wire; cases. Rev. de stomatol. *31:*330–336, June '29

DIEULAFÉ, R.: Suppurative cyst of neck; case. Bordeaux chir. *7:*452–453, Oct '36

DIEZ, J.: Stellectomy in therapy of case of facial paralysis. Bol. y trab., Acad. argent. de cir. *27:*564–566, July 21, '43

DIGGS, L. W.: Plasma therapy in shock. Memphis M. J. *16:*58–61, April '41

DIMEG, O.: Compact splints with new fixation method for maxillary fractures. Ztschr. f. Stomatol. *40:*485–504, July '42

DIMITRIU, A. (see JIANU, I. *et al*) Nov '32

DIMOND, W. B. (see NEFF, E.) June '30

DINGMAN, R. O.: Use of rubber bands in treatment of facial and jaw fractures. J. Am. Dent. A. *26:*173–183, Feb '39

DINGMAN, R. O.: Acute infections of face. Pennsylvania M. J. *42:*499–505, Feb '39

DINGMAN, R. O.: Congenital preauricular sinus. Arch. Otolaryng. *29:*982–984, June '39

DINGMAN, R. O.: Prognathism–open bite deformity; case. J. Oral Surg. *2:*64–70, Jan '44

DINGMAN, R. O.: Bilateral ankylosis of temporomandibular joints with retrusion deformity; case. J. Oral Surg. *2:*71–76, Jan '44
DINGMAN, R. O.: Epithelioid giant cell tumor of tongue, locally malignant; report of case. J. Oral Surg. *2:*77–80, Jan '44
DINGMAN, R. O.: Ameloblastoma (adamantinoma) of mandible; case report. J. Oral Surg. *2:*175–181, April '44
DINGMAN, R. O.: Osteotomy for correction of mandibular malrotation of developmental origin. J. Oral Surg. *2:*239–259, July '44
DINGMAN, R. O.: Surgical correction of mandibular prognathism; improved method. Am. J. Orthodontics (Oral Surg. Sect.) *30:*683–692, Nov '44
DINGMAN, R. O.: Spindle cell sarcoma of mandible with excision and subsequent bone graft; case. J. Oral Surg. *3:*235–240, July '45
DINGMAN, R. O.: Ankylosis of jaws. Am. J. Orthodontics (Oral Surg. Sect.) *32:*120–125, Feb '46
DINGWALL, J. A. III: Clinical test for differentiating second from third degree burns. Ann. Surg. *118:*427–429, Sept '43
DINGWALL, J. A. III AND ANDRUS, W. DEW.: Comparison of various types of local treatment in burns (especially results with sulfonamide-impregnated plastic film) in controlled series of experimental burns in human volunteers. Ann. Surg. *120:*377–386, Sept '44
DINGWALL, J. A., III. AND ANDRUS, W. DEW.: Comparison of various types of local treatment (especially results with sulfonamide-impregnated plastic film) in controlled series of experimental burns in human volunteers. Tr. Am. S. A. *62:*377–386, '44
DINGWALL, J. A. III AND LORD, J. W. JR.: Fluorescein test in management of tubed (pedicle) flaps. Bull. Johns Hopkins Hosp. *73:*129–131, Aug '43
DINGWALL, J. A. III (see ANDRUS, W. DeW.) May '44
DINSMORE, R. S.: Benign lesions of neck. Proc. Interst. Postgrad. M. A. North America (1940) pp. 322–324, '41
DINTENFASS, H.: New and simple plastic-flap method in radical mastoid operation. Atlantic M. J. *30:*426–428, April '27
DIONISI, H. AND YORNET, H.: Artifical vagina, creatin in congenital absence. Bol. y trab., Soc. de cir. de Cordoba *4:*40–59, '43
DISQUE, T. L.: Exstrophy of bladder, operation by Bergenhem method. Pennsylvania M. J. *33:*546, May '30
DIVELEY, R. L. (see DICKSON, F. D.) Jan '32
DIVINE, D. (see DENNISON, W. M.) July '41
DIVNOGORSKIY, B. F. AND GLUSCHCHENKO, V. T.: Fractures of digital phalanges and their treatment. Sovet. khir. *4:*214–226, '33
DIX, C. R.: Problems of plastic surgery of face. Wisconsin M. J. *44:*593–596, June '45
DIX, C. R. (see NEW, G. B.) March '40
DIX, C. R. (see HAVENS, F. Z.) March '42
DIX, C. R. (see FIGI, F. A. *et al*) Sept '43
DIXON, C. F.: Ureteral transplantation in exstrophy of bladder. Proc. Staff. Meet., Mayo Clin. *4:*33, Jan 30, '29
DIXON, C. F. AND BENSON, R. E.: Surgical management of large tumors of neck; unusual case (mixed tumor) Am. J. Surg. *69:*384–390, Sept '45
DIXON, C. F. (see MAYO, C. H.) Feb '30
DIXON, C. W.: Closed fractures and contusions of fingers; therapy with procaine hydrochloride infiltrations. Clinica, Bogota *1:*139–145, Sept '44
DIXON, O. J.: New postoperative pack for submucous resection. Ann. Otol., Rhin. and Laryng. *45:*1184–1185, Dec '36
DIXON, O. J.: Hemangioma of ear; new method for control of hemorrhage. Ann. Otol., Rhin, and Laryng. *54:*415–420, June '45
DJERASSI, J.: Occurrence and therapy of osteomyelitis of jaw. Ztschr. f. Stomatol. *33:*458–461, April 26, '35
DMITRIEVA, AND IORDANSKIY: Fractures of end phalanges of fingers. Sovet. khir. (no. 6) *6:*870–875, '34
DO AMARAL, A. C.: Traumatic shock. Rev. med.-cir. do Brasil *48:*667–680, Nov '40
DOBELLE, M. AND PROCTOR, S. E.: Operative position for transposition of ulnar nerve. Am. J. Surg. *64:*254–256, May '44
DOBES, W. L., AND KEIL, H.: Cryotherapy (slush method using carbon dioxide snow) for acne. Arch. Dermat and Syph. *42:*547–558, Oct '40
DOBRESCU, D. (see PLACINTEANU, G.) Feb '42
DOBRITZ, O.: Plastic surgery of breast hypertrophy during pregnancy; case. Zentralbl. f. Chir. *65:*1993, Sept 3, '38
DOBRITZ, O.: Epispadias; case. Ztschr. f. Urol. *32:*622–624, '38
DOBRZANIECKI, W.: Plastic and esthetic surgery of face. Polska gaz. lek. *7:*519–524, July 8, '28 also: Paris chir. *20:*129–142. July–Aug '28
DOBRZANIECKI, W.: A new procedure for execution of intra-dermal suture. Paris chir. *21:*19–23, Jan–Feb '29
DOBRZANIECKI, W.: Operative treatment of ear deformities. Ann. d. mal. de l'oreille, du larynx *48:*998–1003, Oct '29
DOBRZANIECKI, W.: Homotransplantation and several blood groups; epidermal grafts made by Thiersch method. Ann. Surg. *90:*926–938, Nov '29

DOBRZANIECKI, W.: Restoration of subseptal portion of nose. Ann. Surg. *90:*974–977, Dec '29

DOBRZANIECKI, W.: Influence of ablation of sympathetic ganglions on evolution of different forms of skin grafts; experimental study. Lyon chir. *27:*537–578, Sept–Oct '30

DOBRZANIECKI, W.: Effect of removal of sympathetic ganglia on cutaneous autoplastic and homoplastic transplants (skin). Polska gaz. lek. *10:*262, April 5; 287, April 12, '31

DOBRZANIECKI, W.: Plastic surgery of face. Rev. de chir. plastique, pp. 182–200, Oct '31

DOBRZANIECKI, W.: Resection and reconstruction of mandible; 2 cases. Arch. ital. di chir. *35:*207–217, '33

DOBRZANIECKI, W.: Reconstruction of epispadias controlled by urethrography; case. J. d'urol. *40:*320–326, Oct '35

DOBRZANIECKI, W.: Surgical correction of bulldog nose; case. J. de chir. *48:*191–196, Aug '36

DODD, H.: Management of septic hand. Practitioner *148:*219–225, April '42

DODDS, G. E.: Case showing partial deficient fusion of maxillary process with lateral nasal process on one side. Brit. J. Ophth. *27:*414–415, Sept '43

DODDS, P.: Responsibility of public health agencies in cleft palate Am. J. Orthodontics (Oral Surg. Sect.) *32:*665–666, Nov '46

DÖDERLEIN, W.: Submucous resection; methods of preventing post-operative fluttering and perforation. Hals-, Nasen-u. Ohrenarzt (Teil 1) *30:*273–275, July '39

DODGE, W. M. JR.: Improved eyelid crutch for ptosis. Arch. Ophth. *14:*989–990, Dec '35

DODSON, A. I.: Transplants from scrotum for repair of urethral defects. Tr. Am. A. Genito-Urin. Surgeons (1940) *33:*11–220, '41

DOERFLER, H.: Distribution and therapy of hand infections. Fortschr. d. Therap. *8:*80, Feb 10; 116, Feb 25, '32

D'OFFAY (see: OFFAY)

DOGLIOTTI, A. M.: Surgical therapy of facial paralysis. Riforma med. *52:*1489–1492, Oct 31, '36

DOGLIOTTI, A. M.: Surgery of facial nerve. Arch. ed atti d. Soc. ital. di chir. *43:*537–691, '37

DOGLIOTTI, A. M. (see ROASENDA, G.) 1934

DOHERTY, J. A.: Jaw fractures. New England J. Med. *216:*425–428, March 11, '37

DOHERTY, J. A.: Jaw fractures. Am. J. Orthodontics *24:*165–170, Feb '38

DOHERTY, J. A.: Fractures of mandible; statistical study of 100 cases. J. Am. Dent. A. *27:*735–737, May '40

DOHERTY, J. A.: Practical points in diagnosis and treatment of jaw fractures. Surg., Gynec. and Obst. *72:*96–98, Jan '41

DOHERTY, J. A.: Fractures of edentulous mandible. J. Oral Surg. *1:*157–161, April '43

DOHERTY, J. A.: Fractures of condyle of mandible. U. S. Nav. M. Bull. *42:*641–643, March '44

DOHERTY, J. A. (see DOHERTY, J. L.) Jan '37

DOHERTY, J. A. (see DOHERTY, J. L.) Dec '37

DOHERTY, J. A. (see DOHERTY, J. L.) May '39

DOHERTY, J. A. (see DOHERTY, J. L.) June '40

DOHERTY, J. A. (see MCGRAIL, F. R.) April '41

DOHERTY, J. L. AND DOHERTY, J. A.: Jaw fractures and treatment. Surg., Gynec. and Obst. *64:*69–73, Jan '37

DOHERTY, J. L. AND DOHERTY, J. A.: Dislocations of mandible. Am. J. Surg. *38:*480–484, Dec '37

DOHERTY, J. L. AND DOHERTY, J. A.: Zygomatic fractures. J. Am. Dent. A. *26:*30–733, May '39

DOHERTY, J. L. AND DOHERTY, J. A.: Jaw fractures. Am. J. Surg. *48:*576–581, June '40

DOLJANSKY, J.: Biologic processes in bone transplantation. Zentralbl. f. Chir. *53:*2523–2526, Oct 2, '26

DOLLAR, J. M. (see BLAINE, G. *et al*) 1945

DOLLFUS, M. A.: Symptomatology and therapy of cancer of eyelids. Bull. med., Paris *51:*375–380, May 29, '37

DOMBROVSKY, A. I.: Megalosyndactylia; case. Munchen. med. Wchnschr. *75:*1503, Aug 31, '28

DOMENECH-ALSINA, F. (see BROGGI, M.) Jan '43

DOMENICI, F.: Facial scars; evaluation in medicolegal expertise. Boll. d. Soc. med.-chir., Pavia *53:*41–55, '39

DONALD, J.: Observations upon operation for deflection of nasal septum. Practitioner *106:*250, April '21

DONLEY, D. E.: Facial hemiatrophy associated with epilepsy; case. J. Nerve. and Ment. Dis. *82:*33–39, July '35

DONNELL, N. R.: Perithelioma of upper eyelid. Arch. Ophth. *53:*411–415, Sept '24

DONNELLY, J. C.: New method of operation for congenital atresia of posterior nares. Arch. Otolaryng. *28:*112–125, July '38

DONOHUE, E. S.: Use of delayed bone grafts in ununited fractures. J. Iowa M. Soc. *35:*8–10, Jan '45

DONOVAN, E. J.: Transplantation of ureters into sigmoid in exstrophy. S. Clin. North America *11:*511–512, June '31

DONOVAN, S. J. AND CARR, F. J. JR.: Extensive

(60 percent) burn; case. U. S. Nav. M. Bull. *41:*1410–1412, Sept '43

DOOLIN, W.: Congenital clefts of lip and palate. Irish J. M. Sc., pp. 708–720, Nov '38

DORDU, F.: Autoplasty for pre-scrotal hypospadias in adult. Arch. franco-belges de chir. *25:*282–286, Dec '21 (illus.)

DORDU, F.: Heteroplasties and autoplasties. Arch. franco-belges de chir. *31:*601–608, July '28

DORE, R.: Anaplasty of skin; case. Union med. du Canada *57:*710–713, Dec '28

DORE, R.: Differential diagnosis of neck tumors. Union med. du Canada *73:*269–271, March '44

DORFFEL, J. AND NOSSEN, H.: Prosthetic surgery in lupus (Hennig-Zinsser method); total rhinoneoplasty. Med. Welt *5:*1172–1174, Aug 15, '31

DORIA, J. R. DA C.: Case of epispadias in man. Brazil-med. *2:*84–86, Aug 15, '25

DORIGO, L.: Use of electric bistury for removing rhinophyma; case. Bollettino *11:*62–72, '37

DOROCHENKO, I. T.: Autoplasty of alae vasi (nose). Acta otolaryng. *25:*147–149, March-April '37

DOROFEEV, V. N.: Surgical therapy of paralytic lagophthalmos in leprosy patients. Vestnik oftal. (no. 1) *14:*69–76, '39

DORON, G.: Ocular complications from local anesthesia in resection of upper jaw. Zentralbl. f. Chir. *54:*2966–2969, Nov 19, '27

DOROSCHENKO, I. T.: New method of plastic surgery of fistulas of dorsal portion of ear. Acta oto-laryng. *22:*105–106, '35

DOROSCHENKO, I. T.: Facial paralysis; improvement by surgery. Monatschr. f. Ohrenh. *70:*1303–1314, Nov '36

DOROSCHENKO, I. T.: Plastic surgery of nasal injuries. Arch. f. Ohren-, Nasen-u. Kehlkopfh. *141:*5–11, '36

DOROSCHENKO, I. T.: New method of plastic surgery in acquired atresia. Arch. f. Ohren-, Nasen-u. Kehlkopfh. *141:*249–251, '36

DOROSCHENKO, I. T.: Surgical therapy of facial paralysis by intra-oral neurotization. Acta oto-laryng. *26:*702–709, '38

DOROSCHENKO, J. T.: New method of plastic surgery in complicated deformities of pinna; cat's ear and coloboma in 2 cases. Monatschr. f. Ohrenh. *70:*718–721, June '36

DOROSCHENKO, J. T.: New plastic method of repairing nasal septal perforation. Acta oto-laryng. *23:*553–554, '36

DORRANCE, G. M.: Etiology, pathology and treatment of cysts of jaws. J.A.M.A. *77:*1883, Dec 10, '21

DORRANCE, G. M.: Double lip. Ann. Surg. *76:*776–777, Dec '22 (illus.)

DORRANCE, G. M.: Lengthening soft palate in cleft palate operations. Ann. Surg. *82:*208–211, Aug '25

DORRANCE, G. M.: Cleft palate. Atlantic M. J. *31:*351–355, Feb '28

DORRANCE, G. M.: Congenital insufficiency of cleft palate. Arch. Surg. *21:*185–248, Aug '30

DORRANCE, G. M.: Osteoperiosteal bone grafts. Ann. Surg. *92:*161–168, Aug '30

DORRANCE, G. M.: Cleft palate repair; palatine insertion of superior constrictor muscle of pharynx and its significance in cleft palate, with remarks on "push-back operation." Ann. Surg. *95:*641–658, May '32

DORRANCE, G. M.: Oral surgical problems of interest to rhinologists. (including cleft palate). New York State J. Med. *32:*1226–1228, Nov. 1, '32

DORRANCE, GEORGE M.: *The Operative Story of Cleft Palate*. W. B. Saunders Co., Phila., 1933

DORRANCE, G. M.: "Push-back operation" of palate. Ann. Surg. *101:*445–459, Jan '35

DORRANCE, G. M. AND BRANSFIELD, J. W.: Burns, with special reference to acetic acid treatment. S. Clin. N. America *2:*299–307, Feb '22

DORRANCE, G. M. AND BRANSFIELD, J. W.: Disfiguring scars; prevention and treatment. Am. J. M. Sc. *165:*562–567, April '23 (illus.)

DORRANCE, G. M. AND BRANSFIELD, J. W.: Treatment of webbed fingers, congenital or acquired. Ann. Surg. *78:*532–533, Oct '23 (illus.)

DORRANCE, G. M. AND BRANSFIELD, J. W.: Immediate covering of denuded area of skull. Am. J. Surg. *58:*236–239, Nov '42

DORRANCE, G. M. AND BRANSFIELD, J. W.: Cleft palate. Ann. Surg. *117:*1–27, Jan '43

DORRANCE, G. M. AND LOUNDENSLAGER, P. E.: Fractures of bones of face. S. Clin. North America *15:*71–83, Feb '35

DORRANCE, G. M. AND LOUNDENSLAGER, P. E.: Hypermotility of upper lip, surgery of. Surg., Gynec. and Obst. *75:*790–791, Dec '42

DORRANCE, G. M. AND MC SHANE, J. K.: Cancer of tongue and floor of mouth. Ann. Surg. *88:*1007–1021, Dec '28

DORRANCE, G. M. AND SHIRAZY, E.: Role of push-back operation in surgery of cleft palate. J. Am. Dent. A. *22:*1108–1117, July '35

DORRANCE, G. M. AND WAGONER, G. W.: Osteoperiosteal bone graft; experimental and clinical data concerning its application for repair of bone defect and extra-articular ankylosis. J.A.M.A. *87:*1433–1435, Oct 30, '26

DORRANCE, G. M.; WEBSTER, D. AND MCWILLIAMS, H.: Arthroplasty upon temporomandibular joint. Ann. surg. *79:*485–487, April '24

Dorrance Operation

Cleft palate procedures in surgery; experiences with Veau and Dorrance technic. IVY, R. H. AND CURTIS, L. Ann. Surg. *100:*502–511, Sept '34

DORRIS, J. M.: Diagnosis of hand infections. Memphis M. J. *15:*142–143, Sept '40

DORRONSORO, D. A.: Surgical treatment of facial paralysis; recovery. Siglo med. *83:*637–638, April 27, '29

DORSET, R. F.: Severe gunshot wound of face. Mil. Surgeon *80:*429–431, June '37

DORSEY, B. M. (see BAY, R. P.) Dec '38

DOSHOYANTS, S. L.: Autotransfusion of blood to counteract shock. Sovet. khir. (no. 1) *6:*57–58, '34

DOSKAROVA, V.: Calcedral (suprarenal preparation) in severe burns. Ceska dermat. *19:*141–145, '40

DOSNE, C.: Traumatic shock and its interpretation. Rev. de med. y aliment. *6:*107–114, April–July '44

DOSNE, C. (see SELYE, H.) July '40

DOSNE DE PASQUALINI, C.: Shock; problem in war and laboratory. Rev. san. mil., Buenos Aires *44:*1405–1417, Oct '45

DOSTER, J. T. JR. Cysts and sinuses of neck. Mississippi Doctor *22:*205–210, Jan '45

DOSTROVSKY, A. AND SAGHER, F.: Problem of burn therapy. Harefuah *24:*114, April 1, '43

DOTTI, E.: Late results of Segond operation for exstrophy of bladder. Gior. veneto di sc. med. *8:*730–739, July '34

DOTTI, S.: Congenital case of recto-urethral fistula with imperforate anus. Gazz. med. lomb. *86:*41–44, March 25, '27

DOUADY, D. (see LECHELLE, P. *et al*) May '27

DOUBLEDAY, F. N.: Cases of gunshot wounds of jaws treated 1914–1918. Guy's Hosp. Gaz. *54:*358–360, Dec 14, '40

DOUGLAS, B.: Skin grafting by exact pattern, a report of cosmetic results obtained without employment of sutures. Ann. Surg. *77:*223–227, Feb '23 (illus.)

DOUGLAS, B.: Treatment of burns with epinephrin. Compt. rend. Soc. de biol. *92:*267–268, Feb 6, '25

DOUGLAS, B.: Sieve graft – stable transplant for covering large skin defects. Surg., Gynec. and Obst. *50:*1018–1023, June '30

DOUGLAS, B.: Radical repair of large skin defects with particular reference to leg ulcers. (grafts). South. M.J. *24:*53–58, Jan '31

DOUGLAS, B.: Conservative and radical measures for treatment of ulcer of leg; critical study of healing in experimental and human wounds under elastic adhesive plaster. Arch. Surg. *32:*756–775, May '36

DOUGLAS, B.: Aids in surgery of harelip. Ann. Surg. *106:*293–296, Aug '37

DOUGLAS, B.: Plastic surgery, with report of original operation for advancement of nasolabial fold. South. M. J. *31:*1047–1052, Oct '38

DOUGLAS, B.: Treatment of x-ray and radium burns by radical excision and grafting. J. Tennessee M. A. *34:*220–224, June '41

DOUGLAS, B.: Therapy of burns with special emphasis on transparent jacket system. Surgery *15:*96–143, Jan '44

DOUGLAS, B., AND BUCHHOLZ, R. R.: Circulation in pedicle flaps; accurate test ("temperature-return test") for determining its efficiency. Ann. Surg. *117:*692–709, May '43

DOUGLAS, B. AND LANIER, L. H.: Changes in cutaneous localization in pedicle flap. Arch. Neurol. & Psychiat. *32:*756–762, Oct '34

DOUGLAS, J. P. (see ANDERSON, C. B. C.) March '38

DOUGLAS, R. A.: Hand injuries. J. Tennessee M. A. *22:*177–178, Sept '29

DOUGLAS, S. J.: Cancer of lips. Brit. J. Radiol. *17:*185–189, June '44

DOUGLASS, M.: Construction of artificial vagina by tube graft method. Am. J. Obst. and Gynec. *35:*675–680, April '38

DOUGLASS, M. D.: Reconstruction of vagina; employment of flap transplantation method in one stage with favorable anatomical result. Surg., Gynec. and Obst. *58:*982–985, June '34

DOUGLASS, R.: Two cases of interest; septic dementia; avulsion of scalp. China M. J. *40:*463–464, May '26

DOUZAIN. (see CAUSSADE, L. *et al*) March '38

DOWD, C. N.: Surgical treatment of cleft palate. Ann. Surg. *81:*573–584, March '25

DOWD, C. N.: Details in repair of circatricial contractures of neck. Surg., Gynec. and Obst. *44:*396–399, March '27

DOWKONTT, C. F.: Operation for pendulous breasts. M. J. and Rec. *130:*624–627, Dec 4, '29

DOWKONTT, C. F.: Modification of double circle operation for pendulous breasts. New York State J. Med. *31:*264–266, March 1, '31

DOWKNOTT, C. F.: Pendulous and hypertrophied breasts; operative treatment. New York State J. Med. *37:*643–644, April 1, '37

DOWKONTT, C. F.: Plastic surgery of breast. M. Rec. *155:*132–133, Feb 18, '42.

DOWMAN, C. E. (see BALKIN, S. G. *et al*) May '45

DOWNS, T. M.: Comparison of certain drugs (tannic acid and gentian violet) used as local applications. (Burns) U. S. Nav. M. Bull. *40:*936–938, Oct '42
DRACHTER, R.: Treatment of exstrophy of bladder. Arch. f. klin. Chir. *120:*291–297, '22 (illus.) abstr: J.A.M.A. *79:*1370, Oct. 14, '22
DRACKLE, W.: Tar burns; case. Deutsche med. Wchnschr. *60:*1961–1962, Dec 21, '34
DRAGANESCO. (see MARINESCO, G. *et al*) May '28
DRAGER, G. A. (see POTH, E. J. *et al*) Nov '45
DRAGISIC, B.: Congenital aural fistulas and differential diagnostic significance in children. Wien. med. Wchnschr. *86:*748–750, July 4, '36
DRAGOMIR, L. (see URECHIA, C. I.) Oct '35
DRAGONETTI, M.: Dystrphic disorders due to lesions of nerves in spinomedullary trauma; clinical and therapeutic study. Gazz. internaz. med.-chir. *47:*416–421, July 15, '37
DRAGSTEDT, L. R. AND WILSON, H.: Modified sieve graft; full thickness graft for covering large defects. Surg., Gynec. and Obst. *65:*104–106, July '37
DRAGUTSKY, D. (see SCHWARTZMAN, J. *et al*) Oct '42
DRAKE, T. G. H. (see BROWN, A.) Oct '24
DREOSTI, A. E.: Triple dye treatment of burns and scalds. South African M. J. *16:*181, May 9, '42
DRESCHKE: Nasal septal perforation in workers with arsenic. Med. Klin. *29:*1378, Oct 6, '33

Dressings

Intranasal operations with special reference to post-operative packing. MILLER, J. W. New York M. J. *113:*456, March 16, '21
Substitute for adhesive plaster bandage in hare-lip operations. FRÜND, H. Zentralbl. f. Chir. *48:*1426, Oct 1, '21
Bandage for plastic operatons on face. ESSER, J. F. S. Arch. f. klin. Chir. *117:*438–443, '21 (illus.)
Tamponing nose. (after surgery). SCHMIDT, C. Schweiz. med. Wchnschr. *52:*540–541, May 25, '22 (illus.)
Application of dental molding compound for maintenance of skin grafts in middle ear and mastoid cavities. ISRAEL, J. Ann. Otol. Rhinol. and Laryngol. *31:*543–545, June '22
Tamponing after operations on nose. RÉTHI, L. Wien. klin. Wchnschr. *35:*637–638, July 20, '22
Paraffin spray in burns. REBAUDI, L. Munchen. med. Wchnschr. *70:*179, Feb. 9, '23
Bandaging after harelip operation. RANFT, G. Zentralbl. f. Chir. *50:*598–600, April 14, '23 (illus.)

Dressings—Cont.

Use of paraffin as primary dressing for skin grafts. COLLER, F. A. Surg., Gynec. and Obst. *41:*221–225, Aug '25
Pressure bags for skin grafting. SMITH, F. Surg., Gynec. and Obst. *43:*99, July '26
Post-operative endo-nasal tamponade with cotton sachets. (in nasal surgery) LAVAL, F. Ann. d. mal. de l'oreille, du larynx *46:*377–379, April '27
Dressing for burns. FIST, H. S. J.A.M.A. *88:*1483, May 7, '27 addendum, 1922.
Postoperative care of Ollier-Thiersch skin grafts; advisability of daily surgical dressings. RULISON, E. T. Surg., Gynec. and Obst. *45:*708–710, Nov '27
Adhesive plaster bandage for plastic operations of nose. FISHBEIN, J. N. Laryngoscope *38:*128, Feb '28
Rational way of bandaging palmar arches. SHARGORODSKAY, I. I. Vestnik khir. (nos. 37–38) *13:*150–157, '28
Bandaging of hand wounds. KIAER, S. Ugesk. f. laeger *92:*347–351, April 10, '30
Plastic operation for restoration of chin, lower lip, and part of cheeks; method of applying dressing. KRAUSS, F. Zentralbl. f. Chir. *57:*1915–1916, Aug 2, '30
Extra-oral emergency bandage in fractures of lower jaw. CHATZKELSON, B. Munchen. med. Wchnschr. *78:*98, Jan 16, '31
Method of nasal packing following submucous resection which allows free nasal respiration. ROTH, E. Arch. Otolaryng. *13:*732, May '31
Use of packing in postoperative treatment in nasal surgery. WOODBURN, J. J., M. J. Australia *2:*390–392, Sept 26, '31
Elastic bandage in fracture of mandible. SPANIER, F. Chirurg *3:*891–893, Oct 15, '31
Fixative bandage in corrective nasal plastic surgery. ERCZY, M. Orvosi hetil. *76:*657–658, July 23, '32
Method of placing dressing in order to relieve tension of suture after operation for harelip. PORZELT, W. Zentralbl. f. Chir. *59:*2165–2167, Sept 3, '32
Question of tamponade after nasal operations. (Comment on von Liebermann's article). KREBS, G. Ztschr. f. Hals-, Nasen- u. Ohrenh. *30:*684–685, '32
New technic of bandaging of epidermic grafts; application in therapy of ulcers of leg. RIOU, M. Bull. Soc. path. exot. *26:*1296–1301, '35
Combination of cod liver oil and plaster bandage in therapy of injuries with tissue loss of fingers. LÖHR, W. Chirurg *6:*5–11, Jan 1, '34

Dressings – Cont.

Trypaflavine (acridine dye) compresses in burns. SOSODORO-DJATIKOESOEMO, R. Geneesk. tijdschr. v. Nederl.-Indie *74:*759-760, June 5, '34

Cod liver oil salve treatment of burns with and without use of plaster of paris cast. LÖHR, W. Zentralbl. f. Chir. *61:*1686-1695, July 21, '34

First bandage in hand injuries. VOSKRESENSKIY, N. V. Sovet. khir. (no. 1) *7:*171-172, '34

Decubitus ulcer, treatment with elastic adhesive plaster. CARTY, T. J. A. Brit. M. J. *1:*105-106, Jan 19, '35

Use of medicated gauze dressing (tulle gras) in plastic and esthetic surgery. CODAZZI AGUIRRE, J. A. Rev. med. del Rosario *25:*441-446, April '35

Use of ambrine (paraffin dressing) in burns. BALTODANO BRICENO, E. Med. de los ninos *36:*300-304, Oct '35

Burn in children and their therapy with powdered chalk dressings. TERNOVSKIY, S. D. Vestnik khir. *39:*3-8, '35

Good dressing for wounds produced by electrocoagulation. HOLLANDER, L. Arch. Dermat. and Syph. *33:*730, April '36

Cod liver oil and cod liver oil bandage in therapy of hand injuries. LÖHR, W. Ztschr. f. arztl. Fortbild. *33:*421-427, Aug 1, '36

Pressure bag in skin grafting. TAYLOR, F. Am. J. Surg. *33:*328-329, Aug '36

Permanent functional results of use of cod liver oil and plaster of paris cast after injury or loss of fingertip. FLIMM, W. Zentralbl. f. Chir. *63:*2500-2506, Oct 17, '36

Paraffin dressing for transplanted grafts. TRUEBLOOD, D. V. West. J. Surg. *44:*578, Oct '36

New postoperative pack for submucous resection. DIXON, O. J. Ann. Otol., Rhin. and Laryng. *45:*1184-1185, Dec '36

Practical bandage for finger. BEHNCKE. Deutsche med. Wchnschr. *63:*558-559, April 2, '37

Biologic therapy of burns; rest and immobilization with plaster of paris bandaging. ZENO, L. An. de cir. *3:*228-232, Sept '37

Plaster of paris bandage in therapy of burns of extremities. ZENO, L. AND BARENBOYM, S. Novy khir. arkhiv *38:*485, '37

Plaster of paris bandages in treatment of burns of extremities. ZENO, L. AND KAPLAN, A. V. Vestnik khir. *51:*16-18, '37

Therapy of burns of extremities with plaster of paris bandages. GORBAN, I. A. Vestnik khir. *56:*100, July '38

Dressings – Cont.

Use of celluloid to cover operations for harelip. COELST. Rev. de chir. structive *8:*99-101, Aug '38

Zeno method of burn therapy by immobilization in plaster cast. AFONSO, J. Arq. brasil. de cir. e ortop. *6:*302-309, Sept-Dec '38

Skin grafts with film bandage. OLESEN, M. Ugesk. f. laeger *101:*144-147, Feb 2, '39

Therapy of simple and complicated burns by means of plaster casts. ZENO, L. Arch. urug. de med., cir. y especialid. *14:*322-324, March '39

Barrel bandage in jaw fractures. FRY, W. K. Brit. M. J. *2:*1086, Dec 2, '39

Use of medicated paper dressing in facial surgery. COELST. Bull. Soc. belge d'otol., rhinol, laryng., pp. 319-320, '39

Thiersch skin grafting; use of collodion-gauze technic. SZUTU, C. AND CHEN, C. Y. Chinese M. J. *57:*535-545, June '40

Burn treatment (with paraffin dressing). ZEISS, C. R. Illinois M. J. *78:*540-544, Dec '40

Immovable bandage in free cutaneous graft. (extremities) VORONCHIKHIN, S. I. Novy khir. arkhiv. *45:*244-247, '40

Bag bandage for hand burns. STRECKFUSS, H. Chirurg *13:*96, Feb 1, '41

Collodion as dressing for skin grafting of granulating wounds. ELLIS, S. S. AND VON WEDEL, C., J. Oklahoma M. A. *34:*103-105, March '41

Perforated oiled silk in burns. STOPFORD-TAYLOR, R. Brit. M. J. *1:*403-404, March 15, '41

Hess operation; new bandage substitute (eyelid ptosis) PEREIRA, R. F. Arch. de oftal. de Buenos Aires *16:*241-242, May '41

Closed-plaster burn treatment. ROULSTON, T. J. Brit. M. J. *2:*611-613, Nov 1, '41

Plaster casts in local burn therapy. BALESDENT, E. Hospital, Rio de Janeiro *21:*753-768, May '42

Dressings after submucous resection of septum. PRUVOT, M. Rev. de laryng. *63:*196-199, June-July '42

Use of sulfanilamide and gauze packing following intranasal operation. KERN, E. C. Arch. Otolaryng. *36:*134, July '42

Practical concept for major and minor burns (including use of sulfathiazole, sulfanilamide derivative, emulsion and "sulfamesh" dressing); importance of timing therein. GURD, F. B. *et al.* Ann. Surg. *116:*641-657, Nov '42

"Prefabricated eschar" or bandage, containing sulfonamide. CLARK, W. G. *et al.* Journal-Lancet *62:*455-456, Dec '42

Dressings – Cont.

Burn therapy with special reference to use of cats. ZENO, L. An. de cir. *8:*265–280, Dec '42

Treatment of acute stage of burns (with alcohol compressed.) COMPTON, W. C. Cincinnati J. Med. *23:*540-547, Jan '43

Plastic film (containing sulfonamides) in treatment of experimental burns. SKINNER, H. G. AND WAUD, R. A. Canad. M. A. J. *48:*13–18, Jan '43

Compression treatment of burns. BRANTIGAN, O. C., AND HEBB, D. Bull. School Med. Univ. Maryland *28:*12–20, July '43

Handy bandage for jaw fractures. BROWNSON, H. N., J. Oral Surg. *1:*271, July '43

Closed-plaster method of burn therapy, with certain physiologic considerations implicit in success of this technic. GLENN, W. W. L. *et al.* J. Clin. Investigation *22:*609-625, July '43

Treatment of hand burns with close fitting plaster of paris casts. LEVENSON, S. M. AND LUND, C. C., J.A.M.A. *123:*272-277, Oct 2, '43

Pressure dressings in burns. OWENS, N., S. Clin. North America *23:*1354-1366, Oct '43

Effect of plaster bandages and local cooling on hemoconcentration and mortality rate in burns. SELLERS, E. A. AND WILLARD, J. W. Canad. M.A.J. *49:*461-464, Dec '43

Use of stents in skin grafting in mouth. BEDER, O. E., J. Oral Surg. *2:*32–38, Jan '44

Therapy of burns with special emphasis on transparent jacket system. DOUGLAS, B. Surgery *15:*96–143, Jan '44

Report on management of burns with sulfathiazole emulsion using occlusive compression dressing. ACKMAN, D. *et al.* Ann. Surg. *119:*161–177, Feb '44

Modified nonadherent gauze pressure treatment of burns. MARSHALL, W. AND GREENFIELD, E. Am. J. Surg. *63:*324–328, March '44

Emergency dressing for burns of extermities. McGRAW, A. B. Hosp. Corps Quart. (no. 2) *17:*40–44, March '44

Elimination of intranasal pack by topical use of thrombin. STEVENSON, H. N. Ann. Otol., Rhin. and Laryng. *53:*159-162, March '44

Cod liver oil, sulfanilamide-sulfathiazole (sulfonamides) powder dressing in burns. FLAX, H. J. Bol. Assoc. med. de Puerto Rico *36:*208–214, May '44

Interlocking finger bandage which needs no anchor. POOL, H. H., J. Michigan M. Soc. *43:*406, May '44

Dressings – Cont.

Effect of plaster confinement applied at varying intervals after burning. ALRICH, E. M. AND LEHMAN, E. P. Surgery *15:*899-907, June '44

Early plastic care of deep burns (including use of pressure dressing with sulfathiazole, sulfonamide) GURD, F. B. AND GERRIE, J. W., J.A.M.A. *125:*616-621, July 1, '44

Analysis of modern treatment (especially with closed plaster) of severe burns. DRINKER, C. K., J. Oklahoma M. A. *37:*339-346, Aug '44

New type of hand dressing to improve function. COX, F. J. *et al.* M. Bull. Mediterranean Theat. Op. *2:*168–169, Dec '44

Plaster of paris bandage in therapy of gunshot wounds of fingers. RYZHIKH, A. N. Khirurgiya, no. 4, pp. 65–69, '44

Effect of applying pressure to experimental thermal burns. CAMERON, G. R. *et al.* J. Path. and Bact. *57:*37–46, Jan '45

Vaseline gauze contact fixation of split thickness (Padgett) skin grafts. ROBERTS, W. M. and SCHAUBEL, H. J. Am. J. Surg. *67:*16–22, Jan '45

"Cellophane" (medicated with sulfanilamide, sulfonamide) treatment of burns. FARR, J. D. Rev. san. mil. Buenos Aires *44:*313–317, March '45

Local treatment of burns with pressure dressing and films containing sulfonamide. REESE, E. C. Am. J. Surg. *67:*524–529, March '45

New medicated gauze for use in nasal operations. SELTZER, A. P. Eye, Ear, Nose and Throat Monthly *24:*189, April '45

Streamlined finger dressings. DURRANT, M. M. Brit. J. Phys. Med. *8:*88–89, May–June '45

Nylon backing for dermatome grafts. GREEN, R. W. *et al.* New England J. Med. *233:* 268–270, Aug 30, '45

Maxillofacial bandage. KINCAID, C. J. Bull. U. S. Army M. Dept. *4:*475–477, Oct '45

New dressing for burns (medicated ointment in perforated cellophane envelope). KING, G. S. Indust. Med. *14:*796–797, Oct '45

"Cellophane" dressing for second degree burns. BLOOM, H. Lancet *2:*559, Nov 3, '45

Dermatome skin grafts in patients prepared with dry dressings and with and without penicillin. LEVENSON, S. M. AND LUND, C. C. New England J. Med. *233:*607-612, Nov. 22, '45

Bandage for Perthes operation (tendon transplant). NIKIFOROVA, E. K. Khirurgiya, no. 6, p. 94, '45

Dressing—Cont.
Acceleration of healing by pressure application to experimental thermal burns. Cameron, G. R. *et al.* J. Path. and Bact. *58:*1-9, Jan '46
Plaster casts in burns. de Moraes Leme, J. Rev. paulista de Med. *28:*109-125, Feb '46
Plaster bandages in burns. Faura, C. Actas dermo-sif. *37:*705-707, Feb '46
Rayon, ideal surgical dressing for surface wounds. Owens, N. Surgery *19:*482-485, April '46
Nonadherent surgical dressings (especially nylon surgical gauze). Bingham, R. Arch. Surg. *52:*610-618, May '46
Burn dressing (cellophane). Kings, G. S. New York State J. Med. *46:*1567, July 15, '46
Free graft in form of cutaneous "bandage;" use in severe burns. Marino, H. Bol. y trab. Acad. argent. de cir. *30:*451-459, July 17 '46
Use of cellophane in treatment of wounds Chistyakov, N. L. Am. Rev. Soviet Med. *3:*490-493, Aug '46
Treatment of burns under plexiglass covers Erusalimskiy, A. L. Vrach. delo (nos. 7-8) *26:*549-552, '46

Dressler, L.: Principles of prophylaxis and therapy of surgical shock. Harefuah *26:*5, Jan 1, '44; 24, Jan 16, '44 (in Hebrew)
Dreuschuch, F.: Roentgen diagnosis of hand infections. and injuries. Rozhl. v chir. a gynaek. (cast chir.) *14:*24-34, '35
Drevermann, E. B. (see Bick, M.) June '41
Drevon. (see Roudil, G. *et al*) April '36
Drew, C. R.: Early recognition and treatment of shock. Anesthesiology *3:*176-194, March '42
Dreyer: Case of cavernous angioma (facial nevus). Munchen. med. Wchnschr. *74:*563, April 1, '27
Dreyfus, G. (see Weissenbach, R. J. *et al*) April '35
Dreyfus, J. R.: Camptodactylia in children. Jahrb. f. Kinderh. *148:*336-345, '37
Dreyfus, J. R.: Blocking on tendons of both thumbs; comparison with syndrome described by Notta (trigger finger). Schweiz. med. Wchnschr. *68:*650-654, May 28, '38
Dreyfuss, M.: Congeital "windmill sail" position of fingers. Ztschr. f. Orthop. *65:*205-225, '36
Driessen, H. E.: Modern therapy of burns in war. Nederl. tijdschr. v. geneesk. *90:*497-500, May 18 '46
Driessens, J. (see Lambert, O.) May '37
Driessens, J. (see Lambert, O. *et al*) July '38
Drinker, C. K.: Analysis of modern treatment (especially with closed plaster) of severe burns. J. Oklahoma M. A. *37:*339-346, Aug '44
Drinker, C. K. (see Glenn, W. W. L. *et al*) Nov '42
Drinker, C. K. (see Glenn, W. W. L. *et al*) July '43
Drinnenberg, A.: Clubhand resulting from congenital absence of radius; 3 cases. Ztschr. f. orthop. Chir. *63:*297-307, '35
Driscoll, W. P.: Shock in pregnancy and labor. Anesth. and Analg. *7:*113-120, March-April '28
Driscoll, W. P. (see Bailey, H.) March '26
Driver, J. R. and Mac Vicar, D. N.: Melanomas of skin; clinical study of 60 cases. J.A.M.A. *121:*413-420, Feb 6, '43
Driver, S.: Volkmann's contracture. South. M. J. *23:*953-956, Oct '30
Drobyshev, G. I.: Treatment of penetrating war wounds of neck. Khirurgiya, no. 2, pp. 49-54, '44
Droogleever Fortuyn, A. B.: Inheritance of harelip and cleft palate in man. Genetica *17:*349-366, '35
Drum, B. C. (see Leech, C. H. *et al*) Oct '46
Drummond, A. C.: Treatment of burns of external genitalia. J. Urol. *50:*497-502, Oct '43
Drummond, N. R. (see Kimball, G. H.) April '40
Drummond, N. R. (see Kimball, G. H.) Aug '40
Drummond, N. R. (see Kimball, G. H.) Jan '41
Drummond, W. B.: Case of hyperterlorism. Arch. Dis. Childhood *1:*166-170, June '26
Drury, R. B. and Schwarzell, H. H.: Congenital absence of penis. Arch. Surg. *30:*236-242, Feb '35
Druss, J. G. and Allen, B.: Congenital fistula of neck communicating with middle ear (with aural malformations). Arch. Otolaryng. *31:*437-443, March '40
Duarte Cardoso, A.: Tubular graft in therapy of ulcers of legs. Arq. de cir. clin. e exper. *6:*251-260, April-June '42
Duarte Cardoso, A.: New material (vinylite) in plastic surgery; preliminary report. Rev. brasil. de oto-rino-laring. *10:*319-327, May-June '42
Duarte Cardoso, A.: Therapy of hemangiomas of auricular pavilion; case. Rev. paulista de med. *23:*347-352, Dec '43
Duarte Cardoso, A.: Nasal fractures; cases. Rev. brasil. de oto-rino-laring. *12:*284-296, July-Oct '44
Duarte Cardoso, A.: Total rhinoplasty following destruction of leishmaniasis; case. Rev.

med. e cir. de Sao Paulo *5:*271–277, Sept–Dec '45

DUBE, E.: Harelip with special reference to therapy. Ann. med.-chir. de l'Hop. Sainte-Justine, Montreal *3:*89–93, May '41

DUBE, E.: Sulfanilamide and its derivatives in burns. Union med. du Canada *71:*1062–1066, Oct '42

DUBE, P.: Physical therapy following suture of nerves. M. Clin. North America *27:*1091-1096, July '43

DUBECQ, X. J.: Fractured jaw caused by depression of upper jaw; case. J. de med. de Bordeaux *112:*43–44, Jan 20, '35

DUBECQ, X. J.: Fractures of upper part of face necessitating cranial support; author's device. J. de med. de Bordeaux *113:*817–820, Nov. 30, '36

DUBECQ, X. J.: Morphologic, physiologic and clinical study of mandibular meniscus; habitual luxation and temporomaxillary cracking. J. de med. de Bordeaux *114:*125–178, Jan 30, '37 also: Rev, d'odonto-stomatol. *1:*1–54, Jan '37

DUBECQ, X. J. AND BOIVIN, J.: Surgical therapy of war wounds to face due to projectile. Progres med. *68:*56–58; 63, Jan 20, '40

DU BOIS, C.: Treatment of hairy nevi. Rev. med. de la Suisse Rom *41:*769–772, Dec '21 (illus.) abstr: J.A.M.A. *78:*690, March 4, '22

DU BOIS, C.: Successful radiotherapy of cicatrices and keloids with case report. Rev. med. de la Suisse Rom *44:*705–713, Nov '24

DUBOIS, F. (with C. MONTANT): *Chirurgie plastique des seins*. Maloine, Paris, 1933.

DUBOIS-ROQUEBERT: Radium treatment of cancer of lip. Paris med. *12:*110–112, Feb 4, '22

DUBOST, T. (see GUILLEMINET, M.) Jan–Apr '46

DUBOUCHER, H. (see CANGE, A.) MARCH '31

DUBOV, M. D.: Primary bone suture in fracture of lower jaw. Novy khir. arkhiv *31:*89–95, '34

DUBOV, M. D.: Transplantation of thick skin flap in plastic surgery of face. Sovet. khir. (nos. 3–4) *6:*489–502, '34

DUBOV, M. D.: External injuries of nose. Sovet. khir. (no. 4) *7:*670–680, '34

DUBOV, M. D.: Injuries of jaws and face in farm laborers. Sovet. khir., no. 3, pp. 98–102, '35

DUBOV, M. D.: Frequency of bilateral ankylosis of temporomaxillary joint. Sovet. khir., no. 9, pp. 106–113, '35

DUBOV, M. D.: Fracture of zygomatic arch; case. Vestnik khir. *41:*189–190, '35

DUBOV, M. D.: Injuries of jaws and face among agricultural workers. Novy khir. arkhiv *38:*378–383, '37

DUBROV, Y. G.: Plastic surgery of flexor tendons of hand. Ortop. i travmatol. (no. 5) *9:*109–120, '35

DUBROV, Y. G.: Plastic repair of flexor tendons of fingers. Ortop. i travmatol. (no. 1) *15:*66–74, '41

DUBS, J.: Atrophy of bone (Sudeck) following burns. Munchen. med. Wchnschr. *68:*1141, Sept. 9, '21

DUC, C. (see PETTERINO PATRIARCA, A.) March–April '36

DUCHANGE: Apparatus for treatment of jaw fractures, with loss of substance. Rev.d'hyg. *49:*608–613, Oct '27

DUCHANGE, R.: Study and treatment of fractures of malar bone and xygoma. J. de med. de Bordeaux *95:*557–561, Aug 10, '23 (illus.)

DUCHET, G.: Treatment of loss skin substance in surgery of extremities. Semaine d. hop. Paris *22:*1671–1680, Sept 21, '46

DUCKETT, J. W. (see FLYNN, C. W.) April '36

DUCOURTIOUX: Technic of diathermic epilation in hypertrichosis. Rev. d'actinol. *10:*14–19, Jan–Feb '34

DUCOURTIOUX, M.: Rhinophyma and its treatment. Presse med. *47:*799–800, May 24, '39

DUCOURTIOUX, M. (see AUBRY, M.) July–Sept '44

DUCOURTIOUX, M. (see SÉZARY, A. *et al*) Feb '33

DUCUING, (see ESCAT, *et al*) 1930

DUCUING, J.: Surgical therapy of secondary adenopathies of neck in buccopharyngeal cancer. Ars med., Barcelona *11:*353–359, Sept '35

DUCUING, L.: Bifid uvula. Rev. de laryng. *52:*76–80, Jan 31, '31

DUDLEY, H. D.: Dupuytren's contracture. Northwest Med. *38:*138–139, April '39

DUEL, A. B.: Surgical treatment of facial palsy; Ballance-Duel method. Laryngoscope *42:*579–587, Aug '32

DUEL, A. B.: Clinical experiences in surgical treatment of facial palsy by autoplastic grafts; Ballance-Duel method. Arch. Otolaryng. *16:*767–788, Dec '32

DUEL, A. B.: History and development of surgical treatment of facial palsy (including grafts). Surg., Gynec. and Obst. *56:*382–390, Feb (No. 2A) '33

DUEL, A. B.: Advanced methods in surgical treatment of facial paralysis (Mütter lecture) (nerve transplants.). Ann. Otol., Rhin. and Laryng. *43:*76–88, March '34

DUEL, A. B.: Clinical presentation of improvement in surgical repair of facial nerve (transplant). Laryngoscope *44:*599–611, Aug '34

DUEL, A. B.: Operative treatment of facial palsy (transplant). Brit. M. J. *2:*1027-1031, Dec 8, '34

DUEL, A. B.: Surgical treatment of facial paralysis. Acta oto-laryng. *22:*373–381, '35

DUEL, A. B., AND TICKLE, T. G.: Surgical repair of facial paralysis. Ann. Otol., Rhin. and Laryng. *45:*3–27, March '36

DUEL, A. B. (see BALLANCE, C.) 1931

DUEL, A. B. (see BALLANCE, C.) Jan '32

Duel-Ballance Operation

Duel-Ballance nerve graft for cure of complete traumatic facial paralysis; case. HORGAN, J. B. Irish J. M. Sc., pp. 196–198, May '41

Duel, Operation (See Ballance-Duel Operation)

DUEÑO, F. P.: see PEREZ DUEÑO, F.

DUERTO, J.: Correction of deviation of nasal septum: case. Rev. espan. de med. y cir. *12:*600–603, Oct '29

DUESBERG, R.: So-called wound shock; physiopathology of posthemorrhagic states. Deut. Militerarzt *7:*69, Feb '42 also: Bull. War Med. *3:*149–150, No '42 (abstract)

DUFFY, J. J.: Cervical lymph nodes in intraoral carcinoma. Radiology *9:*373–379, Nov '27

DUFFY, J. J.: Treatment of bulky lesions of lips by combination of external and interstitial irradiation. Am. J. Cancer *15:*246–254, Jan '31

DUFFY, J. J.: Conservative procedure in care of cervical lymph nodes in intra-oral carcinoma. Am. J. Roentgenol. *29:*241–247, Feb '33

DUFFY, J. J.: New developments in study of hygroma. J. Iowa M. Soc. *27:*205–208, May '37

DUFOUR, A.: Extensive burns. Hopital *24:*187–190, March (B) '36

DUFOUR, A.: Modern treatment of severe burns. Hopital *25:*643–647, Dec (A) '37

DUFOURMENTEL, L.: Surgical treatment of prognathism. Presse med. *29:*235, March 23, '21 abstr: J. A. M. A. *76:*1284, April 30, '21

DUFOURMENTEL, L.: Facial surgery in 1921. Medecine *3:*57, Oct. '21 abstr: J. A. M. A. *77:*2152, Dec 31, '21

DUFOURMENTEL, L.: Reconstruction of upper lip. Presse med. *30:*344–346, April 22, '22 (illus.) abstr: J. A. M. A. *78:*1851, June 10, '22

DUFOURMENTEL, L.: Surgery of head without scars. Medecine *5:*52, Oct '23

DUFOURMENTEL, L.: Surgery of deformities of nose. Arch. franco-belges de chir. *28:*273–292, April '25

DUFOURMENTEL, L.: Irreducible deviation of the inferior jaw treated by orthopedic resection of condyle. Rev. odont. *48:*162–164, April '27

DUFOURMENTEL, L.: Double recidivant luxation of the inferior jaw; operated. Paris chir. *19:*134–136, May–June '27

DUFOURMENTEL, LÉON: *Chirurgie de l'articulation temporomaxillaire*. Masson et Cie, Paris, 1928

DUFOURMENTEL, L.: Indications and advantages of areolar incision in breast surgery. Bull. et mem. Soc. de chir. de Paris *20:*9–14, Jan 6, '28

DUFOURMENTEL, L.: Progress in plastic surgery. Arch. franco-belges de chir. *31:*126–132, Feb '28

DUFOURMENTEL, L.: Surgery of temporomaxillary joint in its relation to odontostomatology. Odontologie *66:*330–338, May '28

DUFOURMENTEL, L.: Aesthetic correction of facial paralysis; case. Bull. et mem. Soc. de chir. de Paris *20:*531, June 1, '28

DUFOURMENTEL, L.: Etiology and symptoms of closed temporomaxillary fractures. Bull. et. mem. Soc. de chir. de Paris *20:*557–565, June 15, '28

DUFOURMENTEL, L.: Condylar hypertrophy of inferior maxilla. Bull. et mem. Soc. de chir. de Paris *20:*886, '28

DUFOURMENTEL, LÉON: *Chirurgie correctrice du nez*. University Press of France, Paris, 1929

DUFOURMENTEL, L.: The surgical treatment of mandibular atrophy. Odontologie *67:*582–588, Aug '29

DUFOURMENTEL, L.: Wounds and injuries of face and immediate, aesthetic surgery. Bull. med., Paris *43:*942–948, Aug 31, '29

DUFOURMENTEL, L.: Immediate treatment of facial injuries. Bull. et mem. Soc. de med. de Paris, no. 16, pp. 369–373, No. 23, '29

DUFOURMENTEL, L.: Jaw deformity; treatment by orthopedic resection of condyles. Bull. et mem. Soc. de chir. de Paris *21:*424–431, '29

DUFOURMENTEL, L.: Methods of treatment of facial bone fractures. Clinique, Paris *25:*225, June (B) '30

DUFOURMENTEL, L.: Orthopedic resection of condyles in treatment of prognathism. Rev. de stomatol. *32:*519–527, June '30

DUFOURMENTEL, L.: Temporomaxillary ankylosis of obstetric origin. Bull. et mem. Soc. de chir. de Paris *22:*502–507, July 4, '30

DUFOURMENTEL, L.: Treatment of prognathism by orthopedic excision of condyles. Schweiz. Monatschr. f. Zahnh. *40:*673–681, Nov '30

DUFOURMENTEL, L.: Cancer of upper jaw; 4 cases. Bull. et mem. Soc. de chir. de Paris *22:*745–751, Dec 5, '30

DUFOURMENTEL, L.: Treatment of fractures of temporomaxillary joint. Rev. odont. *52:*517–526, July–Aug '31

DUFOURMENTEL, L.: Complications of minor endo-nasal operations. Paris med. *2:*203–206,

Sept 5, '31

Dufourmentel, L.: Satisfactory operation for pendulous breasts. Bull. med., Paris *46:*194-195, March 12, '32

Dufourmentel, L.: Complications of minor nasal operations. Rev. de laryng. *53:*447-474, April '32

Dufourmentel, L.: Sinking of nasal bone following submucous resection. Oto-rhino-laryng. internat. *16:*233-234, May '32

Dufourmentel, L.: Extirpation of condyle in therapy of subluxation of temporo-maxillary joint. Bull. et mem. Soc. d. chirurgiens de Paris *24:*558-559, Dec 2, '32

Dufourmentel, L.: Furuncles of nose and upper lip. Prat. med. franc. *14:*171-178, March (A) '33

Dufourmentel, L.: Application of auto-, homo- and heterografts in reconstructive surgery. Bull. et mem. Soc. d. chirurgiens de Paris *25:*269-282, May 5, '33

Dufourmentel, L.: Large scalp wound treated by total homoplastic graft of large cellulocutaneous flap. Bull. et mem. Soc. d. chirurgiens de Paris *25:*724-726, Dec 15, '33

Dufourmentel, L. Respective value of autografts, homografts and heterografts. Bull. med., Paris *47:*175-176, March 11, '33

Dufourmentel, L.: Surgery of face in South America. Paris med. (annexe) *1:*i-viii, Feb 18, '33

Dufourmentel, L.: Technic and late results of mastopexy. Bull. et mem. Soc. d. chirurgiens de Paris *25:*292-295, May 5, '33

Dufourmentel, L.: Retractile scars. Bull. med., Paris *48:*85, Feb 10, '34

Dufourmentel, L.: Postoperative cicatrices in otorhinolaryngologic surgery. Prat. med. franc. *15:*243-247, April (B) '34

Dufourmentel, L.: Mission to U. S. S. R. to study plastic surgery. Bull. et mem. Soc. d. chirurgiens de Paris *26:*571-590, Nov 2, '34

Dufourmentel, L.: Nasal fractures. Bull. med., Paris *48:*811-814, Dec 29, '34

Dufourmentel, L.: Autoplastic osseous and cutaneous grafts in destruction of lower jaw. Bull. et mem. Soc. d chirurgiens de Paris *27:*82-85, Feb 1, '35

Dufourmentel, L.: Deep epitheliomas of benign evolution; 6 cases. Bull. et mem. Soc. d. chirurgiens de Paris *27:*586-596, Dec 6, '35

Dufourmentel, L.: New surgical technics; Limberg pterygoid displacement in cleft palate. Bull. et mem. Soc. d. chirurgiens de Paris *27:*130-135, March 1, '35 also: Prat. med. franc. *17:*339-345, June (A-B) '36

Dufourmentel, L.: Cirsoid craniofacial angiomas; cases. Bull. et mem. Soc. d. chirurgiens de Paris *28:*103-109, March 6, '36.

Dufourmentel, L.: Cavernous angioma of face. Oto-rhino-laryng. internat. *20:*297-300, May '36

Dufourmentel, L.: Facial inclusion tumors. Mem. Acad. de chir. *62:*793-798, June 3, '36

Dufourmentel, L.: Study of favorable conditions for cicatrix formation; practical application in skin grafting. Bull. et mem. Soc. d chirurgiens de Paris *28:*401-423, June 19, '36

Dufourmentel, L.: Free skin grafts. Oto-rhino-laryng. internat. *20:*354-355, June '36

Dufourmentel, L.: Late complications of nasal fractures. Paris med. *2:*152-155, Sept 5, '36

Dufourmentel, L.: The fate of free grafts. Rev. de chir. structive, pp. 371-383, Dec '36

Dufourmentel, L.: Extirpation of tumors of parotid gland; technic to avoid injury to facial nerve. Oto-rhino-laryng. internat. *21:*75-.6, Feb '37

Dufourmentel, L.: Emergency surgery of facial wounds (with fractures). Presse med. *45:*387-390, March 13, '37

Dufourmentel, L.: Free full thickness skin grafts. Bull. et mem. Soc. d. chirurgiens de Paris *29:*306-317, June 18, '37

Dufourmentel, L.: The different application of free grafts in oto-rhino-laryngology. Prat. med. franc. *18:*187-195, June '37

Dufourmentel, L.: Cartilage homografts. Oto-rhino-laryng. internat. *21:*461-462, Aug '37

Dufourmentel, L.: Topographic varieties of free skin grafts. Rev. de chir. structive, pp. 259-263, Dec '37

Dufourmentel, L.: Total free skin grafts. Rev. de chir., Paris *76:*37-53, Jan '38

Dufourmentel, L.: Angiomas of face; therapy. Bull. et mem. Soc. de med. de Paris *142:*271-281, March 26, '38

Dufourmentel, L.: Reconstruction of pavilion using skin grafts (ear); case. Rev. de laryng. *59:*517-518, May '38 also: Oto-rhino-laryng. internat. *22:*395-396, July '38

Dufourmentel, L.: New route of approach to temporomaxillary articulation; case. Bull. et mem. Soc. d. chirurgiens de Paris *30:*420-424, No. 4-18, '38

Dufourmentel, L.: Irreducible luxation of lower jaw; case. Bull. et mem. Soc. d. chirurgiens de Paris *30:*485-488, Dec 2-16, '38

Dufourmentel, L.: Advantages, inconveniences and limits of free grafts of whole skin. Presse med. *47:*1336-1337, Sept 13, '39

Dufourmentel, L.: Surgery of face; graft by bipedicled flaps. Oto-rhino-laryng. internat. *23:*528-529, Oct '39

Dufourmentel, L.: Indications for emergency facial surgery. Mem. Acad. de chir. 65:1132-1138, Oct 25-Nov 8, '39

Dufourmentel, L.: Total craniofacial disjunction; case. Bull. et men. Soc. d. chirurgiens de Paris *32:*69–71, '41

DUFOURMENTEL, L. (see SEBILEAU, P.) Aug '27

DUFOURMENTEL, L. (see SEBILEAU, P.) Aug-Sept '27

DUFOURMENTEL, L. AND DARCISSAC, M.: Attempt at treatment of retrognathism; case. Bull. et mem. Soc. de chir. de Paris *20:*750–753, Nov 2, '28

DUFOURMENTEL, L. AND DARCISSAC, M.: Unilateral and bilateral condyloid resections in deviations of lower jaw and prognathism. Rev. de stomatol. *34:*340–346, June '32

DUFOURMENTEL, L. AND DARCISSAC, M.: Fracture of lower jaw in edentulous patient; reduction and immobilization by transosseous metallic loops with external extension splints. Bull. et mem. Soc. d. chirurgiens de Paris *25:*304–309, May 5, '33

DUFOURMENTEL, L. AND DARCISSAC, M.: Prognathism of lower jaw treated by bicondylar resection; 2 cases. Bull. et mem. Soc. d. chirurgiens de Paris *25:*583–589, Oct 20, '33

DUFOURMENTEL, L. AND DARCISSAC, M.: Reconstruction in crushing of facial bones. Bull. et mem. Soc. d. chirurgiens de Paris *26:*315–330, May 4, '34

DUFOURMENTEL, L. AND DARCISSAC, M.: Surgical and orthopedic prosthetic correction of depression of middle portion of face due to automobile accidents; cases. Rev. de stomatol. *36:*447–457, July '34

DUFOURMENTEL, L. AND DARCISSAC, M.: Surgical therapy of temporomaxillary ankylosis; 100 cases. Bull. et mem. Soc. d. chirurgiens de Paris *27:*149–161, March 15, '35

DUFOURMENTEL, L. AND DARCISSAC, M.: Fractures of neck of maxillary condyle, with special reference to therapy; cases. Bull. et mem. Soc. d. chirurgiens de Paris *31:*72–96, '39

DUFOURMENTEL, L., DARCISSAC, M. AND HENNION: Horizontal fracture of upper jaw consolidated in defective position and resulting in total malocclusion; functional and esthetic restoration by surgical and prosthetic therapy. Bull. et mem. Soc. d. chirurgiens de Paris *24:*555–558, Dec 2, '32

DUFOURMENTEL, L., DARCISSAC, M. AND HENNION: Consolidation of horizontal maxillary fracture in vicious position with total loss of dental articulation. Rev. de stomatol. *35:*339–342, June '33

DUFOURMENTEL, LÉON, AND FRISON, LÉON: *Diagnostic, Traitement, et Expertise des Sequelles des Accidents des Regions Maxillofaciales*. J. B. Baillière et fils, Paris, 1922

DUFOURMENTEL, LÉON (with PIERRE SEBILEAU): *Correction chirurgicale des difformités congenitale et acquises de la pyramide nasale*. Arnette, Paris, 1927

Dufourmentel Operation

Dufourmentel operation in therapy of prognathism of lower jaw. JULLIARD, C. Schweiz. med. Wchnschr. *68:*609–611, May 21, '38

DUFRESNE, E.: Total avulsion of scalp; therapy of case. Union med. du Canada *70:*825–829, Aug '41

DUGAL, L. P. (see DESAULNIERS, L.) 1945

DUGAN, W. M. AND UPSON, W. O.: Unusual anomaly of pelvis with exstrophy of bladder. J. Michigan M. Soc. *29:*512–515, July '30

DUGOUJON, F.: Epithelioma of pinna. Rev. de laryng. *57:*439–501, April '36

DUJARDIN, E.: New method of partial rhinoplasty. Ugesk. f. Laeger *90:*384–386, April 26 '28 also: Lancet *1:*1280–1281, June 23 '28

DUJARDIN, E.: Partial cheiloplasty by transplantation from one person to another. Ugesk. f. Laeger *94:*382–383, April 14, '32

DUJARDIN, E.: Treatment of disfiguring scars (keloids), defects and malformations. Hospitalstid. *79:*524–533, May 19, '39

DUJARDIN, E.: Process of healing after free transplantation of skin. Ugesk. f. laeger *98:*1073, Oct 29, '36

DUJARDIN, E. Electrocoagulation in treatment of cavernous hemangioma. Ugesk. f. laeger *99:*1257 – 1258, Nov 25, '37

DUJARDIN, E.: Free transplantation of cartilage in rhinoplasty. Ugesk. f. laeger *99:*1292, Dec. 2, '37

DUJARDIN, E.: Plastic correction of boxer's ears and nose. Ugesk. f. laeger *100:*115, Feb 3, '38

DUJARDIN, E.: Blocking and forming of nose in child aged 4. Ugesk. f. laeger *101:*211–212, Feb 16, '39

DUJARDIN, E.: Plastic surgery in therapy of facial scars. (grafts) Ugesk. f. laeger *102:*222, Feb 29, '40

DUJARDIN, E: Rhinoplastic surgery combined with paraffin prosthesis in correction of saddle nose. Ugesk. f. laeger *103:*404–405, March 27, '41

Dujardin-Beaumetz Operation

Dujardin-Beaumetz operation in accidental lesions of fingers for functional restoration of mutilated hands. FORGUE, E. Progres med., pp. 305–309, Feb 22, '36

DUJARIER, C. AND BOURGUIGNON: Rupture of tendon of thumb cured by tendinous graft. Bull. et mem. Soc. nat. de chir. *53:*532–535, April 9, '27

DUJOVICH, A.: Shock therapy. Dia med. *12:*418–421, May 20, '40
DUKEN, J.: Congenital ankylosis of finger joints (Comment on Brügger's article.). Munchen. med. Wchnschr. *70:*986, July 27, '23
DUMALLE, G. AND HOUOT, A.: Bilateral congenital branchial fistulas; case. Ann. Fac. franc. de med. et de pharm. de Beyrouth *7:*129–133, '38
DUMAS, J. M. R.: Phagedenic ulcer of lower leg with subjacent osteitis and extensive tissue loss; cure by autodermic graft and later anesthesia of articular ligaments according to Leriche; case. Marseille-med. *1:*553–556, April 25, '32
DUMITRESCU, D. (see JIANU, I. *et al*) Nov '32
DUMITRESCU, J. (see TETU, I.) Feb '35
DUNBAR, J.: Review of burn cases treated in Glasgow Royal Infirmary during past hundred years (1833–1933), with some observations on present-day treatment. Glasgow M. J. *122:*239–255, Dec '34
DUNCAN, C. S.: Common precanceroses of skin West Virginia M. J. *42:*299–301, Dec '46
DUNCAN, G. W. AND BLALOCK, A.: Shock produced by crush injury; effects of administration of plasma and local application of cold. Arch. Surg. *45:*183–194, Aug '42
DUNCAN, G. W. (see BLALOCK, A.) Oct '42
DUNCAN, R. D. (see SKINNER, H. L.) Dec '43
DUNDAS-GRANT, J.: Surgery of throat, nose and ear. Practitioner *110:*11–25, Jan '23
DUNE, M. V.: Traumatic loss of skin of penis. Vestnik khir. *53:*51, '37
DUNET, (see BÉRARD, L.) Aug–Sept '29
DUNLAP, H. J. (see SOMMER, G. N. J. Jr. *et al*) Aug '43
DUNLAP, S. E.: Hand infections. Surg. J. *34:*18–20, Sept–Oct '27
DUNLOP, G. R. AND HUMBERD, J. D.: Arm board for navy operating table. U. S. Nav. M. Bull. *44:*171–172, Jan '45
DUNLOP, J.: Use of index finger for thumb, some interesting points in hand surgery. J. Bone and Joint Surg. *5:*99–103, Jan '23 (illus.)
DUNN, E. P.: Rational treatment of burns (including tannic acid). Am. J. Surg. *6:*519–521, April '29
DUNN, F. S.: Fractures of jaw. Am. J. Surg. *36:*83–87, April '37
DUNN, N.: Surgery of muscle and tendon in relation to paralysis and injury. Post-Grad. M. J. *13:*374–380, Oct '37
DUNN, R. (see DAVIS, A. D.) April '33
DUNNE, R. E.: Cancer of lips. Connecticut M. J. *6:*175–176, March '42
DUNNING, H. S.: Jaw fractures. Internat. J. Med. and Surg. *47:*277–286, July–Aug '34
DUNNING, H. S.: Plastic surgery of mouth. Laryngoscope *50:*532–434, June '40
DUNNING, H. S. (see MCWILLIAMS, C. A.) Jan '23
DUNNING, W. M.: Submucous resection of nasal septum. Am. J. Surg. *35:*1, Jan '21
DUNNINGTON, J. H.: Treatment of wounds of eyelids. Virginia M. Monthly *69:*473–475, Sept '42
DUNPHY, E. B.: Treatment of eyes in exophthalmic goiter. S. Clin. N. America *4:*1439–1442, Dec '24
DUNPHY, J. E.: Surgical shock – practical aspects; medical progress. New England J. Med. *224:*903–908, May 22, '41
DUNPHY, J. E.: Shock, therapy, Lessons from military surgery. Post-Grad. M. J. *21:*111–116, April '45
DUNPHY, J. E. AND GIBSON, J. G. JR.: Effect of replacement therapy (especially with plasma or saline) in experimental shock. Surgery *10:*108–118, July '41
DUPERTUIS, S. M.: Actual growth of young cartilage transplants in rabbits; experimental studies. Arch. Surg. *43:*32–63, July '41
DUPERTUIS, S. M. AND HENDERSON, J. A.: Rehabilitation; plastic and reconstructive surgery of stumps. U. S. Nav. M. Bull. (supp.) pp. 65–77, Mar '46

Duplay Operation

Repair of urethra with hypospadias by single operation (Duplay's method). MARTIN, Bull. Soc. Franc. J. d'urol. *7:*242–244, Nov. 19, '28 also: J. d'urol. *26:*564–567, Dec '28
Penoscrotal hypospadias; satisfactory results of Duplay operation with hypogastric derivation of urine; case. SALLERAS, J. Rev. Assoc. med. argent. *46:*988–990, Sept '32
Therapy of penile, penoscrotal and perineoscrotal hypospadias by Duplay operation. ELBIM. A. J. d'urol. *40:*484–498, Dec '35

DUPONNOIS, (see ETIENNE, E.) March '28
DUPONNOIS, (see MASSABUAU, *et al*) Aug '27
DUPONT, R.: Cancer in exstrophy of bladder. J. d'urol. *13:*433–444, June '22 (illus.) abstr: J. A. M. A. 79:855, Sept. 2, '22
DUPUY DE FRENELLE: Treatment of radial paralysis by tendon anastomosis. Paris chir. *19:*20–27, Jan '27
DUPUY DE FRENELLE: Suture of superficial sectioned tendon. Hopital *15:*198–200, March (B)'27
DUPUY DE FRENELLE: Technic of conservative amputation after hand injuries. Tech. Chir. *27:*109–122, May–July '35

DUPUY-DUTEMPS, L.: Restoration of completely destroyed eyelid by cutaneous and tarso-conjunctival grafts from other lid; 3 cases. Ann. d'ocul. *164:*915–926, Dec '27

DUPUY-DUTEMPS, L.: Eyelid surgery, technic; case. Bull. Soc. d'opht. de Paris, pp. 315–318, July '28

DUPUY-DUTEMPS, L.: Regeneration of destroyed eyelid by cutaneous and tarsoconjunctival graft taken from other lid; case. Monde med., Paris *38:*705–711, Sept, 1, '28

DUPUY-DUTEMPS, L.: Congenital eyelid ptosis with Gunn's phenomenon; case. Bull. Soc. d'opht. de Paris, pp. 136–140, March '29

DUPUY-DUTEMPS, L.: Progressive atrophy of eyelids with coloboma and facial hemiatrophy; case. Bull. Soc. d'opht. de Paris, pp. 181–187, April '29

DUPUY-DUTEMPS, L.: Repair of entirely destroyed eyelid by cutaneous and tarso-conjunctival graft taken from other eyelid. Bull. med., Paris *43:*935–938, Aug. 31, '29

DUPUY-DUTEMPS, L.: Plastic surgery of eyelid using cervical flap with tubular pedicle; case. Ann. d'ocul. *167:*895–907, Nov '30 also: Bull. et mem. Soc. franc. d'opht. *43:*451–458, '30

DUPUY-DUTEMPS, L.: Statistics on 1000 plastic dacryocystotomies. Bull. Soc. d'opht. de Paris, pp. 392–399, June '32

DUPUY-DUTEMPS, L.: Observations on 1000 plastic dacryocystotomies. Ann. d'ocul. *170:*361–384, May '33

DUPUY-DUTEMPS, L.: Marginal cutaneous blepharopexy in plastic surgery. Ann. d'ocul. *174:*312–317, May '37

DUPUY-DUTEMPS, L. AND BOURGUET: Closure of large nasal breach by grafts of frontal and cervicothoracic flaps placed side by side; case. Bull. Soc. d'opht. de Paris, pp. 435–442, Oct '30

Dupuy-Dutemps Operation

Dupuy-Dutemps and Bourguet's plastic dacryocystorhinostomy in chronic dacryocystitis. HUSSON, A. AND JEANDELIZE, P. Medecine *5:*256–259, Jan '24

Surgical relief of chronic dacryocystitis and epiphora; Dupuy-Dutemps et Bourguet technique; direct anastomosis of tear sac with nasal mucous membrane. CORBETT, J. J., M. J. and Rec. *128:*158–160, Aug 15, '28 also: New England J. Med. *199:*459–461, Sept 6, '28 also: Am. J. Ophth. *11:*774–778, Oct '28

Dacryocystorhinostomy by method of Dupuy-Dutemps and Bourguet. POTIQUET, H. Ann. d'ocul. *166:*470–487, June '29

Dupuy-Dutemps and Bourguet technic in dacryocystotomy. BARBEROUSSE, Bull. Soc. d'opht. de Paris, p. 226, March '31

Dupuy-Dutemps Operation – Cont.

Dacryocystorhinostomy, Dupuy-Dutemps method; 25 cases. GONZÁLEZ LLANOS, N. Rev. de especialid. *6:*237, May '31

Dupuy Operation (See Bourguet-Dupuy-Dutemps Operation

DUPUYTREN, G.: Permanent retraction of fingers, produced by affection of palmar fascia. M. Classics *4:*142–150, Oct '39 (Reprint). also: M. Classics *4:*127–141, Oct '39 (Reprint; in French).

Dupuytren's Contracture: See Contracture, Dupuytren's

DURAN RODRIGUEZ, C.: Bilateral congenital ptosis of eyelids treated by Traynor operation. Vida nueva *53:*245–249, May '44

DURAND: Therapy of small cutaneous angiomas by systematic association of cryotherapy with carbon dioxide snow and diathermy. Bull. Soc. franc. de dermat. et syph. (Reunion dermat.) *41:*587–589, April '34

DURAND, M.: Present status of bone transplantation. Lyon med. *130:*473, June 10, '21

DURAND, P.: Traumatic amputation of child's finger by rabbit bite. Presse med. *46:*907, June 8, '38

DURANTE, L.: Extirpation of lymphatics with lip cancer. Arch. ital. di chir. *8:*201–208, Oct '23

DURANTE, L.: Volkmann's retraction; surgical treatment; case. Arch. ital. di chir. *25:*429–439, '30

DURBAN, K.: Subcutaneous ruptures of extensor tendons of fingers. Zentralbl. f. Chir. *53:*2773–2774, Oct 30, '26

DUREN, N. (see SINGLETON, A. O.) April '41

DURLING, E. J.: Compound and comminuted fractures of ramus of mandible; case. J. Am. Dent. A. *28:*1832–1835, Nov '41

DURMAN, D. C.: Conservatism in treatment of hand injuries. J. Michigan M. Soc. *25:*381–383, Aug '26

DUROUX, E.: Technic of grafting living nervous tissue. Rev. tech. chir. *24:*21–26, Jan–Feb '32

DUROUX, E. AND DUROUX, P. E.: Late results of double heterogenous graft performed in 1911. Progres med. *70:*140–145, March 7, '42

DUROUX, P. E. (see DARGENT, M.) Aug '46

DUROUX, P. E. (see DUROUX, E.) March '42

DURRANT, M. M.: Streamlined finger dressings. Brit. J. Phys. Med. *8:*88–89, May–June '45

DUSATTI, C.: Pathogenic study of case of Dupuytren's contracture. Minerva med. *2:*79–80, July 28, '36

DUSCHL, L.: New instrument for grasping tendons. Chirurg *12:*756, Dec 15, '40

DUSSELDORP, M.: Resection of orbicularis oculi

in therapy of spasmodic entropion. Rev. Asoc. med. argent. *48:*296–298, March–April '34 also: Rev. oto-neuro-oftal. *9:*207–209, June '34

Dutemps Operation: See Bourguet-Dupuy-Dutemps Operation; Dupuy-Dutemps Operation

DUTTA, P. C.: Operation for utilising middle finger as "trigger" finger. Indian M. Gaz. *66:*676–677, Dec '31

DUTTO, U.: Dupuytren's contracture, cases. Gazz. med. di Roma *54:*198, Oct '28

DUVAL, P.: Rapid death due to extensive burns. Dia med. *10:*877–880, Aug 29, '38

DUVAL, P. AND MOURGUE-MOLINES, E.: Pathologic physiology and therapy of recent extensive cutaneous burns. J. de chir. *50:*471–488, Oct '37

DUVAL, P. AND REDON, H.: Technic of total or subtotal extirpation of parotid gland with conservation of superior branch of facial nerve in so-called mixed tumors; clinical results. J. de chir. *39:*801–808, June '32

Duval Operation

Extirpation of parotid gland by Duval method. FIORILLO, J. F. Prensa med. argent. *22:*150–152, Jan 16, '35

Malignant tumor of parotid gland treated by Duval operation, with transplantation of digastric muscle to relieve resulting paralysis (Cadenat operation); case. MIRIZZI, P. L. AND URRUTIA, J. M. Bol. y trab., Soc. de cir. de Cordoba (no. 4) *1:*52–55, '40

Parotidectomy with conservation of superior facial nerve (Duval operation); 2 cases. COGNIAUX, P. J. de chir. et ann. Soc. belge de chir. *38-36:*370–372, Dec '39

DWORKIN, R. M. (see ANTOS, R. J. *et al*) Oct '44

DYCHNO, A.: Comparative value of different sutures in tendon surgery, with presentation of 2 new technics. Lyon chir. *34:*290–303, May-June '37

DYKES, S. N.: Rupture of extensor longus pollicis tendon. Brit. M. J. *1:*387–388, March 11, '22

DYKHNO, A. M.: Two new methods of tendon suture. Novy khir. arkhiv *37:*403–416, '36

DYNIEWICZ, H. A. (see FANTUS, B.) July '37

DZBANOVSKIY, V. P.: New method for plastic correction of defects of lower jaw and chin. Sovet. khir. (no. 4) *7:*654–661, '34

DZBANOVSKIY, V. P.: Transplantation of toe to replace thumb; Nicoladoni method. Vestnik khir. *55:*626–629, May '38

DZBANOVSKIY, V. P.: Plastic reconstruction of fingers. Khirurgiya no. 4, pp. 92–94, '45

DZHANELIDZE, U. U.: Restoration of flexion of fingers by Sterling Bunnel's method. Vestnik khir. (nos. 56-57) *19:*39-53, '30

DZHANELIDZE, Y. Y.: Suture of tendons of hand. Novy khir, arkiv *36:*497-507, '36

DZIOB, J. M. (see BROWN, R. K.) Oct '42

E

E. M. S. memorandum: Treatment of burns. M. J. Australia *1:*356, March 21, '42

EADIE, C. M.: Rib implant for depressed bridge of nose. M. J. Australia *2:*137–139, Aug 1, '25

EADIE, N. M.: Modification of Davis gag. J. Laryng. and Otol. *43:*531, July '28

Earlobes

Technic for correcting deformities of ears among natives of Dutch East Indies acquired from wearing heavy things in ear lobes. WAAR, C. A. H. Nederlandsch Tijdschr. v. Geneesk. *2:*32–35, July 7, '23 (illus.)

Making lobule of ear smaller. EITNER, E. Wien. klin. Wchnschr. *39:*1423–1424, Dec 2, '26

Dangers of puncturing ear lobes of children for purpose of inserting earrings. FRIEDJUNG, J. K. Wien. med. Wchnschr. *85:*203, Feb 16, '35

Keloid formation in ear lobe. SPRENGER, W. Monatschr. f. Ohrenh. *70:*188–194, Feb '36

Technic of reparation of ear lobe by tubular skin grafts. GONZALEZ ULLOA, M. Rev. mex. de cir., ginec. y cancer *5:*33–41, Jan '37

Nodules due to ear-rings; case. GUILLEMIN, A. Rev. med. de Nancy *66:*292–294, April 1, '38

Plastic surgery of ear lobule. EITNER, E. Wien. med. Wchnschr. *88:*774–775, July 11, '38

Deformities of ear lobe and their surgical correction. MALBEC, E. F. Semana med. *2:*623–631, Sept 15, '38

Plastic reconstruction of ear lobe with circular pedicled flap from neck. SCHUCHARDT, K. Zentralbl. f. Chir. *69:*345, Feb 28, '42

Plastic correction of deformities of ear lobe in leprosy. SILVEIRA, L. M. Arq. de. cir. clin. e exper. *6:*485–488, April–June '42

Keloid formation in both ear lobes. WEAVER, D. F. Arch. Otolaryng. *44:*212–213, Aug '46

Ears (See also Otoplasty; Earlobes)

Use of paraffin and wax in ear and nose surgery. STAHLMAN, T. M. Pennsylvania M. J. *24:*875, Sept '21

5 years of surgery of ear and nose. HAAG, H.

Ears – Cont.

Schweiz. med. Wchnschr. *52:*498–504, May 25, '22

Surgery of throat, nose and ear. DUNDAS-GRANT, J. Practitioner *110:*11–25, Jan '23

Use of dental stent in skin grafts of middle ear and mastoid cavities. DE RIVER, J. P. M. J. and Rec. *122:*63–64, July 15, '25

Two new instruments; septum needle and thread-holder for ear surgery. POLLAK, E. Monatschr. f. Ohrenh. *61:*1252, Nov '27

Plastic surgery of ear. BONDY, G. Monatschr. f. Ohrenh. *62:*1227, Oct '28

Kubo's aurograph for tracing form of concha. KUBO, I. Ztschr. f. Hals-, Nasen-u. Ohrenh. *22:*320–322, Nov 10, '28

Plastic operation on auditory canal after complete opening of middle ear with chisel. UFFENORDE, W. Ztschr. f. Hals-, Nasen-u. Ohrenh. *23:*317, Sept 10, '29

Plastic surgery of ear. HEERMANN, H. Ztschr. f. Hals-, Nasen-u. Ohrenh. *26:*35–41, May 6, '30

New method of primary plastic surgery after antro-atticotomy (ear). LEO, E. Valsalva *6:*388–398, June '30

Plastic surgery of ear. LOCKWOOD, C. D., S. Clin. North America *10:*1103–1108, Oct '30

Use of tubular stem in transplantation from ear to defect of ala. VETCHTOMOFF, A. A. Vestnik khir. (no. 55) *20:*143–150, '30

Auricular epicanthus. FRINDENBERG, P. Presse med. *39:*584, April 18, '31

Plastic surgery with bridge flap for correction of retroauricular defects. CLAUS, G. Deutsche med. Wchnschr. *57:*1779–1780, Oct 16, '31

Plastic surgery of ear. SANVENERO-ROSSELLI, G. Rev. de chir. plastique, pp. 27–52, April '32

Closure of persistent retro-auricular opening by means of Hungarian method of using semicircular flaps. SZOKOLIK, E. Monatschr. f. Ohrenh. *66:*1058–1059, Sept '32

Correction of postauricular defect by implantation of fascia lata. GRIFFITH, C. M. AND SCHATTNER, A. Laryngoscope *43:*280–281, April '33

Progress in plastic surgery of ear and nose. FRUEHWALD, V. Rev. de chir. plastique, pp. 155–167, Oct '33

Technic of radical operation in plastic surgery of ear. POGÁNY, O. Gyogyaszat *74:*38, Jan 21, '34

Development of keloids from trifling causes (case following puncture of ear during delivery). VON LORMAYER, G. Zentralbl. f. Chir. *61:*253, Feb 3, '34

Repair of postauricular fistula following radical mastoidectomy (grafting). STRAATSMA, C. R. Arch. Otolaryng. *19:*616–618, May '34

Otoplasty for dermatitis congelationis (frostbite). LIGGETT, H. M. Rec. *142:*278–279, Sept 18, '35

Histopathologic changes in freely transplanted tissue from human auricle. KYANDSKIY, A. A. Sovet. khir., no. 9, pp. 66–69, '35

Experimental studies on transplantation of cartilage (ear) to cover tracheal defect. MORI, S. Okayama-Igakkai-Zasshi *48:*516, March '36

Congenital aural fistulas and differential diagnostic significance in children. DRAGISIC, B. Wien. med. Wchnschr. *86:*748–750, July 4, '36

Transplantation of cartilage (ear) in surgical therapy of strabismus. DUBINOV, O. A. Sovet. vestnik oftal. *8:*250–255, '36

Plastic surgery of ear pavilion. MALBEC, E. F. Semana med. *1:*994–1001, May 5, '38

Repair of permanent cavity behind left ear, following petromastoid evident; excision of concha of ear; case. COELST. Rev. de chir. structive *8:*113–115, Aug '38

Recent advances in plastic and reconstructive surgery (of ears, nose and throat). GUTTMAN, M. R. Am. J. M. Sc. *196:*875–882, Dec '38

Diseases of ear in patients with cleft palate. MEISSNER, K. Hals-, Nasen-u. Ohrenarzt (Teil 1) *30:*6–20, Jan '39

Fractures of malar bone and zygoma with eye, ear, nose and throat complications. MEYER, M. F. New Orleans M. and S. J. *92:*90–94, Aug '39

Technical modifications in operation for strabismus by transplanting auricular cartilage. IVANOV, A. I. Vestnik oftal. (no. 2) *15:*43–45, '39

Rare complication following peritomy and transplantation of auricular cartilage in therapy of pannus. MITSKEVICH, L. D. Vestnik oftal. (no. 1) *14:*118–119, '39

Argyrosis of auricles with certain practical observations on plastic operations. KESSEL, O. Hals-, Nasen-u. Ohrenarzt (Teil 1) *31:*250–252, Dec '40

Plastic surgery of auricle; postoperative care and errors committed during surgery. MALBEC, E. F. Semana med. *1:*219–221, Jan 23, '41

Progress of surgery of head (including face, ears, nose, mouth, etc.) and throat (esophagus and larynx); review of literature for 1940. REBELO NETO, J. Rev. brasil. de otorino-laring. *9:*37–46, Jan–Feb '41

Ears – Cont.

Plastic surgery of external ear; case (and nose). MALBEC, E. F. Prensa med. argent. *28:*1700–1702, Aug 20, '41

Bleeding from external auditory meatus following fracture of mandible. SUGGIT, S. J. Laryng. and Otol. *56:*364–367, Oct '41

Practice model for plastic surgery of auditory canal. SCHÜTZ, W. Ztschr. f. Hals-. Nasen-u. Ohrenh. *47:*388–389, '41

New plastic flap for use in endaural radical mastoidectomy. SHAMBAUGH, G. E. JR. Ann. Otol., Rhin. and Laryng. *51:*117–121, March '42

Burns of ear, nose, mouth and adjacent tissues (with special reference to therapy with hydrosulphosol, sulfhydryl solution). CRUTHIRDS, A. E. Laryngoscope *53:*478–494, July '43

Burns of ear, nose, mouth and adjacent tissues (including use of hydrosulphosol, sulfhydryl solution). CRUTHIRDS, A. E. Tr. Am. Laryng., Rhin. and Otol. Soc., pp. 219–235, '43

Temporomandibular ankylosis; surgical therapy of case in child following otitis with mastoiditis. OREGGIA, J. C. Arch. de pediat. d. Uruguay *15:*223–234, April '44

Plastic surgery of ear; case. HERNANDEZ, A. Prensa med. argent. *31:*2367–2373, Nov 22, '44

Ears, Avulsion

Ear reconstruction; conservation of avulsed portion. GREELEY, P. W. U. S. Nav. M. Bull. *42:*1323–1325, June '44

Ears, Cancer (See also Cancer, Basal Cell; Cancer, Squamous; Skin Cancer)

Caustic treatment of superficial cancer of ear and nose. CITELLI, AND CALICETI. Tumori *8:*165, Aug '21 abstr: J.A.M.A. *77:*1139, Oct 1, '21

A study of 63 cases of epithelioma of ear. BRODERS, A. C. S. Clin. N. Amer. *1:*1401, Oct '21

Carcinoma of external ear; combined surgical and radium treatment. BECK, E. G. Internat. Clinics *1:*29, '21

Epithelioma of face and ear. YOUNG, W. J. Kentucky M. J. *20:*367–368, May '22

Epithelioma of auricle. MONTGOMERY, D. W. AND CULVER, G. D. Arch. Dermat. and Syph. *7:*472–478, April '23

Prosthesis after removal of auricle for carcinoma. FENTON, R. A. AND LUPTON, I. M. Northwest Med. *22:*212, June '23 (illus.)

Electrocoagulation and radiation therapy in malignant disease of ear, nose and throat. PFAHLER, G. E., J.A.M.A. *85:*344–347, Aug 1, '25

Ears, Cancer – Cont.

Radium treatment of epithelioma of ear. KENNEDY, W. H. Radiology *7:*249–252, Sept '26

Results of surgical and diathermic-surgical treatment of cancer of concha of ear. GIESE, A. Ztschr. f. Laryng., Rhin. *19:*414–423, July '30

Personal and practical experiences with neoplasms about head and neck, with special reference to ear, nose and throat. BECK, J. C. Pennsylvania M. J. *34:*467–469, April '31

Epithelioma of auricle and its therapy. DESAIVE, P. Cancer, Bruxelles *12:*273–286, '35

Epithelioma of pinna. DUGOUJON, F. Rev. de laryng. *57:*439–501, April '36

Basocellular epithelioma of ear treated surgically. BATTISTA, A. Rinasc. med. *6:*31–34, Jan 15, '29

Ears, Cauliflower

Hematoma of external ear. LEROUX, L. Medecine *8:*306–309, Jan '27

Treatment for acute traumatic hematoma of external ear. BRITTON, H. A., J.A.M.A. *89:*111–112, July 9, '27

Window operation for hematoma auris and perichondritis, with effusion. HOWARD, R. C. Laryngoscope *39:*590–594, Sept '29

Dressing for hematoma of ear. FERGUSON, L. K., J.A.M.A. *100:*736, March 11, '33

Hematoma auris. CARSON, L. D. AND BROWN, J. L., U. S. Nav. M. Bull. *32:*204–205, April '34

Window operation for hematoma and perichondritis with effusion of ear. HOWARD, R. C. Laryngoscope *45:*81–105, Feb '35

Plastic correction of boxer's ears and nose. DUJARDIN, E. Ugesk. f. laeger *100:*115, Feb 3, '38

Therapy of perichondritis of auricle. HERRMANN. Ztschr. f. Hals-, Nasen-u. Ohrenh. *44:*373–377, '38

Surgical therapy of perichondritis of auricle. TOBECK, A. Ztschr. f. Hals-, Nasen-u. Ohrenh. *44:*368–373, '38

Ears, Cryptotia (See also Ears, Deformity)

Pouch ear; case. NOGUCHI, M. AND KOTAKE, Y. Oto-rhino-laryng. *9:*820, Sept '36

Pouch ear; case. OTSUKA, H. Oto-rhino-laryng. *9:*813, Sept '36

"Pocket ear"; case. YAMANAKA, K. Oto-rhino-laryng. (abstr. sect) *13:* n.p., Feb '40

Ears, Cysts and Fistulas

Congenital fistula of ear and atresia of external meatus. ERFURTH, W. Monatschr. f. Kinderh. *22:*55–59, Oct '21 (illus.)

Salivary fistula behind ear; 2 cases. KAUSCH, W. Zentralbl. f. Chir. *52:*914–917, April 25, '25

Pre-auricular fistulae. STAMMERS, F. A. R. Brit. J. Surg. *14:*359–363, Oct '26

Congenital aural fistula; case. RUTTIN, E. Wien. med. Wchnschr. *77:*1019, July 30, '27

Congenital fistula of external ear; case. BREUER, F. Deutsche Ztschr. f. Chir. *202:*278–282, '27

Congenital fistula of external ear; 2 cases. STEINER, A. Dermat. Wchnschr. *86:*325–328, March 10, '28

So-called fistula auris congenita. SEIFERT, E. Deutsche Ztschr. f. Chir. *209:*118–124, '28

Heredity of fistula auris congenita. SCHÜLLER, J. Munchen. med. Wchnschr. *76:*160–162, Jan 25, '29

Congenital preauricular fistula. FISCHER, H. J. de med. de Bordeaux *59:*711–714, Sept 10, '29

Congenital auricular fistula; 3 cases in same family. MONTGOMERY, M. L., S. Clin. North America *11:*141–148, Feb '31

Repair of postauricular fistula by means of free fat graft. STRAATSMA, C. R. AND PEER, L. A. Arch. Oto-laryng. *15:*620–621, April '32

Fistula auris congenita; surgical therapy; 2 cases. BARAJAS VILCHES, F. Rev. med. de Canarias *1:*243–244, June '32

Retro-auricular salivary fistula; therapy. BORKOWSKI, J. Warszawskie czasop. lek. *9:*653, July 14, '32

Human congenital auricular and juxta-auricular fossae, sinuses and scars (including so-called aural and auricular fistulae) and bearing of their anatomy upon theories of their genesis. CONGDON, E. D. *et al.* Am. J. Anat. *51:*439–463, Nov '32

Congenital auriculo-hyoid fistula; medical therapy; case. BERGARA, R. AND BERGARA, C. An. de oto-rino-laring. d. Uruguay *2:*117–130, '32

Erroneous diagnoses in cases of aural and cervical fistulas and cysts. ZÖLLNER, F. Ztschr. f. Hals-, Nasen-u. Ohrenh. *32:*54–61, '32

Cure of mastoid fistula with fat graft; case. BENNETT, A. B. M. Ann. District of Columbia *2:*117–118, May '33

Bilateral congenital preauricular fistula, with report of case in congenital syphilitic. BERGARA, R. A. AND BERGARA, C. Rev. Asoc. med. argent. *48:*44–50, Jan '34

Ears, Cysts and Fistulas—Cont.

Sinus preauricularis (fistula preauricularis congenita). BECKER, S. W. AND BRUNSCHWIG, A. Am. J. Surg. *24:*174–177, April '34

Repair of postauricular fistula following radical mastoidectomy (grafting). STRAATSMA, C. R. Arch. Otolaryng. *19:*616–618, May '34

Preauricular fistula; development of external ear. JONES, F. W. AND WEIN, I. C., J. Anat. *68:*525–533, July '34

Typical and atypical forms of aural fistulae; review of literature. GUYOT, R. Ann. d'otolaryng., pp. 1227–1248, Dec '34

Congenital aural fistula. SELKIRK, T. K. Am. J. Dis. Child. *49:*431–447, Feb '35

Preauricular fistulae; two cases. KLABER, R. Proc. Roy. Soc. Med. *28:*1553–1554, Oct '35

Congenital fistula of ear lobe; case. SCALORI, G. Valsalva *11:*606–622, Oct 1, '35

New method of plastic surgery of fistulas of dorsal portion of ear. DOROSCHENKO, I. T. Acta oto-laryng. *22:*105–106, '35

Extirpation following paraffin injections into congenital aural fistula. KUBO, K. Otorhino-laryng. *9:*101, Feb '36

Congenital aural fistulas and differential diagnostic significance in children. DRAGISIC, B. Wien. med. Wchnschr. *86:*748–750, July 4, '36

Congenital aural fistula in marines; statistical study. TOYOSHIMA, Y. Oto-rhino-laryng. *9:*825, Sept '36

Familial congenital aural fistula; case. SÖDERLUND, S. Finska lak.-sallsk. handl. *80:*71–77, Jan '37

Postauricular sinus; case. FLETT, R. L. J. Laryng. and Otol. *53:*458, July '38

Aural fistula; retropharyngeal abscess with fistulization into external auditory canal; report of 2 cases. MERKLIN, L. Arch. Pediat. *55:*395–399, July '38

Congenital preauricular sinus. DINGMAN, R. O. Arch. Otolaryng. *29:*982–984, June '39

Congenital preauricular sinus; treatment. HAVENS, F. Z. Arch. Otolaryng. *29:*985–986, June '39

Three generations of ear pits. WHITNEY, D. D. J. Hered. *30:*323–324, Aug '39

Congenital fistulas of lacrimal sac combined with congenital aural fistulas and anosmia. REH, H. Klin. Monatsbl. f. Augenh. *104:*55–59, Jan '40

Congenital fistula of neck communicating with middle ear (with aural malformations). DRUSS, J. G., AND ALLEN, B. Arch. Otolaryng. *31:*437–443, March '40

Operation for cure of postauricular fistula; 8

Ears, Cysts and Fistulas – Cont.

consecutive cases. GREENFIELD, S. D. Laryngoscope *50:*312–325, April '40

Congenital preauricular fistula. MARTIN, J. D. JR. J. M. A. Georgia *29:*411–413, Aug '40

Ear pit and its inheritance; fistula auris congenita, described in 1864, still genetic and embryologic puzzle. QUELPRUD, T. J. Hered. *31:*379–384, Sept '40

Skin graft in closure of retro-auricular fistulas. MATIS, I. Medicina, Kaunas *21:*1027–1031, Dec '40

Preauricular fistula. KHANNA, M. N. Indian M. Gaz. *76:*72–75, Feb '41

Symptoms of aural fistula. HASEGAWA, T. Oto-rhino-laryng. *14:*691–696, Sept '41 (in Japanese)

Congenital aural fistula. FOX, M. S. Arch. Otolaryng. *35:*431–433, March '42

Congenital preauricular sinus. HARDING, R. L. Am. J. Orthodontics (Oral Surg. Sect.) *28:*399–401, July '42

Congenital preauricular cysts and fistulas. PASTORE, P. N. AND ERICH, J. B. Arch. Otolaryng. *36:*120–125, July '42

Differential diagnosis between thymic duct fistulas and branchial cleft fistulas; case of bilateral aural fistulas and bilateral thymic duct fistulas. BAUMGARTNER, C. J. AND STEINDEL, S. Am. J. Surg. *59:*99–103, Jan '43

Congenital auricular fistula. BECKER, F. T. Arch. Dermat. and Syph. *48:*520–522, Nov '43

Congenital fistula of external ear; case. AUSTIN, E. R. Proc. Staff Meet. Clin., Honolulu *10:*1–4, Jan '44

Preauricular sinuses; diagnosis and treatment. PENICK, R. M. JR. South. M. J. *38:*103–105, Feb '45

Congenital sinuses of external ear. EWING, M. R., J. Laryng. and Otol. *61:*18–23, Jan '46

Preauricular congenital sinuses. WEAVER, D. F. Laryngoscope *56:*246–251, May '46

Ear-pit (congenital aural and preauricular fistula) AIRD, I. Edinburgh M. J. *53:*498–507, Sept '46

Ears, Deformity (See also Ears, Cryptotia; Ears, Reconstruction; Otoplasty)

Congenital fistula of ear and atresia of external meatus. ERFURTH, W. Monatschr. f. Kinderh. *22:*55–59, Oct '21 (illus.)

Accessory external ear. BOSE, P. Indian M. Gaz. *57:*139–140, April '22

Case of macrotia, with occlusion of left external auditory canal; operated with satisfactory results. SHEMELEY, W. G. Laryngoscope *33:*841–844, Nov '23 (illus.)

Congenital absence of right ear with cleft of left upper eyelid. ANZINGER, F. P. Ohio State M. J. *19:*869–870, Dec '23

Anatomy, psychology, diagnosis and treatment of congenital malformation and absence of ear. BECK, J. C. Laryngoscope *35:*813–831, Nov '25

Surgical treatment of flopping ear. EITNER, E. Wien. klin. Wchnschr. *39:*868, July 22, '26

Congenital malformation of ears; case. HOFMANN, L. Monatschr. f. Ohrenh. *61:*509–512, May–June '27

Abnormalities of auricle; 2 cases. KRUPSKY, A. Ztschr. f. Laryng., Rhin. *16:*255–258, Feb '28

Congenital defects of radius and ear with facial paralysis; case. ESSEN-MÖLLER, E. Ztschr. f. d. ges. Anat. (Abt. 2) *14:*52–70, March 28, '28

Unusual malformation of external ear. JACQUES, P. AND ROIG, A. Compt. rend. Soc. de biol. *98:*1135–1137, April 27, '28 also: Ann. d. mal. de l'oreille, du larynx *47:*545–549, June '28

Complete absence (anotia) of ear with tonsillar aplasia. SERCER, A. Ztschr. f. Hals-, Nasen-u. Ohrenh. *22:*75–78, June 16, '28

Rare case of congenital malformation of external ear. BOTTURA, G. Ann. di laring., Otol. *29:*323–328, Nov '28

Role of nervous system in causation of congenital malformations of external and middle ear. BENESI, O. Handb. d. Neurol. d. Ohres (Teil 1) *2:*89–112, '28

Faulty anlage and defects of ear. STEIN, C. Handb. d. Neurol. d. Ohres (Teil 1) *2:*113–150, '28

Dissemblance of external ear in uniovular male twins of 17 years. VARIOT, G. Bull. et mem. Soc. d'anthrop. de Paris *9:*94, '28

Heterotopy of pinna of ear and congenital facial paralysis; case. CASTERÁN, E. Rev. de especialid. *4:*1035–1038, Sept '29

Operative treatment of ear deformities. DOBRZANIECKI, W. Ann. d. mal. de l'oreille, du larynx *48:*998–1003, Oct '29

Anomalies of outer ear. PIRES DE LIMA, J. A. Ann. d'anat. path. *7:*377–378, March '30

Congenital deformities of external ear; their mental effect. STRAATSMA, C. R. Arch. Otolaryng. *11:*609–613, May '30

Hypertrophy of ear; case and fingers. MORAZA, M. Med. ibera *2:*630–633, Dec 6, '30

Ears, Deformity—Cont.

Plastic surgery in abnormalities of direction, convolution and flexion of external ear. BOURGUET, J. Monde med., Paris *41:*483-492, April 1, '31

Congenital abnormalities of external ear. WATSON-WILLIAMS, E. Bristol Med.-Chir. J. *48:*273-274, '31

Infant with deformed ears (case). WAKELEY, C. P. G. Proc. Roy. Soc. Med. *25:*421, Feb '32

Deformed fetus complicating clubhands and microtia. FUKE, T. Jap. J. Obst. and Gynec. *15:*255-258, June '32

Plastic surgery of ear deformities. FERRARI, R. C. AND FIORINI, J. M. Rev. de chir. plastique, pp. 150-156, July '32

Surgical therapy of abnormalities of external ear. BOURGUET, J. Bull. Acad. de med., Paris *109:*602-604, April 25, '33

Plastic surgery in correction of ear deformities. EHRENFELD, H. Gyogyaszat *73:*374, June 11, '33

Auricular dyschondrogenesis; technic of surgical correction. TORELLÓ CENDRA, M. But. Soc. catalana de pediat. *6:*193-198, July-Aug '33

Abnormalities of external ear and their surgical correction. EITNER, E. Chirurg *5:*618-625, Aug 15, '33

Unilateral malformations of ear associated with cyclopia. HAGENS, E. W. Arch. Otolaryng. *18:*332-338, Sept '33

Surgical correction of deformed external ear and nose; case. REBELLO NETO, J. Rev. med. de Pernambuco *3:*285-290, Oct '33

Surgical therapy of congenital abnormalities of external ear. PIERI, G. Valsalva *9:*842-846, Nov '33

Cosmetic correction of Darwin's ear. EITNER, E. Ztschr. f. Hals-, Nasen-u. Ohrenh. *33:*564-567, '33

Dysplasias of external ear. ROQUES-SATIVO, R. Rev. de laryng. *57:*304-371, March '36

New method of plastic surgery in complicated deformities of pinna; cat's ear and coloboma in 2 cases. DOROSCHENKO, J. T. Monatschr. f. Ohrenh. *70:*718-721, June '36

Abnormally large mouth with ear abnormality on same side; case. EITNER, E. Monatschr. f. Ohrenh. *70:*714-717, June '36

New method of plastic surgery in acquired external ear atresia. DOROSCHENKO, I. T. Arch. f. Ohren-, Nasen-u. Kehlkopfh. *141:*249-251, '36

Combined developmental abnormalities of outer ear. MANKEL, W. Hals-, Nasen-u. Ohrenarzt (Teil 1) *27:*354-363, '36

Ears, Deformity—Cont.

Congenital atrophy of lower eyelids, both auricles and lower jaw; case. VAN LINT, A. AND HENNEBERT, P. Bull. Soc. belge d'opht., no. 73, pp. 51-61, '36

Congenital malformation of external ear; 2 cases. MARTILLOTTI, F. Pediatria *45:*337-344, April '37

Congenital atrophy of lower eyelids, both auricles and lower jaw; case. VAN LINT, A. AND HENNEBERT, P. Bruxelles-med. *17:*1065-1070, May 16, '37

Treatment of ear deformities. HINDMARSH, J. Nord. med. tidskr. *16:*1178-1181, July 23, '38

Deformation of auricular pavilion and its surgical corrections. CORA ELISEHT, F. AND AUBONE, J. Rev. argent. de oto-rino-laring. *7:*411-421, Nov-Dec '38

Unilateral gigantic development of auricle; case. PODGAETSKIY, G. B. Zhur. ush., nos. i gorl. bolez. *15:*551-552, '38

Surgical correction of too large auricles. VOGEL, K. Ztschr. f. Hals-, Nasen-u. Ohrenh. *44:*366-367, '38

Congenital absence of one tonsil; microtia and polydactylism in same patient. GERRIE, J. W. Arch. Otolaryng. *29:*378-381, Feb '39

Heredity of ear malformations. GAUS, W. Erbbl. f. d. Hals-, Nasen-u. Ohrenarzt, Hft. 1-2, pp. 20-30, March '39; in Hals-, Nasen-u. Ohrenarzt (Teil 1) *30:*March '39

Congenital deformities of ear. COE, H. E. Northwest Med. *38:*135-136, April '39

Supernumerary ears. COSTELLO, M. J. AND SHEPARD, J. H. Arch. Otolaryng. *29:*695-698, April '39

Congenital deformation of ear; rare case. GOPENCHAJM, I. Polska gaz. lek. *18:*400-402, April 30, '39

Malformations of ear pavilion. LASKIEWICZ, A. Rev. de laryng. *60:*332-344, April '39

Psychology of plastic surgery of ear. BERNDORFER, A. Gyogyaszat *79:*349-351, June 4, '39

Plastic surgery; psychic repercussion and social aspects of deformed ears. MALBEC, E. F. Semana med. *2:*1506-1509, Dec 28, '39

Congenital abnormalities (with surgical therapy of prominent ear). FOUCAR, H. O. Canad. M. A. J. *43:*26-27, July '40

Harmful effects of malformed ears in school; plastic surgery of protruding ears. CODAZZI AGUIRRE, J. A. Semana med. *1:*456-462, Feb 20, '41

Plastic surgery for positional anomalies of ear. EITNER, E. Wien. med. Wchnschr. *91:*140-142, Feb 22, '41

Ears, Deformity—Cont.

Congenital ptosis of ear. SERCER, A. Arch. f. Ohren-, Nasen-u. Kehlkopfh. *149:*298–308, '41

New classification of congenital auricular malformations. URZUA, C. C., R. Arq. de cir. clin. e exper. *6:*479–484, April–June '42

Management of nasal deformities in infants and small children. And ear, eyelids, lips and palate deformities. PEER, L. A. Dis. Eye, Ear, Nose and Throat *2:*166–176, June '42

Malformation involving external, middle and internal ear, with otosclerotic focus. KELEMEN, G. Arch. Otolaryng. *37:*183–198, Feb '43

Rare case of deformed ear. GRAU BARBERA, L. Actas dermo-sif. *35:*52–55, Oct '43

Associated malformations of eyes and ears. FRANCESCHETTI, A. AND VALERIO, M. Confinia neurol. *6:*255–257, '45

Ears, Electrical Injuries

Ear injury by electric current; 2 cases. CALICETI, P. Ann. di laring., otol. *29:*16–21, Jan '28

Ear injuries due to electricity. NAGER, F. R. AND RÜEDI, L. Rassegna ital. di oto-rino-laring. *5:*129–140, Jan–Dec '31

Injuries of ear by electricity. PETZAL, E. Internat. Zentralbl. f. Ohrenh. *34:*65–76, July '31

Ear injury due to electric discharge; case. BRUZZONE, C. Ann. di laring., otol. *34:*147–150, '34

Injuries to ear due to electric current. HAARMANN, H. Hals-, Nasen-u. Ohrenarzt (Teil 1) *28:*49–58, Feb '37

Injuries of external and middle ear in lightning stroke clinical study of case. CRESPI REGHIZZI, A. Arch. ital. di otol. *52:*49–60, Feb '40

Electric injury to ear. MIKHLIN, E. G. Sovet. med. (no. 23) *4:*29–30, '40

Ears, Injuries

Immediate transplantation on defects of ear and nose due to accident; 2 cases. AUFRICHT, G. Arch. Otolaryng. *17:*769–773, June '33

Plastic repair of mutilated ear. ESSER, J. F. S. Rev. de chir. structive, pp. 269–271, June '36

War injuries of ear, nose and throat. VOSS, O. Med. Klin. *35:*1589–1591, Dec 15, '39

Some minor nasal and aural injuries in recreations. MACARTNEY, C. J. Roy. Nav. M. Serv. *26:*139–143, April '40

Accidental severing of ear and its suturing; case. CSILLAG, S. Budapesti orvosi ujsag *38:*268–269, June 6, '40

Injuries to nose, paranasal sinuses, mouth and ears. CANFIELD, N. Connecticut M. J. *6:*796–798, Oct '42

Ear wounds and injuries among battle casualties of Western Desert. COLLINS, E. G. J. Laryng. and Otol. *59:*1–15, Jan '44

Wounds in ear and mastoid region. WHITTAKER, R. J. Laryng. and Otol. *59:*205–217, June '44

Plastic reconstruction of acquired defects of external ear, with case reports. SURACI, A. J. Am. J. Surg. *66:*196–202, Nov '44

Wounds of eye, ear, nose and throat. SMART, F. P., U. S. Nav. M. Bull. *44:*1231-1233, June '45

Care of injured ear. WEBSTER, G. V. Surgery *18:*515–521, Oct '45

Ears, Prostheses

Replacement of nose and ear by gelatin prosthesis. STRAUSS. Schweiz. med. Wchnschr. *56:*464–465, May 15, '26

Case of surgical prosthesis of ear. AXT, E. F. Dental Cosmos *69:*828–830, Aug '27

Prosthetic aids in reconstructive surgery about head; presentation of new methods (including ear.) nose. LEDERER, F. L. Arch. Otolaryng. *8:*531–554, Nov '28

Preparation and adjustment of prosthesis in loss of auricular substance. CHENET, H. Odontologie *68:*861–870, Dec '30 also: Ann. d'oto-laryng., pp. 1-9, Jan '31

Artificial ear, replacement of entire auricle. GULEKE. Chirurg *4:*274–278, April 1, '32

Chenet technic in prosthesis of ear deformities. GRIMAUD, *et al.* Rev. med. de l'est. *61:*485–486, July 1, '33

Loss of external ear and its artificial replacement. HARTMANN, E. Nord. med. tidskr. *11:*728–729, May 2, '36

Elastic prosthesis for defects of nose and ear. BERING, F. Muchen. med. Wchnschr. *86:*253–254, Feb 17, '39 (Comment on Siemens' article)

Psychologic aspects of problem of artificial ear, with critical comment on rigid permanent prosthesis and elastic temporary prosthesis. FUNK, F. Dermat. Wchnschr. *109:*1402-1407, Dec 30, '39

Artificial ear and nose. BULBULIAN, A. H. Hygeia *18:*980–982, Nov '40

Prosthetic reconstruction of nose and ear with latex compound. BULBULIAN, A. H. J. A. M. A. *116:*1504–1506, April 5, '41

Congenital and postoperative loss of ear; re-

Ears, Prostheses – Cont.
construction by prosthetic method. BULBULIAN, A. H., J. Am. Dent. A. *29:*1161-1168, July 1, '42
Paraffinoma, harelip, cicatrices, auricular prosthesis in plastic surgery. GONCALVES, G. Arq. de cir. clin. e exper. *6:*307-316, April-June '42

Ears, Reconstruction
Reconstruction of ears. DAY, H. F. Boston M. and S. J. *185:*146, Aug 4, '21
Total reconstruction of external ear. ESSER, J. F. S. Munchen. med. Wchnschr. *68:*1150, Sept 9, '21
Reconstruction of ear. ESSER, J. F. S. AND AUFRICHT, G. Arch. f. klin, Chir. *120:*518-525, '22 (illus.) abstr: J. A. M. A. *79:*1887, Nov 25, '22
Plastic reconstruction of ear with pedunculated tube flap. VAN DIJK, J. A. Nederl. Tijdschr. v. Geneesk. *1:*895-900, Feb 21, '25
Anatomy, psychology, diagnosis and treatment of congenital malformation and absence of ear. BECK, J. C. Laryngoscope *35:*813-831, Nov '25
Reconstruction of totally lost ear by "tubed pedicle flap" method. VAN DIJK, J. A. Acta oto-laryng. *10:*121-129, '26
Experimental transplantation of cartilage and skin for repair of concha. GUSSIO, S. Valsalva *3:*58-77, Feb '27
Restoration of auricle. DE RIVER, J. P. California and West. Med. *26:*654-656, May '27
Use of foreign bodies in ear, nose and throat surgery. POLLOCK, H. L. Ann. Otol. Rhin. and Laryng. *36:*463-471, June '27
Reconstruction of completely destroyed auricle; case report. GRAHAM, H. B. California and West. Med. *27:*518-519, Oct '27
Entire restoration of auricle after complete traumatic separation; case. OLDENSTAM, R. A. Nederl. Tijdschr. v. Geneesk. *1:*1097, March 2, '29
Reconstruction of external ear. PIERCE, G. W. Surg., Gynec. and Obst. *50:*601-605, March '30
Reconstruction of ear; case. NEW, G. B. Proc. Staff Meet., Mayo Clin. *6:*97, Feb 18, '31
Atrophy of external ear with hemiatrophy of face and paresis of lower facial nerve; case. ROCHER, H. L., J. de med. de Bordeaux *108:*231, March 20, '31
Autoplastic surgery of ear. OMBRÉDANNE, L. Presse med. *39:*982-983, July 4, '31
Plastic replacement of upper rim of ear. EITNER, E. Monatschr. f. Ohrenh. *67:*222-225, Feb '33

Ears, Reconstruction – Cont.
Plastic reconstruction of external auditory meatus. PALMER, F. E. AND REIFSNEIDER, J. S. Laryngoscope *43:*618-621, Aug '33
Modified technic in plastic surgery for correction of atresia and stenosis of external ear developing after otitis media. PREOBRASCHENSKI, B. S. Otolaryng. slavica *4:*249-255, Aug '33
Third grade hypoplasia of right auricle, absence of auditory canal and malformation of tympanic cavity. RICCI, B. Boll. d. mal. d. orecchio, d. gola, d. naso *52:*57-70, Feb '34
Total reconstruction of ear; original technic. BETTMAN, A. G. Rev. de chir. plastique, pp. 3-13, May '34
Otoneoplasty. PRUDENTE, A. Rev. oto-laring. de Sao Paulo *2:*388-391, Sept-Oct '34
Plastic reconstruction of auricle. EITNER, E. Deutsche Ztschr. f. Chir. *242:*797-801, '34
New and simple method for plastic surgery in congenital or accidental absence of ear. ESSER, J. F. S. Presse med. *43:*325-326, Feb 27, '35
Microtia with meatal atresia, with description of operation for its correction; 2 cases. HUME, J. R. AND OWENS, N. Ann. Otol., Rhin. and Laryng. *44:*213-219, March '35
Complete atresia of auditory canal due to trauma; plastic repair; case. SAES, P. Rev. oto-laring. de Sao Paulo *4:*83-86, March-April '36
Plastic reconstruction of large portion of pavilion of ear by new method. GUCCIARDELLO, S. Riv. san. siciliana *24:*640-642, June 15, '36
Total reconstruction of external ear. NATTINGER, J. K. Northwest Med. *36:*172-174, May '37
Complete avulsion of scalp and loss of right ear; reconstruction by pedunculated tube grafts and costal cartilage. CAHILL, J. A. JR. AND CAULFIELD, P. A. Surg., Gynec. and Obst. *66:*459-465, Feb (no. 2A) '38
Repair for partial loss of auricle. THOMAS, C. H. J. Laryng. and Otol. *53:*259-260, April '38
Ear reconstruction. MONEY, R. A., M. J. Australia *1:*819-820, May 7, '38
Reconstruction of pavilion using skin grafts (ear); case. DUFOURMENTEL, L. Rev. de laryng. *59:*517-518, May '38 also: Oto-rhino-laryng. internat. *22:*395-396, July '38
Free full thickness graft in restoration of loss of substance of auricle; case. COELST. Rev. de chir. structive *8:*111-112, Aug '38
Total reconstruction of auricle. PADGETT, E.

Ears, Reconstruction – Cont.

C. Surg., Gynec. and Obst. *67:*761–768, Dec '38

Use of full thickness free grafts in surgical therapy of microtia; case. COELST, M. Rev. de chir. structive *8:*155–159, '38

Ear reconstruction. (graft). MACOMBER, D. Rocky Mountain M. J. *36:*37–40, Jan '39

Restoration of partial defect of auricle by free transplantation. ERCZY, M. Gyogyaszat *79:*319–320, May 21, '39

Plastic reconstruction of auricle. GNILORYBOV, T. E. Novy khir. arkhiv *45:*148–156, '39

Microtia and congenital atresia of external auditory canal; demonstration of external auditory canal by means of tomography. CAMP, J. D. AND ALLEN, E. P. Am. J. Roentgenol. *43:*201–203, Feb '40

Use of preserved cartilage in ear reconstruction. KIRKHAM, H. L. D. Ann. Surg. *111:*896–902, May '40

Autoplastic methods for surgical restoration of congenital agenesis of ear. VEINTEMILLAS, F. Rev. brasil. de oto-rino-laring. *8:*413–418, Nov–Dec '40

Surgery of auricle, including total reconstruction and protuberant ears. COX, G. H. Laryngoscope *51:*791–797, Aug '41

Reconstruction of external ear. NEWMAN, J. Surg., Gynec. and Obst. *73:*234–235, Aug '41

Reconstructive otoplasty (by transplantation of cartilage). GREELEY, P. W. Surgery *10:* 457–461, Sept '41

Plastic surgery in loss of ear and nose substance. MALBEC, E. F. Semana med. *2:*714–716, Sept 18, '41

Bone (iliac) and cartilage transplants to ear and nose; use and behavior. MOWLEM, R. Brit. J. Surg. *29:*182–193, Oct '41

Technic in construction of auricle. GILLIES, H. Tr. Am. Acad. Ophth. (1941) *46:*119–121, Jan–Feb '42

Use of meniscus of knee in plastic surgery (ear). DELLEPIANE RAWSON, R. Prensa med. argent. *29:*654–658, April 22, '42

Auriculoplasty for hypoplasia of pavilion using tubular skin graft; case. ZENO, L. Bol. y trab., Acad. argent. de cir. *26:*807–812, Sept 16, '42

Plastic method to correct occlusions of meatus and auditory canal. CITELLI, S. Oto-rino-laring. ital. *12:*300–305, '42

Complete reconstruction of auricle. BERSON, M. I. Am. J. Surg. *60:*101–104, April '43

Atresia of auditory canal. COHEN, L. AND FOX, S. L. Arch. Otolaryng. *38:*338–346, Oct '43

Ears, Reconstruction – Cont.

Present status of complete reconstruction of external ear. PEER, L. A. Tr. Am. Soc. Plastic and Reconstructive Surg. *12:*11–16, '43

Reconstructive plastic surgery of absent ear with necrocartilage; original method. LAMONT, E. S. Arch. Surg. *48:*53–72, Jan '44

Imperforate auditory canal in connection with congenital malformations of auricle. OMBREDANNE, M. Ann. d'oto-laryng., pp. 1–5, Jan–March '44

Ear reconstruction; conservation of avulsed portion. GREELEY, P. W., U. S. Nav. M. Bull. *42:*1323–1325, June '44

Microtia; therapeutic problem. CORA ELISERT, F.; *et al.* Prensa med. argent. *31:*1671–1673, Aug 23, '44

Imperforation of external auditory canal with aplasia of auricle; results of operation. OMBREDANNE, M. Arch. franc. pediat. *2:*73–74, '44

External agenesis of ear treated surgically by Humberto and Ricardo Bisi. IVANISSEVICH, O. Bol. y trab., Acad. argent. de cir. *29:*666–668, Aug 1, '45

Total loss of pavilion of ear and its plastic repair; technic in case. ASIS, R. Actas Soc. de cir. de Madrid *5:*131–136, Jan–Mar '46

Atresia of external auditory canal occurring in military service; correction of this condition in 10 cases. CONLEY, J. J. Arch. Otolaryng. *43:*613–622, June '46

Reconstructive otoplasty; further observations; utilization of tantalum wire mesh support. GREELEY, P. W. Arch. Surg. *53:*24–31, July '46

Recent cases of agenesia of ears. VEINTEMILLAS, F. Prensa med. La Paz (nos. 7–8) *6:*1–6, Jul–Aug '46

Ears, Tumors

Tumors of nose, throat and ear; review of literature. NEW, G. B. Arch. Otolaryng. *1:*545–552, May '25

Angioma of auricle; case. PAGE, J. R. Ann. Otol. Rhin. and Laryng. *37:*358–360, March '28

Benign tumors of external ear: condyloma, hemangioma; cases. TURTUR, G. Valsalva *6:*97–104, Feb '30

Radium treatment of angioma of external ear in infant. DHALLUIN, M. Gaz. med. de France (supp. radiol.) no. 6, pp. 136–138, Oct 1, '31

Angioma of auricle; case. TAKEZAWA, N. AND NAKAJIMA, K. Oto-rhino-laryng. *11:*406, May '38

Ears, Tumors – Cont.
Hemangioma of ear. KEPES, P. Monatschr. f. Ohrenh. *72:*798–808, Aug '38
Therapy of hemangiomas of auricular pavilion; case. DUARTE CARDOSO, A. Rev. paulista de med. *23:*347–352, Dec '43
Hemangioma of ear; new method for control of hemorrhage. DIXON, O. J. Ann. Otol., Rhin. and Laryng. *54:*415–420, June '45

EASTMAN, J. R.: Prophylaxis of malignant growths of mouth, face and jaws. J.A.M.A. *79:*118–120, July 8, '22
EATON, A. G. (see DAVIS, H. A.) Jan '42
EATON, A. G. (see DAVIS, H. A.) March '42
EBA, M. (see KIKUCHI, R.) Dec '39
EBENIUS, B.: Clinical study of 778 cases of cancer of lips with particular regard to predisposing factors and radium therapy. Acta radiol., supp. 48, pp. 1–232, '43
EBERBACH, C. W.: Traumatic shock. Wisconsin M. J. *42:*225–228, Feb '43
EBERBACH, C. W. AND PIERCE, J. M.: Pregnancy terminated by caesarean section after ureteral transplantation into sigmoid for exstrophy of bladder. Surg., Gynec. and Obst. *47:*540–542, Oct '28
EBERT, E. C. AND BOYDEN, R. C.: Improved method of lip fixation in harelip. U. S. Nav. M. Bull. *36:*501, Oct '38
EBERT, R. V. (see EMERSON, C. P. JR.) Nov '45
EBRARD, D. (see DESMAREST, E.) Feb '26
EBY, J. D.: Structures of face in case of ankylosis of jaws before and after treatment. Internat. J. Orthodontia *17:*848–853, Sept '31
ECK, F. (see FONTAINE, R.) Jan–Apr '46
ECKELBERRY, N. E.: Relation of trauma of hand to occupation. Am. J. Surg. *41:*51–56, July '38
ECKERT, C. T. AND PETRY, J. L.: Lip carcinoma. S. Clin. North America *24:*1064–1076, Oct '44
ECKERT, G. A. AND MADER, J. W.: "Solace" (hospital ship) in action (burns) U. S.Nav. M. Bull. *40:*552–557, July '42
ECKHARDT, G.: Use of flaps from avulsed scalp and skin grafts in repair of total avulsion. Zentralbl. f. Chir. *66:*2337–2340, Oct 28, '39
ECKHOFF, N.: Prognosis of hand infections. Lancet *1:*1369, June 13, '36; 1425, June 20, '36
ECKHOFF, N.: Tumors and swellings of hand. Guy's Hosp. Gaz. *51:*199–204, May 8, '37
ECKHOFF, N.: Plastic surgery. Guy's Hosp. Gaz. *51:*440–448, Oct 23, '37
ECKHOFF, N. L.: Hand infections. Lancet *1:*1276–1281, June 17, '33
ECKHOFF, N. L.: Hand infections. Guy's Hosp. Gaz. *48:*246–253, June 9, '34
ECKHOFF, N. L.: (Facial bone fractures.) Injuries to face. Guy's Hosp. Gaz. *54:*300–305, Oct 19, '40
ECKHOFF, N. L.: Injuries to face (soft tissues). (with burns) Guy's Hosp. Gaz. *54:*345–350, Nov 30, '40
ECKHOFF, N. L.: Hand infections. Guy's Hosp. Gaz. *57:*67–70, March 20, '43
ECKHOFF, N. L.: Burns. Guy's Hosp. Gaz. *57:*156–162, July 24, '43
ECKINGER, W.: Aspects of so-called symbrachydactylia. Arch. f. orthop. u. Unfall-Chir. *38:*662–669, '38
ECKSTEIN, H.: Resection of bone to remedy finger contracture. Zentralbl. f. Chir. *49:*547–548, April 22, '22 abstr: J.A.M.A. *79:*598, Aug. 12 '22
ECKSTEIN, H.: Three decades of plastic use of paraffin. Arch. f. klin. Chir. *169:*646–674, '32
EDBERG, E.: Harelip and cleft palate operation. Acta chir. Scandinav. *55:*1–26, '22 (in English) abstr: J.A.M.A. *79:*1562, Oct 28, '22
EDBERG, E.: Therapy of harelip and cleft palate. Hygiea *94:*529–558, July 31, '32
EDBERG, E.: Experiences in treatment of children with harelip and cleft palate. Nord. med. *1:*89–92, Jan 14, '39
EDLING, L.: Acrocephalo-syndactylia, a general malformation of bony system. Acta radiol., supp. 3, pars 2, pp. 70–71, '29
EDMONDSON, E. E.: Symptoms and treatment of deviations of nasal septum. Illinois M. J. *43:*208–210, March '23
EDMUNDS, A.: Pseudo-hermaphroditism and hypospadias; their surgical treatment. Lancet *1:*323–327, Feb 13, '26
EDMUNDS, A.: Treatment of hypospadias. M. Press *194:*456–462, May 12, '37
EDMUNDS, A.: Treatment of superficial granulating surfaces (burns). Lancet *2:*130, Aug 2, '41
EDWARDS, B.: Artist's approach to restorative prosthetics. Mil. Surgeon *92:*197–201, Feb '43
EDWARDS, F. R.: Shock treatment in air raid casualties. M. Press *208:*3–5, July 1, '42
EDWARDS, F. R.: Form of bovine serum suitable for plasma substitute in treatment of shock. Proc. Roy. Soc. Med. *36:*337, May '43
EDWARDS, H. C.: Amputation of fingers. Brit. M. J. *2:*631–633, Sept 17, '38
EDWARDS, H. G. F.: Vascular birthmarks. South. M. J. *34:*717–724, July '41
EFFLER, L. R.: Near-fatal postoperative secondary hemorrhage in nasal surgery. Laryngoscope *42:*201–206, March '32
EFTIMIE, C.: Surgical treatment of phlegmons of palms and fingers. Spitalul *48:*226–227, June '28

EGBERT, H. L. (see TRUSLER, H. M. *et al*) Dec '39

EGEBERG, B. (see WILSON, J. A.) Sept '42

EGGER, F.: Therapy of fractured jaws. Schweiz. med. Wchnschr. *64:*1044–1047, Nov 17, '34

EGGERS, G. W. N.: Ankylosis of jaws. South. Surgeon *10:*1–7, Jan '41

EGGERS, G. W. N.: Arthroplasty of temporomandibular joint in children with interposition of tantalum foil; preliminary report. J. Bone and Joint Surg. *26:*603–606, July '46

EGGSTON, A. A.: Nasal tumors. New York State J. Med. *43:*2403–2412, Dec 15, '43

EGIDI, G.: Total plastic reconstruction of esophagus using transverse colon and tubal graft; case. Policlinico (sez. prat.) *42:*1287–1289, July 1, '35

EGOROV, M. A.: Ligature of nerve in prevention of neuroma of amputation-stump. Khirurgiya, no. 4, pp. 38–42, '44

EGÜES, A.: Thyroglossal fistula; classification, clinical aspects, surgical treatment; cases. Bol. Inst. de clin. quir. *4:*313–367, '28

EHALT, W.: Possible uses of Reverdin skin flap for plastic surgery, primarily for covering skin defects, and secondarily for scar contractures. Munchen. med. Wchnschr. *82:*669–671, April 25, '35

EHALT, W.: Conservative surgical therapy of almost completely severed arm. Chirurg. *7:*519–522, Aug. 1, '35

EHALT, W.: Replacement of large amounts of skin. Zentralbl. f. Chir. *64:*70–73, Jan. 9, '37

EHLER, F.: Plastic surgery of lower lip. Casop. lek. cesk. *66:*141–144, Jan. 21, '27

EHLER, F.: Plastic operation for avulsion of scalp. Casop. lek. cesk. *70:*1525; 1555; 1578, '31

EHLERS, G.: Burns and explosions in anesthesia. Deutsche Ztschr. f. Chir. *255:*485–522, '42

EHRENCLOU, A. H. (see WOLFF, H. G.) March '27

EHRENFELD, H.: Transplantation of strip of cheek and naris in harelip therapy. Arch. F. klin. Chir. *144:*486–488, '27

EHRENFELD, H.: Plastic method of covering large loss of substance of face. Arch. f. klin. Chir. *147:*633–636, '27

EHRENFELD, H.: Plastic surgery of cleft lip. Gyogyaszat *71:*607, Sept. 27, '31

EHRENFELD, H.: Plastic surgery of face. Gyogyaszat *72:*186–189, March 20, '32

EHRENFELD, H.: Plastic surgery of face. Gyogyaszat *72:*675–676, Oct. 30, '32

EHRENFELD, H.: Deformities of breast and their correction by plastic surgery. Gyogyaszat *73:*90–94, Feb. 5, '33

EHRENFELD, H. Plastic surgery in correction of ear deformities. Gyogyaszat *73:*374, June 11, '33

EHRENFELD, H.: New points of view in regard to corrective surgery of pendulous breasts, together with description of new method. Zentralbl. f. Chir. *62:*628–634, March 16, '35

EHRENFELD, H.: New ideas with regard to plastic surgery of pendulous cheeks with description of new method. Zentralbl. f. Chir. *64:*202–205, Jan. 23, '37

EHRENFELD, H.: Cosmetic operation for protruding ears. Zentralbl. f. Chir. *65:*1236–1239, May 28, '38

EHRENFELD, H. J.: Method of determining correct seat of nipples in plastic surgery for pendulous breasts; new instrument to facilitate it. M. Rec. *154:*92–94, Aug. 6, '41

EHRENFELD, H. J.: Modification of facial characteristics through remodelling of nose. M. Rec. *155:*5–8, Jan. 7, '42

EHRENFELD, H. J.: Symposium on neuropsychiatry; changing character through corrective surgery. M. Rec. *155:*531–533, Dec '42

EHRICKE, A.: Prosthetic therapy of acquired palatal defects. Med. Welt *12:*775–776, May 28, '38

EIBRINK JANSEN, G. A. H.: Right hemihypertrophy and left hemiatrophy of jaw; case. Tijdschr. v. tandheelk. *35:*131–134, Feb. 15, '28

EICHENBERG, S.: Nascent iodine in therapy of osteomyelitis of lower jaw. An. Fac. de med. de Porto Alegre *2:*189–212, July-Sept '40

EICHHOFF, E.: Uranoplasty at several sittings. Chirurg *3:*595–599, July 1, '31

EICHHOFF, E.: Most favorable time for surgical correction of cleft palate. Chirurg *5:*263–265, April 1, '33

EICHHOFF, E. AND HELLMANN, K.: Cleft palate operation with multiple mobilization. Beitr. z. klin. Chir. *143:*290–319, '28

EIGER, J.: Iodine iontophoresis in keloid occurring after furuncle. Munchen. med. Wchnschr. *76:*1297, Aug. 2, '29

Eiger

Comment on article by Eiger on keloid therapy by iodine iontophoresis. WIRZ, F. Munchen. med. Wchnschr. *76:*1515, Sept. 6, '29

EILERS: Subcutaneous ruptures of extensor tendons of fingers in buttonhole dislocation of first interphalangeal joint. Deutsche Ztschr. f. Chir. *223:*317–327, '30

EIMAN, J. (see SCULL, C. W.) June '42

EINARSSON, F.: Treatment of Dupuytren's contracture Acta chir. Scandinav. *93:*1–22, '46

EINHAUSER, M.: Therapy of severe burns with cortical suprarenal hormone and vitamin C; animal experiments. Klin. Wchnschr. *17:*127–134, Jan. 22, '38

EISBACH, E. J.: Cartilaginous septum in reconstruction of nose; modified procedure. Arch. Otolaryng. *44:*207–211, Aug '46

EISBERG, H. B. AND SONNENSCHEIN, H. D.: Primary repair of lacerated tendons and nerves. Am. J. Surg. *3:*582–587, Dec '27

EISELSBERG, A.: Prosthetic appliance in jaw surgery. Internat. Clin. *4:*220, Dec' 26

EISELBERG, A.: Transplantation of skin, fat, blood vessels, nerves, etc. Wien. med. Wchnschr. *80:*50–55, Jan. 4, '30

EISELSBERG, A.: Thiersch grafts. Wien. klin. Wchnschr. *46:*1179, Sept. 29, '33

EISELSBERG, A.: Plastic repair of defect of cheek. Schweiz. med. Wchnschr. *65:*25–26, Jan. 12, '35

EISELSBERG, A. AND PICHLER, H.: Reconstruction of jaw and chin. Arch. f. klin. Chir. *122:*337–369, '22 (illus.) abstr: J.A.M.A. *80:*732, March 10, '23

EISENKLAM, D.: Case of carcinomatous degeneration of rhinophyma, with remarks on treatment of rhinophyma. Wien. klin. Wchnschr. *44:*1407–1408, Nov. 6, '31

EISENKLAM, I.: Treatment of ganglion of back of hand. Wien. klin. Wchnschr. *41:*740–741, May 24, '28

EISENKLAM, I.: Reply to Eitner's comments on article on plastic surgery for large and protruding ears. Wien. klin. Wchnschr. *43:*1377, Nov. 6, '30

EISENKLAM, J.: Plastic surgery for large and protruding ears. Wien. klin. Wchnschr. *43:*1176, Sept. 18, '30

EISENSTODT, L. W.: Technic of secondary resection of nasal septum demonstrating regeneration of cartilage. Laryngoscope *54:*190–197, April '44

EISENSTODT, L. W.: Complete avulsion of scalp; review of literature and case report. Am. J. Surg. *68:*376–382, June '45

EISENSTODT, L. W.: Skin grafting in moribund patients. Am. J. Surg. *69:*168–176, Aug '45

EISENSTODT, L. W.: Surgical correction of chin malformations. Am. J. Surg. *71:*491–501, Apr '46

EISNER: Carbon dioxide snow in injuries of skin due to x-ray. Zentralbl. f. Haut-u. Geschlechtskr. *24:*580, Oct. 5, '27

EITNER, E.: Operations to reduce size of nose. Med. Klin. *17:*908, July 24, '21 abstr: J.A.M.A. *77:*1215, Oct. 8, '21

EITNER, E.: Correction of flaring ears. Med. Klinik *18:*1117–1118, Aug. 27, '22

EITNER, E.: Plastic correction for nose deformities. Med. Klinik *19:*238–239, Feb. 25, '23

EITNER, E.: Correction of sunken noses. Med. Klinik *20:*1000–1001, July 20, '24

EITNER, E.: Shortening the nose. Med. Klin. *22:*999, June 25, '26

EITNER, E.: Surgical treatment of flopping ear. Wien. klin. Wchnschr. *39:*868, July 22, '26

EITNER, E.: Making lobule of ear smaller. Wien. klin. Wchnschr. *39:*1423–1424, Dec. 2, '26

EITNER, E.: Treatment of hypertrichosis with electrocoagulation. Wien. klin. Wchnschr. *40:*460, April 7, '27

EITNER, E.: Subcutaneous plastic operation of deformed end of nose. Wien. klin. Wchnschr. *40:*916, July 14, '27

EITNER, E.: Operative removal of skin folds for cosmetic purposes. Wien. med. Wchnschr. *77:*1006, July 23, '27

EITNER, E.: Forceps for inserting grafts in corrective operations of nose. Munchen. med. Wchnschr. *74:*1876, Nov. 4, '27

EITNER, E.: Plastic surgery of pendulous breast. Wien. med. Wchnschr. *77:*1572, Nov. 12, '27

EITNER, E.: Subcutaneous plastic correction of rhinokyphosis. Wien. klin. Wchnschr. *40:*1449–1450, Nov. 17, '27

EITNER, E.: Cosmetic treatment of small nevus. Wien. med. Wchnschr. *78:*366, March 10, '28

EITNER, E.: Cosmetic treatment of facial scars. Urol. and Cutan. Rev. *32:*282, May '28

EITNER, E.: Indications and technic of cosmetic correction of facial wrinkles. Wien. klin. Wchnschr. *41:*1281–1283, Sept. 6, '28

EITNER, E.: Reply to comment by Halla on cosmetic correction of facial wrinkles. Wien. klin. Wchnschr. *41:*1530, Nov. 1, '28

EITNER, E.: Plastic operations for wry-nose. Med. Klin. *25:*600, April 12, '29

EITNER, E.: Cosmetic correction of deviations of tip of nose. Wien. klin. Wchnschr. *43:*1260, Oct. 9, '30

EITNER, E.: Plastic surgery for large and protruding ears. (Comment on Eisenklan's article). Wien. klin. Wchnschr. *43:*1377, Nov. 6, '30

EITNER, E.: Ivory in cosmetic operations of nose. Med. Welt *4:*1615, Nov. 8, '30

EITNER, E.: Cosmetic correction of convex nasal profile. Med. Klin. *26:*1924, Dec. 24, '30

EITNER, E.: Plastic treatment of facial hemiatrophy by transplantation of fat tissues. Med. Klin. *27:*624–625, April 24, '31

EITNER, ERNST: *Kosmetische Operationen.* Springer-Verlag, Berlin, 1932

EITNER, E.: Defects of tip of nose; surgical correction. (Comment on Wodak's article). Med. Klin. *28:*49–50, Jan. 8, '32

EITNER, E.: Cosmetic correction of pinna which turns forward in abnormal fashion. Wien. klin. Wchnschr. *45:*1537 1538, Dec. 9, '32

EITNER, E.: Cosmetic correction of Darwin's

ear. Ztschr. f. Hals-, Nasen-u. Ohrenh. *33:*564–567, '33

EITNER, E.: Plastic correction of nasal deformities after operation for harelip. Deutsche Ztschr. f. Chir. *238:*644–646, '33

EITNER, E.: Plastic replacement of upper rim of ear. Monatschr. f. Ohrenh. *67:*222–225, Feb '33

EITNER, E.: Plastic replacement of tip of nose. Med. Klin. *29:*358, March 10, '33

EITNER, E.: Double lips. Wien. med. Wchnschr. *83:*429–430, April 8, '33

EITNER, E.: Cosmetic correction of wry-nose. Wien. med. Wchnschr. *83:*739–740, June 24, '33

EITNER, E.: Abnormalities of external ear and their surgical correction. Chirurg *5:*618–625, Aug. 15, '33

EITNER, E.: Cosmetic corrections of abnormalities of septal cartilage. Ztschr. f. Laryng., Rhin., Otol. *25:*40–45, '34

EITNER, E.: Plastic reconstruction of auricle. Deutsche Ztschr. f. Chir. *242:*797–801, '34

EITNER, E.: Nasal injuries and their cosmetic therapy. Wien. med. Wchnschr. *84:*307–309, March 10, '34

EITNER, E.: Cosmetic therapy of facial cicatrices. Wien. med. Wchnschr. *84:*555–556, May 12, '34

EITNER, E.: Cosmetic corrections of form of external ear. Wien. med. Wchnschr. *84:*810–811, July 14, '34

EITNER, E.: Cosmetic correction of defects of tip of nose. Ztschr. f. Laryng., Rhin. Otol. *26:*46–53, '35

EITNER, E.: Cosmetic surgery of facial wrinkles. Wien. med. Wchnschr. *85:*244, Feb. 23, '35

EITNER, E.: Use of skin flaps for cosmetic plastic surgery of breast. Zentralbl. f. Chir. *62:*625–627, March 16, '35

EITNER, E.: Plastic surgery of pendulous breasts. Wien. med. Wchnschr. *85:*586, May 18, '35

EITNER, E.: Shortening and lengthening of nose. Wien. klin. Wchnschr. *48:*799–800, June 7, '35

EITNER, E.: Abnormally large mouth with ear abnormality on same side; case. Monatschr. f. Ohrenh. *70:*714–717, June '36

EITNER, E.: Cosmetic correction of convex nasal profile. Chirurg *8:*528–532, July 1, '36

EITNER, E.: Cosmetic shortening of broad nose bridge. Monatschr. f. Ohrenh. *71:*313–315, March '37

EITNER, E.: Cosmetic surgery in facial hemiatrophy. Wien. med. Wchnschr. *87:*362–363, March 27, '37

EITNER, E.: Cosmetic correction of ptosis of lower eyelid. Wien. med. Wchnschr. *87:*423–424, April 10, '37

EITNER, E.: Therapy of old nasal fractures; 3 cases. Zentralbl. f. Chir. *64:*1096–1101, May 8, '37

EITNER, E.: Simple method for correction of protruding ears. Wien. klin. Wchnschr. *50:*1206, Aug. 20, '37

EITNER, E.: Plastic surgery of ear lobule. Wien. med. Wchnschr. *88:*774–775, July 11, '38

EITNER, E.: Correction of cleft nose. Deutsche Ztschr. f. Chir. *252:*507–510, '39

EITNER, E.: Plastic correction of lips. Wien. med. Wchnschr. *89:*89–90, Jan. 28, '39

EITNER, E.: Rhinophyma: cosmetic surgery in primary stage. Wien. med. Wchnschr. *89:*442–443, April 29, '39

EITNER, E.: Plastic surgery for positional anomalies of ear. Wien. med. Wchnschr. *91:*140–142, Feb. 22, '41

Eitner

Reply to Eitner's comments on article about nasal tip defects. and Halla's comments. WODAK, E. Med. Klin. *28:*50, Jan. 8, '32

EITZEN, A. C.: Fractures of lower margin of orbit.; reduction and visualization by x-ray. J. Kansas M. Soc. *39:*15, Jan '38

EL BAKLY, M. A.: Operation for repair of coloboma of upper eyelid. Bull. Ophth. Soc. Egypt *28:*26–28, '35

ELBIM. A.: Therapy of penile, penoscrotal and perineoscrotal hypospadias by Duplay operation. J. d'urol. *40:*484–498, Dec '35

Elbim Operation

Recurrent temporomaxillary luxation; osteoplastic abutment (Elbim method); case. POLLOSSON, E. AND FREIDEL, Lyon chir. *35:*460–463, July-Aug '38

EL DIWANY, M. A. M.: New technic (application of hot air immediately after spraying with tannic acid) of burn therapy. J. Egyptian M. A. *17:*112–114, Jan '34

Electrotherapy

Electric-ionisation and nose operations. PRADHAN, K. N. Indian M. Gaz. *57:*137–138, April '22

Cancer of lip treated by electrocoagulation and radiation. PFAHLER, G. E. Arch. Dermat. and Syph. *6:*428–433, Oct. '22 also: Tr. Sect. Dermat. and Syphilol., A. M. A. pp. 213–219, '22

Electrotherapy – Cont.

Small apparatus for diathermy and electrocoagulation depilation treatment of hypertrichosis in women. LANZI, G. Gior. ital. d. ma. ven. *65:*1718–1720, Oct '24

Diathermy as rapid and effectual means of permanent depilation. KATZ, T. Dermat. Wchnschr. *79:*1492–1493, Nov. 15, '24

Iontophoresis in treatment of deforming or adherent scars. BOURGUIGNON, G. Paris med. *2:*515–520, Dec. 20, '24 abstr: J.A.M.A. *84:*404, Jan. 31, '25

Electrocoagulation of desiccation in treatment of keratoses and malignant degeneration which follow radiodermatitis. PFAHLER, G. E. Am. J. Roentgenol. *13:*41–48, Jan '25

Treatment of angiomas with carbon dioxide snow and electrolysis. TRIER, K. Hospitalstid. *68:*117–118, Feb. 5, '25

Cancer of lip; its treatment by means of electrothermic coagulation, radium and roentgen rays. STEVENS, J. T. Radiology *4:*372–377, May '25

Epilation with diathermy; preliminary report. ROSTENBERG, A., M. J. and Rec. *121:*751, June 17, '25

Electrocoagulation and radiation therapy in malignant disease of ear, nose and throat. PFAHLER, G. E., J.A.M.A. *85:*344–347, Aug. 1, '25

Electrocoagulation and desiccation of surface malignancies. PLANK, T. H. Physical Therap. *44:*363–367, July '26

Diathermy in treatment of shock. CRADDOCK, F. H. AND WHETSTONE, G. South. M. J. *19:*812–813, Nov '26

Treatment of nevocarcinoma by diathermocoagulation. RAVAUT, P. AND FERRAND, M. Bull. Soc. franc. de dermat. et syph. *34:*96–105, Feb '27

Permanent destruction of hair by diathermy in facial hypertrichosis. VAN PUTTE, P. J. Nederl. Tijdschr. v. Geneesk. *1:*924–928, Feb. 19, '27

Diathermy in shock; case. COTTLE, G. F., U. S. Nav. M. Bull. *25:*340–343, April '27

Treatment of hypertrichosis with electrocoagulation. EITNER, E. Wien. klin. Wchnschr. *40:*460, April 7, '27

Keloid removal by electro-coagulation. PEEPLES, D. L. Am. J. Phys. Therapy *4:*160, July '27

New electrical epilation apparatus. MEZEI, K. Dermat. Wchnschr. *85:*1107, Aug. 6, '27

New needle-holder for use in diathermic epilation in hypertrichosis. KENDE, B. Wien. klin. Wchnschr. *41:*382, March 15, '28

Treatment of nevi, with particular reference to high frequency current. KLAUDER, J. V. J.A.M.A. *90:*1763–1768, June 2, '28

Extensive epithelioma of cheek and lower jaw treated by diathermy. HARRISON, W. J. Brit. M. J. *2:*102, July 21, '28

Electro-coagulation (diathermy) for facial cancer. LALVANI, P. P. Indian M. Gaz. *63:*640, Nov '28

Diathermic treatment of rhinophyma; 2 cases. BEHADJET, H. Dermat. Wchnschr. *88:*129–130, Jan 26, '29

Roentgenotherapy and electrotherapy of keloids. LEPENNETIER, F. Rev. d'actinol. *5:*69, Jan-Feb '29

Electrodesiccation and electro-coagulation in neoplastic and allied diseases of oral cavity and adjacent parts; clinical, physical, historical and photographic studies based upon 20 years' experience. CLARK, W. L. Am. J. Surg. *6:*257–275, March '29

Multiple epilation with diathermy by simultaneous use of several needles. MEZEI, K. Dermat. Wchnschr. *88:*720, May 18, '29

Electro-coagulation (surgical diathermy) in multiple angiomata of head. LALVANI, P. P. Indian M. Gaz. *64:*387–388, July '29

Comment on article by Eiger on keloid therapy by iodine iontophoresis. WIRZ, F. Munchen. med. Wchnschr. *76:*1515, Sept. 6, '29

Electrothermic surgery of cancer of lips. STEVENS, J. T. Am. J. Surg. *7:*831–835, Dec '29

Treatment of congenital fistula of neck with diathermy (electrocoagulation). HOFER, G. Arch. f. klin. Chir. *156:*274–283, '29

Electrolysis as cosmetic treatment of keloids. and nevus pigmentosus. MARQUE, A. M. AND LANARI, E. Semana med. *1:*159–164, Jan 16, '30

Low voltage currents in contractures of hand. GRIES, L. Arch. Physical Therapy *11:*10–13, Jan '30

Diathermo-surgical treatment of septal malformations. JOUFFRAY, Rev. d'actinol. *6:*35–39, Jan–Feb '30

Effective use of electric coagulation in rhinophyma. BORDIER, H. Presse med. *38:*538–539, April 19, '30

Hemo-aspiration and trephining with aid of electric apparatus in dacryocystorhinostomy. SUBILEAU, J. M. Ann. d'ocul. *167:*301–306, April '30

Results of surgical and diathermic-surgical treatment of cancer of concha of ear. GIESE, A. Ztschr. f. Laryng., Rhin. *19:*414–423, July '30

Fractional cauterization of large cicatricial

Electrotherapy – Cont.
keloids. HENKELS, P. Deutsche tierarztl. Wchnschr. *38:*501-504, Aug 9, '30
Surgical diathermy of cancer of nose. HESSE, W. Deutsche med. Wchnschr. *56:*1479-1481, Aug 29, '30
Electrocoagulation of cancer of cheek. CLAIRMONT, P. AND SCHÜRCH, O. Deutsche Ztschr. f. Chir. *227:*115-125, '30
Electrotherapy of tuberous angioma of face. GERONIMI, E. Schweiz. med. Wchnschr. *61:*589-593, June 20, '31
Electrocoagulation therapy of subcutaneous angiomas. DE QUERVAIN, F. Schweiz. med. Wchnschr. *61:*1169-1170, Dec 5, '31
Plastic surgery of face following electrocoagulation treatment of malignant tumors of nose and accessory sinuses. ÖHNGREN, G. Acta oto-laryng. *16:*292-305, '31
Closure of lymph vessels in electrocoagulation; significance in prevention of shock. ZSCHAU, H. Deutsche Ztschr. f. Chir. *233:*109-120, '31
Technic of diathermic epilation. BORDIER, H. Am. J. Phys. Therapy *8:*273-274, Jan '32 also: Monde med., Paris *42:*78-81, Feb 1, '32
Diathermy in treatment of rhinophyma. PÉRI, M. Practicien du Nord de l'Afrique *5:*150-151, March 15, '32
Keloids, radium therapy; case, with suggestions of other physiotherapeutic methods (electrolysis, electropuncture, ionization, cryotherapy, electrocoagulation and roentgenotherapy). TRÉPAGNE, D. Ann. de med. phys. *25:*291-297, '32
New technic designed for electrocoagulation of vascular tumors. TYLER, A. F. Nebraska M. J. *18:*6-9, Jan '33
Electrocoagulation of melanomas and its dangers. AMADON, P. D. Surg., Gynec. and Obst. *56:*943-946, May '33
Hypertrichosis in women and its therapy, with special reference to diathermocoagulation. DE PAGANETTO, M. J. T. Semana med. *1:*1792-1794, May 25, '33
Diethermic recanalization of lacrimonasal canal. SPINELLI, F. Klin. Monatsbl. f. Augenh. *91:*202-207, Aug '33
Pagnelin cautery in therapy of furunculosis. WINCKLER, E. Munchen. med. Wchnschr. *80:*1974-1975, Dec 15, '33
Technic of diathermic epilation in hypertrichosis. DUCOURTIOUX, Rev. d'actinol. *10:*14-19, Jan-Feb '34
Diathermocoagulation in rhinophyma; case. FIUMICELLI, F. Dermosifilografc *9:*35-38, Jan '34 also: Minerva med. *1:*228-229, Feb 17, '34

Electrotherapy – Cont.
Results of treatment of cancer of lips by electrocoagulation and irradiation. PFAHLER, G. E. AND VASTINE, J. H. Pennsylvania M. J. *37:*385-389, Feb '34
Cautery pencil in treatment of furunculosis. SCHÜLE, A. Med. Welt *8:*407, March 24, '34
Diathermic depilation in hypertrichosis. SOLLA, L. Actas dermo-sif. *26:*445-449, March '34
Therapy of small cutaneous angiomas by systematic association of cryotherapy with carbon dioxide snow and diathermy. DURAND, Bull. Soc. franc. de dermat. et syph. (Reunion dermat.) *41:*587-589, April '34
Large angiomas of upper eyelid treated with surgical diathermy. CARAMAZZA, F. Boll. d'ocul. *13:*742-753, June '34
Shock, collapse and electrosurgery. SCHÖRCHER, F. Deutsche Ztschr. f. Chir. *243:*225-273, '34
Technic of cosmetic electrolysis of hair removal. GOODMAN, H. Am. Med. *41:*35-36, Jan '35
Therapy of mandibular epithelial cancers by electrocoagulation followed by curietherapy. GERNEZ, L.; *et al.* Bol. Liga contra el cancer *10:*293-308, Oct '35
Diathermocoagulation as only therapy for nevocarcinoma. JOLY, M. Bull. et mem. Soc. de med. de Paris *140:*70-71, Jan 25, '36
Question of electrolysis or diathermocoagulation in therapy of vascular tumors of face; experimental study. POCHY-RIANO, R. Arch. di radiol. *12:*121-133, March-April '36
Good dressing for wounds produced by electrocoagulation. HOLLANDER, L. Arch. Dermat. and Syph. *33:*730, April '36
Treatment of rhinophyma by electrodesiccation. KLAUDER, J. V. Arch. Dermat. and Syph. *33:*885, May '36
Thermocauterization in therapy of facial cancer. MERIC, A. J. L. Rev. de laryng. *57:*768-802, July-Aug '36
Electrocoagulation therapy of hemangiomas. MICHALOWSKI, E. Munchen. med. Wchnschr. *84:*101, Jan 15, '37
Treatment of epithelioma of lip by electrodesiccation; technic and preliminary report of results during past 5 years. MORROW, H.; *et al.* Arch. Dermat. and Syph. *35:*821-830, May '37
Injuries following epilation by electrolysis or roentgen rays. (Further comment on Nobl's article). KARPELIS, E. Wien. med. Wchnschr. *87:*685, June 19, '37
Electrocoagulation in treatment of cavernous

Electrotherapy – Cont.
hemangioma. DUJARDIN, E. Ugesk. f. laeger *99:*1257-1258, Nov. 25, '37
Diathermocoagulation in therapy of congenital imperforation of choanae; 2 cases. GIGNOUX, A. Lyon med. *160:*652-654, Dec 12, '37
Use of electric bistury for removing rhinophyma; case. DORIGO, L. Bollettino *11:*62-72, '37
Surgical diathermy in cicatricial stenosis of larynx. BOMBELLI, U. Oto-rhino-laryng. internat. *22:*16-24, Jan '38
Results of electrocoagulation therapy of congenital fistulas of neck. SPITZY, M. Zentralbl. f. Chir. *65:*114-117, Jan 15, '38
Diathermy applied to facial lymphangiomas; cases. VAN DEN WILDENBERG, Oto-rhino-laryng. internat. *22:*5-10, Jan '38
Jaw cancer; electrosurgery; segmental bone resection without interruption of continuity. KROEFF, M. Hospital, Rio de Janeiro *14:*337, Aug; 595, Sept; 1007, Oct '38
Facial hypertrichosis in female; local therapy by diathermocoagulation, with special reference to technic. LUMER, M. Semana med. *2:*891-897, Oct 20, '38
Electrolysis for hair removal; discussion of equipment, method of operation, indications, contraindications and warnings concerning its use. CIPOLLARO, A. C., J. A. M. A. *111:*2488-2491, Dec 31, '38
Hair removal; electrolysis; surgical procedure. CIPOLLARO, A. C. New York State J. Med. *39:*1475-1480, Aug 1, '39
New type of forceps used as accessory element in depilation by diathermocoagulation. CATEULA, J. Semana med. *2:*628, Sept 14, '39
Iontophoresis in treatment of Dupuytren's contracture and keloids. NIJKERK, M. Nederl. tijdschr. v. geneesk. *83:*5135-5140, Oct 28, '39
Diathermosurgery for furunculosis. ALESSANDRINI, Rev. med. de Chile *67:*1348-1352, Dec '39
Essentials in art of epilation for hypertrichosis (electrolysis). LERNER, C., M. Rec. *151:*193-194, March 20, '40
Congenital atresia of postnasal orifices; simple, effective office technic for treatment by electrocoagulation. MORGENSTERN, D. J. Arch. Otolaryng. *31:*653-662, April '40
Treatment of hypertrichosis by improved apparatus and technic (electrolysis). MARTON, M. H. Arch. Phys. Therapy *21:*678-683, Nov '40
High frequency current in treatment of hypertrichosis. KARP, F. L. Arch. Dermat. and Syph. *43:*85-91, Jan '41
Septic branchial cyst eradicated by electrical cauterization; case. BERGE, C. A., J. Michigan M. Soc. *40:*189-191, March '41
Hypertrichosis with particular reference to electrolysis. REQUE, P. G. South. Med. and Surg. *103:*376-379, July '41
Cauterization in therapy of rectal prolapse, with report of cases. NOVOA, A. N. Prensa med. mex. *6:*120-121, Aug 15, '41
"Thimble forceps" for epilation (during electrolysis). SHELTON, J. M. Arch. Dermat. and Syph. *44:*260, Aug '41
Treatment of hypertrichosis by electrocoagulation. LERNER, C. New York State J. Med. *42:*879-882, May 1, '42
Electrolysis; introduction of instrument for relatively painless treatment in hair removal. HAND, E. A. Arch. Dermat. and Syph. *45:*1094-1100, June '42
Superfluous hair; removal with monopolar diathermy needle. ERDOS-BROWN, M. Arch. Dermat. and Syph. *46:*496-501, Oct '42
Hair removal, nonsurgical reparative dermatology, or electromedical cosmetology. GOODMAN, H. Urol. and Cutan. Rev. *46:*726-727, Nov '42
Use of diathermy in submucous resection. JONES, A. C. Tr. Am. Laryng., Rhin. and Otol. Soc. *48:*331-332, '42
Removal of superfluous hair with cutting current. ROSENBERG, W. A. AND SMITH, E. M. JR. Arch. Phys. Therapy *24:*277-279, May '43
Treatment of acne vulgaris with comedos by monoterminal electrodesiccation. NOMLAND, R. Arch. Dermat. and Syph. *48:*302-304, Sept '43
Use of diathermy in submucous resection. JONES, A. C. Arch. Otolaryng. *38:*445-446, Nov '43
Counterstroke electrocoagulation of buccal mucosa during treatment of facial lesions. BARMAN, J. M. Rev. argent. dermatosif. *28:*191-192, June '44
Plastic repair after electrothermal operations. (cancer) VIANNA, J. B. Med. cir. farm., pp. 598-606, Nov '44
New method of treatment of parotid fistula; cauterization and silence cure. COSTANTINI, H. Afrique franc. chir., nos. 3-4, pp. 65-68, May-Aug '45
Epilation; fifteen year comparative evaluation of electrolysis and electrocoagulation. NIEDELMAN, M. L. Arch. Phys. Med. *26:*290-296, May '45

Electrotherapy – Cont.

Therapy of anorectal cancers exteriorized to perineum by diathermocoagulation; subsequent plastic operation. Moulonguet, P. Mem. Acad. de chir. *71:*298–300, June 13–20, '45

Diathermal depilation in therapy of hypertrichosis. Barman, J. M. Rev. med. de Rosario *35:*703–709, Aug '45

Use of cautery in plastic operations of eyelids. Simpson, D. Brit. M. J. *2:*424–425, Sept 29, '45

Treatment of sebaceous cysts by electrosurgical marsupialization. Danna, J. A. Ann. Surg. *123:*952–956, May '46

Elephantiasis: See Lymphedema

Eletskaya, O. I.: Therapy of purulent tendovaginitis and phlegmon. Novy khir. arkhiv *46:*3–8, '40

Eliason, E. L.: Fractures of fingers. Am. J. Surg. *6:*501–505, April '29

Eliassow, A.: Unusual types of skin cancer with remarks on its genesis. Dermat. Wchnschr. *78:*365–370, March 29 '24

El-Katib, A.: Ectopia vesicae; full report of case treated by transplantation of ureters into recto-sigmoid and complete cystectomy. J. Egyptian M. A. *16:*3–16, Jan '33

Elkin, D. C.: Hereditary ankylosis of proximal phalangeal joints. J. A. M. A. *84:*509, Feb 14, '25

Elkin, M. A.: Therapy of traumatic exfoliation of skin. Khirurgiya, no. 1, pp. 60–62, '39

Elkins, C. W. and Cameron, J. E.: Cranioplasty with acrylic plates. J. Neurosurg. *3:*199–205, May '46

Elkins, C. W. (see Barker, D. E. *et al*) 1946

Elkins, C. W. (see Barker, D. E.) April '46

Elkinton, J. R.: Systemic disturbances in severe burns and their treatment. Bull. Ayer Clin. Lab., Pennsylvania Hosp. *3:*279–292, Dec '39

Elkinton, J. R., Wolff, W. A. and Lee, W. E.: Plasma transfusion in treatment of fluid shift in severe burns. Ann. Surg. *112:*150–157, July '40

Elkinton, J. R. (see Lee, W. E. *et al.*) June '41

Eller, J. J.: Simple procedure for cure of rhinophyma. New York State J. Med. *33:*741–743, June 15, '33

Eller, J. J. and Wolff, S.: Skin peeling and scarification in treatment of pitted scars, pigmentations and certain facial blemishes. J. A. M. A. *116:*2208, May 10, '41

Elliot, H.: Easily made "drop-wrist" splint. Canad. M. A. J. *47:*363, Oct '42

Elliot, H. L. and Arrowood, J. G.: Anesthesia (topical anesthesia and administration of pentothal sodium, barbital derivative, before intratracheal use of nitrous oxide and oxygen) for oral surgery in presence of cautery and diathermy. Anesthesiology *6:*32–38, Jan '45

Elliot, J.: Blood plasma in shock therapy. South. Med. and Surg. *103:*252–254, May '41

Elliott, R. H. E. Jr. (see Scudder, J.) Dec '42

Ellis, B. E.: Surgical treatment of facial paralysis. Tr. Indiana Acad. Ophth. and Otolaryng. *20:*22–27, '36

Ellis, B. E.: Follow-up report on facial nerve repair. Tr. Indiana Acad. Ophth. and Otolaryng. *21:*22–27, '37

Ellis, B. E.: Treatment of facial paralysis. North Carolina M. J. *3:*130–132, March '42

Ellis, E. L. H.: Hermaphroditism, case and its treatment. Lancet *2:*17–18, July 3, '37

Ellis, J. D.: New splint for finger tip fractures. Am. J. Surg. *5:*508, Nov '28

Ellis, J. D. (see Mock, H. E.) Oct '27

Ellis, O. H.: Ptosis of eyelids; combined operation. Tr. Pacific Coast Oto-Ophth. Soc. *27:*159–166, '42

Ellis. O. H.: Combined operation for ptosis of eyelids. Am. J. Ophth. *26:*1048–1053, Oct '43

Ellis, S. S. and von Wedel, C.: Indications, results and reasons for use of different types of skin grafts. J. Oklahoma M. A. *33:*8–14, Dec '40

Ellis, S. S. and von Wedel, C.: Collodion as dressing for skin grafting of granulating wounds. J. Oklahoma M. A. *34:*103–105, March '41

Ellis, V. H.: Minor fractures in hand. Proc. Roy. Soc. Med. *35:*710–711, Sept '42

Ellis Ribeiro, F.: Therapy of shock. Rev. brasil. de cir. *5:*171–174, April '36

Ellis Ribeiro, F.: Burn therapy. Rev. med.-cir. do Brasil *51:*255–286, April-June '43

Ellmer, G. and Schmincke, A.: Successful 15½ year old homeoplastic bone graft in man. Zentralbl. f. Chir. *52:*562–565, March 14, '25 abstr: J. A. M. A. *84:*1463, May 9, '25

Elman, R.: Therapeutic significance of plasma protein replacement in severe burns. J. A. M. A. *116:*213–216, Jan 18, '41

Elman, R.: Acute protein deficiency (hypoproteinemia) in shock due to severe hemorrhage and in burns, intestinal obstruction and general peritonitis, with special reference to use of plasma and hydrolized protein (amigen). J. A. M. A. *120:*1176–1180, Dec 12, '42

Elman, R.: Early mortality as influenced by rapid tanning and by transfusions in burns. Ann. Surg. *117:*327–331, March '43

ELMAN, R.: Influence of ether, morphine and nembutal (Pentobarbital) on mortality in experimental burns. Ann. Surg. *120:*211-213, Aug '44

ELMAN, R. *et al*: Severe burns; clinical findings with simplified plan of early treatment. Surg, Gynec. and Obst. *83:*187-199, Aug '46

ELMAN, R. (see LISCHER, C. E.) May '43

ELMAN, R. (see LISCHER, C. *et al*) Jan '44

ELMAN, R. (see WEINER, D. O. *et al*) May '36

ELOESSER, L: Plastic operations. Surg., Gynec. and Obst. *34:*532-537, April '22 (illus.)

ELSCHNIG, A.: Entropion in new-born. Monatschr. f. Kinderh. *31:*439-440. Dec-Jan '26

ELTERICH, T. O.: Talipomanus (congenital club hand). Atlantic M. J. *31:*953-954, Sept '28

EL-TOBGY, A. F: Plastic operations for restoration of lower eyelid. Bull. Ophth. Soc. Egypt *26:*1-7, '33

EL-TOBGY, A. F.: Plastic operations for restoration of upper eyelid. Bull. Ophth. Soc. Egypt *28:*21-25, '35

ELVIDGE, A. AND BAXTER, H.: Treatment of multiple fractures of face with external pin fixation splint. McGill M. J. *13:*469-475, Dec '44

ELY, J. O. AND ANGULO, A. W.: Gelatin-glucose-salts solution; influence on hemoconcentration of experimental burns. J. Franklin Inst. *235:*197-204, Feb '43

ELY, L. W.: Dupuytren's contraction. S. Clin. N. Amer. *6:*421-424, April '26

Embryonal Tissue Grafts, Cancer in

Growth of transplanted embryonal tissue and origin of neoplasms. SKUBISREWSKI, L. Compt. rend. Soc. de biol. *93:*1398-1400, Dec 4, '25

Possibility of producing tumors by subcutaneous inoculation of normal, particularly embryonal tissue; experimental study. LÖWENTHAL, K. Med. Klin. *24:*1263-1268, Aug 17, '28

Growth of transplanted embryonal tissue and its significance with regard to origin of tumors. SKUBISZEWSKI, L. Ztschr. f. Krebsforsch. *26:*308-329, '28

Production of malignant tumors by transplantation of embryonal tissues. KLEE-RAWIDOWWICZ, E. Deutsche med. Wchnschr. *58:*1439-1440, Sept 9, '32

EMERSON, C.: Technic for ideal skin-graft, with report of extensive lymphangioma pigmentosa verrucosa. Nebraska, M. J. *13:*214-216, June '28

EMERSON, C. P. JR. AND EBERT, R. V.: Shock in battle casualties; measurements of blood volume changes occurring in response to therapy. Ann. Surg. *122:*745-772, Nov '45

EMERSON, D. (see PIERCE, G. W. *et al*) Jan '44

EMILIADIS, K.: Rare case of cornu cutaneum humanum of forehead. Zentralbl. f. Chir. *64:*727-728, March 27, '37

EMILIANI, C. M. (see BISI, R. H.) Sept '38

EMILIANI, C. M. (see MARFORT, A. *et al*) Oct '37

EMILIANI, C. M. (see MARFORT, A.) April '38

EMILIANI C. M. (see VON SOUBIRON, N. *et al*) June '38

EMORY, L.: Temporary prosthesis as aid in treatment of war injuries of face. Mil. Surgeon *99:*105-109, Aug '46

ENGEL, D.: Proposal to prevent necrosis of tabula externa of skull denuded of periosteum (scalping). Brit. M. J. *1:*185, Feb 5, '44

ENGEL, L. P.: Infections of upper lip. J. Kansas M. Soc. *24:*44-46, Feb '24

ENGLAND, M. C.: Plastic operations of nose. J. Oklahoma M. A. *33:*10-12, Jan '40

ENLOE, G. R.: Jaw fractures. Texas State J. Med. *27:*27-29, May '31

ENNIS, W. N. AND HUBER, H. S.: Traumatic amputations of fingers. S. Clin. North America *18:*305-319, April '38

Enophthalmos

Four cases of unusual eye injuries; eyelash in iris; horsehair in lens; ink pencil injury; traumatic enophthalmos. HORAY, G. Klin. Monatsbl. f. Augenh. *80:*202-208, Feb 24, '28

Progress with tarsal graft of Müller's muscle in pseudoptosis due to enophthalmos. GALLENGA, R. Rassegna ital. d'ottal. *3:*626-636, July-Aug '34

Traumatic enophthalmos. PFEIFFER, R. L. Arch. Ophth. *30:*718-726, Dec '43

ENSEIME, J. AND TRINTIGNAC, P.: Action on general ossification with bone transplantation. Lyon chir. *36:*434-436, July-Aug '39

ENTIN, D. A.: First aid for maxillary injuries. Vrach. delo (nos. 11–12) *22:*727-730, '40

ENTIN, D. A.: Closure of granulating wounds of face by means of button sutures. Am. Rev. Soviet. Med. *1:*351-354, April '44

ENTWISLE, R. M. AND GARDNER, J. A.: Fractures of mandible. Atlantic M. J. *28:*515-518, May '25

EPES, B. M. (see IVY, R. H.) March '27

Epicanthus

Congenital deformity in formation of inner corners of eyelids; 2 cases. GALA, A. Bratisl. lekar. listy *9:*1248-1251, Dec '29

Hereditary eyelid ptosis with epicanthus;

Epicanthus – Cont.

case with pedigree extending over 4 generations. McIlroy, J. H. Proc. Roy. Soc. Med. (sect. Ophth.) *23:*17–20, Jan '30

Congenital epicanthus and ptosis of eyelid transmitted through 4 generations. Ross, N. Brit. M. J. *1:*378–379, Feb 27, '32

Correction of epicanthus and eyelid ptosis. Blair, V. P., Brown, J. B., and Hamm, W. G. Arch. Ophth. *7:*831–846, June '32

Therapy of epicanthus tarsalis. Oláh, E. Klin. Monatsbl. f. Augenh. *90:*233–234, Feb '33

Epidermolysis Bullosa

Epidermolysis bullosa dystrophica; etiopathogenic study of case following burn in tuberculous child. Ciaccio, I. Arch. ital. di dermat., sif. *12:*326–344, May '36

Epilation

Technic of diathermic epilation. Bordier, H. Am. J. Phys. Therapy *8:*273–274, Jan '32. also: Monde med., Paris *42:*78–81, Feb 1, '32

Technic of diathermic epilation in hypertrichosis. Ducourtioux, Rev. d'actinol. *10:*14–19, Jan–Feb '34

Symposium on question of permanent epilation of excessive hair for cosmetic purposes (Dauerepilation an kosmetisch wichtigen Korperstellan). Various authors. Dermat. Wchnschr. *98:*275–287, March 3, '34

Comment on article by various authors on permanent epilation for cosmetic purposes. Zoon, J. J. Dermat. Wchnschr. *98:*501, April 21, '34

Permanent epilation of hair for cosmetic purposes. (Reply to Zoon) Hoede, K. Dermat. Wchnschr. *99:*932, July 14, '34

Permanent epilation of hair for cosmetic purposes. (Reply to Zoon). Wucherpfennig, V. Dermat. Wchnschr. *99:*933–934, July 14, '34

Injuries following epilation by electrolysis or roentgen rays. (Further comment on Nobl's article). Karpelis, E. Wien. med. Wchnschr. *87:*685, June 19, '37

Short wave epilation. Derow, D. Arch. Phys. Therapy *20:*101–102, Feb '39

Hair removal; electrolysis; surgical procedure. Cipollaro, A. C. New York State J. Med. *39:*1475–1480, Aug 1, '39

Essentials in art of epilation for hypertrichosis (electrolysis). Lerner, C. M. Rec. *151:*193–194, March 20, '40

How to remove superfluous hair. Costello, M. J. Hygeia *18:*584–586, July '40

Epispadias (See also Bladder, Exstrophy)

Operative cure of incontinence of urine in epispadias by Goebell-Stoeckel operation. Reifferscheid, K. Zentralbl. f. Gynak. *45:*97, Jan 22, '21

New operation for total epispadia. Melchoir, E. Zentralbl. f. Chir. *48:*220, Feb 19, '21

Operation for cure of incontinence associated with epispadias. Young, H. H., J. Urology *7:*1–32, Jan '22

Treatment of hypospadias and epispadias. Sanchez-Covisa, I. Arch. espan. de pediat. *6:*577–613, Oct '22 (illus.) abstr: J. A. M. A. *80:*285, Jan 27, '23

Operative treatment of epispadias in the female. Liek, E. Zentralbl. f. Gynak. *47:*604–606, April 14, '23

Case of epispadias associated with complete incontinence treated by rectus transplantation. Thompson, A. R. Brit. J. Child. Dis. *20:*146–151, July–Sept '23

Epispadias in women, report of case. Lower, W. E., J. Urology *10:*149–157, Aug '23 (illus.)

Operative treatment of epispadias. Gaza, W. v. Arch. f. klin. Chir. *126:*510–514, '23

Treatment of epispadias in women. Potel, G. Gynec. et Obst. *10:*94–101, Aug '24

Epispadias in male. Mullen, T. F. Northwest Med. *24:*63–67, Feb '25

Case of true epispadias. MacEwen, J. A. C. Brit. M. J. *1:*454, March 7, '25

Case of epispadias in man. Doria, J. R. da C. Brazil-med. *2:*84–86, Aug 15, '25

Epispadias in female, transplantation of gracilis muscle for incontinence. Deming, C. L., J. A. M. A. *86:*822–825, March 20, '26

Case of complete epispadias associated with incontinence of urine cured by operation; 4 additional cases. Muschat, M., J. Urol. *18:*177–185, Aug '27

Unusual developmental abnormalities (including imperforate anus). (epispadias). Thomas, A. K. Brit. M. J. *2:*985–986, Nov 26, '27

Epispadias in women; case report. Sexton, W. G., J. Urol. *18:*663–666, Dec '27

Epispadias in females, surgical treatment. Davis, D. M. Surg. Gynec. and Obst. *47:*680–696, Nov '28. abstr. J. Urol. *20:*673–678, Dec '28

Treatment of case of male epispadias. Cecil, A. B., S. Clin. N. Amer. *8:*1351–1356, Dec '28

Repair of epispadias and exstrophy of bladder. Rockey, E. W., S. Clin. N. Amer. *8:*1503–1509, Dec '28

Epispadias—Cont.
Epispadias; operation. DANZIGER, F. Ztschr. f. urol. Chir. *25:*21-24, '28
Late results of Subbotin's operation for complete epispadias with urinary incontinence; 2 cases. PETROV, N. Arch. f. klin. Chir. *149:*762-768, '28
Surgical treatment of epispadias of second degree. BOEMINGHAUS, H. Chirurg *2:*11-14, Jan 1, '30
Plastic operations for epispadias and hypospadias. CABOT, H. Proc. Staff Meet., Mayo Clin. *5:*315, Nov 5, '30
Hypospadias and epispadias, indications for and technique of their operative correction. BLAIR, V. P. Tr. South. S. A. (1929) *42:*163-165, '30
Plastic operation for epispadias by means of temporary suturing into scrotum; case. SPRINGER, C. Zentralbl. f. Chir. *58:*1047-1051, April 25, '31
Epispadias as cause of incontinence in woman; case. SEYNSCHE, K. Zentralbl. f. Gynak. *55:*3585-3591, Dec 12, '31
Surgery of hypospadias and epispadias in male. CECIL, A. B. Tr. Am. A. Genito-Urin. Surgeons *24:*253-302, '31. also: J. Urol. *27:*507-537, May '32
Surgery of hypospadias and epispadias in male. CECIL, A. B. West. J. Surg. *40:*297-315, June '32
Hypospadias and epispadias; philological note. BREMER, J. L. New England J. Med. *207:*537-539, Sept 22, '32
Epispadias in women; technic of surgical therapy. ESTELLA, J. Progresos de la clin. *40:*541-549, Sept '32
Surgical therapy of epispadias in women. MERCIER, O. Union med. de Canada *61:*1004-1009, Sept '32
Surgical therapy of epispadias in male. FASSRAINER, S. Deutsche Ztschr. f. Chir. *237:*537-548, '32
Trifid ureter and epispadias in girl 10 years old. FRANCK, A. Bull. Soc. franc.d'urol., pp. 107-112, Feb 20, '33
Epispadias totalis. HARRISON, F. G. Pennsylvania M. J. *36:*589-590, May '33
Correction of epispadias. and scrotal hypospadias. BLAIR, V. P.; *et al.* Surg., Gynec. and Obst. *57:*646-653, Nov '33
Operative treatment of complete epispadias. DE QUERVAIN, F. Ztschr. f. urol. Chir. *36:*237-242, '33
Cure of grave epispadias by vesico-urethral plication; case in boy 5 years old. GAUTIER, J. Bull. et mem. Soc. nat. de chir. *60:*219-221, Feb 10, '34

Epispadias—Cont.
Ureteral transplantation to rectosigmoid for exstrophy of bladder, complete epispadias and other urethral abnormalities with total urinary incontinence; 85 cases operated. WALTERS, W. AND BRAASCH, W. F. Am. J. Surg. *23:*255-270, Feb '34
Subsymphyseal female epispadias; case. GRIMALDI, F. E. AND RUBI, R. A. Semana med. *1:*1748-1749, June 7, '34
Ureterosigmoidal transplantation for exstrophy and complete epispadias with absent urinary sphincters. WALTERS, W. Am. J. Surg. *24:*776-792, June '34
Epispadias, personal technic for cure in women. MERCIER, O. Brit. J. Urol. *6:*313-319, Dec '34
Author's technic for cure of female epispadias. MERCIER, O. J.de l'Hotel-Dieu de Montreal *4:*84-90, March-April '35
Implantation of ureters into large intestine in treatment of epispadias. BANGERTER, J. Schweiz. med. Wchnschr. *65:*747-748, Aug 17, '35
Cure of epispadias; further report. CECIL, A. B. J. Urol. 34:278-283, Sept '35
Reconstruction of epispadias controlled by urethrography; case. DOBRZANIECKI, W. J. d'urol. *40:*320-326, Oct '35
New operation for epispadias. BRANDT, G. Arch. f. klin. Chir. *183:*607-610, '35
Therapy of grave incontinence of urethral origin by vesico-urethral fold (epispadias). GAUTIER, J., J. d'urol. *44:*55-68, July '37
Unusual obstetric injury causing detachment of bladder and urethra from symphysis pubis and complete epispadias. HUNNER, G. L. Am. J. Obst. and Gynec. *34:*840-854, Nov '37
Epispadias; treatment in male. CABOT, H. Proc. Staff Meet., Mayo Clin. *12:*793-795, Dec 15, '37
Surgical therapy of epispadias. LUBMANN, K. Beitr. z. klin. Chir. *165:*376-381, '37
Surgical therapy of epispadias. LEPOUTRE, C. Bull. Soc. franc. d'urol., pp. 31-35, Jan 17, '38
Clinical anatomy of cases of epispadias and extroversion of bladder. THOMPSON, A. R. Brit. J. Child. Dis. *35:*36-43, Jan-March '38
Epispadias; surgical therapy; case. LEPOUTRE, C., J. d'urol. *46:*466-472, Nov '38
Hypospadias and epispadias (surgical correction). BLAIR, V. P. AND BYARS, L. T. J. Urol. *40:*814-825, Dec '38
Epispadias; casc. DOBRITZ, O. Ztschr. f. Urol. *32:*622-624, '38

Epispadias–Cont.
Exstrophy of bladder and masculine epispadias; treatment by prerectal pelvic transposition of bladder. GODARD, H., J. d'urol. *47:*97–109, Feb '39
Exstrophy of bladder and epispadias (surgical technic). LADD, W. E. AND LANMAN, T. H. New England J. Med. *222:*130–134, Jan 25, '40
Plastic surgery of urethra and penis in total epispadias. VOZNESENSKIY, V. P. Novy khir. arkhiv *47:*281–283, '40
Simplified technic of plastic repair of epispadias. FRUMKIN, J., J. Urol. *46:*690–692, Oct '41
Epispadias with incontinence in male. DEES, J. E. Surgery *12:*621–630, Oct '42
Epispadias in women. KEPP, R. K. Chirurg *15:*332, June 1, '43
Plastic surgery (modified Ombredanne operation) in therapy of epispadias with urinary incontinence; case. DE BRUIN, T. R. Nederl. tijdschr. v. geneesk. *90:*1127–1129, Sept 7, '46

EPPINGER, H.: Postoperative shock. Wien. klin. Wchnschr. *44:*65–71, Jan 16, '31
EPPINGER, H.: Postoperative syndrome (shock and collapse). Klin. Wchnschr. *11:*618–622, April 9, '32
EPSTEIN, (see GILLERSON, A. B.) Dec '28
EPSTEIN, I.: Free transplantation of bone. Bucursti. med. *7:*138–146, '35
EPSTEIN, J.: Ectopia of the urinary bladder in an infant. M. J. and Rec. *121:*151–152, Feb 4, '25
EPSTEIN, J. (see TARLOV, I. M.) Jan '45
ERB, I. H., MORGAN, E. M. AND FARMER, A. W.: Pathologic picture as revealed at autopsy in series of 61 fatal burn cases treated (with and without tannic acid) at Hospital for Sick Children, Toronto, Canada. Ann. Surg. *117:*234–255, Feb '43
ERB, W. H. (see ELIASON, E. L) Feb '37
ÉRCZY, M.: Narrowing of wide alae of nose by reimplantation of cartilage from tip of nose. Ztschr. f. Hals-, Nasen-u. Ohrenh, *26:*194–197, July 3, '30
ÉRCZY, M.: Fixative bandage in corrective nasal plastic surgery. Orvosi hetil. *76:*657–658, July 23, '32
ÉRCZY, M.: Cosmetic surgery of incomplete (operated) harelip and nasal deformities combined with harelip. Gyogyaszat *72:*719–721, Nov 20, '32
ÉRCZY, M.: Anesthesia in plastic surgery of nose. Orvosi hetil. *79:*641–643, June 8, '35
ÉRCZY, M.: Plastic surgery of pendulous breast. Gyogyaszat *77:*324–326, May 23, '37
ÉRCZY, M.: Development of plastic surgery. Gyogyaszat *78:*207–210, March 27, '38
ÉRCZY, M.: Corrective operations of nose and development of plastic surgery. Gyogyaszat *78:*272–276, April 24, '38
ÉRCZY, M.: Corrective operations and development of plastic surgery. Gyogyaszat *78:*454–456, July 17–24, '38
ÉRCZY, M.: Corrective operations and development of plastic surgery. (including breast). Gyogyaszat *78:*495–498, Aug. 14–21, '38
ÉRCZY, M.: Restoration of partial defect of auricle by free transplantation. Gyogyaszat *79:*319–320, May 21, '39
ERDOS-BROWN, M.: Superfluous hair; removal with monopolar diathermy needle. Arch. Dermat. and Syph. *46:*496–501, Oct '42
EREN, N. O.: Cryotherapy of hemangioma. Turk. tib cem. mec. *6:*139–141, '40
ERFURTH, W.: Congenital fistula of ear and atresia of external meatus. Monatschr. f. Kinderh. *22:*55–59, Oct '21 (illus.)
ERICH, J. B.: Recent traumatic injuries of face. Proc. Staff Meet., Mayo Clin. *15:*166–169, March 13, '40
ERICH, J. B.: Cysts; sebaceous, mucous, dermoid and epidermoid. Am. J. Surg. *50:*672–677, Dec '40
ERICH, J. B.: Facial bone fractures. Mil. Surgeon *88:*637–639, June '41
ERICH, J. B.: Treatment of fractures of upper jaw. J. am. Dent. A. *29:*783–793, May '42
ERICH, JOHN B., AND AUSTIN, LOUIE T.: *Traumatic injuries of facial bones*. W. B. Saunders Co., Phila., 1944
ERICH, J. B. (see NEW, G. B.) July '37
ERICH, J. B. (see NEW, G. B.) 1938
ERICH, J. B. (see NEW, G. B.) Dec '38
ERICH, J. B. (see NEW, G. B.) Feb '39
ERICH, J. B. (see NEW, G. B.) June '39
ERICH, J. B. (see NEW, G. B. *et al*) Aug '39
ERICH, J. B. (see NEW, G. B.) Jan '40
ERICH, J. B. (see NEW, G. B.) May '40
ERICH, J. B. (see NEW, G. B.) July '40
ERICH, J. B. (see NEW, G. B.) March '41
ERICH, J. B. (see NEW, G. B.) July '41
ERICH, J. B. (see NEW, G. B.) Nov '41
ERICH, J. B. (see NEW, G. B.) Feb '44
ERICH, J. B. (see NEW, G. B.) Aug '44
ERICH, J. B. (see PASTORE, P. N.) July '42

Erich Operation: See New-Erich Operation

ERICKSEN, L. G: Curability of carcinoma of skin of nose. J. Iowa M. Soc. *25:*309–311, June '35
ERKES, F.: Homeoplastic skin grafts. Deutsche Ztschr. f. Chir. *234:*852–854, '31
ERLACHER, P.: Correction of deformed hand in congenital syphilis. Arch. f. klin. Chir. *125:*776–789, '23

ERLER, F.: Treatment of stumps in accidental amputation of finger tips. Munchen. med. Wchnschr. *88:*1287, Nov 28, '41

ERMOLAEV, P. E.: Shock following injuries of extremities; procaine hydrochloride block of vagus nerve. Khirurgiya, no. 6, pp. 45–46, '45

ERNST, F.: Plastic operations on hard palate; comment on Rosenthal's article. Zentralbl. f. Chir. *52:*464–470, Feb 28, '25

ERNST, F.: Surgical therapy of harelip and cleft palate; possibilities of results. Kinderarztl. Praxis *5:*120–128, March '34

ERNST, F.: Harelip. and cleft palate. Med. Welt *11:*1061–1064, July 31, '37

Ernst Operation

Plastic operation of cleft palate according to Ernst method. STANČIUS, P. Medicina, Kaunas *18:*558–562, July '37

ERRECART, P. L.: Congenital facial paralysis. Rev. de especialid. *5:*930–935, July '30

ERRECART, P. L.: Death of patient after Killian operation for deformed septum. Rev. Asoc. med. argent. (50): 974–977, June '36

ERRECART, P. L. (see SAMENGO, L.) Oct '28

ERRECART, P. L. (see SAMENGO, L.) Nov '28

ERSNER, M. S.: Reconstruction of deformed septum; critical evaluation of orthodox submucous resection from anatomophysiologic standpoint. Arch. Otolaryng. *39:*476–484, June '44

ERSNER, M. S.: Wounds and injuries of nose and their implications. Pennsylvania M. J. *49:*840–844, May '46

ERSNER, M. S. AND MYERS, D.: Variation of pedicle flap for epitheliation of radical mastoidectomy cavity. Arch. Otolaryng. *23:*469–474, April '36

ERTL, J.: Regenerative-reconstructive operations and late results of bone and tissue transplantations. Budapesti orvosi ujsag *36:*949–953, Nov 3, '38

ERUSALIMSKIY, A. L.: Treatment of burns under plexiglass covers. Vrach. delo (nos. 7–8) *26:*549–552, '46

ESAT, A.: Formation of artificial vagina. Turk tip cem. mec. *1:*15–20, Jan 1, '35

ESAU, P.: Two rare congenital anomalies; 1. hydro-encephalocel; 2. intra-uterine adhesion of tip of tongue to hard palate. Arch. f. klin. Chir. *118:*817–820, '21

ESAU, P.: Thiersch grafts. Zentralbl. f. Chir. *57:*1780–1783, July 19, '30

ESCAT, DUCUING, AND RIGAUD: Results of radium therapy in cancer of larynx; 150 cases. Cancer, Bruxelles *7:*121–126, '30

ESCAT, E.: Surgical treatment of facial paralysis attributed to cold. Ann. d. mal. de l'oreille, du larynx *46:*213–221, March '27

ESCAT, E.: Surgical treatment of facial paralysis from cold; cases. Rev. de stomatol. *30:*614–624, Oct '28

ESCAT, M.: Congenital atresia of pyriform orifice as cause of respiratory insufficiency; surgical correction. Oto-rhino-laryng. internat. *22:*65–74, Feb '38

ESCAT, M.: Sinusofacial wounds in war surgery with report of cases. Oto-rhino-laryng. internat. *24:*241–252, Sept '40

ESCAT, M. (see VIÉLA, A.) Nov '28

ESCH, A.: Surgical therapy of cicatrical stenosis and atresia of vestibule and interior of nose. Ztschr. f. Hals-, Nasen-u. Ohrenh. *48:*41–46, '41

ESCHER, F.: Surgical treatment of war injuries of nasal accessory sinuses. Schweiz. med. Wchnschr. *73:*715, May 29, '43. abstr. Bull. War Med. *4:*278, Jan '44

ESKES, T. J.: Simple treatment of maxillary fracture. Nederl. tijdschr. v. geneesk. *76:*670–674, Feb. 13, '32

Esmarch Operation

Ankylosis of temporomandibular joints; cure by Esmarch operation. MILLER, I. D. Australian and New Zealand J. Surg. *8:*406–407, April '39

Esophagus

Statistics on 1,323 operations on mouth, pharynx and esophagus for cancer. SIMEONI, V. Valsalva *5:*86–89, Feb '29

Two modifications of technic in making use of skin flaps in esophagoplasty. POKOTILO, W. L. Zentralbl. f. Chir. *57:*2295–2300, Sept 13, '30

Mandibular hypoplasia with atresia of esophagus; case. SOER, J. J. Maandschr. v. kindergeneesk. *1:*309–310, March '32

Technic of closure of esophageal fistula; significance in surgical treatment of laryngoesophageal cancer. PORTMANN, G. AND DESPONS, J. Bordeaux chir. *3:*252–261, July '32

Closure of esophageal defect after laryngectomy with help of movable flap (Filatov operation). SOLOWJEW, L. M. Acta oto-laryng. *21:*219–221, '34

Anterior thoracic esophagoplasty by means of skin graft; case. VAZA, D. L. Klin. med. (no. 1) *12:*121–124, '34

Total plastic reconstruction of esophagus using transverse colon and tubal graft; case. EGIDI, G. Policlinico (sez. prat.) *42:*1287–1289, July 1, '35

Antethoracic esophagoplasty using loop of small intestine and tubal skin graft in cica-

Esophagus – Cont.
tricial inflammatory stenosis of esophagus; case. COSTANTINI, H. Bull. et mem. Soc. nat. de chir. *61:*1312-1315, Dec 7, '35
Fate of flap in esophagoplasty after circular resection of cervical part of esophagus. PALCHEVSKIY, E. I. AND POLYAK, S. O. Vestnik khir. *53:*113-115, '37
Perforated esophagus with burns. ROBSON, L. C. Brit. M. J. *1:*414, April 3, '43
Prethoracic esophagoplasty by new esthetic method with enclosed epithelial graft. RAPIN, M. Helvet. med. acta *8:*429-435, Aug '41

ESPERABÉ Y GONZÁLEZ, J. M.: Pathogenesis and treatment of Volkmann contracture; Med. ibera *2:*285-294, Sept 5, '31
ESPERNE, P. (see MARINO, H.) Feb '41
ESPINOSA ROBLEDO, M. (see ROGERS, S. P.) July-Sept '35
ESSEN-MÖLLER, E.: Congenital defects of radius and ear with facial paralysis; case. Ztschr. f. d. ges. Anat. (Abt. 2) *14:*52-70, March 28, '28
ESSER, E.: Median fissure of nose; surgical therapy of cases. Plast. chir. *1:*40-50, '39
ESSER, E.: Congenital absence of vagina; choice of operative procedure. J. Internat. Coll. Surgeons *6:*496-499, Sept-Oct '43
ESSER, J. F. S.: Bandage for plastic operations on face. Arch. f. klin. Chir. *117:*438-443, '21 (illus.)
ESSER, J. F. S.: Pedunculated flaps without skin pedicle in plastic surgery. Arch. f. klin. Chir *117:*477-491, '21 (illus.) abstr: J.A.M.A. *78:*1009, April 1, '22
ESSER, J. F. S.: Correction of displaced canthus. Arch. f. klin. Chir. *115:*704, March '21
ESSER, J. F. S.: Operation on nose without incision skin. Deutsche Ztschr. f. Chir. *164:*211, June '21. abstr: J. A. M. A. *77:*898, Sept 10, '21
ESSER, J. F. S.: Total reconstruction of external ear. Munchen. med. Wchnschr. *68:*1150, Sept 9, '21
ESSER, J. F. S. AND AUFRICHT, G.: Reconstruction of ear. Arch. f. klin. Chir. *120:*518-525, '22 (illus.) abstr: J. A. M. A. *79:*1887, Nov 25, '22
ESSER, J. F. S.: Constructive surgery. Munchen. med. Wchnschr. *69:*502-503, April 7, '22 (illus.)
ESSER, J. F. S.: Arterial flaps and epithelial inserts in plastic surgery. Munchen. med. Wchnschr. *69:*669-671, May 5, '22 (illus.)
ESSER, J. F. S.: Rotation of cheek in plastic surgery. Munchen. med. Wchnschr. *69:*780-781, May 26, '22 (illus.)
ESSER, J. F. S.: Incisions in plastic surgery. Munchen. med. Wchnschr. *69:*818-819, June 2, '22
ESSER, J. F. S.: Source of material for plastic operations. Munchen. med. Wchnschr. *69:*888, June 16, '22
ESSER, J. F. S.: Constructive surgery. Med. Klinik *18:*793-796, June 18, '22. abstr: J.A.M.A. *79:*2043, Dec 9, '22
ESSER, J. F. S.: Foundation in plastic surgery. Munchen. med. Wchnschr. *69:*966-967, June 30, '22
ESSER, J. F. S.: Inlays in plastic nasal operations. Munchen. med. Wchnschr. *69:*1154-1155, Aug 4, '22
ESSER, J. F. S.: Use of tissues for various plastic purposes. Munchen. med. Wchnschr. *69:*1186-1187, Aug 11, '22
ESSER, J. F. S.: Reconstruction of face by Esser's method of Thiersch flaps fitted on dentist's cast. Zentralbl. f. Chir. *49:*1217-1219, Aug 19, '22 (illus.)
ESSER, J. F. S.: Facial autoplasty. Paris chirurg. *18:*263, Nov '26
ESSER, J. F. S.: Biological skin flaps for pronounced scars. Zentralbl. f. Chir. *60:*1639-1641, July 15, '33
ESSER, J. F. S.: Preservation of innervation and circulation supply in plastic restoration of upper lip. Ann. Surg. *99:*101-111, Jan '34
ESSER, J. F. S.: Biological or artery flaps; general observations and technic. Rev. de chir. plastique, pp. 275-286, Jan '34
ESSER, J. F. S.: Frontal flaps of lips; special practice of biological or artery flaps. Rev. de chir. plastique, pp. 288-294, Jan '34
ESSER, J. F. S.: Eyelid flaps. Rev. de chir. plastique, pp. 295-297, Jan '34
ESSER, J. F. S.: Cheek rotation. Rev. de chir. plastique, pp. 298-299, Jan '34
ESSER, J. F. S.: Biologic flap to form 2 eyelids at same time; case. Rev. espan. de cir. *17:*1-3, Jan-Feb '35
ESSER, J. F. S.: New and simple method for plastic surgery in congenital or accidental absence of ear. Presse med. *43:*325-326, Feb 27, '35
ESSER, J. F. S.: Use of moulages in application of skin grafts; 2 cases. Presse med. *43:*1286-1288, Aug. 14, '35
ESSER, J. F. S.: Value of epithelial inlays in general surgery. Tech. chir. *27:*125-129, Aug-Sept '35
ESSER, J. F. S.: Difficulties in technic of epithelial inlay. Rev. de chir. structive, pp. 127-132, Dec '35
ESSER, J. F. S.: Plastic repair of mutilated ear. Rev. de chir. structure, pp. 269-271, June '36
ESSER, J. F. S.: Epithelial inlay in cases of

refractory ectropion. Arch. Ophth. *16:*55–57, July '36

ESSER, J. F. S.: Rotation of cheek to remake face; case. Tech. chir. *28:*293–296, Dec '36

ESSER, J. F. S.: Multiple stage operation for difficult saddle nose, avoidance of scar. Surg., Gynec. and Obst. *64:*102, Jan '37

ESSER, J. F. S.: Pedicle breast flap for amputation-stump; structive surgery applied to amputation stump at knee. Ann. Surg. *105:*469–472, March '37

ESSER, J. F. S.: Resection for prognathism of upper jaw; case. An. de cir. *3:*364–368, Dec '37

ESSER, J. F. S.: Serious case of roentgen necrosis of face and mandible. Rev. de chir. structive *8:*1–3, May '38

ESSER, J. F. S.: Correction of bird's face (jaw deformity). Am. J. Orthodontics *24:*791–794, Aug '38

ESSER, J. F. S.: Biologic frontal flaps in eyelid surgery. Am. J. Ophth. *21:*963–967, Sept '38

ESSER, J. F. S.: Rotation of cheek in ophthalmology. Arch. Ophth. *20:*410–416, Sept '38

ESSER, J. F. S.: Dangers of roentgenotherapy of hypertrichosis of chin; 2 cases. An. de cir. *4:*260–262, Sept '38

ESSER, J. F. S. Epithelial inlay graft in dentistry. Am. J. Orthodontics *24:*1083–1090, Nov '38

ESSER, J. F. S. Use of skin of female breast in plastic surgery. Brit. M. J. *2:*1256–1257, Dec. 17, '38

ESSER, J. F. S.: Epithelial inlay for scars in neck dragging lower jaw downwards. Am. J. Surg. *45:*148–149, July '39

ESSER, J. F. S.: Biologic scrotal flaps—new approach. J. Internat. Coll. Surgeons *5:*168–170, March–April '42

ESSER, J. F. S.: Esser inlays as practical auxillary operation. J. Internat. Coll. Surgeons *6:*208–211, May–June '43

ESSER, J. F. S.: Use of preputial skin in "structive" surgery. J. Internat. Coll. Surgeons *7:*469–470, Nov–Dec '44

ESSER, J. F. S. AND RANSCHBURG, P. Reconstruction of hand and 4 fingers by transplantation of middle part of foot and 4 toes. Ann. Surg. *111:*655–659, April '40

ESSER, J. F. S. AND RAOUL: Epithelial inlay in therapy of syndactylia. Rev. de chir. plastique, pp. 21–32, May '34

ESSER, J. F. S. (see PENHALE, K. W.) Aug '42

Esser-Wheeler Operation

Reconstruction of orbit by Esser-Wheeler technic. SVERDLICK, J. AND FERNANDEZ, L. L. Semana med. *2:*142–144, July 26, '45

ESSEX, H. E. AND DE REZENDE, N. T.: Injury and repair of peripheral nerves (importance of blood supply as shown by transparent chamber technic). Am. J. Physiol. *140:*107–114, Oct '43

ESSEX, H. E. (see KENDRICK, D. B. JR. *et al*) May '40

ESTEBAN, M.: Cause of failure of dacryocystorhinostomy. Rev. cubana de oto-neuro-oftal. *5:*99–100, May–June '36

ESTEBAN ARANJUEZ, M.: Treatment of blepharoptosis. Arch. de med., cir. y. espec. *26:*696–700, June 4, '27

ESTELLA, J.: Epispadias in women; technic of surgical therapy. Progresos de la clin. *40:*541–549, Sept '32

ESTELLA, J. AND MORALES, L.: Operative technic in congenital branchial fistulas. Arch. de med., cir. y espec. *33:*73–84, July 26, '30

ESTELLA Y BERMÚDEZ DE CASTRO, J.: Clinical aspects and treatment of harelip. Clin. y lab. *12:*177–199, Sept '28

ESTELLA Y BERMÚDEZ DE CASTRO, J.: Surgical treatment of congenital facial malformation. Clin. y lab. *12:*276, Oct.; 364, Nov.; 456, Dec. '28

ESTES, W. L.: Implantation of both ureters into rectum; prolongation of life 24 years (exstrophy of bladder). Ann. Surg. *99:*223–226, Jan '34

Esthetic Surgery

Review of 25 years' observation in plastic surgery, with special reference to rhinoplasty. BECK, J. C. Laryngoscope *31:*487, July '21

Cosmetic surgery of face, neck and breast. BOOTH, F. A. Northwest. Med. *21:*170–172, June '22 (illus.)

Surgery of skin without disfigurement; esthetic surgery. GIMENO Y RODRÍGUEZ JAÉN, V. AND PULIDO, A. Siglo med. *71:*503–506, May 26 ; 532–534, June 2; 555–558, June 9; 582–585, June 16; 603–607, June 23; 629–632, June 30, '23

Rhinoplastic surgeon versus rhinologist. BERNE, L. P. Tr. Sect. Laryng., Otol. and Rhin., A. M. A., pp. 118–121, '23

Cosmetic Surgery: The Correction of Featural Imperfections, by Charles C. Miller. F. A. Davis Co., Phila., 1924

Cannula Implants and Review of Implantation Technics in Esthetic Surgery, by Charles C. Miller. Oak Printing and Pub. Co., Chicago, 1926

Correction chirurgicale des difformités congenitales et acquises de la pyramide na-

Esthetic Surgery – Cont.
sale, by Pierre Sebileau and Léon Dufourmentel. Arnette, Paris, 1927
Cosmetic paraffin injections in facial surgery. STEIN, R. O. Wien. klin. Wchnschr. *40:*830, June 23, '27
Nasenplastik und sonstige Gesichtsplastik. Nebst einem Anhang über Mammaplastik, by Jacques Joseph. C. Kabitsch, Leipzig, 1928
Chirurgie esthétique; le sein, by M. Virenque. Maloine, Paris, 1928
Plastic and esthetic surgery of face. DOBRZANIECKI, W. Polska gaz. lek. *7:*519–524, July 8, '28 also: Paris chir. *20:*129–142, July-Aug '28
Technic in aesthetic surgery of breast, face. LIBERA, D. Med. ital. *9:*629–636, Oct '28
Cosmetic operations. MONCORPS, C.: Zentralbl. f. Haut-u. Geschlechtskr. *28:*1–14, Oct. 5, '28
La chirurgie esthétique – nouveaux procedes de correction du prolapses mammaire. Noël, S., and Martinez, L.: Le Concour Medical, No. 46 (October 27, 1928)
Chirurgie correctrice du nez, by Léon Dufourmentel. University Press of France, Paris, 1929
Moderne Kosmetik unter besonderer Berücksichtigung der chirurgischen Kosmetik, by Martin Bab. Karger, Basel, 1929
Conservative cosmetic correction of legs. HARTWICH, A. Wien. med. Wchnschr. *79:*368–370, March 16, '29
Limits of esthetic surgery. PANGLOSS: Policlinico (sez. prat.) *36:*1087, July 29, '29
Medical responsibility in practice of cosmetic surgery. ROJAS, N. Rev. de especialid. *4:*520–527, July '29
Cosmetic operations. FRISCH, O. Wien. med. Wchnschr. *79:*1575–1577, Dec 7, '29
Die Förmfehler und die plastischen Operationen der weiblichen Brüst, by Erna Gläsmer. F. Enke, Stuttgart, 1930
Chirurgie esthétique pure, by Raymond Passot. Gaston Doin et Cie, Paris, 1930
Surgical sculpturing. BAMES, H. O., J. Coll. Surgeons, Australasia *3:*104–109, July '30
Esthetic surgery of pendulous breast, abdomen and arms in female. THOREK, M. Illinois M. J. *58:*48–57, July '30
Esthetic surgery. BAMES, H. O. California and West. Med. *33:*588–591, Aug '30
Cosmetic considerations in plastic surgery. KURTZAHN, Deutsche med. Wchnschr. *56:*1897–1900, Nov. 7, '30
Making of a Beautiful Face, or Face-Lifting Unveiled, by J. Howard Crum. Walton Book Co., New York, 1931

Esthetic Surgery – Cont.
Nasenplastik und sonstige Gesichtsplastik. Nebst einem Anhang über Mammaplastik und einege weitere Operationen as dem Gebiete der äusseren Körperplastik, by Jacques Joseph. C. Kabitsch, Leipzig, 1931
Chirurgische und konservative Kosmetik der Gesichtes, by Leander Pohl (editor). Urban and Schwarzenberg, München, 1931
Chirurgia plastica del naso, by Gustavo Sanvenero-Rosselli. Luigi Pozzi, Rome, 1931
Possibilities of esthetic remodeling of human form. THOREK, M. Tri-State M. J. *3:*621–622, July '31
Demonstrations of cosmetic surgery. SIMON, H. Beitr. z. klin. Chir. *154:*174–177, '31
Propos sur la chirurgie esthétique, by Charles Claoué. Maloine, Paris, 1932
Kosmetische Operationen, by Ernst Eitner. Springer-Verlag, Berlin, 1932
Korrektiv-cosmetische Chirurgie der Näse, der Ohren, und den Gesichts, by Victor Frühwald. Wilhelm Maudrich, Vienna, 1932 (Also English edition, translated by Geoffrey Morey)
La chirurgie esthétique, son role social, by A. Noél. Masson et Cie, Paris, 1926 (German translation by A. Hardt published by Barth, Leipzig, 1932)
Cosmesis and surgery. ÖHNGREN, G. Nord. med. tidskr. *4:*342–345, May 21, '32
Cosmetic corrections of the legs. BIESENBERGER, H. Wien. med. Wchnschr. *82:*735–738, June 4, '32
Technic of sutures in cosmetic surgery. KAPP, J. F. Fortschr. d. Med. *50:*967–968, Nov 11, '32
Chirurgie plastique des seins, by C. Montant and F. Dubois. Maloine, Paris, 1933
Social role of esthetic surgery. PALACIO POSSE, R. Semana med. *1:*330–335, Jan 26, '33
Cosmetic surgery in Dutch East Indies. RADO, T. Geneesk. tijdschr. v. Nederl.-Indie *73:*291–295, Feb 28 '33
Plastic operations of face, breast. HABERLAND, H. F. O. Zentralbl. f. Chir. *60:*746–748, March 31, '33
Esthetic surgery (face). BOURGUET, J. Bull. et mem. Soc. d. chirurgiens de Paris *25:*282–288, May 5, '33
Correction esthetique veineuses des mains. A. Noël. Bull. Medical, 14 Octobre, 1933
Development and present status of cosmetic surgery. RODRÍGUEZ BERCERUELO, S. Siglo med. *92:*436, Oct 21, '33
Esthetic surgery. GRACIA SIERRA, S. Clin. y lab. *23:*996–1000, Nov '33

Esthetic Surgery – Cont.

Sculpture in the Living, by Jacques W. Maliniak. Lancet Press, New York, 1934

Facts and fallacies of cosmetic surgery (paraffin injections, hair removal, face-lifting, nose-remodeling, etc.). MALINIAK, J. W. Hygeia *12:*200–202, March '34

Successful operative procedure for reshaping lower limbs. BLACKBURNE, G., J. M. Soc. New Jersey *31:*214–215, April '34

Facial and nasal plastic surgery from esthetic point of view. VILARDOSA LLUBES, E. Rev. de cir. de Barcelona *8:*1, July–Aug; 99, Sept–Dec '34

Corrective Rhinoplastic Surgery, by Joseph Safian. Paul Hoeber Co., New York, 1935

Esthetic surgery and its development. CODAZZI AGUIRRE, J. A. Semana med. *1:*1245–1248, April 25, '35

Restorative surgery of breast and face. MALINIAK, J. W. Bull. Assoc. d. med. de lang. franc. de l'Amerique du Nord *1:*199–206, April '35

Fundamental principles of esthetic surgery. MUNOZ ARENOS, J. M. Arch. de med., cir. y especialid. *38:*756–760, Nov 30, '35

Responsibility of surgeon in esthetic surgery; case. MANNA, A. Rev. de chir. structive, pp. 149–151, Dec '35

La véritable chirurgie esthétique du visage, by Julien Bourguet. Librairie Plon, Paris, 1936

Plastique mammaire, by Charles Claoué and Irene Bernard. Maloine, Paris, 1936

Chirurgie réparatrice: Plastique et esthétique de la poitrine, des seins, et de l'abdomen, by L. Dartigues. Lépine, Paris, 1936

Plastic Surgery of the Nose, by J. Eastman Sheehan. Paul Hoeber Co., New York, 1925. Second Edition, 1936

New Faces – New Futures: Rebuilding Character with Plastic Surgery, by Maxwell Maltz. Richard R. Smith, New York, 1936

Living Canvas: A Romance of Aesthetic Surgery, by Elisabeth Margetson. Methuen, London, 1936

Advances in plastic surgery (abdomen). HABERLAND, H. F. O. Zentralbl. f. Chir. *63:*154–156, Jan 18, '36

Esthetic surgery; cases. MALBEC, E. F. Semana med. *1:*31–51, Jan 2, '36

Progress of plastic and esthetic surgery in Buenos Aires. CODAZZI AGUIRRE, J. A. Semana med. *1:*464–467, Feb 6, '36

Further application of author's method of outlay on celluloid frame. (facial surgery). COELST. Rev. de chir. structive, pp. 195–198, March '36

Esthetic Surgery – Cont.

Esthetic surgery (of nose); cases. MALBEC, E. F. Semana med. *2:*1632–1643, Dec 10, '36

New method of plastic surgery in acquired external ear atresia. DOROSCHENKO, I. T. Arch. f. Ohren-, Nasen-u. Kehlkopfh. *141:*249–251, '36

Il viso. Igiene cutanea, terapia estetica, chirurgia plastica, by Libero Donato. Hoepli, Milan, 1938

As Others See You: The Story of Plastic Surgery, by Henry J. Schireson. Macauley, New York, 1938

Field of activity and methods of modern plastic surgery including cosmetic surgery. RAGNELL, A. Nord. med. tidskr. *15:*361–370, March 5, '38

Esthetic and psychologic principles of plastic surgery of nose, ear and face. WODAK, E. Monatschr. f. Ohrenh. *72:*424, April; 490, May '38

Esthetic and psychologic principles of plastic surgery (ear). (face). (nose) WODAK, E. Monatschr. f. Ohrenh. *72:*288–303, March '38

Esthetics of plastic surgery (face). BERNDORFER, A. Gyogyaszat *78:*638–641, Oct 30, '38

Use of celluloid in facial surgery. COELST, M. Rev. de chir. structive *8:*161–162, '38

Plastic and esthetic surgery of ear, nose and face; cases. MALBEC, E. F. Semana med. *1:*83–95, Jan 12, '39

Esthetic surgery; criteria or artistic precepts (nose). SCAVUZZO, R. Semana med. *1:*144–146, Jan 19, '39

Plastic and esthetic surgery; cases. CASTELLANO, J. L. and GIGANTI, I. J. Semana med. *1:*1337–1343, June 8, '39

Technical details of esthetic surgery. STAPLER, D. Ann. paulist. de med. e cir. *38:*101–108, Aug '39

Plastic surgery and esthetic feeling. ZENO, L. An. de cir. *5:*199–211, Sept '39

Chirurgie plastique abdominale; cure chirurgicale de ptose cutaneé abdominale, ventre en tablier, by Charles Claoué. Maloine, Paris, 1940

Esthetic surgery for elimination of sequals of smallpox of face in girl 18 years old. KANKAT, C. T. Turk tib cem. mec. *6:*260–266, '40

Plastic Surgery of the Breast and Abdominal Wall, by MAX THOREK. C C Thomas Co., Springfield, Ill., 1942

Economic considerations of cosmetic surgery. RENIE, R. O. Am. J. Surg. *55:*126–130, Jan '42

References to esthetic surgery in work of Hip-

Esthetic Surgery—Cont.
pocrates. CODAZZI AGUIRRE, J. A. Arq. de cir. clin. e exper. *6:*137-144, April-June, '42
Esthetic surgery and care of accident cases. MALBEC, E. F. Prensa med. argent. *30:*2359-2361, Dec 8, '43
Rural esthetic surgery. QUIROGA, P. Semana med. *2:*1454-1456, Dec. 30, '43
Cirugía estética, by Ramon Palacio Posse. El Ateñeo Press, Buenos Aires, 1946

ESTIÚ, M.D.: (see GIUSTINIAN, V.) July '32
ESTIENNY, E. (see GALY-GASPARROU, *et al*) March '28

Estlander Operation
Modification of Estlander's operation for lip defect. TWYMAN, E. D. Surg., Gynec. and Obst. *38:*824-825, June '24
Plastic method of correcting microstomia, particularly of type following Estlander cheiloplastic operation. TUOMIKOSKI, V. Acta chir. Scandinav. *70:*353-362, '33
Cheiloplasty by Estlander technic. ALFREDO, J. Rev. med. de Pernambuco *5:*233-237, June '35

ESTOR, E.: Exstrophy of bladder; junction of ureters with upper part of rectum; results 24 years after operation. J. d'urol. *22:*242-243, Sept '26
ETCHEVERRY, M.: Facial paralysis and its surgical correction; study apropos of promising result. Bol. y trab., Soc. argent. de cirujanos *6:*302-308, '45 also: Rev. Assoc. med. argent. *59:*844-846, July 30, '45
ETIENNE: Sydactylism; case. Arch. Soc. d. sc. med. et biol. de Montpellier *9:*409, Sept '28
ETIENNE, LAPEYRIE, AND PASSEBOIS: Creation of new bladder with aid of loop of small intestine in case of exstrophy. Arch. Soc. d. sc. med. et biol. de Montpellier *20:*285-291, June '39
ETIENNE, E. AND Déjean, C.: Enormous harelip with deep oblique fissure accompanied by coloboma of eyelid and iris; case. Arch. Soc. d. sc. med. et biol. de Montpellier *13:*94-99, Feb '32
ETIENNE, E. AND DUPONNOIS: Irreducible, metacarpophalangeal dislocation of index finger; presence of abnormal sesamoid; case. Arch. Soc. d. sc. med. et biol. de Montpellier *9:*106, March '28
ETZEL, E.: Gum acacia in shock; 80 cases. Rev. de cir. de Buenos Aires *14:*691-705, Dec '35
ETZEL, E. (see CORRÊA NETTO, A.) Nov '33
ETZEL, E. (see CORREIA NETTO, A.) Dec '35
EUVRARD, (see SARGNON) March '32
EUZIÈRE, J. *et al:* Acrocephalosyndactylia, microcephaly, ptosis of eyelids and infantilism; addition of acute spasmodic paraplegia. Arch. Soc. d. sc. med. et biol. de Montpellier *14:*110-119, March '33
EUZIÈRE, J.; VIDAL, J. AND MAS, P.: Facial and lingual hemiatrophy; case. Arch. Soc. d. sc. med. et biol. de Montpellier *15:*501-510, Aug '34
EVANS, E. I.: Plastic surgery; early repair of skin defects caused by severe burns. Bull. Am. Coll. Surgeons. *28:*142-143, June '43
EVANS, E. I. AND AIM, T. J. Plastic surgery of severe burns. Virginia M. Monthly *71:*342-350, July '44
EVANS, E. I. AND BIGGER, I. A.: Rationale of whole blood therapy in severe burns; clinical study. Ann. Surg. *122:*693-705, Oct '45
EVANS, E. I. AND HOOVER, M. J.: Sulfanilamide (sulfonamide) ointment treatment of severe burns. Surg., Gynec. and Obst. *77:*367-375, Oct '43
EVANS, E. I.; HOOVER, M. J. AND JAMES, G. W. III.: Sulfonamides (in ointment base); absorption from burn surface. Surg. Gynec. and Obst. *80:*297-302, March '45
EVANS, E. I.; JAMES, G. W. III. AND HOOVER, M. J.: Traumatic shock; restoration of blood volume in—Surgery *15:*420-431, March '44
EVANS, E. I. AND RAFAL, H. S.: Traumatic shock; treatment of clinical shock with gelatin. Tr. South. S. A. (1944) *56:*94-110, '45
EVANS, E. I. AND RAFAL, H. S.: Traumatic shock; treatment of clinical shock with gelatin (as plasma substitute). Ann. Surg. *121:*478-494, April '45
EVANS, G.: Trophic necrosis, skin grafting and vitamin C (in 2 cases of leg ulcers). Brit. M. J. *1:*788, June 26, '43
EVANS, J. G.: Sano tissue glue skin grafting. J. Internat. Coll. Surgeons *8:*424-425, Sept-Oct '45
EVANS, J. P. (see KREDEL, F. E.) June '33
EVANS, S. S.: Fractures about orbit. South. M. J. *26:*548-549, June '33
EVANS, W. A. AND LEUCUTIA, T.: Treatment of pigmented moles. and malignant melanomas. Am. J. Roentgenol. *26:*236-259, Aug '31
EVANS, W. J.: Tumors of eyelids. China M. J. *39:*145-146, Feb '25
EVERSOLE, U. H.: Anesthesia for surgery about head. J.A.M.A. *117:*1760-1764. Nov 22, '41
EVRARD, (see BÉRARD, *et al*) May '33
EVRARD, H. (see ISELIN, M.) Dec '31
EWALD, C.: Therapy of decubitus ulcers. Med. Klin. *33:*1202-1205, Sept. 3, '37
EWALD, P.: Treatment of rupture of extensor tendons of fingers. Zentralbl. f. Chir. *57:*714-715, March 22, '30

Ewig, W.: Shock and collapse. Zentralbl. f. inn. Med. *54:*690–704, Aug. 5, '33

Ewig, W. Collapse following burns. Verhandl. d. deutsch. Gesellsch. f. Kreislaufforsch., pp. 148–157, '38

Ewig, W. and Klotz, L.: Postoperative shock. Deutsche Ztschr. f. Chir. *235:*681–710, '32 also: Klin. Wchnschr. *11:*932–936, May 28, '32

Ewing, J.: Cancer of nose and mouth with special reference to treatment by irradiation. Radiology *9:*359–365, Nov '27

Ewing, M. R.: Congenital sinuses of external ear. J. Laryng. and Otol. *61:*18–23, Jan '46

Ewing Operation

Modified Ewing operation for cicatricial entropion. Smith, J. E. and Siniscal, A. A. Am. J. Ophth. *26:*382–389, April '43

Exophthalmos

Treatment of eyes in exophthalmic goiter. Dunphy, E. B., S. Clin. N. America *4:* 1439–1442, Dec '24

Exophthalmos, treatment by plastic surgery. Bourguet, J. Monde med., Paris *42:*104–113, Feb 15, '32

Surgical treatment of progressive exophthalmos following thyroidectomy. Naffziger, H. C. and Jones, O. W. Jr. J.A.M.A. *99:*638–642, Aug 20, '32

Surgical treatment of exophthalmos. Weeks, W. W. New York State J. Med. *33:*78–83, Jan. 15, '33

Traumatic exophthalmos and its treatment. Schie, E. Nord. med. (Norsk mag. f. laegevidensk.) *7:*1275–1283, July 27, '40

Decompressive trephining for malignant basedowian exophthalmos. Welti, H. and Offret, G. Mem. Acad. de chir. *68:*379–384, Oct. 28-Nov. 4, '42

Intractable and non-intractable exophthalmus; casues and surgical treatment. Poppen, J. L. Proc. Interst. Postgrad. M. A. North American (1942) pp. 266–269, '43

Diagnosis and surgical treatment of intractable cases of exophthalmus. Poppen, J. L. Am. J. Surg. *64:*64–79, April '44

Unilateral exophthalmos; case report of unusual result. Budetti, J. A. Ann. Otol. Rhin. and Laryng. *55:*434–439, June '46

Exposito, L.: Premature synostosis in children Rev. cubana pediat. *18:*497–508, Aug '46

Extremities (See also Burns; Contractures; Hands; Feet; Leg Ulcers; Lymphedema; War Injuries; Wringer Injuries)

Webbing of left arm. Manson, J. S. Lancet *1:*1182, June 4, '21

Extremities – Cont.

Operation for relief of flexion-contracture in forearm. Page, C. M., J. Bone and Joint Surg. *5:*233–234, April '23

Plastic repair of face and limbs. Shaw, J. J. M. Tr. Medico-Chir. Soc. Edinburgh, pp. 110–116, '22–'23 (illus.) in Edinburgh M. J., June '23

Treatment of weblike dermatogenic contractures of large joints. Loeffler, F. Zentralbl. f. Chir. *51:*681–683, March 29, '24

Plastic surgery in treatment of compound injuries of extremities. Garlock, J. H. Ann. Surg. *87:*321–354, March '28 abstr: Bull. New York Acad. Med. *4:*36–41, Jan '28

Replacement of scar over tibia and os calcis by tube pedicle transplant from abdomen. Jones, H. T., S. Clin. N. Amer. *9:*936–938, Aug '29

End results of covering amputation stumps with free fascia transplants. Ritter, C. Zentralbl. f. Chir. *56:*2565–2566, Oct. 12, '29

Plastic repair of extremities and face. Shaw, J. J. M. Tr. Roy. Med. -Chir. Soc., Glasgow (1927–1928) *22:*151, '29

Cleft palate and bilateral lack of development of upper extremities; case. Ryll-Nardzewska, J. Ginek. polska *11:*678–683, July–Sept '32

Skin-grafting of arm wound; successful outcome despite unusual difficulties. Salvin, A. A. Am. J. Surg. *26:*572–574, Dec '34

Congenital deformities of forearm, hand, and leg. Harris, H. E. Jr. Brit. M. J. *1:*711, April 19, '24

Skin flap methods in upper extremity deformities. Steindler, A., J. Bone & Joint Surg. *7:*512–527, July '25

Reconstructive surgery; case of congenital absence of arms. Mock, H. E., J.A.M.A. *86:*541–544, Feb 20, '26

Braun's skin grafting after amputations. Lihotzky, Med. Klin. *22:*1757–1758, Nov. 12, '26

Phalangization of stumps of forearm amputations (Putti-Krukenberg operation); 13 cases. Birckel, A. Strasbourg-med. (pt. 2) *85:*437–447, Dec 20, '27

Skin grafts on extremities. Pieri, G. Arch. ital. di chir. *18:*607–621, '27

Symmetric polydactylia and macromelia of upper and lower extremities. Shneyder, S. L. Sovet. khir. (no. 6) *6:*889–894, '34

Conservative surgical therapy of almost completely severed arm. Ehalt, W. Chirurg *7:*519–522, Aug 1, '35

Syndrome characterized by bilateral clubfoot and clubhand associated with special type

Extremities – Cont.
of amyotrophy of upper and lower extremities, dating from birth; case. THOMAS, A. AND HUC, G. Rev. neurol. *64:*918–925, Dec '35
Plastic surgery of elbow after transplantation of skin in ankylosis with cicatricial contracture; case. VON SEEMEN, H. Zentralbl. f. Chir. *63:*946–950, April 18, '36
Surgical treatment of congenital webbed skin across joints. MATOLCSY, T. Orvosi hetil. *80:*1159–1161, Dec 5, '36
Absence of hands and feet in Brazilian family; question of heredity of congenital abnormalities. KOEHLER, O. Ztschr. f. menschhl. Vererb. -u. Konstitutionslehre *19:*670–690, '36
Pedicle breast flap for amputation-stump; structive surgery applied to amputation stump at knee. ESSER, J. F. S. Ann. Surg. *105:*469–472, March '37
Plastic surgery of cutaneous lesion of leg due to amniotic adhesions. ZENO, L. An. de cir. *4:*14–15, March '38
Kineplastic surgery for amputated arms. MULVIHILL, D.A., S. Clin. North America *18:*467–481, April '38
Plastic surgery of amputation stumps. WEBSTER, J. P., S. Clin. North America *18:*441–466, April '38
Construction of the amputated shoulder in order to fit a prosthesis with a mechanical arm. COELST, Rev. de chir. structive *8:*117–122, Aug '38
Avulsion injuries to extremities in skiing. PETITPIERRE, M. Helvet. med. acta *6:*968–973, March '40
Amputation-plastic surgery with bone reversal. SCHÜRCH, O. Helvet. med. acta *6:*874, March '40
Diffuse phlemons of hand and forearm. MUNOZ ARENOS, J. M. Semana med. espan. *4:*167–171, Feb 15, '41
Reparative surgery of upper limb (in contractures of hands or arms) COLE, P. P Brit. J. Surg. *28:*585–607, April '41
Contracture therapy, extension treatment of shoulder joint. JORDE, A. AND MAGNUSSON, R. Nord. med. (Hygiea) *11:*2471–2474, Aug 30, '41
Crushing of extremities with resulting shock. CARVALHO LUZ, F. Brasil-med. *56:*35–41, Jan 17, '42
Surgical technic employed in therapy of extremely short stumps in amputations of thigh; preliminary report. DAINELLI, M. Policlinico (sez. prat.) *49:*377–383, Mar 16, '42

Extremities – Cont.
Therapy of flexion contracture of leg stumps. CORSI, G. Arch. ortop. *57:*320–340, Jul-Aug '42
Mangled forearm; treatment in skeleton splint with fixed skeletal traction. BROWN, D. Brit. M. J. *2:*425–426, Oct 10, '42
Surgical therapy of local gigantism of one leg resulting from congenital vascular abnormality. SCHERWITZ, K. Chirurg. *15:*263, May 1, '43
Giant epithelioma of lower extremity; roentgenotherapy and Reverdin grafts; case. CAMPOS MARTIN, R. AND USUA MARINE, J. Actas dermo-sif. *34:*747–750, June '43
Practical application of plastic surgery to extremities. MACEY, H. B., S. Clin. North America *32:*1030–1058, Aug '43
Reconstructive surgery following traumatic deformities of upper extremity. STEINDLER, A. Am. Acad. Orthop. Surgeons, Lect., pp. 268–279, '43
Management of injuries and infections of upper extremities. SILER, V. E., J.A.M.A. *124:*408–412, Feb 12, '44
Symposium on reparative surgery; cineplastic amputations. KESSLER, H. H., S. Clin. North America *24:*453–466, April '44
Symposium on reparative surgery after amputation. MOORHEAD, J. J., S. Clin. North America *24:*435–452, April '44
Open abdominal flaps for repair of surface defects of upper extremity. SHAW, D. T., S. Clin. North America *24:*293–308, April '44
Surface repair of compound injuries of extremities. BROWN, J. B., J. Bone and Joint Surg. *26:*448–454, July '44
Reconstructive surgery of extremities today; introduction. DAVIS, A. G., J. Bone and Joint Surg. *26:*435–436, July '44
Amputation surgery and plastic repair. THOMPSON, T. C. AND ALLDREDGE, R. H., J. Bone and Joint Surg. *26:*639–644, Oct '44
Adherent scars of lower extremity. WEBSTER, G. V., U.S. Nav. M. Bull. *43:*878–888, Nov '44
Use of flaps and pedicles in repair of hand and arm defects. KISKADDEN, W. S. Am. Acad. Orthop. Surgeons, Lect., pp. 180–183, '44
Skin defects of extremities. LEWIS, G. K. Am. Acad. Orthop. Surgeons, Lect., pp. 229–245, '44
Grave trauma of hand and forearm; biologic therapy of case. ZENO, L. Bol. y trab., Soc. argent. de cirujanos *5:*583–595, '44
Conservative treatment in grave trauma of arm and forearm. CEBALLOS, A. AND CAL-

Extremities – Cont.

ZETTA, J. C. Prensa med. argent. *32:*31–34, Jan 5, '45

Symposium on amputation from Naval Amputation Center, U.S. Naval Hospital, Mare Island, California; plastic surgery of stumps. O'CONNOR, G. B. AND KESSLER, H. H., U.S. Nav. M. Bull. *44:*1167–1180, June '45

Scar problem in compound injuries of lower leg. WEBSTER, G. V. Stanford M. Bull. *3:*109–113, Aug '45

Kineplasty of forearm. DE FARIA VAZ, J. Med. cir. farm. pp. 584–589, Oct '45

Bilateral complicated harelip with bilateral palpebral coloboma and left iridic coloboma; total ectromelia of right upper extremity. ROCHER, H. L. AND PESME. J. de med. de Bordeaux *121–122:*493–494, Oct '45

New plastic procedures for covering stumps. RAPIN. Mem. Acad. de chir. *71:*488, Nov 28–Dec 19, '45

Shock following injuries of extremities; procaine hydrochloride block of vagus nerve. ERMOLAEV, P. E. Khirurgiya, no. 6, pp. 45–46, '45

Use of tubular flap in amputations of extremities. KUKIN, N. I. Khirurgiya No. 6, pp. 83–86, '45

Present status of reconstructive surgery of organs of support and locomotion. NOVACHENKO, N. P. Vrach. delo (nos. 11–12) *25:*587–592, '45

Skin graft to cover defects in short stump of leg; modified technic. SMIRNOVA, L. A. Khirurgiya, No. 1, pp. 27–28, '45

Contiguous skin flaps for wounds of extremities. RUBIN, L. R. Am. J. Surg. *71:*36–54, Jan '46

Principles of cineplastic operations. BERGMANN, E. J. Internat. Coll. Surgeons *9:*99–103, Jan–Feb '46

Conditions involving elbow, forearm, wrist and hand; progress in orthopedic surgery for 1944. BLOUNT, W. P. Arch. Surg. *52:*197–209, Feb '46

Rehabilitation; plastic and reconstructive surgery of stumps. DUPERTUIS, S. M. AND HENDERSON, J. A., U.S. Nav. M. Bull. (supp.) pp. 65–77, Mar '46

Repair of surface defects of arms. SHAW, D. T. AND PAYNE, R. L. JR. Ann. Surg. *123:*705–730, May '46

Dermoepidermal grafts in grave traumas of upper extremity; case. BULFARO, J. A. H. Bol. y trab. Soc. argent. de cirujanos *7:*340–343, '46 also: Rev. Asoc. med. argent. *60:*605–606, July 15, '46

Extremities – Cont.

Case of tumors resembling hemangiomatosis of lower extremity. KING, D. J., J. Bone and Joint Surg. *28:*623–628, July '46

Treatment of loss skin substance in surgery of extremities. DUCHET, G. Semaine d. hop. Paris *22:*1671–1680, Sept 21, '46

Cineplastic forearm amputations and prostheses. RANK, B. K. AND HENDERSON, G. D. Surg. Gynec. and Obst. *83:*373–386, Sept '46

Covering defects of popliteal space with skin grafts. SCHURCH, O. Schweiz. med. Wchnschr. *76:*1040–1041, Oct 5, '46

Guillotine amputation modified to preserve skin flaps. MEYER, N. C., U.S. Nav. Bull. *46:*1844–1847, Dec '46

Repair of surface defects of upper extremity. SHAW, D. T. AND PAYNE, R. L., JR. Tr. South. S. A. (1945) *57:*243–268, '46

Eye, Burns of

Treatment of lime burn of eye. BARKAN, O. AND BARKAN, H., J.A.M.A. *83:*1567–1569, Nov 15, '24

Phenol burns of left eyelids, eyeball, upper face and temporal area. SHEEHAN, J. E. Laryngoscope *35:*55, Jan '25

Case after operation for extensive burn of left lids, eyeball, upper face and temporal area. SHEEHAN, J. E., M. J. and Rec. *121:*291–292, March 4, '25

Treatment of lime burns of cornea by 10 per cent neutral ammonium tartrate. WOLFF, E. Brit. J. Ophth. *10:*196–197, April '26

Favorable results of iridectomy in case of ammonia burn of eyes. THIES, O. Klin. Monatsbl. f. Augenh. *79:*534–536, Oct 28, '27

Transplantation of oral mucosa in diseases of cornea and burns of eyes. DENIG, R. Arch. f. Ophth. *118:*729–737, '27

Acid and alkali burns of eyes; experimental study. COSGROVE, K. W. AND HUBBARD, W. B. Ann. Surg. *87:*89–94, Jan '28

Ammonia burns of eyes. THIES, O. Zentralbl. f. Gewerbehyg. *5:*83–88, March '28

Early plastic operation (transplantation of oral mucosa) in caustic injuries of eye. THIES, O. Arch. f. Ophth. *123:*165–170, '29

Destruction of capsule of crystalline lens by fire. KRAUPA, E. Klin. Monatsbl. f. Augenh. *87:*397, Sept '31

Plastic surgery in cicatrices of eyelid caused by burn; case. ROY, J. N. Bull. med. de Quebec *32:*322–328, Oct '31

Extensive cicatrix of face; reconstruction of both eyelids and of both lips by tubular

Eye, Burns of–Cont.
grafts. Rocher, H. L. Bull. et mem. Soc. de chir. de Bordeaux et du Sud-Ouest, pp. 154–156, '32
Early grafting of mucous membrane in burns of eye. O'Connor, G. B. Arch. Ophth. *9:*48–51, Jan '33
Burns due to sulfur dioxide of eyes; 2 cases. Detroy. Echo med. du Nord *4:*742bis-743, Oct 27, '35
Application of grafts early in burns of eye. O'Connor, G. B. Rev. de chir. structive, pp. 273–277, June '36
Immediate treatment of eye injuries including burns. Ruedemann, A. D., S. Clin. North America *16:*979–989, Aug '36
Chemical burns to eyes. Moss, O. W. New Orleans M. and S. J. *89:*302–306, Dec '36
Chemical burns to eyes. Berezinskaya, D. I. Sovet. vestnik oftal. *8:*319–332, '36
Burns to eyes with sulfuric acid. Coppez, J. H. and Brenta, Mme. Bull. Soc. belge d'opht., no. 72, pp. 88–100, '36
Alkali burns to eyes; experimental study. Vinogorov, D. R. and Kopit, R. Z. Sovet. vestnik oftal. *8:*333–347, '36
Denig operation for burns of eyes. Avizonis, V. Medicina, Kaunas *19:*309–315, April '38
Caustic burns of eyes. Hubbard, W. B. Arch. Ophth. *19:*968–975, June '38
Management of burns of cornea. Culler, A. M. Ohio State M. J. *34:*873–878, Aug '38
Role of paracentesis in therapy of chemical burns to eyes. Berezinskaya, D. I. Vestnik oftal. *13:*361–367, '38
Reasons for early operation in cases of severe burns of eyes. Thies, O. Arch. f. Ophth. *138:*686–692, '38
Paraffin film treatment of burns of eyelids. Shuman, G. H. Pennsylvania M. J. *42:*907–909, May '39
Phenol burns of both eyes and their general sequels; therapy of chemical burns. Winkler, A. Klin. Monatsbl. f. Augenh. *102:*810–815, June '39
First aid in case of burns of eye due to lime. Kaplan, Y. D. Vestnik oftal. (nos. 2–3) *14:*114–118, '39
Therapy of ocular burns by transplantation of conjunctiva from cadaver. Zenkina, L. V. Vestnik oftal. (no. 2) *15:*28–29, '39
Mucosal graft in therapy of corneoconjunctival burns. von Grolman, G. Arch. de oftal. de Buenos Aires *15:*429–434, Sept '40 also: Rev. med. y cien. afines *2:*629–632, Sept 30, '40
Rational therapy of chemical burns to eyes. Bursuk, G. G. and Shults, V. A. Vestnik oftal. *17:*55–56, '40

Eye, Burns of–Cont.
Surgical therapy of chemical burns to eyes. Dashevskiy, A. I. and Marmorshteyn, F. F. Vestnik oftal. *16:*415–420, '40
Bilateral burns to eyes; case. Fink, M. V. Vestnik oftal. *16:*509–510, '40
Chemical burns to eyes. Rameev, R. S. Vestnik oftal. *16:*381–383, '40
Local application of cod liver oil in therapy of burns of eyes. Tikhova, V. A. Vestnik oftal. *17:*396–397, '40
Severe chemical burns to eyes. Thies, O. Klin. Monatsbl. f. Augenh. *106:*47–56, Jan '41
Conjunctival burn due to ammonia treated by Denig method (excision of tissue and graft of buccal mucosa); case. von Grolman, G. Prensa med. argent. *28:*839–840, April 16, '41
Burn of eyes caused by brilliant green. Krückels, H. Klin. Monatsbl. f. Augenh. *106:*571–574, May '41
Electric accidents to eyes; shock, burns and glare injuries. Fisher, H. E. Arch. Phys. Therapy *22:*611–617, Oct '41
Lime burns to eyes; use of rabbit peritoneum to prevent severe delayed effects; experimental studies and report of cases. Brown, A. L. Arch. Ophth. *26:*754–769, Nov '41
Lime burns to eye; use of rabbit peritoneum to prevent severe delayed effects; experimental studies and report of cases. Brown, A. L. Tr. Sect. Ophth., A.M.A., pp. 40–57, '41
Treatment of burns of eyes and face with sulfhydryl solution (hydrosulphosol). Cruthirds, A. E. Indust. Med. *11:*109–112, March '42
Ophthalmic injuries (including burns) of war. Matthews, J. L. War Med. *4:*247–261, Sept '43
Discussion on burns of eyelids and conjunctiva. Wakeley, C. P. G. *et al.* Proc. Roy. Soc. Med. *37:*29–33, Nov '43
Buccal mucous membrane grafts in treatment of burns of eye. Siegel, R. Arch. Ophth. *32:*104–108, Aug '44
Burn of cornea and conjunctiva; how to prevent symblepharon. Pavia, J. L. Rev. otoneuro-oftal. *19:*159–171, Nov-Dec '44 also: Semana med. *2:*1117–1122, Dec 7, '44
Early transplantation of buccal mucosa and conjunctiva in chemical burns of eyes. Pavisic, Z. Ophthalmologica *108:*297–304, Dec '44
Improved treatment for chemical burns of eye. Oaks, L. W. Am. J. Ophth. *28:*370–373, April '45

Eye, Burns of – Cont.

Transplantation of mucous membrane (Denig operation) in severe burns of eyes. MITERSTEIN, B. AND KORNBLUETH, W. Harefuah *29:*152, Oct 1, '45

Eye Prostheses

Articulated prosthesis of eye, nose and upper lip; case. PONT, A. AND LAPIERRE, V. Rev. de chir. structive, pp. 38–41, March '37

Prostheses for eye and orbit. BROWN, A. M. Arch. Ophth. *32:*208–212, Sept '44

Eyelid surgery for partial contraction of socket. GREEVES, R. A. Tr. Ophth. Soc. U. Kingdom *47:*101–106, '27

Enucleation of eye-ball and cartilage transplantation as basis for prosthesis. FABER, A. Beitr. z. klin. Chir. *141:*524–527, '27

Operative treatment for sunken upper lid following enucleation. LÖWENSTEIN, A. Klin. Monatsbl. f. Augenh. *80:*233–236, Feb 24, '28

Transplantation of fat in enucleation of eye. LINDBERG, J. G. Finska lak.-sallsk. handl. *70:*898–902, Nov '28

Reconstruction of conjunctival culdesac and eyelid in patients after enucleation of eye; technic. DAMEL, C. S. Rev. Asoc. med. argent. *47:*2733–2738, June '33

Construction of artificial conjunctival sac by free transplantation of epidermis as preliminary to prosthesis. HERSCHENDÖRFER, A. Ztschr. f. Augenh. *84:*284–292, Nov '34

Free skin grafts in restoration of defects of conjunctival oral mucous membranes and cutaneous defects of nasal fossae. LIMBERG, A. A. Sovet. khir. (nos. 3–4) *6:*462–482, '34

Fixation of artificial eye in conjunctival sac made of skin graft. CSAPODY, I. Budapesti orvosi ujsag *33:*337–343, April 11, '35

New method for construction of artificial conjunctival sac by transplantation of skin flap divided into 2 parts. VON CSAPODY, I. Ztschr. f. Augenh. *87:*114–130, Sept '35

Reconstruction of orbital cavity for wearing prosthesis long after exenteration of orbit. LOTIN, A. V. Sovet. vestnik oftal. *7:*402, '35

Restoration of orbit and repair of conjunctival defects, with grafts from prepuce and labia minora. CLAY, G. E. AND BAIRD, J. M. Tr. Sect., Ophth. A.M.A., pp. 252–259, '36

Skin grafting after enucleation of eye; case. MOERS. Rev. de chir. structive, pp. 119–120, June '37

Plastic construction of artificial conjunctival sac using skin flaps. CSAPODY, I. Orvosi hetil. *81:*1217–1219, Dec 4, '37

Total symblepharon after enucleation of eye; remaking of orbital cavity for ocular prosthesis by means of dermo-epidermic graft; case. JEANDELIZE, P. AND THOMAS, C. Bull. Soc. d'opht. de Paris *50:*272, May '38

Transplantation of conjunctiva from cadaver. ROZENTSVEYG, M. G. Vestnik oftal. (nos. 2–3) *14:*26–36, '39

New method for formation of stump after enucleation by transplantation of cadaver's cartilage into Tenon's capsule of eye. SVERDLOV, D. G. Vestnik oftal. (nos. 5–6) *19:*45–50, '41

Reconstruction of contracted eye socket. HUGHES, W. L. Tr. Am. Soc. Plastic and Reconstructive Surg. *12:*25–28, '43

Plastic surgery of eye cavity. LECH, JR. Arq. Inst. Penido Burnier *7:*30–56, Dec '45

Fascia lata transplant for retrotarsal atrophy of upper lid following enucleation. CUTLER, N. L. Am. J. Ophth. *29:*176–179, Feb '46

Plastic restoration of upper lid and socket. LUC, J. Brit. J. Ophth. *30:*665–668, Nov '46

Eyebrows

Vertical skin-grafts for reconstruction of eyebrows. BUNNELL, S. Surg., Gynec. and Obst. *53:*239–240, Aug '31

Grafting of hairy skin with aid of pedunculated flap for formation of eyebrows, mustache and beard. PARIN, V. N. Vestnik khir. (nos. 73–74) *24:*10–12, '31

Destruction of skin of face by irradiation of birthmark in early life; restoration of nose by rhinoplasty, correction of lip by plastic operation, restoration of eyebrow by implantation of narrow flap from hairy scalp, restoration of upper eyelid by full-thickness graft from thigh. BABCOCK, W. W., S. Clin. North America *12:*1409–1410, Dec '32

Eyebrow alopecias and their therapy. PIGNOT, M. Presse med. *46:*843–844, May 25, '38

Rare congenital malformation of eyelid, eyebrow, scalp and of eyeball; case. VALERIO, M. Ann. di ottal. e clin. ocul. *67:*704–714, Sept '39

Living graft of eyebrows in leprosy. ARAUJO, D. G. AND BERTI, A. Rev. brasil. de leprol. (num. espec.) *8:*7–13, '40

Free graft of scalp in repair of alopecia of eyebrows. SILVEIRIA, L. M. Arq. de cir. clin. e exper. *6:*689–692, April – June '42

Successful modern plastic surgery in serious disfiguration due to scalping; reconstruction of eyelids and eyebrows and replacement of total skin of forehead and temples.

Eyebrows – Cont.
von Seemen, H. Zentralbl. f. Chir. *69:*1280–1287, Aug 1, '42

Eyelids (See also Blepharoplasty; Blepharoptosis; Blepharospasm; Enophthalmos; Epicanthus; Exophthalmos; Lacrimal Apparatus; Lagophthalmos)

Correction of scar tissue deformities by epithelial grafts, report of 5 cases. (including eyelids) Spaeth, E. B. Arch. Surg. *2:*176, Jan '21
Plastic surgery of eyelids and orbit. Waldron, C. W. Minnesota Med. *4:*504, Aug '21
New principles in plastic operations of eyelids and face. Imre, J. Jr. J. A. M. A. *76:*1293, May 7, '21
Plastic repair of eyelids by pedunculated skin grafts. Cross, G. H., J. A. M. A. *77:*1233, Oct 15, '21
Plastic surgery in and about eyelids. Nutting, R. J. California State J. Med. *20:*15–16, Jan '22
Use of epidermic graft in plastic eye surgery. Wheeler, J. M. Internat. Clinics *3:*292–302, '22 (illus.)
Plastic operation for palpebro-facial deformity. Lehrfeld, L. Am. J. Ophth. *6:*895–898, Nov '23 (illus.)
Newer Methods of Ophthalmic Plastic Surgery, by Edmund B. Spaeth. Blakiston Co., Phila., 1925
Autoplastic skin implant in blepharoplasty. d'Alessandro, Semana med. *2:*1531–1534, Dec 17, '25
Plastic operations on face, in region of eye. Various Authors Proc. Roy. Soc. Med. (sect. Ophth.) *19:*14–38, June '26
Autoplastic operation on lower margin of tarsus for ingrown eyelash. Shimkin, N. Klin. Monatsbl. f. Augenh. *77:*538–546, Oct 30, '26
Ophthalmic plastic surgery; clinical procedure in certain cases. Parker, W. R. Am. J. Ophth. *10:*109–113, Feb '27
Utilization of skin of upper eyelid for repair of small facial defects. Sheehan, J. E. Arch. Otolaryng. *6:*107–111, Aug '27
Ocular complications from local anesthesia in resection of upper jaw. Doron, G. Zentralbl. f. Chir. *54:*2966–2969, Nov. 19, '27
Round movable pedicles in complicated plastic operations on eyelids and face. Filatow, W. P. Arch. f. klin. Chir. *146:*609–614, '27
Corrective surgery of eyelids. and nose. Atkinson, D. T. J. Ophth., Otol. and Laryng. *32:*73–82, March '28

Eyelids – Cont.
Plastic repair of right lower eyelid. McKee, S. H. Canad. M. A. J. *18:*307–308, March '28
Transplantation of eyelid tissue. von Gernet, R. Klin. Monatsbl. f. Augenh. *80:*496, April 27, '28
Eyelid surgery, technic; case. Dupuy-Dutemps, L. Bull. Soc. d'opht. de Paris, pp. 315–318, July '28
Plastic surgery about eyes. Bettman, A. G. Ann. Surg. *88:*994–1006, Dec '28
Circumcorneal transplantation of oral mucosa as curative measure in diseases of eye. Denig, R. Arch. Ophth. *1:*351–357, March '29
Two cases of eyelid repair. McKee, S. H. Canad. M. A. J. *20:*506–508, May '29
Treatment of eyelid abnormalities by plastic surgery. Bourguet, J. Monde med., Paris *39:*725–731, July 1, '29
Plastic surgery of eyelid. Menestrina, G. Boll. d'ocul. *8:*667–685, July '29
Machine for shaping skinflaps in anaplasty of eyelids. Lénárd, E. Klin. Monatsbl. f. Augenh. *83:*526–530, Oct–Nov '29
Palpebrosuperciliary autoplasty; case. Agnantis, C. Ann. d'ocul. *167:*226–229, March '30
Plastic surgery of eyelid using cervical flap with tubular pedicle; case. Dupuy-Dutemps, L. Ann. d'ocul. *167:*895–907, Nov '30 also: Bull. et mem. Soc. franc. d'opht. *43:*451–458, '30
How an eye was saved by plastic surgery. Mauldin, L. O., J. South Carolina M. A. *26:*299–300, Dec '30
Autoplastic graft of conjunctiva and of eyelid; 2 cases. Déjean, C. Arch. Soc. d. sc. med. et biol. de Montpellier *12:*23–25, Jan '31
Two new methods of plastic surgery of eyelids. Blanco, T. Arch. de oftal. hispano-am. *31:*79–84, Feb '31
Skin grafts in repair of ocular lesions from pemphigus (eyelids). Terrien, F. *et al* Arch. d'opht. *48:*275–281, April '31
Plastic operation for denudation of nasolacrimal region. Favaloro, G. Rassegna ital. d'ottal. *1:*197–209, March–April '32
New eyelid clamp. Cruickshank, M. M. Indian M. Gaz. *67:*82–83, Feb '32 also: Am. J. Ophth. *15:*349, April '32
Pedicled flap in plastic surgery of eyelids. Spaeth, E. B. Pennsylvania M. J. *35:*560–562, May '32
Biological principles which underlie plastic surgery of eyelids. Spaeth, E. B. Am. J. Ophth. *15:*589–603, July '32

Eyelids – Cont.
Repairs and adjustments of eyelids. BLAIR, V. P., J. A. M. A. *99:*2171–2176, Dec 24, '32
Repairs and adjustments of eyelids. BLAIR, V. P. Tr. Sect. Ophth., A. M. A., pp. 328–341, '32
Argumosa blepharoplastic methods. MÁRQUEZ, M. Arch. de oftal. hispano-am. *33:*1–8, Jan '33
Therapy of positional abnormalities of eyelids. ONKEN, T. Klin. Monatsbl. f. Augenh. *90:*78–79, Jan '33
Partial cryptophthalmos with epicanthus and congenital ptosis of upper eyelid; author's technic for surgical correction; 2 cases. SATANOWSKY, P. Arch. de oftal. hispano-am. *33:*643–652, Nov '33
Plastic surgery of eyelids. GLEZEROV, S. Y. Sovet. vestnik oftal. *3:*305–307, '33
Homotransplantation of mucous membrane in ophthalmic surgery. MITSKEVICH, L. D. Sovet. vestnik oftal. *3:*299–302, '33
Eyelid flaps. ESSER, J. F. S. Rev. de chir. plastique, pp. 295–297, Jan '34
Reconstructive surgery in ophthalmology and otolaryngology. GILL, W. D. Texas State J. Med. *29:*616–622, Feb '34
Correction of ocular disfigurements. WIENER, M. Surg., Gynec. and Obst. *58:*390–394, Feb (no. 2A) '34
Plastic surgery in removal of excessive cutaneous tissues obstructing vision. KAHN, K. New York State J. Med. *34:*781–783, Sept 1, '34
Plastic repair of congenital and acquired deformities of palpebral margin by means of cartilage from auricle. LÖWENSTEIN, A. Klin. Monatsbl. f. Augenh. *93:*320–323, Sept '34
Radium as adjuvant to operation in case of deformity of eyelids from burn with keloid scars. HUDSON, A. C. Proc. Roy. Soc. Med. *27:*1611, Oct '34
Closure of defects of lower eyelid on side nearest to nose by means of skin grafts from nose. KRAUPA, E. Ztschr. f. Augenh. *84:*216–217, Oct '34
Operations on eyelids in Foville syndrome; case. COPPEZ, J. H. J. belge de neurol. et de psychiat. *35:*206–208, April '35
External canthal ligament in surgery of lower eyelid. HILDRETH, H. R. Am. J. Ophth. *18:*437–439, May '35
Extensive destruction of eyelids and skin of face caused by lupus and syphilis; surgical therapy. RAUH, W. Ztschr. f. Augenh. *86:*193–199, June '35
Plastic surgery of eyelids. GILLIES, H. D. Tr. Ophth. Soc. U. Kingdom *55:*357–373, '35

Eyelids – Cont.
Comparative evaluation of marginoplastic operations of eyelids. LUZHINSKIY, G. F. Sovet. vestnik oftal. *7:*137–142, '35
Euroblepharon; case. WEVE, H. Nederl. tijdschr. v. geneesk. *80:*1213–1217, March 21, '36
Lesions of eye with permanent disfigurement of face; medicolegal study of case. CUCCO, A. Riv. san. siciliana *24:*137–141, Feb 1, '36
Restoration of orbit and repair of conjunctival defects, with grafts from prepuce and labia minora. CLAY, G. E. AND BAIRD, J. M. J. A. M. A. *107:*1122–1125, Oct 3, '36
Sources of grafts for plastic surgery about eyes. WHEELER, J. M. New York State J. Med. *36:*1372–1376, Oct 1, '36
Surgical therapy of cicatricial trachoma. ABDULAEV, G. G. Sovet. vestnik oftal. *8:*712–715, '36
Instruments for eyelid treatment. HEATH, P. Tr. Sect. Ophth., A. M. A., pp. 272–273, '36 also: Arch. Ophth. *17:*894–895, May '37
Fate of implanted tissue in eyelid after Schneller operation. RYBNIKOVA, O. I. Sovet. vestnik oftal. *9:*324–325, '36
Marginal cutaneous blepharopexy in plastic surgery. DUPUY-DUTEMPS, L. Ann. d'ocul. *174:*312–317, May '37
Use of mucous membrane in ophthalmic surgery. SPAETH, E. B. Am. J. Ophth. *20:*897–907, Sept '37
Skin grafts in certain cutaneous diseases and corneal transplants. FILATOV, V. P. Med. zhur. *7:*743–753, '37 also: Vestnik oftal. *11:*295–310, '37
Technic of median nonmutilating blephorrhaphy. KLEEFELD, G. Bull. Soc. belge d'opht., no. 74, pp. 16–21, '37
Autoplasty of eyelids. LEONARDI. Bull. et mem. Soc. franc. d'opht. *50:*20–24, '37
Blepharoplasty by means of free transplants of skin. LEVITSKIY, M. A. Vestnik oftal. *11:*798–802, '37
Experimental studies on transplantation of conjunctiva from eye of cadaver; preliminary report. ROZENTSVEVG, M. G. Vestnik oftal. *11:*311–316, '37
Plastic surgery of eyelids; use of pedicled flaps with handle. VON SEEMEN, H. Deutsche Ztschr. f. Chir. *248:*411–419, '37
New experiences with plastic construction of artificial conjunctival sac, using flaps. VON CSAPODY, I. Ztschr. f. Augenh. *94:*23–33, Jan '38
Pedicled dermomuscular blepharoplasty; 12 cases. CHARAMIS, J. S. Arch. d'opht. *2:*206–218, March '38

Eyelids – Cont.
Paradental cyst of upper maxillary sinus with fistulization into lower eyelid; case. (Palpebral fistula). PIQUET, J. AND DETROY, L. Echo med. du Nord *9:*337–339, June 30, '38
Plastic surgery of eyelids. KREIBIG, W. Ztschr. f. Augenh. *95:*269–275, Aug '38
Advantages of use of coagulants, especially in plastic operations on eyes. BUSACCA, A. Arch. Ophth. *20:*406–409, Sept '38
Biologic frontal flaps in eyelid surgery. ESSER, J. F. S. Am. J. Ophth. *21:*963–967, Sept '38
Review of some modern methods for plastic surgery of eyes. SPAETH, E. B. Am. J. Surg. *42:*89–100, Oct '38
Use of orbicularis palpebrarum muscle in eyelid surgery. WHEELER, J. M. Am. J. Surg. *42:*7–9, Oct '38
Plastic operation of eyelids. IMRE, J. Tr. Ophth. Soc. U. Kingdom (pt. 2, 1937) *57:*494–508, '38
Technic of Millingen-Sapezhko operation (eyelid). MITSKEVICH, L. D. Vestnik oftal. *13:*848–849, '38
Hemiatrophy of face with eye complications. BAKER, H. Proc. Roy. Soc. Med. *32:*364–365, Feb '39
Discussion on plastic surgery of eyelids. KILNER, T. P. AND IMRE, J. Proc. Roy. Soc. Med. *32:*1247–1260, Aug '39
Operation in patient with large eyelids and maintained levator function. FAZAKAS, A. Klin. Monatsbl. F. Augenh. *103:*621–624, Dec '39
Modification of Millingen-Sapezhko operation (eyelids). MINEEV, P. Vestnik oftal. (no. 2) *15:*40–42, '39
Plastic surgery about eye and orbit. SPAETH, E. B. Tr. Indiana Acad. Ophth. and Otolaryng. *23:*81–83, '39
Free full-thickness grafts of skin to eyelids; cases. ZENO, L. Bol. Soc. de cir. de Rosario *7:*127–135, May '40 also: An. de cir. *6:*156–164, June '40
History of total transplantation of eyeball. AYRES, F. Arq. brasil. de oftal. *3:*305–310, Dec '40
Plastic surgery of eyelids. SHANKS, J. M. Rec. *152:*408, Dec 4, '40
Placenta as plastic material in eye surgery. BARKHASH, S. A. Vestnik oftal. *17:*758–761, '40
New studies on brephoplastic grafts. MAY, R. M. Arch. d'anat. micr. *35:*147–199, '40
Elimination of cicatricial ectropion by free Thiersch graft. MÜLLER, P. Schweiz. med. Wchnschr. *71:*5–6, Jan 4, '41

Eyelids – Cont.
Plastic repair of deformities of eyelids. MORGAN, A. L. Canad. M. A. J. *44:*560–562, June '41
Further data on therapeutic value of preserved tissue, especially in ocular diseases; transplantation of tissues and use of placental microclusters; preliminary report. FILATOV, V. P. Gaz. clin. *39:*292–295, Aug '41
Transplantation of conjunctiva of cadaver; clinical and histologic aspects. SIE BOEN LIAN. Geneesk. tijdschr. v. Nederl.-Indie *81:*2097–2101, Sept 30, '41
Some phases of plastic surgery about eye. Mc LEAN, J. M. Mississippi Doctor *19:*335–339, Dec '41
Tubed pedicle skin graft to eyelids. SIE BOEN LIAN. Geneesk. tijdschr. v. Nederl.-Indie *81:*2781–2784, Dec 30, '41
Measuring force of elevation of upper eyelid and its clinical significance; description of apparatus. MULLER, H. K. AND LANGGUTH, H. Arch. f. Ophth. *144:*234–246, '41
Successful modern plastic surgery in serious disfiguration due to scalping; reconstruction of eyelids and eyebrows and replacement of total skin of forehead and temples. VON SEEMEN, H. Zentralbl. f. Chir. *69:*1280–1287, Aug 1, '42
Plastic surgery of eyelids. AJO, A. Nord. med. *15:*2437–2440, Sept 5, '42
Cure of depression of lower eyelid following reinsertion of inferior rectus muscle; case. INCIARDI, J. A. Arch. Ophth. *28:*464–466, Sept '42
Use of Padgett dermatome in ophthalmic plastic surgery. SMITH, B. Arch. Ophth. *28:*484–489, Sept '42
Synkinesis between third and seventh pairs of cranial nerves (of musculus levator palpebrae superioris and of musculus zygomaticus respectively); similarity to Marcus Gunn phenomenon; case. AZZOLINI, U. Riv. oto-neuro-oftal. *19:*398–412, Nov-Dec '42
Recent advances in eyelid surgery. HAGUE, E. B. Dis. Eye, Ear, Nose and Throat *2:*353–359, Dec '42
"Pocket-flap" as method for total restoration of eyelid; preliminary report. KURLOV, I. N. Vestnik oftal. (nos. 1–2) *20:*12–19, '42
Operations for trachomatous eversion of eyelids and trichiasis. MAKHLIN, I. M. Sovet. med. (nos. 1–2) *6:*22–23, '42
Resection of left inferior oblique muscle at its scleral attachment for postoperative left hypotropia and left pseudoptosis. BERENS,

Eyelids – Cont.

C. AND LOUTFALLAH, M. Am. J. Ophth. *26:*528–533, May '43

Useful plastic procedures of eyes. PIERCE, G. W. Tr. Am. Acad. Ophth. (1943) *48:*309–322, May–June '44

Plastic surgery of eyelids. SUAREZ VILLAFRANCA, M. R. Arch. Soc. oftal. hispano-am. *4:*816–838, Sept–Oct '44

Minor surgery of eyelids. ALVIS, B. Y. Tr. Indiana Acad. Ophth. and Otolaryng. *28:*78–93, '44

Restoration of vision after crossing of optic nerves and after contralateral transplantation of eye. SPERRY, R. W., J. Neurophysiol. *8:*15–28, Jan '45

Two rare cases of homoplastic surgery of eyelids. SHIMKIN, N. I. Brit. J. Ophth. *29:*363–369, July '45

Plastic surgical repair about eyes with free grafts. SCHULTZ, A. AND JAECKLE, C. E. Arch. Ophth. *34:*103–106, Aug '45

Use of cautery in plastic operations of eyelids. SIMPSON, D. Brit. M. J. *2:*424–425, Sept 29, '45

Plastic procedures of eyelids. PUNTENNEY, I. Illinois M. J. *88:*238–242, Nov '45

Factor in repair of wounds of eyelids. RANKIN, C. A. Pennsylvania M. J. *49:*258–259, Dec '45

Conjunctival palpebral autoplasty. BELFORT MATTOS, W. Arq. brasil. de oftal. *8:*103–109, '45

Surgery of eyelids. LODGE, W. O., J. Internat. Coll. Surgeons *9:*383–388, May–June '46

Repair of eyelids and periorbital structures. RANK, B. K. Tr. Ophth. Soc. Australia (1944) *4:*84–97, '46

Eyelids, Cancer

Carcinoma of eyelids treated with radium. WITHERS, S. Am. J. Ophth. *4:*8, Jan '21

Case of epithelioma of outer canthus of eye. MEYER, H. W., S. Clin. N. Amer. *1:*1643, Dec '21

Transplantation flap repair of lower eyelid following removal of epithelioma. MINCHEW, B. H., J. M. A. Georgia *11:*110–111, March '22

Case of sarcoma of eyelids. FISHER, J. A. Am. J. Ophth. *7:*619–620, Aug '24

Buediner's modification of Dieffenbach's operation for early epithelioma of lower lid. WRIGHT, R. E. Brit. J. Ophth. *8:*58–61, Feb '24

Sarcoma of eyelid. SATANOWSKY, P. Semana med. *2:*169–177, July 23, '25 abstr: J. A. M. A. *85:*1264, Oct 17, '25

Eyelids, Cancer – Cont.

Treatment of epithelioma of face and eyelid. SIMPSON, C. A. Virginia M. Monthly *52:*337–340, Sept '25

Skin grafting in 2 cases of epithelioma of eyelids. MORAX, V. Ann. d'ocul. *164:*6–15, Jan '27

Superiority of radium to surgery in cancer of eyelids; cures without risk of recurrence, mutilation or pain. DEGRAIS, P. AND BELLOT, A. Bull. Soc. d'opht. de Paris, no. 9, pp. 536–544, '27 also: Clinique, Paris *22:*397–403, Oct (B) '27

Cancer in right eye; unsuccessful radium therapy; extended exeresis and graft of medio-frontal, pediculated flap; 2 photographs. NIDA. Bull. Soc. d'opht. de Paris, no. 9, pp. 532–536, '27

Cancer of eyelid; radium therapy; case. CAPIZZANO, N. Bol. Inst. de med. exper. para el estud. y trat. del cancer *4:*139, April '28

Professional epithelioma of lower eyelid following burn by hot tar; case. MILIAN, G. AND GARNIER, G. Bull. Soc. franc. de dermat. et syph. *35:*793, Nov '28

Treatment of cancer of eyelids. BENEDICT, W. L. AND ASBURY, M. K. New York State J. Med. *29:*675–677, June 1, '29

Cancer of upper eyelid; plastic operation; case. FROTHINGHAM, G. E., J. Michigan M. Soc. *28:*632–633, Sept '29

Epithelioma of eyelids; indications for radium treatment and surgical intervention. VILLARD, H. Medecine *11:*19–23, Jan '30

Radium treatment of epitheliomas of eyelids. APPELMANS, M. Rev. belge sc. med. *2:*829–840, Dec '30

Epithelioma of eyelid; case. CORBETT, J. J. New England J. Med. *204:*774–776, April 9, '31

Recurrence after roentgenotherapy and then after excision of epithelioma of internal angle and of upper right eyelid; case. COSTE, J. Bull. Soc. franc. de dermat. et syph. (Reunion dermat., Lyon) *38:*501–504, April '31

Epithelioma of eyelid; excision. CASTROVIEJO, R. JR. Am. J. Ophth. *14:*634–635, July '31

Epithelioma of eyelid. LEHMANN, C. F. Texas State J. Med. *27:*422–426, Oct '31

Radiotherapy of epithelioma of eyelids; aesthetic results. ARCELIN, F. Lyon med. *149:*289–292, March 6, '32

Therapy of cancer of eyelid by evisceration followed by plastic surgery; case. AGUILAR, H. AND ZAVALETA, D. Hosp. argent. *4:*506–512, Jan 15, '34

Eyelids, Cancer—Cont.

Pigmented basocellular epithelioma of palpebral skin. SEDAN, J. Bull. Soc. d'opht. de Paris, pp. 341-348, April '36

Cancer of face, especially in region of eye; method of treatment. ALBRIGHT, H. L. Am. J. Surg. *33:*176-179, Aug '36

Excision of cancer of eyelids and autoplastic surgery according to Imre technic. DE SAINT-MARTIN, Bull. Soc. d'opht. de Paris *49:*36-40, Jan '37

Symptomatology and therapy of cancer of eyelids. DOLLFUS, M. A. Bull. med., Paris *51:*375-380, May 29, '37

Nevocarcinoma of eyelids and conjunctiva. VEIL, P. Bull. med., Paris *51:*371-375, May 29, '37

Successfully operated basalioma of eyelid; case. LOTIN, A. V. Vestnik oftal. *10:*891-892, '37

Plastic surgery of eyelid following removal of epithelioma caused by irradiation. LAUBER, H. Ophthalmologica *97:*312-316, July '39

Conservative autoplasty for malignant melanoma of upper eyelid; case. BADEAUX, F. AND PERRON, L. Union med. du Canada *70:*1065-1066, Oct '41

Partial resection of eyelid and plastic repair for epithelioma involving margin of lid. REESE, A. B. Arch. Ophth. *32:*173-178, Sept '44

Eyelids, Canthoplasty

Correction of displaced canthus. ESSER, J. F. S. Arch. f. klin. Chir. *115:*704, March '21

Surgery of inner canthus and related structures. BLAIR, V. P. *et al.* Am. J. Ophth. *15:*498-507, June '32

Canthoplasty. BURSUK, G. G. Vestnik oftal. *16:*243-245, '40

Eyelids, Colobomas of

Congenital eyelid coloboma; case. SANDER, P. Ztschr. f. Augenh. *61:*180-183, Feb '27

Congenital eyelid coloboma. ISAKOWITZ, J. Klin. Monatsbl. f. Augenh. *78:*509-512, April '27

Progressive atrophy of eyelids with coloboma and facial hemiatrophy; case. DUPUY-DUTEMPS, L. Bull. Soc. d'opht. de Paris, pp. 181-187, April '29

Congenital coloboma of upper eyelid with dermoids on cornea; case. HORNER, W. D. AND CORDES, F. C. Am. J. Ophth. *12:*959-964, Dec '29

Enormous harelip with deep oblique fissure accompanied by coloboma of eyelid and

Eyelids, Colobomas of—Cont.

iris; case. ETIENNE, E. AND DÉJEAN, C. Arch. Soc. d. sc. med. et biol. de Montpellier *13:*94-99, Feb '32

Coloboma (Morian's second type) with extensive facial malformations; anatomic study of case in infant 6 months old. ROCHER, H. L. *et al.* Ann. d'anat. path. *9:*487-498, May '32

Congenital bilateral coloboma of upper eyelid. BONNET, P. *et al.* Bull. Soc. d'opht. de Paris, pp. 229-232, March '34

Bilateral facial colobomas, with oculopalpebral adhesions and eye complications. MAZZI, L. Arch. di ottal. *41:*148-157, March '34

Repair of coloboma of upper eyelid. PEER, L. A. Arch. Ophth. *11:*1028-1031, June '34

Congenital bilateral palpebral coloboma complicated by corneal ulcer with hypopyon; case. VILA ORTIZ, J. M. JR. Arch. de oftal. hispano-am. *34:*315-319, June '34

Tooth in eyelid and palpebral coloboma; case. VAN DER STRAETEN, AND APPELMANS, M. Arch d'opht. *51:*417-425, July '34

Operation for repair of coloboma of upper eyelid. EL BAKLY, M. A. Bull. Ophth. Soc. Egypt *28:*26-28, '35

Plastic correction of coloboma of eyelid. DERKAC, V. Klin. Monatsbl. f. Augenh. *96:*102-104, Jan '36

Coloboma of eyelid; cases. WILSON, C. A. California and West. Med. *44:*484-486, June '36

Surgical therapy of congenital coloboma of eyelids. CHARAMIS, J. Ann. d'ocul. *173:*810-819, Oct '36

Congenital coloboma of eyelids. SHERSHEVSKAYA, O. I. Vestnik oftal. *13:*822-828, '38

Congenital coloboma and incomplete development of meibomian glands in Japanese. HIROSE, K. Arch. d'opht. *3:*673-689, Aug '39

Correction of massive defects of both eyelids. SPAETH, E. B. Pennsylvania M. J. *43:*663-668, Feb '40

Congenital colobomata of lower eyelid. SPAETH, E. B. Am. J. Ophth. *24:*186-190, Feb '41

New procedure for treating congenital colobomata. FAHMY, A. Y. Bull. Ophth. Soc. Egypt *34:*51-56, '41

Bilateral congenital coloboma of upper eyelids; case. POTTER, W. B. Am. J. Ophth. *26:*1087-1089, Oct '43

Bilateral complicated harelip with bilateral palpebral coloboma and left iridic coloboma; total ectromelia of right upper ex-

Eyelids, Colobomas of–Cont.

tremity. ROCHER, H. L. AND PESME. J. de med. de Bordeaux *121-122:*493–494, Oct '45

Congenital coloboma of upper eyelid; cases GAUFFRE, R. Arch. d'opht. *5:*342–343, '45

Eyelids, Congenital Deformities

Congenital absence of right ear with cleft of left upper eyelid. ANZINGER, F. P. Ohio State M. J. *19:*869–870, Dec '23

Congenital bilateral anophthalmos and polydactylism with report of case. HEINBERG, C. J., J. Florida M. A. *12:*253–256, April '26

Lips and teeth and cyclopia and harelips. BOLK, L. Ztschr. f. d. ges. Anat. (Abt. 1) *85:*762–783, May 21, '28

Absence of palpebral fissure of eyelids. McRITCHIE, P. Am. J. Ophth. *12:*744–745, Sept '29

Unilateral malformations of ear associated with cyclopia. HAGENS, E. W. Arch. Otolaryng. *18:*332–338, Sept '33

Anomalies of eye and orbit in acrocephalosyndactylia (Apert syndrome). WAARDENBURG, P. J. Maandschr. v. kindergeneesk. *3:*196–212, Feb '34

Tooth in eyelid and palpebral coloboma; case. VAN DER STRAETEN, AND APPELMANS, M. Arch d'opht. *51:*417–425, July '34

Peculiar form of craniofacial malformation (acrocephalosyndactylia with facial asymmetry and ophthalmoplegia); case. KREINDLER, A. AND SCHACHTER, M. Paris med. *2:*102–105, Aug 4, '34

Relation between hereditary abnormalities of eyes and partially developed fingers and toes. KARSCH, J. Ztschr. f. Augenh. *89:*274–279, July '36

Teeth in cyclopia and congenital cleft of face. BRECKWOLDT, H. Beitr. z. path. Anat. u. z. allg. Path. *98:*115–135, '36

Congenital atrophy of lower eyelids, both auricles and lower jaw; case. VAN LINT, A. AND HENNEBERT, P. Bruxelles-med. *17:*1065–1070, May 16, '37

Rare congenital malformation of nose and lower eyelid. GRITTI, P. Boll. d. mal. d. orecchio, d. gola, d. naso *55:*321–334, Sept '37

Familial eyelid and ophthalmoplegia of supranuclear type. SCHARF, J. Klin. Monatsbl. f. Augenh. *101:*71–76, July '38

Congenital facial hemihypertrophy with ocular anomalies; 2 cases. GÖZBERK, R. Ann. d'ocul. *176:*624–630, Aug '39

Rare congenital malformation of eyelid, eyebrow, scalp and of eyeball; case. VALERIO, M. Ann. di ottal. e clin. ocul. *67:*704–714, Sept '39

Eyelids, Congenital Deformities–Cont.

Unilateral microphthalmia with congenital anterior synechiae and syndactyly. BERLINER, M. L. Arch. Ophth. *26:*653–660, Oct '41

Deficiency of malar bones with defect of lower eyelids. JOHNSTONE, I. L. Brit. J. Ophth. *27:*21–23, Jan '43

Deficiency of malar bones with defect of lower eyelids. MANN, I. AND KILNER, T. P. Brit. J. Ophth. *27:*13–20, Jan '43

Congenital bilateral anophthalmos vera with unilateral polydactyly and cleft palate; case. APPLEBAUM, A. AND MARMELSTEIN, M. Arch. Ophth. *29:*258–265, Feb '43

Bilateral ptosis and atypical slant eyes associated with unilateral syndactylia, adactylia and brachyphalangia. GIRI, D. V. Proc. Roy. Soc. Med. *37:*360–361, May '44

Ascher syndrome (blepharochalasis, double upper lip and goiter), with report of case GALLINO, J. A. AND CORA ELISEHT, F. Prensa med. argent. *32:*2423–2426, Dec 7, '45

Associated malformations of eyes and ears. FRANCESCHETTI, A. AND VALERIO, M. Confinia neurol. *6:*255–257, '45

Eyelids, Deformity

Partial cryptophthalmus with epicanthus and congenital ptosis of upper eyelid; authors' technic for surgical correction; 2 cases. SATANOWSKY, P. Semana med. *1:*1953–1958, June 15, '33. abstr: Rev. Assoc. med. argent. *47:*2718–2724, June '33

Bilateral congenital epicanthus inversus and ptosis; case. LUO, T. H. Chinese M. J. *48:*814–818, Sept '34

Surgical correction of traumatic epicanthus. VERDERAME, F. Klin. Monatsbl. f. Augenh. *103:*436–441, Oct–Nov '39

Vertical shortening deformities of eyelids; plastic and reconstructive surgical correction. KIRBY, D. B., S. Clin. North America *24:*348–369, April '44

Eyelids, Ectropion

Simple operation for relief of mild types of entropion and ectropion of lower lid. JENNINGS, J. E., J.A.M.A. *83:*1329–1331, Oct 25, '24

So-called lacrymal or senile ectropion of lower eyelid, and its treatment. AUBARET, Medecine *7:*261–262, Jan '26

Technic of total ectropion operation. VERNON, E. L. Am. J. Ophth. *9:*598–600, Aug '26

Surgical treatment of senile ectropion. DE ROSA, G. Arch. di ottal. *34:*15–19, Jan '27

Eyelids, Ectropion – Cont.
Senile form of ectropion. RICCIARDI, M. Ann. di ottal. e clin. ocul. *55:*51-57, Jan-Feb '27
Acquired ectropium uveae. REESE, A. B. Am. J. Ophth. *10:*586-593, Aug '27
Ectropion of lower eyelids following burns and scalds; new early pathognomonic sign. BERKOW, S. G., J.A.M.A. *90:*1708-1709, May 26, '28
Repair of cicatricial ectropion by free dermic graft. TAYLOR, J. W. South M. J. *22:*634-637, July '29
Easy and successful operation for over-eversion of eyelids. BAKRY, M. Bull. Ophth. Soc. Egypt *22:*20-23, '29
Resection of orbicular muscle in ectropion paralysis. HOLLÓS, L. Orvosi hetil. *74:*1094-1095, Oct 25, '30 also: Ztschr. f. Augenh. *73:*27-31, Dec '30
Plastic operation for cicatricial ectropion of eyelids resulting from burn. WEINGOTT, L. Arch. d'opht. *48:*505-507, July '31
Surgical therapy of ectropion of upper lid; case. MULLER, P. Clinique, Paris *27:*124-125, April (A) '32
Good esthetic and functional results in correction of cicatricial ectropion by means of plastic graft operation. ORZALESI, F. Boll. d'ocul. *12:*906-931, Sept '33
Autoplastic skin grafts in therapy of cicatricial ectropion; 5 cases. SENÁ, J. A. Rev. Asoc. med. argent. *48:*298-306, March-April '34 also: Semana med. *2:*489-498, Aug 16, '34
Truc operation in ectropion; technic and review of cases. DELORD, E.; *et al.* Arch. d'opht. *51:*763-774, Dec '34
Modification of ectropion operation according to Kuhnt-Szymanowsky method. KESTENBAUM, A. Klin. Monatsbl. f. Augenh. *95:*51-53, July '35
Operation for senile ectropion. IMRE, J. Klin. Monatsbl. f. Augenh. *95:*303-305, Sept '35
New method of blepharoplastic operation for cicatricial ectropion using free transplant from ear flap. GOLDFEDER, A. E. Sovet. vestnik. oftal. *6:*173-177, '35
Surgery for trachomatous ectropion. KITAEVA, A. Sovet. vestnik oftal. *7:*387-388, '35
Modification of Panas operation for cicatricial ectropion. PARADOKSOV, L. F. Sovet. vestnik oftal. *7:*381-383, '35
Ectropion; problem for eye surgeons. WHEELER, J. M. South M. J. *29:*377-382, April '36
Cicatricial ectropion as result of mucocele of frontal sinus; plastic repair. McLEOD, J.

Eyelids, Ectropion – Cont.
AND LUX, P. Arch. Ophth. *15:*994-997, June '36
Epithelial inlay in cases of refractory ectropion. ESSER, J. F. S. Arch. Ophth. *16:*55-57, July '36
Plastic surgery in ectropion or loss of substance, with special reference to Hungarian method. DE SAINT-MARTIN. Rev. med. de Nancy *64:*879-903, Dec 1, '36 also: Bull. Soc. d'opht. de Paris, pp. 648-671, Oct '36
Mimical ectropion of upper eyelids. HOLTH, S. Acta ophth. *14:*340, '36
Mimical ectropion or entropion of one or both eyelids. HOLTH, S. Norsk mag. f. laegevidensk. *98:*938-940, July '37
New technic in therapy of eversion of lacrimal point and ectropion of lower lid; preliminary report. POKHISOV, N. Vestnik oftal. *11:*218-222, '37
Operation for correction of eversion of inferior lacrimal point. TIKHOMIROV, P. E. Vestnik oftal. *11:*216-217, '37
Cicatricial ectropion of upper eyelid and contracture of lower lip following burn; blepharoplasty and labioplasty; case. ROY, J. N. Rev. de chir. structive *8:*85-90, Aug '38
Ectropion and entropion of eyelids. WEEKS, W. W. Am. J. Surg. *42:*78-82, Oct '38
Surgical treatment of ectropion and entropion. BAKER, C. B., J. Oklahoma M. A. *31:*418-420, Dec '38
Reconstruction of 4 eyelids for ectropion resulting from cicatrix of severe facial burn, by means of free cutaneous grafts; case. DE LIETO VOLLARO, A. Arch. ital. di chir. *51:*588-595, '38
Author's modification of van Millingen-Sapejko operation for ectropion and trichiasis. LOSEV, N. A. Vestnik oftal. *12:*573-579, '38
Imre operation for ectropion of lower eyelid. ZATS, L. B. Vestnik oftal. *13:*554-557, '38
Simple rapid surgical technic for cure of paralytic ectropion. DE LIETO VOLLARO, A. Boll. d'ocul. *18:*769-780, Oct '39
Ectropion and its therapy. COVARRUBIAS ZENTENO, R. Rev. med. de Chile *68:*1187-1190, Sept '40
Cicatricial ectropion; therapy by free grafts; case. MARINO, H. Rev. med. -quir. de pat. fem. *16:*231-236, Sept '40
Elimination of cicatricial ectropion by free Thiersch graft. MÜLLER, P. Schweiz. med. Wchnschr. *71:*5-6, Jan 4, '41
Therapy of cicatricial ectropion. BURMISTROVA, E. Vestnik oftal. *18:*89, '41
Principles of plastic surgery in cicatricial ec-

Eyelids, Ectropion – Cont.
tropion of lower eyelid. GLEZEROV, S. Y. Vestnik oftal. *18:*397-400, '41
Operations for trachomatous eversion of eyelids and trichiasis. MAKHLIN, I. M. Sovet. med. (nos. 1-2) *6:*22-23, '42
Congenital ectropion associated with bilateral ptosis – case. GORDON, S. AND CRAGG, B. H. Brit. J. Ophth. *28:*520-521, Oct '44
Surgical technic for correction of spastic entropion and senile ectropion. SANCHEZ BULNES, L. Arch. Asoc. para evit. ceguera Mexico *2:*125-135, '44
Subcutaneous splitting of eyelid in operative treatment of senile ectropion. LYTTON, H. Brit. J. Ophth. *29:*378-380, July '45
Full-thickness skin grafts from neck for function and color in eyelid. BROWN, J. B. AND CANNON, B. Ann. Surg. *121:*639-643, May '45
Full-thickness skin grafts from neck for function and color in eyelid. BROWN, J. B. AND CANNON, B. Tr. South. S. A. (1944) *56:*255-259, '45
Ectropion due to ichthyosis of both upper and lower lids on child corrected by homoplastic grafting of skin from child's mother. SHIMKIN, N. I. Harefuah *29:*155, Oct 1, '45
Importance of repositioning of lacrimal openings in treating senile ectropion. TORRES ESTRADA, A. Gac. med. de Mexcio *75:*336-351, Oct 31, '45

Eyelids, Entropion
Entropion following influenza, with new surgical procedure. CLAPP, C. A. Am. J. Ophth. *5:*542-544, July '22 (illus.)
Surgical treatment of entropion by method of Panas. CANGE, A. Medecine *4:*261-262, Jan '23 abstr: J.A.M.A. *80:*1183, April 21, '23
Case of spastic entropion. CAMPOS, E. Brazil-med. *1:*309, May 31, '24
Simple operation for relief of mild types of entropion and ectropion of lower lid. JENNINGS, J. E., J.A.M.A. *83:*1329-1331, Oct 25, '24
Modification of Maher's operation for entropion. ARKIN, V. Klin. Monatsbl. f. Augenh. *77:*677-680, Nov '26
Entropion in new-born. ELSCHNIG, A. Monatschr. f. Kinderh. *31:*439-440, Dec–Jan '26
Modification of Maher's operation (entropion). VON GERNET, R. Klin. Monatsbl. f. Augenh. *78:*73, Jan '27
Operative procedure in trachomatous entropion of upper lid. OLÁH, E. Klin. Monatsbl. f. Augenh. *79:*388, Sept 30, '27

Eyelids, Entropion – Cont.
Webster's operation for entropion of upper lid. MACRAE, A. Brit. J. Ophth. *12:*25-30, Jan '28
Congenital entropion; 2 cases. AUBINEAU, E. Ann. d'ocul. *165:*161-169, March '28
Wedge-shaped implantation of oral mucosa into intermarginal border of eyelid in trichiasis. KREIKER, A. Klin. Monatsbl. f. Augenh. *80:*386-389, March 23, '28
Case of entropion of lower eyelid and case of spastic entropion of upper lid. LIPOWITZ, N. S. Klin. Monatsbl. f. Augenh. *80:*353-356, March 23, '28
Treatment of spastic entropion by Weeker's method. ZBOROWSKY, W. F. Klin. Monatsbl. f. Augenh. *80:*648-651, May 25, '28
Margino-tarsal graft in treatment of trichiasis and cicatricial entropion of both eyelids. VITALE, F. Gior. di ocul. *9:*61-65, June '28
Spontaneous entropion. BRINITZER, W. Med. Klin. *24:*1310, Aug 24, '28
Spastic entropion after total tarsectomy of upper lid cured by tarsal homoplasty; 3 cases. SHIMKIN, N. Klin. Monatsbl. f. Augenh. *82:*360-364, March 22, '29
Transplantation of cartilage from auricle into eyelid in trachomatous cicatricial entropion. GOLDFEDER, A. E. Klin. Monatsbl. f. Augenh. *82:*809-813, June 21, '29
Congenital entropion; cases. GÓMEZ MÁRQUEZ, J. Clin. y lab. *15:*11-23, Jan '30
Congenital entropion. GÓMEZ-MÁRQUES, J. Arch. de oftal. hispano-am. *30:*187-198, April '30
New method in correction of cicatricial entropion. SALVATI, G. Ann. d'ocul. *167:*311-314, April '30
Alcohol injection in blepharospasm and spastic entropion. SAFAR, K. Ztschr. f. Augenh.*71:*135-141, May '30
Marginotarsal graft in correction of cicatricial entropion of lower eyelid. VITALE, F. Cultura med. mod. *9:*588-592, July 31, '30
Marginoplasty by means of cartilage of auricle without skin in partial trichiasis of eyelid. GOLDFEDER, A. E. Klin. Monatsbl. f. Augenh. *86:*218-225, Feb '31
New marginoplastic method of operation in trichiasis of eyelids. POCHISSOFF, N. Klin. Monatsbl. f. Augenh. *86:*213-218, Feb '31
Congenital entropion due to epiblepharon. MÜLLER, H. K. Klin. Monatsbl. f. Augenh. *87:*184-190, Aug '31
Surgical therapy of entropion and trichiasis. LAUTERSTEIN, M. Ztschr. f. Augenh. *75:*183, Sept '31

Eyelids, Entropion – Cont.

Removal of cartilage in trachomatous entropion. WARSCHAWSKI, J. Klin. Monatsbl. f. Augenh. *87:*378–382, Sept '31

Surgical therapy of trichiasis and entropion of upper eyelid. CHRONIS, P. Cong. internat. de med. trop. et d'hyg., Compt. rend. (1928) *3:*755–757, '31

New surgical technic in entropion musculare and trichiasis of lower eyelid. CHRONIS, P. Cong. internat. de med. trop. et d'hyg., Compt. rend. (1928) *3:*759, '31

Entropion spasticum after tarsectomia totalis of upper eyelid cured by homoplastica tarsi; 3 cases. SHIMKIN, N. Cong. internat. de med. trop. et d'hyg., Compt. rend. (1928) *3:*743–751, '31

Congenital entropion; case. VON BARTHA, E. Klin. Monatsbl. f. Augenh. *88:*517–520, April '32

Therapy of spasmodic entropion with palpebral injections of alcohol associated with canthotomy. WEEKERS, L. Bull. Soc. belge d'opht., no. 64, pp. 34–38, '32 also: Arch. d'opht. *49:*427–430, July '32

Low tarsotomy and horizontal suture in trachomatous entropion of upper eyelid. JUNÈS, E. Ann. d'ocul. *169:*704–717, Sept '32

Lip-graft operation for trichiasis of eyelid. ALEXANDER, G. F. Tr. Ophth. Soc. U. Kingdom *52:*162–169 '32

Lagleys operation for trachomatous entropion. KHAVANSKIY, K. I. Sovet. vestnik oftal. *1:*159–160, '32

Operation of choice in trachomatous entropion of upper eyelid. JUNÈS, E. Bull. et mem. Soc. franc. d'opht. *45:*70–85, '32

Radical operation in therapy of trichiasis and entropion of upper eyelid. CHRONIS, P. Folia ophth. orient. *1:*187–190, Feb '33

Correction of entropion in trachoma by modified Chronis method. BATALIN, A. K. Sovet. vestnik oftal. *3:*398–399, '33

Modification of operation for trachomatous entropion (trichiasis) by means of free transplant. BURSUK, G. G. Sovet. vestnik oftal. *2:*251–252, '33

Sie-Boen-Lian operation in entropion. KANTOR, D. V. Sovet. vestnik oftal. *2:*292–295, '33

Therapy of trachomatous entropion. MEDVEDEV, N. I. Sovet. vestnik oftal. *3:*36–42, '33

New technic of operation in case of hypertrophy of tarsal plate, with trichiasis as complication. TSHERNOFF, L. Hebrew Physician *2:*55, '33

Eyelids, Entropion – Cont.

Resection of orbicularis oculi in therapy of spasmodic entropion. DUSSELDORP, M. Rev. Assoc. med. argent. *48:*296–298, March-April '34 also: Rev. oto-neuro-oftal. *9:*207–209, June '34

Double blepharostat of varying width for entropion operation. WERNER, S. Finska lak.-sall sk. handl. *76:*275–277, March '34

Internal plastic surgery of tarsus in posttrachomatous entropion and trichiasis. WORONYTSCH, N. Ztschr. f. Augenh. *84:*58–72, Aug '34

Entropion in newborn and its treatment. CHOW, K. V. Chinese M. J. *48:*830–832, Sept '34

Cuénod and Nataf modification of Saunders' operation for trichiasis and entropion. CUNNINGHAM, E. R. Chinese M. J. *48:*819–829, Sept '34

External tarsorrhaphy in therapy of spontaneous entropion of lower eyelid. HAMBRESIN, L. Bull. Soc. belge d'opht., no. 68, pp. 68–71, '34

Double blepharostat of varying widths for entropion operation. WERNER, S. Acta ophth. *12:*149–152, '34

Late results of Snellen and Millingen-Sapezhko operations for correction of trachomatous entropion. ZAKHAROV, A. P. Sovet. vestnik oftal. *4:*491–497, '34

Surgical therapy of entropion of external angular origin. POULARD, A. Ann. d'ocul. *172:*97–105, Feb '35

Correction of trachomatous entropion of upper eyelid. BALDINO, S. Rassegna ital. d'ottal. *4:*212–217, March-April '35

Correction of entropion according to Vogt method. SCHLÄPFER, H. Klin. Monatsbl. f. Augenh. *94:*610–611, May '35

Correction of trichiasis of eyelids by transplantation of cartilage from auricle. CHEPURIN, N. S. Sovet. vestnik oftal. *7:*368–373, '35

Operation for spastic entropion. POKHISOV, N. Y. Sovet. vestnik oftal. *6:*131–135 '35

Removal of tarsal section of orbicular muscle of upper eyelid in therapy of entropion and trichiasis and for prevention of recurrence of trachomatous processes. BUSACCA, A. Ztschr. f. Augenh. *88:*100–106, Jan '36

Surgical therapy of entropion and trichiasis according to Maher method. GALEWSKA, S. AND LITAUER, R. Rev. internat. du trachome *13:*41–47, Jan '36

Surgical therapy of incoercible senile spasmodic entropion. BORGES DE SOUZA, A. Lisboa med. *13:*169–177, March '36

Eyelids, Entropion – Cont.

Surgical therapy of entropion and trichiasis in trachoma patients. IFY, I. Budapesti orvosi ujsag *34:*774–776, Sept 17, '36

Satisfactory operation for entropion of upper eyelid. GODDARD, F. W. Chinese M. J. *50:*1505, Oct '36

Method for correction of entropion in trachomatous patients, with particular attention to esthetic results. BUSACCA, A. Arch. Ophth. *16:*822–828, Nov '36

Linear incision for entropion or trichiasis due to trachoma. LÜTFÜ, Ö. AND BASTUG, K. Ö. Deutsche med. Wchnschr. *62:*2014–2015, Dec 4, '36

Modification of Millingen-Sapezhko operation for trachomatous entropion. SERGIEVA, M. Sovet. vestnik oftal. *8:*244–245, '36

Mimical ectropion or entropion of one or both eyelids. HOLTH, S. Norsk mag. f. laegevidensk. *98:*938–940, July '37

Operation for cicatricial entropion of lower eyelid. KIPARISOV, N. M. Vestnik oftal. *11:*223–225, '37

Vertical section and flat incisions of cartilage of eyelids in therapy of trachomatous entropion. SHEVELEV, M. M. Vestnik oftal. *11:*383–386, '37

Transplanted conchae auriculae as new method of correcting spastic entropion of upper eyelid following total tarsectomy. SHIMKIN, N. I. Rev. internat. du trachome *15:*15–20, Jan '38 also: Brit. J. Ophth. *22:*282–287, May '38

Effective operation for entropion in trachoma. HARBERT, F. Am. J. Ophth. *21:*268–271, March '38

Surgical treatment of trachoma (complicated by entropion). RAMBO, V. C. Am. J. Ophth. *21:*277–285, March '38

Simple surgical method in post-trachomatous entropion and trichiasis. MIRIC, B. Klin. Monatsbl. f. Augenh. *101:*381–386, Sept '38

Ectropion and entropion of eyelids. WEEKS, W. W. Am. J. Surg. *42:*78–82, Oct '38

Surgical treatment of ectropion and entropion. BARKER, C. B., J. Oklahoma M. A. *31:*418–420, Dec '38

Author's modification of van Millingen-Sapejko operation for ectropion and trichiasis. LOSEV, N. A. Vestnik oftal. *12:*573–579, '38

Surgical therapy of cicatricial entropion of lower eyelid. PARADOKSOV, L. F. Vestnik oftal. *13:*550–551, '38

Simplified taroplastic in cicatricial entropion. KREIKER, A. Ophthalmologica *97:*69–78, May '39

Eyelids, Entropion – Cont.

Spastic entropion correction by orbicularis transplantation. WHEELER, J. M. Am. J. Ophth. *22:*477–483, May '39

Transplantation of conjunctiva in surgical therapy of trichiasis. KLAUBER, E. Ann. d'ocul. *176:*476–477, June '39

New knife for Van Millingen grafting operation (ingrown eyelashes). KAMEL, S. Bull. Ophth. Soc. Egypt *32:*73–78, '39

Correcting spastic entropion of upper lid following total tarsectomy, by transplanting a shaving from concha auriculae. ANAND, H. L. Indian J. Ophth. *1:*20–23, Jan '40

Inversion of tarsus as surgical procedure in correction of granulous entropion. NIZETIC, Z. Ann. d'ocul. *177:*211–217, June '40

Operation for spastic entropion. MEEK, R. E. Arch. Ophth. *24:*547–551, Sept '40

Technic of operation for correction of trachomatous entropion. NIZETIC, Z. Klin. Monatsbl. f. Augenh. *105:*641–647, Dec '40

Modification of Hotz operation for entropion due to trachoma. MAXWELL, J. S. Am. J. Ophth. *24:*298–302, March '41

Treatment of spastic entropion. ROBBINS, A. R. Arch. Ophth. *25:*475–476, March '41

Spasmodic entropion; new surgical technic in therapy. TORRES ESTRADA, A. Bol. d. Hosp. oftal. de Ntra. Sra. de la Luz *1:*265–272, Nov–Dec '41

New surgical technic for treating spasmodic entropion. TORRES ESTRADA, A. Cir. y cirujanos *9:*559–569, Dec. 31, '41

Best operation against spastic entropion. HABACHI, S. Bull. Ophth. Soc. Egypt *34:*57–63, '41

Author's modification of Sie Boen Lian operation for trachomatous entropion and its late results. KANTOR, D. V. Vestnik oftal. *18:*301–305, '41

Transgrafting operation for trichiasis and entropion of upper eyelid. PATHAN, H. A. H. Indian M. Gaz. *77:*204–206, April '42

Paganelli's modification of operation for entropion. PAGANELLI, T. R. Dis. Eye, Ear, Nose and Throat *2:*347–349, Nov '42

Modified Ewing operation for cicatricial entropion. SMITH, J. E. AND SINISCAL, A. A. Am. J. Ophth. *26:*382–389, April '43

Simple procedure for relief of entropion (device attached to spectacle frame). WIENER, A. Arch. Ophth. *29:*634, April '43

Treatment of cicatricial entropion. BERKLEY, W. L., U. S. Nav. M. Bull. *41:*729–736, May '43

Operation for entropion of trachoma. COCKBURN, C. Brit. J. Ophth. *27:*308–310, July '43

Eyelids, Entropion – Cont.

Surgical technic for correction of spastic entropion and senile ectropion. SANCHEZ BULNES, L. Arch. Asoc. para evit. ceguera Mexico *2:*125–135, '44

New treatment of entropion. MACDONALD, A. E. Tr. Am. Ophth. Soc. *43:*372, '45

Eyelids, Injuries of

Fracture of maxillary sinus plus emphysema of lower eyelid. MOREAU, J. Arch. franco-belges de chir. *25:*421–424, Feb '22 (illus.)

Diplopia in fracture of upper and lower maxillary and of malar bones; case. PAOLI, M. Rev. de stomatol. *41:*548–552, July '39

Fractures of malar bone and zygoma with eye ear, nose and throat complications. MEYER, M. F. New Orleans M. and S. J. *92:*90–94, Aug '39

Injuries to eyelids. KIRBY, D.B., S. Clin. North America *20:*573–587, April '40

Treatment of wounds of eyelids. DUNNINGTON, J. H. Virginia M. Monthly *69:*473–475, Sept '42

Surgical repair of recent lacerations of eyelids; intramarginal splinting suture. MINSKY, H. Surg., Gynec. and Obst. *75:*449–456, Oct '42

Eyelid suture in injuries. KROL, A. G. Sovet. med. (nos. 11–12) *6:*25–26, '42

Injuries of eyes and eyelids. KIRBY, D. B. AND TOWN, A. E., S. Clin. North America *23:*404–438, April '43

Lacerations of eyelids. CLARK, C. P., J. Indiana M. A. *36:*245–247, May '43

Injuries to eyes, with remarks on plastic surgery. KNAPP, A. A., U. S. Nav. M. Bull. *42:*651–653, March '44

Late complications and sequels following blunt trauma to eye and orbital wall. NEBLETT, H. C. South. Med. and Surg. *106:*436–437, Nov '44

Wounds of eye, ear, nose and throat. SMART, F. P., U. S. Nav. M. Bull. *44:*1231–1233, June '45

Eyelids, Reconstruction

One-stage plastic reconstruction of upper eyelid together with muscle fibers and eyelashes. KAZ, R. Zentralbl. f. Chir. *48:*1239, Aug. 27, '21

Reconstruction of lower eyelid. JIMÉNEZ LÓPEZ, C. AND RIBÓN, V. Semana med. *2:*832, Oct 19, '22 (illus.)

Reconstruction of eyelids. JOSEPH, H. Beitr. z. klin. Chir. *131:*52–65, '24

Formation of new upper eyelid from auricle. ROCHAT, G. F. Nederl. Tijdschr. v. Geneesk. *2:*709, Aug 6, '27

Eyelids, Reconstruction – Cont.

Restoration of completely destroyed eyelid by cutaneous and tarso-conjunctival grafts from other lid; 3 cases. DUPUY-DUTEMPS, L. Ann. d'ocul. *164:*915–926, Dec '27

Hungarian method of forming lower eyelid. SZOKOLIK, E. Klin. Monatsbl. f. Augenh. *80:*652–655, May 25, '28

Regeneration of destroyed eyelid by cutaneous and tarso-conjunctival graft taken from other lid; case. DUPUY-DUTEMPS, L. Monde med., Paris *38:*705–711, Sept. 1, '28

Plastic restoration of all 4 eyelids, with use of skin from arm in 3 cases. PAYR, E. Arch. f. klin. Chir. *152:*532–540, '28

Repair of entirely destroyed eyelid by cutaneous and tarso-conjuctival graft taken from other eyelid. DUPUY-DUTEMPS, L. Bull. med., Paris *43:*935–938, Aug 31, '29

Surgery and plastic replacement of eyelids. BÜCKLERS, M. Chirurg *5:*460–472, June 15, '33

Removal of eyelid, with plastic repair. HUGHES, W. L. Arch. Ophth. *10:*198–201, Aug '33

Plastic operations for restoration of lower eyelid. EL-TOBGY, A. F. Bull. Ophth. Soc. Egypt *26:*1–7, '33

Principles of plastic surgery of eyelids, with special reference to Hungarian school. KATZ, D. Arch. Ophth. *12:*220–227, Aug '34

Biologic flap to form 2 eyelids at same time; case. ESSER, J. F. S. Rev. espan. de cir. *17:*1–3, Jan–Feb '35

Plastic operations for restoration of upper eyelid. EL TOBGY, A. F. Bull. Ophth. Soc. Egypt *28:*21–25, '35

Indications and comparative evaluation of Hungarian method of blepharoplasty. KOPP, I. F. Sovet. vestnik oftal. *7:*603–609, '35

Total blepharoplasty. BLASKOVICS, L. Orvosi hetil. *81:*1050–1055, Oct. 16, '37

Eyelid surgery; about sliding-flap, known also as Hungarian plastic. CZUKRASZ, I. Tr. Ophth. Soc. U. Kingdom (pt. 2) *58:*561–575, '38

Results of reconstruction of eyelids following loss of substance due to grave trauma. NICOLATO, A. Ann. di ottal. e clin. ocul. *67:*81–92, Feb '39

Hughes procedure for rebuilding lower eyelid. GIFFORD, S. R. Arch. Ophth. *21:*447–452, March '39

Technic of plastic reconstruction in toto of eye. KURLOV, N. I. Vestnik oftal. (nos. 3–4) *15:*103–112, '39

Plastic reconstruction of upper eyelid. Mc-

Eyelids, Reconstruction – Cont.

LEAN, J. M. Am. J. Ophth. *24:*46–48, Jan '41

Hughes operation for total loss of lower eyelid. DELLEPIANE RAWSON, R. Arq. de cir. clin. e exper. *6:*235–251, April–June '42

Hughes operation for total loss of lower eyelid. DELLEPIANE RAWSON, R. Dia med. *14:*461, May 25, '42

Plastic reconstruction of lower and upper eyelids. RAPIN, M. Ophthalmologica *105:*233–239, May '43

Tarsoconjunctival sliding-graft technics for reconstruction of eyelids. SUGAR, H. S. Am. J. Ophth. *27:*109–123, Feb '44

Reconstruction of ablated lower eyelid. WHALMAN, H. F. Arch. Ophth. *32:*66–67, July '44

Reconstruction of lower eyelid by Hughes method. FOSTER, J. Brit. J. Ophth. *28:*515–519, Oct '44

Reconstructive surgery of eyelids; case. CASTROVIEJO, R. Arch. Asoc. para evit. ceguera Mexico *2:*189–194, '44

Surgical reconstruction of upper eyelid. HAGUE, E. B. Am. J. Ophth. *28:*886–889, Aug '45

Total reconstruction of upper lid (blepharopoiesis) HUGHES, W. L. Am. J. Ophth. *28:*980–992, Sept '45

Reconstruction of eyelids. HUGHES, W. L. Am. J. Ophth. *28:*1203–1211, Nov '45

Methods of repair and reconstruction. (eyelids) FOX, S. A. Am. J. Ophth. *29:*452–458, Apr '46

Eyelids, Symblepharon

Skin-grafting in acute symblepharon (eyelids). BALL, J. M. Lancet *1:*863, April 24, '26

Plastic preparation for prosthesis in extensive symblepharon. LIJÓ PAVÍA, J. Rev. Especialid. *1:*75–82, '26

Treatment for traumatic symblepharon. HUGHES, E. N. Brit. J. Ophth. *11:*337–338, July '27

Repair of conjunctival fornix by Reverdin-Thiersch graft. SALVATI, G. Gior. di ocul. *9:*56, May '28

Symblepharon of eyelids; treatment by Thiersch and mucous membrane grafting. GILLIES, H. D. AND KILNER, T. P. Tr. Ophth. Soc. U. Kingdom *49:*470–479, '29

Morax operation in correction of symblepharon orbitale. CHISTYAKOV, P. I. Vestnik oftal. *11:*795–797, '37

New technic for mucous graft in ophthalmology. KOLEN, A. A. Vestnik oftal. (nos. 3–4) *15:*100–102, '39

Eyelids, Symblepharon – Cont.

Paralysis of lower eyelid, scleral scars and grafts. BLAIR, V. P., AND BYARS, L. T. Surg., Gynec., and Obst. *70:*426–437, Feb '40

Plastic surgery of adherent eyelid; case. MATHIEU, C. J. de l'Hotel-Dieu de Montreal *9:*156–159, May–June '40

Surgical therapy of symblepharon. GRAUE Y GLENNIE, E. Bol. d. Hosp. oftal. de Ntra. Sra. de la Luz *1:*101–105, July–Aug '40

Recidivating symblepharon in leper treated with conjunctival transplant; case. BEAUJON, O. Arch. venezol. Soc. de oto-rino-laring., oftal., neurol. *2:*23–27, March '41

Plastic operations of total defect of eyelids and symblephara orbitalia. INOUE, S. Far East. Sc. Bull. *1:*3, April '41 (abstract)

Use of palpebral conjunctiva in reconstruction of inferior fornix. PUGA, R. Amatus *2:*207–211, Mar '43

New technic for correcting symblepharon. PANNETON, P. Union med. du Canada *73:*42–44, Jan '44

Surgical therapy of very extensive symblepharon. CHULIA, V. Arch. soc. oftal. hispano-am. *4:*1070–1071, Nov–Dec '44

Burn of cornea and conjunctiva; how to prevent symblepharon. PAVIA, J. L. Rev. oto-neuro-oftal. *19:*159–171, Nov–Dec '44 also: Semana med. *2:*1117–1122, Dec 7, '44

Buccal mucosa grafts in therapy of total symblepharon. BERTOTTO, E. V. Rev. med. de Rosario *35:*317–322, April '45

Eyelids, Tumors

Treatment of xanthoma of eyelid. NOBL, G. Med. Klinik *19:*1631–1633, Dec 16, '23 abstr: J. A. M. A. *82:*344, Jan 26, '24

Unusual dermoid cyst of eyelid. GRADLE, H. S. AND STEIN, J. C. Arch. Ophth. *53:*254–257, May '24

Perithelioma of upper eyelid. DONNELL, N. R. Arch. Ophth. *53:*411–415, Sept '24

Case of diffuse angioma of eyelid cured by electrolysis. CAMPOS, E. Brazil-med. *2:*233, Oct 18, '24

Tumors of eyelids. EVANS, W. J. China M. J. *39:*145–146, Feb '25

Two cases of cavernous angioma of eyelid and case of lymphangioma of bulbar conjunctiva. RAY, V. Ohio State M. J. *21:*720–722, Oct '25

Plastic repair of eyelid after excision of tumor. MORAX, V. Bull. Soc. d'opht. de Paris, pp. 411, Oct '26

Multiple fibromata of eyelid and forehead; removal; case. BAKRY, M. Bull. Ophth. Soc. Egypt *22:*78, '29

Eyelids, Tumors—Cont.
Comparative results of bipolar electrolysis and radium therapy in angioma of eyelids in infants; 2 cases. MARÍN AMAT, M. Arch. de oftal. hispano-am. *32:*604–613, Nov '32
Hemangioma of eye; excision by high-frequency knife. BABCOCK, W. W., S. Clin. North America *12:*1411–1412, Dec '32
Large angiomas of upper eyelid treated with surgical diathermy. CARAMAZZA, F. Boll. d'ocul. *13:*742–753, June '34
Angiomas of eyelids; therapy by sclerosing injections. WEEKERS, L. AND LAPIERRE, S. Bull. Soc. belge d'opht., no. 68, pp. 23–36, '34
Angiomas of eyelids; therapy by sclerosing injections; technic, indications and results; 4 cases. WEEKERS, L. AND LAPIERRE, S. Arch. d'opht. *52:*14–22, Jan '35
Technic in using trichloroacetic acid for removal of moles from eyelids. MURPHY, F. G., J. Iowa M. Soc. *26:*147–148, March '36
Treatment of angioma of eyelid by injection of sclerosing solutions. MALKIN, B. Arch. Ophth. *16:*578–584, Oct '36
Removal of adjacent nevi of eyelids. CALLAHAN, A. Am. J. Ophth. *29:*563–565, May '46

EYKMAN VAN DER KEMP, P. H. (see DE JOSSELIN DE JONG, R.) Feb '28
EYMER, H.: Instrument for obtaining Thiersch grafts. Deutsche med. Wchnschr. *61:*1954–1955, Dec 6, '35

F

FABER, A.: Enucleation of eye-ball and cartilage transplantation as basis for prosthesis. Beitr. z. klin. Chir. *141:*524–527, '27
FABER, A.: Technic and results of tendon translocations. Verhandl. d. deutsch. orthop. Gesellsch., Kong. 27, pp. 331–333, '33
FABER, H. K. (see MERRITT, K. K. *et al*) March '37
FABER, K.: Facial hemiatrophy associated with vitiligo and myxedema; case. Ugesk. f. laeger *95:*1207–1211, Nov 9, '33
FABER, K.: Pathogenesis of hemiatrophy, vitiligo and myxedema appearing successively in face of same patient. Acta med. Scandinav. *82:*419–432, '34
FABIAN, A.: Syphilitic deformities of nose. Bratisl. lekar. listy 15:749–768, June '35
FABRE, A. (see COUDANE, R.) July–Sept '44
FABRE, J. (see GALY-GASPARROU, *et al*) March '28
FABRE, M.: Unilateral amastia; case. Bull. Soc. franc. de dermat. et syph. (Reunion dermat., Lyon) *40:*1072–1074, July '33
FABRICIUS-MOLLER, J. AND KJAERHOLM, H.: First aid for jaw fractures. Ugesk. f. laeger *103:*1307–1311, Oct 9, '41
FABRIKANT, M. B.: Early plastic reconstruction of defects following gunshot wounds. Khirurgiya, no. 3, pp. 27–29, '44
FABRY, J.: Treatment of grave roentgen burns of hands with radium and Doramad ointment. Med. Klinik *21:*1498, Oct. 2, '25

Face: See Facial

Face, Anatomy of
Anatomie medico-chirurgicale, Fascicles 2 and 3, La Face, by PHILIPPE B. BELLOCQ. Masson et Cie, Paris, 1926
Medicosurgical anatomy of face. LIMA, E. Rev. med.-cir. do Brasil *51:*287–304, April–June '43

Face, Burns (See also Burns)
Phenol burns of left eyelids, eyeball, upper face and temporal area. SHEEHAN, J. E. Laryngoscope *35:*55, Jan '25
Case after operation for extensive burn of left lids, eyeball, upper face and temporal area. SHEEHAN, J. E., M. J. and Rec. *121:*291–292, March 4, '25
Contractures due to burns of face, neck and body. BEHREND, M., S. Clin. N. America *6:*237–243, Feb '26
Treatment of burns of face without dressings; 2 cases. SASSARD, P. Lyon med. *147:*43, Jan 11, '31
Reconstructive surgery and old facial burns. UPDEGRAFF, H. L., J. A. M. A. *101:*1138–1140, Oct 7, '33
Surgical restoration by means of grafts in severe burns of face with cicatrix. SANVENERO-ROSSELLI, G. Bull. et mem. Soc. d. chirurgiens de Paris *27:*391–403, July 5, '35
Plastic surgery for deformity and contractures after nitric acid burns to face (case). MONEY, R. A., M. J. Australia *2:*848–853, Dec 19, '36
Choice method in plastic restoration of face following extensive burns causing cicatricial disfigurement. DANTRELLE, M. Rev. de chir. structive, pp. 108–109, June '37
Chemical burns of face. BECK, W. C., S. Clin. North America *18:*13–20, Feb '38
Esthetic results of grafts of Anglo-Russian type in facial burn; case. CODAZZI AGUIRRE, J. A. Semana med. *1:*651–655, March 14, '40
Treatment of burns of eyes and face with sulfhydryl solution (hydrosulphosol). CRUTHIRDS, A. E. Indust. Med. *11:*109–112, March '42

Face, Burns—Cont.

Esthetic repair of face (after burn) by free grafts of skin; case. ROCHER, H. L. Bordeaux chir. *3-4:*98–100, July–Oct '44

Local therapy including facial, interdigital and perineal burns; preliminary report. ZORRAQUIN, G. AND ZORRAQUIN, G. F. Dia med. *17:*329–331, April 16, '45

Face, Cancer of (See also Cancer; Melanoma; etc.)

Treatment of basal epithelioma of face. YOUNG, W. J. Kentucky M. J. *19:*154, April '21

Malignancy of face and jaws. FORT, F. T. Kentucky M. J. *19:*456, Aug '21

Extensive epitheliomatous ulcer of side of face. MCKILLOP, L. M., M. J. Australia *2:*456, Nov 19, '21

Epitheliomas of face and their treatment with radium. MORROW, H. AND TAUSSIG, L. Arch. Dermat. and Syph. *5:*73–87, Jan '22 (illus.)

Carcinoma of cheek, case report. SHERRILL, J. G. Kentucky M. J. *20:*284–285, April '22

Epithelioma of face and ear. YOUNG, W. J. Kentucky M. J. *20:*367–368, May '22

Prophylaxis of malignant growths of mouth, face and jaws. EASTMAN, J. R., J. A. M. A. *79:*118–120, July 8, '22

Carcinoma of lip and cheek; general principles involved in operation and results obtained at Presbyterian, Memorial, and Roosevelt Hospitals. BREWER, G. E. Surg., Gynec. and Obst. *36:*169–184, Feb '23

Radiotherapy in treatment of superficial malignant disease of face. JOSSELYN, R. B., J. Maine M. A. *13:*279–284, June '23 (illus.)

Epithelioma of face. BOWEN, W. W., J. Iowa M. Soc. *14:*154–157, April '24

Treatment of malignant growths about the face. WITHERS, S. AND RANSON, J. R. Colorado Med. *21:*92–97, April '24

Suggestion for relief of pain from carcinoma of mouth and cheek. GRANT, F. C. Ann. Surg. *81:*494–498, Feb '25

Radium treatment of epithelioma of face. KENNEDY, W. H., J. Radiol. *6:*52–55, Feb '25

Radium treatment of cancer of face. TRUEHART, M., J. Kansas M. Soc. *25:*70–73, March '25

Surgical relief of pain in deep carcinoma of face and neck. FAY, T. Am. J. Roentgenol. *14:*1–5, July '25

Case report of plastic repair of mutilating operations of lip and cheek following radical removal of carcinoma. COPP, F. A., J. Florida M. A. *12:*29–35, Aug '25

Treatment of epithelioma of face and eyelid.

Face, Cancer—Cont.

SIMPSON, C. A. Virginia M. Monthly *52:*337–340, Sept '25

Relief for pain in carcinoma of face. GRANT, F. C., J. A. M. A. *86:*173–176, Jan 16, '26

Epithelioma of face and buccal cavity. WETZEL, J. O. New York State J. Med. *26:*634–639, July 15, '26

Radio-active substances; their therapeutic uses and applications; radiation of cancer of cheek. MUIR, J. Radiology *7:*131–136, Aug '26

Repair of defects caused by surgery and radium in cancer of hand, mouth and cheek. BLAIR, V. P. Am. J. Roentgenol. *17:*99–100, Jan '27

Treatment of advanced carcinoma of skin of face with radium. BRADLEY, R. A. AND SNOKE, P. O., S. Clin. N. Amer. *7:*165–168, Feb '27

Basal-cell carcinoma of face. SCHAMBERG, J. F., S. Clin. N. Amer. *7:*113–115, Feb '27

Cancer of skin of face and neck. LOUNSBERRY, C. R. California and West. Med. *26:*800–801, June '27

Treatment of adenopathies which accompany cancer of lower half of face. MARQUIS, E. Bull. et mem. Soc. nat. de chir. *53:*760–767, June 4, '27

Plastic operation for ulcerative epithelioma of upper lip and cheek. ZAGNI, L. Stomatol. *25:*591–594, July '27

Radium treatment in 13 cases of cancer of face. FRUCHAUD, H. AND MARY, A. Gazettes med., Paris, pp. 465–471, Aug 15, '27

Epithelioma of lip and face. BONDURANT, C. P., J. Oklahoma M. A. *20:*252–256, Sept '27

Treatment of baso-cellular epithelioma of face. MARIN, A. Union med. du Canada *56:*489–500, Sept '27

New method of treating carcinoma of cheek. PATTERSON, N. Lancet *2:*703, Oct 1, '27

Treatment of cancer of mucosa of cheek. HÜNERMANN, T. Deutsche Ztschr. f. Chir. *203-204:*332–336, '27

Carcinoma of mucosa of cheek treated surgically; 10 cases. SERAFINI, G. AND ANTONIOLI, G. M. Gior. d. r. Accad. di med. di Torino *91:*51–56, Jan–March '28 also: Minerva med. (pt. 2) *8:*599–610, Sept 15, '28

Relief of pain of facial cancer. MIXTER, W. J. AND GRANT, F. C. Tr. Am. S. A. *45:*473–482, '27 also: Ann. Surg. *87:*179–185, Feb '28

Multiple epitheliomata of face developed from keratoma senile. WIENER, E. Nederl. Tijdschr. v. Geneesk. *1:*614–616, Feb 4, '28

Treatment of facial cancer by irradiation.

Face, Cancer—Cont.
KAPLAN, I. I. Am. J. Roentgenol. *19:*437-439, May '28
Treatment of epithelioma about face, mouth and jaws. PADGETT, E. C., J. Missouri M. A. *25:*190-194, May '28
Extensive epithelioma of cheek and lower jaw treated by diathermy. HARRISON, W. J. Brit. M. J. *2:*102, July 21, '28
Cancer of face. MEYER, H. W. Am. J. Surg. *5:*352-357, Oct '28
Epithelioma of face treated by grattage and radiotherapy. BELOT, J. AND LEPENNETIER, F. Bull. et mem. Soc. de radiol. med. de France *16:*227, Nov '28
Electro-coagulation (diathermy) for facial cancer. LALVANI, P. P. Indian M. Gaz. *63:*640, Nov '28
Multiple dermal cancer in face and on neck; case. ODQVIST, H. Acta radiol. *9:*302-304, '28
X-ray treatment of epithelioma of face. MARTIN, J. M. Proc. Inter-State Post-Grad. M. Assemb., North America (1927) *3:*303-305, '28
Roentgen therapy in inoperable epithelioma of face. SCADUTO, G. Urol. and Cutan. Rev. *33:*28-35, Jan '29
Neglected treatment of cancer of face; case. HEILBRONN, S. Munchen. med. Wchnschr. *76:*374, March 1, '29
Primary double epithelioma of face; case. ABERNETHY, D. A. Brit. J. Surg. *16:*687-689, April '29
Relief of pain with cancer of face. GRANT, F. C. Pennsylvania M. J. *32:*548-551, May '29
Diagnosis of cutaneous cancer of face. RAMOND, L. Presse med. *37:*951-952, July 20, '29
Spreading epitheliomas, recurring after radium therapy; cure by surgical treatment (face). BÉRARD, L. AND DUNET. Lyon chir. *26:*562-565, Aug-Sept '29
Basocellular epithelioma of face with clinical syndrome simulating scleroderma. BERTANZI, R. Gior. ital. di dermat. e sifil. *70:*1344-1348, Oct '29
Biologic aspects of cancer of face in view of results of treatment. VON DOELINGER DA GRACA. Folha med. *10:*384-386, Nov 5, '29
Epithelioma of cheek from drop of carbon disulphide; case. GOUGEROT, H. AND BURNIER. Bull. Soc. franc. de dermat. et syph. *36:*1041, Nov '29
Plastic surgery of lip, chin and cheek in man after resection for cancer. CAVINA, C. Arch. ed atti d. Soc. ital. di chir. *35:*526-541, '29

Face, Cancer—Cont.
Value of radium in treatment of cancer of face. LARKIN, A. J. Am. J. Surg. *8:*164-165, Jan '30
Use of small amounts of radium at distance in treatment of cancer of face. PETTIT, R. T. Radiology *14:*55-59, Jan '30
Etiology of cancer of face; prevention. DARIER, J. Monde med., Paris *40:*65-73, Feb 1, '30
Recurring epithelioma of face. FIGI, F. A., S. Clin. N. Amer. *10:*105-107, Feb '30
Treatment of surface cancers of face with scraping and roentgen therapy; value in relation to other methods. BELOT, J. AND BUHLER, Y. E. Rev. d'actinol. *6:*91-107, March-April '30
Unusual case of cancer of face. WILLIS, R. A. J. Coll. Surgeons, Australasia *2:*417-421, March '30
Treatment of large epitheliomas after failure of radiotherapy (on face). BÉRARD, L. AND CREYSSEL, J. Paris med. *1:*237-243, March 15, '30
Spinocellular epithelioma of cheek in patient with old lupus. VIGNE, P. Marseille med. *2:*369-371, Dec 15, '30
Electrocoagulation of cancer of cheek. CLAIRMONT, P. AND SCHÜRCH, O. Deutsche Ztschr. f. Chir. *227:*115-125, '30
Plastic operations on cheeks and nose for cancer. WOLF, H. Arch. f. klin. Chir. *160:*105-117, '30
Epithelioma of face; treatment and subsequent surgical reconstruction. NEW, G. B. AND HAVENS, F. Z., J. A. M. A. *97:*687-690, Sept 5, '31
Epithelioma of face secondary to extensive epithelioma of eyelids; three-stage operation; removal of tumor, skin graft and restoration of eyelids. TIXIER, L. AND BONNET, P. Lyon chir. *28:*719-722, Nov-Dec '31
Epithelioma of face; treatment and subsequent surgical reconstruction. NEW, G. B. AND HAVENS, F. Z. Tr. Sect. Surg., Gen. and Abd., A. M. A., pp. 166-176, '31
Plastic surgery of face following electrocoagulation treatment of malignant tumors of nose and accessory sinuses. ÖHNGREN, G. Acta oto-laryng. *16:*292-305, '31
Surgery for cancer of face and lip. TRUEBLOOD, D. V. West. J. Surg. *40:*401-404, Aug '32
Destruction of nose and part of face by squamous-celled carcinoma of rodent ulcer type. RIDOUT, C. A. S. Proc. Roy. Soc. Med. *25:*1767, Oct '32
Carcinoma of mucosa of cheek treated by

Face, Cancer – Cont.
irradiation only; patient living and free of disease 5 years, 3 months. MARTIN, H. E. S. Clin. North America *13:*442–443, April '33
Management of facial teguments in extensive exeresis for cancers of inferior maxilla, of floor of mouth, of tonsils and of pharynx. BERNARD, R. Presse med. *41:*748–751, May 10, '33
Squamous cell epitheliomata of face; 26 cases. TRAUB, E. F. AND TOLMACH, J. A. New York State J. Med. *33:*875–881, July 15, '33
Cancer of cheek, with special reference to results of surgical therapy. THEODORESCO, D. AND HOFFER, O. Presse med. *42:*2040–2043, Dec 19, '34
Cancer of cheek and neighboring bone. BLAIR, V. P.; *et al.* Am. J. Surg. *30:*250–253, Nov '35
Cancer of cheek and neighboring bone. BLAIR, V. P.; *et al.* Internat. J. Orthodontia *22:*183–188, Feb '36
Repair of postoperative defects involving lips and cheeks secondary to removal of malignant tumors. NEW, G. B. AND FIGI, F. A. Surg., Gynec. and Obst. *62:*182–190, Feb '36
Terebrant cancers of face. IMBERT, R. Rev. de chir., Paris *74:*331–373, May '36
Thermocauterization in therapy of facial cancer. MERIC, A. J. L. Rev. de laryng. *57:*768–802, July–Aug '36
Plastic repair of defects resulting from radical extirpation of facial cancer. OWENS, N. South. M. J. *29:*654–664, July '36
Cancer of face, especially in region of eye; method of treatment. ALBRIGHT, H. L. Am.J. Surg. *33:*176–179, Aug '36
Reparation of loss of substance due to electrosurgical therapy of nasofacial cancer. PRUDENTE, A. Rev. oto-laring. de Sao Paulo (no. 5, bis) *4:*749–810, Sept–Oct '36
Reconstruction following ablation of cancer of face. PRUDENTE, A. Bull. et mem. Soc. d. chirurgiens de Paris *28:*485–496, Nov 6, '36
Results of roentgen rays, radium, diathermocoagulation and surgery in therapy of cutaneous epithelioma (face); 14 cases. MARTIN, J. Arch. d'electric med. *44:*444–460, Dec '36
Neglected and recurrent basal cell epitheliomas of face. MEYER, H. W. Surg., Gynec. and Obst. *64:*675–683, March '37
Carcinoma of cheek; original method of treatment, with reports on 10 cases. PATTERSON, N. Brit. J. Surg. *25:*330–336, Oct '37

Face, Cancer – Cont.
Treatment of epitheliomas of nasolabial fold. MELAND, O. N. Am. J. Roentgenol. *38:*730–739, Nov '37
Five year end-results in treatment of cancer of tongue, lip and cheek. MARTIN, H. E. Surg., Gynec. and Obst. *65:*793–797, Dec '37
Indications for and limits of surgical therapy in extensive cancers of buccofacial region; 3 cases. BERARD, L.; *et al.* Lyon chir. *35:*318–327, May–June '38
Ulcerating epithelioma of cheek; case treated with 500,000 volt therapy. MERSHON, H. F. South. Surgeon *7:*262, June '38
Experiences in reconstruction in surgical treatment of malignant diseases of face with skin grafts. KILNER. Rev. de chir. structive *8:*170–180, '38
Repair of deformities following surgical removal of malignant tumors of face with grafting. MCINDOE, A. H. Rev. de chir. structive *8:*181–186, '38
Plastic surgery for mutilations of face resulting from exeresis of malignant tumors from soft parts. SANVENERO ROSSELLI, G. Arch. ital. di chir. *54:*491–501, '38
Role of plastic surgery in treatment of malignancies about face. BURTON, J. F. South. M. J. *32:*67–68, Jan '39
Plastic reconstruction after therapy for facial cancer. SCHÜRCH, O. Plast. chir. *1:*60–70, '39
Malignant disease of face, buccal cavity, pharynx and larynx in first three decades of life. HERTZ, C. S. Proc. Staff Meet., Mayo Clin. *15:*152–156, March 6, '40
Cancer of face. BLAIR, V. P. AND BYARS, L. T. Mississippi Valley M. J. *62:*90–93, May '40
Cancer of face. NEW, G. B. Proc. Staff Meet., Mayo Clin. *16:*71–72, Jan 29, '41
Cancer of lips and cheeks. FIGI, F. A. Proc. Staff Meet., Mayo Clin. *16:*280–282, April 30, '41
Treatment of cancer of face, including reconstructive surgery. NEW, G. B., S. Clin. North America *21:*969–978, Aug '41
Metastasizing basal cell carcinoma of face. DE NAVASQUEZ, S. J. Path. and Bact. *53:*437–439, Nov '41
Cancer of the Face and Mouth. BLAIR, V. P., MOORE, S., AND BYARS, L. T., C. V. Mosby Co., St. Louis, 1942
Principles of plastic surgery in treatment of malignant tumors of face. CONWAY, H. Surg., Gynec. and Obst. *74:*449–457, Feb (no. 2A) '42
Plastic reconstruction of cheek after exten-

Face, Cancer—Cont.

sive epithelioma. Flynn, R., M. J. Australia *1:*555–556, May 9, '42

Full thickness defects of cheek (cancer) involving angle of mouth; method of repair. MacFee, W. F. Surg., Gynec. and Obst. *76:*100–105, Jan '43

Cancer of mouth. (and face) Blair, V. P. and Byars, L. T. Texas State J. Med. *38:*641-645, March '43

Surgical treatment of pain; malignant lesions of face, nose and mouth. Robertson, J. S. Tr. Roy. Med.-Chir. Soc. Glasgow, pp. 29–31, '43–'44 in Glasgow M. J. May '44

Basal cell lesions of nose, cheek and lips. Davis, W. B. Ann. Surg. *119:*944–948, June '44

Large carcinoma of cheek. Nathanson, I. T. Am. J. Orthondontics (Oral Surg. Sect.) *31:*284–286, April '45

Clinical and statistical study of 1062 cases of facial cancer. de Cholnoky, T. Ann. Surg. *122:*88–101, July '45

Subtotal replacement of skin of face for actinodermatitis due to roentgenotherapy with multiple areas of squamous cell carcinoma. Jenkins, H. P. Ann. Surg. *122:*1042–1048, Dec '45

Face, Congenital Deformities (See also Cleft Lips; Facial Cleft; and Other Specific Deformities)

Congenital salivary fistula in cleft cheek. Pommrich, W. Deutsche Ztschr. f. Chir. *191:*136–142, '25

Congenital absence of vomer and causes of septal deformities. Menzel, K. M. Wien. med. Wchnschr. *77:*1081–1083, Aug 13, '27

Unilateral absence of intermaxillary bone without cleft; case. Kozlik, F. Anat. Anz. *88:*91–100, April 3, '39

Deficiency of malar bones with defect of lower eyelids. Mann, I. and Kilner, T. P. Brit. J. Ophth. *27:*13–20, Jan '43

Face, Infections of

Treatment of progressive pyogenic processes of face; injection of own blood. Läwen, A. Zentralbl. f. Chir. *50:*1018–1024, June 30, '23 abstr: J. A. M. A. *81:*1155, Sept 29, '23

Progressive furuncle of face. Rieder, W. Zentralbl. f. Chir. *50:*1024–1025, June 30, '23 abstr: J. A. M. A. *81:*1155, Sept 29, 23

Treatment of malignant furuncle of face by incision and circular injection of patient's own blood. Läwen, A. Zentralbl. f. Chir. *50:*1468–1471, Sept 29, '23

Treatment of furuncles on face. Hofmann,

Face, Infections of—Cont.

W. Arch. f. klin. Chir. *123:*51-66, '23 (illus.) abstr: J.A.M.A. *80:*1420, May 12, '23

Treatment of furuncles on face by "chemical incision" with phenol. Perret, C. A. Schweiz. med. Wchnschr. *55:*469–470, May 28, '25 abstr: J.A.M.A. *85:*393, Aug 1, '25

Furuncles on face and their treatment. Morian, R. Deutsche Ztschr. f. Chir. *193:*45–58, '25 abstr: J.A.M.A. *85:*1437, Oct 31, '25

Treatment of furuncles of face. Melchior, E. Beitr. z. klin. Chir. *135:*681–695, '26

Surgical therapy of facial furuncle. Schmid, W. Chirurg *6:*447–456, June 15, '34

Infections of lip and face. Coller, F. A. and Yglesias, L. Surg., Gynec. and Obst. *60:*277–290, Feb (no. 2A) '35

Naphthalene in therapy of gangrene following grave trauma of face due to bullet wounds. Palazzi, S. Gior. di med. mil. *85:*944–952, Sept '37

Acute infections of face. Dingman, R. O. Pennsylvania M. J. *42:*499–505, Feb '39

Incision of facial furunculosis. Klapp, R. Zentralbl. f. Chir. *67:*1618-1619, Aug 31, '40

Treatment of facial furuncles. Sittenauer, L. Med. Klin. *36:*1385-1388, Dec 13, '40

Infections of masticator space. Hall, C. and Morris, F. Ann. Otol., Rhin. & Laryng. *50:*1123-1133, Dec '41

Furuncle of face; modification of continuous sutures. de Souza, A. R. Folha med. *25:*60, April 25, '44

Therapy of furunculosis of face. Salleras Llinares, V. and Sagrera, J. M. Med. clin. Barcelona *7:*36–44, July '46

Face, Surgery of

Restoration of cheek and temporal region by pedicled and sliding grafts of skin and muscle. Whitham J.D. J.A.M.A. *76:*448, Feb 12, '21

Plastic operation on protruding cheek. Joseph, J. Deutsche med. Wchnschr. *47:*287, March 17, '21

New principles in plastic operations of eyelids and face Imre, J. Jr. J.A.M.A. *76:*1293, May 7, '21

Plastic and cosmetic surgery of head, neck and face (including keloids). Tieck, G. J. E. and Hunt, H. L. Am. J. Surg. *35:*173, June '21; 355, Nov '21

Technic for reconstruction of face. Molinié, J. Paris med. *11:*89, July 30, '21 abstr: J.A.M.A. *77:*1053, Sept 24, '21

Plastic and cosmetic surgery of head, face and neck; correction of nasal deformities.

Face, Surgery of–Cont.
TIECK, G. J. E. AND HUNT, H. L. Am. J. Surg. *35:*234, Aug '21
Plastic operation on face and lips. BULLOCK, H., M. J. Australia *2:*220, Sept 17, '21
Delayed transfer of long pedicle flaps in plastic surgery (face). BLAIR, V. P. Surg., Gynec. & Obst. *33:*261, Sept '21
Repair of major defects of face. BLAIR, V. P. Texas State J. Med. *17:*301, Oct '21
Scalp flaps in reconstruction of face. MOURE, P. Presse med. *29:*1021–1022, Dec 4, '21 (illus.) Abstr: J.A.M.A. *78:*470, Feb 11, '22
Bandage for plastic operations on face. ESSER, J. F. S. Arch. f. klin. Chir. *117:*438–443, '21 (illus.)
Case of facial fistula due to submaxillary sialolithiasis. CAHN, L. R. AND LEVY, J. Am. J. Surg. *36:*11, Jan '22 (illus.)
Plastic surgery, tube skin-flap in plastic surgery of face. PICKERILL, H. P. AND WHITE, J. R. Brit. J. Surg. *9:*321–333, Jan '22 (illus.)
Plastic surgery of head, face and neck, local anesthesia in operations upon head, face and neck. TIECK, G. J. E.; *et al.* Am. J. Surg. *36:*29–42, Feb '22 (illus.)
Plastic operations on face. SCHLAEPFER, K. Schweiz. med. Wchnschr. *52:*383–386, April 20, '22
Rotation of cheek in plastic surgery. ESSER, J. F. S. Munchen. med. Wchnschr. *69:*780–781, May 26, '22
Some plastic operations on face. IVANISSEVICH, O. Semana med. *1:*382–389, March 9, '22 (illus.) abstr: J.A.M.A. *78:*1672, May 27, '22
Reconstruction surgery of face. BLAIR, V. P. Surg., Gynec. and Obst. *34:*701–716, June '22 (illus.)
Reconstruction of face. LINDEMANN, A. Deutsche Ztschr. f. Chir. *170:*182–208, '22 (illus.) abstr: J.A.M.A. *79:*250, July 15, '22
Plastic operations for defects of face due to noma. HORSLEY, J. S. Southern M. J. *15:*557-561, July '22 (illus.)
Plastic repair of face and hand. SHAW, J. J. M. Brit. J. Surg. *10:*47–51, July '22 (illus.)
Present status of plastic surgery of nose and face. DA SILVA, S. C. Brazil-med. *2:*96–97, Aug 12, '22
Reconstruction of face by Esser's method of Thiersch flaps fitted on dentist's cast. ESSER, J. F. S. Zentralbl. f. Chir. *49:*1217–1219, Aug 19, '22 (illus.)
Plastic surgery of face. HIGHSMITH, E. DEW. Ann. Surg. *76:*129–132, Aug '22 (illus.)
Correction of facial defects with special reference to nutrition of skin flaps and planning

Face, Surgery of–Cont.
of repair. COLEMAN, C. C. Virginia M. Monthly *49:*301-306, Sept '22 (illus.)
Reconstruction of face, new successes of plastic surgery. IVANISSEVICH, O. Semana med. *2:*692–700, Oct 5, '22 (illus.)
Delayed pedicle flap in plastic surgery of face and neck. NEW, G. B. Minnesota Med. *6:*721–724, Dec '22 (illus.)
Plastic and reconstructive surgery of face. IVY, R. H. Surg., Gynec. and Obst. (Internat. Abstract Surg.) *36:*1–7, Jan '23
Rhinoplasty and cheek, chin, and lip plastics with tubed, temporal-pedicled, forehead flaps. MCWILLIAMS, C. A. AND DUNNING, H. S. Surg., Gynec. and Obst. *36:*1–10, Jan '23 (illus.)
Some diseases of mouth, jaws, and face surgically treated. FEDERSPIEL, M. N. Journal-Lancet *43:*267–275, June 1; 297–301, June 15, '23
Plastic repair of face and limbs. SHAW, J. J. M. Tr. Medico-Chir. Soc. Edinburgh, pp. 110–116, '22–'23 (illus.) in Edinburgh M. J., June '23
Surgical reconstruction of face. GIOVACCHINI, L. U. Rev. Asoc. med. argent. *36:*312–315, July '23 (illus.) abstr: J.A.M.A. *81:*1826, Nov 24, '23
Reconstruction of face. MOURE, P., J. de chir. *21:*414–422, April '23 (illus.) abstr: J.A.M.A. *81:*78, July 7, '23
Reconstruction of cheek. POTOTSCHNIG, G. Arch. ital. di chir. *8:*209–224, Oct '23
Plastic operation for palpebro-facial deformity. LEHRFELD, L. Am. J. Ophth. *6:*895–898, Nov '23 (illus.)
Plastic surgery of face and neck. SHEEHAN, J. E. New York M. J. *118:*676–678, Dec 5, '23 (illus.)
Visor scalp flap reconstruction of face. PERTHES, G. Arch. f. klin. Chir. *127:*165–177, '23 (illus.) abstr: J.A.M.A. *81:*2155, Dec 22, '23
Gersuny's pedunculated flaps for reconstruction of face. MOSZKOWICZ, L. Arch. f. klin. Chir. *130:*796–798, '24
Injuries to nerves from surgical treatment of diseases of face and neck. BABCOCK, W. W. J.A.M.A. *84:*187-192, Jan 17, '25
Repair of acquired defects of face (and nose). IVY, R. H., J.A.M.A. *84:*181–185, Jan 17, '25
Case of extensive plastic repair of face and neck with "visor flap." GOLDSCHMIDT, T. Zentralbl. f. Chir. *52:*688–691, March 28, '25
Plastic surgery about face, head and neck. BECK, J. C., J. Indiana M. A. *18:*167–184, May '25

Face, Surgery of—Cont.

Combined satchel handle or tubed pedicle and large delayed whole skin pedicle flaps in case of plastic surgery of face, neck and chest. ALDEN, B. F. Surg., Gynec. and Obst. *41:*493–496, Oct '25

New procedures and method in plastic surgery of face and neck. NEW, G. B. South. M. J. *19:*138–140, Feb '26

Plastic operations on face, in region of eye. VARIOUS AUTHORS. Proc. Roy. Soc. Med. (sect. Ophth.) *19:*14–38, June '26

Facial disfigurements. MCWILLIAMS, C. A. Am. J. Surg. *1:*76–79, Aug '26

Plastic repair of facial defects. MULLEN, T. F. Northwest Med. *25:*408–416, Aug '26

Facial autoplasty. ESSER, J. F. S. Paris chirurg. *18:*263, Nov '26

Facial reconstructive surgery with presentation of cases and lantern slide demonstration. MALINIAK, J. Laryngoscope *37:*157–169, March '27 also: M. Times, New York *55:*57; 72, March '27 also: J. M. Soc. New Jersey *24:*349–355, June '27

Technic of plastic surgery of face and nose. VAN DEN BRANDEN, J. Bruxelles-med. *7:*917–920, May 15, '27

Plastic surgery of face. GATEWOOD. S. Clin. N. Amer. *7:*539–549, June '27

Plastic surgery of face (including nose). IVY, R. H. Atlantic M. J. *30:*572–575, June '27

Plastic covering of facial defects. KUKULIES, C. Deutsche Monatschr. f. Zahnh. *45:*494–496, June 1, '27

Surgical correction of cervicofacial scars of dental origin. MAUREL, G., J. de med. de Paris *46:*577–583, July 21, '27

Utilization of skin of upper eyelid for repair of small facial defects. SHEEHAN, J. E. Arch. Otolaryng. *6:*107–111, Aug '27

Correction of some facial disfigurements. STRAITH, C. L., J. Michigan M. Soc. *26:* 506–515, Aug '27

Facial deformities. HIGHSMITH, E. D. South. M. J. *20:*688–689, Sept '27

Correction of facial deformities. MALINIAK, J. M. Rev. of Rev. *33:*571–578, Dec '27

Epithelialized flap from forehead to reconstruct lower lip and cheek. NEW, G. B., S. Clin. N. Amer. *7:*1481–1483, Dec '27

Facial deformities of mid face. VIRCHOW, H. Ztschr. f. d. ges. Anat. (abt. 1) *84:*555–596, Dec 28, '27

Plastic surgery of face, neck and chest skin losses. BLAIR, V. P. Tr. Am. S. A. *45:*190–199, '27

Plastic method of covering large loss of substance of face. EHRENFELD, H. Arch. f. klin. Chir. *147:*633–636, '27

Face, Surgery of—Cont.

Round movable pedicles in complicated plastic operations on eyelids and face. FILATOV, W. P. Arch. f. klin. Chir. *146:*609–614, '27

Restoration of face. BERCOWWITSCH, G. G. Dental Cosmos *70:*167–170, Feb '28

Progress in reparative surgery of face. SHEEHAN, J. E. Arch. franco-belges de chir. *31:*122–125, Feb '28

Reparative facial surgery. SHEEHAN, J. E. M. J. and Rec. *127:*245–246, March 7, '28

Functional restoration as element in facial repair and nose. SHEEHAN, J. E. Bull. New York Acad. Med. *4:*416–421, March '28

Functional restoration as chief concern in repair of facial defects. SHEEHAN, J. E., S. Clin. N. Amer. *8:*293–307, April '28

Plastic surgery of face. DE RIVER, J. P. California and West. Med. *28:*651–655, May '28

Cosmetic treatment of facial scars. EITNER, E. Urol. and Cutan. Rev. *32:*282, May '28

"Transport" plastic operations of face. MATTI, H. Schweiz. med. Wchnschr. *58:*669–673, July 7, '28

Plastic surgery of face and harelip and nose and cleft palate. JOBSON, G. B. Atlantic M. J. *31:*716–723, July '28

Correction of frontal depression by inclusion of celluloid; case. BALDENWECK. Ann. d. mal. de l'oreille, du larynx *47:*757, Aug '28

Functional restoration as element in facial repair. SHEEHAN, J. E. Am. J. Surg. *5:*164–166, Aug '28

Repair of facial defects. ASPINALL, A. J., J. Coll. Surgeons, Australasia *1:*230–232, Nov '28

Surgical treatment of congenital facial malformation. ESTELLA Y BERMÚDEZ DE CASTRO, J. Clin. y. lab. *12:*276, Oct; 364, Nov; 456, Dec '28

Technic of facial surgery. CHIAROLANZA, R. AND CAVINA, C. Arch. ed. atti d. Soc. ital. di chir. (1927) *34:*cxvi, '28

Free transplants of skin in plastic surgery of face and neck. SANVENERO-ROSSELLI, G. Arch. ital. di chir *21:*245–265, '28

Methods and results of plastic surgery of face. SANVENERO-ROSSELLI, G. Bruxelles-med. *9:*476–482, Feb. 24, '29 abstr: Bruxelles med. (supp.) *9:*63, '28

Extensive facial reconstructive surgery; 2 cases. REINBERG, H. Zentralbl. f. Chir. *56:*530–534, March 2, '29

Cartilage graft to malar bone. MOOREHEAD, F. B., S. Clin. N. Amer. *9:*331–332, April '29

Facial deformities caused by abnormalities of jaw; operative and dental treatment; cases. POHL, L. Rev. odont. *50:*134–150, April '29

Face, Surgery of–Cont.

Plastic and reconstructive surgery of face and jaws. Ivy, R. H. Virginia M. Monthly *56:*174–180, June '29

Treatment of traumatic and acquired deformities of face. Straith, C. L., J. Michigan M. Soc. *28:*431–443, June '29

Plastic surgery of face; cases. Figuras, V. Gac. med. de Mexico *60:*353–381, Aug '29

General principles of plastic surgery of face. Mirizzi, P. L. Schweiz. med. Wchnschr. *59:*1011–1019, Oct 5, '29

Plastic surgery of nose, ear, face. Davis, A. D. Arch. Otolaryng. *10:*575–584, Dec '29

Bridging of osseous defects of forehead, using metal models as guides for shaping cartilage transplants. Rush, L. V.; *et al.* Am. J. Surg. *7:*805–807, Dec '29

Principles of plastic surgery of importance to general practitioners (for face). Brown, G. V. I. Proc. Internat. Assemb. Inter-State Post-Grad. M. A., North America (1928), pp. 542–547, '29

Covering defects of face by double skin transplantation from abdomen to forearm and face. Ivanitzkyi, G. Ukrain. m. visti *5:*41–42, '29

Covering disfiguring cuts on face by method of skin transplantation from abdomen to forearm and face. Khartzieff. Ukrain. m. visti *5:*42–46, '29

Plastic repair of extremities and face. Shaw, J. J. M. Tr. Roy. Med.-Chir. Soc., Glasgow (1927–1928) *22:*151, '29

Plastic surgery of face. Horsley, J. S. Jr. West Virginia M. J. *26:*1–8, Jan '30

Plastic restorations after specific lesions of face. Pickerill, P., M. J. Australia *1:*414–417, March 29, '30

Eliminating facial scars. Bames, H. O. M. J. and Rec. *131:*348–350, April 2, '30

Correction of facial deformities. Rhinoplasty, a few statistical data. Maliniak, J. W. Eye, Ear, Nose and Throat Monthly *9:*194–198, June '30 also: Laryngoscope *40:*495–501, July '30

Cancrum oris with recovery; subsequent repair of defect by plastic operation. Goodall, E. W. Brit. J. Child. Dis. *27:*204–208, July–Sept '30

Plastic operation for restoration of chin, lower lip, and part of cheeks; method of applying dressing. Krauss, F. Zentralbl. f. Chir. *57:*1915–1916, Aug 2, '30

Reparation of loss of facial substance with tubular graft; case. Kroeff, M. Folha med. *11:*325–327, Oct 5, '30

Plastic surgery of face. Schreiber, F. Ztschr. f. Laryng., Rhin. *20:*1–9, Oct '30

Face, Surgery of–Cont.

Treatment of harelip and other facial fissures. Härtel, F. F. Chirurg *2:*1057–1061, Dec 1, '30

Physiologic troubles in patients with old wounds and injuries of face. Bertein, P. Bull. med., Paris *44:*947–949, Dec 27, '30

Plastic surgery by Rehn's method of shifting soft parts to cover defect of face. Fohl, T. and Killian, H. Deutsche Ztschr. f. Chir. *222:*309–320, '30

Plastic method for correcting depression after external operations of frontal sinus; celluloids plates. Stupka, W. Monatschr. f. Ohrenh. *65:*39–56, Jan '31

Tube flaps in reconstructive surgery of face. Peer, L. A., J. M. Soc. New Jersey *28:*86–89, Feb '31

Plastic surgery in malignant syphilis of face and nasal fossae; case. Portmann, G. Rev. de laryng. *52:*199–208, March 31, '31

Facial abnormalities, fancied and real; reaction of patient; attempted correction (including nose). Blair, V. P. Proc. Inst. Med., Chicago *8:*217–223, April 15, '31

Facial plastic surgery; cases. Klapp, R. Chirurg *3:*353–357, April 15, '31

Plastic surgery of face. Poggi, J. Bol. do coll. brasil. de cir. *2:*91–99, April–Nov '31

Maintenance of facial form after removal of right half of mandible. Anderson, G. M. Internat. J. Orthodontia *17:*860–864, Sept '31

Plastic surgery of face. Dobrzaniecki, W. Rev. de chir. plastique, pp. 182–200, Oct '31

Simplified method for correction of dishface. Maliniak, J. W. Laryngoscope *41:*715–717, Oct '31

Problem of cartilage implant (face). Updegraff, H. L. Am. J. Surg. *14:*492–498, Nov '31

Plastic surgery of different parts of face. Bourguet, J. Cong. internat. de med. trop. et d'hyg., Compt.rend (1928) *3:*347–351, '31

Use of pedicled flaps in reconstructive surgery of face. New, G. B. Tr. Am. Laryng., Rhin. and Otol. Soc. *37:*485–491, '31

Reparative surgery in relation to face. Sheehan, J. E. and Barsky, A. J. Proc. Internat. Assemb. Inter-State Post-Grad. M. A., North America (1930) *6:*434–437, '31

Cystic disease of pilosebaceous system of face. Favre, M. Bull. Soc. franc. de dermat. et syph. (Reunion dermat.) *39:*93–96, Jan '32

Plastic surgery of face. Ehrenfeld, H. Gyogyaszat *72:*186–189, March 20, '32

Important factors in surgery of common fa-

Face, Surgery of—Cont.
cial deformities. MALINIAK, J. W. Eye, Ear, Nose and Throat Monthly *11:*95-99, April '32
Important factors in surgery of acquired and congenital facial deformities. MALINIAK, J. W., J. M. Soc. New Jersey *29:*314-323, April '32
Planning plastic operation of face. RUSH, H. L. AND RUSH, L. V. New Orleans M. and S. J. *84:*948-953, June '32
Lined pedicled flaps in reconstructive surgery of face; modification of technic. HAVENS, F. Z. S. Clin. North America *12:*955-957, Aug '32
Use of pedicled flaps and skin grafts in reconstructive surgery of (face) and head and neck. FIGI, F. A. Nebraska M. J. *17:*361-365, Sept '32
Plastic surgery of face. EHRENFELD, H. Gyogyaszat *72:*675-676, Oct 30, '32
Extensive cicatrix of face; reconstruction of both eyelids and of both lips by tubular grafts. ROCHER, H. L. Bull. et mem. Soc. de chir. de Bordeaux et du Sud-Ouest, pp. 154-156, '32
Methods and results of plastic surgery of face. SANVENERO-ROSSELLI, G. Boll. e mem. Soc. piemontese di chir. *2:*1024-1050, '32
Surgery of face in South America. DUFOURMENTEL, L. Paris med. (annexe) *1:*i-viii, Feb 18, '33
Surgical correction of facial deformities. PEUGNIEZ. Bull. et mem. Soc. d. chirurgiens de Paris *25:*315-318, May 19, '33
Technic of incisions and sutures in plastic surgery (face). DANTRELLE. Rev. de chir. plastique, pp. 75-108, Aug '33
Traumatic facial scarring; removal. FIGI, F. A., S. Clin. North America *13:*882-884, Aug '33
Transplantation of pedicled skin flap to face; case. KANEMATSU, T. Okayama-Igakkai-Zasshi *45:*2099-2100, Sept '33
Plastic surgery of face. BROWN, J. B. Internat. Abstr. Surg., pp. 297-311, Oct '33
Cheek rotation. ESSER, J. F. S. Rev. de chir. plastique, pp. 298-299, Jan '34
Plastic repair of face; case. SMYTH, G. J. C. South African M. J. *8:*181-182, March 10, '34
Reconstruction in crushing of facial bones. DUFOURMENTEL, L. AND DARCISSAC, M. Bull. et mem. Soc. d. chirurgiens de Paris *26:*315-330, May 4, '34
Cosmetic therapy of facial cicatrices. EITNER, E. Wien. med. Wchnschr. *84:*555-556, May 12, '34

Face, Surgery of—Cont.
Plastic repair of face by means of skin transplantation; case. BARROS LIMA. Arq. de cir. e ortop. *1:*386-394, June '34
Replacement of tissues of forehead and scalp. NEW. G. B.; *et al.* S. Clin. North America *14:*607-613, June '34
Surgical and orthopedic prosthetic correction of depression of middle portion of face due to automobile accidents; cases. DUFOURMENTEL, L. AND DARCISSAC, M. Rev. de stomatol. *36:*447-457, July '34
Traumatism of face and jaws with special reference to complications. KAZANJIAN, V. H., J. Am. Dent. A. *21:*1138-1152, July '34
New operative technic for facial salivary cyst of traumatic nature. MIHĂILESCU, S. P. Rev. de chir., Bucuresti *37:*713-715, Sept-Dec '34
Use of reconstructive surgery in certain types of facial deformities and nasal. NEW, G. B. AND FIGI, F. A., J.A.M.A. *103:*1434-1438, Nov 10, '34
Facial plastic surgery; cases. LÓPEZ VILLORIA, L. Gac. med. de Caracas *41:*338-344, Nov 30 '34
Facial plastic surgery; cases. ALFREDO, J. Rev. med. de Pernambuco *4:*277-301, Dec '34
Transplantation of thick skin flap in plastic surgery of face. DUBOV, M. D. Sovet. khir. (nos. 3-4) *6:*489-502, '34
Use of reconstructive surgery in certain types of deformities (face) (nose). NEW, G. B. AND FIGI, F. A. Tr. Sect. Laryng., Otol. and Rhin., A.M.A., pp. 52-63, '34
Celluloid prosthesis in cosmetic correction after disfiguring surgery of frontal sinus. STUPKA, W. Arch. f. Ohren-Nasen-u. Kehlkopfh. *138:*79-86, '34
Plastic repair of defect of cheek. EISELSBERG, A. Schweiz. med. Wchnschr. *65:*25-26, Jan 12, '35
Recent advances in plastic surgery with special reference to vascularization of implants (face). GOLDEN, H. M. Illinois M. J. *67:*175-181, Feb '35
Plastic surgery of facial defects. BURIAN, F. Casop. lek. cesk. *74:*261-263, March 8, '35
Fundamental principles of plastic surgery including grafts (face). FORD, J. F. Texas State J. Med. *30:*761-763, April '35
Fissural cyst of cheek; case. CROCQUEFER. Rev. de Stomatol. *37:*513-518, Aug '35
Correction of deformities of forehead and nose; presentation of 2 patients. NEW, G. B. Proc. Staff Meet., Mayo Clin. *10:*519-521, Aug 14, '35
Plastic surgery of face; interesting cases.

Face, Surgery of–Cont.

O'SULLIVAN, T. J. Maine M. J. *26:*167-173, Nov '35

Possibility of reconstructing whole face by full thickness, free cutaneous grafts, using several flaps. COLELST. Rev. de chir. structive, pp. 105-125, Dec '35

Plastic operation of face following noma. SMYRNOFF, S. S., M. Rec. *143:*186-188, March 4, '36

Modern plastic surgery (face). ALFREDO, M. Rev. med. de Pernambuco *6:*109-118, April '36

Plastic surgery of face. JULLIARD, C. Helvet. med. acta *3:*136-142, May '36

Cartilage transplants in facial surgery. BAMES, H. O. Rev. de chir. structive, pp. 281-285, June '36

Plastic replacement of extensive mucosal defects of cheek. HOFER, O. Wien. klin. Wchnschr. *49:*990-992, July 31, '36

Plastic surgery of ears; cases (and face) (and nose). MALBEC, E. F. Semana med. *2:*718-728, Sept 10, '36

Surgical care of injuries and deformities of nose, lip and premaxilla, with report of cases. FEDERSPIEL, M. N. Internat. J. Orthodontia *22:*1054-1068, Oct '36

Rotation of cheek to remake face; case. ESSER, J. F. S. Tech. chir. *28:*293-296, Dec '36

Repair of facial defects with special reference to source of skin grafts. MALINIAK, J. W. Rev. de chir. structive, pp. 431-439, Dec '36 also: Arch. Surg. *34:*897-908, May '37

Skin, cartilage and bone grafts to face. NEW, G. B. Proc. Staff Meet., Mayo Clin. *11:*791-794, Dec 9, '36

Alloplastic and heteroplastic grafts in reconstruction of facial defects; use of ivory and cartilage. SPANIER, F. Rev. de chir. structive, pp. 391-401, Dec '36

Late results after transplantation of mammary gland in closure of facial defect. IGNATEV, S. S. Vestnik khir. *47:*103, '36

Traumatic origin of late angioneurotic condition in region of nose and cheek; 3 cases. SEMRAU, J. Hals-, Nasen-u. Ohrenarzt (Teil 1) *27:*363-370, '36

Plastic repair of frontal deformity using hump from nose. STRAATSMA, C. R. Tr. Am. Acad. Ophth. *41:*625-626, '36

New ideas with regard to plastic surgery of pendulous cheeks with description of new method. EHRENFELD, H. Zentralbl. f. Chir. *64:*202-205, Jan 23, '37

Treatment of old traumatic boney lesions of face. McINDOE, A. H. Surg., Gynec. and Obst. *64:*376-386, Feb (no. 2A) '37

Traumatic deformities of nose and other bones of face. NEW, G. B. Surg., Gynec. and Obst. *64:*532-537, Feb (no. 2A) '37

Role of intra-oral and intranasal grafts in contour restoration of face. KILNER, T. P. Rev. de chir. structive, pp. 1-3, March '37

Scars of facial wounds. STRAITH, C. L. Am. J. Surg. *36:*88-90, April '37

Skin grafts for plastic surgery of face. SANCHEZ ARBIDE, A. Semana med. *2:*1281-1286, Dec 2, '37

Reconstructive surgery (face). ADAMS, W. M. Mississippi Doctor *15:*23-28, Feb '38

Method of obliterating depressions of face; case. MALBEC, E. F. Semana med. *1:*600-602, March 17, '38

Plastic repair of facial deformations. BAMES, H. O. Bol. y trab. de la Soc. de cir. de Buenos Aires *22:*116-119, May 4, '38

Procedure for removing sebaceous cysts of face with conservative excision. UGGERI, C. Gazz. d. osp. *59:*456-458, May 1, '38

Facial asymmetry; plastic surgery (including jaws). ZENO, L. An. de cir. *4:*134-136, June '38

Plastic surgery of face cases. CHIAROLANZA, R. Chir. plast. *4:*114-123, July-Sept '38

Rotation of cheek in ophthalmology. ESSER, J. F. S. Arch. Ophth. *20:*410-416, Sept '38

Plastic surgery (face) (nose). KING, E. D., J. Med. *19:*348-354, Sept '38

Plastic surgery, with report of original operation for advancement of nasolabial fold. DOUGLAS, B. South. M. J. *31:*1047-1052, Oct '38

Refrigerated cartilage isografts in facial surgery. O'CONNOR, G. B. AND PIERCE, G. W. Surg., Gynec. and Obst. *67:*796-798, Dec '38

Flat skin graft in restoration of extensive facial defects. NIKANOROV, A. M. Novy khir. arkhiv *40:*255-258, '38

Plastic surgery for mutilations of face resulting from exeresis of malignant tumors from soft parts. SANVENERO-ROSSELLI, G. Arch. ital. di chir. *54:*491-501, '38

Total restoration of lower half of face. SOKOLOV, N. N. Novy khir. arkhiv *40:*426-437, '38

Plastic surgery of face. THEODORESCO, D. Rev. de chir., Bucuresti *42:*365-372, May-June '39

Plastic surgery for Hutchinson's facies and various accompanying ptoses. BOURGUET, J. Monde med., Paris *49:*659-667, June 15, '39

Plastic and reconstructive surgery about face and head–then and now. BECK, J. C. Illinois M. J. *76:*237-242, Sept '39

Face, Surgery of–Cont.

Surgery of face; graft by bipedicled flaps. DUFOURMENTEL. Oto-rhino-laryng. internat. *23:*528–529, Oct '39

Modern changes in plastic and reconstructive surgery of face and neck. GUTTMAN, M. R. Illinois M. J. *76:*349–351, Oct '39

Use of medicated paper dressing in facial surgery. COELST. Bull. Soc. belge d'otol., rhinol. laryng., pp. 319–320, '39

Plastic surgery of face (including harelip and cleft palate). HAGENTORN. A. Arch. f. klin. Chir. *195:*455–488, '39

Tubular graft (Gillies-Filatov Anglo-Russian graft) in repair of facial defects; cases. CODAZZI AGUIRRE, J. A. Rev. med. de Rosario *30:*208–218, Feb '40

Plastic surgery in therapy of facial scars (grafts). DUJARDIN, E. Ugesk. f. laeger *102:*222, Feb 29, '40

Repair of defects of frontal bone. NEW, G. B. and DIX, C. R. Surg., Gynec. and Obst. *70:*698–701, March '40

Cervicofacial arc, apparatus for isolating surgical field. BERTOLA, V. J. Prensa med. argent. *27:*997–998, May 8, '40

Sulfathiazole (sulfanilamide derivative) used with cartilage implants for repair of facial defects. CHILDREY, J. H. Ann. Otol., Rhin. and Laryng. *49:*709–712, Sept '40

Plastic surgery of face. GINGRASS, R. P. Am. J. Orthodontics *26:*961–967, Oct '40

Retractile scars of cervicofacial region; biologic fundamentals for plastic reconstruction. ZENO, L. Bol. Soc. de cir. de Rosario *7:*446–454, No. '40 also: An. de cir. *6:*341–349, Dec '40 also: Dia med. *13:*264–266, April 14, '41

Plastic surgery of face. SIURKUS, T. Medicina, Kaunas *22:*90–96, Jan '41

Facial structure in relationship to fractures. JAMES, W. W. AND FICKLING, B. W. Proc. Roy. Soc. Med. *34:*205–211, Feb '41

Plastic surgery of face and head. JENKINS, H. P., S. Clin. North America *21:*37–53, Feb '41

Facial autoplasty; cases. KROEFF, M. Hospital, Rio de Janeiro *19:*559–570, April '41

Use of iliac bone in facial and cranial repair. SHEEHAN, J. E. Am. J. Surg. *52:*55–61, April '41

Facial autoplasty in nasal surgery; cases. KROEFF, M. Hospital, Rio de Janeiro *19:*773–781, May '41; *20:*11, July '41

Grafts of preserved cartilage in restorations of facial contour. STRAITH, C. L. AND SLAUGHTER, W. B., J.A.M.A. *116:*2008–2013, May 3, '41

Plastic surgery of face and nose. KING, E. D. West Virginia M. J. *37:*293–297, July '41

Tubed pedicle graft in facial reconstruction; superiority when subcutaneous loss is present. WILMOTH, C. L. Am. J. Surg. *53:*300–305, Aug '41

Plastic surgery of face; 2 cases. MALBEC, E. F. Semana med. *2:*1311–1313, Nov. 27, '41

Method to prevent fresh cartilage grafts from warping (facial surgery). NEW, G. B. AND ERICH, J. B. Am. J. Surg. *54:*435–438, Nov '41

Plastic surgery of face, with report of cases. ZENO, L. Bol. Soc. de cir. de Rosario *8:*469–476, Nov '41 also: An. de cir. *7:*287–294, Dec '41

Preserved human cartilage in reconstructive surgery of face. IGLAUER, S. Ann. Otol., Rhin. and Laryng. *50:*1072–1078, Dec '41

Chirurgie de la face et de la région maxillo-faciale, by MAURICE AUBRY AND CHARLES FREIDEL. Masson et Cie, Paris. 1942

Plastic surgery of face; 5 cases. MALBEC, E. F. Arq. de cir. clin. e exper. *6:*503–512, April–June '42

Use of implants in plastic surgery of face. RIVAS, C. I. *et al.* Arq. de cir. clin. e exper. *6:*621–638, April–June '42

Soft tissue repair in injuries about face and head. MARCKS, K. M. Pennsylvania M. J. *45:*801–806, May '42

Symposium on industrial surgery; fractures of jaws and injuries of face, mouth and teeth. THOMAS, E. H., S. Clin. North America *22:*1029–1048, Aug '42

Successful modern plastic surgery in serious disfiguration due to scalping; reconstruction of eyelids and eyebrows and replacement of total skin of forehead and temples. VON SEEMEN, H. Zentralbl. f. Chir. *69:*1280–1287, Aug 1, '42

Refinements in reconstructive surgery of face. SMITH, F., J.A.M.A. *120:*352–358, Oct 3, '42

Plastic surgery of face. DELLEPIANE RAWSON, R. Dia med. *14:*1052–1055, Oct 12, '42

Free skin grafts versus flaps in surface defects of face and neck. MALINIAC, J. W. Am. J. Surg. *58:*100–109, Oct '42

Plastic surgery of face. ZENO, L. An. de cir. *8:*139–151, Sept '42

Use of tubular flaps in repair of defects of face. RAPIN, M. Helvet. med. acta *9:*787–792, Dec '42

Plastic surgery of face; synthesis. DELLEPIANE RAWSON, R. Dia med. *15:*638–640, June 21, '43

Sebaceous cysts of face; extirpation. FINOCHIETTO, R. Prensa med. argent. *30:*1876–

Face, Surgery of–Cont.
1877, Sept 29, '43
Facial reconstruction and speech. HIGLEY, L. B., J. Am. Dent. A. *30:*1716–1725, Nov 1, '43
Use of one flap to restore extensive losses of middle third of face. BARSKY, A. J. Ann. Surg. *118:*998–999, Dec '43
Use of one flap to restore extensive losses of middle third of face. BARSKY, A. J. Tr. Am. Soc. Plastic and Reconstructive Surg. *12:*29–41, '43
Reconstruction of deformities of forehead and frontal bone. KAZANJIAN, V. H. Tr. Am. Soc. Plastic and Reconstructive Surg. *12:*83–97, '43
Deformities of face and their correction. DAVIS, W. B. Surgery *15:*43–55, Jan '44
Evaluation of pedicle flaps versus skin grafts in reconstruction of surface defects and scar contractures of chin, cheeks and neck. AUFRICHT, G. Surgery *15:*75–84, Jan '44
Symposium on plastic surgery; planning the reconstruction of the face. SMITH, F. Surgery *15:*1–15, Jan '44
Sculpturally molded synthetic implants (methyl methacrylate) in plastic surgery of face. BROWN, A. M. Arch. Otolaryng. *39:*179–183, Feb '44
Repair of bony and contour deformities of face. IVY, R. H. Surgery *15:*56–74, Jan '44 also: Am. J. Orthodontics (Oral Surg. Sect.) *30:*76–94, Feb '44
Closure of granulating wounds of face by means of button sutures. ENTIN, D. A. Am. Rev. Soviet. Med. *1:*351–354, April '44
Cast and precast cartilage grafts; use in restoration of contour of face. YOUNG, F. Surgery *15:*735–748, May '44
Counterstroke electrocoagulation of buccal mucosa during treatment of facial lesions. BARMAN, J. M. Rev. argent. dermatosif. *28:*191–192, June '44
Reconstruction after radical operation for osteomyelitis of frontal bone; experience in 38 cases. KAZANJIAN, V. H. AND HOLMES, E. M. Surg., Gynec. and Obst. *79:*397–411, Oct '44
Stomatoplasty in loss of cheek due to gangrene. MENDIZABAL, P. Cir. y. cirujanos *12:*427–431, Oct–Nov '44
Plastic reconstruction of soft tissues of face during period of secondary suture. BALON, L. R. Khirurgiya, no. 3, pp. 30–31, '44
Secondary suture of granulating wounds of face. FELDMAN, S. P. AND GROSSMAN, S. Y. Sovet. med. (no. 6) *8:*22–23, '44
Acrylic resin as implant for correction of facial deformities. PENHALE, K. W. Arch.

Face, Surgery of–Cont.
Surg. *50:*233–239, May '45
Problems of plastic surgery of face. DIX, C. R. Wisconsin M. J. *44:*593–596, June '45
Davis grafts in reparative surgery of face. FERRIE, J. Ophthalmologica *110:*292–299, Nov–Dec '45
Plastic surgery in congenital deformities about face. LAMONT, E. S. Eye, Ear, Nose and Throat Monthly *24:*571, Dec '45; *25:*25 Jan; 85, Feb '46
Pedicle grafts from arm for reconstructions about face. JENKINS, H. P., S. Clin. North America *26:*20–32, Feb '46
Rebuilding bony depressions of face and skull. BERSON, M. I., J. Internat. Coll. Surgeons *9:*243–247, Mar–Apr '46
Repair of defects (using tantalum), with special reference to periorbital structures and frontal sinus. TURNER, O. A. Arch. Surg. *53:*312–326, Sept '46

Face, Tumors of (See also Specific Tumor; Face, Cancer of; Face, Surgery of)

Hypertrophic capillary angioma of cheek; removal; plastic replacement of skin, case. WEICHERT, M. Beitr. z. klin. Chir. *145:*718–720, '20
Clinical history of tumors of face and jaws as guide to their correct diagnosis and proper treatment. GATCH, W. D., J. Indiana M. A. *15:*251–255, Aug '22
Angiomas of parotid region. SCHENK, P. Mitt. a. d. Grenzgeb. d. Med. u. Chir. *37:*51–55, '23
Primary tumors of facial bones. DELLEPIANE RAWSON, R. Semana med. *1:*652–654, March 19, '25
Angioma cavernosum; report of case of face treated with radium. FRAZIER, C. N. Arch. Dermat. and Syph. *12:*506–508, Oct '25
Angioma of left temporal and malar regions. REDER, F., S. Clin. N. America *5:*1303–1311, Oct '25
Treatment of extensive subcutaneous angiomas of face. by Morestin's method. MARAGLIANO, D. Arch. ital. di chir. *12:*603–615, '25
Ulcerating angioma of face; case. MILIAN, G. AND DELARUE, J. Bull. Soc. franc. de dermat. et syph. *34:*189–192, March '27
Case of cavernous angioma (facial nevus). DREYER. Munchen. med. Wchnschr. *74:*563, April 1, '27
Lipoma of cheek and neck. DALEPPA, K. Indian M. Gaz. *62:*385–386, July '27

Face, Tumors of–Cont.

Removal of tumor of cheek and temporal region with secondary plastic operation. NEW, G. B., S. Clin. N. Amer. *7:*1479–1481, Dec '27

Results of cryotherapy in angiomas of face in nurslings and in angiomas of eyelids. LORTAT-JACOB, L. Bull. et mem. Soc. med. d. hop. de Paris *52:*527–528, March 29, '28

Cavernous angioma of cheek; case. QUARTERO. Nederl. Tijdschr. v. Geneesk. *1:*1997, April 21, '28

Treatment of angioma of face. KOVALSKY, N. P. Vestnik khir. (no. 40) *14:*30–38, '28

Cavernous angioma of face with homolateral glaucoma; case. OHNO, T. Jap. J. Dermat. and Urol. *29:*33, May '29

Multiple fibromata of eyelid and forehead; removal; case. BAKRY, M. Bull. Ophth. Soc. Egypt *22:*78, '29

Multiple pigmented papillary nevi of face. (pigmented mole) FIGI, F. A., S. Clin. N. Amer. *10:*101–103, Feb '30

Electrotherapy of tuberous angioma of face. GERONIMI, E. Schweiz. med. Wchnschr. *61:*589–593, June 20, '31

Plastic and esthetic surgery in hemangioma (face). DESELAERS. Rev. de chir. plastique, pp. 70–73, April '32

Cavernous lymphangioma of forehead; extirpation and cure. MARTÍNEZ VARGAS, A. Med. de los ninos *33:*89–100, April '32

Radium therapy of giant angiomas of face; 3 cases. LLORENS SUQUE, A. J. de radiol. et d'electrol. *16:*211–213, May '32

Massive congenital cervicofacial cavernous hemangioma; case. GIUSTINIAN, V. AND ESTIÚ, M. D. Semana med. *2:*245–246, July 28, '32

New method of surgical therapy of subcutaneous angiomas of face. BARDANZELLU, T. Arch. di ottal. *39:*520–543, Nov–Dec '32

Tumor of cheek and problem of surgical restoration. CHAVANNAZ, G., J. de med. de Bordeaux *110:*7–9, Jan 10, '33

Sebaceous nevus of face; case. REDAELLI, E. Gior. ital. di dermat. e sif. *74:*122–129, Feb '33

Multiple cutaneous horns; removal and skin graft. FIGI, F. A., S. Clin. North America *13:*880–881, Aug '33

Congenital recurrent lymphangioma of cheek. FRIEDMAN, M. Eye, Ear, Nose & Throat Monthly *12:*334–335, Sept '33

Congenital angiomas with nasofacial localization; case. FRANCHINI, Y. AND RICCITELLI, E. An. de oto-rino-laring. d. Uruguay *3:*193–203, '33

Angiomas of face and mouth. CLARK, C. M. Ohio State M. J. *30:*438–441, July '34

Success of surgical therapy of angiomas on face of nurslings; 2 cases. VALLINO, M. T. AND SERFATY, M. Rev. Asoc. med. argent. *48:*1463–1465, Dec '34

Pediculated vascular tumor developed on large nevus of face; case. NICOLAS, J. AND ROUSSET, J. Bull. Soc. franc. de dermat. et syph. (Reunion dermat., Lyon) *42:*1050–1051, July '35

Vascular tumors of face; 2 cases. DE CERQUEIRA FALCAO, E. Rev. oto-laring. de Sao Paulo *3:*533–538, Nov–Dec '35 also: Brasil-med. *50:*134–139, Feb 15, '36

Cirsoid craniofacial angiomas; cases. DUFOURMENTEL, L. Bull. et mem. Soc. d. chirurgiens de Paris *28:*103–109, March 6, '36

Question of electrolysis or diathermocoagulation in therapy of vascular tumors of face; experimental study. POCHY-RIANO, R. Arch. di radiol. *12:*121–133, March–April '36

Cavernous angioma of face. DUFOURMENTEL, L. Oto-rhino-laryng. internat. *20:*297–300, May '36

Surface angioma of face treated with cryotherapy and radium. MARIN, A. Union med. du Canada *65:*446–449, May '36

Facial inclusion tumors. DUFOURMENTEL, L. Mem. Acad. de chir. *62:*793–798, June 3, '36

Angiomas of face; treatment. FIGI, F. A. Arch. Otolaryng. *24:*271–281, Sept '36

Cavernous angiomas of face in children; late results of radium therapy. PERUSSIA, F. Strahlentherapie *57:*109–120, '36

Angioma of face; treatment. FIGI, F. A. Proc. Staff Meet., Mayo Clin. *12:*437–442, July 14, '37

Diathermy applied to facial lymphangiomas; cases. VAN DEN WILDENBERG. Oto-rhino-laryng. internat. *22:*5–10, Jan '38

Angiomas of face; therapy. DUFOURMENTEL, L. Bull. et mem. Soc. de med. de Paris *142:*271–281, March 26, '38

Tumor of lower lip and right cheek; extirpation followed by pedicled skin graft from head. PORUMBARU, I. Rev. de chir., Bucuresti *41:*714–721, Sept–Oct '38

Extensive congenital angioma of face obliterated by injections of sodium salicylate. FILDERMAN, L. Bull. et mem. Soc. de med. de Paris *142:*576–578, Oct 22, '38

Therapy of cavernous angioma of face; cases. NOEL. Rev. de chir. structive *8:*199–203, '38

Therapy of facial naevus flammeus with new mercury high pressure lamp (intensol lamp). LOMHOLT, S. Dermat. Wchnschr. *109:*898–900, July 29, '39

Face, Tumors of—Cont.

Facial angioma with macrocheilia; case. KIKUCHI R. AND EBA, M. Oto-rhino-laryng. *12:*1018, Dec '39

Surgical therapy of extensive facial tumors, and plastic restoration (grafts). VON SEEMEN, H. Arch. f. klin. Chir. *200:*553–566, '40

Surgical removal of hemangioma of face with grafting. BERSON, M. I. Am. J. Surg. *51:*362–365, Feb '41

Tumors of head and face. WOLFER, J. A. Indust. Med. *10:*59–60, Feb '41

Extensive mole of face and scalp; excision and full thickness skin graft. FIGI, F. A. Proc. Staff Meet., Mayo Clin. *16:*280–282, April 30, '41

Hypertrophic angioma of cheek; case. MUKASA, H. Oto-rhino-laryng. *14:*487, July '41

Cavernous hemangioma of nose, nasal septum and forehead. SALINGER, S. Ann. Otol., Rhin. and Laryng. *51:*268–272, March '42

Angioma arteriale racemosum of face and tongue; surgical therapy; case. PAVLOVSKY, A. J. Bol. y trab., Acad. argent. de cir. *26:*670–672, Aug 19, '42

Tumors of head, face and neck. WOLFER, J. A. Indust. Med. *11:*528–529, Nov '42

Cavernous hemangioma of face in infant treated with radium; case. JACOBS, A. W. Am. J. Roentgenol. *49:*816–818, June '43

Extensive destructive ulcerating angioma of face, 5 years after treatment. KAPLAN, I. I. Urol. & Cutan. Rev. *47:*545, Sept '43

Lipoma of forehead; surgical therapy of case. URIBURU, J. V. JR. Prensa med. argent. *30:*2451–2452, Dec 22, '43

Facial (See Face)

Facial Bones, Fractures of (See also Jaws, Fractures of)

Signs of fracture of orbit. KEHL, H. Beitr. z. klin. Chir. *123:*203, '21 abstr: J.A.M.A. *77:*1292, Oct 15, '21

Complete separation of facial bones from base of skull. ASPINALL, A., M. J. Australia *1:*292–294, March 17, '23 (illus.)

Study and treatment of fractures of malar bone and zygoma. DUCHANGE, R., J. de med. de Bordeaux *95:*557–561, Aug 10, '23 (illus.)

Plastic repair of depressed fracture of lower orbital rim. GOLDTHWAITE, R. H., J.A.M.A. *82:*628–629, Feb 23, '24

Splint for unusual break of face. BOYCE, W. A. Laryngoscope *36:*266–269, April '26

Facial Bones—Cont.

Facial bone fractures. TITTERINGTON, P. F. Radiology *11:*207–212, Sept '28

Fractures of facial bones involving nasal accessory sinuses. NAFTZGER, J. B. Tr. Am. Laryng., Rhin. and Otol. Soc. *34:* 383–394, '28

Methods of treatment of facial bone fractures. DUFOURMENTEL, L. Clinique, Paris *25:*225, June (B) '30

Surgical treatment of accidental wounds of mouth and face, with special reference to those complicated by bone injury. IVY, R. H., J. Am. Dent. A. *17:*967–974, June '30

Typical case of Guerin fracture of upper jaw. GIOIA, T. Bol. y trab. de la Soc. de cir. de Buenos Aires *14:*976–982, Nov 26, '30 also: Semana med. *2:*1982–1985, Dec 25, '30

Multiple facial fractures. PARISH, B. B. AND WHITAKER, L. W., U. S. Vet. Bur. M. Bull. *7:*162–163, Feb '31

Prognosis of fractures of frontal sinus. BONNET, P. Bull. Soc. d'opht. de Paris, pp. 327–328, May '32

Chronic maxillary sinusitis; fatal complications of traumatic fracture of wall of sinus in patient with sinusitis. FEUZ, J. Rev. med. de la Suisse Rom. *52:*347–354, May 25, '32

Injuries of facial bones and soft tissues. IVY, R. H. Pennsylvania M. J. *35:*761–763, Aug '32

Fractures of bones of face; management. SHEA, J. J. Tri-State M. J. *5:*1160, Sept '33 also: J.M.A. Alabama *3:* 125–128, Oct '33

Open treatment of facial bone fractures. SHEA, J. J., J. Tennessee M. A. *27:*15–21, Jan '34

Facial bone fractures, especially orbits and sinuses. GILL, W. D. South. M. J. *27:*197–205, March '34

Reconstruction in crushing of facial bones. DUFOURMENTEL, L. AND DARCISSAC, M. Bull. et mem. Soc. d. chirurgiens de Paris *26:*315–330, May 4, '34

Treatment of fractures of maxilla, mandible and other bones of face. AUFDERHEIDE, P. J., J. Am. Dent. A. *21:*950–961, June '34

Nasal fractures in connection with fracture of facial cranium. CSILLAG, S. Monatschr. f. Ohrenh. *68:*663–669, June '34 also: Orvosi hetil. *78:*586–588, June 30, '34

Complex fracture (craniofacial disjunction and vertical fractures) of upper jaw and double fracture of lower jaw; simplified therapy of case. PONROY, *et al.* Rev. de stomatol. *36:*470–471, July '34

Fractures of bones of face. DORRANCE, G. M.

Facial Bones – Cont.

AND LOUDENSLAGER, P. E., S. Clin. North America *15:*71–83, Feb '35

Compound comminuted depressed fracture of frontal bone and orbit, with recovery. LOVE, J. G. Proc. Staff Meet., Mayo Clin. *10:*291-293, May 8, '35

Clinical cases in stomatology (including fractures). BOISSON, R. Rev. de stomatol. *38:*625-662, Sept '36

Fractures of upper part of face necessitating cranial support; author's device. DUBECQ, X. J., J. de med. de Bordeaux *113:*817-820, Nov 30, '36

Treatment of facial bone fractures. COX, G. H. New York State J. Med. *37:*52–58, Jan 1, '37

Emergency surgery of facial wounds (with fractures). DUFOURMENTEL, L. Presse med. *45:*387-390, March 13, '37

Facial bone fractures. GILL, W. D. Ann. Otol., Rhin. and Laryng. *46:*228-236, March '37

Avertin (tribrom-ethanol) in reduction of facial fractures. FENNELLY, W. A., J. Am. Dent. A. *24:*1089–1104, July '37

Traumatic craniofacial disjunctions; clinical study. FREIDEL, C.; *et al.* J. de chir. *50:*27–43, July '37

Treatment of facial fractures. PATTERSON, R. J. Tennessee M. A. *30:*273–279, Aug '37

Fracture of skull involving paranasal sinuses. COLEMAN, C. C., J.A.M.A. *109:* 1613–1616, Nov 13, '37

Immediate treatment of facial fractures. GORDON, S. Canad. M.A.J. *37:*440–443, Nov '37

Surgical treatment of fractures of bones of face. RISDON, F. Canad. M.A.J. *38:*33-36, Jan '38

Multiple open fractures of cranial and facial bones; 2 cases with recovery after operation. COVALI, N. AND TROCMAIER, C. Rev. de chir., Bucuresti *41:*284-287, March–April '38

Primary treatment of facial fractures. GILLIES, H. Practitioner *140:*414–425, April '38

Management of fractures of bones of face (and wounds). OSBORN, C. H., M. J. Australia *2:*41-49, July 9, '38

Prevention and correction of disfigurement in facial fractures. BLAIR, V. P.; BROWN, J. B., AND BYARS, L. T. Am. J. Surg. *42:*536–541, Dec '38

Craniofacial disjunction; case. BOBBIO, A. Boll. e mem. Soc. piemontese di chir. *8:*515-520, '38

Fractures involving frontal sinus; 2 cases.

Facial Bones – Cont.

BONNET, P. Bull. Soc. d'opht. de Paris *51:*83–84, Jan '39

Facial bone fractures. BROWN, J. B. Surg., Gynec. and Obst. *68:*564–573, Feb. (no. 2A) '39 also: Am. J. Orthodontics *25:*432–446, May '39

Use of rubber bands in treatment of facial and jaw fractures. DINGMAN, R. O., J. Am. Dent. A. *26:*173–183, Feb '39

Symposium on automobile fractures (including facial). SMITH, G. W. Rocky Mountain M. J. *36:*238–240, April '39

Treatment of facial fractures and nose. WHITHAM, J. D. Laryngoscope *49:*394–400, May '39

Treatment of malar and zygomatic fractures. RICHISON, F. A., U. S. Nav. M. Bull. *37:*566-571, Oct '39

Fractures and dislocations of jaws and wounds of face. BELLINGER, D. H. Am. J. Surg. *46:*535-541, Dec '39

Maxillofacial fractures. HAUTANT, A. Ann. d' oto-laryng., pp. 169-194, March–April '40

Treatment of facial fractures. DANIEL, R. A. JR. J. Tennessee M. A. *33:*419-426, Nov '40

Facial fractures; pericranial anchorage utilizing lining of French soldier's helmet; model B.B.V. 236. FREIDEL, C. Rev. de stomatol. *41:*867-872, '40

Facial structure in relationship to fractures. JAMES, W. W. AND FICKLING, B. W. Proc. Roy. Soc. Med. *34:*205-211, Feb '41

Management of facial fractures. SHEA, J. J. Mississippi Doctor *18:*498-502, Feb '41 also: Memphis M. J. *16:*75-76, May '41

Method of dealing with fractures through infraorbital margin. LAW, T. B., M. J. Australia *1:*666-667, May 31, '41

Facial bone fractures. ERICH, J. B. Mil. Surgeon *88:*637-639, June '41

Total craniofacial disjunction; case. DUFOURMENTEL, L. Bull. et men. Soc. d. chirurgiens de Paris *32:*69–71, '41

Multiple facial fractures; case. RICHISON, F. A., J. Am. Dent. A. *29:*3–6, Jan '42

Facial fractures; treatment by wiring fixation. ADAMS, W. M. Mississippi Doctor *19:*427-435, Feb '42

Facial fractures involving nasal accessory sinuses. NAFTZGER, J. B. Ann. Otol., Rhin. and Laryng. *51:*414-423, June '42

Reduction of faciocranial fractures. SMITH, G. C., J. Missouri M. A. *39:*178–180, June '42

Fractures of bones of face. TILLOTSON, R. S. California and West. Med. *57:*137-141, Aug '42

Facial Bones – Cont.

Facial fractures; internal wiring fixation. ADAMS, W. M. Surgery *12:*523–540, Oct '42

Management of facial fractures involving paranasal sinuses. SHEA, J. J., J.A.M.A. *120:*745–749, Nov 7, '42

Treatment of facial fractures (description of extra-oral fixation appliance). ADAMS, W. M. J. Tennessee M. A. *35:*469–475, Dec '42

Fractures involving nasal accessory sinuses. NAFTZGER, J. B. Tr. Am. Laryng., Rhin. and Otol. Soc. *48:*333–341, '42

Desirability of early proper treatment of facial fractures. BLAIR, V. P. AND BYARS, L. T. Texas State J. Med. *38:*533–537, Jan '43

Care of military and civilian injuries; internal wiring fixation of facial fractures. ADAMS, W. M. Am. J. Orthodontics (Oral Surg. Sect.) *29:*111–130, Feb '43

Care of military and civilian injuries; fractures of mandible, maxilla, zygoma and other facial bones; statistical study of 1,149 cases. LYONS, D. C. Am. J. Orthodontics (Oral Surg. Sect.) *29:*67–76, Feb '43

Lagrange's law of indirect ocular war injuries (facial fractures). SOUDAKOFF, P. S. Am. J. Ophth. *26:*293–296, March '43

Wire suturing in treatment of facial fractures. GORDON, S. D. Canad. M.A.J. *48:*406–409, May '43

Plastic as substitute for metal in fracture appliances in facial fractures. FREEMAN, J. J. Oral Surg. *1:*241–245, July '43

Instrument for manipulation of central middle third of face fractures. MCINDOE, A. H. Brit. M.J. *1:*14, Jan 1, '44

Facial bone fractures. RANK, B. K. Australian and New Zealand J. Surg. *13:*184–198, Jan '44

Compound fronto-orbital fractures; 8 cases. SCHORSTEIN, J. Brit. J. Surg. *31:*221–230, Jan '44

Technic for building head cast fracture appliances from coat hangers for facial fractures. VAN ZILE, W. N., U. S. Nav. M. Bull. *42:*200–207, Jan '44

Removable plaster headcap for facial fractures. WOODARD, D. E., J. Oral Surg. *2:*23–31, Jan '44

Fractures of middle third of face in civil and military practice according to British experience. CASTRO O'CONNOR, R. Dia med. *16:*361–367, April 17, '44

Surgical management of compound depressed fracture of frontal sinus, cerebrospinal rhinorrhea and pneumocephalus. GURDJIAN, E. S. AND WEBSTER, J. E. Arch. Otolaryng. *39:*287–306, April '44

Facial Bones – Cont.

Method of fixation in fractures involving maxillary antrum. SCHARFE, E. E. Canad. M.A.J. *50:*435–437, May '44

Treatment of multiple fractures of face with external pin fixation splint. ELVIDGE, A. AND BAXTER, H. McGill M. J. *13:*469–475, Dec '44

Instrument for anchoring fractures of face. STEVENSON, H. N. Arch. Otolaryng. *40:*503, Dec '44

Fractures of middle third of face. THOMA, K. H.; *et al.* Am. J. Orthodontics (Oral Surg. Sect.) *31:*226–234, Apr '45

Modified traction and fixation splint for fractures of facial bones. WACHSBERGER, A. Arch. Otolaryng. *42:*53–55, July '45

Headpiece for face wounds and fractures. JORDAN, C. E., U. S. Nav. M. Bull. *45:*330, Aug '45

Control of bone fragments in maxillofacial surgery. WEISS, L. R., J. Oral Surg. *3:*271–285, Oct '45

Fracture of frontal and nasal bones. GONZALEZ ULLOA, M. Vida nueva *56:*195–201, Dec '45

Management of fractures into nasal sinuses. SHEA, J. J. Laryngoscope *56:*22–25, Jan '46

Fractures involving frontal air sinuses, due to localized violence; 30 cases. SARTORIUS, K. South African M. J. *20:*202–208, April 27, '46

Fractures involving frontal air sinuses due to localized violence; 30 cases. SARTORIUS, K. South African M. J. *20:*234–237, May 11 '46

Fractures of malar-zygomatic compound; treatment by improved methods and myoplasty. STEWART, M. B. AND CONLEY, J. J. Arch. Otolaryng. *44:*443–451, Oct '46

Facial Bones, Osteomyelitis

Septic osteomyelitis of bones of skull and face; plea for conservative treatment. BLAIR, V. P. AND BROWN, J. B. Ann. Surg. *85:*1–26, Jan '27

Osteomyelitis of bones of face; diagnosis and treatment. THOMAS, E. H., J. Am. Dent. A. *20:*614–621, April '33

Osteomyelitis of bones of face in a severe diabetic with recovery and plastic reconstruction (case). HOSMER, M. N.: *et al.* California and West. Med. *53:*165–168, Oct '40

Reconstruction after radical operation for osteomyelitis of frontal bone; experience in 38 cases. KAZANJIAN, V. H. AND HOLMES, E. M. Surg., Gynec. and Obst. *79:*397–411, Oct '44

Facial Clefts

Congenital facial clefts. BLAIR, V. P. Surg., Gynec. and Obst. *37:*530-533, Oct '23

Care of facial fissure in nurslings. KEJŘ, O. Casop. lek. cesk. *66:*258-260, Feb 11, '27

Facial coloboma with complete, unilateral, velopalatine fissure; case. ROCHER, H. L. AND PESME, P., J. de med. de Bordeaux *107:*763, Oct 10, '30

Enormous harelip with deep oblique fissure accompanied by coloboma of eyelid and iris; case. ETIENNE, E. AND DÉJEAN, C. Arch. Soc. d. sc. med. et biol. de Montpellier *13:*94-99, Feb '32

Genesis of facial clefts. PETER, K. Kinderarztl. Praxis *4:*335-339, July '33

Congenital clefts of face and jaws; 350 cases in which operation was performed. RITCHIE, H. P. Arch. Surg. *28:*617-658, April '34

Median cleft of lower lip and mandible, cleft sternum and absence of basihyoid (inferior gnathoschisis); case. MORTON, C. B. AND JORDAN, H. E. Arch. Surg. *30:*647-656, April '35

Unilateral secondary facial cleft with excess tooth and bone formation. RUSHTON, M. A. AND WALKER, F. A. Proc. Roy. Soc. Med. *30:*79-82, Nov '36

Origin of facial cleft, harelip and cleft palate. POLITZER, G. Monatschr. f. Ohrenh. *71:*63-73, Jan '37

Facial cleft or fissural cysts. THOMA, K. H. Internat. J. Orthodontia *23:*83-89, Jan '37

Case of malformation from persistence of oblique fissure of face; method of plastic reparation. FOCOSI, M. Boll. d'ocul. *17:*255-269, April '38

New experiences with cleft of face in man and animals. FLEISCHMANN, A. Sitzungsb. d. phys.-med. Soz. zu Erlangen (1937) *69:*315-324, '38

Fissures of face, apropos of case of unusual labiogenal malformation. PREVOT, M. Rev. de chir. structive *8:*196-198, '38

Congenital clefts of face and jaws; report of operations used and discussion of results. RITCHIE, H. P. Surg., Gynec. and Obst. *73:*654-670, Nov '41

Fissural cyst of nose (facial cleft). ROSENBERGER, H. C. Arch. Otolaryng. *40:*288-290, Oct '44

Secondary oblique facial cleft; case. MELLICK, A. Brit. J. Ophth. *30:*221-224, Apr '46

Facial Deformities (See also Face, Congenital Deformities; Facial Hemiatrophy; Facial Hypertrophy; Facial Lesions; Hypertelorism)

Congenital deformities of mouth and face. VON WEDEL, C., J. Oklahoma M. A. *15:*46-49, Feb '22 (illus.)

Congenital malformations of face. HERTZBERG, R. F. AND HERTZBERG, G. R. R., M. J. and Rec. *120:*5-8, July 2, '24

New procedure for relief of facies scaphoidea—dish face. COUGHLIN, W. T. Surg., Gynec. and Obst. *40:*109-111, Jan '25

Case of facial deformity (jaw also). BEYERS, C. F. AND BERRY, T. B., M. J. S. Africa *21:*127-131, Dec '25

Case of hyperostosis of one-half of face. DEREUX, J. Bull. et mem. Soc. med. d. hop. de Paris *50:*307-311, Feb 26, '26 abstr: J.A.M.A. *86:*1486, May 8, '26

Hare-lip and other developmental lesions of face. RANKIN, W. Glasgow M. J. *106:*350-358, Dec '26

Complete harelip and cleft palate on left side, with absence of left half of intermaxillary bone, of philtrum and of cartilaginous portion of nasal septum. BERG, A. Arch. f. klin. Chir. *140:*168-171, '26

Glossoptosis and facial deformity. LAUMONIER, J. Gaz. d. hop. *100:*848-850, June 25, '27

Abnormalities along median line of face. CADENAT, E. Bruxelles-med. *7:*1151-1153, July 10, '27

Maxillofacial dystrophies. MEYER, J. AND NICOLLE. Rev. franc. de pediat. *3:*304-340, July '27

Bird-face (opisthogenia). ABELS. Wien. med. Wchnschr. *77:*1208, Sept 3, '27

One of the fundamental factors concerned in etiology of dentofacial deformities. HELLMAN, M. J. Am. Dent. A. *14:*1674-1679, Sept '27

Reconstruction of smaller defects and lesions of face. PICKERILL, P., M. J. Australia *2:*605-610, Oct 29, '27

Causes of facial asymmetry in muscular wryneck and jaw dislocations. BECK, O. Ztschr. f. orthop. Chir. *49:*424-449, May 18, '28

Role of hereditary syphilis in maxillo-facial dystrophies. MEYER, J. Ann. d. mal. ven. *23:*494-505, July '28

Developmental anomalies of face and neck and their surgical significance (also cleft palate). SINGLETON, A. O. Texas State J. Med. *25:*659-663, Feb '30

Meningo-encephaloma of right nasofrontal

Facial Deformities—Cont.

region with malformation of nose and forehead; case. ROCHER, H. L., J. de med. de Bordeaux *107:*571–573, July 20, '30

Diagnosis of dento-maxillo-facial deformities. MUZII, E. Stomatol. *28:*821–865, Oct '30

Facial coloboma with complete, unilateral, velopalatine fissure; case. ROCHER, H. L. AND PESME, P., J. de med. de Bordeaux *107:*763, Oct 10, '30

Coloboma (Morian's second type) with extensive facial malformations; anatomic study of case in infant 6 months old. ROCHER, H. L.; *et al.* Ann. d'anat. path. *9:*487–498, May '32

Congenital transverse fissure of cheek. FRICKE, K. F. Beitr. z. Anat. Physio., Path. u. Therap. d. Ohres *30:*282–297, '32

Unusual familial developmental disturbance of face (acrocephalosyndactylia, craniofacial dysostosis and hypertelorism). CHOTZEN, F. Monatschr. f. Kinderh. *55:*97–122, '32

Facial deformities caused by congenital syphilis. WATRY. Bruxelles-med. *14:*471–484, Feb 4, '34

Familial aplasia of upper jaw, new type of facial dysostosis. SENDRAIL, M. Prat. med. franc. *15:*127–130, Feb (B) '34

Bilateral facial colobomas, with oculopalpebral adhesions and eye complications. MAZZI, L. Arch. di ottal. *41:*148–157, March '34

Differential diagnosis of certain types of facial deformities and their treatment (including jaws). ROSE, J. E. Internat. J. Orthodontia *20:*222–228, March '34

Congenital facial malformation; case. TARTAKOWSKY, A. Folia oto-laryng. orient. *2:*46–51, Jan '35

Congenital facial deformities; types found in series of 1,000 cases. DAVIS, W. B. Surg., Gynec. AND Obst. *61:*202–209, Aug '35

Hypertelorism, case with unusual congenital malformation of external portion of nose, double overlapping external parts. VAN VOORTHUYSEN, D. G. W. Acta oto-laryng. *22:*540–544, '35

Commonest deformities of face presenting themselves for correction, and their correctibility. BAMES, H. O. Rev. de chir. structive, pp. 219–232, March '36

Maxillofacial dysmorphism; 5 cases. PEYRUS, J. Rev. de stomatol. *38:*393–409, May '36

Rare case of cornu cutaneum humanum of forehead. EMILIADIS, K. Zentralbl. f. Chir. *64:*727–728, March 27, '37

Harelip, cleft palate; congenital deformities

Facial Deformities—Cont.

of mouth and face. KIMBALL, G. H., J. Oklahoma M. A. *31:*85–89, March '38

Correction of bird's face (jaw deformity). ESSER, J. F. S. Am. J. Orthodontics *24:*791–794, Aug '38

Complications of dento-maxillo-facial malformations; importance of correction. FAUCONNIER, H. J. AND PATCAS, H. Liege med. *32:*1–9, Jan 1, '39

Origin and nature of certain malformations of face, head and foot. KEITH, A. Brit. J. Surg. *28:*173–192, Oct '40

Familial combination of deformities in region of first visceral arch. DEBUSMANN. Arch. f. Kinderh. *120:*133–139, '40

Rare congenital malformation of face; median harelip with dissociation without deformation of 2 halves of nose (double nose); case. STEFANI, F. Plast. chir. *1:*162–166, '40

Eugenic aspect of cleft palate and other facial deformities. OLINGER, N. A., J. Am. Dent. A. *31:*1431–1434, Nov 1, '44

New syndrome; mandibulofacial dysostosis. FRANCESCHETTI, A. Bull. schweiz. Akad. d. med. Wissensch. *1:*60–66, '44

Classification of dentofacial anomalies. MAYORAL, J. Am. J. Orthodontics *31:*429–439, Sept '45

The asymmetrical face. MARINO, H. Prensa med. argent. *33:*1242–1247, June 14, '46

Facial Deformities, Medicolegal Aspects

Plastic surgery of face in relation to identification. REBELLO NETTO, J. Arq. de med. leg. e ident. (no. 10) *4:*87–93, '34

Injuries and plastic surgery of face from medicolegal point of view. DANTRELLE, A. Rev. de chir. structive, pp. 133–147, Dec '35

Lesions of eye with permanent disfigurement of face; medicolegal study of case. CUCCO, A. Riv. san. siciliana *24:*137–141, Feb 1, '36

Facial scars; evaluation in medicolegal expertise. DOMENICI, F. Boll. d. Soc. med.-chir., Pavia *53:*41–55, '39

Facial Deformities, Psychological Aspects

Treatment of facial scars, with remarks on their psychological aspects. HUNT, H. L. Am. J. Surg. *4:*313–320, March '28

Social sequels of maxillo-facial wounds received in war. REGNART, R. L. F. Rev. odont. *51:*372–378, Sept–Oct '30

Your child's face and future. MALINIAK, J. W. Hygeia *13:*410–413, May '35

Plastic surgery of head, face and neck;

Facial Deformities Psychological Aspects – Cont.
psychic reactions. Blair, V. P., J. Am. Dent. A. *23:*236–240, Feb '36
Social importance of facial surgery. Alfredo, J. Rev. med. de Pernambuco *6:*317–320, Sept '36
Plastic surgery from point of view of mental hygiene (face). Roy, J. N. Rev. san. mil., Bucuresti *35:*1070–1076, Oct '36
Minor plastic surgery (face) and its relation to inferiority complex. McClelland, E. S. M. Rec. *146:*419–424, Nov 17, '37
Psychic repercussion of facial defects; value of plastic surgery. Malbec, E. F. Semana med. *2:*94–99, July 13, '39
Improving mental attitude by means of plastic surgery of face. Richison, F. A., J. Am. Dent. A. *28:*437–441, March '41
Facial deformity and change in personality following corrective surgery. MacKenzie, C. M. Northwest Med. *43:*230–231, Aug '44
Orofacial cripple. Beder, O. E. and Saporito, L. A. Am. J. Orthodontics (Oral Surg. Sect.) *32:*351–358, Jun '46

Facial Hemiatrophy (See also Facial Hypertrophy)

Progressive hemiatrophy of face. Očenášek, M. Cas. lek. cesk. *61:*378–382, April 29, '22
Morphea associated with hemiatrophy of face. Osborne, E. D. Arch. Dermat. and Syph. *6:*27–34, July '22 (illus.)
Hemihypertrophy of face. Léri, A. and Sartre. Bull. et mem. Soc. med. d. hop. de Par. *48:*690–693, May 16, '24
Hemiatrophy of face and scleroderma. Ben, F. Dermat. Wchnschr. *83:*1366–1371, Sept 11, '26
Case of hemihypertrophy of face with buphthalmos. Süss, H. Ztschr. f. Kinderh. *41:*404–408, '26
Hemiatrophy of face with visual disturbances. Mezzatesta, F. Riv. oto-neuro-oftal. *4:*315–327, March–June '27
Trophic disorders of central origin; report of case of progressive facial hemiatrophy, associated with lipodystrophy and other metabolic derangements. Wolff, H. G. and Ehrenclou, A. H., J.A.M.A. *83:*991–994, March 26, '27
Peripheral facial paralysis and progressive facial hemiatrophy as sequels of teeth extraction. Bönheim, E. Deutsche Monatschr. f. Zahnh. *45:*353–366, April 15, '27
Case of facial hemiatrophy. Vázquez Rodríguez, A. Pediat. espan. *16:*135–138, May '27

Facial Hemiatrophy – Cont.
Progressive facial hemiatrophy; case in child. Bost, C. Arch. Pediat. *44:*497–501, Aug '27
Congenital torticollis with unilateral facial atrophy; case. di Vestea, D. Rassegna internaz. di clin. e terap. *9:*16–29, Jan '28
Unilateral facial atrophy; 2 cases. Marinesco, G.; *et al.* Rev. d'oto-neuro-opht. *6:*405–407, May '28
Progressive facial hemiatrophy; case with other signs of disease of central nervous system. Wolff, H. G. Arch. Otolaryng. *7:*580–582, June '28
Right facial hemiatrophy following thyroidectomy. Manthey, P. Ztschr. f. d. ges. Neurol. u. Psychiat. *114:*192–199, '28
Progressive facial hemiatrophy; case with convulsions and anisocoria. Wolff, H. G. J. Nerv. and Ment. Dis. *69:*140–144, Feb '29
Progressive atrophy of eyelids with coloboma and facial hemiatrophy; case. Dupuy-Dutemps, L. Bull. Soc. d'opht. de Paris, pp. 181–187, April '29
Hemiatrophia alternans facialis progressiva with hemilateral alopecia; pigment displacement and atrophy of skin; case. Bernstein, E. Dermat. Wchnschr. *90:*235–237, Feb 15, '30
Treatment of facial hemiatrophy by means of transplantation of fat tissues. Moszkowicz, L. Med. Klin. *26:*1478, Oct 3, '30
Facial hemiatrophy. Surat, W. S. Monatschr. f. Psychiat. u. Neurol. *77:*202–216, Oct '30
Reconstructive surgery in progressive facial hemiatrophy. Updegraff, H. L. Am. J. Surg. *10:*439–443, Dec '30
Pathogenesis of facial hemiatrophy and heterochromia of iris. Budina, R. Y. Sovrem. psikhonevrol. *11:*316–323, '30
Role of sympathetic nervous system in pathogenesis of facial hemiatrophy with report of case of hemiatrophy of one side of face and other side of body. Marinesco, G.; *et al.* Paris med. *1:*269–275, March 26, '32 also: Bull. sect. scient. Acad. roumaine (nos. 6–8) *14:*155–166, '31
Atrophy of external ear with hemiatrophy of face and paresis of lower facial nerve; case. Rocher, H. L., J. de med. de Bordeaux *108:*231, March 20, '31
Progressive facial hemiatrophy. Wagenhals, F. C. Ohio State M.J. *27:*217–219, March '31
Plastic treatment of facial hemiatrophy by transplantation of fat tissues. Eitner, E. Med. Klin. *27:*624–625, April 24, '31
Progressive facial hemiatrophy; 3 cases. Archambault, L. and Fromm, N. K. Arch.

Facial Hemiatrophy – Cont.

Neurol. and Psychiat. *27:*529–584, March '32

So-called facial hemiatrophy; case. BRÜCKNER, S. AND OBSTÄNDER, E. Psychiat.-neurol. Wchnschr. *34:*448–451, Sept 10, '32

Progressive facial hemiatrophy; case. YATER, W. M. AND CAVANAGH, J. R., M. Ann. District of Columbia *1:*236–239, Sept '32

Clinical and etiologic study of progressive facial hemiatrophy; case in woman with dental focus of infection; regression after therapy of infection. MOLLARET, P. Rev. neurol. *2:*463–474, Nov '32

Etiology of facial hemiatrophy. CHASANOW, M. Ztschr. f. d. ges. Neurol. u. Psychiat. *140:*473–485, '32

Partial atrophy of right side of face. FLINT, G. Tr. Ophth. Soc. U. Kingdom *52:*308–309, '32

Hemiatrophy of face. CAMPBELL, D. Fortschr. a. d. Geb. d Rontgenstrahlen *47:*198–202, Feb '33

Symmetrical facial atrophy with segmentary adiposis dolorosa; case. LÉCHELLE, *et al.* Rev. neurol. *1:*182–186, Feb '33

Hemiatrophy on left side of face with circumscribed scleroderma; case. TRUFFI, G. Dermosifilografo *8:*90–99, Feb '33

Atypical facial hemiatrophy of sympathetic origin. WORMS, G. Rev. d'oto-neuro-opht. *11:*99–103, Feb '33

Progressive atrophy of facial bones with complete atrophy of mandible; case. THOMA, K. H., J. Bone and Joint Surg. *15:*494–501, April '33

Progressive facial hemiatrophy treated by means of expansion prosthesis of oral cavity; case. BØE, H. W. Med. rev., Bergen *50:*212–225, May '33

Facial hemiatrophy; case. BENEDEK, L. AND KULCSÁR, F. Gyogyaszat *73:*356–357, June 4, '33

Facial hemiatrophy associated with vitiligo and myxedema; case. FABER, K. Ugesk. f. laeger *95:*1207–1211, Nov 9, '33

Facial hemiatrophy; autopsy findings; case. STIEF, S. Ztschr. f. d. ges. Neurol. u. Psychiat. *147:*573–593, '33

Progressive hemiatrophy of face, shoulder girdle and hand; case. VASILEVSKIY, M. V. Sovet. nevropat. psikhiat. i. psikhogig. (no. 7) *2:*78–79, '33

Progressive facial hemiatrophy (Romberg's disease); case. GINANNESCHI, G. Pensiero med. *23:*157–160, May '34

Surgical aspects of progressive unilateral facial atrophy. BAKÁCS, G. Orvosi hetil. *78:*590–593, June 30, '34

Facial Hemiatrophy – Cont.

Facial and lingual hemiatrophy; case. EUZIÈRE, J.; *et al.* Arch. Soc. d. sc. med. et biol. de Montpellier *15:*501–510, Aug '34

Facial hemiatrophy (Romberg's disease). VINAŘ, J. Casop. lek. cesk. *73:*865–867, Aug 3, '34

Progressive facial hemiatrophy. LAZARESCU, D. AND LAZARESCU, E. Ann. d'ocul. *171:*1004–1011, Dec '34

Facial hemiatrophia progressiva treated with expansion prosthesis in mouth; case. BØE, H. W. Acta psychiat. et neurol. *9:*1–27, '34

Pathogenesis of hemiatrophy, vitiligo and myxedema appearing successively in face of same patient. FABER, K. Acta med. Scandinav. *82:*419–432, '34

Pathogenesis of facial hemiatrophy. JONESCO-SISESTI, N. Vol. jubilaire, Parhon, pp. 219–232, '34

Bilateral progressive facial hemiatrophy. STIEFLER, G. Jahrb. f. Psychiat. u. Neurol. *51:*277–292, '34

Facial hemiatrophy. PICKERILL, H. P. Australian and New Zealand J. Surg. *4:*404–406, April '35

Facial hemiatrophy, with description of 3 cases. COX, L. B. AND MACLURE, A. F. Australian and New Zealand J. Surg. *5:*68–76, July '35

Facial hemiatrophy associated with epilepsy; case. DONLEY, D. E., J. Nerv. and Ment. Dis. *82:*33–39, July '35

Sympathetic disturbances in course of facial hemiatrophy; case. THOMAS, A. Presse med. *43:*1339–1340, Aug 24, '35

Progressive facial hemiatrophy; early case. BRAGMAN, L. J. Arch. Pediat. *52:*686–688, Oct '35

Secretion of sweat in Romberg's progressive facial hemiatrophy. RAKONITZ, J. Orvosi hetil. *79:*1369–1372, Dec 28, '35

Facial asymmetry; unilateral atrophy and facial hypertrophy; cases. MASTEN, M. G. Arch. Neurol. and Psychiat. *35:*136–145, Jan '36

Facial hemiatrophy. MEYER, H. E. Med. Klin. *32:*352–354, March 13, '36

Right facial hemiatrophy with muscular atrophy of left upper extremity; case. URECHIA, C. I. AND RETEZEANU, MME. Bull. et mem. Soc. med. d. hop. de Paris *52:*398–402, March 16, '36

Congenital hemiatrophy of face with facial paralysis and microphthalmos; case. BOISSERIE-LACROIX, J., J. de med. de Bordeaux *113:*419–420, May 30, '36

Congenital bony temporomandibular anky-

Facial Hemiatrophy – Cont.

losis and facial hemiatrophy; review of literature and report of case. BURKET, L. W. J.A.M.A. *106:*1719–1722, May 16, '36

Progressive facial hemiatrophy; case. RIN, K. Taiwan Igakkai Zasshi *35:*1156, May '36

Progressive facial hemiatrophy; case. ISHIKAWA, K. Oto-rhino-laryng. *9:*518, June '36

Congenital atrophy of lower eyelids, both auricles and lower jaw; case. VAN LINT, A. AND HENNEBERT, P. Bull. Soc. belge d'opht., no. 73, pp. 51–61, '36

Progressive facial hemiatrophy (Romberg's disease), case. GAREISO, A., AND ALVAREZ, G. Rev. Asoc. med. argent. *50:*91–100, Jan '37

Cosmetic surgery in facial hemiatrophy. EITNER, E. Wien. med. Wchnschr. *87:*362–363, March 27, '37

Progressive facial hemiatrophy; 2 cases with cerebral calcification. MERRITT, K. K.; *et al.* J. Pediat. *10:*374–395, March '37

Facial hemiatrophy and its therapy. ZATLOUKAL, F. Casop. lek. cesk. *76:*553–563, May 7, '37

Hemiatrophy of face complicated by spontaneous fracture of jaw; case. ROCCIA, B. Stomatol. *35:*448–458, July '37

Unusual complication (facial hemi-atrophy) following Caldwell-Luc operation. FULLER, T. E., J. Arkansas M. Soc. *34:*94, Oct '37

Progressive facial hemiatrophy; case. MONTANARO, J. C. AND PIERINI, L. E. Semana med. *1:*704–710, March 31, '38

Unusual complication of radical antrum operation (hemiatrophy of face following Caldwell-Luc operation). FULLER, T. E. South. M. J. *31:*1094–1095, Oct '38

Congenital hemiatrophy of face with Claude Bernard-Horner syndrome; case. VELASCO BLANCO, L. AND WAISBEIN, S. Arch. am. de med. *14:*74–76, '38

Hemiatrophy of face; 2 cases. WALSH, F. B. Am. J. Ophth. *22:*1–10, Jan '39

Hemiatrophy of face with eye complications. BAKER, H. Proc. Roy. Soc. Med. *32:*364–365, Feb '39

Hemiatrophia faciei progressiva. TAUBER, E. B. AND GOLDMAN, L. Arch. Dermat. and Syph. *39:*696–704, April '39

Progressive hemiatrophy of face; case in boy 13 years old. BABONNEIX, L. AND HOUZEL, G. Gaz. d. hop. *112:*1069, Aug 9, '39

Progressive facial hemiatrophy; case with attacks of syncope and gynandromorphism. WOLFE, M. O. AND WEBER, M. L. J. Nerv. and Ment. Dis. *91:*595–607, May '40

Facial hemiatrophy. SCHAFER, D. P. H., M.

Facial Hemiatrophy – Cont.

J. Australia *1:*901–902, June 29, '40

Progressive facial and crossed hemiatrophy complicated by transient hypoglycemia. PREVITALI, G. AND JACOBZINER, H. Am. J. Dis. Child. *60:*116–129, July '40

Surgical treatment of hemiatrophy of face. KAZANJIAN, V. H. AND STURGIS, S. H. J.A.M.A. *115:*348–354, Aug 3, '40

Facial hemiatrophy. WERBA, D. H., M. Bull Vet. Admin. *17:*291–292, Jan '41

Progressive facial hemiatrophy; case with attacks of syncope and gynandromorphism. WOLFE, M. O. AND WEBER, M. L., M. Bull. Vet. Admin. *17:*283–290, Jan '41

Associated facial, lingual and velopalatine hemiatrophy and Basedow's disease; case. DECOURT, J.; *et al.* Rev. neurol. *73:*135–140, March–April '41

Hemiatrophy of face coexisting with diffuse cutaneous neurofibromatosis; case. GUILLAIN, G.; *et al.* Rev. neurol. *74:*87–88, Jan–Feb '42

Hemiatrophy of face; graft of fat in therapy. ZENO, L. An. de cir. *8:*52–57, March–June '42

Progressive hemiatrophy of face. VRAA-JENSEN, G. F. Nord. med. (Hospitalstid.) *14:*1861–1865, June 20, '42

Hemiatrophy of face. CERNEA AND LAMBERT. Rev. de stomatol. *43:*185–187, Nov–Dec '42

Progressive hemiatrophy of face (following injuries); case. FULCHER, O. H. AND LANE, W. Z., U. S. Nav. M. Bull. *41:*192–196, Jan '43

Progressive facial hemiatrophy; total hemiatrophy; case. AUSTREGESILO, A.; *et al.* Arch. brasil, de med. *33:*387–408, Nov–Dec '43

Progressive hemiatrophies combined with scleroderma; pathogenic study. ALVAREZ, G. Arch. argent. de pediat. *21:*83–94, Feb '44

Progressive hemiatrophy of face with scleroderma, vitiligo and canities; case. GAREISO, A.; *et al.* Arch. argent. de pediat. *22:*416–425, Nov '44

Congenital hemiatrophy. ZONDEK, L. H. Arch. Dis. Childhood *20:*35–43, March '45

Facial progressive hemiatrophy; facioabdominocrural hemidystrophic form; case. BULLO, J. Dia med. *17:*444–445; 448, May 14, '45

Progressive hemiatrophy of face. SIMON, H. E. AND KAYE, B. Arch. Neurol. and Psychiat. *53:*437–438, June '45

Progressive hemiatrophy (facial). WARTENBERG, R. Arch. Neurol. and Psychiat. *54:*75–96, Aug '45

Facial Hypertrophy (See also Facial Hemiatrophy)

Case of facial hemihypertrophy. LÉRI, A. AND SARTRE. Arch. de med. d. enf. *27:*747–749, Dec '24

Enlargement of bones of half of face. LÉRI, A. AND LAYANI, F. Bull. et mem. Soc. med. d. hop. de Par. *49:*1013-1018, July 3, '25

Case of hyperostosis of one-half of face. DEREUX, J. Bull. et mem. Soc. med. d. hop. de Paris *50:*307–311, Feb. 26, '26 abstr: J.A.M.A. *86:*1486, May 8, '26

Pringle's disease with hemifacial hyperplasia (of cheeks, lips, conjunctiva and concha of ear), but without any psychoneurologic symptoms. HERMAN, E. AND MERENLENDER, J. Acta dermat.-venereol. *16:*276–291, Oct '35

Craniofacial hemihypertrophy; case. LEREBOULLET, P. AND ECTORS, MME. M. L. Arch. de med. d. enf. *39:*37–39, Jan '36

Facial asymmetry; unilateral atrophy and facial hypertrophy; cases. MASTEN, M. G. Arch. Neurol. and Psychiat. *35:*136–145, Jan '36

Congenital facial hemihypertrophy; case. GÖZBERK, R. A. Turk tib cem. mec. *3:*210–212, '37

Congenital facial hemihypertrophy with ocular anomalies; 2 cases. GÖZBERK, R. Ann. d'ocul. *176:*624–630, Aug '39

Rightsided hemihypertrophy of face; case. KEIZER, D. P. R. Geneesk. tijdschr. v. Nederl.-Indie *81:*1931–1934, Sept. 9, '41

Unilateral gigantism of face and teeth; case. MILES, A. E. W. Brit. Dent. J. *77:*197–199, Oct. 6, '44

Partial gigantism of face with neurologic complications. KARNOSH, L. J. AND GARDNER, W. J. Cleveland Clin. Quart. *12:*43–47, April '45

Facial Injuries

Plastic repair of soft tissue injuries of face. WHITHAM, J. D. Mil. Surgeon *48:*65, Jan '21

Injuries to face and jaws. COUGHLIN, W. T. Southwestern Med. *6:*356–359, Oct '22

Early treatment of facial injuries. JOHNSON, L. W., U. S. Nav. M. Bull. *24:*508–515, July '26

Plastic surgery, facio-maxillary; case reports. HARTER, J. H. Northwest Med. *25:*404–408, Aug '26

Injuries to jaws and face; outline of treatment. CLEWER, D., J. Roy. Army M. Corps

Facial Injuries – Cont.

*48:*286–295, April '27

Treatment of injuries of upper part of face. KAZANJIAN, V. K., J. Am. Dent. A. *14:*1607–1618, Sept '27

Cases illustrating maxillo-facial and plastic surgery. JOHNSON, L. W., U. S. Nav. M. Bull. *26:*843–861, Oct '28

Wounds and injuries of face and immediate aesthetic surgery. DUFOURMENTEL, L. Bull. med., Paris *43:*942–948, Aug. 31, '29

Maxillofacial surgery. BUTOIANU, S. AND STOIAN, C. Rev. san. mil., Bucuresti *28:*344–355, Sept '29

Maxillofacial surgery; cases. MAUREL, G. Rev. odont. *50:*377–407, Oct '29

Immediate treatment of facial injuries. DUFOURMENTEL, L. Bull. et mem. Soc. de med. de Paris, no. 16, pp. 369–373, Nov 23, '29

Immediate treatment of facial injuries. FRISON. Rev. odont. *51:*11–16, Jan '30

Facial injuries. BUTLER, E. Am. J. Surg. *8:*336–337, Feb '30

Surgical treatment of accidental wounds of mouth and face, with special reference to those complicated by bone injury. IVY, R. H., J. Am. Dent. A. *17:*967–974, June '30

Physiologic troubles in patients with old wounds and injuries of face. BERTEIN, P. Bull. med., Paris *44:*947–949, Dec. 27, '30

Relation of traumatic lesions of sense organs to maxillofacial surgery. LACAZE. Rev. odont. *52:*87–99, Feb '31

Facial injuries and scalp. RHEA, B. S., J. Tennessee M. A. *24:*41–42, Feb '31

Treatment of automobile accidents in cases where nose and face are involved. CARTER, W. W. Ann. Otol., Rhin. and Laryng. *41:*571–575, June '32

Injuries of facial bones and soft tissues. IVY, R. H. Pennsylvania M. J. *35:*761–763, Aug '32

Treatment of automobile injuries of face and jaws. KAZANJIAN, V. H., J. Am. Dent. A. *20:*757–773, May '33

Injuries to face and jaws in automobile accidents. KAZANJIAN, V. H. Tr. Am. Acad. Ophth. *38:*275–308, '33

Principles governing first aid of facial injuries. YAVLINSKIY, A. L. Ortop. i travmatol. (no. 1) *7:*43–45, '33

Maxillo-facial injuries. FEDERSPIEL, M. N. Wisconsin M. J. *33:*561–568, Aug '34

Maxillo-facial injuries. GINGRASS, R. P. Wisconsin M. J. *33:*568–571, Aug '34

Traumatic surgery of facial structures.

Facial Injuries – Cont.

HUME, E. C. Kentucky M. J. *32:*520-522, Oct '34

Surgical repair of facial injuries and harelip and cleft palate deformities. RISDON, E. F. Canad. M. A. J. *32:*51-54, Jan '35

Treatment of facial wounds in automobile accidents. STRAITH, C. L., J. Michigan M. Soc. *34:*64-70, Feb '35

Laceration of face with traumatic avulsion of entire maxilla; case. STUMPF, F. W. J. Am. Dent. A. *22:*1206-1208, July '35

Therapeutics of Cook County Hospital; therapy of facial injuries; outline by J. E. Schaeffer and M. B. Skinner. FANTUS, B. J.A.M.A. *105:*1679-1682, Nov. 23, '35

Injuries of jaws and face in farm laborers. DUBOV, M. D. Sovet. khir., no. 3, pp. 98-102, '35

Fractures of jaw and allied traumatic lesions of facial structures. WEISENGREEN, H. H. AND LEVIN, W. N. Ann. Surg. *103:*428-437, March '36

Results of immediate surgical therapy in grave trauma to face; case. MAROTTOLI, O. R. An. de cir. *2:*273-279, Aug '36

Management of facial injuries in automobile accidents. STRAITH, C. L., J.A.M.A. *108:* 101-105, Jan. 9, '37 also: Rev. de chir. structive, pp. 403-412, Dec '36

Early local care of facial wounds. BLAIR, V. P.; *et al.* Surg., Gynec. and Obst. *64:*358-371, Feb (no. 2A) '37 also: Internat. J. Orthodontia *23:*515-533, May '37

Emergency surgery of facial wounds (with fractures). DUFOURMENTEL, L. Presse med. *45:*387-390, March 13, '37

Management of injuries of face and jaws, with special reference to common automobile injury. PADGETT, E. C., J. Kansas M. Soc. *38:*240-248, June '37

Automobile injuries (face). STRAITH, C. L. J.A.M.A. *109:*940-945, Sept 18, '37

Acute purulent parotitis caused by facial trauma; case. YAMASAKI, Y. Oto-rhino-laryng. *10:*1027, Nov '37

Maxillofacial injuries. BOWER, R. L., J. Missouri M. A. *34:*448-449, Dec '37

Injuries of jaws and face among agricultural workers. DUBOV, M. D. Novy khir. arkhiv *38:*378-383, '37

Facial injuries. IVANISSEVICH, O. Dia med. *10:*11-13, Jan. 3, '38

New developments in application of plastic surgery to accident cases involving the face. PEARLMAN, R. C. Kentucky M. J. *36:*30-34, Jan '38

Facial Injuries – Cont.

Facial lacerations. PHILIPS, W. P. Dallas M. J. *24:*41-43, March '38

Treatment of facial wounds and cut throat. TAYLOR, J. Brit. M. J. *1:*792-795, April 9, '38

Early management of facial injuries. GINGRASS, R. P., J. Am. Dent. A. *25:*693-699, May '38

First aid in facial injuries. BICHLMAYR, A. Munchen. med. Wchnschr. *85:*1267-1275, Aug. 19, '38

Plastic surgery in relation to automobile accidents (face). LANGE, W. A., J. Michigan M. Soc. *37:*787-792, Sept '38

Care of compound injuries of face. BROWN, J. B. South. M. J. *32:*136-144, Feb '39 also: New Orleans M. and S. J. *91:*474-480, March '39

Acute lacerations of face. ADAMS, W. M. Mississippi Doctor *17:*139-142, Aug '39

Indications for emergency facial surgery. DUFOURMENTEL. Mem. Acad. de chir. *65:*1132-1138, Oct. 25-Nov 8, '39

Role of plastic surgery in facial injuries. VON WEDEL, C. South. M. J. *32:*1118-1120, Nov '39

Treatment of wounds of face. MIKHELSON, N. M. Khirurgiya, no. 1, pp. 33-40, '39

Care of automobile injuries to face. NEW, G. B. AND ERICH, J. B. Minnesota Med. *23:*1-8, Jan '40

Treatment and primary suture of facial wounds. DAVIS, E. D. D. Brit. M. J. *1:*381-383, March 9, '40

Recent traumatic injuries of face. ERICH, J. B. Proc. Staff Meet., Mayo Clin. *15:*166-169, March 13, '40

Maxillofacial surgery. IMBERT, L. Marseille-med. *1:*121-124, March 15, '40

Severe facial injuries; diagnosis and treatment. FOSTER, A. K. JR. Am. J. Surg. *48:*391-397, May '40

Care of severe injuries of face and jaws. BROWN, J. B. AND MCDOWELL, F. Journal-Lancet *60:*260-267, June '40

Therapy of facial injuries. IVANISSEVICH, O. Rev. med.-cir. do Brasil *48:*359-366, June '40 also: Rev. mex. de cir., ginec. y cancer *8:*241-255, June '40

Immediate treatment of facial injuries preparatory to plastic repair. PASSE, E. R. G. J. Roy. Nav. M. Serv. *26:*273-275, July '40

Two hundred sixteen sutures in face. GONZALEZ ULLOA, M. Dia med. *12:*844, Sept. 16, '40

Immediate care of automobile injuries to face

Facial Injuries – Cont.

at scene of accident. New, G. B. Proc. Staff Meet., Mayo Clin. *15:*728–729, Nov 13, '40

Injuries to face (soft tissues) (with burns). Eckhoff, N. L. Guy's Hosp. Gaz. *54:*345–350, Nov 30, '40

Feeding and care of patients with maxillofacial wounds. Aks, L. V. Ortop. i. travmatol. (no. 1) *14:*90–96, '40

Care of fresh wounds of face and jaws. Uebermuth, H. Arch. f. klin. Chir. *200:*546–552, '40

Maxillofacial injuries; important considerations. Ivory, J., J. Indust. Med. *10:*52–54, Feb '41

Primary care of facial injuries and jaws. Kazanjian, V. H. Surg., Gynec. and Obst. *72:*431–436, Feb (no. 2A) '41

Late care of severe facial injuries and jaw. Padgett, E. C. Surg., Gynec. and Obst. *72:*437–452, Feb. (no. 2A) '41 also: Am. J. Orthodontics (Oral Surg. Sect) *27:*190–207, April '41

Severe facial injuries and jaws. Padgett, E. C. Am. J. Surg. *51:*829–846, March '41

Unusual hand injuries and face. Poka, L. Orvosi hetil. *85:*105–107, March 1, '41

Immediate therapy for facial injuries; essential concepts. Gabarro, P. Rev. Fac. de med., Bogota *9:*717–727, April '41

Traumatic wounds of soft tissues of face, with preliminary report on new azochloramid (hypochlorite derivative) solution, and new modified sulfanilamide solution. Kintz, F. P. Mil. Surgeon *89:*60–70, July '41

Primary care of facial wounds. Kazanjian, V. H. Am. J. Orthodontics (Oral Surg. Sect) *27:*448–457, Aug '41

Management of facial injuries. Owens, N. and Vincent, R. W. New Orleans M. and S. J. *94:*221–232, Nov '41

Total craniofacial disjunction; case. Dufourmentel, L. Bull. et mem. Soc. d. chirurgiens de Paris *32:*69–71, '41

Maxillofacial injuries. Fox, C. Mil. Surgeon *90:*61–72, Jan '42 Also: Am. J. Orthodontics (Oral Surg. Sect) *28:*202–212, April '42

Treatment of traumatic injuries of face. Hume, E. C. Kentucky M. J. *40:*89–93, March '42

Treatment of facial wounds. Beall, L. L. Mississippi Doctor *19:*370–372, April '42

Panel discussions; treatment of injuries to face. Brown, J. B. Bull. Am. Coll. Surgeons *27:*132–134, April '42

Plastic correction of depressed deformities of facial bones, especially by means of traction apparatus. Rego, G. Arq. de cir. clin. e exper. *6:*200–234, April–June '42

Facial Injuries – Cont.

Treatment of wounds to face due to explosions. Straith, C. L., J. Michigan M. Soc. *41:*484–487, June '42

Early care of facial wounds. Amaral, O. and Vieira Filho, O. Rev. med. brasil. *13:*111–116, July '42

Plastic surgery in case of severe wound of cranium and face. de Vasconcelos Marques, A. Amatus *1:*612–615, July '42

Surgical treatment of recent facial wounds. Maltz, M., J. Internat. Coll. Surgeons *5:*334–342, July–Aug '42

New ideas in reconstructive maxillofacial surgery. Virenque. Rev. de stomatol. *43:*149–158, Sept–Oct, '42

Injuries to soft tissues of face. Claiborn, L. N. Connecticut M. J. *6:*793–795, Oct '42

Facial injuries; care and treatment. Williams, P. E. Mil. Surgeon *91:*650–659, Dec '42

Immediate and later care of facial injuries. New, G. B. Tr. Pacific Coast Oto-Ophth. Soc. *27:*14–16, '42

Organizational problem of nutrition in maxillofacial trauma. Pyatnitskiy, F. A. Klin. med. (nos. 3–4) *20:*22–28, '42

Modern therapy of facial injuries. Gonzalez Ulloa, M. Rev. mex. de cir., ginec. y cancer *11:*51–74, Feb '43

Maxillofacial reconstruction. Soderberg, N. B. Mil. Surgeon *92:*268–276, March '43

Special considerations in repair of facial injuries. Gurdin, M. Hawaii M. J. *2:*199–200, March–April '43

Early care of facial injuries. Boyne, H. N. Nebraska M. J. *28:*111–113, April '43

Severe facial injury of unusual etiology; case. Johnston, L. R., J. Oral Surg. *1:*179–181, April '43

Facial wounds and their plastic repair. Panneton, P. Union med. du Canada *72:*392–397, April '43

Plastic surgery of facial injuries. Kazanjian, V. H. Bull. Am. Coll. Surgeons *28:*140–141, June '43

Early treatment of facial wounds (and neck). New, G. B. Minnesota Med. *26:*619–622, July '43

Modern therapy of facial injuries. Gonzalez Ulloa, M. Rev. brasil. de cir. *12:*547–564, Sept '43 also: Vida nueva *53:*42–61, Feb '44

Early treatment of facial wounds. Mullen, T. F., S. Clin. North America *23:*1458–1464, Oct '43

Maxillofacial wounds; prophylaxis and therapy of pulmonary complications. Badylykes, S. O. Sovet. med. (no. 10) *7:*15–16, '43

Facial Injuries – Cont.

Treatment of crushing injuries of face. STRAITH, C. L. Proc. Interst. Postgrad. M. A. North America (1942) pp. 292–294, '43

Traumatic Injuries of Facial Bones, by John B. Erich and Louie T. Austin. W. B. Saunders Co., Phila., 1944

Maxillofacial injuries. STREICHER, C. J. AND ROSEDALE, R. S. Ohio State M. J. *40:*38–40, Jan '44

Suturing infected wounds of the face. GUILBERT, H. D., J. Internat. Coll. Surgeons *7:*44–48, Jan–Feb '44

Surgical treatment of recent wounds of face. MALTZ, M. Eye, Ear, Nose and Throat Monthly *23:*60–68, Feb '44

Maxillofacial injuries; extracts from case histories. GRAHAM, M. P. Brit. Dent. J. *76:*339–341, June 16, '44

Present therapy of facial injury. GONZALEZ ULLOA, M. Prensa med. argent. *31:* 1863–1876, Sept 20, '44

Notes from maxillofacial centers, Warwick, October, 1642. BROWN, O. F. Brit. Dent. J. *77:*195–197, Oct. 6, '44

Maxillofacial injuries. CHRISTIANSEN, G. W. M. Ann. District of Columbia *14:*76–77, Feb '45

Definitive treatment of maxillofacial injuries. PARKER, D. B., J. Oral Surg. *3:*320–325, Oct '45

Maxillofacial injuries. BLOCKER, T. G. JR. AND WEISS, L. R., J. Indiana M. A. *39:*60–63, Feb '46

Early management of facial injuries. SLAUGHTER, W. B. AND WONG, W., S. Clin North America *26:*2–19, Feb '46

Therapy of acute maxillofacial wounds. HENDERSON, J. A. Dia med. *18:*183–184, March 4, '46

Facial injuries. HILGER, J. A. Minnesota Med. *29:*235, Mar '46

Trismus in relation to maxillofacial surgery. LOADER, G. S. Brit. Dent. J. *81:*193–196, Sept 20, '46

Surgical technic for lacerations of face. VANDER VELDE, K. M., U. S. Nav. M. Bull. *46:*1451–1452, Sept '46

Rationale of treatment in maxillofacial injuries, with report of 4 cases. MAXWELL, M. M.; *et al.* J. Oral Surg. *4:*269–303, Oct '46

Reparative operation for maxillary ankylosis and labiofacial destruction due to noma. KANKAT, C. T. Turk tip cem. mec. *12:*163–168, '46

Facial Injuries, Tracheotomy in

Tracheotomy for grave subcutaneous emphysema following cervicofacial trauma; cases. CASTELNAU, M. Oto-rhino-Laryng. internat. *22:*195–196, April '38

Emergency treatment of smashed-in face; value of tracheotomy and laryngotomy. PATEY, D. H. AND RICHES, E. W. Lancet *2:*161–162, Aug. 7, '43

Facial Lesions

Lesions of hand and face caused by colored copying pencil. BETTAZZI, G. Policlinico (sez. chir.) *35:*501–505, Oct '28

Trophic postencephalitic ulcerations of outer nose and of cheek. SCHLITTLER, E. Schweiz. med. Wchnschr. *59:*1121–1122, Nov 9, '29

Permanent enlargement of lips and face secondary to recurring swellings and associated with facial paralysis; clinical entity. NEW, G. B. AND KIRCH, W. A., J.A.M.A. *100:*1230–1233, April 22, '33

Osteitis deformans affecting bones of face. NEW, G. B. AND HARPER, F. R. Proc. Staff Meet., Mayo Clin. *8:*465–466, Aug 2, '33

Permanent enlargement of lips and face, secondary to recurring swellings and associated with facial paralysis; clinical study. NEW, G. B. Tr. Am. Laryng. A. *55:*43–50, '33

Pneumatization of bones of face in Crouzon's disease, Apert's syndrome and oxycephaly; 13 cases. DE GUNTEN, P. Schweiz. med. Wchnschr. *68:*268–270, March 12, '38

Differential diagnosis of swellings of face and neck. WINTER, L. Am. J. Orthodontics *25:*1087–1116, Nov '39

Etiology and treatment of common diseases of face and scalp (acne). BARBER, H. W. Guy's Hosp. Gaz. *53:*397–399, Dec 16, '39 *53:*381, Dec 2, '39

Elephantiasis of face cured with rubiazol (sulfonamide); case. MILIAN, G. Ann. de dernat. et syph. (Bull. Soc. dranc. de dermat. et syph) *2:*106–108, Feb '42

Oral and genital aphthae of mutilating character; case. DEGAUDENZI, C. Dermosifilografo *17:*520–526, Sept '42

Intermaxilloparotid cellular space; abscesses formed there. PONS-TORTELLA, E. AND BROGGI, M. Med. Clin., Barcelona *5:*273–277, Oct '45

Facial Paralysis

Prosthesis to correct facial paralysis. SICARD, J. A. Bull. et mem. Soc. med. d. hop. de Paris *45:*612, May 6, '21 abstr: J.A.M.A. *76:*1862, June 25, '21

Facial Paralysis – Cont.

Correction of facial paralysis. OMBRÉDANNE, L. Presse med. *29:*636, Aug. 10, '21 abstr: J.A.M.A. *77:*1053, Sept 24, '21

Spinofacial anastomosis for facial paralysis. TITONE, M. Lyon chir. *18:*601–605, Sept–Oct '21 (illus.) abstr: J.A.M.A. *78:*249, Jan 21, '22

Facial paralysis. GIBSON, A. Surg., Gynec. and Obst. *33:*472, Nov '21

Correction of deformity from facial paralysis. BURIAN, F. Rev. de chir. *59:*52, '21

Experimental artificial neurotization of paralyzed muscle. JINNAKA, S. Mitt. a. d. med. Fakult. d. k. Univ. zu Tokyo *25:*367–441, '21

Facial palsy and its treatment by nerve anastomosis. DE PAIVA MEIRA, S. Internat. Clinics *2:*241, '21

Facial paralysis and surgical repair of facial nerve. NEY, K. W. Laryngoscope *32:*327–347, May '22 (illus.)

Surgical treatment of facial paralysis. COLEMAN, C. C. Virginia M. Monthly *49:*180–188, July '22 (illus.)

Case of facio-hypoglossal anastomosis for facial palsy. STONEY, R. A. Irish J. M. Soc. pp. 404–408, Nov '22

Anastomosis of seventh and eleventh cranial nerves to correct facial paralysis. NIX, J. T. New Orleans M. and S. J. *77:*123–126, Sept '24

Nerve grafting versus musculoplasty in paralysis of facial nerve. PERTHES, G. Zentralbl. f. Chir. *51:*2073–2076, Sept 20 '24

Treatment of central and peripheral paralysis of facial nerve. FUCHS, A. AND PFEFFER, M. Wien. klin. Wchnschr. *37:*1008–1010, Oct. 2, '24 abstr: J.A.M.A. *83:*1546, Nov 8, '24

Operative correction of paralysis of lower lip. SCHMERZ, H. Arch. f. klin. Chir. *131:*353–360, '24 abstr: J.A.M.A. *83:*1464, Nov 1, '24

Surgical treatment of facial paralysis. ADSON, A. W. Arch. Otolaryng. *2:*217–249, Sept '25 also: Tr. Sect. Laryng. Otol. and Rhin., A. M. A., pp. 187–211, '25

Operative correction of facial paralysis. BLAIR, V. P. South. M. J. *19:*116–120, Feb '26

Treatment of facial paralysis. FUCHS, A. Wien. klin. Wchnschr. *39:*248–250, Feb 25, '26; 277–279, March 4, '26

Results of hypoglossofacial anastomosis for facial paralysis in 2 cases. BROWN, A. Surg., Gynec. and Obst. *42:*608–613, May '26

Surgical treatment of facial paralysis. BRUNNER. Ztschr. f. Hals-, Nasen-u. Ohrenh. *15:*379–382, Oct. 6, '26

Immediate results of operations for facial paralysis. TAVERNIER, L. Bull. et mem. Soc. nat. de chir. *52:*992–994, Nov 20, '26

Plastic operations for paralysis of facial nerve. BRUNNER, H. Arch. f. klin. Chir. *140:*85–100, '26

Contractures in peripheral facial paralysis. LESCHTSCHENKO, G. D. Ztschr. f. d. ges. Neurol. u. Psychiat. *104:*586–595, '26

Facial paralysis treated by spino-facial anastomosis; 2 cases. ANTONIOLI, G. M. Gior. d. r. Accad. di med. di Torino *33:*80–88, Feb '27

Surgical treatment of facial paralysis attributed to cold. ESCAT, E. Ann. d. mal. de l'oreille, du larynx *46:*213–221, March '27

Cervical sympathectomy in traumatic peripheral facial paralysis. JIANU, I. AND BUZOIANU, G. Bull. et mem. Soc. med. d. hop. de Bucarest *9:*35–39, March '27

Surgical treatment of facial paralysis. ZAHRADNICEK, J. Casop. lek. cesk. *66:*592–594, March 28, '27

Peripheral facial paralysis and progressive facial hemiatrophy as sequels of teeth extraction. BÖNHEIM, E. Deutsche Monatschr. f. Zahnh. *45:*353–366, April 15, '27

Treatment of traumatic facial paralysis. BUZZARD, E. F. Proc. Roy. Soc. Med. (Sect. Otol.) *20:*35–39, May '27

Rational treatment of Bell's palsy. COHEN, M. A. AND FELDMAN, L. Am. J. Phys. Therapy *4:*59–61, May '27

Treatment of traumatic facial paralysis. BUZZARD, E. F., J. Laryng. and Otol. *42:*437–439, July '27

Facial paralysis; causes, symptoms and treatment. SIEMERLING, E. Deutsche med. Wchnschr. *53:*1467–1470, Aug 26, '27

Treatment of facial paralysis due to exposure. BERTWISTLE, A. P. Brit. M. J. *2:*494, Sept 17, '27

Remarks on 1008 cases of facial paralysis. MARQUE, A. M. Rev. de especialid. *2:*1195–1199, Dec '27 also: Rev. oto. neuro-oftal. *2:*1–4, Jan '28

Surgical treatment of paralysis of face, vocal cords, and diaphragm. BALLANCE, C. Tr. Roy. Med.-Chir. Soc., Glasgow *21:*90–102, '27

Leriche's operation for traumatic peripheral facial paralysis as compared with other operative procedures. JIANU, J. AND BUZOIANU, G. Lyon chir. *25:*10–21, Jan–Feb '28

Surgery of traumatic facial paralysis. ANTONIOLI, G. M. Clin. chir. *31:*81–104, Feb '28

Facial Paralysis – Cont.

Congenital defects of radius and ear with facial paralysis; case. ESSEN-MÖLLER, E. Ztschr. f. d. ges. Anat. (Abt. 2) *14:*52–70, March 28, '28

Rational treatment of facial paralysis; with special reference to Bell's palsy. FELDMAN, L. Am. J. Phys. Therapy *4:*539–544, March '28

Peripheral facial paralysis; 1,008 cases. MARQUE, A. M. Semana med. *1:*946–949, April 19, '28

Facial paralysis, palatal repair and some other plastic operations. PICKERILL, P., M. M. J. Australia *1:*543–548, May 5, '28

Endoral plastic correction of results of paralysis of facial nerve. BRUNNER, H. Wien. klin. Wchnschr. *41:*876–877, June 21, '28

Aesthetic correction of facial paralysis; case. DUFOURMENTEL, L. Bull. et mem. Soc. de chir. de Paris *20:*531, June 1, '28

Treatment of facial paralysis. KOCH, C. F. A. Nederl. Tijdschr. v. Geneesk. *2:*3628–3632, July 21, '28

Fasciaplasty in treatment of facial paralysis. MOSZKOWICZ, L. Wien. klin. Wchnschr. *41:*1151–1153, Aug. 9, '28

Mechanism involved in return of contractility of facial muscles when cervical sympathectomy is performed for facial paralysis. LERICHE, R. AND FONTAINE, R. Compt. rend. Soc. de biol. *99:*858–860, Sept 18, '28

Surgical treatment of facial paralysis from cold; cases. ESCAT, E. Rev. de stomatol. *30:*614–624, Oct '28

Resection of superior cervical sympathetic ganglion for facial paralysis; case. ALBERT, R., J de chir, et ann. Soc belge de chir. *27:*285–291, '28

Surgical treatment of facial deformity due to paralysis. VREDEN, R. R. Vestnik khir. (nos. 43–44) *14:*11–13, '28

Simple method for raising corner of mouth in facial paralysis BLUME, AND SCHOLZ. Deutsche med. Wchnschr. *55:*272, Feb 15, '29

Traumatic facial paralysis; treatment by free transplantation of fascia lata. FISCHER, H. Ann. Surg. *89:*334–339, March '29

Facial palsies and their management. ROSENHECK, C., M. J. and Res *129:*266–269, March 6, '29

Treatment of facial paralysis by excision of cervical sympathetic ganglion; case. ALBERT, F. Liege med. *22:*592–599, April 28, '29

Surgical treatment of facial paralysis; recovery. DORRONSORO, D. A. Siglo med. *83:*637–638, April 27, '29

Facial Paralysis – Cont.

Facial nerve anastomosis in paralysis. BALLANCE, C., J. Egyptian M. A. *12:*63–68, May '29

Heterotopy of pinna of ear and congenital facial paralysis; case. CASTERÁN, E. Rev. de especialid. *4:*1035–1038, Sept '29

Paralysis of intrapetrosal portion of facial nerve; clinical forms, treatment. SARGNON, A. AND BERTEIN, P., J. de med. de Lyon *10:*539–560, Sept 5, '29

Bilateral congenital facial paralysis; review of literature and classification. BONAR, B. E. AND OWENS, R. W. Am. J. Dis. Child. *38:*1256–1272, Dec '29

Peripheral facial paralysis; kinesthetic treatment; 10 cases. FERNÁNDEZ, O. C. Semana med. *2:*1718–1734, Dec 12, '29

Plastic operation for facial paralysis. LODGE, W. O. Brit. J. Surg. *17:*422–423, Jan '30

Treatment of facial paralysis. CAHALL, W. L. Arch. Physical Therapy *11:*78–81, Feb '30

Classification of peripheral facial paralyses. ZIMMERN, A. AND CHAVANY, J. A. Medecine *11:*453–457, June '30

Congenital facial paralysis. ERRECART, P. L. Rev. de especialid. *5:*930–935, July '30

Further observation upon compensatory use of live tendon strips in facial paralysis. BLAIR, V. P. Ann. Surg. *92:*694–703, Oct '30

Postoperative facial paralysis treated with Leriche operation, excision of upper cervical sympathetic ganglion; case. DELLA TORRE, P. L. Cervello *9:*299–312, Nov 15, '30

Compensatory use of live tendon strips; further observations in facial paralysis. BLAIR, V. P. Tr. Am. S. A. *48:*369–378, '30

Facial paralysis; causes; treatment by neurosurgery (muscular neurotization). ROSENTHAL, W. Deutsche Ztschr. f. Chir. *223:*261–270, '30

Surgical therapy of facial paralysis. WERTHEIMER, P. Lyon chir. *28:*111–113, Jan–Feb '31

Facial nerve anastomosis for relief of paralysis. BROWN, A. Illinois M. J. *59:*130, Feb '31

Atrophy of external ear with hemiatrophy of face and paresis of lower facial nerve; case. ROCHER, H. L., J. de med. de Bordeaux *108:*231, March 20, '31

Peripheral facial paralysis following frostbite; case. ROY, J. N. Union med. du Canada *60:*223–229, April '31

Surgical therapy of peripheral facial paralysis. WERTHEIMER, P. AND CARCASSONNE, F. Lyon chir. *28:*560–570, Sept–Oct '31

Facial Paralysis – Cont.

Operative treatment of facial palsy by introduction of nerve grafts into fallopian canal and by other intratemporal methods. BALLANCE, C. AND DUEL, A. B. Tr. Am. Otol. Soc. *21:*288–295, '31

Operative treatment of facial palsy by introduction of nerve grafts into fallopian canal and by other intratemporal methods. BALLANCE, C. AND DUEL, A. B. Arch. Otolaryng. *15:*1-70, Jan '32

Operative treatment of facial paralysis; with account of animal experiments. BALLANCE, C. Brit. M. J. *1:*787–788, April 30, '32

Keloid therapy; clinic in reparative surgery, unilateral facial paralysis. SHEEHAN, J. E. S. Clin. North America *12:*341–356, April '32

Old-standing facial paralysis treated by removal of inferior cervical ganglion of sympathetic (case). WAKELEY, C. P. G. Proc. Roy. Soc. Med. *25:*795, April '32

Successful treatment of postoperative facial paralysis. ARWINE, J. T., M. Bull., Vet. Admin. *8:*404, May '32

Anastomosis of hypoglossal and facial nerves 10 months after operation; presentation of case. LEARMONTH, J. R. Proc. Staff Meet., Mayo Clin. *7:*389–390, July 6, '32

Correction of unilateral facial paralysis. SHEEHAN, J. E., J. M. Soc. New Jersey *29:*556–560, July '32

Surgical treatment of facial palsy; Ballance-Duel method. DUEL, A. B. Laryngoscope *42:*579–587, Aug '32

Removal of deformity of facial paralysis. HALLE, M. Med. Welt *6:*1279–1280, Sept. 3, '32

Peripheral facial paralysis; electrologic, diagnostic and therapeutic technic. NICOLLE, A. Rev. d'actinol. *8:*510–524, Nov–Dec '32

Clinical experiences in surgical treatment of facial palsy by autoplastic grafts; Ballance-Duel method. DUEL, A. B. Arch. Otolaryng. *16:*767–788, Dec '32

Correction of disfigurement in facial paralysis. HALLE, M. Ztschr. f. Hals-, Nasen-u. Ohrenh. *31:*554–560, '32

Facial paralysis treated by fascial grafts; case. BROOKE, R. Brit. J. Surg. *20:*523–526, Jan '33

Fascia lata grafts in facial paralysis. WARDILL, W. E. M. Newcastle M. J. *13:*35–38, Jan '33

Therapy of peripheral facial paralysis by resection of superior cervical sympathetic ganglion. WERTHEIMER, P. Bull. et mem. Soc. nat. de chir. *59:*4–7, Jan. 14, '33

Facial Paralysis – Cont.

History and development of surgical treatment of facial palsy (including grafts). DUEL, A. B. Surg., Gynec. and Obst. *56:*382–390, Feb (no. 2A) '33

Permanent enlargement of lips and face secondary to recurring swellings and associated with facial paralysis; clinical entity. NEW, G. B. AND KIRCH, W. A., J.A.M.A. *100:*1230–1233, April 22, '33

Removal of deformity of facial paralysis. HALLE. Rev. de chir. plastique, pp. 3–15, May '33

Therapy of postoperative facial paralysis. HJELMMAN, G. Acta Soc. med. fenn. duodecim (Ser. B, fasc. 3, art. 6) *17:*1–11, '33

Permanent enlargement of lips and face, secondary to recurring swellings and associated with facial paralysis; clinical study. NEW, G. B. Tr. Am. Laryng. A. *55:*43–50, '33

Advanced methods in surgical treatment of facial paralysis (Mütter lecture) (nerve transplants). DUEL, A. B. Ann. Otol., Rhin. and Laryng. *43:*76–88, March '34

Surgical therapy of facial paralysis with free aponeurotic graft. DE ANDRADE, P. C. Bol. coll. brasil. de cirurgioes *5:*39–40, June–July '34

Plastic use of fascia in treatment of facial paralysis. DEMEL, R. Zentralbl. f. Chir. *61:*1445–1448, June 23, '34

Facial paralysis from gunshot wound caused by attempted suicide; therapy by resection of superior cervical sympathetic ganglion and suspension of corners of mouth. ROQUES, P. Bull. et mem. Soc. nat. de chir. *60:*981–984, July 21, '34

Operative treatment of facial palsy, with observations on prepared nerve graft. BALLANCE, C. Proc. Roy. Soc. Med. *27:*1367–1372, Aug '34 also: J. Laryng. and Otol. *49:*709–718, Nov '34

Experience with fascia lata grafts in operative treatment of facial paralysis. GILLIES, H. Proc. Roy. Soc. Med. *27:*1372–1378, Aug '34 also: J. Laryng. and Otol. *49:*743–756, Nov '34

Buccal-facial anastomosis in facial nerve injury. PONS TORTELLA, E. Rev. de cir. de Barcelona *8:*82–89, Sept–Dec '34

Surgical relief of lagophthalmos following seventh nerve paralysis in cases of leprosy. GASS, H. H. Leprosy Rev. *5:*178–180, Oct '34

Surgical treatment of facial paralysis by autoplastic nerve graft. SULLIVAN, J. A. Canad. M. A. J. *31:*474–479, Nov '34

Facial Paralysis – Cont.

Operative treatment of facial palsy (transplant). DUEL, A. B. Brit. M. J. *2:*1027-1031, Dec 8, '34

Results of resection of superior cervical ganglion and of part of trunk of cervical sympathicus in peripheral facial paralysis of long standing; case. ROASENDA, G. AND DOGLIOTTI, A. M. Boll. e mem. Soc. piemontese di chir. *4:*980-990, '34

Bilateral spinofacial anastomosis and resection of superior cervical ganglion for bilateral facial paralysis; case. COSTANTINI, H. AND CURTILLET, E. Lyon chir. *32:*291-305, May-June '35

Results of stellectomy in facial paralysis due to section of nerve involved in parotid tumor; case. CAEIRO, J. A. Bol. y trab. de la Soc. de cir. de Buenos Aires *19:*392-403, June 26, '35

Autoplastic grafts in facial palsy. FOSTER, J. H. Ann. Otol., Rhin. and Laryng. *44:*521-526, June '35

Plastic surgery of deformities due to facial paralysis; further study. HALLE, M. Rev. de chir. structive, pp. 35-38, July '35

Surgical treatment of facial paralysis. DUEL, A. B. Acta oto-laryng. *22:*373-381, '35

Muscle-nerve graft in paralysis of facial nerve. YARITSYN, A. A. Vestnik-khir. *39:*132-134, '35

Results of stellectomy in facial paralysis due to section of facial nerve involved in parotid tumor; case. CAEIRO, J. A. Semana med. *1:*572-579, Feb 20, '36

Treatment of facial paralysis. VERBRUGGHEN, A., S. Clin North America *16:*223-229, Feb '36

Surgical repair of facial paralysis. DUEL, A. B. AND TICKLE, T. G. Ann. Otol., Rhin. and Laryng. *45:*3-27, March '36

Congenital hemiatrophy of face with facial paralysis and microphthalmos; case. BOISSERIE-LACROIX, J., J. de med. de Bordeaux *113:*419-420, May 30, '36

Method for correcting paralysis of lower part of face due to nerve injury in extirpation of benign parotid tumors. CADENAT, F. M. Mem. Acad. de chir. *62:*961-962, June 17, '36

Surgical treatment of facial paralysis. DAVIS, L. AND CLEVELAND, D. West. J. Surg. *44:*313-317, June '36

Resection of superior cervical ganglion (Leriche operation) in therapy of peripheral facial paralysis; 3 cases. BERTOLA, V.; *et al.* Prensa med. argent. *23:*2414-2427, Oct 21, '36

Facial Paralysis – Cont.

Surgical therapy of facial paralysis. DOGLIOTTI, A. M. Riforma med. *52:*1489-1492, Oct. 31, '36

Extirpation of benign parotid tumors; use of digastric muscle as guide during operation and in correction of facial paralysis. CADENAT, F. M., J. de chir. *48:* 625-629, Nov '36

Facial paralysis; improvement by surgery. DOROSCHENKO, I. T. Monatschr. f. Ohrenh. *70:*1303-1314, Nov '36

Resection of superior cervical ganglion in therapy of peripheral facial paralysis caused by injury to cranium; case. HUARD, P. Bull. Soc. med.-chir. de l'Indochine *14:*1289-1293, Nov '36

Surgical treatment of facial paralysis (with nerve grafting). MORRIS, W. M. Lancet *2:*1172-1174, Nov. 14, '36

Surgical treatment of facial paralysis. ELLIS, B. E. Tr. Indiana Acad. Ophth. and Otolaryng. *20:*22-27, '36

Surgical therapy of facial paralysis; case. SOHMA, T. AND IMAMURA, T. Mitt. a. d. med. Akad. zu Kioto *16:*1403-1404, '36

Modification of Ballance-Duel technic in treatment of facial paralysis. SULLIVAN, J. A. Tr. Am. Acad. Ophth. *41:*282-299, '36

Problem of facial paralysis. TUMARKIN, I. A. J. Laryng. and Otol. *52:*107-115, Feb '37

Surgical repair in facial paralysis. BUNNELL, S. Arch. Otolaryng. *25:*235-259, March '37

Mechanism and therapy of facial paralysis. DE MUNTER, L. AND BARAKIN, M. Liege med. *30:*415-434, April 4, '37

Nerve transplantation in facial paralysis. CAWTHORNE, T. Tr. M. Soc. London *60:*171-177, '37

Treatment of facial paralysis. CRITCHLEY, M. AND GILLIES, H. Tr. M. Soc. London *60:*166-171, '37

Surgical treatment of Bell's palsy. MORRIS, W. M. Lancet *1:*429-431, Feb. 19, '38

Facial paralysis and methods for correction. HALLE, M. Laryngoscope *48:*225-235, April '38

Plastic surgery in therapy of irreparable facial paralyses; Lexer-Rosenthal method. SCHMID, B. Zentralbl. f. Chir. *65:*1296-1297, June 4, '38

Plastic surgery in therapy for postoperative facial paralysis; case. COELST. Rev. de chir. structive *8:*107-109, Aug '38

Skin grafts and suspension of labial commissure by skin sutures for facial paralysis. ZENO, L. An. de chir. *4:*187-189, Sept '38 Also: Bol. Soc. de cir. de Rosario *5:*412-414, Oct '38

Facial Paralysis – Cont.

Transplantation of nerves in facial palsy. BAUER, G. Acta chir. Scandinav. *81:*130–138, '38

Surgical therapy of facial paralysis by intraoral neurotization. DOROSCHENKO, I. T. Acta oto-laryng. *26:*702–709, '38

Spinofacial anastomosis for bilateral traumatic facial paralysis; late results. COSTANTINI, H. AND CURTILLET, E. Lyon chir. *36:*50–53, Jan–Feb '39

Nerve (hypoglossal-facial) anastomosis in treatment of facial paralysis. TRUMBLE, H. C., M. J. Australia *1:*300–302, Feb. 25, '39

Utilization of temporal muscle and fascia for facial paralysis. BROWN, J. B. Ann. Surg. *109:*1016–1023, June '39

Preservation of muscle function in Bell's palsy with splint. LEWIN, P., J.A.M.A. *112:*2273, June 3, '39

Plastic reconstruction for facial paralysis. STRAATSMA, C. R. Laryngoscope *49:*482–483, June '39

Nerve transplant for facial paralysis. TICKLE, T. G. Laryngoscope *49:*475–481, June '39

Facial paralysis; recent treatment with case report (nerve graft). JUERS, A. L. Kentucky M. J. *37:*368–371, Aug '39

Surgical treatment of facial paralysis; review of 46 cases (nerve transplant). MORRIS, W. M. Lancet *2:*558–561, Sept 2, '39

Facial paralysis treated by incision of sheath of facial nerve. HORGAN, J. B. Brit. M. J. *2:*768, Oct 14, '39

Unusual case of facial paralysis and new operation. AYMARD, J. L. Brit. M. J. *2:*1185–1186, Dec 16, '39

Facial paralysis treatment; collective review from 1932 to 1938. CLEVELAND, D. Internat. Abstr. Surg. *69:*545–555, '39; in Surg., Gynec. and Obst., Dec '39

Modification of Vreden operation in therapy of paralytic facial deformity. KORSUNSKIY, P. D. Khirurgiya, no. 10, pp. 35–38, '39

Utilization of temporal muscle and fascia in facial paralysis. BROWN, J. B. Am. J. Orthodontics *26:*80–87, Jan '40

Measures to protect eye in facial paralysis. OBERHOFF, K. Munchen. med. Wchnschr. *87:*33, Jan 12, '40

Intratemporal repair of facial nerve for facial paralysis (Ballance-Duel operation). CASSIDY, W. A. Nebraska M. J. *25:*47–50, Feb '40

Etiology and treatment of facial paralysis. McCASKEY, C. H. Ann. Otol., Rhin. and Laryng. *49:*199–210, March '40

Facial Paralysis – Cont.

Results of facio-hypoglossal anastomosis in treatment of facial paralysis. COLEMAN, C. C. Ann. Surg. *111:*958–970, June '40

Facial paralysis and its operative treatment (Hunterian lecture abridged). COLLIER, J. Lancet *2:*91–94, July 27, '40

Possible new operation for therapy of definitive paralysis; anastomosis of facial and sympathetic nerves. LERICHE, R. Presse med. *48:*721–722, Sept 17, '40

Recent experiences with operation on facial nerve (including 2 cases of paralysis following mastoidectomy). MARTIN, R. C. Arch. Otolaryng. *32:*1071–1075, Dec '40

Etiology and treatment of facial paralysis. McCASKEY, C. H. Tr. Am. Laryng., Rhin. and Otol. Soc. *46:*285–295, '40

Malignant tumor of parotid gland treated by Duval operation, with transplantation of digastric muscle to relieve resulting paralysis (Cadenat operation); case. MIRIZZI, P. L. and URRUTIA, J. M. Bol. y trab., Soc. de cir. de Cordoba (no. 4) *1:*52–55, '40

Duel-Ballance nerve graft for cure of complete traumatic facial paralysis; case. HORGAN, J. B. Irish J. M. Sc., pp. 196–198, May '41

Therapy of facial paralysis. KOWARSCHIK, J. Wien. klin. Wchnschr. *54:*494–498, June 6, '41

Discussion on limitations of operative treatment in traumatic facial paralysis. COLLIER, D. J.; *et al.* Proc. Roy. Soc. Med. *34:*575–584, July '41, also: J. Laryng. and Otol. *56:*207–222, June '41

Correction of facial paralysis (muscle transplant). ALEXANDER, R. J. Rocky Mountain M. J. *38:*713–716, Sept '41

Late result of hypoglossofacial anastomosis: inadaptation of centers. BOURGUIGNON, G. Rev. neurol. *73:*601–603, Nov–Dec '41

Excision of superior cervical ganglion in therapy of peripheral paralysis (facial). PLACINTEANU, G. AND DOBRESCU, D. Zentralbl. f. Chir. *69:*323, Feb 21, '42

Treatment of facial paralysis. ELLIS, B. E. North Carolina M. J. *3:*130–132, March '42

Relation between sympathetic phenomena and contracture in facial paralysis; therapeutic conclusions. PONTHUS, P.; *et al.* Presse med. *50:*308–309, April 20, '42

Treatment of facial paralysis. LATHROP, F. D. Lahey Clin. Bull. *3:*20–27, July '42

Paralysis of seventh cranial pair; 2 cases. LURASCHI, J. C. E. AND PORRINI, E. A. Dia med. *14:*1214–1216, Nov. 16, '42

Combined plastic surgery on facial and fa-

Facial Paralysis – Cont.

cial-hypoglossal nerves for facial paralysis. BERGGREN, S. AND FROSTE, N. Acta otolaryng. *30:*325–327, '42

Peripheral facial paralysis, based upon 50 observations. ADLER, E. Acta med. orient. *2:*1–9, Dec '42–Jan '43

Facial palsy of otitic origin, with special regard to its prognosis under conservative treatment and possibilities of improving results by active surgical intervention; account of 264 cases subjected to reexamination. KETTEL, K. Arch. Otolaryng. *37:*303–348, March '43

Facial paralysis following mastoid surgery; 3 cases treated successfully. MCCALL, J. W. AND GARDINER, F. S. Laryngoscope *53:* 232–239, April '43

Stellectomy in therapy of case of facial paralysis. DIEZ, J. Bol. y trab., Acad. argent. de cir. *27:*564–566, July 21, '43

Facial paralysis; diagnosis and therapy. BARRAQUER FERRE, L. Med. clin., Barcelona *1:*334–338, Nov '43

Treatment of lip and cheek in cases of facial paralysis (by plastic lip cradle). DAHLBERG, A. A., J.A.M.A., *124:*503–504, Feb 19, '44

Plastic surgery of facial paralysis (including fascial transplant) with modification in technic. LAMONT, E. S. Arch. Otolaryng. *39:*155–163, Feb '44

Paralysis of seventh cranial pair; study apropos of 2 cases. LURASCHI, J. C. E. AND PORRINI, E. A. Semana med. *1:*218–220, Feb 3, '44

Cervical sympathectomy in therapy of facial paralysis. ALBANESE, A. R. Prensa med. argent. *31:*415–417, March 1, '44

Procedure to correct facial paralysis (by spinofacial anastomosis and fascial strips). HANRAHAN, E. M. AND DANDY, W. E. J.A.M.A. *124:*1051–1053, April 8, '44

New technic for repair of facial paralysis with tantalum wire. SCHUESSLER, W. W. Surgery *15:*646–652, April '44

Facial paralysis; intraoral splint. ALLEN, A. G. AND NORTHFIELD, D. W. C. Lancet *2:*172–173, Aug 5, '44

Surgical therapy of otogenic facial paralysis according to Ballance-Duel and Bunnell: 35 cases. KETTEL, K. Nord. med. (Hospitalstid.) *24:*1783–1795, Oct 6,'44

Surgical therapy of facial paralysis. VON SEEMEN, H. Arch. f. klin. Chir. *205:*598, '44

Facial paralysis and its surgical correction; study apropos of promising result. ETCHEVERRY, M. Bol. y. trab., Soc. argent. de cirujanos *6:*302–308, '45, also: Rev. Asoc. med. argent. *59:*844–846, July 30, '45

Facial Paralysis – Cont.

Intraoral splint for facial palsy. ALLEN, A. G. AND NORTHFIELD, D. W. C. Brit. Dent. J. *79:*213–215, Oct 19, '45

Early treatment of Bell's palsy. PICKERILL, H. P. AND PICKERILL, C. M. Brit. M. J. *2:*457–459, Oct 6, '45

Support of the paralyzed face by fascia. BROWN, J. B. AND MCDOWELL, F. Arch. Surg., *53:*420, Dec '45

Surgical correction of facial paralysis; results in cases. COTTINI, G. F. Bol. y. trab., Soc. argent. de cirujanos *6:*443–448, '45

Unilateral facial paralysis; correction with tantalum wire; preliminary report on 8 cases. SHEEHAN, J. E. Lancet *1:*263–264, Feb 23, '46

Effect of facial paralysis on growth of skull of rat and rabbit. WASHBURN, S. L. Anat. Rec. *94:*163–168, Feb '46

Facial splint for treatment of Bell's palsy. PRACY, J. P. Brit. M. J. *1:*528, April 6, '46

Facial Prostheses: See Prostheses

Facial Spasm

Surgical treatment of facial spasm. COLEMAN, C. C. Ann. Surg. *105:*647–657, May '37

Treatment of clonic facial spasm by nerve anastomosis. PHILLIPS, G., M. J. Australia *1:*624–626, April 2, '38

Surgical treatment of spasmodic facial tic. GERMAN, W. J. Surgery *11:*912–914, June '42

Facial Surgery, Anesthesia for

Rectal anesthesia in facial surgery. JACOD, M. Ann. d. mal. de l'oreille, du larynx *46:*583–586, June '27

New methods of anesthetizing jaws and face. LINDEMANN, A. Narkose u. Anaesth. *1:*3–16, Jan 15, '28

Accidents of local anesthesia in cranio-facial region; pathogenesis. HAMANT, A. AND BODART, M. Rev. med. de l'est. *56:*610–616, Sept 15, '28

Anesthesia in operations on face and neck. GUISEZ, J. Ann. d. mal. de l'oreille, du larynx *49:*516–524, May '30

Deep block anesthesia of second and third divisions of fifth nerve. BROWN, J. B. Internat. J. Orthodontia *18:*193–199, Feb '32

Inhalation anesthesia with chlorylene (trichloroethylene) in plastic surgery of face. KELLER, P. Dermat. Wchnschr. *95:*973–985, July 2, '32

Facial Surgery, Anesthesia for—Cont.

Rectal anesthesia with tribrom-ethanol in cervicofacial surgery; indications, technic, results and experimental studies. MOULONGUET, A. AND LEROUX-ROBERT, J. Ann. d'oto-laryng., pp. 283-304, March '34

Rectal anesthesia with mixture of ether, tribrom-ethanol and oil in cervicofacial surgery. JACOD, M. Lyon chir. *32:*35-42, Jan-Feb '35

Rectal anesthesia with mixture of ether, tribrom-ethanol and oil in cervicofacial surgery. JACOD, M. Ann. d'oto-laryng., pp. 802-808, July '35

Potassium bromide as anesthetic in facial orbital surgery. KHRAMELASHVILI, N. G. Sovet. vrach. zhur., pp. 677-678, May 15, '36

Vinethene (vinyl ether) burn of face. LYONS, S. S., J.A.M.A. *111:*1284-1285, Oct 1, '38

Anesthesia for faciomaxillary surgery. MUSHIN, W. W. Post-Grad. M. J. *16:*245-246, July '40

Preanesthetic medication with special consideration of problems in maxillofacial surgery. LYMAN, E. E. Mil. Surgeon *88:*57-62, Jan '41

Procaine hydrochloride block of phrenic nerve in therapy of postoperative complications, with report of case of autoplastic repair of face. PENIDO BURNIER, E. M. Rev. med.-cir. do Brasil *49:*53-68, Feb '41

Review of local anesthesia in maxillofacial cases. O'HARA, D. M. Mil. Surgeon *89:*652-656, Oct '41

General anesthesia in treatment of maxillofacial cases. FISCHER, T. E. Mil. Surgeon *89:*877-892, Dec '41

Block of branches of trigeminal nerve in surgery. PLAZA, F. L. Jorn. neuro-psiquiat. panam., actas (1939) *2:*104-112, '41

Choice of anesthesia for maxillofacial surgery in war and civilian injuries. MARVIN, F. W. Am. J. Orthodontics (Oral Surg. Sect) *28:*254-257, May '42

Anesthesia of recent injuries of jaw and face. ROCHE, G. K. T. Anesthesiology *7:*233-254, May '46

Facial Surgery, Dental Aspects of

Procedures which extend field of dentofacial orthopedics. FEDERSPIEL, M. N., J. Am. Dent. A. *14:*2143-2157, Dec '27

New method of morphologic analysis in dentofacial orthopedics. DE COSTER. Rev. de stomatol. *32:*552-564, June '30

Prognathism; study in development of face. TODD, T. W., J. Am. Dent. A. *19:*2172-2184, Dec '32

Facial Surgery, Dental Aspects of—Cont.

Treatment of facial fractures of special interest to dental surgeon. MAXWELL, M. M. U.S. Nav. M. Bull. *36:* 501-507, Oct '38

Responsibility of orthodontist in treatment of traumatic injuries of face and jaws. FAIRBANK, L. C. Am. J. Orthodontics *27:*414-422, Aug '41

Dentofacial musculature. DEWEL, B. F. Am. J. Orthodontics *27:*469-488, Sept '41

Dentists and first surgical care of face and jaw injuries on battlefield. SQUIRRU, C. M. Rev. san. mil., Buenos Aires *41:*457-469, July '42

Dental aspect of maxillofacial surgery. GOLDIE, H. South African M. J. *18:*224-225, July 8, '44

Dentofacial orthopedics; effect on development of child. LEBOURG, L. AND LAMBERG. Semaine d. hop Paris *21:*544-547, May 28, '45

Medical and dental relationship in maxillofacial team. RANKOW, R. M. Ann. Dent. *4:*164-166, Mar '46

Facial Surgery, Reviews of

Facial surgery in 1921. DUFOURMENTEL, L. Medecine *3:*57, Oct '21, abstr: J.A.M.A. *77:*2152, Dec 31, '21

Plastic surgery of face; recent contributions, present status. HARTER, J. H. Northwest Med. *28:*185-187, April '29

Developments in plastic surgery of face and neck. NEW, G. B. Wisconsin M. J. *32:*243-246, April '33

Congenital defects and deformities of face; review of literature for 1936. IVY, R. H. Internat. Abstr. Surg. *64:*433-442, '37; in Surg., Gynec. and Obst. May '37

Facial surgery; review of literature, 1939. IVY, R. H. AND MILLER, H. A. Arch. Otolaryng. *32:*159-176, July '40

Review of reconstructive surgery of face. MCDOWELL, F. AND BROWN, J. B. Laryngoscope *50:*1117-1138, Dec '40

Progress of surgery of head (including face, ears, nose, mouth, etc.) and throat (esophagus and larynx); review of literature for 1940. REBELO NETO, J. Rev. brasil. de oto-rino-laring. *9:*37-46, Jan-Feb '41

Review of reconstructive surgery of face—1940-1942. BROWN, J. B. AND MCDOWELL, F. Laryngoscope *52:*489-504, June '42

Surgery of face, mouth and jaws, 30 years ago and now. IVY, R. H., J. Oral Surg. *1:*95-99, April '43

Review of reconstructive surgery of face, 1942-1943. MCDOWELL, F. Laryngoscope *53:*433-439, June '43

FAÇON, E. (see MARINESCO, G. *et al*) 1931
FAEHRMANN, J.: Vaginal formation from sigmoid flexure; case. Zentralbl. f. Chir. *56:*1989–1993, Aug 10, '29
FAGARASANO, J. (see FAGARASANU, I.)
FAGARASANU, I.: Cranioplasty using parallel split costal grafts (protective grille). Tech. chir. *29:*57–64, May–June '37
FAGGE, C. H.: Branchial cysts and fistulae. Clin. J. *57:*421–423, Sept 5, '28
FAGGE, C. H.: Harelip. Australian and New Zealand J. Surg. *5:*359–365, April '36
FAHEY, J. J. (see SIEGLING, J. A.) April '36
FAHLUND, G. T. R.: Suture of posterior tibial nerve below knee, with follow-up study of clinical results. J. Neurosurg. *3:*223–233, May '46
FAHMY, A. Y.: New procedure for treating congenital colobomata. Bull. Ophth. Soc. Egypt *34:*51–56, '41
FAIRBANK, L. C.: Short history of treatment of maxillary fractures. Mil. Surgeon *78:*95–103, Feb '36
FAIRBANK, L. C.: Responsibility of orthodontist in treatment of traumatic injuries of face and jaws. Am. J. Orthodontics *27:*414–422, Aug '41
FAIRBANK, L. C.: Care of face and jaw casualties in United States Army. War Med. *2:*223–229, March '42
FAIRBANK, L. C. AND IVY, R. H.: Emergency treatment and primary apparatus for jaw fractures in warfare. Mil. Surgeon *86:*124–134, Feb '40
FAIRCHILD, F. R.: Cancer of lower lip; operative technic in plastic repair. Arch. Surg. *17:*630–640, Oct '28
FAIRCHILD, R. D. (see GHORMLEY, R. K.) May '40
FALCONE, R.: Surgical treatment of elephantiasic conditions in legs by Kondoleon's method. Arch. ital. di chir. *13:*662–669, '25
FALCONE, R.: Hypospadias, treatment by new operative process. Arch. ital. di chir. *18:*497–514, '27
FALDINO, G.: Grafts of embryonal tissue. Chir. d. org. di movimento *9:*1–27, Dec '24, abstr: J.A.M.A. *84:*786, March 7, '25
FALENI, R. A.: Congenital fistulas of neck. Prensa med. argent. *21:*882, May 9; 932, May 16; 980, May 23, '34
FALK, P.: Studies on effect of pressure on plastic bodies and their application to living tissue. Ztschr. f. Hals-, Nasen-u. Ohrenh. *46:*251–267, '39
FALLIS, L. S. (see MCCLURE, R. D. *et al*) Sept '44
FALLIS, R. J.: Use of bone grafts in reconstructing mandible. Mil. Surgeon *90:*535–545, May '42
FALLS, F. H.: Simple method for construction of artificial vagina. Am. J. Obst. and Gynec. *40:*906–917, Nov '40
FALSÍA, M. V.: Postpartum shock; case. Folha med. *9:*269–273, Aug 15, '28, Semana med. *2:*625–631, Sept 6, '28
FALTIN, R.: Surgical construction of vagina; 2 cases. Acta obst. et gynec. Scandinav. *9:*124–131, '30
FALTIN, R.: Plastic repair of tip of nose, alae and septum with T-shaped round skin flap (Limberg method); case. Acta chir. Scandinav. *68:*254–265, '31
FALTIN, R.: Extension method of Faltin for fractures of lower jaw. Vestnik khir. *35:*221–223, '34
FALTIN, R.: Treatment of cleft palate. Finska lak.-sallsk. handl. *76:*961–984, Nov '34
FALTIN, R.: History of plastic surgery in Finland. Finska lak.-sallsk. handl. *78:*188–238, '35
FALTIN, R.: Typical method for reconstruction of nasal tip, septum and median portion of alae nasi. Acta chir. Scandinav *78:*492–511, '36
FALTIN, R.: History of plastic surgery in Finland. Finska lak.-sallsk. handl. *80:*97–124, Feb '37
FALTIN, R.: Phalangization of first metacarpal bone combined with round stylus plastic surgery in case of loss of thumb and skin on both hands. Nord. med. (Finska lak.-sallsk. handl.) *2:*1412–1415, May 13, '39
FALTIN, R.: Therapy of maxillofacial gunshot wounds. Acta chir. Scandinav. *91:*434–447, '44
FANJEAUX (see RICARD) Jan '46
FANTUS, B.: Burn therapy of Cook County Hospital. J.A.M.A. *103:*1446–1447, Nov 10, '34
FANTUS, B.: Decubitus ulcer, therapy of Cook County Hospital. J.A.M.A. *104:*46–48, Jan 5, '35
FANTUS, B.: Therapeutics of Cook County Hospital; therapy of facial injuries; outline by J. E. Schaeffer and M. B. Skinner. J.A.M.A. *105:*1679–1682, Nov 23, '35
FANTUS, B.: Therapy of Cook County Hospital; therapy of acute peripheral circulation failure; syncope, shock and collapse, in collaboration with L. Seed. J.A.M.A. *114:*2010–2015, May 18, '40
FANTUS, B. AND DYNIEWICZ, H. A.: Compound solution of tannic acid in burn therapy. J.A.M.A. *109:*200–203, July 17, '37
DE FARIA, J.: Small burns, with special reference to use of amertam (tannic acid preparation). Rev. brasil. de cir. *5:*503–516, Nov '36

de Faria Vaz, J.: Kineplasty of forearm. Med. cir. farm. pp. 584–589, Oct '45

de Faria Voz, J.: Trigger finger; surgical therapy of case. Arq. brasil. de cir. e ortop. *12:*157–163, '44

Farina, R.: Pedicled grafts versus free grafts. Sao Paulo med. *2:*125–132, Aug '44

Farina, R. C. (see Paolini Landa, J.) Dec '42

Faris, A. M. (see Robertson, R. C.) Jan '46

Farjat, F. P. (see Marfort, A. *et al*) Oct '37

Farmer, A. W.: Treatment of avulsed flaps. Ann. Surg. *110:*951–959, Nov '39

Farmer, A. W.: Burn therapy. Bull. Vancouver M. A. *18:*333-336, Aug '42

Farmer, A. W.: Hypospadias. Surgery *12:*462–470, Sept '42

Farmer, A. W.: Burn experience at Hospital for Sick Children. Am. J. Surg. *59:*195–209, Feb '43

Farmer, A. W.: Whole skin removal and replacement; operative procedure of value for salvage of skin undermined by trauma, or for recovering areas from which resection of extensive subcutaneous tissue has been necessary. S. Clin. North America *23:*1440–1447, Oct '43

Farmer, A. W.: Problems of surface restoration in Royal Canadian Air Force. Am. Acad. Orthop. Surgeons, Lect. pp. 226–229, '44

Farmer, A. W.: Early treatment of burns. Surgery *15:*144–152, Jan '44 also: Am. J. Orthodontics (Oral Surg. Sect.) *30:*146–153, March '44

Farmer, A. W., Webster, D. R. and Woolhouse, F. M.: Medical report on St. John's conflagration. Canad. M. A. J. *48:*191–195, March '43

Farmer, A. W. and Woolhouse, F. M.: Resurfacing of dorsum of hand following burns. Ann. Surg. *122:*39–47, July '45

Farmer, A. W. (see Erb, I. H. *et al*) Feb '43

Farquharson, E. L.: Fractures and dislocations of wrist and hand. Practitioner *144:*598–608, June '40

Farr, J.: "Cellophane" (medicated with sulfanilamide, sulfonamide) treatment of burns. Brit. M. J. *1:*749-750, June 3, '44

Farr, J. D.: "Cellophane" (medicated with sulfanilamide, sulfonamide) treatment of burns. Rev. san. mil. Buenos Aires *44:*313–317, March '45

Farr, R. E.: Treatment of congenital cleft lip and palate. Minnesota Med. *8:*149–153, March '25

Farr, R. E.: Cleft lip and palate; correction of late deformities resulting from neglect or improper treatment. Minnesota Med. *8:*561–568, Sept '25

Farr, R. E.: Shortcomings in surgery of cleft lip and palate, with suggestions for meeting them. Minnesota Med. *10:*70–76, Feb '27

Farrell, H. J.: Cutaneous melanomas with special reference to prognosis. Arch. Dermat. and Syph. *26:*110–124, July '32

Farrell Operation: See Lyman-Farrell Operation

Fasal, P.: Prophylaxis of tetanus following burns. Wien. klin. Wchnschr. *48:*181–182, Feb 8, '35

Fasal, P.: Present status of problem of burn therapy. Klin. Wchnschr. *16:*697, May 15, '37; 729, May 22, '37

Fasal, P.: Burn management and therapy, with special reference to use of tannin. Chirurg *10:*454–462, July 1, '38

Fasano, M.: Old ankylosis of temporomaxillary articulation. Arch. ital. di chir. *8:*575–588, Dec '23

Fascia

Fascia implant to correct respiratory sinking in of nasal wings. Boecker, W. Zentralbl. f. Chir. *48:*1796–1797, Dec 10, '21

Application of fascia lata in plastic surgery. Cuff, C. H. Brit. M. J. *1:*599–600, April 15, '22

Clinical and experimental study of free transplantation of fascia and tendon. Gallie, W. E. and Le Mesurier, A. B., J. Bone and Joint Surg. *4:*600–612, July '22 (illus.)

Tendon and fascia autografts drawn through channel in bone or joint. Bertocchi, A. and Bianchetti, C. F. Chir. d. org. di movimento *7:*225–243, June '23 (illus.) abstr: J.A.M.A. *81:*964, Sept 15, '23

Fascial bands as supports to relaxed facial tissue. Miller, C. C. Ann. Surg. *82:*603–608, Oct '25

Functions of isolated fascia of jejunum tenia used in operation for artificial vagina by Baldwin's method. Vakar, A. A. Russk. Klin. *7:*19–34, Jan '27

New method of obtaining autogenous fascial grafts without extensive incision. Rowlands, J. S. Practitioner *119:*321–326, Nov '27

Fascial Grafting in Principle and Practice, By H. C. Orrin. Oliver and Boyd, Ltd., London, 1928

Correction of eyelid ptosis by fascia lata hammock. Derby, G. S. Am. J. Ophth. *11:*352–354, May '28

Surgical treatment of spastic adductor contraction of thumb by dorsal suspension of metacarpus of thumb by fascial sling.

Fascia – Cont.
HENSCHEN, C. Schweiz. med. Wchnschr. *58:*621-625, June 23, '28
Fasciaplasty in treatment of facial paralysis. MOSZKOWICZ, L. Wien. klin. Wchnschr. *41:*1151-1153, Aug 9, '28
Traumatic facial paralysis; treatment by free transplantation of fascia lata. FISCHER, H. Ann. Surg. *89:*334-339, March '29
End results of covering amputation stumps with free fascia transplants. RITTER, C. Zentralbl. f. Chir. *56:*2565-2566, Oct 12, '29
Subcutaneous fascial stripper. GRACE, R. V. Ann. Surg. *90:*1109-1110, Dec '29
Metaplastic formation of bone in transplanted connective tissue. LEXER, E. Deutsche Ztschr. f. Chir. *217:*1-32, '29
Autotransplantation of fascia by cutaneous flaps with tubulate pedicles. MOURE, P. Rev. odont. *51:*5-10, Jan '30
Use of fascia lata in repair of disability at wrist. LOWMAN, C. L., J. Bone and Joint Surg. *12:*400-402, April '30
Fascia as suture material. WOLFSOHN, G. Chirurg *2:*475-477, May 15, '30
Instrument for subcutaneous removal of fascia lata strips for suture purposes. BATE, J. T. Ann. Surg. *95:*313-314, Feb '32
Facial paralysis treated by fascial grafts; case. BROOKE, R. Brit. J. Surg. *20:*523-526, Jan '33
Fascia lata grafts in facial paralysis. WARDILL, W. E. M. Newcastle M. J. *13:*35-38, Jan '33
Use of fasciae in reconstructive surgery, with special reference to operative technic. GRATZ, C. M. Eye, Ear, Nose and Throat Monthly *12:*27-29, Feb '33
Ox fascia (dead fascia) graft. GLASSER, S. T. Am. J. Surg. *19:*542-544, March '33
Correction of postauricular defect by implantation of fascia lata. GRIFFITH, C. M. AND SCHATTNER, A. Laryngoscope *43:*280-281, April '33
Use of fascia in reconstructive surgery, with special reference to operative technic. GRATZ, C. M. Ann. Surg. *99:*241-245, Feb '34
Surgical therapy of facial paralysis with free aponeurotic graft. DE ANDRADE, P. C. Bol. coll. brasil. de cirurgioes *5:*39-40, June-July '34
Plastic use of fascia in treatment of facial paralysis. DEMEL, R. Zentralbl. f. Chir. *61:*1445-1448, June 23, '34
Facial paralysis from gunshot wound caused by attempted suicide; therapy by resection of superior cervical sympathetic ganglion

Fascia – Cont.
and suspension of corners of mouth. ROQUES, P. Bull. et mem. Soc. nat. de chir. *60:*981-984, July 21, '34
Experience with fascia lata grafts in operative treatment of facial paralysis. GILLIES, H. Proc. Roy. Soc. Med. *27:*1372-1378, Aug '34 also: J. Laryng. and Otol. *49:*743-756, Nov '34
Plastic repair of patulous anus by means of fascia lata strips. CATO, E. Australian and New Zealand J. Surg. *4:*315-317, Jan '35
Sutures or reconstruction (using fascia lata) of sectioned hand tendons; 3 cases. MASMONTEIL, F. Bull. et mem. Soc. d. chirurgiens de Paris *28:*379-384, June 5, '36
Eyelid ptosis, superior-rectus fascia-lata sling in correction. DICKEY, C. A. Am. J. Ophth. *19:*660-664, Aug '36
Correction by 2 strips of fascia lata, eyelid ptosis. MAGNUS, J. A. Brit. J. Ophth. *20:*460-464, Aug '36
Tendinoplasty of flexor tendons of hand; use of tunica vaginalis in reconstructing tendon sheaths. WILMOTH, C. L., J. Bone and Joint Surg. *19:*152-156, Jan '37
Ox-fascia-transplant operation in eyelid ptosis. HILDRETH, H. R. South. M. J. *30:*471-473, May '37
Plastic repair of eyelid hernia with fascia lata. SAKLER, B. R. Am. J. Ophth. *20:*936-938, Sept '37
New suture for tendon and fascia repair. GRATZ, C. M. Surg., Gynec. and Obst. *65:*700-701, Nov '37
Correction of eyelid ptosis by transplantation of fascia lata. TSITOVSKIY, M. L. Vestnik oftal. *11:*373-377, '37
Complete rectal prolapse; fascial repair. MAYO, C. W. West. J. Surg. *46:*75-77, Feb '38
Use of fascia and ribbon catgut in harelip and cleft palate repair. BRENIZER, A. G. Ann. Surg. *107:*692-700, May '38
Instrument for subcutaneous stripping of lengths of fascia lata. FINOCHIETTO, R. Prensa med. argent. *26:*69-70, Jan 4, '39
Utilization of temporal muscle and fascia for facial paralysis. BROWN, J. B. Ann. Surg. *109:*1016-1023, June '39
Utilization of temporal muscle and fascia in facial paralysis. BROWN, J. B. Am. J. Orthodontics *26:*80-87, Jan '40
Fascia lata transplant in eyelid ptosis. ROSENBURG, S. Am. J. Surg. *47:*142-148, Jan '40
Skin and fascia grafting. BRENIZER, A. G. Am. J. Surg. *47:*265-279, Feb '40

Fascia – Cont.

New instrument for passing portions of tendons and fasciae latae. MACEY, H. B. Am. J. Surg. *47:*686, March '40

Results with fascia plastic operation for incontinence of anus. STONE, H. B. AND MCLANAHAN, S. Ann. Surg. *114:*73–77, July '41

Plastic surgery of rectal prolapse with fascia ring by Thiersch method. POHL, W. Beitr. z. klin. Chir. *171:*520–523, '41

Plastic surgery of facial paralysis (including fascial transplant) with modification in technic. LAMONT, E. S. Arch. Otolaryng. *39:*155–163, Feb '44

Procedure to correct facial paralysis (by spinofacial anastomosis and fascial strips). HANRAHAN, E. M. AND DANDY, W. E. J.A.M.A. *124:*1051–1053, April 8, '44

Modified sling operation for correction of ptosis (eye). LAVAL, J. Arch. Ophth. *33:*482–483, June '45

Fascia lata transplant for rectrotarsal atrophy of upper lid following enucleation. CUTLER, N. L. Am. J. Ophth. *29:*176–179, Feb '46

Nasal perforation; free transplantation; experiments with fascia lata. BEHRMAN, W. Acta oto-laryng. *34:*78–81, '46

FASSRAINER, S.: Surgical therapy of epispadias in male. Deutsche Ztschr. f. Chir. *237:*537–548, '32

FASTING, G. F.: Carbon tetrachloride; new and important applications in medical therapy of burns. New Orleans M. and S. J. *96:*439–445, April '44

Fat Grafts

Technic of free fat flap transplantation. HAMMESFAHR, C. Zentralbl. f. Chir. *48:*117, Jan 29, '21

Plastic operations on face by means of fat grafts. ROY, J. N. Laryngoscope *31:*65, Feb '21

Transplants of fat tissue. PENNISI, A. Policlinico (sez. chir.) *28:*62, Feb '21, abstr: J.A.M.A. *76:*1202, April 23, '21

Plastic operations on face by means of fat grafts. ROY J. N. Laryngoscope *31:*65, Feb '21

Pedicled flaps aided by free fat transplantation in plastic surgery. VAN HOOK, W. Med. Rec. *101:*625–626, April 15, '22

Deformity of neck treated by transplantation of fat. MCGUIRE, S., S. Clin. N. America *2:*1259–1261, Oct. '22

Transplantation of fat tissue previously

Fat Grafts – Cont.

treated with fixation fluid. BERTOCCHI, A. Arch. ital. di chir. *12:*621–625, '25

Heterotransplantation of cartilage and fat tissue and reaction against heterotransplants in general. LOEB, L. AND HARTER, J. S. Am. J. Path. *2:*521–537, Nov '26

Free fat transplantation in therapy of cleft palate. v. GAZA, W. Arch. f. klin. Chir. *142:*590–599, '26

Plastic surgery; depressed forehead following Kilian operation; repaired by fat grafts. HARTER, J. H. Northwest Med. *26:*313–314, June '27

Late results of fat transplantation in breast surgery. WREDE, L. Deutsche Ztschr. f. Chir. *203–204:*672–685, '27

Histological results after experimental free transplantation of fat tissue. HILSE, A. Beitr. z. path. Anat. u. z. allg. Path. *79:*592–624, April 16, '28

Transplantation of fat in enucleation of eye. LINDBERG, J. G. Finska lak.-sallsk. handl. *70:*898–902, Nov '28

Transplantation of skin, fat, blood vessels, nerves, etc. EISELSBERG, A. Wien. med. Wchnschr. *80:*50–55, Jan 4, '30

Reconstruction of atrophic mammary gland by means of autotransplantation of fat. PASSOT, R. Presse med. *38:*627–628, May 7, '30

Treatment of facial hemiatrophy by means of transplantation of fat tissues. MOSZKOWICZ, L. Med. Klin. *26:*1478, Oct 3, '30

Plastic treatment of facial hemiatrophy by transplantation of fat tissues. EITNER, E. Med. Klin. *27:*624–625, April 24, '31

Depression of frontal region of face, fat transplant. FIGI, F. A., S. Clin. North America *11:*831–833, Aug '31

Plugging of tuberculous cavities with transplants of fatty tissue. TSANOV, A. I. Kazanskiy med. j. *28:*203–206, Feb–March '32

Repair of postauricular fistula by means of free fat graft. STRAATSMA, C. R. AND PEER, L. A. Arch. Oto-laryng. *15:*620–621, April '32

Grafts of fixed fat tissues. CIERI, G. Rassegna di terap. e pat. clin. *4:*587–597, Oct '32

Cure of mastoid fistula with fat graft; case. BENNETT, A. B., M. Ann. District of Columbia *2:*117–118, May '33

Technic of fat grafts. COTTON, F. J. New England J. Med. *211:*1051–1053, Dec 6, '34

Free fat transplants in facial plastic surgery. VON BRANDIS, H. J. Deutsche Ztschr. f. Chir. *244:*228–232, '34

Clinical, experimental and histologic studies

Fat Grafts – Cont.

in connection with subcutaneous injections of homogeneous and heterogeneous fat; morphologic changes of subcutaneous cells. Kapitsa, L. M. Vestnik khir. *45:*3–8, '36

Extensive loss of substance in subhyoid region; recovery after fat transplantation. Stepleanu-Horbatzky. Rev. de chir., Bucuresti *41:*512–515, July–Aug '38

Grafts of adipose tissue and their use in correction of depressed cicatrices of face. Urzua, R. Rev. Asoc. med. argent. *53:*647–649, July 30, '39

Filling of osteomyelitis cavities by means of fat transplants. Leonte, C. Rev. de chir., Bucuresti *43:*801–805, Nov–Dec '40

Free transplantation of fat for bronchopulmonary cavity; case. Neuhof, H. Ann. Surg. *113:*153–155, Jan '41

Graft of fat in correction of cicatricial depressions. Zeno, L. An. de cir. *7:*47–51, March–June '41, also: Bol. Soc. de cir. de Rosario *8:*1–5, April '41

Transplantation of fat in correction of cicatricial depressions. Zeno, L. Semana med. *1:*1324–1327, June 5, '41

Histology of fat transplantation. Burkhardt, L. Deutsche Ztschr. f. Chir. *254:*372–378, '41

Hemiatrophy of face; graft of fat in therapy. Zeno, L. An. de cir. *8:*52–57, March–June '42

Correction of depressed cicatrices with grafts of fatty tissue. Urzua, C. C. R., Arq. de cir. clin. e exper. *6:*269–272, April–June '42

Free transplant of areola preliminary to amputation of breast for benign tumor; free fat graft; case. Zeno, L. An. de cir. *10:*190–194, Sept–Dec '44

Fauconnier, H. J. and Patcas, H.: Complications of dento-maxillo-facial malformations; importance of correction. Liege med. *32:*1–9, Jan 1, '39

Faugeron, P. (see Boppe, M.) June '39

Faulkner, E. R.: Plastic operations developed by Dr. Mackenty in field of otorhinolaryngology. Laryngoscope *43:*103–105, Feb '33

Faura, C.: Plaster bandages in burns. Actas dermo-sif. *37:*705–707, Feb '46

Faure, J. L.: Medicolegal aspects of esthetic surgery. Presse med. *41:*1677–1678, Oct 28, '33

Faure, Mme. (see Marriq) Feb–March '35

Faurel (see Sicard, A.) July '46

Faust, H.: Reviten in prophylaxis and therapy of shock. Monatschr. f. Unfallh. *40:*282–286, June '33

Favaloro, G.: Plastic operation for denudation of nasolacrimal region. Rassegna ital. d'ottal. *1:*197–209, March–April '32

Favata, B. V. (see Young, F.) March '44

Favre, M.: Cystic disease of pilosebaceous system of face. Bull. Soc. franc. de dermat. et syph. (Reunion dermat.) *39:*93–96, Jan '32

Favreau, J. C.: Recurrent luxation of mandible and its surgical therapy; case. Union med. du Canada *66:*271–277, March '37

Favreau, J. C.: Acute synovitis of hand. Union med. du Canada *68:*513–514, May '39

Favreau, J. C.: Modern therapy of burns. Union med. du Canada *68:*1329–1330, Dec '39

Favreau, M.: Surgical therapy of total absence of vagina. Gynecologie *33:*5–14, Jan '34, also: J. d'obst. et de gynec. prat. *5:*3–16, Jan '34

Faxon, N. W. and Churchill, E. D.: Cocoanut Grove disaster in Boston; preliminary account. J.A.M.A. *120:*1385–1388, Dec 26, '42

Faxon, N. W. and Churchill, E. D.: Burn therapy; Cocoanut Grove disaster in Boston; preliminary account. Hospitals *17:*13–18, Jan '43

Fay, T.: Surgical relief of pain in deep carcinoma of face and neck. Am. J. Roentgenol. *14:*1–5, July '25

Fayn, I. E.: Necessity for examination of corneal sensitivity before operating for congenital eyelid ptosis. Sovet. vestnik oftal. *9:*905, '36

Fazakas, A.: Operation in patient with large eyelids and maintained levator function. Klin. Monatsbl. f. Augenh. *103:*621–624, Dec '39

Fazakas, S.: Surgical correction of eyelid ptosis. Orvosi hetil. *82:*492–494, May 21, '38

de Fazio, M.: Malocclusion resulting from pathologic fracture and deforming callus in mandibular osteitis; therapy; case. Riforma med. *50:*851–858, June 2, '34

Feder, A. (see Vorhaus, M. G. *et al*) Feb '43

Federspiel, M. N.: Harelip and cleft palate. Laryngoscope *32:*909–928, Dec '22 (illus.)

Federspiel, M. N.: Some diseases of mouth, jaws, and face surgically treated. Journal-Lancet *43:*267–275, June 1; 297–301, June 15, '23

Federspiel, Matthew N.: *Harelip and Cleft Palate*. C. V. Mosby Co., St. Louis, 1927

Federspiel, M. N.: Procedures which extend field of dentofacial orthopedics. J. Am. Dent. A. *14:*1243–1257, Dec '27

Federspiel, M. N.: Value of orthodontic appliances to immobilize jaw fractures. Internat. J. Orthodontia *14:*185–196, March '28

Federspiel, M. N.: Rhinophyma, with report of case. Wisconsin M. J. *29:*75–79, Feb '30

FEDERSPIEL, M. N.: Rhinophyma, with report of case. Internat. J. Orthodontia *18:*92–98, Jan '32

FEDERSPIEL, M. N.: Extreme cleft of hard and soft palate closed with use of author's tension plates. Wisconsin M. J. *32:*172–177, March '33

FEDERSPIEL, M. N.: Maxillo-facial injuries. Wisconsin M. J. *33:*561–568, Aug '34

FEDERSPIEL, M. N.: Surgical care of injuries and deformities of nose, lip and premaxilla, with report of cases. Internat. J. Orthodontia *22:*1054–1068, Oct '36

FEDERSPIEL, M. N.: Incomplete and complete ankylosis of jaws. J. Am. Dent. A. *26:*585–594, April '39

FEDERSPIEL, M. N.: Extensive plastic repair for restoration of lower lip; report of procedure in case in which lower lip was entirely removed for eradication of epithelioma. Am. J. Orthodontics (Oral Surg. Sect) *28:*163–166, March '42

FEDOROVICH, D. P.: Blood transfusion in burn therapy. Sovet. med. (no. 9) *7:*28, '43

FEHR, A. (see SCHÜRCH, O.) 1939

FEIGENBAUM, A.: Simple procedure of advancement of levator combined with tarsectomy in trachomatous as well as in congenital ptosis. Folia ophth. orient. *2:*50–58, '35

FEIGL, E. (see DEMEL, R.) 1931

FEIGUES, I. (see MACERA, J. M.) Sept '29

FEIL (see BOURGEOIS, P. *et al*) March '33

FEIL, A. (see LÉVY-VELENSI) Jan '30

FELDERMAN, L.: Principles of rhinoplasty. Pennsylvania M. J. *47:*13–20, Oct '43

FELDMAN, L.: Rational treatment of facial paralysis; with special reference to Bell's palsy. Am. J. Phys. Therapy *4:*539–544, March '28

FELDMAN, L. (see COHEN, M. A.) May '27

FELDMAN, M. H.: Jaw fracture in epileptic patient. Internat. J. Orthodontia *15:*381, April '29

FELDMAN, S. P. AND GROSSMAN, S. Y.: Secondary suture of granulating wounds of face. Sovet. med. (no. 6) *8:*22–23, '44

FELDMANN, E.: Fundamentals in treatment of protruding intermaxillary bone in bilateral harelip. Zentralbl. f. Chir. *62:*434–437, Feb. 23, '35

FELDSTEIN, E.: Nasal fractures in clinical practice. Rev. gen. de clin. et de therap. *49:*388–390, June 15, '35

FELDSTEINAS, L.: Therapy of cutaneous burns according to Davidson method. Medicina, Kaunas *20:*875–881, Oct–Nov '39

FELIX, W.: Neurotization of paralyzed muscles in nerve transplant. Arch. f. klin. Chir. *162:*681–692, '30

FELSENREICH, F.: Value of Böhler's wire-finger-splint in treatment of severe injuries of fingers. Wien. klin. Wchnschr. *42:*1046–1048, Aug 8, '29

FELSTEAD, R.: Formation of artificial vagina. J. Coll. Surgeons, Australasia *3:*112–114, July '30

FENDER, F. A.: Lymphatic pathology in relation to "toxin" of burns. Surg., Gynec. and Obst. *57:*612–620, Nov '33

FENGER, M.: Treatment of fracture of phalanges of hand. Ugesk. f. Laeger *90:*935, Sept 27, '28

FENGER, M.: Treatment of fractures of fingers. Ugesk. f. laeger *93:*169–173, Feb 19, '31

FENKNER, W.: Traumatic shock. Med. Welt *10:*1869–1872, Dec 26, '36

FENNEL, E. A.: Shock, without or with hemorrhage, and burns. Hawaii, M. J. *1:*385–389, July '42

FENNEL, E. A.: Skin grafting with "human glue" (coagulum-contact method); supplementary note on some technical details. Proc. Staff. Med. Clin., Honolulu *10:*19–22, Feb '44

FENNELLY, W. A.: Avertin (tribrom-ethanol) in reduction of facial fractures. J. Am. Dent. A. *24:*1089–1104, July '37

FENNER, E. D.: When and how should cleft palate be treated? New Orleans M. and S. J. *81:*718–722, April '29

FENTON, R. A.: Indications, contraindications and preparation for dacrycystorhinostomy. Ann. Otol., Rhin. and Laryng. *32:*67–83, March '23 (illus.)

FENTON, R. A.: Osteomyelitis of mandible, etiology, treatment and results. J. Iowa M. Soc. *15:*560–562, Oct '25

FENTON, R. A. AND LUPTON, I. M.: Prosthesis after removal of auricle for carcinoma. Northwest Med. *22:*212, June '23 (illus.)

FERBER, E. W.: Combined intraoral and dental fixation in fracture of mandibular angle with considerable displacement. J. Am. Dent. A. *30:*906–910, June 1, '43

FERGUS, A. F.: Mr. Percival Pott on treatment of lacrimal fistula. Proc. Roy. Soc. Med. (Sect. Ophth.) *20:*60–64, Aug '27

FERGUSON, L. K.: Dressing for hematoma of ear. J.A.M.A. *100:*736, March 11, '33

FERGUSON, L. K.: Burn therapy. Bull. New York Acad. Med. *21:*127–144, March '45

FERGUSON, L. K.; BUSH, L. F. AND KUEHNER, H. G.: Round-table conference on office surgery of hand. Pennsylvania M. J. *44:*433–439, Jan '41

FERGUSON, L. K. (see RAVDIN, I. S.) Feb '25

FERGUSON, L. K. (see SHAAR, C. M. *et al*) Oct '42

FERNANDES, J. F. JR.: Clinical and physiopathologic study of burns. Rev. med. brasil.

*11:*117-133, Aug '41

FERNANDES, M.: Furuncle of upper lip; case. Rev. med. de Pernambuco *9:*137-145, May '39

FERNANDEZ, B.: Tumors of jaw with report of cases. Rev. med. de Rosario *34:*340, April; 442, May '44

FERNANDEZ, E. B. (see POTH, E. J.) May '44

FERNANDEZ, E. B. (see POTH, E. J. *et al*) Nov '45

FERNANDEZ, J. C.: Successful surgical therapy of Dupuytren's contracture, 2 cases. Semana med. *1:*260-262, Jan 28, '37

FERNANDEZ, J. C.: Protruding ears; original technic of surgical therapy. Bol. y trab., Soc. argent. de cirujanos *4:*768-772, '43, also: Rev. Asoc. med. argent. *57:*1019-1020, Nov 30, '43

FERNANDEZ, J. C.: Protruding ears; author's technic of correction. Dia med. *18:*1052-1053, Aug 5, '46

FERNANDEZ, L. L.: Protruding ears; technical detail of surgical correction. Semana med. *2:*89-90, July 11, '40

FERNANDEZ, L. L.: Cancer of chin; extirpation in case. Prensa med. argent. *31:*291-292, Feb. 9, '44

FERNANDEZ, L. L.: Metacarpophalangeal luxation of thumb; surgical reduction. Prensa med. argent. *32:*1395-1398, July 20, '45

FERNANDEZ, L. L.: Ulcer of dorsum pedis; free graft on granulation tissue. Prensa med. argent. *32:*1601-1604, Aug 17, '45

FERNANDEZ, L. L. (see SVERDLICK, J.) July '45

FERNÁNDEZ, O. C.: Peripheral facial paralysis; kinesthetic treatment; 10 cases. Semana med. *2:*1718-1734, Dec 12, '29

FERNÁNDEZ SARALEGUI, A.: Jaw ankylosis; treatment by Murphy's arthroplastic operation; case. Bol. y trab. de la Soc. de cir. de Buenos Aires *13:*165-171, May 29, '29

FERNANDEZ DEL VALLE, A.: Industrial burns and their therapy by tannic acid or silver nitrate. Rev. d. trab. *4:*203-207, Aug '39

FERNICOLA, C.; PALAZZO, R. AND MARQUEZ, D. E.: Bilocular branchiogenic cyst of neck; case. Bol. Soc. de cir. de Rosario *9:*511-519, Sept '42

FERRAND, M. (see RAVAUT, P.) Feb '27

FERRANDO, M. (see GIANOTTI, M.) 1939

FERRANNINI, L.: Intravenous injection of caffeine in therapy of shock. Policlinico (sez. prat.) *44:*1648-1650, Aug 30, '37

FERRARI. (see COSTANTINI) Oct '36

FERRARI, A. (ADOLFO): Clinical and etiopathogenetic study of 2 rare cases of Dupuytren's contracture. Minerva med. *2:*230-235, Dec 1, '45

FERRARI, R. A. AND BRUZZONE, I. A.: Sacral eschar occurring early in puerperium; case. Semana med. *2:*1977-1979, Dec 21, '33

FERRARI, R. C.: Injuries of hand caused by bread making machine; new case with complication of gangrene demanding amputation of arm. Bol. Inst. de clin. quir. *5:*263, '29 also: Semana med. *2:*1734-1735, Dec 12, '29

FERRARI, R. C.: Plastic reconstruction of fingers by Italian method of skin graft; case. Semana med. *2:*1104-1105, Oct 12, '33

FERRARI, R. C. AND FIORINI, J. M.: Plastic surgery of ear deformities. Rev. de chir. plastique, pp. 150-156, July '32

FERRARI, R. C. AND VIACAVA, E. P.: Therapy of external cancer by extirpation and Padgett grafts. Bol. y trab., Acad. argent. de cir. *28:*959-970, Oct 18, '44

FERRARI, R. C. (see ARCE, J. *et al*) 1929

FERRARI, R. C. (see IVANISSEVICH, O.) 1927

FERRARI, R. C. (see IVANISSEVICH, O.) May '28

FERRARI, R. C. (see IVANISSEVICH, O.) 1930

FERRARI, R. C. (see IVANISSEVICH, O.) April '30

FERRARI, R. C. (see IVANISSEVICH, O.) April '35

FERRARI, R. C. (see IVANISSEVICH, O. *et al*) Jan-March '40

FERRARI, R. C. (see IVANISSEVICH, O.) Aug '40

FERRARI, R. C. (see IVANISSEVICH, O.) Oct '40

FERRARI, R. C. (see IVANISSEVICH, O.) June '43

FERRARI, R. C. (see IVANISSEVICH, O. *et al*) Oct-Dec '45

FERRARINI, G.: Rectal incontinence relieved by plastic operation. Arch. ital. di chir. *10:*85-107, '24 abstr: J.A.M.A. *83:*1544, Nov 8, '24

FERRARINI, M.: Dupuytren's contracture; pathologic anatomy and etiopathogenesis; review of literature and report of cases. Arch. ital. di chir. *57:*1-110, '39

FERRARINI, M.: Pathologic anatomy and etiopathogenesis of Dupuytren's contracture; review. Gior. d. r. Accad. di med. di Torino (parte seconda) *102:*40-51, Jan-March '39

FERRARINI, M.: Dupuytren's contracture can be considered as occupational disease. Rassegna di med. indust. *11:*70-97, Feb '40

FERRAZ ALVIM, J.; MONTENEGRO, J. AND BUENO DOS REIS, J. D.: Gunshot wound of upper third of arm with complete section of ulnar nerve and compression of median nerve; late suture of ulnar nerve. Rev. otoneuro-oftal. *9:*44-52, Feb '34

FERRÉ, R. L.: Plastic reparation of heel by grafts. Semana med. *2:*2049-2053, Dec 27, '34

FERRE, R. L.: Surgical therapy of chronic rheumatism. Rev. Asoc. med. argent. *58:*324-330, May 30, '44

FERRE, R. L. (see PINEIRO SORONDO, J.) May '44

Ferreira, F.: Miotic ptosis; case of Fuchs' progressive muscular dystrophy in man. Brasil-med. *53:*1087–1088, Dec 2, '39

Ferreira, F.: Eyelid ptosis; cases. Rev. med. Bahia *8:*9–13, Jan '40

Ferrie, J.: Davis grafts in reparative surgery of face. Ophthalmologica *110:*292–299, Nov–Dec '45

Ferriman, D.: Genetics of acrocephalosyndactylia. Proc. Internat. Genet. Cong. (1939) *7:*120, '41

Ferro, A.: Massive hypertrophy of breast in puerperium. Riv. d'ostet. e ginec. prat. *15:*198–203, May '33

Ferro, G.: Coramin therapy of preoperative and postoperative shock. Sett. med. *27:*361–364, March 23, '39

Fessler, A.: Pigmentation and transplantation of skin. Brit. J. Dermat. *53:*201–214, July '41

Fessler, J.: Plastic operations on corner of mouth. Deutsche Ztschr. f. Chir. *172:*427–429, '22 (illus.)

Fetisova, E. V.: Surgical therapy of combined injuries of peripheral nerves and bones. Khirurgiya, No. 2, pp. 55–58, '45

Fetter, T. R. and Gartman, E.: Traumatic rupture of penis; case. Am. J. Surg. *32:*371–372, May '36

Feuerstein, B. L.: Radium therapy in birthmarks. Mississippi Valley M. J. *62:*77, May '40

Feurstein, J. G.: Radium therapy in Dupuytren's contracture. Wien. klin. Wchnschr. *49:*1090–1092, Sept 4, '36

Feuz, J.: Chronic maxillary sinusitis; fatal complications of traumatic fracture of wall of sinus in patient with sinusitis. Rev. med. de la Suisse Rom. *52:*347–354, May 25, '32

Feuz, J.: Correction of saddle nose; 3 cases. Rev. med. de la Suisse Rom. *53:*801–819, Nov 25, '33

Fevre, M.: Spring fingers and flexion contracture due to blockage of digital tendons. Rev. d'orthop. *23:*137–142, March '36

Fevre, M.: Anatomic lesion of camptodactylic supernumerary finger. Ann. d'anat. path. *13:*1018–1023, Nov '36

Fevre, M.: Coffey operation for exstrophy of bladder; cases. Mem. Acad. de chir. *64:*1114–1123, Oct 26, '38

Fevre, M.: Blockage of tendon of flexor pollicis longus. Presse med. *50:*754–755, Dec 12, '42

Fevre, M. and Bricage, R.: Congenital irregular hypertrophy of fingers; case due to lymphangiomas. Ann. d'anat. path. *13:*337–341, March '36

Fèvre, M.; Kaufmann, R. and Lecoeur, P.: Backward dislocation of metacarpophalangeal joint of thumb. Ann. d'anat. path. *8:*294–295, March '31

Feyeux, A. (see Froment) March–April '39

Feygin, N.: Rare congenital malformations of nose; case histories, and treatment: (1) fibrolipoma of septum, harelip; (2) bull-dog nose, fibrolipoma of dorsum of nose. Zentralbl. f. Chir. *53:*1686, July 3, '26

Fichardt, T.: X-ray or radium burn. South African M. J. *15:*403–405, Oct 25, '41

Fick: First aid in burns, with special consideration of conditions prevailing in air raids. Ztschr. f. arztl. Fortbild. *36:*584–592, Oct 1, '39

Fickling, B. W. (with W. Warwick James): *Injuries of the Jaws and Face*. Bale, London, 1940

Fickling, B. W.: Initial treatment of jaw injuries (with special reference to air raid casualties). M. Press *206:*203–208, Sept 10, '41

Fickling, B. W.: Severe retrusion of mandible treated by buccal inlay and dental prosthesis. Proc. Roy. Soc. Med. *37:*7–10, Nov '43

Fickling, B. W.: Advances in construction and use of splints in treatment of jaw fractures. Brit. Dent. J. *80:*8–13, Jan 4, '46

Fickling, B. W. (see James, W. W.) Feb '41

Field, H. J. and Ackerman, A. A.: Fulminating osteomyelitis of mandible with pathologic fracture. J. Am. Dent. A. *23:*448–450, March '36

Fieschi, D.: Grafts of long bones and joints. Chir. d. org. di movimento *5:*359, Aug '21 abstr: J.A.M.A. *77:*1373, Oct 22, '21

Fieschi, D.: Syndactylia; therapy of case. Arch. ital. di chir. *37:*204–208, '34

Fieschi, D.: Use of rubber sponge (new flesh) over period of 25 years. Arch. ital. di chir. *46:*221–251, '37

Fieschi, D.: Plastic surgery; use of rubber (nuova carne); results in various cases after 25 years. Rev. de chir., Paris *76:*1–36, Jan '38

Fifield, Lionel R.: *Infections of the Hand*. H. K. Lewis & Co., London, 1926. Second Edition, 1939

Figarella, J.: Section of flexor tendons of hand; suture with recovery after physiopathic phenomena; case. Marseille-med. *1:*725–727, May 25, '36

Figi, F. A.: Radium in treatment of multilocular lymph cysts (cystic hygromas) of neck in children. Am. J. Roentgenol. *21:*473–480, May '29

Figi, F. A.: Partial reconstruction of nose. S. Clin. N. Amer. *9:*923–928, Aug '29

Figi, F. A.: Stenosis of nasopharynx. Arch. Otolaryng. *10:*480–490, Nov '29

Figi, F. A.: Multiple pigmented papillary nevi

of face. (pigmented mole) S. Clin. N. Amer. *10:*101–103, Feb '30
FIGI, F. A.: Recurring epithelioma of face. S. Clin. N. Amer. *10:*105–107, Feb '30
FIGI, F. A.: Treatment of malignant tumors of mouth and throat. Am. J. Roentgenol. *23:*648–653, June '30
FIGI, F. A.: Early diagnosis and treatment of cancer of lips and mouth. Minnesota Med. *13:*788–792, Nov '30
FIGI, F. A.: Depression of frontal region of face, fat transplant. S. Clin. North America *11:*831–833, Aug '31
FIGI, F. A.: Loss of nasal ala and upper lip reconstruction. S. Clin. North America *11:*834–837, Aug '31
FIGI, F. A.: Stenosis of larynx; laryngofissure and skin graft. S. Clin. North America *11:*837–840, Aug '31
FIGI, F. A.: Actinodermatitis (roentgen-ray burn) of entire neck; replacement with tubed flap from thorax. S. Clin. North America *12:*947–949, Aug '32
FIGI, F. A.: Traumatic scarring and depressed fracture of right malar bone and orbital border; cartilage implant. S. Clin. North America *12:*949–951, Aug '32
FIGI, F. A.: Recurring epithelioma of lower lip and chin; diathermy and cautery excision; reconstruction of lower lip. S. Clin. North America *12:*951–954, Aug '32
FIGI, F. A.: Use of pedicled flaps and skin grafts in reconstructive surgery of (face) head and neck. Nebraska M. J. *17:*361–365, Sept '32
FIGI, F. A.: Jaw fractures. Surg., Gynec. & Obst. *55:*762–770, Dec '32
FIGI, F. A.: Jaw fractures. Proc. Staff Meet., Mayo Clin. *8:*135–138, March 1, '33
FIGI, F. A.: Multiple cutaneous horns; removal and skin graft. S. Clin. North America *13:*880–881, Aug '33
FIGI, F. A.: Traumatic facial scarring; removal. S. Clin. North America *13:*882–884, Aug '33
FIGI, F. A.: Epithelioma of lower lip; results of treatment. Surg., Gynec. & Obst. *59:*810–819, Nov '34
FIGI, F. A.: Skin grafting in mouth; 2 cases. Proc. Staff Meet., Mayo Clin. *9:*740–742, Dec 5, '34
FIGI, F. A.: Cancer of mouth. S. Clin. North America *15:*1233–1240, Oct '35
FIGI, F. A.: Selection of treatment of cancer of pharynx. Radiol. Rev. & Mississippi Valley M. J. *58:*13–19, Jan '36
FIGI, F. A.: Cancer of mouth. J. Am. Dent. A. *23:*216–224, Feb '36
FIGI, F. A.: Transplantation of parotid (Stensen's) duct in cancer of antrum. Proc. Staff Meet., Mayo Clin. *11:*241–243, April 15, '36
FIGI, F. A.: Angiomas of face; treatment. Arch. Otolaryng. *24:*271–281, Sept '36
FIGI, F. A.: Angioma of face; treatment. Proc. Staff Meet., Mayo Clin. *12:*437–442, July 14, '37
FIGI, F. A.: Plastic repair after removal of extensive malignant tumors of antrum. Arch. Otolaryng. *28:*29–41, July '38
FIGI, F. A.: Plastic repair following removal of neoplasms about head. Nebraska M. J. *25:*165–171, May '40
FIGI, F. A.: Chronic laryngeal stenosis, with special consideration of skin grafting. Ann. Otol., Rhin. & Laryng. *49:*394–409, June '40
FIGI, F. A.: Cancer of lips and cheeks. Proc. Staff Meet., Mayo Clin. *16:*280–282, April 30, '41
FIGI, F. A.: Extensive mole of face and scalp; excision and full thickness skin graft. Proc. Staff Meet., Mayo Clin. *16:*280–282, April 30, '41
FIGI, F. A.: Excision of amyloid tumor of larynx and skin graft; case. Proc. Staff Meet., Mayo Clin. *17:*239–240, April 15, '42
FIGI, F. A.: Treatment of pigmented nevi of neck. S. Clin. North America *23:*1059–1075, Aug '43
FIGI, F. A.; NEW G. B. AND DIX, C. R.: Radiodermatitis of head and neck, with discussion of its surgical treatment (skin grafting). Surg., Gynec. & Obst. *77:*284–294, Sept '43
FIGI, F. A. AND NEW, G. B.: Carcinoma of larynx in young. Tr. Am. Laryng., Rhin. & Otol. Soc. *35:*350–357, '29
FIGI, F. A. AND NEW, G. B.: Cancer of larynx in young. Arch. Otolaryng. *9:*386–391, April '29
FIGI, F. A. (see NEW, G. B.) Oct '24
FIGI, F. A. (see NEW, G. B.) Nov '24
FIGI, F. A. (see NEW, G. B.) March '25
FIGI, F. A. (see NEW, G. B.) June '31
FIGI, F. A. (see NEW, G. B.) Dec '31
FIGI, F. A. (see NEW, G. B.) 1934
FIGI, F. A. (see NEW, G. B. *et al*) June '34
FIGI, F. A. (see NEW, G. B.) Nov '34
FIGI, F. A. (see NEW, G. B.) Feb '35
FIGI, F. A. (see NEW, G. B.) Feb '36
FIGUEROA, L. AND LAVIERI, F. J.: Use of pectin (as substitute for whole blood or plasma) and other agents in shock prevention. Surg., Gynec. & Obst. *78:*600–605, June '44
FIGUEROA ALCORTA, L.: Therapy of para-urethral fistulas with glacial acetic acid. Rev. de especialid. *6:*1125–1137, Nov '31 also: Med. argent. *11:*1239–1243, Feb '32
FIGURAS, V.: Plastic surgery of face; cases. Gac. med. de Mexico *60:*353–381, Aug '29
FIKH, E.: Comment on phonetic education in

palatal fissures in article by Fiorini. Semana med. *2:*735–738, Sept 6, '34
FILATOFF, W.: Priority in plastic surgery. Presse med. *31:*1061-1062, Dec 19, '23
FILATOV, A.: Mistakes, dangers and unforeseen complications in burn therapy. Chirurg *4:*568–576, July 15, '32
FILATOV, V. P.: Skin grafts in certain cutaneous diseases and corneal transplants. Med. zhur. *7:*743–753, '37 also: Vestnik oftal. *11:*295–310, '37
FILATOV, V. P.: Tissue transplantation in intraocular diseases. Vestnik oftal. *12:*157–159, '38
FILATOV, V. P.: Therapeutic homoplastic transplantation of conserved mucous membrane. Vestnik oftal. *12:*307–310, '38
FILATOV, V. P.: Therapeutic transplantation of tissue. Acta med. URSS *1:*412–439, '38 Vrach. delo *20:*813–822, '38
FILATOV, V. P.: Therapeutic transplantation of tissues. Probl. tuberk., no. 6, pp. 8–13, '39
FILATOV, V. P.: Skin grafts in certain cutaneous diseases. Gaz. clin. *37:*61-64, Feb '39
FILATOV, V. P.: Further data on therapeutic value of transplantation of preserved tissue; preliminary report. Sovet. med. (nos. 13–14) *4:*5–8, '40
FILATOV, V. P.: Further data on therapeutic value of preserved tissue, especially in ocular diseases; transplantation of tissues and use of placental microclysters; preliminary report. Gaz. clin. *39:*292–295, Aug '41
FILATOV, V. P.: Transplantation tissue therapy in certain diseases. Sovet. med. (no. 10) *7:*1–3, '43
FILATOV, V. P.: Transplantation tissue therapy. Vrach. delo (nos. 11–12) *25:*499–510, '45
FILATOW, W. P.: Round movable pedicles in complicated plastic operations on eyelids and face. Arch. f. klin. Chir. *146:*609–614, '27
FILDERMAN: Continued improvement of Dupuytren's contracture after injections of patient's own blood mixed with testicular extract. Bull. et mem. Soc. de med. de Paris, no. 4, pp. 115–117, Feb 28, '31
FILDERMAN, J.: Metallic crowns and bridges in maxillofacial orthopedics. Rev. odont. *52:*5–12, Jan '31
FILDERMAN, L.: Extensive congenital angioma of face obliterated by injections of sodium salicylate. Bull. et mem. Soc. de med. de Paris *142:*576–578, Oct 22, '38
FILHO, A. P.: Plastic dacryocystorhinostomy. Rev. oto-laring. de Sao Paulo (no. 5, bis) *4:*731-747, Sept-Oct '36
FILIPATO, A. J. J.: Sulfamide therapy in burns due to occupational accidents. Prensa med. argent. *31:*119-121, Jan 12, '44
FILIPS, L.: Practical observations of keloids and potential keloids. M. Rec. *150:*418–422, Dec 20, '39
FILLINGER, F. (see MELTZER, H.) May '36
FILLIOL, L. (see RAVAUT, P.) Dec '28
FILLMORE, R. S.: Chronic leg ulcers (rationale of treatment). Texas State J. Med. *35:*281–286, Aug '39
FINALY, R.: Surgical therapy of elephantiasis. Nederl. tijdschr. v. geneesk. *79:*5298-5301, Nov 16, '35 also: Zentralbl. f. Chir. *63:*389–394, Feb 15, '36
FINCKE, B.: Burns and scalds in infants and children. Monatschr. f. Kinderh. *86:*73–95, '41
FINCKH: Heredity of syndactylia in one family during period of 100 years. Med. Welt *8:*705, May 19, '34
FINDLAY, R. T.: Burns of scalp in women. Am. J. Surg. *8:*389–396, Feb '30
FINDLAY, R. T.: Conservative treatment vs. immediate amputation in severe crushing injuries of hand and forearm. S. Clin. North America *18:*297–303, April '38
FINE, A.: Twilight sleep in plastic surgery. Eye, Ear, Nose & Throat Monthly *22:*342–343, Sept '43
FINE, J.: FISCHMANN, J. AND FRANK, H. A.: Effect of adrenal cortical hormones in hemorrhage and shock. Surgery *12:*1–13, July '42
FINE, J.; FRANK, H. A. AND SELIGMAN, A. M.: Traumatic shock incurable by volume replacement therapy; summary of further studies including observations on hemodynamics, intermediary metabolism and therapeutics. Ann. Surg. *122:*652–662, Oct '45
FINE, J. AND SELIGMAN, A. M.: Traumatic shock; study of problem of "lost plasma" in hemorrhagic shock by use of radioactive plasma protein. J. Clin. Investigation *22:*285–303, March '43
FINE, J. (see FRANK, H. A. *et al*) July '45
FINESILVER, E. M.: Nomenclature in plastic surgery. Am. J. Surg. *35:*549–553, March '37
FINESILVER, E. M. (see DAVIS, J. S.) June '32
FINESILVER, E. M. (see GERMAN, W. *et al*) Jan '33

Fingernails

Replacement of thumb nail. SHEEHAN, J. E. J.A.M.A. *92:*1253–1255, April 13, '29
Treatment of traumatic hematoma of fingernails. BEER, H. Munchen. med. Wchnschr. *76:*1635, Sept 27, '29
Treatment of split fingernails. CARTER, W. W., M. J. & Rec. *131:*599–600, June 18, '30
Differential diagnosis of subungual melanomas; 4 cases. ADAIR, F. E.; *et al*. Bull.

Fingernails – Cont.

Assoc. franc. p. l'etude du cancer *19:*549–566, July '30

Treatment of chronically recurring paronychias and related ungual diseases by excision and by Thiersch grafts. RUDOFSKY, F. Med. Klin. *30:*198, Feb 9, '34

Method of bloodless removal of splinter from under nail. LADYZHENSKIY, M. E. Sovet. vrach. zhur., pp. 217–218, Feb 15, '36

Cosmetic autotransplantation of nails. KO, G. Taiwan Igakkai Zasshi *35:*1072, May '36

Glomus tumor: arterial angioneuromyoma of Masson. COLE, H. N. AND SROUB, W. E. J.A.M.A. *107:*428–429, Aug 8, '36

Use of small skin grafts for treating recent injuries of nail bed. RÖPER, W. Zentralbl. f. Chir. *64:*2679–2681, Nov 20, '37

Malignant melanomas, with particular reference to subungual type. NEWELL, C. E. South. M. J. *31:*541–547, May '38

Subungual melanoma; differential diagnosis of tumors of nail bed. PACK, G. T. AND ADAIR, F. E. Surgery *5:*47–72, Jan '39

Anatomy, pathology and treatment of infections of finger tip and nail. TENDLER, M. J. Memphis M. J. *15:*139–140, Sept '40

Total graft of nail and of matrix; case. IVANISSEVICH, O. AND RIVAS, C. I. Bol. d. Inst. clin. quir. *18:*640–642, Sept '42

Radical operation with plastic closure, for cure of ingrowing nails. BENNETT, L. C. Mil. Surgeon *94:*361–364, June '44

Simple treatment for hemorrhage into nail bed. SCHWAB, W. J. AND FOLEY, F. A., U.S. Nav. M. Bull. *43:*371, Aug '44

Suture in crushing injuries of finger nails. HAMRICK, W. H., U.S. Nav. M. Bull. *46:*225–228, Feb '46

Therapy of injuries in fingernail region. VERAART, B. Nederl. tijdschr. v. geneesk. *90:*743–745, June 29 '46

Split thickness graft as covering following removal of fingernail. HANRAHAN, E. M. Surgery *20:*398–400, Sept '46

Fingertips

Treatment of infections of the terminal phalanges of hand. PROBSTEIN, J. G. AND BROOKES, H. S. JR., J. MISSOURI M. A. *21:*307–309, Sept '24

Plastic operation for repair of traumatic amputation of end of finger. GILCREEST, E. L. S. Clin. N. Amer. *6:*555–556, April '26

Experiences with decapitation finger cap. BLOND, K. Zentralbl. f. Gynak. *50:*2907–2909, Nov 6, '26

Necrosis of terminal phalanx of finger;

Fingertips – Cont.

method of treatment. BEARSE, C. Boston M. & S. J. *197:*1083–1086, Dec 8, '27

Treatment of injuries of finger tips. KRECKE, A. Munchen. med. Wchnschr. *75:*571, March 30, '28

Distal anterior closed space infections of fingers. CARP, L. Surg., Gynec. & Obst. *46:*484–495, April '28

Common injuries to finger tips and their care. LICHTENSTEIN, M. E. Illinois M. J. *55:*125–127, Feb '29

Treatment of acute paronychia. KIAER, S. Ugesk. f. laeger *92:*425–427, May 1, '30

Skin grafts in changing of fingerprints. UPDEGRAFF, H. L. Am. J. Surg. *26:*533–534, Dec '34

Permanent results of plastic surgery of finger tips. MELTZER, H. AND FILLINGER, F. Chirurg *8:*397–404, May 15, '36

Necrosis of finger tips following use of local anesthetic in operation for contracture; study of epinephrine toxicity. HANKE, H. Chirurg *8:*684–687, Sept 1, '36

Permanent functional results of use of cod liver oil and plaster of paris cast after injury or loss of fingertip. FLIMM, W. Zentralbl. f. Chir. *63:*2500–2506, Oct 17, '36

Injuries to finger tips caused by stamping press. BEHRENS, B. Med. Welt *12:*1706–1710, Nov 26, '38

Finger tip reconstruction; new operation (using bone and skin grafts). LAUTEN, W. F. Indust. Med. *8:*99–100, March '39

Wounds with loss of distal phalangeal substance of fingers. PINTO DE SOUZA, O. Rev. Assoc. paulista de med. *14:*219–226, April '39

Unusual fracture of terminal phalanx. WISE, R. A., J. Bone & Joint Surg. *21:*467–469, April '39

Immediate full thickness grafts to finger tips. REED, J. V. AND HARCOURT, A. K. Surg., Gynec. & Obst. *68:*925–929, May '39

Anatomy, pathology and treatment of infections of finger tip and nail. TENDLER, M. J. Memphis M. J. *15:*139–140, Sept '40

Treatment of stumps in accidental amputation of fingertips. ERLER, F. Munchen. med. Wchnschr. *88:*1287, Nov 28, '41

Method for closing traumatic defect of finger tip. (graft) JONES, R. A. Am. J. Surg. *55:*326–338, Feb '42

Traumatic amputation of finger tips (with special reference to tank door accident; value of skin grafts.) TERHUNE, S. R. AND CAMP, M. N. South. Surgeon *11:*646–651, Sept '42

Fingertips—Cont.
Immediate skin grafting for traumatic amputation of finger tips. ZADIK, F. R. Lancet *1:*335–336, March 13, '43
Method for repair of finger amputation. KUTLER, W. Ohio State M. J. *40:*126, Feb '44
Immediate repair by means of free total graft in flat (guillotine) mutilation of fingers. DE SOUZA RAMOS, R. Med. cir. Farm. pp. 339–341, June '46
Immediate application of free full-thickness skin graft for traumatic amputation of finger. MCCARROLL, H. R., J. Bone & Joint Surg. *26:*489–494, July '44
Celluloid splint in traumatic amputation of distal phalanges. O'TOOLE, J. B. JR., U.S. Nav. M. Bull. *42:*460–461, Feb '44

Finger, Trigger

Etiology and mechanism of snapping finger. KÖNIG, E. Med. Klin. *17:*434, April 10, '21
Snapping finger. HOOGVELD, W. P. J. Nederlandsch Tijdschr. v. Geneesk. *1:*2663, May 14, '21 abstr: J.A.M.A. *77:*416, July 30, '21
Tendovaginitis and snapping finger. HAUCK, G. Arch. f. klin. Chir. *123:*233–258, '23 (illus.)
Snapping finger in polyarthritis. HELWEG, J. Ugesk. f. Laeger *86:*546–547, July 17, '24 abstr: J.A.M.A. *83:*1042, Sept 27, '24
Snapping finger in polyarthritis. HELWEG, J. Klin. Wchnschr. *3:*2383–2384, Dec 23, '24 abstr: J.A.M.A. *84:*560, Feb 14, '25
Snapping finger and its treatment. MONBERG, A. Hospitalstid. *68:*295–300, April 2, '25
Contracture of thumb in infants following symptoms of snapping finger. GÖHLER, W. Deutsche med. Wchnschr. *51:*1200, July 17, '25
Snapping finger and stenosis from tendovaginitis of flexor tendons. KROH, F. Arch. f. klin. Chir. *136:*240–276, '25
Stenosing tendovaginitis of long abductor and of short extensor of thumb. LAROYENNE, AND BOUYSSET. Arch. franco-belges de chir. *30:*98–104, Feb '27 also: Lyon med. *140:*573–575, Nov 27, '27
Strangulation of long abductor and short extensor of thumb; treatment. LAROYENNE, AND TREPOZ. Lyon med. *142:*394, Sept 30, '28
Snapping finger. PEIPER, H. Arch. f. klin. Chir. *150:*496–505, '28
Treatment of snapping thumb. OTTENDORF. Zentralbl. f. Chir. *57:*1273, May 24, '30
Causes, pathology, diagnosis and therapy of stenosing tendovaginitis of thumb. LANDOIS, F. Med. Klin. *26:*927-929, June 20, '30

Finger, Trigger—Cont.
Anatomic grounds for clinical treatment of tendovaginitis of palm. KHAITZISS, G. M. Vestnik khir. (nos. 56–57) *19:*356–362, '30
Operative treatment in inflamation of digital tendon sheaths. CADENAT, F. M. Bull. et mem. Soc. nat. de chir. *57:*522, April 25, '31
Operative technic in inflammation of digital tendon sheaths. ISELIN, M. Bull. et mem. Soc. nat. de chir. *57:*456–465, April 4, '31
Digital tendovaginitis. ISELIN, M. Schweiz. med. Wchnschr. *62:*1159–1163, Dec 10, '32
Bilateral snapping thumbs. COMPERE, E. L. Ann. Surg. *97:*773–777, May '33
Snapping thumb in childhood; 8 cases. HUDSON, H. W. JR. New England J. Med. *210:*854–857, April 19, '34
Snapping finger (intermittent reflex contraction) in electric welders. VEGER, A. M. Novy khir. arkhiv *30:*321–325, '34
Etiology of "snapping finger"; simultaneous appearance in uniovular twins. CAMERER, J. W. AND SCHLEICHER, R. Med. Klin. *31:*245–246, Feb 22, '35
Snapping thumb; tendovaginitis stenosans. ZELLE, O. L. AND SCHNEPP, K. H. Am. J. Surg. *33:*321–322, Aug '36
Trigger finger in children. JAHSS, S. A. J.A.M.A. *107:*1463–1464, Oct 31, '36
Tendovaginitis stenosans of extensor pollicis longus sinister. POHL, H. Med. Klin. *32:*1596–1597, Nov 20, '36
Snapping thumb in young children. HARRENSTEIN, R. J. Nederl. tijdschr. v. geneesk. *81:*1237–1241, March 20, '37
Blocking of tendons of both thumbs; comparison with syndrome described by Notta (trigger finger). DREYFUS, J. R. Schweiz. med. Wchnschr. *68:*650–654, May 28, '38
Surgical therapy of trigger finger. SPISIC, B. Zentralbl. f. Chir. *67:*157–159, Jan 27, '40
Snapping of finger joints due to injury to tendons. SCHÖRCHER, F. Zentralbl. f. Chir. *67:*627–628, April 6, '40
Tendovaginitis stenosans of finger. SPISIC, B. Lijecn. vjes. *62:*246–248, May '40
Snapping fingers due to tendosynovitis; case. SANDBERG, I. R. Nord. med. (Hygiea) *9:*707–709, March 8, '41
Blockage of tendon of flexor pollicis longus. FEVRE, M. Presse med. *50:*754–755, Dec 12, '42
Stenosing tenosynovitis of flexors; treated cases. (hand) ALJAMA, V. Rev. espan. cir., traumatol. y ortop. *1:*373–374, Nov '44
Trigger finger; surgical therapy of case. DE FARIA VOZ, J. Arq. brasil. de cir. e ortop. *12:*157–163, '44

Finger, Trigger—Cont.

Bilateral trigger thumb in infants. ROSE, T. F., M. J. Australia *1:*18–20, Jan 5, '46

Fingers, Amputations of

Case of minor surgery of hand; accidental amputation of finger with preservation of terminal phalanx. TOMB, J. W. Lancet *2:*930, Oct 27, '23
Soft parts in finger amputations. PORZELT, W. Zentralbl. f. Chir. *51:*1343–1345, June 21, '24
Plastic operation for repair of traumatic amputation of end of finger. GILCREEST, E. L. S. Clin. N. Amer. *6:*555–556, April '26
Severe laceration of hand with traumatic amputation of two fingers. LOEB, M. J. J.A.M.A. *86:*1345–1347, May 1, '26
Unusual amputation of finger and tendon. ADAMS, J. C., U. S. Nav. M. Bull. *27:*379–380, April '29
Full thickness skin grafts in finger amputations. O'MALLEY, T. S. Wisconsin M. J. *33:*337–340, May '34
Value of amputation after trauma of fingers and hand. CARCASSONNE, F. AND LÉNA, A. Marseille-med. *2:*643–651, Nov 25, '34
Amputation of fingers. WILLEMS, J. D. Surg., Gynec. and Obst. *62:*892–894, May '36
Comparative evaluation of methods for amputation of fingers. AFANASEVA, A. V. Vestnik khir. *42:*232–239, '36
Evaluation of degree of invalidity in amputation of various segments of fingers. OLIVIER, E.; *et al.* Ann. de med. leg. *17:*883–888, Oct '37
Traumatic amputations of fingers. ENNIS, W. N. AND HUBER, H. S., S. Clin. North America *18:*305–319, April '38
Traumatic amputation of child's finger by rabbit bite. DURAND, P. Presse med. *46:*907, June 8, '38
Digital mutilations. LUQUET, G. H., J. de psycholmnorm. et path. *35:*548–598, July–Dec '38
Amputation of fingers. EDWARDS, H. C. Brit. M. J. *2:*631–633, Sept 17, '38
Injuries to finger tips caused by stamping press. BEHRENS, B. Med. Welt *12:*1706–1710, Nov 26, '38
Wounds with loss of distal phalangeal substance of fingers. PINTO DE SOUZA, O. Rev. Assoc. Paulista de med. *14:*219–226, April '39
Indications for amputation of fingers. ZUR VERTH, M. Deutsche med. Wchnschr. *65:*1795–1797, Dec 15, '39
Technic of application of Filatov flaps in plastic operations on amputation-stumps of hands and fingers. YUSEVICH, M. S. Ortop. i travmatol. (no. 3) *14:*50–56, '40

Fingers, Amputations of—Cont.

Amputation of fingers. ROGERS, L. J. Roy. Nav. M. Serv. *27:*137–141, April '41
Simple plastic procedure of fingers for conserving bony tissue and forming soft tissue pad (after traumatic amputation). DE JONGH, E. Am. J. Surg. *57:*346–347, Aug '42
Method for repair of finger amputation. KUTLER, W. Ohio State M. J. *40:*126, Feb '44
Surgical treatment of pain in peripheral nervous system (following amputations of fingers). PARKES, A. R. Tr. Roy. Med.-Chir. Soc. Glasgow, pp. 23–25, '43–'44; in Glasgow M. J. May '44
Principles of amputations of fingers and hand. SLOCUM, D. B. AND PRATT, D. R., J. Bone and Joint Surg. *26:*535–546, July '44
Treatment of tendons in finger amputations and description of new instrument. WEBSTER, G. V. Surgery *17:*102–108, Jan '45
Treatment of simple and compound finger fractures; finger amputations. CURRY, G. J. Am. J. Surg. *71:*80–83, Jan '46
Immediate repair by means of free total graft in flat (guillotine) mutilation of fingers. DE SOUZA RAMOS, R. Med. cir. Farm. pp. 339–341, June '46
Finger amputations. CURRY, G. J. Amer. J. Surg. *72:*40–42, July '46
Disarticulations and amputations of fingers and toes. GIORDANENGO, G. Minerva chir. *1:*165–166, July '46

Fingers, Ankylosis

Limitation of movement at metacarpophalangeal joints; its causes and treatment. GLISSAN, D. J., M. J. Australia *2:*257, Oct '21
Prevention of stiff fingers. KRECKE, A. Munchen. med. Wchnschr. *68:*1296–1297, Oct 7, '21
Stiff fingers. COTTON, F. J. AND SAWYER, E. J. Boston M. and S. J. *186:*183–185, Feb 9, '22 (illus.)
Operative mobilization of stiff fingers. HESSE, E. Arch. f. klin. Chir. *119:*1–19, '22 (illus.) abstr: J.A.M.A. *78:*1173, April 15, '22
Congenital ankylosis of finger joints. BRÜGGER. Munchen. med. Wchnschr. *70:*874–875, July 6, '23 (illus.)
Congenital ankylosis of finger joints (Comment on Brügger's article). DUKEN, J.

Fingers, Ankylosis – Cont.

Munchen. med. Wchnschr. *70:*986, July 27, '23

Mobilization of stiff metacarpophalangeal joints. HEYMAN, C. H. Surg., Gynec. and Obst. *39:*506–507, Oct '24

Ankylosis of fingers; pathologic study. RISAK, E. Deutsche Ztschr. f. Chir. *211:*86–115, '28

Congenital ankylosis and osseous fusion of phalanges; familial disease. PERVÈS, J. Rev. d'orthop. *19:*628–632, Nov–Dec '32

Development of stiffness of fingers (congenital and hereditary). MOSENTHAL. Verhandl. d. deutsch. orthop. Gesellsch. (1931) Kong. 26, pp. 66–68, '32

Carpometacarpal arthroplasty of thumb. PATTERSON, R., J. Bone and Joint Surg. *15:*240–241, Jan '33

Treatment of stiffening of fingers and hand with and without muscular paralysis. LANGE, M. Munchen. med. Wchnschr. *81:*894–897, June 15, '34

Hereditary multiple ankylosing arthropathy (congenital stiffness of finger joints). BLOOM, A. R. Radiology *29:*166–171, Aug '37

Arthroplasty of fingers; 2 cases. GUILLEMINET, M. Lyon chir. *35:*117–119, Jan–Feb '38

Surgical therapy of post-traumatic functional disturbance of proximal joint of thumb. MONDRY, F. Zentralbl. f. Chir. *67:*1532–1535, Aug 17, '40

Vitallium cap arthroplasty of metacarpophalangeal and interphalangeal joints of fingers. BURMAN, M. S. Bull. Hosp. Joint Dis. *1:*79–89, Oct '40

Traumatic rigidity of fingers. GEBAUER, T. Arch. Soc. cirujanos hosp., num. espec., pp. 57–64, Dec '41

Excision of ankylosed sesamoid of thumb. MILCH, H. M. Rec. *156:*541–542, Sept '43

Nylon fabric arthroplasty of carpometacarpal joint of thumb. BURMAN, M. Bull. Hosp. Joint Dis. *4:*74–78, Oct '43

Use of plastics in reconstructive surgery; lucite in arthroplasty; tissue tolerance for lucite, its use as interposition mold in arthroplasty of phalangeal joints; 3 cases. BURMAN, M. AND ABRAHAMSON, R. H. Mil. Surgeon *93:*405–414, Nov '43

Arthroplastic reconstruction in joints. CHARRY, R. Rev. d'orthop. *31:*186–194, Sept–Dec '45

New arthroplasty for small joints. CROSBY, E. H. AND GALASINSKI, R. E. Connecticut M. J. *9:*926–928, Dec '45

Mobilization of hand following loss of all fingers. PARIN, B. V. Khirurgiya no. 3, p. 89, '45 (comment on Geymanovich's article)

Fingers, Arachnodactylia

Arachnodactylia; case. ROEDERER, C. Bull. Soc. de pediat. de Paris *35:*225–231, April '37

Arachnodactylia, kyphoscoliosis, patent interventricular septum and ectopy of crystalline lens (Marfan syndrome); case. ROCH, M. Presse med. *45:*1429–1430, Oct 9, '37

Fingers, Avulsion Injuries

Avulsion of tendon of extensor pollicis. KIRCHENBERGER, A. Med. Klin. *22:*1640–1641, Oct 22, '26

Avulsion of tendon of musculus flexor pollicis longus from muscle; case. GONTERMANN, C. Monatschr. f. Unfallh. *36:*546–549, Dec '29

Muscular (tendinous) avulsion of flexor profundus of middle finger of right hand; case. MARINUCCI, C. L. Riforma med. *48:*1834–1838, Nov 26, '32

Traumatic avulsion of ungual phalanx of thumb and of its flexor tendon. MOUCHET, A. Bull. et mem. Soc. nat. de chir. *59:*1244–1247, Oct 28, '33

Complete tearing of right thumb from joint by electric hand drill; rare case. SCHWERDTFEGER, H. Zentralbl. f. Chir. *64:*741–742, March 27, '37

Complete tearing of ungual phalanx of ring finger and of its extensor tendon; case. RAFFO, J. M. AND ARCONE, R. Rev. ortop. y traumatol. *7:*29–31, July '37

Avulsion of so-called extensor aponeurosis of thumb. GOLLA, F. Zentralbl. f. Chir. *65:*1803–1807, Aug 13, '38

Avulsion of last 2 phalanges of forefinger and 15 cm. of 2 flexor tendons in child 7 years old; case. ROCHER, H. L. AND POUYANNE, L., J. de med. de Bordeaux *115:*175–176, Aug 20–27, '38

Traumatic tearing off of fifth finger and of corresponding flexor tendon; case. BOTERO JARAMILLO, L. E. Colombia med. *2:*82–85, March–April '40

Rare trauma of hand; tearing off of part of index finger with 20 cm. of flexor tendon; case. SGROSSO, J. A. Bol. Soc. de cir. de Rosario *10:*172–174, June '43

Traumatic amputation of terminal phalanx of second finger of left hand with tearing out of tendon of flexor digitorum profundus muscle; case. IBSEN, B. Ugesk. f. laeger *105:*707, July 15, '43

Bloodless treatment of avulsion of extensor tendon of finger. LEDERGERBER, E. Schweiz. med. Wchnschr. *75:*1088–1089, Dec 8, '45

Fingers, Baseball Injuries (See also: Fingers, Splints)

Mallet finger. FOSTER, W. J. Brit. N. J. *1:*226, Feb 11, '22

Treatment of rupture of extensor tendon of third phalanx. SONNTAG. Munchen. med. Wchnschr. *69:*1333–1334, Sept 15, '22 (illus.)

"Baseball finger" cured by operation. STEPHENS, R., J. Bone and Joint Surg. *6:*469–470, April '24

Simple splint for baseball finger. LEWIN, P. J.A.M.A. *85:*1059, Oct 3, '25

Typical finger injuries in baseball. MANDL, F. Wien. med. Wchnschr. *77:*965, July 16, '27

Rupture of extensor tendon at terminal phalanx of finger. (comment on Glass' article) SONNTAG, E. Zentralbl. f. Chir. *55:*410, Feb 18, '28

Improved splint for baseball finger. LEWIN, P., J.A.M.A. *90:*2102, June 30, '28

Suture of avulsion of extension tendon of last phalanx. HAUCK, G. J. Med. Welt *3:*1657, Nov 16, '29

Treatment of torn extensor tendons of terminal phalanges. SCHLOFFER, H. Zentralbl. f. Chir. *57:*1053–1055, April 26, '30

Improved splint for baseball finger. LEWIN, P., J.A.M.A. *90:*2102, June 30, '28

Surgical or nonsurgical treatment of rupture of extensor tendons of terminal phalanx of finger. HORWITZ, A. Deutsche med. Wchnschr. *57:*445–448, March 13, '31

Treatment of disrupted extensor tendon from terminal phalanx of finger by means of simple splint. DALSGAARD, S. Ugesk. f. laeger *96:*273–274, March 8, '34 abstr: Acta chir. Scandinav. *74:*429, '34

Spontaneous healing of subcutaneous rupture of tendons in terminal phalanx of finger. LINDENSTEIN, L. Zentralbl. f. Chir. *62:*2961, Dec 14, '35

Bilateral rupture of extensor aponeurosis of terminal phalanx of finger and its treatment. GOLLA, F. Beitr. z. klin. Chir. *162:*594–600, '35

Complete repair of "mallet finger". MERRIMAN, B. Brit. M. J. *2:*760, Oct 17, '36

Mallet finger. SMILLIE, I. S. Brit. J. Surg. *24:*439–445, Jan '37

Mallet or baseball finger. KAPLAN, E. B. Surgery *7:*784–791, May '40

Technic for repair of "baseball" finger. SAYPOL, G. M. Am. J. Surg. *61:*103–104, July '43

Fingers, Boutonniere Deformity of

Luxation of tendons of extensor digitorum. LEVY, W. Zentralbl. f. Chir. *48:*482, April 9, '21

Luxation of tendons of extensores digitorum. HABERERN, J. P. Zentralbl. f. Chir. *48:*1080, July 30, '21

Traumatic dislocation of extensor tendon of second finger. RAZEMON, P. Ann. d'anat. path. *7:*238–241, Feb '30

Traumatic dislocation of extensor tendons of fingers; case. RAZEMON, P. Echo m. du nord *34:*213–216, May 3, '30

Buttonhole rupture of extensor tendon of finger at point of insertion into terminal phalanx. KALLIUS, H. U. Zentralbl. f. Chir. *57:*2432–2435, Sept 27, '30

Subcutaneous ruptures of extensor tendons of fingers in buttonhole dislocation of first interphalangeal joint. EILERS. Deutsche Ztschr. f. Chir. *223:*317–327, '30

Button-hole rupture of extensor tendon of finger. MILCH, H. Am. J. Surg. *13:*244–245, Aug '31

"Buttonholed" extensor expansion of finger. BINGHAM, D. L. C. AND JACK, E. A. Brit. M. J. *2:*701–702, Oct 9, '37

Joining dorsal aponeurosis and tendons in therapy of injuries to extensor tendons of fingers; cases. JOHNER, T. Schweiz. med. Wchnschr. *68:*111–113, Jan 29, '38

Rupture and luxation of dorsal (extensor) tendons of fingers at first interphalangeal articulation; physiologic and clinical study. MONTANT, R. AND BAUMANN, A. Rev. d'orthop. *25:*5–22, Jan '38

Lateral luxation of portion of extensor tendon of finger. DE ROUGEMONT, J. Presse med. *47:*1197, Aug 2, '39

Luxation of extensor tendons. STRAUS, F. H. Ann. Surg. *111:*135–140, Jan '40

Buttonhole rupture-luxation of extensor tendon of fingers. CASANUEVA DEL C., M. AND CROQUEVIELLE G., A. Rev. med. de Chile *70:*57–63, Jan '42

Fingers, Burns of (See also Burn Contractures)

Typical finger injuries received while working with mangle. GROSS, W. Zentralbl. f. Chir. *60:*2790–2791, Dec 2, '33

Therapy of cicatricial contracture of hand and fingers after burns. BAKUSHINSKIY, R. N. Ortop. i travmatol. (no. 2) *12:*76–83, '38

Hand and finger contracture due to burns. HOHMANN, G. Chirurg. *14:*289, May 15, '42

Finger exerciser for burned hands. OLDFIELD,

Fingers, Burns of—Cont.

M. C. AND KING, C. J. Lancet *2:*109, July 22, '44

Local therapy including facial, interdigital and perineal burns; preliminary report. ZORRAQUIN, G. AND ZORRAQUIN, G. F. Dia med. *17:*329-331, April 16, '45

Fingers, Camptodactylism

Familial symmetrical finger contracture (camptodactylia). HEERUP, L. Ugesk. f. laeger *91:*1072-1075, Nov 28, '29

Camptodactylism and its variable expression. MOORE, W. G. AND MESSINA, P. J. Hered. *27:*27-30, Jan '36

Family with camptodactylia. RITTERSKAMP, P. Munchen. med. Wchnschr. *83:*724-725, May 1, '36

Anatomic lesion of camptodactylic supernumerary finger. FEVRE, M. Ann. d'anat. path. *13:*1018-1023, Nov '36

Familial ankylosis of finger joints (camptodactylia). NOWAK, H. Deutsche med. Wchnschr. *63:*937-938, June 11, '37

Camptodactylia in children. DREYFUS, J. R. Jahrb. f. Kinderh. *148:*336-345, '37

Note on Dupuytren's contracture, camptodactylia and knuckle-pads. WEBER, F. P. Brit. J. Dermat. *50:*26-31, Jan '38

Bilateral symmetric contractures of hand and phalanges; case. SPISIC, B. Ztschr. f. Orthop. *75:*33, '44

Fingers, Contractures

Resection of bone to remedy finger contracture. ECKSTEIN, H. Zentralbl. f. Chir. *49:*547-548, April 22, '22 abstr: J.A.M.A. *79:*598, Aug 12, '22

Orthopedic treatment of hand and finger contractures. REY, J. Ztschr. f. orthop. Chir. *48:*21-31, Feb 11, '27

Surgical treatment of spastic adductor contraction of thumb by dorsal suspension of metacarpus of thumb by fascial sling. HENSCHEN, C. Schweiz. med. Wchnschr. *58:*621-625, June 23, '28

Slow screw extension in contractures of fingers. WOLF, J. Monatschr. f. Unfallh. *36:*447-451, Oct '29

Successful therapy of severe contractures of fingers and hand by cotton redressments. ŠPIŠIČ, B. Ztschr. f. orthop. Chir. *57:*195-202, '32

Orthopedic treatment of contraction of fingers. HOHMANN, G. Munchen. med. Wchnschr. *83:*2088-2089, Dec 18, '36

Diagnosis and treatment of contractures of fingers. THOMSEN, W. Arch. f. orthop. u. Unfall-Chir. *39:*201-205, '38

Pathology and operative correction of finger deformities due to contractures of extensor digitorum tendon. KAPLAN, E. B. Surgery *6:*451, Sept '39

Flexor contracture of little finger, typical late tertiary symptom of tropical frambesia. PRONK, K. J. Geneesk. tijdschr. v. Nederl.-Indie *81:*1403-1407, July 1, '41

Correction of disabling flexion contracture of thumb. KAPLAN, E. B. Bull. Hosp. Joint Dis. *3:*51-54, April '42

Contractures of fingers and toes after war wounds. SQUIRE, C. M. Proc. Roy. Soc. Med. *36:*665-666, Oct '43

Fingers, Deformity (See also specific deformities and also Fingers, Reconstructive Surgery of; Syndactylism)

Rare malformation of hands, polydactylia, syndactylia and thumb with 3 phalanges. DHALLUIN, A. Arch. franco-belges de chir. *25:*931-933, July '22 (illus.)

Case of macrodactylia. VAN NECK, M. Arch. franco-belges de chir. *26:*895-898, Sept '23 (illus.)

Heredity of malformations especially harelip and polydactylism. LÜCKER, F. C. Monatschr. f. Geburtsh. u. Gynak. *66:*327-336, July '24 abstr: J.A.M.A. *83:*882, Sept 13, '24

Hereditary ankylosis of proximal phalangeal joints. ELKIN, D. C., J.A.M.A. *84:*509, Feb 14, '25

Dactylomegaly, bilateral affection; only case reported. KILLINGER, R. R., J. Florida M. A. *12:*6-10, July '25

Aplasia of joints in fingers. STECHER, L. Arch. f. klin. Chir. *134:*818-825, '25

Congenital familial finger contracture and associated familial knee-joint subluxation. MURPHY, D. P., J.A.M.A. *86:*395-397, Feb 6, '26

Congenital bilateral anophthalmos and polydactylism with report of case. HEINBERG, C. J., J. Florida M. A. *12:*253-256, April '26

Case of multiple anomaly of phalanges of hands in girl aged 15. SHORE, L. R., J. Anat. *60:*420-425, July '26

Plastic reconstruction of fingers with particular regard to formation of cleft hand. ZOLLINGER, A. Deutsche Ztschr. f. Chir. *196:*271-287, '26

Bilateral absence of thumb; case. VAN DEN BROEK, A. J. P. Nederl. Tijdschr. v. Geneesk. *1:*1452-1456, March 19, '27

Fingers, Deformity – Cont.
Congenital absence of fifth finger. WRETE, M. Upsala Lakaref. Forh. *32:*285–294, March '27
Thumb with 3 phalanges. GRYNKRAUT, B. J. de radiol. et d'electrol. *11:*325, June '27
Double phalangx in thumb of acromegalic subject. BORDONI, L. Radiol. med. *14:*775–781, Sept '27
Congenital bilateral club hand with absence of thumbs; case. PETRIDIS, P. A. Rev. d'orthop. *14:*419–421, Sept '27
Finger abnormalities. GILMORE, E. R. W. Brit. M. J. *2:*935–936, Nov. 19, '27
Congenital atrophy of fingers; 19 cases. PIRES DE LIMA, J. A. Arq. de anat. *10:*401–429, '27
Hypertrophied thumb; case. RALLO, A. Ann. di med. nav. *1:*257–273, May–June '28
Megalosyndactylia; case. DOMBROVSKY, A. I. Munchen. med. Wchnschr. *75:*1503, Aug. 31, '28
Bifid and supernumerary fingers. ZAMPA, G. Chir. d. org. di movimento *13:*195–212, Dec '28
Congenital contractures of fingers and clinodactyly; 4 cases. TOMESKU, I. Arch. f. Orthop. *26:*126–137, '28
Thumb with 3 phalanges; case. CAMPBELL, D. Fortschr. a. d. Geb. d. Rontgenstrahlen *39:*479–481, March '29
Megalodactylia; case. KAUFMANN, M. Med. Klin. *25:*907–908, June 7, '29
Three-jointed thumbs; case. SCHRADER, E. Fortschr. a. d. Geb. d. Rontgenstrahlen *40:*693, Oct '29
Ectrodactylia of last 4 fingers; case. LÉVY-VALENSI, AND FEIL, A. Semaine d. hop. de Paris *6:*61–62, Jan 31, '30
Supernumerary distal phalanx of thumb; case. WEINGROW, S. M. Am. J. Roentgenol. *23:*206–207, Feb '30
Case having thumbs with 3 phalanges simulating fingers. FRERE, J. M. South. M. J. *23:*536–537, June '30
Congenital bilateral absence of radius and thumb. D'ABREU, A. R. Indian M. Gaz. *65:*505–507, Sept '30
Symphalangism. MUSSER, J. H. New Orleans M. and S. J. *83:*325–326, Nov '30
Hypertrophy of ear; case and fingers. MORAZA, M. Med. ibera *2:*630–633, Dec 6, '30
Absence of several fingers and fibroma of middle finger of right hand in new-born infant. BRUNETTI, F. Rinasc. med. *9:*7–8, Jan 1, '32
Bilateral absence of radius and thumb. D'ABREU, A. R. Indian M. Gaz. *67:*266–267, May '32

Fingers, Deformity – Cont.
Congenital stiffness of digital joints. ROCHLIN, D. G. AND SIMONSON, S. G. Fortschr. a. d. Geb. d. Rontgenstrahlen *46:*193–204, Aug '32
Inheritance of doublejointedness in thumb. WHITNEY, L. F., J. Hered. *23:*425–426, Oct '32
Spontaneous amputation of human supernumerary digits; pedunculated postminimi. CUMMINS, H. Am. J. Anat. *51:*381–416, Nov '32
Isolated case of craniofacial dysostosis (Crouzon's disease) with ectrodactylia. GARCIN, R.; *et al.* Bull. et mem. Soc. med. d. hop. de Paris *48:*1458–1466, Nov 28, '32
Congenital ulnar deviation of fingers of familial occurrence. LUNDBLOM, A. Acta orthop. Scandinav. *3:*393–404, '32
Congenital absence of right thumb; attempt at functional restoration. BONZON. Scalpel *86:*799–801, May 27, '33
Isolated case of craniofacial dysostosis (Crouzon's disease) with ectrodactylia. GARCIN, R.; *et al.* Arch. de med. d. enf. *36:*359–365, June '33
Macrodactyl; pathogenesis and surgical therapy; case. IMAZ, J. I. Hosp. argent. *3:*1100–1103, June 15, '33
Congenital variations in numbers of fingers. RONNEAUX, G. AND BRUNEL. Bull. et mem. Soc. de radiol. med. de France *21:*712–718, Nov '33
Congenital megalodactylia; case. VARA LÓPEZ, R. Progresos de la clin. *42:*96–99, Feb '34
Congenital macrodactyly; case. TATAFIORE, E. Pediatria *42:*405–412, April '34
Heredity of ectrodactylia. GORIAINOWA, R. W. Fortschr. a. d. Geb. d. Rontgenstrahlen *50:*289–294, Sept '34
Cleft hands and cleft feet with oligodactylia. KELLNER, A. W. Klin. Wchnschr. *13:*1507–1509, Oct 20, '34
Symmetric polydactylia and macromelia of upper and lower extremities. SHNEYDER, S. L. Sovet. khir. (no. 6) *6:*889–894, '34
Congenital craniofacial aplasia and malformation of toes (Apert syndrome); case. GUÉRIN, R. J. de med. de Bordeaux *112:*171–173, March 10, '35
Pseudarthrosis of first phalanx of right thumb; operative therapy; case. GIULIANI, G. M. Chir. d. org. di movimento *20:*31–435, May '35
Resection of phalanges as method of treating skin defects of fingers. ZEBOLD, A. Vestnik khir. *39:*204–205, '35

Fingers, Deformity – Cont.

Favorable results of surgical therapy of aplasia of opponens muscle of thumb by transplantation of tendons of flexor digitalis sublimis V; survey of methods. GÖBELL, R. AND FREUDENBERG, K. Arch. f. orthop. u. Unfall-Chir. *35:*675–677, '35

Congenital irregular hypertrophy of fingers; case due to lymphangiomas. FEVRE, M. AND BRICAGE, R. Ann. d'anat. path. *13:*337–341, March '36

Unusual case of absence of phalanges and wrist bones. ALEXANDROW, G. N. Zentralbl. f. Chir. *63:*1110–1111, May 9, '36

Macrodactylia. DAMBRIN, L. Rev. d'orthop. *23:*215–229, May '36

Plastic repair of giant finger by stretching nerve of finger, shortening by excision, and excision of soft parts. HENSCHEN, C. Helvet. med. acta *3:*166–176, May '36

Multiple congenital malformations including hand with 5 fingers and no thumb. PICHON, E. AND WIRZ, S. Bull. Soc. de pediat. de Paris *34:*310–311, June '36

Relation between hereditary abnormalities of eyes and partially developed fingers and toes. KARSCH, J. Ztschr. f. Augenh. *89:*274–279, July '36

Genealogical study of case of symmetrical congenital brachydactylia. STECHER, W. R. M. Rec. *144:*5–8, July 1, '36

Syndrome characterized by fracture of radius, hematoma of forearm, dyskinesia of flexor muscles of fingers, with fingers in permanent extension; surgical therapy of case. DESVERNINE, C. M. Cron. med.-quir. de la Habana *62:*343–349, Aug '36

Congenital malformation with fingers and toes in flexion; new case. LICEAGA, F. J. Semana med. *2:*421–425, Aug 13, '36

Arachnodactylia in children; 3 cases. WESTENDORFF, E. G. Kinderarztl. Praxis *7:*393–399, Sept '36

Osteochondritis deformans juvenilis of fingers with brachyphalangia; case. THIES, O. Chirurg *8:*807–813, Oct 15, '36

Hereditary anarthrosis of index finger, with associated abnormalities in proportions of fingers; case. DANIEL, G. H. Ann. Eugenics *7:*281–297, Nov '36

Congenital "windmill sail" position of fingers. DREYFUSS, M. Ztschr. f. Orthop. *65:*205–225, '36

Dyscephalodactylia (Vogt) and developmental abnormalities of uvea. INCZE, K. Arch. f. Augenh. *109:*562–566, '36

Triphalangeal thumb. MÜLLER, W. Arch. f. klin. Chir. *185:*377–386, '36

Fingers, Deformity – Cont.

Congenital anomalies of fingers. PTIC, D. Polski przegl. radjol. *10–11:*65–70, '36

Problem of abnormal thumbs and thumbs with 3 phalanges. BELLELLI, F. Riforma med. *53:*320, Feb 27, '37

Macrodactylism. BLOOM, J. D. New Orleans M. and S. J. *90:*29–30, July '37

Hyperphalangism of middle finger with bilateral partial brachydactylia (involving first to third fingers). LOSSEN, H. Fortschr. a. d. Geb. d. Rontgenstrahlen *56:*428–438, Sept '37

Polydactylia and oligophalangia. AKSELRUD, S. S. Ortop. i travmatol. (no. 4) *11:*66–75, '37

Concomitance of muscular torticollis and contracture of fingers. DECKNER, K. Zentralbl. f. Chir. *65:*1192–1195, May 21, '38

Pedigree of symphalangism. STILES, K. A. AND WEBER, R. A., J. Hered. *29:*199–202, May '38

Brachyphalangia; rare case. MANABE, K. Bull. Mav. M. A., Japan (Abstr. Sect.) *27:*37, June 15, '38

Hereditary transmission of rare deformity of thumb. PALTRINIERI, M. AND DE LUCCHI, G. Bull. d. sc. med., Bologna *110:*158–167, May–June '38

Congenital hypoplasia of thumb. HAYD, F. W. Deutsche med. Wchnschr. *64:*1041–1042, July 15, '38

Contracture of middle fingers as new occupational deformation in milkers; case. ALKIEWICZ, J. Dermat. Wchnschr. *107:*1233–1234, Oct 15, '38

Congenital mutilating lesions of fingers; roentgen and clinical aspects at age of 30; case. LOUYOT, P. Rev. med. de Nancy *66:*822–826, Oct 1, '38

Aspects of so-called symbrachydactylia. ECKINGER, W. Arch. f. orthop. u. Unfall-Chir. *38:*662–669, '38

Congenital bilateral deformation of thumbs. GULYAEVA, N. M. Ortop. i travmatol. (no. 3) *12:*73–76, '38

Flexion contracture of thumb in small children, typical phenomenon. RUSCHENBERG, E. Ztschr. f. Orthop. *68:*172–178, '38

Congenital absence of one tonsil; microtia and polydactylism in same patient. GERRIE, J. W. Arch. Otolaryng. *29:*378–381, Feb '39

Megalodactylia and megalosyndactylia. DE ARAUJO, A. Rev. brasil. de orthop. e traumatol. *1:*341–368, May–June, '40

Monodactylomegaly; surgical therapy of case. DE LARA, I. Rev. mex. de cir., ginec. y cancer *8:*375–380, Sept '40

Fingers, Deformity—Cont.

Congenital contracture of thumb. Beck, W. Arch. f. orthop. u. Unfall-Chir. *40:*318–325, '40

Macrodactyly; case. Annecchino, A. Pediatria *49:*162–166, March '41

Dactylomegaly; case. Brinitzer, W. Indian M. Gaz. *76:*286–287, May '41

Macrodactyly; case. Austin, W. E. Canad: M. A. J. *45:*158, Aug '41

Macrodactyly and associated peripheral nerve changes. Moore, B. H., J. Bone and Joint Surg. *24:*617–631, July '42

Congenital bilateral anopthalmos vera with unilateral polydactyly and cleft palate; case. Applebaum, A. and Marmelstein, M. Arch. Ophth. *29:*258–265, Feb '43

Triphalangeal thumb; 6 cases. Lapidus, P. W.; *et al.* Surg., Gynec. and Obst. *77:*178–186, Aug '43

Macrodactyly; case. Timoney, F. X. Ann. Surg. *119:*144–147, Jan '44

Bilateral ptosis and atypical slant eyes associated with unilateral syndactylia, adactylia and brachyphalangia. Giri, D. V. Proc. Roy. Soc. Med. *37:*360–361, May '44

Triphalangeal bifid thumb; 6 cases. Lapidus, P. W. and Guidotti, F. P. Arch. Surg. *49:*228–234, Oct '44

Fingers, Dislocations

Dislocation of fingers. Borelli, E. Policlinico (sez. prat.) *28:*115, Jan 24, '21 abstr: J.A.M.A. *76:*826, March 19, '21

Operative treatment of dislocation of thumb, "monkey hand." Kortzeborn, A. Arch. f. klin. Chir. *133:*465–478, '24

Dislocation of thumb. Guibal, A. Montpel. med. *48:*382, Sept 1, '26

Multiple carpo-metacarpal dislocations, with report of case. Metz, W. R. New Orleans M. and S. J. *79:*327–330, Nov '26

Forward dislocations of phalangeal joints. Bonneau, R. Rev. gen. de clin. et de therap. *40:*824, Dec 4, '26

Dorsal dislocation of proximal phalanx of second to fifth fingers. Proske, R. Beitr. z. klin. Chir. *136:*528–536, '26

Dislocations of phalanges of thumb on both sides. Hofmann, A. H. Zentralbl. f. Chir. *54:*788, March 26, '27

Congenital club hand with subluxation of phalanges; case. Gruca, A. Rev. d'orthop. *14:*407–412, Sept '27

Compound dislocation fracture of distal phalanx of finger; report of case. Boies, L. R. Minnesota Med. *10:*773–775, Dec '27

Irreducible, metacarpophalangeal dislocation of index finger; presence of abnormal

Fingers, Dislocations—Cont.

sesamoid; case. Etienne, E. and Duponnois, Arch. Soc. d. sc. med. et biol. de Montpellier *9:*106, March '28

Metacarpophalangeal dislocations of thumb. Garling-Palmer, R. Presse med. *36:*885–886, July 14, '28

Clinical aspects and treatment of forward, metacarpophalangeal dislocations of thumb. Garling Palmer, R. Gaz. d. hop. *102:*146–149, Jan 26, '29

Recurrent dislocations of thumb; capsulorrhaphy. Milch, H. Am. J. Surg. *6:*237–239, Feb '29

Dislocation of thumb; surgical treatment. Charbonnel, and Masse. Arch. franco-belges de chir. *32:*229–230, March '30

Boxer's thumb (dislocation). Lloyd-Williams, I. H. Brit. M. J. *2:*9, July 5, '30

Pseudosubluxation of carpo-metacarpal joint of thumb. Kleinhaus, E. Rontgenpraxis *2:*804–806, Sept 1, '30

Old luxation of fifth finger with double pseudarthrosis. Contaidès, X. J. Ann. d'anat. path. *7:*1011–1013, Nov '30

Backward dislocation of metacarpophalangeal joint of thumb. Fèvre, M. *et al.* Ann. d'anat. path. *8:*294–295, March '31

Dislocation of 2 joints on same finger. Scholle, W. Munchen. med. Wchnschr. *78:*1337–1338, Aug 7, '31

Dislocations of 2 joints of same finger; case. Schörcher, F. Chirurg *4:*150–151, Feb 15, '32

Therapy of traumatic dislocations of digital phalanges. Shkurov, B. I. Ortop. i travmatol. (no. 3) *9:*99–103, '35

Cause of irreducibility of metacarpophalangeal joint of index finger in palmar luxation; 6 cases. Scheggi, S. Chir. d. org. di movimento *20:*142–148, July '35

Technic for surgical reduction of palmar metacarpophalangeal luxation of thumb and index finger. Scheggi, S. Chir. d. org. di movimento *22:*281–284, Aug '36

Surgical therapy of dorsal luxation of thumb. Shatunovskiy, L. Y. Ortop. i travmatol. (no. 1) *11:*58–63, '37

Traumatic irreducible posterior luxation of metacarpophalangeal articulation of thumb. Mosoteguy, C. and Sammartino, E. S. Dia med. *10:*462–464, May 30, '38

Dislocations and fractures of thumb and fingers. Trevor, D. Brit. m. J. *2:*461, Aug 27, '38; 583, Sept 10, '38

Minor displacements of phalanges. Cyriax, E. Brit. J. Phys. Med. *2:*21–22, Jan '39

Metacarpophalangeal luxation of index finger; case. Schena, A. T. Dia med. *11:*267–269, April 3, '39

Fingers, Dislocations—Cont.

Dislocations of fingers in children, and fractures. BISSON, C. Ann. med.-chir. de l'Hop. Sainte-Justine, Montreal *3:*36–43, May '39

Habitual dislocation of digital extensor tendons. FITZGERALD, R. R. Ann. Surg. *110:*81–83, July '39

Irreducible buttonhole dislocations of fingers. SELIG, S. AND SCHEIN, A., J. Bone and Joint Surg. *22:*436–441, April '40

Traumatic luxation of extensor tendon of middle finger. MOUCHET, A. Presse med. *50:*455, July 11, '42

Exposed interphalangeal luxations of hand; cases. MALLO HUERGO, E. AND QUIRNO LAVALLE, R. Prensa med. argent. *29:*1367–1370, Aug 26, '42

Dislocations of thumb. ANDERSON, W. D. M. Press *208:*158, Sept 2, '42

Complete compound dislocation, without fracture, of distal joint of ring finger. SALMON, D. D. Radiology *40:*79–80, Jan '43

Recidivating interphalangeal luxation; therapy. GARCIA CAPURRO, R. AND RUSSI, J. C. Arch. urug. de med., cir. y especialid. *23:*134–137, Aug '43

Recidivating interphalangeal luxation; therapy. GARCIA CAPURRO, R. AND RUSSI, J. C. Bol. Soc. cir. d. Uruguay *14:*36–39, '43

Metacarpophalangeal luxation of index finger. NUNZIATA, A. Prensa med. argent. *31:*1760–1762, Sept 6, '44

Luxation of thumb; therapy in rural practice. WERNECK, C. Rev. brasil. med. *1:*782–783, Sept '44

Metacarpophalangeal luxation of thumb; surgical reduction. FERNANDEZ, L. L. Prensa med. argent. *32:*1395–1398, July 20, '45

Screwing as treatment of choice in trapezoid-metacarpal subluxations complicating fractures of thumb of Bennett or Rolando type. FONTAINE, R. AND ECK, F. Rev. d'orthop. *32:*76–80, Jan–Apr '46

Treatment of fracture-dislocation of interphalangeal joints of hand. ROBERTSON, R. C.; *et al*. J. Bone and Joint Surg. *28:*68–70, Jan '46

Metacarpophalangeal luxations of thumb. GIORDANENGO, G. Minerva chir. *1:*92–94, May '46

Treatment of fracture-dislocations of proximal interphalangeal joints of fingers. SCHULZE, H. A. Mil. Surgeon *99:*190–191, Sept '46

Operation for habitual luxation of thumb. VON STAPELMOHR, S. Acta chir. Scandinav. *94:*379–382, '46

Fingers, Dressings for

Combination of cod liver oil and plaster bandage in therapy of injuries with tissue losses of fingers. LÖHR, W. Chirurg *6:*5–11, Jan 1, '34

Practical bandage for finger. BEHNCKE. Deutsche med. Wchnschr. *63:*558–559, April 2, '37

Cod liver oil and plaster of paris cast therapy of injuries of fingers and hand. HERLYN, K. E. Beitr. z. klin. Chir. *165:*278–282, '37

Interlocking finger bandage which needs no anchor. POOL, H. H., J. Michigan M. Soc. *43:*406, May '44

Plaster of paris bandage in therapy of gunshot wounds of fingers. RYZHIKH, A. N. Khirurgiya, no. 4, pp. 65–69, '44

Streamlined finger dressings. DURRANT, M. M. Brit. J. Phys. Med. *8:*88–89, May–June '45

Fingers, Drumstick

Drumstick fingers from freezing. SABATUCCI, F. Policlinico (sez. med.) *28:*233, June '21 abstr: J.A.M.A. *77:*580, Aug 13, '21

Congenital drumstick fingers. LEWY, E. Med. Klin. *17:*845, July 10, '21

Fingers, Fractures

Fractures of fingers and toes. MOCK, H. E. Am. J. Surg. *35:*109, May '21

Fracture of terminal phalanx of finger with rupture of common extensor tendon. BURNHAM, C. Brit. M. J. *1:*141, Jan 28, '22

Traction splint for fractured metacarpals and phalanges. HAWK, G.W., J.A.M.A. *78:*106, Jan 14, '22 (illus.)

Fracture of end phalanx of finger with rupture of common extensor tendon. LAIRD, J. N. Brit. M. J. *1:*101, Jan 21, '22

Treatment of fractures of metacarpals and phalanges of fingers. WHEELER, R. H. J.A.M.A. *78:*422–423, Feb 11, '22 (illus.)

Simple finger splint. FRANKE, F. Munchen. med. Wchnschr. *69:*468, March 31, '22 (illus.)

Fracture at base of terminal phalanx of finger. ZUR VERTH. Arch. f. klin. Chir. *118:*630–644, '21 (illus.) abstr: J.A.M.A. *78:*852, March 18, '22

Fracture of terminal phalanx of finger. BRAIMBRIDGE, C. V. Brit. M. J. *1:*838, May 27, '22

Pathology, prognosis and treatment of fractures of phalanges and metacarpal bones. SCHUM, H. Deutsche Ztschr. f. Chir. *188:*234–272, '24

Fingers, Fractures—Cont.
Apparatus for treatment of fractures of fingers. VALLET, E. Presse med. *33:*590–591, May 6, '25 abstr: J.A.M.A. *84:*1966, June 20, '25
Treatment of finger fractures. LANGE, F. Munchen. med. Wchnschr. *72:*1522–1524, Sept 4, '25
Fractures of bones of hand and fingers. SCHUM, H. Deutsche Ztschr. f. Chir. *193:*132–139, '25
Fracture of finger; bone cyst. THIBONNEAU. Bull. et mem. Soc. de radiol. med. de France *14:*197, Dec '26
Fracture of sesamoid bone of thumb; case. HERZBERG, B. Zentralbl. f. Chir. *54:*1807–1809, July 16, '27
Treatment of fractures of fingers and metacarpals with description of authors' finger caliper. MOCK, H. E. AND ELLIS, J. D. Surg., Gynec. and Obst. *45:*551–556, Oct '27
Compound dislocation fracture of distal phalanx of finger; report of case. BOIES, L. R. Minnesota Med. *10:*773–775, Dec '27
New traction finger splint for fractures. DAVIDOFF, R. B. New England J. Med. *198:*79–80, March 1, '28
Fracture of base of first phalanx of thumb resulting in fragment resembling sesamoid bone; difficulty in interpreting radiograph. MOUCHET, A. AND DESFOSSES, P., J. de radiol. et d'electrol. *12:*331–333, July '28
Treatment of fracture of phalanges of hand. FENGER, M. Ugesk. f. Laeger *90:*935, Sept. 27, '28
New splint for finger tip fractures. ELLIS, J. D. Am. J. Surg. *5:*508, Nov '28
Finger fractures. MAGNUSON, P. B., J.A.M.A. *91:*1339–1340, Nov. 3, '28
Thomas finger splint for fractures. MILCH, H. M. J. and Rec. *128:*473, Nov. 7, '28
Finger fractures. MAGNUSON, P. B. Tr. Sect. Surg., General and Abd. A.M.A., pp. 79–84, '28
Fractures of finger with infections. Physical Therap. *47:*91–94, Jan 26, '29
Fractures of fingers. ELIASON, E. L. Am. J. Surg. *6:*501–505, April '29
Finger fractures, and hand. ADAMS, B. S. Minnesota Med. *12:*515–520, Sept '29
Treatment of finger fractures. FORRESTER, C. R. G. AND MCLEAN, D. R. Am. J. Surg. *8:*384–386, Feb '30
Simplified method of traction for finger fractures. ROBINSON, W. H. Am. J. Surg. *8:*791–792, April '30
Splint for fractures of phalanges. KNOWLES, J. R., J.A.M.A. *94:*2065, June 28, '30

Fingers, Fractures—Cont.
Treatment of fractures of fingers. FENGER, M. Ugesk. f. laeger *93:*169–173, Feb 19, '31
Treatment of fractures, ischemic contractures, cicatricial contractures and nerve injuries to fingers. BRANDI, B. Chirurg *3:*263–269, March 15, '31
Avulsion fracture of flexor side of terminal phalanx of left little finger. BRANDENBURG, E. Zentralbl. f. Chir. *58:*1065–1067, April 25, '31
Extension treatment for fractures of fingers. ADAMS, B. S. Journal-Lancet *51:*283–284, May 1, '31
Avulsion fracture of flexor side of terminal phalanx of left little finger. BRANDENBURG, E. Zentralbl. f. Chir. *58:*1065–1067, April 25, '31
Treatment of fractures of fingers. GOURDON, R. AND JEANNE, H. Bull. med., Paris *45:*321–326, May 9, '31
Safetypin "tongs" for fractured fingers, with report of case FOWLER, E. B. Illinois M. J. *59:*438–439, June '31
New splint for finger traction in fractures. LANGAN, A. J. California and West. Med. *35:*377, Nov '31
Traction with rustless steel wire in finger fractures. HALL, E. S. Maine M. J. *23:*11, Jan '32
Therapy of fractures of fingers and middle hand. MELTZER, H. Chirurg *4:*58–64, Jan 15, '32
Apparatus for treatment of finger fractures by skeletal traction. PAGE, C. M. Lancet *1:*986, May 7, '32
Wire extension treatment of fractures of fingers. MELTZER, H. Surg., Gynec. and Obst. *55:*87–89, July '32
Extension apparatus for therapy of fractures of phalangeal and metacarpal bones. ZAHUMENSZKY, E. Orvosi hetil. *76:*629–630, July 16, '32
Fractures of metacarpals and phalanges. MCNEALY, R. W. AND LICHTENSTEIN, M. E. Surg., Gynec. and Obst. *55:*758–761, Dec '32
Fracture of fingers during baseball game. MUSKAT, G. Deutsche med. Wchnschr. *58:*2032–2033, Dec. 23, '32
Reactions of soft parts and periosteum after fractures without displacement and contusion of fingers. MONTANT. Bull. et mem. Soc. d. chirurgiens de Paris *25:*60–67, Jan 20, '33
Modification of extension treatment in fractures of fingers. CHRISTOFFERSEN, A. K. Ugesk. f. laeger *95:*1239–1240, Nov 16, '33

Fingers, Fractures – Cont.

Fractures of digital phalanges and their treatment. DIVNOGORSKIY, B. F. AND GLUSHCHENKO, V. T. Sovet. khir. *4:*214–226, '33

Fractures of digital phalanges. ZAYCHENKO, I. L. Ortop. i travmatol. (no. 2) *7:*34–48, '33

Fractures of fingers. GHETTI, L. Arch. di ortop. *50:*557-645, June 30, '34

Finger and hand fractures treated by skeletal traction. HAGGART, G. E., S. Clin. North America *14:*1203–1210, Oct '34

Fractures of end phalanges of fingers. DMITRIEVA, AND IORDANSKIY. Sovet. khir. (no. 6) *6:*870–875, '34

Chronic osteomyelitis of spine as result of injury to thumb; case. JORNS, G. Arch. f. orthop. u. Unfall-Chir. *34:*451–457, '34

Healing of 100 consecutive phalangeal fractures. SMITH, F. L. AND RIDER, D. L. J. Bone and Joint Surg. *17:*91–109, Jan '35

Fractures of metacarpals and phalanges. MCNEALY, R. W. AND LICHTENSTEIN, M. E. West. J. Surg. *43:*156–161, March '35

Treatment of fractures of fingers. ROMBACH, K. A. Nederl. tijdschr. v. geneesk. *79:*1112–1113, March 16, '35

Avulsion fracture of terminal phalanx due to pull on flexor tendon. VON OPPOLZER, R. Zentralbl. f. Chir. *62:*2907–2910, Dec 7, '35

Splint for extension and immobilization of digital fractures. LESER, A. J. Zentralbl. f. Chir. *63:*795–797, April 4, '36

Fractures of proximal phalanges; alignment and immobilization. JAHSS, S. A., J. Bone and Joint Surg. *18:*726–731, July '36

Open fractures of fingers and their treatment. Rozov, V. I. Sovet. khir., no. 7, pp. 119–122, '36

Bennett fracture of thumb. WHEELER, W. I. DE C., J. Bone and Joint Surg. *19:*520–521, April '37

Fractures of ungual phalanx of fingers. PERSCHL, A. Munchen. med. Wchnschr. *84:*810, May 21, '37

Pseudarthroses in fractures of terminal phalanx. SCHIFFMANN, H. Rontgenpraxis *9:*394–399, June '37

New type of finger splints (for fractures). MIKKELSEN, O. Ugesk. f. laeger *99:*790–791, July 22, '37

Fractures of proximal phalanx of thumb; treatment. JAHSS, S. A., J. Bone and Joint Surg. *19:*1124–1125, Oct '37

New splint with surface for supporting injured fingers. BOECKER, P. Zentralbl. f. Chir. *64:*2134–2137, Sept 11, '37

Finger fractures. RIDER, D. L. Am. J. Surg. *38:*549–559, Dec '37

Fingers, Fractures – Cont.

Fracture of proximal phalanx of thumb. VERNON, S. Am. J. Surg. *39:*130–132, Jan '38

Simple wire extension for use in therapy of metatarsal and metacarpal fractures and in fractures of fingers and toes. STEBER, F. Munchen. med. Wchnschr. *85:*480–481, March 31, '38

Technic of wire extension in fractures of fingers. THOMSEN, W. Chirurg *10:*145–148, March 1, '38

Treatment of fractures of fingers. FONIO, A. Schweiz. med. Wchnschr. *68:*563, May 14, '38

Fractures of phalanges of hand and metacarpals. ROBERTS, N. Proc. Roy. Soc. Med. *31:*793–798, May '38

Dislocations and fractures of thumb and fingers. TREVOR, D. Brit. M. J. *2:*461, Aug 27, '38; 583, Sept 10, '38

Fractures of phalanges. WIER, C. K., J. Kansas M. Soc. *39:*501–504, Dec '38

Unusual fracture of terminal phalanx. WISE, R. A., J. Bone and Joint Surg. *21:*467–469, April '39

Dislocations of fingers in children, and fractures. BISSON, C. Ann. med.-chir. de l'Hop. Sainte-Justine, Montreal *3:*36–43, May '39

Caliper for reduction of phalangeal and metacarpal fractures by skeletal traction. CARR, R. W. South. M. J. *32:*543–546, May '39

Simple standard apparatus for treatment of compound fractures of hand, fingers and wrist; report of case and evaluation of end result. FOSTER, A. K. JR. Arch. Surg. *39:*214–230, Aug '39

Fractures of phalanges of fingers, with report of cases. CAVALCANTI, J. Arq. brasil. de cir. e ortop. *7:*326–337, Dec '39

Fractures of sesamoid of thumb. SINBERG, S. E., J. Bone and Joint Surg. *22:*444–445, April '40

Therapeutic technic in Bennett fracture of thumb. THOMSEN, W. Chirurg *12:*520–522, Sept 1, '40

Treatment of fractures and dislocations of hand and fingers; technic of unpadded casts for carpal, metacarpal and phalangeal fractures. KAPLAN, L., S. Clin. North America *20:*1695–1720, Dec '40

Tautening arch for wire traction in therapy of fractures of phalanges. URRUTIA, J. M. Bol. y trab., Soc. de cir. de Cordoba (no. 1) *1:*54–58, '40

Fractures of fingers. LAMB, E. D. Journal-Lancet *61:*372–374, Sept '41

Crush fracture of sesamoid bone of thumb. SCOBIE, W. H. Brit. M. J. *2:*912, Dec 27, '41

Fingers, Fractures – Cont.

Fractures of fingers in work accidents. VERGARA, R. G. Arch. Soc. cirujanos hosp., num. espec. pp. 50–56, Dec '41

Two small wire splints for treatment by traction of fractures and deformities of fingers and metacarpal bones. LYFORD, J. III. J. Bone and Joint Surg. *24:*202–203, Jan '42

Modification of banjo splint for finger fractures. WILSON, C. S. Canad. M. A. J. *46:*585–586, June '42

Fractures of metacarpals and proximal phalanges. JAHSS, S. A. Bull. Hosp. Joint Dis. *3:*79–92, July '42

Treatment of fractures of hands and fingers caused by gunshot wounds. GUSYNIN, V. J.A.M.A. *121:*952, March 20, '43

Two small supplementary devices for author's extension apparatus for fractured fingers. THOMSEN, W. Chirurg. *15:*311, May 15, '43

Compound fracture of fingers. SMITH, C. H. Ann. Surg. *119:*266–273, Feb '44

Closed fractures and contusions of fingers; therapy with procaine hydrochloride infiltrations. DIXON, C. W. Clinica, Bogota *1:*139–145, Sept '44

Splint for treatment of fractured fingers requiring traction. SAYPOL, G. M. Mil. Surgeon *95:*226–228, Sept '44

Treatment of fractures of metacarpals and proximal phalanx by skeletal traction. KAPLAN, E. B. Bull. Hosp. Joint Dis. *5:*99–109, Oct '44

Treatment of simple and compound finger fractures; finger amputations. CURRY, G. J. Am. J. Surg. *71:*80–83, Jan '46

Screwing as treatment of choice in trapezoid-metacarpal subluxations complicating fractures of thumb of Bennett or Rolando type. FONTAINE, R. AND ECK, F. Rev. d'orthop. *32:*76–80, Jan–Apr '46

Treatment of fracture-dislocation of interphalangeal joints of hand. ROBERTSON, R. C.; *et al.* J. Bone and Joint Surg. *28:*68–70, Jan '46

Treatment of fracture-dislocations of proximal interphalangeal joints of fingers. SCHULZE, H. A. Mil. Surgeon *99:*190–191, Sept '46

Novel method of digital traction in fractures MACLEOD, K. M. Brit. M. J. *2:*614, Oct 26, '46

Fingers, Grease Gun Injuries

Penetration of tissue (of finger) by grease under pressure of 7,000 pounds. SMITH, F. H., J.A.M.A. *112:*907–908, March 11, '39

Fingers, Grease Gun Injuries – Cont.

Grease-gun finger; 2 cases. BROOKE, R. AND ROOKE, C. J. Brit. M. J. *2:*1186, Dec 16, '39

Wounds of fingers due to jets of oil under high pressure; case with review of cases previously reported. HEPP, J. Arch. d. mal. profess. *2:*565–573, '40

Wound of fingers by Diesel oil under pressure. DE LACERDA FILHO, N. Bahia med. *12:*63–66, April '41

Penetration of tissue of finger by Diesel oil under pressure. HUGHES, J. E., J.A.M.A. *116:*2848–2849, June 28, '41

Grease gun injuries to fingers. BYRNE, J. J. J.A.M.A. *125:*405–407, June 10, '44

Fingers, Infection

Treatment of finger infections of physicians. HONIGMANN, F. Munchen. med. Wchnschr. *69:*160–161, Feb 3, '22

Treatment of suppuration in fingers. HÄRTEL, F. Klin. Wchnschr. *1:*484–487, March 4, '22

Office treatment of acute inflammation of fingers. HENRICHS, R. Med. Klinik *18:*764–765, June 11, '22

Treatment of infections of the terminal phalanges of hand. PROBSTEIN, J. G. AND BROOKES, H. S. JR. J. Missouri M. A. *21:*307–309, Sept '24

Treatment of finger infections. CARTER, R. M. Wisconsin M. J. *24:*312–315, Nov '25

Infected hand followed by loss of power in extensors of fingers and thumb. CORBET, G. G. Canad. M. A. J. *16:*1502, Dec '26

Importance of cellular spaces of hand and fingers in infections. ISELIN, M. Ann. d'anat. path. *4:*603–613, June '27

Distal anterior closed space infections of fingers. CARP, L. Surg., Gynec. and Obst. *46:*484–495, April '28

Phlegmon of flexor tendon of thumb; vaccinotherapy; case. DELBET, P. Bull. et mem. Soc. nat. de chir. *54:*666–672, May 12, '28

Surgical treatment of phlegmons of palms and fingers. EFTIMIE, C. Spitalul *48:*226–227, June '28

Treatment of suppurative arthritis of fingers by resection of joint. ISELIN, M. Union med. du Canada *57:*385–393, July '28

Fractures of fingers with infections. BROOKE, C. R. Physical Therap. *47:*91–94, Jan 26, '29

Phlegmon of synovial sheath of finger; treatment without incision; case. LAROYENNE, AND MEYSSONNIER. Lyon med. *143:*259–261, March 3, '29

Actual surgery in digitopalmar infections.

Fingers, Infection – Cont.
POPESCU, S. AND BUZOIANU, G. V. Romania med. *7:*51–52, March 1, '29
d'Herelle's bacteriophage in paronychia and wounds of hand; cases. RAIGA, A. Progres med. *44:*415–429, March 9, '29
Treatment of synovial and lymphangitic phlegmonata; practical importance of anatomic data on cellular spaces of hand and fingers. PAITRE, F. Bull. med., Paris *43:*1171–1177, Nov 2, '29
Hand infections, and fingers. BECK, C. Am. J. Surg. *8:*301–304, Feb '30
Treatment of acute paronychia. KIAER, S. Ugesk. f. laeger *92:*425–427, May 1, '30
Treatment of suppurations of fingers and hands. SOKOLOV, S. Arch. f. klin. Chir. *161:*89–116, '30
Panaris and phlegmon of hand. LORIN, H. Hospital *19:*416–420, June (A) '31
Therapy of phlegmons of digitopalmar tendon sheaths. VIALLE, P. Arch. med.-chir. de Province *21:*412–423, Dec '31
Mummifying gangrene following phlegmons on finger and hand. BÜDINGER, K. Wien. klin. Wchnschr. *45:*1093, Sept 2, '32
Conservation of fingers in injuries and infections. RICE, E. R. Internat. J. Med. and Surg. *46:*105–108, March '33
Statistics on injuries and infections of fingers and hands based on accident insurance records. JAROŠ, M. Rozhl. v chir. a gynaek. (cast chir.) *13:*270–288, '34
Symptoms and therapy of acute purulent diseases of hands and fingers. ZAYTSEV, G. P. Sovet. vrach. zhur., pp. 422–428, March 30, '36
Method of splinting septic fingers. HUNT, A. H. Lancet *2:*370–371, Aug 15, '36
Infections of fingers and hand. HANDFIELD-JONES, R. M. Lancet *2:*833–836, Oct 10, '36
Relation of suppurative processes of hands and fingers to minor trauma. KORABELNIKOV, I. D. Sovet. khir., no. 3, pp. 488–490, '36
Infections of fingers and hands. BELLO, E. Rev. med. peruana *9:*169–178, April '37
Hand and fingers infections. MONSERRATE, D. N. M. Bull. Vet. Admin. *13:*321–326, April '37
Infections of fingers and palm. KOCH, S. L. Pennsylvania M.J. *40:*597–604, May '37
Pulp-space infection of fingers. HARDMAN, J. Brit. M.J. *2:*156–160, July 24, '37
Atypical osteomyelitis with multiple localizations following metacarpophalangeal suppurative arthritis due to Staphylococcus aureus; case. FRANCAIS, AND BOUROULLEC.

Fingers, Infection – Cont.
Bull. et mem. Soc. d. chirurgiens de Paris *30:*149–156, March 4–18, '38
Infections of hand and fingers. LAKE, N. C. Brit. M.J. *2:*715, Oct 1; 754, Oct 8; 798, Oct 15, '38
Anatomy, pathology and treatment of infections of finger tip and nail. TENDLER, M. J. Memphis M.J. *15:*139–140, Sept '40
X-ray treatment of acute osteomyelitis of fingers; preliminary report. MARCUS, A. AND GROH, J. A. Indust. Med. *9:*551–554, Nov '40
Anterior closed space infections of finger (surgical treatment). MILCH, H. M. Rec. *152:*361–362, Nov 20, '40
Osteomyelitis of ungual phalanges of fingers. OVNATANYNA, K. T. Sovet. med. (no. 4) *4:*18–20, '40
Deep paronychias of hand. GOLDHAHN, R. Ztschr. f. arztl. Fortbild. *39:*319–323, July 15, '42
Acute suppurative infection in flexor tendon sheaths of hand, with particular reference to late results after operation with transverse finger incisions according to K. G. Holm. GRETTVE, S. Acta chir. Scandinav. (supp. 91) *90:*1–63, '44
Septic puncture of fingers in industry. DESPLAS, B. Arch. d. mal. profess. *6:*231–232, '44–'45
Therapy of osteomyelitis of hand and fingers at evacuation hospitals. KONONENKO, I. F. Vrach. delo (nos. 7–8) *25:*341–346, '45
Treatment of suppurative tenosynovitis in fingers. BURT, L. I., M. J. Australia *1:*399, Mar 23, '46

Fingers, Injuries of (See also Fingers, Amputations of; Fingers, Avulsion Injuries; Fingers, Baseball Injuries; Fingers, Boutonniere Deformity; Fingers, Burns of; Fingers, Dislocations of; Fingers, Fractures of; Fingers, Grease Gun Injuries; Finger Injuries, Immediate Skin Grafting for; Fingers, Ring Injuries of; Fingers, Tendon Ruptures; Fingers, Tendon Surgery; Fingers, Vascular Injuries)

Severe industrial injuries to fingers and their treatment. ROMAN, C. L. Canad. M.A.J. *13:*633–635, Sept '23
Strangulation of finger and penis by long hair. GROSSE. Munchen. med. Wchnschr. *72:*1887–1888, Oct 30, '25
Lesions of hands and fingers from aniline pencils. ISELIN, M. Presse med. *35:*467–469, April 13, '27

Fingers, Injuries of—Cont.
Cuts and punctures of fingers; treatment. CADENAT, F. M. Semaine d. hop. de Paris *4:*395–408, July 15, '28
Traumatic deformity "en coup de vent," preventing extension of hand and fingers; case. HANNS, *et al.* Strasbourg-med. (pt. 2) *88:*392, Dec 20, '28
Harmful effects of hot water in open finger and hand injuries. SCHNEK, F. Munchen. med. Wchnschr. *76:*57–58, Jan 11, '29
Wounds of hand, particularly of thumb in miners; statistics. PORCU-MACCIONI, G. Rassegna d. previd. soc. *16:*8–17, Feb '29
Sprains and injuries of fingers. THOMPSON, H. A. Am. J. Surg. *6:*522–523, April '29
Injuries to fingers caused by aniline pencils; surgical treatment. BUZZI, A. *et al.* Semana med. *2:*1064–1068, Oct 10, '29
Arthroplasty of interphalangeal joint for correction of "hammer finger." CAEIRO, J. A. Semana med. *2:*1346–1347, Nov. 7, '29
Treatment of injuries of fingers. STEINDL, H. Wien. klin. Wchnschr. *42:*1631–1636, Dec 19, '29
Removal of foreign bodies from hand, fingers and feet. GOLDBLATT, D. Am. J. Surg. *8:*324–327, Feb '30
Treatment of new injuries of fingers. MELTZER, H. Munchen. med. Wchnschr. *77:*498–503, March 21, '30
Procedure to be followed in treatment of minor injuries and diseases of fingers by general practitioner. HIRSCH, M. Wien. klin. Wchnschr. *43:*883–885, July 10, '30
Restoration of flexion of fingers by Sterling Bunnel's method. DZHANELIDZE, U. U. Vestnik khir. (nos. 56–57) *19:*39–53, '30
Treatment of fractures, ischemic contractures, cicatricial contractures and nerve injuries to fingers. BRANDI, B. Chirurg *3:*263–269, March 15, '31
Diagnosis and treatment of joint injuries in wounds of dorsal surface of fingers. POLLOSSON, AND DE ROUGEMONT. Lyon chir. *28:*227–230, March-April '31
Treatment of serious injuries of fingers. VEYRASSAT, J. Rev. med. de la Suisse Rom. *51:*193–211, March 25, '31
Finger injuries with injury of peripheral nerves. TURNER, G. I. Vestnik khir. (nos. 65–66) *22:*49–55, '31
Advisable therapeutic measures in finger and hand injuries. GOLD, E. Wien. klin. Wchnschr. *45:*308–309, March 4, '32
Therapy of open injuries of fingers. BLENCKE, B. Ztschr. f. arztl. Fortbild. *29:*301–302, May 15, '32

Fingers, Injuries of—Cont.
Rare injury to fingers from bite of monkey; case. FRANKENTHAL, L. Munchen. med. Wchnschr. *79:*1641–1643, Oct 7, '32
Conservative therapy of crushing injuries of fingers. PETROVA, A. A. Ortop. i travmatol. (nos. 3–4) *6:*53–58, '32
Conservation of fingers in injuries and infections. RICE, E. R. Internat. J. Med. and Surg. *46:*105–108, March '33
Sprains of fingers. CARCASSONNE, F. AND DARGENT. Lyon med. *152:*5–8, July 2, '33
Conservative therapy in crushing of thumb and index finger; late result. COGNIAUX, P. AND MARIQUE, P. Scalpel *86:*995–996, July 1, '33
Crushing of right hand and wrist; conservation of useful "grip" formed from thumb and small portion of index finger. DESJACQUES, R. Rev. d'orthop. *20:*315–318, July-Aug '33
Post-traumatic epidermoid cysts of hands and fingers. KING, E. S. J. Brit. J. Surg. *21:*29–43, July '33
Therapy of injuries to fingers and hands. VOGELER, K. Med. Welt *7:*1097–1100, Aug 5, '33
Surgical treatment of injuries of hand and finger, with exception of fractures. SCHMORELL, H. Med. Klin. *29:*1382, Oct 6; 1414, Oct 13, '33
Surgical treatment of injuries of hand and fingers, with exception of bone fractures. SCHMORELL, H. Med. Klin. *29:*1449–1450, Oct 20, '33
Phalangization of metacarpals for functional restoration of hand of workman deprived of all fingers. VENEZIAN, E. Rassegna d. previd. sociale *20:*38–46, Nov '33
Therapy of recent wounds of hands and fingers in miners. BELOT, F. Scalpel *86:*1272–1276, Dec 2 '33
Articular lesions due to crushing of fingers. D'ARMAN, S. Gior. veneto di sc. med. *8:*597–603, June '34
Common injuries to joints of fingers and wrist. BUXTON, ST. J. D. Clin. J. *63:*270–274, July '34
Statistics on injuries and infections of fingers and hands based on accident insurance records. JAROŠ, M. Rozhl. v chir. a gynaek. (cast chir.) *13:*270–288, '34
Traumatic lesions of frequent occurrence to fingers and their treatment, especially after-treatment. WULFF, H. Ugesk. f. laeger *97:*405–411, April 4, '35
Acrodystonia following injury to thumb;

Fingers, Injuries of—Cont.
case. VICTORIA, M. Rev. oto-neur-oftal. *10:*180–183, July '35
Wounds of hands and fingers; immediate therapy. DE FOURMESTRAUX, J. AND FREDET, M. Arch. med.-chir. de Province *25:*341–348, Oct '35
Open method in therapy of finger wounds. and hand. FISANOVICH, A. L. Sovet. khir., no. 3, pp. 28–33, '35
Primary suture in finger injuries. and hand. SHCHERBINA, I. A. Sovet. khir., no. 3, pp. 22–27, '35
Restoration of function of hand after loss of 4 fingers. VAKULENKO, M. V. Sovet. khir., no. 8, p. 135, '35
Extension deformities of proximal interphalangeal joints of fingers; anatomic study. KAPLAN, E. B., J. Bone and Joint Surg. *18:*781–783, July '36
Prevention of hand and finger injuries in industry. VOLKMANN, J. Monatschr. f. Unfallh. *43:*417–425, Sept '36
Instrument for insertion of Kirschner wire in phalanges for skeletal traction. MEEKISON, D. M., J. Bone and Joint Surg. *19:*234, Jan '37
Injuries of thumb. STEINMANN, B. Casop. lek. cesk. *76:*963–965, June 11, '37
Digital injury in infant from silk wool blanket. DETWILER, R. H. Arch. Pediat. *54:*625–626, Oct '37
Treatment of finger injuries. LAARMANN, A. Deutsche med. Wchnschr. *63:*1651–1654, Oct 29, '37
Primary treatment of wounds of hand and fingers. MAZUROVA, N. A. AND MASHKARA, K. I. Sovet. vrach. zhur. *41:*1809–1814, Dec 15, '37
Therapy of finger injuries. HOCKS, A. Deutsche med. Wchnschr. *64:*169, Jan 28, '38
Zoster of left arm following injury to thumb; case. JADASSOHN, W. Schweiz. med. Wchnschr. *68:*93, Jan 22, '38
Wounds of fingers during work. BEVILACQUA, E. Gazz. d. osp. *59:*506–510, May 15, '38
Unusual finger accident. MOORE, T. Brit. J. Surg. *26:*198–199, July '38
Elective traumatism of extensor digitorum and flexor digitorum profundus in injury to forearm; reflex inhibition of extension; infiltration of stellate ganglion; Volkmann contracture; tendinous transmutation. FROMENT, J. AND MALLET-GUY, P. Lyon chir. *35:*623–629, Sept–Oct '38
Functioning false joint of finger following severe trauma. MANGANO, J. L. Am. J. Surg. *42:*659–661, Dec '38
Evaluation of pluridigital lesions (injuries). BIANCALANI, A. Rassegna d. previd. sociale *26:*40–44, Sept '39
Therapy of injuries of hands and fingers. SOUBRANE. J. de med. et chir. prat. *110:*533–542, Oct 10–25, '39
Needle fragments in finger. GOLD, S. Canad. M.A.J. *42:*269–270, March '40
Minor injuries to fingers. CARTER, D. M. Guy's Hosp. Gaz. *54:*142–144, May 18, '40
War wounds of fingers. OLDHAM, J. B. M. Press *204:*476–480, Dec 18, '40
Traumatic implantation of epithelial cyst in phalanx. YACHNIN, S. C. AND SUMMERILL, F. J.A.M.A. *116:*1215–1218, March 22, '41
Finger injuries. BUFFINGTON, C. B. West Virginia M. J. *37:*499–502, Nov '41
Finger surgery; analysis of 1000 cases. SIMON, L. G. Indust. Med. *11:*517–518, Nov '42
Injuries of fingers and hand from point of view of state accident insurance. KONIG, F. Munchen. med. Wchnschr. *90:*509, Aug 27, '43
Industrial injuries to fingers. TOLAND, J. J. JR. AND KORNBLUEH, I. H. Pennsylvania M. J. *47:*466–473, Feb '44
Wounds of fingers (and hand). KAGANOVICH-DVORKIN, A. L. AND RYSKINA, Z. B. Khirurgiya no. 3, pp. 45–48, '45
Trauma to sesamoid bones of thumb. REITZ, G. B. Am. J. Surg. *72:*284–285, Aug '46
Treatment of wounds of fingers. PARK, W. D. M. Press *216:*26–262, Oct 9, '46

Fingers, Injuries, Immediate Skin Grafting for
Thiersch's skin grafting in fresh industrial mutilations of fingers. STOLZE, M. AND MELTZER, H. Chirurg *1:*1068–1072, Oct 15, '29
Skin transplantation in fresh wounds of fingers. BAGER, B. Chirurg *2:*169–171, Feb 15, '30
Primary skin graft in fresh injuries of hand and fingers. BASS, Y. M. AND ZHOLONDZ, A. M. Sovet. khir. (nos. 3–4) *6:*350–357, '34
Immediate flap grafts following trauma (of fingers). DAY, H. F. New England J. Med. *218:*758–759, May 5, '38
Immediate skin grafts on finger injuries. READ, F. L. AND HASLAM, E. T., U. S. Nav. M. Bull. *42:*183–186, Jan '44

Fingers, Mallet: See Fingers, Baseball Injuries

Fingers, Miscellaneous Topics

Transplants in fingers, fate of joint transplants. OEHLECKER, F. Beitr. z. klin. Chir. *126:*135-181, '22 (illus.) abstr: J.A.M.A. *79:*778, Aug 26, '22

Necrosis of terminal phalanx of finger; method of treatment. BEARSE, C. Boston M. and S. J. *197:*1083-1086, Dec 8, '27

Neotonocain (procaine preparation) in surgery of fingers. STEOPOE, V. Romania med. *7:*245, Nov 15, '29

Pseudo-atrophy of fingers or Ledderhose-Secrétan syndrome. BELLELLI, F. Riforma med. *46:*257-258, Feb 17, '30

Opposition of thumb; explanation based on muscular physiology; therapy of loss of opposition. GRÜNKORN, J. Ztschr. f. orthop. Chir. *57:*517-530, '32

Elephantiasis of plastic skin graft on thumb. WICHMANN, F. W. Arch. f. klin. Chir. *169:*783-788, '32

Regional anesthesia with solution of procaine hydrochloride and epinephrine in surgery of fingers. DE ROUGEMONT, J. AND CARCASSONNE, F. Presse med. *41:*218-220, Feb 8, '33

"Tulip fingers". BERTWISTLE, A. P. Brit. M. J. *2:*255, Aug 10, '35

Thumb of man. TROXELL, E. L. Scient. Monthly *43:*148-150, Aug '36

Late gangrene of finger after electrical injuries; case. SCHNETZ, H. Ztschr. f. klin. Med. *132:*120-127, '37

Opposition of thumb. BUNNELL, S. J. Bone and Joint Surg. *20:*269-284, April '38

Hallomegaly; surgical therapy of case. LIMA, E. J. *et al.* Semana med. *1:*1098-1102, May 19, '38

Surgical treatment of pain (painful fingers). TAYLOR, J. Lancet *2:*1151-1154, Nov 19, '38

Fibroid osteitis of phalanx; therapy of case. VOTTA, E. A. Rev. Asoc. med. argent. *54:*299-302, April 15-30, '40

Valgism of third phalanx of finger; therapy of case. MARINO, H. Prensa med. argent. *27:*1798-1799, Aug 28, '40

Diagnosis of skin diseases of hand and fingers. KRANTZ, W. Med. Klin. *38:*29, Jan 9, '42; 54, Jan 16, '42; 98, Jan 30, '42

Excision of ankylosed sesamoid of thumb. MILCH, H. M. Rec. *156:*541-542, Sept '43

Pollex varus; 2 cases. MILLER, J. W. Univ. Hosp. Bull., Ann Arbor *10:*10-11, Feb '44

Mobilization of hand following loss of all fingers. GEYMANOVICH, Z. Khirurgiya, no. 6, pp. 82-84, '44

Functional significance of insertions of extensor communis digitorum in man. KAPLAN, E. B. Anat. Rec. *92:*293-303, July '45

Fingers, Paralysis of

Tendon substitution to restore function of extensor muscles of fingers and thumb. MERRILL, W. J., J.A.M.A. *78:*425-426, Feb 11, '22 (illus.)

Surgical treatment of so-called paralysis of opponens muscle. WEIL, S. Klin. Wchnschr. *5:*650-651, April 9, '26

Loop operation for paralysis of adductors of thumb. ROYLE, N. D., J.A.M.A. *111:*612-May '27

Flexor plasty of thumb in thenar palsy. STEINDLER, A. Surg., Gynec. and Obst. *50:*1005-1007, June '30

Paralysis of extensors of hand and fingers in persons working with lead. TELEKY, L. Deutsche med. Wchnschr. *59:*723-724, May 12, '33

Bunnell operation to repair loss of grasping power of thumb (paralysis of opponens pollicis) after infantile paralysis; case. (transplantation of tendon). INCLAN, A. AND RODRIGUEZ, R. Cir. ortop. y traumatol., Habana *6:*140-145, July-Sept '38

Operation for paralysis of intrinsic muscles of thumb. ROYLE, N. D. J.A.M.A. *111:*612-613, Aug 13, '38

Surgery for opposition of thumb. BUNNELL, S. J. Bone and Joint Surg. *20:*1072, Oct '38

Plastic surgery of flexor tendon of hand, with special reference to paralysis of opponens pollicis. PACHER, W. Arch. f. orthop. u. Unfall-Chir. *40:*93-101, '39

New method (transplantation of flexor pollicis longus tendon) for relief of paralysis of opponens pollicis. SCHECK, M. Indian M. Gaz. *75:*464-466, Aug '40

Surgery of intrinsic muscles other than those producing opposition of thumb. BUNNELL, S., J. Bone and Joint Surg. *24:*1-31, Jan '42

Transplants to thumb to restore function of opposition; end results. IRWIN, C. E. South. M. J. *35:*257-262, March '42

Modified operation for opponens paralysis. THOMPSON, T. C., J. Bone and Joint Surg. *24:*632-640, July '42

Flexion of distal phalanx of thumb in lesions of median nerve. SUNDERLAND, S. Australian and New Zealand J. Surg. *13:*157-159, Jan '44

Significance of hypothenar elevation in movements of opposition of thumb. SUNDERLAND, S. Australian and New Zealand J. Surg. *13:*155-156, Jan '44

Muscle transplants; opposition of thumb. BUNNELL, S. Am. Acad. Orthop. Surgeons, Lect., pp. 283-288, '44

Tendon transplant in paralysis of extensors of hand and fingers; case in boy 5 years old.

Fingers, Paralysis of–Cont.
GUILLEMINET, M. AND DUBOST, T. Rev. d'orthop. *32:*72–75, Jan–Apr '46

Fingers, Reconstructive Surgery of

Plastic operation on contracted finger. RAHM, H. Beitr. z. klin. Chir. *127:*214–217, '22 (illus.) abstr: J.A.M.A. *79:*1726, Nov 11, '22

Treatment of contracture of fingers. CIACCIA, S. Chir. d. org. di movimento *6:*666–684, Nov '22 (illus.) abstr: J.A.M.A. *80:*513, Feb 17, '23

Typical cicatricial bridges between fingers of dairymaids. PICHLER, K. Wien. klin. Wchnschr. *36:*850–851, Nov 29, '23 (illus.)

Contractures of thumbs in children. HAUCK, G. Med. Klinik *20:*1465–1466, Oct 19, '24

Plastic surgery of fingers. MÜHSAM, E. Zentralbl. f. Chir. *53:*585–588, March 6, '26

Flexion contracture of fingers. REICH, W. Zentralbl. f. Chir. *53:*1503–1504, June 12, '26

Plastic repair of finger defects without hospitalization. GATEWOOD. J.A.M.A. *87:*1479, Oct 30, '26

Flexion contracture of fingers. SEBENING, W. Zentralbl. f. Chir. *53:*2526–2527, Oct 2, '26

Plastic surgery of thumb. DEGA, W. Rev. d'orthop. *13:*497–501, Nov '26

Unusual case of congenital naevus of forefinger and thumb. BRAITHWAITE, L. R. Brit. J. Surg. *14:*538–540, Jan '27

Scar contracture of flexor sublimis digitorum. KOVACS, R. Physical Therap. *45:*383–384, Aug '27

Plastic surgery of fingers and hand. SEIFFERT, K. Arch. f. Orthop. *28:*370–375, May 6, '30

Thumb contractures in children. STRACKER, O. Wien. klin. Wchnschr. *44:*197–199, Feb 6, '31

Operation for utilising middle finger as "trigger" finger. DUTTA, P. C. Indian M. Gaz. *66:*676–677, Dec '31

Primary plastic operations on fingers. SCHOSSERER, W. Deutsche Ztschr. f. Chir. *233:*434–440, '31

Syndactylizing fingers preliminary to skin grafting. BETTMAN, A. G. Northwest Med. *31:*70–71, Feb '32

Which finger deformities are more amenable to surgical than to conservative therapy? STRACKER, O. Wien. klin. Wchnschr. *45:*1541–1542, Dec 9, '32

Primary plastic surgery in injuries of fingers, hands and forearms. TUOMIKOSKI, V. Duodecim *48:*393–411, '32

Fingers, Reconstructive Surgery of–Cont.

Plastic reconstruction of fingers by Italian method of skin graft; case. FERRARI, R. C. Semana med. *2:*1104–1105, Oct 12, '33

Cicatricial adhesive contracture of thumb with surface of hand; surgical therapy. SITTERLI, A. Ztschr. f. orthop. Chir. *59:*142–144, '33

New plastic operation for avulsion of skin of thumb; utilization of scrotal skin. MAYANTS, I. A. Arch. f. klin. Chir. *181:*303–310, '34 abstr.: Novy khir. arkhiv. *32:*180–184, '34

Functional therapy of finger contractures. ORBACH, E. Arch. f. orthop. u. Unfall-Chir. *34:*572–579, '34

Phalangeal autografts in restoration of fingers. JIANU, I. Rozhl. v chir. a gynaek. (čast chir.) *14:*122–124, '35

Contracture of fingers due to cicatrices on back of hand. NAPALKOV, N. Ortop. i. travmatol. (no. 6) *9:*43–47, '35

Resection of phalanges as method of treating skin defects of fingers. ZEBOLD, A. Vestnik khir. *39:*204–205, '35

Dujardin-Beaumetz operation in accidental lesions of fingers for functional restoration of mutilated hands. FORGUE, E. Progres med., pp. 305–309, Feb 22, '36

Plastic surgery of thumb and of thenar region. ANGLESIO, B. Boll. e mem. Soc. piemontese di chir. *6:*64–72, '36

Bilateral plastic surgery of second phalanx of thumbs almost severed in industrial accident; functional and anatomic recovery of case. BIOLATO, D. Boll. e mem. Soc. piemontese di chir. *6:*277–285, '36

Plastic restoration for loss of all fingers of both hands. HAAS, S. L. Am. J. Surg. *36:*720–723, June '37

Metacarpolysis in mutilation of thumb; illustrative cases. GARCIA DIAZ, F. Semana med. *1:*658–660, March 24, '38

Plastic surgery of thumb. PALMSTIERNA, K. Nord. med. (Hygiea) *1:*243–244, Jan 28, '39

Covering cutaneous defect after avulsion of skin of thumb. ZAMOSHCHIN, M. B. Novy khir. arkhiv *46:*260–262, '40

Etiology and therapy of contracture of fingers. BECKER, J. Zentralbl. f. Chir. *68:*2070–2072, Nov 1, '41

Full thickness skin grafts in injured fingers; 2 cases. ANDERSON, W. S. Memphis M. J. *17:*23–24, Feb '42

Operation for increasing range of independent extension of ring finger for pianists. BATTY-SMITH, C. G. Brit. J. Surg. *29:*397–400, April '42

Fingers, Reconstructive Surgery of—Cont.
Fusion of metacarpals of thumb and index finger to maintain functional position of thumb. THOMPSON, C. F., J. Bone and Joint Surg. *24:*907-911, Oct '42
Restoration of lost fingers. PARIN, B. V. Trudy Molotovsk. gos. med. Inst. *21:*125-142, '42
Stabilization of articulation of greater multangular and first metacarpal. SLOCUM, D. B., J. Bone and Joint Surg. *25:* 626-630, July '43
Orientation in etiology of permanent retraction of fingers. MAY, J. An. Fac. de med. de Montevideo *28:*675-685, '43
Plastic surgery of flexed fingers; semeiologic and therapeutic study. PEDEMONTE, P. V. Bol. Soc. cir. d. Uruguay *14:*318-344, '43
Plastic surgery of hand; fingers in flexion contracture; semeiologic and therapeutic study. PEDEMONTE, P. V. Arch. urug. de med., cir. y especialid. *24:*249-274, Mar '44
Contracture of fingers and hand following gunshot wounds. FRIDLAND, M. O. Khirurgiya, no. 8, pp. 56-61, '44
Operations for correction of locking of proximal interphalangeal joint in hyperextension. BATE, J. T., J. Bone and Joint Surg. *27:*142-144, Jan '45
Plastic reconstruction of fingers. DZBANOVSKIY, V. P. Khirurgiya no. 4, pp. 92-94, '45
Operation for irreducible contractures of fingers. ZATSEPIN, T. S. Khirurgiya, No. 5, pp. 81-83, '45
Therapy of cicatrices of fingers by "pocketbook" graft. CASCO, C. M. Dia med. *18:*788-789, June 24, '46
Reconstruction of fingers. PARIN, B. V. Bull. War Med. *6:*524, Aug '46 (Abstract)
Plastic operations on thumb. KALLIO, K. E. Acta chir. Scandinav. *93:*231-253, '46

Fingers, Ring Injuries
Method of removing tight ring from finger. BHAVE, Y. M. Indian M. Gaz. *75:*354, June '40
Removal of constricting foreign body (metallic ring). (fingers) IGNATEV, S. S. Vestnik khir. *60:*196-197, Sept '40
String method of removing tight ring from swollen finger. ARBUCKLE, M. F. Mil. Surgeon *90:*184, Feb '42
Ring injuries to fingers. SIMON, H. E. AND ALBAN, H. Mil. Surgeon *97:*506-508, Dec '45
Danger of finger rings in injuries. THOMPSON, C. M., U. S. Nav. M. Bull. *46:*1273-1274, Aug '46

Fingers, Splints for (See also Fingers, Baseball Injuries
Extension apparatus for crooked fingers. SCHMIDT, L. Deutsche med. Wchnschr. *47:*564, May 19, '21
Splint for tendon of extensor digitorum. STAUB, H. A. Munchen. med. Wchnschr. *69:*119-120, Jan 27, '22 (illus..)
Simple finger splint. FRANKE, F. Munchen. med. Wchnschr. *69:*468, March 31, '22 (illus.)
Useful appliances in treatment of common finger injury. WEGEFORTH, H. M. AND WEGEFORTH, A. California and West. Med. *23:*1590, Dec '25
Splint for overcoming contractures of fingers. MONTGOMERY, A. H. Surg., Gynec. and Obst. *44:*404-405, March '27
Use of splints in wounds of fingers. SCHNEK, F. Munchen. med. Wchnschr. *74:*977-979, June 10, '27
Metal finger splints for injuries received in athletic games. GLASS, E. Zentralbl. f. Chir. *55:*601-602, March 10, '28
Metal splint for injuries of extensor tendons of fingers. (reply to Glass) FRANKE, F. Zentralbl. f. Chir. *55:*852-853, April 7, '28
Practical metal finger splint for injured finger. GLASS, E. Deutsche med. Wchnschr. *54:*1121, July 6, '28
Coaptation splint for immobilization of thumb in abduction. LESTER, C. W. J.A.M.A. *91:*96-97, July 14, '28
Value of Böhler's wire-finger-splint in treatment of severe injuries of fingers. FELSENREICH, F. Wien. klin. Wchnschr. *42:*1046-1048, Aug 8, '29
Curved metal finger splint. GLASS, E. Zentralbl. f. Chir. *56:*2459-2460, Sept 28, '29
New finger splint. MYERS, T. Minnesota Med. *13:*840, Nov '30
Treatment of disrupted extensor tendon from terminal phalanx of finger by means of simple splint. DALSGAARD, S. Ugesk. f. laeger *96:*273-274, March 8, '34, abstr: Acta chir. Scandinav. *74:*429, '34
Slow screw extension in contractures of fingers. WOLF, J. Monatschr. f. Unfallh. *36:*447-451, Oct '29
Correction appliance for contracture of fingers and wrist. HOWITT, F. Lancet *2:*1394-1395, Dec 22, '34
Simple instrument for finger extension. BROCK, R. C. Lancet *1:*382, Feb 16, '35
Useful splints for hand and finger. ZUR VERTH, M. Zentralbl. f. Chir. *62:*2270-2274, Sept 21, '35
Practical and easily prepared finger splint.

Fingers, Splints for–Cont.

Andersson, O. J. Svenska lak.-tidning. *32:*1776–1777, Dec 20, '35

Splint bandage with lever in treatment of rupture of extensor aponeurosis of terminal digital phalanx. Saxl, A. Zentralbl. f. Chir. *63:*394–395, Feb 15, '36

Simple and efficient finger splint. Hart, V. L., J. Bone and Joint Surg. *19:*245, Jan '37

Splint for correction of finger contracture. Oppenheimer, E. D., J. Bone and Joint Surg. *19:*247–248, Jan '37

Simple pliable finger splint. Burch, J. E. J.A.M.A. *108:*2036–2037, June 12, '37

New splint with surface for supporting injured fingers. Boecker, P. Zentralbl. f. Chir. *64:*2134–2137, Sept 11, '37

Splint for therapy of lesions of extension tendons of fingers. Rozov, V. I. Ortop. i travmatol. (no. 2) *11:*98–100, '37

Method for skeletal traction to digits. Taylor, G. M. and Neufeld, A. J. J. Bone and Joint Surg. *20:*496–497, April '38

Finger splint for extension or flexion. Shnayerson, N., J.A.M.A. *110:*2070–2071, June 18, '38

Pin and stirrup for finger and toe traction. Reed, E. N., J. Bone and Joint Surg. *20:*786, July '38

New banjo splint (for extension of contractures of metacarpophalangeal and interphalangeal joints). Cozen, L. Mil. Surgeon *85:*67–68, July '39

Tensor and digital tractor (Ferres). Schwartz, M. Dia med. *12:*433–434, May 20, '40

Splints for fingers and thumb. Wheeler, W. I. deC. Lancet *2:*546–547, Nov 2, '40

Finger splint that will not impair hand function. Jelsma, F. Am. J. Surg. *50:*571–572, Dec '40

Extension splint for fingers. Madsen, E. Nord. med. (Hospitalstid.) *14:*1650, May 30, '42

Opponens thumb wire splint. Horwitz, T. Am. J. Surg. *58:*460, Dec '42

Splint for control of ulnar deviation of fingers in rheumatoid arthritis. Bodenham, D. C. Lancet *2:*354–355, Sept 18, '43

Celluloid splint in traumatic amputation of distal phalanges. O'Toole, J. B. Jr. U. S. Nav. M. Bull. *42:*460–461, Feb '44

Splint for correction of extension contractures of metacarpophalangeal joints. Nachlas, I. W., J. Bone and Joint Surg. *27:*507–512, July '45

Improvised finger splint. Palmen, A. J. Nord. med. *27:*1960, Sept 28, '45

Fingers, Splints for–Cont.

Metal finger splint. Packard, J. W. Jr. U. S. Nav. M. Bull. *45:*769–770, Oct '45

Improved finger splint. Charbonneau, L. O. Hosp. Corps Quart. (no. 12) *18:*57, Dec '45

Small type skeletal traction apparatus (fingers). Bond, B. J., U. S. Nav. M. Bull. *46:*124–126, Jan '46

Corrective splint for paralysis of thenar muscles. Napier, J. R. Brit. M. J. *1:*15, Jan 5, '46

Knuckle bender splint. Bunnell, S. Bull. U. S. Army M. Dept. *5:*230–231, Feb '46

Plastic splint for oppenens pollicis paralysis. Cholmeley, J. A. Brit. M. J. *1:*357, March 9, '46

Finger traps for banjo splint. Aldred-Brown, G. R. P. Brit. M. J. *1:*652, Apr 27, '46

Splint for treatment of mallet finger. Schaubel, H. G. and Smith, E. W. J. Bone and Joint Surg. *28:*394–395, Apr '46

Fingers, Spring

Congenital nodules of tendons; etiology of spring thumbs. Van Neck, M. Arch. franco-belges de chir. *29:*924–927, Oct '26

Rupture of tendon of thumb cured by tendinous graft. Dujarier, C. and Bourguignon. Bull. et mem. Soc. nat. de chir. *53:*532–535, April 9, '27

Rare case of tendon rupture of thumb. Suermondt, W. F. Deutsche Ztschr. f. Chir. *201:*400–402, '27

Late rupture of extensor pollicis longus tendon; case. Lülsdorf, F. Ztschr. f. orthop. Chir. *51:*191–199, Jan 11, '29

Treatment of rupture of extensor tendons of fingers. Kaefer, N. Zentralbl. f. Chir. *56:*389, Feb 16, '29

Late rupture of extensor pollicis longus tendon after fracture of radius. Lassen, E. Hospitalstid. *72:*460–464, April 25, '29

Rupture of subcutaneous tendon of thumb; case. Nuboer, J. F. Nederl. tijdschr. v. geneesk. *2:*5645–5649, Nov 30, '29

Treatment of rupture of extensor tendons of phalanges of hand. Silfverskiöld, N. Zentralbl. f. Chir. *56:*3210, Dec 21, '29

Spontaneous rupture of extensor pollicis longus tendon. van der Lee, H. S. and Scheffelaar Klots, T. Geneesk. gids *7:*1141, Dec 13; 1171, Dec 20, '29

Explanation of late rupture of extensor pollicis longus following fracture of radius. Kleinschmidt, K. Beitr. z. klin. Chir. *146:*530–535, '29

Treatment of rupture of extensor tendons of

Fingers, Spring—Cont.

fingers. EWALD, P. Zentralbl. f. Chir. *57:*714-715, March 22, '30

Rupture of tendons of hand; with study of extensor tendon insertions in fingers. MASON, M. L. Surg., Gynec. and Obst. *50:*611-624, March '30

Cause of rupture of extensor pollicis longus tendon in typical fracture of radius. COENEN, H. Arch. f. Orthop. *28:*193-206, May 6, '30

Treatment of rupture of extensor tendons of fingers. HORWITZ, A. Zentralbl. f. Chir. *57:*1463-1464, June 14, '30

Comment on article by Horwitz on rupture of extensor tendons of fingers. GLASS, E. Zentralbl. f. Chir. *57:*2063, Aug 16, '30

Late rupture of tendon of extensor pollicis longus. KHURGIN, M. A. Ortop. i travmatol. (nos. 5-6) *4:*47-50, '30

Treatment of rupture of extensor tendon of terminal phalanx of finger. STRACKER, O. Zentralbl. f. Chir. *58:*727-730, March 21, '31

Late rupture of tendon of extensor pollicis longus following fracture of radius. SIMON, W. V. Zentralbl. f. Chir. *58:*1298-1301, May 23, '31

Rupture of extensor longus of thumb in fractures of lower extremity of radius; case. FROELICH, M. Rev. d'orthop. *18:*584-597, Sept '31

Late subcutaneous rupture of tendon of extensor pollicis longus after fracture of radius and other bone changes in region of injury. HORWITZ, A. Deutsche Ztschr. f. Chir. *234:*710-722, '31

Subcutaneous rupture of extensor pollicis longus simulating partial radial paralysis; case. CROUZON, O. *et al.* Bull. et mem. Soc. med. d. hop. de Paris *48:*1043-1046, June 27, '32

Pathologic rupture of tendon of extensor pollicis longus. BIZARD, G. *et al.* Echo med. du nord. *36:*368-369, July 30, '32

Subcutaneous rupture of tendon in finger injuries. ROMBACH, K. A. Nederl. tijdschr. v. geneesk. *77:*2938-2939, June 24, '33

Functional prognosis in rupture of tendons of fingers. VON ZWEIGBERGK, J. O. Svenska lak.-tidning. *32:*1064-1070, July 26, '35

So-called late rupture of tendon of extensor pollicis longus in connection with wrist fractures. VON STAPELMOHR, S. Nord. med. tidskr. *11:*174-178, Jan 31, '36

Spring fingers and flexion contracture due to blockage of digital tendons. FEVRE, M. Rev. d'orthop. *23:*137-142, March '36

Fingers, Spring—Cont.

Congenital bilateral flexion contracture of thumb (spring finger) in children. REGELE, H. Munchen. med. Wchnschr. *83:*391-392, March 6, '36

Spring finger and Dupuytren's contracture; case in woman. RUIZ MORENO, A. Semana med. *1:*939-946, March 19, '36

Spontaneous rupture of extensor pollicis longus tendon associated with Colles fracture. MOORE, T. Brit. J. Surg. *23:*721-726, April '36

Treatment of subcutaneous rupture of extensor tendons of distal phalanges of fingers. VAN REE, A. Nederl. tijdschr. v. geneesk. *80:*1999-2000, May 9, '36

Subcutaneous rupture of tendon of long extensor of thumb; case. AIMES, A. Progres med., pp. 1533-1534, Oct 3, '36

Treatment of subcutaneous rupture of extensor tendons of terminal phalanges of fingers. KANTALA, J. Duodecim *52:*31-45, '36

Late rupture of extensor pollicis longus tendon; rare and peculiar complication of trauma of wrist. STRØM, R. Norsk mag. f. laegevidensk. *98:*346-359, April '37

Late rupture of extensor pollicis longus tendon following Colles' fracture. BLOUNT, W. P. Wisconsin M. J. *37:*912-916, Oct '38

Subcutaneous rupture of long extensor tendon of thumb; case. CORRET, P. Rev. med. de Nancy *66:*867-870, Oct 15, '38

Late rupture of tendon of extensor pollicis longus after fracture of radius; case. CLEMETSEN, N. Norsk. mag. f. laegevidensk. *99:*1322-1328, Dec '38

Subcutaneous rupture of tendon of extensor pollicis longus; case. ROQUES, P. AND SOHIER, H. Rev. d'orthop. *26:*230-235, May '39

So-called late rupture of extensor pollicis longus tendon after fracture of radius. ARONSSON, H. Nord. med. (Hygiea) *2:*1985-1987, June 30, '39

Rupture of tendon of extensor pollicis longus as sequel of fracture of lower end of radius; case. CAGNOLI, H. Arch. urug. de med., cir. y especialid. *19:*598-603, Dec '41

High "late rupture" of tendon of extensor pollicis longus. VON STAPELMORH, S. Acta chir. Scandinav. *86:*110-128, '42

Subcutaneous rupture of tendon of extensor pollicis longus after fracture of inferior epiphysis of radius; case. MICHANS, J. R. AND GARCIA FRUGONI, A. Prensa med. argent. *30:*1221-1235, July 7, '43 also: Bol. y trab., Acad. argent. de cir. *27:*288-298, June 9, '43 (abstr)

Fingers, Tendon Ruptures in

Rupture of thumb tendon (drummer's paralysis). LEVY, W. Zentralbl. f. Chir. *49:*15–18, Jan 7, '22

Rupture of extensor pollicis longus tendon. DYKES, S. N. Brit. M. J. *1:*387–388, March 11, '22

Rupture of extensor pollicis longus tendon. GARDNER, F. G. Brit. M. J. *1:*476, March 25, '22

Operation for rupture of thumb tendon and fracture of radius. HAUCK, G. Arch. f. klin. Chir. *124:*81–91, '23 (illus.)

Rupture of tendon of extensor pollicis longus following a Colles' fracture. ASHHURST, A. P. C. Ann. Surg. *78:*398–400, Sept '23

Rupture of tendon of long extensor of thumb occurring late after injury. HONIGMANN, F. Med. Klin. *22:*728–731, May 7, '26 abstr: J.A.M.A. *87:*133, July 10, '26

Spontaneous rupture of extensor pollicis longus. BARNES, C. K., J.A.M.A. *87:*663, Aug 28, '26

Subcutaneous ruptures of extensor tendons of fingers. DURBAN, K. Zentralbl. f. Chir. *53:*2773–2774, Oct 30, '26

Blockage of digital tendons causing spring fingers; 4 cases. GRINDA, J. P. Mem. Acad. de chir. *68:*34–38, Jan 14–21, '42

Spring finger due to partial hernia of flexor tendon. BEAUX, A. R. Prensa med. argent. *29:*1694–1698, Oct 21, '42

Simple treatment of spring finger. LASSERRE, C., J. de med. de Bordeaux *121-122:*375–376, July '45

Fingers, Tendon Surgery (See also Fingers, Injuries of; Fingers, Tendon Ruptures; Fingers, Avulsion Injuries

Suture of tendon in hand or finger. KAUFMANN, C. Schweiz. med. Wchnschr. *51:*601, June 30, '21 abstr: J.A.M.A. *77:*653, Aug 20, '21

Repair of tendons in fingers. BUNNELL, S. Surg., Gynec. and Obst. *35:*88–97, July '22 (illus.)

Laceration of tendons of thumb. MOORHEAD, J. J., S. Clin. N. America *5:*170–173, Feb '25

Repair of wounds of flexor tendons of hand. GARLOCK, J. H. Ann. Surg. *83:*111–122, Jan '26

Tendon transplantations for division of extensor tendon of fingers. MAYER, L., J. Bone and Joint Surg. *8:*383–394, April '26

Treatment of wounds of tendons of hand and fingers. ISELIN, M. AND TAILHEFER, A. Gaz. d. hop. *100:*961–964, July 20, '27

Fingers, Tendon Surgery – Cont.

Repair of cut flexor tendons of fingers. ISELIN, M., J. de chir. *20:*531–540, Nov '27

Importance of tendinous union in lesion of extensor tendons of fingers. PRATI, M. Arch. ital. di chir. *17:*597–610, '27

Primitive suture of 2 flexor tendons of fourth finger in palmar region; suture of deep flexor of index in same region; case. TAILHEFER, A. Bull. et mem. Soc. nat. de chir. *54:*827–829, June 16, '28

Section of 2 extensor tendons of fingers; delayed suture; case. BLANC, H. Bull. et mem. Soc. de chir. de Paris *21:*42, Jan 4, '29

Plastic operations on tendon flexors of fingers; technic. BLOCH, J. C. AND TAILHEFER, A. Gaz. d. hop. *102:*5, Jan 2, '29

Modification of incision for reparation of flexor tendons on fingers. ISELIN, M. Presse med. *37:*124–126, Jan 26, '29

Treatment of section of tendons of fingers. CHATON, M. Rev. gen. de clin. et de therap. *43:*289–296, May 4, '29

Evolution and treatment in wounds of tendons of hands and fingers. CAZIN, M. Paris chir. *21:*179–190, Sept–Oct '29

Wound of flexor tendon of thumb; perfect functional cure. BONNET, P. AND MICHON, L. Lyon chir. *26:*849–852, Nov–Dec '29

Suture of tendon of flexor digitorum profundus; case. RIVARD, J. H. Union med. du Canada *59:*28–30, Jan '30

Treatment of cuts of flexor tendons of fingers by tendinous graft. ALBERT, F. Liege med. *23:*1069–1077, Aug 10, '30 also: Ann. Soc. med.-chir. de Liege *63:*18–21, Sept '30

Free tendon grafts in fingers; case. MORRIS, K. A., J. Florida M.A. *17:*161–164, Oct '30

Results of suture of flexor tendon of thumb after healing of wound; case. BONNET, P. AND DELAYE. Lyon chir. *28:*189–190, March–April '31

Functional results of section of extensor tendons of third and fourth fingers; 2 cases. FOGLIANI, U. Policlinico (sez. prat.) *38:*1431–1433, Sept 28, '31

Reparative surgery of flexor tendons of fingers. ISELIN, M. Bull. et mem. Soc. nat. de chir. *57:*1227–1231, Oct 31, '31

Acute suppurative synovitis of tendon sheath following wound of right index finger; excellent function after surgical therapy; case. TIXIER, L. *et al.* Lyon chir. *28:*714–717, Nov–Dec '31

Use of silk in plastic construction of tendons of fingers. COENEN, H. Deutsche Ztschr. f. Chir. *234:*699–709, '31

Plastic replacement of flexor tendons of fin-

Fingers, Tendon Surgery – Cont.
ger. LEXER, E. Deutsche Ztschr. f. Chir. *234:*688–698, '31
Pathologic anatomy and therapy of wounds of flexor tendons of hands. ISELIN, M. Presse med. *40:*606–610, April 20, '32
Section of flexor tendons of middle finger of left hand through palmar wound; primary suture and cure. ANDREASEN, A., J. Bone and Joint Surg. *14:*700–701, July '32
Recovery after late suture of flexor tendon of index finger. CORNET, J. Scalpel *85:*1296–1297, Oct 22, '32
Section of flexor tendons of index and middle fingers in palm of hand. DE LEEUW, E. Scalpel *85:*1269–1271, Oct 15, '32
Restoration of digital portion of flexor tendon and sheath. CLEVELAND, M., J. Bone and Joint Surg. *15:*762–765, July '33
Primary suture of accidentally sectioned flexor tendons of fingers. DE LA MARNIERRE. Bull. et mem. Soc. nat. de chir. *59:*1314–1317, Nov 18, '33
Section of flexor tendons of finger treated by reinsertion; case. LYONNET, J. H. AND MOREDA, J. J. Rev. Asoc. med. argent. *48:*260–264, March–April '34
Result of graft of extensor tendon of left index finger in repair of flexor tendon of same finger. BURTY. Bull. et mem. Soc. d. chirurgiens de Paris *26:*659–660, Dec 7, '34
Technic for repair of flexor tendons of fingers. INTROINI, L. A. Rev. med. del Rosario *25:*1191–1200, Nov '35
Physiological method of repair of damaged finger tendons; preliminary report on reconstruction of destroyed tendon sheath. MAYER, L. AND RANSOHOFF, N. S. Am. J. Surg. *31:*56–58, Jan '36
Therapy of digital wounds of flexor tendons; St. Bunnell operation using tendon graft; technic and results; 14 cases. BLOCH, J. C. AND ZAGDOUN, J., J. de chir. *47:*376–391, March '36
Late sequels of finger tendon sutures. VON ZWEIGBERGK, J. O. Chirurg *8:*243–247, April 1, '36
Therapy of lesions of extensor tendons of fingers. PEDOTTI, F. Helvet. med. acta *3:*161–165, May '36
Reconstruction of digital tendon sheath; contribution to physiological method of repair of damaged finger tendons. MAYER, L. AND RANSOHOFF, N. J. Bone and Joint Surg. *18:*607–616, July '36
Repair of flexor tendons of fingers. THATCHER, H. V. Northwest Med. *36:*259–263, Aug '37

Fingers, Tendon Surgery – Cont.
Repair of laceration of flexor pollicis longus tendon (by faucet handle). MURPHY, F. G. J. Bone and Joint Surg. *19:*1121–1123, Oct '37
Injuries of extensor tendons of fingers and their therapy. ROZOV, V. I. Vestnik khir. *54:*95–105, '37
Management of recent wound of tendons of fingers. ISELIN, M. Presse med. *46:*499–500, March 30, '38
Primary and secondary suture of flexor tendons of wrist and fingers. ROZOV, V. I. Novy khir. arkhiv *41:*490–504, '38
Unusual tendon injuries to fingers; 3 cases. LEVIN, J. J. South African M. J. *13:*29–33, Jan 14, '39
Personal restorative technic of section of flexor tendons of fingers. MONTANT, R., J. de chir. *53:*768–774, June '39
Reconstruction of tendons of fingers. NIKIFOROVA, E. K. Vestnik khir. *58:*255–260, Sept '39
Plastic repair of flexor tendons of fingers. DUBROV, Y. G. Ortop. i travmatol. (no. 1) *15:*66–74, '41
Device for measuring length of tendon graft in flexor tendon surgery. KAPLAN, E. B. Bull. Hosp. Joint Dis. *3:*97–99, July '42
Results of repair of flexor tendons of wrist, hand and fingers. IVANISSEVICH, O. AND RIVAS, C. I. Bol. y trab., Acad. argent. de cir. *27:*576–583, July 28, '43
Division of flexor tendons within digital sheath. KOCH, S. L. Surg., Gynec. and Obst. *78:*9–22, Jan '44
Successful suture of finger flexor tendon. JONES, R. M. Lancet *2:*111, July 22, '44
Use of nylon sheath in secondary repair of torn finger flexor tendons. BURMAN, M. S. Bull. Hosp. Joint Dis. *5:*122–133, Oct '44
Cut tendons of fingers with special reference to flexor tendon cut within its digital sheath. KINMONTH, J. B. St. Thomas's Hosp. Gaz. *42:*154–158, Dec '44
Surgery of divided digital tendons. STONHAM, F. V. Indian M. Gaz. *81:*225–227, June–July '46

Fingers, Transplantation of Toe to Finger or Thumb
Big toe as substitute for thumb. TROELL, A. Hygiea *86:*407–413, June 30, '24
Successful thumb plasty from big toe from opposite side $4^1/_2$ years after unsuccessful transplantation. PORZELT, W. Arch. f. klin. Chir. *135:*340–355, '25
Autotransplantation of toe for traumatic loss

Fingers, Transplantation of Toe to Finger or Thumb—Cont.

of finger. FULD, J. E., J.A.M.A. *86:*1281-1282, April 24, '26

Substitution of great toe for traumatically amputated thumb. HALLBERG, K. Hygiea *90:*452-456, June 15, '28

Transplantation of second toe on stump of thumb. KLEINSCHMIDT, O. Arch. f. klin. Chir. *164:*809-811, '31

Plastic reconstruction of fingers by transplantation of toes. BECK, C. AND BECK, W. C., S. Clin. North America *14:*763-767, Aug '34

Autografts of phalanges of toes in reconstruction of fingers. JIANU, I. Rev. de chir., Bucuresti *37:*761-763, Sept-Dec '34

Surgical substitution of toes for missing fingers. LABUNSKAYA, O. V. Sovet. khir. (nos. 3-4) *6:*503-505, '34

Transplantation of toes for fingers. LABUNSKAYA, O. V. Ann. Surg. *102:*1-4, July '35

Transplantation of toes for fingers. BORISOV, M. V. Sovet. khir., no. 10, pp. 136-140, '35

Late results of transplantation of large toe to replace lost thumb. OEHLECKER, F. Arch. f. klin. Chir. *189:*674-680, '37

Transplantation of toe to replace thumb; Nicoladoni method. DZBANOVSKIY, V. P. Vestnik khir. *55:*626-629, May '38

Total transplantation of large toe to replace thumb. NOVITSKIY, S. T. Vestnik khir. *57:*352-361, Feb-March '39

Plastic reconstruction of fingers by means of transplantation of toes. APETROSYAN, K. A. Ortop. i travmatol. (no. 1) *13:*74-78, '39

Transplantation of large toe to replace thumb; case. SORALUCE, J. A. Semana med. espan. *3:*81-84, Jan 20, '40

Reconstruction of hand and 4 fingers by transplantation of middle part of foot and 4 toes. ESSER, J. F. S. AND RANSCHBURG, P. Ann. Surg. *111:*655-659, April '40

Toe to finger transplant. BLAIR, V. P. AND BYARS, L. T. Ann. Surg. *112:*287-290, Aug '40

Transplantation of toe for missing finger; end-result. NEUHOF, H. Ann. Surg. *112:*291-293, Aug '40

Transplantation of toes for fingers. YOUNG, F. Surg. *20:*117-123, July '46

Fingers, Tumors

Tumors of fingers; with report of cases. THOREK, M., M. J. and Rec. *122:*443-446, Oct 21, '25

Isolated giant cell xanthomatic tumors of fingers and hand. MASON, M. L. AND WOOLSTON, W. H. Arch. Surg. *15:*499-529, Oct '27

Hemangioma of skin of fingers; perforating through epidermis. FRANKENTHAL, L. Zentralbl. f. Chir. *59:*2619-2620, Oct 22, '32

Tumor of neuro-myo-arterial glomus in left index finger; anatomicopathologic and histologic study. COSTA, A. J. Bol. y trab. de la Soc. de cir. de Buenos Aires *16:*1514-1524, Nov 30, '32

Hemangioma of skin of fingers perforating through epidermis. (Comment on Frankenthal's article.) GROSS, W. Zentralbl. f. Chir. *60:*154, Jan 21, '33

Hyperplastic angioma of fingers; 7 cases. DESJARDINS, E. J. de l'Hotel-Dieu de Montreal *2:*99-114, March-April '33

Subungual glomus tumor causing hemihyperthermia; complete cure after surgical removal; case. PAULIAN, D. E. *et al.* Ann. d'anat. path. *10:*271-276, March '33

Angioneuromyomas of tactile region of finger; cases. DE LUCIA, P. Arch. ital. di anat. e istol. pat. *7:*106-112, Jan '36

Congenital irregular hypertrophy of fingers; case due to lymphangiomas. FEVRE, M. AND BRICAGE, R. Ann. d'anat. path. *13:*337-341, March '36

Chondrosarcoma of fingers; case. ALLENDE, G. Rev. ortop. y tramatol. *6:*71-81, July '36

Benign tumors of hand and fingers. DESJARDINS, E. Union med. du Canada *70:*999-1001, Sept '41

Osteochondromata of tendon sheaths; case arising from flexor sheath of index finger. SHEPHERD, J. A. Brit. J. Surg. *30:*179-180, Oct '42

Glomus tumor of fingers; case. LOEB, M. J., J. Florida M. A. *29:*372-374, Feb '43

Glomus tumor or glomangioma of fingers; case. SCULLY, J. C., J. Michigan M. Soc. *42:*118-121, Feb '43

Fingers, Vascular Injuries

Strangulation of finger and penis by long hair. Grosse. Munchen. med. Wchnschr. *72:*1887-1888, Oct 30, '25

Contracture of fingers (ischemic myositis). OEHLECKER, F. Beitr. z. klin. Chir. *149:*333-364, '30

Method of restoring function to finger stiffened by venous phlegmon of hand. MACKUTH, E. Arch. f. klin. Chir. *185:*370-372, '36

Post-traumatic arteriospasms in fingers. MIKKELSEN, O. Hospitalstid. *80:*177-184, Feb 16, '37

Fingers, Vascular Injuries—Cont.
Influence of trauma of small portion of finger pad on rate of blood flow in distal segment of finger. TURNER, R. H. Tr. A. Am. Physicians *57:*182-183, '42
Arterial occlusion in hands and fingers associated with repeated trauma. BARKER, N. W. AND HINES, E. A. JR. Proc. Staff Meet., Mayo Clin. *19:*345-349, June 28, '44

FINK, M. V.: Bilateral burns to eyes; case. Vestnik oftal. *16:*509-510, '40
FINK, W. H.: Surgical management of eyelid ptosis. Journal-Lancet *60:*245-246, May '40
FINKEL, Z. I.: Neurotization of nerve transplants. J. nevropat. i psikhiat. (no. 8) *24:*24-31, '31
FINKELSTEIN, H.: Stenosing tendovaginitis at radial styloid process. J. Bone and Joint Surg. *12:*509-540, July '30
FINKELSTEIN, H. (see HABOUSH, E. J.) Oct '32
FINNERUD, C. W.: Epithelioma of lip. M. Clin. North America *14:*1148-1150, March '31
FINOCHIETTO, E.: Rhinoplasty; result 25 years after operation. Prensa med. argent. *25:*897-901, May 11, '38
FINOCHIETTO, E.; CASTILLO ODENA, I. AND TESONE, J. D.: Aberrant manifestations; retraction of palmar aponeurosis. Prensa med. argent. *27:*1421-1424, July 10, '40
FINOCHIETTO, R.: Exuberance of labial mucosa. Semana med. *1:*1159-1162, May 12, '27
FINOCHIETTO, R.: Instrument for subcutaneous stripping of lengths of fascia lata. Prensa med. argent. *26:*69-70, Jan 4, '39
FINOCHIETTO, R.: Sebaceous cysts of face; extirpation. Prensa med. argent. *30:*1876-1877, Sept 29, '43
FINOCHIETTO, R.: Anesthesia by procaine hydrochloride block of cervical plexus in neck surgery. Prensa med. argent. *31:*1757-1760, Sept 6, '44
FINOCHIETTO, R. AND DICKMANN, G. H.: Technic of local anesthesia for total extirpation of parotid gland. Semana med. *2:*1349-1352, Nov 7, '35
FINOCHIETTO, R. AND MARINO, H.: Plastic surgery of soft parts of chin, with report of case treated by scalp graft. Prensa med. argent. *21:*1672-1685, Sept 5, '34
FINOCHIETTO, R. AND MARINO, H.: Zygoma fractures; with report of 2 cases. Prensa med. argent. *22:*2101-2110, Oct 30, '35
FINOCHIETTO, R. AND MARINO, H.: Progenia (anteposition of lower jaw); surgical therapy. Prensa med. argent. *25:*1087-1092, June 8, '38
FINOCHIETTO, R. AND MARINO, H.: Progenism of jaw; surgical therapy. Bol. Acad. nac. de med. de Buenos Aires pp. 528-537, Sept-Nov '45
FINOCHIETTO, R.; MARINO, H. AND RADICE, J. C.: Histology of harelip. Bol. Acad. nac. de med. de Buenos Aires, pp. 627-636, Nov '42
FINOCHIETTO, R.; MARINO, H. AND ZAVALETA, D.: Extirpation of parotid gland with complete conservation of facial nerve. Rev. med. munic. *2:*790-803, Dec '41
FINOCHIETTO. R. AND TURCO, N. B.: Osteomyelitis of lower jaw, with special reference to therapy. Prensa med. argent. *23:*667-681, March 11, '36
FINOCHIETTO, R.; TURCO, N. B. AND CANALE, A.: Hemiresection of lower jaw; immediate prosthesis with later iliac bone graft. Semana med. (tomo cincuent., fasc. 1) pp. 65-71, '44
FINOCHIETTO, R. AND VEPPO, A. A.: Technic for extirpation of thyroglossal fistulas. Prensa med. argent. *26:*1920-1926, Oct 4, '39
FINOCHIETTO, R. AND ZAVALETA, D. E.: Local anesthesia of distal half of forearm and of hand. Rev. med. y cien. afines *2:*295-297, May 30, '40
FIRER, S. L.: Transplantation of nerves treated with formalin (solution of formaldehyde). Sovet. med. (nos. 4-5) *8:*19, '44
FIRESTONE, C.: Two improved instruments for use in plastic surgery of nose. Laryngoscope *48:*356-357, May '38
FIRESTONE, C.: Positive method for ablation of septoturbinal synechiae. Arch. Otolaryng. *31:*976-978, June '40
FIRESTONE, C.: Cosmetic surgery of nose. Northwest Med. *44:*213-216, July '45
FIRESTONE, C.: Cosmetic reduction of full, everted lower lip. Northwest Med. *45:*499-501, July '46
FIRESTONE, C.: Boiled cartilage implants. Am. J. Surg. *72:*153-160, Aug '46
FIORILLO, J. F.: Extirpation of parotid gland by Duval method. Prensa med. argent. *22:*150-152, Jan 16, '35
FIORINI, J. M.: Phonetic education of patients with palatal fissures. Semana med. *1:*1985-1997, June 21, '34. Comment by FIKH. Semana med. *2:* 735-738, Sept 6, '34
FIORINI, J. M. (see FERRARI, R. C.) July '32
FISANOVICH, A. L.: Open method in therapy of finger wounds and hand. Sovet. khir., no. 3, pp. 28-33, '35
FISCHEL, E.: Rational therapy for cancer of lower lip. Tr. South. S. A. (1929) *42:*306-321, '30
FISCHEL, E.: Treatment of cancer of lips. Colorado Med. *28:*57-61, Feb '31
FISCHEL, E.: Rational therapy for lower lip cancer. Am. J. Cancer *15:*1321-1337, July '31
FISCHEL, E.: Surgical treatment of metastases

to cervical lymph nodes from intra-oral cancer. Am. J. Roentgenol. *29:*237–240, Feb '33

Fischel, E.: Surgery as applied to lymph nodes of neck in cancer of lip and buccal cavity; statistical study. Am. J. Surg. *24:*711–731, June '34

Fischel, E.: Standard methods of treatment of cancer of lips by surgery and radiation. Surg., Gynec. and Obst. *60:*505–512, Feb (no. 2A) '35

Fischer, A.: Operation for hypospadias and defect of pendulous portion of urethra. Zentralbl. f. Chir. *49:*399–401, March 25, '22

Fischer, A.: Reply to Nagel's remarks on my article, "Operation for hypospadias." Zentralbl. f. Chir. *49:*1748, Nov 25, '22

Fischer, A.: Principles of prosthetic treatment in cleft palate. Ugesk. f. Laeger *91:*108–110, Feb 7, '29

Fischer, A. W.: Plastic surgery of anal canal after unsuccessful Whitehead operation. Zentralbl. f. Chir. *61:*157–159, Jan 20, '34

Fischer, E.: New operation for athermoma. Arch. f. klin. Chir. *150:*549, '28

Fischer, H.: Temporo-maxillary ankylosis; case. Ann. d'anat. path. *4:*223, Feb '27

Fischer, H.: Traumatic facial paralysis; treatment by free transplantation of fascia lata. Ann. Surg. *89:*334–339, March '29

Fischer, H.: Congenital preauricular fistula. J. de med. de Bordeaux *59:*711–714, Sept 10, '29

Fischer, H.: Experimental studies on homeotransplantation. Arch. f. klin. Chir. *156:*224–250, '29

Fischer, H. (see Rocher, H. L.) July '29

Fischmann, J. (see Fine, J. *et al*) July '42

Fischer, T. E.: General anesthesia in treatment of maxillofacial cases. Mil. Surgeon *89:*877–892, Dec '41

Fishbein, J. N.: Double-end arrow elevator for nasal plastic operations and submucous resections. Laryngoscope *38:*97, Feb '28

Fishbein, J. N.: Adhesive plaster bandage for plastic operations of nose. Laryngoscope *38:*128, Feb '28

Fishbein, J. N.: Choanal atresia; case. Rhode Island M. J. *14:*180–182, Nov '31

Fisher, A. A.: Removal of accidental vaccination scar by blistering doses of ultraviolet rays. J.A.M.A. *110:*642–643, Feb 26, '38

Fisher, A. G. T.: Principles of orthopedic and surgical treatment in rheumatoid arthritis. J. Bone and Joint Surg. *19:*657–666, July '37

Fisher, A. G. T.: Orthopedic and surgical aspects of chronic rheumatism. Practitioner *143:*286–296, Sept '39

Fisher, D.: Insulin-glucose treatment of shock. Surg., Gynec. and Obst. *43:*224–229, Aug '26

Fisher, D. and Mensing, E.: Insulin-glucose treatment of surgical shock and non-diabetic acidosis. Surg., Gynec. and Obst. *40:*548–555, April '25

Fisher, D. and Snell, M. W.: Treatment of shock with glucose infusions and insulin. J.A.M.A. *83:*1906–1908, Dec 13, '24

Fisher, G. A.; Schauffler, G. C.; Gurney, C. E. and Bendshadler, G. H.: Massive hypertrophy breast (approximate weight 35 pounds) in adolescence; notable case. West. J. Surg. *51:*349–355, Sept '43

Fisher, H. C. (see Burch, J. C.) April '46

Fisher, H. E.: Electric accidents to eyes; shock, burns and glare injuries. Arch. Phys. Therapy *22:*611–617, Oct '41

Fisher, J. A.: Case of sarcoma of eyelids. Am. J. Ophth. *7:*619–620, Aug '24

Fisher, J. E.: Roentgen ray in treatment of skin disease, with special reference to acne vulgaris. Ohio State M. J. *23:*374–378, May '27

Fisher, J. H.: Case of ureteral transplantation (Peters' operation) for exstrophy of bladder surviving 22 years. Brit. J. Urol. *10:*241–244, Sept '38

Fishman, L. Z. and Fishman, V. P.: Plastic surgery for outstanding ears; simple surgical procedure. Bull. Pract. Ophth. *16:*19–21, July '46

Fishman, V. P. (see Fishman, L. Z.) July '46

Fist, H. S.: Dressing for burns. J.A.M.A. *88:*1483, May 7, '27 addendum, 1922

Fitchet, S. M.: Imperforate anus; surgical treatment of cases of maldevelopment of terminal bowel and anus. Boston M. and S. J. *195:*25–31, July 1, '26

Fitzgerald, L. M.: Treatment of acute osteomyelitis of jaws. Dental Cosmos *72:*259–266, March '30

Fitzgerald, L. M.: Diagnosis and treatment of malignancy of mouth. J. Am. Dent. A. *24:*763–770, May '37

Fitzgerald, R. R.: Cleft palate operation supplemented by obturator in treatment. Brit. J. Surg. *25:*816–825, April '38

Fitzgerald, R. R.: Habitual dislocation of digital extensor tendons. Ann. Surg. *110:*81–83, July '39

Fitzgerald, R. R. (see Leigh, M. D.) Oct '36

Fitzgibbon, J. H.: Duodenal ulcer following skin burns; 2 cases with recovery. Northwest Med. *31:*427–430, Sept '32

Fitz-Gibbon, J. J.: Correction of congenital cleft-palate speech by appliances. Dental Cosmos *72:*231–238, March '30

Fitz-Gibbon, J. J.: Fitz-Gibbon's prosthesis for correcting phonetic troubles in congenital cleft palate. Odontologie *69:*760–767, Nov '31

FITZ-GIBBON, J. J.: Cooperation necessary in treatment of cleft palate. Ann. Dent. *5:*143-153, Sept '38

FITZ-HUGH, G. S. (see WOODWARD, F. D.) Nov '42

FITZWILLIAMS, D. C. L.: Nevi in children and their treatment. Practitioner *107:*153, Sept '21

FIUMICELLI, F.: Diathermocoagulation in rhinophyma; case. Dermosifilografo *9:*35-38, Jan '34 also: Minerva med. *1:*228-229, Feb 17, '34

FLACK, F. L.: Fascial space and bursal infections of hand. J. Oklahoma M. A. *27:*314-318, Sept '34

FLACK, H. L.; CLARKE, D. A. AND TICE, L. F.: Preliminary report of new gelatin product used in burns (containing sulfadiazine, sulfonamide)-sulfagel. J. Am. Pharm. A. (Scient. Ed.) *34:*187-190, July '45

Flaps: See Composite Flaps; Skin Flaps

FLARER, F. AND GRILLO, V.: Results of homologous skin transplantation in lepers. Arch. ital. di dermat., sif. *12:*309-325, May '36

FLAX, H. J.: Cod liver oil, sulfanilamide-sulfathiazole (sulfonamides) powder dressing in burns. Bol. Asoc. med. de Puerto Rico *36:*208-214, May '44

FLEISCHER-HANSEN, C. C.: Lesions of tendons and their prognosis with respect to hand function. Nord. med. (Hospitalstid.) *9:*88-98, Jan 11, '41

FLEISCHMANN, A.: New experiences with cleft of face in man and animals. Sitzungsb. d. phys.-med. Soz. zu Erlangen (1937) *69:*315-324, '38

FLEISHER, M. S.: Leukocytic and fibroblastic reactions about transplanted tissues. J. M. Research *42:*163, Nov '20-Jan '21

FLEISHER, M. S.: Immunity in relation to transplanted tissue. J. M. Research *43:*145-153, April-May '22

FLEMING, B. L.: Cystic hygroma of neck. J.A.M.A. *110:*1899-1900, June 4, '38

FLEMMING, C.: Combination of burns and wounds; treatment. Proc. Roy. Soc. Med. *34:*53, Nov '40

FLEMMING, C. W.: Impending Volkmann's ischaemic contracture treated by incision of deep fascia; case. Lancet *2:*293, Aug 8, '31

FLEMMING, C. W.: Plea for simplicity in burn treatment. Brit. M. J. *2:*314-316, Sept 8, '45

FLEMMING, P. N.: Saddle nose deformity. Dis. Eye, Ear, Nose and Throat *2:*244-245, Aug '42

FLESCH-THEBESIUS, M. AND WEINSHEIMER, K.: Pendulous abdomen, surgical treatment. Chirurg *3:*841-846, Oct 1, '31

FLESHER, R. E. (see SIMPSON, F. E.) 1925

FLESHER, R. E. (see SIMPSON, F. E.) Aug '27

FLESHER, R. E. (see SIMPSON, F. E.) May '28

FLESHER, R. E. (see SIMPSON, F. E.) July '28

FLETCHER, E. (see NEW, G. B.) Nov '32

FLETCHER, E. M. (see NEW, G. B.) 1932

FLETCHER, W. M. A.: Congenital absence of abdominal wall. M. J. Australia *1:*435-436, April 7, '28

FLETT, R. L.: Postauricular sinus; case. J. Laryng. and Otol. *53:*458, July '38

FLEURY. (see BERCHER, J. *et al*) Oct '27

FLEURY, R.: Fractures of lower jaw; case. Rev. de stomatol. *32:*84-87, Feb '30

FLICK, K.: Technic for securing large flaps of epidermis. Deutsche Ztschr. f. Chir. *222:*302-305, '30

FLICK, K.: Use of Thiersch skin flaps in treatment of recent wounds of arms. Deutsche Ztschr. f. Chir. *222:*331-334, '30

FLICK, K. AND TRAUM, E.: Plastic method of repairing defects in soft coverings of cranium due to trauma. Zentralbl. f. Chir. *59:*908-909, April 2, '32

FLIMM, W.: Permanent functional results of use of cod liver oil and plaster of paris cast after injury or loss of fingertip. Zentralbl. f. Chir. *63:*2500-2506, Oct 17, '36

DE FLINES, E. W.: Nasal plastic surgery; 7 cases. Nederl. Tijdschr. v. Geneesk. *1:*1984, April 21, '28

FLINKER, A.: Acrocephalosyndactylia; case. Virchows Arch. f. path. Anat. *280:*546-553, '31

FLINT, G.: Partial atrophy of right side of face. Tr. Ophth. Soc. U. Kingdom *52:*308-309, '32

FLÖRCKEN, H.: Treatment of frost-bite. Therap. Halbmonatsch. *35:*430, July 15, '21

FLÖRCKEN, H.: Treatment of burns. Therap. Halbmonatsch. *35:*460, Aug 1, '21

FLÖRCKEN, H.: Operative treatment of scrotal hypospadias. Ztschr. f. Urol. Chir. *10:*119-121, July '22 (illus.) abstr: J.A.M.A. *79:*1187, Sept 30, '22

FLÖRCKEN, H.: War burns. Chirurg *12:*89-92, Feb 15, '40

FLORES, A.: Plastic surgery of simple harelip. Rev. med. peruana *13:*55-58, Feb '41

FLORESCO, A.: Tannic acid in burns. Gaz. d. hop. *100:*1281-1285, Sept 28, '27

FLORIS, M.: Hereditary transmission of harelip. Boll. d. Soc. eustachiana *37:*25-32, '39

FLOSDORF, E. W. (see MUDD, S.) Nov '41

FLUHMANN, D. G. (see CASANUEVA DEL C., M.) Dec '44

FLURIN, H. AND MAGDELEINE, J.: Burns of larynx. Ann. d. mal. de l'oreille, du larynx *46:*1207-1221, Dec '27

FLYNN, C. W. AND DUCKETT, J. W.: Plastic

operations for construction of artificial vagina. Surg., Gynec. and Obst. *62:*753–756, April '36

Flynn, J. E.: Anatomic investigations of deep fascial space infections in hand. Am. J. Surg. *55:*467–475, March '42

Flynn, J. E.: Acute suppurative tenosynovitis of hand. Surg., Gynec. and Obst. *76:*227–235, Feb '43

Flynn, J. E.: Surgical significance of middle palmar septum. Surgery *14:*134–141, July '43

Flynn, J. E.: Medical progress; grave infections of hand. New England J. Med. *230:*45, Jan 13, '44

Flynn, R.: Infections of anterior aspect of hand. M. J. Australia *2:*262–268, Aug 25, '34

Flynn, R.: Hypospadias treated by Ombredanne technic. M. J. Australia *2:*479, Sept 18, '37

Flynn, R.: Restoration of scalp avulsion. M. J. Australia *2:*525–526, Sept 25, '37

Flynn, R.: Suggested aid in treatment of cleft palate in older children or adults. Australian and New Zealand J. Surg. *8:*82–84, July '38

Flynn, R.: Plastic reconstruction of cheek after extensive epithelioma. M. J. Australia *1:*555–556, May 9, '42

Flynn, S. E.: Insulin in burn therapy. U. S. Nav. M. Bull. *38:*538–540, Oct '40

Foa, C.: Substitutes for human plasma in combatting shock. Resenha clin.-cient. *13:*157–169, April 1, '44

Fogh-Andersen, Poul (See also Andersen, Fogh and Andersen, V. F.)

Fogh-Andersen, Poul: *Inheritance of Harelip and Cleft Palate*. NYT Nordisk Forlag, Arnold Busch, Copenhagen, 1942

Focosi, M.: Case of malformation from persistence of oblique fissure of face; method of plastic reparation. Boll. d'ocul. *17:*255–269, April '38

Foged, J.: Operative treatment of breast hypertrophy. Bibliot. f. Laeger *119:*xlvii–lvi, Feb '27

Foged, J.: Plastic surgery of breast hypertrophy. Nord. med. tidskr. *8:*954–961, July 21, '34

Foged, J.: Surgical therapy of prognathism. Hospitalstid. (Supp., Festskr. Bisp. Hosp.) *81:*55–83, '38

Fogliani, U.: Functional results of section of extensor tendons of third and fourth fingers; 2 cases. Policlinico (sez. Prat.) *38:*1431–1433, Sept 28, '31

Fohl, T.: Transplantation of cartilage; experiments. Arch. f. klin. Chir. *155:*232–243, '29

Fohl, T. and Killian, H.: Plastic surgery by Rehn's method of shifting soft parts to cover defect of face. Deutsche Ztschr. f. Chir. *222:*309–320, '30

Fohr, O.: Construction of artificial vagina; mortality rate. Zentralbl. f. Gynak. *45:*1332, Sept 17, '21 abstr: J.A.M.A. *77:*2154, Dec 31, '21

Foley, F. A. (see Schwab, W. J.) Aug '44

Folk, M. L.: Plastic surgery of orbit. Illinois M. J. *70:*419–424, Nov '36

Folliasson, A. and Béchet, A.: Phlegmon of superficial palmar space; method of therapy; case. Ann. d'anat. path. *9:*825–826, July '32

Follmann, E.: Epithelioma of nose in girl of 15. Dermat. Wchnschr. *85:*940–943, July 2, '27

Fomon, S.: Treatment of old unreduced nasal fractures. Ann. Surg. *104:*107–117, July '36

Fomon, S.: Surgical treatment of idiopathic breast hypertrophy. Arch. Surg. *33:*253–266, Aug '36

Fomon, Samuel: *The Surgery of Injury and Plastic Repair*. Wm. Wood and Co., New York, 1939

Fomon, S.: Role of plastic surgery in field of otolaryngology. Arch. Otolaryng. *39:*518–520, June '44

Fomon, S. *et al*: Rhinoplastic analysis. Eye, Ear, Nose and Throat Monthly *24:*19–24, Jan '45

Fomon, S. *et al*: Cancellous bone transplants for correction of saddle nose. Ann. Otol. Rhin.and Laryng. *54:*518–533, Sept '45

Fomon, S. *et al*: Plastic repair of deflected septum of nose. Arch. Otolaryng. *44:*141–156, Aug '46

Fomon, S. (see Gorney, H. S. *et al*) May '42

Fonio, A.: Treatment of fractures of fingers. Schweiz. med. Wchnschr. *68:*563, May 14, '38

Fonseca e Castro: Treatment of lymphangiomas with sclerosing injections of sodium citrate; cases. Arch. de med. d. enf. *41:*798–802, Dec '38

Fontaine, R. and Eck, F.: Screwing as treatment of choice in trapezoidmetacarpal subluxations complicating fractures of thumb of Bennett or Rolando type. Rev. d'orthop. *32:*76–80, Jan–Apr '46

Fontaine, R. (see Leriche, R.) April '28

Fontaine, R. (see Leriche, R.) Sept '28

Fontaine, R. (see Leriche, R.) Jan–Feb '33

Fontaine, R. (see Leriche, R. *et al*) May '35

Fontaine, R. (see Simon, R. *et al*) March '25

Fonts, E.: Deductions from 191 cases of cancer of lips. Bol. de la Liga contra el cancer *3:*4–9, Jan 1, '28

Foot

Reconstructive surgery of traumatic foot and ankle deformities. COTTON, A. J. Orthop. Surg. *3:*196, May '21

Congenital deformity of hands and feet. GAZZOTTI, L. G. Chir. d. org. di movimento *6:*265-280, July '22 (illus.) abstr: J.A.M.A. *79:*1084, Sept 23, '22

Congenital ankylosis of joints of hands and feet. MILLER, E. M., J. Bone and Joint Surg. *4:*560-569, July '22 (illus.)

Two cases of congenital deformities of hands and feet. SMITH, N. F. Lancet *1:*802, April 19, '24

Loss of tendo achillis and overlying soft tissues by trauma; plastic reconstruction. JONES, H. T., S. Clin. N. Amer. *7:*1452-1456, Dec '27

Transplantation of skin in amputations of foot. BLENCKE, A. Zentralbl. f. Chir. *56:*2050-2054, Aug 17, '29

Factors in foot reconstruction. CARLTON, C. H. Lancet *2:*605-606, Sept 21, '29

Loss of substance of sole of foot; treatment by autoplastic grafts from ischiatic region. COSTANTINI, H. AND CURTILLET, É. Rev. de chir., Paris *67:*515-539, '29

Rare congenital osseous abnormalities of hands and feet in same patient; case. TESCOLA, C. Riv. di radiol. e fis. med. *5:*570-576, '31

Abnormalities of hands and feet. KOENNER, D. M., J. Hered. *25:*329-334, Aug '34

Congenital malformations of hands and feet; roentgen study of 12 cases. ZUPPA, A. Pediatria *42:*943-966, Aug '34

Plastic reparation of heel by grafts. FERRÉ, R. L. Semana med. *2:*2049-2053, Dec 27. '34

Plantar warts, flaps and grafts. BLAIR, V. P. *et al.* J.A.M.A. *108:*24-27, Jan 2, '37

Pedicle graft of sole of foot. WHITE, W. C. Ann. Surg. *105:*472-473, March '37

Complete syndactylia of hands and feet associated with other deformities; case. LICEAGA, F. J. Arch. de med. d. enf. *40:*448-452, July '37 Abstr.: Bull. Soc. de pediat. de Paris *35:*141-146, Feb '37

Congenital deformities of hands and feet (case). CALLUM, E. N. Brit. M. J. *2:*991, Nov 12, '38

Typical combination of congenital abnormalities of hand and foot. BRAUN, K. Ztschr. f. menschl. Vererb.-u. Konstitutionslehre *23:*510-515, '39

Origin and nature of certain malformations of face, head and foot. KEITH, A. Brit. J. Surg. *28:*173-192, Oct '40

Foot—Cont.

Secondary plastic surgery of soles and restoration of soft tissues. KRASOVITOV, V. K. Vestnik khir. *60:*593-598, Dec '40

Dupuytren's contracture in both hands and both feet. HOHMANN, G. Ztschr. f. Orthop. *73:*45, '41

Therapy of neuropathic ulcers of foot (mal perforant) by implantation of sensory nerves. NORDMANN, O. Chirurg *14:*116-122, Feb 15, '42

Late evolution in case of "scalping" of heel (with skin grafting). LANDIVAR, A. F. AND IPARRAGUIRRE, C. A. Dia med. *14:*202-203, March 16, '42

Indications, technic and results of skin grafting in third degree frostbite of foot. MARZIANI, R. Boll. e mem. Soc. piemontese chir. *12:*277-279, '42

Treatment of perforating ulcer of foot. MUIR, E. Leprosy Rev. *14:*49, July '43

Total loss of skin and subcutaneous cellular tissue of heel; monopedicled graft; case. PEDEMONTE, P. V. Arch. urug. de med., cir. y especialid. *23:*154-157, Aug '43

Total loss of skin and of subcutaneous cellular tissue of heel; monopedicled graft; case. PEDEMONTE, P. V. Bol. Soc. cir. d. Uruguay *14:*57-60, '43

Ankylosing operations in therapy of hallux rigidus; after-examination. STAHL, F. Acta orthop. Scandinav. *14:*97-126, '43

Congenital malformations of hands and feet. DE SOUSA DIAS, A. GONCALO. Amatus *3:*325-329, May '44

Use of untubed pedicle grafts in repair of deep defects of foot and ankle; technic and results. GHORMLEY, R. K. AND LIPSCOMB, P. R., J. Bone and Joint Surg. *26:*483-488, July '44

Retractile cicatrix causing pes planopronatovalgus; plastic surgery in therapy of case. ZENO, L. An. de cir. *10:*179-182, Sept-Dec '44

Repair of surface defects of foot. BROWN, J. B. AND CANNON, B. Ann. Surg. *120:*417-430, Oct '44

Repair of surface defects of foot. BROWN, J. B. AND CANNON, B. Tr. Am. S. A. *62:*417-430, '44

Repair of deep skin defects of foot and ankle. GHORMLEY, R. K. Am. Acad. Orthop. Surgeons, Lect., pp. 107-112, '44

Cleft foot. GOTTLIEB, A. West. J. Surg. *53:*157-158, May '45

FOOT – Cont.
Ulcer of dorsum pedis; free graft on granulation tissue. FERNANDEZ, L. L. Prensa med. argent. *32:*1601–1604, Aug 17, '45
Reconstructive surgery in patients with war fractures of ankle and foot. SNEDECOR, S. T. J. Bone and Joint Surg. *28:*332–342, Apr '46
Early covering of extensive traumatic deformities of hand and foot. MCDONALD, J. J. AND WEBSTER, J. P. Plast. and Reconstruct. Surg. *1:*49–57, July '46

FOOTE, J. A.: Malnutrition in infants with cleft palate, with description of new external obturator. Am. J. Dis. Child. *30:*343–346, Sept '25
FORBES, A. M.: Cleft palate; clinical study of method for its treatment. Canad. M. A. J. *17:*76–78, Jan '27
FORBES, A. M.: Cleft palate. Surg., Gynec. and Obst. *47:*707–709, Nov '28
FORBES, G.: Case of congenital clubhand (and absence of radius) with review of etiology of condition. Anat. Rec. *71:*181–199, June 25, '38
FORBES, S. B.: General anesthesia for nasal surgery. South. M. J. *23:*305–308, April '30
FORD, J. F.: Fundamental principles of plastic surgery including grafts (face). Texas State J. Med. *30:*761–763, April '35
FORD, J. F.: Plastic operation for lengthening congenitally short upper lip; preliminary report. J. Oral Surg. *2:*260–265, July '44
FORD, R. (see BAILEY, O. T.) Nov '46
FORERO, A.: Technic of cosmetic surgery of nose. Semana med. *2:*1461–1474, Nov 21, '29
FORERO, A.: Plastic surgery of nose. Semana med. *1:*187–191, Jan 15, '31
FORERO, A.: Plastic surgery in correction of crooked noses; technic and report of cases. Semana med. *2:*1631–1637, Dec 1, '32
FORERO, A.: Question of age for operating on simple or complicated harelip. Rev. argent. de oto-rino-laring. *8:*191–206, May–June '39
FORESTIER, J. (see COSTE, F. *et al*) May '37
FORGUE, E.: Question of advantages of use of loop of small intestine, of segment of rectum or Thiersch grafts in colpoplasty for congenital absence of vagina. Paris med. *2:*479–486, Dec 15, '34
FORGUE, E.: Dujardin-Beaumetz operation in accidental lesions of fingers for functional restoration of mutilated hands. Progres med., pp. 305–309, Feb 22, '36
FORMBY, R. H.: Shock; treatment in the field. M. J. Australia *1:*357–368, April 22, '44
FORNARI, G. B.: Study of keloids, with description of case of cicatricial keloid in mastoid area. Oto-rino-laring. ital. *4:*552–565, Nov '34
FORNELL, C. H.: Resector for removing shaped piece of rib cartilage for nasal transplant. Laryngoscope *38:*733–734, Nov '28
FORRESTER, C. R. G.: Author's method for repair of ankylosed joint of hand. Am. J. Surg. *33:*101–103, July '36
FORRESTER, C. R. G.: End results of early and delayed suture of tendon wounds. Am. J. Surg. *39:*552–556, March '38
FORRESTER, C. R. G.: Peripheral nerve injuries, with results of early and delayed suture. Am. J. Surg. *47:*555–572, March '40
FORRESTER, C. R. G. AND MCLEAN, D. R.: Treatment of finger fractures. Am. J. Surg. *8:*384–386, Feb '30
FORRESTER-BROWN, M. F.: Possibilities of suture after extensive nerve injury. J. Orthop. Surg. *3:*277, June '21
FORRESTER-BROWN, M. F.: Study of some methods of bone-grafting. Brit. J. Surg. *9:*179, Oct '21
FORSHELL, Y. P.: Exstrophy of bladder; surgery and later complications; case. Acta path. et microbiol. Scandinav., supp. 16, pp. 350–357, '33
FORSTER, W.: Tetanus after burn from high power current. Munchen. med. Wchnschr. *68:*1655, Dec 23, '21
FORT, F. T.: Malignancy of face and jaws. Kentucky M. J. *19:*456, Aug '21
FOSSATARO, E.: To prevent disability after trauma of hand. Policlinico (sez. chir.) *28:*1, Jan '21 abstr: J.A.M.A. *76:*968, April 2, '21
FOSSATI, A.: Elephantiasis of penis and scrotum; study apropos of case treated surgically. Bol. Soc. cir. d. Uruguay *14:*355–364, '43
FOSSATI, A.: Elephantiasis of penis and scrotum; clinical study of case treated surgically. Arch. urug. de med., cir. y especialid. *24:*285–294, March '44
FOSTER, A. D. JR.; NEUMANN, C. AND ROVENSTINE, E. A.: Peripheral circulation during anesthesia, shock and hemorrhage; digital plethysmograph as clinical guide. Anesthesiology *6:*246–257, May '45
FOSTER, A. K. JR.: Simple standard apparatus for treatment of compound fractures of hand, fingers and wrist; report of case and evaluation of end result. Arch. Surg. *39:*214–230, Aug '39
FOSTER, A. K. JR.: Severe facial injuries; diagnosis and treatment. Am. J. Surg. *48:*391–397, May '40
FOSTER, G. C.: Structive surgery as carried on in North Dakota. Journal-Lancet *63:*62–66, March '43
FOSTER, G. V.: Ureteral transplantations in exstrophy of bladder. Pennsylvania M. J. *39:*874–877, Aug '36

FOSTER, G. S.: Surgical shock. J. Missouri M. A. *28:*424–427, Sept '31

FOSTER, J.: Reconstruction of lower eyelid by Hughes method. Brit. J. Ophth. *28:*515–519, Oct '44

FOSTER, J. H.: Autoplastic grafts in facial palsy. Ann. Otol., Rhin. and Laryng. *44:*521–526, June '35

FOSTER, W. J.: Mallet finger. Brit. M. J. *1:*226, Feb 11, '22

FOTIADE, V.: Burns of larynx from swallowing sodium hydroxide; 2 cases. Arch. internat. de laryng. *34:*22–30, Jan '28

FOUCAR, H. O.: Harelip. Canad. M. A. J. *28:*373–376, April '33

FOUCAR, H. O.: Congenital abnormalities (with surgical therapy of prominent ear). Canad. M. A. J. *43:*26–27, July '40

FOUCHE, F. P.: Reconstruction surgery of Imperial and Union Defense Force. Am. Acad. Orthop. Surgeons, Lect. pp. 542–546, '44

FOULDS, G. S.: Historical data on ureteral transplantation in exstrophy; Peters operation. Am. J. Surg. *22:*217–219, Nov '33

FOULDS, G. S. AND ROBINSON, T. A.: Late results of Peters operation for exstrophy. Brit. J. Urol. *4:*20–26, March '32

FOULDS, G. S. (see ROBINSON, T. A.) Jan '27

DE FOURMESTRAUX, J. AND FREDET, M.: Wounds of hands and fingers; immediate therapy. Arch. med.-chir. de Province *25:*341–348, Oct '35

Fournier's Syndrome

Spontaneous gangrene (Fournier's gangrene). MANSFIELD, O. T. Brit. J. Surg. *33:*275–277, Jan '46

Foville Syndrome

Operations on eyelids in Foville syndrome; case. COPPEZ, J. H., J. belge de neurol. et de psychiat. *35:*206–208, April '35

FOWLER, A.: Case showing anatomical and functional reproduction of metacarpal by bone-graft. Brit. J. Surg. *14:*675–676, April '27

FOWLER, E. B.: Safetypin "tongs" for fractured fingers, with report of case. Illinois M. J. *59:*438–439, June '31

FOWLER, F. E. (see WAFFLE, E. B.) March '26

FOWLER, L. H. AND HANSON, W. A.: Megacolon, with report of traumatic case (anal stricture due to burn), treated by left lumbar sympathectomy. Minnesota Med. *18:*646–655, Oct '35

FOWLER, S. B. (see BROCKWAY, A.) Aug '42

FOX, C.: Maxillofacial injuries. Mil. Surgeon *90:*61–72, Jan '42 Also: Am. J. Orthodontics (Oral Surg. Sect) *28:*202–212, April '42

FOX, C. L.: Sulfonamides in war wounds and burns. Spec. Libraries *34:*244–247, July–Aug '43

FOX, C. L. JR.: Sulfonamides in treatment of war burns. Smithsonian Inst. Annual Rep. (1943) pp. 569–574, '44

FOX, C. L. JR.: Oral sodium lactate in burn shock. J.A.M.A. *124:*207–212, Jan 22, '44

FOX, C. L. JR. AND KESTON, A. S.: Mechanism of shock from burns and trauma traced with radiosodium. Surg., Gynec. and Obst. *80:*561–567, June '45

FOX, C. L. JR. (see BULLOWA, J. G. M.) 1943

FOX, E. C.: Therapy of birthmarks. Urol. and Cutan. Rev. *40:* 20–823, Nov '36

FOX, H. R. (see REUBEN, M. S.) Feb '28

FOX, M. S.: Congenital aural fistula. Arch. Otolaryng. *35:*431–433, March '42

FOX, S. A.: Methods of repair and reconstruction (eyelids). Am. J. Ophth. *29:*452–458, Apr '46

FOX, S. L.: Nasal fractures. Eye, Ear, Nose and Throat Monthly *24:*286–287, June '45

FOX, S. L. (see COHEN, L.) Oct '43

FOX, T. A.: Newer concepts, with suggestions for management of wartime thermal injuries. U. S. Nav. M. Bull. *40:*557–570, July '42

FOX, T. A.: Newer concepts, with suggestions for management of wartime thermal injuries. J. Lab. and Clin. Med. *28:*474–484, Jan '43

FOX, T. A. AND APFELBACH, G. L.: Prevention of decubitus ulcers in fractures. J.A.M.A. *115:*1438–1439, Oct 26, '40

FRAENKEL, L.: Artificial vagina made from skin. Zentralbl. f. Gynak. *48:*193–197, Feb 9, '24

FRAENKEL, L.: Plastic surgery of hypertrophy of breast; case. Zentralbl. f. Gynak. *56:*1506–1510, June 17, '32

FRAMPTON, W. H.: Burn therapy. Indust. Med. *6:*501–503, Sept '37

FRANCAIS, AND BOUROULLEC.: Atypical osteomyelitis with multiple localizations following metacarpophalangeal suppurative arthritis due to Staphylococcus aureus; case. Bull. et mem. Soc. d. chirurgiens de Paris *30:*149–156, March 4–18, '38

FRANCESCHETTI, A.: Chronic dacryocystitis due to fistula resulting from maxillary sinusitis; case. Bull. et mem. Soc. franc. d'opht. *48:*27–34, '35

FRANCESCHETTI, A.: New syndrome; mandibulofacial dysostosis. Bull. schweiz. Akad. d. med. Wissensch. *1:*60–66, '44

FRANCESCHETTI, A. AND VALERIO, M.: Associated malformations of eyes and ears. Confinia neurol. *6:*255–257, '45

FRANCESCHELLI, N.: Behavior of bone transplants; clinical and anatomicopathologic study. Arch. di orthop. *55:*297–320, Sept 30, '39

FRANCHINI, Y. AND RICCITELLI, E.: Congenital angiomas with nasofacial localization; case. An. de oto-rino-laring. d. Uruguay *3:*193–203, '33

FRANCILLON, J. (see RICARD, A. *et al*) Jan-Feb '45

FRANCIS, A. E.: Streptococci resistant to sulfonamide (sulfanilamide and its derivatives) in plastic ward (local application of gramicidin). Lancet *1:*408–409, April 4, '42

FRANCISCO, C. B.: Tendon shifting and tendon transplantation. J. Kansas M. Soc. *27:*274–275, Aug '27

FRANCK, A.: Trifid ureter and epispadias in girl 10 years old. Bull. Soc. franc. d'urol., pp. 107–112, Feb 20, '33

FRANCON, F. (see WEISSENBACH, R. J.) May '31

FRANCON, F. (see WEISSENBACH, R. J.) March '41

FRANGENHEIM, P.: Treatment of congenital fistula of neck. Zentralbl. f. Chir. *57:*259–260, Feb 1, '30

FRANK, H. A.; SELIGMAN, A. M. AND FINE, J.: Traumatic shock; treatment of hemorrhagic shock irreversible to replacement of blood volume deficiency. J. Clin. Investigation *24:*435–444, July '45

FRANK, H. A. (see FINE, J. *et al*) July '42

FRANK, H. A. (see FINE, J. *et al*) Oct '45

FRANK, I.: Recent nasal fractures. Ann. Otol., Rhin. and Laryng. *32:*768—779, Sept '23

FRANK, I. AND STRAUSS, J. S.: An invisible scar method in cosmetic nasal surgery. Ann. Otol., Rhinol. and Laryng. *30:*670, Sept '21

FRANK, L. W.: Congenital defects of lips and mouth. Kentucky M. J. *24:*331-335, July '26

FRANK, L. W.: Cancer of lip and intra-oral mucous membrane. South. Surgeon *4:*444–456, Dec '35

FRANK, M.: Artificial vagina in case of external male pseudohermaphroditism. Monatschr. f. Geburtsh. u. Gynak. *55:*5, July '21 abstr: J.A.M.A. *77:*1215, Oct 8, '21

FRANK, P.: Evaluation of submucous resection; points as to technic. M. Rec. *146:*469–470, Dec 1, '37

FRANK, R. T.: Formation of artificial vagina (Frank-Geist method). S. Clin. North America *12:*305–310, April '32

FRANK, R. T.: Artificial vagina formation without operation. Am. J. Obst. and Gynec. *35:*1053–1055, June '38

FRANK, R. T.: Formation of artificial vagina without operation (by intubation method). New York State J. Med. *40:*1669–1670, Nov 15, '40

FRANK, R. T.: Evolution of treatment for absent vagina. J. Mt. Sinai Hosp. *7:*259–262, Jan-Feb '41

FRANK, R. T. AND GEIST, S. H.: Artificial vagina formation by new plastic technic. Am. J. Obst. and Gynec. *14:*712–718, Dec '27

FRANK, R. T. AND GEIST, S. H.: Additional reports on satchel handle operation for artificial vagina. Am. J. Obst. and Gynec. *23:*256–258, Feb '32

Frank Operation

Formation of artificial vagina without operation by Frank method. HOLMES, W. R. AND WILLIAMS, G. A. Am. J. Obst. and Gynec. *39:*145–146, Jan '40

Frank-Geist Operation

Frank-Geist operation for congenital absence of vagina (skin graft). DANNREUTHER, W. T. Am. J. Obst. and Gynec. *35:*452–468, March '38

Frank Operation: See Geist-Frank Operation

FRANKE, F.: Simple finger splint. Munchen. med. Wchnschr. *69:*468, March 31, '22 (illus.)

FRANKE, F.: Nitroglycerin in surgery for shock. Zentralbl. f. Chir. *50:*1325–1328, Aug 25, '23

FRANKE, F.: Metal splint for injuries of extensor tendons of fingers (reply to Glass). Zentralbl. f. Chir. *55:*852–853, April 7, '28

FRANKE, F.: Comment on article by Levy on surgical treatment of atheroma. Munchen. med. Wchnschr. *77:*1277, July 25, '30. Reply to Franke and Halle on comments about surgical treatment of atheroma. LEVY, S. Munchen. med. Wchnschr. *77:*1845–1846, Oct 24, '30

FRANKENBERG, B.: Artificial vagina formed from sigmoid. Arch. f. Gynak. *140:*226–252, '30

FRANKENBERG, B. E.: Operative improvement of form of breasts in women. Vestnik khir. (no. 61) *21:*67–70, '30

FRANKENBERG, B. E.: Baldwin operation for formation of vagina closely resembling normal one, from vagina septa (bipartite vagina). Zentralbl. f. Chir. *57:*2792–2796, Nov 8, '30

FRANKENBERG, B. E.: Plastic closure of defective hard palate by means of round pedicled flap (Filatov). Sovet. khir. *4:*591–595, '33

FRANKENBERG, B. E.: Proper time and principles of primary treatment of gunshot wounds of face. Vrach. delo (nos. 7–8) *26:*465–470, '46

FRANKENTHAL, L.: Present opinion about malignant melanotic tumors of skin and their most suitable treatment. Arch. f. klin. Chir. *166:*678–693, '31

FRANKENTHAL, L.: Rare injury to fingers from bite of monkey; case. Munchen. med. Wchnschr. *79:*1641–1643, Oct 7, '32

FRANKENTHAL, L.: Hemangioma of skin of fingers; perforating through epidermis. Zentralbl. f. Chir. *59:*2619–2620, Oct 22, '32

FRANKENTHAL, L.: Dupuytren's contracture, covering palmar defects with skin from little finger. Zentralbl. f. Chir. *64:*211–214, Jan 23, '37

FRANKL, Z.: Simplified splinting of jaw fractures. Gyogyaszat *77:*686, Dec 5, 714, Dec 12, '37

FRANKLIN, R. H.: Principles of burn therapy. Practitioner *152:*167–173, March '44

FRANZ, R.: Formation of artificial vagina from rectum in deficiency of vagina. Zentralbl. f. Gynak. *50:*545–547, Feb 27, '26

FRANZETTI, C. O.: Vitamins A and D and camphorated oil in burns; preliminary report. Semana med. *2:*998, Oct 3, '35

FRASER, F. R. (see GILLIES, H.) Jan '35

FRASER, I.: Rare neck cyst. Brit. J. Surg. *18:*338–339, Oct '30

FRASER, J.: Operation shock. Brit. J. Surg. *11:*410–425, Jan '24

FRASER, J.: Burns in children. Brit. M. J. *1:*1089–1092, June 18, '27 also: M. Standard *50:*11–16, Sept '27

FRASER, J.: Cleft palate. Practitioner *125:*203–218, July '30

FRASER, J.: Hand infections. Practitioner *129:*18–32, July '32

FRASER, J. Shock and hemorrhage. War and Doctor, pp. 25–40, '42

FRASER, K. B.: Harelip and cleft palate. M. J. Australia *1:*361–381, March 16, '40

FRASER, N. D.: Reverdin's method of skin grafting; case. China M. J. *41:*364–365, April '27

FRATTIN, G.: Rational treatment of burns. Zentralbl. f. Chir. *53:*201–203, Jan 23, '26

FRASER, J. E. (see BERTWISTLE, A. P.) Jan '25

FRAZIER, C. H.: Surgical treatment of eyelid spasm. Ann. Surg. *93:*1121–1125, June '31

FRAZIER, C. H.: Modern treatment of shock. J.A.M.A. *105:*1731–1734, Nov 30, '35

FRAZIER, C. N.: Angioma cavernosum; report of case of face treated with radium. Arch. Dermat. and Syph. *12:*506–508, Oct '25

FRED, G. B.: Extranasal block anesthesia for submucous resection. Ann. Otol., Rhin. and Laryng. *53:*127–132, March '44

FREDET, M. (see DE FOURMESTRAUX, J.) Oct '35

FREDET, P.: Surgical therapy of Dupuytren's contracture. Bull. et mem. Soc. nat. de chir. *58:*440–444, March 19, '32

FREED, S. C. (see PRINZMETAL, M. *et al*) Feb '44

FREEDLANDER, S. O. AND LENHART, C. H.: Traumatic shock. Arch. Surg. *25:*693–708, Oct '32

FREEDMAN, A. M. AND KABAT, H.: Pressor response in adrenalin in course of traumatic shock. Am. J. Physiol. *130:*620–626, Oct '40

FREEMAN, D. B.: Cancer of lips. Illinois M. J. *87:*94–96, Feb '45

FREEMAN, J.: Plastic as substitute for metal in fracture appliances in facial fractures. J. Oral Surg. *1:*241–245, July '43

FREEMAN, J. T. (see PETERSON, R. G. *et al*) July '45

FREEMAN, L.: Use of visor flaps from chest in plastic operations upon neck, chin and lip. Ann. Surg. *87:*364–368, March '28

FREEMAN, L.: Plastic reconstruction of lower lip. Colorado Med. *26:*160–162, June '29

FREEMAN, N. E.: Cortin (hormone from suprarenal cortex) and traumatic shock. Science *77:*211–212, Feb 24, '33

FREEMAN, N. E.: Mechanism and management of surgical shock. Pennsylvania M. J. *42:*1449–1452, Sept '39

FREEMAN, N. E.: Intravenous fluid therapy in shock; symposium on military surgery. S. Clin. North America *21:*1769–1781, Dec '41

FREEMAN, R. C. (see SHARP, G. S.) Jan '44

FREEMAN, S. (see GRODINS, F. S.) Jan '41

FREIDEL, (see POLLOSSON, E.) July–Aug '38

FREIDEL, C.: Facial fractures; pericranial anchorage utilizing lining of French soldier's helmet; model B.B.V. 236. Rev. de stomatol. *41:*867–872, '40

FREIDEL, CHARLES (With MAURICE AUBRY): *Chirurgie de la face et de la région maxillo-faciale*. Masson et Cie, Paris, 1942

FREIDEL, C.; ARNULF, G. AND ANGIELOWICZ,: Traumatic craniofacial disjunctions; clinical study. J. de chir. *50:*27–43, July '37

FREIDEL, C. (see BERTRAND, P.) Sept–Oct '32

FREIDEL, C. (see BERTRAND, P.) Aug '31

FREITAS, G. DA C.: Shock in military medicine. Rev. med. brasil. *16:*337–351, March '44

FRENCKNER, P. AND SUNDBERG, S.: Plastic and prosthetic therapy after resection of upper jaw for cancer; cases. Acta oto-laryng. *27:*147–158, '39

FRENYÓ, L.: Questions of malignancy of parotid tumors, diagnosis and therapy. Deutsche Ztschr. f. Chir. *235:*130–139, '32

FRERE, J. M.: Case having thumbs with 3 phalanges simulating fingers. South. M. J. *23:*536–537, June '30

FREUD, E.: Reeducation of speech in ablation of

lower jaw; case. Rev. franc. de phoniatrie *7:*119–121, April '39

FREUDENBERG, E.: Cradle suspended from ceiling for quieting infants after surgical therapy for harelip. Kinderarztl. Praxis *3:*213–214, May '32

FREUDENBERG, K. (see GÖBELL, R.) 1935

FREUDENTHAL, P.: Mummification of skin (decubitus). Ugesk. f. laeger *95:*1095–1096, Oct 5, '33

FREUND: Apparatus for restoring shape to sunken nose. Deutsche med. Wchnschr. *48:*1422, Oct 20, '22

FREW, A. L.: Cleft lip and palate. Texas State J. Med. *23:*333–335, Sept '27

FREW, A. L.: Treatment of cleft palate. J. Am. Dent. A. *14:*1857–1859, Oct '27

FREW, A. L.: Cleft lip and palate surgery. J. Am. Dent. A. *21:*251–255, Feb '34

FREW, A. L.: Correction of cleft lip. and palate. J. Am. Dent. A. *23:*29–34, Jan '36

FREY, S.: Plastic surgery of upper lip with skin flaps from chin. Zentralbl. f. Chir. *70:*539, April 10, '43

FREYTES, M. V. AND SUAREZ, A. R.: Reconstruction of nasal tip; case. Bol. y trab., Soc. de cir. de Cordoba *2:*193–205, '41

FRICKE, K. F.: Congenital transverse fissure of cheek. Beitr. z. Anat. Physio., Path. u. Therap. d. Ohres *30:*282–297, '32

FRIDLAND, M. O.: Contracture of fingers and hand following gunshot wounds. Khirurgiya, no. 8, pp. 56–61, '44

FRIEBERG, T.: Progress in dacryocystorhinostomy. Nord. med. tidskr. *12:*1686–1687, Oct 10,'36

FRIEDE, R.: Peripheral neurectomy in blepharospasm. Ztschr. f. Augenh. *72:*299–303, Oct '30

FRIEDJUNG, J. K.: Therapy of vascular nevus in children. Wien. klin. Wchnschr. *46:*1520, Dec 15, '33

FRIEDJUNG, J. K.: Dangers of puncturing ear lobes of children for purpose of inserting earrings. Wien. med. Wchnschr. *85:*203, Feb 16, '35

FRIEDL-MEYER, M.: Formation of artificial vagina by using Thiersch transplants (Henkel modification of Kirschner-Wagner operation). Deutsche Ztschr. f. Chir. *244:*379–386, '35

FRIEDLANDER, H. M.: Failure with cryotherapy (using carbon dioxide slush) in treatment of acne scars. Arch. Dermat. and Syph. *46:*734–736, Nov '42

FRIEDMAN, G. A.: One-stage rhinoplasty for deflected bony nose, with sequelae. M. Rec. *155:*123–124, Feb 18, '42

FRIEDMAN, J.: Jaw fractures. Dental Digest *37:*71–83, Feb '31

FRIEDMAN, M.: Congenital recurrent lymphangioma of cheek. Eye, Ear, Nose and Throat Monthly *12:*334–335, Sept '33

FRIEDMAN, M. (see DANZIS, M. *et al*) Aug '38

FRIEDMANN, L.: Nasal prosthesis with heavy paraffin. Romania med. *15:*186–187, July 1–15, '37

FRIEDRICH, R.: Etiology of cancer of lips. Wien. klin. Wchnschr. *44:*177–179, Feb 6, '31

FRIEND, L. F.: Traction treatment of hand fractures. U. S. Nav. M. Bull. *40:*988–990, Oct '42

FRIEZ, PIERRE: *Les luxations habituelles* sans blocage de l'articulation temporo-maxillaire. Le François, Paris, 1933

FRIEZ, P. (see BERCHER, J.) April '33

FRINDENBERG, P.: Auricular epicanthus. Presse med. *39:*584, April 18, '31

FRISCH, O.: Indications for operation to improve shape of female breast. Wien. klin. Wchnschr. *41:*640–641, May 3, '28

FRISCH, O.: Cosmetic operations. Wien. med. Wchnschr. *79:*1575–1577, Dec 7, '29

FRISON, LÉON (with LÉON DUFOURMENTEL): *Diagnostic, Traitement, et Expertise des Sequelles des Accidents des Regions Maxillofaciales*. J. B. Baillière et fils, Paris, 1922

FRISON: Immediate treatment of facial injuries. Rev. odont. *51:*11–16, Jan '30

FRIST, J.: Plastic operations for pendulous abdomen and pendulous breast; a survey. Med. Klin. *23:*1269–1271, Aug 19, '27

FRITSCHI, U. (see CORDES, F. C.) March–April '44

FRITZELL, K. E.: Hand infections due to human mouth organisms. Journal-Lancet *60:*135–137, March '40

FROELICH, M.: Rupture of extensor longus of thumb in fractures of lower extremity of radius; case. Rev. d'orthop. *18:*584–597, Sept '31

FROES, H.: Technic for autoplastic repair of septum of nose. Brazil-med. *1:*349–352, June 21, '24

FRÖSCHELS, E.: Form of new obturator (meatus obturator) for preventing nasal speech in cleft palate. Ztschr. f. Stomatol. *26:*882–888, Sept '28

FRÖSCHELS, E. AND SCHALIT, H.: Obturators in treatment of rhinolalia aperta. Wien. med. Wchnschr. *78:*840, June 23, '28

FRÖSCHELS, E. AND SCHALIT, A.: New obturator to combat nasalization in patients with cleft of hard palate. Wien. klin. Wchnschr. *42:*1442–1444, Nov 7, '29

FROLOV, V. I.: Plastic reconstruction of skin of scrotum by Filatov grafts. Vestnik khir. *46:*251–252, '36

FROMENT, AND FEYEUX, A.: Phonetic reeducation for velopalatine division; conditions necessary for improving speech. Lyon chir. *36:*201–207, March–April '39

FROMENT, J. AND MALLET-GUY, P.: Elective traumatism of extensor digitorum and flexor digitorum profundus in injury to forearm; reflex inhibition of extension; infiltration of stellate ganglion; Volkmann contracture; tendinous transmutation. Lyon chir. *35:*623-629, Sept-Oct '38

FROMENT, J.; THIERS, H. AND BRUN, J.: Anuria after burn with hypertensive crisis and bradycardia treated successfully by sodium bicarbonate and transfusions of non-citrated blood; case. Lyon med. *158:*412-415, Oct 11, '36

FROMM, G. A.: Treatment of wounds of tendons. Dia med. *16:*1182-1187, Oct 2, '44

FROMM, N. K. (see ARCHAMBAULT, L.) March '32

FROMME, A.: Treatment of jaw ankylosis and micrognathia. Beitr. z. klin. Chir. *144:*195-206, '28

FROMMOLT, G.: Congenital absence of skin above small fontanelle in new-born infant. Ztschr. f. Geburtsh. u. Gynak. *108:*178-179, '34

FRONGIA, L.: Maxillary fractures in relation to dentistry. Rassegna med. sarda *43:*18-41, Jan-Feb '41

FRONK, C. E.: Mammaplasty of pendulous breasts. Hawaii M. J. *5:*23-25, Sept-Oct '45

FRONTEAU, M.: Surgical therapy of permanent constriction of jaw; case. Arch. med. d'Angers *43:*69-72, April '39

FROST, A. D.: Supporting suture in ptosis operations. Am. J. Ophth. *17:*633, July '34

Frostbite (See also War Injuries)

Drumstick fingers from freezing. SABATUCCI, F. Policlinico (sez. med.) *28:*233, June '21 abstr: J.A.M.A. *77:*580, Aug 13, '21

Peripheral facial paralysis following frostbite; case. ROY, J. N. Union med. du Canada *60:*223-229, April '31

Treatment of frost-bite. FLÖRCKEN, H. Therap. Halbmonatsh. *35:*430, July 15, '21

Paraffin therapy of burns produced by heat and cold. and for cicatrices. JOUAN, S.; *et al.* Rev. med. latino-am. *18:*1424-1427, Sept '33

Otoplasty for dermatitis congelationis (frostbite). LIGGETT, H., M. Rec. *142:*278-279, Sept 18, '35

Freezing of parts of face in aviators. DE GAULEJAC, R. Bull. med. Paris *52:*705-707, Oct 1, '38

Burns and frostbite. MICHAËL, P. R. Geneesk. gids *18:*476, May 31, '40; 494, June 7, '40

Indications, technic and results of skin grafting in third degree frostbite of foot. MARZIANI, R. Boll. e mem. Soc. piemontese chir. *12:*277-279, '42

Skin transplantation in surgical after-treatment of amputation-stumps following frostbite of foot. STUDEMEISTER, A. Deutsche Ztschr. f. Chir. *258:*49, '43

Skin grafts to cover defects of stumps after frostbite. GEKTIN, F. L. Khirurgiya, no. 4, pp. 23-27, '44

Frostbite in wartime. TABANELLI, M. Arch. ital. chir. *68:*111-195, '46

FROSTE, N.: Phalangization of first metacarpal bone in surgical therapy of thumb injuries; 2 cases. Svenska lak.-tidning. *30:*337-341, April 7, '33

FROSTE, N. (see BERGGREN, S.) 1942

FROTHINGHAM, G. E.: Cancer of upper eyelid; plastic operation; case. J. Michigan M. Soc. *28:*632-633, Sept '29

FRUCHAUD, H. AND MARY, A.: Radium treatment in 13 cases of cancer of face. Gazettes med., Paris, pp. 465-471, Aug 15, '27

FRUEHWALD, V.: Progress in plastic surgery of ear and nose. Rev. de chir. plastique, pp. 155-167, Oct '33

FRUHMANN, P. AND STERNBERG, H.: Hypospadias, discussion and review of cases. Arch. f. klin. Chir. *160:*633-673, '30

FRÜHWALD, VICTOR: *Korrektiv-cosmetische Chirurgie der Näse, der Ohren, und des Gesichts.* Wilhelm Maudrich, Vienna, 1932. (Also English edition, translated by Geoffrey Morey)

FRUMKIN, A. P. Reconstruction of male genitals. Am. Rev. Soviet Med. *2:*14-21, Oct '44

FRUMKIN, J.: Simplified technic of plastic repair of epispadias. J. Urol. *46:*690-692, Oct '41

FRÜND, H.: Substitute for adhesive plaster bandage in hare-lip operations. Zentralbl. f. Chir. *48:*1426, Oct 1, '21

FRÜND, H.: Schönborn-Rosenthal operation for cleft palate. Zentralbl. f. Chir. *54:*3206-3210, Dec 10, '27

FRÜND, H.: Reich-Matti operation for double harelip. Munchen. med. Wchnschr. *75:*1067-1070, June 22, '28

FRY, W. K.: Dental aspect of treatment of congenital cleft palates. Proc. Roy. Soc. Med. (Sect. Odontology) *14:*57, Oct '21

FRY, W. K.: Treatment of cleft palate. Lancet *2:*1081-1082, Nov 22, '24

FRY, W. K.: Fracture of mandible in, and posterior to, the molar region. Proc. Roy. Soc. Med. (Sect. Odont.) *22:*37-45, March '29

FRY, K.: Fractures of mandible. Guy's Hosp. Gaz. *50:*267-270, July 4, '36

FRY, W. K.: Fractures of mandible and their

treatment. M. Press *197:*108–112, Aug 10, '38
FRY, W. K.: Barrel bandage in jaw fractures. Brit. M. J. *2:*1086, Dec 2, '39
FRY, W. K.: Gunshot wounds of jaws. M. Press *203:*524–527, June 26, '40
FRY, W. K. (see GILLIES, H. D.) March '21
FUCHS, A.: Treatment of facial paralysis. Wien. klin. Wchnschr. *39:*248–250, Feb 25, '26; 277–279, March 4, '26
FUCHS, A. AND PFEFFER, M.: Treatment of central and peripheral paralysis of facial nerve. Wien. klin. Wchnschr. *37:*1008–1010, Oct 2, '24 abstr: J.A.M.A. *83:*1546, Nov 8, '24
FUCHS, E.: Maxillary labial frenum in School Health Service. Brit. Dent. J. *80:*327–329, May 17, '46
FUCHS, V. H.: Nasal fractures and their treatments. New Orleans M. and S. J. *81:*802–806, May '29
FUHS, H.: Radium treatment of cicatricial keloids. Med. Klin. *30:*160–161, Feb 2, '34
FUHS, H.: Skin injuries from incendiary bombs and war chemicals. Wien. klin. Wchnschr. *53:*40–44, Jan 12, '40
FUHS, H.: Decubitus ulcers. Wien. klin. Wchnschr. *56:*145, Feb 26, '43
FUHS, H.: Treatment of burns. Wien. klin. Wchnschr. *57:*120, March 10, '44
FUHS, H. (see ARZT, L.) Jan '32
FUHS, H. (see ARTZ, L.) June '33
FUKAMACHI, T.: Precancerous dermatoses, report of case. Arch. Dermat. and Syph. *10:*714–721, Dec '24
FUKE, T.: Deformed fetus complicating club-hands and microtia. Jap. J. Obst. and Gynec. *15:*255–258, June '32
FUKS, B. I.: Formation of artificial hand. Novy khir. arkhiv. *39:*125–129, '37
FUKS, B. I. (see NIRENBERG, B. B.) 1934
FULCHER, O. H.: Peripheral nerve lesions; experience in South Pacific area. U. S. Nav. M. Bull. *46:*325–334, March '46
FULCHER, O. H.: Use of tantalum for cranioplasties; further studies. U. S. Nav. M. Bull. *46:*1493–1498, Oct '46
FULCHER, O. H. AND LANE, W. Z.: Progressive hemiatrophy of face (following injuries); case. U. S. Nav. M. Bull. *41:*192–196, Jan '43
FULCHER, O. H. AND MAXWELL, M. M.: Tissue reactions to metallic implants. U. S. Nav. M. Bull. *41:*845–847, May '43
FULD, J. E.: Restoration of hand injuries by plastic surgery. New York M. J. *114:*692, Dec 21, '21
FULD, J. E.: Autotransplantation of toe for traumatic loss of finger. J.A.M.A. *86:*1281–1282, April 24, '26
FULD, J. E.: Restoration of function of hand after traumatic injury. Ann. Surg. *99:*195–216, Jan '34
FULLER, E. B.: Exstrophy of bladder, case with operations. J. M. A. South Africa *3:*525–526, Sept 28, '29
FULLER, T. E.: Unusual complication (facial hemi-atrophy) following Caldwell-Luc operation. J. Arkansas M. Soc. *34:*94, Oct '37
FULLER, T. E.: Unusual complication of radical antrum operation (hemiatrophy of face following Caldwell-Luc operation). South. M. J. *31:*1094–1095, Oct '38
FULLER, W. H. A.: First aid and preliminary treatment of maxillofacial injuries. Brit. Dent. J. *78:*106–108, Feb 16, '45
FUNCK-BRENTANO, P.: Intravenous injection of morphine in therapy of shock; case. Mem. Acad. de chir. *66:*615–616, June 5-26, '40
FUNK, F.: Psychologic aspects of problem of artificial ear, with critical comment on rigid permanent prosthesis and elastic temporary prosthesis. Dermat. Wchnschr. *109:*1402–1407, Dec 30, '39
FURSTENBERG, A. C.: Reconstruction of facial nerve (especially in operations on parotid gland). Arch. Otolaryng. *41:*42–47, Jan '45
FÜTH, H.: Artificial vagina made from intestine. Monatschr. f. Geburtsh. u. Gynak. *55:*262–266, Sept '21

Furuncles

Surgical treatment of intractable furunculosis of axilla. BRUNZEL, H. F. Zentralbl. f. Chir. *48:*991, July 16, '21
Surgical treatment of furunculosis of axilla. BOCKENHEIMER, P. Zentralbl. f. Chir. *48:*1317, Sept 10, '21
Treatment of furuncles on face. HOFMANN, W. Arch. f. klin. Chir. *123:*51–66, '23 (illus.) abstr: J.A.M.A. *80:*1420, May 12, '23
Progressive furuncle of face. RIEDER, W. Zentralbl. f. Chir. *50:*1024–1025, June 30, '23 abstr: J.A.M.A. *81:*1155, Sept 29, '23
Treatment of malignant furuncle of face by incision and circular injection of patient's own blood. LÄWEN, A. Zentralbl. f. Chir. *50:*1468–1471, Sept 29, '23
Malignant furuncle of lip. ROEDELIUS, E. Klin. Wchnschr. *2:*2348–2353, Dec 24, '23 abstr: J.A.M.A. *82:*506, Feb 9, '24
Treatment of malignant furuncle of lip. ROEDELIUS, E. Dermat. Wchnschr. *78:*37–42, Jan 12, '24
Treatment of furuncles on face by "chemical incision" with phenol. PERRET, C. A. Schweiz. med. Wchnschr. *55:*469–470, May 28, '25 abstr: J.A.M.A. *85:*393, Aug 1, '25

Furuncles—Cont.
Treatment of furuncles of face. MELCHIOR, E. Beitr. z. klin. Chir. *135:*681-695, '26
Medical and surgical technic in therapy of furunculosis. SIGNORIS, E. Riv. med. *36:*146-148, Oct '28
Therapy of furunculosis by fan-shaped section. THILENIUS. Deutsche med. Wchnschr. *55:*618, April 12, '29
Iodine iontrophoresis in keloid occurring after furuncle. EIGER, J. Munchen. med. Wchnschr. *76:*1297, Aug 2, '29
Surgical treatment of furunculosis. HAYWARD. Med. Klin. *25:*1631-1632, Oct 18, '29
Furuncles of nose and upper lip. DUFOURMENTEL, L. Prat. med. franc. *14:*171-178, March (A) '33
Pagnelin cautery in therapy of furunculosis. WINCKLER, E. Munchen. med. Wchnschr. *80:*1974-1975, Dec 15, '33
Cautery pencil in treatment of furunculosis. SCHÜLE, A. Med. Welt *8:*407, March 24, '34
Surgical therapy of facial furuncle. SCHMID, W. Chirurg *6:*447-456, June 15, '34
Furuncles on face and their treatment. MORIAN, R. Deutsche Ztschr. f. Chir. *193:*45-58, '25 abstr: J.A.M.A. *85:*1437, Oct 31, '25
Furuncles of upper lip and nose. GAUS, W. Therap. d. Gegenw. *77:*75-76, Feb '36
Furuncle of upper lip; case. FERNANDES, M. Rev. med. de Pernambuco *9:*137-145, May '39
Extensive furunculosis of upper lip treated by roentgenotherapy; case. GRIMAUD, R. AND JACOB, P. Rev. med. de Nancy *67:*701-703, Aug 1, '39
Diathermosurgery for furunculosis. ALESSANDRINI. Rev. med. de Chile *67:*1348-1352, Dec '39
Nasal furuncle. MAYER, F. J. Monatschr. f. Ohrenh. *74:*167-182, April '40
Incision of facial furunculosis. KLAPP, R. Zentralbl. f. Chir. *67:*1618-1619, Aug 31, '40
Treatment of facial furuncles. SITTENAUER, L. Med. Klin. *36:*1385-1388, Dec 13, '40
Surgical therapy of furunculosis. BOVENSIEPEN, F. G. Zentralbl. f. Chir. *68:*909-912, May 17, '41
Therapy of furunculosis by means of Thiersch graft. HOELZ, P. Arq. de cir. clin. e exper. *6:*550-558, April-June '42
Therapy of furunculosis of face. SALLERAS LLINARES, V. AND SAGRERA, J. M. Med. clin. Barcelona *7:*36-44, July '46
Complications of malignant furuncle of upper lip and their prevention. CALLILAR, N. Turk tip cem mec *12:*44-50, '46

FUSO, B.: Jaw fractures; therapy by continually applied force. Stomatol. ital. *2:*95-111, Feb '40
FUSS, H.: Surgical therapy of harelip. Arch. f. klin. Chir. *182:*253-272, '35
FUSS, H.: Technic of surgical correction of harelip. Chirurg *7:*372-375, June 1, '35
FUSTE, R. AND MORA MORALES, L.: Malignant degeneration of gigantic pigmented nevus of shoulder; case. Rev. med. cubana *55:*307-314, April '44
FUZII, M. AND MURATA, M.: Amyloid degeneration of transplanted tissues. (in Japanese). Tr. Jap. Path. Soc. *21:*84-88, '31

G

GABARRO, P.: Immediate therapy for facial injuries; essential concepts. Rev. Fac. de med., Bogota *9:*717-727, April '41
GABARRO, P.: Determination of real defect in plastic repair of cicatrix. Rev. san. mil., Buenos Aires *40:*923-926, Oct '41
GABARRO, P.: Use of abdominal skin to correct cervical defect due to burn. Rev. Fac. de med., Bogota *10:*339-342, Oct '41
GABARRO, P.: New method of skin grafting. Brit. M. J. *1:*723-724, June 12, '43
GABARRO, P.: Board for cutting grafts of definite width. Lancet *2:*788, Dec 16, '44
GABARRO, P.: New design for raising tubed pedicle flap. Surgery *18:*732-741, Dec '45
GABRIEL, E.: Replacement of thumb with portion of index finger. Munchen. med. Wchnschr. *83:*1391-1393, Aug 21, '36
GABY, R. E.: Electrical burns and electrical shock. Canad. M.A.J. *17:*1343-1345, Nov '27
DE GAETANO, L.: Congenital cysts and fistulas in neck. Arch. ital. di chir. *4:*265-324, Nov '21 (illus.) abstr: J.A.M.A. *78:*250, Jan 21, '22
DE GAETANO, L.: Resection and arthroplasty in case of lock-jaw from old osseous ankylosis of temporomaxillary articulation. Arch. ital. di chir. *12:*673-712, '25
DE GAETANO, L.: Two cases of congenital complete lateral pharyngo-cervico-sternal fistulas of neck and their extirpation. Riforma med. *41:*889-896, Sept 21, '25
DE GAETANO, L.: Treatment of posttraumatic Volkmann contracture by sympathectomy and shortening of bones of forearm. Ann. ital. di chir. *6:*447-479, May '27
DE GAETANO, L.: Multilocular cystic lymphangioma of neck. Riforma med. *43:*529-532, June 6, '27
DE GAETANO, L.: Surgical treatment of ele-

phantiasis of legs. Riforma med. *44:*1649-1651, Dec 17, '28

DE GAETANO, L.: Congenital median fistula, with report of case. Riforma med. *53:*523-526, April 10, '37

DE GAETANO, L.: Congenital cysts and fistulas of neck. Arch. di ortop. *53:*455-479, Sept 30, '37

DE GAETANO, L.: Correction of sequels of infantile paralysis; technic of osteoperiosteal incision in tendinous transplants. Riforma med. *54:*887-895, June 11, '38

GAFAFER, W. M.: Time changes in relative mortality from accidental burns among children in different geographic regions of United States, 1925-32; studies on fatal accidents of childhood. Pub. Health Rep. *51:*1308-1316, Sept 18, '36

GAGE, E. L.: Splint to prevent contracture in surgery of hand. J.A.M.A. *94:*1063-1064, April 5, '30

GAGLIARDI, P.: Hyperplastic cavernous lymphangioma of forearm; case. Arch. ital. di anat. e istol. pat. *8:*108-612, Sept '38

GAGLIO, V.: Free homoplastic and heteroplastic grafts of periosteum and of bone in sensitized animals. Ann. ital. di chir. *11:*2017-2030, Oct 31, '32

GAGNON, G. (see GUTHRIE, D.) 1946

GAGNON, G. (see GUTHRIE, D.) May '46

GAHLEN, W. (see PROPPE, A.) 1940

GAIDUKOFF, M. F.: Plastic surgery of floor of mouth after excision of malignant tumors. Odessky M. J. *4:*332-334, '29

GAINES, J. A.: Massive puberty hypertrophy of breast. Am. J. Obst. and Gynec. *34:*130-136, July '37

GALA, A.: Congenital deformity in formation of inner corners of eyelids; 2 cases. Bratisl. lekar. listy *9:*1248-1251, Dec '29

GALAKHOFF, E. V.: Artificial vagina; formation from double coil of small intestine. Vrach. gaz. *34:*127-130, Jan 31, '30

GALANTE, E. (see CARANDO, V. *et al*) Jan '37

GALASINSKI, R. E. (see CROSBY, E. H.) Dec '45

GALBRAITH, J. B. D. (see FINDLAY, L.) Jan '23

GALE, C. K.: Lateral osteotomy; anatomic considerations (description of grove on frontal process of maxilla). Am. J. Surg. *63:*368-370, March '44

GALEWSKA, S. AND LITAUER, R.: Surgical therapy of entropion and trichiasis according to Maher method. Rev. internat. du trachome *13:*41-47, Jan '36

GALLAGHER, J. L.: Initial care of wounds from reconstructive viewpoint. Mil. Surgeon *94:*212-216, April '44

GALLAGHER, J. L.: Initial care of wounds from reconstructive viewpoint. Rev. san. mil., Buenos Aires *43:*1629-1636, Dec '44

GALLENGA, R.: Progress with tarsal graft of Müller's muscle in pseudoptosis due to enophthalmos. Rassegna ital. d'ottal. *3:*626-636, July-Aug '34

GALLIE, W. E.: Implantation of tendons. Am. J. Surg. *35:*268, Sept '21

GALLIE, W. E.: Bone transplantation. Brit. M. J. *2:*840-844, Nov 7, '31

GALLIE, W. E.: Further experiences with tendon transplantation. Tr. West. S. A. (1936) *46:*47-57, '37

GALLIE, W. E. AND LE MESURIER, A. B.: Use of living sutures in operative surgery. Canad. M.A.J. *11:*504, July '21

GALLIE, W. E. AND LE MESURIER, A. B.: Clinical and experimental study of free transplantation of fascia and tendon. J. Bone and Joint Surg. *4:*600-612, July '22 (illus.)

GALLIE, W. E. AND LE MESURIER, A. B.: Transplantation of fibrous tissues in repair of anatomical defects. Brit. J. Surg. *12:*289-320, Oct '24

Galliera Operation: See Passaggi-Galliera Operation

GALLINO, J. A. AND CORA ELISEHT, F.: Ascher syndrome (blepharochalasis, double upper lip and goiter), with report of case. Prensa med. argent. *32:*2423:2426, Dec 7, '45

GALLUSSER, E.: Cosmetic operations on nose. Schweiz. med. Wchnschr. *52:*381-383, April 20, '22 (illus.) abstr: J.A.M.A. *78:*1931, June 17, '22

GALT, S.: Use of foille in burns. Dallas M. J. *25:*81-86, July '39

GALTIER: Treatment of partial loss of substance of ala nasi. Semaine d. hop. Paris *21:*491-493, May 14, '45

GALTIER, M.: Total free skin grafts; indications and operative technic. J. de chir. *50:*322-335, Sept '37

GALTIER, M.: Plastic surgery in Great Britain. Presse med. *54:*329-330, May 18, '46

GALVAO, H. (see WANDERLEY FILHO, E.) March '38

GALVAO, L.: Traumatic shock. Hora med., Rio de Janeiro *2:*33-44, Aug '44

GALY-GASPARROU, ESTIENNY, E. AND FABRE, J.: Complete imperfection of anus in newborn; operation. Bull. Soc. d'obst. et de gynec. *17:*335, March '28

GAMARRA ANTEZANA, J.: Burn therapy. Prensa med., La Paz *2:*221-225, Oct '42

GAMBAROW, G.: Artificial vagina formation by Baldwin's method. Monatschr. f. Geburtsh. u. Gynak. *78:*106-108, Jan '28

GAMBAROW, G.: Simple method of construction of artificial vagina. Zentralbl. f. Gynak. *57:*2559–2562, Oct 28, '33

GAMBEE, L. P.: Serious hand infections. West. J. Surg. *43:*449–455, Aug '35

GAMBLE, H. A.: Congenital absence of part of abdominal wall. South. M. J. *25:*771–772, July '32

GAMES, F. AND MERCANDINO, C.: Plastic surgery of nose. Semana med. *1:*727–736, March 3, '32

GAMES, F. (see ARÁUZ, S.) July '32

GAMMAGE, F. V.: New instruments for submucous resection of nasal septum. Arch. Otolaryng. *16:*573–574, Oct '32

Ganglions

Treatment of ganglion of back of hand. EISENKLAM, I. Wien. klin. Wchnschr. *41:*740–741, May 24, '28

Tendovaginitis and tendon nodules, ganglion, hygroma and bursitis. STORCK, H. Med. Welt *10:*522–525, April 11, '36

Treatment of ganglion. SAEGESSER, M. Schweiz. med. Wchnschr. *66:*663–664, July 11, '36

Ganglion of wrist, with special reference to therapy. LUCHETTI, S. E. Semana med. *2:*843–847, Oct 7, '37

Ganglions of tendon sheaths; method of treatment. BEARSE, C., J.A.M.A. *109:*1626, Nov 13, '37

Ganglions and their therapy (of tendon sheath). CHISTYAKOV, N. L. Khirurgiya, no. 5, pp. 84–95, '39

Therapy of so-called ganglia of wrist. VOIGT, H. W. Ztschr. f. arztl. Fortbild. *39:*55–57, Feb 1, '42

Ganglia of tendon sheaths (bursae). NELSON, H. Minnesota Med. *26:*734–737, Aug '43

Ganglion (of wrist); case (treated with sylnasol, fatty acid solution). VAN DEN BERG, W. J. California and West. Med. *60:*24, Jan '44

GANZER, H.: Total plastic reconstruction of orbit. Plast. chir. *1:*72–76, '39

GANZER, H.: Gunshot wounds of jaws. Ztschr. f. arztl. Fortbild. *36:*641–646, Nov 1, '39

GANZER, H.: Technic of bone transplantation in traumatic defects of lower jaw; author's experiences. Plast. chir. *1:*113–154, '40

GANZER, H.: War injuries to jaws. Deut. Militararzt *5:*419–426, Oct '40

GARA, G.: Hypertrichosis; problem and how to handle it as it appears in every-day practice. Urol. and Cutan. Rev. *45:*771–774, Dec '41

GARAVANO, P. H.: Elephantiasis of legs; surgical therapy. Semana med. *2:*1–13, July 7, '38

GARAVANO, P. H.: Indications and results of immediate free grafts to repair extensive loss of substance. Dia med. (sup.) *1:*33–40, July 3, '44

GARAY, P. M. (see IVANISSEVICH, O.) June '41

GARB, J. AND STONE, M. J.: Review of literature and report of 80 cases of keloids. Am. J. Surg. *58:*315–335, Dec '42

GARCIA, C. L.: Embryologic study of case of exstrophy of bladder with umbilical hernia and aplasia of anus and rectum. Semana med. *1:*347–355, Feb 22, '23 (illus.)

GARCIA BIRD, J.: Postpartum traumatic gynatresia, 2 cases. Bol. Asoc. med. de Puerto Rico *37:*205–207, June '45

GARCÍA CAPURRO, R.: Subcutaneous abscesses of palm; preliminary report. Arch. urug. de med., cir. y especialid. *4:*133–139, Feb '34

GARCÍA CAPURRO, R.: Subcutaneous abscesses of palm. Cron. med. mex. *33:*157–161, June '34

GARCÍA CAPURRO, R.: Dermoepidermal grafts. Arch. urug. de med., cir. y especialid. *22:*406–418, April '43

GARCÍA CAPURRO, R. AND RUSSI, J. C.: Recidivating interphalangeal luxation; therapy. Bol. Soc. cir. d. Uruguay *14:*36–39, '43

GARCÍA CAPURRO, R. AND RUSSI, J. C.: Recidivating interphalangeal luxation; therapy. Arch. urug. de med., cir. y especialid. *23:*134–137, Aug '43

GARCIA CASTELLANOS, J. A. AND MAURETTE, R.: Functional surgical therapy of cleft palate. Bol. y trab., Soc. de cir. de Cordoba *4:*141–148, '43

GARCIA DIAZ, F.: Metacarpolysis in mutilation of thumb; illustrative cases. Semana med. *1:*658–660, March 24, '38

GARCIA FRUGONI, A. (see MICHANS, J. R.) July '43

GARCIA LOPEZ, A. (see CARDELLE PENICHET, G.) April–June '41

GARCIA-SALA, J.: Burn therapy with A and D vitaminized oil; case. Rev. clin. espan. *8:*201–202, Feb 15, '43

GARCIA VALCARCEL, A.: Therapy of infected callus (hand). Med. espan. *9:*75–82, Jan '43

GARCIN, R.; THUREL, R. AND RUDAUX, P.: Isolated case of craniofacial dysostosis (Crouzon's disease) with ectrodactylia. Bull. et mem. Soc. med. d. hop. de Paris *48:*1458–1466, Nov 28, '32

GARCIN, R.; THUREL, R. AND RUDAUX, P.: Isolated case of craniofacial dysostosis (Crouzon's disease) with ectrodactylia. Arch. de med. d. enf. *36:*359–365, June '33

GARDINER, F. S. (see MCCALL, J. W.) April '43

GARDINI, G. F.: Cavernous angioma; radium and roentgen therapy; cases. Bull. d. sc. med., Bologna *110:*293–314, Sept–Oct '38

GARDNER, F. G.: Rupture of extensor longus pollicis tendon. Brit. M. J. *1:*476, March 25, '22

GARDNER, J. A. (see ENTWISLE, R. M.) May '25

GARDNER, W. J.: Use of tantalum for repair of defects in infected cases in cranium. Cleveland Clin. Quart. *13:*72–87, Apr '46

GARDNER, W. J. (see KARNOSH, L. J.) April '45

GAREISO, A. AND ALVAREZ, G.: Progressive facial hemiatrophy (Romberg's disease); case. Rev. Asoc. med. argent. *50:*91–100, Jan '37

GAREISO, A. *et al:* Progressive hemiatrophy of face with scleroderma, vitiligo and canities; case. Arch. argent. de pediat. *22:*416–425, Nov '44

GAREISO, A.; VIVIANI, J. E. AND CERDEIRO, A. M.: Acrocephalosyndactylia (Apert syndrome); case. Rev. med. latino-am. *23:*1245–1265, Aug '38

GARELICK, S. (see DEL VALLE, D.) Nov '40

GARFIN, S. W.: Study of 202 cases of laryngeal cancer with end results. New England J. Med. *213:*1109–1123, Dec 5, '35

GARFIN, S. W.: Multiple fractures of skull complicated by fractures of jaws. Am. J. Surg. *52:*460–465, June '41

GARLAND, J. G. AND DAVIES, J. A.: Cancer of lips. Marquette M. Rev. *9:*113–118, June '44

GARLING-PALMER, R.: Metacarpophalangeal dislocations of thumb. Presse med. *36:*885–886, July 14, '28

GARLING PALMER, R.: Clinical aspects and treatment of forward, metacarpophalangeal dislocations of thumb. Gaz. d. hop. *102:*146–149, Jan 26, '29

GARLOCK, J. H.: Hand infections. Surg., Gynec. and Obst. *39:*165–191, Aug '24

GARLOCK, J. H.: Repair of wounds of flexor tendons of hand. Ann. Surg. *83:*111–122, Jan '26

GARLOCK, J. H.: Surgery of flexor tendons of hand. Am. J. Surg. *40:*68–69, March '26

GARLOCK, J. H.: Repair processes in wounds of tendons and in tendon grafts. Ann. Surg. *85:*92–103, Jan '27

GARLOCK, J. H.: Plastic surgery treatment of compound injuries of extremities. Ann. Surg. *87:*321–354, March '28 abstr: Bull. New York Acad. Med. *4:*36–41, Jan '28

GARLOCK, J. H.: Method of reconstruction of axilla for contracture. Surg., Gynec. and Obst. *51:*705–710, Nov '30

GARLOCK, J. H.: Full-thickness graft; field of applicability and technical considerations. Ann. Surg. *97:*259–273, Feb '33

GARLOCK, J. H.: Treatment of persistent bronchial fistula by use of pedicled muscle flap. S. Clin. North America *14:*307–313, April '34

GARLOCK, J. H.: Industrial accidents; management of injuries of tendons and nerve of hand. New York State J. Med. *36:*1740–1748, Nov 15, '36

GARLOCK, J. H.: Recurrent epithelioma of arm; method of covering defect after radical excision illustrating 2 useful types of skin transplantation. J. Mt. Sinai Hosp. *5:*75–78, July–Aug '38

GARLOCK, J. H.: Suppurative tenosynovitis of hand; plan of treatment. J. Mt. Sinai Hosp. *8:*540–542, Jan–Feb '42

GARMSEN, B. M.: Formation of artificial bladder in exstrophy; 3 cases. Zentralbl. f. Chir. *54:*1736–1741, July 9, '27

GARNEAU, P. (see VEZINA, C. *et al*) June '38

GARNIER, G. (see MILLIAN, G.) Nov '28

GARRETSON, W. T.: Reconstruction of nasal bridge by means of auogenous rib cartilage grafts. J. Michigan M. Soc. *26:*36–41, Jan '27

GARRIDO-LESTACHE, J.: Imperforate anus; case. Pediatria espan. *15:*273–275, Sept '26

GARTMAN, E. (see FETTER, T. R.) May '36

GASCO PASCUAL, J.: Burn therapy. Med. espan. *6:*242–251, Sept '41

GASCO PASCUAL, J.: Burn therapy (and physiopathology). Med. espan. *6:*324–337, Oct '41

Gas Gangrene

Gas gangrene of extremities, with special reference to trivalent anaerobic serotherapy. LARSON, E. E. AND PULFORD, D. S. Tr. Sect. Surg., General and Abd., A.M.A., pp. 261–279, '29 also: J.A.M.A. *94:*612–618, March 1, '30

GASKINS, J. H. (see PADGETT, E. C.) 1945

GASKINS, J. H. (see PADGETT, E. C.) Sept '45

GASPARINI, C.: Pathogenesis, diagnosis and treatment of jaw deformities. Stomatol. *27:*950-963, Nov '29

GASS, H. H.: Surgical relief of lagophthalmos following seventh nerve paralysis in cases of leprosy. Leprosy Rev. *5:*178–180, Oct '34

GASSUL, R.: Homoplastic transplantation of adult frog skin. Deutsche med. Wchnschr. *48:*1163–1164, Sept 1, '22 (illus.)

GASTÉLUM, B. J.: Therapy of fractures of horizontal ramus of lower jaw. Gac. med. de Mexico *64:*245–253, May '33

GASTON, E. A.: Cysts and sinuses of neck. Cleveland Clin. Quart. *3:*311–322, Oct '36

GASTON, J. H.: Ethyl chloride spray for freezing donor area for skin grafting. J. M. A. Georgia *33:*151, May '44

GATCH, W. D.: Clinical history of tumors of face and jaws as guide to their correct diagnosis and proper treatment. J. Indiana M. A. *15:*251–255, Aug '22

GATCH, W. D. AND TRUSLER, H. M.: Use of ultraviolet light in preparation of infected granulation tissue for grafting; value of very thick Thiersch grafts. Surg., Gynec. and Obst. *50:*478–482, Feb '30

GATÉ, J. AND MASSIA, G.: Basocellular epithelioma of nose. Bull. Soc. franc. de dermat. et syph. *33:*668–673, Nov '26

GATÉ, J.; MICHEL, P. J. AND THÉVENON, J. A.: Angiomatosis of back of hands. Bull. Soc. franc. de dermat. et syph. (Reunion dermat., Lyon) *39:*1575–1577, Dec '32

GATEWOOD: Plastic repair of finger defects without hospitalization. J.A.M.A. *87:*1479, Oct 30, '26

GATEWOOD: Plastic surgery of face. S. Clin. N. Amer. *7:*539–549, June '27

GATEWOOD: Plastic repair of hypospadias. S. Clin. North America *14:*783–788, Aug '34

GATEWOOD: Simple technic for cure of hypospadias. Surg., Gynec. and Obst. *63:*655–659, Nov '36

GATEWOOD, W. L.: Essential facts in connection with use of local anesthesia in nose and throat surgery. Virginia M. Monthly *54:*163–166, June '27

GATEWOOD, W. L.: Correction of multiple deformities of nose. Virginia M. Monthly *71:*227–231, May '44

GATEWOOD, W. L.: Correction of multiple deformities of nose. Eye, Ear, Nose and Throat Monthly *24:*134–138, March '45

GATTI, G.: Uranostaphylorrhaphy. Surg., Gynec. and Obst. *51:*224–226, Aug '30

GATTI-MANACINI: Nerve trunk anesthesia of nasal cavity. Arch. ital. di otol. *51:*495–512, Oct '39

GAUDIN, H. J. AND CABOT, H.: Partial exstrophy of bladder; embryologic considerations; case. Proc. Staff Meet., Mayo Clin. *13:*216–220, April 6, '38

GAUFFRE, R.: Congenital coloboma of upper eyelid; cases. Arch. d'opht. *5:*342–343, '45

DE GAULEJAC, R.: Freezing of parts of face in aviators. Bull. med., Paris *52:*705–707, Oct 1, '38

GAULTIER, M. (see LAIGNEL-LAVASTINE, *et al*) Dec '34

GAUS, W.: Furuncles of upper lip and nose. Therap. d. Gegenw. *77:*75–76, Feb '36

GAUS, W.: New type of plaster of paris protector for use in therapy of nasal fractures. Hals-, Nasen-u. Ohrenarzt (Teil 1) *28:*94–97, April '37

GAUS, W.: Heredity of ear malformations. Erbbl. f. d. Hals-, Nasen-u. Ohrenarzt, Hft. 1–2, pp. 20–30, March '39; in Hals-, Nasen-u. Ohrenarzt (Teil 1) *30:* March '39

GAUTHIER, F. (see COMTOIS, A. *et al*) May '41

GAUTIER, J.: Cure of grave epispadias by vesico-urethral plication; case in boy 5 years old. Bull. et mem. Soc. nat. de chir. *60:*219–221, Feb 10, '34

GAUTIER, J.: Small exstrophy of bladder in women; case in girl 4½ years old; surgical therapy with use maintained for 5 years. Bull. et mem. Soc. nat. de chir. *61:*708–713, June 1, '35

GAUTIER, J.: Therapy of grave incontinence of urethral origin by vesico-urethral fold (epispadias). J. d'urol. *44:*55–68, July '37

GAUTIER, J.: Infra-red light in burns. Arch. med. d'Angers *43:*65–68, April '39 also: Presse med. *47:*139–141, Jan 28, '39

GAUTRELET, J.: Paralysis of parasympathetic as basis for shock treatment. Medecine *5:*204–206, Dec '23 abstr: J.A.M.A. *82:*424, Feb 2, '24

GAUVAIN, H.: Combination of Finsen light and plastic surgery in lupus of face. Strahlentherapie *45:*19–24, '32

GAXIOLA GANDARA, J.: Extensive skin detachment; therapy. Prensa med. mex. *7:*178–179, Dec 15, '42

GAY, E. C.: Burn therapy. Mil. Surgeon *91:*298–305, Sept '42

GAY, E. C.: Skin dressings (split grafts) in treatment of debrided wounds. Am. J. Surg. *72:*212–218, Aug '46

GAY PRIETO, J. AND CAZORLA ROMERO, J.: Idiopathic (glandular and exfoliative) cheilitis; relation to epithelioma of lower lip; case. Actas dermo-sif. *25:*700–706, May '33

GAYET, R. (see THEVENOT) Sept–Oct '38

GAZA, W. v.: Operative treatment of epispadias. Arch. f. klin. Chir. *126:*510–514, '23

GAZA, W. v.: Treatment of exstrophy of bladder by Makkas-Lengemann technic. Arch. f. klin. Chir. *126:*515–522, '23

GAZA, W. v.: Free fat transplantation in therapy of cleft palate. Arch. f. klin. Chir. *142:*590–599, '26

GAZZOTTI, L. G.: Pedunculated bone grafts. Policlinico (sez. chir.) *28:*548–555, Dec '21 (illus.) abstr: J.A.M.A. *78:*691, March 4, '22

GAZZOTTI, L. G.: Congenital deformity of hands and feet. Chir. d. org. di movimento *6:*265–

280, July '22 (illus.) abstr: J.A.M.A. *79:*1084, Sept 23, '22

GEBAUER, T.: Traumatic rigidity of fingers. Arch. Soc. cirujanos hosp., num. espec., pp. 57–64, Dec '41

GEBHARD, U. E.: Burn therapy. Indust. Med. *7:*622–623, Oct '38

GEBHARD, U. E.: Tendon repair by transfixion. Indust. Med. *13:*38–39, Jan '44

GEE, A. Traumatic aneurysm of ulnar artery. M. J. Australia *1:*395–396, April 21, '45

GEFFNER, S. (see GINI LACORTE, F. D.) Dec '44

GEIST, D. C.: Management of burned patient. Am. J. Surg. *57:*20–25, July '42

GEIST, S. H. (see FRANK, R. T.) Dec '27

GEIST, S. H. (see FRANK, R. T.) Feb '32

Geist-Frank Operation

Formation of artificial vagina (Frank-Geist method). FRANK, R. T., S. Clin. North America *12:*305–310, April '32

GEKTIN, F. L.: Surgical therapy of localized third degree burns. Vestnik khir. *46:*205–208, '36

GEKTIN, F. L.: Method of therapy of cancer of lower lip. Novy khir. arkhiv. *46:*52–59, '40

GEKTIN, F. L.: Skin grafts in reconstructive surgery at base hospitals. Khirurgiya, no. 2, pp. 26–35, '44

GEKTIN, F. L.: Skin grafts to cover defects of stumps after frostbite. Khirurgiya, no. 4, pp. 23–27, '44

GEMMELL, J. A. M.: Construction of simple obturator in cleft palate. Brit. Dent. J. *76:*69–70, Feb 4, '44

GENATIOS, T. (see ALARCON, C. J.) Aug '43

GENDLER, A. V. (see KEVDIN, N. A.) 1944

GENESIO SALLES: Plastic surgery of breast. Bahia med. *5:*623–624, Sept '34

GENET, L.: Repeated inflammation and fistulae treated by excision of lacrimal sac; cases. Lyon med. *143:*178–181, Feb 10, '29

Genetics: See Heredity

DEL GENIO, F.: Autoplastic grafts in rabbits whose skin had been frozen previously. Sperimentale, Arch. di biol. *90:*75–85, '36

Genitalia (See also Bladder Exstrophy: Epispadias; Hypospadias; Penis; Scrotum; Urethra; Vagina)

Elephantiasis nostras of genitalia; report of case and operative treatment. ORR, T. G. S. Clin. N. America *3:*1537–1545, Dec '23 (illus.)

Exstrophy of bladder, case with abnormalities of genitals. PAVLOVSKY, A. J. AND SAVAGE, R. Bol. Soc. de obst. y ginec. *8:*64–74, June 5, '29 also: Semana med. *2:*615–620, Aug 29, '29

Ectopy of bladder, remains of cloacal duct, perineal hernia of caudal gut and apparent doubling of external genitals. GRUBER, G. B. Beitr. z. path. Anat. u. z. allg. Path. *87:*455–465, June 27, '31

Plastic operations of the genitourinary tract. LOWSLEY, O. S. AND HUNT, R. W. South. M. J. *35:*676–687, July '42

Surgery of congenital anomalies of female genitals. SARNOFF, J. AND SARNOFF, S. J. J. Internat. Coll. Surgeons *6:*36–47, Jan–Feb '43

Treatment of burns of external genitalia. DRUMMOND, A. C., J. Urol. *50:*497–502, Oct '43

Medical progress; plastic operations on external genitalia. LOWSLEY, O. S. New York Med. (no. 20) *1:*17, Oct 20, '45

Recurrent aphthous ulceration of oral mucous membrane and genitals associated with recurrent hypopyon iritis (Behcet syndrome); 3 cases. KATZENELLENBOGEN, I. Brit. J. Dermat. *58:*161–172, Jul–Aug '46

GENKIN, I. I.: Traumatic burns in etiology of cancer. Vrach. delo *15:*496–499, '32

GENNER, V.: Hypertrichosis and its treatment with special regard to cosmetically disfiguring forms. Ugesk. f. laeger *103:*1400–1403, Oct 30, '41

Gensoul

Album of Gensoul, maxillary surgeon. LERICHE, R. Lyon chir. *25:*1–9, Jan–Feb '28

GEPFERT, J. R. (see ABBOTT, M. D.) Jan '44

GERALD, H. F.: Substitutes for human blood and plasma in treatment of surgical shock. Nebraska M. J. *29:*77–80, March '44

GERCHUNOFF, G. (see VON SOUBIRON, N. *et al*) June '38

GERGENREDER, F. A.: Total excision of skin of leg in elephantiasis and closure of defect with Thiersch graft. Vestnik khir. *55:*603–609, May '38

GERKE, J.: Orthopedic surgery in treatment of simple fractures of zygomatic arch. Deutsche Ztschr. f. Chir. *247:*398–403, '36

GERKE, J.: Artificial restoration of nasolacrimal duct. Ztschr. f. Augenh. *91:*50–52, Jan '37

GERKE, J.: Multiple cleft formations of maxillofacial region and their combination with other malformations. Munchen. med. Wchnschr. *90:*712, Dec 17, '43

GERLACH, J.: War injuries of nerves of arm. Med. Klin. *38:*173, Feb 20, '42

GERLINGS, P. G. AND DEN HOED, D.: Diagnosis and therapy of malignant tumors of nasopharynx. Nederl. tijdschr. v. geneesk. *81:*581–589, Feb 6, '37

GERMAN, W. J.: War surgery of face and head. Yale J. Biol. and Med. *14:*453–462, May '42

GERMAN, W. J.: Surgical treatment of spasmodic facial tic. Surgery *11:*912–914, June '42

GERMAN, W. J.; FINESILVER, E. M. AND DAVIS, J. S.: Establishment of circulation in tubed skin flaps; experimental study. Arch. Surg. *26:*27–40, Jan '33

GERMAN, W. J. (see DAVIS, J. S.) July '30

GERNEZ, L.; MOULONGUET, P. AND MALLET, L.: Therapy of mandibular epithelial cancers by electrocoagulation followed by curietherapy. Bol. Liga contra el cancer *10:*293–308, Oct '35

GERONIMI, E.: Electrotherapy of tuberous angioma of face. Schweiz. med. Wchnschr. *61:*589–593, June 20, '31

GERRARD, E. A. (see HEGGIE, R. M. *et al*) March '42

GERRIE, J. W.: Fracture of maxillary zygomatic compound. Canad. M.A.J. *38:*535–538, June '38

GERRIE, J. W.: One hundred broken noses. Canad. M.A.J. *39:*433–436, Nov '38

GERRIE, J. W.: Congenital absence of one tonsil; microtia and polydactylism in same patient. Arch. Otolaryng. *29:*378–381, Feb '39

GERRIE, J. W.: Plastic surgery at 72. Canad. M.A.J. *41:*548–549, Dec '39

GERRIE, J. W.: Choice of skin grafts in plastic surgery. Canad. M.A.J. *44:*9–13, Jan '41

GERRIE, J. W.: Prosthetic reconstruction of face. Canad. M.A.J. *50:*104–109, Feb '44

GERRIE, J. W.: New cement for use in cutting skin grafts. Canad. M.A.J. *51:*465–466, Nov '44

GERRIE, J. W. (see GURD, F. B.) July '44

GERRIE, J. W. (see MACLEAN, J. T.) Oct '46

GERRITZEN, P.: Etiology of Dupuytren's contracture; relation to occupation and trauma. Monatschr. f. Unfallh. *42:*545–551, Nov '35

GERRY, R. G.: Simplified technic for fabrication of tantalum plates in cranial surgery. U. S. Nav. M. Bull. *46:*1499–1505, Oct '46

GERSH, I. (see PFEIFFER, C. C. *et al*) May '45

Gersuny Operation

Plastic operation on protruding ears (Gersuny). BIESENBERGER, H. Zentralbl. f. Chir. *51:*1126–1127, May 24, '24

Gersuny's pedunculated flaps for reconstruction of face. MOSZKOWICZ, L. Arch. f. klin. Chir. *130:*796–798, '24

GERY, L.: Causes of abnormal cicatrization. Bull. et mem. Soc. d. chirurgiens de Paris *28:*405–417, June 19, '36

GESCHELIN, A. I.: Congenital malformation of region of pinna; case. Arch. f. Ohren-, Nasen- u. Kehlkopfh. *136:*332–334, '33

GESCHICKTER, C. F.: Hypertrophy of breasts. Surgery *3:*916–949, June '38

GESSE, E. R.: Perineal hypospadias in man who for 26 years was regarded as woman; surgical care. Ztschr. f. urol. Chir. *38:*18–22, '33

GESSNER, H. B.: Thyroglossal cyst and fistula. Southern M. J. *17:*428–430, June '24

GEY, R.: Question of cod liver oil or tannin; comparative study in burns. Deut. Militararzt *6:*287–288, May '41

GEYMANOVICH, Z. I.: Open treatment of fresh hand injuries. Novy khir. arkhiv. *31:*424–430, '34

GEYMANOVICH, Z. I.: Mobilization of hand following loss of all fingers. Khirurgiya, no. 6, pp. 82–84, '44

GHEESLING, G.: Tannic acid in burns. Indust. Med. *6:*306, May '37

GHETTI, L.: Fractures of fingers. Arch. di ortop. *50:*557–645, June 30, '34

GHORMLEY, R. K.: Symposium on acute burns; surgical care. Proc. Staff Meet., Mayo Clin. *8:*126–127, Feb 22, '33

GHORMLEY, R. K.: Emergency care of burns and injuries to skin. Proc. Staff Meet., Mayo Clin. *15:*741, Nov 20, '40

GHORMLEY, R. K.: Surgical treatment of roentgen and radium dermatitis. Proc. Staff Meet., Mayo Clin. *16:*69, Jan 29, '41

GHORMLEY, R. K.: Choice of graft methods in bone and joint surgery. Ann. Surg. *115:*427–434, March '42

GHORMLEY, R. K.: Repair of deep skin defects of foot and ankle. Am. Acad. Orthop. Surgeons, Lect., pp. 107–112, '44

GHORMLEY, R. K. AND CAMERON, D. M.: Tendon transplantation for paralysis of radial nerve. Proc. Staff Meet., Mayo Clin. *15:*537–539, Aug 21, '40

GHORMLEY, R. K. AND FAIRCHILD, R. D.: Surgical treatment of roentgen and radium dermatitis. Surgery *7:*737–752, May '40

GHORMLEY, R. K. AND LIPSCOMB, P. R.: Use of untubed pedicle grafts in repair of deep defects of foot and ankle; technic and results. J. Bone and Joint Surg. *26:*483–488, July '44

GHORMLEY, R. K. AND OVERTON, L. M.: Surgical treatment of severe lymphedema of extremities; study of end results. Proc. Staff Meet., Mayo Clin. *9:*564–566, Sept 19, '34

GHORMLEY, R. K. AND OVERTON, L. M.: Surgical treatment of severe forms of lymphedema of extremities; end-results. Surg., Gynec. and

Obst. *61:*83-89, July '35

Ghormley, R. K. and Stuck, W. G.: Study of experimental transplantation of bone, with special reference to effect of "decalcification." Proc. Staff Meet., Mayo Clin. *8:*253-254, April 26, '33

Ghormley, R. K. and Stuck, W. G.: Experimental bone transplantation, with special reference to effect of "decalcification." Arch. Surg. *28:*742-770, April '34

Ghormley, R. K. (see Allen, E. V.) Nov '35

Ghormley, R. K. (see Brunsting, L. A.) Feb '36

Ghormley, R. K. (see Steenrod, E. J. *et al*) May '37

Ghosh, N.: Case of diffuse hypertrophy of breast. Indian M. Gaz. *61:*395-396, Aug '26

Ghosh, P. K.: Gastrothoracoschisis; rare case of fetal maldevelopment. Calcutta M. J. *41:*10-12, Jan '44

Giacinto, G.: Surgical treatment of elephantiasis of lower limbs. Riforma med. *41:*793-795, Aug 24, '25

Giampaolo, R.: Pathogenesis of death from burns and its relation to anaphylaxis. Policlinico (sez. prat.) *32:*207-208, Feb 9, '25

Gianni, O.: Behavior of cartilage in submucous resection; histopathologic study. Arch. ital. di otol. *47:*487-498, July '35

Gianotti, M. and Ferrando, M.: Comparative study of repair of loss of peripheral nerve substance by interposition of fixed spinal cord or nerve. Boll. e mem. Soc. piemontese di chir. *9:*100-128, '39

Gianturco, G.: Certain fundamental principles of esthetic surgery; with method of plastic reconstruction of lower lip for cicatricial deformity. Rinasc. med. *4:*507, Nov 1, '27

Gianturco, G.: Treatment of some cicatricial deformities of hand. Chir. d. org. di movimento *13:*158-167, Dec '28

Giardino, G.: Grave acute osteomyelitis due to necrosis of dental pulp caused by repeated sport trauma; surgical therapy of case. Riv. di chir. *3:*371-374, July-Aug '37

Gibson, A.: Facial paralysis. Surg., Gynec. and Obst. *33:*472, Nov '21

Gibson, G. G.: Transscleral lacrimal canaliculus transplants. Am. J. Ophthl. *27:*258-269, March '44

Gibson, J. G. Jr. (see Dunphy, J. E.) July '41

Gibson, S. T. (see Woodruff, L. M.) Oct '42

Gibson, S. T. (see Woodruff, L. M.) July '43

Gibson, T. and Medawar, P. B.: Fate of skin homografts in man. J. Anat. *77:*299-310, July '43

Gibson, T. (see Colebrook, L. *et al*) April '44

Giese, A.: Results of surgical and diathermic-surgical treatment of cancer of concha of ear. Ztschr. f. Laryng., Rhin. *19:*414-423, July '30

Gifford, A. C.: Clinical report illustrating application of orthodontic principles in treatment of jaw fractures. Internat. J. Orthodontia *18:*1285-1289, Dec '32

Gifford, H. Jr.: Dacryocystitis; transplantation operation. Tr. Sect. Ophth., A.M.A., pp. 156-161, '44

Gifford, M. F.: Necessity of speech and voice re-education, with special reference to nasality. Laryngoscope *35:*317-323, April '25

Gifford, S. R.: Machek operation in eyelid ptosis. Arch. Ophth. *8:*495-502, Oct '32

Gifford, S. R.: Hughes procedure for rebuilding lower eyelid. Arch. Ophth. *21:*447-452, March '39

Gifford, S. R. and Puntenney, I.: Modification of Dickey operation in eyelid ptosis. Arch. Ophth. *28:*814-820, Nov '42

Giganti, I. J. (see Castellano, J. L.) June '39

Giganti, I. J. (see Castellano, J. L.) Oct '43

Giglio, H. (see Goni Moreno, I.) 1942

Gignoux, A.: Diathermocoagulation in therapy of congenital imperforation of choanae; 2 cases. Lyon med. *160:*652-654, Dec 12, '37

Gigon. (see Sorrel, E. *et al*) Nov '35

Gilbert, H. H. (see Glenn, W. W. L. *et al*) July '43

Gilbert-Dreyfus. (see Lesné, E. *et al*) Dec '28

Gilcreest, E. L.: Plastic operation for repair of traumatic amputation of end of finger. S. Clin. N. Amer. *6:*555-556, April '26

Gile, B. C.: Fractures of nose. Atlantic M. J. *28:*512-515, May '25

Giliberti, P.: Relation between burns and development of anaphylaxis; experimental study. Gior. di batteriol. e immunol. *20:*19-35, Jan '38

Gilkison, C. C. Treatment of maxillomandibular fractures at aid station and at base hospital. Mil. Surgeon *84:*441-451, May '39

Gill, A. B.: Fibrous ankylosis of hand due to prolonged swelling. J.A.M.A. *83:*1137-1139, Oct 11, '24

Gill, A. B.: Operation to make posterior bone block at ankle to limit foot-drop. J. Bone and Joint Surg. *15:*166-170, Jan '33

Gill, A. B.: Surgery of muscles and tendons for contracture. S. Clin. North America *15:*203-212, Feb '35

Gill, A. B.: Dupuytren's contracture. Ann. Surg. *107:*122-127, Jan '38

Gill, E. G.: Correction of nasal deformities by external route. Virginia M. Monthly *52:*578-581, Dec '25

GILL, E. G.: Cysts of neck, nine cases. Virginia M. Monthly *63:*482–487, Nov '36
GILL, E. G.: Implantation of costal cartilage for correction of nasal deformities. Virginia M. Monthly *65:*279–281, May '38
GILL, G. G. (see ABBOTT, L. C.) 1942
GILL, W. D.: Fractures about orbit. South. M. J. *21:*527–534, July '28
GILL, W. D.: Fractures involving orbit and paranasal sinuses, with special reference to diagnosis and treatment. Texas State J. Med. *27:*351–358, Sept '31
GILL, W. D.: Reconstructive surgery in ophthalmology and otolaryngology. Texas State J. Med. *29:*616–622, Feb '34
GILL, W. D.: Facial bone fractures, especially orbits and sinuses. South. M. J. *27:*197–205, March '34
GILL, W. D.: Facial bone fractures. Ann. Otol., Rhin. and Laryng. *46:*228–236, March '37
GILLERSON, A. B. AND EPSTEIN.: Naphthalene ointment in burns. Vrach. gaz. *32:*1645, Dec 15, '28
GILLETTE, C. P.: Inheritable defect of human hand. J. Hered. *22:*189–190, June '31
GILLIES, H. D.: "Eternal (plastic) triangle," simple cure. Lancet *2:*930–931, Oct 27, '23 (illus.)
GILLIES, H. D.: Deformities of syphilitic nose. Brit. M. J. *2:*977–979, Nov 24, '23 (illus.)
GILLIES, H. D.: Design of direct pedicle flaps. Brit. M. J. *2:*1008, Dec 3, '32
GILLIES, H. D.: Experience with fascia lata grafts in operative treatment of facial paralysis. Proc. Roy. Soc. Med. *27:*1372–1378, Aug '34 also: J. Laryng. and Otol. *49:*743–756, Nov '34
GILLIES, H. D.: Plastic surgery of eyelids. Tr. Ophth. Soc. U. Kingdom *55:*357–373, '35
GILLIES, H. D.: Development and scope of plastic surgery (Charles H. Mayo lecture). Northwestern Univ. Bull., Med. School *35:*1–32, Jan 28, '35
GILLIES, H. D.: Experiences with tubed pedicle flaps. Surg., Gynec. and Obst. *60:*291–303, Feb (no. 2A) '35
GILLIES, H. D.: Reconstructive surgery; repair of superficial injuries. Surg., Gynec. and Obst. *60:*559–567, Feb (no. 2A) '35
GILLIES, H. D.: Reconstruction of external ear with special reference to use of maternal ear cartilage as supporting structure (cases). Rev. de chir. structive, pp. 169–179, Oct '37
GILLIES, H. D.: Syphilitic saddle nose. Deutsche Ztschr. f. Chir. *250:*379–401, '38
GILLIES, H. D.: Primary treatment of facial fractures. Practitioner *140:*414–425, April '38
GILLIES, H. D.: Practical uses of tubed pedicle flap. Am. J. Surg. *43:*201–215, Feb '39
GILLIES, H. D.: Autograft of amputated digit; suggested operation. Lancet *1:*1002–1003, June 1, '40
GILLIES, H. D.: Technic in construction of auricle. Tr. Am. Acad. Ophth. (1941) *46:*119–121, Jan–Feb '42
GILLIES, H. D.: Plastic surgery of burns. Rev. Asoc. med. argent. *56:*196–198, April 15-30, '42
GILLIES, H. D.: New free graft (of skin and ear cartilage) applied to reconstruction of nostril. Brit. J. Surg. *30:*305–307, April '43
GILLIES, H. D.: Technique of good suturing. St. Barth. Hosp. J. *47:*170–173, July '43
GILLIES, H. D.: Closure of wounds of the scalp. Lancet *2:*310–311, Sept 2, '44
GILLIES, H. D.: Operative replacement of mammary prominence. Brit. J. Surg. *32:*477–479, April '45

Gillies, H. D.

Sir Harold Gillies, surgeon examplatory. ZENO, L. An. de cir. *7:*315–320, Dec '41 also: Semana med. *2:*1543–1546, Dec 25, '41

GILLIES, H. D. AND FRASER, F. R.: Treatment of lymphedema by plastic operation; preliminary report. Brit. M. J. *1:*96–98, Jan 19, '35
GILLIES, H. D. AND FRY, W. K.: A new principle in surgical treatment of "congenital cleft palate," and its mechanical counterpart. Brit. M. J. *1:*335, March 5, '21
GILLIES, H. D. AND KILNER, T. P.: Symblepharon of eyelids; treatment by Thiersch and mucous membrane grafting. Tr. Ophth. Soc. U. Kingdom *49:*470–479, '29
GILLIES, H. D. AND KILNER, T. P.: Treatment of nasal fractures. Lancet *1:*147–149, Jan 19, '29
GILLIES, H. D. AND KILNER, T. P.: Operations for correction of secondary deformities of cleft lip. Lancet *2:*1369–1375, Dec 24, '32
GILLIES, H. D.; KILNER, T. P. AND STONE, D.: Fractures of malar-zygomatic compound, with description of new X-ray position. Brit. J. Surg. *14:*651–656, April '27
GILLIES, H. D. AND MCINDOE, A. H.: Plastic surgery in chronic radiodermatitis and radionecrosis. Brit. J. Radiol. *6:*132–147, March '33
GILLIES, H. D. AND MCINDOE, A. H.: Late surgical complications of fracture of mandible. Brit. M. J. *2:*1060–1063, Dec 9, '33
GILLIES, H. D. AND MCINDOE, A. H.: Role of plastic surgery in burns due to roentgen rays and radium. Ann. Surg. *101:*979–996, April '35
GILLIES, H. D. AND MCINDOE, A. H.: Technic of

mammaplasty (for hypertrophy). Surg., Gynec. and Obst. *68:*658-665, March '39
GILLIES, H. D. AND MOWLEM, R.: Prognosis in plastic surgery. Lancet *2:*1346-1347, Dec 6, '36
GILLIES, H. D. AND MOWLEM, R.: Prognosis in plastic surgery. Lancet *2:*1411-1412, Dec 12, '36
GILLIES, H. D. (see CRITCHLEY, M.) 1937
GILLIES, H. D. (see JAMES, W. W.) 1933
GILLIES, H. D. (see LEVITT, W. M.) April '42
GILLIES, H. D. (see WAKELEY, C. P. G. *et al*) 1945

Gillies Operation

Plastic surgery of nose according to Gillies. MOE, R. Nord. med. (Norsk mag. f. laegevidensk.) *28:*2329-2332, Nov 2, '45
Treatment of depressed fracture of zygomatic arch by Gillies method. CHRISTIANSEN, G. W. AND BRADLEY, J. L. U. S. Nav. M. Bull. *44:*1066-1068, May '45
Gillies operation for correction of depressed fracture deformities of zygomatic-malar bones. GREELEY, P. W. Illinois M. J. *71:*419-420, May '37
Gillies new method in giving support to depressed nasal bridge and columella. SHEEHAN, J. E. New York M. J. *113:*448, March 16, '21
Nasal deformity of syphilitic type due to injury; loss of mucosa and of supporting bone and cartilage; modified Gillies operation in therapy of case. DELLEPIANE RAWSON, R. AND PEREZ FERNANDEZ, M. Arq. de cir. clin. e exper. *6:*492-503, April-June '42

GILLUM, J. R.: Dacryocystorhinostomy. J. Indiana M. A. *17:*113-116, April '24
GILMAN, P. K.: Cysts and fistulae of thyroglossal duct. Surg., Gynec. and Obst. *32:*141, Feb '21
GILMAN, P. K.: Branchial cysts and fistulas. J.A.M.A. *77:*26, July 2, '21
GILMER, L.: Construction of artificial vagina. Monatschr. f. Geburtsh. u. Gynak. *91:*48-56, May '32
GILMORE, E. R. W.: Finger abnormalities. Brit. M. J. *2:*935-936, Nov 19, '27
GILPATRICK, R. H.: Ankylosis of jaw. Boston M. and S. J. *186:*374-377, March 23, '22 (illus.)
GIMENEZ, A. LEON: Vascular collapse and its therapy. Dia med. *16:*1322-1325, Oct 30, '44
GIMENO Y RODRÍGUEZ JAÉN, V. AND PULIDO, A.: Surgery of skin without disfigurement; esthetic surgery. Siglo med. *71:*503-506, May 26; 532-534, June 2; 555-558, June 9; 582-585, June 16; 603-607, June 23; 629-632, June 30, '23
GINANNESCHI, G.: Progressive facial hemiatrophy (Romberg's disease); case. Pensiero med. *23:*157-160, May '34
GINESTET, G.: Reduction of double fracture of lower jaw by combined action of intermaxillary forces and transosseous loop. Rev. de stomatol. *40:*289-294, May '38
GINESTET, G.: Surgical therapy of mordex apertus and of prognathism. Rev. de stomatol. *41:*4-17, Jan '39
GINESTET, G.: Instruments for maxillofacial and oral surgery. Rev. de stomatol. *43:*121-123, July-Aug '42
GINESTET, G. AND CHEMIN: Bone grafts in pseudoarthrosis and loss of substance of upper jaw. Rev. de stomatol. *47:*137-139, May-June '46
GINESTET, G. AND GINESTET, F.: Surgical treatment under regional anesthesia for harelip. Rev. de stomatol. *31:*12, April '29
GINESTET, G.; ROY, AND HOUPERT, L.: Orthopedic surgery of temporomaxillary joint; cases. Rev. de stomatol. *41:*520-532, July '39
GINESTET, F. (see GINESTET, G.) April '29
GINESTET, G. (see BERCHER, J.) May '34
GINESTIE, J. (see MASSABUAU, *et al*) April '35
GINGRASS, R. P.: Maxillo-facial injuries. Wisconsin M. J. *33:*568-571, Aug '34
GINGRASS, R. P.: Early management of facial injuries. J. Am. Dent. A. *25:*693-699, May '38
GINGRASS, R. P.: Stabilization of mandibular joint by injection of sclerosing solution (sodium psylliate). Wisconsin M. J. *37:*383-384, May '38
GINGRASS, R. P.: Plastic surgery of face. Am. J. Orthodontics *26:*961-967, Oct '40
GINGRASS, R. P.: Submucous cleft palate; traumatic perforation by denture. Am. J. Orthodontics (Oral Surg. Sect) *28:*113-114, Feb '42
GINI LACORTE, F. D. AND GEFFNER, S.: Prontosil (sulfonamide) in burn therapy. Dia med. *16:*1492-1493, Dec 4, '44
GINSBURG, L.: Rhinophyma in woman. Arch. Dermat. and Syph. *32:*468, Sept '35
GINZBERG, M. M.: Data on plastic surgical operations. Sovet. klin. *19:*447-452, '33
GINZBURG, R. L.: Injuries of nerves of upper extremities. Ortop. i travmatol. (no. 3) *12:*105-119, '38
GIOIA, T.: Typical case of Guerin fracture of upper jaw. Bol. y trab. de la Soc. de cir. de Buenos Aires *14:*976-982, Nov 26, '30 also: Semana med. *2:*1982-1985, Dec 25, '30
GIOIA, T.: Therapy of recent fractures of lower jaw; with description of apparatus used. Semana med. *2:*1370-1378, Nov 7, '35
GIOIA, T.: Burns. Semana med. *2:*543-549, Sept 8, '38
GIOIA, T.: Phalangization of first metacarpus to

substitute for thumb, with report of case. Semana med. *1:*490–497, March 4, '43

Gioia, T. (see Ceballos, A.) May '27

Gioia, T. (see Ceballos, A.) June '28

Giordanengo, G.: Metacarpophalangeal luxations of thumb. Minerva chir. *1:*92–94, May '46

Giordanengo, G.: Disarticulations and amputations of fingers and toes. Minerva chir. *1:*165–166, July '46

Giordano, D.: Elephantiasis; surgical treatment. Riforma med. *39:*889–891, Sept 17, '23 (illus.)

Giordano, A. S.: Physiologic pathology as applied to treatment of shock. J. Indiana M. A. *34:*197–200, April '41

Giorgi, C.: Case of zygomatic fracture cured by direct skeletal traction applied with screw. Riv. di chir. *5:*34–39, Jan–Feb '39

Giovacchini, L. U.: Surgical reconstruction of face. Rev. Asoc. med. argent. *36:*312–315, July '23 (illus.) abstr: J.A.M.A. *81:*1826, Nov 24, '23

de Girardier, J.: Halsted-Davis skin grafts; conditions of transplantation and technic. Lyon med. *140:*89–103, July 31, '27

de Girardier, J.: Halsted-Davis skin grafts; indications and results. Lyon med. *140:*117, Aug 7; 145, Aug 14, '27

de Girardier, J.: Complete traumatic section of radial nerve in young girl; rapid regeneration following immediate suture; case. Lyon med. *163:*13–15, Jan 1 '39

de Girardier, J.: Technic needed for correct treatment of panaris and infections of hand. Hopital *27:*213–215, April '39

Giraudeau, and Acquaviva.: Decoloration of flat angioma by application of light containing neither ultraviolet nor infrared rays after sensitization with essence of bergamot. Bull. Soc. franc. de dermat. et syph. *42:*1391, July '35

Girdlestone, G. R.: Some points in reconstructive surgery. Practitioner *109:*456–459, Dec '22

Girdwood, W.: Immobilization and its disastrous effects on hand function. South African M. J. *18:*350–352, Oct 28, '44

Giri, D. V.: Bilateral ptosis and atypical slant eyes associated with unilateral syndactylia, adactylia and brachyphalangia. Proc. Roy. Soc. Med. *37:*360–361, May '44

Girode, C.: Disadvantages of dead bone implants in pseudoarthrosis or fracture of femur. Rev. de chir. *60:*60–80, '22 (illus.) abstr: J.A.M.A. *79:*507, Aug 5, '22

de Gironcoli, F.: Incontinence due to severe hypospadias of female urethra with simultaneous ectopy of ureteral orifice; case. Ztschr. f. urol. Chir. u. Gynak. *42:*152–156, '36

Gismondi, A.: Physiopathology and therapy of recent cutaneous burns. Prat. pediat. *15:*195–197, Nov '37

Gitelson, U. E.: Baldwin operation for artificial vagina; 7 cases. J. akush. i zhensk. boliez. *41:*467–476, '30

Giuliani, G. M.: Pseudarthrosis of first phalanx of right thumb; operative therapy; case. Chir. d. org. di movimento *20:*31–35, May '35

Giuliani, G. M.: Tendon transplantation in therapy of complete paralysis of radial nerve; case. Arch. ital. di chir. *42:*613–616, '36

Giuliani, G. M.: Tendon transplantation in therapy of inverterate radial paralysis. (Comment on Bonola's article.) Chir. d. org. di movimento *23:*102, Oct '37

Giuliano, A.: Local therapy of burns with author's formula containing prontosil (sulfonamide) and tannic acid; preliminary report. Rev. Asoc. med. argent. *57:*254–257, May 15–30, '43 also: Semana med. *1:*1434–1438, June 24, '43

Giurgiu, V. (see Kernbach, M.) July '31

di Giuseppe, F.: Apparatus for immediate treatment and prosthesis in jaw fractures. Giro. ital. di clin. trop. *1:*81, March 31, '37

Giussani, M.: Nasopharyngeal cyst of branchial origin; case. Ann. di laring., otol. *29:*213–226, July '28

Giussani, M. Laryngotracheal reconstruction with free autoplastic cartilaginous grafts. Arch. ital. di chir. *52:*472–483, '38

Giustinian, V. and Estiú, M. D.: Massive congenital cervicofacial cavernous hemangioma; case. Semana med. *2:*245–246, July 28, '32

Givner, I. Reconstruction of floor of orbit; case Am. J. Ophth. *29:*1010–1012, Aug '46

Gizzi, C.: Modifications in Graefe's apparatus for reduction and retention of fractures. Stomatol. *28:*865–870, Oct '30

Gjankovic, H.: Fibrous contracture of head and neck after extensive burns. Lijecn. vjes. *61:*279–284, May '39

Glaesmer, E.

Care, preservation and repair of female breasts; review of Erna Glaesmer's "Die Formfehler und die plastischen Operationen de weiblichen Brust," and H. Biesenberger's "Deformitaten und Operationen de weiblichen Brust." Sellheim, H. Deutsche med. Wchnschr. *58:*1414–1417, Sept 2, '32

Glaesmer, E. and Amersbach, R.: Pathology and surgical treatment of pendulous breast. Munchen. med. Wchnschr. *74:*1171–1176, July 15, '27

GLAESMER, E. AND AMERSBACH, R.: Improved technic for surgical correction of pendulous breast. Munchen. med. Wchnschr. *75:*1547-1549, Sept 7, '28

GLÄSMER, ERNA: *Die Formfehler und die plastischen Operationen der weiblichen Brüst.* F. Enke. Stuttgart, 1930

GLÄSMER, E.: Cosmetic operations of the breast. Med. Welt *4:*630, May 3, '30

GLÄSMER, E.: Method for plastic surgery of hypertrophy of breast. Zentralbl. f. Gynak. *54:*2202-2204, Aug 30, '30

GLÄSMER, E.: Importance of dermatogram for plastic operations of breast. Dermat. Wchnschr. *95:*1713-1718, Nov 26, '32

GLÄSMER, E.: Plastic surgery of breast and preservation of lactating function. Deutsche med. Wchnschr. *63:*559, April 2, '37

GLASCOCK, H. AND GLASCOCK, H. JR.: Repair of traumatic fistulas of Stenson's duct (parotid). Surg., Gynec. and Obst. *65:*355-356, Sept '37

GLASCOCK, H. JR. (see GLASCOCK, H.) Sept '37

GLASER, K.; MEHN, W. H. AND SCHULTZ, L. W.: Congenital hemangioma of parotid gland. J. Pediat. *28:*729-732, June '46

GLASNER, J.: Syndactylia and synphalangism; case. Arq. brasil. de cir. e ortop. *7:*338-344, Dec '39

Glass

Rupture of extensor tendon at terminal phalanx of finger (comment on Glass' article). SONNTAG, E. Zentralbl. f. Chir. *55:*410, Feb 18, '28

GLASS, E.: Appliance for pendulous breasts. Deutsche med. Wchnschr. *51:*660, April 17, '25 abstr: J.A.M.A. *84:*1881, June 13, '25

GLASS, E.: Metal splint for injuries of extensor tendons of fingers. Zentralbl. f. Chir. *54:*3027-3028, Nov 26, '27

GLASS, E.: Metal finger splints for injuries received in athletic games. Zentralbl. f. Chir. *55:*601-602, March 10, '28

GLASS, E.: Practical metal finger splint for injured finger. Deutsche med. Wchnschr. *54:*1121, July 6, '28

GLASS, E.: Curved metal finger splint. Zentralbl. f. Chir. *56:*2459-2460, Sept 28, '29

GLASS, E.: Comment on article by Horwitz on rupture of extensor tendons of fingers. Zentralbl. f. Chir. *57:*2063, Aug 16, '30

GLASSBURG, J. A.: Cleft palate speech. Arch. Otolaryng. *12:*820-821, Dec '30

GLASSER, B. F. AND RICHLIN, P.: Scrape method of skin grafting. Am. J. Surg. *64:*131-134, April '44

GLASSER, S. T.: Ox fascia (dead fascia) graft. Am. J. Surg. *19:*542-544, March '33

GLASSER, S. T. (see HERRLIN, J. O. JR.) June-Oct '42

GLATT, M. A.: Rhinophyma. Illinois M. J. *61:*174-175, Feb '32

GLATZEL, J. AND ZUBRZYCKI, J.: Construction of artificial vagina. Ginek. polska *11:*580, April-June '32

GLATZEL, J. AND ZUBRZYCKI, J.: Kirschner-Wagner operation for artificial vagina. Polska gaz. lek. *12:*577-579, July 29, '33

GLEAVE, H. H.: Prognosis in malignant melanoma; 40 consecutive cases. Lancet *2:*658-659, Sept 28, '29

GLENN, W. W. L.: Physiologic analysis of burns. Ann. Surg. *119:*801-814, June '44

GLENN, W. W. L.: Physiologic analysis of nature and treatment of burns. Prensa med. argent. *32:*1298-1300, July 6, '45

GLENN, W. W. L.; GILBERT, H. H. AND DRINKER, C. K.: Closed-plaster method of burn therapy, with certain physiologic considerations implicit in success of this technic. J. Clin. Investigation *22:*609-625, July '43

GLENN, W. W. L.; PETERSON, D. K. AND DRINKER, C. K.: Flow of lymph from burned tissue, with particular reference to effects of fibrin formation upon lymph drainage and composition. Surgery *12:*685-693, Nov '42

GLEYBERMAN, E. Y.: Transplantation of preserved skin in experimental cutaneous tuberculosis. Med. zhur. *10:*269-275, '40

GLEZEROV, S. Y.: Plastic surgery of eyelids. Sovet. vestnik oftal. *3:*305-307, '33

GLEZEROV, S. Y.: Eyelid ptosis operation. Vestnik oftal. *17:*132-134, '40

GLEZEROV, S. Y.: Principles of plastic surgery in cicatricial ectropion of lower eyelid. Vestnik oftal. *18:*397-400, '41

GLICKMAN, I. (see LANZANSKY, J. P. *et al*) March '46

GLISSAN, D. J.: Limitation of movement at metacarpophalangeal joints; its causes and treatment. M. J. Australia *2:*257, Oct '21

GLISSAN, D. J.: Use of plantaris tendon in certain types of plastic surgery of hand. Australian and New Zealand J. Surg. *2:*64-67, July '32

Glomus Tumors

Glomus tumor: arterial angioneuromyoma of Masson. COLE, H. N. AND SROUB, W. E. J.A.M.A. *107:*428-429, Aug 8, '36

Glomus tumor of fingers; case. LOEB, M. J. J. Florida M. A. *29:*372-374, Feb '43

Glomus tumor or glomangioma of fingers;

Glomus Tumors – Cont.

case. SCULLY, J. C., J. Michigan M. Soc. *42:*118–121, Feb '43

GLOVER, D. M.: Six years of tannic acid treatment in burns. Surg., Gynec. and Obst. *54:*798–805, May '32

GLOVER, D. M.: Evaluation of tannic acid; clinical study of 556 burns so treated over period of 11 years. Ohio State M. J. *33:*146–151, Feb '37

GLOVER, D. M.: Immediate treatment of burns. Proc. Interst. Postgrad. M. A. North America (1940) pp. 98–102, '41

GLOVER, D. M.: Immediate treatment of burn patient (coagulation regime). Australian and New Zealand J. Surg. *12:*91–102, Oct '42

GLOVER, D. M. AND JACOBY, M. W.: Reconstruction of conjunctival sac with Thiersch grafts. Arch. Surg. *26:*617–622, April '33

GLOVER, D. M. AND SYDOW, A. F.: Fifteen years of tannic acid method in burns. Am. J. Surg. *51:*601–619, March '41

GLOWINSKI, M.: Artificial vagina constructed from peritoneum. Ginek. polska *16:*683–687, July–Aug '37

GLOWINSKI, M.: Artificial vagina constructed from Douglas pouch. Zentralbl. f. Gynak. *61:*2440–2442, Oct 16, '37

GLUCK, T.: Experimental and clinical advances during nineteenth century (including plastic surgery). Arch. f. klin. Chir. *167:*626–666, '31

GLUSCHKOV, P.: Method of plastic resection of lower jaw. Vestnik khir. (no. 30) *10:*67–70, '27

GLUSHCHENKO, V. T. (see DIVNOGORSKIY, B. F.) 1933

GNILORYBOV, T. E.: Fixation of movable kidney by implantation of skin. Khirurgiya, no. 11, pp. 114–116, '39

GNILORYBOV, T. E.: Plastic reconstruction of auricle. Novy khir. arkhiv. *45:*148–156, '39

GNILORYBOV, T. E.: Plastic repair of defects of lips and corner of mouth by means of Filatov's tubular flaps. Vestnik khir. *59:*592–599, June '40

GOAR, E. L.: Infantile dacyrostenosis. M. Rec. and Ann. *37:*611–613, July '43

GOBBI, L.: Congenital cysts in neck. Policlinico (sez. chir.) *30:*372–388, July '23 (illus.)

GÖBELL, R.: Osteoplastic repair of congenital and acquired defects of lower jaw. Arch. di chir. inf. *1:*111–125, Jan '34

GÖBELL, R. AND FREUDENBERG, K.: Favorable results of surgical therapy of aplasia of opponens muscle of thumb by transplantation of tendons of flexor digitalis sublimis V; survey of methods. Arch. f. orthop. u. Unfall-Chir. *35:*675–677, '35

GOBICH, E. (see RIVAS, C. I. *et al*) April–June '42

GODARD, H.: Pelvic prerectal transposition in surgical therapy of exstrophy of bladder. Bull. Soc. de pediat. de Paris *33:*408–415, June '35 also: Bull. Soc. franc. d'urol., pp. 291–298, July 9, '35

GODARD, H.: Successful restoration in exstrophy of bladder resulting in continence and enabling urination by natural channels. Bull. Soc. franc. d'urol., pp. 157–160, March 16, '36

GODARD, H.: Urethroplasty for congenital strictures; method of temporary graft of penis to scrotum; case. Rev. de chir., Paris *74:*374–386, May '36

GODARD, H.: Urethroplasty; general review of technic using free or pedicled grafts in restoration of hypospadias. J. d'urol. *42:*105–142, Aug '36

GODARD, H.: Urethroplasty using scrotal grafts; review of various methods. J. d'urol. *43:*201–232, March '37

GODARD, H.: Exstrophy of bladder and masculine epispadias; treatment by prerectal pelvic transposition of bladder. J. d'urol. *47:*97–109, Feb '39

GODARD, H. (see LEVEUF, J.) Sept '36

GODDARD, F. W.: Satisfactory operation for entropion of upper eyelid. Chinese M. J. *50:*1505, Oct '36

GODDU, L. A. O.: Complete disability of hand by relaxed articulation of first metacarpus and trapezium, and slipping of tendon and extensor brevis pollicis; postoperative result. Boston M. and S. J. *192:*666–667, April 2, '25

GODOY MOREIRA, F. E.: Volkmann's contracture; case. Chir. d. org. di movimento *14:*573–582, March '30

GODOY MOREIRA, F. E.: Surgical therapy of paralysis of median nerve caused by section following wound with resultant neuroma formation. Sao Paulo med. *1:*211–215, Jan '33

GODWIN, J. G.: Extraoral plaster splint fixation in treatment of fractures of mandible. J. Am. Dent. A. *31:*76–85, Jan 1, '44

Goebell-Stoeckel Operation

Operative cure of incontinence of urine in epispadias by Goebell-Stoeckel operation. REIFFERSCHEID, K. Zentralbl. f. Gynak. *45:*97, Jan 22, '21

GOEPFERT, see CAUSSADE, L. *et al*) July '37

GOERINGER, C. F. (see GROSS, R. E.) July '39

GOETSCH, E.: Hygroma colli cysticum and hygroma axillare; pathologic and clinical study and report of 12 cases. Arch. Surg. *36:*394–479, March '38

GOETZE, O.: Conservative and operative treatment of arthritis deformans. Med. Welt *5:*81–83, Jan 17, '31

GOETZE, O.: Freezing of facial nerve in treatment of harelip. Zentralbl. f. Chir. *58:*927–930, April 11, '31

GÖHLER, W.: Contracture of thumb in infants following symptoms of snapping finger. Deutsche med. Wchnschr. *51:*1200, July 17, '25

GOFREN, A. G.: Grafts as method of primary therapy of wounds. Khirurgiya, no. 12, pp. 3–14, '37

GOHRBANDT, E.: Plastic operations for keloids. Med. Welt *4:*1510, Oct 18, '30

GOINARD, P.: Therapy of inveterate ulcers of leg by excision followed by immediate dermo-epidermic graft; cases. Algerie med. (Ed. chir.) *42:*75–81, Feb '38

GOINARD, P. AND CURTILLET, A.: Fractures at union of ramus and body of lower jaw; cases. Bull. med., Paris *48:*447–449, July 21, '34

GOLD, E.: Advisable therapeutic measures in finger injuries and hand. Wien. klin. Wchnschr. *45:*308–309, March 4, '32

GOLD, S.: Needle fragments in finger. Canad. M. A. J. *42:*269–270, March '40

GOLDBERG, H. M.: Volkmann contracture; causes and treatment. Kentucky M. J. *31:* 531–533, Nov '33

GOLDBERG, H. C.: Combined epilation needle and forceps handle. Arch. Dermat. and Syph. *44:*1104–1105, Dec '41

GOLDBERG, H.: Extensive burns treated in open irrigation chamber (with sodium hypochlorite solution). Lancet *1:*371–372, March 18, '44

GOLDBERG, R. R. (see ROGERS, W. L. *et al*) May '44

GOLDBERG, S. L. (see SACHS, A. E.) May '43

GOLDBLATT, D.: Study of burns, their classification and treatment. Ann. Surg. *85:*490–501, April '27

GOLDBLATT. D.: Removal of foreign bodies from hand, fingers and feet. Am. J. Surg. *8:*324–327, Feb '30

GOLDEN, H. M.: Recent advances in plastic surgery with special reference to vascularization of implants (face). Illinois M. J. *67:*175–181, Feb '35

GOLDFEDER, A. E.: Transplantation of cartilage from auricle into eyelid in trachomatous cicatricial entropion. Klin. Monatsbl. f. Augenh. *82:*809–813, June 21, '29

GOLDFEDER, A. E.: Marginoplasty by means of cartilage of auricle without skin in partial trichiasis of eyelid. Klin. Monatsbl. f. Augenh. *86:*218–225, Feb '31

GOLDFEDER, A. E.: New method of blepharoplastic operation for cicatricial ectropion using free transplant from ear flap. Sovet. vestnik. oftal. *6:*173–177, '35

GOLDFEDER, A. E. AND BUSHMICH, D. G.: Blaskovics operation for eyelid ptosis. Vestnik oftal. *11:*824–829, '37

GOLDHAHN, R.: Burn therapy. Deutsche med. Wchnschr. *65:*1472–1474, Sept 22, '39

GOLDHAHN, R.: Burn therapy. Med. Welt *14:*107–109, Feb 3, '40

GOLDHAHN, R.: Shock and collapse. Med. Welt *14:*573, June 8, '40; 597, June 15, '40

GOLDHAHN, R.: Deep paronychias of hand. Ztschr. f. arztl. Fortbild. *39:*319–323, July 15, '42

GOLDIE, H.: Dental aspect of maxillofacial surgery. South African M. J. *18:*224–225, July 8, '44

GOLDIE, J. C. (see BELLOSO, R. A.) July '40

GOLDIN, L. B. (see SVERDLOV, D. G.) 1938

GOLDING, H. S.: Fracture of lower jaw due to gunshot wounds in face during Waziristan operations, 1937; 3 cases. J. Roy. Army M. Corps *71:*50–54, July '38

GOLDMAN, H. M.: Case reports of jaw tumors from files of Registry of Dental and Oral Pathology sponsored by American Dental Association. Am. J. Orthodontics (Oral Surg. Sect.) *30:*265–314, May '44

GOLDMAN, I. B.: Prevention and correction of dorsal depressions by septal implants. (nose) Arch. Otolaryng. *32:*524–529, Sept '40

GOLDMAN, L. (see TAUBER, E. B.) April '39

GOLDMAN, L. (see BLACKFIELD, H. M.) June '39

GOLDMAN, M. L. (see BODENHEIMER, M.) Jan–Feb '41

GOLDMANN, H.: Plastic reconstruction of eye socket. Ophthalmologica *107:*60–63, Jan–Feb '44

GOLDSCHMIDT, T.: Case of extensive plastic repair of face and neck with "visor flap." Zentralbl. f. Chir. *52:*688–691, March 28, '25

GOLDSTEIN, M. S.: Development of bridge of nose. Am. J. Phys. Anthropol. *25:*101–117, April–June '39

GOLDTHWAIT, J. E.: "Flat hand" (manus planus): its correction essential to normal function of hand. J. Bone and Joint Surg. *4:*469–480, July '22 (illus.)

GOLDTHWAITE, R. H.: Laryngectomy for cancer of larynx with modified technique and attempted formation of skin tube in place of larynx. Laryngoscope *32:*446–450, June '22

GOLDTHWAITE, R. H.: Plastic repair of nasal displacement and deformity. Mil. Surgeon *51:*42–43, July '22

GOLDTHWAITE, R. H.: Plastic repair of depressed fracture of lower orbital rim.

J.A.M.A. *82:*628–629, Feb 23, '24
GOLJANITZKI, J. A.: Surgical treatment of true hermaphrodism. Arch. f. klin. Chir. *144:*732–751, '27
GOLKIN, M.: Partial rhinoplasty; restoration of nasal tip, alae and septum. Deutsche Ztschr. f. Chir. *199:*354–359, '26
GOLL, H. AND KAHLICH-KOENNER, D. M.: Acrocephalosyndactylia with cleft hand in one of a pair of uniovular twins. Ztschr. f. menschl. Vererb.-u. Konstitutionslehre *24:*516–535, '40
GOLLA, F.: Bilateral rupture of extensor aponeurosis of terminal phalanx of finger and its treatment. Beitr. z. klin. Chir. *162:*594–600, '35
GOLLA, F.: Avulsion of so-called extensor aponeurosis of thumb. Zentralbl. f. Chir. *65:*1803–1807, Aug 13, '38
GOLONZKO, L. Y. (see LARIN, N.) 1933
GOLYANITSKIY, I. A.: New principle for skin grafting. Sovet. vrach. gaz., pp. 588–590, April 15, '35
GÓMEZ, O.: Pseudoarthrosis of upper jaw after fracture of Guerin type; case. Bol. y trab. de la Soc. de cir. de Buenos Aires *12:*393–400, Aug 1, '28
GÓMEZ, O.: Therapy of burns. Bol. y trab. de la Soc. de cir. de Buenos Aires *19:*484–491, July 17, '35
GOMEZ, O. L.: Unusual fracture of superior maxilla; appreciation of incapacity for labor. Rev. de especialid. *3:*511–519, Sept '28
GOMEZ DURAN, M.: Modern concept of traumatic shock. Semana med. espan. *4:*673–681, June 14, '41
GÓMEZ-MÁRQUES, J.: Congenital entropion. Arch. de oftal. hispano-am. *30:*187–198, April '30
GÓMEZ-MÁRQUEZ: Technic in dacryocystorhinostomy. Arch. de oftal. hispano-am. *31:*147–176, March '31
GÓMEZ-MÁRQUEZ: Dacryocystorhinostomies; 517 cases. Klin. Monatsbl. f. Augenh. *86:*620–629, May '31
GÓMEZ MÁRQUEZ, J.: Congenital entropion; cases. Clin. y lab. *15:*11–23, Jan '30
GOMEZ NAVARRO, A. C.: Creation of artificial vagina in girl before marriage. Semana med. *1:*221–224, Jan 23, '41
GOMEZ NAVARRO, A. C.: Artificial vagina, creation before marriage; case. Rev. Asoc. med. argent. *55:*484–486, June 15–30, '41
GOMEZ OLIVEROS, L.: Author's application of Lohr method using cod liver oil in burns. Rev. clin. espan. *2:*170–173, Feb 1, '41
GOMEZ DE ROSAS, N.: New concepts of postoperative secondary shock and its therapy; physiology and general pathology. Vida nueva *48:*283–297, Nov '41
GOMOIU, V.: Practical therapy of burns. Spitalul *54:*302–305, July–Aug '34
GOMPERTZ, M. L. (see VORHAUS, M. G. *et al*) Feb '43
GONALONS, G. P.: Burns by running water; physiopathologic mechanism. Prensa med. argent. *26:*1117–1119, June 7, '39
GONCALVES, G.: Paraffinoma, harelip, cicatrices, auricular prosthesis in plastic surgery. Arq. de cir. clin. e exper. *6:*307–316, April–June '42
GONCALVES BOGADO, L.: War burns. Rev. med.-cir. do Brasil *50:*1087–1098, Dec '42
GONI MORENO, I.: (comment on article by Igarzabel on pendulous abdomen). Semana med. *2:*52–53, July 7, '38
GONI MORENO, I.: Creation of artificial vagina by Baldwin-Mori operation. Bol. y trab., Acad. argent. de cir. *24:*453–460, July 3, '40
GONI MORENO, I.: Artificial vagina; Baldwin-Mori procedure; surgical technic. Prensa med. argent. *27:*2579–2583, Dec 11, '40
GONI MORENO, I. AND GIGLIO, H.: Authors' technic of burn therapy, especially in children. An. Cong. brasil. e am. cir. *3:*375–383, '42
GONI MORENO, I. AND RUSSO, A. G.: Total parotidectomy with conservation of facial nerve; 3 cases. Bol. y trab., Acad. argent. de cir. *28:*722–739, Sept 6, '44
GONI MORENO, I. (see PESSANO, J. E.) May '34
GONTERMANN, C.: Avulsion of tendon of musculus flexor pollicis longus from muscle; case. Monatschr. f. Unfallh. *36:*546–549, Dec '29
GONZALEZ, B. (see SARTORIO RIGANTI, J.) Aug '45
GONZÁLEZ, S.: Surgical therapy of phlegmons and felons of hand. Arch. de med., cir. y especialid. *37:*1182–1184, Oct 27, '34
GONZALEZ N., B.: Congenital fistula of neck; case. Rev. mex. de cir., ginec. y cancer *7:*471–477, Oct '39
GONZALEZ N., B.: Therapy of most frequent fractures of lower jaw. Rev. mex. de cir., ginec. y cancer *9:*331–339, Aug '41
GONZALEZ R., R.: Surgical therapy of case of hermaphroditism. Rev. Fac. de med., Bogota *11:*710–714, June '43
GONZÁLEZ AVILA, E. (see DELLEPIANE RAWSON, R.) Aug '30
GONZÁLEZ AVILA, E. (see DELLEPIANE RAWSON, R.) Oct '30
GONZALEZ CALVO, S. (see MERINO EUGERCIOS, E.) Feb '46
GONZALEZ HURTADO, R.: Autoplastic restoration of scrotum by so-called Hindu method, using flap taken from posterointernal section of thigh; cases. Cir. y cirujanos *6:*359–366, Aug '38

GONZALEZ LIZCANO, J.: Bone implants in treatment of Pott's disease (Albee method). Siglo med. *71:*624-629, June 30, '23; *72:*652-656, July 7; 680-682, July 14; 701-705, July 21; 726-729, July 28; 752-754, Aug 4, '23

GONZÁLEZ LLANOS, N.: Dacryocystorhinostomy, Dupuy-Dutemps method; 25 cases. Rev. de especialid. *6:*237, May '31

GONZÁLEZ LOZA, M.: Plastic surgery of nose; 2 cases. Rev. med. del Rosario *21:*701-706, Jan '31

GONZÁLEZ LOZA, M.: Plastic surgery in nasal reconstruction; classification of deformities. Rev. med. del Rosario *22:*268-282, May '32

GONZÁLEZ LOZA, M.: Therapy of nasal fractures. Rev. med. del Rosario *22:*514-529, July '32

GONZÁLEZ LOZA, M.: Technic of plastic correction of external ear; 3 cases. Rev. med. del Rosario *22:*833-837, Oct '32

GONZÁLEZ LOZA, M.: Correction of dislocation of nasal subseptum from functional and esthetic points of view. Rev. med. del Rosario *22:*929-941, Nov '32

GONZÁLEZ LOZA, M.: Restoration of portion of nostril. Rev. med. del Rosario *23:*217-219, March '33

GONZÁLEZ LOZA, M.: Correction of saddle nose. Rev. med. del Rosario *23:*220-225, March '33

GONZÁLEZ LOZA, M.: Correction of flattened nose without graft; author's technic. Rev. argent. de oto-rino-laring. *6:*147-160, May-June '37

GONZÁLEZ LOZA, M.: Correction of flattened nose without graft; author's technic. Rev. med. de Rosario *28:*388-400, April '38 also: Gol. Soc. de cir. de Rosario *5:*21-32, May '38

GONZÁLEZ LOZA, M.: Correction of flat nose without graft. Arq. de cir. clin. e exper. *6:*145-148, April-June '42

GONZÁLEZ LOZA, M. AND MAISONNAVE, R.: Surgical importance of abnormalities of frontal sinus; result of postoperative plastic correction using vitallium inclusion. Rev. otorrinolaring. d. litoral *2:*298-306, June '43

González Loza Operation

González Loza operation for removing tip of nose. CORA ELISEHT, F. AND BERRI, C. Rev. Asoc. med. argent. *53:*214-215, April 15, '39

Correction of flattened nose without graft, according to González Loza prodecure; author's experience. BERGAGLIO, E. O. Rev. otorrinolaring. d. litoral *1:*373-377, March '42

GONZALEZ ULLOA, M.: Technic of reparation of ear lobe by tubular skin grafts. Rev. mex. de cir., ginec. y cancer *5:*33-41, Jan '37

GONZALEZ ULLOA, M.: Surgical mastopexy in mastoptosis. Rev. mex. de cir., ginec. y cancer *7:*191-202, May '39

GONZALEZ ULLOA, M.: History and possibilities of plastic surgery. Rev. mex. de cir., ginec. y cancer *8:*53-67, Feb '40

GONZALEZ ULLOA, M.: Surgical therapy of scars. Rev. mex. de cir., ginec. y cancer *8:*321-329, Aug '40

GONZALEZ ULLOA, M.: History, possibilities and present status of plastic surgery. Dia med. (Ed. espec., no. 6), p. 120, Aug '40

GONZALEZ ULLOA, M.: Two hundred sixteen sutures in face. Dia med. *12:*844, Sept 16, '40

GONZALEZ ULLOA, M.: Results obtained in use of various materials in plastic surgery. Rev. mex. de cir., ginec. y cancer *8:*463-479, Nov '40

GONZALEZ ULLOA, M.: Use of skin grafts in general surgery. Rev. mex. de cir., ginec. y cancer *9:*91-113, March '41

GONZALEZ ULLOA, M.: Use of bone from cattle in restoration of saddle nose. Rev. mex. de cir., ginec. y cancer *9:*321-329, Aug '41

GONZALEZ ULLOA, M.: New traction and fixation apparatus for fractured nose. Rev. mex. de cir., ginec. y cancer *10:*65-74, Feb '42 also: Rev. brasil. de cir. *11:*215-218, May '42

GONZALEZ ULLOA, M.: Syndactylia; solution to problem. Rev. mex. de cir., ginec. y cancer *10:*157-167, April '42

GONZALEZ ULLOA, M.: Use of bone from cattle in restoration of saddle nose. Arq. de cir. clin. e exper. *6:*535-538, April-June '42

GONZALEZ ULLOA, M.: Modern therapy of facial injuries. Rev. mex. de cir., ginec. y cancer *11:*51-74, Feb '43

GONZALEZ ULLOA, M.: New instrument with needle continuously threaded for suturing. Rev. mex. de cir., ginec. y cancer *11:*123-135, April '43

GONZALEZ ULLOA, M.: Modern therapy of facial injuries. Rev. brasil. de cir. *12:*547-564, Sept '43 also: Vida nueva *53:*42-61, Feb '44

GONZALEZ ULLOA, M.: Fractures of jaw with special reference to therapy. Rev. mex. de cir., ginec. y cancer *12:*89-98, March '44

GONZALEZ ULLOA, M.: Fractures of mandible. Rev. mex. de cir., ginec. y cancer *12:*145-152, May '44

GONZALEZ ULLOA, M.: Fractures of zygoma. Rev. mex. de cir., ginec. y cancer *12:*171-177, June '44

GONZALEZ ULLOA, M.: Present therapy of facial injury. Prensa med. argent. *31:*1863-1876, Sept 20, '44

GONZALEZ ULLOA, M.: Plastic surgery in past and future. Salud y belleza (no. 4) *1:*18-21, Aug-Sept '45

GONZALEZ ULLOA, M.: Fractures of maxilla. Vida nueva *56:*175–182, Dec '45

GONZALEZ ULLOA, M.: Fractures of mandible. Vida nueva *56:*183–189, Dec '45

GONZALEZ ULLOA, M.: Fractures of malar-zygomatic compound. Vida nueva *56:*190–194, Dec '45

GONZALEZ ULLOA, M.: Fracture of frontal and nasal bones. Vida nueva *56:*195–201, Dec '45

GONZALEZ ULLOA, M.: Utilization of cadaver cartilage in surgery. Medicina, Mexico *25:*495–503, Dec 10, '45

GONZALEZ ULLOA, M.: Use of cadaver cartilage in surgery. Rev. brasil. de cir. *14:*663–670, Dec '45 also: Prensa med. argent. *33:*705–709, April 5, '46

GOOD, R. W. AND BOYER, B. E.: Intravenous use of acacia solution in shock. J. Med. *12:*630–636, Feb '32

GOOD, R. W.; MUGRAGE, R. AND WEISKITTEL, R.: Acacia solution in treatment of shock; analysis of 111 case histories. Am. J. Surg. *25:*134–139, July '34

GOODALL, E. W.: Cancrum oris with recovery; subsequent repair of defect by plastic operation. Brit. J. Child. Dis. *27:*204–208, July–Sept '30

GOODHOPE, C. D.: Correction of chordee and hypospadias. Northwest Med. *44:*356–358, Nov '45

GOODMAN, B. A.: Mastitis gargantuan; unusual case of puberty hypertrophy. J.A.M.A. *103:*335–336, Aug 4, '34

GOODMAN, C.: Transplantation of tissues and organs. Internat. Clinics. *3:*54–72, '22

GOODMAN, H.: Technic of cosmetic electrolysis of hair removal. Am. Med. *41:*35–36, Jan '35

GOODMAN, H.: Skin peeling. Hygeia *20:*514, July '42

GOODMAN. H.: Hair removal, nonsurgical reparative dermatology, or electromedical cosmetology. Urol. and Cutan. Rev. *46:*726–727, Nov '42

GOODMAN, J. I. AND CORSARO, J. F.: Topical use of sulfathiazole (sulfanilamide derivative) in decubitus ulcers; preliminary report. Ohio State M. J. *37:*956–958, Oct '41

GOODSELL, J. O.: Use of ordinary small brass hinge as locking device for splints in multiple fractures of jaws. J. Oral Surg. *1:*250–251, July '43

GOODSELL, J. O.: Temporary external salivary drainage (from Stenson's duct) following arthroplasty. J. Oral Surg. *3:*174–176, April '45

GOODSELL, J. O. JR.: Treatment of fractures of edentulous jaws. Dental Cosmos *72:*385–389, April '30

GOODYEAR, H. M.: Use of hollow tube following submucous resection of nasal septum. J.A.M.A. *77:*1103, Oct 1, '21

GOODYEAR, H. M.: Plastic operation for protruding ears. Arch. Otolaryng. *18:*527–530, Oct '33 also: J. Med. *14:*479–480, Nov '33

GOODYEAR, H. M.: Nasopharyngeal atresia; description of operation. Arch. Otolaryng. *29:*974–976, June '39

GOPALAN, N.: Treatment of burns and scalds by sterilized cocoanut oil. Indian M. Gaz. *61:*549, Nov '26

GOPENCHAJM, I.: Congenital deformation of ear; rare case. Polska gaz. lek. *18:*400–402, April 30, '39

GORANSON, E. S. (see SELLERS, E. A.) Aug '44

GORANSON, E. S. (see SELLERS, E. A.) May '45

GORBAN, I. A.: Burns and their treatment; 400 cases. Novy khir. arkhiv *38:*479–482, '37

GORBAN, I. A.: Therapy of burns of extremities with plaster of paris bandages. Vestnik khir. *56:*100, July '38

GORBOUNOFF, V. P.: Data on autoplastic bone grafting and cartilage. Vestnik khir. (nos. 37–38) *13:*71–85, '28

GORBUNOFF, W. P.: Auto- and homotransplantation of bone and cartilage. Arch. f. klin. Chir. *161:*651–670, '30

GORBUNOV, V. P.: Excision as method of treatment of third degree burns. Sovet. vrach. gaz., pp. 637–639, April 30, '34

GORDIENKO, A. N.: Blood changes in shock following burns. Bull. War Med. *6:*473, July '46 (abstract)

GORDIN, A. E.: Electric shock, electric burns and their treatment. Indust. Med. *10:*87–91, March '41

GORDON, A.: Unusual localization of arthropathies (mandibulotemporal and metacarpophalangeal ankylosis), in postencephalitic parkinsonian syndrome and their pathogenesis. M. Rec. *140:*351–353, Oct 3, '34

GORDON, D. (see SIEGEL, S. A. *et al*) Sept '45

GORDON, J. O.: Treatment of hand infections. J. Tennessee M. A. *22:*201–204, Oct '29

GORDON, R. A.: Problems of anesthesia in plastic surgery. Anesthesiology *3:*507–513, Sept '42

GORDON, R. A.: Intravenous novocain (procaine hydrochloride) for analgesia in burns; preliminary report. Canad. M. A. J. *49:*478–481, Dec '43

GORDON, R. A.: Significance of blood changes in treatment of patient with burns. Anesth. and Analg. *24:*78–84, March–April '45

GORDON, R. A.: Anesthesia in Plastic Surgery Unit Canadian Army Overseas. Bull. Acad. Med., Toronto *19:*233–237, Aug '46

GORDON, R. A. AND BOWERS, V. H.: Toxic

blood-level of sulfanilamide from local application in burns. Lancet *2:*484, Oct 24, '42

GORDON, R. A. AND SHACKLETON, R. P. W.: Trichloroethylene anesthesia in plastic surgery. Brit. M. J. *1:*380–381, March 27, '43

GORDON, R. A. (see GORDON, S. D.) April '43

GORDON, R. A. (see GORDON, S. D.) May '44

GORDON, R. M.: Burn therapy with tannic acid. Lancet *1:*336–337, Feb 18, '28

GORDON, S.: Immediate treatment of facial fractures. Canad. M. A. J. *37:*440–443, Nov '37

GORDON, S.: Repair of secondary traumatic defects in mucous membrane of lips. Canad. M. A. J. *38:*382, April '38

GORDON, S.: Fractures of mandible. Canad. M. A. J. *42:*521–525, June '40

GORDON, S.: Chronic recurrent ulceration of leg. Canad. M. A. J. *42:*4–10, Jan '40

GORDON, S.: Maxillary forceps in fractures. Lancet *2:*80, July 15, '44

GORDON, S.: Autograft of amputated thumb. Lancet *2:*823, Dec 23, '44

GORDON, S.: Role of cancellous bone in plastic surgery. Surgery *20:*202–203, Aug '46

GORDON, S. AND CRAGG, B. H.: Congenital ectropion associated with bilateral ptosis—case. Brit. J. Ophth. *28:*520–521, Oct '44

GORDON, S. AND WARREN, R. F.: Reflex vasodilatation in tubed pedicle grafts. Ann. Surg. *123:*436–446, March '46

GORDON, S. D.: Wire suturing in treatment of facial fractures. Canad. M. A. J. *48:*406–409, May '43

GORDON, S. D.: Treatment of gunshot wounds of face. Bull. Acad. Med., Toronto *18:*185–187, July '45

GORDON, S. D.: Repair of deformities of hands. Bull. Vancouver M. A. *21:*279–281, Aug '45

GORDON, S. D.: Mandibular fractures. Bull. Vancouver M. A. *21:*281–283, Aug '45

GORDON, S. D.: Therapy of thermal burns. Bull. Vancouver M. A. *21:*283–286, Aug '45

GORDON, S. D.: Skin transplantation. Bull. Vancouver M. A. *22:*9–11, Oct '45

GORDON, S. D. AND GORDON, R. A.: Thermal burns. Canad. M. A. J. *48:*302–309, April '43

GORDON, S. D. AND GORDON, R. A.: Changes in blood following thermal burns. J. Canad. M. Serv. *1:*312–320, May '44

GORIA, V.: Surgical therapy of penoscrotal hypospadias by author's technic. Rev. argent. de urol. *10:*419–426, July–Aug '41

GORIAINOWA, R. W.: Heredity of ectrodactylia. Fortschr. a. d. Geb. d. Rontgenstrahlen *50:*289–294, Sept '34

GORINEVSKAYA, V. V. AND SAMSONOVA, Z. P.: Burns and their therapy. Sovet. khir., no. 6, pp. 216–224, '35

GORNEY, A. J. (see GORNEY, H. S. *et al*) May '42

GORNEY, H. S.; GORNEY, A. J. AND FOMAN, S.: Creation of mandibular ridge by deepening labial sulcus and lining it with graft. J. Am. Dent. A. *29:*751–754, May '42

GORODINSKIY, D. M.: Makkas operation in exstrophy of bladder. Novy khir. arkhiv *33:*290–294, '35

GORODNER, J.: Cavernous hemangioma of penis; case. Rev. argent. de urol. *11:*413–418, Nov–Dec '42

GOROKHOV, A. V.: Cysts and fistulas of neck. Zhur. ush. nos. i gorl. bolez. *16:*444–447, '39

GORTER, A. J.: Surgical therapy of elephantiasis of lower extremities. Geneesk. tijdschr. v. Nederl.-Indie *77:*1236–1242, May 18, '37

GOSS, E. L.: Burns and their treatment. Journal-Lancet *44:*510–515, Oct 15, '24

GOSSET, A. AND CHARRIER, J.: Fate of nerve grafts. J. de chir. *19:*1–14, Jan '22 abstr: J.A.M.A. *78:*848, March 18, '22

GOSSET, J.: Recent progress in burn treatment. Presse med. *53:*539, Oct 6, '45

GOT, A.: Recent nasal fractures; surgical therapy. Rev. de laryng. *60:*166–171, Feb '39

GOTTLIEB, A.: Deformities of hand acquired after accidents. California State J. Med. *19:*72, Feb '21

GOTTLIEB, A.: Cleft foot. West. J. Surg. *53:*157–158, May '45

GOTTLIEB, A. AND NEWMAN, L. I.: Restoration of function in acquired hand deformities. California State J. Med. *19:*365, Sept '21

GOTTLIEB, F. M.: Urgent therapy of grave burns. Bucuresti med. *6:*109–110, '34

GOTTSCHALK, L. (see OTTENBERG, R.) Jan '25

GOTZE, W. (see TONNIS, W.) April '42

GOTZE, W. (see TONNIS, W.) Dec '42

GOUFAS, G.: Branchioma of right parotid in young girl; extracapsular extirpation and closure of resulting defect by Thiersch graft. Ann. d'oto-laryng., pp. 677–685, July '36

GOUGEROT, H. AND BURNIER: Epithelioma of cheek from drop of carbon disulphide; case. Bull. Soc. franc. de dermat. et syph. *36:*1041, Nov '29

GOUGEROT, H. AND MEYER, J.: Clinically atypical, but histologically typical lupus immediately following burn; case. Bull. Soc. franc. de dermat. et syph. *44:*269–270, Feb '37

GOUGEROT, H. (see TERRIEN, F. *et al*) April '31

GOURDON, J.: Syndactylia. Bull. et mem. Soc. med. et chir. de Bordeaux, pp. 252–255, '32

GOURDON, R. AND JEANNE, H.: Treatment of fractures of fingers. Bull. med., Paris *45:*321–326, May 9, '31

GOUVÉA, J.: Auto-bone implants. Brazil-med.

*35:*61, Jan 29, '21
DE GOUVEIA, G. S.: Rare case of urethral fistula. Hospital, Rio de Janeiro *21:*195–199, Feb '42
GOVOROFF, A. P.: Surgical treatment of elephantiasis of lower limbs. Vrach. dielo *10:*277–278, Feb 28, '27
GOWER, W. E.: Treatment of fresh burns with scarlet red bandage and moist sulfanilamide dressings. J. Iowa M. Soc. *31:*234–237, June '41
DE GOWIN, E. L.: Modern treatment of traumatic shock. J. Iowa M. Soc. *34:*1–7, Jan '44
DE GOWIN, E. L.: Possible role of whole blood transfusions in military medicine (shock). J.A.M.A. *127:*1037–1039, April 21, '45
GOWLAND, W. P.: Recent work in anatomy bearing on surgical practice (transplantation of nerves). Australian and New Zealand J. Surg. *6:*339–349, April '37
GOYDER, F. W.: Two problems in treatment of cleft palate. Brit. M. J. *2:*615, Oct 4, '24
GÖZBERK, R. A.: Congenital facial hemihypertrophy; case. Turk tib cem. mec. *3:*210–212, '37
GÖZBERK, R. A.: Congenital facial hemihypertrophy with ocular anomalies; 2 cases. Ann. d'ocul. *176:*624–630, Aug '39
GOZLAN, A. (see ABOULKER, H.) April '31
GRACE, E. J.: Importance of prickle cell layer in skin grafting. Am. J. Surg. *32:*498, June '36
GRACE, L. G.: Frequency of occurrence of cleft palates and harelips. J. Dent. Research *22:*495–497, Dec '43
GRACE, R. V.: Subcutaneous fascial stripper. Ann. Surg. *90:*1109–1110, Dec '29
GRACIA SIERRA, S.: Cosmetic surgery in correction of saddle nose deformity; case. Clin. y lab. *23:*673–675, Aug '33
GRACIA SIERRA, S.: Esthetic surgery. Clin. y lab. *23:*996–1000, Nov '33
GRAD, H.: Technic of formation of artificial vagina. Surg., Gynec. and Obst. *54:*200–206, Feb '32
GRADLE, H. S. AND STEIN, J. C.: Unusual dermoid cyst of eyelid. Arch. Ophth. *53:*254–257, May '24
GRADMAN, R. (see MEYER, K. A.) May '43

Graefe's Apparatus

Modifications in Graefe's apparatus for reduction and retention of fractures. GIZZI, C. Stomatol. *28:*865–870, Oct '30

GRAF, P.: Methods of formation of artificial vagina. Deutsche Ztschr. f. Chir. *232:*364–374, '31
GRAF, W. J.: Imperforate anus in 12 year-old girl; case. J. Med. *21:*82–83, April '40
GRAFFI, E.: Prognathism. Riv. di antropol. *28:*123–163, '28–'29

Grafts: See Bone Grafts; Cartilage Grafts; Composite Grafts; Dermal Grafts; Fascia Grafts; Fat Grafts; Homografts; Mucosal Grafts; Muscle Transplantation; Nerve Grafts; Skin Grafts; Storage of Grafts; Tendons, Transplantation

GRAHAM, A. J.: Submucosa dissector. Surg., Gynec. and Obst. *40:*709, May '25 also: M. J. and Rec. *122:*527, Nov 4, '25
GRAHAM, H. B.: Reconstruction of completely destroyed auricle; case report. California and West. Med. *27:*518–519, Oct '27
GRAHAM, H. B.: Facial nerve damage; repair. California and West. Med. *40:*174–177, March '34
GRAHAM, H. B.: Plastic surgery of ear. West. J. Surg. *44:*478–480, Aug '36
GRAHAM, J. D. P.: Shock and hemorrhage; rapid replacement of fluid. Brit. M. J. *2:*623–625, Nov 11, '44
GRAHAM, J. G.: Burns; chemotherapy of local suppuration, acriflavine and boric acid compared. Brit. M. J. *2:*826, Nov 7, '25
GRAHAM, J. W.: Mandibular fractures at King County Hospital treated by Roger Anderson skeletal fixation. Northwest Med. *44:*250–252, Aug '45
GRAHAM, M. P.: Maxillofacial injuries; extracts from case histories. Brit. Dent. J. *76:*339–341, June 16, '44
GRAHAM, M. P. (see SMALL, J. M.) Oct '45
GRAHAM, W. C. (see CANNON, B.) Aug '45
GRAHAM-LITTLE, E.: Extensive lupus erythematosus with subsequent carcinoma of lower lip (case). Proc. Roy. Soc. Med. *25:*1741, Oct '32
GRANDI, E.: Surgical therapy of war wounds of jaws; 2 cases. Stomatol. ital. *2:*391–397, May '40
GRANDI, G.: Jaw fractures; clinical aspects and treatment by blockage of maxillae. Stomatol. *27:*94–106, Feb '29
GRANSTRÖM, K. O.: Congenital stenosis of nasolacrimal duct; complications and treatment. Nord. med. tidskr. *16:*1280–1283, Aug 13, '38
GRANT, D. N. W.: Congenital absence of radius and club hand; case. Mil. Surgeon *69:*518–521, Nov '31
GRANT, F. C.: Suggestion for relief of pain from carcinoma of mouth and cheek. Ann. Surg. *81:*494–498, Feb '25
GRANT, F. C.: Relief for pain in carcinoma of face. J.A.M.A. *86:*173–176, Jan 16, '26

GRANT, F. C.: Relief of pain with cancer of face. Pennsylvania M. J. *32:*548–551, May '29

GRANT, F. C. (see MIXTER, W. J.) Feb '28

GRANT, R. T.: Shock in air raid casualties. Guy's Hosp. Gaz. *55:*90–95, April 19, '41

GRANT, R. T.: Memorandum on observations required in cases of wound shock. Brit. M. J. *2:*332–336, Sept 6, '41

GRANT, R. T.; *et al*: Discussion on methods of resuscitation in shock. Proc. Roy. Soc. Med. *35:*445–454, April '42

GRANT, W. W.: Exstrophy of bladder. Southern M. J. *15:*297–302, April '22 (illus.)

GRANT, W. W.: Cancer of mouth. Colorado Med. *20:*248–251, Sept '23 (illus.)

GRASHCHENKOV, N. I. P.: Nerve transplantation. Am. Rev. Soviet Med. *1:*28–31, Oct '43 also: Sovet. med. (no. 9) *6:*8–10, '42

GRASHCHENKOV, N. I. P. AND ANOKHIN, P. K.: Instructions for transplantation of formalized nerve to replace defect of injured nerve. Nevropat. i. psikhiat. (nos. 1–2) *11:*44–45, '42

GRASSI, G.: Italian contribution to plastic surgery; historical study. Riv. di storia d. sc. med. e nat. *27:*215–232, July–Aug '36

GRATTAN, J. F.: Rhinophyma; report of 6 cases cured by radical operations followed by X-ray and acid treatments to relieve associated hypertrophy of skin and to reduce operative scars to state of invisibility. Surg., Gynec. and Obst. *41:*99–102, July '25

GRATTAN, J. F.: Scars; new triple technic for reducing disfiguring cicatrices to degree of invisibility amounting to practical removal. J.A.M.A. *88:*638–641, Feb 26, '27

GRATZ, C. M.: Use of fasciae in reconstructive surgery, with special reference to operative technic. Eye, Ear, Nose and Throat Monthly *12:*27–29, Feb '33

GRATZ, C. M.: Use of fascia in reconstructive surgery; with special reference to operative technic. Ann. Surg. *99:*241–245, Feb '34

GRATZ, C. M.: New suture for tendon and fascia repair. Surg., Gynec. and Obst. *65:*700–701, Nov '37

GRAU BARBERA, L.: Rare case of deformed ear. Actas dermo-sif. *35:*52–55, Oct '43

GRAUBNER, E.: Late results of Maydl operation for congenital ectopy of bladder. Zentralbl. f. Chir. *63:*2657–2658, Nov 7, '36

GRAUE Y GLENIE, E.: Dacryocystorhinostomy; indications and technic; case. An. Soc. mex. de oftal. y oto-rino-laring. *9:*114–116, Jan–March '32

GRAUE Y GLENNIE, E.: Surgical therapy of symblepharon. Bol. d. Hosp. oftal. de Ntra. Sra. de la Luz *1:*101–105, July–Aug '40

GRAVES, J. Q. (see ADAMS, J. L.) Dec '23

GRAVES, W. P.: Method of constructing artificial vagina. S. Clin. N. Amer. *1:*611, June '21

GRAVES-MORRIS, W. M. (see SIMPSON-SMITH, A.) Oct '34

Grawitz Experiments: See Busse-Grawitz Experiments

GRAY, H. K. AND CHAUNCEY, L. R.: Shock, surgical. U. S. Nav. M. Bull. *37:*1–10, Jan '39

GRAY, H. K. (see WALTERS, W. *et al*) Aug '31

GRAZIANI, M.: Buccomaxillofacial prosthesis; artificial nose and palate; case. Rev. brasil. de oto-rino-laring. *9:*217–221, May–June '41

GRECO, A. (see JORGE, J. M.) Sept '40

GRECO, T.: Recurrent cystic lymphangioma of neck in child; case. Sperimentale, Arch. di biol. (no. 2) *86:*viii–xii, '32

GREEF, J. H. H.: Bone transplantation. J. M. A. S. Africa *1:*474–475, Sept 24, '27

DE GREEF, R.: Study of 101 cases of elephantiasis and adenolymphoceles at Negro Hospital, Buta, Belgian Congo, with special reference to surgical technic. Ann. Soc. belge de med. trop. *18:*5–39, March 31, '38

GREELEY, P. W.: Gillies operation for correction of depressed fracture deformities of zygomatic-malar bones. Illinois M. J. *71:*419–420, May '37

GREELEY, P. W.: Types of grafts and their individual application. Illinois M. J. *75:*436–441, May '39

GREELEY, P. W.: Problems in plastic and reconstructive surgery. J. Am. Dent. A. *26:*1954–1965, Dec '39

GREELEY, P. W.: Plastic repair of cutaneous injuries to hand. Indust. Med. *9:*300–303, June '40

GREELEY, P. W.: Reconstructive otoplasty (by transplantation of cartilage). Surgery *10:*457–461, Sept '41

GREELEY, P. W.: Plastic correction of superficial pigmented nevi. Tr. West. S. A. (1941) *51:*398–414, '42

GREELEY, P. W.: Abrasions and accidental tattoos, scars, keloids and scar contractures, and nasal deformities. S. Clin. North America *22:*253–276, Feb '42

GREELEY, P. W.: Plastic repair of extensor hand contractures following healed deep second degree burns. Tr. Am. Soc. Plastic and Reconstructive Surg. *12:*79–82, '43

GREELEY, P. W.: Plastic repair of burned hand. Am. Acad. Orthop. Surgeons, Lect., pp. 169–173, '44

GREELEY, P. W.: Problems of surface restoration (in Navy). Am. Acad. Orthop. Surgeons, Lect. pp. 250–253, '44

GREELEY, P. W.: Plastic repair of extensor hand contractures following healed deep second degree burns. Surgery *15:*173–177, Jan '44

GREELEY, P. W.: Plastic repair of scar contractures. Surgery *15:*224–241, Feb '44

GREELEY, P. W.: Factors influencing choice of skin grafts. U. S. Nav. M. Bull. *42:*659–663, March '44

GREELEY, P. W.: Ear reconstruction; conservation of avulsed portion. U. S. Nav. M. Bull. *42:*1323–1325, June '44

GREELEY, P. W.: Plastic surgery in burns among naval personnel; current experiences. Am. J. Surg. *67:*401–411, Feb '45

GREELEY, P. W.: Plastic repair of radiation ulcers of sole. U. S. Nav. M. Bull. *45:*827–830, Nov '45

GREELEY, P. W.: Plastic correction of superficial pigmented nevi. Surgery *19:*467–481, April '46

GREELEY, P. W.: Reconstruction of thumb. Ann. Surg. *124:*60–70, July '46

GREELEY, P. W.: Reconstructive otoplasty; further observations; utilization of tantalum wire mesh support. Arch. Surg. *53:*24–31, July '46

GREELEY, P. W. AND POUND, A. E.: Plastic and dental prosthetic repair of jaw injuries. Illinois M. J. *89:*216–221, May '46

GREELEY, P. W. AND THRONDSON, A. H.: Arteriovenous aneurysm resulting from application of Roger Anderson splint for fractured jaw. J.A.M.A. *124:*1128, April 15, '44

GREELEY, P. W. (see COLE, W. H.) Sept '42

GREELEY, P. W. (see MEHERIN, J. M.) Dec '43

GREEN, F. H. K.: Local treatment of thermal burns. Prensa med. argent. *33:*94–102, Jan 11, '46

GREEN, H. D. AND BERGERON, G. A.: Effects of environmental temperature on traumatic shock produced by ischemic compression of extremities. Surgery *17:*404–412, March '45

GREEN, H. D. (see ANTOS, R. J. *et al*) Oct '44

GREEN, J. L. JR.: Therapy of burns. Southwestern Med. *15:*194–198, May '31

GREEN, R. M.: Brief review of anatomy, blood and nerve supply of mouth, jaws and teeth. Am. J. Orthodontics (Oral Surg. Sect) *27:*469–471, Sept '41

GREEN, R. W. ; LEVENSON, S. M. AND LUND, C. C.: Nylon backing for dermatome grafts. New England J. Med. *233:*268–270, Aug 30, '45

GREEN, R. W. (see LEVENSON, S. M. *et al*) July '46

GREEN, T. M.: Elephantiasis and the Kondeleon operation. Virginia M. Monthly *48:*196, July '21

GREEN, W. T.: Transplantation of flexor carpi ulnaris for pronation-flexion deformity of wrist. Surg., Gynec. and Obst. *75:*337–342, Sept '42

GREEN-ARMYTAGE, V. B.: Complete exstrophy of bladder with split pelvis; Peter's operation in 1912 with subsequent complication of pregnancy; caesarean section and recovery in 1926. J. Obst. and Gynec. Brit. Emp. *33:*436–438, '26

GREEN-ARMYTAGE, V. B.: Observations on insulin-glucose method in obstetric shock. Indian M. Gaz. *62:*675–680, Dec '27

GREEN-ARMYTAGE, V. B.: Implantation of ureters for inoperable vesico-vaginal fistula and ectopia vesicae; new technic. Brit. J. Surg. *20:*130–138, July '32 also: Indian M. Gaz. *67:*631–636, Nov '32

GREENBERG, L.: Dupuytren's contracture of palmar and plantar fasciae. J. Bone and Joint Surg. *21:*785–788, July '39

GREENBLATT, R. B.; PUND, E. R. AND BERNARD, G. T.: Benign nevus: malignant melanoma; problem of borderline case. South. M. J. *29:*122–129, Feb '36

GREENE, H. S. N.: Heterologous transplantation of embryonic mammalian tissues. Cancer Research *3:*809–822, Dec '43

GREENE, J. S.: Some mouth and jaw conditions responsible for defects in speech. Med. Rec. *100:*8, July 2, '21

GREENFIELD, E. (see MARSHALL, W.) March '44

GREENFIELD, S. D.: Operation for cure of postauricular fistula; 8 consecutive cases. Laryngoscope *50:*312–325, April '40

GREENWOOD, H. H.: Massive breast enlargement. Lancet *1:*232–234, Jan 30, '32

GREEVES, R. A.: Eyelid surgery for partial contraction of socket. Tr. Ophth. Soc. U. Kingdom *47:*101–106, '27

GREEVES, R. A.: Operation for relief of congenital eyelid ptosis. Proc. Roy. Soc. Med. *26:*1478–1482, Sept '33

GREEVES, R. A.: Operation for relief of congenital ptosis of eyelids. Brit. J. Ophth. *17:*741–745, Dec '33

GREGERSEN, M. I. (see NOBLE, R. P.) March '46

GREGORINI, H. (see LIMA, E. J. *et al*) May '38

GREIFENSTEIN: Gunshot wounds of neck. Bull. War Med. *3:*441, April '43 (abstract)

GREIFENSTEIN, A.: Unusual stenoses of larynx and their surgical therapy. Hals-, Nasen-u. Ohrenarzt (Teil 1) *27:*101–130, '36

GREIG, D. M.: Pubertal mammary hypertrophy. Edinburgh M. J. *28:*153–167, April '22 (illus.)

GREIG, D. M.: Hypertelorism; a hitherto undifferentiated congenital cranio-facial deformity. Edinburgh M. J. *31:*560–593, Oct '24

GREIG, M. E. (see LAMSON, P. D. *et al*) March '45

GRET, L. G.: Hand infections, with special reference to therapy. An. Fac. de cien. med. de La Plata *3:*137-144, '38
GRET, L. G.: Hand infections; biologic conception of pathology and therapeutics. Bol. y. trab., Soc. argent. de cirujanos *2:*811-823, '41
GRETTVE, S.: Acute suppurative infection in flexor tendon sheaths of hand, with particular reference to late results after operation with transverse finger incisions according to K. G. Holm. Acta chir. Scandinav. (supp. 91) *90:*1-63, '44
GREUER, W.: Biology of burn lesions. Ztschr. f. d. ges. exper. Med. *111:*120-144, '42
GREVE, K.: Dental prosthesis after resection of lower jaw. Beitr. z. klin. Chir. *142:*747-752, '28
GREVE, K.: Bone suture in treatment of jaw fractures. Beitr. z. klin. Chir. *152:*310-322, '31
GRIDNEV, A.: Evaluation of formation of artificial vagina by Baldwin-Mori operation. Arch. f. Gynak. *162:*397-402, '36
GRIDNEW, A.: Baldwin-Mori operation for artificial vagina; case. Gynec. et obst. *34:*312-314, Oct '36
GRIER, G. W.: Roentgen-ray treatment of keloid. Am. J. Roentgenol. *16:*22-26, July '26
GRIES, L.: Low voltage currents in contractures of hand. Arch. Physical Therapy *11:*10-13, Jan '30
GRIESMAN, B. L.: Muscles and cartilage of nose from standpoint of typical rhinoplasty. Arch. Otolaryng. *39:*334-341, April '44
GRIESMAN, B. L.: Structure of external nose; study from point of view of plastic surgery. Arch. Otolaryng. *42:*117-122, Aug '45
GRIESSMANN, B.: Congenital lateral fistulas of neck. Munchen. med. Wchnschr. *68:*460, April 15, '21
GRIESSMANN, B.: Experiences with corrective plastic surgery of nose. Klin. Wchnschr. *6:*1045, May 28, '27
GRIFFIN. J. R.: Treating fractures of mandible by skeletal fixation. Am. J. Orthodontics (Oral Surg. Sect) *27:*364-376, July '41
GRIFFIN, J. R.: Treating fractures of mandible by skeletal fixation. Rev. san. mil., Buenos Aires *40:*1006-1010, Nov '41
GRIFFITH, C. M. AND SCHATTNER, A.: Correction of postauricular defect by implantation of fascia lata. Laryngoscope *43:*280-281, April '33
GRIFFITH, G. C.: Burn therapy in Presbyterian Hospital of Philadelphia. Internat. Clin. *4:*129-131, Dec '28
GRIFFITHS, D. L. AND CRAWFORD, T.: Neuroma of palmar fascia simulating Dupuytren's contracture. J. Roy. Army M. Corps *84:*130-131, March '45
GRIFFITHS, H. E.: Minor injuries of hand. Practitioner *156:*254-261, Apr '46
GRIFFITHS, S. J. H.: Acute infections and suppurations of hand and arm. Practitioner *125:*721-730, Dec '30

Grigoriu Operation (See also Schubert-Grigoriu Operation)

Grigoriu modification of Schubert method in aplasia vaginae. IUBAS, C. Zentralbl. f. Gynak. *55:*3379-3384, Nov 21, '31
Construction of artificial vagina according to Grigoriu method in case of aplasia. IUBAS, C. Rev. de chir., Bucuresti *38:*170-175, Sept-Dec '35

GRIGOROVSKIY, I. M.: Postoperative shock. Vestnik khir. *55:*129-132, Feb '38
GRIGSBY, B. C.: Sulfanilamide in burns. Virginia M. Monthly *67:*306-307, May '40
GRILLO, V. (see FLARER, F.) May '36
GRIMALDI, F. E. AND BERNARDI, R.: Urethral fistula cured by Landerer-Bidder procedure; case. Prensa med. argent. *28:*1886-1888, Sept 24, '41
GRIMALDI, F. E. AND BERNARDI, R.: Landerer-Bidder operation in cure of large urethral fistula; case. Rev. argent. de urol. *10:*535-539, Sept-Oct '41
GRIMALDI, F. E. AND RUBI, R. A.: Subsymphyseal female epispadias; case. Semana med. *1:*1748-1749, June 7, '34
GRIMAUD, ROSENTHAL, AND TAUB: Chenet technic in prosthesis of ear deformities. Rev. med. de l'est. *61:*485-486, July 1, '33
GRIMAUD (see JACQUES, P.) June '33
GRIMAUD, R. AND JACOB, P.: Extensive furunculosis of upper lip treated by roentgenotherapy; case. Rev. med. de Nancy *67:*701-703, Aug 1, '39
GRIMSON, K. S.: Healing of fractures of mandible and zygoma. J. Am. Dent. A. *24:*1458-1469, Sept '37
GRINCHAR, F. N.: Disturbance in acid-base equilibrium due to burns and its treatment with thiosulfate. Sovet. khir., no. 6, pp. 232-244, '35
GRINDA, J. P.: Blockage of digital tendons causing spring fingers; 4 cases. Mem. Acad. de chir. *68:*34-38, Jan 14-21, '42
GRINDA, M.: Skin grafts. Presse med. *43:*2053-2055, Dec 18, '35
GRINNELL, R. S.: Acute suppurative tenosynovitis of flexor tendon sheaths; review of 125 cases. Ann. Surg. *105:*97-119, Jan '37
GRISANTI, S.: Therapy of syndactylia. Riv. san.

siciliana *21:*1304–1308, Sept 1, '33

GRISANTI, S.: Behavior of homoplastic transplants of bone prophylactically treated with blood serum of host; preliminary report. Riv. san. siciliana *22:*3–18, Jan 1, '34

DE GRISOGONO, A.: Exstrophy of bladder; with report of case in adult. Clin. ostet. *40:*560–569, Nov '38

GRISWOLD, R. A.: Burn therapy. Kentucky M. J. *40:*203–207, June '42

GRISWOLD, R. A. AND WOODSON, W. H.: Brachial plexus block anesthesia of upper extremities. Am. J. Surg. *59:*439–443, Feb '43

GRITTI, P.: Rare congenital malformation of nose and lower eyelid. Boll. d. mal. d. orecchio, d. gola, d. naso *55:*321–334, Sept '37

GRIVOT, M.: Repair of faulty, postoperative cicatrices of mastoid region. Ann. d. mal. de l'oreille, du larynx *48:*666–670, June '29

GRIZAUD, H.: Congenital bilateral clubhand; roentgen study of case. J. de radiol. et d'electrol. *16:*515–516, Oct '32

GROB, M.: Merbromin (mercury compound) in local therapy of second degree burns. Helvet. paediat. acta *1:*267–275, Feb '46

GRODINS, F. S. AND FREEMAN, S.: Traumatic shock. Internat. Abstr. Surg. *72:*1–8, '41; in Surg., Gynec. and Obst. Jan '41

GRODINSKY, M.: Pyogenic infections; lymphatic, tendon sheath and fascial space infections of hand. Nebraska M. J. *27:*13–17, Jan '42

GRODINSKY, M. AND HOLYOKE, E. A.: Fasciae and fascial spaces of palm. Anat. Rec. *79:*435–451, April 25, '41

GRODZKI, M.: Technical mistakes and dangers in plastic surgery of breast. Rev. de chir. structive, pp. 39–57, July '35

GROFF, ROBERT A., AND HOUTZ, SARA J.: *Manual of Diagnosis and Management of Peripheral Nerve Injuries*. J. B. Lippincott, Phila., 1945

GROH, J. A. (see MARCUS, A.) Nov '40

GROHS, R.: Actinomycosis following fracture of lower jaw. Ztschr. f. Stomatol. *32:*427–433, April 27, '34

GROMAKOVSKAYA, M. M. AND KAPLAN, L. E.: Biologic properties of blood and spinal fluid in traumatic shock complicated by burns. Byull. eksper. biol. i med. (no. 6) *15:*12–16, '43

GRONEMANN: Gunpowder burns in munitions factory. Zentralbl. f. Gewerbehyg. *19:*217, Dec '42

DE GROOT, A.: Hydrogen dioxide in treatment of burns. Nederlandsch Tijdschr. v. Geneesk. *2:*354, July 28, '23

GROS, J. C.: Plastic operation in pharyngostoma following laryngectomy; case. Rev. de med. y cir. de la Habana *36:*65–70, Jan 31, '31

GROS, J. C.: Analysis of 137 cases of cancer of lips treated in services of department of laryngology of Instituto del Cancer in Havana. Bol. Liga contra el cancer *8:*8–11, Jan '33

GROS, J. C.: Therapy of epitheliomas of septum of nose. Bol. Liga contra el cancer *12:*148–154, May '37

GROS, J. C.: Early diagnosis and therapy of cancer of nose. Bol. Liga contra el cancer *15:*305–311, Nov '40

GROSS, P. P.: Method of keeping palatal mucoperiosteum against bony structures following surgery. Am. J. Orthodontics (Oral Surg. Sect) *28:*522–524, Sept '42

GROSS, P. P.: Extraoral skeletal fixation of mandibular fractures; cases. Am. J. Orthodontics (Oral Surg. Sect.) *29:*392–400, July '43

GROSS, R. E. AND GOERINGER, C. F.: Cystic hygroma of neck; 27 cases. Surg., Gynec. and Obst. *69:*48–60, July '39

GROSS, R. E. (see LADD, W. E.) Feb '38

GROSS, W.: Operation for complete fistula of neck. Zentralbl. f. Chir. *53:*2076–2080, Aug 14, '26

GROSS, W.: Hemangioma of skin of fingers perforating through epidermis. (Comment on Frankenthal's article.) Zentralbl. f. Chir. *60:*154, Jan 21, '33

GROSS, W.: Typical finger injuries received while working with mangle. Zentralbl. f. Chir. *60:*2790–2791, Dec 2, '33

GROSS, W. A.: Conservatism in surgery as applied to nasal mucosa. Am. J. Phys. Therapy *9:*199–200, Nov '32 also: Eye, Ear, Nose and Throat Monthly *11:*392–393, Nov '32

GROSSE: Strangulation of finger and penis by long hair. Munchen. med. Wchnschr. *72:*1887–1888, Oct 30, '25

GROSSE, O.: New plastic operation of breast. Zentralbl. f. Chir. *60:*8–12, Jan 7, '33

GROSSIORD, A. (see GUILLAIN, G. *et al*) Jan–Feb '42

GROSSMAN, L. (see SCHWARTZMAN, J. *et al*) Oct '42

GROSSMAN, M. O. AND LIGHTFOOT, L. H.: Therapy of decubitus. Hospital, New York *1:*35–36, Aug '45

GROSSMAN, S. Y. (see FELDMAN, S. P.) 1944

GROSSMANN, H.: Construction of artificial vagina by formation of pedicled skin flap. Zentralbl. f. Gynak. *63:*1810–1814, Aug 12, '39

GROTH, K. E.: Experimental studies in decubitus ulcer. Nord. med. (Hygiea) *15:*2423–2428, Aug 29, '42

GROVE, R. C.: Congenital atresia of right posterior naris. Virginia M. Monthly *60:*682–684, Feb '34

GRUBBS, R. H.: Hand infections. Virginia M. Monthly *69:*668-672, Dec '42

GRUBER, G. B.: Ectopy of bladder, remains of cloacal duct, perineal hernia of caudal gut and apparent doubling of external genitals. Beitr. z. path. Anat. u. z. allg. Path. *87:*455-465, June 27, '31

GRUBER, G. B.: Question of double malformations; acrocephalosyndactylia and dysencephalia splanchnocystica. Beitr. z. path. Anat. u. z. allg. Path. *93:*459–476, '34

GRUBER, L. W. AND LYFORD, J. III.: Care of military and civilian injuries; conservative treatment of simultaneous fractures through necks of both mandibular condyles associated with multiple fractures of other parts of mandible. Am. J. Orthodontics (Oral Surg. Sect.) *28:*258–264, May '42

GRUBER, L. W. AND LYFORD, J. III.: Appliance for use in conservative treatment of collum fractures of mandible, in maintaining vertical dimension of jaw, and for overcoming spasm of elevator muscles of mandible. Am. J. Orthodontics (Oral Surg. Sect.) *29:*160-162, March '43

GRUCA, A.: Plastic covering of large defects following breast amputation. Zentralbl. f. Chir. *54:*1293-1297, May 21, '27

GRUCA, A.: Congenital club hand with subluxation of phalanges; case. Rev. d'orthop. *14:*407-412, Sept '27

GRUCA, A. (see MACZEWSKI, S.) April–June '32

GRÜNKORN, J.: Opposition of thumb; explanation based on muscular physiology; therapy of loss of opposition. Ztschr. f. orthop. Chir. *57:*517-530, '32

GRUNEWALD, A. H.: Oral surgeon, prosthodontist and orthopedist as team in difficult fractures of jaw. U. S. Nav. M. Bull. *41:*157-167, Jan '43

GRÜNWALD, B.: Keloid and its treatment. Gyogyaszat *76:*279-280. May 3, '36

GRUSS, J.: Artificial vagina in case of external male pseudohermaphroditism. Deutsche med. Wchnschr. *47:*509, May 5, '21

GRYNKRAUT, B.: Thumb with 3 phalanges. J. de radiol. et d'electrol. *11:*325, June '27

GRZHEBIN, Z. N.: Therapy of skin lesions due to war gases. Klin. med. (no. 6) *17:*83–86, '39

GRZYWA, N.: Plastic surgery of contracture after burns. Geneesk. tijdschr. v. Nederl.-Indie *74:*1539-1540, Nov 6, '34

GUBERN-SALISACHS, L.: Nervous etiology of Dupuytren's contracture; cases. Rev. de cir. de Barcelona *6:*81–115, Sept '33

GUBERN-SALISACHS, L.: Modern burn therapy; 2 cases. Rev. de cir. de Barcelona *9:*325–348, April '35

GUCCIARDELLO, S.: Plastic reconstruction of large portion of pavilion of ear by new method. Riv. san. siciliana *24:*640-642, June 14, '36

GUCCIARDELLO. S.: Hinge mobilization of lower jaw to correct permanent constriction probably due to hypertonia of masticatory muscles; technic and results in case. Riv. san. siciliana *25:*255-263, March 1, '37

GUERIN, J.: Practical treatment of burns. Presse med. *53:*424, Aug 4, '45

GUÉRIN, R.: Congenital craniofacial aplasia and malformation of toes (Apert syndrome); case. J. de med. de Bordeaux *112:*171-173, March 10, '35

GUEULLETTE, R.: Technic of restoration of thumb. J. de chir. *36:*1-23, July '30

GUGEL-MOROZOVA, T. P.: Therapy of traumatic shock according to method of I. R. Petrov. Klin. med. (no. 9) *21:*60-63, '43

GUIBAL. (see MASSABUAU, *et al*) Aug '27

GUIBAL, A.: Dislocation of thumb. Montpel. med. *48:*382, Sept 1, '26

GUICHARD. (see SORREL, E. *et al*) Nov '35

GUICHARD, P.: Orthopedic treatment of fractures of lower jaw. Loire med. *45:*49-61, Feb '31

GUIDI, H. (see CONVERSE, J. M. *et al*) May '44

GUIDOTTI, F. P. (see LAPIDUS, P. W. *et al*) Aug '43

GUIDOTTI, F. P. (see LAPIDUS, P. W.) Oct '44

GUILBERT, H. D.: Suturing infected wounds of the face. J. Internat. Coll. Surgeons *7:*44-48, Jan-Feb '44

GUILD, W. A.: Better local application for first and second degree burns (picric acid in flexible collodion). J. Am. Inst. Homeop. *35:*532-533, Dec '42

GUILERA, L. G.: Deep, cicatricial keloid treated by radium; case. An. Hosp. de Santa Cruz y San Pablo *2:*234, July 15, '28

GUILLAIN, G.; GROSSIORD, A. AND ROUZAUD, M.: Hemiatrophy of face coexisting with diffuse cutaneous neurofibromatosis; case. Rev. neurol. *74:*87-88, Jan-Feb '42

GUILLAUME, J. (see ALAJOUANINE, T. *et al*) Dec '30

GUILLEMIN, A.: Nodules due to ear-rings; case. Rev. med. de Nancy *66:*292-294, April 1, '38

GUILLEMINET: Results of therapy of extensive burns in children. Lyon chir. *36:*476-479, July-Aug '39

GUILLEMINET, AND GUILLET: Surgical therapy of harelip. Lyon chir. *36:*197-201, March-April '39

GUILLEMINET, M.: Arthoplasty of fingers; 2 cases. Lyon chir. *35:*117-119, Jan-Feb '38

GUILLEMINET, M.: Volkmann contracture; case. Lyon chir. *34:*183-187, March-April '37
GUILLEMINET, M. AND DUBOST, T.: Tendon transplant in paralysis of extensors of hand and fingers; case in boy 5 years old. Rev. d'orthop. *32:*72-75, Jan-Apr '46
GUILLERMO, AND TISSANDIE: Urethroperineal fistula, cure by pedicled graft; urethroplasty without preliminary cystostomy; case. Bull. Soc. franc. d'urol. pp. 322-326, Dec 21, '36
GUILLERY, H.: Composition of embryonal tissue fluid; significance for growth of transplanted tissue. Virchows Arch. f. path. Anat. *275:*181-192, '30
GUILLET. (see GUILLEMINET) March-April '39
GUIMARAES, N. A.: Imperforate vagina; case. Med. cir. pharm., pp. 40-41, Jan '42
GUISEZ, J.: Anesthesia in operations on face and neck. Ann. d. mal. de l'oreille, du larynx *49:*516-524, May '30
GUISO, L.: Burn therapy, review of literature. Ann. di med. nav. e colon *44:*149-156, March-April '38
GUISO, L.: Local first aid treatment of burns during naval combat. Ann. di med. nav. e colon *46:*151-154, March-April '40
GUISS, J. M.: Burn physiology applied to modern surgery; symposium; fluid therapy. Northwest Med. *45:*488-491, July '46
GULEKE: Artificial ear, replacement of entire auricle. Chirurg *4:*274-278, April 1, '32
GULYAEVA, N. M.: Congenital bilateral deformation of thumbs. Ortop. i travmatol. (no. 3) *12:*73-76, '38
GUMPERT, M.: Excision of unsightly skin folds. Med. Welt. *4:*219, Feb 15, '30
GUMPERTZ, F.: Nasal lisping and speech in palatoschisis; palatographic study. Wien. med. Wchnschr. *82:*901-903, July 9, '32

Gunn's Phenomenon

Congenital eyelid ptosis with Gunn's phenomenon; case. DUPUY-DUTEMPS, L. Bull. Soc. d'opht. de Paris, pp. 136-140, March '29

GUNN, J. AND HILLSMAN, J. A.: Thermal burns. Ann. Surg. *102:*429-443, Sept '35
GUNN, J. A.: Injuries to forearm and hand. Canad. M.A.J. *13:*627-633, Sept '23
GUNN, J. A. (see HILLSMAN, J. A.) April '38
GUNN, W. D.: Mercurochrome in burns. J. Roy. Nav. M. Serv. *23:*260-261, July '37
GUNSETT, *et al*: Suppurations of maxillary sinus and of orbit with extensive destruction of wall of sinus simulating cancer of upper jaw; case. Bull. et mem. Soc. de radiol. med. de France *24:*170, Feb '36
GUNSETT, A.: Acute, spinocellular epithelioma developed after burn with flaming asphalt; case. Bull. Assoc. franc. p. l'etude du cancer *19:*459-462, June '30
GUNSETT, A.: Late results of fractional roentgenotherapy of intrinsic cancer of larynx; results of 5 years' experience. Gaz. med. de France (supp. radiol.), pp. 173-177, May 1, '32

Gunshot Wounds (See also War Injuries)

Gunshot wound of upper third of arm with complete section of ulnar nerve and compression of median nerve; late suture of ulnar nerve. FERRAZ ALVIM, J.; *et al.* Rev oto-neuro-oftal. *9:*44-52, Feb '34
Severe gunshot wound of face. DORSET, R. F. Mil. Surgeon *80:*429-431, June '37
Naphthalene in therapy of gangrene following grave trauma of face due to bullet wounds. PALAZZI, S. Gior. di med. mil. *85:*944-952, Sept '37
Gunshot wounds of face and jaws. MACLURE, F. M. J. Australia *1:*62-64, Jan 13, '40
Chemotherapy (with sulfonamides) in gunshot wounds of face, neck and jaws. OGLE, M. W. Rev. san. mil., Habana *6:*312-317, Oct-Dec '42
Emergency therapy of gunshot wounds of face with fracture of lower jaw. BROGGI, M. AND DOMENECH-ALSINA, F. Med. espan. *9:*70-74, Jan '43
Early plastic reconstruction of defects following gunshot wounds. FABRIKANT, M. B. Khirurgiya, no. 3, pp. 27-29, '44
Therapy of maxillofacial gunshot wounds. FALTIN, R. Acta chir. Scandinav. *91:*434-447, '44
Extensive plastic reconstruction of shoulder joint following gunshot wound. RIKHTER, G. A. Khirurgiya, no. 8, pp. 79-80, '44
Reconstructive treatment of gunshot wound of face and neck. LEWIN, M. Arch. Otolaryng. *42:*191-197, Sept '45 also: Tr. Am. Acad. Ophth. (1944) *49:*276-282, May-June '45

DE GUNTEN, P.: Pneumatization of bones of face in Crouzon's disease, Apert's syndrome and oxycephaly; 13 cases. Schweiz. med. Wchnschr. *68:*268-270, March 12, '38
GUNTER, J. H. (see MELOY, T. M. JR.) Sept '44
GUNTHER, B.: Physiopathology of shock. Arch. Soc. cirujanos hosp. *15:*369-377, March '45
GÜNTHER, G. W.: Pathology of collapse following burns. Arch. f. klin. Chir. *194:*539-557, '39
GÜNTHER, H.: Anomalies and complex abnormalities of region of first pharyngeal arch. Ztschr. f. menschl. Vererb.-u. Konstitution-

slehre *23:*43-52, '39
GUNTHER, L.: Venopressor mechanism in production of shock (role of muscle tonus); treatment with nikethamide. U. S. Nav. M. Bull. *44:*300-307, Feb '45
GURD, F. B.: Burn therapy. Proc. Interst. Postgrad. M. A. North America (1943) pp. 141-146, '44
GURD, F. B.; ACKMAN, D.; GERRIE, J. W. AND PRITCHARD, J. E.: Practical concept for major and minor burns (including use of sulfathiazole, sulfanilamide derivative, emulsion and "sulfamesh" dressing); importance of timing therein. Ann. Surg. *116:*641-657, Nov '42
GURD, F. B. AND GERRIE, J. W.: Early plastic care of deep burns (including use of pressure dressing with sulfathiazole, sulfonamide). J.A.M.A. *125:*616-621, July 1, '44
GURDIN, M.: Special considerations in repair of facial injuries. Hawaii M. J. *2:*199-200, March-April '43
GURDIN, M.: Early care of nasal fractures. U. S. Nav. M. Bull. *41:*1706-1712, Nov '43
GURDIN, M. M.; BAU, R. G. AND KEVAN, J. E. JR.: Extraoral facial prosthesis; elastic vinyl (vinylite resin) plastic method. U. S. Nav. M. Bull. *42:*644-650, March '44
GURDJIAN, E. S. AND WEBSTER, J. E.: Surgical management of compound depressed fracture of frontal sinus, cerebrospinal rhinorrhea and pneumocephalus. Arch. Otolaryng. *39:*287-306, April '44
GURDJIAN, E. S. AND WILLIAMS, H. W.: Surgical treatment of intractable cases of eyelid spasm. J.A.M.A. *91:*2053-2056, Dec 29, '28
GURNEY, C. E.: Surgical correction of collapsed alar cartilages; case. Arch. Otolaryng. *33:*199-203, Feb '41
GURRIA URGELL, D.: External dacryocystorhinostomy by Torres Estrada technic. Gac. med. de Mexico *69:*336-340, Oct 30, '39
GÜRSEL, A. E.: Coffey operation in exstrophy of bladder. Turk tib cem. mec. *5:*90-91, '39
GURVICH, M. O.: Surgical treatment of smallpox scars. Sovet. vrach. gaz., pp. 421-422, March 15, '35
GUSEV, B. P.: Instrument for transplantation of tendons. Vestnik khir. *58:*590-591, Dec '39
GUSMAO, D. (see AUSTREGESILO, A. *et al*) Nov-Dec '43
GUSSIO, S.: Experimental transplantation of cartilage and skin for repair of concha. Valsalva *3:*58-77, Feb '27
GUSYNIN, V.: Treatment of fractures of hands and fingers caused by gunshot wounds. J.A.M.A. *121:*952, March 20, '43
GUSYNIN, V. A.: Active surgical therapy of traumatic shock. Novy khir. arkhiv. *35:*566-572, '36
GUTHRIE, D.: Surgery of nasal deformities. Edinburgh M. J. *27:*365, Dec '21
GUTHRIE, D.: Nasal disfigurement and its correction. J. Laryng. and Otol. *38:*300-303, June '23 (illus.)
GUTHRIE, D. (DONALD) AND GAGNON, G.: Prevention and treatment of postoperative lymphedema of arm (in breast cancer). Tr. South. S. A. (1945) *57:*460-471, '46
GUTHRIE, D. AND GAGNON, G.: Postoperative lymphedema of arm (in breast cancer); (Beck operation). Ann. Surg. *123:*925-936, May '46
GUTIERREZ, A.: Three cases of snapping temporomaxillary joint. Bol. y trab. de la Soc. de cir. de Buenos Aires *16:*65-74, April 20, '32
GUTIÉRREZ, A.: Baldwin-Mori operation for artificial vagina; case. Bol. y trab. de la Soc. de cir. de Buenos Aires *17:*739-742, Aug 2, '33
GUTIÉRREZ, A.: Local anesthesia in total excision of parotid. Rev. de cir. de Buenos Aires *15:*288-292, May '36
GUTIÉRREZ, A.: Symphysis of both thighs due to burn cicatrix; surgical therapy of case. Rev. de cir. de Buenos Aires *16:*13-21, Jan '37
GUTNER, Y. I.: Salivary fistulas following gunshot wounds to face, and their therapy. Khirurgiya, no. 7, pp. 54-58, '44
GUTTERIDGE, E.: Human cartilage heterografts in plastic surgery. M. J. Australia *1:*9-10, Jan 6, '45
GÜTTICH, A.: Technic of endonasal operation on lacrimal sac. Arch. f. Ohren-, Nasen-u. Kehlkopfh. *143:*233-235, '37
GUTTMANN, E. (see HERZBERG, E.) Nov '29
GUTTMANN, L.: Reestablishment of function of sweat glands in grafted skin. Dermat. Ztschr. *77:*73-77, Feb '38
GUTTMANN, L.: Experimental study on nerve suture with various suture materials. Brit. J. Surg. *30:*370-375, April '43
GUTTMANN, L.: New hope for spinal cord sufferers (with decubitus). M. Times, New York *73:*318-326, Nov '45 also: South African M. J. *20:*141-144, March 23, '46
GUTTMAN, M. R.: Recent advances in plastic and reconstructive surgery (of ears, nose and throat). Am. J. M. Sc. *196:*875-882, Dec '38
GUTTMAN, M. R.: Plastic surgery in Prague, Czechoslovakia; recent experiences. Laryngoscope *49:*291-296, April '39
GUTTMAN, M. R.: Modern changes in plastic and reconstructive surgery of face and neck. Illinois M. J. *76:*349-351, Oct '39
GUTTMAN, M. R. (see BECK, J. C.) Aug '34
GUTTMAN, M. R. (see BECK, J. C.) June '36
GUTZEIT, R.: New instruments for Toti operation (dacryocystorhinostomy). Klin. Monatsbl. f. Augenh. *84:*92, Jan '30

GUTZEIT, R.: "Tendon stretcher" for pulling forward muscle for tenotomy. (Comment on Streiff's article.) Klin. Monatsbl. f. Augenh. *98:*671, May '37

Gutzeit Operation

Dacryocystorhinostomy by modified Gutzeit method. MATA, P. Arch. de oftal. hispano-am. *34:*141-147, March '34

External dacryocystorhinostomy according to Gutzeit method. DIAZ-CANEJA, E. Ann. d'ocul. *170:*384-414, May '33 also: An. Casa de Salud Valdecilla *3:*292-313, '32

GUTZMANN, H.: Speech exercises after cleft palate operation. Chirurg *2:*1019-1027, Nov 15, '30

GUY, L.: Simple dacryocystorhinostomy. Arch. Ophth. *20:*954-957, Dec '38

GUY, L. P.: Construction of lacrimal passage. Arch. Ophth. *29:*575-577, April '43

GUY, L. P. (see HUGHES, W. L. *et al*) Sept '41

GUY, W.: Injuries of jaw. Brit. Dent. J. *49:*904-909, Aug 15, '28

GUYOT, J. AND JEANNENEY, G.: Diagnosis of traumatic shock. Progres med. *36:*199, May 7, '21 abstr: J.A.M.A. *77:*73, July 2, '21

GUYOT, J. AND JEANNENEY, G.: Traumatic shock. Paris med. *11:*157, Aug 27, '21

GUYOT, R.: Typical and atypical forms of aural fistulae; review of literature. Ann. d'oto-laryng., pp. 1227-1248, Dec '34

GYGAX, P.: Ankylosis of jaws, case. Schweiz. Monatschr. f. Zahnh. *40:*179-208, April '30

GYLLENSVÄRD, N.: Operation in case of hermaphroditismus masculinus tubularis et externus with restoration of patient to feminine types. Acta obst. et gynec. Scandinav. *10:*392-409, '30

GYMNICH, W.: Tannic acid in burns. Med. Welt *6:*1646, Nov 12, '32

HAAG, H.: 5 years of surgery of ear and nose. Schweiz. med. Wchnschr. *52:*498-504, May 25, '22

Gynecomastia

Operation for gynecomasty and pendulous breast in male. KURTZAHN, H. Deutsche Ztschr. f. Chir. *209:*403-406, '28

Plastic operation for unusually extensive gynecomastia. ADLER, A. Zentralbl. f. Chir. *64:*889-893, April 10, '37

Plastic surgery in gynecomastia. VOGT, L. G. Chirurg *13:*322-324, May 15 '41

Gynecomastia; new technic of surgical therapy. IVANISSEVICH, O. *et al*. Semana med. *1:*1434-1438, June 19, '41

Gynecomastia; surgical therapy of 2 cases.

Gynecomastia – Cont.

MALBEC, E. F. Semana med. *2:*988-989, Oct 23, '41

Bilateral gynecomastic and its surgical therapy; case. CAMPOS, F. Arq. de cir. clin. e exper. *6:*703-705, April-June '42

Gynecomastia; surgical therapy of 2 cases. MALBEC, E. F. Arq. de cir. clin. e exper. *6:*686-689, April-June '42

Two cases of pseudogynecomastia in male, with surgical reconstruction. MALINIAC, J. W., J. Clin. Endocrinol. *3:*364-366, June '43

Gynecomastia; pathogenesis and therapy. ROSENBLATT, S. Dia med. *15:*1147-1149, Oct 4, '43

Gynecomastia; new surgical technic. MALBEC, E. F. Dia med. *17:*498-500, May 28, '45

Gynecomastia; surgical technic. MALBEC, E. F. Prensa med. argent. *32:*1759-1763, Sept 7, '45

Gynecomastia; surgical technics. MALBEC, E. F. Rev. Fac. de med., Bogota *14:*380-391, Dec '45

Gynecomastia; new surgical technic. MALBEC, E. F., J. Internat. Coll. Surgeons *9:*652-654, Sept-Oct '46

Mastectomy for gynecomastia through semicircular intra-areolar incision. WEBSTER, J. P. Ann. Surg. *124:*557-575, Sept '46

H

HAAG, H.: Five years of surgery of ear and nose. Schweiz. med. Wchnschr. *52:*498-504, May 25, '22

HAAGENSEN, C. D.: Treatment of uncomplicated primary carcinoma of lips. Am. J. Cancer *15:*239-245, Jan '31

DE HAAN, H. R. M.: Peculiar case of purpura developing after burns. Nederl. tijdschr. v. geneesk. *82:*2556-2557, May 21, '38

HAARDT, W.: Prevention of angina after nasal operations. Wien. klin. Wchnschr. *40:*320, March 10, '27

HAARMANN, H.: Injuries to ear due to electric current. Hals-, Nasen-u. Ohrenarzt (Teil 1) *28:*49-58, Feb '37

HAAS, E.: Chisel for dacryocystorhinostomy. Bull. Soc. d'opht. de Paris *50:*468-469, Oct '38

HAAS, E. (see POSER, E.) Nov '43

HAAS, S. L.: Function in relation to transplantation of bone. Arch. Surg. *3:*425, Sept '21

HAAS, S. L.: Spontaneous healing inherent in transplanted bone. J. Bone and Joint Surg. *4:*209-214, April '22 (illus.)

HAAS, S. L.: Ideal bone graft as determined by experimental investigations. S. Clin. N. America *3:*761-763, June '23

HAAS, S. L.: Fractures in transplanted bone.

Surg., Gynec. and Obst. *36:*749–762, June '23 (illus.)
HAAS, S. L.: Importance of periosteum and endosteum in repair of transplanted bone. Arch. Surg. *8:*535–556, March '24
HAAS, S. L.: Further observation on transplantation of epiphyseal cartilage plate. Surg., Gynec. and Obst. *52:*958–963, May '31
HAAS, S. L.: Plastic restoration for loss of all fingers of both hands. Am. J. Surg. *36:*720–723, June '37
HAAS, S. L.: Bilateral complete syndactylism of all fingers. Am. J. Surg. *50:*363–366, Nov '40
HAAS, S. L.: (KOFMANN, S.) New points of view in arthroplasty of jaw; comment on Haas's article. Zentralbl. f. Chir. *53:*1125–1126, May 1, '26
HAASE, E. B.: After-examination of 131 patients who had been operated on according to Caldwell-Luc procedure. Acta oto-laryng. *34:*23–30, '46
HAASE, G.: Leukoplakia of mouth and labial and lingual cancer in smokers. Deutsche Monatschr. f. Zahnh. *49:*881, Sept 15; 929, Oct 1, '31
HAASE, W.: Criticism of ointments and skin-forming preparations, especially in relation to third degree burns. Zentralbl. f. Chir. *68:*350–353, Feb 22, '41
HABABOU-SALA: Infection of surgeon's hand by hemolytic streptococci entering through prick from surgical instrument during operation; successful vaccine therapy. Tunisie med. *26:*78–79, Feb '32
HABACHI, S.: Best operation against spastic entropion. Bull. Ophth. Soc. Egypt *34:*57–63, '41
HABERERN, J. P. Luxation of tendons of extensores digitorum. Zentralbl. f. Chir. *48:*1080, July 30, '21
HABERLAND, H. F. O.: Unsuccessful trials with alloplasty in vascular wounds. Zentralbl. f. Chir. *49:*542–543, April 22, '22
HABERLAND, H. F. O.: Epithelization of skin grafts with roentgen rays. Klin. Wchnschr. *2:*353–354, Feb 19, '23
HABERLAND, H. F. O.: Plastic surgery of breast. Med. Welt *6:*118–120, Jan 23, '32
HABERLAND, H. F. O.: Plastic operations of face, breast. Zentralbl. f. Chir. *60:*746–748, March 31, '33
HABERLAND, H. F. O.: Advances in plastic surgery (abdomen). Zentralbl. f. Chir. *63:*154–156, Jan 18, '36
HABERLAND, H. F. O.: Constantly recurring unsatisfactory end results of plastic surgery in hypertrophy of breast. Zentralbl. f. Chir. *63:*510–511, Feb 29, '36
HABERLAND, H. F. O.: Injury to mammary areola and progressive necrosis after plastic surgery of breast. Arch. f. klin. Chir. *190:*87–95, '37
HABERLER, G.: Therapy of Volkmann's contracture. Zentralbl. f. Chir. *58:*1774–1781, July 11, '31
HÄBERLIN, F.: Funnel chest; successfully operated case. Schweiz. med. Wchnschr. *72:*126–128, Jan 31, '42
HACQUEBORD, P.: Dermoid cysts of dorsum of nose; 3 cases. Geneesk. gids *9:*721–728, July 31, '31
HADDOCK, T. R.: Sulfathiazole (sulfanilamide derivative) in treatment of fractures of mandible. J. Am. Dent. A. *29:*1002–1004, June 1, '42
HADLEY, F. A.: Skull defects repaired by tibial grafts. J. Coll. Surgeons, Australasia *1:*208–213, Nov '28
HAFFNER, H. (see BROWN, J. B.) Dec '39
HAGAN, C. E. JR.: Secondary endaural grafting of cavity resulting from radical mastoidectomy. Arch. Otolaryng. *34:*1029–1035, Nov '41
HAGEDOORN, A.: Plastic restoration of deformity caused by complete exenteration of orbit. Surg., Gynec. and Obst. *70:*193–195, Feb '40
HAGEN, G. L.: Dermotome. J.A.M.A. *82:*1933, June 14, '24
HAGENBACH: Age for surgery of cleft palate. Schweiz. med. Wchnschr. *55:*487–488, May 28, '25
HAGENBACH, E.: Treatment of prominent intermaxillary bone in therapy of harelip and cleft palate. Schweiz. med. Wchnschr. *63:*949–950, Sept 23, '33
HAGENBACH, E.: Plastic surgery of hypoplasia of breast. Helvet. med. acta *3:*811–812, Dec '36
HAGENBACH, E.: Coffey method of ureteral implantation in exstrophy of bladder. Helvet. med. acta *10:*321–324, June '43
HAGENS, E. W.: Unilateral malformations of ear associated with cyclopia. Arch. Otolaryng. *18:*332–338, Sept '33
HAGENS, E. W.: Congenital dermoid cyst and fistula of dorsum of nose; case. Arch. Otolaryng. *28:*399–403, Sept '38
HAGENTORN, A.: Technic of operation for harelip. Deutsche Ztschr. f. Chir. *212:*391–398, '28
HAGENTORN, A.: Harelip operation. Zentralbl. f. Chir. *55:*528–533, March 3, '28
HAGENTORN, A.: Plastic surgery of face (including harelip and cleft palate). Arch. f. klin. Chir. *195:*455–488, '39
HAGENTORN, A.: Cheiloplastic methods. Zen-

tralbl. f. Chir. *56:*3031–3032, Nov 30, '29
'HAGENTORN, A.: Technic of rhinoplasty. Zentralbl. f. Chir. *57:*600–603, March 8, '30
HAGENTORNAS, A.: Operation of harelip. Medicina, Kaunas *10:*917–918, Dec '29
HAGENTORNAS, A.: Surgery of double harelip. Zentralbl. f. Chir. *59:*1460–1463, June 11, '32
HAGGARD, W. D.: Avulsion of scalp, skin grafting for complete. S. Clin. N. Amer. *10:*719–723, Aug '30
HAGGART, G. E.: Finger and hand fractures treated by skeletal traction. S. Clin. North America *14:*1203–1210, Oct '34
HAGGART, W. W. (see MCIVER, M. A.) April '23
HAGGLAND, P. B.: Instrument for pinch grafting. Am. J. Surg. *39:*171, Jan '38
HÄGGSTRÖM, P.: Ekehorn's rectopexy in adults. Upsala Lakaref. Forh. *31:*527–542, Sept '26
HAGNER, F. R.: New method for straightening penis in hypospadias. Tr. South. S. A. *44:*245–246, '31 also: J.A.M.A. *99:*116, July 9, '32
HAGNER, F. R. AND KNEALE, H. B.: Pseudohermaphrodism or complete hypospadias. Surg., Gynec. and Obst. *36:*495–501, April '23 (illus.)
HAGUE, E. B.: Recent advances in eyelid surgery. Dis. Eye, Ear, Nose and Throat *2:*353–359, Dec '42
HAGUE, E. B.: Surgical reconstruction of upper eyelid. Am. J. Ophth. *28:*886–889, Aug '45
HAILES, W. A.: Burn therapy. Australian and New Zealand J. Surg. *12:*30–33, July '42
HAILEY, H.: Radium treatment of early epithelioma of lips. South. M. J. *23:*1121–1125, Dec '30
HAILEY, H.: Squamous-celled epithelioma of lower lip; radium therapy. J. M. A. Georgia *20:*386–388, Oct '31
HAIM, E.: Technic for artificial vagina. Zentralbl. f. Gynak. *48:*2382–2387, Oct 25, '24

Hair

Cosmetic depilation of hair. NOBL, G. Med. Klinik *20:*369–371, March 23, '24 abstr: J.A.M.A. *82:*1575, May 10, '24
Small apparatus for diathermy and electrocoagulation depilation treatment of hypertrichosis in women. LANZI, G. Gior. ital. d. ma. ven. *65:*1718–1720, Oct '24
Diathermy as rapid and effectual means of permanent depilation. KATZ, T. Dermat. Wchnschr. *79:*1492–1493, Nov 15, '24
Epilation with diathermy; preliminary report. ROSTENBERG, A., M. J. and Rec.

Hair – Cont.
*121:*751, June 17, '25
Strangulation of finger and penis by long hair. GROSSE. Munchen. med. Wchnschr. *72:*1887–1888, Oct 30, '25
Alopecia, case cured by phototherapy. JAUSION, *et al.* Bull. Soc. franc. de dermat. et syph. *33:*641–650, Nov '26
Permanent destruction of hair by diathermy in facial hypertrichosis. VAN PUTTE, P. J. Nederl. Tijdschr. v. Geneesk. *1:*924–928, Feb 19, '27
Treatment of hypertrichosis with electrocoagulation. EITNER, E. Wien. klin. Wchnschr. *40:*460, April 7, '27
New electrical epilation apparatus. MEZEI, K. Dermat. Wchnschr. *85:*1107, Aug 6, '27
New needle-holder for use in diathermic epilation in hypertrichosis. KENDE, B. Wien. klin. Wchnschr. *41:*382, March 15, '28
Multiple epilation with diathermy by simultaneous use of several needles. MEZEI, K. Dermat. Wchnschr. *88:*720, May 18, '29
Operative depilation in plastic surgery. RÉTHI, A. Chirurg *1:*695–698, June 15, '29
Cystic tuberous lymphangioma of skin with hypertrichosis. TRÝB, A. Arch. f. Dermat. u. Syph. *158:*468–479, '29
Hemiatrophia alternans facialis progressiva with hemilateral alopecia; pigment displacement and atrophy of skin; case. BERNSTEIN, E. Dermat. Wchnschr. *90:*235–237, Feb 15, '30
Hypertrichosis following burns. BATTISTA, A. Folia med. *16:*1420–1431, Oct 30, '30
Grafting of hairy skin with aid of pedunculated flap for formation of eyebrows, mustache and beard. PARIN, V. N. Vestnik khir. (nos. 73–74) *24:*10–12, '31
Technic of diathermic epilation. BORDIER, H. Am. J. Phys. Therapy *8:*273–274, Jan '32 also: Monde med., Paris *42:*78–81, Feb 1, '32
Alopecia and its treatment. SIBLEY, K. Post-Grad. M. J. *8:*110–113, April '32
Plastic surgery therapy of trichiasis and free skin graft for hemangioma. DESELAERS, H. Rev. espan. de med. y cir. *15:*353–355, July '32
Hypertrichosis in women and its therapy, with special reference to diathermocoagulation. DE PAGANETTO, M. J. T. Semana med. *1:*1792–1794, May 25, '33
Technic of diathermic epilation in hypertrichosis. DUCOURTIOUX. Rev. d'actinol. *10:*14–19, Jan–Feb '34
Diathermic depilation in hypertrichosis.

Hair—Cont.
SOLLA, L. Actas dermo-sif. *26:*445–449, March '34
Symposium on question of permanent epilation of excessive hair for cosmetic purposes (Dauerepilation an kosmetisch wichtigen Korperstellen). VARIOUS AUTHORS. Dermat. Wchnschr. *98:*275–287, March 3, '34
Comment on article by various authors on permanent epilation for cosmetic purposes. ZOON, J. J. Dermat. Wchnschr. *98:*501, April 21, '34
Permanent epilation of hair for cosmetic purposes. (Reply to Zoon) HOEDE, K. Dermat. Wchnschr. *99:*932, July 14, '34
Permanent epilation of hair for cosmetic purposes. (Reply to Zoon). WUCHERPFENNIG, V. Dermat. Wchnschr. *99:*933–934, July 14, '34
Technic of cosmetic electrolysis of hair removal. GOODMAN, H. Am. Med. *41:*35–36, Jan '35
Short wave therapy of alopecia; cases. PETGES, AND WANGERMEZ. Bull. et mem. Soc. de radiol. med. de France *24:*477–478, May '36
New therapeutic procedure in trichiasis. WEISS, A. S. Folia ophth. orient. *2:*143–147, '36
Traumatic alopecias of scalp; different types. RABUT, R. Presse med. *46:*379–380, March 9, '38
Eyebrow alopecias and their therapy. PIGNOT, M. Presse med. *46:*843–844, May 25, '38
Dangers of roentgenotherapy of hypertrichosis of chin; 2 cases. ESSER, J. F. S. An. de cir. *4:*260–262, Sept '38
Facial hypertrichosis in female; local therapy by diathermocoagulation, with special reference to technic. LUMER, M. Semana med. *2:*891–897, Oct 20, '38
Electrolysis for hair removal; discussion of equipment, method of operation, indications, contraindications and warnings concerning its use. CIPOLLARO, A. C., J.A.M.A. *111:*2488–2491, Dec 31, '38
Roentgen epilation. ARONSTEIN, E. Radiology *32:*95–96, Jan '39
Short wave epilation. DEROW, D. Arch. Phys. Therapy *20:*101–102, Feb '39
Alopecia prematura and its surgical treatment (flap-method of plastic surgery). TAUBER, H. J. Ceylon Br., Brit. M. A. *36:*237–242, July '39
Hair removal; electrolysis; surgical procedure. CIPOLLARO, A. C. New York State J. Med. *39:*1475–1480, Aug 1, '39
New type of forceps used as accessory element in depilation by diathermocoagulation. CATEULA, J. Semana med. *2:*628, Sept 14, '39
Clinical and experimental studies on transplantation of living hairs. OKUDA, S. Jap. J. Dermat. and Urol. *46:*135–138, Dec 20, '39
Surgical correction of superciliary alopecia in leprosy. SILVEIRA, L. M. Rev. brasil. de leprol. (num. espec.) *7:*277–281, '39
Essentials in art of epilation for hypertrichosis (electrolysis). LERNER, C. M. Rec. *151:*193–194, March 20, '40
How to remove superfluous hair. COSTELLO, M. J. Hygeia *18:*584–586, July '40
Treatment of hypertrichosis by improved apparatus and technic (electrolysis). MARTON, M. H. Arch. Phys. Therapy *21:*678–683, Nov '40
Late sequels of roentgen depilation of scalp. PROPPE, A. AND GAHLEN, W. Arch. f. Dermat. u. Syph. *108:*155–164, '40
High frequency current in treatment of hypertrichosis. KARP, F. L. Arch. Dermat. and Syph. *43:*85–91, Jan '41
Hypertrichosis with particular reference to electrolysis. REQUE, P. G. South. Med. and Surg. *103:*376–379, July '41
"Thimble forceps" for epilation (during electrolysis). SHELTON, J. M. Arch. Dermat. and Syph. *44:*260, Aug '41
Hypertrichosis and its treatment with special regard to cosmetically disfiguring forms. GENNER, V. Ugesk. f. laeger *103:*1400–1403, Oct 30, '41
Hypertrichosis; problem and how to handle it as it appears in every-day practice. GARA, G. Urol. and Cutan. Rev. *45:*771–774, Dec '41
Treatment of hypertrichosis by electrocoagulation. LERNER, C. New York State J. Med. *42:*879–882, May 1, '42
Electrolysis; introduction of instrument for relatively painless treatment of hair removal. HAND, E. A. Arch. Dermat. and Syph. *45:*1094–1100, June '42
Superfluous hair; removal with monopolar diathermy needle. ERDOS-BROWN, M. Arch. Dermat. and Syph. *46:*496–501, Oct '42
Hair removal, nonsurgical reparative dermatology, or electromedical cosmetology. GOODMAN, H. Urol. and Cutan. Rev. *46:*726–727, Nov '42
Removal of superfluous hair with cutting current. ROSENBERG, W. A. AND SMITH, E. M. JR. Arch. Phys. Therapy *24:*277–279, May '43

Hair–Cont.
Epilation; fifteen year comparative evaluation of electrolysis and electrocoagulation. NIEDELMAN, M. L. Arch. Phys. Med. *26:*290–296, May '45
Diathermal depilation in therapy of hypertrichosis. BARMAN, J. M. Rev. med. de Rosario *35:*703–709, Aug '45
Superfluous hair and acne-cause and cure. KAUFMAN, S. M. Hygeia *24:*272, Apr '46
Hair growth in skin transplanted under skin and into peritoneal cavity in rat. BUTCHER, E. O. Anat. Rec. *96:*101–109, Oct '46

HAIST, R. E. (see HAMILTON, J. I. *et al*) Feb '46
HAJEK, M. AND HEINDL, A.: Statistics on results of 393 surgically treated cases of laryngeal cancer from May 1919 to July 1934 inclusive. Monatschr. f. Ohrenh. *69:*385, April; 583, May '35
HALDEMAN, K. O.: Influence of periosteum on survival of bone grafts. J. Bone and Joint Surg. *15:*302–319, April '33
HALFORD, F. J.: Management of war burns. Hawaii M. J. *1:*191–192, Jan '42
HALKIN, H.: Research on melanomas of skin. Ann. de med. *12:*189–225, Sept '22 (illus.) abstr: J.A.M.A. *79:*1722, Nov 11, '22
HALKIN, H.: Cutaneous epithelioma developed on pigmented nevi. Cancer, Bruxelles *9:*241–247, '32
HALKIN, H.: Epitheliomas developing on pigmented nevi and pigmented epitheliomas; cases. Paris med. *1:*241–249, March 20, '37
HALL, C. AND MORRIS, F.: Infections of masticator space. Ann. Otol., Rhin. and Laryng. *50:*1123–1133, Dec '41
HALL, C. T. (see ROGERS, L. *et al*) Jan '32
HALL, E. S.: Traction with rustless steel wire in finger fractures. Maine M. J. *23:*11, Jan '32
HALL, M. H. (see KOHN, F. *et al*) Jan '43
HALL, R. H.: Whole upper extremity transplant for human beings; general plans of procedure and operative technic. Ann. Surg. *120:*12–23, July '44
HALLA, F.: (WODAK, E.) Reply to Eitner's comments on article about nasal tip defects, and Halla's comments. Med. Klin. *28:*50, Jan 8, '32
HALLA, F.: Indications and technic of cosmetic correction of facial wrinkles. (comment on Eitner's article) Wien. klin. Wchnschr. *41:*1442, Oct 11, '28
HALLA, F.: Correction of hypertrophy of breasts by cosmetic surgery. Med. Klin. *25:*1020–1021, June 28, '29
HALLA, F.: Comment on Kromayer's article on facial wrinkle removal. Deutsche med. Wchnschr. *55:*1262–1263, July 26, '29
HALLA, F.: Simplification of plastic method for hypertrophy of breast. Med. Klin. *25:*1697–1698, Nov 1, '29
HALLA, F.: Two types of operation for hypertrophy of breast. Wien. med. Wchnschr. *80:*417, March 15, '30
HALLA, F.: Comment on article by Levy on surgical treatment of atheroma. Munchen. med. Wchnschr. *77:*1277, July 25, '30
HALLA, F.: Defects of tip of nose; surgical correction. (Comment on Wodak's article.) Med. Klin. *28:*50, Jan 8, '32
HALLAM, J. W.: Inferior alveolar nerve and fractured mandible. Guy's Hosp. Gaz. *57:*22, Jan 23, '43
HALLAM, J. W.: Review of 215 fractures of maxillae. Brit. Dent. J. *76:*181–182, April 6, '44
HALLBERG, K.: Substitution of great toe for traumatically amputated thumb. Hygiea *90:*452–456, June 15, '28
HALLBERG, O. E.: Spreading osteomyelitis of maxilla (use of surgery and penicillin). Minnesota Med. *28:*126–127, Feb '45
HALLE, M.: (LEVY, S.) Reply to Franke and Halle on comments about surgical treatment of atheroma. Munchen. med. Wchnschr. *77:*1845–1846, Oct 24, '30
HALLE, M.: Surgical and phonetic results of late cleft palate operations. Med. Klin. *24:*1976–1979, Dec 21, '28
HALLE, M.: Surgical and phonetic results of late operations for cleft palate. Verhandl. d. Berl. med. Gesellsch. (1928) *59:*267–276, '29
HALLE, M.: Correction of disfigurement in facial paralysis. Ztschr. f. Hals-, Nasen-u. Ohrenh. *31:*554–560, '32
HALLE, M.: Correction of cicatrices from smallpox and acne necrotica. Fortschr. d. Therap. *8:*505–506, Aug 25, '32
HALLE, M.: Removal of deformity of facial paralysis. Med. Welt *6:*1279–1280, Sept 3, '32
HALLE, M.: Therapy of scars after variola and acne necrotica. Rev. de chir. plastique, pp. 293–294, Oct '32
HALLE, M.: Removal of deformity of facial paralysis. Rev. de chir. plastique, pp. 3–15, May '33
HALLE, M.: Securing successful results in surgical therapy of cleft palate. Rev. de chir. plastique, pp. 17–21, May '33
HALLE, M.: Plastic surgery of deformities due to facial paralysis; further study. Rev. de chir. structive, pp. 35–38, July '35
HALLE, M.: Facial paralysis and methods for correction. Laryngoscope *48:*225–235, April '38

Halle Operation

Technic of endonasal dacryocystorhinostomy. (Halle operation); cases. JUST TISCORNIA, B. AND MERCANDINO, C. P. Rev. med. latino-am. *20:*1118–1136, July '35

HALLEY MIRALLES, G.: Rare case of horny epithelioma on burn cicatrix; surgical extirpation and plastic repair of residual defect by free skin graft of Davis type. Bol. Liga, contra el cancer *18:*41–46, Feb '43

HALLMAN, L. F. (see PFEIFFER, C. C. *et al*) May '45

HALLUM, A. V.: Dacryocystorhinostomy; logical treatment of occlusion of lacrimal sac. J. M. A. Georgia *32:*186–189, June '43

HALLUM, J. W.: Gag for dysfunction of temporomandibular joint following mandibular injury. Brit. M. J. *1:*569, May 8, '43

HALSTED, W. S.: (BRODEL, M.) Case of Reverdin skin grafting exhibited in Dr. Halsted's clinic on wound healing. Bull. Johns Hopkins Hosp. *36:*60, Jan '25

HALSTED, W. S.: Elephantiasis chirurgica–its cause and prevention. Bull. Johns Hopkins Hosp. *32:*309, Oct '21

HALSTED, W. S.; REICHERT, E. L. AND MONTREID: Mechanism of surgical elephantiasis. Lyon chir. *19:*369–376, July–Aug '22 abstr: J.A.M.A. *79:*1460, Oct 21, '22

HALTY, M.: Study apropos of 2 cases of elephantiasis with lesions of extraordinary magnitude; therapy. Rev. argent. dermatol-sif. *26:*991–1000, '42

HAM, A. W.: Tannic acid in burn therapy; experimental study with particular reference to its effect on local fluid loss and healing. Ann. Surg. *120:*698–706, Nov '44

HAM, T. H. (see SHEN, S. C.) Nov '43

HÄMÄLÄINEN, M.: Treatment of jaw ankylosis; 7 cases. Acta chir. Scandinav. *64:*493–508, '29

HAMANT, A. AND BODART, M.: Accidents of local anesthesia in cranio-facial region; pathogenesis. Rev. med. de l'est. *56:*610–616, Sept 15, '28

HAMANT, A.; BODART, AND CHALNOT: Autoplasties (grafts). Bull. Soc. franc. de dermat. et syph. (Reunion dermat.) *40:*28–30, Jan '33

HAMANT, A. (see SPILLMANN, L. *et al*) June '34

HAMBRESIN, L.: External tarsorrhaphy in therapy of spontaneous entropion of lower eyelid. Bull. Soc. belge d'opht., no. 68, pp. 68–71, '34

HAMILTON, C. M.: Cancer of lip. J. Tennessee M. A. *15:*190–192, Aug '22

HAMILTON, C. M. (see KING, H.) May '31

HAMILTON, G. J. (see LYNCH, J. M.) 1942

HAMILTON, J. E.: Modern burn treatment with special reference to new dressing, "foille." Indust. Med. *10:*427–432, Oct '41

HAMILTON, J. E.: Local treatment of burns. Kentucky M. J. *40:*207–211, June '42

HAMILTON, J. E.: Comparative study of local burn treatments. Am. J. Surg. *58:*350–364, Dec '42

HAMILTON, J. E. AND BARNETT, L. A.: Therapy of war burns. S. Clin. North America *23:*1575–1588, Dec '43

HAMILTON, J. I.; HOAR, W. S. AND HAIST, R. E.: Comparison of efficacy of different infusion media in shock. Canad. J. Research, Sect. E, *24:*31–35, Feb '46

HAMILTON, R. G.: Operation for chronic dacryocystitis (plastic dacryocystorhinostomy). Pennsylvania M. J. *49:*1327–1330, Sept '46

HAMILTON, T. G.: Conservatism in treatment of hand injuries. Canad. M.A.J. *14:*686–692, Aug '24

HAMILTON, W. F. (see VOLPITTO, P. P. *et al*) Jan '40

HAMLIN, E. JR. (see MARBLE, H. C. *et al*) Feb '42

HAMLIN, H. (see WHITE, J.C.) Sept '45

HAMM, F. C.: Exstrophy of bladder; treatment by uretero-intestinal anastomosis. Brooklyn Hosp. J. *2:*14–24, Jan '40

HAMM, W. G.: Split skin graft. J.M.A. Georgia *26:*495–500, Oct '37

HAMM, W. G.: Jaw fractures. South. Surgeon *10:*185–193, March '41

HAMM, W. G. AND KITE, J. H.: Relief of contractures of knee following extensive burns. South. Surgeon *10:*795–801, Nov '41

HAMM, W. G. (see BLAIR, V. P. *et al*) April '32

HAMM, W. G. (see BLAIR, V. P. *et al*) June '32

HAMM, W. G. (see BLAIR, V. P. *et al*) Dec '32

HAMM, W. G. (see BLAIR, V. P. *et al*) 1932

HAMM, W. G. (see BLAIR, V. P. *et al*) Jan '33

HAMM, W. G. (see BLAIR, V. P. *et al*) Feb '33

HAMM, W. G. (see BLAIR, V. P. *et al*) Nov '33

HAMM, W. G. (see BROWN, J. B.) April '32

HAMM, W. G. (see BROWN, J. B. *et al*) April '33

HAMMATT, H. (see PUESTOW, C. B. *et al*) March '38

HAMMEL, H.: Diagnosis and therapy of fresh fractures of zygoma. Chirurg *8:*964–966, Dec 15, '36

HAMMER, E.: Cancer of sigmoid flexure 10 years after ureteral implantation, for exstrophy of bladder. J. d'urol. *28:*260–263, Sept '29

HAMMER, H.: Malignant tumors of jaw and their differential diagnosis. Med. Welt *12:*261–264, Feb 19, '38

HAMMER, H.: Therapy of maxillary gunshot wounds, with special reference to war wounds. Therap. d. Gegenw. *82:*100-106, March '41

HAMMER, H.: Therapy of gunshot wounds to jaws. Therap. d. Gegenw. *82:*174-177, April '41

HAMMESFAHR, C.: Technic of free fat flap transplantation. Zentralbl. f. Chir. *48:*117, Jan 29, '21

HAMON, J.: Fractures of upper jaw; reduction apparatus with pneumatic cushion. Rev. de stomatol. *38:*518-521, July '36

HAMRICK, D. W.: New combined submucous dissector and suction cannula. Arch. Otolaryng. *9:*655-656, June '29

HAMRICK, W. H.: Suture in crushing injuries of finger nails. U. S. Nav. M. Bull. *46:*225-228, Feb '46

HANCE, G.; BROWN, J. B.; BYARS, L. T. AND McDOWELL, F.: Color matching of skin grafts and flaps with permanent pigment injection. Surg., Gynec. and Obst. *79:*624-628, Dec '44

HANCHETT, M.: Proper drainage in hand infections. J. Iowa M. Soc. *25:*259-262, May '35

HANCOCK, J. D.: Dupuytren's contracture. Kentucky M. J. *38:*290-293, July '40

HAND, E. A.: Electrolysis; introduction of instrument for relatively painless treatment in hair removal. Arch. Dermat. and Syph. *45:*1094-1100, June '42

HAND, E. A. (see WILE, U. J.) Jan '37

HANDFIELD-JONES, R. M.: Hand infections. Lancet *1:*966-967, May 10, '24

HANDFIELD-JONES, R. M.: Infections of fingers and hand. Lancet *2:*833-836, Oct 10, '36

HANDFIELD-JONES, R. M.: Infection of tendons and tendon sheaths. M. Press *211:*53-57, Jan 26, '44

HANDFIELD-JONES, R. M.: *Surgery of the Hand.* E. and S. Livingstone Ltd., Edinburgh, 1946

Hands, Amputations

Severe laceration of hand with traumatic amputation of two fingers. LOEB, M. J. J.A.M.A. *86:*1345-1347, May 1, '26

Injuries of hand caused by bread making machine; new case with complication of gangrene demanding amputation of arm. FERRARI, R. C. Bol. Inst. de clin. quir. *5:*263, '29 also: Semana med. *2:*1734-1735, Dec 12, '29

Value of amputation after trauma of fingers and hand. CARCASSONNE, F. AND LÉNA, A. Marseille-med. *2:*643-651, Nov 25, '34

Technic of conservative amputation after hand injuries. DUPUY DE FRENELLE. Tech. chir. *27:*109-122, May-July '35

Technic of application of Filatov flaps in plastic operations on amputation-stumps of

Hands, Amputations – Cont.

hands and fingers. YUSEVICH, M. S. Ortop. i travmatol. (no. 3) *14:*50-56, '40

Principles of amputations of fingers and hand. SLOCUM, D. B. AND PRATT, D. R., J. Bone and Joint Surg. *26:*535-546, July '44

Learning to write again after mutilation or amputation of right hand. CALLEWAERT, H. Arch. serv. san. Parmée belge *99:*71-77, Mar-Apr '46

Hands, Anatomy of

Anatomic observations in hand surgery. KIAER, S. Ugesk. f. laeger *92:*755-764, Aug 7, '30

Anatomy of hand and surgery of phlegmons of palm; new data on cellular spaces. CORDIER, P. AND COULOUMA, P. Echo med. du nord *1:*513, April 8; 545, April 15, '34

Anatomy of hand and surgery of phlegmons of palm; new data on cellular spaces. CORDIER, P. AND COULOUMA, P. Echo med. du nord *1:*661-674, May 6, '34

New data on cellular space of palm; roentgen study; importance in infections. CORDIER, P. AND COULOUMA, P. Rev. de chir., Paris *53:*563-588, Oct '34

Cavities of hand from surgical point of view. VON STAPELMOHR, S. Nord. med. tidskr. *10:*1341-1344, Aug 31, '35

Collateral circulation in hand after cutting radial and ulnar arteries at wrist. LAWRENCE, H. W. Indust. Med. *6:*410-411, July '37

Fascial spaces of palm; surgical anatomy. SPALDING, J. E. Guy's Hosp. Rep. *88:*432-439, Oct '38

Midpalmar compartment, associated spaces and limiting layers. ANSON, B. J. AND ASHLEY, F. L. Anat. Rec. *78:*389-407, Nov 25, '40

Fasciae and fascial spaces of palm. GRODINSKY, M. AND HOLYOKE, E. A. Anat. Rec. *79:*435-451, April 25, '41

Role of second thoracic spinal segment in preganglionic sympathetic innervation of human hand; surgical implications. ATLAS, L. N. Ann. Surg. *114:*456-461, Sept '41

The Principles of Anatomy as Seen in the Hand, by FREDERIC W. JONES. Baillière, Tindall and Cox, London, 1942

Structure of carpal bones in connection with problem of reconstructive operations. RUBINSHTEYN, A. Y. Khirurgiya, no. 6, pp. 68-72, '44

Surgical anatomy of flexor tendons of wrist. KAPLAN, E. B., J. Bone and Joint Surg. *27:*368-372, July '45

Hands, Burns (See also Burns, War; War Injuries, Hand)

Unusual deformity sequential to a burn of hand. PACK, G. T. AND PARSONS, J. L. Am. J. Surg. *38:*159, June '24

Crush-burns of hand. MACLURE, F., J. Coll. Surgeons, Australasia *1:*233–235, Nov '28

Burns on both forearms and back of hand; treatment by graft from thigh. MIRIZZI, P. L. Bull. et mem. Soc. nat. de chir. *55:*780–785, June 8, '29

Hypertension of hand and fingers from burn; correction by single pedicled skin and fascial flap from anterior abdominal wall. JACKSON, C. AND BABCOCK, W. W., S. Clin. North America *10:*1285–1286, Dec '30

Reconstruction of burned hand (grafts). VON WEDEL, C., J. Oklahoma M. A. *24:*164–165, May '31

Extensive burns on both forearms and back of hand; remote results of resection of retractile scar and pedicled graft from thigh. MIRIZZI, P. L. Bull. et mem. Soc. nat. de chir. *59:*694–695, May 6, '33

Palmar contracture of hand as sequel of burn received in infancy; therapy with Gillies tubular graft at age 17 years. LLUESMA URANGA, E. Cron. med., Valencia *38:*11–14, Jan 15, '34

Autoplasty using digital flap in therapy of stubborn ulcers resulting from burns received in childhood. CHAUVENET, A. Bordeaux chir. *6:*18–25, Jan '35

Therapy of cicatricial contracture of hand and fingers after burns. BAKUSHINSKIY, R. N. Ortop. i travmatol. (no. 2) *12:*76–83, '38

Burn contractures of hand. BLACKFIELD, H. M. Surg., Gynec. and Obst. *68:*1066–1073, June '39

Management of old contractures of hand resulting from third degree burns. JONES, R. JR. Surgery *7:*264–275, Feb '40 also: North Carolina M. J. *1:*148–152, March '40

Treatment of superficial injuries and burns of hand. Allen, H. S., J.A.M.A. *116:*1370–1373, March 29, '41

Burns of hand. MACCOLLUM, D. W. J.A.M.A. *116:*2371–2377, May 24, '41

Hand and finger contracture due to burns. HOHMANN, G. Chirurg *14:*289, May 15, '42

Preservation of function in burnt hand (including description of steering wheel apparatus). AINSWORTH-DAVIS, J. C. Brit. M. J. *1:*724, June 13, '42

Restoration of function in burnt hand. BODENHAM, D. C. Lancet *1:*298–300, March 6, '43

Burn therapy (hands). BARNES, J. M. Brit. M. J. *1:*408–410, April 3, '43

Symposium on management of Cocoanut Grove burns at Massachusetts General Hospital; note on physical therapy (hands). WATKINS, A. L. Ann. Surg. *117:*911–914, June '43

Treatment of hand burns with close fitting plaster of paris casts. LEVENSON, S. M. AND LUND, C. C., J.A.M.A. *123:*272–277, Oct 2, '43

Viacutan (silver dianphthylmethane disulfonate) in burn therapy (hand). PICK, F. AND BARTON, D. Lancet *2:*408–410, Oct 2, '43

Symposium on war surgerv: rehabilitation of burned hand. MEHERIN, J. M. AND GREELEY, P. W., S. Clin. North America *23:*1651–1665, Dec '43

Plastic repair of extensor hand contractures following healed deep second degree burns. GREELEY, P. W. Surgery *15:*173–188, Jan '44

The burned hand. MCINDOE, A. H., M. Press *211:*57–61, Jan 26, '44

Repair of burned hand. PIERCE, G. W.; *et al.* Surgery *15:*153–172, Jan '44

Burns of hands. JAYES, P. H. Brit. J. Indust. Med. *1:*106–109, April '44

Finger exerciser for burned hands. OLDFIELD, M. C. AND KING, C. J. Lancet *2:*109, July 22, '44

Plastic repair of burned hand. GREELEY, P. W. Am. Acad. Orthop. Surgeons, Lect., pp. 169–173, '44

Adaption of structure of hand to disturbed function following deep burns (clawhand). HUDACK, S. S. Am. Acad. Orthop. Surgeons, Lect., pp. 208–211, '44

Plastic considerations of burn scars and contractures of hand and forearm. MACOMBER, W. B. Am. Acad. Orthop. Surgeons, Lect., pp. 174–179, '44

Reconstruction of hand; early surfacing of burns. WOOLHOUSE, F. M. Am. Acad. Orthop. Surgeons, Lect., pp. 187–190, '44

Dermoplasty of healed burned dorsum of hand. PICK, J. F., J. Internat. Coll. Surgeons *8:*217–223, May–June '45

Resurfacing of dorsum of hand following burns. FARMER, A. W. AND WOOLHOUSE, F. M. Ann. Surg. *122:*39–47, July '45

Principles in early reconstructive surgery of severe thermal burns of hand. SMITH, B.; *et al.* Brit. J. Surg. *33:*155–159, Oct '45

Skin grafting burned dorsum of hand. WEBSTER, G. V. AND ROWLAND, W. D. Ann. Surg. *124:*449–462, Aug '46

Hands, Cancer (See also Radiation Injuries)

Epithelioma of hand, with tendency to spontaneous cure. CORLETTE, C. E. AND INGLIS, K. M. J. Australia *1:*250, March 26, '21

Surgical treatment of epithelioma of hand. MANNA, A. Policlinico (sez. prat.) *29:*753-755, June 5, '22 (illus.) abstr: J.A.M.A. *79:*776, Aug 26, '22

Epithelioma of back of hand. MONTGOMERY, D. W. AND CULVER, G. D. New York M. J. *118:*674-676, Dec 5, '23 (illus.)

Repair of defects caused by surgery and radium in cancer of hand, mouth and cheek. BLAIR, V. P. Am. J. Roentgenol. *17:*99-100, Jan '27

Cancer of hand in radiologist, cured by diathermo-coagulation; case. BORDIER, H. Cancer, Bruxelles *4:*328-330, '27

Cancer of back of hand. TOURNEUX, J. P. Progres med., pp. 149-158, Jan 24, '31

Epitheliomas of hand; types and treatment. ADAIR, F. E. S. Clin. North America *13:*423-430, April '33

Hands, Congenital Deformities (See also Club-hand; Syndactylism)

Congenital deformity of hands and feet. GAZZOTTI, L. G. Chir. d. org. di movimento *6:*265-280, July '22 (illus.) abstr: J.A.M.A. *79:*1084, Sept 23, '22

"Flat hand" (manus planus): Its correction essential to normal function of hand. GOLDTHWAIT, J. E., J. Bone and Joint Surg. *4:*469-480, July '22 (illus.)

Congenital ankylosis of joints of hands and feet. MILLER, E. M., J. Bone and Joint Surg. *4:*560-569, July '22 (illus.)

Correction of deformed hand in congenital syphilis. ERLACHER, P. Arch. f. klin. Chir. *125:*776-789, '23

Congenital deformities of forearm, hand, and leg. HARRIS, H. E. JR. Brit. M. J. *1:*711, April 19, '24

Two cases of congenital deformities of hands and feet. SMITH, N. F. Lancet *1:*802, April 19, '24

Congenital malformation of hands. BEADNELL, C. M. Lancet *2:*800, Oct 18, '24

Monograph on the Various Types of Deformities of the Hand and Arm, by CARL BECK. J. B. Lippincott Co., Phila., 1925

Maldevelopment of wrist and hand. ROGERS, L. Edinburgh M. J. *32:*407-409, Aug '25

Case of multiple anomaly of phalanges of hands in girl aged 15. SHOR, L. R. J. Anat. *60:*420-425, July '26

Hands, Congenital Deformities – Cont.

Plastic reconstruction of fingers with particular regard to formation of cleft hand. ZOLLINGER, A. Deutsche Ztschr. f. Chir. *196:*271-287, '26

Inborn crook-hands; case. MESTSCHANINOV, A. Vrach. dielo *10:*1000, July 15, '27

Talipomanus; three cases in one family. MARTMER, E. E. Am. J. Dis. Child. *34:*384-387, Sept '27

Unilateral symbrachydactylia with defect of thoracic wall and amastia; case. STÖHR, F. J. Ztschr. f. Morphol. u. Anthrop. *26:*384-390, '27

Absence of hand; 3 cases. CHIARIELLO, A. Rev. d'orthop. *15:*242-251, May '28

Symmetrical malformation (cleft) of hands and feet. SEROICZKOWSKI, A. Ztschr. f. d. ges. Anat. (Abt. 1) *89:*145-155, March 25, '29

Cleft hand; case. BOORSTEIN, S. W., J. Bone and Joint Surg. *12:*172-176, Jan '30

Bilateral congenital manus vara without defects of bones of forearm; 3 cases. BERNTSEN, A. Acta chir. Scandinav. *67:*61-67, '30

Unusual types of congenital abnormalities of hand. SALAZAR DE SOUSA, C. Arq. de anat. *13:*119-128, '29-'30

Inheritable defect of human hand. GILLETTE, C. P., J. HERED. *22:*189-190, June '31

Operative treatment in Madelung deformity of hand; case. TANCREDI, G. Bull. e atti. d. r. Accad. med. di Roma *57:*153-158, June '31

Hand deformities. MASSIE, G. Guy's Hosp. Gaz. *45:*296-298, July 25, '31

Congenital absence of radius and club hand; case. GRANT, D. N. W. Mil. Surgeon *69:*518-521, Nov '31

Congenital deformities of hands. BRUNET, P. Arch. d'anat., d'histol. et d'embryol. *13:*1-31, '31

Congenital malformations of hand. KANAVEL, A. B. Tr. Sect. Surg., Gen. and Abd., A.M.A., pp. 17-121, '31

Rare congenital osseous abnormalities of hands and feet in same patient; case. TESCOLA, C. Riv. di radiol. e fis. med. *5:*570-576, '31

Bilateral absence of radius and thumb. D'ABREU, A. R. Indian M. Gaz. *67:*266-267, May '32

Partial biphallism (double penis) associated with exstrophy of bladder and multiple abnormalities of hands and feet; case. BAUZÁ, J. A. Arch. de pediat. d. Uruguay *3:*353-355, Aug '32

Congenital malformations of hands. KANA-

Hands, Congenital Deformities – Cont.

VEL, A. B. Arch. Surg. *25:*1, July; 282, Aug '32

Cleft hand; 2 cases. MIKI, Y. Okayama-Igakkai-Zasshi *44:*2295–2296, Aug '32

Rare type of congenital deformity of right hand; case. TATAFIORE, E. Pediatria *40:*829–834, Aug 1, '32

Congenital hypertrophy of right hand; case. MCMURTRIE, K. F., J. Trop. Med. *35:*343–344, Nov 15, '32

Hereditary deformities of hand and foot in members of one family; polydactylia and syndactylia. KEMP, T. AND RAVN, J. Acta psychiat. et neurol. *7:*275–296, '32

Abnormalities of hands and feet. KOENNER, D. M., J. Hered. *25:*329–334, Aug '34

Congenital malformations of hands and feet; roentgen study of 12 cases. ZUPPA, A. Pediatria *42:*943–966, Aug '34

Congenital gigantism of hand. COATE, J. D. Radiog. and Clin. Photog. *11:*16–17, April '35

Familial occurrence of deformities of hands and feet in 5 generations. STRÖER, W. F. H. Genetica *17:*299–312, '35

Bilateral congenital dysmorphosis of wrists (Madelung's disease); roentgen study of case. ROUDIL, G.; *et al.* J. de radiol. et d'electrol. *20:*241–245, April '36

Multiple congenital malformations including hand with 5 fingers and no thumb. PICHON, E. AND WIRZ, S. Bull. Soc. de pediat. de Paris *34:*310–311, June '36

Syndrome of "forked hands and feet" and oligophrenia; 2 cases. MUYLE, G. AND BATSELAERE, R., J. belge de neurol. et de psychiat. *36:*441–455, July '36

Absence of hands and feet in Brazilian family; question of heredity of congenital abnormalities. KOEHLER, O. Ztschr. f. menschl. Vererb.-u. Konstitutionslehre *19:*670–690, '36

Craniofacial dysostosis and congenital malformation of hands; case. KOSTEČKA, F. Ztschr. f. Stomatol. *35:*113–120, Jan 9, '37

Split-hand deformity. POPENOE, P., J. Hered. *28:*174–176, May '37

Rare hand malformation. STACEY, R. S. J. Anat. *72:*456–457, April '38

Ulnar-volar bayonet hand as typical deformity in chondrodysplasia. STEHR, L. Fortschr. a. d. Geb. d. Rontgenstrahlen *57:*587–604, June '38

Congenital deformities of hands and feet (case). CALLUM, E. N. Brit. M. J. *2:*991, Nov 12, '38

Congenital absence of radius with bilateral

Hand, Congenital Deformities – Cont.

manus vara. KAGANOVICH-DVORKIN, A. L. Ortop. i travmatol. (no. 1) *12:*85, '38

Study of family with cleft hands and feet. LIEBENAM, L. Ztschr. f. menschl. Vererb.-u. Konstitutionslehre *22:*136–151, '38

Absence of ulnar derivations of hand; case. BORRI, N. Sett. med. *27:*450–455, April 13, '39

Correction of congenital hand deformations. MEYERDING, H. W. AND DICKSON, D. D. Am. J. Surg. *44:*218–231, April '39

Congenital malformations of hand; attempted classification and report of cases. LONGHI, L. Arch. di ortop. *55:*183–212, June 30, '39

Typical combination of congenital abnormalities of hand and foot. BRAUN, K. Ztschr. f. menschl. Vererb.-u. Konstitutionslehre *23:*510–515, '39

Rare malformation of arm; double humerus with 3 hands and 16 fingers. STEIN, H. C. AND BETTMANN, E. H. Am. J. Surg. *50:*336–343, Nov '40

Multiple deformities of hand. SCHOLTZ, A. Ztschr. f. Orthop. *72:*231–237, '41

Congenital malformations of hands and feet. DE SOUSA DIAS, A. GONCALO. Amatus *3:*325–329, May '44

Hands, Cysts of

Dermoid cysts of palm. JAUREGUI, P. Bol. y trab. de la Soc. de cir. de Buenos Aires *13:*233–239, June 12, '29

Post-traumatic epidermoid cysts of hands and fingers. KING, E. S. J. Brit. J. Surg. *21:*29–43, July '33

Hands, Deformities, Acquired

Deformities of hand acquired after accidents. GOTTLIEB, A. California State J. Med. *19:*72, Feb '21

Correction of deformity of hand. NUZZI, O. Riforma med. *37:*248, March 12, '21 abstr: J.A.M.A. *76:*1435, May 21, '21

Restoration of function in acquired hand deformities. GOTTLIEB, A. AND NEWMAN, L. I. California State J. Med. *19:*365, Sept '21

Fibrous ankylosis of hand due to prolonged swelling. GILL, A. B., J.A.M.A. *83:*1137–1139, Oct 11, '24

Treatment of traumatic deformity of hand. ROUVILLOIS, H. Bull. Acad. de med., Par. *92:*1094–1097, Nov 4, '24 abstr: J.A.M.A. *83:*2050, Dec 20, '24

Operative treatment of dislocation of thumb, "monkey hand." KORTZEBORN, A. Arch. f. klin. Chir. *133:*465–478, '24

Hands, Deformities, Acquired–Cont.

Complete disability of hand by relaxed articulation of first metacarpus and trapezium, and slipping of tendon and extensor brevis pollicis; postoperative result. GODDU, L. A. O. Boston M. and S. J. *192:*666-667, April 2, '25

Pill roller hand deformities due to imbalance of intrinsic muscles; relief by ulnar resection. STEINDLER, A., J. Bone and Joint Surg. *10:*550-553, July '28

Treatment of some cicatricial deformities of hand. GIANTURCO, G. Chir. d. org. di movimento *13:*158-167, Dec '28

"Carpenter's hand." BILLICH, H. U. Mitt. a. d. Grenzgeb. d. Med. u. Chir. *40:*638-647, '28

Hand deformities. VON WEDEL, C., J. Oklahoma M. A. *22:*38-42, Feb '29

Surgical treatment of arthritis. O'FERRALL, J. T. New Orleans M. and S. J. *81:*899-902, June '29

Two cases of hand deformity. MOREAU, L. Ann. d'anat. path. *6:*1132-1133, Nov '29

Surgical treatment of acquired club-hand. RESCHKE, K. Deutsche Ztschr. f. Chir. *232:*458-462, '31

Reconstructive surgery in chronic arthritis. WILSON, P. D. AND OSGOOD, R. B. New England J. Med. *209:*117-125, July 20, '33

Crippled hand. VON WEDEL, C., J. Oklahoma M. A. *26:*320-323, Sept '33

Phalangization of metacarpals for functional restoration of hand of workman deprived of all fingers. VENEZIAN, E. Rassegna d. previd. sociale *20:*38-46, Nov '33

Cicatricial adhesive contracture of thumb with surface of hand; surgical therapy. SITTERLI, A. Ztschr. f. orthop. Chir. *59:*142-144, '33

Restoration of function of hand after loss of 4 fingers. VAKULENKO, M. V. Sovet. khir., no. 8, p. 135, '35

Opera-glass hand in chronic arthritis; "la main en lorgnette" of Marie and Leri. NELSON, L. S., J. Bone and Joint Surg. *20:*1045-1049, Oct '38

Skin grafts in surgical correction of defective cicatrix of hand causing contracture; 2 cases. BARBERIS, J. C. Bol. Soc. de cir. de Rosario *5:*469-477, Nov '38

Absence of hand, two cases. ROCHER, H. L. J. de med. de Bordeaux *116:*115-117, July 22-29, '39

Rigid hand caused by fibrous cicatrix; free graft of full-thickness skin. ZENO, L. An. de cir. *7:*52-56, March-June '41 also: Bol. Soc. de cir. de Rosario *8:*53-58, April '41

Hands, Deformities, Acquired–Cont.

Scar disabilities in hand. RANK, B. K. Australian and New Zealand J. Surg. *12:*191-206, Jan '43

Plastic surgery; advantages and inconveniences of tubular transplants in grave cicatrices of hand. PEDEMONTE, P. V. Bol. Soc. cir. d. Uruguay *14:*114-122, '43 also: Arch. urug. de med., cir. y especialid. *23:*453-461, Nov '43

Spontaneous cicatrization of section of tendon of extensor pollicis longus (biologic therapy); cases. TAULLARD, J. C. Bol. y trab., Soc. argent. de cirujanos *4:*772-776, '43 also: Rev. Asoc. med. argent. *57:*1018-1019, Nov 30, '43

Bilateral symmetric contractures of hand and phalanges; case. SPISIC, B. Ztschr. f. Orthop. *75:*33, '44

Repair of deformities of hands. GORDON, S. D. Bull. Vancouver M. A. *21:*279-281, Aug '45

Hands, Dislocations

Multiple carpo-metacarpal dislocations, with report of case. METZ, W. R. New Orleans M. and S. J. *79:*327-330, Nov '26

Irreducible, metacarpophalangeal dislocation of index finger; presence of abnormal sesamoid; case. ETIENNE, E. AND DUPONNOIS. Arch. Soc. d. sc. med. et biol. de Montpellier *9:*106, March '28

Carpometacarpal dislocation; case. AGRIFOGLIO, M. Arch. di ortop. *46:*615-628, June 30, '30

Dislocation of hand. WOLF, J. Vereinsbl. d. pfalz. Aerzte *44:*1-5, Jan 1, '32

Cause of irreducibility of metacarpophalangeal joint of index finger in palmar luxation; 6 cases. SCHEGGI, S. Chir. d. org. di movimento *(20):*142-148, July '35

Technic for surgical reduction of palmar metacarpophalangeal luxation of thumb and index finger. SCHEGGI, S. Chir. d. org. di movimento *22:*281-284, Aug '36

Neuritis of median nerve due to compression by luxated semilunar bone; case in workman. BRUNI, A. Rassegna d. previd. sociale *24:*42-43, Nov-Dec '37

Volar dislocation of semilunar bone as distinguished from perilunar dorsal dislocation of hand; case. PERSCHL, A. Arch. f. orthop. u. Unfall-Chir. *38:*657-661, '38

Fractures and dislocations of wrist and hand. FARQUHARSON, E. L. Practitioner *144:*598-608, June '40

Treatment of fractures and dislocations of hand and fingers; technic of unpadded casts for carpal, metacarpal and phalan-

Hands, Dislocations – Cont.

geal fractures. KAPLAN, L., S. Clin. North America *20:*1695–1720, Dec '40

Exposed interphalangeal luxations of hand; cases. MALLO HUERGO, E. AND QUIRNO LAVALLE, R. Prensa med. argent. *29:*1367–1370, Aug 26, '42

Metacarpophalangeal luxation of index finger. NUNZIATA, A. Prensa med. argent. *31:*1760-1762, Sept 6, '44

Hands, Dressings for (See also War Injuries, Hand)

Rational way of bandaging palmar arches. SHARGORODSKAY, I. I. Vestnik khir. (nos. 37–38) *13:*150–157, '28

Bandaging of hand wounds. KIAER, S. Ugesk. f. laeger *92:*347–351, April 10, '30

Successful therapy of severe contractures of fingers and hand by cotton redressments. ŠPIŠIĆ, B. Ztschr. f. orthop. Chir. *57:*195–202, '32

First bandage in hand injuries. VOSKRESENSKIY, N. V. Sovet. khir. (no. 1) *7:*171–172, '34

Therapeutic value of cod liver oil combined with vaseline for hand infections and injuries. KŇAZOVICKÝ, J. Rozhl. v. chir. a gynaek. (cast chir.) *14:*93–102, '35

Cod liver oil and cod liver oil bandage in therapy of hand injuries. LÖHR, W. Ztschr. f. arztl. Fortbild. *33:*421–427, Aug 1, '36

Cod liver oil and plaster of paris cast therapy of injuries of fingers and hand. HERLYN, K. E. Beitr. z. klin. Chir. *165:*278–282, '37

Bag bandage for hand burns. STRECKFUSS, H. Chirurg *13:*96, Feb 1, '41

Hands, Fractures

Treatment of fractures of metacarpals and phalanges of fingers. WHEELER, R. H. J.A.M.A. *78:*422–423, Feb 11, '22 (illus.)

Pathology, prognosis and treatment of fractures of phalanges and metacarpal bones. SCHUM, H. Deutsche Ztschr. f. Chir. *188:*234–272, '24

Fractures of bones of hand and fingers. SCHUM, H. Deutsche Ztschr. f. Chir. *193:*132–139, '25

Treatment of fractures of fingers and metacarpals with description of authors' finger caliper. MOCK, H. E. AND ELLIS, J. D. Surg., Gynec. and Obst. *45:*551–556, Oct '27

Operative treatment of fractures of forearm and hand. LAURIE, R. D., J.M.A.S. Africa *1:*585–587, Nov 26, '27

Non-operative treatment of fractures of forearm and hand. WYNNE, F. E., J.M.A.S. Africa *1:*582–584, Nov 26, '27

Hands, Fractures – Cont.

Ball splint for hand fractures. DAVIS, G. G. Internat. Clin. *1:*182–183, March '28

Clinical aspects and treatment of skeletal injuries of hand in industry. BRUNI, A. Rassegna d. previd. soc. *15:*27-41, Dec '28

Finger and hand fractures. ADAMS, B. S. Minnesota Med. *12:*515–520, Sept '29

Therapy of fractures of fingers and middle hand. MELTZER, H. Chirurg. *4:*58–64, Jan 15, '32

Extension apparatus for therapy of fractures of phalangeal and metacarpal bones. ZAHUMENSZKY, E. Orvosi hetil. *76:*629–630, July 16, '32

Fractures of metacarpals and phalanges. MCNEALY, R. W. AND LICHTENSTEIN, M. E. Surg., Gynec. and Obst. *55:*758–761, Dec '32

Finger and hand fractures treated by skeletal traction. HAGGART, G. E., S. Clin. North America *14:*1203–1210, Oct '34

Fractures of metacarpals and phalanges. MCNEALY, R. W. AND LICHTENSTEIN, M. E. West. J. Surg. *43:*156–161, March '35

Fractures of bones of hand. MURRAY, C. R. New York State J. Med. *36:*1749–1761, Nov 15, '36

Hand fractures. NORTHCUTT, E. W. Kentucky M. J. *35:*8–10, Jan '37

Hand fractures; incidence over 5 year period. SHANDS, A. R. JR. AND SCHIEBEL, H. M. Indust. Med. *6:*210–213, April '37

Fractures of bones of hand. OWEN, H. R. Surg., Gynec. and Obst. *66:*500–505, Feb (no. 2A) '38

Simple wire extension for use in therapy of metatarsal and metacarpal fractures and in fractures of fingers and toes. STEBER, F. Munchen. med. Wchnschr. *85:*480–481, March 31, '38

Fractures of phalanges of hand and metacarpals. ROBERTS, N. Proc. Roy. Soc. Med. *31:*793–798, May '38

Principles in treatment of fractures of small bones of hand. SHERIDAN, W. J., J. Tennessee M. A. *31:*263–271, July '38

Caliper for reduction of phalangeal and metacarpal fractures by skeletal traction. CARR, R. W. South. M. J. *32:*543–546, May '39

Simple standard apparatus for treatment of compound fractures of hand, fingers and wrist; report of case. and evaluation of end result. FOSTER, A. K. JR. Arch. Surg. *39:*214–230, Aug '39

Hands, Fractures – Cont.

Traumatic aseptic necrosis of scaphoid bone of right hand. BADE, H. Rontgenpraxis *11:*573–574, Oct '39

The more common hand fractures. TISDALE, A. A. New Orleans M. and S. J. *92:*356–359, Jan '40

Fractures and dislocations of wrist and hand. FARQUHARSON, E. L. Practitioner *144:*598–608, June '40

Treatment of fractures and dislocations of hand and fingers; technic of unpadded casts for carpal, metacarpal and phalangeal fractures. KAPLAN, L., S. Clin. North America *20:*1695–1720, Dec '40

Fractures of hand bones. MCNEALY, R. W. AND LICHTENSTEIN, M. E. Am. J. Surg. *50:*563–570, Dec '40

Hand fractures. HAYES, W. M. South. Surgeon *11:*105–112, Feb '42

Molded plaster splints in treatment of hand fractures. CARRINGTON, G. L. North Carolina M. J. *3:*195–196, April '42

Fractures of metacarpals and proximal phalanges. JAHSS, S. A. Bull. Hosp. Joint Dis. *3:*79–92, July '42

Minor fractures in hand. ELLIS, V. H. Proc. Roy. Soc. Med. *35:*710–711, Sept '42

Fractures of hand. BROWN, R. K. AND DZIOB, J. M. New York State J. Med. *42:*1824–1832, Oct 1, '42

Traction treatment of hand fractures. FRIEND, L. F., U. S. Nav. M. Bull. *40:*988–990, Oct '42

Treatment of fractures of hands and fingers caused by gunshot wounds. GUSYNIN, V. J.A.M.A. *121:*952, March 20, '43

Use of skeletal traction in hand fractures. COBEY, M. C.; *et al.* Army M. Bull. (no. 68) pp. 135–141, July '43

Treatment of fractures of metacarpals and proximal phalanx by skeletal traction. KAPLAN, E. B. Bull. Hosp. Joint Dis. *5:*99–109, Oct '44

Fractures of hand. MORTON, H. S. Canad. M.A.J. *51:*430–434, Nov '44

Displaced fractures of hand. SAYPOL, G. M. AND SLATTERY, L. R. Surg., Gynec. and Obst. *79:*522–525, Nov '44

Hand fractures. CUTTING, C. C. California and West. Med. *62:*21–22, Jan '45 also: Indust. Med. *14:*242, March '45

Hands, Grease Gun Injuries (See also Fingers, Grease Gun Injuries)

Penetration of tissue by fuel oil under high pressure from Diesel engine (hand). REES, C. E., J.A.M.A. *109:*866–867, Sept 11, '37

Hands, Grease Gun Injuries – Cont.

Hand injury due to injection of oil at high pressures. DIAL, D. E., J.A.M.A. *110:*1747, May 21, '38

Grease gun injuries to hand; pathology and treatment of injuries (oleomas) following injection of grease under high pressure. MASON, M. L. AND QUEEN, F. B. Quart. Bull., Northwestern Univ. M. School. *15:*122–132, '41

Hands, Infections

Infections of hand. JACKSON, F. G., J. Indiana M. A. *14:*180, June '21

Etiology and treatment of hand infections. HILL, C. D. New York M. J. *114:*575, Nov 16, '21

Suppurative tenosynovitis of flexor muscles of hand. CLEVELAND, M. Arch. Surg. *7:*661–686, Nov '23 (illus.)

Treatment of acute primary infections of hand. WILKIE, D. P. D. *et al.* Brit. M. J. *2:*1025–1032, Dec 1, '23

Hand infections. HANDFIELD-JONES, R. M. Lancet *1:*966–967, May 10, '24

Hand infections. GARLOCK, J. H. Surg., Gynec. and Obst. *39:*165–191, Aug '24

Surgery of injuries and infections of hand. MARTIN, E. D. New Orleans M. and S. J. *77:*85–89, Aug '24

Some anatomical points relative to infections of hand. THOMPSON, I. M. Canad. M.A.J. *14:*683–686, Aug '24

Splinting and physiotherapy in infections of hand. KANAVEL, A. B., J.A.M.A. *83:*1984–1988, Dec 20, '24

Infections of hand. AIEVOLI, E. Riforma med. *41:*36, Jan 12, '25

Hand infections. ROSS, R. A., M. J. South Africa *20:*84–96, Nov '24

Hand infections. WILSON, G. E. Canad. M.A.J. *15:*715–718, July '25

Hand infections. WOODSON, L. M., J. Tennessee M. A. *18:*112–114, Aug '25

Incision in natural folds of hand; contribution to treatment of cellulitis of sheaths of tendons and calluses. SCHIESSL, M. Munchen. med. Wchnschr. *72:*1728–1730, Oct 9, '25 abstr: J.A.M.A. *85:*1681, Nov 21, '25

Infections of the Hand, by LIONEL R. FIFIELD, H. K. Lewis and Co., London, 1926. Second Edition, 1939

Hand infections; involvement of tendon sheaths and fascial spaces. WEINBERG, J. A. Nebraska M. J. *11:*144–146, April '26

Treatment of hand infections and injuries. OPPEGAARD, M. O. Minnesota Med. *9:*373–375, July '26

Hands, Infections—Cont.
Hand injuries and infections. WALKER, R. H. W. Virginia M. J. *22:*456–460, Sept '26
Infected hand followed by loss of power in extensors of fingers and thumb. CORBET, G. G. Canad. M.A.J. *16:*1502, Dec '26
Infection clinic; infections of hand. KANAVEL, A. B., J. Iowa M. Soc. *17:*4–8, Jan '26
Management of hand infections. LESEUR, H. H. Am. J. Surg. *2:*38–42, Jan '27
Tendon sheath abscess; diagnosis; treatment. CADENAT, F. M. Hopital *15:*106–108, Feb (B) '27
Prevention of contractures following infections of hand, KOCH, S. L., J.A.M.A. *88:*1214–1217, April 16, '27
Importance of cellular spaces of hand and fingers in infections. ISELIN, M. Ann. d'anat. path. *4:*603–613, June '27
Hand infections. KERNS, I. N. Kentucky M. J. *25:*445–449, Aug '27
Hand infections. MANWARING, J. G. R. J. Michigan M. Soc. *26:*554–555, Sept '27
Hand infections. DUNLAP, S. E. Surg. J. *34:*18–20, Sept-Oct '27
Plaies et maladies infectieuses des mains, by MARC ISELIN. Masson et Cie, Paris, 1928. Second Edition, 1932. Third Edition, 1938
Diagnosis and after treatment of severe hand infections. KOCH, S. L., J. Kansas M. Soc. *28:*10–16, Jan '28
Hand infections. MCKIM, L. H. Canad. M.A.J. *18:*17–22, Jan '28
Phlegmon of hand with acute metastatic osteomyelitis of femur, followed by spontaneous fracture at this point; operation; fatal case. AUVRAY. Bull. et mem. Soc. nat. de chir. *54:*592–598, April 28, '28
Case of total phlegmon of left hand flexors; antibrachiopalmar incision; recovery with remarkable functional restitution. BRAINE, J. Bull. et mem. Soc. nat. de chir. *54:*524–529, April 7, '28
Diagnosis and treatment of acute hand infections. KOCH, S. L., J. Indiana M. A. *21:* 137–145, April '28 also: J. Med. *9:*116–124, May '28
Virulent hand infections; treatment by prophylactic chemical and traumatic inflammation. ROEDER, C. A., J.A.M.A. *90:*1371–1373, April 28, '28
Early treatment of hand infections. HOETS, J. M. J. Australia *1:*652–653, May 26, '28
Surgical treatment of phlegmons of palms and fingers. EFTIMIE, C. Spitalul *48:*226–227, June '28
Diagnosis and treatment of some major hand

Hands, Infections—Cont.
infections. KOCH, S. L., J. Iowa M. Soc. *18:*254–261, July '28
Clinical aspects and treatment of hand infections. PAREDAS, J. Med. contemp. *46:*269–274, Aug 19, '28
Hand infections. WILSON, G. E. St. Michael's Hosp. M. Bull. *3:*43–49, Aug '28
Applied anatomy in treatment of hand infections. KNIGHT, H. O. Texas State J. Med. *24:*528–533, Dec '28
Anatomical and clinical study of hand infections. BEST, R. R. Ann. Surg. *89:*359–378, March '29
Actual surgery in digitopalmar infections. POPESCU, S. AND BUZOIANU, G. V. Romania med. *7:*51–52, March 1, '29
d'Herelle's bacteriophage in paronychia and wounds of hand; cases. RAIGA, A. Progres med. *44:*415–429, March 9, '29
Felon, acute lymphangitis and tendon sheath infections of hand; differential diagnosis and treatment. KOCH, S. L., J.A.M.A. *92:*1171–1173, April 6, '29
Hand infections. RAISON, C. A. Am. J. Surg. *6:*530–534, April '29
Treatment of septic hands and feet on shipboard. NEWSOM, R. A. Brit. M. J. *1:*809–810, May 4, '29
Intra-arterial medication of deep diffuse hand phlegmon. BONOLI, U. Policlinico (sez. prat.) *36:*851–853, June 17, '29
Tenosynovitis and fascial space abscesses. SCOTT, R. T. Northwest Med. *28:*317–322, July '29
Intra-arterial medication of deep diffuse phlegmon of hand. (comment on Bonoli's article.) CINQUEMANI, F. Policlinico (sez. prat.) *36:*1395–1396, Sept 30, '29
Treatment of hand infections. GORDON, J. Q. J. Tennessee M. A. *22:*201–204, Oct '29
Treatment of synovial and lymphangitic phlegmonata; practical importance of anatomic data on cellular spaces of hand and fingers. PAITRE, F. Bull. med., Paris *43:*1171–1177, Nov 2, '29
Palm abscess. WASHBURN, B. A. Kentucky M. J. *27:*529–531, Nov '29
Major hand infections; differential diagnosis and treatment. KOCH, S. L., J. Indiana M. A. *22:*510–517, Dec '29
Hand infections, and fingers. BECK, C. Am. J. Surg. *8:*301–304, Feb '30
Streptococcic inflammation of 2 large tendon sheaths of right hand; case. PARIS, M. Liege med. *23:*137–142, Feb 2, '30
Therapy of deep phlegmon of hand by intra-

Hands, Infections – Cont.
arterial injection of colloidal silver (comment on Bonoli's article). SCOLLO, G. Policlinico (sez. prat.) *37:*546-548, April 14, '30
Interesting case of hand infection and injury. MAYER, L. Am. J. Surg. *8:*1087-1088, May '30
Intra-arterial medication with colloidal silver in treatment of deep phlegmon of hand. (Reply to Scollo) BONOLI, U. Policlinico (sez. prat.) *37:*949-950, June 30, '30
Hand infections. CARSCADDEN, W. G. St. Michael's Hosp. M. Bull. *4:*11-26, June '30
Hand infections. PLOUSSARD, C. N. Southwestern Med. *14:*319-322, July '30
Reply to article by Bonoli on hand infections. SCOLLO, G. Policlinico (sez. prat.) *37:*1103, July 28, '30
Suppurative inflammation of milkers' hands. BECKER, E. Chirurg *2:*708-811, Aug 1, '30
Hand infections. OGILVIE, W. H. Guy's Hosp. Gaz. *44:*314-321, Aug 23, '30
Diagnosis and treatment of hand infections. BREA, M. M. Dia med. *3:*357, Nov 24, '30
Human bite infections, with study of route of extension of infection from dorsum of hand. MASON, M. L. AND KOCH, S. L. Surg., Gynec. and Obst. *51:*591-625, Nov '30
Acute infections and suppurations of hand and arm. GRIFFITHS, S. J. H. Practitioner *125:*721-730, Dec '30
Treatment of suppurations of fingers and hands. SOKOLOV, S. Arch. f. klin. Chir. *161:*89-116, '30
Therapy of phlegmons of carpal sheaths by disconnected, lateral incisions. LEIBOVICI, R. AND ISELIN, M., J. de chir. *37:*358-387, March '31
Treatment of acute septic tendovaginitis. PERMAN, E. Hygiea *93:*197-199, March 15, '31
Diagnosis and treatment of hand infections. TORMEY, A. Wisconsin M. J. *30:*176-182, March '31
Improvement of methods of section in treatment of abscesses of tendon sheaths and of palm of hand. KLAPP, R. Zentralbl. f. Chir. *58:*953-954, April 11, '31
Hand infections. OGILVIE, W. H., J. Roy. Army M. Corps *56:*261-274, April '31
Hand infections. CHASE, I. C. Texas State J. Med. *27:*31-34, May '31
Panaris and phlegmon of hand. LORIN, H. Hopital *19:*416-420, June (A) '31
Treatment of hand infections. DE ROUGEMONT, J. Presse med. *39:*1088, July 18, '31
Treatment of phlegmons of hand with bacteriophage, minimizing surgery. PETIT DE LA VILLÉON. Bull. et mem. Soc. d. chirurgiens de Paris *23:*430-434, June 19, '31 also: Cron. med. mex. *30:*435-438, Oct '31
Infection localized in cellular spaces of midpalm. ISELIN, M. AND EVRARD, H. Bull. et mem. Soc. nat. de chir. *57:*1620-1622, Dec 19, '31
Therapy of phlegmons of digitopalmar tendon sheaths. VIALLE, P. Arch. med. -chir. de Province *21:*412-423, Dec '31
Contractures of hand from infections. BUNNELL, S., J. Bone and Joint Surg. *14:*27-46, Jan '32
Diagnosis and treatment of major infections of hand. KOCH, S. L. Minnesota Med. *15:*1-7, Jan '32
Rationalization of treatment of cellulitis of hand. NOBLE, T. B. JR. J. Indiana M. A. *25:*12-16, Jan '32
Distribution and therapy of hand infections. DOERFLER, H. Fortschr. d. Therap. *8:*80, Feb 10; 116, Feb 25, '32
Infection of surgeon's hand by hemolytic streptococci entering through prick from surgical instrument during operation; successful vaccine therapy. HABABOU-SALA. Tunisie med. *26:*78-79, Feb '32
Phlegmons of cellular spaces of hand; 40 cases. ISELIN, M., J. de chir. *39:*331-365, March '32
Case of severe sepsis with hand infection; with some note on general treatment of such conditions. BEATTIE, D. A. St. Barth. Hosp. J. *39:*147-152, May '32
Renal abscess following panaris of sheath of flexor tendon developing from cut of palm; case. MOCK, J. Bull. et mem. Soc. d. chirurgiens de Paris *24:*295-298, May 20, '32
Hand infections and their therapy. VASILE, D. Cluj. med. *13:*317-321, June 1, '32
Surgical treatment of acute hand infections. BONNET. Arch. de med. et pharm. mil. *97:*1-23, July '32
Phlegmon of superficial palmar space; method of therapy; case. FOLLIASSON, A. AND BÉCHET, A. Ann. d'anat. path. *9:*825-826, July '32
Hand infections. FRASER, J. Practitioner *129:*18-32, July '32
Acute nephritis following acute cellulitis of hand and forearm; case. PROWSE, C. B. St. Barth. Hosp. J. *39:*191-193, July '32
Mummifying gangrene following phlegmons on finger and hand. BÜDINGER, K. Wien. klin. Wchnschr. *45:*1093, Sept 2, '32

Hands, Infections—Cont.
Therapy of acute hand infections. SANZ DE FRUTOS, F. Medicina, Madrid *3:*509–548, Oct '32
Vincent's disease following bite of hand. COLBY, F. AND BARR, H. B. Texas State J. Med. *28:*467–470, Nov '32
Phlegmons of 2 carpal sheaths of flexor muscles; excellent function after therapy by disconnected lateral incisions. MALLET-GUY, P. Lyon chir. *29:*736–740, Nov–Dec '32
Development and therapy of phlegmons of hand. PETEL, R. Progres. med., pp. 1873–1881, Nov 5, '32
Common hand infections; etiology and treatment. PRIOLEAU, W. H., J. South Carolina M. A. *28:*276–278, Nov '32
Infections of the Hand, by ALLEN B. KANAVEL. Sixth Edition. Lea and Febiger, Phila., 1933. Seventh Edition, 1939
Severe hand infections. CONNELL, J. E. A. Colorado Med. *30:*17–19, Jan '33
Acute hand infections; surgical therapy. D'HARCOURT, M. Medicina, Madrid *4:*5–42, Jan '33
Therapy of acute hand infections following industrial accidents. PALLARÉS MACHÍ, V. Cron. med., Valencia *37:*31–48, Jan 15, '33
Surgical aspect of therapy in hand infections. MIRIZZI, P. L. Semana med. *1:*1052–1068, March 30, '33
Value of lateral incisions in hand phlegmons. ORY, M. Liege med. *26:*404–411, March 26, '33
Hand infections. ECKHOFF, N. L. Lancet *1:*1276–1281, June 17, '33
Therapy of acute infections of hand and forearm. BRAVO GARCÍA, R. Med. latina *6:*375–394, Aug '33
Subcutaneous abscesses of palm; preliminary report. GARCIA CAPURRO, R. Arch. urug. de med., cir. y especialid. *4:*133–139, Feb '34
Lateral incisions in phlegmons of tendon sheaths of hand. ORY, M. Ann. Soc. med.-chir. de Liege, no. 1, pp. 30–35, '33 abstr: Liege med. *27:*384–387, March 18, '34
Anatomy of hand and surgery of phlegmons of palm; new data on cellular spaces. CORDIER, P. AND COULOUMA, P. Echo med. du nord *1:*513, April 8; 545, April 15, '34
Anatomy of hand and surgery of phlegmons of palm; new data on cellular spaces. CORDIER, P. AND COULOUMA, P. Echo med. du nord *1:*661–674, May 6, '34
Hand infections. ECKHOFF, N. L. Guy's Hosp. Gaz. *48:*246–253, June 9, '34
Subcutaneous abscesses of palm. GARCIA CAPURRO, R. Cron. med. mex. *33:*157–161, June '34
Infections of anterior aspect of hand. FLYNN, R., M. J. Australia *2:*262–268, Aug 25, '34
Probability of existence of diabetes in patients with panaris or phlegmons of hand. DESJACQUES, R. Presse med. *42:*1431–1432, Sept 12, '34
Fascial space and bursal infections of hand. FLACK, F. L., J. Oklahoma M. A. *27:*314–318, Sept '34
Acute rapidly spreading hand infections following trivial injuries. KOCH, S. L. Surg., Gynec. and Obst. *59:*277–308, Sept '34
Black grain mycetoma of hand; case. MAZZINI, O. F. Bol. y trab. de la Soc. de cir. de Buenos Aires *18:*943–946, Sept 19, '34
Gas phlegmon in connection with accidental hand injury. PERNYÉSZ, S. Gyogyaszat *74:*534–536, Sept 16, '34
New data on cellular space of palm; roentgen study; importance in infections. CORDIER, P. AND COULOUMA, P. Rev. de chir., Paris *53:*563–588, Oct '34
Surgical therapy of phlegmons and felons of hand. GONZÁLEZ, S. Arch. de med., cir. y especialid. *37:*1182–1184, Oct 27, '34
Treatment in some minor surgical problems of hand. (infections) HUNTER, J. B. Practitioner *133:*522–528, Oct '34
Problem of septic hand. KENNON, R. Brit. M. J. *2:*1189–1192, Dec 29, '34
Hand infections in surgeons. CHARUGIN, A. I. Novy khir. arkhiv *31:*414–417, '34
Phlegmon of palm as occupational disease of miners. KHEYFETS, A. F. AND SHLEPOV, A. V. Novy khir. arkhiv *31:*408–411, '34
Statistics on injuries and infections of fingers and hands based on accident insurance records. JAROŠ, M. Rozhl. v chir. a gynaek. (cast chir.) *13:*270–288, '34
Classification, prophylaxis and rational treatment of hand infections. MESHCHANINOV, A. I. Novy khir. arkhiv *31:*388–394, '34
Classification of acute inflammatory processes in hand. ZAYTSEV, G. P. Novy khir. arkhiv *31:*394–399, '34
Hand infections in industrial accidents. KANAVEL, A. B. Surg., Gynec. and Obst. *60:*568–570, Feb (no. 2A) '35
Hints on prophylaxis, diagnosis and treatment of deep hand infections. MITCHINER, P. H. St. Thomas's Hosp. Gaz. *35:*10–13, Feb '35
Technic of surgical therapy in diffuse phlegmons of hand and forearm. DIAZ Y GOMEZ, E. Med. ibera *1:*436–442, March 16, '35

Hands, Infections – Cont.
Progress in therapy of suppurative diseases of hand. JEŘÁBEK, V. Casop. lek. cesk. *74:*241-244, March 1, '35
Gonococcal tenosynovitis of hand. MURRAY, D. W. G. AND MORGAN, J. R. E. Canad. M.A.J. *32:*374-375, April '35
Hand infections. CARTER, D. M. Internat. J. Med. and Surg. *48:*187-189, May-June '35
Proper drainage in hand infections. HANCHETT, M., J. Iowa M. Soc. *25:*259-262, May '35
Hand infections. BRANCH, J. L., J. M. A. Alabama *5:*1-3, July '35
Serious hand infections. GAMBEE, L. P. West. J. Surg. *43:*449-455, Aug '35
Hand infections. BUCHANAN, J. S. Tr. Roy. Med.-Chir. Soc. Glasgow, pp. 117-128; 129-130, '34-'35; in Glasgow M. J. Sept, Oct '35
Roentgen diagnosis of hand infections. and injuries. DREUSCHUCH, F. Rozhl. v chir. a gynaek. (cast chir.) *14:*24-34, '35
Therapeutic value of cod liver oil combined with vaseline for hand infections and injuries. KŇAZOVICKÝ, J. Rozhl. v chir. a gynaek. (cast chir.) *14:*93-102, '35
Bacteremia due to Staphylococcus aureus and Streptococcus hemolyticus arising from hand infection. TANZER, R. C. Clin. Misc., Mary I. Bassett Hosp. *2:*69-74, '35
Hand infections and injuries. ROGERS, L. J. Roy. Nav. M. Serv. *22:*2-6, Jan '36
Symptoms and therapy of acute purulent diseases of hands and fingers. ZAYTSEV, G. P. Sovet. vrach. zhur., pp. 422-428, March 30, '36
Treatment of inflammation of hand. AGAFONOV, F. A. Sovet. vrach. zhur., pp. 544-546, April 15, '36
Hand whitlows and infections. LAKE, N. C. Practitioner *136:*376-393, April '36
Soft tissues of hand in infection; microscopic study of pathologic changes produced by deep cellulitis complicated by osteomyelitis. TAYLOR, M. M. Indust. Med. *5:*187-192, April '36
Brucella abortus infection of hand after injury; fatal case. WERTHEMANN, A. Schweiz. med. Wchnschr. *66:*333-335, April 4, '36
Prognosis of hand infections. ECKHOFF, N. Lancet *1:*1369, June 13, '36; 1425, June 20, '36
Diagnosis and treatment of more common infections of hand. POTTER, P. C. S. Clin. North America *16:*763-769, June '36
Necessity for use of splints at certain stages in treatment of hand infections, with demonstration of some of the newer types.

Hands, Infections – Cont.
BROWNE, W. E. New England J. Med. *215:*743-749, Oct 22, '36
Infections of fingers and hand. HANDFIELD-JONES, R. M. Lancet *2:*833-836, Oct 10, '36
Industrial diseases and accidents of hand (also infections). BARBER, R. F. New York State J. Med. *36:*1736-1740, Nov 15, '36
Human bite infections of hand. WELCH, C. E. New England J. Med. *215:*901-908, Nov 12, '36
Deep infections of hand. RUSSELL, E. P. J. Iowa M. Soc. *26:*689, Dec '36
Relation of suppurative processes of hands and fingers to minor trauma. KORABELNIKOV, I. D. Sovet. khir., no. 3, pp. 488-490, '36
Method of restoring function to finger stiffened by venous phlegmon of hand. MACKUTH, E. Arch. f. klin. Chir. *185:*370-372, '36
Osteomyelitis of hands. KOCH, S. L. Surg., Gynec. and Obst. *64:*1-8, Jan '37
Infections of fingers and hands. BELLO, E. Rev. med., peruana *9:*169-178, April '37
Office treatment of hand infections. IASON, A. H. Am. J. Surg. *36:*376-383, April '37
Hand and finger infections. MONSERRATE, D. N., M. Bull. Vet. Admin. *13:*321-326, April '37
Hand infections. OGILVIE, W. H. Guy's Hosp. Gaz. *51:*114, March 13, '37 *51:*177-184, April 24, '37
Hand infections complicating injuries. DAVIS, J. W. Indust. Med. *6:*309-310, May '37
Infections of fingers and palm. KOCH, S. L. Pennsylvania M. J. *40:*597-604, May '37
Pitfalls in management of hand infections. MASON, M. L. Minnesota Med. *20:*485-495, Aug '37
Human bite infections of hand. MAIER, R. L. Ann. Surg. *106:*423-427, Sept '37
Roentgen treatment of infection from human bite of hand. SMITH, R. M. AND MANGES, W. F. Am. J. Roentgenol. *38:*720-725, Nov '37
Therapy of hand phlegmons; cases. CERESETO, P. L. Dia med. *10:*64-68, Jan 24, '38
Atypical osteomyelitis with multiple localizations following metacarpophalangeal suppurative arthritis due to Staphylococcus aureus; case. FRANCAIS, AND BOUROULLEC. Bull. et mem. Soc. d. chirurgiens de Paris *30:*149-156, March 4-18, '38
Hand infections. MOBLEY, H. E., J. Arkansas M. Soc. *34:*269-270, May '38
Surgical principles in treatment of hand infections. KOCH, S. L., J. Indiana M. A.

Hands, Infections—Cont.
*31:*231–232, May '38 also: West. J. Surg. *46:*301–304, June '38
Prognosis of hand infections. Ross, J. P. St. Barth. Hosp. J. *45:*269–270, Aug '38
Infections of hand and fingers. LAKE, N. C. Brit. M. J. *2:*715, Oct 1; 754, Oct 8; 798, Oct 15, '38
Infections of hand; 3 years' experience in clinic for study of whitlow. DEVENISH, E. A. Arch. Surg. *37:*726–734, Nov '38
Hand infection and its treatment. RUTHERFORD, R. Clin. J. *67:*444–452, Nov '38
Surgical principles in care of infections of hand. KOCH, S. L. Ohio State M. J. *34:*1325–1328, Dec '38
Septic hand. WILKIE, D. P. D. Brit. M. J. *2:*1127–1130, Dec 3, '38
Hand infections, with special reference to therapy. GRET, L. G. An. Fac. de cien. med. de La Plata *3:*137–144, '38
Treatment of Hand and Forearm Infections, by A. C. J. BRICKEL. C. V. Mosby Co., St. Louis, 1939
Medial approach to mid-palmar space and ulnar bursa. HENRY, A. K. Lancet *1:*16–18, Jan 7, '39
Surgical principles in treatment of hand infections and injuries. KOCH, S. L., J. Kansas M. Soc. *40:*89–95, March '39
Technic needed for correct treatment of panaris and infections of hand. DE GIRARDIER. J. Hopital *27:*213–215, April '39
Double incisions in therapy of phlegmon of sheath and empyema of joints. KLAPP, R. Zentralbl. f. Chir. *66:*753–758, April 1, '39
Acute synovitis of hand. FAVREAU, J. C. Union med. du Canada *68:*513–514, May '39
Therapy of acute hand infections. ANDREON, E. Arch. urug. de med., cir. y especialid. *14:*567–575, June '39
Hand infections. KINSELLA, V. J., M. J. Australia *1:*856–861, June 10, '39
Osteo-aponeurotic cavities of palm of hand in infections; roentgen study to determine mode of propagation of suppurative processes. BELLONE, A. Arch. di radiol. *15:*491–495, July-Oct '39
Hand infections. MASON, A. New Zealand M. J. *38:*304–315, Oct '39
Hand infections. MAGUIRE, D. L. South. Surgeon *9:*11–20, Jan '40
Hand infections due to human mouth organisms. FRITZELL, K. E. Journal-Lancet *60:*135–137, March '40
Hand infections following human bites. COHN, R. Surgery *7:*546–554, April '40
Nondiffused infections of hand in daily practice. MUNOZ ARENOS, J. M. Semana med. espan. *3:*636–642, May 18, '40
Prognosis and treatment of infections of hand and foot in diabetes. KANAKASABESAN, D. Antiseptic *37:*554–560, June '40
Perisynovial phlegmons in hand; cases. ANDREON, E. Arch. urug. de med., cir. y especialid. *17:*80–83, July '40
Management of acute hand infections. COURTNEY, J. E. Nebraska M. J. *25:*299–301, Aug '40
Anatomy and pathology of hand infections. AVENT, C. H. JR. Memphis M. J. *15:*140–142, Sept '40
Diagnosis of hand infections. DORRIS, J. M. Memphis M. J. *15:*142–143, Sept '40
Treatment of hand infections. KELLY, E. G. Memphis M. J. *15:*143–144, Sept '40
Intra-arterial mercurochrome in hand infections. MASCIOTTRA, E. Rev. med.-quir. de pat. fem. *16:*273–280, Sept '40
Treatment of hand infections. PROBSTEIN, J. G., S. Clin. North America *20:*1457–1472, Oct '40
Principles of management of hand infections. MASON, M. L. Rocky Mountain M. J. *37:*814–824, Nov '40
Hand infections. MOCK, A. E. AND WEBB, C. C., J. Florida M. A. *27:*296–298, Dec '40
Infection of fascial spaces of palm. PEMBERTON, P. A. Am. J. Surg. *50:*512–515, Dec '40
Therapy of purulent tendovaginitis and phlegmon. ELETSKAYA, O. I. Novy khir. arkhiv *46:*3–8, '40
Acute hand infections. LYONNET, J. H. Dia med. *13:*33–39, Jan 20, '41; 53–55, Jan 27, '41
Diffuse phlegmons of hand and forearm. MUNOZ ARENOS, J. M. Semana med. espan. *4:*167–171, Feb 15, '41
Prevention and treatment of hand infections. KOCH, S. L., J.A.M.A., *116:*1365–1367, March 29, '41
Hand infections; intra-arterial mercurochrome. MASCIOTTRA, E. L. Rev. Asoc. med. argent. *55:*271–273, April 15–30, '41
Therapy of hand infections. Prensa med. argent. *28:*1104–1112, May 21, '41
Intra-arterial mercurochrome and sulfanilamide and its derivatives in therapy of phlegmons in hand. IMABLE, J. Rev. Asoc. med. argent. *55:*463–465, June 15–30, '41
Hand infections; dry after-treatment. BAILEY, H. Lancet *2:*189–190, Aug 16, '41
Phlegmons of hand. DESJARDINS, E. Union med. du Canada *70:*1329–1331, Dec '41
Hand infections; biologic conception of pa-

Hands, Infections—Cont.
thology and therapeutics. GRET, L. G. Bol. y. trab., Soc. argent. de cirujanos *2:*811-823, '41
Suppurative tenosynovitis of hand; plan of treatment. GARLOCK, J. H., J. Mt. Sinai Hosp. *8:*540-542, Jan-Feb '42
Pyogenic infections; lymphatic, tendon sheath and fascial space infections of hand. GRODINSKY, M. Nebraska M. J. *27:*13-17, Jan '42
Anatomic investigations of deep fascial space infections in hand. FLYNN, J. E. Am. J. Surg. *55:*467-475, March '42
Management of septic hand. DODD, H. Practitioner *148:*219-225, April '42
Symposium on surgical infections of hand. MASON, M. L., S. Clin. North America *22:*455-477, April '42
Deep paronychias of hand. GOLDHAHN, R. Ztschr. f. arztl. Fortbild. *39:*319-323, July 15, '42
Management of acute hand infections. SILER, V. E. Ohio State M. J. *38:*922-924, Oct '42
Hand infections. GRUBBS, R. H. Virginia M. Monthly *69:*668-672, Dec '42
Surgical infections of hand. RIVAS, C. I. Bol. d. Inst. clin. quir. *18:*917-1382, Dec '42
Significant factors in development of hand infections. MASON, M. L. AND ALLEN, H. S. Quart. Bull., Northwestern Univ. M. School. *16:*42-56, '42
Therapy of infected callus (hand). GARCIA VALCARCEL, A. Med. espan. *9:*75-82, Jan '43
Acute suppurative tenosynovitis of hand. FLYNN, J. E. Surg., Gynec. and Obst. *76:*227-235, Feb '43
Hand infections. ECKHOFF, N. L. Guy's Hosp. Gaz. *57:*67-70, March 20, '43
Prevention and treatment of hand infections. SILER, V. E., J. Indiana M. A. *36:*334-339, July '43
Medical progress; grave infections of hand. FLYNN, J. E. New England J. Med. *230:*45, Jan 13, '44
Treatment of hand infections; necessity for new approach. PATEY, D. H. Practitioner *152:*329-330, May '44
Acute suppurative infection in flexor tendon sheaths of hand, with particular reference to late results after operation with transverse finger incisions according to K. G. Holm. GRETTVE, S. Acta chir. Scandinav. (supp. 91) *90:*1-63, '44
Acute hand infections; surgical concept. RIVAS, C. I. Dia med. *17:*63-66, Jan 22, '45
Bacterial flora of wounds and septic lesions of hand. WILLIAMS, R. E. O. AND MILES, A. A., J. Path. and Bact. *57:*27-36, Jan '45
Sulfathiazole (sulfonamide)-cod liver oil ointment in postoperative care of septic hand. BREZIN, D. Am. J. Surg. *68:*232-233, May '45
Infections of hand and surgery. SNODGRASS, T. J. Wisconsin M. J. *44:*503-507, May '45
Pseudo-gas gangrene of hand (role of magnesium). RUBENSTEIN, A. D.; *et al.* J.A.M.A. *129:*659-662, Nov 3, '45
Therapy of osteomyelitis of hand and fingers at evacuation hospitals. KONONENKO, I. F. Vrach. delo (nos. 7-8) *25:*341-346, '45

Hands, Injuries of (See also Hands, Nerve Ininjuries in; Hands, Reconstructive Surgery of; Hands, Tendon Injuries in; War Injuries, Hand)
Injuries to forearm and hand. GUNN, J. A. Canad. M.A.J. *13:*627-633, Sept '23
Conservatism in treatment of hand injuries. HAMILTON, T. G. Canad. M.A.J. *14:*686-692, Aug '24
Surgery of injuries and infections of hand. MARTIN, E. D. New Orleans M. and S. J. *77:*85-89, Aug '24
Conclusions based on study of 433 hand injuries. HULLSIEK, H. E. Minnesota Med. *7:*670-675, Oct '24
Injuries to small bones of hand and wrist. CRONK, F. Y., J. Oklahoma M. A. *19:*64-66, March '26
Treatment of hand infections and injuries. OPPEGAARD, M. O. Minnesota Med. *9:*373-375, July '26
Conservatism in treatment of hand injuries. DURMAN, D. C., J. Michigan M. Soc. *25:*381-383, Aug '26
Hand injuries and infections. WALKER, R. H. W. Virginia M. J. *22:*456-460, Sept '26
Injuries to hand. RUTHERFORD, A. G., W. Virginia M. J. *23:*83-86, Feb '27
Rare traumatic lesions of wrist and hand. OLLER, A. Arch. de med., cir. y espec. *26:*465-469, April 9, '27
Severe hand injury restored to complete function. SCHNEK, F. Arch. f. Orthop. *26:*308-314, March 22, '28
Medical and surgical treatment of hand injuries. PFAB, B. Monatschr. f. Unfallh. *35:*148-160, May '28
Conservative surgery in hand injury. LAMBOTTE, A. Arch. franco-belges de chir. *31:*759-764, Sept '28
Treatment of hand injuries. ISELIN, M. Medecine *9:*1020-1028, Oct '28

Hands, Injuries of—Cont.
Traumatic lesions of hand. ROMANI, A. Arch. ital. di chir. *22:*1-39, '28
Treatment of hand injuries. BUNNELL, S. California and West. Med. *30:*1-5, Jan '29
Minor injuries resulting in death (including hand). CORBET, G. G. Canad. M. A. J. *20:*40-41, Jan '29
Harmful effects of hot water in open finger and hand injuries. SCHNEK, F. Munchen. med. Wchnschr. *76:*57-58, Jan 11, '29
Hand injuries caused by breadmaking machine; cases of industrial accidents. ARCE, J.; *et al.* Bol. Inst. de clin. quir. *5:*13-46, '29 also: Semana med. *2:*142-160, July 18, '29
Hand injuries. DOUGLAS, R. A., J. Tennessee M. A. *22:*177-178, Sept '29
Accident from compressed air; hand shattered with bony lesions and open fracture of forearm; conservative treatment. COUREAUD. Bull. et mem. Soc. nat. de chir. *55:*1374-1377, Dec 21, '29
Treatment of lacerated wounds of hands. ZACHARINAS, B. Medicina, Kaunas *11:*39-41, Jan '30
Removal of foreign bodies from hand, fingers and feet. GOLDBLATT, D. Am. J. Surg. *8:*324-327, Feb '30
Interesting case of hand infection and injury. MAYER, L. Am. J. Surg. *8:*1087-1088, May '30
Hand injuries. ARMSTRONG, H. G. St. Michael's Hosp. M. Bull. *4:*54-73, June '30
Hand surgery. KANAVEL, A. B. Proc. Internat. Assemb. Inter-State Post-Grad. M. A., North America (1929) *5:*28-34, '30
Immediate treatment of hand injuries. KOCH, S. L. Surg., Gynec. and Obst. *52:*594-601, Feb (No. 2A) '31
Immediate therapy of hand injuries. KOCH, S. L. M. Arts and Indianapolis M. J. *34:*763-771, Dec '31
Advisable therapeutic measures in finger injuries and hand. GOLD, E. Wien. klin. Wchnschr. *45:*308-309, March 4, '32
Technic of surgical therapy of hand injuries. SARROSTE. Arch. de med. et pharm. mil. *97:*24-43, July '32
Injuries to carpal bones. DARNER, L. D. Internat. J. Med. and Surg. *45:*541-546, Dec '32
Hand injuries during boxing. MAYER, F. O. Arch. f. orthop. u. Unfall-Chir. *32:*245-246, '32
Primary plastic surgery in injuries of fingers. hands and forearms. TUOMIKOSKI, V. Duodecim *48:*393-411, '32
Crushing of right hand and wrist; conservation of useful "grip" formed from thumb

Hands, Injuries of—Cont.
and small portion of index finger. DESJACQUES, R. Rev. d'orthop. *20:*315-318, July-Aug '33
Therapy of injuries to fingers and hands. VOGELER, K. Med. Welt *7:*1097-1100, Aug 5, '33
Surgical treatment of injuries of hand and finger, with exception of fractures. SCHMORELL, H. Med. Klin. *29:*1382, Oct 6; 1414, Oct 13, '33
Surgical treatment of injuries of hand and fingers, with exception of bone fractures. SCHMORELL, H. Med. Klin. *29:*1449-1450, Oct 20, '33
Therapy of recent wounds of hands and fingers in miners. BELOT, F. Scalpel *86:*1272-1276, Dec 2, '33
Bilateral fissure of navicular bone of hand from injury; question of aseptic necrosis. (Comment on Reich's article). WETTE, W. Arch. f. orthop. u. Unfall-Chir. *33:*194-199, '33
Injured hand. MILLER, F. M. Internat. J. Med. and Surg. *47:*18, Jan '34
Common injuries to joints of fingers and wrist. BUXTON, ST. J. D. Clin. J. *63:*270-274, July '34
Porcelain faucet handle injuries to hand. MALONEY, H. P., J.A.M.A., *103:*1618-1619, Nov 24, '34
Primary skin graft in fresh injuries of hand and fingers. BASS, Y. M. AND ZHOLONDZ, A. M. Sovet. khir. (nos. 3-4) *6:*350-357, '34
Open treatment of fresh hand injuries. GEYMANOVICH, Z. I. Novy khir. arkhiv. *31:*424-430, '34
Traumatic surgery of hand. COBB, S. A. Maine M. J. *26:*33-36, March '35
Treatment of compound hand injuries. KOCH, S. L. Journal-Lancet *55:*569-572, Sept 1, '35
Wounds of hands and fingers; immediate therapy. DE FOURMESTRAUX, J. AND FREDET, M. Arch. med.-chir. de Province *25:*341-348, Oct '35
Hand injuries. ALBERT, B. Rozhl. v chir. a gynaek. (cast chir.) *14:*3-19, '35
Roentgen diagnosis of hand infections and injuries. DREUSCHUCH, F. Rozhl. v chir. a gynaek. (cast chir.) *14:*24-34, '35
Open method in therapy of finger wounds and hand. FISANOVICH, A. L. Sovet. khir., no. 3, pp. 28-33, '35
Primary suture in finger injuries and hand. SHCHERBINA, I. A. Sovet. khir., no. 3, pp. 22-27, '35
Hand infections and injuries. ROGERS, L. J.

Hands, Injuries of—Cont.
Roy. Nav. M. Serv. *22:*2–6, Jan '36
Injuries to hand. RUTH, V. A., J. Iowa M. Soc. *26:*90–92, Feb '36
Hand surgery. HARMER, T. W. New England J. Med. *214:*613–617, March 26, '36
Hand injuries. KOCH, S. L. Kentucky M. J. *34:*101–109, March '36
Conservative surgery and its limitations in industrial injuries to hands. MORI, A. Rassegna d. previd. sociale *23:*12–30, March '36
Surgical therapy of hand injuries. ZAGAMI, A. Riv. san. siciliana *24:*295–312, March 15, '36
Hand injuries with particular reference to immediate treatment. KOCH, S. L. Nebraska M. J. *21:*281–288, Aug '36
Hand injuries. KOCH, S. L. J.A.M.A. *107:*1044–1049, Sept 26, '36
Prevention of hand and finger injuries in industry. VOLKMANN, J. Monatschr. f. Unfallh. *43:*417–425, Sept '36
Industrial diseases and accidents of hand (also infections). BARBER, R. F. New York State J. Med. *36:*1736–1740, Nov 15, '36
Hand infections complicating injuries. DAVIS, J. W. Indust. Med. *6:*309–310, May '37
Surgical principles involved in treatment of open injuries of hand. MASON, M. L. West. J. Surg. *45:*239–248, May '37
Hand injuries due to shattered porcelain handles of water faucets. STEENROD, E. J.; *et al.* Surg., Gynec. and Obst. *64:*950–955, May '37
Immediate treatment of hand injuries. MASON, M. Indust. Med. *6:*536–538, Oct '37
Surgical emphysema of hand due to use of pneumatic tools (case). PARKER, W. S. J. Roy. Nav. M. Serv. *23:*347–348, Oct '37
Hand injuries and wrist. COLE, W. H. Minnesota Med. *20:*727–730, Nov '37
Localization and removal of metallic bodies in hand. WILLIS, D. A. Surg., Gynec. and Obst. *65:*698–699, Nov '37
Primary treatment of wounds of hand and fingers. MAZUROVA, N. A. AND MASHKARA, K. I. Sovet. vrach. zhur. *41:*1809–1814, Dec 15, '37
Die verletzte Hand, by KARL KRÖMER. Wilhelm Maudrich, Vienna, 1938
Hand injuries. DAVIS, J. W. South. M. J. *31:*251–254, March '38
Conservative treatment vs. immediate amputation in severe crushing injuries of hand and forearm. FINDLAY, R. T., S. Clin. North America *18:*297–303, April '38

Hands, Injuries of—Cont.
Conservative surgery in hand injuries. HOLDER, J. S. Indust. Med. *7:*238–239, May '38
Treatment of hand injuries. SPENCER, J. A. J. Michigan M. Soc. *37:*515–521, June '38
Hand injuries. HARMER, T. W. Am. J. Surg. *42:*638–658, Dec '38
Treatment of compound hand injuries. KOCH, S. L., J. Michigan M. Soc. *38:*27–31, Jan '39
Hand injuries. STOLOFF, I. A. AND SILTEN, A. M. Indust. Med. *8:*16–18, Jan '39
Surgical principles in treatment of hand infections and injuries. KOCH, S. L., J. Kansas M. Soc. *40:*89–95, March '39
Immediate treatment of open hand wounds. MASON, M. L. Mississippi Valley M. J. *61:*136–143, July '39
Hand injuries. ASPINALL, A., M. J. Australia *2:*529–532, Oct 7, '39
Therapy of injuries of hands and fingers. SOUBRANE. J. de med. et chir. prat. *110:*533–542, Oct 10–25, '39
Treatment of hand injuries (with special reference to tendons). TEECE, L., M. J. Australia *2:*532–534, Oct 7, '39
Surface defects of hand. BROWN, J. B. Am. J. Surg. *46:*690–699, Dec '39
Needles in hands and method of extraction. VOSKRESENSKIY, N. V. Khirurgiya, no. 12, pp. 86–91, '39
Problems in minor traumatic surgery of hand. HAYS, S. C., J. South Carolina M. A. *36:*33–37, Feb '40
Injuries to hand in boxing; etiology and prevention. KLAUS, E. J. Munchen. med. Wchnschr. *87:*265–267, March 8, '40
Splitting of thenar eminence with protrusion of muscles due to crushing of hand in industrial accident; therapy of case. SAMMARTINO, E. S. AND PIQUE, J. A. Rev. Asoc. med. argent. *54:*178–180, March 15–30, '40
"Dead hand"; lesion produced by rapid vibration. CUMMINS, R. C. Irish J. M. Sc., pp. 171–175, April '40
Plastic repair of cutaneous injuries to hand. GREELEY, P. W. Indust. Med. *9:*300–303, June '40
Treatment of commoner injuries of hand. NELSON, L. S., J. Kansas M. Soc. *41:*236–239, June '40
Grave wounds of hands; biologic therapy. ALLENDE, C. I. Bol. y trab., Acad. argent. de cir. *24:*714–720, Aug 21, '40
Grave wounds of hands; biologic therapy. ZENO, L. Bol. y trab., Acad. argent. de cir. *24:*639–652, Aug 7, '40

Hands, Injuries of—Cont.

Hand injuries. DAVIS, J. W. Indust. Med. *9:*565-567, Nov '40

Value of immediate treatment of hand injuries. VEREBELY, T. JR. Orvosi hetil. *84:*647-651, Dec 21, '40

Grave hand wounds and their biologic therapy. ZENO, L. Dia med. *12:*1138-1141, Dec 9, '40

Indelible pencil injuries to hands. MASON, M. L. AND ALLEN, H. S. Ann. Surg. *113:*131-139, Jan '41

Plastic surgery and repair of hand, with particular reference to repair of cutaneous defects. MASON, M. L. Indust. Med. *10:*47-52, Feb '41

Treatment of superficial injuries and burns of hand. ALLEN, H. S., J.A.M.A. *116:*1370-1373, March 29, '41

Unusual hand injuries and face. POKA, L. Orvosi hetil. *85:*105-107, March 1, '41

Anatomic diagnosis of hand injuries. WINFIELD, J. M. J.A.M.A. *116:*1367-1370, March 29, '41

Injuries to hands by puncture wounds and foreign bodies. CUTLER, C. W. JR. S. Clin. North America *21:*485-493, April '41

Hand injuries. DAVIS, J. W. South. Med. and Surg. *103:*258-259, May '41

Treatment of hand injuries. KOCH, S. L. New England J. Med. *225:*105-109, July 17, '41

Treatment of hand injuries. TRAVERS, M. P. J. Florida M. A. *28:*66-71, Aug '41

Direction for therapy of hand wounds. SILVEIRA, L. M. Rev. paulista de med. *22:*41-52, Jan '43

Management of traumatic injuries of hand. HUTCHINSON, W. B. Northwest Med. *42:*134-135, May '43

Immediate transfer of pedunculated flap graft to palm; case. SILVIS, R. S., U. S. Nav. M. Bull. *41:*821-824, May '43

Successful repair of severely wounded hand; case. ROA, R. L. Rev. med.-quir. de pat. fem. *22:*456-457, Dec '43

Management of compound injuries of hand. MUELLER, R. F. Minnesota Med. *27:*110-114, Feb '44

Management of hand injuries. MARBLE, H. J. Indust. Hyg. and Toxicol. *26:*189-192, June '44

Grave trauma of hand and forearm; biologic therapy. ZENO, L. Bol. Soc. de cir. de Rosario *11:*221-224, Aug '44 also: Rev. Asoc. med. argent. *58:*938-942, Oct 30, '44

Grave trauma of hand and forearm; biologic therapy of case. ZENO, L. Bol. y trab., Soc. argent. de cirujanos *5:*583-595, '44

Early management of hand wounds. CUTLER, C. W. JR. Bull. U. S. Army M. Dept. (no. 85) pp. 92-98, Feb '45

Injuries of carpal bones. SPEED, K., S. Clin. North America *25:*1-13, Feb '45

Conservative operation for severe injury to hand. POLLOCK, G. A. Brit. J. Surg. *32:*535-536, April '45

Suggestions to improve early treatment of hand injuries. BUNNELL, S. Bull. U. S. Army M. Dept. (no. 88) pp. 78-82, May '45

Wrist bone injuries. SHERRILL, J. D. South. M. J. *38:*306-312, May '45

Late treatment of dorsal injuries associated with loss of skin in hand. CUTHBERT, J. B. Brit. J. Surg. *33:*66-71, July '45

Suggestions to improve early treatment of hand injuries. BUNNELL, S. Arch. Phys. Med. *26:*693-697, Nov '45

Closure of surface defects of hand. MAY, H. Pennsylvania M. J. *49:*116-120, Nov '45

Diagnosis and primary surgical treatment of injuries of hand. BROWNE, W. E. Rhode Island M. J. *28:*875, Dec '45 also: J. Maine M. A. *37:*21, Feb '46

Wounds of fingers (and hand). KAGANOVICH-DVORKIN, A. L. AND RYSKINA, Z. B. Khirurgiya no. 3, pp. 45-48, '45

Wounds and injuries of hands. KOCH, S. L. Quart. Bull., Northwestern Univ. M. School. *19:*265-277, '45

Minor injuries of hand. GRIFFITHS, H. E. Practitioner *156:*254-261, Apr '46

Crushing injury of hand; conservative reparative surgery; case. RUIZ RUBIO, M. Arch. Soc. cirujanos hosp. *16:*398-400, June '46

Discussion on treatment of hand injury. MOORE, F. T. Brit. J. Surg. *34:*70-74, July '46

Medical progress; saving injured hand. CLEVELAND, M. New York Med. (no. 17) *2:*19-22, Sept 5, '46

Hands, Miscellaneous

To prevent disability after trauma of hand. FOSSATARO, E. Policlinico (sez. chir.) *28:*1, Jan '21 abstr: J.A.M.A. *76:*968, April 2, '21

Limitation of movement at metacarpophalangeal joints; its causes and treatment. GLISSAN, D. J., M. J. Australia *2:*257, Oct '21

Certain phases of surgery of hand. HARMER, T. W., S. Clin. N. America *2:*973-994, Aug '22 (illus.)

Disabilities of hand and their physiological treatment. LYLE, H. H. M. Ann. Surg. *78:*816-845, Dec '23 (illus.)

Lesions of hands and fingers from aniline pencils. ISELIN, M. Presse med. *35:*467-469, April 13, '27

Hands, Miscellaneous – Cont.
Lesions of hand and face caused by colored copying pencil. BETTAZZI, G. Policlinico (sez. chir.) *35:*501–505, Oct '28
Necrosis of hand resulting from application of ammonium hydroxide after snake bite. KRAUSS, F. Zentralbl. f. Chir. *56:*459–460, Feb 23, '29
Wounds of hand, particularly of thumb in miners; statistics. PORCU-MACCIONI, G. Rassegna d. previd. soc. *16:*8–17, Feb '29
Chronic traumatic edema of dorsum of hand; 7 cases. KLASSEN, P. Monatschr. f. Unfallh. *36:*289–309, July '29
New incision for ligature of palmar arch. POPOVICI, V. M. Lyon chir. *26:*686–693, Sept-Oct '29 also: Rev. de chir., Bucuresti *21:*437–443, July '29
Amytrophic mutilating sclerodactylia with vasomotor trophic symptoms due to trauma 30 years previously to hand. LHERMITTE, J. AND LÉVY, G. Rev. neurol. *1:*622–631, April '30
Implements for hand injuries. MASLAND, H. C. Am. J. Surg. *12:*142–143, April '31
Traumatic hard edema of hand. BETTMANN, E. JR. Arch. f. orthop. u. Unfall-Chir. *32:*570–575, '33
Progressive hemiatrophy of face, shoulder girdle and hand; case. VASILEVSKIY, M. V. Sovet. nevropat. psikhiat. i psikhogig. (no. 7) *2:*78–79, '33
Device for fixation of hands and arms for certain operative cases. ADAMS, B. D. New England J. Med. *210:*423, Feb 22, '34
Unusual localization of arthropathies (mandibulotemporal and metacarpophalangeal ankylosis), in postencephalitic parkinsonian syndrome and their pathogenesis. GORDON, A., M. Rec. *140:*351–353, Oct 3, '34
Statistics on injuries and infections of fingers and hands based on accident insurance records. JAROŠ, M. Rozhl. v chir. a gynaek. (cast chir.) *13:*270–288, '34
Consequences of hand injuries. NOVAK, V. Rozhl. v chir. a gynaek. (cast chir.) *14:*20–24, '35
Brucella abortus infection of hand after injury; fatal case. WERTHEMANN, A. Schweiz. med. Wchnschr. *66:*333–335, April 4, '36
Contracture of hands with arthropathies in postencephalitic parkinsonism; clinical and anatomicopathologic study of cases. PENNACCHIETTI, M. Minerva med. *1:*423–431, May 5, '36
Lesions of hands of bakers. SEARA, P. Prensa med. argent. *24:*580–583, March 17, '37
Formation of artificial hand. FUKS, B. I. Novy khir. arkhiv *39:*125–129, '37

Hands, Miscellaneous – Cont.
Zoster of left arm following injury to thumb; case. JADASSOHN, W. Schweiz. med. Wchnschr. *68:*93, Jan 22, '38
Air embolism following hand injury; case. KOVACS, H. J. Zentralbl. f. Chir. *65:*180–182, Jan 22, '38
Technical study of accidents to longshoremen of Minatitlan (including hand injuries). CHAVEZ, E. JR. Rev. d. trab. *2:*167–172, May '38
Relation of trauma of hand to occupation. ECKELBERRY, N. E. Am. J. Surg. *41:*51–56, July '38
Manifestations of fatigue (necrosis and pseudarthrosis) of carpal scaphoid bone caused by chronic trauma (work with pneumatic tools). ANDREESEN, R. Fortschr. a. d. Geb. d. Rontgenstrahlen *60:*253–263, Oct '39
Traumatic aseptic necrosis of scaphoid bone of right hand. BADE, H. Rontgenpraxis *11:*573–574, Oct '39
Local anesthesia of distal half of forearm and of hand. FINOCHIETTO, R. AND ZAVALETA, D. E. Rev. med. y cien. afines *2:*295–297, May 30, '40
Therapy of "knuckle pads" with carbon dioxide snow. ASBECK, F. Dermat. Wchnschr. *110:*457–461, June 1, '40
Table for gymnastic after-treatment of hand injuries. KOTILAINEN, T. Duodecim *56:*333–335, '40
Traumatic edema of hand. SCHÖRCHER. Beitr. z. klin. Chir. *171:*176–194, '40
Round-table conference on office surgery of hand. FERGUSON, L. K.; *et al.* Pennsylvania M. J. *44:*433–439, Jan '41
Lesions of tendons and their prognosis with respect to hand function. FLEISCHER-HANSEN, C. C. Nord. med. (Hospitalstid.) *9:*88–98, Jan 11, '41
Hand wounds; medicosocial problem. CASANUEVA DEL C., M. Arch. Soc. cirujanos hosp., num. espec., pp. 39–50, Dec '41
Procaine hydrochloride blocking of stellate ganglion in therapy of traumatic hard edema of hand. LÄWEN, A. Arch. f. klin. Chir. *201:*687–691, '41
The Hand: Its Disabilities and Diseases, by CONDICT W. CUTLER, JR. W. B. Saunders Co., Phila., 1942
Diagnosis of skin diseases of hand and fingers. KRANTZ, W. Med. Klin. *38:*29, Jan 9, '42; 54, Jan 16, '42; 98, Jan 30, '42
Hand hazards. BRUNER, R. A. Hygeia *20:*424, June '42
Chronic edema of back of hand; simulated sequel of trauma for purpose of collecting insurance. JENNY, F. Praxis *31:*365–367, June 25, '42

Hands, Miscellaneous—Cont.

Scar disabilities in hand. RANK, B. K. Australian and New Zealand J. Surg. *12:*191-206, Jan '43

Surgical significance of middle palmar septum. FLYNN, J. E. Surgery *14:*134-141, July '43

Kinetic disabilities of hand and their classification; study in balance and imbalance of hand muscles. BURMAN, M. Am. J. Surg. *61:*167-214, Aug '43

Injuries of fingers and hand from point of view of state accident insurance. KONIG, F. Munchen. med. Wchnschr. *90:*509, Aug 27, '43

Vasomotor disturbances in hand after injuries. RICHARDS, R. L. Edinburgh M. J. *50:*449-468, Aug '43

Immersion hand (peripheral vasoneuropathy after chilling). UNGLEY, C. C. Bull. War Med. *4:*61-65, Oct '43

Significance of hypothenar elevation in movements of opposition of thumb. SUNDERLAND, S. Australian and New Zealand J. Surg. *13:*155-156, Jan '44

Rehabilitation of injured hand. D'OFFAY, T. M. J., M. Press *211:*76-79, Feb 2, '44

Hand retraction piece for hand surgery. RANK, B. K. Brit. M. J. *1:*496, April 8, '44

Use of skeletal traction in hand. COBEY, M. C.; *et al.* South. M. J. *37:*309-313, June '44

Mobilization of hand following loss of all fingers. GEYMANOVICH, Z. Khirurgiya, no. 6, pp. 82-84, '44

Arm board for navy operating table. DUNLOP, G. R. AND HUMBERD, J. D., U. S. Nav. M. Bull. *44:*171-172, Jan '45

Mechanics of synovial joints; hinge-joints and nature of intra-articular displacements. MACCONAILL, M. A. Irish J. M. Sc. pp. 620-626, Sept '46

Two instruments for surgery of hand. HEBRAUD, A. Rev. med. nav. *1:*63-65, '46

Hands, Nerve Injuries in (See also Hands, Injuries of; Hands, Tendon Injuries in)

Tendon transplant for intrinsic hand muscle paralysis. NEY, K. W. Surg., Gynec. and Obst. *33:*342, Oct '21

Insidious paralysis of intrinsic muscles of hand and its operative relief. STOOKEY, B. P., S. Clin. N. America *3:*465-488, April '23 (illus.)

Peripheral nerve lesions of the hand. ALLISON, W. L. Texas State J. Med. *20:*46-51, May '24

Surgical treatment of so-called paralysis of opponens muscle. WEIL, S. Klin. Wchnschr. *5:*650-651, April 9, '26

Hands, Nerve Injuries in—Cont.

Surgery of nerves of hand. BUNNELL, S. Surg., Gynec. and Obst. *44:*145-152, Feb '27

Repair of nerves and tendons of hand and grafting. BUNNELL, S., J. Bone and Joint Surg. *10:*1-26, Jan '28 abstr: Arch. franco-belges de chir. *30:*93-97, Feb '27

Transplantation of tendons of flexor pollicis longus for paralysis of flexor opponens pollicis. SILFVERSKIÖLD, N. Acta chir. Scandinav. *64:*296-299, '28

Flexor plasty of thumb in thenar palsy. STEINDLER, A. Surg., Gynec. and Obst. *50:*1005-1007, June '30

Abnormalities of nerve in palmar region of man. CAPONNETTO, A. Monitore zool. ital. *41:*180-183, '30

Incised wound of palm; severance of median nerve; immediate nerve suture. COHN, I. Internat. Clin. *2:*104-106, June '31

Division of nerves and tendons of hand, with discussion of surgical treatment and its results. KOCH, S. L. AND MASON, M. L. Surg. Gynec. and Obst. *56:*1-39, Jan '33

Paralysis of extensors of hand and fingers in persons working with lead. TELEKY, L. Deutsche med. Wchnschr. *59:*723-724, May 12, '33

Injuries of nerves and tendons of hand (surgical therapy). KOCH, S. L., J. Oklahoma M. A. *26:*323-327, Sept '33

Injuries to nerves and tendons of hand. KOCH, S. L. Pennsylvania M. J. *37:*555-557, April '34

Treatment of stiffening of fingers and hand with and without muscular paralysis. LANGE, M. Munchen. med. Wchnschr. *81:*894-897, June 15, '34

Injuries of nerves and tendons of hand. KOCH, S. L. Wisconsin M. J. *33:*655-661, Sept '34

Retraction of palmar aponeurosis with syringomyelic dissociation of sensitivity; 2 cases. URECHIA, C. I. AND DRAGOMIR, L. Paris med. *2:*274-276, Oct 5, '35

Operation for thenar paralysis. ROYALE, N. D., M. J. Australia *2:*155-156, Aug 1, '36

Severed tendons and nerves of hand and forearm. O'SHEA, M. C. Ann. Surg. *105:*228-242, Feb '37

Recurrent pseudoarthrosis of humerus complicated by irreparable paralysis of radial nerve; curative osteoplasty and functional reconstruction of hand by means of tendon transplants. INCLAN, A. Cir. ortop. y trau-

Hands, Nerve Injuries in – Cont.
matol., Habana *7:*43-53, April–June '39
Extensive primary nerve and tendon suture at wrist; 2 cases. HOWARD, R. N., M. J. Australia *2:*322-323, Aug 26, '39
Wrist-drop; graft of 15 cm. of rabbit's spinal cord and infiltration of stellate ganglion followed by rapid recovery; case. SOUBIRAN. J. de med. de Bordeaux *116:*353-354, Nov 4-25, '39
Plastic surgery of flexor tendon of hand, with special reference to paralysis of opponens pollicis. PACHER, W. Arch. f. orthop. u. Unfall-Chir. *40:*93-101, '39
Traumatic lesions of nerves of wrist and hand. HARMER, T. W. Am. J. Surg. *47:*517-541, Feb '40
Injuries to nerves and tendons of hand. MASON, M. L., J.A.M.A. *116:*1375-1379, March 29, '41
Ascending neuropathy due to injury of hand; predominance and unusual nature of trophic phenomena. COUTO, DEOLINDO. Cultura med. *3:*355-370, Feb '42
Nerve and tendon injuries of hand. MASON, M. L. Indust. Med. *11:*61-66, Feb '42
Modified operation for opponens paralysis. THOMPSON, T. C., J. Bone and Joint Surg. *24:*632-640, July '42
Transplantation of flexor carpi ulnaris for pronation flexion deformity of wrist. GREEN, W. T. Surg., Gynec. and Obst. *75:*337-342, Sept '42
Innervation and function of thenar muscles. HIGHET, W. B. Lancet *1:*227-230, Feb 20, '43
Post-traumatic neuralgia as serious complication of section of tendons of hand in cultivators of sugar cane. OLIVERAS GUERRA, A. Bol. Asoc. med. de Puerto Rico *35:*47-51, Feb '43
Repair of lacerated nerves at wrist. SONNENSCHEIN, H. D., S. Clin. North America *23:*487-496, April '43
Reconstructive orthopedic surgery (tendon transplantation and arthrodesis of wrist) for disabilities resulting from irreparable injuries to radial nerve. ABBOTT, L. C., J. Nerv. and Ment. Dis. *99:*466-474, May '44
Radial paralysis; tenoplasty of extensors. POINOT, J. Bordeaux chir. *3-4:*148-149, July-Oct '45
Tendon transplant in paralysis of extensors of hand and fingers; case in boy 5 years old. GUILLEMINET, M. AND DUBOST, T. Rev. d'orthop. *32:*72-75, Jan-Apr '46
Treatment of injuries, with particular reference to nerve and tendon repair in hand. MASON, M. L. Indust. Med. *15:*323-325, May '46
Trauma to hand; with particular reference to indications for primary and secondary nerve and tendon repair. MASON, M. L. J. Oklahoma M. A. *39:*246-251, June '46
Injuries of nerves and tendons of hand. KOCH, S. L. Cincinnati J. Med. *27:*515-521, Aug '46

Hands, Reconstructive Surgery of
Reconstruction of hand, a new technic in tenoplasty. TAYLOR, R. T. Surg., Gynec. and Obst. *32:*237, March '21
Hand plastic. JOHNSON, L. W., U. S. Nav. M. Bull. *15:*399, April '21
Restoration of hand injuries by plastic surgery. FULD, J. E. New York M. J. *114:*692, Dec 21, '21
Surgery of wrist and hand. LEDDERHOSE, G. Deutsche med. Wchnschr. *48:*943-944, July 14, '22
Plastic repair of face and hand. SHAW, J. J. M. Brit. J. Surg. *10:*47-51, July '22 (illus.)
Transplantation of bone in hand. MICHON, L. J. de chir. *20:*260-273, Sept '22 (illus.) abstr: J. A. M. A. *79:*1884, Nov 25, '22
Use of index finger for thumb, some interesting points in hand surgery. DUNLOP, J., J. Bone and Joint Surg. *5:*99-103, Jan '23 (illus.)
Results of tendon transplantation for intrinsic hand paralysis (Ney's operation). JOHNSTONE, J. G., J. Bone and Joint Surg. *5:* 278-283, April '23 (illus.)
Case of minor surgery of hand; accidental amputation of finger with preservation of terminal phalanx. TOMB, J. W. Lancet *2:*930, Oct 27, '23
Reconstructive surgery of hand. BUNNELL, S. Surg., Gynec. and Obst. *39:*259-274, Sept '24
Surgery of flexor tendons of hand. GARLOCK, J. H. Am. J. Surg. *40:*68-69, March '26
Skin plastics in treatment of traumatic lesions of hand and forearm. LYLE, H. H. M. Ann. Surg. *83:*537-542, April '26
Orthopedic treatment of hand and finger contractures. REY, J. Ztschr. f. orthop. Chir. *48:*21-31, Feb 11, '27
Treatment of old extensive destruction of tendons. (hand) CHIANELLO, C. Cultura med. mod. *6:*104-106, March 1, '27
Case showing anatomical and functional reproduction of metacarpal by bone-graft. FOWLER, A. Brit. J. Surg. *14:*675-676, April '27

Hands, Reconstructive Surgery in – Cont.

Scar contracture of flexor sublimis digitorum. KOVACS, R. Physical Therap. *45:*383–384, Aug '27

Orthopedic reconstruction work on hand; early and late results. STEINDLER, A. Surg., Gynec. and Obst. *45:*476–481, Oct '27

Traumatic luxation of some extensor tendons of hand. SILFVERSKIÖLD, N. Acta chir. Scandinav. *64:*305–310, '28

Examples of restorative surgery and functional adaptation of hand and feet. OLLER, A. Siglo med. *83:*77-82, Jan 5, '29

Surgical treatment of arthritis. O'FERRALL, J. T. New Orleans M. and S. J. *81:*899–902, June '29

Conservative hand surgery. RICARD, A. Lyon chir. *26:*596–599, Aug–Sept '29

Cases of hand surgery. MCWATTERS, R. C. Indian M. Gaz. *65:*276, May '30

Plastic surgery of fingers and hand. SEIFFERT, K. Arch. f. Orthop. *28:*370–375, May 6, '30

Operation for utilising middle finger as "trigger" finger. DUTTA, P. C. Indian M. Gaz. *66:*676–677, Dec '31

Use of plantaris tendon in certain types of plastic surgery of hand. GLISSAN, D. J. Australian and New Zealand J. Surg. *2:*64–67, July '32

Carpometacarpal arthroplasty of thumb. PATTERSON, R., J. Bone and Joint Surg. *15:*240-241, Jan '33

Practical points in hand surgery. SALSBURY, C. R., J. Oklahoma M. A. *26:*315–319, Sept '33

Complicated contractures of hand; their treatment by freeing fibrosed tendons and replacing destroyed tendons with grafts. KOCH, S. L. Ann. Surg. *98:*546–580, Oct '33

Restoration of function of hand after traumatic injury. FULD, J. E. Ann. Surg. *99:*195–216, Jan '34

Plastic surgery of crippled hand and injured hand. BURIAN, F. Rozhl. v chir. a gynaek. (cast chir.) *13:*252–270, '34

Technic of Italian graft in hand injuries. BIAILLE DE LANGIBAUDIERE, M. Bull. Soc. med.-chir. de l'Indochine *13:*387–396, May '35

Favorable results of surgical therapy of aplasia of opponens muscle of thumb by transplantation of tendons of flexor digitalis sublimis V; survey of methods. GÖBELL, R. AND FREUDENBERG, K. Arch. f. orthop. u. Unfall-Chir. *35:*675-677, '35

So-called late rupture of tendon of extensor pollicis longus in connection with wrist fractures. VON STAPELMOHR, S. Nord. med. tidskr. *11:*174–178, Jan 31, '36

Dujardin-Beaumetz operation in accidental lesions of fingers for functional restoration of mutilated hands. FORGUE, E. Progres med., pp. 305–309, Feb 22, '36

Late results of secondary plastic operations on tendons and nerves of hand. KALALOVA-DI LOTTIOVA, V. Bratisl. lekar. listy *16:*162–174, April '36

Sutures or reconstruction (using fascia lata) of sectioned hand tendons; 3 cases. MASMONTEIL, F. Bull. et mem. Soc. d. chirurgiens de Paris *28:*379–384, June 5, '36

Author's method for repair of ankylosed joint of hand. FORRESTER, C. R. G. Am. J. Surg. *33:*101–103, July '36

Tendinoplasty of flexor tendons of hand; use of tunica vaginalis in reconstructing tendon sheaths. WILMOTH, C. L., J. Bone and Joint Surg. *19:*152–156, Jan '37

Plastic restoration for loss of all fingers of both hands. HAAS, S. L. Am. J. Surg. *36:*720–723, June '37

Pedicle flap patterns for reconstruction of hand. PIERCE, G. W. AND O'CONNOR, G. B. Rev. de chir. structive, pp. 85–90, June '37 also: Surg., Gynec. and Obst. *65:*523–527, Oct '37

Treatment of minor hand injuries. ROZHANSKIY, V. I. Khirurgiya, no. 3, pp. 53–59, '37

Spastic hand. BURMAN, M. S., J. Bone and Joint Surg. *20:*133–145, Jan '38

Reconstruction of injured hand. BUNNELL, S. Rocky Mountain M. J. *35:*194–200, March '38

Metacarpolysis in mutilation of thumb; illustrative cases. GARCIA DIAZ, F. Semana med. *1:*658–660, March 24, '38

Surgical repair of long-disabled hand. YOUNG, F. Surg., Gynec. and Obst. *67:*73–81, July '38

Surgery of the Hand, by JOHN H. COUCH. Univ. Toronto Press, Toronto, 1939

Minor surgical conditions of hands. LOVE, R. J. M. Practitioner *142:*261–269, March '39

Plastic repair of cutaneous injuries to hand. GREELEY, P. W. Indust. Med. *9:*300–303, June '40

Treatment and restoration of totally crippled hands. PAYR, E. Arch. f. klin. Chir. *200:*527–545, '40

Fat formation in abdominal skin flap on hand 23 years after grafting. VON MEZÖ, B. Chirurg *13:*18–19, Jan 1, '41

Minor surgical conditions of hand. MASON,

Hands, Reconstructive Surgery in—Cont.
M. L., S. Clin. North America *21:*181-195, Feb '41
Plastic surgery and repair of hand, with particular reference to repair of cutaneous defects. MASON, M. L. Indust. Med. *10:*47-52, Feb '41
Post-traumatic dorsal torsion of hand; late results of surgical therapy; case. DE ARAUJO, A. Rev. brasil. de orthop. e traumatol. *2:*339-355, May-June '41
Skin and tendon transplantation in severe injury to back of right hand by polishing machine. HILLEBRAND, H. Chirurg *13:*521-523, Sept 1, '41
Minor surgery of hand. LAKE, N. C. Practitioner *147:*593-602, Sept '41
Fusion of metacarpals of thumb and index finger to maintain functional position of thumb. THOMPSON, C. F., J. Bone and Joint Surg. *24:*907-911, Oct '42
Transverse palmar incision. MCKIM, L. H. Am. J. Surg. *59:*444-446, Feb '43
Stabilization of articulation of greater multangular and first metacarpal. SLOCUM, D. B., J. Bone and Joint Surg. *25:*626-630, July '43
Surgery of the Hand, by STERLING BUNNELL. J. B. Lippincott Co., Phila., 1944
Reconstruction of the Fingers, by B. V. PARIN. U.S.S.R. "Medgiz" Press, Moscow, 1944
Plastic surgery of hand; fingers in flexion contracture; semeiologic and therapeutic study. PEDEMONTE, P. V. Arch. urug. de med., cir. y especialid. *24:*249-274, Mar '44
Method for fusion of wrist. COLONNA, P. C. South. M. J. *37:*195-199, April '44
Elementary theories on therapy of hand from point of view of plastic surgery. REBELO NETO, J. An. paulist. de med. e cir. *48:*97-118, Aug '44
Conditions involving elbow, forearm, wrist and hand; progress in orthopedic surgery for 1943. BLOUNT, W. P. Arch. Surg. *49:*258-261, Oct '44
Value of tendon transplantation for rapid restoration of function of wrist following injuries. LOMAZOV, M. G. Vrach. delo *24:*51-54, Dec 1, '44
Excision of proximal row of carpus. STAMM, T. T. Proc. Roy. Soc. Med. *38:*74-75, Dec '44
Reconstruction of hand; early surfacing of burns. WOOLHOUSE, F. M. Am. Acad. Orthop. Surgeons, Lect., pp. 187-190, '44
Chirurgie de la main, livre du chirurgien: Chirurgie reparatrice des traumatismes de la main, by MARC ISELIN. Masson et Cie,

Hands, Reconstructive Surgery in—Cont.
Paris, 1945
Conservation of metacarpus by skin and bone grafting in 3 patients. MORONEY, P. B. Brit. J. Surg. *32:*464-466, April '45
Plastic and reconstructive surgery of hand. CANNON, B. AND GRAHAM, W. C. Mil. Surgeon *97:*137-139, Aug '45
New arthroplasty for small joints. CROSBY, E. H. AND GALASINSKI, R. E. Connecticut M. J. *9:*926-928, Dec '45
Surgery of hand. STONHAM, F. V. Indian M. Gaz. *80:*597-601, Dec '45
Mobilization of hand following loss of all fingers. PARIN, B. V. Khirurgiya no. 3, p. 89, '45 (comment on Geymanovich's article)
Surgery of the Hand, by R. M. HANDFIELD-JONES, E. and S. Livingstone Ltd., Edinburgh, 1946
Conditions involving elbow, forearm, wrist and hand; progress in orthopedic surgery for 1944. BLOUNT, W. P. Arch. Surg. *52:*197-209, Feb '46
Late repair of tendons of hand. WEBSTER, G. V. Am. J. Surg. *72:*171-178, Aug '46
Rehabilitation of injured hand. HARDY, S. B. Am. J. Surg. *72:*352-362, Sept '46
Reconstructive surgery of hand. BUNNELL, S. Guy's Hosp. Gaz. *60:*293-296, Oct 26, '46
Use of tantalum in tendon reconstruction of hand. PEARLMAN, R. C., U. S. Nav. M. Bull. *46:*1647-1650, Nov '46

HANDS, S. G.: Treatment of lacrimal fistula following dacrocystectomy. J. Iowa M. Soc. *15:*598-600, Nov '25

Hands, Skin Grafts and Flaps to

Covering of raw surfaces with particular reference to hand. KOCH, S. L. Surg., Gynec. and Obst. *43:*677-686, Nov '26
Surgical treatment of "de-gloved" hand. COLT, G. H. Brit. J. Surg. *14:*560-568, April '27
Contracture of right hand treated by full-thickness skin grafts. JONES, H. T., S. Clin. N. Amer. *9:*939-940, Aug '29
Low voltage currents in contractures of hand. GRIES, L. Arch. Physical Therapy *11:*10-13, Jan '30
Acquired contractures of hand. KOCH, S. L. Am. J. Surg. *9:*413-423, Sept '30
Contracture of hand. KOCH, S. L. Surg., Gynec. and Obst. *52:*367-370, Feb (No. 2A) '31
Contracture of fingers due to cicatrices on back of hand. NAPALKOV, N. Ortop. i. travmatol. (no. 6) *9:*43-47, '35
Glove flap method of dorsal repair in hand

Hands, Skin Grafts and Flaps to – Cont.
surgery. O'CONNOR, G. B. Am. J. Surg. *32:*445–447, June '36
Glove flap method of dorsal hand repair. O'CONNOR, G. B. Rev. de chir. structive, pp. 384–389, Dec '36
Repair of surface defects of hand. BROWN, J. B. Ann. Surg. *107:*952–971, June '38
Skin grafts in surgical correction of defective cicatrix of hand causing contracture; 2 cases. BARBERIS, J. C. Bol. Soc. de cir. de Rosario *5:*469–477, Nov '38
Technic of free graft of whole skin for cicatricial contracture of hand. ZENO, L. Bol. y trab., Soc. de cir. de Buenos Aires *23:*525–531, July 26, '39
Free full thickness skin grafts in hand contracted by cicatrix; technical problems in case. ZENO, L. Rev. ortop. y traumatol. *9:*73–77, July '39
Technic of full thickness free grafts for cicatricial contracture of hand. ZENO, L. Semana med. *2:*829–831, Oct 12, '39
Surface defects of hand. BROWN, J. B. Am. J. Surg. *46:*690–699, Dec '39
Technic of pedicled flaps in plastic surgery of skin; use in treating cicatricial contracture of hand. ZENO, L. Bol. y trab., Acad. argent. de cir. *24:*886–890, Sept 18, '40 also: Semana med. *2:*1058–1061, Nov 7, '40
Transplantation of skin and subcutaneous tissue to hand. KOCH, S. L. Surg., Gynec. and Obst. *72:*157–177, Feb '41
Preservation of tendon function in hand by use of skin flaps. KITLOWSKI, E. A. Am. J. Surg. *51:*653–661, March '41
Rigid hand caused by fibrous cicatrix; free graft of full-thickness skin. ZENO, L. An. de cir. *7:*52–56, March–June '41 also: Bol. Soc. de cir. de Rosario *8:*53–58, April '41
Reparative surgery of upper limb (in contractures of hands or arms). COLE, P. P. Brit. J. Surg. *28:*585–607, April '41
Treatment of injuries to hand requiring skin grafting. HAWKINS, T. L. Am. J. Surg. *59:*383–391, Feb '43
Rare muscular contractures of hand following poisoning with carbon monoxide, phosphorus and ethyl gasoline. BAYR, G. Deut. Militararzt *8:*623, Nov '43
Plastic surgery; advantages and inconveniences of tubular transplants in grave cicatrices of hand. PEDEMONTE, P. V. Bol. Soc. cir. d. Uruguay *14:*114–122, '43 also: Arch. urug. de med., cir. y especialid. *23:*453–461, Nov '43
Plastic repair of extensor hand contractures following healed deep second degree burns. GREELEY, P. W. Tr. Am. Soc. Plastic and Reconstructive Surg. *12:*79–82, '43
Plastic surgery of retractile cicatrix of hand. ZENO, L. An. de cir. *10:*183–185, Sept–Dec '44 also: Bol. Soc. de cir. de Rosario *11:*451–454, Nov '44
Use of flaps and pedicles in repair of hand and arm defects. KISKADDEN, W. S. Am. Acad. Orthop. Surgeons, Lect., pp. 180–183, '44
Skin graft of dorsum of hand; use of large size dermatome to obtain one-piece pattern. CONVERSE, J. M. Ann. Surg. *121:*172–174, Feb '45
Late treatment of dorsal injuries associated with loss of skin in hand. CUTHBERT, J. B. Brit. J. Surg. *33:*66–71, July '45
Closure of surface defects of hand. MAY, H. Pennsylvania M. J. *49:*116–120, Nov '45

Hands, Splints
Traction splint for fractured metacarpals and phalanges. HAWK, G. W., J.A.M.A. *78:*106, Jan 14, '22 (illus.)
Dynamics of functions of hand, with considerations as to methods of obtaining position of function by splints. KANAVEL, A. B. M. J. Australia *2:*598–602, Oct 29, '27
Ball splint for hand fractures. DAVIS, G. G. Internat. Clin. *1:*182–183, March '28
Four splints of value in treatment of disabilities of hand. KOCH, S. L. Surg., Gynec. and Obst. *48:*416–418, March '29
New type of splint for hand fractures. WERTHEIM, W., J.A.M.A. *92:*2171, June 29, '29
Splint to prevent contracture in surgery of hand. GAGE, E. L., J.A.M.A. *94:*1063–1064, April 5, '30
Aluminum splints for fractures of forearm and hand. PERMAN, E. Svenska lak.-tidning. *29:*769–784, July 15, '32
Aluminum splints in hand fractures. PERMAN, E. Acta chir. Scandinav. *72:*331–343, '32
Device for fixation of hands and arms for certain operative cases. ADAMS, B. D. New England J. Med. *210:*423, Feb 22, '34
Useful splints for hand and finger. ZUR VERTH, M. Zentralbl. f. Chir. *62:*2270–2274, Sept 21, '35
Necessity for use of splints at certain stages in treatment of hand infections, with demonstration of some of the newer types. BROWNE, W. E. New England J. Med. *215:*743–749, Oct 22, '36
Making of arm and hand splints. PRO-

Hands, Splints – Cont.
CHAZKA, A. Physiotherapy Rev. *18:*59-64, March-April '38
Purposeful splinting of hand following injuries (including sketch on Hugh Owen Thomas). KOCH, S. L. AND MASON, M. L. Surg., Gynec. and Obst. *68:*1-16, Jan '39
Finger splint that will not impair hand function. JELSMA, F. Am. J. Surg. *50:*571-572, Dec '40
Simple apparatus for relief of palsies of upper extremities. POLYA, E. Surgery *8:*1023, Dec '40
Purposeful splinting of hand following injuries. MARBLE, H. C., J.A.M.A. *116:*1373-1375, March 29, '41
Adjustable volar-flexion splint. COHEN, H. H. J. Bone and Joint Surg. *24:*189-192, Jan '42
Two small wire splints for treatment by traction of fractures and deformities of fingers and metacarpal bones. LYFORD, J. III. J. Bone and Joint Surg. *24:*202-203, Jan '42
Uses and abuses of splints and other instruments in treatment of nerve injuries. McMURRAY, T. P. Brit. J. Phys. Med. *5:*20-25, Feb '42
Easily made "drop-wrist" splint. ELLIOT, H. Canad. M. A. J. *47:*363, Oct '42
Importance of purposeful splinting of hand following injuries. HOY, C. D. Ohio State M. J. *38:*1025, Nov '42
Simple splint in treatment of ulnar paralysis. RAFFLER, K. Zentralbl. f. Chir. *70:*764, May 22, '43
New elastic splint for wrist drop. MAYFIELD, F. H. Bull. U. S. Army M. Dept. (no. 73) pp. 96-97, Feb '44
Splint for radial (musculospiral) nerve palsy. THOMAS, F. B., J. Bone and Joint Surg. *26:*602-605, July '44
Immobilization and its disastrous effects on hand function. GIRDWOOD, W. South African M. J. *18:*350-352, Oct 28, '44
Splint for radial nerve palsies. HERZOG, E. G. Lancet *2:*754, Dec 9, '44
Suggestions on immobilization of hand. PRATT, D. R. Bull. U. S. Army M. Dept. (no. 86) pp. 105-108, March '45
Splint for correction of extension contractures of metacarpophalangeal joints. NACHLAS, I. W., J. Bone and Joint Surg. *27:*507-512, July '45
Utilization of Haynes splint (hand). TEJERA LORENZO, F. Vida nueva *56:*29-34, July '45
Suggestions on immobilization of hand injuries. PRATT, D. R. Arch. Phys. Med. *26:*649-653, Oct '45

Hands, Splints – Cont.
Universal splint for deformities of hand. BATEMAN, J. E., J. Bone and Joint Surg. *28:*169-173, Jan '46
Corrective splint for paralysis of thenar muscles. NAPIER, J. R. Brit. M. J. *1:*15, Jan 5, '46
Splint to correct deformity (clawhand) resulting from injury to ulnar nerve. PRUCE, A. M., J. Bone and Joint Surg. *28:*397, Apr '46
Active splinting of hand. BUNNELL, S. J. Bone and Joint Surg. *28:*732-736, Oct '46

Hands, Tendon Injuries in (See also Hands, Injuries of; Hands, Nerve Injuries in)
Suture of tendon in hand or finger. KAUFMANN, C. Schweiz. med. Wchnschr. *51:*601, June 30, '21 abstr: J. A. M. A. *77:*653, Aug 20, '21
To improve outcome of suture of tendon in hand. RUEF, H. Arch. f. klin. Chir. *130:*757-762, '24 abstr: J. A. M. A. *83:*1379, Oct 25, '24
Repair of wounds of flexor tendons of hand. GARLOCK, J. H. Ann. Surg. *83:*111-122, Jan '26
Treatment of wounds of tendons of hand and fingers. ISELIN, M. AND TAILHEFER, A. Gaz. d. hop. *100:*961-964, July 20, '27
Les techniques et les résultats actuals de la réparation des tendons de la main et des doigts, by ANDRÉ TAILHEFER. Arnette, Paris, 1928
Prevention of adhesions to tendons in hand and wrist, with report of 2 cases. MARSHALL, G. D., J. Bone and Joint Surg. *10:*816-818, Oct '28
Evolution and treatment in wounds of tendons of hands and fingers. CAZIN, M. Paris chir. *21:*179-190, Sept-Oct '29
Injuries of tendons of hand; surgical repair. BLOCH, J. C. AND BONNET, P., J. de chir. *34:*456-474, Oct '29
Evolution and treatment of wounds of tendons of hand. BLOCH, J. J. AND BONNET, P. Gaz. d. hop. *102:*1581, Nov 6, '29
Suture of tendon of flexor digitorum profundus; case. RIVARD, J. H. Union med. du Canada *59:*28-30, Jan '30
Method in exposure of flexor tendons of hand. KHAITZISS, G. M. Vestnik khir. (no. 64) *22:*115-120, '30
Invalidism after cutting of tendons of hand. KIAER, S. Acta orthop. Scandinav. *2:*202-220, '31
Plastic surgery of tendons and nerves of hand. CHIARIELLO, A. G. Policlinico (sez. prat.) *39:*520-525, April 4, '32

Hands, Tendon Injuries in – Cont.
Pathologic anatomy and therapy of wounds of flexor tendons of hands. ISELIN, M. Presse med. *40:*606-610, April 20, '32
Suture of flexor tendon in therapy of hand injury; case. LASSERRE, C., J. de med. de Bordeaux *109:*357-358, May 10, '32
Section of flexor tendons of middle finger of left hand through palmar wound; primary suture and cure. ANDREASEN, A., J. Bone and Joint Surg. *14:*700-701, July '32
Successful suture of extensor tendons of hand sectioned by wounds; case. JARAMILLO ARANGO, J. Repert. de med. y cir. *23:*289-320, July '32
Section of flexor tendons of index and middle fingers in palm of hand. DE LEEUW, E. Scalpel *85:*1269-1271, Oct 15, '32
Treatment of injuries of tendons within synovial sheaths in palm of hand and of flexor tendons of finger by insertion of foreign substance. HESSE, F. Arch. f. klin. Chir. *170:*772-789, '32
Tendons in hand injuries. SALSBURY, C. R. Am. J. Surg. *21:*354-357, Sept '33
Therapy of section of tendons of hand in industrial accidents; 50 cases. ROGERS, S. P. AND ESPINOSA ROBLEDO, M. Cir. ortop. y traumatol. *3:*177-181, July-Sept '35
Plastic surgery of flexor tendons of hand. DUBROV, Y. G. Ortop. i travatol. (no. 5) *9:*109-120, '35
Section of flextor tendons of hand; suture with recovery after physiopathic phenomena; case. FIGARELLA, J. Marseille-med. *1:*725-727, May 25, '36
Primary tenorrhaphy in therapy of section of tendons during cane cutting. OLIVERAS GUERRA, A. Bol. Asoc. med. de Puerto Rico *28:*114-118, June '36
Industrial accidents; management of injuries of tendons and nerve of hand. GARLOCK, J. H. New York State J. Med. *36:*1740-1748, Nov 15, '36
Suture of tendons of hand. DZHANELIDZE, Y. Y. Novy khir. arkhiv *36:*497-507, '36
Injury of hand tendons. STAHEL, W. Schweiz. med. Wchnschr. *67:*51-54, Jan 16, '37
Severed tendons and nerves of hand and forearm. O'SHEA, M. C. Ann. Surg. *105:*228-242, Feb '37
Principles of management of tendon injuries (hand). MASON, M. L. Physiotherapy Rev. *18:*119-123, May-June '38
Late results of surgical therapy in injuries to tendons of hand. DERRA, E. AND RUBERG, G. Monatschr. f. Unfallh. *45:*305-315, June '38

Hands, Tendon Injuries in – Cont.
Repair of severed tendons in hand. MAYER, L. Am. J. Surg. *42:*714-722, Dec '38
Late results of sutures of tendons of arm and hand. HECK, F. Arch. f. orthop. u. Unfall-Chir. *39:*21-28, '38
Primary and secondary suture of flexor tendons of wrist and fingers. ROZOV, V. I. Novy khir. arkhiv *41:*490-504, '38
Hematoma of flexor tendon sheaths following penetrating wounds (hand). DEVENISH, E. A. Lancet *1:*447-448, Feb 25, '39
Treatment and results of 870 severed tendons and 57 severed nerves of hand and forearm (in 362 patients). O'SHEA, M. C. Am. J. Surg. *43:*346-366, Feb '39
Repair of tendons of hand. CLEVELAND, H. E. Journal-Lancet *59:*524-525, Dec '39
Celloidin tube reconstruction of extensor digitorum communis sheath. MAYER, L. Bull. Hosp. Joint Dis. *1:*39-45, July '40
Injuries of flexor tendons of hand. BETTS, L. O., M. J. Australia *2:*457-460, Nov 9, '40
Suturing of flexor tendons (transfixation) in hand. BOVE, C. M. Rec. *153:*94, Feb 5, '41
Treatment of tendons in compound injuries to hand. BUNNELL, S., J. Bone and Joint Surg. *23:*240-250, April '41
Hand tendon injuries; study of 116 cases. HOOKER, D. H. AND LAM, C. R. Am. J. Surg. *54:*412-416, Nov '41
Surgery of intrinsic muscles other than those producing opposition of thumb. BUNNELL, S., J. Bone and Joint Surg. *24:*1-31, Jan '42
Repair of severed tendons of hand and wrist; statistical analysis of 300 cases. MILLER, H. Surg., Gynec. and Obst. *75:*693-698, Dec '42
Post-traumatic hematoma of tendon sheaths. PIULACHS, P. AND ARANDES, R. Rev. clin. espan. *8:*435-436, March 30, '43
Results of repair of flexor tendons of wrist, hand and fingers. IVANISSEVICH, O. AND RIVAS, C. I. Bol. y trab., Acad. argent. de cir. *27:*576-583, July 28, '43
Spontaneous cicatrization of section of tendon of extensor pollicis longus (biologic therapy); cases. TAULLARD, J. C. Bol. y trab., Soc. argent. de cirujanos *4:*772-776, '43 also: Rev. Asoc. med. argent. *57:*1018-1019, Nov 30, '43
Plastic repair of section of flexor tendons of hand and of median nerve; case. MARINO, H. Prensa med. argent. *31:*1305-1308, July 12, '44
Wounds of hand tendons; analysis of 168 cases. CASANUEVA DEL C., M. AND FLUHMANN D., G. Rev. med. de Chile

Hands, Tendon Injuries in—Cont.
*72:*1044–1048, Dec '44
Occupational injury of hand (palmar tendon injury of agricultural workers). CHAN, L. F. Caribbean M. J. (no. 5) *6:*341–342, '44
Tendon surgery of hand. MOBERG, E. Nord. med. (Hygiea) *25:*535–539, March 23, '45
Cutting wound of wrist with section of tendon and radial artery; functional restitution. SEARA, P. Prensa med. argent. *32:*674–675, April 13, '45
Treatment of injuries of tendons of hand. HERTZBERG, J. Nord. med. *31:*1893–1897, Aug 23, '46
Tendon transplantation in hand. MAY, H. Surg., Gynec. and Obst. *83:*631–638, Nov '46

Hands, Tendon Ruptures in

Tardy rupture of tendon with fracture of radius. AXHAUSEN, G. Beitr. z. klin. Chir. *133:*78–88, '25
Late rupture of extensor pollicis longus tendon after fracture of radius. LASSEN, E. Hospitalstid. *72:*460–464, April 25, '29
Treatment of rupture of extensor tendons of phalanges of hand. SILFVERSKIÖLD, N. Zentralbl. f. Chir. *56:*3210, Dec 21, '29
Explanation of late rupture of extensor pollicis longus following fracture of radius. KLEINSCHMIDT, K. Beitr. z. klin. Chir. *146:*530–535, '29
Rupture of tendons of hand; with study of extensor tendon insertions in fingers. MASON, M. L. Surg., Gynec. and Obst. *50:*611–624, March '30
Late subcutaneous rupture of tendon of extensor pollicis longus after fracture of radius and other bone changes in region of injury. HORWITZ, A. Deutsche Ztschr. f. Chir. *234:*710–722, '31
Late rupture of tendon of extensor pollicis longus after fracture of radius; case. CLEMETSEN, N. Norsk mag. f. laegevidensk. *99:*1322–1328, Dec '38

Hands, Tumors of

Isolated giant cell xanthomatic tumors of fingers and hand. MASON, M. L. AND WOOLSTON, W. H. Arch. Surg. *15:*499–529, Oct '27
Angiomatosis of back of hands. GATÉ, J. *et al.* Bull. Soc. franc. de dermat. et syph. (Reunion dermat., Lyon) *39:*1575–1577, Dec '32
Cavernous angiomas of tendons of hands. BOTTO MICCA, A. Riv. san. siciliana *22:*568–577, April 15, '34

Hands, Tumors of—Cont.
Primary new growths involving hand. SCHREINER, B. F. AND WEHR, W. H. Am. J. Roentgenol. *32:*516–523, Oct '34
Synoviomas of tendon sheaths and of serous bursae. ZWAHLEN, P. Bull. Assoc. franc. p. l'étude du cancer *24:*682–707, Dec '35
Treatment of ganglion. SAEGESSER, M. Schweiz. med. Wchnschr. *66:*663–664, July 11, '36
Tumors of hand. MASON, M. L. Surg., Gynec. and Obst. *64:*129–148, Feb '37
Tumors and swellings of hand. ECKHOFF, N. Guy's Hosp. Gaz. *51:*199–204, May 8, '37
Enormous angioma of bones of hand; case. TANGUY, R. Gaz. med. de France (supp. Cah. radiol.) *45:*371–373, Feb 15, '38
Tumors of the Hands and Feet, by GEORGE T. PACK. C. V. Mosby Co., St. Louis, 1939
Tumors of synovia, tendons and joint capsules (hand). BRUNSCHWIG, A. Surgery *5:*101–111, Jan '39
Angiomas of hands and feet. OUGHTERSON, A. W. AND TENNANT, R. Surgery *5:*73–100, Jan '39
Hemangioma of hand muscles. SORENSEN, F. Klin. Wchnschr. *20:*222–224, March 1, '41
Benign tumors of hand and fingers. DESJARDINS, E. Union med. du Canada *70:*999–1001, Sept '41
Hemangioma of hand, involving phalangeal bones, with distinctive radiologic appearance. HIRSCHFELD, K. Australian and New Zealand J. Surg. *11:*136–139, Oct '41
Therapy of so-called ganglia of wrist. VOIGT, H. W. Ztschr. f. arztl. Fortbild. *39:*55–57, Feb 1, '42
Solitary enchondromas of hand bones; 3 cases treated surgically. AHLBERG, A. Acta chir. Scandinav. *89:*75–80, '43
Ganglion (of wrist); case (treated with sylnasol, fatty acid solution). VAN DEN BERG, W. J. California and West. Med. *60:*24, Jan '44
Mixed tumor of salivary gland type on left hand. HIGHMAN, B. Arch. Path. *37:*387–388, June '44
Pigmented mole of hand. STOUT, A. P. Texas State J. Med. *41:*579–580, Mar '46

Hands, Vascular Injuries of

Treatment of ischemic contracture of wrist. RESCHKE, K. Beitr. z. klin. Chir. *147:*302–307, '29
Traumatic thrombosis of deep palmar vein (case). SNYDER, M. H. AND SNYDER, W. H. JR. J. A. M. A. *111:*2007–2008, Nov 26, '38
Arterial occlusion in hands and fingers asso-

Hands Vascular Injuries of–Cont.
ciated with repeated trauma. BARKER, N. W. AND HINES, E. A. JR. Proc. Staff Meet., Mayo Clin. *19:*345–349, June 28, '44
Aneurysm of palmar arteries; case. Mil. Surgeon *97:*486–489, Dec '45

HANELIN, H. A.: Modern treatment of traumatic shock. J. Michigan M. Soc. *40:*876–881, Nov '41
HANKE, H.: Necrosis of finger tips following use of local anesthetic in operation for contracture; study of epinephrine toxicity. Chirurg *8:*684–687, Sept 1, '36
HANNAY, J. W.: Burn therapy with envelope irrigation (with electrolytic sodium hypochlorite solution). Brit. M. J. *2:*46–48, July 12, '41
HANNETT, J. W.: Autogenous bone inlay; its indications and advantages. Southwestern Med. *5:*1, Dec '21
HANNS, CHAUMERLIAC, J. AND WALTER, E. V.: Traumatic deformity "en coup de vent," preventing extension of hand and fingers; case. Strasbourg-med. (pt. 2) *88:*392, Dec 20, '28
HANRAHAN, E. M.: Split thickness graft as covering following removal of fingernail. Surgery *20:*398–400, Sept '46
HANRAHAN, E. M. AND DANDY, W. E.: Procedure to correct facial paralysis (by spinofacial anastomosis and fascial strips). J. A. M. A. *124:*1051-1053, April 8, '44
HANRAHAN, E. M. JR. Surgical treatment of rhinophyma, with report of case. Bull. Johns Hopkins Hosp. *32:*49, Feb '21
HANSEN, H. C. (see COBEY, M. C. *et al*) July '43
HANSEN, H. C. (see COBEY, M. C. *et al*) June '44
HANSEN, P.: Tannic acid in burns. Ugesk. f. laeger *97:*1–6, Jan 3, '35
HANSEN, T. L.: Burn therapy. Indust. Med. *9:*251–254, May '40
HANSON, A. M.: Costo-chondral graft for the repair of skull defects. Minnesota Med. *7:*610–612, Sept '24
HANSON, A. M.; *et al*.: Costochondral graft for repair of skull defects. Mil. Surgeon *48:*691, June '21
HANSON, R. Tendovaginitis or tendinitis stenosans. Acta chir. Scandinav. *60:*281–286, '26 (in English)
HANSON, W. A. (see FOWLER, L. H.) Oct '35
HANSSEN, S. A.: Exstrophy of bladder, ureteral transplantation. Hospitalstid *79:*285–292, March 24, '36
HARBERT, F.: Effective operation for entropion in trachoma. Am. J. Ophth. *21:*268–271, March '38
HARBERT, F.: Correction of saddleback deformities of nose by specially cut cartilage from ear. Arch. Otolaryng. *31:*339–341, Feb '40
HARBERT, F.: Correction of lateral displacement of free border of nasal septal cartilage. Arch. Otolaryng. *31:*341–343, Feb '40
HARBIN, M. AND LIBER, K. E.: Behavior of transplanted bone; clinical consideration. Surg., Gynec. and Obst. *59:*149–160, Aug '34
HARBIN, M. AND MORITZ, A. R.: Autogenous free cartilage transplanted into joints; experimental study. Arch. Surg. *20:*885–896, June '30
HARBIN, M. (see McGAW, W. H.) Oct '34
HARBISON, S. P. AND ODEN, L. H., JR.: Split skin grafts in early closure of wounds. Bull. U. S. Army M. Dept. *6:*88–90, July '46
HARBITZ, H. F.: Staphylopharyngoplasty by Rosenthal's method. Norsk. Mag. f. Laegevidensk. *90:*13–16, Jan '29
HARCOURT, A. K. (see REED, J. V.) May '39
D'HARCOURT, J.: Substitute tenoplasties in therapy of radial paralysis. Pasteur *1:*121–127, June 15, '43
D'HARCOURT, M.: Acute hand infections; surgical therapy. Medicina, Madrid *4:*5–42, Jan '33
HARDGROVE, M.: Recent advances in use of human serum and plasma in shock. Wisconsin M. J. *42:*298–302, March '43
HARDIE, D.: Case of myasthenia gravis operated on for eyelid ptosis by Hess's method. Brit. J. Ophth. *12:*31–33, Jan '28
HARDIN, P. C.: Cod liver oil in burns. North Carolina M. J. *1:*82–91, Feb '40
HARDIN, P. C.: Cod liver oil in burns. South. Surgeon *10:*301–338, May '41
HARDIN, P. C.: Cod liver oil in burns. South. Surgeon *11:*691–728, Oct '42
HARDING, R. L.: Congenital preauricular sinus. Am. J. Orthodontics (Oral Surg. Sect.) *28:*399–401, July '42
HARDMAN, J.: Pulp-space infection of fingers. Brit. M. J. *2:*156–160, July 24, '37
HARDWICK, R. S. (see RANDALL, L. M.) June '34
HARDY, E. A.: Cleft palate and harelip; adolescent case treated orthodontically in conjunction with lip-stretching device and skin grafting of labial sulcus. Internat. J. Orthodontia *20:*750–758, Aug '34
HARDY, E. A.: New Cupid's-bow operation (in harelip). Lancet *1:*361, Feb 24, '40
HARDY, E. A.: Epithelial inlays to labial sulcus of mandible. Proc. Roy. Soc. Med. *38:*645–646, Sept '45 (Comment on Fickling's article)
HARDY, S. B.: Rehabilitation of injured hand. Am. J. Surg. *72:*352–362, Sept '46
HARDY, S. B. AND McNICHOL, J. W.: Use of small pieces of film-covered skin grafts. S. Clin. North America *24:*281–292, April '44

HARET: Rhinophyma; case cured by radiotherapy. Bull. et mem. Soc. de radiol. med. de France *16:*236, Nov '28

HARKINS, C. S.: Responsibility of prosthodontist in treatment of cleft palate. Am. J. Orthodontics (Oral Surg. Sect.) *32:*684-687, Nov '46

HARKINS, H. N.: Rate of fluid shift and its relation to onset of shock in severe experimental burns. Arch. Surg. *31:*71-85, July '35

HARKINS, H. N.: Bleeding volume in severe burns. Ann. Surg. *102:*444-454, Sept '35

HARKINS, H. N.: Correlation of clinical treatment of burns with recent experimental studies. Illinois M. J. *70:*332-338, Oct '36

HARKINS, H. N. Surgical shock from burns, freezing and similar traumatic agents. Colorado Med. *33:*871-876, Dec '36

HARKINS, H. N.: Hemangioma of tendon or tendon sheath; report of case with study of 24 cases from literature. Arch. Surg. *34:*12-22, Jan '37

HARKINS, H. N.: Recent advances in study of burns. Surgery *3:*430-465, March '38

HARKINS, H. N.: Acute ulcer of duodenum (Curling's ulcer) as complication of burns; relation to sepsis; report of case with study of 107 cases collected from literature, 94 with necropsy, 13 with recovery; experimental studies. Surgery *3:*608-641, April '38

HARKINS, H. N.: Recent advances in study and management of traumatic shock. Surgery *9:*231, Feb; 447, March; 607, April '41

HARKINS, H. N.: Treatment of shock in wartime (Theodore A. McGraw memorial lecture). War Med. *1:*520-555, July '41

HARKINS, HENRY: *Treatment of Burns.* C C Thomas Co., Springfield, Ill., 1942

HARKINS, H. N.: Shock from war injuries. J. Michigan M. Soc. *41:*287-293, April '42

HARKINS, H. N.: Burn therapy in wartime. (Ernest Edward Irons lecture). J.A.M.A. *119:*385-390, May 30, '42

HARKINS, H. N.: Local treatment of thermal burns. Ann. Surg. *115:*1140-1151, June '42

HARKINS, H. N.: Local treatment of burns. Clinics *1:*6-24, June '42

HARKINS, H. N.: Shock and anesthesia. Anesth. and Analg. *21:*273-279, Sept-Oct '42

HARKINS, H. N.: Burn therapy. Proc. Interst. Postgrad. M. A. North America (1942) pp. 245-246, '43

HARKINS, H. N.: Physiologic aspects of burn therapy. Am. Acad. Orthop. Surgeons, Lect., pp. 186-188, '43

HARKINS, H. N.: New type of relaxing incision—dermatome-flap method. Am. J. Surg. *59:*79-82, Jan '43

HARKINS, H. N.: Treatment of shock. Illinois M. J. *83:*325-331, May '43

HARKINS, H. N.: Burn therapy. Illinois M. J. *84:*103-106, Aug '43 (abstract) also: S. Clin. North America *23:*1233-1258, Oct '43

HARKINS, H. N.: Local treatment of burns. Dia med. *16:*30-34, Jan 10, '44

HARKINS, H. N.: Problem of thermal burns: 1944. J.A.M.A. *125:*533-536, June 24, '44

HARKINS, H. N.: Burn therapy. J. South Carolina M. A. *41:*27-30, Feb '45

HARKINS, H. N.: General care of burn patient. Nebraska M. J. *30:*175-176, May '45

HARKINS, H. N.: Cutis grafts. Clinical and experimental studies on use as reinforcing patch in repair of large ventral and incisional hernias. Ann. Surg. *122:*996-1015, Dec '45

HARKINS, H. N. AND HARMON, P. H.: Plasma exudation; loss of plasma-like fluid in various conditions resembling surgical shock; experimental study. Ann. Surg. *106:*1070-1083, Dec '37

HARKINS, H. N.; HARMON, P. H. AND HUDSON, J. E.: Lethal factors in bile peritonitis; "surgical shock." Arch. Surg. *33:*576-608, Oct '36

HARKINS, H. N.; LAM, C. R. AND ROMENCE, H.: Plasma in severe burns. Surg., Gynec. and Obst. *75:*410-420, Oct '42

HARKINS, H. N. AND LONG, C. N. H.: Metabolic changes in shock after burns. Am. J. Physiol. *144:*661-668, Oct '45

HARKINS, H. N. AND MCCLURE, R. D.: Present status of intravenous fluid treatment of traumatic and surgical shock. Ann. Surg. *114:*891-906, Nov '41

HARKINS, H. N. *et al*: Fluid and nutritional therapy in burns. J.A.M.A. *128:*475-479, June 16, '45

HARKINS, H. N. AND ROOME, N. W.: Concealed hemorrhage into tissues and its relation to traumatic shock. Arch. Surg. *35:*130-139, July '37

HARKINS, H. N.; WILSON, E. C. AND STEWART, C. P.: Depressor action of extracts of burned skin. Proc. Soc. Exper. Biol. and Med. *32:*913-914, March '35

HARKINS, H. N. (see KANTHAK, F. F.) Dec '38

HARKINS, H. N. (see LAM, C. R.) April '42

HARKINS, H. N. (see SWENSON, S. A. JR.) Dec '43

HARMER, T. W.: Certain phases of surgery of hand. S. Clin. N. America *2:*973-994, Aug '22 (illus.)

HARMER, T. W.: Hand surgery. New England J. Med. *214:*613-617, March 26, '36

HARMER, T. W.: Hand injuries. Am. J. Surg. *42:*638-658, Dec '38

HARMER, T. W.: Traumatic lesions of nerves of wrist and hand. Am. J. Surg. *47:*517-541, Feb '40

HARMON, P. H. (see HARKINS, H. N. *et al*) Oct '36

HARMON, P. H. (see HARKINS, H. N.) Dec '37

HARPER, F. R. (see NEW, G. B.) Aug '33

HARPER, H. D.: Use of cotter key in intermaxillary ligation allowing quick release in case of nausea and vomiting. Am. J. Orthodontics *29:*373–382, July '43

HARPER, R. A. K. (see BROWN, A.) July '46

HARPER, R. A. K. (see HARTLEY, H.) Nov '37

HARPER, W. F.: Distribution of palmar aponeurosis in relation to contracture of thumb. J. Anat. *69:*193–195, Jan '35

HARRELL, G. T. AND VALK, A. DET.: Autogenous transplantation of fibrosarcoma during application of full-thickness skin graft. Ann. Surg. *111:*285–291, Feb '40

HARRENSTEIN, R. J.: Double penis and scrotum (diphallus); case. Beitr. z. klin. Chir. *154:*308–314, '31

HARRENSTEIN, R. J.: Surgical therapy of harelip in children. Nederl. tijdschr. v. geneesk. *76:*5557–5566, Dec 3, '32

HARRENSTEIN, R. J.: Angiomas of skin in infants; therapy. Maandschr. v. kindergeneesk. *3:*388–395, July '34

HARRENSTEIN, R. J.: Syndactylia and its therapy. Maandschr. v. kindergeneesk. *6:*131–147, Jan '37

HARRENSTEIN, R. J. Snapping thumb in young children. Nederl. tijdschr. v. geneesk. *81:*1237–1241, March 20, '37

HARRENSTEIN, R. J.: Burns in children. Maandschr. v. kindergeneesk. *7:*179–191, Feb '38

HARRENSTEIN, R. J.: Therapy of hypospadias. Nederl. tijdschr. v. geneesk. *82:*2963–2974, June 11, '38

HARRENSTEIN, R. J.: Therapy of anus atresia. Nederl. tijdschr. v. geneesk. *90:*698–700, June 22, '46

HARRIS, E. (see BLOCK, L. S.) March '42

HARRIS, H. E. (see MOORE, P. M. JR.) Dec '40

HARRIS, H. E. JR.: Congenital deformities of forearm, hand, and leg. Brit. M. J. *1:*711, April 19, '24

HARRIS, H. I.: Advantages of split graft following tonsillectomy. Ann. Otol., Rhin. and Laryng. *47:*1045–1048, Dec '38

HARRIS, H. I.: Heterogenous grafts by coagulum contact method. Am. J. Surg. *65:*315–320, Sept '44

HARRIS, H. I.: New technic for correction of macrostomia. J. Oral Surg. *3:*156–163, April '45

HARRIS, L. W. AND CHRISTIANSEN, G. W.: Fracture of mandible at angle; appliance to depress posterior fragment. J. Oral Surg. *3:*212–214, July '45

HARRIS, M.: Role of humoral antagonism (due to cytotoxins) in heteroplastic transplantation in mammals. J. Exper. Zool. *93:*131–145, June '43

HARRIS, M. H.: Burn therapy in home (tannic acid). Virginia M. Monthly *65:*403–404, July '38

HARRIS, M. H. AND WOODHALL, B.: Plastic closure of defect of cranium; case report illustrating use of tantalum plate and pedicle-tube graft. Surgery *17:*422–428, March '45

HARRIS, M. M.: Free grafts in plastic surgery. Semana med. *2:*841–844, Oct 7, '43

HARRIS, M. M. (see PAVLOVSKY, A. J.) Sept '42

HARRIS, M. M. (see PAVLOWSKY, A. J. *et al*) Feb '46

HARRIS, R. I.: Haemorrhage into suprarenal capsule and haemorrhage from duodenal ulcer in burns; case. Clin. J. *59:*150–152, March 26, '30

HARRIS, W. AND WRIGHT, A. D.: Treatment of clonic facial spasm; alcohol injection; nerve anastomosis (with hypoglossal). Lancet *1:*657–662, March 26, '32

HARRISON, F. G.: Epispadias totalis. Pennsylvania M. J. *36:*589–590, May '33

HARRISON, G. A. AND PICKEN, L. E. R.: Quantitative aspects of transfusion in shock. Lancet *1:*685–686, May 31, '41

HARRISON, R. S.: Surgical and radiotherapy of cancer of lips. Strahlentherapie *46:*401–434, '33 Abstr.: Schweiz. med. Wchnschr. *63:*159–162, Feb 18, '33

HARRISON, W. G. JR.: Clinical types of circulatory failure and their treatment. J. M. A. Alabama *8:*305–309, March '39

HARRISON, W. J.: Extensive epithelioma of cheek and lower jaw treated by diathermy. Brit. M. J. *2:*102, July 21, '28

HARRISON, W. J.: Traumatic stenosis of trachea treated by skin grafting. Brit. M. J. *2:*811, Oct 24, '36

HARROLD, T. JR.: Tannic acid in burns. J. M. A. Georgia *17:*286–288, July '28

HARROWER, J. G.: Treatment of cystic hygroma by sodium morrhuate. Brit. M. J. *2:*148, July 22, '33

HARRYMAN, W. K. (see SNEDECOR, S. T.) Sept '40

HART, A.: Ureterointestinal anastomosis by Reimer method; preliminary results in case of exstrophy in boy. Zentralbl. f. Chir. *69:*1485–1495, Sept 12, '42

DEHART, R. M.: Gentian violet in burns. Virginia M. Monthly *62:*594–595, Jan '36

HART, V. K.: Dermoid cyst of dorsum of nose; citation of case. Laryngoscope *37:*760–763, Oct '27

HART, V. L.: Fundamental principles of bone transplantation. J. Michigan M. Soc. *31:*184-187, March '32

HART, V. L.: Simple and efficient finger splint. J. Bone and Joint Surg. *19:*245, Jan '37

HÄRTEL, F.: Treatment of suppuration in fingers. Klin. Wchnschr. *1:*484-487, March 4, '22

HÄRTEL, F.: Unilateral harelip; fundamental principles of operation. Beitr. z. klin. Chir. *144:*313-319, '28

HÄRTEL, F. F.: Treatment of harelip and other facial fissures. Chirurg *2:*1057-1061, Dec 1, '30

HARTER, J. H.: Plastic surgery, facio-maxillary; case reports. Northwest Med. *25:*404-408, Aug '26

HARTER, J. H.: Plastic surgery; depressed forehead following Kilian operation; repaired by fat grafts. Northwest Med. *26:*313-314, June '27

HARTER, J. H.: Plastic surgery of face; recent contributions, present status. Northwest Med. *28:*185-187, April '29

HARTER, J. H.: Plastic surgery; convex nose in women. Northwest Med. *30:*74-77, Feb '31

HARTER, J. S. (see LOEB, L.) Nov '26

HARTLEY, H. AND HARPER, R. A. K.: Elephantiasis; lymphangioplasty—fate of silk. Brit. M. J. *2:*1066-1067, Nov 27, '37

HARTMAN, F. W. AND ROMENCE, H. L.: Liver necrosis in burns. Ann. Surg. *118:*402-416, Sept '43

HARTMAN, F. W. AND SCHELLING, V.: Studies on hexyl-chloro-m-cresol and other carbocyclic antiseptics (for use with tannic acid) in burns. Am. J. Surg. *46:*460-467, Dec '39

HARTMAN, F. W., *et al*: Pectin solution as blood substitute in shock therapy. Ann. Surg. *114:*212-225, Aug '41

HARTMAN, F. W., *et al*: Relative value of pectin solution in shock therapy. J.A.M.A. *121:*1337-1342, April 24, '43

HARTMANN, E.: Loss of external ear and its artificial replacement. Nord. med. tidskr. *11:*728-729, May 2, '36

HARTMANN, H.: Formation of artificial vagina. Gynec. et obst. *25:*401-403, May, '32

HARTMANN, M.: Importance of department for plastic surgery and advisory center for disfigurations at dermatologic clinic. Dermat. Wchnschr. *111:*1089-1091, Dec 21, '40

HARTSTEIN, S. D.: Simplified maxillary anesthesia. Am. Dent. Surgeon *48:*90, Feb '28

HARTTUNG, H.: Burns and their treatment. Therap. Hallomonatsh. *35:*464, Aug 1, '21

HARTTUNG, H.: Artificial vagina made from rectum (Schubert's method). Zentralbl. f. Gynak. *46:*1610-1612, Oct 7, '22

HARTTUNG, H.: Total avulsion of scalp with comment on treatment of wound; case. Zentralbl. f. Chir. *66:*951-953, April 22, '39

HARTTUNG, H.: Burn therapy. Med. Klin. *37:*129-132, Feb 7, '41

HARTUNG, F.: Hemorrhage in nasal septal resection. Rev. oto-laring. de Sao Paulo *6:*379-382, Sept-Oct '38

HARTWICH, A.: Conservative cosmetic correction of legs. Wien. med. Wchnschr. *79:*368-370, March 16, '29

HARTZELL, J. B.: Restoration of rectum after injury. U. S. Nav. M. Bull. *42:*1151-1155, May '44

HARVEY, S. C.: Modification of operation of Bucknall for hypospadias. Ann. Surg. *77:*572-579, May '23 (illus.)

HARVEY, S. C. (see CONNOR, G. J.) 1944

HARVEY, S. C. (see CONNOR, G. J.) Sept '44

HARVEY, S. C. (see CONNOR, G. J.) Nov '46

HARWELL, W. R.: Radium treatment of hemangiomata. New Orleans M. and S. J. *92:*576-580, April '40

HASAMA, T. (see YOKOTA, K.) 1935

HASEGAWA, T.: Symptoms of aural fistula. Oto-rhino-laryng. *14:*691-696, Sept '41 (in Japanese)

HASENBALG, A.: Prontosil (sulfonamide) in burns; cases. Semana med. *2:*755-756, Oct 12, '44

HASHIMOTO, T. (see MAEKAWA, S.) Sept '41

HASLAM, E. T. (see READ, F. L.) Jan '44

HASS, J.: Transplantation of tendons in paralysis of radial nerve. Wien. klin. Wchnschr. *42:*642-644, May 9, '29

HASS, J.: Surgical treatment of syndactylia. Zentralbl. f. Chir. *56:*1413-1416, June 8, '29

HASSON (see TERRIEN, F. *et al*) April '31

HAUBENREISSER, W.: Lymph drainage in elephantiasis. Zentralbl. f. Chir. *49:*474-475, April 8, '22 abstr: J.A.M.A. *79:*511, Aug 5, '22

HAUCK, G.: Tendovaginitis and snapping finger. Arch. f. klin. Chir. *123:*233-258, '23 (illus.)

HAUCK, G.: Operation for rupture of thumb tendon and fracture of radius. Arch. f. klin. Chir. *124:*81-91, '23 (illus.)

HAUCK, G.: Injury, regeneration and suture of tendons. Arch. f. klin. Chir. *128:*568-585, '24

HAUCK, G.: Contractures of thumbs in children. Med. Klinik *20:*1465-1466, Oct 19, '24

HAUCK, G. J.: Suture of avulsion of extension tendon of last phalanx. Med. Welt *3:*1657, Nov 16, '29

HAUENSTEIN, K.: Gunshot wounds to jaws; therapy and prognosis. Med. Welt *14:*1189-1193, Nov 23, '40

HAUGEN, F. P.: General anesthesia for jaw casualties. Mil. Surgeon *89:*70-80, July '41

HAUN, E.: Surgical shock. J. Tennessee M. A.

*37:*57-61, Feb '44
HÄUPL, K.: Modern principles in maxillary orthopedics. Wien. klin. Wchnschr. *54:*131-132, Feb 14, '41
HAUSER, G.: Traumatic tendovaginitis crepitans; case. Deutsche Ztschr. f. d. ges. gerichtl. Med. *15:*242-245, May 18, '30
HAUSMANN, R.: Question of external or internal dacryocystorhinostomy. Arch. f. Ohren-, Nasen-u. Kehlkopfh. *149:*309-316, '41
HAUTANT, A.: Maxillofacial fractures. Ann. d'oto-laryng., pp. 169-194, March-April '40
HAUTANT, A. AND LANOS: Lymphangioma of nose. Ann. d. mal. de l'oreille, du larynx *46:*1235, Dec '27
HAUTANT, A. AND MONOD, O.: Operative treatment of radium resistant epitheliomata; cases. (of nose.) Ann. d. mal. de l'oreille, du larynx *49:*394-410, April '30
HAUTANT, A.; MONOD, O. AND VERGER, G.: Surgery associated with radium in treatment of epitheliomas of upper jaw. J. de chir. *28:*257-274, Sept '26
HAVENS, F. Z.: Multiple fractures of upper and lower jaws. Proc. Staff Meet., Mayo Clin. *7:*433-434, July 27, '32
HAVENS, F. Z.: Lined pedicled flaps in reconstructive surgery of face; modification of technic. S. Clin. North America *12:*955-957, Aug '32
HAVENS, F. Z.: Simplified method of local anesthesia for removal of sebaceous cysts. S. Clin. North America *15:*1230-1232, Oct '35
HAVENS, F. Z.: Congenital preauricular sinus; treatment. Arch. Otolaryng. *29:*985-986, June '39
HAVENS, F. Z.: Preoperative and postoperative care in skin grafts. S. Clin. North America *20:*1087-1092, Aug '40
HAVENS, F. Z.: Reconstruction of columella nasi; method advantageous for female patient. S. Clin. North America *25:*877-879, Aug '45
HAVENS, F. Z. AND DIX, C. R.: Axillary-iliac tubed flap in neck surgery. Proc. Staff Meet., Mayo Clin. *17:*167-169, March 18, '42
HAVENS, F. Z. (see JUDD, E. S. JR.) Nov '43
HAVENS, F. Z. (see NEW, G. B.) 1931
HAVENS, F. Z. (see NEW, G. B.) Sept '31
HAVENS, F. Z. (see NEW, G. B. *et al*) June '34
HAWK, G. W.: Traction splint for fractured metacarpals and phalanges. J.A.M.A. *78:*106, Jan 14, '22 (illus.)
HAWKINS, G. (see SHREVES, H. B.) Jan '46
HAWKINS, T. L.: Treatment of injuries to hand requiring skin grafting. Am. J. Surg. *59:* 383-391, Feb '43
HAWN, C. V. *et al*: Fibrinogen and thrombin in surface treatment of burns. J. Clin. Investigation *23:*580-585, July '44
HAXTHAUSEN, H.: Pathogenesis of allergic eczema elucidated by transplantation experiments on identical twins. Acta dermat.-venereol. *23:*438-454, Jan '43
HAY, A. W. S.: Cancer of lip and mouth. Manitoba M. A. Rev. *18:*231-234, Dec '38
HAYASHI, Y.: Submucous cleft of palate. Otorhino-laryng. (Abstr. Sect) *13:*60, Nov '40
HAYD, F. W.: Congenital hypoplasia of thumb. Deutsche med. Wchnschr. *64:*1041-1042, July 15, '38
HAYDEN, R.: Burn therapy; activities of Naval Hospital at Pearl Harbor following Japanese air raid of December 7, 1941; comments on care of battle casualties. Am. J. Surg. *60:*161-181, May '43
HAYDEN, R.: Summary of present burn treatment. New York State J. Med. *43:*1213-1219, July 1, '43
HAYDEN, R.: Experiences with burns at Naval Hospital, Pearl Harbor during and after Japanese air raid of December 7, 1941. J. Internat. Coll. Surgeons *6:*259-268, July-Aug '43
HAYDEN, R.: Present treatment of burns. J. Internat. Coll. Surgeons *7:*179-190, May-June '44
HAYES, B. A.: Treatment of urethral fistula. J. Oklahoma M. A. *31:*33-35, Feb '38
HAYES, W. M.: Hand fractures. South. Surgeon *11:*105-112, Feb '42
HAYLLAR, B. L. (see STRUMIA, M. M. *et al*) Nov '41
HAYMANN, L.: Septal structural changes; sequels and therapy. Med. Klin. *35:*1365-1368, Oct 20. '39
HAYNEN, A. S.: Statistical report of series of fractures of jaw. Am. J. Orthodontics *25:*478-480, May '39
HAYNEN, A. S.: Mandibular resection. Am. J. Orthodontics *26:*793-796, Aug '40
HAYNER, J. C. (see TARLOV, I. M. *et al*) Nov '46
HAYNES, L. K.: Wounds and deformities of orbital region. Mil. Surgeon *91:*83-90, July '42
HAYS, H.: Relationship between otolaryngologist and plastic surgeon. Am. J. Surg. *31:*38-47, Jan '36
HAYS, H. W. (see SWINGLE, W. W. *et al*) May '44
HAYS, S. C.: Problems in minor traumatic surgery of hand. J. South Carolina M. A. *36:*33-37, Feb '40
HAYWARD: Treatment of decubitus. Med. Klin. *25:*1328-1329, Aug 23, '29
HAYWARD: Repair of cutaneous defects. Med. Klin. *25:*1365, Aug 30; 1397, Sept 6, '29

HAYWARD: Technic and value of Thiersch's method of skin grafting. Med. Klin. *25:*1435-1437, Sept 13, '29

HAYWARD: Burn therapy. Med. Klin. *25:*1501-1511, Sept 27, '29

HAYWARD: Surgical treatment of roentgen ray burns. Med. Klin. *25:*1548-1550, Oct 4, '29

HAYWARD: Surgical treatment of furunculosis. Med. Klin. *25:*1631-1632, Oct 18, '29

HAYWARD: Surgical treatment of atheroma. Med. Klin. *26:*668-669, May 2, '30

HAYWARD: Surgical treatment of diseases of lymphatic apparatus. Med. Klin. *27:*96-97, Jan 16, '31

HAYWARD: Surgical treatment of Volkmann's contracture. Med. Klin. *27:*473-474, March 27, '31

HAYWARD: Surgical treatment of tendovaginitis crepitans and abscesses of sheaths. Med. Klin. *27:*1321-1322, Sept 4, '31

HAYWARD: Treatment of gonorrhea of tendon sheaths. Med. Klin. *27:*1683-1684, Nov 13, '31

HAYWARD: Surgical treatment of Dupuytren's contracture. Med. Klin. *27:*1721-1722, Nov 20, '31

HAZEN, H. H.: Roentgen-ray treatment of keloids. Am. J. Roentgenol. *11:*547-549, June '24

HAZEN, S. F.: Total rhinoplasty; cases. Proc. Staff Meet., Mayo Clin. *5:*69-71, March 12, '30

Head

Plastic and cosmetic surgery of head, neck and face. (including keloids). TIECK, G. J. E. AND HUNT, H. L. Am. J. Surg. *35:*173, June '21; 355, Nov '21

Plastic and cosmetic surgery of head, face and neck; correction of nasal deformities. TIECK, G. J. E. AND HUNT, H. L. Am. J. Surg. *35:*234, Aug '21

Plastic surgery of head, face and neck, local anesthesia in operations upon head, face and neck. TIECK, G. J. E. *et al.* Am. J. Surg. *36:*29-42, Feb '22 (illus.)

Plastic surgery of head and neck. RISDON, F. Canad. M.A.J. *12:*797-798, Nov '22

Surgery of head without scars. DUFOURMENTEL, L. Medecine *5:*52, Oct '23

Plastic surgery about face, head and neck. BECK, J. C., J. Indiana M. A. *18:*167-184, May '25

Principles in plastic surgery about head and neck (and nose). BECK, J. C. Illinois M. J. *48:*194-202, Sept '25

Electro-coagulation (surgical diathermy) in multiple angiomata of head. LALVANI, P. P. Indian M. Gaz. *64:*387-388, July '29

Head – Cont.

End-results in 20 cases of primary skin grafts in radical mastoidectomies. CUNNING, D. S. Laryngoscope *41:*484-486, July '31

Treatment of head scars in Japan. MAYEDA, T. Ztschr. d. japan. chirurg. Gesellsch. *35:*59-60, '34

Operative treatment of extensive angioma of head. SHILOVTSEV, S. P. Arch. f. klin. Chir. *184:*179-182, '35

Plastic surgery of head, face and neck; psychic reactions. BLAIR, V. P., J. Am. Dent. A. *23:*236-240, Feb '36

Surgical therapy of extensive angioma of head. SHILOVTSEV, S. P. Vestnik khir. *45:*236-239, '36

Tumors of head and neck. JORSTAD, L. H., J. Missouri M. A. *34:*82-84, March '37

Cancer of head and neck; management of lesions with borderline operability and curability. KIME, E. N. Arch. Phys. Therapy *20:*282-287, May '39

Plastic and reconstructive surgery about face and head – then and now. BECK, J. C. Illinois M. J. *76:*237-242, Sept '39

Progress of plastic surgery of head (including ears, mouth, jaws, nose, etc.); review of literature for 1939. REBELO NETO, J. Rev. brasil. de oto-rino-laring. *8:*111-120, March-April '40

Plastic repair following removal of neoplasms about head. FIGI, F. A. Nebraska M. J. *25:*165-171, May '40

Origin and nature of certain malformations of face, head and foot. KEITH, A. Brit. J. Surg. *28:*173-192, Oct '40

Plastic surgery of face. and head. JENKINS, H. P., S. Clin. North America *21:*37-53, Feb '41

Tumors of head and face. WOLFER, J. A. Indust. Med. *10:*59-60, Feb '41

Concepts of anatomy of head and neck. BUCHANAN, A. R. Am. J. Orthodontics *28:*152-166, March '42

Soft tissue repair in injuries about face and head. MARCKS, K. M. Pennsylvania M. J. *45:*801-806, May '42

Surgical progress; head and throat; review of literature for 1941. REBELO NETO, J. Rev. brasil. de oto-rino-laring. *10:*347-357, May-June '42

Tumors of head, face and neck. WOLFER, J. A. Indust. Med. *11:*528-529, Nov '42

Surgery of head, progress of plastic surgery; review of literature for 1942. REBELO NETO, J. Rev. brasil. de oto-rino-laring. *11:*173-185, March-April '43

Heald, C. B. (see Hobhouse, N.) April '36
Heath, P.: Instruments for eyelid treatment. Tr. Sect. Ophth., A. M. A., pp. 272-273, '36 also: Arch. Ophth. *17:*894-895, May '37
Heatley, T. F.: Surgical treatment of burns. Internat. J. Med. and Surg. *42:*360, July '29
Heatly, M. D.: Use of thromboplastin fixation in skin grafts. Texas State J. Med. *42:*275-278, Aug '46
Hebb, D. (see Brantigan, O. C.) July '43
Hebraud, A.: Two instruments for surgery of hand. Rev. med. nav. *1:*63-65, '46
Hecht, H.: Cutaneous epithelioma developing rapidly on upper lip after diathermic treatment of supposed verruca carnea; case. Dermat. Wchnschr. *88:*501-502, April 6, '29
Hechter, O.; Bergman, H. C. and Prinzmetal, M.: Comparison of therapeutic effectiveness of serum and sodium chloride in scald shock. Am. Heart J. *29:*484-492, April '45
Hechter, O.; Bergman, H. C. and Prinzmetal, M.: Role of renal pressor system in shock of burns. Am. Heart J. *29:*493-498, April '45
Hechter, O. *et al*: Liver principle which is effective against burn shock; further studies. Am. Heart J. *29:*499-505, April '45
Hechter, O. (see Bergman, H. C. *et al*) April '45
Hechter, O. (see Pinzmetal, M. *et al*) Dec '44
Heck,F.: Late results of sutures of tendons of arm and hand. Arch. f. orthop. u. Unfall-Chir. *39:*21-28, '38
Heckel, E. B.: Blepharochalasis with ptosis; report of case. Am. J. Ophth. *4:*273, April '21
Hecker, I. W.: Therapy of malformations and acquired lesions of palate. Rev. de stomatol. *35:*412-420, July '33
Hed, H.: Orthopedic-prosthetic therapy of fractures of condyloid process of mandible. Nord. med. (Hygiea) *18:*789-793, May 8, '43
Hedin, R. F.: Immediate and subsequent treatment of burns. Minnesota Med. *21:*229-236, April '38
Hedin, R. F. and Karp, M.: Pressure infusion; method of treating persistent shock. Anesth. and Analg. *18:*148-149, May-June '39
Hedin, R. F. (see Kabat, H.) May '42
Heermann, H.: Correction of bony wry and flat nose. Ztschr. f. Hals-, Nasen-u. Ohrenh. *23:*133-136, June 10, '29
Heermann, H.: Plastic surgery of ear. Ztschr. f. Hals-, Nasen-u, Ohrenh. *26:*35-41, May 6, '30
Heerup, L.: Familial symmetrical finger contracture (camptodactylia). Ugesk. f. laeger *91:*1072-1075, Nov 28, '29
Heesch, K.: Therapy of war wounds of eyelids and their surrounding area. Deut. Militararzt *8:*699, Dec '43
Heggie, J. F. and Heggie, R. M.: Antiseptic analgesic tannic acid jelly in burns. Lancet *2:*391, Sept 28, '40
Heggie, J. F. (see Heggie, R. M. *et al*) March '42
Heggie, J. F. (see Heggie, R. M.) Dec '42
Heggie, R. M.; Gerrard, E. A. and Heggie, J. F.: Superficial granulating areas treated with antiseptic emulsions in burns. Lancet *1:*347-350, March 21, '42
Heggie, R. M. and Heggie, J. F.: Infected burns in naval personnel. Lancet *2:*664-667, Dec 5, '42
Heggie, R. M. (see Heggie, J. F.) Sept '40
Heidenhain, L.: Abdominal skin flap after amputation of breast. Zentralbl. f. Gynak. *48:*2649-2650, Nov 29, '24
Heidler, H.: Total inversion of bladder; case. Wien. med. Wchnschr. *86:*1007-1009, Sept 5, '36
Heidrich, L.: Surgery in cancer of mouth and throat. Beitr. z. klin. Chir. *128:*310-347, '23 abstr: J.A.M.A. *80:*1348, May 5, '23
Heidt, E. (see Maxwell, M. M.) Oct '46
Heijl, C.: Malformations of mammary glands and their surgical correction. Hygiea (Festband) *100:*118-127, '38
Heilbronn, S.: Neglected treatment of cancer of face; case. Munchen. med. Wchnschr. *76:*374, March 1, '29
Heim, K.: Life and growth processes in explanted normal and malignant human tissue. Arch. f. Gynak. *134:*250-309, '28
Heim, W.: Modern views on etiology and therapy of syndactylia. Med. Welt *14:*481-483, May 11, '40
Heinberg, C. J.: Congenital bilateral anophthalmos and polydactylism with report of case. J. Florida M. A. *12:*253-256, April '26
Heinberg, C. J. (see Lischkoff, M. A.) Oct '26
Heindl, A. (see Hajek, M.) April, May '35
Heinemann, K.: Question of "cellular tissue decomposition" or wandering of leukocytes; testing of Busse-Grawitz experiments. Beitr. z. path. Anat. u. z. allg. Path. *106:*525-534, '42
Heinemann, O.: Plastic surgery of septum on account of saddle nose. Med. Klin. *26:*1188, Aug 8, '30
Heinemann, O.: Scarless reconstruction of nose broken in childhood. Med. Klin. *28:*1427-1428, Oct 7, '32
Heinsius, F.: Fate of patient in whom exstrophy of bladder was cured by Trendelenburg operation (synchondroseotomy). Zentralbl. f.

Gynak. *55:*322–332, Feb 7, '31 abstr.: Ztschr. f. Geburtsh. u. Gynak. *99:*187–191, '30

Heitz-Boyer-Hovelacque Operation

Exstrophy of bladder, treatment by Heitz-Boyer-Hovelacque operation; 9 cases. RIVAROLA, R. A. Semana med. *2:*1023–1027, Oct 20, '27

Heitz Operation: See: Marion-Heitz-Boyer Operation

HEJDUK, B.: Artificial vagina from sigmoid. Casop. lek. cesk. *70:*1458–1461, Oct 30, '31

HEJDUK, B.: Construction of vagina with loop from sigmoid. Bratisl. lekar. listy *15:*241–251, March '35

HEJDUK, B.: Plastic surgery of vagina aplasia, using portion of sigmoid flexure; review of literature and report of 2 personal cases. Zentralbl. f. Gynak. *63:*1298–1309, June 10, '39

HELBING, C.: Operative treatment of harelip and cleft palate. Allg. deutsche Hebam.-Ztg. *42:*193, July 1, '27

HELDERWEIRT, G.; SCHIEVERS, J. AND SIMONART, A.: Attempts at therapy after extensive burns; consideration of blood volume. Arch. internat. de pharmacodyn. et de therap. *60:*462–465, Dec 31, '38

HELFRICH, L. S.; CASSELS, W. H. AND COLE, W. H.: Cortical extract in treatment of shock; preliminary report. Am. J. Surg. *55:*410–426, Feb '42

HELLE: Extensive nevus covering nearly whole body. Deutsche med. Wchnschr. *48:*1316, Sept 26, '22 (illus.)

HELLENTHAL: Plastic replacement of tip of nose. Chirurg *10:*359–361, May 15, '38

HELLER, E. Bed frame for severe decubitus and sacral wounds. Zentralbl. f. Chir. *67:*1530–1532, Aug 17, '40

HELLER, P. Formation of artificial vagina by Wagner-Kirschner operation; case. Zentralbl. f. Gynak. *56:*2494, Oct 8, '32

HELLMAN, M.: One of the fundamental factors concerned in etiology of dentofacial deformities. J. Am. Dent. A. *14:*1674–1679, Sept '27

HELLMAN, M.: Orthodontic treatment and result of case of malocclusion of teeth brought by conditions associated with congenital cleft palate and harelip; case. Internat. J. Orthodontia *15:*135–138, Feb '29

HELLMANN, K. (see EICHHOFF, E.) 1928

HELLSTADIUS, A.: Ability of bone tissue (including "os novum") to survive in pedicled grafts. Acta chir. Scandinav. *86:*85–109, '42

HELLSTRÖM, J.: Exstrophy of bladder, transplantation of ureters into intestine (Coffey operation). Ztschr. f. urol. Chir. *41:*522–528, '36

HELMHOLZ, H. F. JR. (see KENDRICK, D. B. JR. *et al*) May '40

HELWEG, J.: Snapping finger in polyarthritis. Ugesk. f. Laeger *86:*546–547, July 17, '24 abstr: J.A.M.A. *83:*1042, Sept 27, '24

HELWEG, J.: Snapping finger in polyarthritis. Klin. Wchnschr. *3:*2383–2384, Dec 23, '24 abstr: J.A.M.A. *84:*560, Feb 14, '25

HELWIG, F. C.: Imperforate anus, with exit through prostatic urethra; 3 cases. Am. J. Dis. Child. *38:*559–561, Sept '29

HELWIG, K.: Speech training without obturator in children with cleft palate who have not had operations. Ztschr. f. Kinderforsch. *36:*178–194, Jan 18, '30

Hemangiomas

Hypertrophic capillary angioma of cheek; removal; plastic replacement of skin, case. WEICHERT, M. Beitr. z. klin. Chir. *145:*718–720, '20

Treatment of vascular nevi with radium. RULISON, R. H. AND MCLEAN, S. Am. J. Dis. Child. *25:*359–370, May '23 (illus.)

Radium therapy of vascular nevi. MORROW, H. AND TAUSSIG, L. R. Am. J. Roentgenol. *10:*867–871, Nov '23

Angiomas of parotid region. SCHENK, P. Mitt. a. d. Grenzgeb. d. Med. u. Chir. *37:*51–55, '23

Case of diffuse angioma of eyelid cured by electrolysis. CAMPOS, E. Brazil-med. *2:*233, Oct 18, '24

Hemangioma of nose. ROSENTHAL, M. Laryngoscope *35:*54, Jan '25

Treatment of angiomas with carbon dioxide snow and electrolysis. TRIER, K. Hospitalstid. *68:*117–118, Feb 5, '25

Treatment of angiomata in infancy and early childhood. MCLEAN, S. AND CANNON, A. B. Internat. Clinics *3:*40–45, Sept '25

Angioma cavernosum; report of case of face treated with radium. FRAZIER, C. N. Arch. Dermat. and Syph. *12:*506–508, Oct '25

Two cases of cavernous angioma of eyelid and case of lymphangioma of bulbar conjunctiva. RAY, V. Ohio State M. J. *21:*720–722, Oct '25

Angioma of left temporal and malar regions. REDER, F., S. Clin. N. America *5:*1303–1311, Oct '25

Treatment of extensive subcutaneous angiomas of face. by Morestin's method. MARAGLIANO, D. Arch. ital. di chir. *12:*603–615, '25

Hemangiomas – Cont.
Cavernous hemangioma of upper lip. TAVARES, A. Ann. d'anat. path. *3:*147–150, Feb '26
Surgical removal and pathological study of massive squamous cell epithelioma associated with angioma of scalp. PULFORD, D. S. AND ADSON, A. W. Surg., Gynec. and Obst. *42:*846–848, June '26
Carbon dioxide snow in treatment of angiomas. VENTURELLI, G. Riforma med. *42:*1039–1041, Nov 1, '26
Giant hemangiofibroma of nose; case. BAYMA, F. Ann. paulist. de med. e cir. *18:*1–10, Jan '27
Ulcerating angioma of face; case. MILIAN, G. AND DELARUE, J. Bull. Soc. franc. de dermat. et syph. *34:*189–192, March '27
Case of cavernous angioma (facial nevus). DREYER. Munchen. med. Wchnschr. *74:*563, April 1, '27
Angioma of upper lip; case. DIEULAFÉ, L. Rev. de stomatol. *29:*390–392, July '27
Large cavernous angioma with tumors of thyroid structure in lateral region of neck. LORETI, M. Valsalva *3:*353–363, Aug '27
Radium in removal of "birthmarks." SIMPSON, F. E. AND FLESHER, R. E. Clin. Med. and Surg. *34:*605–607, Aug '27
Radium treatment of haemangiomata, lymphangiomata and naevi pigmentosi. Experiences from "Radium-hemmet," 1909–1924. ANDREN, G. Acta radiol *8:*1–45, '27
Angioma of lower lip reduced by injections of quinine urethane. AUGÉ, A. AND COTSAFTIS, G. G. Arch. Soc. d. sc. med. et biol. de Montpellier *9:*84–86, Feb '28
Results of cryotherapy in angiomas of face in nurslings and in angiomas of eyelids. LORTAT-JACOB, L. Bull. et mem. Soc. med. d. hop. de Paris *52:*527–528, March 29, '28
Angioma of auricle; case. PAGE, J. R. Ann. Otol. Rhin. and Laryng. *37:*358–360, March '28
Cavernous angioma of cheek; case. QUARTERO. Nederl. Tijdschr. v. Geneesk. *1:*1997, April 21, '28
Angioma of nose following erysipelas; radium therapy proposed; case. WALLON, E. Bull. Soc. franc. de dermat. et syph. *35:*406–408, May '28
Treatment of angioma of face. KOVALSKY, N. P. Vestnik khir. (no. 40) *14:*30–38, '28
Cavernous hemangioma in adult. NEW, G. B. S. Clin. N. Amer. *9:*78–80, Feb '29
Birthmarks. KLAUDER, J. V. Hygeia *7:*351–352, April '29
Cavernous angioma of face with homolateral glaucoma; case. OHNO, T. Jap. J. Dermat. and Urol. *29:*33, May '29

Hemangiomas – Cont.
Indications for technic of radium treatment of cutaneous angiomas. WALLON, E. Presse med. *37:*803–804, June 19, '29
Electro-coagulation (surgical diathermy) in multiple angiomata of head. LALVANI, P. P. Indian M. Gaz. *64:*387–388, July '29
Plastic repair of severe radium burns and angioma of face. STRAATSMA, C. R. New York J. Med. *30:*9–10, Jan 1, '30
Benign tumors of external ear: condyloma, hemangioma; cases. TURTUR, G. Valsalva *6:*97–104, Feb '30
Treatment of vascular nevi in children with roentgen and radium therapy. COTTENOT, P. Med. inf. *37:*72–83, March '30 also: J. de med. de Paris *50:*376–378, May 1, '30
Electrotherapy of tuberous angioma of face. GERONIMI, E. Schweiz. med. Wchnschr. *61:*589–593, June 20, '31
Therapy of angiomas from surgical viewpoint. HEYMANN, E. Med. Welt *5:*991–994, July 11, '31
Therapy of angiomas from dermatologic viewpoint. HOFFMANN, C. A. Med. Welt *5:*990, July 11, '31
Angioma of nose; case. PLEWKA. Ztschr. f. Hals-, Nasen-u. Ohrenh. *28:*560–564, Aug 20, '31
Radium treatment of angioma of external ear in infant. DHALLUIN, M. Gaz. med. de France (supp. radiol.) no. 6, pp. 136–138, Oct 1, '31
Electrocoagulation therapy of subcutaneous angiomas. DE QUERVAIN, F. Schweiz. med. Wchnschr. *61:*1169–1170, Dec 5, '31
Surgical therapy of angiomas. HEYMANN, E. Rev. de chir. plastique, pp. 253–262, Jan '32
Plastic and esthetic surgery in hemangioma. (face). DESELAERS. Rev. de chir. plastique, pp. 70–73, April '32
Radium therapy of giant angiomas of face; 3 cases. LLORENS SUQUE, A., J. de radiol. et d'electrol. *16:*211–213, May '32
Plastic surgery in therapy of trichiasis, and free skin graft for hemangioma. DESELAERS, H. Rev. espan. de med. y cir. *15:*353–355, July '32
Massive congenital cervicofacial cavernous hemangioma; case. GIUSTINIAN, V. AND ESTIÚ, M. D. Semana med. *2:*245–246, July 28, '32
Irradiation treatment of red birth-marks; experiences in over 200 cases. KROMAYER, E. Deutsche med. Wchnschr. *58:*1199–1201, July 29, '32 also: Urol. and Cutan. Rev. *36:*524–527, Aug '32
Hemangioma of nose; late results of radiotherapy. PANNETON, J. E. Union med. du Canada *61:*940–944, Aug '32

Hemangiomas – Cont.

Cavernous hemangioma of skin; radium therapy in infants. RATTI, A. Gior. ital. di dermat. e sif. *73:*1430–1436, Aug '32

Cavernous angioma of tendon sheaths; case. DELLA MANO, N. Policlinico (sez. chir.) *39:*593–612, Oct '32

Hemangioma of skin of fingers; perforating through epidermis. FRANKENTHAL, L. Zentralbl. f. Chir. *59:*2619–2620, Oct 22, '32

New method of surgical therapy of subcutaneous angiomas of face. BARDANZELLU, T. Arch. di ottal. *39:*520–543, Nov–Dec '32

Comparative results of bipolar electrolysis and radium therapy in angioma of eyelids in infants; 2 cases. MARÍN AMAT, M. Arch. de oftal. hispano-am. *32:*604–613, Nov '32

Hemangioma of eye; excision by high-frequency knife. BABCOCK, W. W., S. Clin. North America *12:*1411–1412, Dec '32

Angiomatosis of back of hands. GATÉ, J. *et al.* Bull. Soc. franc. de dermat. et syph. (Reunion dermat., Lyon) *39:*1575–1577, Dec '32

Radium therapy of giant angiomatous nevi. LLORENS SUQUE, A. Strahlentherapie *45:*457–460, '32

Hemangioma of skin of fingers perforating through epidermis. (Comment on Frankenthal's article.) GROSS, W. Zentralbl. f. Chir. *60:*154, Jan 21, '33

Radium therapy of cutaneous angiomas. LABORDE, S. Presse med. *41:*103–104, Jan 18, '33

New technic designed for electrocoagulation of vascular tumors. TYLER, A. F. Nebraska M. J. *18:*6–9, Jan '33

Therapy of cutaneous angiomas with sclerosing injections of quinine and urea hydrochloride associated with cryotherapy with carbon dioxide snow. SÉZARY, A. *et al.* Presse med. *41:*260, Feb 15, '33

Therapy of tuberous angiomas with sclerosing injections of sodium salicylate. TOURAINE, A. AND RENAULT, P. Presse med. *41:*259, Feb 15, '33

Hyperplastic angioma of fingers; 7 cases. DESJARDINS, E., J. de l'Hotel-Dieu de Montreal *2:*99–114, March–April '33

Radium treatment of angiomas. TYLER, A. F. Radiol. Rev. and Chicago M. Rec. *55:*51–54, March '33

Should vascular nevi be treated? TRAUB, E. F. Arch. Pediat. *50:*272–278, April '33

Present status of therapy of hemangioma. VENETIANER, P. Gyogyaszat *73:*499–500, Aug 13, '33

Therapy of vascular nevus in children. FRIEDJUNG, J. K. Wien. klin. Wchnschr. *46:*1520, Dec 15, '33

Hemangiomas – Cont.

Congenital angiomas with nasofacial localization; case. FRANCHINI, Y. AND RICCITELLI, E. An. de oto-rino-laring. d. Uruguay *3:*193–203, '33

Angiomas of skin; therapy. PÉRIN, L. Rev. franc. de dermat. et de venereol. *10:*27–39, Jan '34

Cavernous angiomas of tendons of hands. BOTTO MICCA, A. Riv. san. siciliana *22:*568–577, April 15, '34

Treatment of hemangiomata by excision. DAVIS, J. S. AND WILGIS, H. E. South. M. J. *27:*283–290, April '34

Therapy of small cutaneous angiomas by systematic association of cryotherapy with carbon dioxide snow and diathermy. DURAND. Bull. Soc. franc. de dermat. et syph. (Reunion dermat.) *41:*587–589, April '34

Large angiomas of upper eyelid treated with surgical diathermy. CARAMAZZA, F. Boll. d'ocul. *13:*742–753, June '34

Treatment of angiomas with carbon dioxide snow pencil. SEMON, H. C. Lancet *1:*1167–1169, June 2, '34

Angiomas of face and mouth. CLARK, C. M. Ohio State M. J. *30:*438–441, July '34

Angiomas of skin in infants; therapy. HARRENSTEIN, R. J. Maandschr. v. kindergeneesk. *3:*388–395, July '34

Is cryotherapy treatment of choice for angiomas? LORTAT-JACOB, E. Monde med., Paris *44:*781–782, July 1, '34

Ocular neoplasms (orbital hemangiomas) among Chinese; brief clinicopathologic report of 82 cases with discussions. LING, W. P. Chinese M. J. *48:*982–986, Sept '34

Therapy of birthmarks. CASKEY, C. R. California and West. Med. *41:*385–388, Dec '34

Success of surgical therapy of angiomas on face of nurslings; 2 cases. VALLINO, M. T. AND SERFATY, M. Rev. Asoc. med. argent. *48:*1463–1465, Dec '34

Angiomas of eyelids; therapy by sclerosing injections. WEEKERS, L. AND LAPIERE, S. Bull. Soc. belge d'opht., no. 68, pp. 23–36, '34

Angiomas of eyelids; therapy by sclerosing injections; technic, indications and results; 4 cases. WEEKERS, L. AND LAPIERRE, S. Arch. d'opht. *52:*14–22, Jan '35

Decoloration of flat angioma by application of light containing neither ultraviolet nor infrared rays after sensitization with essence of bergamot. GIRAUDEAU, AND ACQUAVIVA. Bull. Soc. franc. de dermat. et syph. *42:*1391, July '35

Vascular tumors of face; 2 cases. DE CERQUEIRA FALCO, E. Rev. oto-laring. de Sao

Hemangiomas – Cont.
Paulo *3:*533–538, Nov–Dec '35 also: Brasil-med. *50:*134–139, Feb 15, '36
Operative treatment of extensive angioma of head. SHILOVTSEV, S. P. Arch. f. klin. Chir. *184:*179–182, '35
Angioneuromyomas of tactile region of finger; cases. DE LUCIA, P. Arch. ital. di anat. e istol. pat. *7:*106–112, Jan '36
Cirsoid craniofacial angiomas; cases. DUFOURMENTEL, L. Bull. et mem. Soc. d. chirurgiens de Paris *28:*103–109, March 6, '36
Question of electrolysis or diathermocoagulation in therapy of vascular tumors of face; experimental study. POCHY-RIANO, R. Arch. di radiol. *12:*121–133, March–April '36
Voluminous angioma of upper lip; treatment by intratumoral quinine injections followed by extirpation of tumor. SORREL, E. Bull. Soc. de pediat. de Paris *34:*210–215, April '36
Cavernous angioma of face. DUFOURMENTEL, L. Oto-rhino-laryng. internat. *20:*297–300, May '36
Surface angioma of face treated with cryotherapy and radium. MARIN, A. Union med. du Canada *65:*446–449, May '36
Glomus tumor: arterial angioneuromyoma of Masson. COLE, H. N. AND SROUB, W. E. J.A.M.A. *107:*428–429, Aug 8, '36
Vascular nevi and their treatment. BLAISDELL, J. H. New England J. Med. *215:*485–488, Sept 10, '36
Angiomas of face; treatment. FIGI, F. A. Arch. Otolaryng. *24:*271–281, Sept '36
Treatment of angioma of eyelid by injection of sclerosing solutions. MALKIN, B. Arch. Ophth. *16:*578–584, Oct '36
Therapy of birthmarks. FOX, E. C. Urol. and Cutan. Rev. *40:*820–823, Nov '36
Development of saddle nose and formation of small multiple hemangiomas of mucous membrane of nose and pharynx complicating diffuse scleroderma; case. MENZEL, K. M. Monatschr. f. Ohrenh. *70:*1409–1418, Dec '36
Cavernous angiomas of face in children; late results of radium therapy. PERUSSIA, F. Strahlentherapie *57:*109–120, '36
Surgical therapy of extensive angioma of head. SHILOVTSEV, S. P. Vestnik khir. *45:*236–239, '36
Hemangioma of tendon or tendon sheath; report of case with study of 24 cases from literature. HARKINS, H. N. Arch. Surg. *34:*12–22, Jan '37

Hemangiomas – Cont.
Electrocoagulation therapy of hemangiomas. MICHALOWSKI, E. Munchen. med. Wchnschr. *84:*101, Jan 15, '37
New method of surgical therapy of angioma racemosum capitis. VON HEDRY, N. Zentralbl. f. Chir. *64:*22–26, Jan 2, '37
Angiomatous tumor of nasal fossae; ligature of external carotid and Rogue-Denker operation; case. PIQUET, J. AND BECUWE. Ann. d'oto-laryng., pp. 393–397, May '37
Angioma of face; treatment. FIGI, F. A. Proc. Staff Meet., Mayo Clin. *12:*437–442, July 14, '37
Electrocoagulation in treatment of cavernous hemangioma. DUJARDIN, E. Ugesk. f. laeger *99:*1257–1258, Nov 25, '37
Cavernous hemangioma of orbit successfully removed by Krönlein's operation. STALLARD, H. B. Lancet *1:*131–133, Jan 15, '38
Interstitial radiation treatment of hemangiomata. BROWN, J. B. AND BYARS, L. T. Am. J. Surg. *39:*452–457, Feb '38
Enormous angioma of bones of hand; case. TANGUY, R. Gaz. med. de France (supp. Cah. radiol.) *45:*371–373, Feb 15, '38
Angiomas of face; therapy. DUFOURMENTEL, L. Bull. et mem. Soc. de med. de Paris *142:*271–281, March 26, '38
Vascular birthmarks; treatment with injection of sclerosing solution. KAESSLER, H. W., J.A.M.A. *110:*1644–1647, May 14, '38
Massive angioma of scalp; rapid growth; case. PAUTRIER, L. M. AND ROEDERER, J. Bull. Soc. franc. de dermat. et syph. (Reunion dermat., Strasbourg) *45:*692–694, May '38
Angioma of auricle; case. TAKEZAWA, N. AND NAKAJIMA, K. Oto-rhino-laryng. *11:*406, May '38
Congenital angioma of nasal tip; case. MATSUDA, E. Oto-rhino-laryng. *11:*608, July '38
Hemangioma of ear. KEPES, P. Monatschr. f. Ohrenh. *72:*798–808, Aug '38
Hemangioma and its treatment. PEYTON, W. T. Minnesota Med. *21:*590–593, Aug '38
Cavernous angioma; radium and roentgen therapy; cases. GARDINI, G. F. Bull. d. sc. med., Bologna *110:*293–314, Sept–Oct '38
Therapy of keloids and angiomas. REISNER, A. Med. Klin. *34:*1233–1235, Sept 16, '38
Extensive congenital angioma of face obliterated by injections of sodium salicylate. FILDERMAN, L. Bull. et mem. Soc. de med. de Paris *142:*576–578, Oct 22, '38
Cryotherapy of cutaneous tuberous angioma and injections of sclerosing substances in

Hemangiomas – Cont.
subcutaneous forms. LORTAT-JACOB, E. Gaz. med. de France *45:*1061-1062, Dec 1, '38
Radium therapy of hemangiomas. BAENSCH, W. Strahlentherapie *63:*496-505, '38
Therapy of cavernous angioma of face; cases. NÖEL. Rev. de chir. structive *8:*199-203, '38
Angiomas of hands and feet. OUGHTERSON, A. W. AND TENNANT, R. Surgery *5:*73-100, Jan '39
Pediculate hemangioma of lower lip; case. KABASHIMA, T. Oto-rhino-laryng. *12:*293, April '39
Treatment of hemangiomas and lymphangiomas in infants and children. HODGES, F. M. *et al.* Virginia M. Monthly *66:*263-266, May '39
Radium treatment of angiomas in children. PATERSON, R. AND TOD, M. C. Am. J. Roentgenol. *42:*726-730, Nov '39
Facial angioma with macrocheilia; case. KIKUCHI, R. AND EBA, M. Oto-rhino-laryng. *12:*1018, Dec '39
Treatment of hemangiomas of skin in children by carbon dioxide snow. WRONG, N. M. Canad. M.A.J. *41:*571-572, Dec '39
Radium treatment of cutaneous cavernous haemangiomas, using surface application of radium tubes in glass capsules. STRANDQVIST, M. Acta radiol. *20:*185-211, '39
Carbon dioxide snow in therapy of hemangioma. CREMER, G. Nederl. tijdschr. v. geneesk. *84:*520-524, Feb 10, '40
Treatment (radium) of infected hemangiomata. POHLE, E. A. Am. J. Roentgenol. *43:*408-415, March '40
Radium treatment of hemangiomata. HARWELL, W. R. New Orleans M. and S. J. *92:*576-580, April '40
Five years' experience with radium therapy of hemangiomas. MÜLLER, R. Munchen. med. Wchnschr. *87:*538-541, May 17, '40
Treatment of hemangiomas in children. KAPLAN, I. I. Urol. and Cutan. Rev. *44:*397-400, June '40
Cryotherapy of hemangioma. EREN, N. O. Turk. tib cem. mec. *6:*139-141, '40
Experiences with thorium-x needles in therapy of hemangiomas. HOEDE, K. AND SCHAEFER, F. Strahlentherapie *67:*23-38, '40
Surgical removal of hamangioma of face with grafting. BERSON, M. I. Am. J. Surg. *51:*362-365, Feb '41
Hemangioma of hand muscles. SORENSEN, F.

Hemangiomas – Cont.
Klin. Wchnschr. *20:*222-224, March 1, '41
Hemangioma of upper lip; case. COMTOIS, A. *et al.* Ann. med.-chir. de l'Hop. Sainte-Justine, Montreal *3:*80-88, May '41
Vascular birthmarks. EDWARDS, H. G. F. South. M. J. *34:*717-724, July '41
Deep cavernous hemangioma of neck; case. LAIRD, E. G. Am. J. Surg. *53:*158-162, July '41
Hypertrophic angioma of cheek; case. MUKASA, H. Oto-rhino-laryng. *14:*487, July '41
Radiation treatment of hemangioma of skin. SPENCER, J. Am. J. Roentgenol. *46:*220-223, Aug '41
Hemangioma of hand, involving phalangeal bones, with distinctive radiologic appearance. HIRSCHFELD, K. Australian and New Zealand J. Surg. *11:*136-139, Oct '41
Use of cold air blast on precancerous skin lesions and hamangiomas. POPPE, J. K. Surgery *11:*460-465, March '42
Cavernous hemangioma of nose, nasal septum and forehead. SALINGER, S. Ann. Otol., Rhin. and Laryng. *51:*268-272, March '42
Angioma arteriale racemosum of face and tongue; surgical therapy; case. PAVLOVSKY, A. J. Bol. y trab., Acad. argent. de cir. *26:*670-672, Aug 19, '42
Cavernous hemangioma of penis; case. GORODNER, J. Rev. argent. de urol. *11:*413-418, Nov-Dec '42
Treatment of congenital hemangiomata of skin. JOHNSON, G. S. AND LIGHT, R. A. Ann. Surg. *117:*134-139, Jan '43
Amputation of buttock for eradication of cavernous hemangioma. WEAVER, J. B. AND RUMOLD, M. J. Am. J. Surg. *60:*149-150, April '43
Cavernous hemangioma of face in infant treated with radium; case. JACOBS, A. W. Am. J. Roentgenol. *49:*816-818, June '43
Extensive destructive ulcerating angioma of face, 5 years after treatment. KAPLAN, I. I. Urol. and Cutan. Rev. *47:*545, Sept '43
Treatment of birthmarks. BAILEY, W. AND KISKADDEN, W. California and West. Med. *59:*265-268, Nov '43
Therapy of hemangiomas of auricular pavilion; case. DUARTE CARDOSO, A. Rev. paulista de med. *23:*347-352, Dec '43
Blood and lymph vessel tumors involving mouth. BELLINGER, D. H., J. Oral Surg. *2:*141-151, April '44
Angiomatous nevus; cases in infants. RUEDA, P. Rev. Soc. pediat. d. litoral *9:*139-142,

Hemangiomas – Cont.
May-Aug '44
Treatment of unusual hemangioma (in Negro) of lip. KAPLAN, I. I. Urol. and Cutan. Rev. *48:*290-291, June '44
Sclerosing agent in treatment of subluxation of mandible and hemangiomas. SALMAN, I. U. S. Nav. M. Bull. *44:*361-369, Feb '45
Discussion of angiomata and pigmented nevi. BIVINGS, L. South. M. J. *38:*241-244, April '45
Hemangioma of ear; new method for control of hemorrhage. DIXON, O. J. Ann. Otol., Rhin. and Laryng. *54:*415-420, June '45
Hemangioma of lip. BURFORD, W. N. AND ACKERMAN, L. V. Am. J. Orthodontics (Oral Surg. Sect.) *31:*559-560, Sept '45
Cavernous hemangioma of orbit successfully removed by Shugrue operation. PAUL, M. Brit. J. Ophth. *30:*35-41, Jan '46
Sclerosing injections in therapy of hemangiomas. VIANNA, J. B. Med. cir. farm. pp. 139-150, Feb-Mar '46
Congenital hemangioma of parotid gland. GLASER, K. *et al.* J. Pediat. *28:*729-732, June '46
Case of tumors resembling hemangiomatosis of lower extremity. KING, D. J., J. Bone and Joint Surg. *28:*623-628, July '46
Angiomatoid formations in genital organs with tumor formation. MOREHEAD, R. P. Arch. Path. *42:*56-63, July '46

HEMBERGER, A. J.: Early treatment of fractures of mandible. Mil. Surgeon *90:*424-428, April '42
HEMBERGER, A. J.: Fractures of mandible. Ann. Dent. *1:*51-58, Sept '42
HEMPEL-JØRGENSEN, E.: Tannic acid in burns. Ugesk. f. laeger *96:*625-626, June 14, '34
HENDERSON, G. D. (see RANK, B. K.) Sept '46
HENDERSON, J. A.: Therapy of acute maxillofacial wounds. Dia med. *18:*183-184, March 4, '46
HENDERSON, J. A. (see DUPERTUIS, S. M.) March '46
HENDERSON, M. S.: Autogenous bone transplantation. J.A.M.A. *77:*165, July 16, '21
HENDERSON, M. S.: Nonunion in fractures; massive bone graft. J.A.M.A. *81:*463-468, Aug 11, '23 (illus.)
HENDERSON, M. S.: Massive bone graft in fracture. J.A.M.A. *107:*1104-1107, Oct 3, '36
HENDERSON, M. S. (see POLLOCK, G. A.) July '40
HENDERSON, M. S. (see SWART, H. A.) June '34
HENDERSON, R. L. V.: Acrylic resin splints for jaw fractures. J. Roy. Nav. M. Serv. *29:*268, Oct '43
HENDERSON, Y.: Acapnia as factor in post-operative shock. J.A.M.A. *95:*572-575, Aug 23, '30
HENDRICK, J. W.: Management of cysts and fistulas (thyroglossal). Texas State J. Med. *32:*34-36, May '36
HENDRICKS, L. J.: Operation on punctum lacrimale; indications. Arch. Ophth. *32:*496, Dec '44
HENDRICKS, W. A.: Exstrophy of bladder (day in Dr. Charles H. Mayo's clinic). Internat. Clin. *1:*182-184, March '26
HENDRICKS, W. A. (see MAYO, C. H.) Aug '26
HENKEL, M.: Construction of artificial vagina with aid of Thiersch transplants. Ztschr. f. Geburtsh. u. Gynak. *104:*36-45, '32

Henkel Operation
Formation of artificial vagina by using Thiersch transplants (Henkel modification of Kirschner-Wagner operation). FRIEDL-MEYER, M. Deutsche Ztschr. f. Chir. *244:*379-386, '35

HENKELS, P.: Fractional cauterization of large cicatricial keloids. Deutsche tierarztl. Wchnschr. *38:*501-504, Aug 9, '30

Henle Operation
Volkmann contracture of hand; therapy by Henle operation; case. SÁNCHEZ TOLEDO, P. Cir. ortop. y traumatol. *1:*113-118, April '33

HENLEY, R. B.: Use of Padgett dermatome. Permanente Found. M. Bull. (no. 2) *1:*1-6, Oct '43
HENNEBERT, P. AND TAISNY, E. Plastic operation on breast; case. Scalpel *86:*1929-1932, Dec 30, '33
HENNEBERT, P. (see VAN LINT, A.) 1936
HENNEBERT, P. (see VAN LINT, A.) May '37

Hennig-Zinsser Operation
Prosthetic surgery in lupus (Hennig-Zinsser method); total rhinoneoplasty. DÖRFFEL, J. AND NOSSEN, H. Med. Welt *5:*1172-1174, Aug 15, '31

HENNION. (see DUFOURMENTEL, L. *et al.*) Dec '32
HENNION. (see DUFOURMENTEL, L. *et al*) June '33
HENNY, F. A.: Fractures of mandible. J. Am. Dent. A. *29:*1840-1845, Oct 1, '42
HENNY, F. A. (see BELLINGER, D. H. *et al*) Jan '43
HENRICHS, R.: Office treatment of acute inflammation of fingers. Med. Klinik *18:*764-765, June 11, '22

HENRY, A. K.: Kondeleon operation for elephantiasis. Brit. J. Surg. *9:*111, July '21

HENRY, A. K.: Simple method of performing arthroplasty in true ankylosis of jaws. Lancet *2:*650–651, Sept 29, '28

HENRY, A. K.: Hinged bone-graft. Brit. M. J. *1:*737–738, April 19, '30

HENRY, A. K.: Plastic surgery methods. Cong. internat. de med. trop. et d'hyg., Compt. rend. (1928) *3:*293–301, '31

HENRY, A. K.: Medial approach to mid-palmar space and ulnar bursa. Lancet *1:*16–18, Jan 7, '39

HENRY, A. K.: Conservation of useful thumb after complete phalangeal necrosis. Lancet *1:*1123, June 22, '40

HENRY, G.: Surgical therapy of exstrophy of bladder; case. J. belge d'urol. *11:*538–545, Dec '38

HENRY, H. B.: New treatment for burns (use of hydrogen peroxide and electric lamp attachment); cases. M. Bull. Vet. Admin. *16:*143–145, Oct '39

Henry, L. M. J.: Results of intranasal dacryocystorhinostomy (West operation). Brit. J. Ophth. *17:*550–552, Sept '33

HENSCHEN, C.: Surgical treatment of spastic adductor contraction of thumb by dorsal suspension of metacarpus of thumb by fascial sling. Schweiz. med. Wchnschr. *58:*621–625, June 23, '28

HENSCHEN, C.: Plastic repair of giant finger by stretching nerve of finger, shortening by excision and excision of soft parts. Helvet. med. acta *3:*166–176, May '36

HENSCHEN, C.: Protection of heels of bedridden patients with half-shells of oranges, lemons or grapefruit. Zentralbl. f. Chir. *66:*782–785, April 8, '39

HENSCHEN, C.: Suggestions for war surgery of facial injuries; use of wire cradle and fixation of tongue, facial flaps and bone fragments by means of safety pin in patients with jaw fractures. Schweiz. med. Wchnschr. *70:*711–715, July 30, '40

HENSCHEN, C.: Burn therapy in peacetime and war. Helvet. med. acta *8:*77–148, April '41

HENSCHEN, C. AND SCHWARZ, R.: Operative treatment of prognathism based on cephalometry. Chirurg *1:*56–66, Nov 20, '28

HENSEL, G. C.: Management of fracture of mandible. Surg., Gynec. and Obst. *55:*238–243, Aug '32

HENSEL, G. C.: Surgical correction of mandibular protraction and retraction (also fractures of ascending rami). Surgery *2:*92–119, July '37 also: Internat. J. Orthodontia *23:*814–839, Aug '37

HENSKE, J. A.: Importance of pediatric care in operative treatment of harelip and cleft palate. J.A.M.A. *89:*1666–1670, Nov 12, '27

HENSON, E. B.: Buried skin grafts of burned children; new use of old method of grafting. West Virginia M. J. *26:*557–559, Sept '30

HENZE, K.: Arrhinencephaly with incomplete development of nose; case. Beitr. z. prakt. u. theoret. Hals-, Nasen-u. Ohrenh. *31:*241–247, '34

HEPLER, A. B.: Ureterorectoneostomy by transfixion suture method in exstrophy of bladder, Coffey's technic 3. S. Clin. North America *13:*1387–1391, Dec '33

HEPP, J.: Wounds of fingers due to jets of oil under high pressure; case with review of cases previously reported. Arch. d. mal. profess. *2:*565–573, '40

HERBIG, B.: Late results of surgical therapy of nerves. Beitr. z. klin. Chir. *166:*414–436, '37

HERBST, R.: Experimental studies on traumatic shock. Arch. f. klin. Chir. *176:*98–122, '33

HERCOG, P.: Septicemia due to Micrococcus catarrhalis after resection of nasal septum; case. Gior. di clin. med. *19:*315–318, April 10, '38

Heredity

Heredity in Dupuytren's contracture. LÖWY, J. Zentralbl. f. inn. Med. *44:*51–52, Jan 27, '23 abstr: J.A.M.A. *80:*1279, April 28, '23

Hereditary ptosis of eyelids. KILLIAN, H. Klin. Wchnschr. *2:*2286, Dec 10, '23

Heredity of malformations, especially harelip and polydactylism. LÜCKER, F. C. Monatschr. f. Geburtsh. u. Gynak. *66:*327–336, July '24 abstr: J.A.M.A. *83:*882, Sept 13, '24

Heredity of complete rectal prolapse. OTTENBERG, R. AND GOTTSCHALK, L., J.A.M.A. *84:*335–336, Jan 31, '25

Hereditary ankylosis of proximal phalangeal joints. ELKIN, D. C., J.A.M.A. *84:*509, Feb 14, '25

Hereditary contracture of palmar fascia; efficiency of radium emanation. APERT, E. Bull. et mem. Soc. med. d. hop. de Paris *49:*1502–1505, Nov 27, '25 abstr: J.A.M.A. *86:*380, Jan 30, '26

Four generations of harelip. MASON, R. J. Hered. *17:*52, Feb '26

Congenital familial finger contracture and associated familial knee-joint subluxation. MURPHY, D. P., J.A.M.A. *86:*395–397, Feb 6, '26

Problem of heredity of Dupuytren's contracture. SPROGIS, G. Compt. rend. Soc. de biol. *94:*631–632, March 12, '26 abstr: J.A.M.A. *87:*131, July 10, '26

Heredity – Cont.
Hereditary nature of harelip and cleft palate. BIRKENFELD, W. Arch. f. klin. Chir. *141:*729–753, '26
Theory of heredity of Dupuytren's contracture. SPROGIS, G. Deutsche Ztschr. f. Chir. *194:*259–263, '26
Family tree of hereditary transmission of Dupuytren's contracture. KARTSCHIKJAN, S. I. Ztschr. f. orthop. Chir. *48:*36–38, Feb 11, '27
Combined acrocephaly and syndactylism occurring in mother and daughter; case report. WEECH, A. A. Bull. Johns Hopkins Hosp. *40:*73–76, Feb '27
Talipomanus; three cases in one family. MARTMER, E. E. Am. J. Dis. Child. *34:*384–387, Sept '27
Study of twins with cleft lip, jaw, and palate from standpoint of pathologic heredity. BIRKENFELD, W. Beitr. z. klin. Chir. *141:*257–267, '27
Pedigree of anomalies in first and second branchial cleft, inherited according to laws of Mendel, and contribution to technique of extirpation of congenital lateral fistulae coli. PŘECECHTĚL, A. Acta oto-laryng. *11:*23–30, '27
Peculiarities of hereditary polydactylia and syndactylia; supplement to author's original article. THOMSEN, O. Acta med. Scandinav. *66:*588–590, '27
Peculiarities of hereditary polydactylia and syndactylia. THOMSEN, O. Acta med. Scandinav. *65:*609–644, '27 also: Hospitalstid. *70:*789–819, Aug 25, '27
Syndactylism in 4 generations. PERKOFF, D. Brit. M. J. *2:*341–342, Aug 25, '28
Hereditary transmission of branchial fistulas; case. STARKENSTEIN, E. Med. Klin. *24:*701, May 4, '28
Heredity of fistula auris congenita. SCHÜLLER, J. Munchen. med. Wchnschr. *76:*160–162, Jan 25, '29
New pedigrees of hereditary disease; polydactylism and syndactylism. BELL, J. Ann. Eugenics *4:*41–48, April '29
Hereditary polysyndactylia; case. LEGORBURU, R. Arch. de med., cir. y espec. *30:*745–752, June 29, '29
Hereditary hypertelorism without mental deficiency. MONTFORD, T. M. Arch. Dis. Childhood *4:*381–384, Dec '29
Familial predisposition to Dupuytren's contracture. CSÖRSZ, K. Budapesti orvosi ujsag *28:*59–61, Jan 16, '30
Hereditary eyelid ptosis with epicanthus; case with pedigree extending over 4 generations. MCILROY, J. H. Proc. Roy. Soc. Med. (sect. Ophth.) *23:*17–20, Jan '30
Congenital fistula of lower lip; embryologic and hereditary factors in pathogenesis of rare congenital abnormalities of face; operative treatment; cases. RUBALTELLI, E. Arch. ital. di otol. *41:*141–154, April '30
Family of eighteenth century with eyelid ptosis; hereditary aspect. VAN SETERS, W. H. Nederl. tijdschr. v. geneesk. *74:*1775–1779, April 5, '30
Congenital auricular fistula; 3 cases in same family. MONTGOMERY, M. L., S. Clin. North America *11:*141–148, Feb '31
Hereditary aspect of harelip and cleft palate. COENEN, H. Chirurg *3:*501–505, June 1, '31
Inheritable defect of human hand. GILLETTE, C. P., J. Hered. *22:*189–190, June '31
Heredity and Dupuytren's contracture. MANSON, J. S. Brit. M. J. *2:*11, July 4, '31
Hereditary aspect of cleft lip and palate. SCHRÖDER, C. H. Arch. f. Rassen-u. Gesellsch.-Biol. *25:*369–394, Nov 25, '31
Congenital epicanthus and ptosis of eyelid transmitted through 4 generations. ROSS, N. Brit. M. J. *1:*378–379, Feb 27, '32
Familial syndactylia. ČÍPEK, J. Casof. lek. cesk. *71:*806–811, June 24, '32
Inheritance of doublejointedness in thumb. WHITNEY, L. F., J. Hered. *23:*425–426, Oct '32
Hereditary deformities of hand and foot in members of one family; polydactylia and syndactylia. KEMP, T. AND RAVN, J. Acta psychiat. et neurol. *7:*275–296, '32
Heredofamilial eyelid ptosis. LYUBARSKAYA, T. E. Sovet. nevropat., psikhiat. i psikhogig. (no. 3) *2:*103–104, '33
Familial aplasia of upper jaw, new type of facial dysostosis. SENDRAIL, M. Prat. med. franc. *15:*127–130, Feb (B) '34
Familial occurrence of hypoplasia of jaws. KLEY, H. Med. Welt *8:*311, March 3, '34
Heredity of Dupuytren's contracture. SCHRÖDER, C. H. Zentralbl. f. Chir. *61:*1056–1059, May 5, '34
Heredity of syndactylia in one family during period of 100 years. FINCKH. Med. Welt *8:*705, May 19, '34
Roentgen study of polydactylia and syndactylia in 3 generations of family. JAUBERT DE BEAUJEU, A. Bull. et mem. Soc. de radiol. med. de France *22:*339–342, June '34
Heredity of ectrodactylia. GORIAINOWA, R. W. Fortschr. a. d. Geb. d. Rontgenstrahlen *50:*289–294, Sept '34
Inheritance of harelip and cleft palate.

Heredity—Cont.
SANDERS, J. Genetica *15:*433–510, '34
Hereditary congenital eyelid ptosis; report of pedigree and review of literature. RODIN, F. H. AND BARKAN, H. Am. J. Ophth. *18:*213–225, March '35
Inheritance of harelip and cleft palate in man. DROOGLEEVER FORTUYN, A. B. Genetica *17:*349–366, '35
Heredity of submucous cleft of palate. MAHLSTEDT, H. Ztschr. f. Laryng., Rhin., Otol. *26:*347–352, '35
Studies on heredity of harelip and cleft palate, with particular regard to mode of transmission. SCHRÖDER, C. H. Arch. f. klin. Chir. *182:*299–330, '35
Familial occurrence of deformities of hands and feet in 5 generations. STRÖER, W. F. H. Genetica *17:*299–312, '35
Familial appearance of Dupuytren's contracture; case. IMBER, I. Note e riv. di psichiat. *65:*209–222, April–June '36
Family tree showing hereditary syndactylia. KIRCHMAIR, H. Munchen. med. Wchnschr. *83:*605–606, April 10, '36
Family with camptodactylia. RITTERSKAMP, P. Munchen. med. Wchnschr. *83:*724–725, May 1, '36
Familial occurrence of keloids. WOLF, M. Wien. med. Wchnschr. *86:*722–723, June 27, '36
Relation between hereditary abnormalities of eyes and partially developed fingers and toes. KARSCH, J. Ztschr. f. Augenh. *89:*274–279, July '36
Pedigree of four generations of hereditary congenital ptosis affecting only one eye and pedigree of one generation of congenital ptosis with epicanthus. RODIN, F. H. Am. J. Ophth. *19:*597–599, July '36
Genealogical study of case of symmetrical congenital brachydactylia. STECHER, W. R. M. Rec. *144:*5–8, July 1, '36
Heredity of hypospadias. STEINER, F. Munchen. med. Wchnschr. *83:*1271, July 31, '36
Hereditary character of eyelid ptosis. BIRO, E. Arch. d'opht. *53:*685–693, Sept '36
Hereditary anarthrosis of index finger, with associated abnormalities in proportions of fingers; case. DANIEL, G. H. Ann. Eugenics *7:*281–297, Nov '36
Absence of hands and feet in Brazilian family; question of heredity of congenital abnormalities. KOEHLER, O. Ztschr. f. menschhl. Vererb.-u. Konstitutionslehre *19:*670–690, '36
Heredity of concealed syndactylic polydactylia. SCHATZKI, P. Arch. f. orthop. u. Unfall-Chir. *36:*613, '36
Pedigree of syndactyly. WIGHTMAN, J. C. J. Hered. *28:*421–423, Dec '37
Hereditary transmission of rare deformity of thumb. PALTRINIERI, M. AND DE LUCCHI, G. Bull. d. sc. med., Bologna *110:*158–167, May–June '38
Pedigree of symphalangism. STILES, K. A. AND WEBER, R. A., J. Hered. *29:*199–202, May '38
Study of family with cleft hands and feet. LIEBENAM, L. Ztschr. f. menschl. Vererb.-u. Konstitutionslehre *22:*136–151, '38
Study of family with syndactylia. LUEKEN, K. G. Ztschr. f. menschl. Vererb.-u. Konstitutionslehre *22:*152–159, '38
Harelip and cleft palate from eugenic point of view. UEBERMUTH, H. Arch. f. klin. Chir. *193:*224–229, '38
Heredity of ear malformations. GAUS, W. Erbbl. f. d. Hals-, Nasen-u. Ohrenarzt, Hft. 1–2, pp. 20–30, March '39; in Hals-, Nasen-u. Ohrenarzt (Teil 1) *30:*March '39
Factor of heredity in harelip. LITTLE, J. L. Canad. M.A.J. *40:*482–483, May '39
Three generations of ear pits. WHITNEY, D. D., J. Hered. *30:*323–324, Aug '39
Bilateral Dupuytren's contracture in three children of one family; case. RIEDL, L. Casop. lek. cesk. *78:*1114–1115, Oct 6, '39
Hereditary cleidocranial dysostosis with features of ocular hypertelorism; 2 cases. RUBENS, E. Arch. Pediat. *56:*771–780, Dec '39
Hereditary transmission of harelip. FLORIS, M. Boll. d. Soc. eustachiana *37:*25–32, '39
Harelip with cleft jaw and palate in relation to law on prevention of hereditary defects. LEHMANN, W. AND RITTER, R. Ztschr. f. menschl. Vererv.-u. Konstitutionslehre *23:*1–16, '39
Studies on family groups with harelip and clefts of jaw and palate. MENGELE, J. Ztschr. f. menschl. Vererb.-u. Konstitutionslehre *23:*17–42, '39
Congenital cardiac defects and harelip with clefts of jaw and palate in twins. RABL, R. AND SCHULZ, F. Virchows Arch. f. path. Anat. *305:*505–520, '39
Hereditary relations between harelip and cleft palate and other malformations, especially of spine. SCHRÖDER, C. H. Beitr. z. klin. Chir. *169:*402–413, '39
Effect of certain experimental conditions on development of hereditary harelip in mice. STEINIGER, F. Ztschr. f. menschl. Vererb.-u. Konstitutionslehre *24:*1–12, '39

Heredity – Cont.

Hereditary etiology of syndactylia; remarkable association of polydactylia and syndactylia in case. DE LUCA, R. Minerva med. *2:*324–327, Sept 29, '40

Surgical problems in hereditary polydactylism and syndactylism. SNEDECOR, S. T. AND HARRYMAN, W. K., J. M. Soc. New Jersey *37:*443–449, Sept '40

Harelip inheritance in man. MATHER, K. AND PHILIP, U. Ann. Eugenics *10:*403–416, Dec '40

Heredopathology of fissures of lips, jaws and palate; report on unselected series of 41 pairs of twins. IDELBERGER, A. AND IDELBERGER, K. Ztschr. f. menschl. Vererb.-u. Konstitutionslehre *24:*417–479, '40

Study of anatomy and heredity of cleft foot and hand deformities in siblings. KLAGES, F. AND JACOB, R. Ztschr. f. Orthop. *70:*265–281, '40

Heredity of congenital fossette of lip in conjunction with clefts of upper jaw. TRAUNER, R. Wien. klin. Wchnschr. *54:*427–429, May 16, '41 addendum: *54:*454, May 23, '41

Genetics of acrocephalosyndactylia. FERRIMAN, D. Proc. Internat. Genet. Cong. (1939) *7:*120, '41

Significance of occult spina bifida in heredity of harelip and cleft palate. SCHRODER, C. H. AND HILLENBRAND, H. J. Arch. f. klin. Chir. *203:*328–342, '42

"Heteropenetration" and twin discordance in hereditary harelip and cleft palate. STEINIGER, F. AND VEIT, G. Ztschr. f. menschl. Vereb-. u.Konstitutionslehre *26:*75–92, '42

Three generations of mucous cysts occurring with harelip and cleft palate. STRAITH, C. L. AND PATTON, H. S., J.A.M.A. *123:*693–694, Nov 13, '43

HERFF, F. P.: Elephantiasis treated by Kondoleon operation. Surg., Gynec. and Obst. *34:*758–760, June '22 (illus.)

HERLYN, K. E.: Technic of suture of cleft palate. Beitr. z. klin. Chir. *165:*276–277, '37

HERLYN, K. E.: Cod liver oil and plaster of paris cast therapy of injuries of fingers and hand. Beitr. z. klin. Chir. *165:*278–282, '37

HERLYN, K. E.: New approach in plastic operations of cleft palate and harelip. Zentralbl. f. Chir. *64:*815–818, April 3, '37

HERLYN, K. E.: Results of cleft palate operation. Beitr. z. klin. Chir. *169:*397–401, '39

HERMAN, A. L.: Double branchial cysts complicated by carcinoma of larynx. Minnesota Med. *14:*555–557, June '31

HERMAN, E. AND MERENLENDER, J.: Pringle's disease with hemifacial hyperplasia (of cheeks, lips conjunctiva and concha of ear), but without any psychoneurologic symptoms. Acta dermat.-venereol. *16:*276–291, Oct '35

HERMAN, M. (see ORNSTEIN, G. G. *et al*) April '39

HERMANS, A. G. J.: Strangulation of penis; 3 cases. Nederl. tijdschr. v. geneesk. *90:*810–816, July 13, '46

Hermaphrodism (See also Hypospadias)

Artificial vagina in case of external male pseudohermaphroditism. GRUSS, J. Deutsche med. Wchnschr. *47:*509, May 5, '21

Case of pseudohermaphrodismus masculinus, showing hypospadias, greatly enlarged utricle, abdominal testis and absence of seminal vesicles. YOUNG, H. H. AND CASH, J. R., J. Urology *5:*405, May '21

Artificial vagina in case of external male pseudohermaphroditism. FRANK, M. Monatschr. f. Geburtsh. u. Gynak. *55:*5, July '21 abstr: J.A.M.A. *77:*1215, Oct 8, '21

Treatment of pseudohermaphroditism. MARIQUE. Arch. franco-belges de chir. *25:*280–281, Dec '21 (illus.)

Pseudohermaphrodism or complete hypospadias. HAGNER, F. R. AND KNEALE, H. B. Surg., Gynec. and Obst. *36:*495–501, April '23 (illus.)

Pseudo-hermaphroditism and hypospadias; their surgical treatment. EDMUNDS, A. Lancet *1:*323–327, Feb 13, '26

True hermaphrodism in man; report of case with critical review of literature. KWARTIN, B. AND HYAMS, J. A., J. Urol. *18:*363–383, Oct '27

Surgical treatment of true hermaphrodism. GOLJANITZKI, J. A. Arch. f. klin. Chir. *144:*732–751, '27

Operations on hermaphrodites. MOSZKOWICZ, L. Med. Klin. *25:*517–519, March 28, '29

Operations on hermaphrodites. (comment on Moszkowicz's article). MEIXNER, K. Med. Klin. *25:*986, June 21, '29

Reply to Meixner's comments on article about operations on hermaphrodites. MOSZKOWICZ, L. Med. Klin. *25:*986, June 21, '29

Rare case of pseudohermaphroditism of internal male type subjected to surgical treatment. SZÉKELY, L. Zentralbl. f. Chir. *57:*3168–3171, Dec 20, '30

Operation in case of hermaphroditismus masculinus tubularis et externus with restoration of patient to feminine types. GYLLENSVÄRD, N. Acta obst. et. gynec. Scandinav. *10:*392–409, '30

Hermaphrodism – Cont.
Androgynous pseudohermaphroditism; surgical correction of perineal and penile urethra. MARTIN, L. AND BONNIOT. Bull. Soc. franc. d'urol., pp. 227-235, June 20, '32
Medicosocial problem of false hermaphroditism; case with hypospadias and ectopic testicles. TORRES TORIJA, J. Gac. med. de Mexico *64:*534-542, Dec '33
Surgical intervention for purpose of feminization of hermaphrodite. KAKUSCHKIN, N. Arch. f. Frauenk. *19:*150-160, '33
Surgical and hormonal therapy of true hermaphroditism. NAUJOKS. Arch. f. Gynak. *156:*93-96, '33
True (lateral) hermaphroditism; complete restoration of masculine habitus after removal of female organs; case. WOLF, C. Endokrinologie *15:*225-232, '35
Ectopia vesicae, imperforate rectum and anus, true hermaphroditism and other anomalies. POTTER, A. H. Am. J. Surg. *31:*172-178, Jan '36
True hermaphrodite, case. LINDVALL, S. AND WAHLGREN, F. Nord. med. tidskr. *11:*635-641, April 18, '36
Surgical treatment of hermaphroditism. SCHMIDT, A. Orvosi hetil. *80:*719-722, Aug 1, '36
Surgical adaptation of female pseudohermaphrodite to true sex; case. PEREIRA, A. Rev. urol. de S. Paulo *4:*169-177, May-June '37
Hermaphroditism, case and its treatment. ELLIS, E. L. H. Lancet *2:*17-18, July 3, '37
Complete lateral alternate bisexual hermaphroditism; surgical therapy of case. QUIROZ, F. Cir. y cirujanos *5:*299-307, July '37
External masculine pseudohermaphroditism with mistake in sex; surgical therapy of case. BARBERIS, J. C. Bol. Soc. de cir. de Rosario *5:*125-150, June '38
Baldwin operation in case of pseudohermaphroditism and vulviform hypospadias. CABANES, E. AND XICLUNA, R. Algerie med. *43:*333-336, July '39
Operative treatment of true hermaphroditism and new technic for curing hypospadias. YOUNG, H. H. Arch. Surg. *41:*557-568, Aug '40
Spurious biglandular hermaphroditism. VONDRACEK, V. AND NEDVED, M. Casop. lek. cesk. *80:*293-295, Feb 28, '41
General norms of surgical conduct; case of gynandroid with clitoris-penis. VIANNA DE PAULA, H. AND VIANNA DE PAULA, G. Rev. de ginec. e d'obst. *1:*402-414, June '41
Hermaphroditism, pseudo- and true; surgical possibilities. CAPRIO, G. An. d. ateneo clin. quir. *7:*414-429, Aug '41
Surgical therapy of hermaphroditism. SCHMIDT, A. Ztschr. f. Urol. *35:*152-169, '41
Error in determination of sex; study on pseudohermaphroditism based on case with perineal hypospadias. SIMARRO PUIG, J. *et al.* Rev. clin. espan. *6:*39-42, July 15, '42
Pseudohermaphroditism; 2 cases. KOZOLL, D. D. Arch. Surg. *45:*578-595, Oct '42
Surgical correction of hermaphroditism. OMBREDANNE, L. Clinics *1:*615-630, Oct '42
Case of hermaphroditism; operation and end result. SENGER, F. L. AND MORGAN, E. K. J. Urol. *48:*658-664, Dec '42
Surgical therapy of case of hermaphroditism. GONZALEZ R., R. Rev. Fac. de med., Bogota *11:*710-714, June '43
Exstrophy bladder in pseudohermaphrodite; case. LOEWEN, S. L. AND RUPE, L. O. J. Kansas M. Soc. *44:*186-189, June '43
Male pseudohermaphroditism with perineal pseudovaginal hypospadias; technic for surgical correction; case. HERNANDEZ IBANEZ, J. A. Vida nueva *53:*263-273, May '44
Female pseudohermaphroditism with hypospadias limited to glans; anomaly due to cessation of development; case. LORDY, C. An. brasil. de ginec. *18:*87-93, Aug '44
Intersexuality; case. SHARMAN, A. Glasgow M. J. *142:*40-44, Aug '44
Pregnancy following surgical intervention in gynandroid with closed scrotum. COTTE, G. AND BARDONNET. Gynec. et obst. *44:*12, '44
Female pseudohermaphroditism with hypospadias limited to glans; anomaly due to cessation of development; plastic correction of case. SPINA, V. Rev. de obst. e ginec. de Sao Paulo *7:*195-208, June-Aug '45

HERNANDEZ, A.: Plastic surgery of ear; case. Prensa med. argent. *31:*2367-2373, Nov 22, '44
HERNANDEZ IBANEZ, J. A.: Male pseudohermaphroditism with perineal pseudovaginal hypospadias; technic for surgical correction; case. Vida nueva *53:*263-273, May '44
HERNANDEZ RAMIREZ, S.: Corrective surgery in war; progress, advantages and possibilities. Pasteur *2:*15-18, July 15, '43
HERNANDEZ RAMIREZ, S.: Do corrective operations of nose cause pathologic disorders? Pasteur *2:*35-37, Aug 15, '43
HERON, D. F. (see MUNSON, F. T.) Aug '41
HERPIN, A.: Fracture of lower jaw, with special reference to therapy. Rev. gen. de clin. et de therap. *49:*641-645, Oct 5, '35
HERRLIN, J. O. JR. AND GLASSER, S. T.: Sympo-

sium on medical aspects of chemical warfare; treatment of burns (including thermal and electric). Bull. New York M. Coll., Flower and Fifth Ave. Hosps. *5:*79–84, June–Oct '42

HERRMANN: Therapy of perichondritis of auricle. Ztschr. f. Hals-, Nasen-u. Ohrenh. *44:*373–377, '38

HERRMANN, J. B. (see ADAIR, F. E.) Sept '46

HERRMANN, M.: Origin and therapy of accidental jaw fractures, with evaluation of compensation. Monatschr. f. Unfallh. *46:*448–457, Aug '39

HERSCHENDÖRFER, A.: Construction of artificial conjunctival sac by free transplantation of epidermis as preliminary to prosthesis. Ztschr. f. Augenh. *84:*284–292, Nov '34

HERSH, J. H.: Management of fractures of bony vault of nose. Ann. Otol., Rhin. and Laryng. *54:*534–553, Sept '45

HERTZ, C. S.: Malignant disease of face, buccal cavity, pharynx and larynx in first three decades of life. Proc. Staff Meet., Mayo Clin. *15:*152–156, March 6, '40

HERTZBERG, G.: Burn therapy; with special reference to tannin salve. Kinderarztl. Praxis *10:*364–370, Aug '39

HERTZBERG, G. R. R. (see HERTZBERG, R. F.) July '24

HERTZBERG, J.: Treatment of injuries of tendons of hand. Nord. med. *31:*1893–1897, Aug 23, '46

HERTZBERG, R. F. AND HERTZBERG, G. R. R.: Congenital malformations of face. M. J. and Rec. *120:*5–8, July 2, '24

HERZ, L. F.: Rapid epithelization (following use of scarlet red ointment); case, without skin grafting in extensive third degree burns. M. Rec. *149:*43–44, Jan 18, '39

HERZ, M.: Practical results of tendon transplantation. Chirurg *1:*555–559, May 1, '29

HERZBERG, B.: Fracture of sesamoid bone of thumb; case. Zentralbl. f. Chir. *54:*1807–1809, July 16, '27

HERZBERG, E. AND GUTTMANN, E.: Heteroplastic implantation of tissues. Munchen. med. Wchnschr. *76:*1922–1923, Nov 15, '29

HERZFELD, G.: Treatment of burns and scalds by tannic acid. Practitioner *122:*106–111, Feb '29

HERZOG, E. G.: Splint for radial nerve palsies. Lancet *2:*754, Dec 9, '44

Hess Operation

Hess operation; new bandage substitute (eyelid ptosis). PEREIRA, R. F. Arch. de oftal. de Buenos Aires *16:*241–242, May '41

Case of myasthenia gravis operated on for eyelid ptosis by Hess's method. HARDIE, D. Brit. J. Ophth. *12:*31–33, Jan '28

HESSE, E.: Operative mobilization of stiff fingers. Arch. f. klin. Chir. *119:*1–19, '22 (illus.) abstr: J.A.M.A. *78:*1173, April 15, '22

HESSE, E. (see GESSE, E. R.)

HESSE, F.: Treatment of injuries of tendons within synovial sheaths in palm of hand and of flexor tendons of finger by insertion of foreign substance. Arch. f. klin. Chir. *170:*772–789, '32

HESSE, G.: Surgical therapy of osteomyelitis of jaws. Ztschr. f. Stomatol. *31:*359, March 24; 434, April 14, '33

HESSE, W.: Surgical diathermy of cancer of nose. Deutsche med. Wchnschr. *56:*1479–1481, Aug 29, '30

HEWITT, W. R.: Burn therapy. J. Missouri M. A. *38:*191–195, June '41

HEYER, E.: Cure of complete incontinentia alvi following Schubert's operation for plastic formation of vagina; case. Zentralbl. f. Gynak. *54:*1238–1240, May 17, '30. Comment by MELZNER, E.

HEYL, J. T. AND JANEWAY, C. A.: Use of human albumin in military medicine; theoretic and experimental basis for use (shock). Army M. Bull. (no. 68) pp. 227–233, July '43

HEYMAN, C. H.: Mobilization of stiff metacarpophalangeal joints. Surg., Gynec. and Obst. *39:*506–507, Oct '24

HEYMANN, E.: Therapy of angiomas from surgical viewpoint. Med. Welt *5:*991–994, July 11, '31

HEYMANN, E.: Surgical therapy of angiomas. Rev. de chir. plastique, pp. 253–262, Jan '32

HEYMAN, J. A. AND CONNER, P. K.: Suture of ulnar nerve. Texas State J. Med. *26:*861–864, April '31

HEYMAN, J. A.: Construction of artificial vagina. Texas State J. Med. *37:*30–33, May '31

HEYN, A.: Diffuse hypertrophy of mamma at puberty. Zentralbl. f. Gynak. *47:*263–265, Feb 17, '23 (illus.)

HEYN, W.: Maydl operation in child $1^1/_2$ years old for exstrophy. Zentralbl. f. Gynak. *64:*194–198, Feb 3, '40

HEYNEN, U.: Plastic repair of hypospadias. Ztschr. f. Urol. *26:*338–359, '32

HEYNINX, A.: Resection under local anesthesia of lower part of jaw, with integrity of nasal membrane; case. Ann. d. mal. de l'oreille, du larynx *47:*996, Nov '28

HICKEN, N. F. AND POPMA, A. M.: Tumors of neck; diagnosis and treatment, cervical cysts and fistulas. Nebraska M. J. *23:*209–212, June '38

HICKEY, H. L.: Lesions associated with fistula of frontal sinus. Ann. Otol., Rhin. and Laryng. *54:*143–158, March '45

HICKEY, M. J.: Care of military and civilian

injuries (burns). Am. J. Orthodontics (Oral Surg. Sect.) *28:*177-182, April '42

Hidradenitis

Surgical treatment of intractable furunculosis of axilla. BRUNZEL, H. F. Zentralbl. f. Chir. *48:*991, July 16, '21

Surgical treatment of furunculosis of axilla. BOCKENHEIMER, P. Zentralbl. f. Chir. *48:*1317, Sept 10, '21

HIGGINS, C. C.: Transplantation of ureters into rectum in exstrophy. Ohio State M. J. *27:*705-708, Sept '31

HIGGINS, C. C.: Aseptic uretero-intestinal anastomosis in exstrophy. Surg., Gynec. and Obst. *57:*359-361, Sept '33 also: Am. J. Surg. *22:*207-209, Nov '33

HIGGINS, C. C.: Ureteral transplantation for exstrophy of bladder and carcinoma. Cleveland Clin. Quart. *2:*32-42, Oct '35

HIGGINS, C. C.: Transplantation of ureters in infants with exstrophy of bladder. J. Urol. *41:*464-472, April '39

HIGGINS, C. C.: Transplantation of ureters into rectosigmoid in infants with exstrophy of bladder; review of 19 cases. J. Urol. *50:*657-666, Dec '43

HIGGINS, C. C.: Exstrophy of bladder in twins. Cleveland Clin. Quart. *11:*25, Jan '44

HIGHET, W. B.: Splintage of peripheral nerve injuries. Lancet *1:*555-558, May 9, '42

HIGHET, W. B.: Innervation and function of thenar muscles. Lancet *1:*227-230, Feb 20, '43

HIGHET, W. B. AND HOLMES, W.: Peripheral nerve traction injuries after suture. Brit. J. Surg. *30:*212-233, Jan '43

HIGHET, W. B. AND SANDERS, F. K.: Effects of stretching nerves after suture. Brit. J. Surg. *30:*355-369, April '43

HIGHMAN, B.: Mixed tumor of salivary gland type on left hand. Arch. Path. *37:*387-388, June '44

HIGHSMITH, E. DEW.: Plastic surgery of face. Ann. Surg. *76:*129-132, Aug '22 (illus.)

HIGHSMITH, E. D.: Facial deformities. South. M. J. *20:*688-689, Sept '27

HIGHSMITH, E. D.: New method of covering denuded areas with surrounding skin. Surg., Gynec. and Obst. *45:*823-824, Dec '27

HIGHLEY, L. B.: Facial reconstruction and speech. J. Am. Dent. A. *30:*1716-1725, Nov 1, '43

HILAROWICZ, H.: Epithelium pulp in epithelium grafting. Zentralbl. f. Chir. *51:*2192-2193, Oct 4, '24

HILBERT, J. W.: Whirlpool baths and posterior splinting to overcome contractures in burns. J.A.M.A. *95:*1021, Oct 4, '30

HILD, J.: Surgical therapy of cryptorchidism with pedicled flap from thigh. Beitr. z. klin. Chir. *170:*387-397, '39

HILDANUS, F.: History of burns in connection with Fabricius Hildanus' book published in 1610. RUBASHEV, S. M. Vestnik khir. *56:*876-880, Dec '38

HILDRETH, H. R.: External canthal ligament in surgery of lower eyelid. Am. J. Ophth. *18:*437-439, May '35

HILDRETH, H. R.: Ox-fascia-transplant operation in eyelid ptosis. South. M. J. *30:*471-473, May '37

HILDRETH, H. R.: Eyelid ptosis; insertions of levator palpebrae muscle. Am. J. Ophth. *24:*749-758, July '41

HILGENFELDT, O.: Burn therapy. Med. Klin. *29:*490-492, April 7, '33

HILGENFELDT, O.: Burn therapy. Ergebn. d. Chir. u. Orthop. *29:*102-210, '36

HILGENREINER, H.: Three cases of congenital fistulas, mucous membrane pouches on lower lip; nature and cause of malformation, with review of 46 cases on record. Deutsche Ztschr. f. Chir. *188:*273-309, '24

HILGER, J. A.: Facial injuries. Minnesota Med. *29:*235, Mar '46

HILL: Short review of treatment of service burns during the war. M. Bull. Bombay *14:*13-15, Jan 28, '46

HILL, B. G. (see WILLIAMS, J. L. D.) Aug '44

HILL, C. D.: Etiology and treatment of hand infections. New York M. J. *114:*575, Nov 16, '21

HILL, D. K.; MCMICHAEL, J. AND SHARPEY-SCHAFER, E. P.: Effects of serum and saline infusions in shock; quantitative studies in man. Lancet *2:*774-776, Dec 21, '40

HILL, F. T.: Reflections on hazards of nasal surgery in person with senile changes. Ann. Otol., Rhin. and Laryng. *36:*503-510, June '27

HILL, H. G.: Autogenous bone graft. Memphis M. J. *7:*21-25, Feb '30

HILL, J. M. AND MUIRHEAD, E. E.: Concentrated plasma; use in treatment of shock. Tri-State M. J. *15:*2844-2849, Dec '42

HILL, J. M. *et al*: Desiccated plasma in shock therapy. J.A.M.A. *116:*395-402, Feb 1, '41

HILL, J. M. (see MUIRHEAD, E. E.) Feb '42

HILL, J. M. (see MUIRHEAD, E. E. *et al*) June '42

HILL, J. M. (see MUIRHEAD, E. E. *et al*) July '42

HILL, J. M. (see MUIRHEAD, E. E.) Dec '42

HILL, L. V.: Immediate treatment of severely injured; general traumatism – shock. J. Kansas M. Soc. *31:*119-121, April '30

HILL, M. (see BENTLEY, F. H.) Oct '36

HILL, M. (see BENTLEY, F. H.) Sept '40

HILL, R. H.: Diagnosis and treatment of shock. J. M. Soc. New Jersey *40:*51–54, Feb '43

HILL, ROBERT T.: *Anatomy of the Head and Neck*. Lea and Febiger Co., Phila., 1946

HILLE, K.: Schubert's operation for artificial vagina. Monatschr. f. Geburtsh. u. Gynak. *76:*288–293, June '27

HILLEBRAND, H.: Skin and tendon transplantation in severe injury to back of right hand by polishing machine. Chirurg *13:*521–523, Sept 1, '41

HILLENBRAND, H. J. (see SCHRODER, C. H.) 1942

HILLENBRAND, K.: Development, structure and changes of form of human nasal septum in fetal life. Arch. f. Ohren-, Nasen-u. Kehlkopfh. *135:*1–24, '33

HILLER, F. (see DAVIS, L.) 1944

HILLSMAN, J. A. AND GUNN, J. A.: Traumatic shock and burns. Manitoba M. A. Rev. *18:*65–68, April '38

HILLSMAN, J. A. (see BRANDSON, B. J.) June '32

HILLSMAN, J. A. (see GUNN, J.) Sept '35

HILSE, A.: Histological results after experimental free transplantation of fat tissue. Beitr. z. path. Anat. u. z. allg. Path. *79:*592–624, April 16, '28

HILZE, A.: Skin grafting and its compensatory growth. Latvijas Arstu z., no. 3–4, pp. 61–66, March–April '27

HINDMARSH, J.: Treatment of ear deformities. Nord. med. tidskr. *16:*1178–1181, July 23, '38

HINES, E. A. JR. (see BARKER, N. W.) June '44

HINES, H. M.: Effects of immobilization and activity on neuromuscular regeneration (after injury). J.A.M.A. *120:*515–517, Oct 17, '42

HINRICHSMEYER, C.: Snapping hand. Zentralbl. f. Chir. *58:*834–837, April 4, '31

HINTON, J. W.: Prevention and treatment of surgical shock. S. Clin. North America *15:*287–293, April '35

HINTZE, A.: Keloid tumor and its cure by radiotherapy. Strahlentherapie *57:*224–240, '36

Hippocrates

References to esthetic surgery in work of Hippocrates. CODAZZI AGUIRRE, J. A. Arq. de cir. clin. e exper. *6:*137–144, April–June '42

References to nasal and auricular esthetic surgery in work of Hippocrates. CODAZZI AGUIRRE, J. A. Semana med. *1:*445–449, Feb 25, '43

HIROSE, K.: Congenital coloboma and incomplete development of meibomian glands in Japanese. Arch. d'opht. *3:*673–689, Aug '39

HIROTA, K.: Changes in Golgi apparatus of kidney, liver and suprarenal cells produced by burning. Nagasaki Igakkwai Zassi *12:*1143–1144, Aug 25, '34

HIRSCH, C. AND KIRCHHOFF, W.: Construction of parts of jaw to be used after plastic surgery. Acta oto-laryng. *12:*488–496, '28

HIRSCH, M.: Procedure to be followed in treatment of minor injuries and diseases of fingers by general practitioner. Wien. klin. Wchnschr. *43:*883–885, July 10, '30

HIRSCHBERG, O.: Instrument for grasping ends of ruptured tendon during suture. Schweiz. med. Wchnschr. *66:*514–515, May 23, '36

HIRSHFELD, J. W. *et al*: Significance of nitrogen loss in exudate from surface burns. Surgery *15:*766–773, May '44

HIRSCHFELD, J. W. *et al*: Alterations following thermal burns; effect of variations in food intake on nitrogen balance of burned patients. Arch. Surg. *50:*194–200, April '45

HIRSHFELD, J. W. *et al.*: Penicillin and skin grafting in burns. J.A.M.A. *125:*1017–1019, Aug 12, '44

HIRSHFELD, J. W.; PILLING, M. A. AND MAUN, M. E.: Comparison of effects of tanning agents (especially tannic acid) and of vaseline gauze on fresh wounds of man (donor sites for skin grafts). Surg., Gynec. and Obst. *76:*556–561, May '43

HIRSHFELD, J. W.; PILLING, M. A. AND MAUN, M. E.: Bio-dyne ointment in burns. J.A.M.A. *123:*476, Oct 23, '43

HIRSCHFELD, K.: Hemangioma of hand, involving phalangeal bones, with distinctive radiologic appearance. Australian and New Zealand J. Surg. *11:*136–139, Oct '41

HIRSHLAND, H.: Congenital defect of scalp. Atlantic M. J. *28:*684–685, July '25

HIRST, O. C.: Osteomyelitis of superior maxilla; treatment with penicillin. Arch. Otolaryng. *41:*351–352, May '45

HISSINK, L. A. G.: Therapy of traumatic shock. Nederl. tijdschr. v. geneesk. *90:*335–336, April 20, '46

History of Plastic Surgery

Harelip operation in 1808. VAN DER HOEVEN, J. Nederl. Tijdschr. v. Geneesk. *1:*44–51, Jan 3, '25

Album of Gensoul, maxillary surgeon. LERICHE, R. Lyon chir. *25:*1–9, Jan–Feb '28

Frühe Plastik in Griechenland und Vorderasien (rund 3000 bis 600 v. Christ), by VALENTIN MÜLLER. B. Filsner, Augsburg, 1929

History and development of plastic surgery.

History of Plastic Surgery – Cont.
Poggi, J. Folha med. *10:*241–243, July 25, '29
Rhinophyma; representations in art and literature. Dieckmann, F. Dermat. Ztschr. *62:*20–31, Sept '31
Experimental and clinical advances during nineteenth century (including plastic surgery). Gluck, T. Arch. f. klin. Chir. *167:*626–666, '31
Rhinoplasty; past and present. Palmer, A. Eye, Ear, Nose and Throat Monthly *11:*58–62, March '32
Rhinoplastic surgery through ages. Clery, A. B. Irish J. M. Sc., pp. 170–176, April '32
Development and present status of cosmetic surgery. Rodríguez Berceruelo, S. Siglo med. *92:*436, Oct 21, '33
Dermo-epidermal grafts; history, technic and indications. Verrière, and Barneville. Arch. de med. et pharm. mil. *100:*173–192, Feb '34
One hundred years after Dupuytren; interpretation. Powers, H. J. Nerv. and Ment. Dis. *80:*386–409, Oct '34
Development and scope of plastic surgery (Charles H. Mayo lecture). Gillies, H. D. Northwestern Univ. Bull., Med. School *35:*1–32, Jan 28, '35
History of plastic surgery in Finland. Faltin, R. Finska lak.-sallsk. handl. *78:*188–238, '35
Short history of treatment of maxillary fractures. Fairbank, L. C. Mil. Surgeon *78:*95–103, Feb '36
Italian contribution to plastic surgery; historical study. Grassi, G. Riv. di storia d. sc. med. e nat. *27:*215–232, July–Aug '36
History of plastic surgery in Finland. Faltin, R. Finska lak.-sallsk. handl. *80:*97–124, Feb '37
Development of plastic surgery. Erczy, M. Gyogyaszat *78:*207–210, March 27, '38
History of burns in connection with Fabricius Hildanus' book published in 1610. Rubashev, S. M. Vestnik khir. *56:*876–880, Dec '38
Plastic surgery in Mississippi Valley; David Prince. Black, C. E. Tr. West. S. A. (1937) *47:*287–309, '38
History of transplantation in general and orthopedic surgery. Orr, H. W. Am. J. Surg. *43:*547–553, Feb '39
Fall and rise of plastic surgery. Updegraff, H. L. Am. J. Surg. *43:*637–656, Feb '39
Augustin Belloste and treatment for avulsion of scalp; old history of operation in head surgery. Strayer, L. M. New England J. Med. *220:*901–905, June 1, '39

History of Plastic Surgery – Cont.
Story (historical sketch) of plastic surgery. Wolfe, M. M. Ann. Otol., Rhin. and Laryng. *48:*473–483, June '39
Plastic and reconstructive surgery about face and head – then and now. Beck, J. C. Illinois M. J. *76:*237–242, Sept '39
Healed fractures of lower jaw, from early Bronze Age. Breitinger, E. Arch. f. Gesch. d. Med. *32:*103–110, '39
History and possibilities of plastic surgery. Gonzalez Ulloa, M. Rev. mex. de cir., ginec. y cancer *8:*53–67, Feb '40
Esthetic and plastic surgery; historical review. Malbec, E. F. Semana med. *1:*1141–1147, May 9, '40
Skin transplantation (including brief historical review). Leven, N. L. Bull. Minnesota M. Found. *1:*77–79, June '40
History, possibilities and present status of plastic surgery. Gonzalez Ulloa, M. Dia med. (Ed. espec., no. 6), p. 120, Aug '40
History of total transplantation of eyeball. Ayres, F. Arq. brasil. de oftal. *3:*305–310, Dec '40
Transplantation of skin and subcutaneous tissue (history of plastic surgery and surgeons). Koch, S. L. Surg., Gynec. and Obst. *72:*1–14, Jan '41
History of plastic surgery. Seltzer, A. P. Laryngoscope *51:*256–262, March '41
Address of president; story of plastic surgery. Davis, J. S. Ann. Surg. *113:*641–656, May '41
Operation on huge scrotal elephantiasis performed by Casimiro Saez y Garcia in 1882. Muller, F. Rev. de med. y cir. Habana *46:*373–383, Aug 31, '41
History of plastic surgery. Davis, J. S. Bol. d. Inst. clin. quir. *18:*34–48, Jan–April '42
References to esthetic surgery in work of Hippocrates. Codazzi Aguirre, J. A. Arq. de cir. clin. e exper. *6:*137–144, April–June '42
Plastic surgery possibilities; development in Cuba; historical study. de Lara, M. J. Arq. de cir. clin. e exper. *6:*325–333, April–June '42
Plastic surgery, Latin American bibliography. Rebelo Neto, J. Arq. de cir. clin. e. exper. *6:*721–776, April–June '42
Plastic surgery, historical background. Penn, J. Leech *13:*23, June '42
References to nasal and auricular esthetic surgery in work of Hippocrates. Codazzi Aguirre, J. A. Semana med. *1:*445–449, Feb 25, '43
Brief panoramic study of nasal surgery. Petit, A. M. Vida nueva *51:*138–145, April '43
Review of reconstructive surgery – 1943–

History of Plastic Surgery–Cont.
1945. McDowell, F. Laryngoscope *55:*239-276, June '45
Plastic surgery in past and future. Gonzalez Ulloa, M. Salud y belleza (no. 4) *1:*18-21, Aug-Sept '45
Evolution of Plastic Surgery, by Maxwell Maltz. Froben Press, New York, 1946
Plastic surgery in World War I and in World War II. Davis, J. S. Ann. Surg. *123:*610-621, April '46
Development of plastic surgery in United States. Aufricht, G. Plast. and Reconstruct. Surg. *1:*3-25, July '46
Plastic surgery in World War I and in World War II. Davis, J. S. Tr. South. S. A. (1945) *57:*141-152, '46

Hitchcock, H. H. and Reynolds, T. E.: Shock therapy by warmed air (use of Sweetland cast-dryer). California and West Med. *44:*98-99, Feb '36
Hjelmman, G.: Therapy of postoperative facial paralysis. Acta Soc. med. fenn. duodecim (Ser. B, fasc. 3, art. 6) *17:*1-11, '33
Hlaváček, V.: Median cervical fistulae. Casop. lek. Cesk. *66:*511-514, March 28, '27
Hoar, W. S. (see Hamilton, J. I. *et al*) Feb '46
Hobhouse, N. and Heald, C. B.: Wrist drop, case of posterior interosseous paralysis. Brit. M. J. *1:*841, April 25, '36
Hoche, L. and Roy: Epithelioma of mucous membrane of lower lip; recovery after radium therapy complicated by partial necrosis of inferior maxilla; case. Bull. Assoc. franc. p. l'etude du cancer *21:*381-384, May '32
Hoche, O.: First aid for thermal war injuries. Med. Klin. *35:*1532, Dec 1; 1563, Dec 8, '39 *36:*39, Jan 12; 67, Jan 19; 94, Jan 26; 154, Feb 9; 239, March 1; 265, March 8; 291, March 15, '40
Hocks, A.: Therapy of finger injuries. Deutsche med. Wchnschr. *64:*169, Jan 28, '38
Hodge, C. C. (see Strumia, M. M.) June '45
Hodge, G. B. (see Cooper, G. R. *et al*) June '43
Hodges, F. M.: Radiation therapy of keloid and keloidal scars. Am. J. Roentgenol. *31:*238-243, Feb '34
Hodges, F. M.; Snead, L. O. and Berger, R. A.: Treatment of hemangiomas and lymphangiomas in infants and children. Virginia M. Monthly *66:*263-266, May '39
Hodgson, N.: Fractures of zygoma. Newcastle M. J. *9:*227-230, July '29
Hodgson, N.: Treatment of Volkmann's contracture by transplantation of internal epicondyle. Brit. J. Surg. *17:*317-318, Oct '29
den Hoed, D. (see Gerlings, P. G.) Feb '37
Hoede, K.: Permanent epilation of hair for cosmetic purposes. (Reply to Zoon) Dermat. Wchnschr. *99:*932, July 14, '34
Hoede, K. and Schaefer, F.: Experiences with thorium-x needles in therapy of hemangiomas. Strahlentherapie *67:*23-38, '40
Hoelz, P.: Therapy of furunculosis by means of Thiersch graft. Arq. de cir. clin. e exper. *6:*550-558, April-June '42
Hoen, T. I.: Peripheral nerve lesions; repair. Am. J. Surg. *72:*489-495, Sept '46
Hoepke, H. and Maurer, H.: Harelip in embryo. Ztschr. f. Anat. u. Entwcklngsgesch. *108:*768-774, '38 (Comment on Fleischmann's and Veau's articles).
Hoets, J.: Early treatment of hand infections. M. J. Australia *1:*652-653, May 25, '28
Hofer, G.: Treatment of congenital fistula of neck with diathermy (electrocoagulation). Arch. f. klin. Chir. *156:*274-283, '29
Hofer, O.: Spontaneous fractures of lower jaw. Arch. f. klin. Chir. *140:*141-162, '26
Hofer, O.: Opportune time and method for cosmetic and functional repair of congenital cleft palate and harelip. Wien. klin. Wchnschr. *43:*1184, Sept 18, '30
Hofer, O.: Plastic replacement of extensive mucosal defects of cheek. Wien. klin. Wchnschr. *49:*990-992, July 31, '36
Hofer, O.: Vertical osteotomy for lengthening lower jaw which has been raised and shortened as result of old trauma; case. Ztschr. f. Stomatol. *34:*826-830, July-Aug '36
Hofer, O. (see Theodorescu, D.) Dec '34
Hoff, H. E. (see Winkler, A. W.) Sept '43
Hoffer, O.: Prognathism of lower jaw; etiology, pathogenesis, prophylaxis and therapy. Stomatol. ital. *1:*657-664, July '39
Hoffman, J. M.: Burns and scalds; etiology and prognosis. Am. J. Surg. *56:*463-468, May '42
Hoffman, W. (see Tarlov, I. M. *et al*) Nov '46
Hoffman, W. J.: Therapy of keloids. Arch. Phys. Therapy *18:*135-138, March '37
Hoffman, W. S. (see Kozoll, D. D.) 1944
Hoffmann, C. A.: Therapy of angiomas from dermatologic viewpoint. Med. Welt *5:*990, July 11, '31
Hoffmann, J. N.: Indications and contraindications for submucous resection of nasal septum. Laryngoscope *33:*13-15, Jan '23
Hoffmann, K. F.: Cosmetic surgery of face. Med. Welt *4:*185-187, Feb 8, '30
Hoffmann, P.: Stenosing tendovaginitis at radial styloid process. J. Bone and Joint Surg. *13:*89-90, Jan '31
Hoffmann, R.: Thiersch grafts; 2 technical points. Schweiz. med. Wchnschr. *56:*816-817, Aug 21, '26

HOFFMANN, R.: Device for external transcutaneous fixation of mandibular fractures. Helvet. med. acta *11:*521–524, June '44

HOFFMANN, V.: Autoplastic bone transplantation from viewpoint of biology and architectonic. Arch. f. klin. Chir. *135:*413–485, '25

HOFMANN, A. H.: Dislocations of phalanges of thumb on both sides. Zentralbl. f. Chir. *54:*788, March 26, '27

HOFMANN, H. M.: Sawdust beds—summary of 7 years' experience (measure for prevention and treatment of bedsores). Mod. Hosp. *56:*49–50, March '41

HOFMANN, L.: Congenital malformation of ears; case. Monatschr. f. Ohrenh. *61:*509–512, May–June '27

HOFMANN, M.: Reconstruction of lower lip. Arch. f. klin. Chir. *131:*338–342, '24

HOFMANN, W.: Treatment of furuncles on face. Arch. f. klin. Chir. *123:*51–66, '23 (illus.) abstr: J.A.M.A. *80:*1420, May 12, '23

HOGAN, M.: Treatment of burns. J. Kansas M. Soc. *25:*35–37, Feb '25

HOGEWIND, F.: Favorable time for reposition of nasal fractures. Geneesk. gids *16:*781, July 15, '38

HOGG, B. M.: General care and treatment of burns. Air Surgeon's Bull. (no. 1) *1:*19–21, Jan '44

HOHMANN, G.: Orthopedic treatment of contraction of fingers. Munchen. med. Wchnschr. *83:*2088–2089, Dec 18, '36

HOHMANN, G.: Dupuytren's contracture in both hands and both feet. Ztschr. f. Orthop. *73:*45, '41

HOHMANN, G.: Hand and finger contracture due to burns. Chirurg *14:*289, May 15, '42

HOHMEIER, F.: Operation for cleft palate and hare-lip. Deutsche med. Wchnschr. *52:*1604–1606, Sept 17, '26

HOLBROOK, J. S.: Construction of vagina from loop of small bowel. Minnesota med. *10:*55, Jan '27

HOLDEN, W. B.: Plastic surgery of penis. S. Clin. N. Amer. *8:*1409–1410, Dec '28

HOLDER, J. S.: Conservative surgery in hand injuries. Indust. Med. *7:*238–239, May '38

HOLLÄNDER, E.: Surgical treatment of hypertrophy of breast. Deutsche med. Wchnschr. *50:*1400–1402, Oct 10, '24. Comment by LEXER, E. Deutsche med. Wchnschr. *51:*26, Jan 2, '25 abstr: J.A.M.A. *83:*1721, Nov 22, '24

HOLLÄNDER, E.: Treatment of hypertrophic breast; reply to Lexer. Deutsche med. Wchnschr. *51:*26, Jan 2, '25

HOLLAND, C. A. (see SANO, M. E. *et al*) Dec '43

HOLLAND, C. L.: Cleft palate. W. Virginia M. J. *23:*262–263, May '27

HOLLAND, D. J. (see STURGIS, S. H.) Jan '44

HOLLAND, D. J. (see STURGIS, S. H.) March '44

HOLLAND, D. J. JR. (see STURGIS, S. H.) Oct '46

HOLLAND, N.: Treatment of maxillofacial casualties in B.L.A. Brit. Dent. J. *78:*78–80, Feb 2, '45

HOLLAND, N. W. A.: Use of cheek wires in treatment of fractures of maxilla. Brit. Dent. J. *79:*333–340, Dec 21, '45

HOLLANDER, L.: Treatment of carcinoma of lip. Arch. Phys. Therapy *17:*17–24, Jan '36

HOLLANDER, L.: Good dressing for wounds produced by electrocoagulation. Arch. Dermat. and Syph. *33:*730, April '36

HOLLANDER, L.: Cancer of lip and oral cavity and skin. Pennsylvania M. J. *40:*749–750, June '37

HOLLANDER, L. AND SHELTON, J. M.: Replacement skin grafts in surgical treatment of lupus vulgaris. Arch. Dermat. and Syph. *40:*263–267, Aug '39

HOLLANDER, L. AND SHELTON, J. M.: Evaluation of cryotherapy of post-acne scars. Pennsylvania M. J. *45:*226–228, Dec '41

HOLLANDER, L. AND SHELTON, J. M.: Replacement skin graft in surgical treatment of lupus vulgaris. Arch. Dermat. and Syph. *49:*60, Jan '44

Holländer's Operation

Plastic surgery by Holländer's operation for breasts. SONNTAG, E. Arch. f. klin. Chir. *164:*812–824, '31

HOLLENDER, A. R.: Delayed healing of septal resections due to Vincent's infection; 3 cases. Arch. Otolaryng. *9:*422–424, April '29

HOLLENDER, A. R.: Fallacious views and factors influencing more successful results in nasal surgery. J. Florida M. A. *28:*27–29, July '41

HOLLENDER, A. R.: Critical review of causes of unsuccessful end results of nasal surgery. South. M. J. *35:*363–372, April '42

HOLLENDER, A. R.: Critical review of causes of unsuccessful end results in nasal surgery. Eye, Ear, Nose and Throat Monthly *22:*21–26, Jan '43

HOLLÓS, L.: Resection of orbicular muscle in ectropion paralysis. Orvosi hetil. *74:*1094–1095, Oct 25, '30 also: Ztschr. f. Augenh. *73:*27–31, Dec '30

HOLLOWAY, J. B. JR. (see PICKERELL, K. L. *et al*) Oct '46

HOLMAN, E.: Protein sensitization in isoskingrafting; is the latter of practical value? Surg., Gynec. and Obst. *38:*100–106, Jan '24

HOLMAN, E.: Restoration of scalp; management of skin grafts. J.A.M.A. *84:*350-352, Jan 31, '25
HOLMAN, E.: Placement of neck incisions. Surg., Gynec. and Obst. *78:*533-534, May '44
HOLMES, A. D.: External use of cod liver oil in burns; review. Indust. Med. *6:*77-83, Feb '37
HOLMES, E. M. (see KAZANJIAN, V. H.) Sept '46
HOLMES, H. B.: Severe burns; case. M. J. Australia *2:*465-466, Dec 22, '45
HOLMES, R. L. JR. AND MIMS, A. T.: Use of desiccated red blood cells in treatment of ulcers of skin. Dallas M. J. *31:*138-144, Nov '45
HOLMES, W. AND YOUNG, J. Z.: Nerve regeneration after immediate and delayed suture. J. Anat. *77:*63-96, Oct '42
HOLMES, W. (see HIGHET, W. B.) Jan '43
HOLMES, W. (see SEDDON, H. J. *et al*) April '42
HOLMES, W. (see SEDDON, H. J.) Oct '44
HOLMES, W. (see YOUNG, J. Z. *et al*) Aug '40
HOLMES, W. E. (see TYLER, A. F.) April '39
HOLMES, W. R. AND WILLIAMS, G. A.: Formation of artificial vagina without operation by Frank method. Am. J. Obst. and Gynec. *39:*145-146, Jan '40
HOLMGREN, B.: Burn therapy. Nord. med. tidskr. *9:*413-420, March 16, '35
HOLMGREN, H. (see CAMITZ, H. *et al*) 1934
HOLMS, S. (see BADENOCH, A. W.) Dec '45
HOLT, R. L.; SLOME, D. AND DALE, H.: Discussion on traumatic shock. Proc. Roy. Soc. Med. *28:*1473-1496, Sept '35
HOLTERMANN, C.: Plastic surgery of anus; using fatty flap of bulbocavernosus muscle, in therapy of incontinence of feces, following transplantation of vestibular anus; case. Zentralbl. f. Gynak. *63:*60-66, Jan 7, '39
HOLTERS, O. R.: Experiences with "Hindenburg" patients and review of cutaneous burns. J. M. Soc. New Jersey *34:*545-548, Sept '37
HOLTH, S.: Mimical ectropion of upper eyelids. Acta ophth. *14:*340, '36
HOLTH, S.: Mimical ectropion or entropion of one or both eyelids. Norsk mag. f. laegevidensk. *98:*938-940, July '37
HOLTON, H. M. (see LUND, C. C.) April '33
HOLTON, H. M. (see LUND, C. C.) July '33
HOLYOKE, E. A. (see GRODINSKY, M.) April '41
HOLZBACH, E.: Treatment of surgical shock with ephetonin (synthetic ephedrine). Zentralbl. f. Gynak. *53:*1106-1110, May 4, '29
HOLZBACH, E.: Nature and treatment of surgical shock and postoperative collapse. Fortschr. d. Therap. *7:*169-172, March 25, '31
HOLZKNECHT, G.: Burns of roentgenologists; therapy. Fortschr. a. d. Geb. d. Rontgenstrahlen *44:*78-81, July '31
HOMANS, J.: Elephantiasis of legs; therapy; preliminary report. New England J. Med. *215:*1099-1104, Dec 10, '36
HOMME, O. H.: Adjustable nasal elevator. Arch. Otolaryng. *20:*711, Nov '34

Homografts

Partial cheiloplasty by transplantation from one person to another. DUJARDIN, E. Ugesk. f. laeger *94:*382-383, April 14, '32
Cranioplasty by sterilized grafts from human cadaver. DAMBRIN, L. AND DAMBRIN, P. Bordeaux chir. *7:*279-286, July '36
Experimental studies on transplantation of conjunctiva from eye of cadaver; preliminary report. ROZENTSVEVG, M. G. Vestnik oftal. *11:*311-316, '37
Therapy of trachomatous pannus by transplantation of mucous membrane from cadaver conserved in cold. KOSTENKO, F. M. Med. zhur. *8:*533-542, '38
Transplantation of mucous membrane from lips of cadavers in Millingen-Sapezhko operation. ALEKSEEV, S. A. Vestnik oftal. (no. 6) *15:*77-79, '39
Cadaver cartilage as material for free transplantation. MIKHELSON, N. M. Khirurgiya, no. 10, pp. 29-34, '39
Therapy of ocular burns by transplantation of conjunctiva from cadaver. ZENKINA, L. V. Vestnik oftal. (no. 2) *15:*28-29, '39
Transplantation of conjunctiva of cadaver; clinical and histologic aspects. SIE BOEN LIAN. Geneesk. tijdschr. v. Nederl.-Indie *81:*2097-2101, Sept 30, '41
Transplantation of cartilage from cadaver according to Mikhelson method in correction of nasal deformities. LITINSKIY, A. M. Novy khir. arkhiv. *48:*211-214, '41
New method for formation of stump after enucleation by transplantation of cadaver's cartilage into Tenon's capsule of eye. SVERDLOV, D. G. Vestnik oftal. (nos. 5-6) *19:*45-50, '41
Massive repairs of burns with thick split skin grafts; emergency dressings with homografts. BROWN, J. B. AND MCDOWELL, F. Ann. Surg., *115:*658, Apr '42
Epithelial healing and the transplantation of skin. BROWN, J. B. AND MCDOWELL, F. Ann. Surg., *115:*1166, June '42. Also in Trans. American Surgical Assn., *60:*1166, June '42. Also in Digest of Treatment, *6:*481, Jan '43. Also in Anales de Cirugia, pp. 272, 1942
Defense of human body against living mam-

Homografts – Cont.
malian cells; address of president. STONE, H. B. Ann. Surg. *115:*883-891, June '42
Experiments on cadaver nerve graft and "glue" suture of divided nerves. DE REZENDE, N. New York State J. Med. *42:*2124-2128, Nov 15, '42
Reconstructive plastic surgery of absent ear with necrocartilage; original method. LAMONT, E. S. Arch. Surg. *48:*53-72, Jan '44
Cadaver cartilage banks. NUNN, L. L. Bull. U. S. Army M. Dept. (no. 74) pp. 99-101, March '44
Transplantation of nerves from cadavers in human surgery. DE REZENDE, N. Rev. brasil. de cir. *13:*245-258, May '44
Preparation and storage of autopsy nerve grafts. SACCOMANNO, G. *et al.* Science *100:*436, Nov 10, '44
Graft of cadaver skin; preliminary report. BIANCHI, R. G. Dia med. *17:*1168, Oct 8, '45 also: Prensa med. argent. *32:*1997, Oct 12, '45
Utilization of cadaver cartilage in surgery. GONZALEZ ULLOA, M. Medicina, Mexico *25:*495-503, Dec 10, '45
Use of cadaver cartilage in surgery. GONZALEZ ULLOA, M. Rev. brasil. de cir. *14:*663-670, Dec '45 also: Prensa med. argent. *33:*705-709, April 5, '46

HOMPES, J. J.: Case report of repair of nasal septal perforation. Tr. Am. Laryng., Rhin. and Otol. Soc. *33:*565-568, '27
HONAN, M. S.: The adrenals and shock. M. Press *213:*13-14, Jan 3, '45
HONIGMANN, F.: Treatment of finger infections of physicians. Munchen. med. Wchnschr. *69:*160-161, Feb 3, '22
HONIGMANN, F.: Rupture of tendon of long extensor of thumb occurring late after injury. Med. Klin. *22:*728-731, May 7, '26 abstr: J.A.M.A. *87:*133, July 10, '26
HOOGVELD, W. P. J.: Snapping finger. Nederlandsch Tijdschr. v. Geneesk. *1:*2663, May 14, '21 abstr: J.A.M.A. *77:*416, July 30, '21
HOOK, F. R. AND TAYLOR, R. W.: Surgical treatment of prognathism; case. U. S. Nav. M. Bull. *40:*157-158, Jan '42
HOOKER, D. H. AND LAM, C. R.: Absorption of sulfanilamide from burned surfaces. Surgery *9:*534-537, April '41
HOOKER, D. H. AND LAM, C. R.: Hand tendon injuries; study of 116 cases. Am. J. Surg. *54:*412-416, Nov '41
HOOPES, B. F.: Chemical burn of penis. U. S. Nav. M. Bull. *44:*846-847, April '45
HOOVER, J. E.: Plastic surgery and criminals; surgeon's responsibility. Am. J. Surg. *28:*156, April '35
HOOVER, J. E.: Practitioner's responsibility when fugitives attempt to conceal identity by means of surgery. J.A.M.A. *104:*1663-1664, May 4, '35
HOOVER, M. J. (see EVANS, E. I.) Oct '43
HOOVER, M. J. (see EVANS, E. I. *et al*) March '44
HOOVER, M. J. (see EVANS, E. I. *et al*) March '45
HOOVER, W. B.: Dacryocystorhinostomy (Mosher-Toti operation). S. Clin. North America *16:*1695-1699, Dec '36
HOOVER, W. B.: Clinical conditions arising from anomalies or maldevelopments of branchial arches and clefts. Ann. Otol., Rhin. and Laryng. *50:*834-849, Sept '41
HOOVER, W. B.: Nasal surgery – local anesthesia; technic and practical considerations. S. Clin. North America *22:*661-673, June '42
HOOVER, W. B. AND POPPEN, J. L.: Surgical repair of seventh cranial nerve. S. Clin. North America *20:*685-695, June '40
HÖRA, J.: Revival of "slumbering cells" theory; criticism of Busse-Grawitz' experiments claiming vitality of various tissues in subcutaneous implantations. Ztschr. f. d. ges. exper. Med. *108:*757-771, '41
HORAN, F. P.: Dichloramine T treatment of burns. Illinois M. J. *40:*123, Aug '21
HORAY, G.: Four cases of unusual eye injuries; eyelash in iris; horsehair in lens; ink pencil injury; traumatic enophthalmos. Klin. Monatsbl. f. Augenh. *80:*202-208, Feb 24, '28
HORGAN, E.: Nerve suture and muscle repair; primary suture of ulnar nerve and secondary reconstruction of extensor tendons of forearm. Ann. Surg. *95:*93-100, Jan '32
HORGAN, J. B.: Facial paralysis treated by incision of sheath of facial nerve. Brit. M. J. *2:*768, Oct 14, '39
HORGAN, J. B.: Duel-Ballance nerve graft for cure of complete traumatic facial paralysis; case. Irish J. M. Sc., pp. 196-198, May '41
HÖRHAMMER, C.: Reposition of dislocated mandible in local anesthesia. Munchen. med. Wchnschr. *73:*446-447, March 12, '26
HÖRHAMMER, C.: Surgical therapy of hypospadias in male. Chirurg *10:*159-161, March 1, '38
HORNBAKER, R. W.: Hemorrhage, shock and their treatment (including teaching principles for naval personnel). Hosp. Corps Quart. (no. 1) *18:*27-31, Jan '45
HORNER, W. D. AND CORDES, F. C.: Congenital coloboma of upper eyelid with dermoids on cornea; case. Am. J. Ophth. *12:*959-964, Dec '29

HORSCH, K.: Underwater douche for decubitus ulcers. Balneologe *4:*512-517, Nov '37

HORSLEY, J. S.: Surgical treatment of extensive basal cell carcinoma. J.A.M.A. *78:*412-416, Feb 11, '22 (illus.)

HORSLEY, J. S.: Plastic operations for defects of face due to noma. Southern M. J. *15:*557-561, July '22 (illus.)

HORSLEY, J. S. JR.: Basal-cell carcinoma of skin. S. Clin. N. America *2:*1247-1257, Oct '22

HORSLEY, J. S. JR.: Transplantation of distant skin flaps for cure of intractable basal-cell carcinoma. Ann. Surg. *82:*14-29, July '25

HORSLEY, J. S. JR.: Harelip and cleft palate. Virginia M. Monthly *53:*782-787, March '27

HORSLEY, J. S. JR.: End-results after harelip operations. Virginia M. Monthly *54:*753-757, March '28

HORSLEY, J. S. JR.: Plastic surgery of face. West Virginia M. J. *26:*1-8, Jan '30

HORSLEY, J. S. JR.: Double harelip. South. Med. and Surg. *94:*197-201, April '32

HORSLEY, J. S. JR.: Full thickness grafts (with special reference to Douglas "sieve graft"). Internat. S. Digest *16:*67-82, Aug '33

HORTOLOMEI, N.: Construction of artificial vagina from small intestine, 4 cases. Zentralbl. f. Chir. *50:*259-262, Feb 17, '23 abstr: J.A.M.A. *80:*1110, April 14, '23

HORTOLOMEI, N.: Baldwin-Mori operation for congenital absence of vagina. Rev. de chir., Bucuresti *42:*136-138, Jan-Feb '39

HORTON, W. S. S.: Implant skin grafting; case in burns. Am. J. Surg. *55:*597-599, March '42

HORWITZ, A.: Treatment of phlegmonous tendovaginitis. Munchen. med. Wchnschr. *73:*1987-1989, Nov 19, '26

HORWITZ, A.: Treatment of rupture of extensor tendons of fingers. Zentralbl. f. Chir. *57:*1463-1464, June 14, '30. Comment by GLASS, E. Zentralbl. f. Chir. *57:*2063, Aug 16, '30

HORWITZ, A.: Late subcutaneous rupture of tendon of extensor pollicis longus after fracture of radius and other bone changes in region of injury. Deutsche Ztschr. f. Chir. *234:*710-722, '31

HORWITZ, A.: Surgical or nonsurgical treatment of rupture of extensor tendons of terminal phalanx of finger. Deutsche med. Wchnschr. *57:*445-448, March 13, '31

HORWITZ, M. T. (see DAVIDSON, A. J.) April '39

HORWITZ, T.: Dupuytren's contracture; consideration of anatomy of fibrous structures of hand in relation to this condition, with interpretation of histology. Arch. Surg. *44:*687-706, April '42

HORWITZ, T.: Effect of sulfanilamide crystals, used topically, on fate of transplanted bone; experimental and clinical observations. Surgery *11:*690-697, May '42

HORWITZ, T.: Opponens thumb wire splint. Am. J. Surg. *58:*460, Dec '42

HOSMER, A. J.: Immobilizing cage in burn therapy and skin grafts. Am. J. Surg. *3:*23-30, July '27

HOSMER, M. N.; BURNHAM, DEW. K. AND DAVIS, A. D.: Osteomyelitis of bones of face in a severe diabetic with recovery and plastic reconstruction (case). California and West. Med. *53:*165-168, Oct '40

HOSOMI, E.: Bilateral anterior nasal atresia; cure; case. Oto-rhino-laryng. *10:*329, April '37

HOSOMI, K.: Experimental and clinical study of transplantation of tissues preserved in alcohol or formalin solution. Deutsche Ztschr. f. Chir. *209:*14-30, '28

HOTTA, H.: Protective prosthesis for plastic operation on palate. Ztschr. d. japan, chirurg. Gesellsch. *36:*100-101, '35

HOTTA, H.: Protective prosthesis for plastic operations of palate. Nagoya J. M. Sc. *10:*280-284, Dec '36

Hotz Operation

Modification of Hotz operation for entropion due to trachoma. MAXWELL, J. S. Am. J. Ophth. *24:*298-302, March '41

HOUCK, J. S.: Forum on therapy of wartime injuries (burns). New York State J. Med. *43:*226-228, Feb 1, '43

HOULIÉ: Surgical treatment of abnormal flaring of ears. Progres med. *38:*85-86, Feb 24, '23 (illus.)

HOUOT, A.: Grave burn in girl 6 years old; death on fifty-second day due to progressive emaciation; role of adrenal insufficiency. Union med. du Canada *72:*25-27, Jan '43

HOUOT, A.: Grave burn in infant; case with recovery after therapy with cortin (adrenal preparation) associated with tannic acid and silver nitrate (Bettmann). Union med. du Canada *72:*169-171, Feb '43

HOUOT, A.: Cortin (adrenal preparation) in burn therapy. Union med. du Canada *74:*289-296, March '45

HOUOT, A.; LAOUENAN, P. AND KHOURY, B.: Results of new therapies for serious recent burns, with special reference to tannin. Ann. Fac. franc. de med. et de pharm. de Beyrouth *8:*32-54, Jan-Feb '39

HOUOT, A. (see DUMALLE, G.) 1938

HOUPERT, L. (see GINESTET, G. *et al*) July '39

HOUSER, K. M.: Submucous resection followed by complications of acute otitis, mastoiditis and sinus thrombosis. Arch. Otolaryng. *7:*631-634, June '28

HOUSER, K. M.: Vincent's ulceration of soft palate. Tr. Am. Laryng. A. *64:*141-143, '42

HOUTZ, SARA J. (with Robert A. Groff): *Manual of Diagnosis and Management of Peripheral Nerve Injuries*. J. B. Lippincott Co., Phila., 1945

HOUZEL, G. (see BABONNEIX, L.) Aug '39

Hovelacque Operation: See Heitz-Boyer-Hovelacque Operation

HOWARD, A. J. (see THOMSON, D. *et al*) March '41

HOWARD, E. F.: Topical application of cocaine in nose. New Orleans M. and S. J. *80:*162-167, Sept '27

HOWARD, J. C. JR. (see WIBLE, L. E.) Aug '46

HOWARD, N. J.: Burn therapy. Stanford M. Bull. *1:*34-36, Aug '42

HOWARD, R. C.: Window operation for hematoma auris and perichondritis, with effusion. Laryngoscope *39:*590-594, Sept '29

HOWARD, R. C.: Window operation for hematoma and perichondritis with effusion of ear. Laryngoscope *45:*81-105, Feb '35

HOWARD, R. N.: Extensive primary nerve and tendon suture at wrist; 2 cases. M. J. Australia *2:*322-323, Aug 26, '39

HOWARTH, W.: Tumors and ulcers of palate and fauces (Semon lecture, abstract). Lancet *2:*1139-1142, Nov 14, '36

HOWARTH, W. AND DAVIS, E. D. D.: Discussion on complications of intranasal surgery. Proc. Roy. Soc. Med. *32:*1238-1246, Aug '39 also: J. Laryng. and Otol. *54:*627-640, Oct '39

HOWE, H. D. (see THOMA, K. H. *et al*) April '45

HOWELL, E. B.: Jaw fractures. U. S. Nav. M. Bull. *33:*76-77, Jan '35

HOWES, A. E.: Malocclusion produced by formation of scar tissue (from burn). Internat. J. Orthodontia *21:*1141-1143, Dec '35

HOWES, W. E. AND LA ROSA, F. J.: Carcinoma of lower lip; interval statistical survey of end-results in all cases treated at Brooklyn Cancer Institute, 1930 to 1939 inclusive. Am. J. Roentgenol. *47:*39-49, Jan '42

HOWITT, F.: Correction appliance for contracture of fingers and wrist. Lancet *2:*1394-1395, Dec 22, '34

HOWLAND, J. W. (see MAHONEY, E. B. *et al*) Feb '42

HOWLAND, J. W. (see MAHONEY, E. B.) Feb '43

HOWLAND, J. W. (see MAHONEY, E. B.) July '43

HOWLETT, H.: Intravenous therapy for postoperative shock. Internat. Clin. *3:*26-29, Sept '30

HOY, C. D.: Importance of purposeful splinting of hand following injuries. Ohio State M. J. *38:*1025, Nov '42

HRAD, O.: Acetylsulfanilamide ointment in local therapy of burns. Deutsche med. Wchnschr. *67:*1147-1150, Oct 17, '41

HRAD, O.: Sulfonamide (sulfacetimide) ointment; local treatment of burns. Bull. War Med. *3:*542-543, June '43 (abstract)

HSU, H. A.: Cosmetic results obtained by use of Thiersch technic of skin grafting. Chinese M. J. *50:*939-944, July '36

HSU, Y. H. (see LIU, J. H.) April '39

HU, M. L.: Depression of bridge of nose (case following abscess of septum) and its plastic treatment. Chinese M. J. *54:*563-567, Dec '38

HUARD, P.: Resection of superior cervical ganglion in therapy of peripheral facial paralysis caused by injury to cranium; case. Bull. Soc. med.-chir. de l'Indochine *14:*1289-1293, Nov '36

HUARD, P. AND BOUTAREAU: Wounds of median nerve with surgical therapy in 5 cases; interest of external route of access; anatomic possibility of anastomosis of anterior branch of radial with peripheral end of median in extended loss of nerve substance. Bull. Soc. med.-chir. de l'Indochine *13:*1856-1873, Dec '35

HUARD, P. AND LONG, M.: Restoration of thumb using bone and skin grafts. Bull. Soc. med.-chir. de l'Indochine *15:*855-860, Aug-Sept '37

HUBBARD, W. B.: Caustic burns of eyes. Arch. Ophth. *19:*968-975, June '38

HUBBARD, W. B. (see COSGROVE, K. W.) Jan '28

HÜBENER, A. W.: Operative treatment of hypertrophied breasts. Deutsche Ztschr. f. Chir. *181:*40-47, '23 (illus.) abstr: J.A.M.A. *81:*1566, Nov 3, '23

HUBER, H. S.: Application of general principles in tendon suture. S. Clin. North America *19:*499-518, April '39

HUBER, H. S. (see ENNIS, W. N.) April '38

HUBER, J. P.: Dermoepidermal grafts in early treatment of severe war burns. Semaine d. hop. Paris *21:*741-747, July 21, '45 also: Bull. internat. serv. san. *18:*197-209, Aug '45

HUBER, M.: Speech re-education following palatal reconstruction. Canad. M.A.J. *46:*325-326, April '42

HUBINGER, H. L.: Ununited fractures of symphysis of mandible. Mil. Surgeon *91:*320-324, Sept '42

HUC, G. (see THOMAS, A.) Dec '35

HUDACK, S. S.: Adaption of structure of hand to disturbed function following deep burns (clawhand). Am. Acad. Orthop. Surgeons, Lect., pp. 208–211, '44

HUDSON, A. C.: Radium as adjuvant to operation in case of deformity of eyelids from burn with keloid scars. Proc. Roy. Soc. Med. *27:*1611, Oct '34

HUDON, F. AND PARADIS, B.: Pervitin (d-desoxyephedrine) therapy in shock. Laval med. *10:*110–128, Feb '45

HUDSON, H. W. (see WHITE, J. C. *et al*) Sept '45

HUDSON, H. W. JR.: Snapping thumb in childhood; 8 cases. New England J. Med. *210:*854–857, April 19, '34

HUDSON, J. E. (see HARKINS, H. N. *et al*) Oct '36

HUDSON, O. C.: Fractures of zygoma. J. Bone and Joint Surg. *14:*958–962, Oct '32

HUDSON, R. T.: Surgical procedures in treatment of arthritis. Kentucky M. J. *35:*373–375, Aug '37

HUDSON, R. V.: Burn therapy by coated silk fabric (including envelopes); report upon conclusion drawn from treatment of 82 cases (by irrigation with electrolytic sodium hypochlorite solution). Brit. M. J. *2:*7–12, July 5, '41

HUDSON, R. V.: Principles governing design and details of first aid Stannard glove. Bull. War Med. *4:*193–195, Dec '43 (abstract)

HUDSON, R. V. (see WAKELEY, C. P. G. *et al*) 1945

HUEPER, W. C.; MARTIN, G. J. AND THOMPSON, M. R.: Methyl cellulose solution as plasma substitute in shock. Am. J. Surg. *56:*629–635, June '42

HUET, P. C.: Aims of early treatment of nasal fractures. Medecine *9:*317–318, Jan '28

HUET, P. C.: Early treatment of nasal fractures. J. de chir. *31:*649–658, May '28

HUET, P. C.: Pathogenesis and treatment of nasal fractures. Ann. d. mal. de l'oreille, du larynx *47:*797–833, Sept '28

HUEY, W. B. (see DAVIS, G. G.) Aug '35

HUFFMAN, L. D.: Intravenous use of solutions of gum arabic (acacia). Proc. Staff Meet., Mayo Clin. *2:*84, April 20, '27

HUFFMAN, L. D.: Solution of acacia and sodium chloride; effects of intravenous administration in shock. J.A.M.A. *93:*1698–1702, Nov 30, '29

HUGHES, E. N.: Treatment for traumatic symblepharon. Brit. J. Ophth. *11:*337–338, July '27

HUGHES, G. K.: Boric-butyn-petrolatum gauze treatment in burns. J. Michigan M. Soc. *41:*653–656, Aug '42

HUGHES, J. E.: Penetration of tissue of finger by Diesel oil under pressure. J.A.M.A. *116:*2848–2849, June 28, '41

HUGHES, J. R. (see ATTWATER, H. L.) Sept '38

HUGHES, R. P. AND SMITH, L. M.: Injection treatment of chronic sinuses; case of infected thyroglossal duct cured by copper sulfate injections. Southwestern Med. *23:*187, June '39

HUGHES, W. H.: Immunologic connection with burn sepsis. Lancet *2:*670–672, Sept 17, '38

HUGHES, W. L.: Removal of eyelid, with plastic repair. Arch. Ophth. *10:*198–201, Aug '33

HUGHES, W. L.: Eye socket reconstruction; new form and method of handling skin graft. Arch. Ophth. *26:*965–968, Dec '41

HUGHES, W. L.: Reconstruction of contracted eye socket. Tr. Am. Soc. Plastic and Reconstructive Surg. *12:*25–28, '43

HUGHES, W. L.: Total reconstruction of upper lid (blepharopoiesis). Am. J. Ophth. *28:*980–992, Sept '45

HUGHES, W. L.: Reconstruction of eyelids. Am. J. Ophth. *28:*1203–1211, Nov '45

HUGHES, W. L.; GUY, L. P. AND BOGART, D. W.: Dacryocystorhinostomy. Surg., Gynec. and Obst. *73:*375–380, Sept '41

Hughes Operation

Hughes procedure for rebuilding lower eyelid. GIFFORD, S. R. Arch. Ophth. *21:*447–452, March '39

Hughes operation for total loss of lower eyelid. DELLEPIANE RAWSON, R. Arq. de cir. clin. e exper. *6:*235–251, April–June '42

Reconstruction of lower eyelid by Hughes method. FOSTER, J. Brit. J. Ophth. *28:*515–519, Oct '44

Hughes operation for total loss of lower eyelid. DELLEPIANE RAWSON, R. Dia med. *14:*461, May 25, '42

HUGONOT. (see CLAVELIN, C.) Nov '36

HUGUENIN, R. (see ROUSSY, G. *et al*) Feb '42

HUIZINGA, E.: Case of lateral fistula of neck. Nederl. Tijdschr. v. Geneesk. *2:*1775–1777, Oct 16, '26

HUIZINGA, E.: Lateral cervical fistula; case. Laryngoscope *37:*878–879, Dec '27

HULBERT, K. F. (see ROSS, J. A.) Nov '40

HULBERT, K. F. (see ROSS, J. A.) April '41

HULL, H. C.: Burns of thermal origin. (with shock) Arch. Surg. *45:*235–252, Aug '42

HULLSIEK, H. E.: Conclusions based on study of 433 hand injuries. Minnesota Med. *7:*670–675, Oct '24

HULLSIEK, H. E.: Skin grafts. Am. Mercury *17:*456–459, Aug '29

HULLSTRUNG, H.: Burn after-treatment. Med. Klin. *40:*164, March 17, '44

Hulsman Operation: See Murray-Nelson-Hulsman Operation

Human Bite Injuries

Human bite infections, with study of route of extension of infection from dorsum of hand. MASON, M. L. AND KOCH, S. L. Surg., Gynec. and Obst. *51:*591–625, Nov '30

Vincent's disease following bite of hand. COLBY, F. AND BARR, H. B. Texas State J. Med. *28:*467–470, Nov '32

Hand infections following human bites. COHN, R. Surgery *7:*546–554, April '40

Human bites of hand. MILLER, H. AND WINFIELD, J. M. Surg., Gynec. and Obst. *74:*153–160, Feb '42

Human bites of hand; analysis of 90 (chiefly delayed and late) cases from Charity Hospital of Louisiana at New Orleans. BOYCE F. F. South. M. J. *35:*631–638, July '42

HUMBERD, J. D. (see DUNLOP, G. R.) Jan '45

HUMBY, G.: Advantage of production and fixation of nearly full thickness skin graft. Rev. de chir. structive, pp. 274–276, Dec '37

HUMBY, G.: Nostril in secondary harelip. Lancet *1:*1275, June 4, '38

HUMBY, G.: One-stage operation for hypospadias. Brit. J. Surg. *29:*84–92, July '41

HUME, E. C.: Traumatic surgery of facial structures. Kentucky M. J. *32:*520–522, Oct '34

HUME, E. C.: Treatment of nasal fractures. Am. J. Orthodontics (Oral Surg. Sect) *27:*105, Feb '41

HUME, E. C.: Treatment of traumatic injuries of face. Kentucky M. J. *40:*89–93, March '42

HUME, E. C.: Treatment of jaw fractures. Kentucky M. J. *40:*297–298, Aug '42

HUME, J. R. AND OWENS, N.: Microtia with meatal atresia, with description of operation for its correction; 2 cases. Ann. Otol., Rhin. and Laryng. *44:*213–219, March '35

HUMPHREY, H. D. (see WELLS, D. B. *et al*) April '42

HUMPHREY, W. R. (see KETCHAM, A. H.) 1927

HUMPHREYS, E. M. (see ORTMAYER, M.) Jan '41

HUMPHRIES, S. V.: "Islet" method of wiring fractures of mandible. Clin. Proc. *5:*154–160, June '46

HUMPHRIES, S. V.: Severe septic wound of left lower leg treated with small deep grafts; case. South African M. J. *20:*472–473, Aug 24, '46

HUMPLIK, H.: Technic of free skin grafts; indications. Wien. med. Wchnschr. *96:*265–269, July 15, '46

HUNDEMER, W.: Grafts of pedicled soft tissue flaps in therapy of osseous fistulas following gunshot fractures. Munchen. med. Wchnschr. *91:*154, March 24, '44

HÜNERMANN, T.: Treatment of cancer of mucosa of cheek. Deutsche Ztschr. f. Chir *203–204:*332–336, '27

Hungarian Operation for Eyelid

Hungarian method of forming lower eyelid. SZOKOLIK, E. Klin. Monatsbl. f. Augenh. *80:*652–655, May 25, '28

Closure of persistent retro-auricular opening by means of Hungarian method of using semicircular flaps. SZOKOLIK, E. Monatschr. f. Ohrenh. *66:*1058–1059, Sept '32

Principles of plastic surgery of eyelids, with special reference to Hungarian school. KATZ, D. Arch. Ophth. *12:*220–227, Aug '34

Indications and comparative evaluation of Hungarian method of blepharoplasty. KOPP, I. F. Sovet. vestnik oftal. *7:*603–609, '35

Plastic surgery in ectropion or loss of substance, with special reference to Hungarian method. DE SAINT-MARTIN. Rev. med. de Nancy *64:*879–903, Dec 1, '36 also: Bull. Soc. d'opht. de Paris, pp. 648–671, Oct '36

Eyelid surgery; about sliding-flap, known also as Hungarian plastic. CZUKRASZ, I. Tr. Ophth. Soc. U. Kingdom (pt. 2) *58:*561–575, '38

Skin autoplasty by Hungarian method. AUBRY, M. Semaine d. hop. Paris *21:*488–491, May 14, '45

HUNNER, G. L.: Unusual obstetric injury causing detachment of bladder and urethra from symphysis pubis and complete epispadias. Am. J. Obst. and Gynec. *34:*840–854, Nov '37

HUNT, A. H.: Method of splinting septic fingers. Lancet *2:*370–371, Aug 15, '36

HUNT, H. B.: Prophylaxis, diagnosis and treatment of cancer of lips. Nebraska M. J. *25:*133, April; 187, May '40

HUNT, H. B.: Treatment of large protruding carcinomas of skin and lip by irradiation and surgery. Am. J. Roentgenol. *44:*254–264, Aug '40

HUNT, H. LYONS: *Plastic Surgery of the Head, Face, and Neck*. Lea and Febiger Co., Phila., 1926

HUNT, H. L.: Treatment of facial scars, with remarks on their psychological aspects. Am. J. Surg. *4:*313–320, March '28

HUNT, H. L.: Cheloids. Am. Med. *23:*337–341, May '28

HUNT, H. L.: Rhinophyma, case. Laryngoscope *43:*282, April '33

HUNT, H. L.: Task of plastic surgeon. Am. Med. *40:*361-362, Sept '34
HUNT, H. L. (see TIECK, G. J. E.) June, Nov '21
HUNT, H. L. (see TIECK, G. J. E.) Aug '21
HUNT, H. L. (see TIECK, G. J. E. *et al*) Feb '22
HUNT, J. H. AND SCOTT, P. G.: Burn therapy in out-patients with reinforced tannic acid dressings. Lancet *2:*774-776, Oct 8, '32
HUNT, R. W. (see LOWSLEY, O. S.) July '42

Hunt-Tansley Operation

Unilateral congenital eyelid ptosis corrected by Hunt-Tansley operation. LOEB, C. Am. J. Ophth. *7:*216-217, March '24
Bilateral eyelid ptosis cured by Hunt-Tansley operation. LOEB, C. Am. J. Ophth. *10:*191-192, March '27

HUNTER, A. F.: Roentgen therapy of hypertrophic scars and keloids. Radiology *39:*400-409, Oct '42
HUNTER, A. F.: Roentgen therapy of hypertrophic scars and keloids. Rev. radiol. y fisioterap. *10:*101-109, May-June '43
HUNTER, A. R.: Present status of problem of shock. M. Press. *212:*350-351, Nov 29, '44
HUNTER, J.: Severe and extensive burn treated with solution of tannic acid. Canad. M.A.J. *17:*1357-1358, Nov '27
HUNTER, J. B.: Cleft palate. Guy's Hosp. Gaz. *46:*102-109, March 19, '32
HUNTER, J. B.: Treatment in some minor surgical problems of hand (infections). Practitioner *133:*522-528, Oct '34
HUNTER, J. T.: Practical points in anesthesia at maxillofacial unit. Anesth. and Analg. *21:*233-228, July-Aug '42
HURLEY, T. E. V.: General principles of treatment of high explosive and bomb injuries and shock hemorrhage, and of resuscitation. M. J. Australia *2:*740-742, Nov 11, '39
HUSSERL, E.: Nature and significance of gnathophysiometry and gnathophore method according to Viggo Andersen in diagnosis of protrusions of lower and upper jaws. Ztschr. f. Stomatol. *36:*532, May 13; 591, May 27, '38
HUSSON, A. AND JEANDELIZE, P.: Dupuy-Dutemps and Bourguet's plastic dacryocystorhinostomy in chronic dacryocystitis. Medecine *5:*256-259, Jan '24
HUTCHENS, D. K. (see WOODEN, W.) Oct '27
HUTCHINS, A. F. (see HUTCHINS, E. H.) June '23
HUTCHINS, E. H. AND HUTCHINS, A. F.: Exstrophy of bladder with successful transplantation of ureters into rectum, report of 2 cases. Surg., Gynec. and Obst. *36:*731-741, June '23 (illus.)
HUTCHINSON, R. H.: Fractures of mandible and maxilla; treatment. Maine M. J. *23:*53-57, March '32
HUTCHINSON, W. B.: Management of traumatic injuries of hand. Northwest Med. *42:*134-135, May '43

Hutchinson Syndrome

Plastic surgery for Hutchinson's facies and various accompanying ptoses. BOURGUET, J. Monde med., Paris *49:*659-667, June 15, '39

HUTTER, F.: Technic of submucous resection. Monatschr. f. Ohrenh. *66:*584-585, May '32
HUTTON, A. J.: Tannic acid in burn therapy. Glasgow M. J. *112:*1-8, July '29
HUTTON, A. J.: Plastic replacement of upper lip in case of epitheliomatous ulcer resulting from x-ray treatment of sycosis barbae. Glasgow M. J. *117:*225-230, May '32
HYAMS, J. A. (see KWARTIN, B.) Oct '27
HYATT, C. N.: Hygroma cysticum colli; case report with review of literature. J. Iowa M. Soc. *22:*406-408, Aug '32
HYDE, T. L.; SELLERS, E. D. AND OWEN, M.: Thymic cyst; case. Texas State J. Med. *39:*539-540, Feb '44

Hygroma: See Cystic Hygroma

HYNDMAN, O. R.: Clinicopathologic analysis of 77 cases of cancer of lips and suggestion for rational plan of treatment. Arch. Surg. *27:*250-266, Aug '33
HYNDMAN, O. R.: Treatment of major cranial wounds; cerebral fungus; skin grafting. Surgery *11:*466-471, March '42
HYNDMAN, O. R. AND LIGHT, G.: Embryologic origin and pathologic changes to which the branchial apparatus gives rise, with presentation of familial group of fistulas. Arch. Surg. *19:*410-452, Sept '29
HYNDMAN, O. R. AND LIGHT, G.: Pathologic changes, with presentation of familial group of branchial fistulas. J. Iowa M. Soc. *20:*260-262, June '30

Hyperhidrosis

Plastic surgery upon axilla in certain cases of persistent bromhidrosis. KAHN, K. New York State J. Med. *45:*1555-1558, July 15, '45

Hypertelorism

Hypertelorism; a hitherto undifferentiated congenital cranio-facial deformity. GREIG, D. M. Edinburgh M. J. *31:*560-593, Oct '24

Hypertelorism—Cont.

Case of hypertelorism. MUIR, D. C. Brit. J. Child. Dis. *22:*102–109, April–June '25

Hypertelorism. COMBY, J. Arch. de med. d. enf. *28:*570–573, Sept '25

Hypertelorism. COCKAYNE, E. A. Brit. J. Child. Dis. *22:*265–274, Oct–Dec '25

Case of hypertelorism without mental defect. ALLEN, F. M. B. Arch. Dis. Childhood. *1:*171–174, June '26

Case of hypertelorism. DRUMMOND, W. B. Arch. Dis. Childhood *1:*166–170, June '26

Case of hypertelorism described, relation of hypertelorism to mongolism. BRAITHWAITE, J. V. C. Arch. Dis. Childhood *1:*369–372, Dec '26

Scaphocephaly, oxycephaly and hypertelorism, with reports of cases. OGILVIE, A. G. AND POSEL, M. M. Arch. Dis. Childhood *2:*146–154, June '27

Hypertelorism in several generations. ABERNETHY, D. A. Arch. Dis. Childhood *2:*361–365, Dec '27

Hypertelorism. REUBEN, M. S. AND FOX, H. R. Arch. Pediat. *45:*105–115, Feb '28

Congenital craniofacial deformity (hypertelorism); case. BABONNEIX, L. *et al.* Bull. Soc. de pediat. de Paris *26:*118, March '28

Unilateral hypertelorism, case. LIGHTWOOD, R. C. AND SHELDON, W. P. H. Arch. Dis. Childhood *3:*168–172, June '28

Acrocephalosyndactylia and ocular hypertelorism; 2 cases. JANSEN, M. Nederl. Tijdschr. v. Geneesk. *2:*5864–5867, Nov 24, '28

Hereditary hypertelorism without mental deficiency. MONTFORD, T. M. Arch. Dis. Childhood *4:*381–384, Dec '29

Ocular hypertelorism. REGNAULT, F. AND CROUZON, O. Ann. d'anat. path. *7:*571–576, May '30

Congenital ocular hypertelorism; case. DELLEPIANE RAWSON, R. AND GONZÁLEZ AVILA, E. Rev. de especialid. *5:*1090–1096, Aug '30 also: Semana med. *2:*1206–1209, Oct 16, '30

Hypertelorism, four cases. REILLY, W. A. J.A.M.A. *96:*1929–1933, June 6, '31

Hypertelorism in girl 4 years old. KRÜGER, E. Ztschr. f. Kinderh. *54:*785–787, '33

Hypertelorism, case. TOZER, F. H. W. Roy. Berkshire Hosp. Rep., pp. 17–21, '33

Hypertelorism, case with unusual congenital malformation of external portion of nose, double overlapping external parts. VAN VOORTHUYSEN, D. G. W. Acta oto-laryng. *22:*540–544, '35

Ocular hypertelorism. SLO-BODKIN, S. G. Arch. Pediat. *53:*191–196, March '36

Hypertelorism—Cont.

Encephalocele associated with hypertelorism and cleft palate. OLDFIELD, M. C. Brit. J. Surg. *25:*757–764, April '38

Notes on 3 cases of hypertelorism. PICKERILL, H. P. Brit. J. Surg. *26:*588–592, Jan '39

Hereditary cleidocranial dysostosis with features of ocular hypertelorism; 2 cases. RUBENS, E. Arch. Pediat. *56:*771–780, Dec '39

Ocular hypertelorism with cleft palate and giant-cell tumor. POSNER, I. AND PIATT, A. D. Radiology *35:*79–81, July '40

Hypertelorism; case with median nasal fissure. ZENO, L. An. de cir. *8:*37–39, March–June '42 also: Bol. Soc. de cir. de Rosario *9:*59–62, May '42

True total hemihypertrophy; case. SCHWARTZMAN, J. *et al.* Arch. Pediat. *59:*637–645, Oct '42

Left total congenital hemihypertrophy; case. TOUSSAINT ARAGON, E. Rev. mex. de pediat. *12:*343–356, Oct 10, '42

Hypertelorism with facies bovinia. CALLISTER, A. C. Rocky Mountain M. J. *40:*36–40, Jan '43

Hypertelorism associated with median nasal cleft; case. ZENO, L. An. argent. de oftal. *4:*3–5, Jan–March '43

Hypertelorism. BERKOVE, A. B. Arch. Otolaryng. *38:*587–589, Dec '43

Craniofacial dysostosis; significance of ocular hypertelorism. BROWN, A. AND HARPER, R. A. K. Quart. J. Med. *15:*171–181, July '46

Hypospadias

Treatment of fistulas into male urethra by inversion of skin. SALLERAS PAGÉS, J. Semana med. *28:*602, May 26, '21 Abstr: J.A.M.A. *77:*580, Aug 13, '21

Case of pseudohermaphrodismus masculinus, showing hypospadias, greatly enlarged utricle, abdominal testis and absence of seminal vesicles. YOUNG, H. H. AND CASH, J. R., J. Urology *5:*405, May '21

Plastic treatment of hypospadias. NIEDERMAYR, R. Munchen. med. Wchnschr. *68:*773, June 24, '21

Ombredanne's method for grave hypospadias. RIVAROLA, R. A. Rev. Asoc. med. argent. *35:*634, Aug '21

Treatment of anterior balanic and penile hypospadias with Beck-von Hacker operation. MADIER, J., J. de chir. *18:*234–242, Sept '21 (illus.) J.A.M.A. *78:*688, March 4, '22 (abstr.)

Autoplasty for pre-scrotal hypospadias in adult. DORDU, F. Arch. franco-belges de chir. *25:*282–286, Dec '21 (illus.)

Hypospadias – Cont.

Operation for hypospadias and defect of pendulous portion of urethra. FISCHER, A. Zentralbl. f. Chir. *49:*399-401, March 25, '22

Correction of balanic hypospadias. SALLERAS PAGÉS, J. Semana med. *1:*797-798, May 18, '22 (illus.) abstr: J.A.M.A. *79:*924, Sept 9, '22

Operative treatment of scrotal hypospadias. FLÖRCKEN, H. Ztschr. f. Urol. Chir. *10:*119-121, July '22 (illus.) abstr: J.A.M.A. *79:*1187, Sept 30, '22

"New operation for hypospadias." NAGEL, Z. Zentralbl. f. Chir. *49:*982-984, July 8, '22

Treatment of hypospadias and epispadias. SANCHEZ-COVISA, I. Arch. espan. de pediat. *6:*577-613, Oct '22 (illus.) abstr: J.A.M.A. *80:*285, Jan 27, '23

New treatment of hypospadias. CAMERA, U. Arch. ital. di chir. *6:*277-296, Nov '22 (illus.) abstr: J.A.M.A. *80:*436, Feb 10, '23

Reply to Nagel's remarks on my article, "Operation for hypospadias." FISCHER, A. Zentralbl. f. Chir. *49:*1748, Nov 25, '22

Case of "hypospadias perinealis." CHELLIAH, S. Internat. A. M. Museums Bull., pp. 162-164, Dec '22

Correction of balanic hypospadias. MARION, G., J. d'urol. *14:*473-478, Dec '22 (illus.) abstr: J.A.M.A. *80:*1032, April 7, '23

Hypospadias. DAVISON, C. Internat. Clinics *2:*10-16, '22 (illus.)

Les hermaphrodites et la chirurgie, by L. OMBREDANNE. Masson et Cie, Paris, 1923

Pseudohermaphrodism or complete hypospadias. HAGNER, F. R. AND KNEALE, H. B. Surg., Gynec. and Obst. *36:*495-501, April '23 (illus.)

Modification of operation of Bucknall for hypospadias. HARVEY, S. C. Ann. Surg. *77:*572-579, May '23 (illus.)

Hypospadias. MORALES, A. Siglo med. *71:*549-550, June 9, '23

Technic for operative treatment of perineoscrotal hypospadias. JEANBRAU, E. J. d'urol. *18:*405-409, Nov '24

Treatment of hypospadias; analysis of 28 cases. BIDGOOD, C. Y. Virginia M. Monthly *51:*634-642, Jan '25

Operative treatment of balanic hypospadias. POTEL, G. J. d'urol. *19:*236-239, March '25

Pseudo-hermaphroditism and hypospadias; their surgical treatment. EDMUNDS, A. Lancet *1:*323-327, Feb 13, '26

Hypospadias, relation to abnormalities of penis. SIEVERS, R. Deutsche Ztschr. f. Chir. *199:*286-306, '26

Hypospadias – Cont.

Well marked hypospadias; case. WEST, C. M. Irish J. M. Sc. pp. 29-33, Jan '27

Use of appendix veriformis in formation of urethra in hypospadias. MCGUIRE, S. Ann. Surg. *85:*391-399, March '27

Hypospadias scrotalis. TARABUCHIN, M. Vrach. dielo *10:*442, March 30, '27

Treatment of hypospadias by method of Nové-Josserand. MICHELSON, J. M. Arch. d. mal. d. reins *2:*513-517, April 1, '27

Operative treatment of hypospadias in man. BIRKENFELD, W. Arch. f. klin. Chir. *145:*445-454, '27

Hypospadias, treatment by new operative process. FALCONE, R. Arch. ital. di chir. *18:*497-514, '27

Operation of case of bulbo-scrotal hypospadias. TROELL, A. Ztschr. f. urol. Chir. *22:*372-376, '27

Urethroplasty in hypospadias. VAN CAPPELLEN, D. Nederl. Tijdschr. v. Geneesk. *1:*356-358, Jan 21, '28

Twelve cases of hypospadias in young boys; operation; immediate and excellent results. MATHIEU, P. Arch. d. mal. d. reins *3:*224-230, Feb '28

Hypospadias; case. PICKERILL, P., M. J. Australia *1:*527-528, April 28, '28

Repair of urethra with hypospadias by single operation (Duplay's method). MARTIN. Bull. Soc. franc. d'urol. *7:*242-244, Nov 19, '28 also: J. d'urol. *26:*564-567, Dec '28

Treatment of case of male hypospadias. CECIL, A. B., S. Clin. N. Amer. *8:*1343-1350, Dec '28

Operative treatment of severe forms of hypospadias in male. BORCHERS, E. Ztschr. f. Urol. *22:*808-822, '28

Hypospadias operation. ZECHEL, G. Arch. f. klin. Chir. *153:*491-494, '28

Abnormalities of hind end of body (including hypospadias). MCKELVEY, J. L., J. Coll. Surgeons, Australasia *1:*285-302, March '29

Urethroplasty for scrotal hypospadias. NISSEN, R. Zentralbl. f. Chir. *56:*962-964, April 20, '29

Von Hacker's operation for hypospadias. MAYET, H. Bull. et mem. Soc. de chir. de Paris *21:*394-403, May 17, '29 also: Paris chir. *21:*149-154, July-Aug '29

New plastic operation for hypospadias. MEYER, H. Arch. f. klin. Chir. *155:*588-596, '29

Method for plastic construction of a urethra in penoscrotal hypospadias by means of flap of mucosa of bladder. ROSENSTEIN, P.

Hypospadias – Cont.
Ztschr. f. Urol. *23:*627-637, '29
Perineal hypospadias; surgical treatment. Schüppel, A. Ztschr. f. Urol. *23:*753-761, '29
Operative treatment for extensive hypospadias. McWhorter, G. L., S. Clin. N. Amer. *10:*275-282, April '30
Ball of hair in urethra; late complication of Bucknall operation for hypospadias. Vermooten, V. New England J. Med. *202:*658-660, April 3, '30
Hypospadias, correction by plastic surgery of urethra by Marion's operation. Salleras, J. Rev. de especialid. *5:*1385-1389, Oct '30 also: Semana med. *1:*10-11, Jan 1, '31
Plastic operations for epispadias and hypospadias. Cabot, H. Proc. Staff Meet., Mayo Clin. *5:*315, Nov 5, '30
Hypospadias; treatment with cutaneous flap in single operation. Mathieu, P. Bull. et mem. Soc. nat. de chir. *56:*1314-1316, Nov 29, '30
Modification of Nissen's operation in hypospadias. Kaïris, Z. Zentralbl. f. Chir. *57:*3047-3048, Dec 6, '30
Hypospadias and epispadias, indications for and technique of their operative correction. Blair, V. P. Tr. South. S. A. (1929) *42:*163-165, '30
Hypospadias, discussion and review of cases. Frühmann, P. and Sternberg, H. Arch. f. klin. Chir. *160:*633-673, '30
Atresia of urethral orifice with penoscrotal hypospadias. Schönfeld, M. Casop. lek. cesk. *70:*921-923, June 26, '31
Hypospadias, cure by transplantation of bladder mucosa; 2 cases. Rosenstein, P. Zentralbl. f. Chir. *58:*1874-1880, July 25, '31
Hypospadias, case with double channel urethra. Bhandari, S. L. Indian M. Gaz. *66:*444, Aug '31
Plastic surgery of urethra and prepuce in surgical treatment of perineal hypospadias. Kurtzahn, H. Zentralbl. f. Chir. *58:*1945-1948, Aug 1, '31
Surgery of hypospadias and epispadias in male. Cecil, A. B. Tr. Am. A. Genito-Urin. Surgeons *24:*253-302, '31 also: J. Urol. *27:*507-537, May '32
New method for straightening penis in hypospadias. Hagner, F. R. Tr. South. S. A. *44:*245-246, '31 also: J.A.M.A. *99:*116, July 9, '32
Congenital polyps of urethra with peno-scrotal hypospadias. Ottow, B. Ztschr. f. urol. Chir. *32:*64-68, '31

Hypospadias – Cont.
Plastic surgery of penobalanic and penoscrotal hypospadias. Sanchís Perpiñá, V. Actas Soc. de cir. de Madrid *1:*197-229, Jan-March '32
Technic of one-stage operation for balanic or juxtabalanic hypospadias. Mathieu, P. J. de chir *39:*481-486, April '32
Surgery of hypospadias and epispadias in male. Cecil, A. B. West. J. Surg. *40:*297-315, June '32
Hypospadias and epispadias; philological note. Bremer, J. L. New England J. Med. *207:*537-539, Sept 22, '32
Hypospadias, hydronephrosis and infected congenital hydro-ureter; case. Knappig, T. Orvosi hetil. *76:*864-866, Sept 24, '32
Penoscrotal hypospadias; satisfactory results of Duplay operation with hypogastric derivation of urine; case. Salleras, J. Rev. Assoc. med. argent. *46:*988-990, Sept '32
Plastic repair of hypospadias. Heynen, U. Ztschr. f. Urol. *26:*338-359, '32
Treatment of hypospadias. Wade, R. B. Australian and New Zealand J. Surg. *2:*417-418, April '33
Hypospadias of penis in uniovular twins. Voûte, P. A. Nederl. tijdschr. v. geneesk. *77:*2431-2433, May 27, '33
Ombredanne-Lyle operation for hypospadias; case. Walters, W. Proc. Staff Meet., Mayo Clin. *8:*467-469, Aug 2, '33
Plastic surgery of penobalanic and penoscrotal hypospadias. Sanchis Perpiñá, V. Arch. de med., cir. y especialid. *36:*989-1002, Sept 2, '33
Ombredanne's pouch operation in hypospadias. Lyle, H. H. M. Ann. Surg. *98:*513-519, Oct '33
Surgical therapy of hypospadias. Pettinari, V. Arch. ital. di urol. *10:*555-588, Oct '33
Correction of epispadias and scrotal hypospadias. Blair, V. P. *et al.* Surg., Gynec. and Obst. *57:*646-653, Nov '33
Medicosocial problem of false hermaphroditism; case with hypospadias and ectopic testicles. Torres Torija, J. Gac. med. de Mexico *64:*534-542, Dec '33
Perineal hypospadias in man who for 26 years was regarded as woman; surgical care. Gesse, E. R. Ztschr. f. urol. Chir. *38:*18-22, '33
Plastic methods for surgical correction of penobalanic and penoscrotal hypospadias. Sanchís Perpiñá, V. Zentralbl. f. Chir. *61:*209-216, Jan 27, '34
Question of surgical therapy of hypospadias. Moszkowicz, L. Chirurg *6:*401-402, June

Hypospadias – Cont.
1, '34
When should hypospadias be operated on? RUBRITIUS, H. Chirurg *6:*402-403, June 1, '34
Plastic repair of hypospadias. GATEWOOD. S. Clin. North America *14:*783-788, Aug '34
Results of surgical therapy of severe forms of hypospadias by means of plastic transplantation of epidermis. ZENKER, R. Chirurg *6:*576-578, Aug 15, '34
Surgical therapy of penoscrotal hypospadias. PIERI, G. Urologia *1:*140-143, Sept 1, '34
Repair of urethra by temporary joining of penis and scrotum (hypospadias). LEVEUF, J. Bull. et mem. Soc. nat. de chir. *61:*30-31, Jan 19, '35
Principles of treatment of hypospadias. CABOT, H. *et al.* J. Urol. *33:*400-407, April '35
Replacement of missing urethra in patient with scrotal hypospadias by pedicled flaps from bladder wall; case. ZELLER, O. Med. Welt *9:*565-567, April 20, '35
Congenital implantation of penis with hypospadias in perineum between scrotum and anus; case. SISTO HONTAN, E. Pediatria espan. *24:*344-347, Sept '35
Perineal hypospadias; case, treatment by tunnelling and skin graft. BEGG, R. C. New Zealand M. J. *34:*378-383, Dec '35
Improved operation for hypospadias. CABOT, H. Proc. Staff. Meet., Mayo Clin. *10:*796-798, Dec 11, '35
Therapy of penile, penoscrotal and perineoscrotal hypospadias by Duplay operation. ELBIM, A., J. d'urol. *40:*484-498, Dec '35
Hypospadias, case. YOKOTA, K. AND HASAMA, T. Mitt. a. d. med. Akad. zu Kioto *15:*906, '35
Hypospadias operation. BROWNE, D. Lancet *1:*141-143, Jan 18, '36
Hypospadias treatment in theory and practice. CABOT, H. New England J. Med. *214:*871-876, April 30, '36
Successful operations for hypospadias. WALTERS, W. Ann. Surg. *103:*949-958, June '36
Heredity of hypospadias. STEINER, F. Munchen. med. Wchnschr. *83:*1271, July 31, '36
Urethroplasty; general review of technic using free or pedicled grafts in restoration of hypospadias. GODARD, H., J. d'urol. *42:* 105-142, Aug '36
Temporary graft of penis to scrotum in therapy of hypospadias; technic and report of cases. LEVEUF, J. AND GODDARD, H., J. de chir. *48:*328-341, Sept '36
Urethroplasty; general review of technics us-

Hypospadias – Cont.
ing free or pedicled grafts in restoration of hypospadias or of loss of substance of masculine urethra. (Comment on Godard's article.) RICHER, V., J. d'urol *42:*339-340, Oct '36
Imperforate anus, bowel opening into urethra; hypospadias; presentation of new plastic methods. YOUNG, H. H., J.A.M.A. *107:*1448-1451, Oct 31, '36
Simple technic for cure of hypospadias. GATEWOOD. Surg., Gynec. and Obst. *63:*655-659, Nov '36
Ombredanne operation in hypospadias; case. BIANCALANA, L. Boll. e mem. Soc. piemontese di chir. *6:*18-25, '36
Incontinence due to severe hypospadias of female urethra with simultaneous ectopy of ureteral orifice; case. DE GIRONCOLI, F. Ztschr. f. urol. Chir. u. Gynak. *42:*152-156, '36
Operation for cure of adult hypospadias. McINDOE, A. H. Brit. M. J. *1:*385-386, Feb 20, '37
Treatment of hypospadias. EDMUNDS, A. M. Press *194:*456-462, May 12, '37
Effects, symptoms and treatment of hypospadias; review of 101 cases. THOMPSON, A. R. Lancet *2:*429-432, Aug 21, '37
Hypospadias treated by Ombredanne technic. FLYNN, R., M. J. Australia *2:*479, Sept 18, '37
Surgical treatment of hypospadias. McINDOE, A. H. Am. J. Surg. *38:* 176-185, Oct '37
Urethroplasty in penoscrotal hypospadias using Passaggi-Galliera technic. TORRE, D. Ann. ital. di chir. *16:*841-854, Oct '37
Congenital absence of one vas deferens with aplasia of left kidney and hypospadias. VORSTOFFEL, E. Zentralbl. f. Chir. *64:*2825-2826, Dec 11, '37
Posterior hypospadias cured by Ombredanne operation; case. BIANCALANA, L. Boll. e mem. Soc. piemontese di chir. *7:*325-327, '37
Unusual urethral calculus containing hair; use of scrotal skin in restoration of hypospadias as probable cause; case. BORN, R. Ztschr. f. Urol. *31:*552-554, '37
Three-stage operation for hypospadias repair; cases. LOWSLEY, O. S. AND BEGG, C. L. J.A.M.A. *110:*487-493, Feb 12, '38
Surgical therapy of hypospadias in male. HÖRHAMMER, C. Chirurg *10:*159-161, March 1, '38
Operative treatment of hypospadias, with report of 13 cases. CREEVY, C. D. Surgery

Hypospadias – Cont.
*3:*719-731, May '38
Vulviform hypospadias; case. CHIODIN, L. Bol. Soc. de cir. de Rosario *5:*151-160, June '38
Therapy of hypospadias. HARRENSTEIN, R. J. Nederl. tijdschr. v. geneesk. *82:*2963-2974, June 11, '38
Surgical procedure for correction of hypospadias. SMITH, C. K., J. Urol. *40:*239-247, July '38
Congenital anomalies with particular reference to cryptorchidism, hypospadias and congenital absence of vagina (surgical treatment). COUNSELLER, V. S., J. Michigan M. Soc. *37:*689-697, Aug '38
Complete hypospadias; case. MURRAY, J. J. AND BOOKHALTER, S. Brit. M. J. *2:*659-660, Sept 24, '38
Hypospadias and epispadias (surgical correction). BLAIR, V. P. AND BYARS, L. T. J. Urol. *40:*814-825, Dec '38
Hypospadias as cause of error in determining sex. PIRES DE LIMA, J. A., J. de sif. e urol. *10:*35-39, Feb '39
Discussion of subject of hypospadias from viewpoint of reconstructive surgery and report of use of depilated scrotal flap. RITCHIE, H. P. Surgery *5:*911-931, June '39
Baldwin operation in case of pseudohermaphroditism and vulviform hypospadias. CABANES, E. AND XICLUNA, R. Algerie med. *43:*333-336, July '39
Treatment of hypospadias. YOUNG, H. H. J. Urol. *42:*470-473, Sept '39
Epidermal grafts in correction of severe forms of hypospadias; further study. BORCHERS, E. Chirurg *11:*713-722, Oct 15, '39
Surgical correction of hypospadias. McKENNA, C. M., J.A.M.A. *113:*2138-2143, Dec 9, '39
Operative treatment of true hermaphroditism; and new technic for curing hypospadias. YOUNG, H. H. Arch. Surg. *41:*557-568, Aug '40
Association of hypospadias with gonococcal infections in male. LAMBERSON, H. H. Rocky Mountain M. J. *37:*668-671, Sept '40
Straightening hypospadiac penis. CREEVY, C. D. Surgery *8:*777-780, Nov '40
Hypospadias. MEYER, H. W. Surgery *8:*781-790, Nov '40
Pedicle tube-graft in surgical treatment of hypospadias in male, with new method of closing small fistulas. DAVIS, D. M. Surg., Gynec. and Obst. *71:*790-796, Dec '40
Operation for penoscrotal hypospadias. LEVI, D. Lancet *2:*777, Dec 21, '40

Hypospadias – Cont.
Hypospadias in girl 4 years old. SORRENTINO, M. Rinasc. med. *18:*65-66, Feb 15, '41
Use of stainless steel wire in operation for hypospadias. COE, H. E. Urol. and Cutan. Rev. *45:*297-298, May '41
Plastic procedure for correction of hypospadias. NESBIT, R. M., J. Urol. *45:*699-702, May '41
Surgical therapy of penoscrotal hypospadias by author's technic. GORIA, V. Rev. argent. de urol. *10:*419-426, July-Aug '41
One-stage operation for hypospadias. HUMBY, G. Brit. J. Surg. *29:*84-92, July '41
Scrotal hypospadias treated by Nove-Josserand-Borchers procedure. MARTIN VIVALDI, J. Rev. clin. espan. *4:*358-359, March 15, '42
Surgical therapy of hypospadias. BUDDE, W. Zentralbl. f. Chir. *69:*1080, June 27, '42
Error in determination of sex; study on pseudohermaphroditism based on case with perineal hypospadias. SIMARRO PUIG, J. *et al.* Rev. clin. espan. *6:*39-42, July 15, '42
Hypospadias. WILLIAMS, L. R. Bull. Vancouver M. A. *18:*348-349, Aug '42
Hypospadias. FARMER, A. W. Surgery *12:*462-470, Sept '42
Therapy of penal and penoscrotal hypospadias; supplementary notes on Ombredanne operation. BARCAT, J. R., J. de chir. *58:*418-426, '41-'42
Unusual anomaly associated with hypospadias. McKENNA, C. M. AND KIEFER, J. H. Urol. and Cutan. Rev. *47:*14-20, Jan '43
Hypospadias. CHARNOCK, D. A. AND KISKADDEN, W. S., J. Urol. *49:*444-449, March '43
Hypospadias. WEHRBEIN, H. L., J. Urol. *50:*335-340, Sept '43
Experiences with Ombredanne operation for hypospadias. MUSCHAT, M., J. Urol. *51:*437-438, April '44
Male pseudohermaphroditism with perineal pseudovaginal hypospadias; technic for surgical correction; case. HERNANDEZ IBANEZ, J. A. Vida nueva *53:*263-273, May '44
Female pseudohermaphroditism with hypospadias limited to glans; anomaly due to cessation of development; case. LORDY, C. An. brasil. de ginec. *18:*87-93, Aug '44
New operation for midscrotal hypospadias. DAVIS, D. M., J. Urol. *52:*340-345, Oct '44
Female pseudohermaphroditism with hypospadias limited to glans; anomaly due to cessation of development; plastic correction of case. SPINA, V. Rev. de obst. e ginec. de Sao Paulo *7:*195-208, June-Aug '45

Hypospadias – Cont.

Correction of chordee and hypospadias. GOODHOPE, C. D. Northwest Med. *44:*356-358, Nov '45

New operation for midscrotal hypospadias. DAVIS, D. M. Tr. Am. A. Genito-Urin. Surgeons (1944) *37:*27-33, '45

Repair of hypospadias and fistula. CECIL, A. B., J. Urol. *56:*237-242, Aug '46

Surgical therapy of hypospadias. LEVEUF, J. J. de chir. *62:*90-98, '46

HYSLOP, V. B.: Principles to be observed in treatment of congenital harelip and cleft palate. Wisconsin M. J. *32:*246-248, April '33

HYSLOP, V. B.: Cleft palate repair technic affording better speech results. Wisconsin M. J. *36:*540-543, July '37

I

IACOBOVICI, I.: Postoperative parathyroid tetany treated by autoplastic and homoplastic bone graft. Rev. de chir., Bucuresti *42:*567-570, July-Aug '39

IACOBOVICI, I. AND ONACA: Epithelioma of lips; 385 cases. Rev. de chir., Bucuresti *38:*1-16, March-April '35

IADEVAIA, F.: Clinical study of therapy of exstrophy of bladder. Clinica *7:*33-46, Jan '41

IASON, A. H.: Office treatment of hand infections. Am. J. Surg. *36:*376-383, April '37

IBARRA PEREZ, R.: Rhinophyma and hypertrophic acne; treatment by means of cold (high frequency) knife. Vida nueva *52:*231-236, Nov '43

IBBOTSON, W.: Treatment of nasal fractures. M. Press *197:*8-12, July 6, '38

IBSEN, B.: Traumatic amputation of terminal phalanx of second finger of left hand with tearing out of tendon of flexor digitorum profundus muscle; case. Ugesk. f. laeger *105:*707, July 15, '43

Ichthyosis

Surgical treatment of ichthyosis hystrix. KAZANJIAN, V. H. Plast. and Reconstruct. Surg. *1:*91-97, July '46

IDELBERGER, A. AND IDELBERGER, K.: Heredopathology of fissures of lips, jaws and palate; report on unselected series of 41 pairs of twins. Ztschr. f. menschl. Vererb.-u. Konstitutionslehre *24:*417-479, '40

IDELBERGER, K. (see IDELBERGER, A.) 1940

IDEMITSU, K.: Scalds of pharynx in small children. Oto-rhino-laryng. *10:*1047, Nov '37

IFY, I.: Surgical therapy of entropion and trichiasis in trachoma patients. Budapesti orvosi ujsag *34:*774-776, Sept 17, '36

IGAMBERDIEV, Z.: Neck wounds; clinical and roentgenologic analysis. Khirurgiya, no. 8, pp. 65-68, '44

IGARZABAL, J. E.: Pendulous abdomen, surgical therapy. Semana med. *1:*1361-1365, June 16, '38 comment by Goni Moreno *2:*52-53, July 7, '38 reply by Igarzabal *2:*152-153, July 21, '38

IGLAUER, S.: Electrically driven nasal saw and rasp. Laryngoscope *35:*78, Jan '25

IGLAUER, S.: Use of negocoll and hominit in making moulages of face as aid in plastic surgery. Laryngoscope *42:*774-778, Oct '32

IGLAUER, S.: Lowering floor of mouth; new operation to provide additional support for lower denture; case. J. Med. *14:*507-509, Dec '33

IGLAUER, S.: Preserved human cartilage in reconstructive surgery of face. Ann. Otol., Rhin. and Laryng. *50:*1072-1078, Dec '41

IGNATEV, S. S.: Late results after transplantation of mammary gland in closure of facial defect. Vestnik khir. *47:*103, '36

IGNATEV, S. S.: Removal of constricting foreign body (metallic ring) (fingers). Vestnik khir. *60:*196-197, Sept '40

IGNATOV, M. G.: Peripheral nerve injuries; basic methods of surgical therapy. Nevropat. i psikhiat. (no. 4) *11:*73, '42

IKEDA, Y.: Anatomic examination of human hemicephalic fetus 10 months old with harelip, cleft palate, hyperdactylia, syndactylia, etc. Arb. a. d. anat. Inst. d. kaiserlich-japan. Univ. zu Sendai, Hft. 15, pp. 61-212, '33

IKLÉ, C.: Histology and pathogenesis of Dupuytren's contracture. Deutsche Ztschr. f. Chir. *212:*106-118, '28

ILABACA LEON, L.: Surgical therapy of prognathism of lower jaw. Rev. med. de Chile *67:*1352-1355, Dec '39

ILABACA L., L. (see VARGAS SALCEDO, L.) Oct '36

ILINSKIY, V. P.: Plastic operations of penis. Khirurgiya, no. 1, pp. 142-143, '37

ILLYIN, G. A.: Use of portion of scapula to fill bony defects of cranium. Vestnik khir. (nos. 68-69) *23:*84-94, '31

IMABLE, J.: Intra-arterial mercurochrome and sulfanilamide and its derivatives in therapy of phlegmons in hand. Rev. Asoc. med. argent. *55:*463-465, June 15-30, '41

IMAKITA, T.: Implantation of skin grafts into muscular tissue. Acta dermat. *20:*137-138, '32

IMAKITA, T.: Significance of mitosis of epithelial cells of implanted tissue. Acta dermat. *20:*138-139, '32

IMAMURA, T. (see SOHMA, T.) 1936

IMAZ, J. I.: Macrodactyly; pathogenesis and surgical therapy; case. Hosp. argent. *3:*1100-1103, June 15, '33

IMBER, I.: Familial appearance of Dupuytren's contracture; case. Note e riv. di psichiat. *65:*209-222, April-June '36

IMBERT, L.: Research on autoplastics. J. de chir. *18:*113-129, Aug '21 (illus.) abstr: J.A.M.A. *78:*688, March 4, '22

IMBERT, L.: Treatment of ankylosis of temporomaxillary articulation. Lyon chir. *18:*572-578, Sept-Oct '21 (illus.)

IMBERT, L.: Bone grafts. Bull. Acad. de med., Par. *90:*174-182, Oct 16, '23 abstr: J.A.M.A. *82:*163, Jan 12, '24 also: Bull. Acad. de med., Par. *91:*371-375, March 18, '24

IMBERT, L.: Fragment method in bone grafts. Bull. Acad. de med., Par. *92:*1285-1290, Dec 2, '24

IMBERT, L.: Bone transplantation with devitalized grafts. Bull. Acad. de med., Par. *93:*204-214, Feb 24, '25 abstr: J.A.M.A. *84:*1240, April 18, '25

IMBERT, L.: Experimental bone grafts; homogenous grafts. Bull. Acad. de med., Paris *94:*1086-1090, Dec 1, '25

IMBERT, L.: Research on bone graft; heterotopic autografts. Bull. Acad. de med., Paris *95:*538-542, May 25, '26

IMBERT, L.: Experimental research on bone grafting. J. de chir. *27:*710-724, June '26

IMBERT, L.: Late results of bone grafts; microscopic study. Ann. d'anat. path. *7:*291-315, March '30

IMBERT, L.: Maxillofacial surgery. Marseille-med. *1:*121-124, March 15, '40

IMBERT, L. AND COTTALORDA, J.: Pathogenesis and treatment of ankylosis of jaws. Acta chir. Scandinav. *54:*515-529, June '22 (illus.) abstr: J.A.M.A. *79:*926, Sept 9, '22

IMBERT, R.: Alternating life of tissues; importance in bone transplantation. Paris med. *1:*267-270, March 25, '33

IMBERT, R.: Terebrant cancers of face. Rev. de chir., Paris *74:*331-373, May '36

IMMENKAMP, A.: Results of bridge plastic (Axhausen) operation for cleft palate in 45 cases. Deutsche Ztschr. f. Chir. *249:*326-336, '37

IMPERATI, L.: Autoplastic skin grafts in man; histologic study. Riforma med. *49:*1133-1134, July 29, '33

IMPERATI, L.: Question of fixed grafts in relation to probable regenerative processes of host. Ann. ital. di chir. *12:*903-914, July 31, '33

IMPERATI, L.: Present status of burn treatment; review of literature. Gior. ital. chir. (No. 2) *1:*51-53, Aug '45

IMPERATORI, C. J.: Carcinoma of larynx and laryngopharynx treated with radium; analysis of 30 cases. Arch. Otolaryng. *4:*151-159, Aug '26

IMPERATORI, C. J.: Branchiogenetic cyst of larynx removed by thyrotomy. Laryngoscope *39:*679-683, Oct '29

Implants

Use of paraffin and wax in ear and nose surgery. STAHLMAN, T. M. Pennsylvania M. J. *24:*875, Sept '21

Source of material for plastic operations. ESSER, J. F. S. Munchen. med. Wchnschr. *69:*888, June 16, '22

Experiments on implantation of dead preserved tissue. REGOLI, G. Policlinico (sez. chir.) *29:*559-574, Oct '22 (illus.)

Depressed nasal deformities, comparison of prosthetic values of paraffin, bone, cartilage and celluloid, with report of cases corrected with celluloid implants by author's method. LEWIS, J. D. Ann. Otol., Rhin. and Laryng. *32:*321-365, June '23 (illus.)

Comparative study of ivory and organic transplants in rhinoplasty; endo-nasal operative technic of some nasal deformities with report of cases. MALINIAK, J. Laryngoscope *34:*882-900, Nov '24

Use of ivory in rhinoplasty. MALINIAK, J. Arch. Otolaryng. *1:*599-611, June '25

Rhinoplasty over silver frame. BOGORODIZKY, W. A. Zentralbl. f. Chir. *52:*2830-2835, Dec 12, '25

Use of gold-wire splints in intranasal plastic surgery. CARTER, W. W. Laryngoscope *35:*942-943, Dec '25

Rhinoplasty with ivory transplant. LUNDON, A. E. Canad. M.A.J. *16:*561-562, May '26

Ivory in alloplasty of nasal fossae. BASAVILBASO, J. Prensa med. argent. *13:*597-598, Nov 30, '26 also: Rev. de especialid. *1:*564-567, '26

Implantation of silk in plastic repair of tissues. SPITZY. Wien. med. Wchnschr. *77:*394-396, March 19, '27

Use of foreign bodies in ear, nose and throat surgery. POLLOCK, H. L. Ann. Otol. Rhin. and Laryng. *36:*463-471, June '27

Cosmetic paraffin injections in facial surgery. STEIN, R. O. Wien. klin. Wchnschr. *40:*830, June 23, '27

Technic of temporary craniectomy and of plastics in cranium defects. SOKOLOV, V. Vestnik khir. (no. 32) *11:*115-116, Nov 5, '27

Cosmetic operations of nose; paraffin injections. BLEGVAD, N. R. Ugesk. f. Laeger *89:*1141-1144, Dec 8, '27

Implants – Cont.

Cartilage and ivory in plastic surgery of nose. SALINGER, S. Arch. Otolaryng. *6:*552–558, Dec '27

Silk tendons and joint ligaments; results of plastic operations. LANGE, F. Munchen. med. Wchnschr. *75:*39–42, Jan 6, '28

Cosmetic operations on nose and paraffin injections; 6 cases. BLEGVAD, N. R. Ugesk. f. Laeger *90:*286–290, March 29, '28

Use of autogenous transplants vs. foreign bodies in correction of nasal deformities. CARTER, W. W. Am. Med. *23:*363–366, May '28

Correction of frontal depression by inclusion of celluloid; case. BALDENWECK. Ann. d. mal. de l'oreille, du larynx *47:*757, Aug '28

Use of rubber in plastic operations on tendons and nerves, in repairing defects in abdominal wall, in hernia and in fractures with loss of substance. DELBET, P. Rev. de chir. *66:*181–213, '28

Ivory implant in atrophic rhinitis. BERNHEIMER, L. B. Illinois M. J. *55:*420–422, June '29

Plastic surgery of nose with bone graft and paraffin. CHÉRIDJIAN, Z. Rev. med. de la Suisse Rom. *49:*751–753, Oct 25, '29

Cork as prosthesis in correction of nasal defects. PRISSELKOFF, P. V. Vrach. gaz. *34:*534–536, April 15, '30

Ivory in cosmetic operations of nose. EITNER, E. Med. Welt *4:*1615, Nov 8, '30

Plastic method for correcting depression after external operations of frontal sinus; celluloid plates. STUPKA, W. Monatschr. f. Ohrenh. *65:*39–56, Jan '31

Cork as plastic material for correction of saddle noses. DAHMANN, H. Ztschr. f. Laryng., Rhin. *20:*451–457, March '31

Implantation of ivory in ozena of nose; approved technic; further observations. KEMLER, J. I. Arch. Otolaryng. *13:*726–731, May '31

Ivory implants for saddle nose; results in 50 cases. SALINGER, S. Ann. Otol., Rhin. and Laryng. *40:*801–808, Sept '31

Use of silk in plastic construction of tendons of fingers. COENEN, H. Deutsche Ztschr. f. Chir. *234:*699–709, '31

Correction of nasal deformities with use of tricoplast. LOEBELL, H. Ztschr. f. arztl. Fortbild. *29:*329–330, June 1, '32

Implants in nasal deformities; history and uses. POLLOCK, H. L. Ann. Otol., Rhin. and Laryng. *41:*1103–1107, Dec '32

Three decades of plastic use of paraffin. ECKSTEIN, H. Arch. f. klin. Chir. *169:*646–674, '32

Implants – Cont.

Treatment of injuries of tendons within synovial sheaths in palm of hand and of flexor tendons of finger by insertion of foreign substance. HESSE, F. Arch. f. klin. Chir. *170:*772–789, '32

Ox fascia (dead fascia) graft. GLASSER, S. T. Am. J. Surg. *19:*542–544, March '33

Cartilage and ivory; indications and contraindications for their use as nasal support. MALINIAK, J. W. Arch. Otolaryng. *17:*649–657, May '33

Treatment (with ivory implants) of atrophic rhinitis. BERNSTEIN, J. J. Laryng. and Otol. *48:*603–607, Sept '33

Results of implantations of porous gold in plastic surgery of nose. THIELEMANN. Ztschr. f. Laryng., Rhin., Otol. *24:*175–180, '33

Facts and fallacies of cosmetic surgery (paraffin injections, hair removal, face-lifting, nose-remodeling, etc.). MALINIAK, J. W. Hygeia *12:*200–202, March '34

Surgical correction of uncomplicated saddle nose by partial inclusion of ivory. PRUDENTE, A. Rev. Assoc. paulista de med. *5:*75–78, Aug '34

Problem of inclusions in surgical therapy of saddle nose; answers to questionnaire (Le probleme des inclusions). VARIOUS AUTHORS. Rev. de chir. plastique, pp. 132–141, Oct '34

Correction of saddle nose, with special reference to implantation of ivory. CLAUS, G. Ztschr. f. Hals-, Nasen-u. Ohrenh. *35:*198–211, '34

Recent advances in plastic surgery with special reference to vascularization of implants (face). GOLDEN, H. M. Illinois M. J. *67:*175–181, Feb '35

Problem of inclusions in surgical therapy of saddle nose; answers to questionnaire (Le probleme des inclusions). VARIOUS AUTHORS. Rev. de chir. structive, pp. 59–64, July '35

Treatment of stenosis of lacrimal ducts by insertion of spiral shaped cannula. ALKIO, V. V. Duodecim *51:*1076, '35; *52:*51, '36 Abstr: Klin. Monatsbl. f. Augenh. *96:*319–324, March '36

Rectal prolapse treated by constricted (rubber) band; case. ANDERSON, J. K. AND BORLAND, V. G. Journal-Lancet *56:*382, July '36

Costal graft and ivory inclusions in reconstruction of saddle nose by transsupraciliary route. ALVES, O. Rev. oto-laring. de Sao Paulo (no. 5, bis) *4:*843–863, Sept–Oct '36

Implants – Cont.
Development and surgical applications of absorbable tubular membrane; preliminary report. BOWEN, A. Am. J. Surg. *34:*122-124, Oct '36
Skin grafting in therapy of paraffinomas due to self-mutilation during World War. CAFORIO, L. Riforma med. *52:*1414-1417, Oct 17, '36
Alloplastic and heteroplastic grafts in reconstruction of facial defects; use of ivory and cartilage. SPANIER, F. Rev. de chir. structive, pp. 391-401, Dec '36
Dangers of paraffin injections in plastic surgery. KARFIK, V. Casop. lek. cesk. *76:*1145-1151, July 2, '37
Elephantiasis; lymphangioplasty – fate of silk. HARTLEY, H. AND HARPER, R. A. K. Brit. M. J. *2:*1066-1067, Nov 27, '37
Saddle nose; ivory and cartilage implants. SALINGER, S. Illinois M. J. *72:*412-417, Nov '37
Treatment of acquired defects of skull (especially use of celluloid plates). PRINGLE, J. H. Brit. M. J. *2:*1105-1107, Dec 4, '37
Use of rubber sponge (new flesh) over period of 25 years. FIESCHI, D. Arch. ital. di chir. *46:*221-251, '37
Plastic surgery; use of rubber (nuova carne); results in various cases after 25 years. FIESCHE, D. Rev. de chir., Paris *76:*1-36, Jan '38
Structure and reabsorption of parchment; histology, sterilization and bacteriologic control. BAIOCCHI, P. Folia med. *24:*1068-1084, Oct 15, '38
Technic of ivory implant for correction of saddle nose. WOLFE, M. M. Arch. Surg. *37:*800-807, Nov '38
New approach for nasal implants. COHEN, S. Ann. Otol., Rhin. and Laryng. *47:*1101-1106, Dec '38
Use of celluloid in facial surgery. COELST, M. Rev. de chir. structive *8:*161-162, '38
Use of stainless steel rods to canalize flexor tendon sheaths. THATCHER, H. V. South. M. J. *32:*13-18, Jan '39
Use of cellophane as permanent tendon sheath. WHEELDON, T. F., J. Bone and Joint Surg. *21:*393-396, April '39
Epithelial inlay with Kerr-material to form eye socket. CZUKRASZ, I. Brit. J. Ophth. *23:*343-347, May '39
Phalangization of first metacarpal bone combined with round stylus plastic surgery in case of loss of thumb and skin on both hands. FALTIN, R. Nord. med. (Finska lak.-sallsk. handl.) *2:*1412-1415, May 13, '39

Implants – Cont.
Marble prosthesis in correcting saddle nose; 2 cases. MALBEC, E. F. Semana med. *1:*1136-1138, May 18, '39
Repair of cranial defects with celluloid. NEY, K. W. Am. J. Surg. *44:*394-399, May '39
Marble prosthesis in correction of saddle nose. ZENO, L. Bol. y trab. de la Soc. de cir. de Buenos Aires *23:*332-338, June 21, '39 also: An. de cir. *5:*111-122, June '39
Marble implantation by transsuperciliary route in saddle nose; case. ALVES, O. Rev. brasil. de oto-rino-laring. *7:*347-350, July-Aug '39
Use of marble in correction of nasal deformities. MALBEC, E. F. Semana med. *2:*1266-1270, Nov 30, '39
Marble prosthesis in correction of saddle nose. ZENO, L. Dia med. (Ed. espec., no. 9), pp. 170-171, Nov '39
Studies on effect of pressure on plastic bodies and their application to living tissue. FALK, P. Ztschr. f. Hals-, Nasen-u. Ohrenh. *46:*251-267, '39
Use of glass for rhinoplastic purposes. LYANDE, V. S. Zhur. ush., nos. i gorl. bolez. *16:*322-324, '39
Treatment of fractures of mandible with vitallium screws. BIGELOW, H. M., M. Bull. Vet. Admin. *17:*54-56, July '40
Celloidin tube reconstruction of extensor digitorum communis sheath. MAYER, L. Bull. Hosp. Joint Dis. *1:*39-45, July '40
Vittallium cap arthroplasty of metacarpophalangeal and interphalangeal joints of fingers. BURMAN, M. S. Bull. Hosp. Joint Dis. *1:*79-89, Oct '40
Paraffinoma of nose; surgical therapy of case. ZENO, L. Bol. Soc. de cir. de Rosario *7:*415-418, Oct '40
Grafts and inclusions in nasal surgery. ADLER, D. Rev. brasil. de oto-rino-laring. *8:*679-682, Nov-Dec '40
Results obtained in use of various materials in plastic surgery. GONZALEZ ULLOA, M. Rev. mex. de cir., ginec. y cancer *8:*463-479, Nov '40
Partial rhinoplasty using marble prosthesis; cases. MALBEC, E. F. Semana med. *2:*1173-1182, Nov 21, '40
Use of various materials for isolation of suture to prevent adhesion in tendon surgery; experimental study. NIKOLAEV, G. F. Ortop. i travmatol. (no. 4) *14:*18-26, '40
Vitallium for skeleton support of nose. KIMBALL, G. H. AND DRUMMOND, N. R., J. Oklahoma M. A. *34:*9-12, Jan '41
Rhinoplastic surgery combined with paraffin prosthesis in correction of saddle nose. DU-

Implants – Cont.
JARDIN, E. Ugesk. f. laeger *103:*404–405, March 27, '41
Paraffinoma of nose; surgical therapy; cases. ZENO, L. An. de cir. *7:*41–45, March–June '41
Duraluminum in plastic surgery of nose. MALBEC, E. F. Semana med. *1:*1016–1019, May 1, '41
Prosthetic inclusions. ZENO, L. Bol. Soc. de cir. de Rosario *8:*158–169, June '41
Facial reconstruction with acrylic resin. MUNSON, F. T. AND HERON, D. F. Am. J. Surg. *53:*291–295, Aug '41
Prosthetic inclusions in plastic surgery. ZENO, L. An. de cir. *7:*108–118, Sept '41
Implants in plastic surgery. REBELO NETO, J. AND MALBEC, E. F. Arq. de cir. clin. e exper. *5:*245–314, Oct '41
Marble inclusion by trans-supraciliary route in saddle nose. ALVES, O. Arq. de cir. clin. e exper. *6:*512–517, April–June '42
Paraffinoma, harelip, cicatrices, auricular prosthesis in plastic surgery. GONCALVES, G. Arq. de cir. clin. e exper. *6:*307–316, April–June '42
Use of implants in plastic surgery of face. RIVAS, C. I. *et al.* Arq. de cir. clin. e exper. *6:*621–638, April–June '42
Care of military and civilian injuries; implantation method of setting fractured mandibles. BERRY, H. C. Am. J. Orthodontics (Oral Surg. Sect) *28:*292–306, May '42
New material (vinylite) in plastic surgery; preliminary report. DUARTE CARDOSO, A. Rev. brasil. de oto-rino-laring. *10:*319–327, May–June '42
Method of fractional implantation and other systematic implantation experiments. BUSSE GRAWITZ, P. Ztschr. d. d. ges. exper. Med. *111:*1–19, '42 (Reply to Hora)
Materials for corrective plastic surgery of nose. RAPIN, M. Pract. oto-rhino-laryng. *4:*133–141, '42
Histologic studies on reaction of alveolar bone to vitallium implants (preliminary report). BERNIER, J. L. AND CANBY, C. P. J. Am. Dent. A. *30:*188–197, Feb 1, '43
Vitallium bone screws and appliances for fracture of mandible. BIGELOW, H. M., J. Oral Surg. *1:*131–137, April '43
Tissue reactions to metallic implants. FULCHER, O. H. AND MAXWELL, M. M., U. S. Nav. M. Bull. *41:*845–847, May '43
Surgical importance of abnormalities of frontal sinus; result of postoperative plastic correction using vitallium inclusion. GONZALEZ LOZA, M. AND MAISONNAVE, R. Rev. otorrinolaring. d. litoral *2:*298–306, June '43

Implants – Cont.
Nylon fabric arthroplasty of carpometacarpal joint of thumb. BURMAN, M. Bull. Hosp. Joint Dis. *4:*74–78, Oct '43
Use of plastics in reconstructive surgery; lucite in arthroplasty; tissue tolerance for lucite, its use as interposition mold in arthroplasty of phalangeal joints; 3 cases. BURMAN, M. AND ABRAHAMSON, R. H. Mil. Surgeon *93:*405–414, Nov '43
Tantalum in plastic surgery. BAXTER, H. McGill M. J. *12:*287–291, Dec '43
Symposium on war surgery; use of tantalum wire and foil in repair of peripheral nerves. SPURLING, R. G., S. Clin. North America *23:*1491–1504, Dec '43
Inhibition of coagulation necrosis of implants by means of oxalate and enzyme poisons. CAIN, H. Frankfurt. Ztschr. f. Path. *58:*171, '43
Sculpturally molded synthetic implants (methyl methacrylate) in plastic surgery of face. BROWN, A. M. Arch. Otolaryng. *39:*179–183, Feb '44
Implant material; production of fibrous tissue around fibers of cotton and other foreign material implanted subcutaneously in rats. SEARCY, H. B. *et al.* South M. J. *37:*149–150, March '44
New technic for repair of facial paralysis with tantalum wire. SCHUESSLER, W. W. Surgery *15:*646–652, April '44
Prosthetic restorations of breast; technic using sponge rubber. BROWN, A. M. Arch. Surg. *48:*388–394, May '44
Inert metals in direct fixation of mandibular fractures. STROCK, A. E. Surg., Gynec. and Obst. *78:*527–532, May '44
Sutureless reunion of severed nerves with elastic cuffs of tantalum. WEISS, P., J. Neurosurg. *1:*219–225, May '44
"Cerlage" of anus with wire in rectal prolapse. FAIMBERG WASSERMAN, I. Dia med. *16:*628, June 12, '44
Tantalum in plastic surgery; glimpse of surgical future. OLSON, C. T. Indust. Med. *13:*738, Sept '44
Use of nylon sheath in secondary repair of torn finger flexor tendons. BURMAN, M. S. Bull. Hosp. Joint Dis. *5:*122–133, Oct '44
Breast tissue as new source for heterogenous implants; preliminary report. LA ROE, E. K. Am. J. Surg. *66:*58–67, Oct '44
Characteristics of local reaction following implantation of tissues preserved in formalin (solution of formaldehyde). LEBEDIN-

Implants—Cont.
SKAYA, S. I. Khirurgiya, no. 4, pp. 18-23, '44
Experimental observations of use of absorbable and nonabsorbable plastics. BLUM, G. Proc. Roy. Soc. Med. *38:*169-171, Feb '45
Plastic closure of defect of cranium; case report illustrating use of tantalum plate and pedicle-tube graft. HARRIS, M. H. AND WOODHALL, B. Surgery *17:*422-428, March '45
Correction of saddle nose by inclusion of vitallium. LINHARES, F. Rev. brasil. de cir. *14:*159-164, March '45
Acrylic resin as implant for correction of facial deformities. PENHALE, K. W. Arch. Surg. *50:*233-239, May '45
Correction of deformities of tip of nose with implantations of paladon. RIVAS, C. I. AND IZURIETA, F. A. Bol. y trab., Acad. argent. de cir. *29:*240-247, May 9, '45
Cranioplasty with tantalum, case. MOUNT, L. A. Rev. argent. de neurol. y psiquiat. *10:*127-131, June '45
Open operation and tantalum plate insertion for fracture of mandible. CHRISTIANSEN, G. W., J. Oral Surg. *3:*194-204, July '45
Acrylic resin (methyl methacrylate) for closure of defects; preliminary report. SMALL, J. M. AND GRAHAM, M. P. Brit. J. Surg. *33:*106-113, Oct '45
Tantalum plates in repair of osseous defects. LE BEAU, J. Rev. neurol. *77:*307-308, Nov-Dec '45
Extradural pneumatocele following tantalum cranioplasty. WOODHALL, B. AND CRAMER, F. J., J. Neurosurg. *2:*524-529, Nov '45
Restoration of patency of nasolacrimal duct by means of vitallium tube; preliminary report. MULDOON, W. E. Am. J. Ophth. *28:*1340-1345, Dec '45
Synthetic resins as tissue implants. AUBRY, M. Ann. d'oto-laryng. *13:*10-13, Jan-Feb '46
Tantalum cranioplasty. BAKODY, J. T. Ohio State M. J. *42:*29-33, Jan '46
Cranioplasty; metallic inserts. WOOLF, J. I. AND WALKER, A. E. Rev. oto-neuro-oftal. *21:*16-18, Jan-Feb '46
Screwing as treatment of choice in trapezoid-metacarpal subluxations complicating fractures of thumb of Bennett or Rolando type. FONTAINE, R. AND ECK, F. Rev. d'orthop. *32:*76-80, Jan-Apr '46
Unilateral facial paralysis; correction with tantalum wire; preliminary report on 8 cases. SHEEHAN, J. E. Lancet *1:*263-264,

Implants—Cont.
Feb 23, '46
Plastic aspects of neurosurgery, with special reference to use of tantalum. CONTRERAS, M. V. AND ROCCA, E. D. Arch. Soc. cirujanos hosp. *16:*353-358, Mar '46
Use of tantalum for repair of defects in infected cases in cranium. GARDNER, W. J. Cleveland Clin. Quart. *13:*72-87, Apr '46
Cranioplasty with acrylic plates. ELKINS, C. W. AND CAMERON, J. E., J. Neurosurg. *3:*199-205, May '46
Failure in early secondary repair of cranial defects with tantalum. BRADFORD, F. K. AND LIVINGSTON, K. E., J. Neurosurg. *3:*318-328, July '46
Arthroplasty of temporomandibular joint in children with interposition of tantalum foil; preliminary report. EGGERS, G. W. N. J. Bone and Joint Surg. *26:*603-606, July '46
Reconstructive otoplasty; further observations; utilization of tantalum wire mesh support. GREELEY, P. W. Arch. Surg. *53:*24-31, July '46
Experimental observations on use of stainless steel for cranioplasty; comparison with tantalum. SCOTT, M. AND WYCIS, H. T. J. Neurosurg. *3:*310-317, July '46
Cranioplasty with tantalum plate in postwar period. BAKER, G. S., S. Clinics North America *26:*841-845, Aug '46
Use of plastic materials in plastic surgery. BLAINE, G., M. Press *216:*223-224, Sept 25, '46 also: Lancet *2:*525-528, Oct 12, '46
Use of tantalum for cranioplasties; further studies. FULCHER, O. H., U. S. Nav. M. Bull. *46:*1493-1498, Oct '46
Simplified technic for fabrication of tantalum plates in cranial surgery. GERRY, R. G. U. S. Nav. M. Bull. *46:*1499-1505, Oct '46
Tissue reactions induced by series of fibrogen plastics implanted in abdominal wall of guinea pigs. BAILEY, O. T. AND FORD, R. Arch. Path. *42:*535-542, Nov '46
Use of tantalum in tendon reconstruction of hand. PEARLMAN, R. C., U. S. Nav. M. Bull. *46:*1647-1650, Nov '46

IMRE, J.: Operation for senile ectropion. Klin. Monatsbl. f. Augenh. *95:*303-305, Sept '35
IMRE, J.: Plastic operation of eyelids. Tr. Ophth. Soc. U. Kingdom (pt. 2, 1937) *57:*494-508, '38
IMRE, J. (see KILNER, T. P.) Aug '39
IMRE, J. JR.: New principles in plastic operations of eyelids and face. J.A.M.A. *76:*1293, May 7, '21

IMRE, JOSEF: *Lidplastik und plastische Operationen anderer Weichteile des Gesichts*. Studium, Budapest, 1928

Imre Operation

Excision of cancer of eyelids and autoplastic surgery according to Imre technic. DE SAINT-MARTIN, Bull. Soc. d'opht. de Paris *49:*36–40, Jan '37

Imre operation for ectropion of lower eyelid. ZATS, L. B. Vestnik oftal. *13:*554–557, '38

INCIARDI, J. A.: Cure of depression of lower eyelid following reinsertion of inferior rectus muscle; case. Arch. Ophth. *28:*464–466, Sept '42

INCLAN, A.: Clinical evolution of bone grafts. Cir. ortop. y traumatol. *3:*161–173, July–Sept '35

INCLAN, A.: Recurrent pseudoarthrosis of humerus complicated by irreparable paralysis of radial nerve; curative osteoplasty and functional reconstruction of hand by means of tendon transplants. Cir. ortop. y traumatol., Habana *7:*43–53, April–June '39

INCLAN, A.: Therapy of fractures of edentulous mandibles by external skeletal fixation, with report of case. Cir. ortop. y traumatol., Habana *9:*158–164, Oct–Dec '41

INCLAN, A.: Use of preserved bone graft in orthopedic surgery. J. Bone and Joint Surg. *24:*81–96, Jan '42

INCLAN, A.: Zygoma fractures and their therapy; cases. Cir. ortop. y traumatol., Habana *10:*14–29, Jan–March '42

INCLAN, A. AND RODRIGUEZ, R.: Bunnell operation to repair loss of grasping power of thumb (paralysis of opponens pollicis) after infantile paralysis; case (transplantation of tendon). Cir. ortop. y traumatol., Habana *6:*140–145, July–Sept '38

INCLAN, A. JR.: Haynes splint in case of bone graft of lower jaw. Cir. ortop. y traumatol. Habana *12:*132–137, July–Sept '45

INCZE, K.: Dyscephalodactylia (Vogt) and developmental abnormalities of uvea. Arch. f. Augenh. *109:*562–566, '36

Infection

Digestion of keloids, cicatrices and buboes with pepsinhydrochloric acid. AHLSWEDE, E. Arch. Dermat. and Syph. *3:*142, Feb '21

Orbital phlegmons as sequels of endonasal operations. BACHMANN, R. Med. Klin. *17:*192, Feb 13, '21

Luetic perforation of hard palate with surgical closure. LOCY, F. E., U. S. Nav. M. Bull. *18:*86–87, Jan '23 (illus.)

Infection – Cont.

Prevention of angina after nasal operations. HAARDT, W. Wien. klin. Wchnschr. *40:*320, March 10, '27

Bone grafting into infected field. BLANC FORTACÍN, J. Siglo med. *82:*117–120, Aug 11, '28

Extrabuccal scarlet fever after burns; cases. BYTCHKOFF, V. S. AND ALEXEEFF, O. A. Mosk. med. j. (no. 1) *9:*23–30, '29

Frequent occurrence of scarlet fever following cleft palate operations. SCHEPPOKAT. Deutsche Ztschr. f. Chir. *218:*383–386, '29

Use of ultraviolet light in preparation of infected granulation tissue for grafting; value of very thick Thiersch grafts. GATCH, W. D. AND TRUSLER, H. M. Surg., Gynec. and Obst. *50:*478–482, Feb '30

Treatment of acute osteomyelitis of jaws. FITZGERALD, L. M. Dental Cosmos *72:*259–266, March '30

Gas gangrene of extremities, with special reference to trivalent anaerobic serotherapy. LARSON, E. E. AND PULFORD, D. S. Tr. Sect. Surg., General and Abd., A.M.A., pp. 261–279, '29 also: J.A.M.A. *94:*612–618, March 1, '30

Epidemiology and prophylaxis of scarlet fever after burns. MINKEWITSCH, I. Med. Welt *4:*1397, Sept 27, '30

Course of infectious process in burns. SMORODINTZEFF, A. A. AND TOGUNOVA, E. F. Microbiol. j. *13:*27–35, '31

Actinomycosis following fracture of lower jaw. GROHS, R. Ztschr. f. Stomatol. *32:*427–433, April 27, '34

Agranulocytosis associated with surgical infections; case report with comments. MACY, J. W., S. Clin. North America *14:*1271–1277, Oct '34

Bacterial infection in burns. CRUICKSHANK, R. Tr. Roy. Med.-Chir. Soc. Glasgow, pp. 79–82, '34–'35; in Glasgow M. J., July '35 also: J. Path. and Bact. *41:*367–369, Sept '35

Parahyoid cellulitis following fracture of lower jaw. DECHAUME, M. Rev. de stomatol. *38:*457–458, June '36

Successful primary suture of nerves in seriously infected wounds. SEIFFERT, L. Zentralbl. f. Chir. *63:*1890–1892, Aug 8, '36

Infections and burns. MCELROY, T., J. Oklahoma M. A. *29:*443–446, Dec '36

Unguentolan (cod liver oil ointment) in therapy of decubitus and postoperative fistula and wound infection; 15 cases. WEBER, H. Wien. med. Wchnschr. *87:*219–221, Feb 20, '37

Infection – Cont.
Treatment (especially tannic acid) of infected burns. MURLESS, B. C. Brit. M. J. *1:*51-53, Jan 13, '40
Hand infections due to human mouth organisms. FRITZELL, K. E. Journal-Lancet *60:*135-137, March '40
Nascent iodine in therapy of osteomyelitis of lower jaw. EICHENBERG, S. An. Fac. de med. de Porto Alegre *2:*189-212, July-Sept '40
"Hospital infection" in plastic surgery ward. SPOONER, E. T. C., J. Hyg. *41:*320-329, Nov '41
Streptococci resistant to sulfonamide (sulfanilamide and its derivatives) in plastic ward (local application of gramicidin). FRANCIS, A. E. Lancet *1:*408-409, April 4, '42
Histophilic asepsis (in plastic surgery). TISCORNIA, A. Minerva med. *1:*481-485, June 16, '42
Total bimaxillary necrobiosis; case with recovery after surgical therapy aided especially by extract of calf jawbone (vaduril). SOLDANO, H. A. O. Prensa med. argent. *30:*1945-1947, Oct 6, '43
Chemotherapy in prevention and treatment of infection in burns; panel discussion; introduction. MELENEY, F. L. Am. Acad. Orthop. Surgeons, Lect., pp. 314-316, '43
Surgery and penicillin in mandibular infection. MOWLEM, R. Brit. M. J. *1:*517-519, April 15, '44
Elimination of cross-infection; experimental (special hospital for infants undergoing plastic surgery). PICKERILL, H. P. AND PICKERILL, C. M. Brit. M. J. *1:*159-160, Feb 3, '45
Statistical analysis of study of prevention of infection in burns, with special reference to sulfonamides. MELENEY, F. L. AND WHIPPLE, A. O. Surg. Gynec. and Obst. *80:*263-296, March '45
Extensive infected burns. MARINO, H. Gac. med., Lima *1:*177-178, June '45 also: Rev. san. de policia *5:*185-196, July-Aug '45
Acute spontaneous infectious gangrene. TVEDT, A. Nord. med. (Norsk mag. f. laegevidensk.) *27:*1750-1753, Sept 7, '45
Use of penicillin therapy in conjunction with free bone grafting in infected areas. ABBOTT, L. C. *et al.* Surg. Gynec. and Obst. *83:*101-106, July '46
Cancellous grafts for infected bone defects; single stage procedure. COLEMAN, H. M. *et al.* Surg. Gynec. and Obst. *83:*392-398, Sept '46

Infection – Cont.
Complications of malignant furuncle of upper lip and their prevention. CALLILAR, N. Turk tip cem mec *12:*44-50, '46
Question of permissibility of bone plastic reamputation in patients with infected wounds. GDALEVICH, I. N. Vrach. delo (nos. 7-8) *26:*459-464, '46

INGEBRIGTSEN, R.: Plastic surgery of nose. Norsk Mag. f. Laegevidensk. *90:*169-175, Feb '29
INGEBRIGTSEN, R.: Rhinoplasty. Lyon chir. *26:*548-553, Aug-Sept '29
INGIANNI, G.: Fistulized tuberculous trochanteritis with extensive bone loss; immediate transplantation of pedicled cutaneous flap into residual cavity; case with recovery. Arch. ed atti d. Soc. ital. di chir. *44:*873-875, '38
INGIANNI, G.: Dermo-epidermal grafts and pedicled tubular grafts in surgical therapy of osteomyelitis. Arch. ed atti d. Soc. ital. di chir. *45:*724-730, '39
INGIANNI, G.: Technical results of grafting skin into cavity of bone after surgical therapy of osteomyelitis. Accad. med., Genova *54:*25-33, Jan '39
INGIANNI, G.: Autoplastic therapy of tuberculous and nontuberculous trochanteritis using free and pedicled flaps; cases. Accad. med., Genova *54:*446-453, May '39
INGLIS, J. V.: Course of instruction in treatment of maxillofacial injuries, Ballochmyle E. M. S. Hospital. Brit. Dent. J. *78:*242-243, April 20, '45
INGLIS, K. (see CORLETTE, C. E.) March '21
INGRAHAM, F. C. AND MATSON, D. D.: Spina bifida and cranium bifidium; unusual nasopharyngeal encephalocele (with cleft palate). New England J. Med. *228:*815-820, June 24, '43
INOUE, S.: Plastic operations of total defect of eyelids and symblephara orbitalia. Far East. Sc. Bull. *1:*3, April '41 (abstract)

Instruments
New perichondrium elevator for resection of nasal septum. CAMPBELL, C. A. Laryngoscope *31:*973, Dec '21 (illus.)
Mouth gag and tongue depressor combination. WOLF, G. D. Tr. Sect. Laryng. Otol. and Rhin., A.M.A. p. 287, 1921
A knife for harelip and cleft palate operations. CATES, B. B. Am. J. Surg. *36:*70, March '22
New instruments used in nose and throat and plastic surgery. SHEEHAN, J. E. New York

Instruments – Cont.
M. J. *115:*493–494, April 19, '22 (illus.)
New nasal septal chisel. BARKER, C. J.A.M.A. *79:*216, July 15, '22 (illus.)
Combined gag and tongue retractor. BOYLE, H. E. G. Lancet *2:*1130, Nov 25, '22 (illus.)
An instrument (drill) to facilitate correction of certain types of external deformities of nose. ISRAEL, S. J.A.M.A. *80:*690, March 10, '23 (illus.)
Automatic gag and tongue holder. SAMENGO, L. Semana med. *1:*734–738, April 19, '23 (illus.)
New nasal septal chisel. OLSHO, S. L. Laryngoscope *33:*308, April '23 (illus.)
Nasal drill for removal of septal spur. YOUNG, H. H., J.A.M.A. *80:*1216, April 28, '23 (illus.)
Improved septal punch forceps. LEWIS, J. D. Laryngoscope *33:*862–864, Nov '23 (illus.)
Method of holding septal membranes in apposition after a submucous resection without use of packing, description and demonstration of instruments and method of use. SIMPSON, H. L., J. Michigan M. Soc. *23:*64–67, Feb '24
Guarded septum chisel. RUSKIN, S. L. Laryngoscope *34:*288–289, April '24
Dermotome. HAGEN, G. L. J.A.M.A. *82:*1933, June 14, '24
New elevator for submucous resection. MYERSON, M. C. Laryngoscope *34:*660, Aug '24
Modification of Davis Boyle gag. BROWN, R. G. Lancet *2:*756, Oct 11, '24
Small apparatus for diathermy and electrocoagulation depilation treatment of hypertrichosis in women. LANZI, G. Gior. ital. d. ma. ven. *65:*1718–1720, Oct '24
Electrically driven nasal saw and rasp. IGLAUER, S. Laryngoscope *35:*78, Jan '25
Submucosa dissector. GRAHAM, A. J. Surg., Gynec. and Obst. *40:*709, May '25 also: M. J. and Rec. *122:*527, Nov 4, '25
Technic for submucous resection, with presentation of membrane elevator. JONES, M. F. Laryngoscope *35:*406–408, May '25
Special periostetomes for cleft palate work. CATES, B. B. Boston M. and S. J. *193:*728–729, Oct 15, '25
New rhinoplastic instruments. MALTZ, M. Laryngoscope *36:*54–60, Jan '26
Peroral endoscopy; its use in complications following operations on nose and throat. TUCKER, G. Arch. Otolaryng. *5:*321–333, April '27
New Thiersch graft razor. BETTMAN, A. G. J.A.M.A. *89:*451, Aug 6, '27
New electrical epilation apparatus. MEZEI,

Instruments – Cont.
K. Dermat. Wchnschr. *85:*1107, Aug 6, '27
Treatment of fractures of fingers and metacarpals with description of authors' finger caliper. MOCK, H. E. AND ELLIS, J. D. Surg., Gynec. and Obst. *45:*551–556, Oct '27
New instrument for use in skin grafting. BORS, E. Zentralbl. f. Chir. *54:*2890–2891, Nov 12, '27
Forceps for inserting grafts in corrective operations of nose. EITNER, E. Munchen. med. Wchnschr. *74:*1876, Nov 4, '27
Two new instruments; septum needle and thread-holder for ear surgery. POLLAK, E. Monatschr. f. Ohrenh. *61:*1252, Nov '27
Dangers of Whitehead mouth-gag used on young children. TRENDTEL. Klin. Wchnschr. *6:*2436–2437, Dec 17, '27
Double-end arrow elevator for nasal plastic operations and submucous resections. FISHBEIN, J. N. Laryngoscope *38:*97, Feb '28
Simple instrument for inverted or retracted nipples. BIVINGS, L., J. M. A. Georgia *17:*120–121, March '28
New needle-holder for use in diathermic epilation in hypertrichosis. KENDE, B. Wien. klin. Wchnschr. *41:*382, March 15, '28
Sound for dilating strictures of naso-lacrimal duct. SCHMIDT, P. Klin. Monatsbl. f. Augenh. *80:*390, March 23, '28
New method of cutting large skin grafts (instrument). JOYNT, R. L. Lancet *1:*816, April 21, '28
Adjustable mouthgag tongue depressor. LEWIS, E. R. Arch. Otolaryng. *7:*636, June '28
Modified nasal septal forceps. TAKAHASHI, K. Ztschr. f. Hals-, Nasen-u. Ohrenh. *22:*130, June 16, '28
Modification of Davis gag. EADIE, N. M. J. Laryng. and Otol. *43:*531, July '28
Esthetic reduction of nasal fractures with new apparatus; case. PROBY, H. Arch. internat. de laryng. *34:*866–868, July–Aug '28
New rhinoplastic instrument. SAFIAN, J. Arch. Otolaryng. *8:*78, July '28
New instrument for intranasal suture. TAKAHASHI, K. Ztschr. f. Laryng., Rhin. *17:*211–216, Sept '28
Resector for removing shaped piece of rib cartilage for nasal transplant. FORNELL, C. H. Laryngoscope *38:*733–734, Nov '28
Subcutaneous plates and knives for cutting large Thiersch grafts for plastic surgery. JOYNT, R. L. Irish J. M. Sc., pp. 700–702, Nov '28

Instruments – Cont.

Kubo's aurograph for tracing form of concha. KUBO, I. Ztschr. f. Hals-, Nasen-u. Ohrenh. *22:*320–322, Nov 10, '28

Endonasal surgery with aid of new instrument; simplified technic. WACHSBERGER, A. Arch. Otolaryng. *8:*712–714, Dec '28

Apparatus for localization of transplanted areolae of breast in plastic surgery. DARTIGUES. Bull. et mem. Soc. de chir. de Paris *21:*43, Jan 4, '29

New combined submucous dissector and suction cannula. HAMRICK, D. W. Arch. Otolaryng. *9:*655–656, June '29

New instrument for reduction of nasal fractures. SALINGER, S. Arch. Otolaryng. *9:*657–658, June '29

Screw curet; use in curettage and in excision of fistulous tracts. YOUNG, H. H., J.A.M.A. *93:*110–113, July 13, '29

Osteotome for resection of mandible. ROCCIA, B. Minerva med. (pt. 2) *9:*700, Nov 3, '29

Subcutaneous fascial stripper. GRACE, R. V. Ann. Surg. *90:*1109–1110, Dec '29

Nasal suturing instrument. CAMPBELL, C. A. Arch. Otolaryng. *11:*95–96, Jan '30

Improved nasofrontal rasp. SPRATT, C. N. Arch. Otolaryng. *11:*783, June '30

New instrument for use in longstanding dislocations of jaws. TAYLOR, A. B., J. M. A. South Africa *4:*326, June 14, '30

Modifications in Graefe's apparatus for reduction and retention of fractures. GIZZI, C. Stomatol. *28:*865–870, Oct '30

Submucous septum punch. REAVES, R. G. Tr. Am. Acad. Ophth. *35:*475, '30

Three new instruments for fronto-ethmosphenoid operation. SMITH, F. Ann. Otol., Rhin. and Laryng. *40:*198–200, March '31

Implements for hand injuries. MASLAND, H. C. Am. J. Surg. *12:*142–143, April '31

New instrument for taking skin grafts. ALTRUDA, J. B., M. J. and Rec. *133:*348, April 1, '31

Self-retaining anaesthetic and post-anaesthetic gag and tongue tractor. MILTON, W. T. Indian M. Gaz. *66:*298, May '31

New instrument for detachment of sac in dacryocystectomy. NEUSCHULER, I. Arch. d'opht. *48:*829–831, Dec '31

Instrument for subcutaneous removal of fascia lata strips for suture purposes. BATE, J. T. Ann. Surg. *95:*313–314, Feb '32

New eyelid clamp. CRUICKSHANK, M. M. Indian M. Gaz. *67:*82–83, Feb '32 also: Am. J. Ophth. *15:*349, April '32

Modification of Lowenstein clamp used in transplantation of lip mucosa. STEIN, R. Klin. Monatsbl. f. Augenh. *88:*370–371, March '32

Forceps for skin grafts. WRIGHT, A. D. Lancet *1:*840, April 16, '32

Submucous flap punch for nasal septal surgery. REAVES, R. G. Arch. Otolaryng. *15:*754, May '32

Forceps for skin grafts. WRIGHT, A. D. Indian M. Gaz. *67:*479–480, Aug '32

New instruments for submucous resection of nasal septum. GAMMAGE, F. V. Arch. Otolaryng. *16:*573–574, Oct '32

Improved gag. WADE, R. Lancet *2:*1220, Dec 3, '32

Cutting hook and inverse hammer for nasal surgery. VAN DER HOEVEN, LEONHARD, J. Oto-rhino-laryng. internat. *17:*27–31, Jan '33

Extreme cleft of hard and soft palate closed with use of author's tension plates. FEDERSPIEL, M. N. Wisconsin M. J. *32:*172–177, March '33

Suture needle for nasal surgery. MALONE, J. Y. Arch. Otolaryng. *17:*562, April '33

New instruments for use of rib cartilage grafts in rhinoplasty. MALINIAK, J. W. Arch. Otolaryng. *18:*79–82, July '33

New mouth gag with interchangeable and adjustable tongue depressors and anesthetizing tube. STUPKA, W. Laryngoscope *43:*585–588, July '33

Cautery pencil in treatment of furunculosis. SCHÜLE, A. Med. Welt. *8:*407, March 24, '34

Double blepharostat of varying width for entropion operation. WERNER, S. Finska lak.-sallsk. handl. *76:*275–277, March '34

Knife for submucous resection. MILLER, A. Lancet *1:*1395, June 30, '34

New mouth gag for cleft palate operation. NEWKIRK, H. D. Laryngoscope *44:*587, July '34

Cleft palate and harelip; adolescent case treated orthodontically in conjunction with lip-stretching device and skin grafting of labial sulcus. HARDY, E. A. Internat. J. Orthodontia *20:*750–758, Aug '34

Adjustable nasal elevator. HOMME, O. H. Arch. Otolaryng. *20:*711, Nov '34

Retractor for intra-oral operations. JOHNSON, B. Lancet *2:*1052, Nov 10, '34

New knife for dacryocystorhinostomy. MEURMAN, Y. Acta otolaryng. *21:*343–345, '34

Instruments for restoration of severed flexor tendons of fingers according to Bunnell method. Rozov, V. I. Sovet. khir. (nos. 3–4) *6:*458–461, '34

Instruments – Cont.
Double blepharostat of varying widths for entropion operation. WERNER, S. Acta ophth. *12:*149-152, '34
Simple instrument for finger extension. BROCK, R. C. Lancet *1:*382, Feb 16, '35
Instrument for skin grafts. SHAFIROFF, B. G. P. Ann. Surg. *101:*814-815, Feb '35
New instruments for nasal reconstructive surgery. BARSKY, A. J. Arch. Otolaryng. *22:*487-490, Oct '35
Two instruments for modelling transplanted cartilage in closure of laryngeal and tracheal defects. MAYER, F. J. Monatschr. f. Ohrenh. *69:*1193-1196, Oct '35
Therapy of recent fractures of lower jaw; with description of apparatus used. GIOIA, T. Semana med. *2:*1370-1378, Nov 7, '35
Instrument for obtaining Thiersch grafts. EYMER, H. Deutsche med. Wchnschr. *61:*1954-1955, Dec 6, '35
Application of Vorschutz lever screw in fractures of lower jaw. STEINKAMM, J. Chirurg *7:*820-824, Dec 1, '35
Further application of author's method of outlay on celluloid frame (facial surgery). COELST. Rev. de chir. structive, pp. 195-198, March '36
Instrument for grasping ends of ruptured tendon during suture. HIRSCHBERG, O. Schweiz. med. Wchnschr. *66:*514-515, May 23, '36
New type nasal rasp in plastic surgery. ISRAEL, S. Laryngoscope *46:*388-389, May '36
New instrument for correction of hump nose. PIERI, P. F. Boll. d. mal. d. orecchio, d. gola, d. naso *54:*180-187, May '36
Compass for symmetrical measured tracing in plastic surgery of breast. BERTOLA, V. J. Semana med. *2:*197-198, July 16, '36
Oblique-angled knife for resetting lower end of dislocated septal cartilage and operations on harelip and cleft palate. METZENBAUM, M. Arch. Otolaryng. *24:*199, Aug '36
Instruments for eyelid treatment. HEATH, P. Tr. Sect. Ophth., A.M.A., pp. 272-273, '36 also: Arch. Ophth. *17:*894-895, May '37
Instrument for insertion of Kirschner wire in phalanges for skeletal traction. MEEKISON, D. M., J. Bone and Joint Surg. *19:*234, Jan '37
Apparatus for immediate treatment and prosthesis in jaw fractures. DI GIUSEPPE, F. Gior. ital. di clin. trop. *1:*81, March 31, '37
"Tendon stretcher" for pulling forward muscle for tenotomy. (Comment on Streiff's article). GUTZEIT, R. Klin. Monatsbl. f. Augenh. *98:*671, May '37

Instruments – Cont.
New profilometer (instrument for plastic surgery of nasal deformities). STRAITH, C. L. Rev. de chir. structive, pp. 156-157, June '37
Plastic surgery of nose; technic and instruments. CLAOUE. Ztschr. f. Hals-, Nasen-u. Ohrenh. *40:*660-662, '37
Apparatus for reducing fractures of zygomatic arch. LIMBERG, A. A. Vestnik khir. *50:*194-197, '37
Instrument for pinch grafting. HAGGLAND, P. B. Am. J. Surg. *39:*171, Jan '38
Two improved instruments for use in plastic surgery of nose. FIRESTONE, C. Laryngoscope *48:*356-357, May '38
Modified Brigg's retractor for dacryocystorhinostomy. STALLARD, H. B. Brit. J. Ophth. *22:*361, June '38
Turbinotome for "ab externo" dacryocystorhinostomy. RAVERDINO, E. Rassegna ital. d'ottal. *7:*499-503, July-Aug '38
New suction elevator for otorhinolaryngologic operations. YOSHIDA, S. Oto-rhino-laryng. *11:*651, July '38
Chisel for dacryocystorhinostomy. HAAS, E. Bull. Soc. d'opht. de Paris *50:*468-469, Oct '38
Badly consolidated fracture of upper jaw; reduction by osteotomy and elastic traction apparatus. THEODORESCO, D. Rev. de chir., Bucuresti *41:*918-926, Nov-Dec '38
Technical improvements on Glatzel's mirror for examination of width of nose. JOCHIMS, J. Ztschr. f. Kinderh. *60:*147-153, '38
Instrument for subcutaneous stripping of lengths of fascia lata. FINOCHIETTO, R. Prensa med. argent. *26:*69-70, Jan 4, '39
Construction of ideal nose with aid of masks and measurements. BERSON, M. I., M. Rec. *149:*80-82, Feb 1, '39
New mouth gag for surgery of cleft palate. LUHMANN, K. Zentralbl. f. Chir. *66:*243-244, Feb 4, '39
Caliper for reduction of phalangeal and metacarpal fractures by skeletal traction. CARR, R. W. South. M. J. *32:*543-546, May '39
Tailor-made chin retractor (for mandibular protrusion). STOFT, W. E. Am. J. Orthodontics *25:*461-466, May '39
New mouth gag for operation of cleft palate. LUHMANN, K. Therap. d. Gegenw. *80:*284-285, June '39
New periosteotome for hard palate. BERTOLA, V. J. Prensa med. argent. *26:*1853-1854, Sept 20, '39
New type of forceps used as accessory ele-

Instruments – Cont.
ment in depilation by diathermocoagulation. CATEULA, J. Semana med. *2:*628, Sept 14, '39
Instrument for transplantation of tendons. GUSEV, B. P. Vestnik khir. *58:*590-591, Dec '39
New technic for cutting skin grafts, including description of new instruments. POTH, E. J. Surgery *6:*935-939, Dec '39
Emergency treatment and primary apparatus for war fractures of jaw (reports of various countries). DEDONCKER *et al.* Internat. Cong. Mil. Med. and Pharm. *2:*206-218, '39
New knife for Van Millingen grafting operation (ingrown eyelashes). KAMEL, S. Bull. Ophth. Soc. Egypt *32:*73-78, '39
Apparatus for fixation of skin flap during epithelization of wound cavity after resection of upper jaw. KHARI, A. P. Novy khir. arkhiv *43:*328-330, '39
Use of knitting needle for suture of conjunctiva in rhinostomy. KURLOV, I. N. AND MILOVIDOVA, A. N. Vestnik oftal. (no. 2) *15:*38-39, '39
New instrument for conservative operations on nasal septum. TSYPIN, M. Y. Zhur. ush., nos. i gorl. bolez. *16:*141-145, '39
Emergency treatment and primary apparatus for jaw fractures in warfare. FAIRBANK, L. C. AND IVY, R. H. Mil. Surgeon *86:*124-134, Feb '40
New instrument for passing portions of tendons and fasciae latae. MACEY, H. B. Am. J. Surg. *47:*686, March '40
Nasal septum trephine. BOILER, W. F. Laryngoscope *40:*438-439, June '40
New type of tissue forceps. BROWN, J. B. Am. J. Surg. *49:*397, Aug '40
Bed frame for severe decubitus and sacral wounds. HELLER, E. Zentralbl. f. Chir. *67:*1530-1532, Aug 17, '40
Improved instruments and postoperative splint for nasal plastic operations; combined chisel and periosteal elevator. PEARLMAN, L. M. Arch. Otolaryng. *32:*338-340, Aug '40
Treatment of hypertrichosis by improved apparatus and technic (electrolysis). MARTON, M. H. Arch. Phys. Therapy *21:*678-683, Nov '40
New instruments for use in rhinoplastic surgery. CINELLI, J. A. Arch. Otolaryng. *32:*1102-1106, Dec '40
New instrument for grasping tendons. DUSCHL, L. Chirurg *12:*756, Dec 15, '40
New devices for reduction of maxillary fractures. WOODWARD, C. M. Mil. Surgeon

Instruments – Cont.
*87:*525-531, Dec '40
Double-edged knife for removing mucous membrane and skin grafts. BERENS, C. Tr. Sect. Ophth., A.M.A., p. 291, '40
New drills for dacryocystorhinostomy. CRAMER, F. E. K. AND BALZA, J. Semana med. *1:*294-295, Jan 30, '41
Dermoepidermal grafts; autostabilizing retractor. MARINO, H. AND ESPERNE, P. Rev. med.-quir. de pat. fem. *17:*137-140, Feb '41
Constriction of mandible; report of case and presentation of new dilator apparatus. VATTEONE, A. L. Dia med. *13:*688-692, July 21, '41
Method of determining correct seat of nipples in plastic surgery for pendulous breasts; new instrument to facilitate it. EHRENFELD, H. J., M. Rec. *154:*92-94, Aug 6, '41
"Thimble forceps" for epilation (during electrolysis). SHELTON, J. M. Arch. Dermat. and Syph. *44:*260, Aug '41
Submucous elevator. METZENBAUM, M. F. Arch. oto-laryng. *34:*847, Oct '41
Combined epilation needle and forceps handle. GOLDBERG, H. C. Arch. Dermat. and Syph. *44:*1104-1105, Dec '41
First aid appliance for treatment of jaw fractures. SORRELS, T. W. Am. J. Orthodontics *27:*714-716, Dec '41
Measuring force of elevation of upper eyelid and its clinical significance; description of apparatus. MULLER, H. K. AND LANGGUTH, H. Arch. f. Ophth. *144:*234-246, '41
Three-fourths graft and other thicknesses cut with dermatome. PADGETT, E. C. AND SODERBERG, N. B. Dia med. *14:*8-11, Jan 5, '42
Self-retaining illuminating palate retractor. DALTON, S. E. Tr. Am. Acad. Ophth. (1941) *46:*151, Jan-Feb '42
Fractures of maxilla; simplified appliance for craniomaxillary support and fixation. WALDRON, C. W. AND BALKIN, S. G. Surgery *11:*183-194, Feb '42
Light aspirator in surgery of palatine fissure and in general surgery. MARINO, H. Prensa med. argent. *29:*481-483, March 18, '42
Retractor for use in neck surgery. BEATTY, H. G. Arch. Otolaryng. *35:*651-652, April '42
Technical devices in surgical therapy of harelip and velopalatine fissures, with report of cases. REBELO NETO, J. Arq. de cir. clin. e exper. *6:*343-358, April-June '42
Canaliculus dilator in eye. BERENS, C. Am. J. Ophth. *25:*725-726, June '42
Electrolysis; introduction of instrument for relatively painless treatment in hair re-

Instruments – Cont.
moval. HAND, E. A. Arch. Dermat. and Syph. *45:*1094–1100, June '42
Simple instrument for cutting Thiersch flaps. MULLER-MEERNACH, O. Munchen. med. Wchnschr. *89:*591, June 26, '42
Device for measuring length of tendon graft in flexor tendon surgery. KAPLAN, E. B. Bull. Hosp. Joint Dis. *3:*97–99, July '42
Instruments for maxillofacial and oral surgery. GINESTET, G. Rev. de stomatol. *43:*121–123, July–Aug '42
Advantages of Padgett dermatome. PIERCE, G. W. California and West. Med. *57:*16–18, July '42
Use of Padgett dermatome to obtain grafts. ZENO, L. AND VERDAGUER, J. F. Bol. Soc. de cir. de Rosario *9:*211–214, July '42
Simple method for preparing dacryocystorhinostomy needles. BALOD, K. Klin. Monatsbl. f. Augenh. *108:*626, Sept–Oct '42
New mouth retractor for oral surgery. BALOGH, K. Ztschr. f. Stomatol. *40:*669–671, Sept 11, '42
Instruments to facilitate mucosal suture in dacryocystorhinostomy. BANGERTER, A. Ophthalmologica *104:*171–174, Sept '42
Dermoepidermal grafts using Padgett dermatome; detail of technic. MARINO, H. Dia med. *14:*912–914, Sept 7, '42
Free grafts (called intermediate or transchorionic) using Padgett dermatome. PAVLOVSKY, A. J. AND HARRIS, M. M. Semana med. *2:*709–713, Sept 24, '42
Use of Padgett dermatome in ophthalmic plastic surgery. SMITH, B. Arch. Ophth. *28:*484–489, Sept '42
New set of automatic retractors for nasal surgery. VELLOSO VIANNA, E. Rev. brasil. de oto-rino-laring. *10:*533–550, Sept–Oct '42
Needle and needle holder for intranasal use. SIMPSON, R. K. Am. J. Ophth. *25:*1368–1369, Nov '42
Angled bistoury with retrograde uniform cutting edge for use in plastic surgery of nose. DELLEPIANE RAWSON, R. AND JAROLAVSKY, N. N. Dia med. *14:*1280, Dec 7, '42
New type of relaxing incision – dermatome-flap method. HARKINS, H. N. Am. J. Surg. *59:*79–82, Jan '43
"Transplantation microtome" new apparatus for obtaining uniformly thick epidermal and cutaneous grafts. SACHARIEW, G. Chirurg. *15:*94, Feb 1, '43
Prevention of contracture deformities following burns by use of Padgett dermatome. THOMPSON, H. A. South. Med. and Surg. *105:*51–55, Feb '43
Prevention of nasal deformity in corrective rhinoplasty (description of rhinometer). BERSON, M. I. Laryngoscope *53:*276–287, April '43
New instrument with needle continuously threaded for suturing. GONZALEZ ULLOA, M. Rev. mex. de cir., ginec. y cancer *11:*123–135, April '43
Gag for dysfunction of temporomandibular joint following mandibular injury. HALLUM, J. W. Brit. M. J. *1:*569, May 8, '43
Shock; new needle for treatment by sternal infusion. JONES, R. M. Surg., Gynec. and Obst. *76:*587–588, May '43
Two small supplementary devices for author's extension apparatus for fractured fingers. THOMSEN, W. Chirurg. *15:*311, May 15, '43
Modified calibrated grafting knife. MARCKS, K. M. Mil. Surgeon *92:*653–654, June '43
Use of cotter key in intermaxillary ligation allowing quick release in case of nausea and vomiting. HARPER, H. D. Am. J. Orthodontics *29:*373–382, July '43
Dermatome for cutting small grafts. WEBSTER, G. V., U.S. Nav. M. Bull. *41:*1145–1151, July '43
Grafts using Padgett dermatome. COVARRUBIAS ZENTENO, R. Rev. med. de Chile *71:*729–741, Aug '43
Use of Padgett dermatome. HENLEY, R. B. Permanente Found. M. Bull. (no. 2) *1:*1–6, Oct '43
New needle holder for plastic surgery. WEBSTER, G. V., U.S. Nav. M. Bull. *41:*1434–1439, Sept '43
Principles governing design and details of first aid Stannard glove. HUDSON, R. V. Bull. War Med. *4:*193–195, Dec '43 (abstract)
Application of dermatome-flap method; use in case of recurrent incisional hernia. SWENSON, S. A. JR. AND HARKINS, H. N. Arch. Surg. *47:*564–570, Dec '43
New rhinometer. BERSON, M. I. Am. J. Surg. *63:*148–149, Jan '44
Instrument for manipulation of central middle third of face fractures. MCINDOE, A. H. Brit. M. J. *1:*14, Jan 1, '44
New instrument for use in rhinoplastic surgery. KAYSER, R. Arch. Otolaryng. *39:*186–188, Feb '44
Improved cutting edge for Padgett dermatome. SHUMACKER, H. B. JR. Surgery *15:*457–459, March '44
Hand retraction piece for hand surgery. RANK, B. K. Brit. M. J. *1:*496, April 8, '44
Simplified method of treatment of maxillary fractures (use of cap splint). MACGREGOR,

Instruments—Cont.
A. B. Brit. Dent. J. *76:*239-241, May 5, '44
Use of skeletal traction in hand. COBEY, M. C.; *et al.* South. M. J. *37:*309-313, June '44
Device for external transcutaneous fixation of mandibular fractures. HOFFMAN, R. Helvet. med. acta *11:*521-524, June '44
Simplified chin support. THUSS, C. J., J. M. A. Alabama *13:*387-388, June '44
Maxillary forceps in fractures. GORDON, S. Lancet *2:*80, July 15, '44
Fixation of mandibular fractures by means of extraoral apparatus based on pins. MOWLEM, R.; *et al.* Rev. san. mil., Buenos Aires *43:*1055-1058, July '44
Finger exerciser for burned hands. OLDFIELD, M. C. AND KING, C. J. Lancet *2:*109, July 22, '44
Free graft; advantages and inconveniences of dermatome. ZENO, L. Bol. y trab., Acad. argent. de cir. *28:*690-698, Aug 23, '44
New cement for use in cutting skin grafts. GERRIE, J. W. Canad. M. A. J. *51:*465-466, Nov '44
Maxillary fracture appliance of new principle and design. JOHNSTON, B. AND TITZE, L. O. Hosp. Corps Quart. (no. 6) *17:*137-139, Nov '44
Instrument for obtaining split skin grafts. MCCALLA, L. H., J. South Carolina M. A. *40:*228, Nov '44
Board for cutting grafts of definite width. GABARRO, P. Lancet *2:*788, Dec 16, '44
Instrument for anchoring fractures of face. STEVENSON, H. N. Arch. Otolaryng. *40:*503, Dec '44
How to use dermatome. PADGETT, E. Am. Acad. Orthop. Surgeons, Lect., pp. 216-224, '44
New device for suturing skin. DA ROCHA, J. Dia med. *17:*77, Jan 22, '45
Arm board for navy operating table. DUNLOP, G. R. AND HUMBERD, J. D., U.S. Nav. M. Bull. *44:*171-172, Jan '45
Modified calibrated knife in skin grafting; further observations. MARCKS, K. M. Surgery *17:*109-115, Jan '45
Treatment of tendons in finger amputations and description of new instrument. WEBSTER, G. V. Surgery *17:*102-108, Jan '45
Resplitting split-thickness skin grafts with dermatome; method for increasing yield of limited donor sites. ZINTEL, H. A. Ann. Surg. *121:*1-5, Jan '45
Skin graft of dorsum of hand; use of large size dermatome to obtain one-piece pattern. CONVERSE, J. M. Ann. Surg. *121:*172-174, Feb '45
Simple knife for skin grafts for general use.

Instruments—Cont.
WEBSTER, G. V. Am. J. Surg. *67:*569-571, March '45
New nasal tissue clamp used in new method of narrowing columella. SELTZER, A. P., J. Internat. Coll. Surgeons *8:*154-159, March-April '45
Technical details in dermatome grafting. WALLACE, F. T. South. M. J. *38:*380-381, June '45
Device for fixation of Wolfe graft. MICHAELSON, I. C. Brit. M. J. *2:*49, July 14, '45
Nylon backing for dermatome grafts. GREEN, R. W.; *et al.* New England J. Med. *233:*268-270, Aug 30, '45
Instrument to facilitate multiple loop wiring in jaw fractures. KLEIN, D. Bull. U.S. Army M. Dept. *4:*479, Oct '45
Further uses for peripheral bone clamp in jaw fractures. THOMA, K. H.; *et al.* Am. J. Orthodontics (Oral Surg. Sect.) *31:*607-618, Oct '45
Lamination with dermatome and "split" grafts; method for increasing yield of limited donor regions. ZINTEL, H. A. Salud y belleza (no. 5) *1:*10-11; 39, Oct-Dec '45
Instruments for dermoepidermal grafts. DELRIO, J. M. A. AND BULFARO, J. A. Bol. y trab, Soc. argent. de cirujanos *6:*745-748, '45 also: Rev. Asoc. med. argent. *59:*1328-1329, Nov 30 '45
New instruments for dacryocystorhinostomy. SANCHEZ BULNES, L. AND SILVA, D. Arch. Asoc. para evit. ceguera Mexico *3:*249-255, '45
New instruments in rhinoplastic surgery. SUNSHINE, L. Am. J. Surg. *71:*434-435, March '46
Plasma, nutrient dusting powder used to nullify rubber cement used in connection with Padgett dermatome. CLIMO, S., U.S. Nav. M. Bull. *46:*1291-1296, Aug '46
Aids in rhinoplastic procedures. BECKER, O. J. Ann. Otol. Rhin. and Laryng. *55:*562-571, Sept '46
Two instruments for surgery of hand. HEBRAUD, A. Rev. med. nav. *1:*63-65, '46
Dermatome. TAULLARD, J. C. Bol. y trab., Soc. argent. de cirujanos *7:*30-38, '46 also: Rev. Asoc. med. argent. *60:*248-251, April 30, '46

INTROINI, L. A.: Technic for repair of flexor tendons of fingers. Rev. med. del Rosario *25:*1191-1200, Nov '35
IOAN-JONES, D.: Wounds and injuries of tendons. Practitioner *156:*262-266, April '46
IONESCU, N. V.: Congenital median cysts and fistulae of neck. Rev. san. mil., Bucuresti *35:*71-80, Jan '36

IONESCU-MILTIADE, I.: Metrazol-ephedrine in prevention of shock. Romania med. *12:*233-234, Sept 15, '34

IORDANSKIY (see DMITRIEVA) 1934

IOVINO, F.: Muscular autotransplants and nerve connections; experimental study. Ann. ital. di chir. *12:*1521-1546, Dec 31, '33

IOKHELSON, S. A.: Abortive burn therapy with alcohol. Vrach. gaz. *35:*1149-1451, Oct 15, '31

IPOLYI, F.: Late results of operations on septum in cases of obstruction of nasal respiration. Monatschr. f. Ohrenh. *69:*685-689, June '35

IPSEN, J.: Therapy of jaw fractures. Zentralbl. f. Chir. *60:*2840-2841, Dec 9, '33

Ipsen Operation

Treatment of fracture of corpus mandibulae ad modum Ipsen (introduction of Kirschner nails). SØBYE, P. Acta chir. Scandinav. *83:*445-477, '40

IRISH, H. E. AND STEPAN, C. E.: Hyperpyrexia following harelip operation. Am. J. Dis. Child. *58:*320-331, Aug '39

IRWIN, C. E.: Transplants to thumb to restore function of opposition; end results. South. M. J. *35:*257-262, March '42

IRWIN, J. H.: Crampton test (blood pressure and pulse recording in recumbent and erect positions) and surgical shock. J. M. Soc. New Jersey *32:*416-418, July '35

ISAACS, H. J. (see SCHWARTZ, A. A.) April '42

ISAKOWITZ, J.: Congenital eyelid coloboma. Klin. Monatsbl. f. Augenh. *78:*509-512, April '27

ISELIN, H.: Treatment of cutaneous ulcer due to roentgen ray burn. Schweiz. med. Wchnschr. *59:*629-630, June 15, '29

ISELIN, M.: Lesions of hands and fingers from aniline pencils. Presse med. *35:*467-469, April 13, '27

ISELIN, M.: Importance of cellular spaces of hand and fingers in infections. Ann. d'anat. path. *4:*603-613, June '27

ISELIN, M.: Repair of cut flexor tendons of fingers. J. de chir. *30:*531-540, Nov '27

ISELIN, MARC: *Plaies et maladies infectieuses des mains*. Masson et Cie, Paris, 1928. Second Edition, 1932. Third Edition, 1938

ISELIN, M.: Treatment of suppurative arthritis of fingers by resection of joint. Union med. du Canada *57:*385-393, July '28

ISELIN, M.: Treatment of hand injuries. Medecine *9:*1020-1028, Oct '28

ISELIN, M.: Modification of incision for reparation of flexor tendons on fingers. Presse med. *37:*124-126, Jan 26, '29

ISELIN, M.: Operative technic in inflammation of digital tendon sheaths. Bull. et mem. Soc. nat. de chir. *57:*456-465, April 4, '31

ISELIN, M.: Reparative surgery of flexor tendons of fingers. Bull. et mem. Soc. nat. de chir. *57:*1227-1231, Oct 31, '31

ISELIN, M.: Phlegmons of cellular spaces of hand; 40 cases. J. de chir. *39:*331-365, March '32

ISELIN, M.: Pathologic anatomy and therapy of wounds of flexor tendons of hands. Presse med. *40:*606-610, April 20, '32

ISELIN, M.: Digital tendovaginitis. Schweiz. med. Wchnschr. *62:*1159-1163, Dec 10, '32

ISELIN, M.: Management of recent wound of tendons of fingers. Presse med. *46:*499-500, March 30, '38

ISELIN, M.: Value of hemoconcentration in shock phenomena; therapeutic deductions. Presse med. *49:*836-838, July 30-Aug 2, '41

ISELIN, MARC: *Chirurgie de la main, livre du chirurgien: Chirurgie reparatrice des tramatismes de la main*. Masson et Cie, Paris, 1945

ISELIN, M.: Plastic use of muscle in thoracic surgery; study based on 24 cases. Mem. Acad. de chir. *71:*422-424, Oct 31-Nov 21, '45

ISELIN, M. AND BERROCAL URIBE, E.: Crushing wounds of fingers and their complications; therapy. Presse med. *40:*220-223, Feb 10, '32

ISELIN, M. AND EVRARD, H.: Infection localized in cellular spaces of mid-palm. Bull. et mem. Soc. nat. de chir. *57:*1620-1622, Dec 19, '31

ISELIN, M. AND MURAT, J.: Restoration of thumb by transposition of second metacarpal; indications and technic; 2 cases. Presse med. *45:*1099-1102, July 28, '37

ISELIN, M. AND TAILHEFER, A.: Treatment of wounds of tendons of hand and fingers. Gaz. d. hop. *100:*961-964, July 20, '27

ISELIN, M. (see LEIBOVICI, R.) March '31

ISELIN, M. (see MONOD, R.) June '36

ISELIN, M. (see TIERNY, A.) Oct '37

ISELIN, M. (see VERNE, J.) July '41

ISHCHENKO, I. M.: Homotransplantation of skin in relation to blood groups. Med. zhur. *4:*59-68, '34

ISHCHENKO, I. N.: Peripheral nerves; surgical therapy of gunshot wounds. Vrach delo. (nos. 7-8) *26:*429-436, '46

ISHCHENKO, I. N. AND LEBEDEVA, M. P.: Surgical methods in burn therapy. Novy khir. arkhiv *38:*452-456, '37

ISHII, T.: Cosmetic rhinoplasty; 150 cases. Oto-rhino-laryng. *11:*722, Aug '38

ISHIKAWA, K.: Progressive facial hemiatrophy; case. Oto-rhino-laryng. *9:*518, June '36

ISHIZAWA, G.: Causes of early death from scalding. Tohoku J. Exper. Med. *26:*527-545, July 31, '35

ISMAIL, M.: Exstrophy of bladder; case. J. Egyptian M.A. *18:*704–715, Oct '35
ISMAIL, M.: Artificial vagina in case of aplasia. J. Egyptian M. A. *22:*583–586, Oct '39
ISMAIL, M.: Exstrophy of bladder, association with congenital prolapse of uterus; case. J. Egyptian M.A. *22:*587–589, Oct '39
ISNARDI, U.: Urethroperineal fistulas; surgical therapy; technic and results in 4 cases. Semana med. *1:*1668–1672, May 18, '33
ISRAEL, J.: Application of dental molding compound for maintenance of skin grafts in middle ear and mastoid cavities. Ann. Otol. Rhinol. and Laryngol. *31:*543–545, June '22
ISRAEL, S.: New intra-nasal suture set. Laryngoscope *31:*633, Aug '21
ISRAEL, S.: Further observations in correction of external deformities of nose by intranasal route. Texas State J. Med. *17:*302, Oct '21
ISRAEL, S.: Correction of external deformities of nose. Tr. Sect. Laryng. Otol. and Rhin., A.M.A., pp. 111–119, '22 (illus.)
ISRAEL, S.: Rhinophyma, report of case. Laryngoscope *32:*218–219, March '22 (illus.)
ISRAEL, S.: External deformities of nose and their correction by intra-nasal route. Southern M. J. *15:*324–327, April '22 (illus.)
ISRAEL, S.: An instrument (drill) to facilitate correction of certain types of external deformities of nose. J.A.M.A. *80:*690, March 10, '23 (illus.)
ISRAEL, S.: Correction of external deformities of nose. Ann. Otol., Rhin. and Laryng. *32:*504–517, June '23 (illus.)
ISRAEL, S.: External nasal deformities and their correction. South. M. J. *25:*916–919, Sept '32
ISRAEL, S.: External nasal deformities and their correction. Texas State J. Med. *31:*281–284, Aug '35
ISRAEL, S.: New type nasal rasp in plastic surgery. Laryngoscope *46:*388–389, May '36
ISRAEL, S. L.: Vaginal aplasia (with ectopic kidney) and creation of artificial vagina. Am. J. Obst. and Gynec. *30:*273–276, Aug '35
ISSERSON, M.: Formation of artificial bladder in exstrophy of bladder. Vestnik Khir. *10:*245–248, '27

Italian Arm Flap

Plastic surgery of nose by Italian method under general ether anesthesia by peritoneal route with J. B. Abalos' technic; case. NATALE, A. M. AND BARBERIS, J. C. Rev. med. del Rosario *20:*487–489, Oct '30
Plastic surgery of nose by Italian method using tubular grafts. BURIAN, F. Presse med. *39:*1418–1420, Sept 26, '31
Autoplastic graft on elbow by Italian method; case. MAKSUD. Cong. internat. de med. trop.et d'hyg., Compt. rend (1928) *3:*385, '31

Italian Arm Flap—Cont.

Autoplastic graft or flap by Italian method in reconstructive surgery of mouth; case. REBELO NETO, J. Bol. Soc. de med. e cir. de Sao Paulo *16:*94–108, Nov '32
Plastic reconstruction of fingers by Italian method of skin graft; case. FERRARI, R. C. Semana med. *2:*1104–1105, Oct 12, '33
Congenital absence of vagina; reconstruction according to Italian method by grafts from genitocrural fold on each side; case in girl 21 years old. VIOLET, H. Lyon med. *158:*277–282, Sept 13, '36
Rhinoplasties by Italian and Hindu methods. COVARRUBIAS ZENTENO, R. Rev. med. de Chile *68:*1331–1346, Oct '40
Italian method of plastic repair of denuded areas followed by mermaid cast immobilization. MURPHY, F. G. Surgery *12:*294–301, Aug '42

IUBAS, C.: Defective vagina and formation of artificial vagina by Schubert-Grigoriu's method. Cluj. med. *10:*404–408, Aug 1, '29
IUBAS, C.: Grigoriu modification of Schubert method in aplasia vaginae. Zentralbl. f. Gynak. *55:*3379–3384, Nov 21, '31
IUBAS, C.: Construction of artificial vagina according to Grigoriu method in case of aplasia. Rev. de chir., Bucuresti *38:*170–175, Sept–Dec '35
IVANISSEVICH, O.: Some plastic operations on face. Semana med. *1:*382–389, March 9, '22 (illus.) abstr: J.A.M.A. *78:*1672, May 27, '22
IVANISSEVICH, O.: Reconstruction of face, new successes of plastic surgery. Semana med. *2:*692–700, Oct 5, '22 (illus.)
IVANISSEVICH, O.: Reconstructive surgery of nose. Rev. Asoc. med. argent. *36:*197–202, May–June '23
IVANISSEVICH, O.: New method for rhinoplasty. Surg., Gynec. and Obst. *38:*828–829, June '24
IVANISSEVICH, O.: Use of tubular skin grafts. Bol. y trab. de la Soc. de cir. de Buenos Aires *13:*144–145, May 22, '29
IVANISSEVICH, O.: Facial injuries. Dia med. *10:*11–13, Jan. 3, '38
IVANISSEVICH, O.: Therapy of facial injuries. Rev. med.-cir. do Brasil *48:*359–366, June '40 also: Rev. mex. de cir., ginec. y cancer *8:*241–255, June '40
IVANISSEVICH, O.: External agenesis of ear treated surgically by Humberto and Ricardo Bisi. Bol. y trab., Acad. argent. de cir. *29:*666–668, Aug 1, '45
IVANISSEVICH, O. *et al:* Plastic reconstruction

of lower lip; French method. Bol. d. Inst. clin. quir. *19:*345–351, June '43

IVANISSEVICH, O. *et al*: Plastic reconstruction of lower lip (French method). Bol. y trab., Acad. argent. de cir. *27:*353–362, June 23, '43

IVANISSEVICH, O. AND FERRARI, R. C.: Argentine method of rhinoplasty; 3 cases. Bol. Inst. de clin. quir. *3:*103–106, '27

IVANISSEVICH, O. AND FERRARI, R. C.: Treatment of protruding ears. Semana med. *1:*1161–1170, May 10, '28

IVANISSEVICH, O. AND FERRARI, R. C.: Reconstruction of nasal ala by Argentine method; cases. Bol. Inst. de clin. quir. *6:*279–294, '30

IVANISSEVICH, O. AND FERRARI, R. C.: Rhinoplasty. Semana med. *1:*967–974, April 17, '30

IVANISSEVICH, O. AND FERRARI, R. C.: Plastic surgery of nose; 6 cases. Semana med. *1:*973–989, April 4, '35

IVANISSEVICH, O. AND FERRARI, R. C.: Rhinoplasty; Argentine method. Surg., Gynec. and Obst. *71:*187–190, Aug '40

IVANISSEVICH, O. AND FERRARI, R. C.: Mixed tumors of submaxillary gland; extirpation by buccal route. Bol. y trab., Acad. argent. de cir. *24:*1051-1054, Oct 30, '40

IVANISSEVICH, O. AND FERRARI, R. C.: Verrucous hairy nevus of interciliary region; extirpation and free skin graft; case with recovery. Bol. y trab., Acad. argent. de cir. *27:*422–424, June 30, '43

IVANISSEVICH, O.; FERRARI, R. C. AND RIVAS, C. I.: Protruding ears; surgical therapy. Bol. d. Inst. clin. quir. *16:*33–47, Jan–March '40

IVANISSEVICH, O.; FERRARI, R. C. AND RIVAS, C. I.: Precise technic for correcting rhinomegaly and rhinokyphosis. Salud y belleza (no. 5) *1:*12–16, Oct–Dec '45

IVANISSEVICH, O. AND GARAY, P. M.: Surgical therapy of prognathism; case. Bol. y trab., Acad. argent. de cir. *25:*554–559, June 25, '41

IVANISSEVICH, O. AND RIVAS, C. I.: Technic for correcting rhinomegaly and rhinokyphosis. Bol. y trab. de la Soc. de cir. de Buenos Aires *23:*442–451, July 12, '39

IVANISSEVICH, O. AND RIVAS, C. I.: Total graft of nail and of matrix; case. Bol. d. Inst. clin. quir. *18:*640–642, Sept '42

IVANISSEVICH, O. AND RIVAS, C. I.: Results of repair of flexor tendons of wrist, hand and fingers. Bol. y trab., Acad. argent. de cir. *27:*576–583, July 28, '43

IVANISSEVICH, O.; RIVAS, C. I. AND AGUIRRE, J. A.: Therapy of nasal fractures. Bol. y trab. de la Soc. de cir. de Buenos Aires *23:*9–14, April 12, '39

IVANISSEVICH, O.; VELEZ DIEZ CANSECO, J. B. AND RIVAS, C. I.: Gynecomastia; new technic of surgical therapy. Semana med. *1:*1434–1438, June 19, '41

IVANISSEVICH, O. (see ARCE, J. *et al*) 1929

IVANITZKYI, G.: Covering defects of face by double skin transplantation from abdomen to forearm and face. Ukrain. m. visti *5:*41–42, '29

IVY, A. C. (see ROBACK, R. A.) Nov '44

IVANOV, S.: Reverdin-Ollier-Davis method of skin grafting. Vestnik khir. *34:*107–112, '34

IVANOVA, MME. (see AVERBAKH, M.) Nov '35

IVERSON, P. C.: Skin and soft tissue war wounds of hand and forearm. Am. Acad. Orthop. Surgeons, Lect., pp. 184–187, '44

IVINS, H. M.: Origin of nasal septal deflections. J. Iowa M. Soc. *18:*428–432, Nov '28

IVORY, H. S.: Cortical adrenal extract in severe burns. Mil. Surgeon *87:*423–429, Nov '40

IVORY, J. J.: Maxillofacial injuries; important considerations. Indust. Med. *10:*52–54, Feb '41

IVY, R. H.: Practical method of fixation in fractures of mandible. Surg., Gynec. and Obst. *34:*670–673, May '22 (illus.)

IVY, R. H.: Fractures of mandible. J.A.M.A. *79:*295–297, July 22, '22 (illus.)

IVY, R. H.: Plastic and reconstructive surgery of face. Surg., Gynec. and Obst. (Internat. Abstract Surg.) *36:*1–7, Jan '23

IVY, R. H.: Repair of acquired defects of face (and nose). J.A.M.A. *84:*181–185, Jan 17, '25

IVY, R. H.: Swellings of submaxillary regions. Ann. Surg. *81:*605–610, March '25

IVY, R. H.: Plastic and reconstructive surgery; repair of traumatic saddle nose. S. Clin. N. Amer. *6:*245–247, Feb '26

IVY, R. H.: Plastic and reconstructive surgery; total rhinoplasty for syphilitic defect. S. Clin. N. Amer. *6:*248–251, Feb '26

IVY, R. H.: Plastic and reconstructive surgery; sarcoma of mandible. S. Clin. N. Amer. *6:*251–255, Feb '26

IVY, R. H.: Benign bony enlargement of condyloid process of mandible. Ann. Surg. *85:*27–30, Jan '27

IVY, R. H.: Surgical treatment of acquired deformities of mouth and jaws. Dental Cosmos *69:*137–142, Feb '27

IVY, R. H.: Plastic surgery of face (including nose). Atlantic M. J. *30:*572–575, June '27

IVY, R. H.: Plastic surgery of nose. Laryngoscope *37:*486–497, July '27

IVY, R. H.: Tumors and cysts of jaws as disclosed by roentgenograms, and their treatment. J. Am. Dent. A. *14:*2272–2280, Dec '27

IVY, R. H.: Plastic and reconstructive surgery of face and jaws. Virginia M. Monthly *56:*174–180, June '29

IVY, R. H.: Surgical treatment of accidental wounds of mouth and face, with special reference to those complicated by bone injury. J. Am. Dent. A. *17:*967-974, June '30

IVY, R. H.: Injuries of facial bones and soft tissues. Pennsylvania M. J. *35:*761-763, Aug '32

IVY, R. H.: Operative treatment of cysts of jaws and fractures. J. Am. Dent. A. *19:*1516-1527, Sept '32

IVY, R. H.: Surgery of nose in relation to orthodontia and facial harmony. Internat. J. Orthodontia *19:*888-898, Sept '33

IVY, R. H.: Jaw fractures. Surg., Gynec. and Obst. *60:*531-534, Feb (no. 2A) '35

IVY, R. H.: Tumors and cysts of mouth and jaws of interest to otolaryngologist. Tr. Am. Acad. Ophth. *41:*163-185, '36

IVY, R. H.: Congenital defects and deformities of face; review of literature for 1936. Internat. Abstr. Surg. *64:*433-442, '37; in Surg., Gynec. and Obst. May '37

IVY, R. H.: Review of recent literature on cleft lip and palate surgery. Internat. J. Orthodontia *23:*844-849, Aug. '37

IVY, R. H.: Treatment of complications of surgical diseases of the mouth. West J. Surg. *46:*202-208, April '38

IVY, R. H.: Tumors of the jaws (and mouth). Delaware State M. J. *10:*147-152, July '38

IVY, R. H.: Multiple dentigerous cysts of jaw, with special reference to occurrence in siblings. Ann. Surg. *109:*114-125, Jan '39

IVY, R. H.: Experiences in surgery of cleft palate. Ann. Surg. *112:*775-782, Oct '40

IVY, R. H.: Bilateral osseous ankylosis of temporomaxillary joints with marked facial deformity; therapy of case. An. de cir. *6:*383-387, Dec '40

IVY, R. H.: First aid and emergency treatment of gunshot wounds of jaws. Mil. Surgeon *89:*197-201, Aug '41

IVY, R. H.: First aid and emergency treatment of gunshot wounds to jaws. Rev. san. mil., Habana *5:*105-109, July-Dec '41

IVY, R. H.: Symposium on military surgery; plastic and maxillofacial surgery. S. Clin. North America *21:*1583-1592, Dec '41

IVY, R. H.: Early and late treatment of face and jaws as applied to war injuries. South. Surgeon *11:*366-373, May '42

IVY, R. H.: Surgery of face, mouth and jaws, 30 years ago and now. J. Oral Surg. *1:*95-99, April '43

IVY, R. H.: Repair of bony and contour deformities of face. Surgery *15:*56-74, Jan '44 also: Am. J. Orthodontics (Oral Surg. Sect.) *30:*76-94, Feb '44

IVY, R. H.: Plastic surgery in combat and civilian casualties. M. Ann. District of Columbia *13:*45-49, Feb '44

IVY, R. H.: Symposium on traumatic surgery; principles of grafting. Clinics *3:*1623-1640, April '45

IVY, R. H.: Principles of skin grafting. J. Internat. Coll. Surgeons *8:*520-524, Nov-Dec '45

IVY, R. H.: Surgical treatment of vicious cicatrices involving cheek, lip and alveolar process in cleft lip and palate cases. Am. J. Orthodontics (Oral Surg. Sect.) *32:*673-674, Nov '46

IVY, ROBERT H. (with VILRAY P. BLAIR and, in the second and third editions, J. B. BROWN): *Essentials of Oral Surgery*. C. V. Mosby Co., St. Louis, 1923. Second Edition, 1936. Third Edition, 1944

IVY, R. H. AND CURTIS, L.: Orthopedic problems of lower jaw; with special reference to unilateral shortening. J. Bone and Joint Surg. *10:*645-660, Oct '28

IVY, R. H. AND CURTIS, L.: Further observations on fractures of mandible. Dental Cosmos *71:*341-352, April '29

IVY, R. H. AND CURTIS, L.: Complicated fractures of mandible. S. Clin. N. Amer. *10:*1411-1426, Dec '30

IVY, ROBERT H. AND CURTIS, LAWRENCE: *Fractures of the Jaws*. Lea and Febiger, Phila., 1931. Second Edition, 1938. Third Edition, 1945

IVY, R. H. AND CURTIS, L.: Operative treatment of losses of substance of mandible, with special reference to fixation of edentulous fragments. Surg., Gynec. and Obst. *52:*849-854, April '31

IVY, R. H. AND CURTIS, L.: Fractures of upper jaw and malar bone. Ann. Surg. *94:*337-346, Sept '31

IVY, R. H. AND CURTIS, L.: Calculi of salivary glands. Ann. Surg. *96:*979-986, Dec '32

IVY, R. H. AND CURTIS, L.: Cleft palate procedures in surgery; experiences with Veau and Dorrance technique. Ann. Surg. *100:*502-511, Sept '34

IVY, R. H. AND CURTIS, L.: Congenital syphilitic osteomyelitis of mandible; 2 analogous cases in sisters. Ann. Surg. *100:*535-538, Sept '34

IVY, R. H. AND CURTIS, L.: Jaw deformities due to loss of substance of mandible following osteomyelitis. Ann. Surg. *103:*149-152, Jan '36

IVY, R. H. AND CURTIS, L.: Zygoma fractures. S. Clin. North America *16:*587-594, April '36

IVY, R. H. AND CURTIS, L.: Metastasis of tumor of rectum to mandible (case). Ann. Dent. *3:*133–137, Sept. '36
IVY, R. H. AND CURTIS, L.: Adamantinoma of jaw. Ann. Surg. *105:*125–134, Jan '37
IVY, R. H. AND CURTIS, L.: Hemorrhagic or traumatic cysts of mandible. Surg., Gynec. and Obst. *65:*640–643, Nov '37
IVY, R. H. AND CURTIS, L.: Permanent therapy of maxillofacial wounds in war surgery. Rev. san. mil., Buenos Aires *41:*638–650, Sept '42
IVY, R. H. AND CURTIS, L.: Recent experiences with skeletal fixation in fractures of mandible. J. Oral Surg. *1:*296–308, Oct '43
IVY, R. H. AND CURTIS, L.: Protrusion of mandible; case. Am. J. Orthodontics (Oral Surg. Sect.) *31:*666–675, Nov '45
IVY, R. H. AND EPES, B. M.: Bone grafting for defects of mandible. Mil. Surgeon *60:*286–293, March '27
IVY, R. H. AND MILLER, H. A.: Plastic surgery; summaries of bibliographic material available in field of otolaryngology, 1936–1938. Arch. Otolaryng. *27:*622–642, May '38
IVY, R. H. AND MILLER, H. A.: Plastic surgery, 1938; summaries of bibliographic material available in field of otolaryngology. Arch. Otolaryng. *30:*99–114, July '39
IVY, R. H. AND MILLER, H. A.: Facial surgery; review of literature, 1939. Arch. Otolaryng. *32:*159–176, July '40
IVY, R. H. AND MILLER, H. A.: Plastic surgery, 1940; sumaries of bibliographic material available in field of otolaryngology. Arch. Otolaryng. *34:*179–192, July '41
IVY, R. H. AND MILLER, H. A.: Plastic surgery; summaries of bibliographic material available in field of otolaryngology. Arch. Otolaryng. *36:*135–148, July '42
IVY, R. H. *et al*: Symposium on war medicine; plastic and reconstruction surgery. Clinics *2:*1165–1193, Feb '44
IVY, R. H. AND STOUT, R. A.: Emergency treatment of war injuries to face. Ann. Surg. *113:*1001–1009, June '41
IVY, R. H. (see FAIRBANK, L. C.) Feb '40

Ivy Operation

Therapy of maxillary fractures according to Ivy. BAKHMUTOVA, E. A. Sovet. med. (no. 4) *4:*38–39, '40

IWATÔ, Y.: Hemorrhagic cyst on side of neck. Okayama-Igakkai-Zasshi *44:*1727–1728, June '32
IZURIETA, F. A. (see RIVAS, C. I.) May '45

J

JACHIA, A.: Extensive butterfly-shaped lupus of face; surgical excision with immediate implantation of Thiersch graft. Boll. e mem. Soc. piemontese di chir. *7:*123–128, '37
JACK, E. A. (see BINGHAM, D. L. C.) Oct '37
JACKSON, A. S.: Lateral or branchial cysts of neck; 13 cases. Wisconsin M. J. *37:*641–646, Aug '38
JACKSON, A. V.: Tannic acid in burn therapy; liver necrosis following therapy. M. J. Australia *2:*352–354, Sept 30, '44
JACKSON, C.: Treatment of laryngeal cancer by laryngofissure. South. Surgeon *1:*223–229, Oct '32
JACKSON, C.: Curability of cancer of larynx by laryngofissure. Surg., Gynec. and Obst. *58:*431–432, Feb (no. 2A) '34
JACKSON, C. AND BABCOCK, W. W.: Hypertension of hand and fingers from burn; correction by single pedicled skin and fascial flap from anterior abdominal wall. S. Clin. North America *10:*1285–1286, Dec '30
JACKSON, C. AND BABCOCK, W. W.: Laryngectomy for cancer. S. Clin. North America *11:*1207–1227, Dec '31
JACKSON, C. AND BABCOCK, W. W.: Elephantiasis of right leg. S. Clin. North America *11:*1243–1244, Dec '31
JACKSON, C. AND BABCOCK, W. W.: Plastic closure of tracheostomic fistula. S. Clin. North America *14:*199–202, Feb '34
JACKSON, C. AND JACKSON, C. L.: Chronic laryngeal stenosis in children. S. Clin. North America *14:*27–37, Feb '34
JACKSON, C. AND JACKSON, C. L.: Treatment of laryngeal cancer by laryngofissure and laryngectomy. Am. J. Surg. *30:*3–17, Oct '35
JACKSON, C. AND JACKSON, C. L.: Cancer of larynx. S. Clin. North America *17:*1791–1795, Dec '37
JACKSON, C. L. (see JACKSON, C.) Feb '34
JACKSON, C. L. (see JACKSON, C.) Oct '35
JACKSON, C. L. (see JACKSON, C.) Dec '37
JACKSON, F. G.: Infections of hand. J. Indiana M. A. *14:*180, June '21
JACKSON, T. (see KILNER, T. P.) July '21
JACOB, A. C. AND MAFFEI, E.: Vitamin B complex therapy of decubital eschars. Rev. med. Rio Grande do Sul *2:*47–49, Sept–Oct '45
JACOB, F. J. Desitin salve in burns. Med. Klin. *23:*1032, July 8, '27
JACOB, P. (see GRIMAUD, R.) Aug '39
JACOB, R. (see KLAGES, F.) 1940
JACOBOVICI, I. (see IACOBOVICI, I.)
JACOBS, A. W.: Epithelioma of lip treated by radiation. M. J. and Rec. *123:*803, June 16, '26

JACOBS, A. W.: Cavernous hemangioma of face in infant treated with radium; case. Am. J. Roentgenol. *49:*816–818, June '43

JACOBS, M. H.: Care of military and civilian injuries; problem of teeth in line of fracture of mandible. Am. J. Orthodontics (Oral Surg. Sect.) *29:*102–110, Feb '43

JACOBS, R. G.: Burn cases off the U.S.S. Wasp. J. Oklahoma M.A. *36:*235–236, June '43

JACOBSEN, H. H. AND BARRON, J. B.: Moulages as aid to maxillofacial restorations. Mil. Surgeon *92:*511–520, May '43

JACOBSON, S. D. AND SMITH, C. J.: Comparative study of effects of human plasma, physiologic saline, pectin and gelatin (4% and 5%) on plasma volume in man. Proc. Central Soc. Clin. Research *17:*45–46, '44

JACOBY, M. W. (see GLOVER, D. M.) April '33

JACOBZINER, H. (see PREVITALI, G.) July '40

JACOD, M.: Rectal anesthesia in facial surgery. Ann. d. mal. de l'oreille, du larynx *46:*583–586, June '27

JACOD, M.: Fistulized preauricular branchial fibrochondroma; case. Lyon med. *151:*613–615, May 14, '33

JACOD, M.: Rectal anesthesia with mixture of ether, tribromethanol and oil in cervicofacial surgery. Lyon chir. *32:*35–42, Jan–Feb '35

JACOD, M.: Rectal anesthesia with mixture of ether, tribromethanol and oil in cervicofacial surgery. Ann. d'oto-laryng., pp. 802–808, July '35

JACQUES: Fracture of nose and its treatment. Paris med. *11:*199, Sept 3, '21 abstr: J.A.M.A. *77:*1289, Oct 15, '21

JACQUES, P.: Repair of syphilitic nasal deformity. Rev. med. de l'est *55:*81–84, Feb 15, '27

JACQUES, P. AND GRIMAUD: Congenital fistula of lateral region of neck. Oto-rhino-laryng. internat. *17:*437–439, June '33

JACQUES, P. AND ROIG, A.: Unusual malformation of external ear. Compt. rend. Soc. de biol. *98:*1135–1137, April 27, '28 also: Ann. d. mal. de l'oreille, du larynx *47:*545–549, June '28

JADASSOHN, W.: Zoster of left arm following injury to thumb; case. Schweiz. med. Wchnschr. *68:*93, Jan 22, '38

JAECKLE, C. E. (see SCHULTZ, A.) Aug '45

JÄGER, F. (see JÄGER, R.) Sept '36

JAEGER, R.: Closure of cranial defects. Plast. and Reconstruct. Surg. *1:*69–78, July '46

JAENSCH, P. A.: Surgical therapy of eyelid ptosis. Klin. Monatsbl. f. Augenh. *94:*183–189, Feb '35

JÄGER, R. AND JÄGER, F.: Therapy of first and second degree burns with taktocut, substance used in tanning. Munchen. med. Wchnschr. *83:*1597–1598, Sept '36

JAGERINK, T. A.: Styloidalgia radii and some other cases of tendovaginitis stensans. Nederl. Tijdschr. v. Geneesk. *1:*3227, June 30, '28

JAGIĆ, N.: Therapy of circulatory insufficiency following surgical interventions. Wien. klin. Wchnschr. *45:*1241–1244, Oct 7, '32

JAHSS, S. A.: Fractures of proximal phalanges; alignment and immobilization. J. Bone and Joint Surg. *18:*726–731, July '36

JAHSS, S. A.: Trigger finger in children. J.A.M.A. *107:*1463–1464, Oct 31, '36

JAHSS, S. A.: Fractures of proximal phalanx of thumb; treatment. J. Bone and Joint Surg. *19:*1124–1125, Oct '37

JAHSS, S. A.: Fractures of metacarpals and proximal phalanges. Bull. Hosp. Joint Dis. *3:*79–92, July '42

JAKABHAZY, I.: Plastic surgery of alveolar process as preparation for artificial plates. Orvosi hetil. *82:*338–340, April 9, '38

JAKABHAZY, I.: New surgical procedure for repair of cleft palate. Gyogyaszat *79:*651–652, Dec 17, '39

JAKOB, M. (see KUBÁNYI, E.) April '27

JAMES, C.: Tropical ulcers; quick and successful method of treatment by excision and skin graft. Lancet *2:*1095–1101, Nov 19, '32

JAMES, G. W. III. (see EVANS, E. I. *et al*) March '44

JAMES, G. W. III (see EVANS, E. I. *et al*) March '45

JAMES, W. D.: Cancer of lips. Am. J. Surg. *8:*593–597, March '30

JAMES, W. WARWICK AND FICKLING, B. W.: *Injuries of the Jaws and Face*. Bale, London, 1940

JAMES, W. W. AND FICKLING, B. W.: Facial structure in relationship to fractures. Proc. Roy. Soc. Med. *34:*205–211, Feb '41

JAMES, W. W. AND GILLIES, H. D.: Fracture of lower jaw. Tr. M. Soc. London *56:*22–36, '33

JAMESON, P. C.: Surgical management of eyelid ptosis, with special reference to use of superior rectus muscle. Arch. Ophth. *18:*547–557, Oct '37

JANCKE, G.: Use of mucosa of lips in Toti operation on lacrimal ducts. Ber. u. d. Versamml. d. deutsch. ophth. Gesellsch. *51:*478–479, '36

JANES, R. M.: Treatment of salivary gland tumors by radical excision. Canad. M. A. J. *43:*554–559, Dec '40

JANES, R. M.: Surgical treatment of salivary gland tumors. S. Clin. North America *23:*1429–1439, Oct '43

JANEWAY, C. A.: Clinical use of products of human plasma fractionation; albumin in shock and hypoproteinemia. J.A.M.A. *126:*674–680, Nov 11, '44

JANEWAY, C. A. *et al*: Concentrated human

serum albumin, safety of albumin, in shock. J. Clin. Investigation *23:*465–490, July '44
JANEWAY, C. A. (see HEYL, J. T.) July '43
JANKOVSKY, P.: Low lateral congenital fistulas of neck. Ann. d'oto-laryng., pp. 1133–1146, Dec '37
JANNUZZI, V. (see REBAUDI, F.) 1945
JANOTA, M. *et al*: Gelatin infusion (as blood substitute) in hemorrhagic shock. Exper. Med. and Surg. *1:*298–303, Aug '43
JANOUŠEK, B.: Treatment of ulcers of thigh and burns with polysan (magnesium hydroxide preparation). Ceska dermat. *9:*154–159, '28
JANSEN, M.: Acrocephalosyndactylia and ocular hypertelorism; 2 cases. Nederl. Tijdschr. v. Geneesk. *2:*5864–5867, Nov 24, '28
JANSEN, M.: Clawhand. Ztschr. f. orthop. Chir. *58:*193–199, '32
JANSSEN, P.: Operation for exstrophy without involving intestine. Zentralbl. f. Chir. *60:*2658–2662, Nov 11, '33
JANTZEN, J.: Rubber plate as support for mouth following cleft palate operation. Deutsche Ztschr. f. Chir. *249:*651–656, '38
JARA ROBLES, R.: Nerve graft from cadaver to repair sectioned nerve; case. Arch. Soc. cirujanos hosp. *13:*214–215, Sept '43
JARAMILLO ARANGO, J.: Successful suture of extensor tendons of hand sectioned by wounds; case. Repert. de med. y cir. *23:*289–320, July '32
JARDENI, J. AND AUERBACH, H.: Orthopedic plate in therapy of jaw deformities. Ztschr. f. Stomatol. *35:*1019–1028, Aug 13, '37
JARMAN, T. F.: Treatment of branchial cleft cysts by aspiration and injection of pure carbolic acid (phenol). Brit. M. J. *1:*953–954, June 22, '46
JARMAN, T. F. (see ARMSTRONG, B.) April '36
JAROLAVSKY, N. N. (see DELLEPIANE RAWSON, R.) Dec '42
JAROŠ, M.: Statistics on injuries and infections of fingers and hands based on accident insurance records. Rozhl. v chir. a gynaek. (cast chir.) *13:*270–288, '34
JAROS, Z.: Congenital fistula and dermoid cyst of nasal dorsum. Casop. lek. cesk. *77:*540–541, April 29, '38
JARVIS, H. G.: Thyroglossal cysts and fistulae. New England J. Med. *205:*987–991, Nov 19, '31
JARZYNKA, F J.: Magnesium burns. Indust. Med. *12:*427–431, July '43
JAUBERT DE BEAUJEU, A.: Roentgen study of polydactylia and syndactylia in 3 generations of family. Bull. et mem. Soc. de radiol. med. de France *22:*339–342, June '34
JAUREGUI, P.: Dermoid cysts of palm. Bol. y. trab. de la Soc. de cir. de Buenos Aires *13:*233–239, June 12, '29
JÁUREGUI, P.: Formation and work of Société Scientifique Française de Chirurgie Réparatrice, Plastique et Esthétique. Semana med. *2:*396–398, July 30, '31
JAUSION; PASTEUR, AND AZAM: Alopecia, case cured by phototherapy. Bull. Soc. franc. de dermat. et syph. *33:*641–650, Nov '26

Jaws, Ankylosis (See also Jaws, Ankylosis, Fibrous; Temporomandibular Joint)

End-results of operations for bony ankylosis of jaw. CARR, W. P. Ann. Surg. *73:*314, March '21
Treatment of ankylosis of temporomaxillary articulation. IMBERT, L. Lyon chir. *18:*572–578, Sept–Oct '21 (illus.)
Ankylosis of lower jaw, surgical treatment. CUMSTON, C. G. Internat. Clinics *1:*65, '21
Ankylosis of jaw. GILPATRICK, R. H. Boston M. and S. J. *186:*374–377, March 23, '22 (illus.)
Treatment of ankylosis of jaw. BOCKENHEIMER. Deutsche med. Wchnschr. *48:*729–730, June 2, '22
Pathogenesis and treatment of ankylosis of jaws. IMBERT, L. AND COTTALORDA, J. Acta chir. Scandinav. *54:*515–529, June '22 (illus.) abstr: J.A.M.A. *79:*926, Sept 9, '22
Correction of ankylosis of jaws. DARCISSAC, M. Paris med. *12:*227–229, Sept 2, '22 (illus.) abstr: J.A.M.A. *79:*1884, Nov 25, '22
Report of cured case of ankylosis of jaw. STERN, W. G. Ohio State M. J. *19:*248–249, April '23 (illus.)
Old ankylosis of temporomaxillary articulation. FASANO, M. Arch. ital. di chir. *8:*575–588, Dec '23
Two cases of ankylosis of left temporo-mandibular joint. CRYMBLE, P. T. Brit. M. J. *1:*996–997, June 7, '24
Resection and arthroplasty in case of lockjaw from old osseous ankylosis of temporomaxillary articulation. DE GAETANO, L. Arch. ital. di chir. *12:*673–712, '25
Case of permanent constriction of jaws; death, autopsy. MALLET-GUY. Lyon med. *138:*628–631, Nov 28, '26
Bilateral temporo-maxillary ankylosis with pleuropneumonia; death; autopsy; case. MALLET-GUY, P. AND JOUVE, P. Ann. d' anat. path. *4:*19–24, Jan '27
Temporo-maxillary ankylosis; case. FISCHER, H. Ann. d'anat. path. *4:*223, Feb '27
Treatment of bilateral case of ankylosis of jaws. JORGE, J. M. Semana med. *2:*711, Sept 15, '27

Jaws, Ankylosis – Cont.
Orthodontic treatment following operation for unilateral ankylosis of temporomaxillary articulation; case report. KETCHAM, A. H. AND HUMPHREY, W. R. Internat. Orthodont. Cong. *1:*479-482, '27
Pathology and treatment of jaw ankylosis. KÖNIG, F. Beitr. z. klin. Chir. *140:*565-576, '27
Consideration of contour as well as function in operations for organic ankylosis of lower jaw. BLAIR, V. P. Surg., Gynec. and Obst. *46:*167-179, Feb '28
Myogenic traumatic ankylosis of jaws; case. BECKER, J. Med. Welt *2:*681, May 5, '28
Treatment of jaw ankylosis by simple section followed by mobilization; case. DE LACERDA, E. Med. contemp. *46:*221-223, July 8, '28
Ankylosis of lower jaw; case. MESA, C. Bol. y trab. de la Soc. de cir. de Buenos Aires *12:*317-326, July 18, '28
Temporomaxillary ankylosis; surgical and prosthetic treatment. DARCISSAC, M., J. de med. et chir. prat. *99:*581-590, Aug 25, '28
Simple method of performing arthroplasty in true ankylosis of jaws. HENRY, A. K. Lancet *2:*650-651, Sept 29, '28
Ankylosis of jaws, case. MESA, C. Semana med. *2:*1178-1181, Nov 1, '28
Constriction of jaw treated by resection of ascending branch; case. LEMAÎTRE AND PONROY. Rev. de stomatol. *30:*734, Dec '28
Treatment of jaw ankylosis and micrognathia. FROMME, A. Beitr. z. klin. Chir. *144:*195-206, '28
Unusual case of jaw ankylosis. UDINE, S. S. Vestnik khir. (no. 35-36) *12:*134-136, '28
Prevention of postoperative recurrence of ankylosis of jaws; case. MUZII, E. Stomatol. *27:*136-147, Feb '29
Jaw ankylosis; treatment by Murphy's arthroplastic operation; case. FERNÁNDEZ SARALEGUI, A. Bol. y trab. de la Soc. de cir. de Buenos Aires *13:*165-171, May 29, '29
Treatment of jaw ankylosis; 7 cases. HÄMÄLÄINEN, M. Acta chir. Scandinav. *64:*493-508, '29
Congenital synosteosis of maxilla and mandible; case. PETHEÖ, J. Ztschr. f. Kinderh. *47:*447-448, '29
Consideration of contour as well as function in operations for organic ankylosis of mandible. BLAIR, V. P. Internat. J. Orthodontia *16:*62-80, Jan '30
Ankylosis of jaws, case. GYGAX, P. Schweiz. Monatschr. f. Zahnh. *40:*179-208, April '30
New method of arthroplasty in bilateral ankylosis of jaws caused by trauma. BENEDETTI-VALENTINI, F. Policlinico (sez. chir) *37:*201-215, May '30
Temporomaxillary ankylosis of obstetric origin. DUFOURMENTEL, L. Bull. et mem. Soc. de chir. de Paris *22:*502-507, July 4, '30
Ankylosis of jaw following smallpox; case. ALLENDE, G. Bol. y trab. de la Soc. de cir. de Buenos Aires *14:*951-959, Nov 26, '30
Temporomaxillary ankylosis; case. CANALS MAYNER, R. Rev. med. de Barcelona *15:*3-21, Jan '31
Bilateral ankylosis of jaws; case. SUERMONDT, W. F. Nederl. tijdschr. v. geneesk. *75:*249, Jan 10, '31
Structures of face in case of ankylosis of jaws before and after treatment. EBY, J. D. Internat. J. Orthodontia *17:*848-853, Sept '31
Beresowski method in surgical treatment of ankylosis of lower jaw. SOKOLOW, N. N. Deutsche Ztschr. f. Chir. *231:*294-298, '31
Therapy of temporomandibular ankylosis. ROCCIA, B. Boll. e mem. Soc. piemontese di chir. *2:*502-518, April 30, '32
Mobilization of ankylosed jaw. CAMPBELL, W. C., J. Am. Dent. A. *19:*1222-1229, July '32
Surgical therapy of ankylosis of temporomaxillary joint; case. JIANU, I. *et al.* Spitalul *52:*433-434, Nov '32
Postpuerperal ankylosing polyarthritis; subluxation of atlas and axis; temporomaxillary and articulatory ankylosis; radiologic and etiologic study. ROCHER, H. L. Bull. et mem. Soc. med. et chir. de Bordeaux, pp. 279-293, '32
Plastic surgery in therapy of maxillotemporal ankylosis; case. DESELAERS, H. Rev. espan. de med. y cir. *16:*114-116, March '33
Bilateral ankylosis of temporomaxillary joint; technic of surgical therapy; case. PAGLIOLI, E. Rev. radiol. clin. *2:*613-620, April '33
Ankylosis of temporomandibular articulation. POLETTI, G. B. Stomatol. *31:*392-429, April '33
Resection of maxillary angle in temporomaxillary ankylosis. DESGOUTTES, L. Tech. chir. *25:*97-102, June '33
Ankylosis of jaws, correction by bilateral resection; case. COUTINHO, A. Rev. brasil. de cir. *2:*469-479, Nov '33
Surgical therapy of posttyphoidal jaw ankylosis. LAPEYRIE AND CABANAC. Montpellier med. *5:*31-37, Jan 15, '34
Complete ankylosis of temporomaxillary joint; surgical therapy; 2 cases. TRAN-

Jaws, Ankylosis – Cont.
QUILLI-LEALI, E. Rassegna d. previd. sociale *21:*8–45, Sept '34
Mandibular automobilizer; use in therapy of postoperative temporomaxillary ankylosis. DARCISSAC, M. Bull. et mem. Soc. d. chirurgiens de Paris *26:*561–568, Oct 19, '34
Unusual localization of arthropathies (mandibulotemporal and metacarpophalangeal ankylosis), in postencephalitic parkinsonian syndrome and their pathogenesis. GORDON, A., M. Rec. *140:*351–353, Oct 3, '34
Ankylosis of jaws. RISDON, F., J. Am. Dent. A. *21:*1933–1937, Nov '34
Surgical and orthopedic treatment of jaw ankylosis. RUSPA, F. Boll. e mem. Soc. piemontese di chir. *4:*130–141, '34
Bilateral ankylosis of mandible; case of traumatic origin; surgical therapy. CAPPA, O. Policlinico (sez. prat.) *42:*59–62, Jan 14, '35
Ankylosis of jaws. TUNG, P. C. AND CHEN, H. I. Chinese M. J. *49:*101–110, Feb '35
Surgical therapy of temporomaxillary ankylosis; 100 cases. DUFOURMENTEL, L. AND DARCISSAC, M. Bull. et mem. Soc. d. chirurgiens de Paris *27:*149–161, March 15, '35
Frequency of bilateral ankylosis of temporomaxillary joint. DUBOV, M. D. Sovet. khir., no. 9, pp. 106–113, '35
Ankylosis of jaws. LUHMANN, K. Beitr. z. klin. Chir. *162:*449–455, '35
Osteotomy and arthroplasty for bony ankylosis of left temporo-mandibular joint of 20 years' duration. LOOP, F. A., J. Indiana M. A. *29:*70–72, Feb '36
Congenital bony temporomandibular ankylosis and facial hemiatrophy; review of literature and report of case. BURKET, L. W. J.A.M.A. *106:*1719–1722, May 16, '36
Surgical therapy of temporomaxillary ankylosis followed by prosthesis of dental arches. VARGAS SALCEDO, L. AND ILABACA L., L. Bol. y trab. de la Soc. de cir. de Buenos Aires *20:*1071–1082, Oct 21, '36
Surgery of ankylosis of jaws. RUTTEN, E. Beitr. z. klin. Chir. *163:*414–415, '36
Hinge mobilization of lower jaw to correct permanent constriction probably due to hypertonia of masticatory muscles; technic and results in case. GUCCIARDELLO, S. Riv. san. siciliana *25:*255–263, March 1, '37
Bilateral bony ankylosis of jaws. WEILER, H. G. West Virginia M. J. *33:*117–120, March '37
New apparatus for producing mechanical movements in cases of ankylosis of jaws. KOCHEV, K. N. Khirurgiya, no. 9, pp. 160–161, '37
Temporomandibular ankylosis. MARFORT, A. AND EMILIANI, C. M. Rev. oto-neuro-oftal. *13:*103–105, April '38
Pathogenesis and surgical therapy of ankylosis of temporomandibular joint. MELA, B. Minerva med. *1:*553–556, May 26, '38
So-called congenital temporomandibular ankylosis. TAVERNIER AND POUZET, F. Lyon chir. *35:*328–332, May–June '38
Ankylosis of temporomandibular joint. KAZANJIAN, V. H. Surg., Gynec. and Obst. *67:*333–348, Sept '38
Right osseous temporomaxillary ankylosis; surgical therapy; case. BIANCHERI, A. Arch. ital. di chir. *50:*396–403, '38
Surgical therapy of ankylosis of jaw; case. DELITALA, F. Gior. veneto di sc. med. *13:*236–237, April '39
Incomplete and complete ankylosis of jaws. FEDERSPIEL, M. N., J. Am. Dent. A. *26:*585–594, April '39
Surgical therapy of permanent constriction of jaw; case. FRONTEAU, M. Arch. med. d'Angers *43:*69–72, April '39
Ankylosis of temporomandibular joints; cure by Esmarch operation. MILLER, I. D. Australian and New Zealand J. Surg. *8:*406–407, April '39
Temporomaxillary ankylosis; resection of mandibular condyle and neck followed by recovery; 2 cases. COSTESCU, P. AND TURAI, I. Rev. de chir., Bucuresti *43:*405–410, May–June '40
Temporomaxillary ankylosis. MARIN, G. M. Med. espan. *3:*406–428, May '40
Temporomandibular ankylosis and its surgical correction. BELLINGER, D. H., J. Am. Dent. A. *27:*1563–1568, Oct '40
Bilateral osseous ankylosis of temporomaxillary joints with marked facial deformity; therapy of case. IVY, R. H. An. de cir. *6:*383–387, Dec '40
Extra-articular bony ankylosis of temporomandibular joint. BERGER, A. Bull. Hosp. Joint Dis. *2:*27–33, Jan '41
Ankylosis of jaws. EGGERS, G. W. N. South. Surgeon *10:*1–7, Jan '41
Cartilage graft restoration of jaw ankylosis; new operation. PICKERILL, H. P. Australian and New Zealand J. Surg. *11:*197–206, Jan '42
New intraoral spring mouth opener for treatment of lockjaw. SCHUCHARDT, K. Ztschr. f. Stomatol. *40:*677–680, Sept 25, '42
Ankylosis of jaw following luxation fracture; case. JONSSON, S. O. Nord. med. (Hygiea) *18:*609–611, April 10, '43
New technic in therapy of temporomandibular ankylosis. SQUIRRU, C. M. Rev. san.

Jaws, Ankylosis – Cont.
mil., Buenos Aires *42:*789–799, Nov '43
Osteotomy of ascending ramus of lower jaw in therapy of ankylosis. STUDEMEISTER, A. Deutsche Ztschr. f. Chir. *258:*358, '43
Temporomandibular ankylosis; surgical therapy in cases. DE ANDRADE, M. A. Med. cir. pharm., pp. 45–58, Jan '44
Bilateral ankylosis of temporomandibular joints with retrusion deformity; case. DINGMAN, R. O., J. Oral Surg. *2:*71–76, Jan '44
Temporomandibular ankylosis; surgical therapy of case in child following otitis with mastoiditis. OREGGIA, J. C. Arch. de pediat. d. Uruguay *15:*223–234, April '44
Temporomandibular ankylosis of osteomyelitic origin; case. MAROTTOLI, O. R. AND BRAGAGNOLO, J. Bol. Soc. de cir. de Rosario *11:*194–201, July '44
Temporomandibular ankylosis. PETTERSSON, G. Nord. med. (Hygiea) *23:*1521–1523, Aug 18, '44
Temporary external salivary drainage (from Stenson's duct) following arthroplasty. GOODSELL, J. O., J. Oral Surg. *3:*174–176, April '45
Ankylosis of jaws. THOMA, K. H. *et al.* Am. J. Orthodontics (Oral Surg. Sect.) *31:*244–248, April '45
Ankylosis of jaw and its treatment in connection with case. ORELL, S. Nord. med. (Hygiea) *29:*83–88, Jan 11, '46
Ankylosis of jaws. DINGMAN, R. O. Am. J. Orthodontics (Oral Surg. Sect.) *32:*120–125, Feb '46
Ankylosis of mandibular joint. THOMA, K. H. Am. J. Orthodontics (Oral Surg. Sect.) *32:*259–272, May '46
Ankylosis and trismus resulting from war wounds involving coronoid region of mandible; 3 cases. BROWN, J. B. AND PETERSON, L. W., J. Oral Surg. *4:*258–266, July '46
Arthroplasty of temporomandibular joint in children with interposition of tantalum foil; preliminary report. EGGERS, G. W. N. J. Bone and Joint Surg. *26:*603–606, July '46
Trismus in relation to maxillofacial surgery LOADER, G. S. Brit. Dent. J. *81:*193–196, Sept 20, '46

Jaws, Ankylosis, Fibrous (See also Jaws, Ankylosis; Temporomandibular Joint)
New plastic operation for chronic cases of contracture of jaws. ROSENTHAL, W. Vrtljschr. f. Zahnh. *42:*499–507, '26
Case of stiff jaw after cancrum oris; surgical interference; cure. MUKERJI, S. N. Indian M. Gaz. *62:*387, July '27
Partial or pseudoankylosis of jaws. CURRAN, J. A. China M. J. *43:*241–244, March '29
Orthopedic treatment of contracture of temporomaxillary joint. KNORR, H. Zentralbl. f. Chir. *56:*1229–1232, May 18, '29
Ankylosis of mandible due to scarring of cheek; restoration of cheek lining with skin graft. KIRCH, W. Proc. Staff Meet., Mayo Clin. *5:*339–341, Nov 26, '30
Diagnosis and treatment of lesions preventing normal opening of mouth; 6 illustrative cases. BROWN, J. B. AND HAMM, W. G. Internat. J. Orthodontia *18:*353–362, April '32
Fracture of zygomatic arch; 2 cases with cicatricial closure of jaws. SCHMUZIGER, P. Schweiz. med. Wchnschr. *65:*721–722, Aug 10, '35
Roentgen ray therapy in fibrous ankylosis of jaws. MACKENZIE, A. R. South. M. J. *30:*816–819, Aug '37
Constriction of mandible; report of case and presentation of new dilator apparatus. VATTEONE, A. L. Dia med. *13:*688–692, July 21, '41
Pseudoankylosis of temporomandibular joint of cicatricial origin; surgical therapy of case. LOZA DIAZ, F. A. Cir. ortop. y traumatol., Habana *9:*129–136, July–Sept '41
Technic of surgical mobilization of lower jaw. KOCHEV, K. N. Sovet. med. (nos. 17–18) *5:*33, '41

Jaws, Bone Grafts to
Plastic surgery, 40 cases of bone-grafted mandibles. CHUBB, G. Lancet *1:*640, March 26, '21
Reconstruction, bone implants for reconstruction of jaw. CAVINA, C. Chir. d. org. di movimento *5:*417, Aug '21 abstr: J.A.M.A. *77:*1374, Oct 22, '21
Traumatic fracture of mandible, preoperative preparation; type of bone-graft; adaption of bone-graft. WOOLSEY, J. H., S. Clin. N. America *2:*333–340, April '22 (illus.)
Bone grafting in pseudoarthrosis of lower jaw. ROUVILLOIS, H. Paris med. *2:*237–245, Sept 26, '25 abstr: J.A.M.A. *85:*1433, Oct. 31, '25
Bone-grafting of mandible, with report of 7 cases. BILLINGTON, W. AND ROUND, H. Brit. J. Surg. *13:*497–505, Jan '26
Bone grafting for defects of mandible. IVY, R. H. AND EPES, B. M. Mil. Surgeon *60:*286–293, March '27
Bone transplantation from crest of ilium for reconstruction of ascending ramus and

Jaws, Bone Grafts to – Cont.

two-thirds of body of lower jaw-bone NEW, G. B., S. Clin. N. America *7:*1483–1486, Dec '27

Free transplantation of bone with periosteum in jaw surgery; 2 cases of excision of tumors. AXHAUSEN, G. Chirurg *1:*23–30, Nov 1, '28

Operative technic of osseous transplantation on lower jaw. CAVINA, C. Arch. ed atti d. Soc. ital. di chir. (1927) *34:*672–675, '28

Bone graft to jaw. MOOREHEAD, F. B., S. Clin. N. Amer. *9:*321–323, April '29

Operations suitable for defects and lack of continuity of inferior maxilla. SUDECK, P. AND RIEDER, W. Beitr. z. klin. Chir. *146:*493–518, '29

Bone-grafting the mandible. BILLINGTON, W. AND ROUND, H. Proc. Roy. Soc. Med. (sect. Odont.) *23:*7–13, March '30

Bone grafting the mandible. BILLINGTON, W. AND ROUND, H. Am. Dent. Surgeon *50:*185–188, May '30

Implantation of bone into lower jaw. AXHAUSEN, G. Deutsche Ztschr. f. Chir. *227:*368–385, '30

Bone transplantation by Axhausen's method in case of pseudoarthrosis of lower jaw resulting from defective healing. NISSEN, R. Deutsche Ztschr. f. Chir. *229:*140–142, '30

Operative treatment of tumors of jaw by Axhausen method of bone transplantation. KLEINSCHMIDT, O. Arch. f. klin. Chir. *164:*205–212, '31

Transplantation of bone and tissues in reconstruction of lower jaw. WEISSENFELS, G. Deutsche Zahnh., Hft. 79, pp. 1–30, '31

Reconstruction of lower jaw with tibial grafts. ROCHER, H. L. Bordeaux chir. *3:*272–277, July '32

Osteoplastic restoration of traumatic defects of lower jaw. KYANDSKITY, A. A. Sovet. khir. (nos. 3–4) *6:*339–349, '34

Autoplastic osseous and cutaneous grafts in destruction of lower jaw. DUFOURMENTEL. Bull. et mem. Soc. d chirurgiens de Paris 27:82–85, Feb 1, '35

Methods of transplanting bone into lower jaw. WASSMUND, M. Deutsche Ztschr. f. Chir. *244:*704–735, '35

Late results of pedicle bone-graft for fractured mandible; 3 cases. COLE, P. Proc. Roy. Soc. Med. *31:*1131–1134, July '38

Therapy of pseudoarthrosis with loss of substance of inferior maxilla. ROUVILLOIS, H. Arch. ital. di chir. *54:*351–356, '38

Pathologic fracture of mandible; nonunion treated with pedicled bone graft. COLE, P. P. Lancet *1:*1044–1045, June 8, '40

Jaws, Bone Grafts to – Cont.

Bone graft of mandible with prosthetic objective. MARTINEZ SUAREZ, M., J. Internat. Coll. Surgeons *3:*260–261, June '40

Therapy of loss of substance of lower jaw by autoplastic bone graft. SANCHEZ GALINDO, J. Med. espan. *4:*35–45, July '40

Bone transplantation in major resections of lower jaw; case of osteofibroma. AXHAUSEN, G. Chirurg *12:*442–444, Aug 1, '40

Technic of bone transplantation in traumatic defects of lower jaw; author's experiences. GANZER, H. Plast. chir. *1:*113–154, '40

Cosmetic and functional aspects of bone grafting in mandibular fractures. MACKENZIE, C. M. AND SHARPLESS, D. H. Northwest Med. *40:*372–374, Oct '41

Use of bone grafts in reconstructing mandible. FALLIS, R. J. Mil. Surgeon *90:*535–545, May '42

Primary bone grafting in resected tumor of mandible. STROMBECK, J. P. Acta chir. Scandinav. *86:*554–560, '42

Bone grafts to mandible. NEW, G. B. AND ERICH, J. B. Am. J. Surg. *63:*153–167, Feb '44

Haynes splint in case of bone graft of lower jaw. INCLAN, A. JR. Cir. ortop. y traumatol. Habana *12:*132–137, July–Sept '45

Fixation of pathologic fractures of mandible. BOURGOYNE, J. R. Am. J. Orthodontics (Oral Surg. Sect.) *31:*492–500, Aug '45

Use of cancellous bone in repair of defects about jaws. BLOCKER, T. G. JR. AND WEISS, L. R. Ann. Surg. *123:*622–638, April '46

Bone grafts in pseudarthrosis and loss of substance of upper jaw. GINESTET AND CHEMIN. Rev. de stomatol. *47:*137–139, May–June '46

Use of cancellous bone in repair of defects of jaw. BLOCKER, T. G. JR. AND WEISS, L. R. Tr. South. S. A. (1945) *57:*153–169, '46

Jaws, Cancer of (See also Cancer; Facial Cancer; Jaws, Tumors of; Jaws, Surgery of; Mouth Cancer; Tongue Cancer)

Malignant disease of superior maxillary bone; continued report. DABNEY, S. G. Kentucky M. J. *19:*125, March '21

Malignancy of face and jaws. FORT, F. T. Kentucky M. J. *19:*456, Aug '21

Malignant tumors of jaws. BERCHER, J. Paris med. *11:*205, Sept 3, '21 abstr: J.A.M.A. *77:*1289, Oct 15, '21

Prophylaxis of malignant growths of mouth, face and jaws. EASTMAN, J. R., J.A.M.A. *79:*118–120, July 8, '22

Treatment of cancer of jaws; observations

Jaws, Cancer of–Cont.
continued since 1918, covering 26 additional cases. Ochsner, A. J. Ann. Surg. *76:*328–332, Sept '22
Atypical operations on jaws for malignant growths. McArthur, L. L., J.A.M.A. *79:*1484–1487, Oct 28, '22
Carcinoma of jaws, tongue, cheek, and lips; general principles involved in operations and results obtained at Cleveland Clinic. Crile, G. W. Surg., Gynec. and Obst. *36:*159–162, Feb '23 (illus.)
Certain difficult problems in treatment of carcinoma of lower jaw. Johnson, F. M. Radiology *5:*280–285, Oct '25
Plastic and reconstructive surgery; sarcoma of mandible. Ivy, R. H., S. Clin. N. Amer. *6:*251–255, Feb '26
Surgery associated with radium in treatment of epitheliomas of upper jaw. Hautant, A. *et al.* J. de chir. *28:*257–274, Sept '26
Resection of lower jaw for removal of cancer of tongue. Krassin, P. M. Zentralbl. f. Chir. *53:*3095–3100, Dec 4, '26
Treatment of epithelioma of lower jaw. Simon, J. Marseille med. *1:*629, May 15, '27
Statistical postoperative prognosis of malignant tumors of upper jaw. Olaison, F. Hygiea *89:*705–710, Sept 30, '27
Cancer of upper maxilla and lip; operation; recovery. Bonnet-Roy, F. Odontologie *66:*39, Jan '28
Treatment of epithelioma about face, mouth and jaws. Padgett, E. C., J. Missouri M. A. *25:*190–194, May '28
Combined surgical and radium treatment of carcinoma of superior maxillary; case. Jentzer, A. Schweiz. med. Wchnschr. *58:*659–662, June 30, '28
Extensive epithelioma of cheek and lower jaw treated by diathermy. Harrison, W. J. Brit. M. J. *2:*102, July 21, '28
Malignant tumors of jaw; 16 cases. Lindemann, A. Deutsche Zahnh., Hft. *73:*15–56, '28
Plastic surgery of lip, chin and cheek in man after resection for cancer. Cavina, C. Arch. ed atti d. Soc. ital. di chir. *35:*526–541, '29
Osteoplastic partial resection of lower jaw by Krassin's method for removal of lingual cancer; 5 cases. Nasarow, N. N. and Kuschewa, M. N. Deutsche Ztschr. f. Chir. *215:*145–146, '29
Malignant tumors of mandible; review of literature. Sudeck, P. and Rieder, W. Ergebn. d. Chir. u. Orthop. *22:*585–678, '29
Results of treatment of cancer of jaws by operation and radiation. Simmons, C. C. Ann. Surg. *92:*681–693, Oct '30
Cancer of upper jaw; 4 cases. Dufourmentel, L. Bull. et mem. Soc. de chir. de Paris *22:*745–751, Dec 5, '30
Recurring epithelioma of lower lip and chin; diathermy and cautery excision; reconstruction of lower lip. Figi, F. A., S. Clin. North America *12:*951–954, Aug '32
Curability of malignant tumors of upper jaw and antrum. New, G. B. and Cabot, C. M. Surg., Gynec. and Obst. *60:*971–977, May '35
Therapy of mandibular epithelial cancers by electrocoagulation followed by curietherapy. Gernez, L. *et al.* Bol. Liga contra el cancer *10:*293–308, Oct '35
Surgical therapy of cancer of jaws. Alteri. Morgagni *77:*1199–1201, Nov 10, '35
Cancer of tongue and lower jaw. New, G. B. Tr. Am. Laryng., Rhin. and Otol. Soc. *41:*610–613, '35
Curability of malignant tumors of upper jaw and antrum. New, G. B. and Cabot, C. M. Tr. Am. Laryng., Rhin. and Otol. Soc. *41:*584–590, '35
Malignant tumors of upper jaw. Portmann, G. and Despons, J. Rev. de laryng. *57:*1–44, Jan '36
Metastasis of tumor of rectum to mandible (case). Ivy, R. H. and Curtis, L. Ann. Dent. *3:*133–137, Sept '36
Results of surgical therapy of carcinoma and sarcoma of lower jaw, some in advanced stage, over last 20 years. Berg, A. Ztschr. f. Stomatol. *35:*933–947, July 23, '37
Hemiresection of lower jaw with immediate osteoperiosteal graft in multilocular cancer; technical study. Prudente, A. Rev. de cir. de Sao Paulo *3:*245–258, Aug '37
Malignant tumors of jaw and their differential diagnosis. Hammer, H. Med. Welt *12:*261–264, Feb 19, '38
Jaw cancer; electrosurgery; segmental bone resection without interruption of continuity. Kroeff, M. Hospital, Rio de Janeiro *14:*337, Aug; 595, Sept; 1007, Oct '38
Cancer of mandible. Thoma, K. H. Am. J. Orthodontics *24:*995–999, Oct '38
Plastic and prosthetic therapy after resection of upper jaw for cancer; cases. Frenckner, P. and Sundberg, S. Acta oto-laryng. *27:*147–158, '39
Cancer of the Face and Mouth. V. P. Blair, S. Moore, and L. T. Byars. C. V. Mosby Co., St. Louis, 1941
Cancer of mouth and jaws (with emphasis on

Jaws, Cancer of–Cont.

therapy). SOMERVELL, T. H. Indian J. Surg. (no. 2) *5:*5–28, June '43

Huge paradental cyst of left upper jaw (giant cell sarcoma with gigantic cystic cavity); surgical therapy of case. DE SOUSA DIAS, J. V. Amatus *2:*552–558, July '43

Malignant tumors of upper jaw; Skinner lecture, 1943. WINDEYER, B. W. Brit. J. Radiol. *16:*362, Dec '43; *17:*18, Jan '44

Secondary carcinoma of mandible; analysis of 71 cases. BUIRGE, R. E. Surgery *15:*553–564, April '44

Recent advances in treatment of carcinoma of jaw. SOMERVELL, T. H. Brit. J. Surg. *32:*35–43, July '44

Malignant tumors of upper jaw. ORSI, J. L. Rev. med. de Rosario *34:*983–1011, Oct '44

Osteogenic tumor of mandible; case. BARATA, E. Brasil-med. *59:*244–247, July 7–14, '45

Spindle cell sarcoma of mandible with excision and subsequent bone graft; case. DINGMAN, R. O., J. Oral Surg. *3:*235–240, July '45

Early diagnosis of malignant tumors of upper jaw. KALLENBERGER, K. Schweiz. med. Wchnschr. *75:*990–995, Nov 10, '45

Osteogenic sarcoma of maxilla; case. BOIES, L. R. *et al.* J. Oral Surg. *4:*56–60, Jan '46; correction *4:*126, Apr '46

Jaws, Cysts

Etiology, pathology and treatment of cysts of jaws. DORRANCE, G. M., J.A.M.A. *77:*1883, Dec 10, '21

Tumors and cysts of jaws as disclosed by roentgenograms, and their treatment. IVY, R. H., J. Am. Dent. A. *14:*2272–2280, Dec '27

Dental cyst in patient operated for harelip; case. ARELLANO, E. R. Cron. med. mex. *29:*337–342, Aug '30

Operative treatment of cysts of jaws and fractures. IVY, R. H., J. Am. Dent. A. *19:* 1516–1527, Sept -32

Tumors and cysts of mouth and jaws of interest to otolaryngologist. IVY, R. H. Tr. Am. Acad. Ophth. *41:*163–185, '36

Surgical therapy of cysts of jaws. ČUPAR, I. Ztschr. f. Stomatol. *35:*1339–1346, Oct 22, '37

Hemorrhagic or traumatic cysts of mandible. IVY, R. H. AND CURTIS, L. Surg., Gynec. and Obst. *65:*640–643, Nov '37

Multiple dentigerous cysts of jaw, with special reference to occurrence in siblings. IVY, R. H. Ann. Surg. *109:*114–125, Jan '39

Fissural cysts of jaws. SAYER, B. AND

Jaws, Cysts–Cont.

SCULLY, J. B. Am. J. Orthodontics (Oral Surg. Sect.) *29:*320–327, June '43

Huge paradental cyst of left upper jaw (giant cell sarcoma with gigantic cystic cavity); surgical therapy of case. DE SOUSA DIAS, J. V. Amatus *2:*552–558, July '43

Traumatic cysts of mandible; case. BENNETT, I. B. AND CHILTON, N. W., J. Am. Dent. A. *32:*51–59, Jan 1, '45

Traumatic cyst of mandible. LAZANSKY, J. P. *et al.* Am. J. Orthodontics (Oral Surg. Sect.) *32:*155–159, Mar '46

Jaws, Deformity

Case of facial deformity (jaw also). BEYERS, C. F. AND BERRY, T. B., M. J. S. Africa *21:*127–131, Dec '25

Duplication of upper jaw. BUMM, E. Arch. f. klin. Chir. *135:*506–519, '25

Patient with only one mandibular condyle. WALLISCH, W. Ztschr. f. Stomatol. *25:*621–626, July '27

Right hemihypertrophy and left hemiatrophy of jaw; case. EIBRINK JANSEN, G. A. H. Tijdschr. v. tandheelk. *35:*131–134, Feb 15, '28

Orthopedic problems of lower jaw; with special reference to unilateral shortening. IVY, R. H. AND CURTIS, L., J. Bone and Joint Surg. *10:*645–660, Oct '28

Hemihypertrophy of jaw. NORD, C. F. L. Tijdschr. v. tandheelk. *35:*811–814, Dec 15, '28

Congenital tendency of nasal septum and intermaxillary bone to abnormal longitudinal growth. PICHLER, H. Ztschr. f. Stomatol. *27:*21–26, Jan '29

Unilateral and congenital agenesis of jaws; cases. ROCHER, H. L. AND FISCHER, H., J. de med. de Bordeaux *59:*611–621, July 30, '29

Progressive atrophy of facial bones with complete atrophy of mandible; case. THOMA, K. H., J. Bone and Joint Surg. *15:*494–501, April '33

Familial occurrence of hypoplasia of jaws. KLEY, H. Med. Welt *8:*311, March 3, '34

Malocclusion produced by formation of scar tissue (from burn). HOWES, A. E. Internat. J. Orthodontia *21:*1141–1143, Dec '35

Congenital atrophy of lower eyelids, both auricles and lower jaw; case. VAN LINT, A. AND HENNEBERT, P. Bull. Soc. belge d'opht., no. 73, pp. 51–61, '36

Rare congenital malformation of right portion of lower and upper jaw (unilateral micrognathia); case. CASTAY. Bull. et

Jaws, Deformity – Cont.
mem. Soc. de radiol. med. de France *25:*125–126, Feb '37
"Norwegian system" of functional orthopedics of jaw deformities. ANDRESEN, V. Ztschr. f. Stomatol. *35:*664–678, May 28, '37
Congenital atrophy of lower eyelids, both auricles and lower jaw; case. VAN LINT, A. AND HENNEBERT, P. Bruxelles-med. *17:*1065–1070, May 16, '37
Maxillary deformities and their orthopedic therapy. CAUHEPE, J. Medecine *18:*657–658, Aug '37
Nature and significance of gnathophysiometry and gnathophore method according to Viggo Andresen in diagnosis of protrusions of lower and upper jaws. HUSSERL, E. Ztschr. f. Stomatol. *36:*532, May 13; 591, May 27, '38
Malformations of profile due to malposition of teeth and deformities of jaws; importance of complete lesional diagnosis. MERLE-BERAL, J., J. de med. de Bordeaux *115:*113–137, Aug 6–13, '38
Congenital absence of ramus of mandible. KAZANJIAN, V. H., J. Bone and Joint Surg. *21:*761–772, July '39
Congenital defect of lower jaw associated with cleft palate (case). SACKS, S. South African M. J. *15:*34, Jan 25, '41
Deformed chin and lower jaw. SCHER, S. L. Ann. Surg. *115:*869–879, May '42
Congenital partial hemihypertrophy jaws involving marked malocclusion. RUDOLPH, C. E. AND NORVOLD, R. W., J. Dent. Research *23:*133–139, April '44
New syndrome; mandibulofacial dysostosis. FRANCESCHETTI, A. Bull. schweiz. Akad. d. med. Wissensch. *1:*60–66, '44

Jaws, Dislocation

Recurrent unilateral subluxation of mandible; excision of interarticular cartilage in cases of snapping jaw. ASHHURST, A. P. C. Ann. Surg. *73:*712, June '21
Habitual dislocation of lower jaw. KONJETZNY, G. E. Arch. f. klin. Chir. *116:*681, Sept '21 abstr: J. A. M. A. *77:*1774, Nov 26, '21
Intramuscular injection of alcohol in treatment of recurring luxation of jaw. SICARD, J. A. Bull. Acad. de med., Par. *89:*271–274, Feb 20, '23
Operative treatment of habitual dislocation of jaw. NIEDEN, H. Deutsche Ztschr. f. Chir. *183:*358–363, '24
Reposition of dislocated mandible after injection of local anesthetics into muscles of

Jaws, Dislocation – Cont.
mastication. WIEDHOPF, O. Munchen. med. Wchnschr. *72:*2007, Nov 20, '25 abstr: J.A.M.A. *86:*78, Jan 2, '26
Reposition of dislocated mandible under local anesthesia. KULENKAMPFF, D. Muchen. med. Wchnschr. *72:*2229, Dec 25, '25
Reposition of dislocated mandible in local anesthesia. HÖRHAMMER, C. Munchen. med. Wchnschr. *73:*446–447, March 12, '26
Nieden's operation for habitual dislocation of lower jaw. LOESSL, J. Zentralbl. f. Chir. *53:*1749–1751, July 10, '26
Crossed dislocation of lower jaw; anatomic and physiologic conception of dislocations of jaw. PODLAHA, J. Zentralbl. f. Chir. *53:*2199–2202, Aug 28, '26
Chronic temporomaxillary subluxation. MORRIS, J. H. Am. J. Surg. *1:*288, Nov '26
Nonsurgical reduction of 50-day old dislocation of lower jaw. KARELL, U. Zentralbl. f. Chir. *53:*3160–3161, Dec 11, '26
Bilateral dislocation of mandible; case. DAS, S. C. Indian M. Gaz. *62:*86, Feb '27
Exarticulation of lower jaw. KLEINSCHMIDT, P. Deutsche med. Wchnschr. *53:*473, March 11, '27
Treatment of irreducible dislocated lower jaw of 98 days' duration; case. WILLCUTTS, M. D., U. S. Nav. M. Bull. *25:*331–336, April '27
Double recidivant luxation of the inferior jaw; operated. DUFOURMENTEL, L. Paris chir. *19:*134–136, May–June '27
Continual dislocation of jaw at temporomaxillary articulation. BERCHER, J. *et al.* Rev. d'hyg. *49:*605–607, Oct '27
Habitual jaw dislocation cured by excision of meniscus; case. COMBIER, V. AND MURARD, J. Bull. et mem. Soc. nat. de chir. *53:*1271, Nov 26, '27
Meniscus injuries of temporomaxillary joint resulting in so-called anterior dislocation. LOTSCH, F. Arch. f. klin. Chir. *149:*40–54, '27
Causes of facial asymmetry in muscular wryneck and jaw dislocations. BECK, O. Ztschr. f. orthop. Chir. *49:*424–449, May 18, '28
Simple wooden appliance for righting horizontal dislocations in treatment of jaw fractures. KUBASSOFF, M. N. Odont. i stomatol. (no. 11) *6:*36–37, '28
Treatment of habitual luxation and so-called habitual subluxation of lower jaw and snapping of temporomaxillary joint. KONJETZNY, G. E. Zentralbl. f. Chir. *56:*3018–3023, Nov 30, '29

Jaws, Dislocation – Cont.

Clicking of temporomaxillary joint and habitual dislocations; cases. VON STAPELMOHR, S. Acta chir. Scandinav. *65:*1–68, '29

Chronic recurring temporomaxillary subluxation; surgical consideration of "snapping jaw" with report of successful operative result. MORRIS, J. H. Surg., Gynec. and Obst. *50:*483–491, Feb '30

New operative method in habitual temporomaxillary dislocations; case. MOCZAR, L. Rev. de stomatol. *32:*129–143, March '30

New instrument for use in longstanding dislocations of jaws. TAYLOR, A. B., J.M.A. South Africa *4:*326, June 14, '30

Rigid fixation of jaws due to forward luxation; arthroplasty. BATTISTA, A. Riforma med. *46:*1122–1127, July 14, '30

Treatment of habitual dislocation of mandible. MÓCZÁR, L. Orvosi hetil. *74:*1081–1084, Oct 25, '30

Nonsurgical treatment of habitual dislocation of lower jaw especially when accompanied by prognathism. REICHENBACH, E. Deutsche Ztschr. f. Chir. *231:*470–476, '31

Surgical therapy of ordinary dislocations of lower jar. SCHMIDT, G. Deutsche Ztschr. f. Chir. *233:*536–542, '31

Fractures and incomplete dislocations of jaws. ROGERS, L. *et al*. Radiology *18:*28–40, Jan '32

Extirpation of condyle in therapy of subluxation of temporo-maxillary joint. DUFOURMENTEL, L. Bull. et mem. Soc. d. chirurgiens de Paris *24:*558–559, Dec 2, '32

Classification of anterior-luxations of temporomaxillary joint. BERCHER, J. AND FRIEZ, P. Presse med. *41:*644–646, April 22, '33

Recurrent dislocation of jaws. MAYER, L., J. Bone and Joint Surg. *15:*889–896, Oct '33

Anatomic changes of bones in chronic, bilateral luxation of mandible. LEDENYI, J. Bratisl. lekar. listy *15:*694–696, April '35

Irreducible luxation of lower jaw; surgical therapy of case. OLIVARES, L. Actas Soc. de circ. de Madrid *4:*279–284, April–June '35

Recurrent dislocation of temporomaxillary joint; therapy with intramuscular alcohol injections. TEMPESTINI, O. Stomatol. *33:*901–912, Oct '35

Habitual temporomaxillary luxation; cure of 3 years duration after meniscopexy; case. CONTIADES, X. J. Mem. Acad. de chir. *62:*18–21, Jan 15, '36

Recurrent dislocation of jaw; bilateral ablation of temporomaxillary menisci; case. SANTY, P. AND BERARD, M. Lyon chir. *33:*75–76, Jan–Feb '36

Morphologic, physiologic and clinical study of mandibular meniscus; habitual luxation and temporomaxillary cracking. DUBECQ, X. J., J. de med. de Bordeaux *114:*125–178, Jan 30, '37, also: Rev. d'odonto-stomatol. *1:*1–54, Jan '37

Recurrent luxation of mandible and its surgical therapy; case. FAVREAU, J. C. Union med. du Canada *66:*271–277, March '37

Luxations of lower jaw; surgical pathology and therapy. PEREIRA DE QUEIROZ, R. Ann. paulist. de med. e cir. *33:*521–527, June '37

Recidivating temporomaxillary subluxation; surgical therapy of case. RODRIGUEZ VILLEGAS, R. AND TAULLARD, J. C. Bol. y trab. de la Soc. de cir. de Buenos Aires *21:*484–492, July 21, '37

Recidivating temporomaxillary luxation; author's experience with therapy. CAMES, O. AND MAROTTOLI, O. R. An. de cir. *3:*274–279, Sept '37

Therapy of recidivating luxation of jaw; authors' experience. CAMES, O. AND MAROTTOLI, O. R. Bol. y trab. de la Soc. de cir. de Buenos Aires *21:*756–763, Sept 8, '37

Treatment for subluxation of temporomandibular joint. SCHULTZ, L. W., J.A.M.A. *109:*1032–1035, Sept 25, '37

Dislocations of mandible. DOHERTY, J. L. AND DOHERTY, J. A. Am. J. Surg. *38:*480–484, Dec '37

Curative treatment for subluxations of temporomandibular joint (injections of sodium psylliate). SCHULTZ, L. W., J. Am. Dent. A. *24:*1947–1950, Dec '37

Fracture-dislocation of mandible. BJERRUM, O. Acta chir. Scandinav. *79:*209–218, '37

Multiple fractures of lower jaw associated with left temporomaxillary luxation; surgical and prosthetic therapy; case. LEVY AND MOATTI. Tunisie med *32:*175–179, May '38

Recurrent temporomaxillary luxation; osteoplastic abutment (Elbim method); case. POLLOSSON, E. AND FREIDEL. Lyon chir. *35:*460–463, July–Aug '38

Habitual temporomaxillary luxation. PINTO DE SOUZA, O. Arq. de cir. clin. e exper. *2:*351–366, Oct '38

Irreducible luxation of lower jaw; case. DUFOURMENTEL, L. Bull. et mem. Soc. d. chirurgiens de Paris *30:*485–488, Dec 2–16, '38

Fracture of lower jaw with bilateral outward dislocation. LINTON, P. Acta chir. Scandinav. *81:*304–308, '38

Reduction of blocked temporomaxillary luxation under regional transmasseteric anesthesia. LEBOURG, L. Presse med. *47:*872, May 31, '39

Jaws, Dislocation – Cont.

Therapy of recidivating luxation of jaws by pre-articular osseous abutment; cases. BREHANT, J. Mem. Acad. de chir. *65:*893-897, June 21, '39

Fractures and dislocations of jaws and wounds of face. BELLINGER, D. H. Am. J. Surg. *46:*535-541, Dec '39

Unreduced unilateral dislocation of jaw; operative correction after 4 years. SCHWARTZ, M., J. Bone and Joint Surg. *22:*176-181, Jan '40

Method of reduction of luxation of temporomaxillary joint. OGNEV, B. V. Sovet. med. (no. 4) *4:*17-18, '40

Bilateral temporomaxillary luxation of 5 months' duration, considered irreducible, but reduced under local anesthesia by elastic traction on transangular metallic loops. DARCISSAC, M. Rev. de stomatol. *43:*5-13, Jan-Feb '42

Procedure for treating habitual or recidivating luxation of temporomaxillary joint. BERTOLA V. J. Prensa med. argent. *29:*536-542, April 1, '42

Ankylosis of jaw following luxation fracture; case. JONSSON, S. O. Nord. Med. (Hygiea) *18:*609-611, April 10, '43

Operation for correction of recurrent dislocation of jaw. SMITH, L. D. Arch. Surg. *46:*762-763, May '43

Reduction of jaw dislocations. WERNECK, C. Rev. Brasil. med. *1:*598-599, July '44

Sclerosing agent in treatment of subluxation of mandible and hemangiomas. SALMAN, I. U. S. Nav. M. Bull. *44:*361-369, Feb '45

Fracture-dislocation of mandible. MEADE, H. S. Irish J. M. Sc. pp. 98-99, March '46

Sclerosing treatment (using sylnasol, fatty acid solution) for subluxation of temporomandibular joint. ROSENBAUM, W. Am. J. Orthodontics *32:*551-571, Oct '46

Jaws, Enlarged Condyle

Benign bony elargement of condyloid process of mandible. IVY, R. H. Ann. Surg. *85:*27-30, Jan '27

Condylar hypertrophy of inferior maxilla. DUFOURMENTEL, L. Bull. et mem. Soc. de chir. de Paris *20:*886, '28

Unilateral hypertrophy of mandibular condyle associated with chondroma. KANTHAK, F. F. AND HARKINS, H. N. Surgery *4:*898-907, Dec '38

Unicondylar hypertrophy; late result after jaw resection; case. BERCHER, J. AND LEPROUST. Rev. de stomatol. *41:*257-262, April '39

Osteoma of mandibular condyle with deviation prognathic deformity; case. WORMAN, H. G. *et al.* J. Oral Surg. *4:*27-32, Jan '46

Jaws, Fractured, Edentulous Fragments

Fractures of toothless mandibles; treatment; 2 cases. WASSMUND, M. AND LABAND, F. Deutsche Monatschr. f. Zahnh. *45:*1009-1015, Dec 15, '27

Simple wooden appliance for righting horizontal dislocations in treatment of jaw fractures. KUBASSOFF, M. N. Odont. i. stomatol. (no. 11) *6:*36-37, '28

Fracture of mandible in, and posterior to, the molar region. FRY, W. K. Proc. Roy. Soc. Med. (Sect. Odont.) *22:*37-45, March '29

Treatment of fractures of edentulous jaws. GOODSELL, J. O. JR. Dental Cosmos *72:*385-389, April '30

Extension treatment of fractures of mandible by combined method (Darcissac-Bruhn-Petroff). TOMIRDIARO, O. Deutsche Monatschr. f. Zahnh. *49:*1112-1116, Nov 15, '31

Use of cranial supports in reduction of fractures of mandibular angle. CROCQUEFER. Rev. de stomatol. *34:*347-351, June '32

Extrabuccal apparatus for immobilization in therapy of fractures of lower jaw. AURÉGAN. Bull. et mem. Soc. d. chirurgiens de Paris *25:*192-197, March 17, '33

Circumferential wiring in fractures of mandible. COLE, P. P. Lancet *1:*749-750, April 8, '33

Fracture of lower jaw in edentulous patient; reduction and immobilization by transosseous metallic loops with external extension splints. DUFOURMENTEL, L. AND DARCISSAC, M. Bull. et mem. Soc. d. chirurgiens de Paris *25:*304-309, May 5, '33

Vertical fractures of mandibular ramus; cases. ACHARD, P. Rev. de stomatol. *36:*321-326, May '34

Osteosynthesis by external fixation apparatus in fractures of lower jaw; technic and description of apparatus. BERCHER, J. AND GINESTET, G. Rev. de stomatol. *36:*294-300, May '34

Fractures at union of ramus and body of lower jaw; cases. GOINARD, P. AND CURTILLET, A. Bull. med., Paris *48:*447-449, Jul 21, '34

Preparation of splint for extra-oral extension in jaw fractures. NIRENBERG, B. B. AND FUKS, B. I. Sovet. khir. (no. 4) *7:*732-734, '34

New method for treatment of fracture of lower jaw (Kirschner wire). MEADE, H. Irish J. M. Sc., pp. 318-319, July '35

Wire extension in treatment of mandibular

Jaws, Fractured, Edentulous Fragments—Cont.
fractures. BROOKE, R. Brit. M. J. *2:*498-499, Sept 14, '35
(Comment to article by Wassmund on Vorschutz method of treatment of jaw fractures.) VORSCHÜTZ, J. Zentralbl. f. Chir. *63:*446, Feb 22, '36
Disadvantages of Vorschütz method of treating complicated fractures and defects of lower jaw with plaster of paris bandage fastened to each side of jaw by screw arm. (Reply to Vorschutz) WASSMUND, M. Zentralbl. f. Chir. *63:*444-445, Feb 22, '36, Further comment by Vorschütz; *63:*446, Feb 22, '36
Therapy of fracture of ascending branch of lower jaw. CANALE, A. Semana med. *2:*381-386, Aug 6, '36
Treatment of nonunion and loss of substance in fracture of edentulous mandible. ADDISON, P. I., J. Am. Dent. A. *25:*1081-1084, July '38
Bilateral fracture of angles of lower jaw; case. WEINBERGER, M. Rev. med.-cir. do Brasil *46:*1112-1118, Nov '38
Fractures of edentulous mandible. JONES, W. I., J. Am. Dent. A. *26:*1360-1361, Aug '39
Treatment of fractures of mandible with vitallium screws. BIGELOW, H. M., M. Bull. Vet. Admin. *17:*54-56, July '40
Orthopedic therapy of fractures of lower jaw; new apparatuses. DE COSTER, L. Rev. de stomatol. *41:*933-947, '40
Treatment of fracture of corpus mandibulae ad modum Ipsen (introduction of Kirschner nails). SØBYE, P. Acta chir. Scandinav. *83:*445-477, '40
New departure from orthodox methods of setting fractured edentulous mandibles. BERRY, H. C., J. Am. Dent. A. *28:*388-392, March '41
Treating fractures of mandible by skeletal fixation. GRIFFIN, J. R. Am. J. Orthodontics (Oral Surg. Sect) *27:*364-376, July '41
Therapy of fractures of edentulous mandibles by external skeletal fixation, with report of case. INCLAN, A. Cir. ortop. y traumatol., Habana *9:*158-164, Oct-Dec '41
External pin fixation for mandible fractures. MOWLEM, R.; *et al.* Lancet *2:*391-393, Oct 4, '41
Extra-oral splinting of edentulous mandible in fractures. POHL, L. Lancet *2:*389-391, Oct 4, '41
Compound and comminuted fractures of ramus of mandible; case. DURLING, E. J., J Am. Dent. A. *28:*1832-1835, Nov '41
Treating fractures of mandible by skeletal

Jaws, Fractured, Edentulous Fragments—Cont.
fixation. GRIFFIN, J. R. Rev. san. mil., Buenos Aires *40:*1006-1010, Nov '41
External skeletal fixation in fractures of mandibular angle. CONVERSE, J. M. AND WAKNITZ, F. W., J. Bone and Joint Surg. *24:*154-160, Jan '42
Internal wire fixation of jaw fractures. BROWN, J. B. AND MCDOWELL, F. Surg., Gynec., and Obst., *74:*227, Feb '42. Also in Am. J. Orthodontics and Oral Surg., *29:*86, Feb '43
Extraoral device for immobilization of mandibular fractures. ALESSANDRINI, I. Rev. med. de Chile *70:*298-299, April '42
Experiences with various methods of skeletal fixation in jaw fractures. MOWLEM, R. Proc. Roy. Soc. Med. *35:*415-426, April '42
Utilization of vitallium appliances to treat edentulous mandible fractures. LOGSDON, C. M., J. Am. Dent. A. *29:*970-978, June 1, '42
Internal wire fixation of jaw fractures; second report. BROWN, J. B. AND MCDOWELL, F. Surg., Gynec., and Obst. *75:*361, Sept '42. Also in Dentistry, A Digest of Practice, *3:*6, Feb '43
Skeletal fixation in treatment of fractures of mandible; review. WALDRON, C. W., J. Oral Surg. 1:59-83, Jan '43
Vitallium bone screws and appliances for fracture of mandible. BIGELOW, H. M., J. Oral Surg. *1:*131-137, April '43
Fractures of edentulous mandible. DOHERTY, J. A., J. Oral Surg. 1:157-161, April '43
External skeletal fixation of mandibles. CONVERSE, J. M., J. Oral Surg. *1:*210-214, July '43
Extraoral skeletal fixation of mandibular fractures; cases. GROSS, P. P. Am. J. Orthodontics (Oral Surg. Sect.) *29:*392-400, July '43
Fracture of lower edentulous jaw; surgical therapy of case. ORIS, J. L. Bol. Soc. de cir. de Rosario *10:*230-235, July '43
Extraoral splinting of mandible. BOURGOYNE, J. R., J. Am. Dent. A. *30:*1390-1392, Sept 1, '43
Mandibular fractures; report of 50 applications of Roger Anderson skeletal fixation appliance. WINTER, L. Am. J. Surg. *61:*367-379, Sept '43
Recent experiences with skeletal fixation in fractures of mandible. IVY, R. H. AND CURTIS, L., J. Oral Surg. *1:*296-308, Oct. '43
Extraoral utilization of screws or pins in immobilization of mandibular fractures. LOGSDON, C. M., J. Am. Dent. A. *30:*1529-

Jaws, Fractured, Edentulous Fragments – Cont.
1540, Oct 1, '43
Horizontal pin fixation for fractures of mandible using pin guide. PINCOCK, D. F. Surg., Gynec. and Obst. *77:*493-496, Nov '43
Extraoral plaster splint fixation in treatment of fractures of mandible. GODWIN, J. G., J. Am. Dent. A. *31:*76-85, Jan 1, '44
Horizontal pin fixation for fractures of mandible using pin guide. PINCOCK, D. F. Am. J. Orthodontics (Oral Surg. Sect.) *30:*67-72, Feb '44
Fractures of mandible; review of experience in 52 patients with particular reference to use of external skeletal fixation. WIESENFELD, I. H. AND MEADOFF, N. Permanente Found. M. Bull. *2:*49-63, March '44
Skeletal fixation in treatment of fractures of mandible. PARKER, D. B., S. Clin. North America *24:*381-391, April '44
Skeletal fixation splint in mandibular fractures as aid to early denture construction. RICHISON, F. A. AND KENNEDY, J. T., J. Am. Dent. A. *31:*646-648, May 1, '44
Inert metals in direct fixation of mandibular fractures. STROCK, A. E. Surg., Gynec. and Obst. *78:*527-532, May '44
Device for external transcutaneous fixation of mandibular fractures. HOFFMANN, R. Helvet. med. acta *11:*521-524, June '44
Fixation of mandibular fractures by means of extraoral apparatus based on pins. MOWLEM, R.; *et al.* Rev. san. mil., Buenos Aires *43:*1055-1058, July '44
Skeletal fixation of pathologic fractures of mandible with extensive loss of substance; 2 cases. MELOY, T. M. JR. AND GUNTER, J. H. Am. J. Orthodontics (Oral Surg. Sect.) *30:*567-571, Sept '44
Three fractures at angle of jaw; one treated by internal wiring, two by internal clamp fixation. THOMA, K. H. Am. J. Orthodontics (Oral Surg. Sect.) *31:*206-220, Apr '45
Extraoral pin fixation for fractures of mandible. MACGREGOR, A. B. Lancet *1:*816, June 30, '45
Open operation and tantalum plate insertion for fracture of mandible. CHRISTIANSEN, G. W., J. Oral Surg. *3:*194-204, July '45
Fracture of mandible at angle; appliances to depress posterior fragment. HARRIS, L. W. AND CHRISTIANSEN, G. W., J. Oral Surg. *3:*212-214, July '45
Method of facilitating insertion of pins in skeletal fixation of jaw fractures. PETERSON, R. G.; *et al.* J. Oral Surg. *3:*258-262, July '45

Jaws, Fractured, Edentulous Fragments – Cont.
Open reduction vs. skeletal fixation in jaw fractures. BOURGOYNE, J. R. Am. J. Orthodontics (Oral Surg. Sect.) *31:*519-532, Aug '45
Mandibular fractures at King County Hospital treated by Roger Anderson skeletal fixation. GRAHAM, J. W. Northwest Med. *44:*250-252, Aug '45
External skeletal fixation of jaw fractures in dental office. SHIPMON, T. H. Am. J. Orthodontics (Oral Surg. Sect.) *31:*486-492, Aug '45
Surgical therapy of mandibular fracture by Kirschner nails; case. CADENAT *et al.* Rev. de stomatol. *46:*130-133, Oct-Dec '45
Further uses for peripheral bone clamp in jaw fractures. THOMA, K. H. *et al.* Am. J. Orthodontics (Oral Surg. Sect.) *31:*607-618, Oct '45
Skeletal fixation of mandibular fractures; 5 cases with 9 fractures. BURKE, H. D. *et al.* Arch. Surg. *51:*279-282, Nov-Dec '45
Control of mandibular fragments by external fixation. ROBERTS, W. R. Brit. Dent. J. *80:*257, April 18, '46; 291, May 3, '46
Fractures of lower jaw; indications for new surgical method of pin fixation. MARONNEAUD, P. L., J. de med. de Bordeaux *123:*201-205, June '46
Fractures of mandible; Mowlem method of external pin fixation. MARINO, H. AND CRAVIOTTO, M. Prensa med. argent. *33:*1823-1827, Sept 6, '46

Jaws, Fractures

Fracture of jaw. NEJROTTI, G. M. Riforma med. *37:*891, Sept 17, '21, abstr: J.A.M.A. *77:*1689, Nov 19, '21
Fractures of jaws. BERCHER, J. Arch. de med. et pharm. mil. *76:*268-282, March '22 (illus.)
Treatment of fractures of jaws. PITTS, A. T. Lancet *2:*1336-1337, Dec 25, '26
Apparatus for treatment of jaw fractures, with loss of substance. DUCHANGE. Rev. d'hyg. *49:*608-613, Oct '27
Successful treatment of jaw fractures by reduction, retention and grafts. CAVINA, C. Rev. de stomatol. *29:*815-842, Nov '27
Permanent reduction of jaw fractures: 7 cases. PONROY, *et al.* Rev. de stomatol. *29:*795-814, Nov '27
Therapy of jaw fractures. JONAS. Deutsche med. Wchnschr. *53:*2203, Dec 23, '27
Value of orthodontic appliances to immobilize jaw fractures. FEDERSPIEL, M. N. In-

Jaws, Fractures – Cont.
ternat. J. Orthodontia *14:*185-196, March '28
Technic of immediate treatment of jaw fractures. BUZZI, A. Rev. de cir. *7:*215, May '28, also: Prensa med. argent. *15:*235-236, July 20, '28
Treatment of jaw fractures. CAVINA, C. Stomatol. *26:*657-678, July '28
Jaw fractures. COUGHLIN, W. T., J. Missouri M. A. *25:*292-296, July '28
Fractures of upper and lower jaw and their correction with dental splint. MOREMEN, C. W., J. Florida M. A. *15:*207-209, Oct '28
Interdental fixation appliance for jaw fractures. WILLETT, R. C. Dental Items Interest *50:*788-799, Oct '28
Jaw fractures; clinical aspects and treatment by blockage of maxillae. GRANDI, G. Stomatol. *27:*94-106, Feb '29
Present status of treatment of jaw fractures. REICHENBACH, E. Munchen. med. Wchnschr. *76:*530-532, March 29, '29
Treatment of jaw fractures. RISDON, F. Canad. M. A. J. *20:*260-262, March '29
Jaw fractures treated by Swiss accident insurance, 1923-1926; 178 cases. SCHMUZIGER, P. Schweiz. Monatschr. f. Zahnh. *39:*234-260, April '29
Jaw fractures, with special reference to treatment. STEADMAN, F. ST. J. Brit. Dent. J. *50:*824-838, July 15, '29
Causes and treatment of jaw fractures. MORAL, H. AND SCHLAMPP, H. Fortschr. d. Zahnheilk. *5:*1055-1076, Nov '29
Principles of treatment of fractures of superior and inferior maxillae. SCHMUZIGER, P. Schweiz. med. Wchnschr. *60:*101-104, Feb 1, '30
Modifications in Graefe's apparatus for reduction and retention of fractures (jaws). GIZZI, C. Stomatol. *28:*865-870, Oct '30
Dental aspect of jaw fractures. MORAL, H. AND SCHLAMPP, H. Fortschr. d. Zahnh *6:*973-994, Nov '30
Treatment of fractures of jaws. MAITLAND, G. R., J. Michigan M. Soc. *29:*915-917, Dec '30
Fractures of the Jaws, by ROBERT H. IVY AND LAWRENCE CURTIS. Lea and Febiger, Phila., 1931. Second Edition, 1938. Third Edition, 1945
Jaw fractures. FRIEDMAN, J. Dental Digest *37:*71-83, Feb '31
Jaw fractures. ENLOE, G. R. Texas State J. Med. *27:*27-29, May '31
Diagnosis and therapy of jaw fractures. MORAL, H. AND SCHLAMPP, H. Fortschr. d. Zahnh. *7:*1017-1038, Nov '31

Jaws, Fractures – Cont.
Bone suture in treatment of jaw fractures. GREVE, K. Beitr. z. klin. Chir. *152:*310-322, '31
Jaw fractures. MICHELSON, N. M. Sovet. khir. *1:*287-290, '31
Fractures of mandible and maxilla; treatment. HUTCHINSON, R. H. Maine M. J. *23:*53-57, March '32
Feeding of liquid diet in jaw fractures. BROWN, J. B. Internat. J. Orthodontia *18:*614-617, June '32
Multiple fractures of upper and lower jaws. HAVENS, F. Z. Proc. Staff Meet., Mayo Clin. *7:*433-434, July 27, '32
Jaw fractures. FIGI, F. A. Surg., Gynec. and Obst. *55:*762-770, Dec '32
Clinical report illustrating application of orthodontic principles in treatment of jaw fractures. GIFFORD, A. C. Internat. J. Orthodontia *18:*1285-1289, Dec '32
Alveolar fractures of jaw. MELCHIOR, M. Ztschr. f. Stomatol. *30:*251-268, '32
Jaw fractures. FIGI, F. A. Proc. Staff Meet., Mayo Clin. *8:*135-138, March 1, '33
Jaw fractures. WALDRON, C. W. Journal-Lancet *53:*317, June 15; 351, July 1, '33
Therapy of jaw fractures. IPSEN, J. Zentralbl. f. Chir. *60:*2840-2841, Dec 9, '33
Special cases of jaw fractures. VORDENBÄUMEN. Arch. f. orthop. u. Unfall-Chir. *32:*608-611, '33
Better method of treating jaw fractures. MOOREHEAD, F. B. J.A.M.A. *102:*1655-1657, May 19, '34
Treatment of fractures of maxilla, mandible and other bones of face. AUFDERHEIDE, P. J., J. Am. Dent. A. *21:*950-961, June '34
Jaw fractures. DUNNING, H. S. Internat. J. Med. and Surg. *47:*277-286, July-Aug '34
Fractured jaw; case. PALAZZI, S. Stomatol. *32:*662-665, July '34
Complex fracture (craniofacial disjunction and vertical fractures) of upper jaw and double fracture of lower jaw; simplified therapy of case. PONROY *et al.* Rev. de stomatol. *36:*470-471, July '34
Therapy of fractured jaws. EGGER, F. Schweiz. med. Wchnschr. *64:*1044-1047, Nov 17, '34
Fractured jaw caused by depression of upper jaw; case. DUBECQ, X. J., J. de med. de Bordeaux *112:*43-44, Jan 20, '35
Jaw fractures. HOWELL, E. B., U.S. Nav. M. Bull. *33:*76-77, Jan '35
Jaw fractures. IVY, R. H. Surg., Gynec. and Obst. *60:*531-534, Feb. (no. 2A) '35
Compound, comminuted fracture of both

Jaws, Fractures—Cont.
maxillae and mandible. BRADSHAW, T. L. Internat. J. Orthodontia *21:*260–262, March '35
Therapy of jaw fractures. VON MADARASZ, E. Ztschr. f. Stomatol. *33:*838–848, July 26, '35
Jaw fractures. WILKINSON, B. Tri-State M. J. *7:*1503–1504, Aug '35
Jaw fractures. BOR, H. A. Geneesk. tijdschr. v. Nederl.-Indie *75:*1530–1536, Sept 3, '35
Fractures of mandible and superior maxilla in time of peace. JELINEK, V. J. Voj.-san. glasnik *6:*513–539, '35
Therapy of jaw fractures. LANDAIS, P. Rev. de stomatol. *38:*65–73, Feb '36
Management of jaw fractures. MOOREHEAD, F. B., S. Clin. North America 16:197–213, Feb '36
Fractures of jaw and allied traumatic lesions of facial structures. WEISENGREEN, H. H. AND LEVIN, W. N. Ann. Surg. *103:*428–437, March '36
Jaw fractures. SONNTAG, E. Monatschr. f. Unfallh. *43:*369–387, Aug '36
Jaw fractures. ARMBRECHT, E. C. Internat. J. Orthodontia *22:*957–975, Sept '36
Gentle means for reducing fracture of jaw. MORGENTHALER, C. F., J. Am. Dent. A. *23:*1736–1738, Sept '36
Jaw fractures. RISDON, F., J. Am. Dent. A. *23:*1639–1641, Sept '36
Jaw fractures and treatment. DOHERTY, J. L. AND DOHERTY, J. A. Surg., Gynec. and Obst. *64:*69–73, Jan '37
Apparatus for immediate treatment and prosthesis in jaw fractures. DI GIUSEPPE, F. Gior. ital. di clin. trop. *1:*81, March 31, '37
Jaw fractures. DOHERTY, J. A. New England J. Med. *216:*425–428, March 11, '37
Fractures of jaw. DUNN, F. S. Am. J. Surg. *36:*83–87, April '37
Occlusal reduction in management of jaw fractures. WRIGHT, C. F. Angle Orthodontist *7:*67–80, April '37
Extension of uniform system of therapy of jaw fractures. VON MADARASZ, E. Ztschr. f. Stomatol. *35:*799–804, June 25, '37
Jaw fractures; types, causes, locations and treatment of 76 recent cases. WOODS, S. H. J. Roy. Army M. Corps *68:*366–378, June '37
Therapy of jaw fractures by simple stomatologic means obtainable by general practitioner. PALAZZI, S. Gior. di med. mil. *85:*833–837, Aug '37
Evaluation of physiotherapeutic modalities in jaw and associated fractures. WEISENGREEN, H. H. West. J. Surg. *45:*537–539,

Jaws, Fractures—Cont.
Oct '37
Simplified splinting of jaw fractures. FRANKL, Z. Gyogyaszat *77:*686, Dec 5; 714, Dec 12, '37
Jaw fractures and their management. MOOREHEAD, F. B. Am. J. Surg. *38:*474–479, Dec '37
Bimaxillary blockage in jaw fractures; compared advantages of 2 orthodontic apparatuses. SENTENAC, E. AND KOEFF, G., J. de med. de Bordeaux *115:*90–96, Jan 29 '38
Jaw fractures. DOHERTY, J. A. Am J. Orthodontics *24:*165–170, Feb '38
Kirschner traction in treatment of maxillary fractures. MAJOR, G., J.A.M.A. *110:*1252–1254, April 16, '38
Jaw fractures. KJAERHOLM, H. Ugesk. f. laeger *100:*659–669, June 16, '38
Fractured maxillae; description of appliance for reduction and fixation with case report. RALPH, H. G. AND MAXWELL, M. M., U.S. Nav. M. Bull. *36:*507–511, Oct '38
Functional therapy of jaw fractures. WUSTROW, P. Ztschr. f. Stomatol. *36:*1171–1190, Oct 28, '38
Jaw fractures. RISDON, F. Canad. M. A. J. *39:*572–573, Dec '38
Technic of preparation and fixation of wire splints with intermaxillary traction. TARNOPOLSKIY, A. I. Ortop. i. travmatol. (no. 6) *12:*71–77, '38
Use of rubber bands in treatment of facial and jaw fractures. DINGMAN, R.O., J. Am. Dent. A. *26:*173–183, Feb '39
Jaw fractures. MURPHY, A. B. Northwest Med. *38:*44–46, Feb '39
Analysis of 115 cases fractured jaw. ASBELL, M. B. Am. J. Orthodontics *25:*282–289, March '39
Statistical report of series of fractures of jaw. HAYNEN, A. S. Am. J. Orthodontics *25:*478–480, May '39
Therapy of complicated jaw fracture in patient with no upper teeth. PAOLI, M. Rev. de stomatol. *41:*398–402, May '39
Jaw fractures. VAN OMMEN, B. Nederl. tijdschr. v. geneesk. *83:*3888–3892, Aug 5, '39
Fractures and dislocations of jaws and wounds of face. BELLINGER, D. H. Am. J. Surg. *46:*535–541, Dec '39
Injuries of the Jaws and Face, by W. WARWICK JAMES AND B. W. FICKLING. Bale, London, 1940
Theory and Treatment of Fractures of the Jaws in Peace and War. HENRY KIMPTON, London, 1940. C. V. Mosby Co., St. Louis, 1941

Jaws, Fractures—Cont.

Jaw fractures; therapy by continually applied force. Fuso, B. Stomatol. ital. *2:*95-111, Feb '40

Fractures of maxillae and mandible. Logsdon, C. M., J. Am. Dent. A. *27:*389-392, March '40

Treatment of fractured jaws. Tratman, E. K., J. Malaya Br., Brit. M. A. *3:*357-373, March '40

Jaw fractures. Kjaerholm, H. Ugesk. f. laeger *102:*321-333, April 4, '40

Application of biologic principles to treatment of jaw fractures. Kloehn, S. J. Angle Orthodontist *10:*94-100, April '40

The care of severe injuries of the face and jaws. Brown, J. B. and McDowell, F. Journal-Lancet (N.S.), *60:*260, June '40

Jaw fractures. Doherty, J. L. and Doherty, J. A. Am. J. Surg. *48:*576-581, June '40

Practical points in diagnosis and treatment of jaw fractures. Doherty, J. A. Surg., Gynec. and Obst. *72:*96-98, Jan '41

Jaw fractures. Hamm, W. G. South. Surgeon *10:*185-193, March '41

Jaw fractures. Curtis, L. Mil. Surgeon *89:*648-652, Oct '41

Treatment of jaw fractures. Watson, R. G. M. Press *206:*458-460, Dec 17, '41

Jaw fractures. Sidorenko, V. I. Sovet. med. (no. 6) *5:*23-24, '41

Synopsis of Traumatic Injuries of the Face and Jaws, by Douglas B. Parker. C. V. Mosby Co., St. Louis, 1942

Fractures of maxillae and mandible; 2 cases (with description of apparatus). Yando, A. H. and Taylor, R. W., U.S. Nav. M. Bull. *40:*155-157, Jan '42

Treatment of jaw fractures. Hume, E. C. Kentucky M. J. *40:*297-298, Aug '42

Symposium on industrial surgery; fractures of jaws and injuries of face, mouth and teeth. Thomas, E. H., S. Clin. North America *22:*1029-1048, Aug '42

Should teeth and comminuted bone be removed in jaw fractures? Walker, D. G. Proc. Roy. Soc. Med. *35:*663-682, Aug '42

Jaw fractures. Stumpf, F. W., J. Am. Dent. A. *29:*1615-1628, Sept 1, '42

Jaw fractures. Anderson, B. G. Connecticut M. J. *6:*799-805, Oct '42

Fractures of the Jaws and Other Facial Bones, by Glenn Major. C. V. Mosby Co., St. Louis, 1943

Teeth in fracture line. Parfitt, G. J.; *et al.* Bull. War Med. *3:*328, Feb '43 (abstract)

Intraoral open reduction for management of certain difficult fractures of jaw. Shearer, W. L., J. Am. Dent. A. *30:*833-834, June 1, '43

Use of ordinary small brass hinge as locking device for splints in multiple fractures of jaws. Goodsell, J. O., J. Oral Surg. *1:*250-251, July '43

Use of cotter key in intermaxillary ligation allowing quick release in case of nausea and vomiting. Harper, H. D. Am. J. Orthodontics *29:*373-382, July '43

Tie-loop wiring of fractured jaws. Peterson, R. G., J. Oral Surg. *1:*246-249, July '43

New method of intermaxillary fixation in patients wearing artificial dentures. Thoma, K. H. Am. J. Orthodontics (Oral Surg. Sect) *29:*433-441, Aug '43

Acrylic resin splints for jaw fractures. Henderson, R. L. V., J. Roy. Nav. M. Serv. *29:*268, Oct '43

Management of fractured jaws. Merrifield, F. W. Radiology *41:*539-542, Dec '43

Fractures of jaw with special reference to therapy. Gonzalez Ulloa, M. Rev. mex. de cir., ginec. y cancer *12:*89-98, March '44

Jaw fractures. Maris, A. M. Bull. U.S. Army M. Dept. (no. 75) pp. 81-88, April '44

History and treatment of fractured jaws from World War I to World War II; collective review. Thoma, K. H. Internat. Abstr. Surg. *78:*281-312, '44; in Surg., Gynec. and Obst. April '44

Fractures of jaw. Maris, A. M. Mil. Surgeon *95:*43-47, July '44

Development of treatment for fractured jaw. Schwartz, L. L., J. Oral Surg. *2:*193-221, July '44

Analysis of 212 cases of fractured jaw. Coakley, W. A. and Baker, J. M. Am. J. Surg. *65:*244-247, Aug '44

Historical review of methods advocated for treatment of fractured jaw; 10 commandments for modern treatment. Thoma, K. H. Am. J. Orthodontics (Oral Surg. Sect.) *30:*399-504, Aug '44

Modern treatment of jaw fractures. Penn, J. and Rand, W. W. Clin. Proc. *3:*455-460, Dec '44

Fractures of interest to dental officer; 3 cases. Maxwell, M. M., U.S. Nav. M. Bull. *44:*353-360, Feb '45

Instrument to facilitate multiple loop wiring in jaw fractures. Klein, D. Bull. U. S. Army M. Dept. *4:*479, Oct '45

Advances in construction and use of splints in treatment of jaw fractures. Fickling, B. W. Brit. Dent. J. *80:*8-13, Jan 4, '46

Treatment of 1,000 fractures (in British

Jaws, Fractures – Cont.
army) of jaw. CLARKSON, P.; *et al.* Ann. Surg. *123:*190–208, Feb '46, also: Brit. Dent. J. *80:*69, Feb 1, '46; 107, Feb 15, '46
Treatment of fractures of superior and inferior maxilla. McNICHOLS, W. A. Illinois M. J. *90:*179–185, Sept '46
Preparation of screw lock sectional splint with mechanical retention for fracture of jaw. McCARTHY, W. D. AND BURNS, S. R. J. Oral Surg. *4:*343–352, Oct '46

Jaws, Fractures, Complications (See also Jaws, Fractures, Infections; Jaws, Fractures, Malunion; Jaws, Fractures, Non-Union)
Fracture and necrosis of mandible; case. BRODY, H. Dental Cosmos *69:*242–247, March '27
Jaw fracture with chronic asthenia. BENON, R., J. de med. et chir. prat. *99:*208–214, March 25, '28
Jaw fracture in epileptic patient. FELDMAN, M. H. Internat. J. Orthodontia *15:*381, April '29
Clinical sequelae of injury to inferior alveolar nerve following fractures of mandible. STEIDL, H. Deutsche Ztschr. f. Chir. *230:*129–146, '31
Odontoma of jaw complicated by surgical fractures; 2 cases. L'HIRONDEL. Rev. de stomatol. *35:*125–139, March '33
Late surgical complications of fracture of mandible. GILLIES, H. AND McINDOE, A. H. Brit. M. J. *2:*1060–1063, Dec 9, '33
Actinomycosis following fracture of lower jaw. GROHS, R. Ztschr. f. Stomatol. *32:*427–433, April 27, '34
Clinical and experimental study of muscle damage in maxillary fractures. LINK, K. H. Arch. f. klin. Chir. *181:*24–77, '34
Diplopia in fracture of upper and lower maxillary and of malar bones; case. PAOLI, M. Rev. de stomatol. *41:*548–552, July '39
Complications associated with treatment of fractures of mandible. SKUES, K. F. Roy. Melbourne Hosp. Clin. Rep. *10:*123–126, Dec '39
Multiple fractures of skull complicated by fractures of jaws. GARFIN, S. W. Am. J. Surg. *52:*460–465, June '41
Bleeding from external auditory meatus following fracture of mandible. SUGGIT, S., J. Laryng. and Otol. *56:*364–367, Oct '41
Inferior alveolar nerve and fractured mandible. HALLAM, J. W. Guy's Hosp. Gaz. *57:*22, Jan 23, '43
Case of undiagnosed cavernous sinus thrombophlebitis; untreated fracture of mandible. CURRAN, M., J. Oral Surg. *2:*7–12, Jan '44
Arteriovenous aneurysm resulting from application of Roger Anderson splint for fractured jaw. GREELEY, P. W. AND THRONDSON, A. H., J.A.M.A. *124:*1128, April 15, '44
Management of jaw fractures complicated by intracranial injuries. KINGSBURY, B. C., U. S. Nav. M. Bull. *42:*915–920, April '44
Fracture of mandible associated with burns of head. KARNES, T. W., J. Oral Surg. *3:*83–86, Jan '45

Jaws, Fractures, First-Aid
Emergency treatment of fractures of mandible. PONROY, *et al.* Paris med. *2:*195–199, Sept 1, '28
First aid in jaw fractures. PROELL, F. Deutsche med. Wchnschr. *65:*1538–1543, Oct 13, '39
Barrel bandage in jaw fractures. FRY, W. K. Brit. M. J. *2:*1086, Dec 2, '39
First aid for jaw fractures. FABRICIUS-MOLLER, J. AND KJAERHOLM, H. Ugesk. f. laeger *103:*1307–1311, Oct 9, '41
First aid appliance for treatment of jaw fractures. SORRELS, T. W. Am. J. Orthodontics *27:*714–716, Dec '41
Stretcher head support in cases of smashed jaw. PAISLEY, J. C. Brit. M. J. *1:*16, Jan 3, '42
First aid splinting of jaw fractures. SPANIER, F., M. Rec. *155:*377, July '42
Simple device for temporary support of fractured mandible. ROMMEL, R. W., U.S. Nav. M. Bull. *40:*977, Oct '42
Handy bandage for jaw fractures. BROWNSON, H. N., J. Oral Surg. *1:*271, July '43
Simplified chin support. THUSS, C. J. J. M. A. Alabama *13:*387–388, June '44

Jaws, Fractures in Children
Fractures of lower jaw in children. DEL CAMPO, R. M. AND SELLERA CASTRO, R. Rev. ortop. y traumatol. *1:*357–371, Jan '32
Treatment of fracture of mandible in child. MURDY, W. F., U. S. Nav. M. Bull. *33:*114–115, Jan '35
Fracture of lower jaw in girl 10 years old; results of therapy. BRUSCHI, F. Stomatol. *35:*17–33, Jan '37
Fractures of lower jaw in children. PETER, K. L. Ztschr. f. Stomatol. *35:*1371–1377, Oct 22, '37
Traumatic injuries to jaws in infants. WEINMANN, J. AND KRONFELD, R. J. Dent. Research *19:*357–366, Aug '40

Jaws, Fractures in Children—Cont.
Fractures of jaw in children. WALDRON, C. W. *et al*. J. Oral Surg. *1:*215-234, July '43

Jaws, Fractures, Infections in

Healing time of fractures of jaw in relation to delay before reduction, infection, syphilis and blood calcium and phosphorus content. WOODARD, D. E., J. Am. Dent. A. *18:*419-442, March '31
Fracture of orbit and superior maxilla followed by subcutaneous and deep emphysema from secondary infection. BONNET, P. Lyon chir. *28:*718-719, Nov-Dec '31
Case of fractured mandible complicated by infection with Streptothrix. CARLTON, C. H. Tr. M. Soc., London *55:*51-53, '32
Maggot therapy in infected wound of comminuted fracture; case. MANZANILLA, M. A. Medicina, Mexico *13:*1-7, Jan 10, '33
Actinomycosis following fracture of lower jaw. GROHS, R. Ztschr. f. Stomatol. *32:*427-433, April 27, '34
Fulminating osteomyelitis of mandible with pathologic fracture. FIELD, H. J. AND ACKERMAN, A. A., J. Am. Dent. A. *23:*448-450, March '36
Parahyoid cellulitis following fracture of lower jaw. DECHAUME, M. Rev. de stomatol. *38:*457-458, June '36
Mandibular fractures, malocclusion and osteomyelitis. SMITH, G. W. Rocky Mountain M. J. *38:*794-798, Oct '41
Sulfathiazole (sulfanilamide derivative) in treatment of fractures of mandible. HADDOCK, T. R., J. Am. Dent. A. *29:*1002-1004, June 1, '42

Jaws, Fractures, Malunion of

Horizontal fracture of upper jaw consolidation in defective position and resulting in total malocclusion; functional and esthetic restoration by surgical and prosthetic therapy. DUFOURMENTEL, L. *et al*. Bull. et mem. Soc. d. chirurgiens de Paris *24:*555-558, Dec 2, '32
Consolidation of horizontal maxillary fracture in vicious position with total loss of dental articulation. DUFOURMENTEL, L. *et al*. Rev. de stomatol. *35:*339-342, June '33
Malocclusion resulting from pathologic fracture and deforming callus in mandibular osteitis; therapy; case. DE FAZIO, M. Riforma med. *50:*851-858, June 2, '34
Therapy of malposition of healed jaw fractures; 2 cases. VANDORY, W. Ztschr. f. Stomatol. *35:*866-871, July 9, '37
Malunited fractures of jaw. MIKHELSON, N. M. Novy khir. arkhiv *38:*549-550, '37

Jaws, Fractures, Malunion of—Cont.
Badly consolidated fracture of upper jaw; reduction by osteotomy and elastic traction apparatus. THEODORESCO, D. Rev. de chir., Bucuresti *41:*918-926, Nov-Dec '38
Late surgical reduction of badly consolidated fracture of mandible by means of osteotomy. ROCCIA, B. Boll. e mem. Soc. piemontese di chir. *8:*643-655, '38
Late surgical therapy of badly consolidated mandibular fracture by means of osteotomy. ROCCIA, B. Stomatol. ital. *1:*197-204, March '39
Therapy of badly consolidated and nonconsolidated jaw fractures. AKS, L. V. Ortop. i travmatol. (no. 1) *13:*30-35, '39
Mandibular fractures, malocclusion and osteomyelitis. SMITH, G. W. Rocky Mountain M. J. *38:*794-798, Oct '41

Jaws, Fractures, Mandible

Double fracture of lower jaw. NEFROTTI, G. M. Riforma med. *37:*438, May 7, '21
Practical method of fixation in fractures of mandible. IVY, R. H. Surg., Gynec. and Obst. *34:*670-673, May '22 (illus.)
Fractures of mandible. IVY, R. H., J.A.M.A. *79:*295-297, July 22, '22 (illus.)
Improvised emergency apparatus for fractured jaw. CANALE, A. Semana med. *2:*1189-1193, Dec 7, '22 (illus.)
Typical mandibular fracture. WALTER, E.L. U.S. Nav. M. Bull. *18:*88-89, Jan '23
Observation on series of 15 fractures of mandible. BROWN, J. L., U.S. Nav. M. Bull. *18:*245-248, Feb '23
Wiring method of treatment for fractures of mandible. TENNENT, E. H., U.S. Nav. M. Bull. *19:*38-42, July '23 (illus.)
Compound and multiple fractures of lower jaw; (case report). SIMMONS, J. W., J.M.A. Georgia *13:*22-23, Jan '24
Fractures of mandible. ENTWISLE, R. M. AND GARDNER, J. A. Atlantic M. J. *28:*515-518, May '25
Fracture of lower jaw; essentials of treatment. BRUHN, C. Tung-chi, Med. Monatschr. *2:*144-150, Jan '27
Fracture and necrosis of mandible; case. BRODY, H. Dental Cosmos *69:*242-247, March '27
Isolated fracture of coronoid apophysis of jaw from direct violence; case. MUCCI, D. Gazz. internaz. med. -chir. *32:*403-407, Nov 30, '27
Fractures of mandible. NERTNEY, E. G., U.S. Vet. Bur. M. Bull. *4:*360-362, April '28
Double fracture of mandible predisposed by

Jaws, Fractures, Mandible–Cont.
impacted third molar. CRICH, W. A. Canad. M.A.J. *19:*207–210, Aug '28
Fractures of mandible. REITER, E. Dental Cosmos *70:*772–782, Aug '28
Fracture of mandible. PAYNE, J. L. Clin. J. *58:*77–84, Feb 13, '29
Further observations on fractures of mandible. IVY, R. H. AND CURTIS, L. Dental Cosmos *71:*341–352, April '29
Treatment of fractures of lower jaw by bone suture with silver wire; cases. DIEULAFÉ, L. Rev. de stomatol. *31:*330–336, June '29
Fracture of lower jaw; prosthetic treatment. ALEMAN. Cluj. med. *10:*378–395, Aug 1, '29
Fractures of lower jaw. LANIER, W. D. JR. U.S. Vet. Bur. M. Bull. *5:*893–895, Nov '29
Osteosynthesis of lower jaw after fracture; cases. RIDARD, L. Rev. de stomatol. *31:*883–888, Dec '29
Fractures of lower jaw; case. FLEURY, R. Rev. de stomatol. *32:*84–87, Feb '30
Splint for fractures of inferior maxilla. MASLAND, H. C., M. Times, New York *58:*75, March '30
Fractures of mandible. COLE, P. P. *et al.* Practitioner *124:*489–505, May '30
Therapy of fractures of lower jaw. SARAVAL, U. Riforma med. *46:*675–678, May 5, '30
Fractures of mandible; analysis of 50 cases. DEAN, H. T., J. Am. Dent. A. *17:* 1074–1085, June '30
Methods of immobilization with mouth open and closed in fracture of lower jaw. RIDARD, L. Rev. gen. de clin. et de therap. *44:*454–456, July 12, '30
Complete fracture of horizontal branch of inferior maxillary bone. PARDO DE TAVERA, V. Semana med. *2:*539–540, Aug 14, '30
Exposed comminuted fracture of inferior maxilla caused by bullet; case. PARDO DE TAVERA, V. Semana med. *2:*598–599, Aug 21, '30
Frequency of fractures of lower jaw due to rebound from blow of fist. ARLOTTA, A. AND LARI, G. L. Stomatol. *28:*1073–1079, Dec '30
Complicated fractures of mandible. IVY, R. H. AND CURTIS, L., S. Clin. N. Amer. *10:*1411–1426, Dec '30
Extra-oral emergency bandage in fractures of lower jaw. CHATZKELSON, B. Munchen. med. Wchnschr. *78:*98, Jan 16, '31
Orthopedic treatment of fractures of lower jaw. GUICHARD, P. Loire med. *45:*49–61, Feb '31
Nonoperative treatment in mandibular fracture. STEFANI, F. Stomatol. *29:*128–134, Feb '31
Metal splint for fractures of mandible.

Jaws, Fractures, Mandible–Cont.
LISTER, C. S., U. S. Vet. Bur. M. Bull. *7:*498, May '31
Rare forms of fractures of mandible. REICHENBACH, E. Ztschr. f. Stomatol. *29:*719–728, June '31
Treatment of fracture of lower jaw without loss of substance. BERTRAND, P. AND FREIDEL, C. Bull. med. Paris *45:*585-587, Aug 22, '31
Elastic bandage in fracture of mandible. SPANIER, F. Chirurg *3:*891–893, Oct 15, '31
Fractures and incomplete dislocations of jaws. ROGERS, L. *et al.* Radiology *18:*28–40, Jan '32
Spontaneous fracture of mandible; case. CURNOCK, J. E. Proc. Roy. Soc. Med. *25:*885, April '32
Fractures of lower jaw; necessity of extracting teeth at point of fracture. TABAR, F. Practicien du Nord de l'Afrique *5:*422–428, July 15, '32
Management of fracture of mandible. HENSEL, G. C. Surg., Gynec. and Obst. *55:*238–243, Aug '32
Operative treatment of cysts of jaws and fractures. IVY, R. H., J. Am. Dent. A. *19:*1516–1527, Sept '32
Therapy and evolution of comminuted fractures of mandible; 2 cases. VAN DER CHINST, J. Arch. med. belges *85:*780–784, Nov '32
Therapy of fractures of horizontal ramus of lower jaw. GASTÉLUM, B. J. Gac. med. de Mexico *64:*245–253, May '33
Fractures of mandible; their treatment. WAHL, J. P. New Orleans M. and S. J. *85:*900–906, June '33
Unusual case of fractured jaw. MELCHIOR, M. Hospitalstid. *76:*829–835, Aug 10, '33
Fractures of mandible. WRIGHT, C. B. West Virginia M. J. *29:*525–526, Dec '33
Fracture of lower jaw. JAMES, W. W. AND GILLIES, H. D. Tr. M. Soc. London *56:*22–36, '33
Diagnosis and therapy of fractures of lower jaw. KALLAY, J. Lijecn. vjes. *55:*248–253, '33
Fractures of mandible. MACK, C. H. AND CONNELLY, J. H., U.S. Nav. M. Bull. *32:* 31–36, Jan '34
Fractures of lower jaw; prosthetic therapy. CITOLER SESÉ, R. Clin. y. lab. *25:*129–132, Aug '34
Treatment of simple fractures of lower jaw. RANGANI, S. Sind M. J. *7:*64–68, Sept '34
Therapy of complicated fractures of lower jaw. VORSCHÜTZ, J. Med. Welt *8:*1474–1475, Oct 20, '34

Jaws, Fractures, Mandible – Cont.
Primary bone suture in fracture of lower jaw. DUBOV, M. D. Novy khir. arkhiv *31:*89–95, '34
Extension method of Faltin for fractures of lower jaw. FALTIN, R. Vestnik khir. *35:*221–223, '34
Mistaken application of Faltin extension in case of fracture of lower jaw. KALINEYKO, I. P. Vestnik khir. *35:*219–220, '34
Therapy of complicated fractures of lower jaw. BICHLMAYR, A. Med. Welt *9:*158–160, Feb 2, '35
Disadvantages of Vorschütz method of treating complicated fractures and defects of lower jaw with plaster of paris bandage fastened to each side of jaw by screw arm. WASSMUND, M. Zentralbl. f. Chir. *62:*914–921, April 20, '35
Therapy of fractures of mandible due to firearms. CAVINA, C. Gior. di med. mil. *83:*713–722, Aug '35
Therapy of extensive fractures of mandible due to firearms. CAVINA, C. Gior. di med. mil. *83:*809, Sept; 923, Oct '35
Fracture of lower jaw, with special reference to therapy. HERPIN, A. Rev. gen. de clin. et de therap. *49:*641–645, Oct 5, '35
Fractures of lower jaw; 2 methods of therapy; 2 cases. ROBERT, AND MERLE-BERAL. Arch. de med. et pharm. nav. *125:*703–715, Oct-Dec '35
Therapy of recent fractures of lower jaw; with description of apparatus used. GIOIA, T. Semana med. *2:*1370–1378, Nov 7, '35
Therapy of complicated fractures of lower jaw (comment on Wassmund's article). VORSCHÜTZ, J. Zentralbl. f. Chir. *62:*2624–2625, Nov 2, '35
Mandibular fracture treated by emergency methods; preliminary report. PALAZZI, S. Stomatol. *33:*1076–1079, Dec '35
Application of Vorschütz lever screw in fractures of lower jaw. STEINKAMM, J. Chirurg *7:*820–824, Dec 1, '35
Therapy of mandibular fractures. ROCCIA, B. Boll. e mem. Soc. piemontese di chir. *5:*1161–1176, '35
Fractures of mandible. FRY, K. Guy's Hosp. Gaz. *50:*267–270, July 4, '36
Orthodontic treatment of jaw fractures and cleft palate. CARTWRIGHT, F. S. Internat. J. Orthondontia *23:*159–163, Feb '37
Fracture of mandible. SHACKELFORD, J. G. Southwestern Med. *21:*96–98, March '37
Fracture of mandible. DELANY, H. B. JR. J. Nat. M.A. *29:*80–82, May '37
Surgical correction of mandibular protraction

Jaws, Fractures, Mandible – Cont.
and retraction. (also fractures of ascending rami). HENSEL, G. C. Surgery *2:*92–119, July '37 also: Internat. J. Orthondontia *23:*814–839, Aug '37
Healing of fractures of mandible and zygoma. GRIMSON, K. S., J. Am. Dent. A. *24:*1458–1469, Sept '37
Reduction of double fracture of lower jaw by combined action of intermaxillary forces and transosseous loop. GINESTET, G. Rev. de stomatol. *40:*289–294, May '38
Fractures of mandible and their treatment. FRY, W. K., M. Press *197:*108–112, Aug 10, '38
Methods of immobilization of fractured mandible. RICHARDS, R. L. Am. J. Orthodontics *24:*973–979, Oct '38
Healing time in fractures of mandible. WELCH, C. C. AND TAYLOR, R. W., U. S. Nav. M. Bull. *36:*513–517, Oct '38
Fractures of lower jaw; therapy by extension; case. BARBERIS, J. C. Bol. Soc. de cir. de Rosario *5:*478–484, Nov '38
Fractures of lower jaw. BAY, R. P. AND DORSEY, B. M. Am. J. Surg. *42:*532–535, Dec '38
Mandibular fracture; symptomatology, evolution and outcome in case involving teeth. BRANCHINI, C. Arch. ital. di chir. *50:*595–600, '38
Fracture of lower jaw with bilateral outward dislocation. LINTON, P. Acta chir. Scandinav. *81:*304–308, '38
Fractures of lower jaw; therapy. APRILE, H. Rev. med. y cien. afines *1:*62–64, May 30, '39
Origin and therapy of accidental jaw fractures, with evaluation of compensation. HERRMANN, M. Monatschr. f. Unfallh. *46:*448–457, Aug '39
Complications associated with treatment of fractures of mandible. SKUES, K. F. Roy. Melbourne Hosp. Clin. Rep. *10:*123–126, Dec '39
Healed fractures of lower jaw, from early Bronze Age. BREITINGER, E. Arch. f. Gesch. d. Med. *32:*103–110, '39
Bone ligation and suture in relation to functional defects and tissue losses in mandible; collective review. WEISENGREEN, H. H. Internat. Abstr. Surg. *68:*450–460, '39; in Surg., Gynec. and Obst., May '39
Fractures of mandible; treatment by so-called maxillary block. WIEL, P. Stomatol. ital. *2:*112–126, Feb '40
Fractures of mandible; statistical study of 100 cases. DOHERTY, J. A., J. Am. Dent. A. *27:*735–737, May '40

Jaws, Fractures, Mandible – Cont.

Wire reposition in linear fractures of lower jaw. REICHENBACH, E. Ztschr. f. Stomatol. *38:*347-357, May 24, '40

Fractures of mandible. GORDON, S. Canad. M.A.J. *42:*521-525, June '40

Possibility and practical value of universal method in therapy of mandibular fractures. BROSCH, F. Ztschr. f. Stomatol. *39:*123-144, Feb 28, '41 comment by Reichenbach *39:*144-147, Feb 28, '41

Fractures of mandible; sign of and method of treatment. COLEMAN, F. Proc. Roy. Soc. Med. *34:*212-214, Feb '41

Fractures of lower jaw; therapy of Böhler method. MONA, C. Policlinico (sez. prat.) *48:*659-666, April 14, '41

Fractures of mandible. STROCK, M. S. Surg., Gynec. and Obst. *72:*1047-1051, June '41

Therapy of most frequent fractures of lower jaw. GONZALEZ, N., B. Rev. mex. de cir., ginec. y cancer *9:*331-339, Aug '41

Early treatment of fractures of mandible. KAZANJIAN, V. H. AND STROCK, M. S., J. Am. Dent. A. *29:*76-83, Jan '42

Internal wire fixation of jaw fractures. BROWN, J. B. AND MCDOWELL, F. Surg. Gynec., and Obst., *74:*227, Feb '42. Also in Am. J. Orthodontics & Oral Surg., *29:*86, Feb '43

Early treatment of fractures of mandible. HEMBERGER, A. J. Mil. Surgeon *90:*424-428, April '42

Fractures of mandible, with special reference to reduction of complicated displacements and subsequent immobilization. WALDRON, C. W. Journal-Lancet *62:*228-240, June '42

Internal wire fixation, with note on external bar fixation. jaw fractures. BROWN, J. B. AND MCDOWELL, F. Surg., Gynec. and Obst. *75:*361-368, Sept '42

Fractures of mandible. HEMBERGER, A. J. Ann. Dent. *1:*51-58, Sept '42

Fractures of mandible. HENNY, F. A., J. Am. Dent. A. *29:*1840-1845, Oct 1, '42

Management of recent faciomaxillary and mandibular fractures. WOODWARD, F. D. AND FITZ-HUGH, G. S. Virginia M. Monthly *69:*612-619, Nov '42

Importance of good technic in therapy of fractures of lower jaw; technic proposed by authors. CORNILLON, A. AND ROJO, J. J. Gac. med. de Mexico *72:*591-597, Dec 31, '42

Combined intraoral and dental fixation in fracture of mandibular angle with considerable displacement. FERBER, E. W., J. Am. Dent. A. *30:*906-910, June 1, '43

Jaws, Fractures, Mandible – Cont.

Correlated fixation of mandibular fractures. KAMRIN, B. B., J. Oral Surg. *1:*235-240, July '43

Fracture of mandible. BROESAMLE, K. M. U.S. Nav. M. Bull. *42:*47-55, Jan '44

Fracture of lower jaw. JIMENEZ PLA, A. Medica, Matanzas *3:*1-6, Jan-Feb '44

Fractures of mandible. GONZALEZ ULLOA, M. Rev. mex. de cir., ginec. y cancer *12:*145-152, May '44

Screw-pin for use in connection with mandibular fractures and grafts. WALKER, F. A. Brit. Dent. J. *78:*266-267, May 4, '45

Simple technic for simple fractures of mandible. LILLY, A. J., U.S. Nav. M. Bull. *45:*135-139, July '45

Mandibular fractures. GORDON, S. D. Bull. Vancouver M.A. *21:*281-283, Aug '45

Fractures of mandible. GONZALEZ ULLOA, M. Vida nueva *56:*183-189, Dec '45

Fracture-dislocation of mandible. MEADE, H. S. Irish J. M. Sc. pp. 98-99, March '46

"Islet" method of wiring fractures of mandible. HUMPHRIES, S. V. Clin. Proc. *5:*154-160, June '46

Jaws, Fractures, Mandibular Condyle

Fracture of condylar region of maxilla; 6 cases. BERCHER, J. Rev. de chir. *61:*200-218, '23 (illus.)

Fractures and dislocation fractures of condyle of lower jaw and its operative treatment. PERTHES, G. Arch. f. klin. Chir. *133:*418-433, '24

Double fractures of articular processes of lower jaw. LINDQVIST, S. Zentralbl. f. Chir. *53:*2777-2778, Oct 30, '26

Fracture of articular process of lower jaw. WALLIN, C. C. Northwest Med. *26:*214, April '27

Fracture of condyle of mandible. RÜEDI, G. Schweiz. Monatschr. f. Zahnh. *38:*727, Nov; 805, Dec '28

Fractures at symphysis and below both condyles of jaw. BRECHOT, AND LEBOURG, L. Odontologie *67:*144-148, March 30, '29

Method for treating fracture of neck of condyle of mandible. RUSSELL, A. Y. Internat. J. Orthondontia *16:*84-86, Jan '30

Treatment of fractures of temporomaxillary joint. DUFOURMENTEL, L. Rev. odont. *52:*517-526, July-Aug '31

Therapy of dislocation fracture of head of mandible. POST, K. Zentralbl. f. Chir. *60:*2118-2121, Sept 9, '33

Dislocation fracture of capitulum of inferior

Jaws, Fractures, Mandibular Condyle – Cont.
maxilla; 5 cases. KAPPIS, M. Zentralbl. f. Chir. *61:*814–821, April 7, '34
Fracture of jaw with luxation of collum mandibulae; surgical treatment. STRÖMBERG, N. Acta chir. Scandinav. *74:*379–404, '34
Therapy of fractures of condyles of jaw; advantages of perifacial arc. LEBOURG, L. Presse med. *44:*360–361, March 4, '36
Double exposed fracture of lower jaw with luxation of one of temporomaxillary articulations; recovery of case after surgical therapy. VES LOSADA, C. AND BRAMBILLA, A. Semana med. *1:*1012–1019, April 8, '37
Fracture-dislocation of mandible. BJERRUM, O. Acta chir. Scandinav. *79:*209–218, '37
Traumatic injury of condyloid process of mandible. THOMA, K. H. New England J. Med. *218:*63–71, Jan 13, '38
Multiple fractures of lower jaw associated with left temporomaxillary luxation; surgical and prosthetic therapy; case. LEVY, AND MOATTI. Tunisie med. *32:*175–179, May '38
Traumatic injury of condyloid process of mandible. THOMA, K. H. Am. J. Orthodontics *24:*774–790, Aug '38
Modern therapy of collum fractures of lower jaw. BØE, H. W. Med. rev., Bergen *55:*627–639, Dec '38
Question of need for resecting basculated condyle in subcondylar fractures (jaw). BERCHER, J. Rev. de stomatol. *41:*196–197, March '39
Fractures of neck of maxillary condyle, with special reference to therapy; cases. DUFOURMENTEL, L. AND DARCISSAC, M. Bull. et mem. Soc. d. chirurgiens de Paris *31:*72–96, '39
Fracture of both condyles of lower jaw; case. CABALLOL Y DE VERA, F. Rev. san. mil., Habana *4:*63–65, Jan-March '40
Mechanism of temporomaxillary fractures. BECK, H. Ztschr. f. Stomatol. *38:*201–221, March 22, '40
Roentgenograms of mandibular condyle and zygomatic arch in jaw fractures. MCGRAIL, F. R. AND DOHERTY, J. A. Am. J. Roentgenol. *45:*637–639, April '41
Fractures of ramus, condyloid and coronoid processes of mandible. WALKER, D. G. Bull. War Med. *3:*147–148, Nov '42 (abstract)
Fractures of mandibular condyle. BELLINGER, D. H. *et al.* J. Oral Surg. *1:*48–58, Jan '43
Appliance for use in conservative treatment of collum fractures of mandible, in maintaining vertical dimension of jaw, and for

Jaws, Fractures, Mandibular Condyle – Cont.
overcoming spasm of elevator muscles of mandible. GRUBER, L. W. AND LYFORD, J. III. Am. J. Orthodontics (Oral Surg. Sect.) *29:*160–162, March '43
Ankylosis of jaw following luxation fracture; case. JONSSON, S. O. Nord. med. (Hygiea) *18:*609–611, April 10, '43
Orthopedic-prosthetic therapy of fractures of condyloid process of mandible. HED, H. Nord. med. (Hygiea) *18:*789–793, May 8, '43
Fractures of mandibular condyle. BERGER, A. J. Am. Dent. A. *30:*819–833, June 1, '43
Bilateral fracture of condyles of edentulous mandible with marked retrusion displacement; case. BALKIN, S. G. AND WALDRON, C. W., J. Oral Surg. *2:*58–63, Jan '44
Fractures of condyle of mandible. DOHERTY, J. A., U.S. Nav. M. Bull. *42:*641–643, March '44
Fracture-dislocations of mandibular condyle; method for open reduction and internal wiring and one for skeletal fixation, with report of thirty-two cases. THOMA, K. H., J. Oral Surg. *3:*3–59, Jan '45
Fractures of condyle of mandible. THOMA, K. H.; *et al.* Am. J. Orthodontics (Oral Surg. Sect). *31:*220–226, Apr '45
Traumatic lesions of head of mandible; treatment. WAKELEY, C. P. G., M. Press *214:*166–168, Sept 12, '45

Jaws, Fractures, Maxilla

Pseudarthrosis of upper jaw after fracture of Guerin type; case. GÓMEZ, O. Bol. y trab. de la Soc. de cir. de Buenos Aires *12:*393–400, Aug 1, '28
Unusual fracture of superior maxilla; appreciation of incapacity for labor. GOMEZ, O. L. Rev. de especialid. *3:*511–519, Sept '28
Compression treatment of fracture of superior maxilla resulting from blow; case. ZARENKO, P. P. Arch. f. klin. Chir. *153:*161–169, '28
Compound fracture of maxilla. MANGOLD, M. W., U.S. Nav. M. Bull. *27:*132–133, Jan '29
Acromioclavicular dislocation; osteosynthesis by kangaroo tendon; fracture of scapula and maxilla. ROCHER, H. L. AND MALAPLATE. J. de med. de Bordeaux *59:*145, Feb 20, '29
Typical case of Guerin fracture of upper jaw. GIOIA, T. Bol. y trab. de la Soc. de cir. de Buenos Aires *14:*976–982, Nov 26, '30 also: Semana med. *2:*1982–1985, Dec 25, '30
Fractures of upper jaw and malar bone. IVY, R. H. AND CURTIS, L. Ann. Surg. *94:*337–346, Sept '31

Jaws, Fractures, Maxilla – Cont.

Fracture of upper jaw; case. PIERI, G. Valsalva *7:*670-673, Sept '31

Simple treatment of maxillary fracture. ESKES, T. J. Nederl. tijdschr. v. geneesk. *76:*670-674, Feb 13, '32

Use of splints in complicated maxillary fracture. WUHRMANN, H. Schweiz. med. Wchnschr. *62:*767-769, Aug 20, '32

Fracture of maxilla through left optic foramen; reduction with Kingsley splint, with restoration of vision. LANGDON, H. M. Arch. Ophth. *9:*980-981, June '33

Treatment of fractures of maxillary bones. BERETTA, A. Gior. di med. mil. *81:*952-956, Nov '33

Surgical therapy of fractures of upper jaw. JEŽEK, K. Bratisl. lekar. listy *14:*243-246, June '34

Splint for fractures of maxillary bones. MORGAN, W. M., J. Am. Dent. A. *21:*1736-1746, Oct '34

Treatment of maxillary fractures. SIMPSON-SMITH, A. AND GRAVES-MORRIS, W. M. Brit. M. J. *2:*632, Oct 6, '34

Fracture of upper jaw; unusual case. MELCHIOR, M. Ztschr. f. Stomatol. *32:*1331-1335, Nov 23, '34

Fractures of upper jaws. ALONSO, J. M. Ann. d'oto-laryng., pp. 1062-1070, Oct '35

Short history of treatment of maxillary fractures. FAIRBANK, L. C. Mil. Surgeon *78:*95-103, Feb '36

Fractures of upper jaw; reduction apparatus with pneumatic cushion. HAMON, J. Rev. de stomatol. *38:*518-521, July '36

Late examination of fractures of upper jaw. LINK, K. H. Zentralbl. f. Chir. *64:*467-469, Feb 20, '37

Treatment of fracture of upper jaw. BLAIR, V. P.; *et al.* Surgery *1:*748-760, May '37

Fractures of upper jaw; treatment. NEUWIRT, F. AND SIMSA, J. Casop. lek. cesk. *76:*1182-1188, July 2, '37

Role of sympathetic in maxillary fractures. DECHAUME, M. Presse med. *46:*714-715, May 4, '38

Technic of reduction of fracture of upper jaw; case. THEODORESCO, D. AND CRISTODULO. Rev. de chir., Bucuresti *41:*496-499, July-Aug '38

Late reduction of fracture of upper jaw. RUSPA, F. Stomatol. ital. *1:*122-130, Feb '39

Therapy of maxillary fractures. BELTRAMI, G. Marseille-med. *1:*32-37, Jan 15, '40

Fractures of maxilla. RICHISON, F. A., J. Am. Dent. A. *27:*558-563, April '40

Management of fractures of maxilla. DAVIDSON, J. B. AND BROWN, A. M. Mil. Surgeon *87:*26-42, July '40

Incomplete fractures of upper maxilla and their sinusal complications. DECHAUME, M. Presse med. *48:*627-628, July 31-Aug 3, '40

New devices for reduction of maxillary fractures. WOODWARD, C. M. Mil. Surgeon *87:*525-531, Dec '40

Therapy of maxillary fractures according to Ivy. BAKHMUTOVA, E. A. Sovet. med. (no. 4) *4:*38-39, '40

Choice of apparatus for reduction and bandaging in maxillary fractures. PONROY, AND PSAUME. Rev. de stomatol. *41:*782-789, '40

Maxillary fractures in relation to dentistry. FRONGIA, L. Rassegna med. sarda *43:*18-41, Jan-Feb '41

Fractures of maxilla; simplified appliance for craniomaxillary support and fixation. WALDRON, C. W. AND BALKIN, S. G. Surgery *11:*183-194, Feb '42

Treatment of fractures of upper jaw. ERICH, J. B., J. Am. Dent. A. *29:*783-793, May '42

Fractures of maxillary bones. PARKER, D. B. Laryngoscope *52:*365-370, May '42

Compact splints with new fixation method for maxillary fractures. DIMEG, O. Ztschr. f. Stomatol. *40:*485-504, July '42

Fractures of upper jaw, malar bone and zygomatic arch. SCHILDT, E. Nord. med. (Hygiea) *16:*3700-3705, Dec 26, '42

Maxillary fractures. PARKER, D. B., J. Oral Surg. *1:*122-130, April '43

Maxillary fractures. STEVENSON, W. B. Am. J. Orthodontics *29:*331-332, June '43

Applicances and attachments for treatment of upper jaw fractures. CRAWFORD, M. J. U.S. Nav. M. Bull. *41:*1151-1157, July '43

Review of 215 fractures of maxillae. HALLAM, J. W. Brit. Dent. J. *76:*181-182, April 6, '44

Simplified method of treatment of maxillary fractures (use of cap splint). MACGREGOR, A. B. Brit. Dent. J. *76:*239-241, May 5, '44

Maxillary forceps in fractures. GORDON, S. Lancet *2:*80, July 15, '44

Maxillary fracture appliance of new principle and design. JOHNSTON, B. AND TITZE, L. O. Hosp. Corps Quart. (no. 6) *17:*137-139, Nov '44

Fractures of upper jaw; 150 cases in overseas maxillofacial center. CLARK, H. B. JR. J. Oral Surg. *3:*286-303, Oct '45

Reduction of complete transverse fracture of edentulous maxilla. STEVENSON, H. N. AND TUOTI, F. A., U.S. Nav. M. Bull. *45:*910-913, Nov '45

Fractures of maxilla. GONZALEZ ULLOA, M.

Jaws, Fractures, Maxilla – Cont.
Vida nueva *56:*175–182, Dec '45
Use of cheek wires in treatment of fractures of maxilla. HOLLAND, N. W. A. Brit. Dent. J. *79:*333–340, Dec 21, '45

Jaws, Fractures, Non-Union of (See also Jaws, Bone Grafts to)

Treatment of nonunion of fractures of mandible by free autogenous bone-grafts. RISDON, F., J.A.M.A. *79:*297–299, July 22, '22
Ununited fracture of mandible. COUGHLIN, W. T., S. Clin. N. America *2:*1609–1626, Dec '22 (illus.)
Ununited fracture of lower jaw with or without loss of bone. ALBEE, F. H., S. Clin. N. America *3:*301–341, April '23 (illus.)
Surgery of jaw in ununited fractures and defects from operation. SUDECK. Deutsche med. Wchnschr. *53:*47, Jan 1, '27
Late surgical complications of fracture of mandible. GILLIES, H. AND MCINDOE, A. H. Brit. M. J. *2:*1060–1063, Dec 9, '33
Ununited fractures of symphysis of mandible. HUBINGER, H. L. Mil. Surgeon *91:*320–324, Sept '42
Nonunion in fracture of mandible, with report of case. SKINNER, H. L. AND ROBINSON, R. L., J. Oral Surg. *1:*162–167, April '43
Alcohol block in delayed consolidation of maxillary fractures. BELSKAYA, V. M. Khirurgiya, no. 7, pp. 46–49, '44
Failure of union in mandibular fracture and its successful nonsurgical treatment. LAZANSKY, J. P. AND WUEHRMANN, A. H. Am. J. Orthodontics (Oral Surg. Sect.) *32:*182–183, March '46
Delayed union of mandibular fractures. CASHMAN, C. J., J. Oral Surg. *4:*166–171, April '46

Jaws, Fractures, Spontaneous

Spontaneous fractures of lower jaw. HOFER, O. Arch. f. klin. Chir. *140:*141–162, '26
Spontaneous fractures of lower jaw; cases. ROCCIA, B. Minerva med. (pt. 1) *9:*701–708, May 12, '29
Osteomyelitis of lower jaw with spontaneous fracture in hereditary syphilitic; case. PACAUD, H. E. L. AND BERGERET, P. M. Rev. de stomatol. *32:*785–790, Oct '30
Hemiatrophy of face complicated by spontaneous fracture of jaw; case. ROCCIA, B. Stomatol. *35:*448–458, July '37
Pathogenesis, therapy and prophylaxis of spontaneous fractures of lower jaw. PRASOL, F. I. Novy khir. arkhiv *40:*414–425, '38

Jaws, Fractures, Spontaneous – Cont.
Fixation of pathologic fractures of mandible. BOURGOYNE, J. R. Am. J. Orthodontics (Oral Surg. Sect). *31:*492–500, Aug '45

Jaws, Fractures, Teamwork

Role of orthodontist and general practitioner in treatment of jaw fractures. RISK, P. A. J. Am. Dent. A. *28:*884–894, June '41
Oral surgeon, prosthodontist and orthopedist as team in difficult fractures of jaw. GRUNEWALD, A. H., U.S. Nav. M. Bull. *41:*157–167, Jan '43

Jaws, Gunshot Injuries (See also War Injuries, Jaws)

Two wounds resulting from firearms, with multiple lesions of jaw bones. CATANIA, V. Stomatol. *31:*179–200, Feb '33
Gunshot fracture of mandible; case. WEISENGREEN, H. H. Am. J. Surg. *39:*133–134, Jan '38
Gunshot wounds of jaws. GANZER, H. Ztschr. f. artztl. Fortbild. *36:*641–646, Nov 1, '39
Compound fracture of mandible due to gunshot wound. CAL, G. AND CAMBGIAGGI, J. E. Rev. san. mil., Buenos Aires *43:*873–875, June '44

Jaws, Infection

Arthroplasty of jaw, with some general remarks on local infection and on formation of new joints. NEFF, J. M. Surg., Gynec. and Obst. *33:*8, July '21
Chronic deep infection of jaws. COLYER, S. Lancet *1:*175–176, Jan 28, '22
Course and treatment of simple osteomyelitis of jaws. BLAIR, V. P. AND BROWN, J. B., S. Clin. N. America *5:*1413–1436, Oct '25
Osteomyelitis of mandible, etiology, treatment and results. FENTON, R. A., J. Iowa M. Soc. *15:*560–562, Oct '25
Total necrosis of mandible from acute osteomyelitis. TORRACA, L. Arch. ital. di chir. *12:*653–672, '25
Diagnosis and treatment of acute and chronic osteomyelitis of mandible and maxilla. MEAD, S. V. Internat. J. Orthodontia *14:*321–340, April '28
Traumatic infection of lower jaw with fracture; necrosing osteitis; operation; regeneration; case. MAUREL, G. AND MARMASSE, A. Rev. odont. *49:*341–357, May '28
Surgical treatment of case of acute osteomyelitis of mandible. MEAD, S. V. Internat. J. Orthondontia *14:*416–424, May '28
Diagnosis and treatment of chronic osteo-

Jaws, Infection – Cont.
myelitis of jaws. MEAD, S. V., J. Am. Dent. A. *15:*2272-2286, Dec '28
Osteomyelitis of superior maxilla in infant; surgical treatment. CAVAZZUTTI, A. M. Semana med. *1:*95-96, Jan 10, '29
Subacute osteomyelitis of jaws; cases. LEMAÎTRE, F. AND RUPPE, C. Rev. de stomatol. *31:*129-135, March '29
Acute osteomyelitis of mandible. MALONY, F. C. Am. Dent. Surgeon *49:*159-162, April '29
Osteomyelitis of lower jaw; cases. LAMAITRE, F. AND RUPPE, C. Arch. internat. de laryng. *35:*773-782, July-Aug '29
Osteomyelitis of jaws. SCHAEFER, J. E., J. Am. Dent. A. *16:*2188-2216, Dec '29
Chronic osteomyelitis of jaws; cases. DECHAUME. Rev. de stomatol. *32:*148-156, March '30
Treatment of acute osteomyelitis of jaws. FITZGERALD, L. M. Dental Cosmos *72:*259-266, March '30
Osteomyelitis of jaws. BLAIR, V. P.; *et al.* J. Missouri M. A. *27:*173-176, April '30
Marginal osteomyelitis of jaws. KIDD, J. D. Lancet *1:*1068, May 17, '30
Osteomyelitis of lower jaw with spontaneous fracture in hereditary syphilitic; case. PACAUD, H. E. L. AND BERGERET, P. M. Rev. de stomatol. *32:*785-790, Oct '30
Osteomyelitis of jaws. BLAIR, V. P. *et al.* Internat. J. Orthodontia *17:*169-175, Feb '31
Osteomyelitis of jaws; cure; case. ROUSSEAU-DECELLE, L. Rev. de stomatol. *33:*86-94, Feb '31
Rare complications in osteomyelitis of lower jaw; Filatov's grafts in defects of oral cavity. STEPANOFF, N. M. Vestnik khir. (nos. 70-71) *24:*233-236, '31
Osteomyelitis of jaws; cases successfully treated by early radical operation. CONNER, W. H., M. Bull. Vet. Admin. *9:*184-186, Oct '32
Case of fractured mandible complicated by infection with Streptothrix. CARLTON, C. H. Tr. M. Soc., London *55:*51-53, '32
Maggot therapy in infected wound of comminuted fracture; case. Jaws. MANZANILLA, M. A. Medicina, Mexico *13:*1-7, Jan 10, '33
Surgical therapy of osteomyelitis of jaws. HESSE, G. Ztschr. f. Stomatol. *31:*359, March 24; 434, April 14, '33
Treatment of suppurative osteomyelitis of mandible. MILTNER, L. J. AND WOLFE, J. J. Surg., Gynec. and Obst. *59:*226-235, Aug '34
Congenital syphilitic osteomyelitis of mandible; 2 analogous cases in sisters. IVY, R. H. AND CURTIS, L. Ann. Surg. *100:*535-538, Sept '34
Osteomyelitis of jaws. BROWN, J. B. AND TUNG, P. C. South. Surgeon *4:*12-26, March '35
Acute osteomyelitis of jaw and its complications. WANAMAKER, F. H. Eye, Ear, Nose and Throat Monthly *14:*56-58, March '35
Acute osteomyelitis of lower jaw. CUTLER, C. W. JR. S. Clin. North America *15:*483-494, April '35
Occurrence and therapy of osteomyelitis of jaw. DJERASSI, J. Ztschr. f. Stomatol. *33:*458-461, April 26, '35
Osteomyelitis of mandible; observations on etiology, pathogenesis and diagnosis. WOLFE, J. J. Chinese M. J. *49:*422-428, May '35
Results of grave inflammations of the jaw and their surgical and orthopedic therapy. LINDEMANN, A. Rev. med. german.-iberoam. *8:*170-176, May-June '35
Osteomyelitis of mandible. CONNER, T., J. Am. Dent. A. *22:*1190-1193, July '35
Osteomyelitis of jaws. BROWN, J. B. AND TUNG, P. C. Internat. J. Orthodontia *22:*69-80, Jan '36
Jaw deformities due to loss of substance of mandible following osteomyelitis. IVY, R. H. AND CURTIS, L. Ann. Surg. *103:*149-152, Jan '36
Fulminating osteomyelitis of mandible with pathologic fracture. FIELD, H. J. AND ACKERMAN, A. A., J. Am. Dent. A. *23:*448-450, March '36
Osteomyelitis of lower jaw, with special reference to therapy. FINOCHIETTO, R. AND TURCO, N. B. Prensa med. argent. *23:*667-681, March 11, '36
Radical treatment for chronic osteomyelitis of jaws. LYONS, D. C., J. Am. Dent. A. *23:*1092-1095, June '36
Osteomyelitis of mandible; surgical therapy. DE SANSON, R. D. Rev. oto-laring. de Sao Paulo *4:*1297-1318, Nov-Dec '36
Gangrenous inflammation of nose and upper jaw of uncertain etiology; 2 cases. JOISTEN, E. Ztschr. f. Hals-, Nasen-u. Ohrenh. *41:*105-128, '36
Grave acute osteomyelitis due to necrosis of dental pulp caused by repeated sport trauma; surgical therapy of case. GIARDINO, G. Riv. di chir. *3:*371-374, July-Aug '37
Therapy of acute invading form of osteomyelitis of lower jaw; author's technic. DARCISSAC, M., J. de med. de Bordeaux *114:*

Jaws, Infection – Cont.

387–408, Oct 30, '37

Osteomyelitis of lower jaw; author's surgical therapy of 3 cases. MARFORT, A. *et al.* Rev. Asoc. med. argent. *51:*386–387, Oct 15, '37

Therapy of osteomyelitis of jaws. DECHAUME, M. Presse med. *46:*265–266, Feb 16, '38

Rational surgical conduct in osteomyelitis of lower jaw; cases. PIAZZA DE ROSENFELD, A. Semana med. *1:*248–249, Feb 3, '38

Nascent iodine in therapy of osteomyelitis of lower jaw. EICHENBERG, S. An. Fac. de med. de Porto Alegre *2:*189–212, July-Sept '40

Mandibular fractures, malocclusion and osteomyelitis. SMITH, G. W. Rocky Mountain M. J. *38:*794–798, Oct '41

Osteomyelitis of jaw; mandibular operation; buccal operation. TURCO N. B. Prensa Med. argent. *30:*2209–2210, Nov 17, '43

Symposium on reparative surgery; osteomyelitis of jaws. BERGER, A., S. Clin. North America *24:*392–403, April '44

Surgery and penicillin in mandibular infection. MOWLEM, R. Brit. M. J. *1:*517–519, April 15, '44

Temporomandibular ankylosis of osteomyelitic origin; case. MAROTTOLI, O. R. AND BRAGAGNOLO, J. Bol. Soc. de cir. de Rosario *11:*194–201, July '44

Spreading osteomyelitis of maxilla (use of surgery and penicillin). HALLBERG, O. E. Minnesota Med. *28:*126–127, Feb '45

Osteomyeltitis of jaw. THOMA, K. H. Am. J. Orthodontics (Oral Surg. Sect.) *31:*235–244, Apr '45

Osteomyelitis of superior maxilla; treatment with penicillin. HIRST, O. C. Arch. Otolaryng. *41:*351–352, May '45

Jaws, Injuries of (See also Jaws)

Injuries to face and jaws. COUGHLIN, W. T. Southwestern Med. *6:*356–359, Oct '22

Injuries to jaws and face; outline of treatment. CLEWER, D., J. Roy. Army M. Corps *48:*286–295, April '27

Injuries of jaw. GUY, W. Brit. Dent. J. *49:*904–909, Aug 15, '28

Jaw injuries. LYONS, D. C. Hygeia *9:*241–244, March '31

Treatment of automobile injuries of face and jaws. KAZANJIAN, V. H., J. Am. Dent. A. *20:*757–773, May '33

Injuries to face and jaws in automobile accidents. KAZANJIAN, V. H. Tr. Am. Acad. Ophth. *38:*275–308, '33

Traumatism of face and jaws with special reference to complications. KAZANJIAN, V. H., J. Am. Dent. A. *21:*1138–1152, July '34

Jaws, Injuries of – Cont.

Injuries of jaws and face in farm laborers. DUBOV, M. D. Sovet. khir., no. 3, pp. 98–102, '35

Industrial injuries of jaw. LINK, K. H. Arch. f. orthop. u. Unfall-Chir. *36:*47–59, '35

Management of injuries of face and jaws, with special reference to common automobile injury. PADGETT, E. C., J. Kansas M. Soc. *38:*240–248, June '37

Injuries of jaws and face among agricultural workers. DUBOV, M. D. Novy khir. arkhiv *38:*378–383, '37

Traumatic lesions of jaws. KOVAL, A. Y. Khirurgiya, no. 12, pp. 41–44, '39

Care of severe injuries of face and jaws. BROWN, J. B. AND McDOWELL, F. Journal-Lancet *60:*260–267, June '40

Care of fresh wounds of face and jaws. UEBERMUTH, H. Arch. f. klin. Chir. *200:*546–552, '40

Severe facial injuries and jaws. PADGETT, E. C. Am. J. Surg. *51:*829–846, March '41

Late care of severe facial injuries. and jaw. PADGETT, E. C. Surg., Gynec. and Obst. *72:*437–452, Feb. (no. 2A) '41 also: Am. J. Orthodontics (Oral Surg. Sect) *27:*190–207, April '41

Maxillary injuries in sport. MATHIS, H. Wien. klin. Wchnschr. *54:*423–427, May 16, '41

Primary care of facial injuries. and jaws. KAZANJIAN, V. H. Surg., Gynec. and Obst. *72:*431–436, Feb (no. 2A) '41

Statistics for years 1936–1940 in clinic for dentistry and maxillary injuries at University of Kiel. TILLMANN, G. Ztschr. f. Stomatol. *40:*61–75, Jan 30, '42

Care of military and civilian injuries of face and jaws. PADGETT, E. C. Am. J. Orthodontics (Oral Surg. Sect.) *28:*213–221, April '42

Trauma to jaw and its sequel. PENALVER, R. Cir. ortop. y traumatol., Habana *11:*73–83, July-Dec '43

Recent advances in treatment of jaw injuries. MACGREGOR, A. B. Proc. Roy. Soc. Med. *38:*201–204, March '45

Plastic and dental prosthetic repair of jaw injuries. GREELEY, P. W., AND POUND, A. E. Illinois M. J. *89:*216–221, May '46

Jaws, Laterognathia (See also Jaws, Deformity; Jaws, Enlarged Condyle; Jaws Miscellaneous; Jaws, Surgery of)

Irreducible deviation of the inferior jaw treated by orthopedic resection of condyle. DUFOURMENTEL, L. Rev. odont. *48:*162–164, April '27

Jaws, Laterognathia—Cont.

Orthopedic problems of lower jaw; with special reference to unilateral shortening. IVY, R. H. AND CURTIS, L., J. Bone and Joint Surg. *10:*645–660, Oct '28

Bicondyloid resection in deviations of lower jaw and prognathism. BOURGUET *et al.* Rev. de stomatol. *33:*715, Dec '31

Subcondyloid osteotomy in therapy of laterognathism of jaw. LANDAIS. Rev. de stomatol. *37:*65–86, Feb '35

Laterally displaced mandible; treatment simplified by aid of splint. LUSSIER, E. F. Internat. J. Orthodontia *22:*139–146, Feb '36

Progressive hypertrophy of half of mandible; case. MELA, B. Boll. e mem. Soc. piemontese di chir. *6:*1070–1087, '36

Rare congenital malformation of right portion of lower and upper jaw (unilateral micrognathia); case. CASTAY. Bull. et mem. Soc. de radiol. med. de France *25:*125–126, Feb '37

Jaws, Micrognathia of

New treatment for undeveloped lower jaw. COUGHLIN, W. T., J. A. M. A. *84:*419–421, Feb 7, '25

Micrognathia. SEIFERT, E. Arch. f. klin. Chir. *135:*726–735, '25

New method of plastic lengthening of mandible in unilateral microgenia and asymmetry of face. LIMBERG, A. A. J. Am. Dent. A. *15:*851–871, May '28

Attempt at treatment of retrognathism; case. DUFOURMENTEL, L. AND DARCISSAC, M. Bull. et mem. Soc. de chir. de Paris *20:*750–753, Nov 2, '28

Treatment of jaw ankylosis and micrognathia. FROMME, A. Beitr. z. klin. Chir. *144:*195–206, '28

The surgical treatment of mandibular atrophy. DUFOURMENTEL, L. Odontologie *67:*582–588, Aug '29

Dangers and treatment of hypotrophy of lower jaw in infants. ROBIN, P. Odontologie *69:*499–505, July '31

Mandibular hypoplasia with atresia of esophagus; case. SOER, J. J. Maandschr. v. kindergeneesk. *1:*309–310, March '32

Micrognathia; suggested treatment for correction in early infancy. DAVIS, A. D. AND DUNN, R. Am. J. Dis. Child. *45:*799–806, April '33

Progressive atrophy of facial bones with complete atrophy of mandible; case. THOMA, K. H., J. Bone and Joint Surg. *15:*494–501, April '33

Glossoptosis in micrognathia; 2 cases. ULLRICH, G. Deutsche med. Wchnschr.

Jaws, Micrognathia of—Cont.

*61:*1033–1036, June 28, '35

Hypoplasia of mandible (micrognathy) with cleft palate; treatment in early infancy by skeletal traction. CALLISTER, A. C. Am. J. Dis. Child. *53:*1057–1059, April '37

Congenital atrophy of lower eyelids, both auricles and lower jaw; case. VAN LINT, A. AND HENNEBERT, P. Bruxelles-med. *17:*1065–1070, May 16, '37

Advancement of receding lower jaw. BABCOCK, W. W. Ann. Surg. *106:*1105–1108, Dec '37

Correction of bird's face (jaw deformity). ESSER, J. F. S. Am. J. Orthodontics *24:*791–794, Aug '38

Receding chin; plastic reconstruction. SAFIAN, J. New York State J. Med. *38:*1331–1335, Oct 15, '38

Factors which control treatment of dwarfed mandible. McCOY, J. D. Am. J. Orthodontics *25:*850–864, Sept '39

Retruded chins; correction by plastic operation. NEW, G. B. AND ERICH, J. B. J. A. M. A. *115:*186–191, July 20, '40

Implantation of bone in chin in severe case of mandibular retraction; case. LUSSIER, E. F. AND DAVIS, A. D. Am. J. Orthodontics *27:*267–274, May '41

Hypoplasia of mandible; report of case, with resume of literature and suggestions for modified form of treatment. LLEWELLYN, J. S. AND BIGGS, A. D. Am. J. Dis. Child. *65:*440–444, March '43

Severe retrusion of mandible treated by buccal inlay and dental prosthesis. FICKLING, B. W. Proc. Roy. Soc. Med. *37:*7–10, Nov '43

Micrognathia; paladon prosthesis in case. MALBEC, E. F., J. Internat. Coll. Surgeons *9:*412–415, May–June '46 Bol. y trab., Acad. argent. de cir. *30:*151–156, May 15 '46

Jaws, Miscellaneous

Some mouth and jaw conditions responsible for defects in speech. GREENE, J. S. Med. Red. *100:*8, July 2, '21

Benign bony enlargement of condyloid process of mandible. IVY, R. H. Ann. Surg. *85:*27–30, Jan '27

Plastic surgery after bicondyloid resection of mandible; case. CABROL. Rev. de stomatol. *33:*720–722, Dec '31

Development of human lower jaw; study of development of fistula of lower lip. SICHER, H. AND POHL, L. Ztschr. f. Stomatol. *32:*552–560, May 25, '34

Progressive hypertrophy of half of mandible;

Jaws, Miscellaneous – Cont.

case. MELA, B. Boll. e mem. Soc. piemontese di chir. *6:*1070–1087, '36

Mandibular "obtusism"; surgical therapy; case. SANTY, P. AND PONT, A. Lyon chir. *35:*727–728, Nov–Dec '38

Reeducation of speech in ablation of lower jaw; case. FREUD, E. Rev. franc. de phoniatrie *7:*119–121, April '39

Effect of abnormalities of occlusion upon temporomandibular joint and associated structures. SCHUYLER, C. H. Proc. Dent. Centen. Celeb., pp. 303–308, '40

Brief review of anatomy, blood and nerve supply of mouth, jaws and teeth. GREEN, R. M. Am. J. Orthodontics (Oral Surg. Sect.) *27:*469–471, Sept '41

Neuromuscular control of mandible. SEAVER, E. P. JR. Am. J. Orthodontics *28:*222–229, April '42

Histologic studies on reaction of alveolar bone to vitallium implants (preliminary report). BERNIER, J. L., AND CANBY, C. P. J. Am. Dent. A. *30:*188–197, Feb 1, '43

Total bimaxillary necrobiosis; case with recovery after surgical therapy aided especially by extract of calf jawbone (vaduril). SOLDANO, H. A. O. Prensa med. argent. *30:*1945–1947, Oct 6, '43

Unusual metastatic manifestations of breast cancer: metastasis to mandible, with report of 5 cases. ADAIR, F. E. AND HERRMANN, J. B. Surg. Gynec. and Obst. *83:*289–295, Sept. '46

Jaws, Osteomyelitis: See Jaws, Infections

Jaws, Prognathism

Surgical treatment of prognathism. DUFOURMENTEL, L. Presse med. *29:*235, March 23, '21 abstr: J.A.M.A. *76:*1284, April 30, '21

Surgical treatment of prognathism. KRUEGER, R. Arch. f. klin. Chir. *118:*261–274, '21 (illus.)

Successful operation for prognathism. ALEMAN, O. Hygiea *84:*239–240, March 31, '22 (illus.)

Surgical treatment of prognathism and of lack of articulation of incisors. ZAHRADNÏČEK, J. Cas. lek. cesk. *62:*1361–1368, Dec. 15, '23

Prognathism from anthropological and orthodontic view-point. OPPENHEIM, A. Ztschr. f. Stomatol. *25:*518–573, June '27

Underdeveloped maxilla and overdeveloped mandible; case report. MCCARTER, W. A. Internat. Orthodont. Cong. *1:*483, '27 also: Internat. J. Orthodontia *13:*625, July '27

Bilateral resection of mandible for prognathism. SCHULTZ, L. Surg., Gynec. and Obst. *45:*379–384, Sept '27

Surgical-orthodontic correction of macromandibular deformity; case report. WILLETT, R. C. Internat. Orthodont. Cong. *1:*458–473, '27

Hapsburg family type of prognathism. BROEKMAN, R. W. Tijdschr. v. tandheelk. *35:*174–186, March 15, '28

Surgical correction of prognathism of lower jaw. PICHLER, H. Wien. klin. Wchnschr. *41:*1333–1334, Sept. 20, '28

Operative treatment of prognathism based on cephalometry. HENSCHEN, C. AND SCHWARZ, R. Chirurg *1:*56–66, Nov. 20, '28

Prognathism from anthropological and orthodontic view-points. OPPENHEIM, A. Dental Cosmos *70:*1092–1110, Nov '28

Prognathism. GRAFFI, E. Riv. di antropol. *28:*123–163, '28–'29

Surgical correction of prognathism; 7 cases. SCHMIDT, G. Deutsche Ztschr. f. Chir. *215:*212–225, '29

Method of determination of prognathism. SERGI, G. Riv. di antropol. *28:*271–279, '28–'29

Surgical correction of prognathism; 2 cases. WYMER, I. Deutsche Ztschr. f. Chir. *215:*226–233, '29

Prognathism from anthropological and orthodontic view-points. OPPENHEIM, A. Ztschr. f. Stomatol. *28:*313–339, April '30 also: Dental Cosmos *72:*645, June; 736, July '30

Orthopedic resection of condyles in treatment of prognathism. DUFOURMENTEL, L. Rev. de stomatol. *32:*519–527, June '30

Treatment of prognathism by orthopedic excision of condyles. DUFOURMENTEL, L. Schweiz. Monatschr. f. Zahnh. *40:*673–681, Nov '30

Surgical and prosthetic interference for correction of excessive protrusion of maxilla. WOODWARD, C. M. Dental Digest *37:*213–218, April '31

Bicondyloid resection in deviations of lower jaw and prognathism. BOURGUET, *et al.* Rev. de stomatol. *33:*715, Dec '31

Prognathism; surgical therapy. KRETZ, R. Deutsche Zahnh., Hft. 81, pp. 28–49, '31

Nonsurgical treatment of habitual dislocation of lower jaw especially when accompanied by prognathism. REICHENBACH, E. Deutsche Ztschr. f. Chir. *231:*470–476, '31

Surgical correction of marked prognathism of the mandible. REINER, J. Internat. J. Orthodontia *18:*271–281, March '32

Unilateral and bilateral condyloid resections in deviations of lower jaw and prognath-

Jaws, Prognathism –Cont.
ism. DUFOURMENTEL, L. AND DARCISSAC, M. Rev. de stomatol. *34:*340–346, June '32
Surgical treatment of prognathism. KAZANJIAN, V. H. Internat. J. Orthodontia *18:*1224–1239, Nov '32
Prognathism and its surgical treatment. KALLAY, J. Lijecn. vjes. *54:*30–33, '32
New surgical procedure for correction of prognathism. PETTIT, J. A. AND WALRATH, C. H., J.A.M.A. *99:*1917–1919, Dec. 3, '32
Prognathism; study in development of face. TODD, T. W., J. Am. Dent. A. *19:*2172–2184, Dec '32
Surgical therapy of prognathism; Jaboulay method of bicondyloid resection; Lane method in section of ascending branch of lower jaw. BOURGUET, M. Rev. de stomatol. *35:*61–79, Feb '33
Care after surgical therapy in prognathism of lower jaw. PONROY, AND CABROL. Rev. de stomatol. *35:*89–95, Feb '33
Superior incisive prognathism; prevention and therapy. MOURGEON, A. Presse med. *41:*1353–1354, Aug. 30, '33
Prognathism of lower jaw treated by bicondylar resection; 2 cases. DUFOURMENTEL, L. AND DARCISSAC, M. Bull. et mem. Soc. d. chirurgiens de Paris *25:*583–589, Oct. 20, '33
Prognathism and its surgical correction by new procedure. PETTIT, J. A. AND WALRATH, C. H., J. Am. Dent. A. *21:*125–129, Jan '34
Surgical therapy of mandibular deformities; prognathism and laterognathism. LANDAIS, P. Rev. de stomatol. *36:*98–103, Feb '34
Surgical therapy of prognathism; bicondyloid resection and osteotomy of ascending branch of lower jaw; critical study. LANDAIS. Rev. de stomatol. *36:*209–227, April '34
Surgical therapy of prognathism; bicondyloid resection and section of ascending branch of lower jaw; cases. BOURGUET, J. Rev. de stomatol. *37:*152–169, March '35
Mandibular macrognathia and its correction. THEODORESCU, D. Rev. de chir., Bucuresti *38:*22–34, March-April '35
Surgical correction of prognathism. SOIVIO, A. Duodecim *51:*702–712, '35
Esthetic surgery in lower jaw prognathism. BOURGUET, J. Monde med., Paris *46:*81–88, Feb. 1, '36
Surgical therapy of prognathism. SCHMUZIGER, P. Helvet. med. acta *3:*834–839, Dec '36
Surgical and orthopedic correction of congenital and false (traumatic) prognathism; 3 cases. MAUREL, G. Rev. de chir. structive, pp. 5–23, March '37
Surgical correction of mandibular protraction and retraction. (also fractures of ascending rami). HENSEL, G. C. Surgery *2:*92–119, July '37 also: Internat. J. Orthodontia *23:*814–839, Aug '37
Surgical correction of prognathism. PETTIT, J. A., J. Am. Dent. A. *24:*1837–1842, Nov '37
Resection for prognathism of upper jaw; case. ESSER, J. F. S. An. de cir. *3:*364–368, Dec '37
Surgical therapy of prognathism. DE QUERVAIN, F. Chirurg *10:*256–260, April 15, '38
Surgico-orthopedic correction of congenital and of false traumatic prognathism. MAUREL, G. Chir. plast. *4:*63, April–June; 97, July-Sept; 171, Oct–Dec '38
Dufourmentel operation in therapy of prognathism of lower jaw. JULLIARD, C. Schweiz. med. Wchnschr. *68:*609–611, May 21, '38
Progenia (anteposition of lower jaw); surgical therapy. FINOCHIETTO, R. AND MARINO, H. Prensa med. argent. *25:*1087–1092, June 8, '38
Surgical therapy of prognathism. FOGED, J. Hospitalstid. (Supp., Festskr. Bisp. Hosp.) *81:*55–83, '38
Operative treatment of progeni in Sweden. RAGNELL, A. Rev. de chir. structive *8:*187–191, '38
Therapy of superior pro-alveolism (superior alveolar prognathism). TSOUCANELIS, A. Stomatol., Athenes *1:*77–90, '38
Surgical therapy of mordex apertus and of prognathism. GINESTET, G. Rev. de stomatol. *41:*4–17, Jan '39
Tailor-made chin retractor (for mandibular protrusion). STOFT, W. E. Am. J. Orthodontics *25:*461–466, May '39
Prognathism of lower jaw; etiology, pathogenesis, prophylaxis and therapy. HOFFER, O. Stomatol. ital. *1:*657–664, July '39
Surgical therapy of prognathism of lower jaw. ILABACA LEON, L. Rev. med. de Chile *67:*1352–1355, Dec '39
Correction of severe mandibular protrusion by osteotomy of rami and orthodontics. WEISS, B. Am. J. Orthodontics *27:*1–8, Jan '41
Surgical therapy of prognathism; case. IVANISSEVICH, O. AND GARAY, P. M. Bol. y trab., Acad. argent. de cir. *25:*554–559, June 25, '41
Surgical correction of mandibular prognath-

Jaws, Prognathism – Cont.
ism. NEW, G. B. AND ERICH, J. B. Am. J. Surg. *53:*2-12, July '41
Surgical treatment of prognathism; case. HOOK, F. R. AND TAYLOR, R. W., U. S. Nav. M. Bull. *40:*157-158, Jan '42
Surgical correction of mandibular prognathism. KITLOWSKI, E. A. Ann. Surg. *115:*647-653, April '42
Therapy of progenism by Lindemann method. MARINO, H. Arq. de cir. clin. e exper. *6:*301-306, April-June '42
Kostecka operation for prognathism; follow up studies on 21 cases. ULLIK, R. Ztschr. f. Stomatol. *40:*255, April 10, '42; 294, April 24, '42
Repair of prognathic and retruded jaws. NEWMAN, J. Am. J. Surg. *58:*35-39, Oct '42
Tratamiento quirúrgico del promentonismo-mandibulo-megalia y otras deformidades mandibulares. Tesis. University Press, Buenos Aires, 1943
Differential analysis and treatment of 2 cases of apparent mandibular protraction. JAY, J. Am. J. Orthodontics *29:*127-133, March '43
Prognathism – open bite deformity; case. DINGMAN, R. O., J. Oral Surg. *2:*64-70, Jan '44
Osteotomy of rami of lower jaw (for prognathism). TRAYNHAM, W. H. JR. Bull. U. S. Army M. Dept. (no. 74) pp. 115-118, March '44
Bilateral osteotomy of rami for marked protrusion of lower jaw; case. TRAYNHAM, W. H. JR. J. Am. Dent. A. *31:*1025-1029, Aug. 1, '44
Surgical correction of mandibular prognathism; improved method. DINGMAN, R. O. Am. J. Orthodontics (Oral Surg. Sect.) *30:*683-692, Nov '44
Progenism of jaw; surgical therapy. FINOCHIETTO, R. AND MARINO, H. Bol. Acad. nac. de med. de Buenos Aires pp. 528-537 Sept-Nov '45
Correction of abnormal mandibular protrusion by intraoral operation. MOOSE, S. M. J. Oral Surg. *3:*304-310, Oct '45
Protrusion of mandible; case. IVY, R. H. AND CURTIS, L. Am. J. Orthodontics (Oral Surg. Sect.) *31:*666-675, Nov '45
Maxillofacial prognathism; surgical therapy of case. BERTOLA, V. J. AND MOREYRA BERNAN, L. Bol. y. trab., Soc. de cir. de Cordoba *6:*59-75, '45
Surgical treatment of mandibular prognathism. WALDRON, C. W.; *et al.* J. Oral Surg. *4:*61-85, Jan '46
Osteotomy for correction of mandibular protrusion. LLOYD, R. S. Am. J. Orthodontics (Oral Surg. Sect.) *32:*445-455, Jul '46
Bilateral osteotomy of mandibular rami for correction of prognathism in edentulous mouth; case. PETERSON, R. G., J. Oral Surg. *4:*203-206, July '46

Jaws, Surgery of
Cosmetic incision of soft parts for temporary division of lower jaw. KÖNIG, F. Zentralbl. f. Chir. *49:*362-363, March 18, '22 (illus.)
Contributions to plastic surgery of jaws and palate. LUXENBURGER, A. Deutsche Ztschr. f. Chir. *172:*384-396, '22 (illus.)
Reconstruction of jaw and chin. EISELSBERG, A. AND PICHLER, H. Arch. f. klin. Chir. *122:*337-369, '22 (illus.) abstr: J.A.M.A. *80:*732, March 10, '23
Some diseases of mouth, jaws, and face surgically treated. FEDERSPIEL, M. N. Journal-Lancet *43:*267-275, June 1; 297-301, June 15, '23
Reconstruction of mandible after resection. PICHLER, H. Wien. klin. Wchnschr. *36:*465-466, June 28, '23
Method of operative attack for central lesions of lower jaw. BLOODGOOD, J. C. New York State J. Med. *24:*379-385, March 21, '24
New method of resection of upper maxillary with lower facial flap. LAUWERS, E. E. Surg., Gynec. and Obst. *39:*499-502, Oct '24
Resection of lower jaw in acromegaly. BLESSING, G. AND ROST, F. Zentralbl. f. Chir. *52:*855-857, April 18, '25
Surgical treatment of acquired deformities of mouth and jaws. IVY, R. H. Dental Cosmos *69:*137-142, Feb '27
Surgical-orthopedical removal of deformations of jaws. BRUHN, C. Internat. J. Orthodontia *13:*65-79, '27
Surgical-orthopedical removal of deformations of jaws. BRUHN, C. Internat. Orthodont. Cong. *1:*245-259, '27
Method of plastic resection of lower jaw. GLUSCHKOV, P. Vestnik khir. (no. 30) *10:*67-70, '27
Reconstructive surgery of jaw necrosis, and after excision. ROSENTHAL, W. Arch. f. klin. Chir. *147:*248-284, '27
Surgical-orthodontic correction of macromandibular deformity; case report. WILLETT, R. C. Internat. Orthodont. Cong. *1:*458-473, '27
New method of plastic lengthening of mandible in unilateral microgenia and asymmetry of face. LIMBERG, A. A., J. Am. Dent. A. *15:*851-871, May '28

Jaws, Surgery of–Cont.

Resection under local anesthesia of lower part of jaw, with integrity of nasal membrane; case. HEYNINX, A. Ann. d. mal. de l'oreille, du larynx *47:*996, Nov '28

Construction of parts of jaw to be used after plastic surgery. HIRSCH, C. AND KIRCHHOFF, W. Acta oto-laryng. *12:*488–496, '28

Use of gnathotome in resection of lower jaw. WOLF, H. Zentralbl. f. Chir. *56:*452–455, Feb. 23, '29

Facial deformities caused by abnormalities of jaw; operative and dental treatment; cases. POHL, L. Rev. odont. *50:*134–150, April '29

Plastic and reconstructive surgery of face and jaws. IVY, R. H. Virginia M. Monthly *56:*174–180, June '29

Plastic covering of defects of jaws. LINDEMANN, A. Chirurg *1:*817–829, Aug. 1, '29

Restoration of width of lower jaw following loss of both condyles; case. TRAUNER, F. Zentralbl. f. Chir. *56:*1986–1989, Aug. 10, '29

Entire resection of lower jaw. VILLARD. Lyon chir. *26:*618–621, Aug–Sept '29

Surgico-orthopedic treatment of congenital and acquired jaw defects. BRUHN, C. Stomatol. *27:*905–926, Nov '29

Pathogenesis, diagnosis and treatment of jaw deformities. GASPARINI, C. Stomatol. *27:*950–963, Nov '29

Osteotome for resection of mandible. ROCCIA, B. Minerva med. (pt. 2) *9:*700, Nov. 3, '29

Jaw deformity; treatment by orthopedic resection of condyles. DUFOURMENTEL, L. Bull. et mem. soc. de chir. de Paris *21:*424–431, '29

Extra-oral splinting to support jaw after resection of middle portion of lower jaw. STAHNKE, E. Deutsche Ztschr. f. Chir. *215:*234–239, '29

Operations suitable for defects and lack of continuity of inferior maxilla. SUDECK, P. AND RIEDER, W. Beitr. z. klin. Chir. *146:*493–518, '29

Plastic surgery of jaw deformities and mouth. WASSMUND, M. Med. Welt *4:*327, March 8, '30

Osteoplastic resection of both alveolar processes according to Kocher. NIKOLSKY, A. M. Ann. Otol., Rhin. and Laryng. *39:*701–719, Sept '30

Jaw resection; plastic and prosthetic surgery. AXHAUSEN, G. Fortschr. d. Zahnh. *6:*917–952, Nov '30

Unusual cases of jaw surgery. SONNTAG. Deutsche Ztschr. f. Chir. *223:*236–260, '30

Plastic repair after operation on upper jaw.

Jaws, Surgery of–Cont.

WOODMAN, E. M. Proc. Roy. Soc. med. (Sect. Laryng.) *24:*11–14, Feb '31 also: J. Laryng. and Otol. *46:*405–409, June '31

Operative treatment of losses of substance of mandible, with special reference to fixation of edentulous fragments. IVY, R. H. AND CURTIS, L. Surg., Gynec. and Obst. *52:*849–854, April '31

Technic in plastic surgery of upper jaw. MAUREL, G. Rev. de chir. plastique, pp. 32–62, April '31

Plastic surgery in loss of substance of alveolar border of incisive region of upper jaw; case. DARCISSAC, M. Bull. et mem. Soc. d. chirurgiens de Paris *23:*507–511, July 3, '31

Maintenance of facial form after removal of right half of mandible. ANDERSON, G. M. Internat. J. Orthodontia *17:*860–864, Sept '31

Spontaneous reconstruction of lower maxilla after total surgical removal; case. ALONSO, J. M. AND QUINTELA, U. An. de oto-rino-laring. d. Uruguay *1:*72–76, '31

Substitute for implantation prosthesis and for osteoplasty in resection of jaw. SPANIER, F. Deutsche Ztschr. f. Chir. *231:*456–469, '31

Tasks and accomplishments of maxillary surgery. AXHAUSEN, G. Deutsche med. Wchnschr. *58:*401–404, March 11, '32

"Open bite"; surgical and prosthetic treatment. SCHMIDT, G. AND REICHENBACH, E. Deutsche Ztschr. f. Chir. *237:*167–176, '32

Lateral expansion of upper jaw in case of marked atresia in patient 30 years old; amelioration of nasal permeability. DARCISSAC, M. Bull. et mem. Soc. d. chirurgiens de Paris *25:*296–300, May 5, '33

Orthopedic measures in surgical reconstruction of defects of lower jaw. BABITSKAYA, E. E. Ortop. i. travmatol. (no. 3) *7:*50–58, '33

Resection and reconstruction of mandible; 2 cases. DOBRZANIECKI, W. Arch. ital. di chir. *35:*207–217, '33

Plastic operation of mandibular region by Clapp's method; case. TSUNODA, E. Mitt. a. d. med. Akad. zu Kioto *8:*131–132, '33

Osteoplastic repair of congenital and acquired defects of lower jaw. GÖBELL, R. Arch. di chir. inf. *1:*111–125, Jan '34

Differential diagnosis of certain types of facial deformities and their treatment (including jaws). ROSE, J. E. Internat. J. Orthodontia *20:*222–228, March '34

Surgery of jaws; review of literature. SEIFERT, E. Chirurg *6:*489–493, July, 1, '34

New method for plastic correction of defects of lower jaw and chin. DZBANOVSKIY, V. P.

Jaws, Surgery of—Cont.
Sovet. khir. (no. 4) *7:*654–661, '34
Osteoplastic restoration of traumatic defects of lower jaw. KYANDSKIY, A. A. Sovet. khir. (nos. 3–4) *6:*339–349, '34
Therapy and prophylaxis of maxillary deformities by immobilization with monobloc. LASSERRE, C. AND MARRONEAUD, P. Arch. franco-belges de chir. *35:*131–134, Feb '36
Surgical correction of jaw deformities and their relationship to orthodontia. KAZANJIAN, V. H. Internat. J. Orthodontia *22:*259–282, March '36
Vertical osteotomy for lengthening lower jaw which has been raised and shortened as result of old trauma: case. HOFER, O. Ztschr. f. Stomatol. *34:*826–830, July–Aug. '36
Orthopedic plate in therapy of jaw deformities. JARDENI, J. AND AUERBACH, H. Ztschr. f. Stomatol. *35:*1019–1028, Aug. 13, '37
Advancement of receding lower jaw. BABCOCK, W. W. Ann. Surg. *106:*1105–1108, Dec '37
Corrective osteotomy of maxilla. AXHAUSEN, G. Deutsche Ztschr. f. Chir. *248:*515–522, '37
Correction of acquired asymmetry caused by osteomyelitis of lower jaw. AXHAUSEN, G. Deutsche Ztschr. f. Chir. *248:*533–551, '37
The Surgery of Oral and Facial Diseases and Malformations, by GEORGE V. I. BROWN. Lea & Febiger, Phila., 1938
Surgical Diseases of the Mouth and Jaws, by EARL C. PADGETT. W. B. Saunders Co., Phila., 1938
Jaw deformities, surgical indications and technic. JORGE, J. M. AND PIAZZA DE ROSENFELD, A. Bol. y trab. de la Soc. de cir. de Buenos Aires *22:*43–48, April 20, '38
Facial asymmetry; plastic surgery (including jaws). ZENO, L. An. de cir. *4:*134–136, June '38
Mandibular "obtusism"; surgical therapy; case. SANTY, P. AND PONT, A. Lyon chir. *35:*727–728, Nov–Dec '38
Deformation of lower jaw corrected by surgical intervention and prosthesis. THEODORESCO, D. Rev. de chir., Bucuresti *41:*926–930, Nov–Dec '38
Therapy of pseudoarthrosis with loss of substance of inferior maxilla. ROUVILLOIS, H. Arch. ital. di chir. *54:*351–356, '38
Jaw reconstruction. KAZANJIAN, V. H. Am. J. Surg. *43:*249–267, Feb '39
Bone ligation and suture in relation to functional defects and tissue losses in mandible; collective review. WEISENGREEN, H.

Jaws, Surgery of—Cont.
H. Internat. Abstr. Surg. *68:*450–460, '39; in Surg., Gynec. and Obst., May '39
Surgical indications and technic in jaw deformities. JORGE, J. M. AND PIAZZA DE ROSENFELD, A. Semana med. *1:*1221–1242, June 1, '39
Surgical treatment of mandibular deformities. SMITH, A. E. AND JOHNSON, J. B., J. Am. Dent. A. *27:*689–700, May '40
Mandibular resection. HAYNEN, A. S. Am. J. Orthodontics *26:*793–796, Aug '40
Resection of lower jaw by oral route. BERTOLA, V. J. Prensa med. argent. *28:*323–327, Feb. 5, '41
Secondary operations for structural and functional correction of post-traumatic deformities of jaws. WOLF, H. Ztschr. f. Stomatol. *39:*157–184, March 14, '41
Technic of surgical mobilization of lower jaw. KOCHEV, K. N. Sovet. med. (nos. 17–18) *5:*33, '41
Osteoplasty of mandibular arch and complementary surgical prosthesis. SOUZA CUNHA, A. Arq. de cir. clin. e exper. *6:*587–593, April–June '42
Function of lower jaw following partial resection. YOUNG, F. Surgery *11:*966–982, June '42
Function of lower jaw following partial resection. YOUNG, F. Am. J. Orthodontics (Oral Surg. Sect) *28:*581–598, Oct '42
Resection of mandible; method that simplified and overcomes defects of cases reported in the past. PEARSON, W. H. Am. J. Orthodontics *29:*141–147, March '43
Surgery of face, mouth and jaws, 30 years ago and now. IVY, R. H., J. Oral Surg. *1:*95–99, April '43
Y-shaped osteotomy for correction of open bite in adults. THOMA, K. H. Surg., Gynec. and Obst. *77:*40–50, July '43 also: Am. J. Orthodontics (Oral Surg. Sect) *29:*465–479, Sept. '43
Correction of jaw deformities. RAGNELL, A. Acta chir., Scandinav. *88:*344–352, '43
Restorative surgery of lower jaw. REINHARD, W. Deutsche Ztschr. f. Chir. *257:*407, '43
Reconstruction of lower jaw; case. MOORE, A. T. AND COOK, W. C., J. South Carolina M. A. *40:*73–75, April '44
Extensive resections of mandible; collaboration with odontologist in temporary functional therapy. JORGE, J. M. AND VIVONE, R. A. Bol. y trab., Acad. argent. de cir. *28:*134–152, May 3, '44
Study of surgical technic in cadaver; hemiresection of lower jaw. MARISCAL, E. Prensa med. mex. *9:*59–61, May 15, '44
Osteotomy for correction of mandibular mal-

Jaws, Surgery of—Cont.
rotation of developmental origin. DINGMAN, R. O., J. Oral Surg. *2:*239–259, July '44
Comparison of 2 methods of treating apertognathia. THOMA, K. H. Am. J. Orthodontics (Oral Surg. Sect.) *31:*248–259, Apr '45
Spontaneous regeneration of bone following excision of section of mandible. KAZANJIAN, V. H. Am. J. Orthodontics (Oral Surg. Sect.) *32:*242–248, April '46
Surgical treatment of jaw deformity. THOMA, K. H. Am. J. Orthodontics *32:*333–339, June '46

Jaws, Surgery, Anesthesia for
Blocking nerve for lower jaw surgery. DE VRIES, J. J. Nederlandsch Tijdschr. f. Geneesk. *1:*197–200, Jan 14, '22
New methods of anesthetizing jaws and face. LINDEMANN, A. Narkose u. Anaesth. *1:*3–16, Jan 15, '28
Local anesthesia with procaine hydrochloride as anesthesia of choice in operations on upper maxilla. AUBRY, M. Presse med. *43:*592, April 10, '35
Selection of anesthetic in cases of jaw fracture. WEISENGREEN, H. H., J. Bone and Joint Surg. *18:*1005–1007, Oct '36
Personal reminiscences of men and methods in field of prosthesis in jaw surgery. STOPPANY, G. A. Ztschr. f. Stomatol. *35:*525–531, April 23, '37
Anesthesia of inferior maxillary nerve by way of zygoma in jaw surgery. POPESCU, G. AND PRICORIU, S. Rev. san. mil., Bucuresti *37:*873–875, Oct '38
Aid to prosthetic restorations of maxilla after excision. WALKER, D. G. Lancet *1:*1209–1210, May 27, '39
General anesthesia for jaw casualties. HAUGEN, F. P. Mil. Surgeon *89:*70–80, July '41
Anatomic considerations in local anesthesia of jaws. PHILLIPS, W. H., J. Oral Surg. *1:*112–121, April '43
Anesthesia in fractures of jaws. SHACKLETON, R. P. W. Lancet *1:*396–398, March 25, '44
Anesthetic management in reconstructive surgery of mandible. PAPPER, E. M. AND ROVENSTINE, E. A. Am. J. Orthodontics (Oral Surg. Sect.) *32:*433–438, Jul '46

Jaws, Surgery, Prostheses in
Present status of prostheses, etc., for jaws. SCHROEDER, H. Arch. f. klin. Chir. *118:*275–297, '21 (illus.)
Prosthetic restoration of portion of mandible, including temporo-mandibular articulation on one side. MITCHELL, V. E. Am. J. Surg. *38:*274–276, Nov '24
Prosthetic appliance in jaw surgery. EISELSBERG, A. Internat. Clin. *4:*220, Dec '26
Dental prosthesis after resection of lower jaw. GREVE, K. Beitr. z. klin. Chir. *142:*747–752, '28
Prosthesis in excision of mandible. LAMÉRIS, H. J. Nederl. Tijdschr. V. Geneesk. *1:*244–246, Jan 12, '29
Resection, plastic surgery and prosthesis of jaw. PICHLER, H. Fortschr. d. Zahnheilk. *5:*1027–1043, Nov '29
Prosthetic treatment of defects of mandible following unilateral exarticulation of mandible for adamantinoma; case. BERGENFELDT, E. Acta chir. Scandinav. *64:*473–492, '29
Immediate maxillary prosthesis. PONT, A. Rev. de chir. plastique, pp. 264–270, Jan '32

Jaws, Tumors of (See also Jaws, Cancer of; Jaws, Surgery of)
Mandibular tumors. PETTIT, J. A., J.A.M.A. *77:*1881, Dec 10, '21
Clinical history of tumors of face and jaws as guide to their correct diagnosis and proper treatment. GATCH, W. D., J. Indiana M. A. *15:*251–255, Aug '22
Adamantinoma of jaw recurs after 45 years. PORZELT, W. Arch. f. klin. Chir. *130:*142–150, '24
Congenital tumors of maxilla; report of case with operation. CUTLER, G. D. AND ROCK, J. C. Boston M. and S. J. *192:*1001–1002, May 21, '25
Tumors and cysts of jaws as disclosed by roentgenograms, and their treatment. IVY, R. H., J. Am. Dent. A. *14:*2272–2280, Dec '27
Value and dangers of radium therapy of tumors of jaws; osteonecrosis; cases. VALLEBONA, A. Minerva med. (pt. 2) *8:*422–440, Aug 25, '28
Operative treatment of tumors of lower jaw. BREITKOPF, E. Beitr. z. klin. Chir. *142:*738–741, '28
Adamantinoma (14 cases with illustrations). SIMMONS, C. C. Tr. Am. S. A. *46:*383–394, '28
Adamantinoma of lower jaw treated with surgical diathermy. NEW, G. B., S. Clin. N. Amer. *9:*80–82, Feb '29
Tumors of jaws and mouth. KAZANJIAN, V. H. New England J. Med. *201:*1200–1201, Dec 12, '29
Prosthetic treatment of defects of mandible following unilateral exarticulation of man-

Jaws, Tumors of–Cont.
dible for adamantinoma; case. BERGENFELDT, E. Acta chir. Scandinav. *64:*473–492, '29
Tumors of lips, tongue, gums and alveolar processes. MITTERMAIER, R. Handb. d. Hals-, Nasen-, Ohrenh. *5:*582–618, '29
Odontoma of jaw complicated by surgical fractures; 2 cases. L'HIRONDEL. Rev. de stomatol. *35:*125–139, March '33
Tumor of upper jaw; surgical therapy with plastic repair; 2 cases. PAVLOVSKY, A. J. AND DI PIETRO, A. Bol. y trab. de la Soc. de cir. de Buenos Aires *19:*384–391, June 26, '35
Adamantinoma of jaw. IVY, R. H. AND CURTIS, L. Ann. Surg. *105:*125–134, Jan '37
Tumors of the jaws (and mouth). IVY, R. H. Delaware State M. J. *10:*147–152, July '38
Retromaxillary tonsillar cysts; removal by predigastric incision; case. LERICHE, R. Lyon chir. *35:*574–575, Sept–Oct '38
Jaw tumors; collective review. THOMA, K. H. Internat. Abstr. Surg. *67:*522–545, '38; in Surg., Gynec. and Obst., Dec '38
Reconstruction of lower jaw after resection for neoplasm (epulis); medico-odontologic collaboration; case. VILLARAN, C. AND SALAS N., E. An. clin. quir. *1:*40–49, May '39
Bone transplantation in major resections of lower jaw; case of osteofibroma. AXHAUSEN, G. Chirurg *12:*442–444, Aug 1, '40
Author's method of plastic reconstruction of palate after removal of huge osteoma of upper jaw. PIERANTONI, L. Plast. chir. *1:*109–112, '40
Treatment of benign tumors of jaw. KAZANJIAN, V. H., J. Am. Dent. A. *28:*208–223, Feb '41
Cystic tumors of jaws; conservative and 2 stage operative procedures to prevent deformity and loss of useful teeth. WALDRON, C. W. Am. J. Orthodontics (Oral Surg. Sect.) *27:*313–322, June '41
Primary bone grafting in resected tumor of mandible. STROMBECK, J. P. Acta chir. Scandinav. *86:*554–560, '42
Tumors of maxilla. ARMBRECHT, E. C. AND APPLE, C. W. Am. J. Orthodontics (Oral Surg. Sect.) *29:*60–64, Jan '43
Surgical therapy of adamantinoma of lower jaw; functional and esthetic problem; 3 cases. JORGE, J. M. AND MEALLA, E. S. Bol. y trab., Acad. argent. de cir. *27:*33–47, April 14, '43
Ameloblastoma (adamantinoma) of mandible; case report. DINGMAN, R. O., J. Oral Surg. *2:*175–181, April '44
Tumors of jaw with report of cases. FERNANDEZ, B. Rev. med. de Rosario *34:*340, April; 442, May '44
Case reports of jaw tumors from files of Registry of Dental and Oral Pathology sponsored by American Dental Association. GOLDMAN, H. M. Am. J. Orthodontics (Oral Surg. Sect.) *30:*265–314, May '44
Tumors of jaws. THOMA, K. H. *et al.* Am. J. Orthodontics (Oral Surg. Sect.) *31:*260–288, Apr '45
Adamantinoma of lower jaw; surgical therapy with immediate prosthesis; case. RONCORONI, E. J. AND CICCHETTI, J. N. Bol. Soc. de cir. de Rosario *12:*27–40, May '45
Embedment of vitallium mandibular prosthesis as integral part of operation for removal of adamantinoma. WINTER, L. *et al.* Am. J. Surg. *69:*318–324, Sept '45
Osteomas of upper jaw. LUSCHER, E. Schweiz. med. Wchnschr. *75:*924–927, Oct 20, '45
Clinic of Dental Department of Massachusetts General Hospital and Department of Oral Surgery of Harvard School of Dental Medicine; miscellaneous case reports of jaw tumors. THOMA, K. H.; *et al.* Am. J. Orthodontics (Oral Surg. Sect.) *31:*619–636, Oct '45
Surgery of mandible; ameloblastoma. BYARS, L. T. AND SARNAT, B. G. Surg., Gynec. and Obst. *81:*575–584, Nov '45
Surgery of mandible; ameloblastoma. BYARS, L. T. AND SARNAT, B. G. Am. J. Orthodontics (Oral Surg. Sect.) *32:*34–46, Jan '46
Myxomatous tumor simulating dentigerous cyst of jaw. MILLHON, J. A. AND PARKHILL, E. M., J. Oral Surg. *4:*129–132, April '46
Ameloblastoma of mandible; case. WILLIAMS, P. E. AND MARCKS, K. M., J. Oral Surg. *4:*133–144, April '46
Fibrin foam and thrombin as used in surgical removal of large fibromyxoma of mandible. WEINER, L. AND WALD, A. H., J. Am. Dent. A. *33:*731–735, June 1, '46

JAY, J.: Differential analysis and treatment of 2 cases of apparent mandibular protraction. Am. J. Orthodontics *29:*127–133, March '43
JAYES, P. H.: Burns of hands. Brit. J. Indust. Med. *1:*106–109, April '44
JEAN, G. (see VILLECHAISE) May '27
JEANBRAU, E.: Technic for operative treatment of perineoscrotal hypospadias. J. d'urol. *18:*405–409, Nov '24
JEANDELIZE, P. AND THOMAS, C.: Total symblepharon after enucleation of eye; remaking of orbital cavity for ocular prosthesis by means of dermo-epidermic graft; case. Bull.

Soc. d'opht. de Paris *50:*272, May '38
JEANDELIZE, P. (see HUSSON, A.) Jan '24
JEANNE: Volkmann's ischemic contracture. Bull. Acad. de med., Par. *92:*1266–1270, Nov 25, '24 abstr: J.A.M.A. *84:*235, Jan 17, '25
JEANNE, H. (see GOURDON, R.) May '31
JEANNENEY, G.: Pathogenesis of traumatic shock. Progres med. *36:*425, Sept 10, '21
JEANNENEY, G.: Treatment of traumatic shock. Arch. franco-belges de chir. *26:*157–175, Feb '23
JEANNENEY, G.: Prognosis of traumatic shock. Paris med. *13:*129–133, Feb 10, '23 abstr: J.A.M.A. *80:*1737, June 9, '23
JEANNENEY, G. AND JUSTIN-BESANCON, L.: New therapeutic methods in traumatic shock. Mem. Acad. de chir. *66:*337–358, March 13–April 3, '40
JEANNENEY, G. AND JUSTIN-BESANCON, L.: States of shock; form for clinical and therapeutic records of military cases. Presse med. *48:*423–424, April 17–20, '40
JEANNENEY, G. AND SOUBIRAN: Continuous bath medicated with tannin in burns. J. de med. de Bordeaux *115:*153–157, Aug 20–27, '38
JEANNENEY, G. (see GUYOT, J.) May '21
JEANNENEY, G. (see GUYOT, J.) Aug '21
JEFFREYS, F. E.: Prosthetic appliance for war injury (maxillofacial injuries). U. S. Nav. M. Bull. *42:*711–714, March '44
JELINEK, K.: Detoxin (glutathione preparation) in therapy of toxinemia in children following burns. Dermat. Wchnschr. *104:*692–695, June 5, '37
JELINEK, V. J.: Fractures of mandible and superior maxilla in time of peace. Voj.-san. glasnik *6:*513–539, '35
JELLIFFE, S. E.: Dupuytren's contracture and the unconscious; preliminary statement of problem. Internat. Clin. *3:*184–199, Sept '31
JELLINEK, S.: Pathology of electric current "burns." Wien. klin. Wchnschr. *34:*239, May 19, '21
JELLINEK, S.: Injury of skin from electric current. Wien. klin. Wchnschr. *36:*157–158, March 1, '23
JELLINEK, S.: Character of skin changes from electric burns. Arch. f. Dermat. u. Syph. *148:*433–440, '25
JELSMA, F.: Finger splint that will not impair hand function. Am. J. Surg. *50:*571–572, Dec '40
JENKINS, H. P. Plastic surgery of face and head. S. Clin. North America *21:*37–53, Feb '41
JENKINS, H. B.: Salivary fistula of submaxillary gland following excision of thyroglossal cyst. Am. J. Surg. *70:*118–120, Oct '45
JENKINS, H. P.: Subtotal replacement of skin of face for actinodermatitis due to roentgenotherapy with multiple areas of squamous cell carcinoma. Ann. Surg. *122:*1042–1048, Dec '45
JENKINS, H. P.: Pedicle grafts from arm for reconstructions about face. S. Clin. North America *26:*20–32, Feb '46
JENKINS, H. P. *et al*: Sulfathiazole (sulfonamide) ointment; further studies on preparation and use. (in burns) Surg. Gynec. and Obst. *80:*85–96, Jan '45
JENNEY, J. (see SHEEHAN, J. E.) Jan '46
JENNEY, J. A.: Modification of plasma fixation method (Sano) by use of bobbinet and mirrow attachment. Am. J. Surg. *67:*3–7, Jan '45
JENNINGS, J. E.: Simple operation for relief of mild types of entropion and ectropion of lower lid. J.A.M.A. *83:*1329–1331, Oct 25, '24
JENNINGS, W. K.: Burn therapy. S. Clin. North America *18:*145–159, Feb '38
JENNY, F.: Chronic edema of back of hand; simulated sequel of trauma for purpose of collecting insurance. Praxis *31:*365–367, June 25, '42
JENSEN, E.: Volkmann's ischemic paralysis. Ugesk. f. Laeger *87:*729–734, Aug 20, '25
JENSEN, E.: Volkmann's ischemic paralysis. Ugesk. f. Laeger *87:*756–759, Aug 27, '25
JENSEN, W.: Epithelization of granulating and fresh wounds with skin from blisters. Zentralbl. f. Chir. *67:*1399–1401, July 27, '40
JENSEN, W. P. (see CONNOLLY, E. A.) July '39
JENTZER, A.: Combined surgical and radium treatment of carcinoma of superior maxilla; case. Schweiz. med. Wchnschr. *58:*659–662, June 30, '28
JENTZER, A.: Therapy of so-called varicose syndrome, with special reference to sympathectomy and grafts. Rev. med. de la Suisse Rom. *53:*482–532, June 25, '33
JENTZER, A.: Surgery of peripheral nerves, including therapy of neurinoma. Schweiz. med. Wchnschr. *68:*1162–1164, Oct 15, '38
JENTZER, A.: Recovery of function with autoplastic bone graft and tubular skin flaps. Schweiz. med. Wchnschr. *73:*1023, Aug 21, '43
JENTZER, A.: Suture of peripheral nerves. Confinia neurol. *6:*257–269, '45
JEPSON, P. N.: Transformation of middle finger into thumb; report of case. Minnesota Med. *8:*552, Aug '25
JEPSON, P. N.: Ischemic contracture; experimental study. Ann. Surg. *84:*785–795, Dec '26
JEŘÁBEK, V.: Progress in therapy of suppurative diseases of hand. Casop. lek. cesk. *74:*241–244, March 1, '35
JEREZ TABLADA, G.: Congenital velopalatine

fissure, with special reference to therapy. Rev. mex. de cir., ginec. y cancer *9:*273–279, July '41
JERVEY, J. W. JR.: Congenital occlusion of both anterior nares. Ann. Otol., Rhin. and Laryng. *53:*182–184, March '44
JESSAMAN, L. W.: Treatment of nasal fractures. New England J. Med. *200:*753–756, April 11, '29
JESSOP, W. H. G. (see DEVENISH, E. A.) Oct '40
JEŽEK, K.: Surgical therapy of fractures of upper jaw. Bratisl. lekar. listy *14:*243–246, June '34
JIANU, A. AND POPESCU, C.: Edema of arms following radical amputation of breast. Rev. de chir., Bucuresti *43:*469–480, July–Aug '40
JIANO, I.: Surgical therapy of elephantiasis. Cong. internat. de med. trop. et d'hyg., Compt. rend. (1928) *3:*353–357, '31
JIANU, I.: Autografts of phalanges of toes in reconstruction of fingers. Rev. de chir., Bucuresti *37:*761–763, Sept–Dec '34
JIANU, I.: Phalangeal autografts in restoration of fingers. Rozhl. v chir. a gynaek. (čast chir.) *14:*122–124, '35
JIANU, I. AND BUZOIANU, G.: Cervical sympathectomy in traumatic peripheral facial paralysis. Bull. et mem. Soc. med. d. hop. de Bucarest *9:*35–39, March '27
JIANU, I. AND BUZOIANU, G.: Study of nerve grafts with case of heterografts of sciatic. Lyon chir. *24:*625–641, Nov–Dec '27
JIANU, I. AND BUZOIANU, G.: Leriche's operation for traumatic peripheral facial paralysis as compared with other operative procedures. Lyon chir. *25:*10–21, Jan–Feb '28
JIANU, I.; DUMITRESCU, D. AND DIMITRIU, A.: Surgical therapy of ankylosis of temporomaxillary joint; case. Spitalul *52:*433–434, Nov '32
JIANO, J. (see JIANU, I.)
JIMÉNEZ LÓPEZ, C. AND RIBÓN, V.: Reconstruction of lower eyelid. Semana med. *2:*832, Oct. 19, '22 (illus.)
JIMENEZ PLA, A.: Fracture of lower jaw. Medica, Matanzas *3:*1–6, Jan–Feb '44
JINNAKA, S.: Experimental artificial neurotization of paralyzed muscle. Mitt. a. d. med. Fakult. d. k. Univ. zu Tokyo *25:*367–441, '21
JIRÁSEK, A.: Surgery of articulation of jaws; 3 cases. Casop. lek. cesk. *73:*169–170, Feb 16, '34
JOACHIM: Dental prosthesis in relation to plastic and reconstructive surgery of face. Rev. de chir. structive *8:*212–215, '38
JOBE, M. C. (see SPIES, J. W. *et al.*) March '34
JOBSON, G. B.: Correction of hump or saddle bridge nose. Arch. Otolaryng. *2:*45–49, July '25
JOBSON, G. B.: Surgical correction of cleft lip and palate. Arch. Otolaryng. *6:*434–445, Nov '27
JOBSON, G. B.: Plastic surgery of face and harelip and nose and cleft palate. Atlantic M. J. *31:*716–723, July '28
JOCHIMS, J.: Technical improvements on Glatzel's mirror for examination of width of nose. Ztschr. f. Kinderh. *60:*147–153, '38
JOHANSSON, H. (see CAMITZ, H. *et al*) 1934
JOHANSSON, S.: Traumatic shock. Nord. med. tidskr. *16:*1767–1771, Nov 12, '38
JOHNER, T.: Joining dorsal aponeurosis and tendons in therapy of injuries to extensor tendons of fingers; cases. Schweiz. med. Wchnschr. *68:*111–113, Jan 29, '38
JOHNS, F. S.: Congenital defect of abdominal wall in newborn (gastroschisis). Tr. South. S. A. (1945) *57:*413–426, '46
JOHNS, F. S.: Congenital defect of abdominal wall in newborn (gastroschisis). Ann. Surg. *123:*886–899, May '46
JOHNS, A. H. G.: Patent branchial cleft. Brit. M. J. *1:*1047, June 7, '30
JOHNSON, B.: Retractor for intra-oral operations. Lancet *2:*1052, Nov 10, '34
JOHNSON, C. A.: Ephedrine sulphate in acute shock from trauma or hemorrhage; clinical use. J.A.M.A. *94:*1388–1390, May 3, '30
JOHNSON, C. A.: Neo-synephrin hydrochloride in acute shock from trauma or hemorrhage. Surg., Gynec. and Obst. *63:*35–42, July '36
JOHNSON, C. A.: Neo-synephrin hydrochloride in treatment of hypotension and shock from trauma or hemorrhage. Surg., Gynec. and Obst. *65:*458–463, Oct '37
JOHNSON, C. C.: Problems in reconstructive surgery. Nebraska M. J. *10:*435–438, Nov '25
JOHNSON, F. M: Certain difficult problems in treatment of carcinoma of lower jaw. Radiology *5:*280–285, Oct '25
JOHNSON, F. M.: Development of carcinoma in scar tissue following burns. Ann. Surg. *83:*165–169, Feb '26
JOHNSON, F. M. (see QUICK, D.) Sept '22
JOHNSON, G. N.: Cutaneous burns. J. Maine M. A. *30:*91–93, May '39
JOHNSON, G. S. AND BLALOCK, A.: Effects of loss of whole blood, of blood plasma and of red blood cells in experimental shock. Arch. Surg. *22:*626–637, April '31
JOHNSON, G. S. AND LIGHT, R. A.: Treatment of congenital hemangiomata of skin. Ann. Surg. *117:*134–139, Jan '43
JOHNSON, G. S. (see BLALOCK, A. *et al*) 1931
JOHNSON, G. S. (see BLALOCK, A. *et al*) Dec '31
JOHNSON, H. F. (see SCHROCK, R. D.) March '34
JOHNSON, J. A.: Branchial cysts and fistulae; report of 5 cases. Minnesota Med. *9:*514–517, Sept '26

JOHNSON, J. B. (see SMITH, A. E.) July '37
JOHNSON, J. B. (see SMITH, A. E.) July '39
JOHNSON, J. B. (see SMITH, A. E.) May '40
JOHNSON, J. R.: Eighty-three percent body surface burn with recovery. U.S. Nav. M. Bull. *45:*163–165, July '45
JOHNSON, L. W.: Hand plastic. U. S. Nav. M. Bull. *15:*399, April '21
JOHNSON, L. W.: Notes on plastic surgery. U. S. Nav. M. Bull. *18:*214–219, Feb '23 (illus.)
JOHNSON, L. W.: Plastic surgery of supra-orbital region. J. A. M. A. *86:*14–16, Jan 2, '26
JOHNSON, L. W.: Early treatment of facial injuries. U. S. Nav. M. Bull. *24:*508–515, July '26
JOHNSON, L. W.: Cases illustrating maxillofacial and plastic surgery. U. S. Nav. M. Bull. *26:*843–861, Oct '28
JOHNSON, L. W.: Plastic surgery in relation to armed forces; past, present and future (Kober lecture). Mil. Surgeon *79:*90–102, Aug '36
JOHNSON, M. R.: Nasal obstruction and impairment of hearing; 46 cases of submucous resection with audiometric studies. Arch. Otolaryng. *33:*536–549, April '41
JOHNSON, M. R.: Symposium on reparative surgery; depressed fracture of orbital rim, with report of case treated by reduction through Caldwell-Luc approach, with maintenance of position of fragment by water-filled balloon. S. Clin. North America *24:*340–347, April '44
JOHNSON, S. C.: Treatment by radiation and gold seed implantation in metastatic nodes in neck from cancer of lips. Am. J. Cancer *15:*254–261, Jan '31
JOHNSON, V. E.: Early care of depressed fractures of malar bone. J. M. Soc. New Jersey *38:*113–117, March '41
JOHNSTON, B. AND TITZE, L. O.: Maxillary fracture appliance of new principle and design. Hosp. Corps Quart. (no. 6) *17:*137–139, Nov '44
JOHNSTON, C. C.: Burn therapy in forward areas. Bull. U. S. Army M. Dept. (no. 76) pp. 109–113, May '44
JOHNSTONE, G. G.: Acrocephalo-syndactylism; case. Lancet *2:*15–16, July 2, '32
JOHNSTONE, I. L.: Deficiency of malar bones with defect of lower eyelids. Brit. J. Ophth. *27:*21–23, Jan '43
JOHNSTONE, J. G.: Results of tendon transplantation for intrinsic hand paralysis (Ney's operation). J. Bone and Joint Surg. *5:*278–283, April '23 (illus.)
JOHNSTON, L. R.: Severe facial injury of unusual etiology; case. J. Oral Surg. *1:*179–181, April '43
JOHNSTON, W.: Simple knot for intranasal sutures. Ann. Otol., Rhin. and Laryng. *32:*201–209, March '23 (illus.)
JOHNSTON, W. H.: Cysts of floor of mouth. Tr. Am. Laryng., Rhin. and Otol. Soc. *48:*83–96, '42
JOHNSTON, W. M.: Surgical operations (on burns) with the Navy Medical Corps in South Pacific. Am. J. Surg. *60:*313–318, June '43
JOHOW, A. AND URZUA, R.: Labiomentothoracic synechia due to burn; plastic repair of case. Rev. med. de Chile *68:*1482–1487, Nov '40

Joint Transplantation

Joint transplantations and arthroplasty. LEXER, E. Surg., Gynec. and Obst. *40:*782–809, June '25

JOISTEN, E.: Gangrenous inflammation of nose and upper jaw of uncertain etiology; 2 cases. Ztschr. f. Hals-, Nasen-u. Ohrenh. *41:*105–128, '36
JOLY, M.: Diathermocoagulation as only therapy for nevocarcinoma. Bull. et mem. Soc. de med. de Paris *140:*70–71, Jan. 25, '36
JOLY, P. AND DE VADDER, A.: Tannin; practical application in burns. Presse med. *48:*171–172, Feb 7–10, '40
JONAS: Therapy of jaw fractures. Deutsche med. Wchnschr. *53:*2203, Dec 23, '27
JONAS, A. D.: Creosote burns. J. Indust. Hyg. and Toxicol. *25:*418–420, Nov '43
JONAS, A. F.: Fate of bone graft. Wisconsin M. J. *20:*407–410, Jan '22
JONES, A. C.: Use of diathermy in submucous resection. Tr. Am. Laryng., Rhin. and Otol. Soc. *48:*331–332, '42
JONES, A. C.: Use of diathermy in submucous resection. Arch. Otolaryng. *38:*445–446, Nov '43
JONES, A. R.: Dupuytren's contracture. M. Press *206:*14–16, July 2, '41
JONES, D. H.: After treatment of submucous resection. New York M. J. *115:*494, April 19, '22
JONES, F. W. AND WEN, I. C.: Preauricular fistula; development of external ear. J. Anat. *68:*525–533, July '34
JONES, FREDERIC W.: *The Principles of Anatomy as Seen in the Hand.* Baillière, Tindall and Cox, London, 1942
JONES, H. T.: Contracture from burn with extensive ulcer in popliteal space; excision and full-thickness skin graft. S. Clin. N. America *7:*1447–1449, Dec '27
JONES, H. T.: Congenital web fingers; addition to Didot's operation for syndactylism. S. Clin. N. Amer. *7:*1450–1452, Dec '27
JONES, H. T.: Loss of tendo achillis and overlying soft tissues by trauma; plastic reconstruction. S. Clin. N. Amer. *7:*1452–1456, Dec '27
JONES, H. T.: Contracture of axilla from burns;

3 cases. Minnesota Med. *11:*210–214, April '28

JONES, H. T.: Anemic ulcer of leg treated by pedicle graft. S. Clin. N. Amer. *9:*933–935, Aug '29

JONES, H. T.: Replacement of scar over tibia and os calcis by tube pedicle transplant from abdomen. S. Clin. N. Amer. *9:*936–938, Aug '29

JONES, H. T.: Contracture of right hand treated by full-thickness skin grafts. S. Clin. N. Amer. *9:*939–940, Aug '29

JONES, H. T.: Z plastic or web splitting operation for relief of scar contractures of extremities. Surg., Gynec. and Obst. *58:*178–182, Feb '34

JONES, H. W. *et al*: Discussion of use of blood and plasma transfusion in shock; method of influencing pH and prothrombin of plasma, intra-marrow injection of concentrated plasma. Delaware State M. J. *14:*137–146, June '42

JONES, H. W. AND ROBERTS, R. E.: Rare type of congenital club hand. J. Anat. *60:*146–147, Jan '26

JONES, H. W. *et al:* 4× concentrated blood plasma intrasternally in treatment of shock. Tr. A. Am. Physicians *57:*88–92, '42

JONES, J. F. X. AND KEEGAN, A. P.: Notes on group of burn cases. M. J. and Record *119:*86–87, Jan 16, '24

JONES, M. F.: Technic for submucous resection, with presentation of membrane elevator. Laryngoscope *35:*406–408, May '25

JONES, O. W. JR. (see NAFFZIGER, H. C.) Aug '32

JONES, R.: Volkmann's contracture, with special reference to treatment. Brit. M. J. *2:*639–642, Oct 13, '28

JONES, R. A.: Method for closing traumatic defect of finger tip (graft). Am. J. Surg. *55:*326–338, Feb '42

JONES, R. M.: Shock; new needle for treatment by sternal infusion. Surg., Gynec. and Obst. *76:*587–588, May '43

JONES, R. M.: Successful suture of finger flexor tendon. Lancet *2:*111, July 22, '44

JONES, R. R. JR.: Management of old contractures of hand resulting from third degree burns. Surgery *7:*264–275, Feb '40 also: North Carolina M. J. *1:*148–152, March '40

JONES, R. R., JR.: Management of old contractures of upper extremity resulting from third degree burns. South. M. J. *34:*789–797, Aug '41

JONES, R. W.: Repair of skull defects by new pedicle bone-graft operation. Brit. M. J. *1:*780–781, May 6, '33

JONES, S. G.: Volkmann contracture. J. Bone and Joint Surg. *17:*649–655, July '35

JONES, W. C.: Prophylaxis of surgical shock. South. M. J. *28:*166–168, Feb '35

JONES, W. I.: Fractures of edentulous mandible. J. Am. Dent. A. *26:*1360–1361, Aug '39

JONESCO-SISESTI, N.: Pathogenesis of facial hemiatrophy. Vol. jubilaire, Parhon, pp. 219–232, '34

DE JONGH, E.: Simple plastic procedure of fingers for conserving bony tissue and forming soft tissue pad (after traumatic amputation). Am. J. Surg. *57:*346–347, Aug '42

JONSSON, S. O.: Ankylosis of jaw following luxation fracture; case. Nord. med. (Hygiea) *18:*609–611, April 10, '43

JOPLIN, R. O.: Newer burn treatment. Kentucky M. J. *36:*134–136, April '38

JORDAN, C. E.: Headpiece for face wounds and fractures. U. S. Nav. M. Bull. *45:*330, Aug '45

JORDAN, H. E. (see MORTON, C. B.) April '35

JORDAN, W. R. (see WARTHEN, H. J.) July '43

JORDE, A. AND MAGNUSSON, R.: Contracture therapy, extension treatment of shoulder joint. Nord. med. (Hygiea) *11:*2471–2474, Aug 30, '41

JORGE: Volkmann's contracture, case. Boll. y trab. de la Soc. de cir. *11:*204, June 1, '27

JORGE, J. M.: Volkmann's ischemic contracture. Semana med. *1:*833–842, May 3, '23

JORGE, J. M.: Case of plastic operation including urethra, bladder and vagina. Semana med. *2:*499–502, Sept 13, '23 (illus.)

JORGE, J. M.: Treatment of bilateral case of ankylosis of jaws. Semana med. *2:*711, Sept 15, '27

JORGE, J. M.: Surgical technic in cleft palate. Bol. y trab. de la Soc. de cir. de Buenos Aires *14:*1019–1025, Dec 3, '30

JORGE, J. M.: Results of nasal decortication performed 20 years ago for rhinophyma; case. Bol. y trab. de la Soc. de cir. de Buenos Aires *20:*472–475, July 1, '36

JORGE, J. M. AND MEALLA, E. S.: Internal prosthesis with autotransplant of bone or cartilage. Arq. de cir. clin. e exper. *6:*539–540, April–June '42

JORGE, J. M. AND MEALLA, E. S.: Surgical therapy of adamantinoma of lower jaw; functional and esthetic problem; 3 cases. Bol. y trab., Acad. argent. de cir. *27:*33–47, April 14, '43

JORGE, J. M. AND PIAZZA DE ROSENFELD, A.: Jaw deformities, surgical indications and technic. Bol. y trab. de la Soc. de cir. de Buenos Aires *22:*43–48, April 20, '38

JORGE, J. M. AND PIAZZA DE ROSENFELD, A.: Surgical indications and technic in jaw deformities. Semana med. *1:*1221–1242, June 1, '39

JORGE, J. M.; SOTO, M. AND STAJANO, C.: Shock

therapy. Rev. Asoc. med. argent. *55:*182–204, March 15–30, '41
JORGE, J. M. AND VIVONE, R. A.: Extensive resections of mandible; collaboration with odontologist in temporary functional therapy. Bol. y trab., Acad. argent de cir. *28:*134–152, May 3, '44
JORNS, G.: Chronic osteomyelitis of spine as result of injury to thumb; case. Arch. f. orthop. u. Unfall-Chir. *34:*451–457, '34
JORSTAD, L. H.: Tumors of head and neck. J. Missouri M. A. *34:*82–84, March '37
JORSTAD, L. H.: Diagnosis and treatment of cancer of lips. Radiol. Rev. and Mississippi Valley M. J. *59:*63–64, March '37
JORY, P.: Treatment of minor degrees of nasal obstruction; deflections of septum. Lancet *1:*147–148, Jan 21, '28
JOSA, L.: Fistulas of first branchial arch. Zentralbl. f. Chir. *63:*1760–1763, July 25, '36
JOSA, L.: Fistulas of first branchial arch. Orvosi hetil. *80:*973–974, Oct 10, '36

Joseph

Reply to article by Joseph on shock therapy. Also, one by Stejskal. SCHÜCK. Zentralbl. f. Chir. *60:*634–635, March 18, '33

JOSEPH. (see LÉCHELLE *et al*) Feb '33
JOSEPH, E.: Intravenous injections of hypertonic solutions in shock. (Comment on Schück's article.) Zentralbl. f. Chir. *59:*2934, Dec 3, '32
JOSEPH, E. S.: Operative treatment of anal stricture (modification of Young operation). Acta med. orient. *4:*312–313, Sept '45
JOSEPH, H.: Reconstruction of eyelids. Beitr. z. klin. Chir. *131:*52–65, '24
JOSEPH, J.: Plastic operation on protruding cheek. Deutsche med. Wchnschr. *47:*287, March 17, '21
JOSEPH, J.: Partial and total rhinoneoplasty. Klin. Wchnschr. *1:*678–680, April 1, '22 (illus.)
JOSEPH, J.: Surgery of hypertrophic breast (mastopexy). Deutsche med. Wchnschr. *51:*1103–1105, July 3, '25 abstr: J. A. M. A. *85:*641, Aug 22, '25
JOSEPH, JACQUES: *Eine Nasenplastik, ausgeführt in Lokalanesthesie. Kinegrammata medica.* (In German, English, French, Italian, Russian, and Spanish text). Pp. 14. G. Stilke, Berlin, 1927
JOSEPH, J.: Plastic surgery of simple and hypertrophied pendulous breasts. Deutsche med. Wchnschr. *53:*1853–1854, Oct 28, '27
JOSEPH, JACQUES: *Nasenplastik und sonstige Gesichtsplastik. Nebst einem Anhang über Mammaplastik.* C. Kabitsch, Leipzig, 1928
JOSEPH, J.: Joseph's improvement of his technic for plastic surgery of pendulous cheeks (meloplasty). Deutsche med. Wchnschr. *54:*567–568, April 6, '28
JOSEPH, JACQUES: *Nasenplastik und sonstige Gesichtsplastik. Nebst einem Anhang über Mammaplastik und . . . Körperplastik.* C. Kabitsch, Leipzig, 1931

Joseph, Jacques

Example of Joseph nose improvement. DANELIUS, B. Acta oto-laryng. *9:*49–52, '26 (in English).
Surgical correction of syphilitic saddle nose by Joseph operation and Filatov graft; case. REBELO NETO, J. Bol. Soc. de med. e cir. de Sao Paulo *16:*123–130, Dec '32
Joseph operation in plastic repair of bulldog nose; case. OHNO, T. Oto-rhino-laryng. *12:*10, Jan '39
Work of Jacques Joseph (1865–1934), especially in plastic surgery. MARINO, H. Prensa med. argent. *31:*449–450, March 1, '44

DE JOSSELIN DE JONG, R. AND EYKMAN VAN DER KEMP, P. H.: Experimental researches on autotransplantation of bones. Beitr. z. path. Anat. u. z. allg. Path. *79:*268–332, Feb 15, '28
JOSSELYN, R. B.: Radiotherapy in treatment of superficial malignant disease of face. J. Maine M. A. *13:*279–284, June '23 (illus.)

Josserand Operation: See Nove-Josserand Operation; Nove-Josserand-Borchers

JOUAN, E. (see JOUAN, S. *et al*) Sept '33
JOUAN, S.; JOUAN, E. AND SCHTARKMAN: Paraffin therapy of burns produced by heat and cold and for cicatrices. Rev. med. latino-am. *18:*1424–1427, Sept '33
JOUFFRAY: Diathermo-surgical treatment of septal malformations. Rev. d'actinol. *6:*35–39, Jan–Feb '30
JOUVE, P. (see MALLET-GUY, P.) Jan '27
JOVČIĆ, M.: Ischemic Volkmann contracture. Chir. narz. ruchu *6:*249–265, Sept '33
JOYCE, J. L.: Results of new operation for substitution of thumb. Brit. J. Surg. *16:*362–369, Jan '29
JOYCE, T. M.; MENNE, F. R. AND ZELLER, W. E. Unusual tumors of cervical region. Arch. Surg. *42:*338–370, Feb '41
JOYNER, A. (see MISCALL, L.) Sept '44
JOYNT, R. L.: New method of cutting large skin grafts (instrument). Lancet *1:*816, April 21, '28
JOYNT, R. L.: Subcutaneous plates and knives for cutting large Thiersch grafts for plastic surgery. Irish J. M. Sc., pp. 700–702, Nov '28

JUARISTI, V.: Remote results of plastic operations. Arch. espan. de pediat. *9:*385–391, July '25 abstr: J. A. M. A. *85:*1262, Oct 17, '25
JUARISTI, V.: Absence of one nostril. Arch. espan. de pediat. *10:*299–300, May '26
JUARISTI, V.: Volkmann's syndrome; treatment by ramisection. Rev. de chir. *6:*760–765, Dec '27
JUARISTI, V.: Problems of surgical therapy of exstrophy of bladder. Arch. espan. de pediat. *18:*385–390, July '34
JUARISTI, V. AND ARRAIZA, D.: Lesions of fingers and hands secondary to roentgen rays. Progresos de la clinica *35:*301–304, April '27
JUDD, E. S. AND NEW, G. B.: Carcinoma of tongue; general principles involved in operations and results obtained at Mayo Clinic. Surg., Gynec. and Obst. *36:*163–169, Feb '23 (illus.)
JUDD, E. S. AND NEW, G. B.: Surgery of cancer of mouth. Radiology *9:*380–383, Nov '27
JUDD, E. S. AND PHILLIPS, J. R.: Curability of cancer of lips. Proc. Staff Meet., Mayo Clin. *8:*637–640, Oct 18, '33
JUDD, E. S. AND THOMPSON, H. L.: Exstrophy of bladder complicated by carcinoma. Arch. Surg. *17:*641–657, Oct '28
JUDD, E. S. JR. AND HAVENS, F. Z.: Traumatic avulsion of skin of penis and scrotum. Am. J. Surg. *62:*246–252, Nov '43
JUDIN, S.: Baldwin operation for formation of artificial vagina; report of 6 cases. Surg., Gynec. and Obst. *44:*530–539, April (pt. 1) '27
JUERS, A. L.: Facial paralysis; recent treatment with case report (nerve graft). Kentucky M. J. *37:*368–371, Aug '39
JUERS, A. L.: Facial nerve repair. Kentucky M. J. *40:*453–455, Nov. '42
JULLIARD, C.: Reconstruction of nasal ala; case. Rev. med. de la Suisse Rom. *54:*463–467, April (25), '34
JULLIARD, C.: Plastic surgery of face. Helvet. med. acta *3:*136–142, May '36
JULLIARD, C.: Dufourmentel operation in therapy of prognathism of lower jaw. Schweiz. med. Wchnschr. *68:*609–611, May 21, '38
JULLIARD, C.: Peripheral nerve injuries; therapy. Praxis *34:*147–148, March 1, '45
JUND, L. (see BRIGGS, R.) May '44
JUNÈS, E.: Operation of choice in trachomatous entropion of upper eyelid. Bull. et mem. Soc. franc. d'opht. *45:*70–85, '32
JUNÈS, E.: Low tarsotomy and horizontal suture in trachomatous entropion of upper eyelid. Ann. d'ocul. *169:*704–717, Sept '32
JUNG, A. (see LERICHE, R.) Dec '30
JUNG, A. (see LERICHE, R.) March–April '33
JUNG, A. (see LERICHE, R. *et al*) May '36
JUNG, J.: Construction of artificial vagina with aid of Thiersch transplants. Rozhl. v chir. a gynaek. (cast gynaek.) *12:*104–109, '33
JUNGANO, M.: Correction of urethroperineal fistula. J. d'urol. *15:*459–462, June '23 (illus.)
JUNGE, W.: Surgical therapy of elephantiasis of legs. Arch. f. Schiffs-u. Tropen-Hyg. *44:*549–562, Dec '40
JUNGERMANN, E. (see LEHMANN, W.) 1920
JUNGHANNS, H. AND JUZBASIC, D. M.: Closure of large hernial apertures by means of skin grafts. Chirurg *12:*742–746, Dec 15, '40
JUNQUEIRA, A.: Skin transplantation in treatment of recidivating hernias. Hospital, Rio de Janeiro *29:*11–16, Jan '46
JURADO, P. (see SANTAS, A. *et al*) Aug '42
JURADO, P. (see SANTAS, A. A. *et al*) Aug '42
JURASZ, A.: Traumatic shock. Lek. wojsk. *34:*80–86, Feb–April '42
JUST, E.: Suture of tendons. Arch. f. klin. Chir. *124:*165–177, '23 (illus.) abstr: J. A. M. A. *81:*1647, Nov 10, '23
JUSTIN-BESANCON, L. (see JEANNENEY, G.) March–April '40
JUST TISCORNIA, B. AND MERCANDINO, C. P.: Technic of endonasal dacryocystorhinostomy. (Halle operation); cases. Rev. med. latino-am. *20:*1118–1136, July '35
JUSTIN-BESANCON, L. (see JEANNENEY, G.) April '40

Juvara Operation: See Delorme-Juvara Operation

JUZBASIC, D. M. (see JUNGHANNS, H.) Dec '40

K

KABASHIMA, T.: Pediculate hemangioma of lower lip; case. Oto-rhino-laryng. *12:*293, April '39
KABAT, H. AND HEDIN, R. F.: Nervous factor in etiology of shock in burns. Surgery *11:*766–776, May '42 also: Proc. Soc. Exper. Biol. and Med. *49:*114–116, Feb '42 (abstract)
KABAT, H. (see FREEDMAN, A. M.) Oct '40
KABAT, H. (see LORBER, V. *et al*) Oct '40
KABELÍK: Theories on therapy of extended burns. Ceska dermat. *12:*313–316, '31
KADANOFF, D.: Histologic observations on regeneration of sensory nerve fibres in skin transplantations. Klin. Wchnschr. *4:*1266, June 25, '25
KAEFER, N.: Treatment of rupture of extensor tendons of fingers. Zentralbl. f. Chir. *56:*389, Feb. 16, '29
KAESSLER, H. W.: Vascular birthmarks; treatment with injection of sclerosing solution. J. A. M. A. *110:*1644–1647, May 14, '38
KAFEMANN, A. W. AND BESELIN, O.: Operative treatment of congenital nasal atresia. Arch.

f. Ohren-, Nasen-u. Kehlkopfh. *116:*116–118, Dec '26

KAGAN, Y. A.: Treatment of trachomatous eyelid ptosis. Sovet. vestnik oftal. *6:*416, '35

KAGANOVICH-DVORKIN, A. L.: Congenital absence of radius with bilateral manus vara. Ortop. i travmatol. (no. 1) *12:*85, '38

KAGANOVICH-DVORKIN, A. L. AND RYSKINA, Z. B.: Wounds of fingers (and hand). Khirurgiya no. 3, pp. 45–48, '45

KAHLICH-KOENNER, D. M. (see GOLL, H.) 1940

KAHN, A.: New method for skin grafting mastoid cavity; new method for closing off Eustachian tube at its tympanic end in radical mastoid operation. Laryngoscope *37:*889–893, Dec '27

KAHN, K.: Humped nose; cosmetic and plastic correction. M. Times and Long Island M. J. *62:*42–44, Feb '34

KAHN, K.: Complete double harelip complicated by protrusion of premaxillae. M. Times and Long Island M. J. *62:*176–178, June '34

KAHN, K.: Plastic surgery in removal of excessive cutaneous tissues obstructing vision. New York State J. Med. *34:*781–783, Sept 1, '34

KAHN, K.: Plastic surgery upon axilla in certain cases of persistent bromidrosis. New York State J. Med. *45:*1555–1558, July 15, '45

KAHN, L.: Treatment of congenital cleft of lip and palate. Am. J. Surg. *39:*142–144, June '25 also: Kentucky M. J. *23:*491–493, Oct '25

KAHN, M.: Infections of lip. J. A. M. A. *82:*1043–1044, March 29, '24

KAHN, W.: New obturator for use in case of unsuccessful uranoplasty, with reference to surgical and prosthetic therapeutic methods in palatine defects. Ztschr. f. Stomatol. *32:*18–27, Jan. 12, '34

KAÏRIS, Z.: Modification of Nissen's operation in hypospadias. Zentralbl. f. Chir. *57:*3047–3048, Dec 6, '30

KAISER, G.: Burn therapy. Zentralbl. f. Gewerbehyg. *19:*201–204, Nov '42

KAKUSCHKIN, N.: Artificial vagina made from rectum. Zentralbl. f. Gynak. *48:*2702–2704, Dec 6, '24

KAKUSCHKIN, N.: Surgical intervention for purpose of feminization of hermaphrodite. Arch. f. Frauenk. *19:*150–160, '33

KÁLALOVÁ, V.: Surgical shock. Cas. lek. cesk. *63:*1867–1878, Dec 22, '24

KALALOVA-DI LOTTIOVA, V.: Late results of secondary plastic operations on tendons and nerves of hand. Bratisl. lekar. listy *16:*162–174, April '36

KALAMBOKAS, A. (see BAHLS, G.) 1937

KALEFF: Simplified modification of external dacryocystorhinostomy. Ztschr. f. Augenh. *91:*140–157, Feb '37

KALIMA, T.: Appearance of bone autotransplant of 2 month's duration; case. Acta chir. Scandinav. *65:*196–208, '29

KALINEYKO, I. P.: Mistaken application of Faltin extension in case of fracture of lower jaw. Vestnik khir. *35:*219–220, '34

KALKOFF, K. W.: Psychology of lupus patients with nasal prostheses. Dermat. Wchnschr. *113:*597–601, July 12, '41

KALLAY, J.: Prognathism and its surgical treatment. Lijecn. vjes. *54:*30–33, '32

KALLAY, J.: Diagnosis and therapy of fractures of lower jaw. Lijecn vjes. *55:*248–253, '33

KALLENBERGER, K.: Early diagnosis of malignant tumors of upper jaw. Schweiz. med. Wchnschr. *75:*990–995, Nov. 10, '45

KALLIO, K. E.: Plastic operations on thumb. Acta chir. Scandinav. *93:*231–253, '46

KALLIUS, H. U.: Buttonhole rupture of extensor tendon of finger at point of insertion into terminal phalanx. Zentralbl. f. Chir. *57:*2432–2435, Sept 27, '30

KALLIUS, H. U.: Causes and prevention of failures in surgical therapy for bilateral harelip. Chirurg *5:*704–712, Sept 15, '33

KALMANOVSKIY, S. M.: Rational treatment of burns. Khirurgiya, no. 1, pp. 63–72, '39

KALMANOVSKIY, S. M. AND ZHAK, E.: Repair of traumatic defects of skin (grafts). Vestnik khir. *55:*375–379, April '38

KALÓ, A. V. AND LIEBERMANN, T. V.: Lobulation of ala nasi. Klin. Wchnschr. *3:*452, March 11, '24

KALT, E.: Technic of blepharoplasty. Bull. Soc. d'opht. de Paris *49:*723–725, Dec '37

KALZ, F.: Technic treating naevus flammeus with infraroentgen (grenz) rays. Strahlentherapie *57:*510–515, '36

KALZ, F.: Infra-roentgen (grenz) rays in therapy of keloids. Dermat. Wchnschr. *103:*1223–1226, Sept 5, '36

KAMEL, S.: New knife for Van Millingen grafting operation (ingrown eyelashes). Bull. Ophth. Soc. Egypt *32:*73–78, '39

KAMEYA, K.: Successful use of disinfecting agents in skin grafts. Zentralbl. f. Chir. *55:*2316–2317, Sept 15, '28

KAMIMURA, S.: Therapy of cleft palate by uranoplasty. Oto-rhino-laryng. *9:*608, July '36

KAMINSKI, D. S.: Transplantation of lip mucosa by Denig method in treatment of trachoma. Klin. Monatsbl. f. Augenh. *87:*60–70, July '31

KAMIO, T. (see KANZAKI, T.) Feb '41

KAMRIN, B. B.: Correlated fixation of mandibular fractures. J. Oral Surg. *1:*235–240, July '43

KANAAR, A. G.: Refrigeration in treatment of trauma (lacerated and almost detached thumb). Anesth. and Analg. *2:*177–190, Sept–Oct '46 *25:*228, Nov–Dec '46

KANAI, T.: Congenital fistula of neck. Taiwan Igakkai Zasshi (Abstr. Sect.) *32:*125, Sept '33

KANAKASABESAN, D.: Prognosis and treatment of infections of hand and foot in diabetes. Antiseptic *37:*554–560, June '40

KANAVEL, A. B.: Plastic procedures for obliteration of cavities with non-collapsible walls. Surg., Gynec. and Obst. *32:*453, May '21

KANAVEL, A. B.: Splinting and physiotherapy in infections of hand. J. A. M. A. *83:*1984–1988, Dec 20, '24

KANAVEL, A. B.: Infection clinic; infections of hand. J. Iowa M. Soc. *17:*4–8, Jan '27

KANAVEL, A. B.: Dynamics of functions of hand, with considerations as to methods of obtaining position of function by splints. M. J. Australia *2:*598–602, Oct. 29, '27

KANAVEL, A. B.: Hand surgery. Proc. Internat. Assemb. Inter-State Post-Grad. M. A., North America (1929) *5:*28–34, '30

KANAVEL, A. B.: Congenital malformations of hand. Tr. Sect. Surg., Gen. and Abd., A. M. A., pp. 17–121, '31

KANAVEL, A. B.: Congenital malformations of hands. Arch. Surg. *25:*1, July; 282, Aug '32

KANAVEL, ALLEN B.: *Infections of the Hand*. Sixth Edition. Lea and Febiger, Phila., 1933. Seventh Edition, 1939

KANAVEL, A. B.: Hand infections in industrial accidents. Surg., Gynec. and Obst. *60:*568–570, Feb (no. 2A) '35

KANAVEL, A. B.; KOCH, S. L. AND MASON, M. L.: Description of palmar fascia, review of literature, and report of 29 surgically treated cases of Dupuytren's contracture. Surg., Gynec. and Obst. *48:*145–190, Feb '29

KANAVEL, A. B. (see KOCH, S. L.) 1928

KANAVEL, A. B. (see KOCH, S. L.) Jan '29

KANEKEVICH, M. I.: Bacterial flora of content of vesicles produced by burns. Ortop. i travmatol. (no. 3) *13:*77–81, '39

KANEKEVICH, M. I.: Immunobiologic state of patients immediately after burns. Eksper. med., no. 2, pp. 17–22, '39

KANEMATSU, T.: Transplantation of pedicled skin flap to face; case. Okayama-Igakkai-Zasshi *45:*2099–2100, Sept '33

KANKAT, C. T.: Esthetic surgery for elimination of sequels of smallpox of face in girl 18 years old. Turk tib cem. mec. *6:*260–266, '40

KANKAT, C. T.: Reparative operation for maxillary ankylosis and labiofacial destruction due to noma. Turk tip cem. mec. *12:*163–168, '46

Kankrov Operation

Kankrov operation in therapy of dacryocystitis. ABDULAEV, G. C. Sovet. vestnik oftal. *8:*710–711, '36

KANTALA, J.: Treatment of subcutaneous rupture of extensor tendons of terminal phalanges of fingers. Duodecim *52:*31–45, '36

KANTER, A. E.: Congenital absence of vagina; simplified operation with report of one case. Am. J. Surg. *30:*314–316, Nov '35

KANTHAK, F. F.: Zygoma fractures. Surgery *7:*796–805, May '40

KANTHAK, F. F.: Dermatome pattern graft and its use in reconstruction (after burns). Surg., Gynec. and Obst. *77:*610–614, Dec '43

KANTHAK, F. F. AND HARKINS, H. N.: Unilateral hypertrophy of mandibular condyle associated with chondroma. Surgery *4:*898–907, Dec '38

KANTOR, A.: Traumatic loss of skin; "skinning" of genitals. Chirurg *8:*972–974, Dec 15, '36

KANTOR, D. V.: Sie-Boen-Lian operation in entropion. Sovet. vestnik oftal. *2:*292–295, '33.

KANTOR, D. V.: Author's modification of Sie Boen Lian operation for trachomatous entropion and its late results. Vestnik oftal. *18:*301–305, '41

KANZAKI, T. AND KAMIO, T.: Congenital closure of anterior nasal aperture and of nasal cavities; 2 cases. Oto-rhino-laryng. (Abst. Sect.) *14:*5, Feb '41

KAPITSA, L. M.: Clinical, experimental and histologic studies in connection with subcutaneous injections of homogeneous and heterogeneous fat; morphologic changes of subcutaneous cells. Vestnik khir. *45:*3–8, '36

KAPLAN, A. D.: Cases of burns of high voltage electricity. Profess. pat. i gig., no. 6, pp. 91–118, '29

KAPLAN, A. V. (see ZENO, L.) 1937

KAPLAN, E. B.: Extension deformities of proximal interphalangeal joints of fingers; anatomic study. J. Bone and Joint Surg. *18:*781–783, July '36

KAPLAN, E. B.: Dupuytren's contracture in connection with palmar fascia. Surgery *4:*415–422, Sept '38

KAPLAN, E. B.: Dupuytren's contracture; operation based on anatomy of palmar fascia. Bull. Russian M. Soc. New York, pp. 78–83, Sept '39

KAPLAN, E. B.: Pathology and operative correction of finger deformities due to contractures of extensor digitorum tendon. Surgery *6:*451, Sept '39

KAPLAN, E. B.: Mallet or baseball finger. Surgery *7:*784–791, May '40

KAPLAN, E. B.: Correction of disabling flexion contracture of thumb. Bull. Hosp. Joint Dis. *3:*51–54, April '42

KAPLAN, E. B.: Device for measuring length of tendon graft in flexor tendon surgery. Bull. Hosp. Joint Dis. *3:*97–99, July '42

KAPLAN, E. B.: Treatment of fractures of metacarpals and proximal phalanx by skeletal traction. Bull. Hosp. Joint Dis. *5:*99–109, Oct '44

KAPLAN, E. B.: Surgical anatomy of flexor tendons of wrist. J. Bone and Joint Surg. *27:*368–372, July '45

KAPLAN, E. B.: Functional significance of insertions of extensor communis digitorum in man. Anat. Rec. *92:*293–303, July '45

KAPLAN, I. I.: Treatment of facial cancer by irradiation. Am. J. Roentgenol. *19:*437–439, May '28

KAPLAN, I. I.: Radiation therapy of cancer of lips. Radiology *28:*533–543, May '37

KAPLAN, I. I.: Treatment of hemangiomas in children. Urol. and Cutan. Rev. *44:*397–400, June '40

KAPLAN, I. I.: Malignant melanoma of nose. Arch. Otolaryng. *35:*85–90, Jan '42

KAPLAN, I. I.: Cancer of floor of mouth. J. Am. Dent. A. *30:*737–740, May 1, '43

KAPLAN, I. I.: Extensive destructive ulcerating angioma of face, 5 years after treatment. Urol. and Cutan. Rev. *47:*545, Sept '43

KAPLAN, I. I.: Treatment of unusual hemangioma (in Negro) of lip. Urol. and Cutan. Rev. *48:*290–291, June '44

KAPLAN, L.: Treatment of fractures and dislocations of hand and fingers; technic of unpadded casts for carpal, metacarpal and phalangeal fractures. S. Clin. North America *20:*1695–1720, Dec '40

KAPLAN, L. E. (see GROMAKOVSKAYA, M. M.) 1943

KAPLAN, S. I. (see THOMA, K. H. *et al*) Oct '45

KAPLAN, Y. D.: First aid in case of burns of eye due to lime. Vestnik oftal. (nos. 2–3) *14:*114–118, '39

KAPP, J. F.: Breast hypertrophies and hypoplasias. Fortschr. d. Med. *50:*652–654, Aug 5, '32

KAPP, J. F.: Technic of sutures in cosmetic surgery. Fortschr. d. Med. *50:*967–968, Nov 11, '32

KAPP, J. F.: New surgical method in hypertrophy of breast. Med. Welt *7:*631–632, May 6, '33

KAPP, J. F.: Breast malformations and suggestions for treatment. M. Rec. *147:*252–253, March 16, '38

KAPPIS, M.: Contracture of underarm; therapy. Zentralbl. f. Chir. *59:*2209–2215, Sept 10, '32

KAPPIS, M.: Dislocation fracture of capitulum of inferior maxilla; 5 cases. Zentralbl. f. Chir. *61:*814–821, April 7, '34

KAPSINOW, R.: Mechanism of production of Curling's ulcer in burns. South. M. J. *27:*500–503, June '34

KARÁSEK, M.: Nasal injuries. Casop. lek. cesk. *69:*92–94, Jan 10, '30

KARELL, U.: Nonsurgical reduction of 50-day old dislocation of lower jaw. Zentralbl. f. Chir. *53:*3160–3161, Dec 11, '26

KARFIK, V.: Plastic surgery of cicatricial contractures of skin. Casop. lek. cesk. *71:*1289–1292. Oct 7, '32

KARFÍK, V.: Esthetic sutures. Rozhl. v chir. a gynaek. (cast chir.) *13:*207–219, '34

KARFIK, V.: Dangers of paraffin injections in plastic surgery. Casop. lek. cesk. *76:*1145–1151, July 2, '37

KARNES, T. W.: Fracture of mandible associated with burns of head. J. Oral Surg. *3:*83–86, Jan '45

KARNOSH, L. J. AND GARDNER, W. J.: Partial gigantism of face with neurologic complications. Cleveland Clin. Quart. *12:*43–47, April '45

KARP, F. L.: High frequency current in treatment of hypertrichosis. Arch. Dermat. and Syph. *43:*85–91, Jan '41

KARP, F. L.; NIEMAN, H. A. AND LERNER, C.: Cryotherapy (with mixture containing carbon dioxide snow) for acne and its scars. Arch. Dermat. and Syph. *39:*995–998, June '39

KARP, M. (see HEDIN, R. F.) May–June '39

KARPELIS, E.: Injuries following epilation by electrolysis or roentgen rays. (Further comment on Nobl's article.) Wien. med. Wchnschr. *87:*685, June 19, '37

KARSCH, J.: Relation between hereditary abnormalities of eyes and partially developed fingers and toes. Ztschr. f. Augenh. *89:*274–279, July '36

KARSTED, A.: Chemical injuries (burns). Am. J. Surg. *8:*360–361, Feb '30

KARTASCHEW, S.: Restoration of lower lip by means of Filatow's tubular skin flap. Deutsche Ztschr. f. Chir. *229:*395–400, '30

KARTASCHEW, S.: Treatment of chronic ulcer of leg by means of skin flap taken from dorsum of foot. Zentralbl. f. Chir. *57:*2472–2475, Oct 4, '30

KARTASCHEW, S. I. Free autoplastic bone transplantation; especially of small bone fragments. Arch. f. klin. Chir. *156:*758–805, '30

KARTASHEFF, Z. I.: Sequels and role of bone transplants. Vestnik khir. (nos. 58–60) *20:*282–296, '30

KARTASHEV, Z. I.: Tubular skin graft in therapy of extensive contracture of neck. Sovet. khir., no. 11, pp. 22–30, '35

KARTSCHIKJAN, S. I.: Family tree of hereditary transmission of Dupuytren's contracture. Ztschr. f. orthop. Chir. *48:*36–38, Feb 11, '27

KARUBE, R. AND KOJIMA, K.: Giant breast; case. J. Orient. Med. (Abst. Sect) *30:*272, June '39

KASARCOGLU: Branchial cyst; case. Turk tib

cem. mec. *4:*182–183, '38

KASHKAROV, S. E.: Treatment of chemical burns in industry. Sovet. khir., no. 8, pp. 3–8, '35

KASMAN, L. P. (see KOSTER, H.) Aug '42

KAST, H.: Pendulous breasts; operation limited to one half of breast without cutting all around areola. Chirurg *10:*472–474, July 1, '38

KAST, H.: One-stage operation for pendulous breasts, using method of peripheral approach in removal of wedge-shaped portion. Zentralbl. f. Chir. *65:*1990–1992, Sept 3, '38

KAST, H.: Technic of surgical therapy of pendulous breasts with incision totally encircling nipple. Chirurg *12:*647–649, Nov 1, '40

KAST, H.: Operation to correct crater nipple; contribution to problem of necrosis of nipple and areola. Chirurg. *14:*181–184, March 15, '42

KATSNELSON, Z. N.: Burn therapy. Sovet. khir., no. 8, pp. 16–20, '35

KATZ, D.: Principles of plastic surgery of eyelids, with special reference to Hungarian school. Arch. Ophth. *12:*220–227, Aug '34

KATZ, L. N.; ASHER, R. AND PERLOW, S.: Shock therapy and observations. J. A. M. A. *122:*197, May 15, '43

KATZ, T.: Diathermy as rapid and effectual means of permanent depilation. Dermat. Wchnschr. *79:*1492–1493, Nov 15, '24

KATZ, T. (see SCHOLE, M. L.) Jan '45

KATZENELLENBOGEN, I.: Recurrent aphthous ulceration of oral mucous membrane and genitals associated with recurrent hypopyon iritis (Behcet syndrome); 3 cases. Brit. J. Dermat. *58:*161–172, Jul–Aug '46

KAUFMAN, I.: Harelip and cleft palate. Am. J. Orthodontics (Oral Surg. Sect.) *32:*47–51, Jan '46

KAUFMAN, J. L.: Facial masks; new technic using newly devised matrix for impression. J. Am. Dent. A. *28:*64–66, Jan '41

KAUFMAN, R.: Esthetic surgery of breasts. Bull. et mem. Soc. de med. de Paris *139:*484–487, Oct 10, '35

KAUFMAN, S. M.: Superfluous hair and acne—cause and cure. Hygeia *24:*272, Apr '46

KAUFMANN, C.: Suture of tendon in hand or finger. Schweiz. med. Wchnschr. *51:*601, June 30, '21 abstr: J. A. M. A. *77:*653, Aug 20, '21

KAUFMANN, M.: Megalodactylia; case. Med. Klin. *25:*907–908, June 7, '29

KAUFMANN, R. (see FÈVRE, M. *et al*) March '31

KAUNE, M. M. (see BYARS, L. T.) April '44

KAUSCH, W.: Salivary fistula behind ear; 2 cases. Zentralbl. f. Chir. *52:*914–917, April 25, '25

KAYASHIMA, K. (see MIYATA, S.) March '43

KAYE, B. (see SIMON, H. E.) June '45

KAYSER, K.: Formation of artificial vagina by Kirschner-Wagner operation. Zentralbl. f. Gynak. *56:*1633–1635, July 2, '32

KAYSER, R.: New instrument for use in rhinoplastic surgery. Arch. Otolaryng. *39:*186–188, Feb '44

KAYSER, R.: New operation for dislocated nasal cartilage. Am. J. Surg. *72:*248–251, Aug '46

KAZ, R.: One-stage plastic reconstruction of upper eyelid together with muscle fibers and eyelashes. Zentralbl. f. Chir. *48:*1239, Aug 27, '21

KAZANJIAN, V. H.: Plastic surgery of lip. J. A. M. A. *77:*1959, Dec 17, '21

KAZANJIAN, V. H.: Treatment of nasal deformities, with special reference to nasal prosthesis. J. A. M. A. *84:*177–181, Jan 17, '25

KAZANJIAN, V. K.: Treatment of injuries of upper part of face. J. Am. Dent. A. *14:*1607–1618, Sept '27

KAZANJIAN, V. H.: Tumors of jaws and mouth. New England J. Med. *201:*1200–1201, Dec 12, '29

KAZANJIAN, V. H.: Surgical treatment of prognathism. Internat. J. Orthodontia *18:*1224–1239, Nov '32

KAZANJIAN, V. H.: Treatment of automobile injuries of face and jaws. J. Am. Dent. A. *20:*757–773, May '33

KAZANJIAN, V. H.: Nasal deformities and their repair. Laryngoscope *43:*955–975, Dec '33

KAZANJIAN, V. H.: Injuries to face and jaws in automobile accidents. Tr. Am. Acad. Ophth. *38:*275–308, '33

KAZANJIAN, V. H.: Dental prosthesis in relation to reparative surgery of face. Surg. Gynec. and Obst. *59:*70–80, July '34

KAZANJIAN, V. H.: Traumatism of face and jaws with special reference to complications. J. Am. Dent. A. *21:*1138–1152, July '34

KAZANJIAN, V. H.: Surgical correction of jaw deformities and their relationship to orthodontia. Internat. J. Orthodontia *22:*259–282, March '36

KAZANJIAN, V. H.: Repair of contractures resulting from burns (grafts). New England J. Med. *215:*1104–1120, Dec 10, '36

KAZANJIAN, V. H.: Plastic repair of deformities about lower part of nose resulting from loss of tissue. Tr. Am. Acad. Ophth. *42:*338–366, '37

KAZANJIAN, V. H.: Lateral pressure splint in nasal fractures. Arch. Otolaryng. *27:*474–475, April '38

KAZANJIAN, V. H.: Ankylosis of temporomandibular joint. Surg., Gynec. and Obst. *67:*333–348, Sept '38

KAZANJIAN, V. H.: Jaw reconstruction. Am. J. Surg. *43:*249–267, Feb. '39

KAZANJIAN, V. H.: Secondary deformities in cleft palate patients. Ann. Surg. *109:*442–467, March '39

KAZANJIAN, V. H.: Congenital absence of ramus of mandible. J. Bone and Joint Surg. *21:*761–772, July '39

KAZANJIAN, V. H.: Interrelation of dentistry and surgery in treatment of harelip. Am. J. Orthodontics (Oral Surg. Sect) *27:*10–30, Jan '41

KAZANJIAN, V. H.: Treatment of benign tumors of jaw. J. Am. Dent. A. *28:*208–223, Feb '41

KAZANJIAN, V. H.: Primary care of facial injuries and jaws. Surg., Gynec. and Obst. *72:*431–436, Feb (no. 2A) '41

KAZANJIAN, V. H.: Primary care of facial wounds. Am. J. Orthodontics (Oral Surg. Sect) *27:*448–457, Aug '41

KAZANJIAN, V. H.: Outline of treatment of extensive comminuted fractures of mandible (based chiefly on experience gained during last war). Am. J. Orthodontics (Oral Surg. Sect) *28:*265–274, May '42

KAZANJIAN, V. H.: Treatment of congenital atresia of choanae. Ann. Otol., Rhin. and Laryng. *51:*704–711, Sept '42

KAZANJIAN, V. H.: Immobilization of wartime, compound, comminuted fractures of mandible. Am. J. Orthodontics (Oral Surg. Sect) *28:*551-560, Oct '42

KAZANJIAN, V. H.: Reconstruction of deformities of forehead and frontal bone. Tr. Am. Soc. Plastic and Reconstructive Surg., *12:*83–97, '43

KAZANJIAN, V. H.: Treatment of extensive loss of mandible and its surrounding tissues. J. Oral Surg. *1:*30–47, Jan '43

KAZANJIAN, V. H.: Plastic surgery of facial injuries. Bull. Am. Coll. Surgeons *28:*140–141, June '43

KAZANJIAN, V. H.: Symposium on plastic surgery; early treatment of gunshot wounds of face and jaws; case histories of patients treated during World War I. Surgery *15:*22–42, Jan '44

KAZANJIAN, V. H.: Treatment of deformity from burns. Connecticut M. J. *8:*661–670, Oct '44

KAZANJIAN, V. H.: Spontaneous regeneration of bone following excision of section of mandible. Am. J. Orthodontics (Oral Surg. Sect.) *32:*242–248, April '46

KAZANJIAN, V. H.: Repair of nasal defects with median forehead flap; primary closure of forehead wound. Surg. Gynec. and Obst. *83:*37–49, July '46

KAZANJIAN, V. H. AND HOLMES, E. M.: Reconstruction after radical operation for osteomyelitis of frontal bone; experience in 38 cases. Surg., Gynec. and Obst. *79:*397–411, Oct '44

KAZANJIAN, V. H. AND HOLMES, E. M.: Nasopharyngeal stenosis and its correction. Arch. Otolaryng. *44:*261–273, Sept '46

KAZANJIAN, V. H.; ROWE, A. T. AND YOUNG, H. A.: Prosthesis of mouth and face. J. Dent. Research *12:*651–693, Oct '32

KAZANJIAN, V. H. AND STROCK, M. S.: Early treatment of fractures of mandible. J. Am. Dent. A. *29:*76–83, Jan '42

KAZANJIAN, V. H. AND STURGIS, S. H.: Surgical treatment of hemiatrophy of face. J. A. M. A. *115:*348–354, Aug 3, '40

KAZANSKIY, V. I.: Blood transfusion in traumatic shock. Sovet. med. (nos. 17–18) *5:*13, '41

KEARNEY, H. L.: Method for maintaining apposition of mucosal flaps after submucous resection. Tr. Am. Laryng., Rhin. and Otol. Soc. *43:*109–110, '37

KEARNS, W. M.: Extroversion of bladder; case. Wisconsin M. J. *36:*820–824, Oct '37

KEARNS, W. M.: Testicular transplantation; successful autoplastic graft following accidental castration. Ann. Surg. *114:*886–890, Nov. '41

KEEGAN, A. P. (see JONES, J. F. X.) Jan '24

KEENAN, H. J.: Preparation of jelly in the field for burn therapy. Hosp. Corps. Quart. *16:*49–50, Jan '43

KEHL, H.: Signs of fracture of orbit. Beitr. z. klin. Chir. *123:*203, '21 abstr: J. A. M. A. *77:*1292, Oct 15, '21

KEIL, H. (see DOBES, W. L.) Oct '40

KEIL, H. (see TRAUB, E. F.) Feb '40

KEILLER, V. H. (see THOMPSON, J. E.) April '23

KEITER, W. E.: Sulfadiazine (sulfanilamide derivative) spray in burns; case. North Carolina M. J. *3:*190–192, April '42

KEITH, A.: Origin and nature of certain malformations of face, head and foot. Brit. J. Surg. *28:*173–192, Oct '40

KEITH, D. Y.: Use of radium in traumatic and postoperative scars. Radiol. Rev. and Chicago M. Rec. *56:*61–63, March '34

KEITH, W. S.: Small bone grafts. J. Bone and Joint Surg. *16:*314–330, April '34

KEIZER, D. P. R.: Rightsided hemihypertrophy of face; case. Geneesk. tijdschr. v. Nederl.-Indie *81:*1931–1934, Sept 9, '41

KEJŘ, O.: Care of facial fissure in nurslings. Casop. lek. cesk. *66:*258–260, Feb 11, '27

KEKWICK, A. *et al:* Diagnosis and treatment of secondary shock; 24 cases. Lancet *1:*99–103, Jan 25, '41

KELEMEN, G.: Embolic infarction of lung after excision of septum of nose. Ztschr. f. Hals-,Nasen-u. Ohrenh. *26:*139–142, July 3,

'30
KELEMEN, G.: Malformation involving external middle and internal ear, with otosclerotic focus. Arch. Otolaryng. *37:*183–198, Feb '43
KELIKIAN, H. AND BINTCLIFFE, E. W.: Functional restoration of thumb; pollicization of the index. Surg. Gynec. and Obst. *83:*807–814, Dec '46
KELLER, P.: Inhalation anesthesia with chlorylene (trichloroethylene) in plastic surgery of face. Dermat. Wchnschr. *95:*973–985, July 2, '32
KELLER, W. I.: Ten years of tunnel graft of skin. Ann. Surg. *91:*924–936, June '30
KELLER, W. L.: Annular stricture of rectum and anus; treatment by tunnel skin graft; preliminary report. Am. J. Surg. *20:*28–32, April '33
KELLNER, A. W.: Cleft hands and cleft feet with oligodactylia. Klin. Wchnschr. *13:*1507–1509, Oct 20, '34
KELLOCK, T. H.: Advantages of two-stage operation for cleft palate. Brit. J. Surg. *9:*290, Oct '21
KELLY, C. C.: Harelip problem and cleft palate. J. Connecticut M. Soc. *3:*490–491, Sept '39
KELLY, D. B.: Congenital occlusion of posterior nasal choanae. Brit. M. J. *1:*157–158, Jan 28, '39
KELLY, E. G.: Treatment of hand infections. Memphis M. J. *15:*143–144, Sept '40
KELLY, J. D.: New technic for plastic operations of nose. Arch. Otolaryng. *8:*433–445, Oct '28
KELLY, J. D.: New method of obtaining costal cartilage for plastic and reconstructive surgery. Surg., Gynec. and Obst. *44:*687–689, May '27
KELLY, J. D.: Nasal fractures. Am. J. Surg. *36:*77–82, April '37
KELLY, M. W.: Two cases avulsion of scalp. Am. J. Surg. *72:*103–109, July '46
KELLY, R. J. (see ANDREWS, G. C.) July '32
KELLY, R. P.: Skin grafting in treatment of osteomyelitic war wounds. J. Bone and Joint Surg. *28:*681–691, Oct '46
KELLY, R. P.; ROSATI, L. M. AND MURRAY, R. A.: Traumatic osteomyelitis; use of grafts; subsequent treatment. Tr. South. S. A. (1945) *57:*219–228, '46
KELLY, R. P.; ROSATI, L. M. AND MURRAY, R. A.: Traumatic osteomyelitis; use of grafts; subsequent treatment. Ann. Surg. *123:*688–697, April '46

Keloids (*See also Scars, Hypertrophic*)

Digestion of keloids, cicatrices and buboes with pepsin-hydrochloric acid. AHLSWEDE, E. Arch. Dermat. and Syph. *3:*142, Feb '21
Pepsin-hydrochloric acid treatment of keloids, further indications. AHLSWEDE, E. H. Arch. Dermat. and Syph. *3:*648, May '21

Keloids – Cont.

Plastic and cosmetic surgery of head, neck and face (including keloids). TIECK, G. J. E. AND HUNT, H. L. Am. J. Surg. *35:*173, June '21; 355, Nov '21
Surgical-physical treatment of keloids. KROMAYER. Deutsche med. Wchnschr. *49:*280–281, March 2, '23
Mixed surgical and radium treatment of prominent keloids. SÁINZ DE AJA. Siglo med. *72:*1185–1187, Dec 8, '23
Treatment of keloids with radium. TAUSSIG, L. R. California State J. Med. *21:*520–522, Dec '23
Keloid of penis. SMITH, E. O., J. Urology *11:*515–524, May '24
Roentgen-ray treatment of keloids. HAZEN, H. H. Am. J. Roentgenol. *11:*547–549, June '24
Successful radiotherapy of cicatrices and keloids with case report. DU BOIS, C. Rev. med. de la Suisse Rom. *44:*705–713, Nov '24
Keloid of forehead. NORTHROP, H. L., S. Clin. N. Amer. *5:*1671, Dec '25
Carbon dioxide snow in treatment of keloids. RAMIREZ, V. Gac. med. de Mexico *57:*318–320, May–June '26
Roentgen-ray treatment of keloid. GRIER, G. W. Am. J. Roentgenol. *16:*22–26, July '26
Simultaneous appearance of acuminate condylomata and warts on face with keloid. MÜHLPFORDT, H. Dermat. Wchnschr. *84:*463–466, April 2, '27
Keloid removal by electro-coagulation. PEEPLES, D. L. Am. J. Phys. Therapy *4:*160, July '27
Keloid in man. SCHRIDDE, H. Klin. Wchnschr. *7:*582–584, March 25, '28
Cheloids. HUNT, H. L. Am. Med. *23:*337–341, May '28
Deep, cicatricial keloid treated by radium; case. GUILERA, L. G. An. Hosp. de Santa Cruz y San Pablo *2:*234, July 15, '28
Radium therapy of keloids. RIETI, E. Arch. di radiol. *4:*941–955, Sept–Dec '28
Etiology and pathogenesis of multiple keloid. BARBAGLIA, V. Gior. ital. di dermat. e sifil. *69:*1573–1596, Dec '28
Treatment of acne-keloid of nape of neck by diathermocoagulation; cases. RAVAUT, P. AND FILLIOL, L. Bull. Soc. franc. de dermat. et syph. *35:*942–946, Dec '28
Roentgenotherapy and electrotherapy of keloids. LEPENNETIER, F. Rev. d'actinol. *5:*69, Jan–Feb '29
Capillary drainage in treatment of keloidal scars. SHEEHAN, J. E., M. J. and Rec. *129:*548–549, May 15, '29

Keloids – Cont.
Iodine iontophoresis in keloid occurring after furuncle. EIGER, J. Munchen. med. Wchnschr. *76:*1297, Aug 2, '29
Comment on article by Eiger on keloid therapy by iodine iontophoresis. WIRZ, F. Munchen. med. Wchnschr. *76:*1515, Sept 6, '29
Electrolysis as cosmetic treatment of keloids and nevus pigmentosus. MARQUE, A. M. AND LANARI, E. Semana med. *1:*159-164, Jan 16, '30
Multiple gigantic keloids; case. NARDUCCI, F. Dermosifilografo *5:*145-156, March '30
Operative treatment of keloids. DE MOSCOSO, A. Rev. brasil. de med. e pharm. *6:*209-218, July-Sept '30
Fractional cauterization of large cicatricial keloids. HENKELS, P. Deutsche tierarztl. Wchnschr. *38:*501-504, Aug 9, '30
Therapy of keloids. BÖHMER, L. Med. Welt *4:*1472-1474, Oct. 11, '30
Plastic operations for keloids. GOHRBANDT, E. Med. Welt *4:*1510, Oct 18, '30
Therapy of keloids by filtered roentgen rays. KILBANE, C. V. New England J. Med. *203:*1238-1241, Dec 18, '30
Radium therapy of postoperative keloids. MÁTYÁS, M. Zentralbl. f. Chir. *57:*3039-3040, Dec 6, '30
Results of therapy of keloids obtained at Instituto de Medicina Experimental in Buenos Aires. ROSNER, S. Bol. Inst. de med. exper. para el estud. y trat. del cancer *7:*1375-1381, Dec '30
Treatment of keloids and hypertrophic scars by introduction of radio-active substances into tissue. SIMONS, A. Strahlentherapie *37:*89-123, '30
Prevention of keloid formation by prophylactic irradiation of fresh operative wound. BAB, M. Deutsche med. Wchnschr. *57:*319-320, Feb 20, '31
Physiotherapy of keloids. BELOT, J. Bull. Soc. franc. de dermat. et syph. (Reunion dermat., Strasbourg) *38:*965-976, July '31
Therapy of keloids. SALLFELD, U. Therap. d. Gegenw. *72:*410-412, Sept '31
Plastic surgery (of keloids). ALHAIQUE, A. Rinasc. med. *9:*25-27, Jan 15, '32
Therapy of keloids. BEELOT, J., J. de med. et chir. prat. *103:*77-87, Feb 10, '32
Radium in therapy of cicatrices and keloids. DEGRAIS, P. AND BELLOT, A. Bull. med., Paris *46:*196-198, March 12, '32
X-ray treatment of keloidal and hypertrophic scars. SHERMAN, B. H. Radiology *18:*754-757, April '32
Keloid therapy; clinic in reparative surgery. Unilateral facial paralysis. SHEEHAN, J. E., S. Clin. North America *12:*341-356, April '32

Keloids – Cont.
Keloid therapy. STEIN, R. O. Wien. klin. Wchnschr. *45:*996-998, Aug 5, '32
Keloids, radium therapy; case, with suggestions of other physiotherapeutic methods (electrolysis, electropuncture, ionization, cryotherapy, electrocoagulation and roentgenotherapy). TRÉPAGNE, D. Ann. de med. phys. *25:*291-297, '32
Keloid in Negro race. ABASCAL, H. Cron. med.-quir. de la Habana *59:*145-155, April '33
Keloids, esthetic therapy, surgical ablation followed immediately by radium irradiation. PASSOT, R. Presse med. *41:*544-546, April 5, '33
Two cases of keloid therapy. DE CARVALHO FRANCO, D. Ann. paulist. de med. e cir. *26:*375-384, Nov '33
Various methods of treating keloids. RABUT, R. Hopital *21:*763-765, Dec (B) '33
Surgical removal followed by radiotherapy of cicatricial keloids. VIALLE, P. Arch. med.-chir. de Province *23:*429-432, Dec '33
Two cases of keloid formation, with comments. BURMAN, C. E. L. Brit. J. Surg. *21:*527-529, Jan '34
Ionization of magnesium chloride in therapy of keloids and keloid cicatrices. CARLU, L. Ann. de dermat. et syph. *5:*162-169, Feb '34 abstr: Bull. et mem. Soc. de med. de Paris *137:*478-481, June 24, '33
Radium treatment of cicatricial keloids. FUHS, H. Med. Klin. *30:*160-161, Feb 2, '34
Radiation therapy of keloid and keloidal scars. HODGES, F. M. Am. J. Roentgenol. *31:*238-243, Feb '34
Development of keloids from trifling causes (case following puncture of ear during delivery). VON LOBMAYER, G. Zentralbl. f. Chir. *61:*253, Feb 3, '34
Keloid of nose; case. TAVANI, E. Boll. d. mal. d. orecchio, d. gola, d. naso *52:*281-288, June '34
Keloid on tip of tongue in trumpeter; case. SCHMIDT, W. Dermat. Wchnschr. *99:*1341-1342, Oct 13, '34
Study of keloids, with description of case of cicatricial keloid in mastoid area. FORNARI, G. B. Oto-rino-laring. ital. *4:*552-565, Nov '34
Scarring of face and neck with keloid from burn treated with radium and plastic operation; case. NEW, G. B. Proc. Staff Meet., Mayo Clin. *10:*283-285, May 1, '35
Surgical and radium therapy of keloids. WEILL, R. Bull. et mem. Soc. de med. de Paris *139:*340-343, May 10, '35

Keloids – Cont.

Keloids, with special reference to curative therapy and prevention. RENAUX, R. Monde med., Paris *45:*702–706, May 15, '35

Nature and significance of keloids. WALTHER, E. Med. Welt *9:*1006–1008, July 13, '35

Keloid formation in ear lobe. SPRENGER, W. Monatschr. f. Ohrenh. *70:*188–194, Feb '36

Treatment of disfiguring scars (keloids), defects and malformations. DUJARDIN, E. Hospitalstid. *79:*524–533, May 19, '36

Keloid and its treatment. GRÜNWALD, B. Gyogyaszat *76:*279–280, May 3, '36

Familial occurrence of keloids. WOLF, M. Wien. med. Wchnschr. *86:*722–723, June 27, '36

Infra-roentgen (grenz) rays in therapy of keloids. KALZ, F. Dermat. Wchnschr. *103:*1223–1226, Sept 5, '36

Keloid tumor and its cure by radiotherapy. HINTZE, A. Strahlentherapie *57:*224–240, '36

Therapy of keloids. HOFFMAN, W. J. Arch. Phys. Therapy *18:*135–138, March '37

Moles, warts and keloids. MORSE, J. L. Am. J. Surg. *36:*137–144, April '37

Roentgen and radium treatment in prevention and therapy of keloids. DEPLAEN, P. Rev. de chir. structive, pp. 99–102, June '37

Keloid and its radium therapy, with report of cases. MOSCARIELLO, T. Arch. di radiol. *13:*317–337, July–Aug '37

Prophylaxis of cicatricial keloid in plastic surgery of breast. SCHWARZMANN, E. AND POLLACZEK, K. F. Wien. med. Wchnschr. *87:*1248–1253, Nov. 27, '37

Radium treatment of keloids. DAVIS, A. H. AND BROWN, W. L. Radiol. Rev. and Mississippi Valley M. J. *60:*67–69, March '38

Therapy of keloids. ASHBURY, H. H. Urol. and Cutan. Rev. *42:*441–444, June '38

Prophylaxis of cicatricial keloid in plastic surgery of pendulous breasts. SCHWARZMANN, E. Rev. de chir. structive *8:*93–98, Aug '38

Therapy of keloids and angiomas. REISNER, A. Med. Klin. *34:*1233–1235, Sept. 16, '38

Iontophoresis in treatment of Dupuytren's contracture and keloids. NIJKERK, M. Nederl. tijdschr. v. geneesk. *83:*5135–5140, Oct. 28, '39

Practical observations of keloids and potential keloids. FILIPS, L., M. Rec. *150:*418–422, Dec. 20, '39

Treatment of x-ray burns and other superficial disfigurements of skin (and keloids). CANNON, A. B. New York State J. Med. *40:*391–399, March 15, '40

Keloids – Cont.

Keloids and their treatment. COSTELLO, M. J. M. Record *154:*205–207, Sept 17, '41

Radiotherapy in prophylaxis and treatment of keloids. LEVITT, W. M. AND GILLIES, H. Lancet *1:*440–442, April 11, '42

Keloids and their treatment. NASON, L. H. New England J. Med. *226:*883–886, May 28, '42

Roentgen therapy of hypertrophic scars and keloids. HUNTER, A. F. Radiology *39:*400–409, Oct '42

Review of literature and report of 80 cases of keloids. GARB, J. AND STONE, M. J. Am. J. Surg. *58:*315–335, Dec '42

Roentgen therapy of hypertrophic scars and keloids. HUNTER, A. F. Rev. radiol. y fisioterap. *10:*101–109, May–June '43

Fibrokeloid cicatrix after attempted removal of pilous nevus; free full thickness skin graft; case. MALBEC, E. F. Dia med. *15:*1100, Sept 13, '43

Tubed pedicle graft in therapy of burn cicatrix; resulting keloids. PEDEMONTE, P. V. Bol Soc. cir. d. Uruguay *14:*106–108, '43 also: Arch. urug. de med., cir. y especialid. *23:*296–298, Sept '43

Case of keloids of unusual size. COSTA, O. G. Arch. Dermat. and Syph. *48:*411–412, Oct '43

Fibrokeloid cicatrix after attempted removal of pilous nevus; free full thickness skin graft; case. MALBEC, E. F. Semana med. *2:*1416–1417, Dec. 23, '43

Pathogenesis of keloids and similar neoplasms in relation to tissue fluid disturbances (and therapy). MARSHALL, W. AND ROSENTHAL, S. Am. J. Surg. *62:*348–357, Dec '43

Disseminated keloid acne; case. MERCADAL PEYRI, J. Actas dermo-sif. *35:*839–849, May '44

Therapy of scars and keloids. MARSHALL, W. New Orleans M. and S. J. *97:*15–17, July '44

Pathogenesis of keloids, with clinical applications in medicine and surgery. MARSHALL, W. Proc. Am. Federation Clin. Research (1943) *1:*25, '44

Importance of keloids to plastic surgeons. REBELO NETO, J. Hospital, Rio de Janeiro *27:*33–43, Jan '45

Keloids and their treatment. STRAND, S. Acta radiol. *26:*397–408, '45

Primary keloids with spontaneous remission. MERINO EUGERCIOS, E. AND GONZALEZ CALVO, S. Actas dermo-sif. *37:*616–622, Feb '46

Therapy of keloids. SILVESTRI, G. Minerva

Keloids – Cont.
chir. *1:*21–22, March '46
Generalized keloids treated by parathroidectomy; case. OLIVER, G. AND BARASCH. Progr. med., Paris *7:*292–293, July 10, '46
Keloid formation in both ear lobes. WEAVER, D. F. Arch. Otolaryng. *44:*212–213, Aug '46

KELSEY, H. E.: Double harelip and cleft palate showing importance of proper surgical and orthodontic treatment of premaxillary lobe or process. Internat. J. Orthodontia *18:*145–147, Feb '32
KEMLER, J. I.: Implantation of ivory in ozena of nose; approved technic; further observations. Arch. Otolaryng. *13:*726–731, May '31
KEMP, T. AND RAVN, J.: Hereditary deformities of hand and foot in members of one family; polydactylia and syndactylia. Acta psychiat. et neurol. *7:*275–296, '32
KEMPER, J. W.: Cleft palate. J. Oral Surg. *2:*227–238, July '44
KEMPER, J. W.: Responsibility of surgeon in treating palatal and related defects. Am. J. Orthodontics (Oral Surg. Sect.) *32:*667–670, Nov '46
KENDALL, A. W.: War burns. M. Press *205:*42–45, Jan. 15, '41
KENDE, B.: New needle-holder for use in diathermic epilation in hypertrichosis. Wien. klin. Wchnschr. *41:*382, March 15, '28
KENDIG, E. I.: Local burn therapy. Virginia M. Monthly *56:*219–222, July '29
KENDRICK, D. B. JR.: Results of intravenous and intra-arterial administration of fluids in traumatic shock produced experimentally. Surgery *6:*520–523, Oct '39
KENDRICK, D. B. JR.: Prevention and treatment of shock in combat zone. Mil. Surgeon *88:*97–113, Feb '41
KENDRICK, D. B. JR.: Shock; prevention and treatment in combat zone. Army M. Bull. (no. 58) pp. 38–60, Oct '41
KENDRICK, D. B. JR.: Prevention and treatment of shock during surgical procedures. Mil. Surgeon *92:*247–253, March '43
KENDRICK, D. B. JR.; ESSEX, H. E. AND HELMHOLZ, H. F. JR.: Investigation of traumatic shock bearing on toxemia theory. Surgery *7:*753–762, May '40
KENDRICK, D. B. JR. AND REICHEL, J. JR.: Practical approach to shock therapy. Anesthesiology *4:*497–507, Sept '43
KENDRICK, D. B. JR.; REICHEL, J. JR. AND MCGRAW, J. J. JR.: Burn therapy with human serum albumin concentrated; clinical indications and dosage. Army M. Bull. (no. 68) pp. 107–112, July '43
KENDRICK, D. B. JR. AND WAKIM, K. G.: Intra-arterial hypertonic saline solution in experimental shock. Proc. Soc. Exper. Biol. and Med. *40:*114–116, Jan '39
KENDRICK, J. I.: Treatment of acute tendon injuries. S. Clin. North America *17:*1469–1474, Oct '37
KENNARD, H. E. (see WHITE, J. C. *et al*) Sept '45
KENNEDY, J. T. (see RICHISON, F. A.) May '44
KENNEDY, J. W.: Differential diagnosis between hemorrhage and shock following abdominal surgery. M. Rec. *140:*420–421, Oct. 17, '34
KENNEDY, R.: Tendon transplants in forearm. An. de Fac. de med., Montevideo *8:*558, May–June '23
KENNEDY, R. D.: Tendon transplantation in forearm. Southwestern Med. *6:*153–154, April '22
KENNEDY, R. H.: Epithelioma of lip, with particular reference to lymph node metastases. Ann. Surg. *99:*81–93, Jan '34
KENNEDY, R. H.: Malignancy and potential malignancy of lower lip. S. Clin. North America *17:*297–301, Feb '37
KENNEDY, R. L. AND LEWIS, F. C. R.: Severe faciomaxillary injury treated at sea. J. Roy. Nav. M. Serv. *31:*36–39, Jan '45
KENNEDY, W. H.: Radium treatment of epithelioma of face. J. Radiol. *6:*52–55, Feb '25
KENNEDY, W. H.: Epithelioma of lip, observations on 150 cases. Radiology *4:*319–324, April '25
KENNEDY, W. H.: Radium treatment of epithelioma of ear. Radiology *7:*249–252, Sept '26
KENNON, R.: Problem of septic hand. Brit. M. J. *2:*1189–1192, Dec. 29, '34
KENNY, T. B. AND MERELLO, M.: Genitoplasty; restitution of skin of penis and of scrotum by autograft; restitution of function after trauma. Prensa med. argent. *15:*1549–1560, May 30, '29
KENTGENS, S. K. (see WEVE, H. J. M.) Feb '37
KENYON, E. L.: Speech complications involved in certain types of inadequate palate, especially congenital short palate, with exhibition of patients. Ann. Otol., Rhin. and Laryng. *34:*887–900, Sept '25
KEPES, P.: Hemangioma of ear. Monatschr. f. Ohrenh. *72:*798–808, Aug '38
KEPP, R. K.: Epispadias in women. Chirurg *15:*332, June 1, '43
KERN, E. C.: Use of sulfanilamide and gauze packing following intranasal operation. Arch. Otolaryng. *36:*134, July '42
KERN, E. C.: Cerebral infarction following submucous resection and turbinectomy. Eye, Ear, Nose and Throat Monthly *23:*29, Jan '44
KERN, R. A. *et al*: Discussion of burns based on

experience with 360 cases seen on board a U. S. hospital ship. U. S. Nav. M. Bull. *41:*1654-1678, Nov '43

KERN, R. A. *et al*: Discussion based on experience with 360 burn cases seen on board a U. S. hospital ship. U. S. Nav. M. Bull. *42:*59-81, Jan '44

KENNEDY, W. H.: Epithelioma of lip, observations on 150 cases. Radiology *4:*319-324, April '25

KERNBACH, M. AND GIURGIU, V.: Determination of fatal cases in burns of skin. Cluj. med. *12:*406-408, July 1, '31

KERNODLE, S. E.: Tannic acid for burns. J. Oklahoma M. A. *22:*384-387, Nov '29

KERNS, I. N.: Hand infections. Kentucky M. J. *25:*445-449, Aug '27

KERNWEIN, G. A.: Combined congenital exstrophy of female bladder and cloaca. Arch. Path. *13:*926-930, June '32 also: Tr. Chicago Path. Soc. *14:*4-9, June 1, '32

KERR, A. B. AND WERNER, H.: Clinical value of growth-promoting substance (H. E. P.) in treatment of indolent wounds. Brit. J. Surg. *32:*281-287, Oct '44

KERR, A. B. AND WERNER, H.: Clinical value of growth-promoting substance (H.E.P.) in treatment of indolent wounds. Rev. san. mil., Buenos Aires *44:*461-475, April '45

KERR, W. G.: Burns and scalds. East African M. J. *19:*274-288, Dec '42

KESSEL, F. K.: Therapy of slowly healing ulcers. Vrach. delo *20:*311-314, '37

KESSEL, O.: Argyrosis of auricles with certain practical observations on plastic operations. Hals-, Nasen-u. Ohrenarzt (Teil 1) *31:*250-252, Dec '40

KESSLER, E. B.: Treatment of burns by actinotherapy. Arch. Physical Therapy *7:*347-354, June '26

KESSLER, H. H. Symposium on reparative surgery; cineplastic amputations. S. Clin. North America *24:*453-466, April '44

KESSLER, H. H. (see O'CONNOR, G. B.) June '45

KESTENBAUM, A.: Modification of ectropion operation according to Kuhnt-Szymanowsky method. Klin. Monatsbl. f. Augenh. *95:*51-53, July '35

KESTON, A. S. (see FOX, C. L. JR.) June '45

KETCHAM, A. H. AND HUMPHREY, W. R.: Orthodontic treatment following operation for unilateral ankylosis of temporomaxillary articulation; case report. Internat. Orthodont. Cong. *1:*479-482, '27

KETELBANT: Branchial fistulas in children. Scalpel *85:*1433-1435, Nov. 26, '32

KETTEL, K.: Homotransplantation based on blood-group determination with special regard to skin transplantation. Bibliot. f. Laeger *121:*204-230, May '29

KETTEL, K.: Facial palsy of otitic origin, with special regard to its prognosis under conservative treatment and possibilities of improving results by active surgical intervention; account of 264 cases subjected to reexamination. Arch. Otolaryng. *37:*303-348, March '43

KETTEL, K.: Surgical therapy of otogenic facial paralysis according to Ballance-Duel and Bunnell: 35 cases. Nord. med. (Hospitalstid.) *24:*1783-1795, Oct. 6, '44

KEVAN, J. E. JR. (see GURDIN, M. M. *et al*) March '44

KEVDIN, N. A. AND GENDLER, A. V.: Transfusion of hypertonic plasma in therapy of shock following acute blood loss. Klin. med. (nos. 10-11) *22:*20-22, '44

KEY, J. A.: Fixation of tendons, ligaments and bone by Bunnell's pull-out wire suture. Tr. South. S. A. (1945) *57:*187-194, '46

KEY, J. A.: Fixation of ligaments by Bunnell's pull-out wire suture. Ann. Surg. *123:*656-663, April '46

KEYES, E. L.: Graft in situ of skin completely avulsed (case). J. Missouri M. A. *37:*75-76, Feb '40

KEYES, H. B.: Stenosing tendovaginitis at radial styloid process (de Quervain's disease). Ann. Surg. *107:*602-606, April '38

KEYSER L. D.: Massive hypertrophy of breast. Surg., Gynec. and Obst. *33:*607, Dec '21

KEYSERLINGK, R.: Construction of vagina (Schubert method). Zentralbl. f. Gynak. *46:*380-381, March 11, '22

KEYSSER: Operative treatment in 14 cases of elephantiasis. Deutsche Ztschr. f. Chir. *203-204:*356-375, '27

Keysser

Keysser's work and plastic surgery of cancer. PRUDENTE, A. Arq. de cir. clin. e exper. *6:* 316-320, April-June '42

KEYZER, A. F.: Plastic correction of saddle nose. Sovet. khir., no. 7, pp. 44-54, '35

KHAITZISS, G. M.: Anatomic grounds for clinical treatment of tendovaginitis of palm. Vestnik khir. (nos. 56-57) *19:*356-362, '30

KHAITZISS, G. M.: Method in exposure of flexor tendons of hand. Vestnik khir. (no. 64) *22:*115-120, '30

KHAN, B.: Shock. J. Indian M. A. *11:*311-316, July '42

KHANDEKAR, K. G.: Noseless man. Indian M. Gaz. *67:*267-268, May '32

KHANNA, M. N.: Preauricular fistula. Indian M. Gaz. *76:*72-75, Feb '41

KHARCHAK, E.: Medial nasal fistula. Acta oto-laryng. *19:*73–76, '33
KHARI, A. P.: Apparatus for fixation of skin flap during epithelization of wound cavity after resection of upper jaw. Novy khir. arkhiv *43:*328–330, '39
KHARTZIEFF: Covering disfiguring cuts on face by method of skin transplantation from abdomen to forearm and face. Ukrain. m. visti *5:*42–46, '29
KHASKELEVICH, M. G.: Primary rhinoplasty. Zhur. ush., nos. i gorl. bolez. *17:*108–112, '40
KHAVANSKIY, K. I.: Lagleys operation for trachomatous entropion. Sovet. vestnik oftal. *1:*159–160, '32
KHEYFETS, A. B. AND SHLEPOV, A. V.: Phlegmon of palm as occupational disease of miners. Novy khir. arkhiv *31:*408–414, '34
KHITROV, F. M.: Free transplant of full thickness graft. Khirurgiya, no. 9, pp. 31–34, '44
KHORANOV, V. M.: Late results of primary suture of tendons. Novy khir. arkhiv *48:*195–199, '41
KHOURY, B. (see HOUOT, A. *et al*) Jan–Feb '39
KHRAMELASHVILI, N. G.: Potassium bromide as anesthetic in facial orbital surgery. Sovet. vrach. zhur., pp. 677–678, May 15, '36
KHRIZMAN, I. A.: Partial rhinoplasty using tissue from auricle on round Filatov pedicle. Sovet. Khir., no. 6, pp. 975–980, '36
KHURGIN, M. A.: Late rupture of tendon of extensor pollicis longus. Ortop. i travmatol. (nos. 5–6) *4:*47–50, '30
KIAER, S.: Bandaging of hand wounds. Ugesk. f. laeger *92:*347–351, April 10, '30
KIAER, S.: Treatment of acute paronychia. Ugesk. f. laeger *92:*425–427, May 1, '30
KIAER, S.: Anatomic observations in hand surgey. Ugesk. f. laeger *92:*755–764, Aug. 7, '30
KIAER, S.: Invalidism after cutting of tendons of hand. Acta orthop. Scandinav. *2:*202–220, '31
KIDD, J. D.: Marginal osteomyelitis of jaws. Lancet *1:*1068, May 17, '30
KIEFER, J. H. (see MCKENNA, C. M.) Jan '43
KIKUCHI, R. AND EBA, M.: Facial angioma with macrocheilia; case. Oto-rhino-laryng. *12:*1018, Dec '39
KILBANE, C. V.: Therapy of keloids by filtered roentgen rays. New England J. Med. *203:*1238–1241, Dec. 18, '30
KILFOY, E. J.: Imperforate anus with persistent cloacal duct. Ann. Surg. *91:*151–154, Jan '30
KILGORE, A. R.: Preparing a wound for skin grafting. S. Clin. N. America *2:*521–524, April '22
KILGORE, A. R. AND TAUSSIG, L. R.: Neck metastases from lip and mouth cancer. S. Clin. North America *11:*1055–1059, Oct '31

Kilian Operation

Plastic surgery; depressed forehead following Kilian operation; repaired by fat grafts. HARTER, J. H. Northwest Med. *26:*313–314, June '27

KILLIAN, H.: Hereditary ptosis of eyelids. Klin. Wchnschr. *2:*2286, Dec. 10, '23
KILLIAN, H. (see FOHL, T.) 1930

Killian Operation

Death of patient after Killian operation for deformed septum. ERRECART, P. L. Rev. Asoc. med. argent. *50:*974–977, Jun '36
Direct incision in submucous resection; modification of Killian operation. TEMPEA, V. Rev. san. mil., Bucuresti *35:*1077–1079, Oct '36
Complications of submucosal resection (Killian operation). CARANDO, V. *et al.* Semana med. *1:*225–227, Jan. 21, '37
Direct incision in submucous resection; modification of Killian operation. TEMPEA, V. Ztschr. f. Hals-, Nasen-u. Ohrenh. *40:*548–552, '37

KILLINGER, R. R.: Dactylomegaly, bilateral affection; only case reported. J. Florida M. A. *12:*6–10, July '25
KILNER: Experiences in reconstruction in surgical treatment of malignant diseases of face with skin grafts. Rev. de chir. structive *8:*170–180, '38
KILNER, T. P.: Principles in plastic surgery. Irish J. M. Sc., pp. 77–81, Feb '26
KILNER, T. P.: Thiersch graft; preparation and uses. Post-Grad. M. J. *10:*176–181, May '34
KILNER, T. P.: Application of Thiersch graft to special areas. Post-Grad. M. J. *10:*317–322, Sept '34
KILNER, T. P.: Full-thickness skin graft. Post-Grad. M. J. *11:*279–282, Aug. '35
KILNER, T. P.: Role of intra-oral and intranasal grafts in contour restoration of face. Rev. de chir. structive, pp. 1–3, March '37
KILNER, T. P.: Cleft lip and palate repair technic. St. Thomas's Hosp. Rep. *2:*127–140, '37
KILNER, T. P.: Treatment of war injuries to face. M. Press *205:*26–29, Jan. 8, '41
KILNER, T. P.: Plastic surgical principles. Practitioner *153:*65–72, Aug '44
KILNER, T. P. AND IMRE, J.: Discussion on plastic surgery of eyelids. Proc. Roy. Soc. Med. *32:*1247–1260, Aug '39
KILNER, T. P. AND JACKSON, T.: Skin-grafting in buccal cavity. Brit. J. Surg. *9:*148, July '21
KILNER, T. P. (see GILLIES, H. D. *et al*) April '27
KILNER, T. P. (see GILLIES, H. D.) 1929

KILNER, T. P. (see GILLIES, H. D.) Jan '29
KILNER, T. P. (see GILLIES, H.) Dec '32
KILNER, T. P. (see MANN, I.) Jan '43
KILNER, T. P. (see NEGUS, V. E.) June '42
KILPATRICK, F. R.: Pseudolaryngocele (aerocele) of neck; case. Guy's Hosp. Rep. *90:*15–20, '40–'41
KIMBALL, G. H.: Harelip; cleft palate; congenital deformities of mouth and face. J. Oklahoma M. A. *31:*85–89, March '38
KIMBALL, G. H.: Surgical treatment of radiation damage to tissue. J. Oklahoma M. A. *34:*285–289, July '41
KIMBALL, G. H. AND DRUMMOND, N. R.: Traumatic affections of nose. J. Oklahoma M. A. *33:*1–3, April '40
KIMBALL, G. H. AND DRUMMOND, N. R.: Experimental and clinical study of cases of exstrophy (technic of Lyman-Farrell operation). J. Oklahoma M. A. *33:*2–8, Aug '40
KIMBALL, G. H. AND DRUMMOND, N. R.: Vitallium for skeleton support of nose. J. Oklahoma M. A. *34:*9–12, Jan '41
KIMBELL, N. K. B. (see COTTER, A. P.) Dec '35
KIMBROUGH, J. W.: Emergency treatment of burns. U. S. Nav. M. Bull. *40:*723, July '42
KIME, E. N.: Cancer of head and neck; management of lesions with borderline operability and curability. Arch. Phys. Therapy *20:*282–287, May '39
KIMURA, H.: Treatment of elephantiasis. Japan M. World *5:*201–211, Aug '25
KINCAID, C. J.: Maxillofacial bandage. Bull. U. S. Army M. Dept. *4:*475–477, Oct '45
KINDERSLEY, C. E.: Reconstruction of thumb. Proc. Roy. Soc. Med. *30:*1260–1262, Aug '37
KINDLER, W.: Dangers of Schönborn-Rosenthal and Ernst-Halle operations; possibility of avoidance. Beitr. z. Anat., Physiol., Path. u. Therap. d. Ohres *27:*187–192, June '28
KING, C. J. (see OLDFIELD, M. C.) July '44
KING, D. J.: Case of tumors resembling hemangiomatosis of lower extremity. J. Bone and Joint Surg. *28:*623–628, July '46
KING, E.: Technic of correcting nasal deformities. Arch. Otolaryng. *14:*483–488, Oct '31
KING, E.: Treatment of cancer of nose. Ohio State M. J. *36:*627–628, June '40
KING, E.: Plastic surgery of nose. Kentucky M. J. *40:*264–266, July '42
KING, E. D.: Plastic surgery of nose. J. Med. *12:*518–524, Dec '31
KING, E. D.: Plastic surgery (face) (nose). J. Med. *19:*348–354, Sept '38
KING, E. D.: Plastic surgery of face and nose. West Virginia M. J. *37:*293–297, July '41
KING, E. S. J.: Post-traumatic epidermoid cysts of hands and fingers. Brit. J. Surg. *21:*29–43, July '33
KING, G. S.: New dressing for burns (medicated ointment in perforated cellophane envelope). Indust. Med. *14:*796–797, Oct '45
KING, G. S.: Burn dressing (cellophane). New York State J. Med. *46:*1567, July 15, '46
KING, H. AND HAMILTON, C. M.: Study of 80 cases of leukoplakia of mouth. South. M. J. *24:*380–383, May '31
KING, J. M.: Cancer of skin and mouth. J. Tennessee M. A. *19:*115–121, Sept '26
KING, M. K.: Burn therapy. Virginia M. Monthly *70:*106–109, Feb '43
KING, M. K.: Immediate grafting following injuries. Surg., Gynec. and Obst. *81:*75–78, July '45
KING, R. A.: Methods of fluid administration in treatment of shock; experimental comparison. Brit. M. J. *2:*485–487, Oct 12, '40
KING, W. E.: Management of severe burns. West Virginia M. J. *40:*83–85, March '44
KINGSBURY, B. C.: Management of jaw fractures complicated by intracranial injuries. U. S. Nav. M. Bull. *42:*915–920, April '44
KINGSLEY, H. D. (see MAHONEY, E. B. *et al*) Feb '42
KINMONTH, J. B.: Cut tendons of fingers with special reference to flexor tendon cut within its digital sheath. St. Thomas's Hosp. Gaz. *42:*154–158, Dec '44
KINNEMAN, R. E.: Peripheral nerve injuries; physical medicine in treatment. M. Clin. North America *27:*1097–1108, July '43
KINSELLA, V. J.: Complete thyroglossal fistulas. Brit. J. Surg. *26:*714–720, April '39
KINSELLA, V. J.: Hand infections. M. J. Australia *1:*856–861, June 10, '39
KINTZ, F. P.: Traumatic wounds of soft tissues of face, with preliminary report on new azochloramid (hypochloride derivative) solution, and new modified sulfanilamide solution. Mil. Surgeon *89:*60–70, July '41
KINZEL, H.: Cleft palate operations. Beitr. z. klin. Chir. *152:*618–624, '31
KIPARISOV, N. M.: Operation for cicatricial entropion of lower eyelid. Vestnik oftal. *11:*223–225, '37
KIRBY, C. K. (see COOK, T. J. *et al*) Oct '45
KIRBY, D. B.: Modified Motais operation for eyelid ptosis. Arch. Ophth. *57:*327–331, July '28
KIRBY, D. B.: Blepharoptosis; technic of surgical correction. Surg., Gynec. and Obst. *70:*438–449, Feb. (no. 2A) '40
KIRBY, D. B.: Injuries to eyelids. S. Clin. North America *20:*573–587, April '40
KIRBY, D. B.: Vertical shortening deformities of eyelids; plastic and reconstructive surgical correction. S. Clin. North America *24:*348–369, April '44

KIRBY, D. B. AND TOWN, A. E.: Injuries of eyes and eyelids. S. Clin. North America *23:*404-438, April '43
KIRCH, W.: Ankylosis of mandible due to scarring of cheek; restoration of cheek lining with skin graft. Proc. Staff Meet., Mayo Clin. *5:*339-341, Nov. 26, '30
KIRCH, W. (see NEW, G. B.) Nov '28
KIRCH, W. (see NEW, G. B.) April '29
KIRCH, W. (see NEW, G. B.) May '30
KIRCH, W. (see NEW, G. B.) April '32
KIRCH, W. A. (see NEW, G. B.) April '33
KIRCH, W. (see NEW, G. B.) March '39
KIRCH, W. (see NEW, G. B. *et al*) Aug '39
KIRCHENBERGER, A.: Avulsion of tendon of extensor pollicis. Med. Klin. *22:*1640-1641, Oct. 22, '26
KIRCHHOFF, W. (see HIRSCH, C.) 1928
KIRCHMAIR, H.: Family tree showing hereditary syndactylia. Munchen. med. Wchnschr. *83:*605-606, April 10, '36
KIRK, N. T.: End results of 158 consecutive autogenous bone grafts for non-union in long bone (A) in simple fractures; (B) in atrophic bone following war wounds and chronic suppurative osteitis (osteomyelitis). J. Bone and Joint Surg. *6:*760-799, Oct '24
KIRKHAM, H. L. D.: Some factors in cleft palate work. Texas State J. Med. *19:*577-579, Feb '24
KIRKHAM, H. L. D.: Preliminary paper on improvement of speech in cleft palate cases. Surg., Gynec. and Obst. *44:*244-246, Feb '27
KIRKHAM, H. L. D.: Plastic surgery. Texas State J. Med. *23:*725-727, March '28
KIRKHAM, H. L. D.: Skin grafts; uses of various types. M. Rec. and Ann. *24:*554, May '30
KIRKHAM, H. L. D.: Management of burns. Texas State J. Med. *29:*636-638, Feb '34
KIRKHAM, H. L. D.: Present day conception of cleft lip and palate surgery. Texas State J. Med. *31:*571-574, Jan '36
KIRKHAM, H. L. D.: Use of preserved cartilage in ear reconstruction. Ann. Surg. *111:*896-902, May '40
KIRKHAM, H. L. D.: Plastic procedures in burn therapy. Am. Acad. Orthop. Surgeons, Lect., pp. 202-208, '43
KIRKHAM, H. L. D.: Plastic procedures in burn therapy. Bull. Am. Coll. Surgeons *28:*144-145, June '43
KIRKHAM, H. L. D.; MILLS, J. T. AND POTTER, L. E.: Plastic surgery as related to war surgery. S. Clin. North America *23:*1603-1611, Dec '43
KIRSCHNER: Transplantation of epidermis (Thiersch grafts). Acta chir. Scandinav. *72:*21-35, '32
KIRSCHNER, M.: Surgical treatment of cleft palate. Arch. f. klin. Chir. *138:*515-533, '25
KIRSCHNER, M.: Surgical shock. Chirurg *10:*249, April 15, '38; 314, May 1, '38
KIRSCHNER, MARTIN (editor): *Allgemeine und spezielle chirurgische Operationslehre. Band III, Die Eingriffe an der Brüst und Brüsthöhle,* by Otto Kleinschmidt. Springer-Verlag, Berlin, 1940
KIRSCHNER, M., AND NORDMANN, O. (editors): *Die Chirurgie: .... Band II, Pp. 393-602, Die plastischen Operationen der Haut,* by K. Tiesenhausen. Urban, Berlin, 1927
KIRSCHNER, M. AND WAGNER, G. A.: New procedure for formation of artificial vagina. Deutsche Ztschr. f. Chir. *225:*242-264, '30 abstr: Zentralbl. f. Gynak. *54:*2690-2696, Oct. 25, '30 Comment by MÜLLER, P. Zentralbl. f. Gynak. *55:*201-203, Jan. 24, '31

Kirschner Operation

Artificial vagina construction by Kirschner method. ZURALSKI, T. Ginek. polska *16:*64-70, Jan-Feb '37

Kirschner-Wagner Operation

Formation of artificial vagina by Kirschner-Wagner operation. VOGT, E. Zentralbl. f. Gynak. *55:*1634-1639, May 16, '31
Formation of artificial vagina by Kirschner-Wagner operation; case. KRAUL, L. Zentralbl. f. Gynak. *55:*2102-2104, July 4, '31
Advantages of Kirschner-Wagner operation for artificial vagina. MILÄNDER, J. Zentralbl. f. Gynak. *55:*2746-2749, Sept. 12, '31
Formation of artificial vagina by Kirschner-Wagner operation. KAYSER, K. Zentralbl. f. Gynak. *56:*1633-1635, July 2, '32
Artificial vagina formation by Kirschner-Wagner operation; case. ALFEROW, M. W. Zentralbl. f. Gynak. *57:*884-885, April 15, '33
Formation of artificial vagina by Kirschner-Wagner operation. KÖHLER, H. Zentralbl. f. Gynak. *57:*1182-1186, May 20, '33
Kirschner-Wagner operation for artificial vagina. GLATZEL, J. AND ZUBRZYCKI, J. Polska gaz. lek. *12:*577-579, July 29, '33
Formation of artificial vagina by Kirschner-Wagner operation. MACZEWSKI, S. Polska gaz. lek. *12:*829-830, Oct. 22, '33
Cure of vaginal aplasia by Kirschner-Wagner operation. WESTMAN, A. Acta obst. et gynec. Scandinav. *13:*269-273, '33
Use of modified Kirschner-Wagner operation in aplasia of vagina and atresia of cervix; case. WESTMAN, A. Zentralbl. f. Gynak. *58:*2843-2845, Dec. 1, '34
Plastic operation for vaginal defect ad

Kirschner-Wagner Operation – Cont.
modum Kirschner-Wagner. NIELSEN, M. Acta obst. et gynec. Scandinav. *14:*314–320, '34
Formation of artificial vagina by using Thiersch transplants (Henkel modification of Kirschner-Wagner operation). FRIEDL-MEYER, M. Deutsche Ztschr. f. Chir. *244:*379–386, '35
Artificial vagina; Kirschner-Wagner operation. BARROWS, D. N. Am. J. Obst. and Gynec. *31:*156–158, Jan '36
Plastic formation of artificial vagina by Kirschner-Wagner operation; case. NIELSEN, M. Acta obst. et gynec. Scandinav. *16:*179–188, '36
Results and indications for Kirschner-Wagner operation in connection with 2 cases of vaginal aplasia. PELKONEN, E. Duodecim *53:*1003–1017, '37
Construction of artificial vagina by Kirschner-Wagner operation. COLOMBINO, C. AND SANVENERO ROSSELLI, G. Atti Soc. ital. di ostet. e ginec. *35:*460–464, Sept-Oct '39

KISCH, H.: Use of muscle grafts in mastoid operations. Post-Grad. M. J. *8:*270–271, July '32
KISKADDEN, W. S.: Newer methods of Thiersch grafting. West. J. Surg. *39:*758–762, Oct '31
KISKADDEN, W. S.: Adherent scars; their treatment (with skin grafts). California and West. Med. *39:*109–113, Aug '33
KISKADDEN, W. S.: Surgical treatment of eyelid ptosis. Am. J. Surg. *27:*499–501, March '35
KISKADDEN, W. S.: Use of flaps and pedicles in repair of hand and arm defects. Am. Acad. Orthop. Surgeons, Lect., pp. 180–183, '44
KISKADDEN, W. S. AND THOLEN, E. F.: Primary and secondary repair of cleft lip. Internat. J. Orthodontia *18:*863–873, Aug '32 also: West. J. Surg. *40:*18–27, Jan '32
KISKADDEN, W. S. (see CHARNOCK, D. A.) March '43
KISKADDEN, W. (see BAILEY, W.) Nov '43
KISNER, W. H. (see RYLANDER, C. M.) Oct '42
KISSEL. (see RICHON, *et al*) March '33
KISSMEYER, A.: Lapis ointment (silver nitrate) in burns. Ugesk. f. laeger *98:*1032–1033, Oct. 22, '36
KISSMEYER, A.: Treatment of burns and scalds with silver nitrate ointment. Lancet *2:*985, Oct. 24, '36
KISSMEYER, M. Silver nitrate ointment in burns. Bull. med., Paris *51:*323, May 15, '37
KITAEVA, A.: Surgery for trachomatous ectropion. Sovet. vestnik oftal. *7:*387–388, '35
KITE, J. H.: Deep burns and contractures. J. M. A. Georgia *33:*139–143, May '44
KITE, J. H. (see HAMM, W. G.) Nov '41
KITLOWSKI, E. A.: Preoperative and postoperative care of congenital clefts of lip and palate. Ann. Surg. *95:*659–666, May '32
KITLOWSKI, E. A.: Preservation of tendon function in hand by use of skin flaps. Am. J. Surg. *51:*653–661, March '41
KITLOWSKI, E. A.: Emergency care of burns. South. Med. and Surg. *104:*189–190, April '42
KITLOWSKI, E. A.: Surgical correction of mandibular prognathism. Ann. Surg. *115:*647–653, April '42
KITLOWSKI, E. A.: Symposium on emergency treatment of burns. S. Clin. North America *22:*1501–1519, Oct '42
KITLOWSKI, E. A. (see DAVIS, J. S.) Dec '31
KITLOWSKI, E. A. (see DAVIS, J. S.) May '33
KITLOWSKI, E. A. (see DAVIS, J. S.) May '34
KITLOWSKI, E. A. (see DAVIS, J. S.) Dec '34
KITLOWSKI, E. A. (see DAVIS, J. S.) Dec '36
KITLOWSKI, E. A. (see DAVIS, J. S.) Dec '37
KITLOWSKI, E. A. (see DAVIS, J. S.) June '39
KJAERHOLM, H.: Jaw fractures. Ugesk. f. laeger *100:*659–669, June 16, '38
KJAERHOLM, H.: Jaw fractures. Ugesk. f. laeger *102:*321–333, April 4, '40
KJAERHOLM, H. (see FABRICIUS-MOLLER, J.) Oct '41
KLABER, R.: Preauricular fistulae; two cases. Proc. Roy. Soc. Med. *28:*1553–1554, Oct '35
KLABUNDE, E. H. (see PIERCE, G. W. *et al*) Jan '44
KLAFF, D. D.: Bilateral congenital atresia of choanae. Arch. Otolaryng. *41:*298–299, April '45
KLAGES, F.: Plastic use of crest of ilium in repair of loss of substance of cranium. Zentralbl. f. Chir. *66:*1580–1587, July 15, '39
KLAGES, F. AND JACOB, R.: Study of anatomy and heredity of cleft foot and hand deformities in siblings. Ztschr. f. Orthop. *70:*265–281, '40
KLAPP, R.: Facial plastic surgery; cases. Chirurg *3:*353–357, April 15, '31
KLAPP, R.: Improvement of methods of section in treatment of abscesses of tendon sheaths and of palm of hand. Zentralbl. f. Chir. *58:*953–954, April 11, '31
KLAPP, R.: Operation for syndactylia. Arch. f. klin. Chir. *177:*688–690, '33
KLAPP, R.: Suture of tendon with central filament. Arch. f. klin. Chir. *177:*690–691, '33
KLAPP, R.: Successful suture of tendon. Sovet. khir. (nos. 1–3) *5:*69–71, '33
KLAPP, R.: Double incisions in therapy of phlegmon of sheath and empyema of joints. Zentralbl. f. Chir. *66:*753–758, April 1, '39
KLAPP, R.: Incision of facial furunculosis. Zentralbl. f. Chir. *67:*1618–1619, Aug. 31, '40

Klapp Operation

Syndactylia operated on according to Klapp method. SCHJØTH-IVERSEN, I. Norsk mag. f. laegevidensk. *97:*700–704, July '36

KLASSEN, P.: Chronic traumatic edema of dorsum of hand; 7 cases. Monatschr. f. Unfallh. *36:*289–309, July '29

KLAUBER, E.: Transplantation of conjunctiva in surgical therapy of trichiasis. Ann. d'ocul. *176:*476–477, June '39

KLAUDER, J. V.: Treatment of nevi, with particular reference to high frequency current. J. A. M. A. *90:*1763–1768, June 2, '28

KLAUDER, J. V.: Birthmarks. Hygeia *7:*351–352, April '29

KLAUDER, J. V.: Treatment of nevi; hazard of insufficient destruction of pigmented nevi. Pennsylvania M. J. *33:*472–477, April '30

KLAUDER, J. V.: Treatment of rhinophyma by electrodesiccation. Arch. Dermat. and Syph. *33:*885, May '36

KLAUDER, J. V. (see BUTTERWORTH, T.) March '34

KLAUS, E. J.: Injuries to hand in boxing; etiology and prevention. Munchen. med. Wchnschr. *87:*265–267, March 8, '40

KLEE-RAWIDOWWICZ, E.: Production of malignant tumors by transplantation of embryonal tissues. Deutsche med. Wchnschr. *58:*1439–1440, Sept. 9, '32

KLEEFELD, G.: Technic of median nonmutilating blepharrhaphy. Bull. Soc. belge d'opht., no. 74, pp. 16–21, '37

KLEIMAN, M.: Rational therapy of shock. Arch. Soc. cirujanos hosp. *14:*596–600, Dec '44

KLEIN, D.: Instrument to facilitate multiple loop wiring in jaw fractures. Bull. U. S. Army M. Dept. *4:*479, Oct '45

KLEINBERG. S.: Traumatic internal derangement of temporomandibular joint. Am. J. Orthodontics (Oral Surg. Sect.) *27:*328–332, June '41

KLEINBERG, W. (see SWINGLE, W. W. *et al*) May '44

DE KLEINE, E. H. (see STRAITH, C. L.) Jan '38

DE KLEINE, E. H. (see STRAITH, C. L.) Dec '38

KLEINER, B.: Gastroschisis in new-born; 2 cases. Monatschr. f. Geburtsh. u. Gynak. *84:*281–293, March '30

KLEINERT, M. N.: Branchial fistula. Arch. Otolaryng. *18:*510–515, Oct '33

KLEINHAUS, E.: Pseudosubluxation of carpometacarpal joint of thumb. Rontgenpraxis *2:*804–806, Sept. 1, '30

KLEINSCHMIDT, K.: Treatment of salivary fistulas. Munchen. med. Wchnschr. *70:*809, June 22, '23 abstr: J. A. M. A. *81:*1245, Oct. 6, '23

KLEINSCHMIDT, K.: Explanation of late rupture of extensor pollicis longus following fracture of radius. Beitr. z. klin. Chir. *146:*530–535, '29

KLEINSCHMIDT, O.: Mammary plastics. Zentralbl. f. Chir. (supp.) *51:*488–493, March 15, '24

KLEINSCHMIDT, O.: Burn therapy. Deutsche med. Wchnschr. *57:*1546–1548, Sept. 4, '31

KLEINSCHMIDT, O.: Ambulant treatment of branchial fistulas. Deutsche med. Wchnschr. *57:*1549–1551, Sept. 4, '31

KLEINSCHMIDT, O.: Operative treatment of tumors of jaw by Axhausen method of bone transplantation. Arch. f. klin. Chir. *164:*205–212, '31

KLEINSCHMIDT, O.: Transplantation of second toe on stump of thumb. Arch. f. klin. Chir. *164:*809–811, '31

KLEINSCHMIDT, O.: Transplantation of skin together with implanted bone to cover defects of soft tissues and bones. Chirurg *14:*737–742, Dec. 15, '42

KLEINSCHMIDT, P.: Exarticulation of lower jaw. Deutsche med. Wchnschr. *53:*473, March 11, '27

KLEITSMAN, R.: Creation of artificial vagina; value of use of vernix caseosa; case. Gynec. et obst. *31:*725–728, May '35

KLEITSMAN, R. AND POSKA-TEISS, L.: Use of vernix caseosa in formation of artificial vagina; histologic examination of vagina some time after operation. Zentralbl. f. Gynak. *59:*755–760, March 30, '35

KLEMME, R. M.; WOOLSEY, R. D. AND DE REZENDE, N. T.: Autopsy nerve grafts in peripheral nerve surgery; clinical application; "glue" suture technic. J. A. M. A. *123:*393–396, Oct. 16, '43

KLEMPERER, P. (see MCCARTHY, J. F.) Oct '25

KLEMPERER, W. W. (see BALKIN, S. G. *et al*) May '45

KLEPSER, R. G. (see VEAL, J. R. *et al*) Dec '41

KLESTADT, W.: Causes of deformities of middle portion of nose. Ztschr. f. Laryng., Rhin. *17:*326–334, Jan '29

KLESTADT, W.: Submucous cleft of palate; case. Ztschr. f. Laryng., Rhin. *19:*279–287, May '30

KLESTADT, W.: Treatment of fresh nasal fractures and nasal sinuses. Med. Klin. *27:*1235–1237, Aug. 21, '31

KLESTADT, W.: Technic of plastic surgery after opening of antrum. Ztschr. f. Laryng., Rhin., Otol. *23:*80–84, '32

KLEY, H.: Familial occurrence of hypoplasia of jaws. Med. Welt *8:*311, March 3, '34

KLICPERA, L.: Surgical correction of protruding ears. Wien. klin. Wchnschr. *52:*536–538, June 2, '39

KLICPERA, L.: Correction of abnormally protruding ears. Ztschr. f. Hals-, Nasen-u. Ohrenh. *46:*367–368, '39

KLICPERA, L.: Plastic correction of cartilaginous crooked nose. Arch. f. Ohren-, Nasen-u. Kehlkopfh. *147:*170–172, '40

KLICPERA, L.: Two-stage plastic operation for nasal deformities. Monatschr. f. Ohrenh. *74:*183–186, April '40

KLIMENKOVA, L. A. (see BALAKHOVSKIY, S. D. *et al*) 1936

KLIMKO, D.: Histologic and biologic value of Schubert operation for vaginal reconstruction after one year; report of case with peritonitis as sequel. Zentralbl. f. Gynak. *63:*1150–1161, May 20, '39

KLIMPEL, W.: Oral and pharyngeal injuries from pointed objects. Ztschr. f. Hals-, Nasen-u. Ohrenh. *45:*328–338, '40

KLINGENSTEIN, P. AND COLP, R.: Congenital cysts and fistulae of neck; review of 42 thyroglossal cysts and fistulae. Ann. Surg. *82:*854–864, Dec '25

KLOEHN, S. J.: Application of biologic principles to treatment of jaw fractures. Angle Orthodontist *10:*94–100, April '40

KLOMPUS, I.: Fractures of toes; simple method of treatment. U. S. Nav. M. Bull. *44:*850–851, April '45

KLOTZ, L. (see EWIG, W.) 1932

KLUG, W.: Tannin solution and other means for treatment of extensive burns. Ztschr. f. arztl. Fortbild. *28:*278–281, May 1, '31

KLUMPP, J. S.: Treatment of third degree burns. West Virginia M. J. *39:*406–414, Dec '43

KLYKOVA, A. L. AND TOKAREVA, B. A.: Blaskovics operation for eyelid ptosis on basis of statistics of Moscow Ophthalmologic Hospital. Vestnik oftal. *12:*495–498, '38

KNAPP, A. A.: Injuries to eyes, with remarks on plastic surgery. U. S. Nav. M. Bull. *42:*651–653, March '44

KNAPP, H. B.: Loose cartilages in temporomandibular articulation. J. Michigan M. Soc. *27:*798–801, Dec '28

KNAPPER, C.: Third-degree burns. Nederl. tijdschr. v. geneesk. *84:*382–387, Feb. 3, '40

KNAPPIG, T.: Hypospadias, hydronephrosis and infected congenital hydro-ureter; case. Orvosi hetil. *76:*864–866, Sept. 24, '32

KNAUS, H.: Artificial vagina, formation from urethra. Zentralbl. f. Gynak. *61:*2540–2545, Oct. 30, '37

KŇAZOVICKÝ, J.: Therapeutic value of cod liver oil combined with vaseline for hand infections and injuries. Rozhl. v chir. a gynaek. (cast chir.) *14:*93–102, '35

KNEALE, H. B. (see HAGNER, F. R.) April '23

KNIGHT, H. O.: Applied anatomy in treatment of hand infections. Texas State J. Med. *24:*528–533, Dec '28

KNIGHT, M. P. AND WOOD, G. O.: Surgical obliteration of cavities following traumatic osteomyelitis (by bone and skin transplantation). J. Bone and Joint Surg. *27:*547–556, Oct '45

KNOBLOCH, J.: Present status of bone transplantation. Rozhl. v. chir. a gynaek. (cast chir.) *13:*191–199, '34

KNOEPP, L. F.: Military burns; analysis of 308 cases. Am. J. Surg. *57:*226–230, Aug '42

KNORR, H.: Present status of traumatic shock. Klin. Wchnschr. *1:*1115–1117, May 27, '22

KNORR, H.: Orthopedic treatment of contracture of temporomaxillary joint. Zentralbl. f. Chir. *56:*1229–1232, May 18, '29

KNOWLES, F. C.: Precancerous eruptions of skin. J. Iowa M. Soc. *14:*403–407, Sept '24

KNOWLES, J. R.: Splint for fractures of phalanges. J. A. M. A. *94:*2065, June 28, '30

KO, G.: Cosmetic autotransplantation of nails. Taiwan Igakkai Zasshi *35:*1072, May '36

KOCH, C. F.: Artificial vagina formed from intestinal segment. Nederl. Tijdschr. v. Geneesk. *1:*214–225, Jan. 8, '27

KOCH, C. F. A.: Treatment of facial paralysis. Nederl. Tijdschr. v. Geneesk. *2:*3628–3632, July 21, '28

KOCH, F.: Occurrence of branchial cysts in neck; case. Monatschr. f. Ohrenh. *66:*1331–1334, Nov '32

KOCH, F.: Injuries due to burns from point of view of naval surgery. Svenska lak.-tidning. *38:*1351–1356, June 13, '41

KOCH, K.: Unsuccessful attempt at plastic surgery of pedunculated scrotal flap. Zentralbl. f. Chir. *55:*587–590, March 10, '28

KOCH, S. L.: Covering of raw surfaces with particular reference to hand. Surg., Gynec. and Obst. *43:*677–686, Nov '26

KOCH, S. L.: Prevention of contractures following infections of hand. J. A. M. A. *88:*1214–1217, April 16, '27

KOCH, S. L.: Therapy of contractures with aid of free full thickness skin-grafts and pedunculated flaps. S. Clin. North America *7:*611–626, June '27

KOCH, S. L.: Diagnosis and after treatment of severe hand infections. J. Kansas M. Soc. *28:*10–16, Jan '28

KOCH, S. L.: Diagnosis and treatment of acute hand infections. J. Indiana M. A. *21:*137–145, April '28 also: J. Med. *9:*116–124, May '28

KOCH, S. L.: Diagnosis and treatment of some major hand infections. J. Iowa M. Soc. *18:*254–261, July '28

KOCH, S. L.: Four splints of value in treatment of disabilities of hand. Surg., Gynec. and Obst. *48:*416–418, March '29

KOCH, S. L.: Felon, acute lymphangitis and

tendon sheath infections of hand; differential diagnosis and treatment. J.A.M.A. *92:*1171–1173, April 6, '29

Koch, S. L.: Major hand infections; differential diagnosis and treatment. J. Indiana M. A. *22:*510–517, Dec '29

Koch, S. L.: Acquired contractures of hand. Am. J. Surg. *9:*413–423, Sept '30

Koch, S. L.: Contracture of hand. Surg., Gynec. and Obst. *52:*367–370, Feb. (No. 2A) '31

Koch, S. L.: Immediate treatment of hand injuries. Surg., Gynec. and Obst. *52:*594–601, Feb. (No. 2A) '31

Koch, S. L.: Immediate therapy of hand injuries. M. Arts and Indianapolis M. J. *34:*763–771, Dec '31

Koch, S. L.: Diagnosis and treatment of major infections of hand. Minnesota Med. *15:*1–7, Jan '32

Koch, S. L.: Dupuytren's contracture. J.A.M.A. *100:*878–880, March 25, '33

Koch, S. L.: Injuries of nerves and tendons of hand (surgical therapy). J. Oklahoma M. A. *26:*323–327, Sept '33

Koch, S. L.: Complicated contractures of hand; their treatment by freeing fibrosed tendons and replacing destroyed tendons with grafts. Ann. Surg. *98:*546–580, Oct '33

Koch, S. L.: Injuries to nerves and tendons of hand. Pennsylvania M. J. *37:*555–557, April '34

Koch, S. L.: Burn contractures of axilla. S. Clin. North America *14:*751–761, Aug '34

Koch, S. L.: Acute rapidly spreading hand infections following trivial injuries. Surg., Gynec. and Obst. *59:*277–308, Sept '34

Koch, S. L.: Injuries of nerves and tendons of hand. Wisconsin M. J. *33:*655–661, Sept '34

Koch, S. L.: Volkmann contracture. Tr. West. S. A. *44:*222–235, '34

Koch, S. L.: Treatment of compound hand injuries. Journal-Lancet *55:*569–572, Sept. 1, '35

Koch, S. L.: Hand injuries. Kentucky M. J. *34:*101–109, March '36

Koch, S. L.: Hand injuries with particular reference to immediate treatment. Nebraska M. J. *21:*281–288, Aug '36

Koch, S. L.: Hand injuries. J.A.M.A. *107:*1044–1049, Sept. 26, '36

Koch, S. L.: Osteomyelitis of hands. Surg., Gynec. and Obst. *64:*1–8, Jan '37

Koch, S. L.: Infections of fingers and palm. Pennsylvania M. J. *40:*597–604, May '37

Koch, S. L.: Surgical principles in treatment of hand infections. J. Indiana M. A. *31:*231–232, May '38 also: West. J. Surg. *46:*301–304, June '38

Koch, S. L.: Surgical principles in care of infections of hand. Ohio State M. J. *34:*1325–1328, Dec '38

Koch, S. L.: Treatment of compound hand injuries. J. Michigan M. Soc. *38:*27–31, Jan '39

Koch, S. L.: Surgical principles in treatment of hand infections and injuries. J. Kansas M. Soc. *40:*89–95, March '39

Koch, S. L.: Surgical principles in repair of divided nerves and tendons. Quart. Bull., Northwestern Univ. M. School *14:*1–8, '40

Koch, S. L.: Transplantation of skin and subcutaneous tissue (history of plastic surgery and surgeons). Surg., Gynec. and Obst. *72:*1–14, Jan '41

Koch, S. L.: Transplantation of skin and subcutaneous tissue to hand. Surg., Gynec. and Obst. *72:*157–177, Feb. '41

Koch, S. L.: Prevention and treatment of hand infections. J. A. M. A. *116:*1365–1367, March 29, '41

Koch, S. L.: Treatment of hand injuries. New England J. Med. *225:*105–109, July 17, '41

Koch, S. L.: Burn therapy. Quart. Bull., Northwestern Univ. M. School *16:*191–196, '42 also: Bull. Am. Coll. Surgeons *27:*106–108, April '42

Koch, S. L. Tendon suturing. Indust. Med. *11:*327–328, July '42

Koch, S. L.: Treatment of raw surfaces. J. Iowa M. Soc. *32:*445–450, Oct '42

Koch, S. L.: Tendon and nerve injuries. New York State J. Med. *42:*1819–1823, Oct. 1, '42

Koch, S. L.: Radial nerve injuries. Quart. Bull., Northwestern Univ. M. School *17:*1–6, '43

Koch, S. L.: Nerve and tendon injuries. Bull. Am. Coll. Surgeons *28:*125–126, June '43

Koch, S. L.: Division of flexor tendons within digital sheath. Surg., Gynec. and Obst. *78:*9–22, Jan '44

Koch, S. L.: Surgical cleanliness, compression, and rest as primary surgical principles in burn therapy. J. A. M. A. *125:*612–616, July 1, '44

Koch, S. L.: Wounds and injuries of hands. Quart. Bull., Northwestern Univ. M. School *19:*265–277, '45

Koch, S. L.: Injuries of nerves and tendons of hand. Cincinnati J. Med. *27:*515–521, Aug '46

Koch, S. L. and Kanavel, A. B.: Contractures due to burns; treatment with free full thickness grafts and pedunculated flaps. Tr. Sect. Surg, General and Abd., A. M. A., pp. 208–227, '28

Koch, S. L. and Kanavel, A. B.: Contracture due to burns; treatment with free full thickness grafts and pedunculated flaps. J.A.M.A. *92:*277–281, Jan. 26, '29

Koch, S. L. and Mason, M. L.: Division of

nerves and tendons of hand, with discussion of surgical treatment and its results. Surg., Gynec. and Obst. *56:*1–39, Jan '33

Koch, S. L. and Mason, M. L.: Purposeful splinting of hand following injuries (including sketch on Hugh Owen Thomas). Surg., Gynec. and Obst. *68:*1–16, Jan '39

Koch, S. L. (see Allen, H. S.) May '42

Koch, S. L. (see Kanavel, A. B. *et al*) Feb '29

Koch, S. L. (see Mason, M. L.) Nov '30

Kocher Operation

Osteoplastic resection of both alveolar processes according to Kocher. Nikolsky, A. M. Ann. Otol., Rhin. and Laryng. *39:*701–719, Sept '30

Kochev, K. N.: New apparatus for producing mechanical movements in cases of ankylosis of jaws. Khirurgiya, no. 9, pp. 160–161, '37

Kochev, K. N.: Technic of surgical mobilization of lower jaw. Sovet. med. (nos. 17–18) *5:*33, '41

Kocsard, E.: Elephantiasis of legs; unusual case. Dermosifilografo *13:*180–185, March '38

Koeff, G. (see Sentenac, E.) Jan '38

Koehler, O.: Absence of hands and feet in Brazilian family; question of heredity of congenital abnormalities. Ztschr. f. menschhl. Vererb.-u. Konstitutionslehre *19:*670–690, '36

Koenner, D. M.: Abnormalities of hands and feet. J. Hered. *25:*329–334, Aug '34

Koepp-Baker, H.: Responsibility of speech correctionist in treatment of patient who has received surgical or prosthetic treatment. Am. J. Orthodontics (Oral Surg. Sect.) *32:*714–717, Nov '46

Kofler, K.: Dacryocystorhinostomy by way of pyriform aperture. Monatschr. f. Ohrenh. *74:*299–306, June '40

Kofmann, S.: New points of view in arthroplasty of jaw; comment on Haas's article. Zentralbl. f. Chir. *53:*1125–1126, May 1, '26

Kogan, A. V. (see Beyul, A. P.) 1937

Kogon, A. I.: Late results of operation for carcinoma of lower lip. Novy khir. arkhiv *37:*227–240, '36

Köhler, H.: Demonstration of value of urea tolerance test as indication of functional condition of kidney in patient with total exstrophy of bladder; case. Zentralbl. f. Chir. *55:*1412–1417, June 9, '28

Köhler, H.: Formation of artificial vagina by Kirschner-Wagner operation. Zentralbl. f. Gynak. *57:*1182–1186, May 20, '33

Köhler, M. Successful plastic operation for aplasia of vagina. Wien. klin. Wchnschr. *40:*1577–1578, Dec. 15, '27

Kohlmayer, H.: Traumatic development of Dupuytren's contracture. Zentralbl. f. Chir. *62:*1928–1931, Aug. 17, '35

Kohlstaedt, K. G. and Page, I. H.: Hemorrhagic hypotension and its treatment by intraarterial and intravenous infusion of blood. Arch. Surg. *47:*178–191, Aug '43

Kohn

Comment on article by Kohn on skin grafting. Neuhäuser, H. Zentralbl. f. Chir. *59:*2532, Oct 15, '32

Kohn, F.; Hall, M. H. and Cross, C. D.: Propamidine for burns at an E. M. S. hospital. Lancet *1:*140–141, Jan 30, '43

Kohn, K. W.: Transplantation of active epithelium. Zentralbl. f. Chir. *59:*1748–1750, July 16, '32

Kohn, S. I.: Treatment of temporomandibular dysfunction accompanied by severe pain syndrome. Am. J. Orthodontics *28:*302–310, May '42

Kohout, J. J.: Prosthetic device for support of eyelids. Bull. U. S. Army M. Dept. *4:*117–118, July '45

Kojima, K. (see Karube, R.) June '39

Kolbe, L.: Congenital absence of skin on skull. Orvosi hetil. *78:*1039–1040, Nov 10, '34

Koldaeff, S. M.: Plastic surgery of lower lip for noma. Vrach. gaz. *32:*1177–1181, '28

Kolen, A. A.: New technic for mucous graft in ophthalmology. Vestnik oftal. (nos. 3–4) *15:*100–102, '39

Kolesov, G. G.: Combined congenital malformation of tongue and hard palate; case. Sovet. khir., no. 9, pp. 524–526, '36

Kolkman, D.: Cysts and fistulas of lateral region of neck. Nederl. tijdschr. v. geneesk. *77:*862–865, Feb. 25, '33

Komissarov, M. K.: Comparative value of closed and open methods of burn therapy. Novy khir. arkhiv *38:*464–468, '37

Kondoleon, E.: Ultimate results of Kondoleon operation for elephantiasic edema. Arch. franco-belges de chir. *27:*104–110, Feb '24 abstr: J.A.M.A. *82:*2087, June 21, '24

Kondoleon Operation

Elephantiasis and the Kondoleon operation. Green, T. M. Virginia M. Monthly *48:*196, July '21

Kondoleon operation for elephantiasis. Henry, A. K. Brit. J. Surg. *9:*111, July '21

Report of end results of Kondoleon operation for elephantiasis. Sistrunk, W. E. Southern M. J. *14:*619, Aug '21

Kondoleon operation for elephantiasis of leg. Pignatti, A. Chir. d. org. di movimento

Kondoleon Operation – Cont.
*6:*49–62, Feb '22 (illus.) abstr: J.A.M.A. *78:*1579, May 20, '22
Elephantiasis treated by Kondoleon operation. HERFF, F. P. Surg., Gynec. and Obst. *34:*758–760, June '22 (illus.)
Results obtained in elephantiasis through Kondoleon operation. SISTRUNK, W. E. Minnesota Med. *6:*173–177, March '23 (illus.)
Kondoleon operation and filariasis. STENHOUSE, H. M., U. S. Nav. M. Bull. *20:*715–716, June '24
Surgical treatment of elephantiasic conditions in legs by Kondoleon's method. FALCONE, R. Arch. ital. di chir. *13:*662–669, '25
Plastic surgery; certain modifications of Kondoleon operation for elephantiasis. SISTRUNK, W. E.: Ann. Surg. *85:*190–193, Feb '27
Kondoleon method of treatment of elephantiasis; 2 cases. MIROLLI, A. Minerva med. *7:*637–649, June 20, '27
Kondoleon operation for elephantiasis. CLUTE, H. M., S. Clin. N. Amer. *8:*119–122, Feb '28
Results in Porto Rico of Kondoleon operations for elephantiasis of extremities. BURKE, G. R. Surg., Gynec. and Obst. *47:*843–847, Dec '28
Elephantiasis of lower extremities successfully treated by Kondoleon's operation. WEINSTEIN, M. Am. J. Surg. *7:*704–710, Nov '29
Non-filarial elephantiasis therapy (Kondoleon operation). SCHOFIELD, J. E. Brit. M. J. *1:*795, May 9, '31
Chronic lymphatic edema and its treatment by Kondoleon operation. MAILER, R. Glasgow M. J. *121:*213–217, June '34
Modified Kondoleon operation for sclerosed leg with ulceration (grafts). BANCROFT, F. W. *et al.* Ann. Surg. *111:*874–891, May '40
Modified Kondoleon operation for chronic leg ulcers. STANLEY-BROWN, M. S. Clin. North America *21:*617–623, April '41
Kondoleon operation for chronic lymphedema. TELFORD, E. D. AND SIMMONS, H. T. Lancet *2:*667, Nov 29, '41

KÖNIG, E.: Etiology and mechanism of snapping finger. Med. Klin. *17:*434, April 10, '21
KÖNIG, E.: Plastic reconstruction of scrotum; case. Arch. f. klin. Chir. *150:*244–250, '28
KÖNIG, E.: Plastic closure of tracheal fistula. Hals-, Nasen-u. Ohrenarzt (Teil 1) *28:*279–282, July '37
KÖNIG, E.: Dupuytren's contracture. Med. Klin. *36:*568–571, May 24, '40
KÖNIG, F.: Plastic operation on lips. Beitr. z. klin. Chir. *122:*288, '21 abstr: J.A.M.A. *77:*656, Aug. 20, '21
KÖNIG, F.: Cosmetic incision of soft parts for temporary division of lower jaw. Zentralbl. f. Chir. *49:*362–363, March 18, '22 (illus.)
KÖNIG, F.: Pathology and treatment of jaw ankylosis. Beitr. z. klin. Chir. *140:*565–576, '27
KÖNIG, F.: Plastic surgery of muscular paralysis; formation of muscular loops. Zentralbl. f. Chir. *62:*2531–2536, Oct. 26, '35
KÖNIG, F.: Injuries of fingers and hand from point of view of state accident insurance. Munchen. med. Wchnschr. *90:*509, Aug. 27, '43
KÖNIG, W.: Shock therapy. Zentralbl. f. Chir. *62:*2862–2873, Nov. 30, '35 Abstr: Med. Welt *9:*1693–1696, Nov. 23, '35
KONJETZNY, G. E.: Habitual dislocation of lower jaw. Arch. f. klin. Chir. *116:*681, Sept '21 abstr: J. A. M. A. *77:*1774, Nov. 26, '21
KONJETZNY, G. E.: Treatment of habitual luxation and so-called habitual subluxation of lower jaw and snapping of temporomaxillary joint. Zentralbl. f. Chir. *56:*3018–3023, Nov. 30, '29
KONJETZNY, G. E.: Treatment of persistent parotid fistulas; 2 cases. Zentralbl. f. Chir. *61:*243–247, Feb. 3, '34
KONONENKO, I. F.: Therapy of osteomyelitis of hand and fingers at evacuation hospitals. Vrach. delo (nos 7–8) *25:*341–346, '45
KOOP, C. E.: Symposium on traumatic surgery; management of shock and hemorrhage. Clinics *3:*1586–1617, April '45
KOPELMAN, H. (see LANDAU, E. *et al*) Aug '42
KOPIT, R. Z. (see VINOGOROV, D. R.) 1936
KOPP, I. F.: Indications and comparative evaluation of Hungarian method of blepharoplasty. Sovet. vestnik oftal. *7:*603–609, '35
KOPP, M. M.: Complications of rhinoplastic surgery. J. Internat. Coll. Surgeons *2:*346–350, Oct '39
KOPP, M. M.: Two congenital deformities; bifid nose and bulldog nose. Laryngoscope *49:*1128–1133, Nov '39
KOPP, M. M.: Deformities of nose due to septal abnormalities. M. Rec. *151:*111–116, Feb 21, '40
KOPP, M. M.: Atrophic rhinitis in plastic surgery. Laryngoscope *50:*510–519, June '40
KOPPÁNYI, T.: Transplantation of organs. Scient. Monthly *27:*502–505, Dec '28
KORABELNIKOV, I. D.: Relation to suppurative processes of hands and fingers to minor trauma. Sovet. khir., no. 3, pp. 488–490, '36
KORKASHVILI, G. L.: Dilatation of lacrimal ducts. Vestnik oftal. *13:*405–406, '38
KORKHOFF, U.: Formation of medial cysts of

neck. Vrach. gaz. *34:*779–781, May 31, '30

KORKHOV, V.: Cases of cancer after skin transplantation. Vestnik khir. (no. 41) *14:*137–142, '28

KORNBLUEH, I. H. (see TOLAND, J. J. Jr.) Feb '44

KORNBLUETH, W. (see MITERSTEIN, B.) Oct '45

KORNEFF, P.: Transplantation and growth of bones. Vestnik khir. (no. 34) *12:*10–61, '27

KORNEW, P. G.: Growth of bone transplants; experimental study. Arch. f. klin. Chir. *154:*499–564, '29

KORNMAN, I. E. AND SMERETCHINSKY, T. M.: Davidson's method in acid burns. Odessky M. J. *4:*13–16, '29

KOROLEV, B. A.: Method for closure of operative wound in cancer of breast; skin grafting. Novy khir. arkhiv. *46:*48–51, '40

KORSUNSKIY, P. D.: Modification of Vreden operation in therapy of paralytic facial deformity. Khirurgiya, no. 10, pp. 35–38, '39

KORTZEBORN, A.: Operative treatment of dislocation of thumb, "monkey hand." Arch. f. klin. chir. *133:*465–478, '24

KORYTKIN-NOVIKOV, L. E.: Brilliant green in burns. Sovet. vrach. gaz., pp. 21–23, Jan 15, '34 also: Zentralbl. f. Chir. *61:*253–256, Feb 3, '34

KORYTKIN-NOVIKOV, L. E.: Brilliant green in burn therapy. Sovet. vrach. zhur., pp. 421–422, March 30, '36 also: Zentralbl. f. Chir. *63:*2427–2430, Oct 10, '36

KOSCH, W.: Plastic surgery of protruding ears. Deutsche med. Wchnschr. *54:*569, April 6, '28

KOSSACK, G.: Cure of nevus flammeus by freezing with ethyl chloride; case. Med. Klin. *23:*2003, Dec 30, '27

KOSTEČKA, F.: Craniofacial dysostosis and congenital malformation of hands; case. Ztschr. f. Stomatol. *35:*113–120, Jan 9, '37

Kostecka Operation

Kostecka operation for prognathism; follow up studies on 21 cases. ULLIK, R. Ztschr. f. Stomatol. *40:*255, April 10, '42; 294, April 24, '42

KOSTER, H. AND KASMAN, L. P.: Effect of desoxycorticosterone acetate (adrenal preparation) in postoperative shock. Arch. Surg. *45:*272–285, Aug '42

KÖSTER, K. H.: Plastic operations in loss of thumb. Acta orthop. Scandinav. *9:*115–131, '38

KOSTER, S.: Unusual case of contracture of palmar fascia of both hands. Nederl. tijdschr. v. geneesk. *79:*674–678, Feb 16, '35 also: Rev. neurol. *63:*281–285, Feb '35

KÖSTLER, J.: Preliminary and substitution operations in treatment of lesions peripheral nerves. Deutsche Ztschr. f. Chir. *259:*1, '44

KOSTRUBALA, J. G.: Skin transplantation. Mil. Surgeon *97:*203–208, Sept '45

KOTAKE, Y. (see NOGUCHI, M.) Sept '36

KOTILAINEN, T.: Table for gymnastic aftertreatment of hand injuries. Duodecim *56:*333–335, '40

KOTSUBEY, L. A.: Application of sollux lamp in skin grafting in plastic surgery. Vestnik khir. *59:*637–639, June '40

KOTZAREFF, A.: Burn therapy. Rev. de chir. *60:*5–29, '22 Abstr: J.A.M.A. *79:*507, Aug 5, '22

KOVACS, A.: Problems in cosmetic surgery of nose. Laryngoscope *47:*92–96, Feb '37

KOVACS, H. J.: Air embolism following hand injury; case. Zentralbl. f. Chir. *65:*180–182, Jan 22, '38

KOVACS, R.: Scar contracture of flexor sublimis digitorum. Physical Therap. *45:*383–384, Aug '27

KOVACS, R.: Peripheral nerve injuries; physical therapy. New York State J. Med. *43:*1403–1408, Aug 1, '43

KOVAL, A. Y.: Traumatic lesions of jaws. Khirurgiya, no. 12, pp. 41–44, '39

KOVALEVA, T. F.: Ectopy of bladder and nephrolithiasis; case. Novy khir. arkhiv *45:*253–255, '40

KOVALSKY, N. P.: Treatment of angioma of face. Vestnik khir. (no. 40) *14:*30–38, '28

KOVANOV, V. V.: Ammargen (silver-ammonia compound) in burn therapy. Sovet. med. (no. 3) *4:*21–22, '40

KOWARSCHIK, J.: Therapy of facial paralysis. Wien. klin. Wchnschr. *54:*494–498, June 6, '41

KOYAMA, M (see TAMIYA, C.) 1929

KOZLIK, F.: Unilateral absence of intermaxillary bone without cleft; case. Anat. Anz. *88:*91–100, April 3, '39

KOZOLL, D. D.: Pseudohermaphroditism; 2 cases. Arch. Surg. *45:*578–595, Oct '42

KOZOLL, D. D. AND HOFFMAN, W. S.: Excretion of intravenously injected gelatin. Proc. Central Soc. Clin. Research *17:*47–48, '44

KOZOLL, D. D. *et al*: Gelatin solutions (as plasma substitute) in human shock. Am. J. M. Sc. *208:*141–147, Aug '44

KOZDOBA, A. Z. (see POKOTILO, V. L.) 1936

KRAATZ, H.: Indications for artificial vagina. Ztschr. f. Geburtsh. u. Gynak. *117:*168–174, '38

KRABBEL, M.: Technic of Mayo-Walters operation in exstrophy of bladder. Zentralbl. f. Chir. *64:*693–696, March 20, '37

KRAEVSKIY, N. A.: Pathologic anatomy and

pathogenesis of shock. Khirurgiya, no. 9, pp. 7-12, '44

KRAFT, A. (see DAVISON, C.) Jan '31

KRAFT, R.: Plastic covering of defects following breast amputation. Deutsche Ztschr. f. Chir. *207:*171-183, '27

KRAFT, R.: Subcutaneous transplantation for ruptured tendons; cases. Arch. f. Orthop. *28:*532-540, July 23, '30

KRAFT, R.: Construction of thumb from first metacarpal in case of absence of all fingers. Deutsche Ztschr. f. Chir. *226:*426-430, '30

KRAGH, J. (see BOSERUP, O.) Nov '23

KRAMER, R.: Lateral cervical fistulae. Laryngoscope *36:*517-522, July '26

KRANTZ, W.: Diagnosis of skin diseases of hand and fingers. Med. Klin. *38:*29, Jan 9, '42; 54, Jan 16, '42; 98, Jan 30, '42

KRASIN, P. M. AND OSIPOVSKIY, V. M.: New methods of free bone autotransplantation. Novy khir. arkhiv *28:*231-235, '33

KRASKE, H.: Operative treatment of hypertrophied mamma. Munchen. med. Wchnschr. *70:*672, May 25, '23 (illus.)

KRASOVITOV, V. K.: Secondary plastic surgery of soles and restoration of soft tissues. Vestnik khir. *60:*593-598, Dec '40

KRASSIN, P. M.: Resection of lower jaw for removal of cancer of tongue. Zentralbl. f. Chir. *53:*3095-3100, Dec 4, '26

KRATOCHVIL, K.: Reverdin grafts in therapy of extensive defects. Deutsche Ztschr. f. Chir. *256:*309-358, '42

KRAUL, L.: Formation of artificial vagina by Kirschner-Wagner operation; case. Zentralbl. f . Gynak. *55:*2102-2104, July 4, '31

KRAUL, L.: Artificial vagina. Zentralbl. f. Gynak. *62:*2099-2102, Sept 17, '38

KRAUPA, E.: Destruction of capsule of crystalline lens by fire. Klin. Monatsbl. f. Augenh. *87:*397, Sept '31

KRAUPA, E.: Closure of defects of lower eyelid on side nearest to the nose by means of skin grafts from nose. Ztschr. f. Augenh. *84:*216-217, Oct '34

KRAUSE, W. H.: Present status of plastic surgery of breast. Chirurg *12:*642-647, Nov 1, '40

Krause Operation

Surgical construction of artificial vagina by Wagner-Kirschner operation and Krause method of using skin flaps. WARNECKE, K. Zentralbl. f. Gynak. *56:*416-418, Feb 13, '32

KRAUSS, F.: Necrosis of hand resulting from application of ammonium hydroxide after snake bite. Zentralbl. f. Chir. *56:*459-460, Feb 23, '29

KRAUSS, F.: Plastic operation for restoration of chin, lower lip, and part of cheeks; method of applying dressing. Zentralbl. f. Chir. *57:*1915-1916, Aug 2, '30

KRAUSS, F.: Gastro-enteroschisis; case. Deutsche med. Wchnschr. *62:*258, Feb. 14, '36

KRAUSS, H.: Surgery of funnel chest. Deutsche Ztschr. f. Chir. *250:*715-726, '38

Krauze

Therapy of nonhealing wounds, ulcers and contractures by transplantation of chemically treated tissues according to Krauze. BLOKHIN, V. N. Khirurgiya No. 6, pp. 3-10, '45

KRAUZE, N. I.: Subcutaneous implantation of chemically treated tissues. Khirurgiya, no. 10, pp. 16-25, '44

KREBS, G.: Question of tamponade after nasal operations. (Comment on von Liebermann's article). Ztschr. f. Hals-, Nasen-u. Ohrenh. *30:*684-685, '32

KRECKE, A.: Prevention of stiff fingers. Munchen. med. Wchnschr. *68:*1296-1297, Oct 7, '21

KRECKE, A.: Treatment of injuries of finger tips. Munchen. med. Wchnschr. *75:*571, March 30, '28

KREDEL, F. E. AND EVANS, J. P.: Recovery of sensation in denervated pedicle and free skin grafts. Arch. Neurol. and Psychiat. *29:*1203-1221, June '33

KREDEL, F. E. AND PHEMISTER, D. B.: Recovery of sympathetic nerve function in skin transplants. Arch. Neurol. and Psychiat. *42:*403-412, Sept '39

KREDEL, F. E. (see CURTIS, G. M.) March '33

KREIBICH, C.: Burn therapy. Med. Klin. *25:*1656-1657, Oct 25, '29

KREIBIG, W.: Plastic surgery of eyelids. Ztschr. f. Augenh. *95:*269-275, Aug '38

KREIKER, A.: Wedge-shaped implantation of oral mucosa into intermarginal border of eyelid in trichiasis. Klin. Monatsbl. f. Augenh. *80:*386-389, March 23, '28

KREIKER, A.: Simplified taroplastic in cicatricial entropion. Ophthalmologica *97:*69-78, May '39

KREIKER, A. AND ORSÓS, J.: Long curve and small triangle flap (plastic surgery). Deutsche Ztschr. f. Chir. *179:*145-159, '23 (illus.) addendum *182:*118, '23 abstr: J.A.M.A. *81:*866, Sept 8, '23

KREINDLER, A. AND SCHACHTER, M.: Peculiar form of craniofacial malformation (acrocephalosyndactylia with facial asymmetry and ophthalmoplegia); case. Paris med. *2:*102-105, Aug 4, '34

KREINDLER, A. (see MARINESCO, G. *et al*) 1931

KREINER, W. (see BRÜDA, B. E.) 1930

KREIS, J.: New plastic operation in case of uterovaginal aplasia. Rev. franc. de gynec. et d'obst. *29:*898-903, Aug '34

KREN, O.: Cosmetic applications of carbon dioxide snow to nevi. Wien. klin. Wchnschr. *40:*1329-1331, Oct 20, '27

KRESS, L. C. (see SCHREINER, B. F.) July '24

KRETCHMAR, H. H.: Shock therapy; biochemical aspects (hematocrit and plasma protein determinations as guide to intravenous infusions). M. J. Australia *2:*305-309, Sept 16, '44

KRETZ, R.: Prognathism; surgical therapy. Deutsche Zahnh., Hft. 81, pp. 28-49, '31

KREYES, H.: Application and technic of autogenous blood dressings in leg ulcers resistant to therapy. Ztschr. f. arztl. Fortbild. *39:*360-362, Aug 15, '42

KRICHEVSKIY, A. M.: Zinc iontophoresis (ion transfer) in hypertrophic scars. Sovet. med. (no. 1) *7:*7-9, '43

KRIDA, A.: Tendon transplantation for irreparable musculo-spiral injury (radial nerve). Am. J. Surg. *9:*331-332, Aug '30

KRIDA, A.: Surgical treatment of chronic arthritis. Hygeia *13:*1117-1119, Dec '35

KRIEG, W.: Critical study of usual methods of burn therapy; cod liver oil, with special reference to third degree burns. Arch. f. klin. Chir. *195:*203-249, '39

KRIGSTEN, W. M. (see HARMON, P. H.) Oct '40

KRIGSTEN, W. M. (see HARMON, P. H.) April '41

KRIKENT, R. K.: Modified Alglav method of skin grafting. Khirurgiya, no. 6, pp. 58-63, '39

KRIKENT, R. K.: Early skin grafts in burns. Ortop. i travmatol. (no. 2) *14:*26-28, '40

KRINITSKIY, Y. M.: Tendoplasty according to Bunnell method. Ortop. i travmatol. (no. 5) *11:*149-151, '37

KRINKE, J.: Surgical and bloodless therapy of Dupuytren's contracture. Rozhl. v chir. a gynaek. (cast chir.) *14:*129-133, '35

KRISTJANSEN, A.: Supernumerary phalanx in thumbs; hyperphalangia pollicis. Hospitalstid. *69:*109-119, Feb 4, '26

KRITZINGER, F. J. (see BERRY, T. B.) Dec '41

KRIVOROTOV, I. A.: Tendon regeneration after plastic operations; experimental study. Novy khir. arkhiv *35:*357-367, '36

KROEFF, M.: Reparation of loss of facial substance with tubular graft; case. Folha med. *11:*325-327, Oct 5, '30

KROEFF, M.: Braun method of skin grafting; 2 cases. Folha med. *12:*145-148, May 5, '31

KROEFF, M.: Jaw cancer; electrosurgery; segmental bone resection without interruption of continuity. Hospital, Rio de Janeiro *14:*337, Aug; 595, Sept; 1007, Oct '38

KROEFF, M.: Facial autoplasty; cases. Hospital, Rio de Janeiro *19:*559-570, April '41

KROEFF, M.: Facial autoplasty in nasal surgery; cases. Hospital, Rio de Janeiro *19:*773-781, May '41; *20:*11, July '41

Kroenlein Operation

Cavernous hemangioma of orbit successfully removed by Kroenlein's operation. STALLARD, H. B. Lancet *1:*131-133, Jan 15, '38

KROGH, A.: Report of the British Medical Research Committee on traumatic shock. Ugesk. f. Laeger *83:*333, March 10, '21

KROGIUS, A.: Pathogenesis of Dupuytren's contracture. Acta chir. Scandinav. *54:*33, '21

KROH, F.: Snapping finger and stenosis from tendovaginitis of flexor tendons. Arch. f. klin. Chir. *136:*240-276, '25

KROL, A. G.: Eyelid suture in injuries. Sovet. med. (nos. 11-12) *6:*25-26, '42

KROMAYER: Surgical-physical treatment of keloids. Deutsche med. Wchnschr. *49:*280-281, March 2, '23

KROMAYER: Removal of facial wrinkles; healing of wound without suture. Deutsche med. Wchnschr. *55:*912-914, May 31, '29

Kromayer

Comment on Kromayer's article on removal of facial wrinkles. SCHLESINGER. Deutsche med. Wchnschr. *55:*1512-1513, Sept 6, '29

KROMAYER, E.: Irradiation treatment of red birth-marks; experiences in over 200 cases. Deutsche med. Wchnschr. *58:*1199-1201, July 29, '32 also: Urol. and Cutan. Rev. *36:*524-527, Aug '32

KRÖMER, KARL: *Die verletzte Hand.* Wilhelm Maudrich, Vienna, 1938

KRONFELD, R. (see WEINMANN, J.) Aug '40

KRONTOVSKY, A. A.: Effect of radium rays on transplanted tissues. Vrach. delo *12:*669-671, May 31, '29

KROSS, I.: Parabiosis and organ transplantation. Surg., Gynec. and Obst. *35:*495-496, Oct '22

KRÜCKELS, H.: Burn of eyes caused by brilliant green. Klin. Monatsbl. f. Augenh. *106:*571-574, May '41

KRUEGER, R.: Surgical treatment of prognathism. Arch. f. klin. Chir. *118:*261-274, '21 (illus.)

KRÜGER, E.: Hypertelorism in girl 4 years old. Ztschr. f. Kinderh. *54:*785-787, '33

KRUGER, H. E. (see PRINZMETAL, M. *et al*) Feb '44

Krukenberg Operation: See Putti-Krukenberg Operation

KRUPSKY, A.: Abnormalities of auricle; 2 cases. Ztschr. f. Laryng., Rhin. *16:*255–258, Feb '28
KRUSEN, F. H. (see MEYERDING, H. W.) March–April '36
KRUSIUS, F. F.: Plastic operations for obtaining nasolacrimal passages. Deutsche med. Wchnschr. *50:*954–955, July 11, '24
KRYAZHEVA, V. I.: Treatment of burns. Sovet. med. (nos. 7–8) *7:*24–25, '43
KRYMOV, A. P.: Transplantation tissue therapy. Sovet. med. (no. 9) *8:*15–16, '44
KUBÁNYI, A.: Blood grouping as guide in skin grafting. Arch. f. klin. Chir. *129:*644–647, '24 abstr: J.A.M.A. *82:*2090, June 21, '24
KUBÁNYI, E.: Provisional storage of tissues to be transplanted (experiments with surviving tissues.) Arch. f. klin. Chir. *161:*502–510, '30
KUBÁNYI, E.: At what age should cleft palate operation be performed? Zentralbl. f. Chir. *65:*1798–1799, Aug. 13, '38
KUBÁNYI, E. AND JAKOB, M.: Biologic study of tissue transplantation. Orvosi hetil. *71:*365–370, April 3, '27
KUBASSOFF, M. N.: Simple wooden appliance for righting horizontal dislocations in treatment of jaw fractures. Odont. i. stomatol. (no. 11) *6:*36–37, '28
KUBERTOVA, E.: Institute of Plastic and Esthetic Surgery in Czechoslovakia. Rev. de chir. structive, pp. 19–33, July '35
KUBO, I.: Kubo's aurograph for tracing form of concha. Ztschr. f. Hals-, Nasen-u. Ohrenh. *22:*320–322, Nov. 10, '28
KUBO, K.: Extirpation following paraffin injections into congenital aural fistula. Oto-rhino-laryng. *9:*101, Feb '36
KUCHERENKO, Y. G.: Formation of antibodies following homotransplantation and heterotransplantation. Med. zhur. *5:*287–294, '35
KUCHERENKO, Y. G.: Homotransplantation of skin on denervated area. Med. zhur. *14:*283–285, '45
KUDRINSKIY, A. A.: Tetanus after burns. Sovet. khir., no. 9, pp. 522–524, '36
KUEHNER, H. G. (see FERGUSON, L. K. *et al*) Jan '41
KUHN, L. P. (see WILLEMS, J. D.) Nov '36

Kuhnt-Szymanowsky Operation

Modification of ectropion operation according to Kuhnt-Szymanowsky method. KESTENBAUM, A. Klin. Monatsbl. f. Augenh. *95:*51–53, July '35

KUKIN, N. I.: Use of tubular flap in amputations of extremities. Kirurgiya No. 6, pp. 83–86, '45
KUKULIES, C.: Plastic covering of facial defects. Deutsche Monatschr. f. Zahnh. *45:*494–496, June 1, '27
KULAKCI, N.: Plastic surgery of nose. Anadolu klin. *5:*199–200, '37
KULCSÁR, F. (see BENEDEK, L.) June '33
KULENKAMPFF, D.: Reposition of dislocated mandible under local anesthesia. Munchen. med. Wchnschr. *72:*2229, Dec 25, '25
KULENKAMPFF, D.: Structural plan of jaw and question of treating projections of intermaxillary bone in harelip. and cleft palate. Zentralbl. f. Chir. *62:*1394–1396, June 15, '35
KULICK, L. R.: Management of mandibular bone loss. M. Bull. North African Theat. Op. *2:*128–132, Nov '44
KULICK, L. R.: Management of mandibular bone loss. J. Am. Dent. A. *32:*866–871, July 1, '45
KULOWSKI, J.: Arm-chest adhesions and their plastic reconstruction by tube flap method. Ann. Surg. *97:*683–692, May '33
KUMM, C.: Treatment of fungus cerebri by skin graft with report of case. China M. J. *40:*1126–1132, Nov '26
KUMMER, W. M. AND LEGG, G. E.: Perspective review of burn therapy. Hahneman. Monthly *79:*175, April; 221, May '44
KUNG, H.: Injury of hard palate by indelible pencil. Arch. f. Ohren-, Nasen-u. Kehlkopfh. *151:*272–274, '42
KUNZE, W.: Use of inverted flaps in plastic surgery. Zentralbl. f. Chir. *56:*1099–1102, May 4, '29
KUNZENDORF, W.: Dental arch of upper jaw as support for apparatus during surgical interventions on head in cases of nasal fractures and corrections, skin grafts of face and mobilization of maxillary ankylosis. Deutsche Ztschr. f. Chir. *258:*348, '43
KUNTZEN, H.: Review of surgical treatment of elephantiasis. Ergebn. d. Chir. u. Orthop. *22:*431–462, '29
KUNTZEN, H.: Surgery of elephantiasis; clinical, histologic and experimental study. Arch. f. klin. Chir. *158:*543–583, '30
KUNTZEN, H.: Surgical treatment of elephantiasis. Chirurg *2:*667–673, July 15, '30
KURLANDER, J. J.: Bone grafting and its clinical application. Ohio State M. J. *17:*816, Dec '21
KURLOV, I. N.: Technic of plastic reconstruction in toto of eye. Vestnik oftal. (nos. 3–4) *15:*103–112, '39
KURLOV, I. N.: "Pocket-flap" as method for total restoration of eyelid; preliminary report.

Vestnik oftal. (nos. 1-2) *20:*12-19, '42

KURLOV, I. N. AND MILOVIDOVA, A. N.: Use of knitting needle for suture of conjunctiva in rhinostomy. Vestnik oftal. (no. 2) *15:*38-39, '39

KURTZAHN: Cheiloplasty of upper lip. Deutsche Ztschr. f. Chir. *218:*378-383, '29

KURTZAHN: Cosmetic considerations in plastic surgery. Deutsche med. Wchnschr. *56:*1897-1900, Nov 7, '30

KURTZAHN: Plastic reconstruction of nose destroyed by lupus. Chirurg *3:*49-52, Jan 15, '31

KURTZAHN: Cosmetic surgery of breast. Chirurg *3:*152-156, Feb 15, '31

KURTZAHN, H.: Growth energy of implanted epithelium. Arch. f. klin. Chir. *138:*534-551, '25

KURTZAHN, H.: Transplantation of fleshy tip of toe to tip of nose. Deutsche Ztschr. f. Chir. *209:*401-402, '28

KURTZAHN, H.: Operation for gynecomasty and pendulous breast in male. Deutsche Ztschr. f. Chir. *209:*403-406, '28

KURTZAHN, H.: One stage plastic surgery after removal of epithelioma of nose and contiguous areas. Beitr. z. klin. Chir. *144:*50-57, '28

KURTZAHN, H.: Plastic surgery of urethra and prepuce in surgical treatment of perineal hypospadias. Zentralbl. f. Chir. *58:*1945-1948, Aug 1, '31

KURTZAHN, H. AND v. BÜLOW, W.: Practical exeriences with some "scar dissolving" substances. Deutsche Gtschr. f. Chir. *198:*43-52, '26

KUSANO, M. (see TAKASHIMA, R.) Jan '36

KUSCHEWA, M. N. (see NASAROW, N. N.) 1929

KUSHNER, ALEXANDER (with FRED. H. ALBEE): *Bone Graft Surgery in Disease, Injury, and Deformity*. Appleton-Century Co., New York, 1940

KUSHNER, A.: Evaluation of Wolff's law of bone formation as related to transplantation. J. Bone and Joint Surg. *22:*589-596, July '40

KUSLIK, M. I.: Transplantation of toe according to method of Nicoladoni; case. Arch. Surg. *32:*123-130, Jan '36

KUSS, H.: Late injuries of roentgen rays. Rontgenpraxis *2:*1133-1136, Dec 15, '30

KÜSTER, H.: Operations for pendulous breast and pendulous abdomen. Monatschr. f. Geburtsh. u. Gynak. *73:*316-341, June '26

KUTLER, W.: Method for repair of finger amputation. Ohio State M. J. *40:*126, Feb '44

KUTTER, A.: Surgical treatment of congenital anal atresia. Beitr. z. klin. Chir. *138:*756-763, '26

KWARTIN, B. AND HYAMS, J. A.: True hermaphrodism in man; report of case with critical review of literature. J. Urol. *18:*363-383, Oct '27

KYANDSKIY, A. A.: Osteoplastic restoration of traumatic defects of lower jaw. Sovet. khir. (nos. 3-4) *6:*339-349, '34

KYANDSKIY, A. A.: Histopathologic changes in freely transplanted tissue from human auricle. Sovet. khir., no. 9, pp. 66-69, '35

L

LAARMANN, A.: Treatment of finger injuries. Deutsche med. Wchnschr. *63:*1651-1654, Oct 29, '37

LABAND, F. (see WASSMUND, M.) Dec '27

LABATE, F. (see OTTOBRINI COSTA, M.) July-Aug '39

LABHARDT, E.: Permanent results of von Eicken operation for choanal atresia. Schweiz. med. Wchnschr. *66:*1153-1154, Nov 21, '36

LABOK, D. M.: Simultaneous osteocutaneous graft in reconstruction of thumb. Khirurgiya, no. 2, pp. 73-75, '44

LABOMBARDA, G.: Modern trends, with special reference to tannic acid and cod liver oil (burns). Clinica *6:*59-76, Feb '40

LABORDE, S.: Radium treatment of vascular nevi. Medecine *2:*696, June '21 abstr: J.A.M.A. *77:*409, July 30, '21

LABORDE, S.: Radium treatment of vascular nevi. Progres med. *36:*531-532, Nov 12, '21

LABORDE, S.: Radium therapy of cutaneous angiomas. Presse med. *41:*103-104, Jan 18, '33

LABRECQUE, R.: Shock due to extensive superficial burns; case. Ann. med.-chir. de l'Hop, Sainte-Justine, Montreal *4:*131-140, May '42

LABUNSKAYA, O. V.: Surgical substitution of toes for missing fingers. Sovet. khir. (nos. 3-4) *6:*503-505, '34

LABUNSKAYA, O. V.: Transplantation of toes for fingers. Ann. Surg. *102:*1-4, July '35

LACASSAGNE, A.: Results of radium treatment of epithelioma of lips; statistics. Arch. d'electric. med. *39:*358-366, Oct '29

LACASSAGNE, A. (see REGAUD, C.) April '27

LACASSAGNE, J. AND ROUSSET, J.: Accidental tattooing by fall; removal by potassium permanganate method; case. Bull. Soc. franc. de dermat. et syph. (Reunion dermat., Lyon) *42:*1518-1520, July '35

LACAZE: Relation of traumatic lesions of sense organs to maxillofacial surgery. Rev. odont. *52:*87-99, Feb '31

DE LACERDA, E.: Treatment of jaw ankylosis by simple section followed by mobilization; case. Med. contemp. *46:*221-223, July 8, '28

DE LACERDA FILHO, N.: Wound of fingers by Diesel oil under pressure. Bahia med. *12:*63-66, April '41

LACHMANN, O.: New plastic operation for male

urethra. Bull. War Med. *4:*393, March '44 (abstract)

Lacrimal Apparatus

Mosher-Toti operation on lacrimal sac. MOSHER, H. P. Laryngoscope *31:*284, May '21
Re-establishing intranasal drainage of lacrimal sac. MOSHER, H. P. Laryngoscope *31:*492, July '21
Results of anastomotic method of treatment of lacrimal obstruction. TOTI. Proc. Roy. Soc. Med. (Sect. Ophth.) *14:*59, Aug '21
Plastic operation on lacrimal canal. BENJAMINS, C. E. AND VAN ROMUNDE, L. H. Nederlandsch Tijdschr. v. Geneesk. *2:*33-35, July 1, '22 (illus.)
Indications, contraindications and preparation for dacryocystorhinostomy. FENTON, R. A. Ann. Otol., Rhin. and Laryng. *32:*67-83, March '23 (illus.)
Dacryocystorhinostomy; combined methods. SAUER, W. E. Ann. Otol., Rhin. and Laryng. *32:*25-43, March '23 (illus.)
Dacryocystorhinostomy. GILLUM, J. R., J. Indiana M. A. *17:*113-116, April '24
Plastic operations for obtaining nasolacrimal passages. KRUSIUS, F. F. Deutsche med. Wchnschr. *50:*954-955, July 11, '24
Treatment of lacrimal fistula following dacrocystectomy. HANDS, S. G., J. Iowa M. Soc. *15:*598-600, Nov '25
Dacryocystorhinoplasty, Mosher's modification of Toti method. COWEN, S. B. Ohio State M. J. *21:*902-905, Dec '25
Toti-Mosher operation; dacryocystorhinostomy; combined endonasal and external technic. SIBBALD, D. AND O'FARRELL, G. Rev. Soc. argent. de Oftal. *1:*79-82, '25
Indications for dacryocystorhinostomy. CASADESÚS CASTELLS, F. Med. ibera *2:*229, Sept 25; 249, Oct 2, '26
Historical observation on improvement of Toti's operation (dacryocystorhinostomy). OHM, J. Klin. Monatsbl. f. Augenh. *77:*825-832, Dec '26
New procedures for tear sac, frontal sinus and endonasal plastic operations. MALTZ, M. Acta oto-laryng. *9:*144-153, '26 (in English)
Toti-Mosher operation; dacryocystorhinostomy. SIBBALD, AND O'FARRELL. Rev. de especialid. *1:*568-573, '26
Toti's dacryocystorhinostomy. WISSELINK, G. W. Klin. Monatsbl. f. Augenh. *78:*550, April '27
Plastic surgery of lacrimal organs. LOPES D'ANDRADE, A. Med. contemp. *45:*137-139, May 1, '27

Lacrimal Apparatus—Cont.

Mr. Percival Pott on treatment of lacrimal fistula. FERGUS, A. F. Proc. Roy. Soc. Med. (Sect. Ophth.) *20:*60-64, Aug '27
Indications for dacryocystorhinostomy. URBANEK, J. Wien. med. Wchnschr. *77:*1109, Aug. 20, '27
Easy method of dacryocystorhinostomy. CLAUS, H. Beitr. z. Anat., Physiol., Path. u. Therap. d. Ohres *26:*121-124, Nov '27
Dacryocystorhinostomy; 2 cases. POLYACK, G. D. Ann. d'ocul. *164:*942-951, Dec '27
Contribution to knowledge of fistula interna sacci lacrymalis. PLOMAN, K. G. Acta ophth. *5:*277-284, '27
Sound for dilating strictures of naso-lacrimal duct. SCHMIDT, P. Klin. Monatsbl. f. Augenh. *80:*390, March 23, '28
Dacryocystorhinostomy; radical cure for lacrimation; MANES, A. J. Semana med. *1:*1020-1027, April 26, '28
Surgical relief of chronic dacryocystitis and epiphora; Dupuy-Dutemps and Bourguet technique; direct anastomosis of tear sac with nasal mucous membrane. CORBETT, J. J., M. J. and Rec. *128:*158-160, Aug 15, '28 also: New England J. Med. *199:*459-461, Sept 6, '28 also: Am. J. Ophth. *11:*774-778, Oct '28
Dacryocystorhinostomy. LARSSON, S. Acta ophth. *6:*193-215, '28
Technic and indications of dacryocystorhinostomy. RUBBRECHT, R. Bull. Soc. belge d'opht., no. 57, pp. 94-106, '28
Repeated inflammation and fistulae treated by excision of lacrimal sac; cases. GENET, L. Lyon med. *143:*178-181, Feb 10, '29
End-results in dacryocystorhinostomy. BASZERRA, J. Med. ibera *1:*545-547, April 27, '29
Reconstruction of destroyed lacrimal excretory apparatus. ASCHER, K. W. Med. Klin. *25:*749-750, May 10, '29
Simplified dacryocystorhinostomy, modification of Toti's method. DE LIETO VOLLARO, A. Boll. d'ocul. *8:*561-574, June '29
Dacryocystorhinostomy by method of Dupuy-Dutemps and Bourguet. POTIQUET, H. Ann. d'ocul. *166:*470-487, June '29
Congenital fistula of lacrimal sac. LEVINE, J. Am. J. Ophth. *12:*745-746, Sept '29
Modification of Toti's dacryocystorhinostomy. POLJAK, G. D. Klin. Monatsbl. f. Augenh. *83:*510-515, Oct-Nov '29
Technical points suggesting dacryocystorhinostomy. ANDINA, M. Rev. cubana de oft. *1:*424-426, Nov '29
New instruments for Toti operation (dacryocystorhinostomy). GUTZEIT, R. Klin. Monatsbl. f. Augenh. *84:*92, Jan '30
Hemo-aspiration and trephining with aid of

Lacrimal Apparatus—Cont.
electric apparatus in dacryocystorhinostomy. SUBILEAU, J. M. Ann. d'ocul. *167:*301-306, April '30
Dacryocystorhinostomy. CILLERUELO. Informacion med. *7:*179-189, Aug '30
Mosher-Toti dacryocystorhinostomy. SPAETH, E. B. Arch. Ophth. *4:*487-496, Oct '30
Persistent fistula of lacrimal sac treated by ultraviolet rays; case. MAXWELL, E. Tr. Ophth. Soc. U. Kingson *50:*648, '30
External dacryocystorhinostomy. LOPES DE ANDRADE. Med. contemp. *49:*21-29, Jan 18, '31
West's dacryocystorhinostomy in 300 cases. ALCAINO, A. AND RODRIGUEZ, D. Arch. de oftal. hispano-am. *31:*65-79, Feb '31
Dupuy-Dutemps and Bourguet technic in dacryocystorhinostomy. BARBEROUSSE. Bull. Soc. d'opht. de Paris, p. 226, March '31
Lacrimal fistula. CANGE, A. AND DUBOUCHER, H. Arch. d'opht. *48:*161-185, March '31
Technic in dacryocystorhinostomy. GÓMEZ-MÁRQUEZ. Arch. de oftal. hispano-am. *31:*147-176, March '31
Dacryocystorhinostomies; 517 cases. GÓMEZ-MÁRQUEZ. Klin. Monatsbl. f. Augenh. *86:*620-629, May '31
Dacryocystorhinostomy, Dupuy-Dutemps method; 25 cases. GONZÁLEZ LLANOS, N. Rev. de especialid. *6:*237, May '31
Grave hemorrhage as late complication of dacryocystorhinostomy, 2 cases. MARÍN AMAT, M. Siglo med. *87:*673-675, June 20, '31 also: Arch. d'opht. *48:*632-638, Sept '31
Technic in external dacryocystorhinostomy. TORRES ESTRADA, A. Gac. med. de Mexico *62:*339-360, Aug '31
Operations on lacrimal ducts. SATTLER, C. H. Ztschr. f. Augenh. *75:*237-239, Oct '31
Severe hemorrhage as late complication of dacryocystorhinostomy. MARÍN-AMAT, M. Bull. et mem. Soc. franc. d'opht. *44:*269-278, '31 also: Arch. de oftal. hispano-am. *31:*629-636, Nov '31
Formation of new lacrimonasal canal after excision of lacrimal sac. MATHEWSON, G. H. Am. J. Ophth. *14:*1252, Dec '31
New instrument for detachment of sac in dacryocystectomy. NEUSCHULER, I. Arch. d'opht. *48:*829-831, Dec '31
Clinical results of intranasal tear sac operation. WEST, J. M. Tr. Sect. Ophth., A. M. A. pp. 69-81, '31
Dacryocystorhinostomy; indications and technic; case. GRAUE Y GLENIE, E. An. Soc. mex. de oftal. y oto-rino-laring. *9:*114-116, Jan-March '32
Congenital fistulas of lacrimal sac. TIRELLI, G. Rassegna ital. d'ottal. *1:*66-75, Jan-Feb '32
Technic of dacryocystorhinostomy. WEEKS, W. W. Arch. Ophth. *7:*443-447, March '32
Technic of external dacryocystorhinostomy. TORRES ESTRADA, A. An. Soc. mex. de oftal. y oto-rino-laring. *9:*131-157, April-June '32
External dacryocystorhinostomy according to Gutzeit method. DIAZ-CANEJA, E. Ann. d'ocul. *170:*384-414, May '33 also: An. Casa de Salud Valdecilla *3:*292-313, '32
Surgery of inner canthus and related structures. BLAIR, V. P. *et al.* Am. J. Ophth. *15:*498-507, June '32
Statistics on 1000 plastic dacryocystotomies. DUPUY-DUTEMPS, L. Bull. Soc. d'opht. de Paris, pp. 392-399, June '32
Congenital fistula of lacrimal sac. COLRAT, A. Bull. Soc. d'opht. de Paris, pp. 60-62, Jan '33
Congenital fistula of lacrimal sac; case. MUSITZ, G. Budapesti orvosi ujsag *31:*28-30, Jan 12, '33
Reconstruction of conjunctival sac with Thiersch grafts. GLOVER, D. M. AND JACOBY, M. W. Arch. Surg. *26:*617-622, April '33
Observations on 1000 plastic dacryocystotomies. DUPUY-DUTEMPS, L. Ann. d'ocul. *170:*361-384, May '33
Reconstruction of conjunctival culdesac and eyelid in patients after enucleation of eye; technic. DAMEL, C. S. Rev. Asoc. med. argent. *47:*2733-2738, June '33
Pathogenesis of congenital fistulas of lacrimal sac. COSMETTATOS, G. F. Ann. d'ocul. *170:*594-599, July '33
Diathermic recanalization of lacrimonasal canal. SPINELLI, F. Klin. Monatsbl. f. Augenh. *91:*202-207, Aug '33
Results of intranasal dacryocystorhinostomy (West operation). HENRY, L. M. J. Brit. J. Ophth. *17:*550-552, Sept '33
Toti-Mosher operation (lacrimal ducts) and its end results. MARTIN, R. C. Tr. Pacific Coast Oto-Ophth. Soc. *21:*50-58, '33
Dacryocystorhinostomy by modified Gutzeit method. MATA, P. Arch. de oftal. hispano-am. *34:*141-147, March '34
External dacryocystorhinostomy. PREOBRAZHENSKIY, V. V. Sovet. vrach. gaz., pp. 388-390, March 15, '34
Result of surgical therapy of suppuration of lacrimal sac after implantation of lower

Lacrimal Apparatus – Cont.
end of lacrimal sac into nose; modified Toti operation. STOCK, W. Klin. Monatsbl. f. Augenh. *92:*433–435, April '34
Dacryocystorhinostomy. WODON. Arch. med. belges *87:*95–97, June '34
New knife for dacryocystorhinostomy. MEURMAN, Y. Acta otolaryng. *21:*343–345, '34
Dacryocystorhinostomy and its clinical results. MOREU, A. Arch. de oftal. hispano-am. *35:*127–139, March '35
External dacryocystorhinostomy. DE AIMEIDA, A. Rev. brasil. de cir. *4:*181–188, April '35
Dacryocystorhinostomy; easy and sure method. WEEKERS, L. Arch. d'opht. *52:*241–246, April '35
Technic of extranasal dacryocystorhinostomy. BASTERRA, J. Cron. med., Valencia *39:*354–363, May 15, '35
Technic of endonasal dacryocystorhinostomy. (Halle operation); cases. JUST TISCORNIA, B. AND MERCANDINO, C. P. Rev. med. latino-am. *20:*1118–1136, July '35
Refinements in tear sac surgery. STOKES, W. H. Nebraska M. J. *20:*388–393, Oct '35
Plastic dacryocystorhinostomy in 1200 cases. AVERBAKH, M. AND IVANOVA, MME. Ann. d'ocul. *172:*913–936, Nov '35
Chronic dacryocystitis due to fistula resulting from maxillary sinusitis; case. FRANCESCHETTI, A. Bull. et mem. Soc. franc. d'opht. *48:*27–34, '35
Question of congenital fistula of lacrimal gland; case. SCHORNSTEIN, T. Arch. f. Augenh. *109:*86–102, '35
Treatment of stenosis of lacrimal ducts by insertion of spiral shaped cannula. ALKIO, V. V. Duodecim *51:*1076, '35; *52:*51, '36 Abstr: Klin. Monatsbl. f. Augenh. *96:*319–324, March '36
Dacryocystorhinostomy by nasal route. PETTERINO PATRIARCA, A. AND DUC, C. Rassegna ital. d'ottal. *5:*205–224, March–April '36
Technic of extranasal dacryocystorhinostomy. BASTERRA, J. Arch. de oftal. hispano-am. *36:*208–216, April '36
Dacryocystorhinostomy according to plastic procedure of Bourguet-Dupuy-Dutemps. VANCEA, P. Rev. san. mil., Bucuresti *35:*393–395, April '36
Cause of failure of dacryocystorhinostomy. ESTEBAN, M. Rev. cubana de oto-neuro-oftal. *5:*99–100, May–June '36
Stricturotomy and injections of iodized oil in therapy of dacryocystitis; results in recent cases. PEYRET, J. A. Arch. de oftal. de Buenos Aires *11:*429–435, July '36

Lacrimal Apparatus – Cont.
Plastic dacryocystorhinostomy. FILHO, A. P. Rev. oto-laring. de Sao Paulo (no. 5, bis) *4:*731–747, Sept–Oct '36
Progress in dacryocystorhinostomy. FRIEBERG, T. Nord. med. tidskr. *12:*1686–1687, Oct 10, '36
Dacryocystorhinostomy. AMSLER, M. Schweiz. med. Wchnschr. *66:*1268–1270, Dec 12, '36
Dacryocystorhinostomy (Mosher-Toti operation). HOOVER, W. B., S. Clin. North America *16:*1695–1699, Dec '36
Kankrov operation in therapy of dacryocystitis. ABDULAEV, G. G. Sovet. vestnik oftal. *8:*710–711, '36
Dacryocystorhinostomy. CHANDLER, P. A. Tr. Am. Ophth. Soc. *34:*240–263, '36
Use of mucosa of lips in Toti operation on lacrimal ducts. JANCKE, G. Ber. u. d. Versamml. d. deutsch. ophth. Gesellsch. *51:*478–479, '36
Surgical therapy of flow of tears after removal of lacrimal sac. TOWBIN, B. G. Arch. f. Ophth. *135:*579–580, '36
Artificial restoration of nasolacrimal duct. GERKE, J. Ztschr. f. Augenh. *91:*50–52, Jan '37
Technic of dacryocystostomy. ZARZYCKI, P. Bull. Soc. d'opht. de Paris *49:*9–12, Jan '37
Simplified modification of external dacryocystorhinostomy. KALEFF. Ztschr. f. Augenh. *91:*140–157, Feb '37
Dacryocystorhinostomy; technic and results. WEVE, H. J. M. AND KENTGENS, S. K. Klin. Monatsbl. f. Augenh. *98:*195–205, Feb '37
Simplification of classic technic of external dacryocystorhinostomy. TORRES ESTRADA, A. Cir. y cirujanos *5:*219–250, May–June '37
Dacrocystorhinostomy. WRIGHT, R. E. Lancet *2:*250–251, July 31, '37
Results of intranasal dacryocystorhinostomy. WALSH, T. E. AND BOTHMAN, L. Am. J. Ophth. *20:*939–941, Sept '37
Congenital fistula of lacrimal gland, with report of case. ALVARO, M. E. AND SAMPAIO DORIA, A. Rev. oto-neuro-oftal. *12:*283–290, Nov '37
Plastic construction of artificial conjunctival sac using skin flaps. CSAPODY, I. Orvosi hetil. *81:*1217–1219, Dec 4, '37
Technic of endonasal operation on lacrimal sac. GÜTTICH, A. Arch. f. Ohren-, Nasen-u. Kehlkopfh. *143:*233–235, '37
Extirpation of lacrimal sac. (Comment on Strakhov's article). POLYAK, B. L. Vestnik oftal. *10:*448–450, '37

Lacrimal Apparatus – Cont.

Extirpation of lacrimal sac. (Reply to comment by Polyak). STRAKHOV, V. P. Vestnik oftal. *10:*450–451, '37

Operation for correction of eversion of inferior lacrimal point. TIKHOMIROV, P. E. Vestnik oftal. *11:*216–217, '37

New experiences with plastic construction of artificial conjunctival sac, using flaps. VON CSAPODY, I. Ztschr. f. Augenh. *94:*23–33, Jan '38

Dacryocystorhinectomy in stenoses of lacrimal sac; new technic. CORNET, E. Rev. med. franc. d'Extreme-Orient *16:*551–554, May '38

Modified Brigg's retractor for dacryocystorhinostomy. STALLARD, H. B. Brit. J. Ophth. *22:*361, June '38

Lacrimal laminaria in surgical therapy of stricture of nasal canal. ZARZYCKI, P. Bull. Soc. d'opht. de Paris *50:*306–310, June '38

Turbinotome for "ab externo" dacryocystorhinostomy. RAVERDINO, E. Rassegna ital. d'ottal. *7:*499–503, July–Aug '38

Congenital stenosis of nasolacrimal duct; complications and treatment. GRANSTRÖM, K. O. Nord. med. tidskr. *16:*1280–1283, Aug 13, '38

Dacryocystorhinostomy by external route; technic. VENCO, L. Rassegna ital. d'ottal. *7:*593–612, Sept–Oct '38

Chisel for dacryocystorhinostomy. HAAS, E. Bull. Soc. d'opht. de Paris *50:*468–469, Oct '38

Dacryocystorhinectomy; new technic. CORNET, E. Ann. d'ocul. *175:*842–845, Nov '38

Dacryocystorhinostomy; criteria of operability, indications, complications and results. VENCO, L. Riv. oto-neuro-oftal. *15:*510–531, Nov–Dec '38

Simple dacryocystorhinostomy. GUY, L. Arch. Ophth. *20:*954–957, Dec '38

Congenital lacrimal fistula. ALVARO, M. E. AND SAMPAIO DORIA, A. Cong. argent. de oftal. (1936) *2:*583–590, '38

Dacryocystorhinostomy by nasal route (West operation) and its results. ARGANARAZ, R.; *et al.* Cong. argent. de oftal. (1936) *2:*491–496, '38

Dilatation of lacrimal ducts. KORKASHVILI, G. L. Vestnik oftal. *13:*405–406, '38

Treatment of congenital atresia of nasolacrimal duct. LARSSON, S. Acta ophth. *16:*271–278, '38

Treatment of epiphora, with special reference of some cases treated by dacryocystorhinostomy. MORGAN, O. G. Tr. Ophth. Soc. U. Kingdom (pt. 1) *58:*163–172, '38

Late results of external dacryocystorhinostomy. TOMKEVICH, A. I. Vestnik oftal. *13:*388–396, '38

Construction of lacrimal passages. NIZETIC, Z. Klin. Monatsbl. f. Augenh. *102:*67–71, Jan '39

Two-stage dacryocystorhinostomy. NIZETIC, Z. Klin. Monatsbl. f. Augenh. *102:*71–76, Jan '39

Present status of surgery of lacrimal sac. RYCHENER, R. O. Surg., Gynec. and Obst. *68:*414–418, Feb (no. 2A) '39

Dacryocystostomy by nasal route. MATSUI, T. Oto-rhino-laryng. *12:*238–241, March '39 (in Japanese)

Surgical technic for construction of pituitary conjunctival canal (artificial lacrimal canal). DA SILVA COSTA, A. Bull. Soc. d'opht. de Paris *51:*385–388, June '39

Transplantation (implantation) of lacrimal sac in chronic dacryocystitis. STOKES, W. H. Arch. Ophth. *22:*193–210, Aug '39

Congenital fistula of lacrimal sac. LAVAL, J. Am. J. Ophth. *22:*1022–1023, Sept '39

External dacryocystorhinostomy by Torres Estrada technic. GURRIA URGELL, D. Gac. med. de Mexico *69:*336–340, Oct 30, '39

Importance of suture of lacrimal sac and nasal mucosa in dacryocystorhinostomy. BALACCO, F. Boll. d'ocul. *18:*876–880, Nov '39

Endonasal tear sac operation. BRYANT, B. L. California and West. Med. *51:*376–378, Dec '39

Use of knitting needle for suture of conjunctiva in rhinostomy. KURLOV, I. N. AND MILOVIDOVA, A. N. Vestnik oftal. (no. 2) *15:*38–39, '39

Use of ocular prosthesis during plastic reconstruction of conjunctival sac with free cutaneous or mucous graft. NEYMAN, V. N. Vestnik oftal. (no. 5) *14:*45–46, '39

Congenital fistulas of lacrimal sac combined with congenital aural fistulas and anosmia. REH, H. Klin. Monatsbl. f. Augenh. *104:*55–59, Jan '40

Dacryocystorhinostomy by way of pyriform aperture. KOFLER, K. Monatschr. f. Ohrenh. *74:*299–306, June '40

Dacryocystorhinostomy; author's experience. PEREIRA, R. F. Arch. de oftal. de Buenos Aires *15:*603–613, Dec '40

New technic for dacryocystorhinostomy. VAQUERO, L. Rev. med. d. Hosp. gen. *3:*244–253, Dec 15, '40

Surgical therapy of obstruction of lacrimal ducts. POKHISOV, N. Y. Vestnik oftal. *16:*356–360, '40

New drills for dacryocystorhinostomy. CRA-

Lacrimal Apparatus—Cont.
MER, F. E. K. AND BALZA, J. Semana med. *1:*294–295, Jan 30, '41
Dacryocystorhinostomy; interesting points on operation. YANES, T. R. Arch. Ophth. *26:*12–20, July '41
Dacryocystorhinostomy. AYUYAO, C. D. AND YAMBAO, C. V., J. Philippine M. A. *21:* 391–393, Aug '41
Dacryocystorhinostomy. HUGHES, W. L.; *et al.* Surg., Gynec. and Obst. *73:*375–380, Sept '41
Operation to drain lacrimal organs into nose some years after ablation of lacrimal sac. BADEAUX, F. AND PELLERIN, R. Union med. du Canada *70:*1063–1064, Oct '41
Question of external or internal dacryocystorhinostomy. HAUSMANN, R. Arch. f. Ohren-, Nasen-u. Kehlkopfh. *149:*309–316, '41
Dacryocystorhinostomy in Venezuela. RHODE, J. Arch. venezol. Soc. de oto-rino-laring., oftal., neurol. *3:*1–56, March '42
Dacryocystorhinostomy versus dacryocystectomy. YANES, T. R. Vida nueva *49:*132–136, April '42
Canaliculus dilator in eye. BERENS, C. Am. J. Ophth. *25:*725–726, June '42
Plastic dacryocystorhinostomy; technic. LATHROP, F. D., S. Clin. North America *22:*675–679, June '42
Simple method for preparing dacryocystorhinostomy needles. BALOD, K. Klin. Monatsbl. f. Augenh. *108:*626, Sept–Oct '42
Instruments to facilitate mucosal suture in dacryocystorhinostomy. BANGERTER, A. Ophthalmologica *104:*171–174, Sept '42
Reconstruction of lacrimal ducts. THIEL, R. Klin. Monatsbl. f. Augenh. *108:*576–583, Sept–Oct '42
Dacryostomy and canaliculorhinostomy. VALLE, D. Arq. brasil. de oftal. *5:*236–251, Oct '42
Construction of lacrimal passage. GUY, L. P. Arch. Ophth. *29:*575–577, April '43
Valle operation (lacrimal), Brazilian contribution. CATALAO, P. V. B. Brasil-med. *57:*213, May 1–15, '43
Intranasal approach to lacrimal sac (transparent dacryocystotomy). MATIS, E. T. Laryngoscope *53:*357–365, May '43
Dacryocystorhinostomy; logical treatment of occlusion of lacrimal sac. HALLUM, A. V., J. M. A. Georgia *32:*186–189, June '43
Infantile dacryostenosis. GOAR, E. L., M. Rec. and Ann. *37:*611–613, July '43
Technical difficulties and complications of dacryocystorhinostomy by external route. CRAMER, F. E. K. Semana med. *2:*604–610,

Lacrimal Apparatus—Cont.
Sept 9, '43
Dacryocystorhinostomy in Venezuela. RHODE, J. Gac. med. de Caracas *50:*231, Nov 30, '43; 241, Dec 15, '43; 251, Dec 31, '43 *51:*261, Jan 15, '44 comment by Lopez Villoria *51:*264, Jan 15, '44; 11, Jan 31, '44
Rhinocanalicular anastomosis with reconstruction of lacrimal sac. BLUMENFELD, L. Arch. Ophth. *31:*248–249, March '44
Transscleral lacrimal canaliculus transplants. GIBSON, G. G. Am. J. Ophth. *27:*258–269, March '44
Simplified technic for dacryocystorhinostomy. TORRES ESTRADA, A., J. Internat. Coll. Surgeons *7:*147–158, March–April '44
Rhinocanalicular anastomosis. WALDAPFEL, R. Arch. Ophth. *31:*432–433, May '44
Simplified external dacryocystorhinostomy. WILLIAMS, J. L. D. AND HILL, B. G. Brit. J. Ophth. *28:*407–410, Aug '44
Repair of lacerations of lacrimal canaliculus. CAMPBELL, M. D. Air Surgeon's Bull. (no. 12) *1:*18, Dec '44
Operation on punctum lacrimale; indications. HENDRICKS, L. J. Arch. Ophth. *32:*496, Dec '44
Dacryocystitis; transplantation operation. GIFFORD, H. JR. Tr. Sect. Ophth., A. M. A., pp. 156–161, '44
Importance of repositioning of lacrimal openings in treating senile ectropion. TORRES ESTRADA, A. Gac. med. de Mexico *75:*336–351, Oct 31, '45
Restoration of patency of nasolacrimal duct by means of vitallium tube; preliminary report. MULDOON, W. E. Am. J. Ophth. *28:*1340–1345, Dec '45
Autoplastic dacryorhinostomy; new process for reconstructing lacrimal organs by means of labial mucosal graft. NIEMEYER, W. Arq. brasil. de oftal. *8:*181–185, Dec '45
New instruments for dacryocystorhinostomy. SANCHEZ BULNES, L. AND SILVA, D. Arch. Asoc. para evit. ceguera Mexico *3:*249–255, '45
Congenital fistula of lacrimal sac; 2 cases. TORTI, M. Rassegna ital. d'ottal. *15:*69–76, Jan–Feb '46
West operation (endonasal dacryocystostomy). MCARTHUR, G. A. D., M. J. Australia *1:*508–510, April 13, '46
Operation for chronic dacryocystitis (plastic dacryocystorhinostomy). HAMILTON, R. G. Pennsylvania M. J. *49:*1327–1330, Sept '46
Cure of nasolacrimal obstruction. MACINDOE, N. M. Tr. Ophth. Soc. Australia (1944) *4:*149, '46

LACROIX, P. G.: Essential in technic of nerve suture; with report of 2 cases. Am. J. Surg. *37:*282–283, Nov '23

LA DAGE, L. H.: Recent developments in plastic surgery. J. Iowa M. Soc. *29:*609–611, Dec '39

LADD, W. E.: Treatment of harelip. Boston M. and S. J. *188:*270–272, March 1, '23 (illus.)

LADD, W. E.: Harelip and cleft palate. Boston M. and S. J. *194:*1016–1025, June 3, '26

LADD, W. E. AND GROSS, R. E.: Congenital branchiogenic anomalies; 82 cases. Am. J. Surg. *39:*234–248, Feb '38

LADD, W. E. AND LANMAN, T. H.: Exstrophy of bladder (treated by ureterosigmoidostomy). New England J. Med. *216:*637–645, April 15, '37

LADD, W. E. AND LANMAN, T. H.: Exstrophy of bladder and epispadias (surgical technic). New England J. Med. *222:*130–134, Jan 25, '40

LADEWIG, P. AND SERT, D.: Branchiogenic malformations of neck region. Schweiz. Ztschr. f. Path. u. Bakt. *7:*1–12, '44

LADYZHENSKIY, M. E.: Method of bloodless removal of splinter from under nail. Sovet. vrach. zhur., pp. 217–218, Feb 15, '36

LAFARGUE, P. AND RIVIERE, M.: Congenital absence of vagina; creation of new vagina by perieotomy; failure of amniotic graft; excellent functional and anatomic results; case. Bull. Soc. d'obst. et de gynec. *26:*278–280, April '37

LAFAYETTE PINTO, I.: Burn therapy. Rev. med. brasil. *8:*211–236, Feb '40

LAFF, H. I.: Deforming and recurring polyps of nose of youth. Arch. Otolaryng. *30:*795–799, Nov '39

LAFFONT, and BONAFOS: Creation of vagina by autoplasty; case. Bull. Soc. d'obst. et de gynec. *23:*637–640, Nov '34

LAGARDE: Plastic surgery of breast. Paris chir. *20:*143–152, July-Aug '28

LAGARDE: Bilateral mastopexy and therapy of mammary prolapse of first degree. Rev. tech. chir. *24:*251–253, Dec '32

LAGARDE M.: Improved technique for removal of wrinkles of face and neck. Am. J. Surg. *3:*132–138, Aug '27 also: Cron. med., Lima *44:*33–42, Feb '27

LAGARDE, M.: Surgical treatment of facial and neck wrinkles; new technics. Arch. franco-belges de chir. *31:*154–163, Feb '28

Lagley's Operation

Lagleys operation for trachomatous entropion. KHAVANSKIY, K. I. Sovet. vestnik oftal. *1:*159–160, '32

DAL LAGO, E.: Congenital bilateral diaphragm of choana; case. Boll. d. mal. d. orecchio, d. gola, d. naso *58:*450–458, Dec '40

Lagophthalmos

Resection of orbicular muscle in ectropion paralysis. HOLLÓS, L. Orvosi hetil. *74:*1094–1095, Oct 25, '30 also: Ztschr. f. Augenh. *73:*27–31, Dec '30

Surgical relief of lagophthalmos following seventh nerve paralysis in cases of leprosy. GASS, H. H. Leprosy Rev. *5:*178–180, Oct '34

Congenital hemiatrophy of face with facial paralysis and microphthalmus; case. BOISSERIE-LACROIX, J., J. de med. de Bordeaux *113:*419–420, May 30, '36

Simple rapid surgical technic for cure of paralytic ectropion. DE LIETO VOLLARO, A. Bull. d'ocul. *18:*769–780, Oct '39

Eyelid paralysis; lagophthalmos in leprosy and its surgical correction. VALLE, S. Arq. Inst. Penido Burnier *5:*238–264, Dec '39

Surgical therapy of paralytic lagophthalmos in leprosy patients. DOROFEEV, V. N. Vestnik oftal. (no. 1) *14:*69–76, '39

Measures to protect eye in facial paralysis. OBERHOFF, K. Munchen. med. Wchnschr. *87:*33, Jan 12, '40

Paralysis of lower eyelid; scleral scars and grafts. BLAIR, V. P. AND BYARS, L. T. Surg., Gynec., and Obst. *70:*426–437, Feb '40

Lagrange's Law

Lagrange's law of indirect ocular war injuries (facial fractures). SOUDAKOFF, P. S. Am. J. Ophth. *26:*293–296, March '43

LAGOS GARCIA, A.: Median harelip and bifid nose; case. Semana med. *2:*237–241, Aug 3, '44

LAHEY, F. H.: Tendon suture which permits immediate motion. Boston M. and S. J. *188:*851–852, May 31, '23 (illus.)

LAHEY, F. H.: Rope (skin) grafts. Boston M. and S. J. *194:*1–5, Jan 7, '26

LAHEY, F. H.: Surgical conditions of neck other than goiter. Proc. Internat. Assemb. Inter-State Post-Grad M. A., North America (1929) *5:*388–392, '30

LAHEY, F. H.: Diagnosis and management of surgical conditions of neck. Proc. Interst. Postgrad. M. A. North America (1944) pp. 102–106, '45

LAHEY, F. H. AND NELSON, H. F.: Branchial cysts and sinuses. Ann. Surg. *113:*508–512, April '41

Lahey Operation

Sacrococcygeal dermoid cysts; Lahey plastic repair using bipedicled flap. BAILA, A. E. Bol. y trab., Soc. argent. de cirujanos *4:*292–293, '43 also: Rev. Asoc. med. argent. *57:*495, July 30, '43

LAIDLEY, J. W. S.: Ectopia vesicae; case. Australian and New Zealand J. Surg. *6:*398–399, April '37

LAIGNEL-LAVASTINE; BONNARD, R. AND GAULTIER, M.: Traumatic Claude Bernard-Horner syndrome associated with Dupuytren's contracture and paroxysmal anxiety (precordial pain) caused by aerophagy; case. Rev. neurol. *2:*784–787, Dec '34

LAIN, E. S.: Treatment of cancer of lip by radiation. Tr. Sect. Dermat. and Syphilol., A. M. A. pp. 220–233, '22 (illus.) also: Arch. Dermat. and Syph. *6:*434–447, Oct '22

LAIRD, A. H.: Bilateral hypertrophy of breasts treated by x-rays. Brit. J. Radiol. *5:*249, March '32

LAIRD, E. G.: Deep cavernous hemangioma of neck; case. Am. J. Surg. *53:*158–162, July '41

LAIRD, J. N.: Fracture of end phalanx of finger with rupture of common extensor tendon. Brit. M. J. *1:*101, Jan 21, '22

LAIRD, W. R. AND WILKERSON, W. V.: "Curling's ulcer" in burns, with report of case. West Virginia M. J. *27:*128–130, March '31

LAIRES, L.: Shock therapy. Amatus *1:*463–480, May '42

LAIRES, L.: Physiopathogenesis and therapy of shock. Amatus *3:*265–299, May '44

LAKE, N. C.: Hand whitlows and infections. Practitioner *136:*376–393, April '36

LAKE, N. C.: Infections of hand and fingers. Brit. M. J. *2:*715, Oct 1; 754, Oct 8; 798, Oct 15, '38

LAKE, N. C.: Minor surgery of hand. Practitioner *147:*593–602, Sept '41

LAKOS, T. Z.: Influence of nasal bacteria on healing process of surgical wounds. Ztschr. f. Hals-, Nasen-u. Ohrenh. *23:*426–435, Sept 10, '29

LAL, K. M.: Congenital absence of penis; case. Indian M. Gaz. *78:*152, March '43

LAL, R. B.: Complete bilateral cleft palate; case. Indian M. Gaz. *66:*268, May '31

LALVANI, P. P.: Electro-coagulation (diathermy) for facial cancer. Indian M. Gaz. *63:*640, Nov '28

LALVANI, P. P.: Electro-coagulation (surgical diathermy) in multiple angiomata of head. Indian M. Gaz. *64:*387–388, July '29

LAM, C. R.: Amputated limbs as source for nerve graft. J.A.M.A. *123:*1067, Dec 18, '43

LAM, C. R.: General care of burn patient. J.A.M.A. *125:*543–546, June 24, '44

LAM, C. R.: Recent advances in burn therapy. Indust. Med. *14:*610, July '45

LAM, C. R. AND HARKINS, H. N.: Panel discussions on burn therapy. Bull. Am. Coll. Surgeons *27:*109–110, April '42

LAM, C. R. AND MCCLURE, R. D.: Penicillin as adjunct in skin grafting of severe burns. Proc. Am. Federation Clin. Research *1:*56, '44

LAM, C. R. AND PUPPENDAHL, M.: Pyruvic acid method of burn slough removal; experimental investigation. Ann. Surg. *121:*866–871, June '45

LAM, C. R. (see HARKINS, H. N. *et al*) Oct '42

LAM, C. R. (see HOOKER, D. H.) April '41

LAM, C. R. (see HOOKER, D. H.) Nov '41

LAM, C. R. (see MCCLURE, R. D.) April '40

LAM, C. R. (see MCCLURE, R. D.) May '40

LAM, C. R. (see MCCLURE, R. D.) July '43

LAM, C. R. (see MCCLURE, R. D. *et al*) 1944

LAM, C. R. (see MCCLURE, R. D. *et al*) Sept '44

LAMACHE, A. (see MICHAUX, J. *et al*) May '25

LAMAITRE, F. AND RUPPE, C.: Osteomyelitis of lower jaw; cases. Arch. Internat. de laryng. *35:*773–782, July–Aug '29

LAMAS, A.: Construction of vagina; 2 cases. An. de Fac. de med., Montevideo *8:*1–6, Jan '23

LAMB, E. D.: Fractures of fingers. Journal-Lancet *61:*372–374, Sept '41

LAMBADARIDIS, A. (see CHRYSSICOS, J.) 1937

LAMBECK, A.: Study of improvement of speech after operation for cleft hard palate; case. Ztschr. f. Kinderforsch. *42:*369–384, '33

LAMBERG (see LEBOURG, L.) May '45

LAMBERSON, H. H.: Association of hypospadias with gonococcal infections in male. Rocky Mountain M. J. *37:*668–671, Sept '40

LAMBERT (see CERNEA) Nov–Dec '42

LAMBOTTE, A.: Technic in plastic operation on big toe. Paris chir. *20:*33–36, March–April '28

LAMBOTTE, A.: Conservative surgery in hand injury. Arch. franco-belges de chir. *31:*759–764, Sept '28

LAMBRET, O. AND DRIESSENS, J.: Humorotissular syndrome in extensive burns; pathogenesis and therapy. Rev. de chir., Paris *75:*319–354, May '37

LAMBRET, O.; DRIESSENS, J. AND CORNILLOT, M.: Action of infra-red irradiation on humorotissular syndrome in extensive burns. Rev. de chir., Paris *76:*478–502, July '38

LAMBRINUDI, C.: Plastic operation for congenital absence of thumb. Proc. Roy. Soc. Med. *31:*181–183, Jan '38

LAMÉRIS, H. J.: Prosthesis in excision of mandible. Nederl. Tijdschr. v. Geneesk. *1:*244–246, Jan 12, '29

LAMON, J. D. AND ALEXANDER, E. JR.: Secondary closure of ulcers with aid of penicillin. J.A.M.A. *127:*396, Feb 17, '45

LAMONT, E. S.: Reconstructive plastic surgery of absent ear with necrocartilage; original method. Arch. Surg. *48:*53–72, Jan '44

LAMONT, E. S.: Plastic surgery of facial paralysis (including fascial transplant) with modification in technic. Arch. Otolaryng. *39:*155–163, Feb '44

LAMONT, E. S.: Reconstructive surgery in congenital deformity, injury and disease of nose. Am. J. Surg. *65:*17–45, July '44

LAMONT, E. S.: Plastic surgery in reconstructing partially absent nose; original technic. Ann. Otol., Rhin. and Laryng. *53:*561–568, Sept '44

LAMONT, E. S.: Plastic surgery in reconstructing enlarged breasts; one-stage mastopexy. Surgery *17:*379–396, March '45

LAMONT, E. S.: Reparative plastic surgery of secondary cleft lip and nasal deformities. Surg., Gynec. and Obst. *80:*422–434, April '45

LAMONT, E. S.: Plastic surgery of nasal fractures. Am. J. Surg. *69:*144–154, Aug '45

LAMONT, E. S.: Plastic surgery in congenital deformities about face. Eye, Ear, Nose and Throat Monthly *24:*571, Dec '45; *25:*25, Jan; 85, Feb '46

LAMONT, E. S.: Two-stage mastopexy in plastic surgery of markedly enlarged breasts. Ann. Surg. *124:*111–117, July '46

LAMONT, E. S.: Physiology of nose and its relation to plastic surgery. Am. J. Surg. *72:*238–245, Aug '46

LAMONT, H. A.: Early skin grafting of war wounds. U. S. Nav. M. Bull. *42:*654–658, March '44

LAMONTAGNE, H.: Clinical aspect of surgical shock. Manitoba M. Rev. *23:*119–122, May '43

LAMPRECHT, V. L.: Baldwin's operation with Constantini's modification for artificial vagina; case. J. akush. i zhensk. boliez. *39:*916–918, '28

LAMSON, P. D.; ROBBINS, B. H. AND GREIG, M. E.: Shock induced by hemorrhage; hemoglobin solutions as blood substitutes in therapy. J. Pharmacol. and Exper. Therap. *83:*225–234, March '45

LAMY (see BABONNEIX, L. *et al*) March '28

LAMY, L.: De Quervain's chronic stenosing tendovaginitis; 3 cases. Bull. et mem. Soc. d. chirurgiens de Paris *24:*373–377, June 3, '32

LANA MARTINEZ, F. AND LANA SALARRULLANA, F.: Plastic induration of penis and Dupuytren's contracture; cases. Med. espan. *7:*450–456, May '42

LANA SALARRULLANA, F. (see LANA MARTINEZ, F.) May '42

LANARI, E. (see MARQUE, A. M.) Jan '30

LANCE, P. (see MERLE D'AUBIGNE, R.) Sept '46

LANCE, P. (see MERLE D'AUBIGNE, R. *et al*) Sept '46

LANDA, G. I.: Therapy of extensive hypertrophic cutaneous scars by application of mud and injection of turpentine. Klin. med. *16:*99–102, '38

LANDAIS: Surgical therapy of prognathism; bicondyloid resection and osteotomy of ascending branch of lower jaw; critical study. Rev. de stomatol. *36:*209–227, April '34

LANDAIS: Subcondyloid osteotomy in therapy of laterognathism of jaw. Rev. de stomatol. *37:*65–86, Feb '35

LANDAIS, P.: Surgical therapy of mandibular deformities; prognathism and laterognathism. Rev. de stomatol. *36:*98–103, Feb '34

LANDAIS, P.: Therapy of jaw fractures. Rev. de stomatol. *38:*65–73, Feb '36

LANDAU, E.; LOGUE, V. AND KOPELMAN, H.: Pholedrine (veritol) in prevention of operative shock. Lancet *2:*210–212, Aug 22, '42

LANDAUER, W.: Supernumerary nipples; congenital hemihypertrophy and congenital hemiatrophy of breast. Human Biol. *11:*447–472, Dec '39

Landerer-Bidder Operation

Urethral fistula cured by Landerer-Bidder procedure; case. GRIMALDI, F. E. AND BERNARDI, R. Prensa med. argent. *28:*1886–1888, Sept 24, '41

Landerer-Bidder operation in cure of large urethral fistula; case. GRIMALDI, F. E. AND BERNARDI, R. Rev. argent. de urol. *10:*535–539, Sept–Oct '41

LANDHAM, J. W.: Squamous cell carcinoma of lower lip; case. Piedmont Hosp. Bull. *4:*32–35, July–Aug '27

LANDIVAR, A. F. AND LEONI IPARRAGUIRRE, C. A.: Late evolution in case of "scalping" of heel (with skin grafting). Dia med. *14:*202–203, March 16, '42

LANDOIS, F.: Causes, pathology, diagnosis and therapy of stenosing tendovaginitis of thumb. Med. Klin. *26:*927–929, June 20, '30

LANDOIS, F.: Technic and some unsuccessful results of various methods of plastic repair of congenital absence of vagina; case. Arch. f. klin. Chir. *170:*178–187, '32

LANDS, A. M.: Physiology and treatment of shock. Mod. Hosp. *61:*110, Nov '43

LANE, F. F.: Method of local anesthesia for intranasal operations. U. S. Nav. M. Bull. *33:*55–59, Jan '35

LANE, W. Z. (see FULCHER, O. H.) Jan '43

LANG, C.: Pathologic and clinical study of lamellar cysts of neck. Arch. f. klin. Chir. *185:*527–536, '36

LANG, G. F.: Traumatic shock. Klin. med. (nos. 5–6) *20:*3; (no. 7) *20:*3, '42

LANG, H.: Ulnar paralysis due to holding of tool handle. Zentralbl. f. Chir. *67:*301-302, Feb 17, '40

LANG, K.: Functional prognosis of suture of tendons. Med. Klinik *19:*530–533, April 22, '23 (illus.)

LANG, M.: Technic for epithelisation with grafts in cases of skin defects. Dermat. Wchnschr. *91:*1478–1483, Oct 4, '30

LANGAN, A. J.: New splint for finger traction in fractures. California and West. Med. *35:*377, Nov '31

LANGDON, H. M.: Fracture of maxilla through left optic foramen; reduction with Kingsley splint, with restoration of vision. Arch. Ophth. *9:*980–981, June '33

LANGE, F.: Treatment of finger fractures. Munchen. med. Wchnschr. *72:*1522–1524, Sept 4, '25

LANGE, F.: Tendon transplantation. Surg., Gynec. and Obst. *44:*455–462, April (pt. 1) '27

LANGE, F.: Technic of tendon surgery. Tungchi, Med. Monatschr. *2:*462–469, Aug '27

LANGE, F.: Silk tendons and joint ligaments; results of plastic operations. Munchen. med. Wchnschr. *75:*39–42, Jan 6, '28

LANGE, F.: Technic of tendon transplantation. Wien. med. Wchnschr. *79:*927-929, July 13, '29

LANGE, H. J. AND CAMPBELL, K. N.: Treatment of severely burned patient; outline of present policies. Univ. Hosp. Bull., Ann Arbor *11:*90–96, Nov '45

LANGE, H. J.; CAMPBELL, K. N. AND COLLER, F. A.: Present policies in treatment of severely burned patient; outline of treatment including use of whole blood transfusions. J. Michigan M. Soc. *45:*619–633, May '46

LANGE, K.: Vascular prerequisites of successful grafting; new method (using fluorescein) for immediate determination of adequacy of circulation in ulcers, skin grafts and flaps. Surgery *15:*85–89, Jan '44

LANGE, M.: Treatment of stiffening of fingers and hand with and without muscular paralysis. Munchen. med. Wchnschr. *81:*894–897, June 15, '34

LANGE, W. A.: Plastic surgery in relation to automobile accidents (face). J. Michigan M. Soc. *37:*787–792, Sept '38

LANGEMAK, O.: Technic for suturing nerves. Zentralbl. f. Chir. *49:*1253–1255, Aug 26, '22 (illus.)

LANGER, M.: Results of tannic acid therapy in children in burns. Wien. klin. Wchnschr. *46:*689-690, June 2, '33

LANGGUTH, H. (see MULLER, H. K.) 1941

LANGMANN, A. G.: Acrocephaly associated with syndactylism, with report of case. Arch. Pediat. *41:*699–706, Oct '24

LANIER, L. H. (see DOUGLAS, B.) Oct '34

LANIER, W. D. JR.: Fractures of lower jaw. U.S. Vet. Bur. M. Bull. *5:*893–895, Nov '29

LANMAN, T. H. (see LADD, W. E.) April '37

LANMAN, T. H. (see LADD, W. E.) Jan '40

LANOS (see HAUTANT, A.) Dec '27

LANZA CASTELLI, R. A.: Nasal septal operation; technic to avoid postoperative tamponade. Rev. otorrinolaring. d. litoral *2:*112-128, Dec '42

LANZI, G.: Small apparatus for diathermy and electrocoagulation depilation treatment of hypertrichosis in women. Gior. ital. d. ma. ven. *65:*1718–1720, Oct '24

LAOUENAN, P. (see HOUOT, A. *et al*) Jan–Feb '39

LAPEYRE, J. L.: Etiology, pathogenesis and therapy of tropical elephantiasis. J. de chir. *49:*682–717, May '37

LAPEYRIE AND CABANAC: Surgical therapy of posttyphoidal jaw ankylosis. Montpellier med. *5:*31–37, Jan 15, '34

LAPEYRIE (see ETIENNE, *et al*) June '39

LAPIDUS, P. W. AND GUIDOTTI, F. P.: Triphalangeal bifid thumb; 6 cases. Arch. Surg. *49:*228–234, Oct '44

LAPIDUS, P. W.; GUIDOTTI, F. P. AND COLETTI, C. J.: Triphalangeal thumb; 6 cases. Surg., Gynec. and Obst. *77:*178–186, Aug '43

LAPIÉRRE, S. (see WEEKERS, L.) 1934

LAPIÉRRE, S. (see WEEKERS, L.) Jan '35

LAPIERRE, V.: Maxillofacial prosthesis of cellulose acetate. Odontologie *68:*634–653, Sept '30

LAPIERRE, V.: Facial prosthesis with cellulose acetate, technic. Rev. de chir. plastique, pp. 168–217, Oct '33

LAPIERRE, V. (see PONT, A.) May '36

LAPIERRE, V. (see PONT, A.) March '37

LAPP, F. W. AND NEUFFER, H.: Method of drying surface of wound before application of Thiersch grafts. Zentralbl. f. Chir. *58:*1634–1635, June 27, '31

LAQUA, K.: Preliminary serum treatment before skin grafting. Klin. Wchnschr. *2:*1360–1362, July 16, '23 abstr: J.A.M.A. *81:*1478, Oct 27, '23

LAQUEUR, B.: Anesthetization in burns. Therap. d. Gegenw. *73:*144, March '32

DE LARA, I.: Monodactylomegaly; surgical therapy of case. Rev. mex. de cir., ginec. y cancer *8:*375–380, Sept '40

DE LARA, M. J.: Plastic surgery possibilities; development in Cuba; historical study. Arq. de cir. clin. e exper. *6:*325–333, April–June

'42
LARI, G. L. (see ARLOTTA, A.) Dec '30
LARICHELLIERE, R.: Surgical therapy in burns. Union med. du Canada *71:*491–494, May '42
LARIN, N. AND GOLONZKO, L. Y.: Ultraviolet rays in burn therapy. Sovet. khir. *4:*44–50, '33
LARKIN, A. J.: Value of radium in treatment of cancer of face. Am. J. Surg. *8:*164–165, Jan '30
LAROCHELLE, J. L.: Burn therapy. Laval med. *9:*413–419, June '44
LA ROE, E. K.: Breast tissue as new source for heterogenous implants; preliminary report. Am. J. Surg. *66:*58–67, Oct '44
LA ROE, E. K.: Failures in mammaplastic surgery for hypertrophy of breast. Am. J. Surg. *66:*339–345, Dec '44
LA ROE, E. K.: Evaluation of common procedures in mammaplasty and new technic. Am. J. Surg. *72:*641–655, Nov '46
LA ROSA, F. J. (see HOWES, W. E.) Jan '42
LAROYENNE AND BOUYSSET: Stenosing tendovaginitis of long abductor and of short extensor of thumb. Arch. franco-belges de chir. *30:*98–104, Feb '27 also: Lyon med. *140:*573–575, Nov 27, '27
LAROYENNE AND MEYSSONNIER: Phlegmon of synovial sheath of finger; treatment without incision; case. Lyon med. *143:*259–261, March 3, '29
LAROYENNE AND TREPOZ: Strangulation of long abductor and short extensor of thumb; treatment. Lyon med. *142:*394, Sept 30, '28
LAROYENNE, L. AND BRUN, M.: Acute forms of de Quervain's stenosing tendovaginitis; 2 cases. Lyon med. *151:*3–9, Jan 1, '33
LARROUDÉ, C.: Chondrosarcoma of ethmoid; surgical therapy; radiotherapy and autoplasty with tubular flap. Rev. de chir. plastique, pp. 239–245, Oct '33
LARROUDÉ, C.: Surgical therapy of nasal deformities; 2 cases. Rev. de chir. plastique, pp. 246–250, Oct '33
LARSON, A. B.: Zygomatic fracture; case. U. S. Nav. M. Bull. *45:*1151–1154, Dec '45
LARSON, C. B. (see SMITH-PETERSEN, M. N. *et al*) May '43
LARSON, E.: Branchiogenetic cysts. California and West. Med. *47:*244–248, Oct '37
LARSON, E. E. AND PULFORD, D. S.: Gas gangrene of extremities, with special reference to trivalent anaerobic serotherapy. Tr. Sect. Surg., General and Abd., A. M. A., pp. 261–279, '29 also: J.A.M.A. *94:*612–618, March 1, '30
LARSSON, S.: Dacryocystorhinostomy. Acta ophth. *6:*193–215, '28
LARSSON, S.: Treatment of congenital atresia of nasolacrimal duct. Acta ophth. *16:*271–278, '38

Larynx, Cancer of

Laryngectomy for cancer of larynx with modified technique and attempted formation of skin tube in place of larynx. GOLDTHWAITE, R. H. Laryngoscope *32:*446–450, June '22
Statistics and technique in treatment of malignant neoplasms of larynx. QUICK, D. A. AND JOHNSON, F. M. Am. J. Roentgenol. *9:*599–606, Sept '22
Surgical treatment of laryngeal cancer with an analysis of 70 cases. MACKENTY, J. E. New York State J. Med. *22:*456–462, Oct '22
Radical operation for extrinsic carcinoma of larynx. BLAIR, V. P. Ann. Otol., Rhin. and Laryng. *33:*373–378, June '24
Carcinoma of larynx. NEW, G. B. Minnesota Med. *9:*365–368, July '26
Carcinoma of larynx and laryngopharynx treated with radium; analysis of 30 cases. IMPERATORI, C. J. Arch. Otolaryng. *4:*151–159, Aug '26
Ten years' experience with radium therapy of cancer of larynx. SARGNON, A., J. de radiol. et d'electrol. *10:*553–555, Dec '26
Intrinsic cancer operated on by laryngo-fissure; immediate and ultimate results. THOMSON, ST. C. Eye, Ear, Nose and Throat Monthly *7:*266–270, June '28 also: Arch. Otolaryng. *8:*377–385, Oct '28
Two stage laryngectomy. NEW, G. B. Proc. Staff Meet., Mayo Clin. *3:*221, July 25, '28 also: Surg., Gynec. and Obst. *47:*826–830, Dec '28
Unusual complication (suppuration of sternoclavicular joint) following laryngectomy. COLLEDGE, L., J. Laryng. and Otol *43:*661–663, Sept '28
Management of malignancies of antrum, superior maxilla, pharynx and larynx at Radium Institute of University of Paris. PACK, G. T. Ann. Otol. Rhin. and Laryng. *37:*967–973, Sept '28
Extrinsic epithelioma of larynx. NEW, G. B. S. Clin. N. Amer. *9:*84–87, Feb '29
Cancer of larynx in young. FIGI, F. A. AND NEW, G. B. Arch. Otolaryng. *9:*386–391, April '29
Intrinsic laryngeal cancer; lasting cure in 76 per cent of cases by laryngo-fissure. THOMSON, ST. C. Canad. M. A. J. *21:*4–8, July '29

Larynx, Cancer of—Cont.
Intrinsic laryngeal cancer; lasting recovery in 76 per cent of cases of laryngofissure. THOMSON, ST. C. Ann. d. ma. de l'oreille, du larynx *48:*1079–1088, Nov '29 also: Union med. du Canada *59:*5–16, Jan '30
Carcinoma of larynx in young. FIGI, F. A. AND NEW, G. B. Tr. Am. Laryng., Rhin. and Otol. Soc. *35:*350–357, '29
Results of radium therapy in cancer of larynx; 150 cases. ESCAT, *et al.* Cancer, Bruxelles *7:*121–126, '30
Double branchial cysts complicated by carcinoma of larynx. HERMAN, A. L. Minnesota Med. *14:*555–557, June '31
Laryngectomy for cancer. JACKSON, C. AND BABCOCK, W. W., S. Clin. North America *11:*1207–1227, Dec '31
Status of thyrotomy in cancer of larynx. NEW, G. B. Tr. Am. Laryng., Rhin. and Otol. Soc. *37:*241–247, '31
Late results of fractional roentgenotherapy of intrinsic cancer of larynx; results of 5 years' experience. GUNSETT, A. Gaz. med. de France (supp. radiol.), pp. 173–177, May 1, '32
Technic of closure of esophageal fistula; significance in surgical treatment of laryngo-esophageal cancer. PORTMANN, G. AND DESPONS, J. Bordeaux chir. *3:*252–261, July '32
Treatment of laryngeal cancer by laryngofissure. JACKSON, C. South. Surgeon *1:*223–229, Oct '32
Selection of treatment of cancer of larynx. NEW, G. B. AND FLETCHER, E., J.A.M.A. *99:*1754–1758, Nov 19, '32
Selection of treatment of cancer of larynx. NEW, G. B. AND FLETCHER, E. M. Tr. Sect. Laryng., Otol. and Rhin., A.M.A., pp 27–42, '32
Statistical report on 5 year cures of cancer of larynx. LEWIS, F. O. Surg., Gynec. and Obst. *56:*466–467, Feb (No. 2A) '33
Radium therapy of cancer of larynx; results in 150 cases. CAPIZZANO, N. Bol. Inst. de med., exper. para el estud. y trat. del cancer *10:*575–579, Oct '33
Laryngectomy for cancer of larynx; results in 140 cases. CETRÁ, C. M. Bol. Inst. de med. exper. para el estud. y trat. del cancer *10:*564–573, Oct '33
Curability of cancer of larynx by laryngofissure. JACKSON, C. Surg., Gynec. and Obst. *58:*431–432, Feb (no. 2A) '34
Curability of cancer of larynx. NEW, G. B. AND WAUGH, J. M. Surg., Gynec. and Obst. *58:*841–844, May '34

Larynx, Cancer of—Cont.
Analysis of 58 cases cancer of larynx treated with laryngofissure. CLERF, L. H. Arch. Otolaryng. *19:*653–659, June '34
Observations in 200 consecutive cases of cancer of larynx. TUCKER, G. Arch. Otolaryng. *21:*1–8, Jan '35
Five year cures of cancer of larynx; and mouth and pharynx. NEW, G. B. AND FIGI, F. A. Surg., Gynec. and Obst. *60:*483–484, Feb (no. 2A) '35
Laryngectomy for carcinoma in aged patient; case. NEW, G. B. Proc. Staff Meet., Mayo Clin. *10:*186–187, March 20, '35
Statistics on results of 393 surgically treated cases of laryngeal cancer from May 1919 to July 1934 inclusive. HAJEK, M. AND HEINDL, A. Monatschr. f. Ohrenh. *69:*385, April; 583, May '35
Cancer of larynx and its therapy. DE SANSON, R. D. Rev. oto-laring. de Sao Paulo *3:*197–214, May–June '35 also: Rev. de laryng. *56:*964–985, Sept–Oct '35
Study of 133 cases of laryngeal cancer. MULLIN, W. V. AND DARSIE, L. L., S. Clin. North America *15:*851–858, Aug '35
Treatment of laryngeal cancer by laryngofissure and laryngectomy. JACKSON, C. AND JACKSON, C. L. Am. J. Surg. *30:*3–17, Oct '35
Study of 202 cases of laryngeal cancer with end results. GARFIN, S. W. New England J. Med. *213:*1109–1123, Dec 5, '35
Treatment of carcinoma of larynx. NEW, G. B. AND FIGI, F. A. Surg., Gynec. and Obst. *62:*420–423, Feb (no. 2A) '36
Diagnosis and surgical cure of cancer of larynx. TUCKER, G. Delaware State M. J. *8:*80–82, May '36
Surgical therapy of cancer of larynx; 200 cases. CETRÁ, M. C. Bol. Inst. de med. exper. para el estud. y trat. d. cancer *14:*169–188, April '37
Results of roentgenotherapy of cancer of larynx after 5 and 10 years of control. COUTARD, H., J. de radiol. et d'electrol. *21:*402–409, Sept '37
Cancer of larynx. JACKSON, C. AND JACKSON, C. L., S. Clin North America *17:*1791–1795, Dec '37
Results of surgical therapy and radiotherapy of epitheliomas of mouth, tongue and larynx. CHRYSSICOS, J. AND LAMBADARIDIS, A. Ztschr. f. Hals-, Nasen-u, Ohrenh. *40:*410–413, '37
Surgical treatment of cancer of larynx. LOOPER, E. A. South. M. J. *31:*367–374, April '38

Larynx, Cancer of—Cont.

Surgical treatment of cancer of larynx. NEW, G. B. Surg., Gynec. and Obst. *68:*462–466, Feb (no. 2A) '39

Surgical treatment of cancer of larynx; results. ORTON, H. B. Mississippi Doctor *17:*128–135, Aug '39

Comparison of results obtained by surgery and radiation therapy, in cancer of larynx. ARBUCKLE, M. F. South. M. J. *32:*1008–1014, Oct '39

Surgical therapy of laryngopharyngeal cancer. AUBRY, M. Ann. d'oto-laryng., pp. 905–908, Nov–Dec '39

Therapy of cancer of larynx. ALONSO, J. M. An. de oto-rino-laring. d. Uruguay *9:*215–232, '39

Surgical treatment of laryngeal cancer. MCCREADY, J. H. Radiology *34:*146–148, Feb '40

Malignant disease of face, buccal cavity, pharynx and larynx in first three decades of life. HERTZ, C. S. Proc. Staff Meet., Mayo Clin. *15:*152–156, March 6, '40

Diagnosis and surgical treatment of cancer of larynx. LOOPER, E. A. South Surgeon *9:*513–521, July '40

Results of treatment of malignant tumors of larynx and hypopharynx. WOODWARD, F. D. AND ARCHER, V. W. Virginia M. Monthly *67:*751–755, Dec '40

Surgical solution to carcinoma of larynx. CETRA, M. Rev. otorrinolaring. d. litoral *3:*99–117, Jan–June '44

Surgical management of carcinoma of larynx. SHERWIN, C. F., S. Clin. North America *24:*1089–1099, Oct '44

Larynx, Miscellaneous

Plastic correction of defects in larynx and trachea. PFEIFFER, C. Zentralbl. f. Chir. *48:*965, July 9, '21

Plastic reconstruction of larynx and trachea. SCHMIDT, C. Schweiz. med. Wchnschr. *52:*539–540, May 25, '22

Burns of larynx. FLURIN, H. AND MAGDELEINE, J. Ann. d. mal. de l'oreille, du larynx *46:*1207–1221, Dec '27

Burns of larynx from swallowing sodium hydroxide; 2 cases. FOTIADE, V. Arch. internat. de laryng. *34:*22–30, Jan '28

Plastic covering of large defects in laryngeal tube; case. ZANGE, J. Ztschr. f. Hals-, Nasen-u. Ohrenh. *21:*638–651, May 10, '28

Branchiogenetic cyst of larynx removed by thyrotomy. IMPERATORI, C. J. Laryngoscope *39:*679–683, Oct '29

Branchiogenic anomalies (cysts and fistulas)

Larynx, Miscellaneous—Cont.

associated with larynx. ROSENAUER, F. Deutsche Ztschr. f. Chir. *226:*304–307, '30

Plastic operation in pharyngostoma following laryngectomy; case. GROS, J. C. Rev. de med. y cir. de la Habana *36:*65–70, Jan 31, '31

Massive electrical burns with destruction of part of larynx and trachea. BABCOCK, W. W., S. Clin. North America *12:*1415–1417, Dec '32

Plastic operations in laryngostomy; 2 cases. CARRARI, G. Arch. ital. di otol. *44:*731–737, Dec '33

Chronic laryngeal stenosis in children. JACKSON, C. AND JACKSON, C. L., S. Clin. North America *14:*27–37, Feb '34

Pharyngolaryngeal burns and scalds; prognosis, complications and therapy. AGUERRE, J. A. JR. Arch. de pediat. d. Uruguay *5:*181–190, May '34

Plastic closure of laryngostomic fistulas and enlargement of lumen of trachea or larynx by implantation of chondrocutaneous flap. BABCOCK, W. W. Arch. Otolaryng. *19:*585–589, May '34

Two instruments for modelling transplanted cartilage in closure of laryngeal and tracheal defects. MAYER, F. J. Monatschr. f. Ohrenh. *69:*1193–1196, Oct '35

Laryngotracheoplasty by Mangoldt technic in therapy of laryngotracheal fistula. LASKIEWICZ, A. Rev. de laryng. *59:*463–471, May '38

Laryngotracheal reconstruction with free autoplastic cartilaginous grafts. GIUSSANI, M. Arch. ital. di chir. *52:*472–483, '38

Wounds of larynx due to burns during childhood. RIECKE, H. G. Hals-, Nasen-u. Ohrenarzt (Teil 1) *30:*111–118, March '39

Pseudolaryngocele (aerocele) of neck; case. KILPATRICK, F. R. Guy's Hosp. Rep. *90:*15–20, '40–'41

Death due to shock after scalding of pharynx and larynx. TANAKA, H. Oto-rhino-laryng. (Abstr. Sect.) *13:*45–46, Oct '40

Wounds of neck and lesions of larynx, trachea and esophagus in war surgery. DE ANDRADE MEDICIS, J. Arq. brasil. de cir. e ortop. *10:*155–179, '42

Cervicolaryngeal cyst of branchial origin; case. MARTIN CALDERIN, A. Semana med. espan. *6:*91, Jan 23, '43

Wounds of neck and larynx. LEWIS, R. S. Lancet *1:*781–784, June 17, '44

Restorative surgery of the larynx. RUEDI, L. Pract. oto-rhino-laryng. *7:*186–197, '45

Tubular graft in laryngotracheal fistula.

Larynx, Miscellaneous—Cont.

VIANA ROSA, A. Rev. med. Rio Grande do Sul *2:*167-172, Jan-Feb '46

Total laryngectomy with right hemipharyngectomy; plastic surgery to reconstruct pharynx using laryngeal flap from left vestibular zone. LEYRO DIAZ, J. Bol. y trab., Acad. argent. de cir. *30:*815-833, Sept 11, '46

Larynx, Stenosis of

Operative treatment of cicatricial stenosis of larynx; case. RETHI, A. Ztschr. f. Laryng., Rhin. *16:*215-224, Nov '27

Surgical treatment of chronic stenosis of larynx; 148 cases. CHARSCHAK, M. J. Monatschr. f. Ohrenh. *65:*57-80, Jan '31

Stenosis of larynx; laryngofissure and skin graft. FIGI, F. A., S. Clin. North America *11:*837-840, Aug '31

Unusual stenoses of larynx and their surgical therapy. GREIFENSTEIN, A. Hals-, Nasen-u. Ohrenarzt (Teil 1) *27:*101-130, '36

Surgical diathermy in cicatricial stenosis of larynx. BOMBELLI, U. Oto-rhino-laryng. internat. *22:*16-24, Jan '38

Surgical treatment of chronic cicatricial stenosis of larynx. Semon lecture. SCHMIEGELOW, E., J. Laryng. and Otol. *53:*1-14, Jan '38

Use of hyoid bone as graft in laryngeal stenosis. LOOPER, E. A. Arch. Otolaryng. *28:*106-111, July '38

Treatment of chronic laryngeal stenosis, with special reference to skin grafting. NEGUS, V. E. Ann. Otol., Rhin. and Laryng. *47:*891-901, Dec '38

Treatment of chronic laryngeal stenosis, with special reference to skin grafting. NEGUS, V. E. Tr. Am. Laryng. A. *60:*82-92, '38

Chronic laryngeal stenosis, with special consideration of skin grafting. FIGI, F. A. Ann. Otol., Rhin. and Laryng. *49:*394-409, June '40

Plastic procedure in correction of laryngotracheostenosis with dermoepidermic skin grafts. RAPIN, M. Pract. oto-rhino-laryng. *4:*88-91, '42

Skin grafting in case of chronic laryngeal stenosis. MOORE, P. M. Cleveland Clin. Quart. *11:*5-8, Jan '44

Larynx, Tumors of

Benign tumors of larynx; 722 cases. NEW, G. B. AND ERICH, J. B. Arch. Otolaryng. *28:*841-910, Dec '38

Larynx, Tumors of—Cont.

Benign tumors of larynx; study of 722 cases. NEW, G. B. AND ERICH, J. B. Tr. Sect. Laryng., Otol. and Rhin., A. M. A., pp. 17-96, '38

Excision of amyloid tumor of larynx and skin graft; case. FIGI, F. A. Proc. Staff Meet., Mayo Clin. *17:*239-240, April 15, '42

LASAGNA, F.: Surgery of labio-maxillo-palatine fissure. Arch. ital. di chir. *20:*661-679, '28

LASCOMBE, J. (see VEAU, V.) Feb '22

LASKIEWICZ, A.: Laryngotracheoplasty by Mangoldt technic in therapy of laryngotracheal fistula. Rev. de laryng. *59:*463-471, May '38

LASKIEWICZ, A.: Malformations of ear pavilion. Rev. de laryng. *60:*332-344, April '39

LASSEN, E.: Late rupture of extensor pollicis longus tendon after fracture of radius. Hospitalstid. *72:*460-464, April 25, '29

LASSEN, E.: Stenosing tendovaginitis of first portion of styloid process of radius; its nature and treatment. Ugesk. f. laeger *91:*837-840, Oct 3, '29

LASSERRE, C.: Therapy of trophic disturbances (ulcer) following injury of limb by resection of neuroma of posterior tibial nerve and by autotransplantation of nervous tissue. Bull. et mem. Soc. nat. de chir. *58:*500-502, April 16, '32

LASSERRE, C.: Suture of flexor tendon in therapy of hand injury; case. J. de med. de Bordeaux *109:*357-358, May 10, '32

LASSERRE, C.: Simple treatment of spring finger. J. de med. de Bordeaux *121-122:*375-376, July '45

LASSERRE, C. AND MARRONEAUD, P.: Therapy and prophylaxis of maxillary deformities by immobilization with monobloc. Arch. franco-belges de chir. *35:*131-134, Feb '36

LASZLO, A. F.: Practical points on submucous resection; pitfalls and corrections. Laryngoscope *46:*840-847, Nov '36

Lateral Cervical Fistula (See also Branchial Cysts and Fistulas)

Congenital lateral cervical fistula. LEVINGER. Munchen. med. Wchnschr. *68:*304, March 11, '21

Congenital lateral fistulas of neck. GRIESSMANN, B. Munchen. med. Wchnschr. *68:*460, April 15, '21

Congenital median and lateral fistulas in neck. BLAESEN, C. Deutsche Ztschr. f. Chir. *167:*60-64, '21

Fistulae and congenital cysts of lateral region of neck; 3 personal cases. SIMON, R.; *et al.* Arch. franco-belges de chir. *28:*203-

Lateral Cervical Fistula–Cont.
258, March '25
Case of lateral fistulas in neck. MÜLLER, S. Deutsche Ztschr. f. Chir. *193:*401–408, '25
Lateral cervical fistulae. KRAMER, R. Laryngoscope *36:*517–522, July '26
Case of lateral fistula of neck. HUIZINGA, E. Nederl. Tijdschr. v. Geneesk. *2:*1775–1777, Oct 16, '26
Lateral cervical fistula; case. HUIZINGA, E. Laryngoscope *37:*878–879, Dec '27
Lateral, congenital, cervical fistula; clinical aspects, histogenesis operative technic; case. SANTORO, E. Ann. ital. di chir. *8:*59–71, Jan '29
Congenital cyst of thymic origin in neck. PEZCOLLER, A. Clin. chir. *32:*272–284, March '29
Genesis of congenital lateral cervical fistulas and cysts. NYLANDER, P. E. A. Deutsche Ztschr. f. Chir. *215:*139–145, '29
Lateral cervical fistula; paraffin injection as aid to excision. CHRISTOPHER, F., S. Clin. N. Amer. *10:*351–353, April '30
Pathogenesis of lateral fistulae and cysts of neck. MOATTI, L. Ann. d'oto-laryng., pp. 11–41, Jan '31
Congenital cartilaginous remains in neck; relation to lateral cervical fistulas. NIEDEN, H. AND ASBECK, C. Beit. z. klin. Chir. *153:*47–59, '31
Congenital fistula of lateral region of neck. JACQUES, P. AND GRIMAUD. Oto-rhino-laryng. internat. *17:*437–439, June '33
Lateral congenital neck fistula; 2 cases. CORNEJO SARAVIA, E. Bol. y trab. de la Soc. de cir. de Buenos Aires *17:*1224–1237, Nov 22, '33
Lateral congenital fistula of neck. CARNEVALE-RICCI, F. Arch. ital. di otol. *45:*473–482, July '34
Modifying liquids in therapy of congenital fistulas of lateral region of neck; new case with recovery. BERGARA, R. A.; *et al.* Rev. Asoc. med. argent. *48:*1212–1215, Oct '34
Low lateral congenital fistulas of neck. JANKOVSKY, P. Ann. d'oto-laryng., pp. 1133–1146, Dec '37
Problems of congenital origin of lateral fistulas and cysts of neck. MARX, J. Beitr. z. klin. Chir. *168:*435–447, '38 also: Orvosi hetil. *82:*891–895, Sept 10, '38
Differential diagnosis between thymic duct fistulas and branchial cleft fistulas; case of bilateral aural fistulas and bilateral thymic duct fistulas. BAUMGARTNER, C. J. AND STEINDEL, S. Am. J. Surg. *59:*99–103, Jan '43
Thymic cyst; case. HYDE, T. L.; *et al.* Texas State J. Med. *39:*539–540, Feb '44
Lateral congenital fistula of neck; case. CISNEROS, R. Bol. y trab., Acad. argent. de cir. *29:*247–259, May 9, '45
Lateral cervical (branchial) cysts and fistulas; clinical and pathologic study. NEEL, H. B. AND PEMBERTON, J. DE J. Surgery *18:*267–286, Sept '45

LATHROP, F. D.: Plastic dacryocystorhinostomy; technic. S. Clin. North America *22:*675–679, June '42
LATHROP, F. D.: Treatment facial paralysis. Lahey Clin. Bull. *3:*20–27, July '42
LATHROP, F. D.: Facial nerve lesions due to war injuries and their repair. J. Laryng. and Otol. *60:*257–266, June '45
LATHROP, F. D.: Facial nerve lesions due to war injuries and their repair. Proc. Roy. Soc. Med. *38:*629–634, Sept '45
LATHROP, F. D.: Facial nerve; repair of traumatic lesions secondary to war wounds. S. Clin. North America *26:*763–773, June '46
LATIMER, E. O.: Treatmént of decubitus ulcers with tannic acid. J.A.M.A. *102:*751–752, March 10, '34
LAUB, G. R.: Nasal septal abscess. South. Med. and Surg. *106:*374, Oct '44
LAUBER, H.: Plastic surgery of eyelid following removal of epithelioma caused by irradiation. Ophthalmologica *97:*312–316, July '39
LAUBER, H. J.: Surgical therapy of syndactylia. Chirurg. *7:*598–599, Sept 1, '35
LAUER, A. (see REINHARD, W.) 1941
LAUMONIER, J.: Glossoptosis and facial deformity. Gaz. d. hop. *100:*848–850, June 25, '27
LAURENS (see CADENAT *et al*) Oct–Dec '45
LAURIE, R. D.: Operative treatment of fractures of forearm and hand. J.M.A.S. Africa *1:*585–587, Nov 26, '27
LAUTEN, W. F.: Finger tip reconstruction; new operation (using bone and skin grafts). Indust. Med. *8:*99–100, March '39
LAUTENSCHLÄGER, A.: Operation for bony wrynose. Chirurg *1:*260–263, Feb 1 '29
LAUTERSTEIN, M.: Surgical therapy of entropion and trichiasis. Ztschr. f. Augenh. *75:*183, Sept '31
LAUWERS, E. E.: New method of resection of upper maxillary with lower facial flap. Surg., Gynec. and Obst. *39:*499–502, Oct '24
LAUX, MME. (see MASSABUAU, *et al*) April '35
LAUWERS, E. E.: *Introduction à la chirurgie réparatrice*. Masson et Cie, Paris, 1934
LAVAL, F.: Post-operative endo-nasal tamponade with cotton sachets (in nasal surgery). Ann. d. mal. de l'oreille, du larynx *46:*377–379, April '27
LAVAL, J.: Congenital fistula of lacrimal sac.

Am. J. Ophth. *22:*1022-1023, Sept '39

LAVAL, J.: Modified sling operation for correction of ptosis (eye). Arch. Ophth. *33:*482-483, June '45

LAVAND' HOMME, P.: Late cancer of artificial vagina formed from rectum (Schubert operation); case. Bruxelles-med. *19:*14-15, Nov 6, '38

LAVEDAN, J. (see NYKA, W.) March '33

LAVENDER, H. J.: Burns and their treatment. J. Med. *11:*635-643, Feb '31

LAVENDER, H. J.: Treatment and management of burn cases (with special reference to bath procedure). Am. J. Surg. *45:*534-538, Sept '39

LAVENDER, H. J.: Burn management in children; analytic study of 250 cases. J.A.M.A. *118:*344-349, Jan 31, '42

LAVIERI, F. J. (see FIGUEROA, L.) June '44

LAW, T. B.: Method of dealing with fractures through infraorbital margin. M. J. Australia *1:*666-667, May 31, '41

LÄWEN, A.: Treatment of progressive pyogenic processes of face; injection of own blood. Zentralbl. f. Chir. *50:*1018-1024, June 30, '23 abstr: J.A.M.A. *81:*1155, Sept 29, '23

LÄWEN, A.: Treatment of malignant furuncle of face by incision and circular injection of patient's own blood. Zentralbl. f. Chir. *50:*1468-1471, Sept 29, '23

LÄWEN, A.: Early operation for severe burns. Zentralbl. f. Chir. *63:*1576-1581, July 4, '36

LÄWEN, A.: Procaine hydrochloride blocking of stellate ganglion in therapy of traumatic hard edema of hand. Arch. f. klin. Chir. *201:*687-691, '41

LAWRENCE, E. A. AND BREZINA, P. S.: Carcinoma of oral cavity; 10 year survery in general hospital. J.A.M.A. *128:*1012-1016, Aug 4, '45

LAWRENCE, E. A. AND OUGHTERSON, A. W.: Cancer of lips at New Haven Hospital, 1921-1940, inclusive. Connecticut M. J. *8:*353-357, June '44

LAWRENCE, H. W.: Collateral circulation in hand after cutting radial and ulnar arteries at wrist. Indust. Med. *6:*410-411, July '37

LAWRIE, R.: Primary closure of battle wounds of face. Lancet *1:*625-626, May 19, '45

LAWRIE, R. S. (see CLARKSON, P. *et al*) Feb '46

LAWRIE, R. S. (see CLARKSON, P.) Apr '46

LAWSON, H.: Secondary vascular shock. Kentucky M. J. *36:*281-284, July '38

LAWWILL, S.: Deviated nasal septum. J. Tennessee M. A. *19:*284-286, Feb '27

LAYANI, F. (see LÉRI, A.) July '25

LAYTON, T. B. *et al*: Discussion on choice and technic of anesthetics for nasal surgery. J. Laryng. and Otol. *52:*501-512, July '37

LAZANSKY, J. P.; WUEHRMANN, A. H. AND GLICKMAN, I.: Traumatic cyst of mandible. Am. J. Orthodontics (Oral Surg. Sect.) *32:*155-159, Mar '46

LAZANSKY, J. P. AND WUEHRMANN, A. H.: Failure of union in mandibular fracture and its successful nonsurgical treatment. Am. J. Orthodontics (Oral Surg. Sect.) *32:*182-183, March '46

LAZARESCU, D. AND LAZARESCU, E.: Progressive facial hemiatrophy. Ann. d'ocul. *171:*1004-1011, Dec '34

LAZARESCU, E. (see LAZARESCU, D.) Dec '34

LAZAREV, E. G.: New modification of operation for eyelid ptosis. Vestnik oftal. *11:*76-80, '37

LAZIER, W. A. (see MATTOCKS, A. M.) Sept '46

LAZYNSKA, W.: Cutaneous burns. Pediatria polska *18:*340-343, June '38

LAZZARINI, L.: Transplants of living bones. Arch. ital. di chir. *11:*109-138, '25 abstr: J.A.M.A. *85:*155, July 11, '25

LAZZARINI, L.: Action of periosteum and connective tissue of host in grafts of bone without periosteum. Arch. di ortop. *43:*65-72, '27

LAZZARINI, L.: Comparison of various forms of bone transplantation. Gazz. d. osp. *49:*97-100, Jan 29, '28

LEADBETTER, W. F.: Urethra; repair of complete tear of membranous portion; case report and suggested new technic for operation. M. Bull. North African Theat. Op. (no. 4) *2:*70-74, Oct '44

LEAL JR.: Congenital ptosis of upper lid. Brazil-med. *2:*179-180, Sept 20, '24 abstr: J.A.M.A. *83:*1626, Nov 15, '24

LEAMER, B. V.: Intranasal procaine anesthesia in nasal surgery. U. S. Nav. M. Bull. *36:*498-499, Oct '38

LEARMONTH, J. R.: Anastomosis of hypoglossal and facial nerves 10 months after operation; presentation of case. Proc. Staff Meet., Mayo Clin. *7:*389-390, July 6, '32

LEARMONTH, J. R.: Technic for transplanting ulnar nerve. Surg., Gynec. and Obst. *75:*792-793, Dec '42

LEARMONTH, J. R.: Personal experience of exploration and reexploration of injured nerves. Proc. Roy. Soc. Med. *37:*553-556, Aug '44

LEARMONTH, J. R. AND WALLACE, A. B.: Plastic problems in surgery of peripheral nerves. Surg., Gynec. and Obst. *76:*106-109, Jan '43

LE BEAU, J.: Tantalum plates in repair of osseous defects. Rev. neurol. *77:*307-308, Nov-Dec '45

LEBEDEFF, V.: Formation of artificial vagina from segment of small intestine. Monatschr. f. Geburtsh. u. Gynak. *76:*294-296, June '27

LEBEDENKO, V. V.: Peripheral nerve lesions; time element in restorative surgery. Am. Rev. Soviet Med. *1:*23-27, Oct '43 also: Khi-

rurgiya, no. 10, pp. 48-52, '42
LEBEDEV, V. F.: Formation of artificial vagina according to Baldwin technic. Sovet. khir., no. 2, pp. 351-354, '36
LEBEDEVA, M. P.: Burn therapy. Med. zhur. *6:*535-538, '36
LEBEDEVA, M. P. (see ISHCHENKO, I. N.) 1937
LEBEDINSKAYA, S. I.: Characteristics of local reaction following implantation of tissues preserved in formalin (solution of formaldehyde). Khirurgiya, no. 4, pp. 18-23, '44
LEBOURG, L.: Therapy of fractures of condyles of jaw; advantages of perifacial arc. Presse med. *44:*360-361, March 4, '36
LEBOURG, L.: Reduction of blocked temporomaxillary luxation under regional transmasseteric anesthesia. Presse med. *47:*872, May 31, '39
LEBOURG, L.: Migraine due to war injury to nose, with recovery following resection of cicatrix. Rev. de stomatol. *43:*27-28, Jan-Feb '42
LEBOURG, L. AND LAMBERG: Dentofacial orthopedics; effect on development of child. Semaine d. hop. Paris *21:*544-547, May 28, '45
LEBOURG, L. (see BRECHOT) March '29
LECÈNE, P.: Early clinical and therapeutic study of invasion of lymphatic nodes in pavement epitheliomas of lips and tongue; 8 cases. Prat. med. franc. *7:*219-227, May (A) '28
LECH, JR.: Plastic surgery of eye cavity. Arq. Inst. Penido Burnier *7:*30-56, Dec '45
LÉCHELLE; THÉVENARD, A. AND JOSEPH: Symmetrical facial atrophy with segmentary adiposis dolorosa; case. Rev. neurol. *1:*182-186, Feb '33
LÉCHELLE, P.; BARUK, H. AND DOUADY, D.: Association of scleroderma and Dupuytren's disease in syphilitic. Bull. et mem. Soc. med. d. hop. de Paris *51:*622-629, May 19, '27
LECLERC, G.: Rhinoplasty by cartilaginous grafts. Bull. et mem. Soc. nat. de chir. *53:*671-678, May 21, '27
LECLERC, G. (see POUZET, F.) March-April '37
LECOEUR, P. (see FÈVRE, M. *et al*) March '31
LECOUTURIER: Spinofacial anastomosis; result after 16 years. Arch. franco-belges de chir. *28:*308-312, April '25
LEDDERHOSE, G.: Surgery of wrist and hand. Deutsche med. Wchnschr. *48:*943-944, July 14, '22

Ledderhose-Secrétan Syndrome

Pseudo-atrophy of fingers or Ledderhose-Secrétan syndrome. BELLELLI, F. Riforma med. *46:*257-258, Feb 17, '30

LEDENYI, J.: Anatomic changes of bones in chronic, bilateral luxation of mandible. Bratisl. lekar. listy *15:*694-696, April '35
LEDERER, F. L.: Prosthetic aids in reconstructive surgery about head; presentation of new methods (including ear) nose. Arch. Otolaryng. *8:*531-554, Nov '28
LEDERER, L.: Accidents to septum in anesthesia with novacain (procaine hydrochloride) in nose. Arch. f. Ohren-, Nasen-u. Kehlkopfh. *150:*162-167, '41
LEDERGERBER, E.: Bloodless treatment of avulsion of extensor tendon of finger. Schweiz. med. Wchnschr. *75:*1088-1089, Dec 8, '45
LEDERMAN, M. (see COLE, P. P.) Sept '41
LEDO, E.: Technic of plastic surgery for rhinophyma. Actas dermo-sif. *27:*249-254, Nov '34
LEE, B. J.: Modern conception and treatment of shock. Am. J. Surg. *36:*166-169, July '22
LEE, C. O. (see MEREDITH, D. T.) June '39
LEE, F. C.: Underlying principles in repair of double harelip. J. M. A. Georgia *23:*383-389, Oct '34
LEE, F. C.: Orbicularis oris muscle in double harelip. Arch. Surg. *53:*407-413, Oct '46
LEE, Q. B. AND MAST, J. R.: Clinical discussion of malignant melanoma. South. Surgeon *9:*437-441, June '40
LEE, W. E.: Surgical treatment of burns. Internat. J. Med. and Surg. *40:*189-194, May '27
LEE, W. E.: Surgical treatment of burns. S. Clin. N. Amer. *8:*901-909, Aug '28
LEE, W. E.; ELKINTON, J. R. AND WOLFF, W. A.: Management of shock and toxemia in severe burns. Pennsylvania M. J. *44:*1114-1117, June '41
LEE, W. E. AND RHOADS, J. E.: Tannic acid method of burn therapy; present status. J.A.M.A. *125:*610-612, July 1, '44
LEE, W. E.; *et al*: Recent advances in burn therapy. Pennsylvania M. J. *48:*563-565, March '45
LEE, W. E.; *et al*: Recent trends in burn therapy. Ann. Surg. *115:*1131-1139, June '42
LEE, W. E. (see ELKINTON, J. R. *et al*) July '40
LEE, W. E. (see RHOADS, J. E. *et al*) June '41
LEE, W. E. (see RHOADS, J. E. *et al*) Oct '42
LEE, W. E. (see SALTONSTALL, H.) May '44
LEE, W. E. (see WOLFF, W. A. *et al*) Nov '42
LEECH, C. H.; DRUM, B. C. AND OSTERHAGEN, H. F.: Management of plastic maxillofacial wounds in evacuation hospital. Surg. Gynec. and Obst. *83:*462-473, Oct '46
LEECH, J. V.; SMITH, L. W. AND CLUTE, H. M.: Aberrant thyroid glands in neck. Am. J. Path. *4:*481-492, Sept '28

Leech Method

Tubular flaps transferred by dermal inclusion (leech method). CLAOUE. Monde med., Paris *50:*149-152, May '40

LEEDS, C. R. D. (see NESBITT, B. E.) April '45

DE LEEUW, E.: Section of flexor tendons of index and middle fingers in palm of hand. Scalpel *85:*1269-1271, Oct 15, '32

LEFEBVRE, C.: Surgical treatment of elephantiasis. J. de chir. *21:*434-458, April '23 (illus.) abstr: J.A.M.A. *81:*78, July 7, '23

LEFRANCOIS, C.: Perifemoral sympathectomy and skin grafts in therapy of leg ulcers; cases. Union med. du Canada *65:*214-219, March '36

LE FUR, R.: Results of 11 cases of bone grafts. Bull. et mem. Soc. d. chirurgiens de Paris *25:*187-192, March 17, '33

Leg Ulcers (See also Ulcers)

Skin grafts in treatment of chronic leg ulcer. TIXIER, L. AND BIZE, P. R. Monde med., Paris *37:*449-455, April 1, '27

Good results of combined periarterial sympathectomy and skin grafts on leg; 24 cases. LERICHE, R. AND FONTAINE, R. Strasbourgh-med. (pt. 2) *86:*101-105, April 20, '28

Extensive chronic ulceration on leg; successful treatment by autoplastic skin grafts. SANTY, P. Lyon chir. *26:*456-457, May-June '29

Anemic ulcer of leg treated by pedicle graft. JONES, H. T., S. Clin. N. Amer. *9:*933-935, Aug '29

Covering of recurrent crural ulcers by means of plastic use of skin flap from thigh of other leg. PETERS, A. Deutsche med. Wchnschr. *55:*1458-1461, Aug 30, '29

Treatment of chronic ulcer of leg by means of skin flap taken from dorsum of foot. KARTASCHEW, S. Zentralbl. f. Chir. *57:*2472-2475, Oct 4, '30

Radical repair of large skin defects with particular reference to leg ulcers (grafts). DOUGLAS, B. South. M. J. *24:*53-58, Jan '31

Phagedenic ulcer of lower leg with subjacent osteitis and extensive tissue loss; cure by autodermic graft and later anesthesia of articular ligaments according to Leriche; case. DUMAS, J. M. R. Marseille-med. *1:*553-556, April 25, '32

Therapy of slowly-healing crural ulcers by "circumcision," i.e. by transplantation of active epithelium. BÜTTNER, G. Zentralbl. f. Chir. *59:*2530-2531, Oct 15, '32

Therapy of slowly-healing crural ulcers by "circumcision," i.e., by transplantation of active epithelium. BÜTTNER, G. Zentralbl. f. Chir. *59:*3092, Dec 29, '32 (Addendum)

Therapy of so-called varicose syndrome, with special reference to sympathectomy and grafts. JENTZER, A. Rev. med. de la Suisse Rom. *53:*482-532, June 25, '33

Surgical treatment of trophic ulcers of leg

Leg Ulcers – Cont.

and foot; autoplastic operation by Italian method, periarterial sympathectomy, lumbar sympathetic ganglionectomy and ramisection. ROMITI, C. Tr. Roy. Soc. Trop. Med. and Hyg. *27:*185-194, July '33

Ulcer of leg, resistant to therapy, cured by cutaneous autotransplant; case. RODRÍGUEZ DE MATA. Actas Soc. de cir. de Madrid *3:*53-56, Oct-Dec '33

New technic of bandaging of epidermic grafts; application in therapy of ulcers of leg. RIOU, M. Bull. Soc. path. exot. *26:*1296-1301, '33

Traumatic ulcer of leg resisting all therapy, finally cured by autoplastic skin graft; case. RODRÍGUEZ DE MATA. Rev. espan. de cir *16:*105-108, March-April '34

Therapy of large ulcers of leg with Thiersch grafts. ORTHNER, F. Wien. klin. Wchnschr. *47:*1047-1048, Aug 24, '34

Unique "skinning" accident involving the leg. UNKNOWN. Brit. J. Surg. *22:*395, Oct '34

Late results of therapy of leg ulcers by sympathectomy combined with skin grafts; study based on 52 cases. LERICHE, R.; *et al.* J. de chir. *45:*689-710, May '35

Perifemoral sympathectomy and skin grafts in therapy of leg ulcers; cases. LEFRANCOIS, C. Union med. du Canada *65:*214-219, March '36

Conservative and radical measures for treatment of ulcer of leg; critical study of healing in experimental and human wounds under elastic adhesive plaster. DOUGLAS, B. Arch. Surg. *32:*756-775, May '36

Repair of ulcerations of lower extremity with thick split skin grafts. BROWN, J. B.; *et al.* Surg., Gynec. and Obst. *63:*331-340, Sept '36

Treatment of chronic varicose ulcers of lower extremities (grafting). OWENS, N. New Orleans M. and S. J. *89:*483-491, March '37

Perifemoral sympathectomy associated with dermoepidermal grafts in therapy of varicose ulcers; 7 cases. ARDOINO, A. Policlinico (sez. prat.) *44:*1265-1267, June 28, '37

Therapy of inveterate ulcers of leg by excision followed by immediate dermo-epidermic graft; cases. GOINARD, P. Algerie med. (Ed. chir.) *42:*75-81, Feb '38

Ulceration of lower extremities and grafts. BROWN, J. B.; *et al.* Am. J. Surg. *43:*452-457, Feb '39

Chronic leg ulcers (rationale of treatment). FILLMORE, R. S. Texas State J. Med. *35:*281-286, Aug '39

Plastic repair of leg ulcers (skin grafting).

Leg Ulcers – Cont.

BURSTEIN, T., M. Rec. *150:*307–308, Nov 1, '39

Transplantation of conserved skin according to Filatov method in therapy of chronic crural ulcers; preliminary report. BROVER, B. I. Vrach. delo *21:*105–110, '39

Chronic recurrent ulceration of leg. GORDON, S. Canad. M. A. J. *42:*4–10, Jan '40

Modified Kondoleon operation for sclerosed leg with ulceration (grafts). BANCROFT, F. W.; *et al*. Ann. Surg. *111:*874–891, May '40

Modified Kondoleon operation for chronic leg ulcers. STANLEY-BROWN, M., S. Clin. North America *21:*617–623, April '41

Braun graft in therapy of varicose ulcers; histopathologic evolution of graft. DE OLIVEIRA MATOS, J. Arq. de cir. clin. e exper. *6:*653–669, April–June '42

Tubular graft in therapy of ulcers of legs. DUARTE CARDOSO, A. Arq. de cir. clin. e exper. *6:*251–260, April–June '42

Application and technic of autogenous blood dressings in leg ulcers resistant to therapy. KREYES, H. Ztschr. f. arztl. Fortbild. *39:*360–362, Aug 15, '42

Treatment of large stasis ulcers by pinch grafts. RINGROSE, E. J., J. Iowa M. Soc. *33:*175–178, April '43

Plastic closure of tissue defects in region of lower leg. ANDINA, F. Zentralbl. f. Chir. *70:*682, May 8, '43

Trophic necrosis, skin grafting and vitamin C (in 2 cases of leg ulcers). EVANS, G. Brit. M. J. *1:*788, June 26, '43

Dermoepidermal grafts in therapy of ulcers of legs. ALARCON, C. J. AND GENATIOS, T. Rev. san. y asist. social *8:*783–796, Aug '43

Penicillin for ulcers of leg treated by pinch grafts. NOMLAND, R. AND WALLACE, E. G. J.A.M.A. *130:*563–564, March 2, '46

Severe septic wound of left lower leg treated with small deep grafts; case. HUMPHRIES, S. V. South African M. J. *20:*472–473, Aug 24, '46

Venous surgery (skin transplantation for stasis ulcers). CARROLL, W. W. Quart. Bull., Northwestern Univ. M. School *20:*373–379, '46

Legal Aspects

Dupuytren's disease from traumatic cause; medicolegal testimony in case. MASCIOTRA, A. A. Semana med. *2:*1615–1617, Dec 24, '25

French law and aesthetic surgery. DARTIGUES. Vie med. *10:*289–298, March 25, '29

Medicolegal aspects of plastic surgery. PEYTEL, A. Paris med. (annexe) *1:*viii–x, May 9, '31

Legal Aspects – Cont.

Plastic surgery from medicolegal point of view. PEYTEL, A. Paris med. (annexe) *1:*ix, May 16; vi, May 30; xiv, June 6, '31

Legal responsibility in plastic surgery; advisability of establishing regulations protecting both physician and patient. RIBEIRO, L. Folha med. *13:*175–178, May 25, '32

Cosmetic surgery in relation to legal liability. REBELO NETO, J. Rev. oto-laryng. de Sao Paulo *1:*23–45, Jan–Feb '33

Legal responsibility in plastic surgery. REBELLO NETO, J. Rev. med. de Pernambuco *3:*204, July; 244, Aug; 271, Sept '33

Medicolegal aspects of esthetic surgery. FAURE, J. L. Presse med. *41:*1677–1678, Oct 28, '33

True and false Dupuytren contracture in relation to traumatic etiogenesis of condition; interest from medicolegal viewpoint. MACAGGI, D. Policlinico (sez. chir.) *40:*743–759, Dec '33

Authorization of physician to perform plastic, and particularly cosmetic operations. WULLE, H. Med. Welt *8:*132, Jan 27; 171, Feb 3, '34

Legal and illegal aspects of plastic surgery. MALINIAK, J. W., M. Times and Long Island M. J. *62:*165–170, June '34

Legal responsibility of plastic surgeons. REBELLO NETO, J. Arch. Soc. de med. leg. e criminol. de S. Paulo *4:*81–109, '34

Plastic surgery and criminals; surgeon's responsibility. HOOVER, J. E., Am. J. Surg. *28:*156, April '35

Practitioner's responsibility when fugitives attempt to conceal identity by means of surgery. HOOVER, J. E., J.A.M.A. *104:*1663–1664, May 4, '35

Medicolegal responsibility for failures in plastic surgery; case. WARNEYER. Chirurg *7:*294–298, May 1, '35

Plastic surgeon and crime. MALINIAK, J. W. J. Crim. Law and Criminol. *26:*594–600, Nov '35

Injuries and plastic surgery of face from medicolegal point of view. DANTRELLE, A. Rev. de chir. structive, pp. 133–147, Dec '35

Lesions of eye with permanent disfigurement of face; medicolegal study of case. CUCCO, A. Riv. san. siciliana *24:*137–141, Feb 1, '36

Duodenal ulcer following burns; medicolegal importance, with report of case following industrial accident. TORCHIANA, L. Policlinico (sez. prat.) *43:*2105–2112, Nov 23, '36

Lawful character of plastic surgery; medicolegal aspects. PERREAU, E. H. Paris med. (annexe) *2:*iv–vii, Sept 18, '37

Retraction of palmar aponeurosis or Dupuytren's disease due to industrial trauma;

Legal Aspects – Cont.
medicolegal expertise in case. MASCIOTRA, A. A. Semana med. *1:*1063–1066, May 12, '38
Harelip and cleft palate in relation to eugenic sterilization, according to German law. MARTINY. Ztschr. f. Stomatol. *36:*947, Aug 26; 1004, Sept 9, '38
Medicolegal aspects in plastic surgery. SCHNEIDER, P. Wien. klin. Wchnschr. *52:*1029–1031, Nov 17, '39
Facial scars; evaluation in medicolegal expertise. DOMENICI, F. Boll. d. Soc. med. chir., Pavia *53:*41–55, '39
Medicolegal aspects of plastic surgery. ALFREDO, J. Rev. med. de Pernambuco *14:*173–180, Aug '44

LEGG, G. E. (see KUMMER, W. M.) April, May '44
LEGORBURU, R.: Hereditary polysyndactylia; case. Arch. de med., cir. y espec. *30:*745–752, June 29, '29
LEHMAN, E. P. (see ALRICH, E. M.) June '44
LEHMANN, C. F.: Epithelioma of eyelid. Texas State J. Med. *27:*422–426, Oct '31
LEHMANN, J. C.: Depression fracture of zygomatic arch. Zentralbl. f. Chir. *51:*2016–2017, Sept 13, '24 abstr: J.A.M.A. *83:*1629, Nov 15, '24
LEHMANN, W. AND JUNGERMANN, E.: Sensibility of flap in remote plastic operations. Mitt. a. d. Grenzgeb. d. Med. u. Chir. *32:*653–658, '20
LEHMANN, W. AND RITTER, R.: Harelip with cleft jaw and palate in relation to law on prevention of hereditary defects. Ztschr. f. menschl. Vererv.- u. Konstitutionslehre *23:*1–16, '39
LEHMANN, W. AND TAMMANN, H.: Transplantation and vital storage. Beitr. z. klin. Chir. *135:*259–302, '25 abstr: Klin. Wchnschr. *4:*2342–2343, Dec 3, '25 abstr: J.A.M.A. *86:*316, Jan 23, '26
LEHNER, R.: Treatment of gunshot fractures of jaw at advanced first aid posts. Deut. Militararzt *7:*98, Feb '42 also: Rev. san. mil., Buenos Aires *41:*542–549, Aug '42 also: Bull. War Med. *3:*146–147, Nov '42 (abstract)
LEHRFELD, L.: Plastic operation for palpebrofacial deformity. Am. J. Ophth. *6:*895–898, Nov '23 (illus.)
LEIBOVICI, R.: Modern burn therapy, with special reference to use of tannin. J. de med. de Paris *54:*765–766, Sept 6, '34
LEIBOVICI, R.: Burn therapy with special reference to tannin. J. de med. de Paris *58:*177–178, March 3, '38
LEIBOVICI, R. AND ISELIN, M.: Therapy of phlegmons of carpal sheaths by disconnected, lateral incisions. J. de chir. *37:*358–387, March '31
LEIGH, A. M.: Extensive burn of body with recovery. Kentucky M. J. *26:*477–478, Sept '28
LEIGH, M. D. AND FITZGERALD, R. R.: Endotracheal anesthesia supplementing avertin (tribrom-ethanol) in cleft palate operations. Canad. M. A. J. *35:*427–428, Oct '36
LEIGHTON, W. E.: Surgical treatment of carcinoma of lower lip. J. Missouri M. A. *20:*90–95, March '23 (illus.)
LEITHAUSER, D. J.: Technic for care of Ollier-Thiersch grafts. Ann. Surg. *97:*311–313, Feb '33
LEIX, R.: Practical suggestions on therapy of maxillary wounds at front. Deut. Miltararzt *9:*48, Jan '44
LELAND, G. A.: Carcinoma of mouth and lip. New England J. Med. *201:*1196–1199, Dec 12, '29
LEMARIÉE, P.: Local actinotherapy in burns. Rev. d'actinol. *5:*371–390, May–June '29
LEMARIÉE, P.: Actinotherapy in burns. Paris med. *2:*161–164, Aug 23, '30
LEMARIÉE, P.: Localized light therapy in burns. Arch. d'electric. med. *39:*269, July '31
LEMAÎTRE: Centers for restorative surgery and prosthesis after war wounds. Mem. Acad. de chir. *65:*1143–1147, Oct 25–Nov 8, '39
LEMAÎTRE, AND PONROY: Constriction of jaw treated by resection of ascending branch; case. Rev. de stomatol. *30:*734, Dec '28
LEMAÎTRE, F.: Maxillo-facial centers. Mil. Surgeon *57:*242–255, Sept '25
LEMAÎTRE, F. AND RUPPE, C.: Subacute osteomyelitis of jaws; cases. Rev. de stomatol. *31:*129–135, March '29
LEMBERK, B. E.: Cleft palate; cases. Odont. i. stomatol. (no. 12) *6:*16–22, '28
LEMERE, H. B.: Persistent bucconasal membrane in new-born. J.A.M.A. *109:*347–348, July 31, '37
LEMESURIER, A. B.: Operative repair of cleft palate. Canad. M.A.J. *33:*150–157, Aug '35
LEMESURIER, A. B.: Operative treatment of cleft palate. Am. J. Surg. *39:*458–469, Feb '38
LEMESURIER, A. B. (see GALLIE, W. E.) July '21
LEMESURIER, A. B. (see GALLIE, W. E.) July '22
LEMESURIER, A. B. (see GALLIE, W. E.) Oct '24
LEMOINE, J.: New treatment of palatopharyngeal synechiae of traumatic origin. Ann. d'oto-laryng., pp. 404–410, April '32
LEMOINE, J.: Skin grafts in évidement cavity with proud flesh; case. Ann. d'oto-laryng., pp. 1085–1088, Nov '38
LEMPKE, H.: Facial burns from electric current

in small children and use of plastic surgery in therapy; 4 cases. Deutsche Ztschr. f. Chir. *251:*331–342, '38
LEMPKE, H. (see LINDEMANN,) Feb '41
LÉNA, A. (see CARCASSONNE, F.) Nov '34
LÉNÁRD, E.: Machine for shaping skinflaps in anaplasty of eyelids. Klin. Monatsbl. f. Augenh. *83:*526–530, Oct–Nov '29
LENDON, A. A. AND NEWLAND, H. S.: Extroversion of bladder. Brit. M. J. *2:*38, July 9, '21 also: M. J. Australia *2:*103, Aug 6, '21
LENEBACH, M. (see SCHOTTER, H.) Sept '24

Lengemann Operation: See Makkas-Langemann Operation

LENGGENHAGER, K.: Simple method of therapy of congenital cervical fistulas. Schweiz. med. Wchnschr. *76:*607–609, July 6, '46
LENHART, C. H. (see FREEDLANDER, S. O.) Oct '32
LENORMANT, C.: Avulsion of scalp and its treatment. J. de chir. *17:*9, '21 abstr: J.A.M.A. *76:*553, Feb 19, '21
LENTH, V.: Epithelioma of lips; radium therapy. Radiol. Rev. and Chicago M. Rec. *51:*132–135, March '29
LENTZ, M. J. (see WEISS, B. *et al*) Jan '41
LEO, E.: New method of primary plastic surgery after antro-atticotomy (ear). Valsalva *6:*388–398, June '30
DE LEO, F.: Pathogenesis of Volkmann contracture. Chir. d. org. di movimento *30:*90–105, Jan–Mar '46
LEON, A. P.: Inversion of inhibition phenomenon by tetanus toxin; application to therapy of shock; experimental study. Medicina, Mexico *16:*505–513, Nov 10, '36
LEONARDI: Autoplasty of eyelids. Bull. et mem. Soc. franc. d'opht. *50:*20–24, '37
LEONENKO, P. M.: Phototherapy of burns. Am. Rev. Soviet Med. *1:*340–343, April '44 also: Khirurgiya, no. 7, pp. 42–46, '42
LEONI IPARRAGUIRRE, C. A.: Treatment of burns with tanning agents, with special reference to tannic acid. Rev. Asoc. med. argent. *57:*862–866, Oct 30, '43
LEONI IPARRAGUIRRE, C. A. (see LANDIVAR, A. F.) March '42
LEONTE, C.: Filling of osteomyelitis cavities by means of fat transplants. Rev. de chir., Bucuresti *43:*801–805, Nov–Dec '40
LEOTTA: Plastic surgery for extensive loss of bone substance of cranium after passage of electric current; case. Arch. ed atti d. Soc. ital. di chir. *37:*633–639, '31
LEOZ ORTÍN, G.: Plastic surgery; practice and biology. Med. ibera *2:*213–223, Aug 22, '31
LEOZ ORTÍN, G.: Technic and biology of plastic surgery. Arch. de oftal. hispano-am. *31:*593–617, Nov '31
LEPENNETIER, F.: Roentgenotherapy and electrotherapy of keloids. Rev. d'actinol. *5:*69, Jan–Feb '29
LEPENNETIER, F. (see BELOT, J.) Nov '28
LEPICARD: First aid in cases of severe burns. Gaz. med. de France *45:*733–734, July 1–15, '38
LEPOUTRE, C.: Surgical therapy of epispadias. Bull. Soc. franc. d'urol., pp. 31–35, Jan 17, '38
LEPOUTRE, C.: Epispadias; surgical therapy; case. J. d'urol. *46:*466–472, Nov '38

Leprosy

Surgical relief of lagophthalmos following seventh nerve paralysis in cases of leprosy. GASS, H. H. Leprosy Rev. *5:*178–180, Oct '34
Results of homologous skin transplantation in lepers. FLARER, F. AND GRILLO, V. Arch. ital. di dermat., sif. *12:*309–325, May '36
Restorative surgery following surgical or pathologic loss of substance in cancer and leprosy. PRUDENTE, A. Rev. de chir. structive, pp. 148–154, June '37
Eyelid paralysis; lagophthalmos in leprosy and its surgical correction. VALLE, S. Arq. Inst. Penido Burnier *5:*238–264, Dec '39
Surgical therapy of paralytic lagophthalmos in leprosy patients. DOROFEEV, V. N. Vestnik oftal. (no. 1) *14:*69–76, '39
Surgical correction of superciliary alopecia in leprosy. SILVEIRA, L. M. Rev. brasil. de leprol. (num. espec.) *7:*277–281, '39
Surgical correction of deformities due to leprosy in nose. PRUDENTE, A. Presse med. *48:*156–158, Feb 6, '40
Surgical correction of hyptertrophy of auricular lobe in leprosy. SILVEIRA, L. M. Rev. brasil. de leprol. *8:*1–3, March '40
Recidivating symblepharon in leper treated with conjunctival transplant; case. BEAUJON, O. Arch. venezol. Soc. de oto-rino-laring., oftal., neurol. *2:*23–27, March '41
Plastic correction of deformities of ear lobe in leprosy. SILVEIRA, L. M. Arq. de cir. clin. e exper. *6:*485–488, April–June '42
Problem of nasal deformity in leprosy. SILVEIRA, L. M. Arq. de cir. clin. e exper. *6:*531–535, April–June '42

LEPROUST (see BERCHER, J.) April '39
LEPUKALN, A. F.: Ephedrine therapy of traumatic shock; experimental study. Khirurgiya, no. 9, pp. 46–53, '37
LEPUKALN, A. F.: Intravenous drop infusion of ephedrine in therapy of traumatic shock.

Vrach. delo *20:*353–358, '38
LEREBOULLET, P. AND ECTORS, MME. M. L.: Craniofacial hemihypertrophy; case. Arch. de med. d. enf. *39:*37–39, Jan '36
LÉRI, A. AND LAYANI, F.: Enlargement of bones of half of face. Bull. et mem. Soc. med. d. hop. de Par. *49:*1013–1018, July 3, '25
LÉRI, A. AND SARTRE: Hemihypertrophy of face. Bull. et mem. Soc. med. d. hop. de Par. *48:*690–693, May 16, '24
LÉRI, A. AND SARTRE: Case of facial hemihypertrophy. Arch. de med. d. enf. *27:*747–749, Dec '24
LERICHE, R.: Album of Gensoul, maxillary surgeon. Lyon chir. *25:*1–9, Jan–Feb '28
LERICHE, R.: Late result of grafts of heterogenous bone tissue. Mem. Acad. de chir. *61:*1341–1343, Dec 14, '35
LERICHE, R.: Immediate application of tannic acid for extensive burns; death in 7 days due to anuria and progressive azotemia; case. Rev. de chir., Paris *75:*143–144, Feb '37
LERICHE, R.: Retromaxillary tonsillar cysts; removal by predigastric incision; case. Lyon chir. *35:*574–575, Sept–Oct '38
LERICHE, R.: Possible new operation for therapy of definitive paralysis; anastomosis of facial and sympathetic nerves. Presse med. *48:*721–722, Sept 17, '40
LERICHE, R. AND FONTAINE, R.: Good results of combined periarterial sympathectomy and skin grafts on leg; 24 cases. Strasbourgh-med. (pt. 2) *86:*101–105, April 20, '28
LERICHE, R. AND FONTAINE, R.: Mechanism involved in return of contractility of facial muscles when cervical sympathectomy is performed for facial paralysis. Compt. rend. Soc. de biol. *99:*858–860, Sept 18, '28
LERICHE, R. AND FONTAINE, R.: Ulcerous radiodermatitis of 16 years' duration cured by periarterial sympathectomy and skin grafts; case. Lyon chir. *30:*107–108, Jan–Feb '33
LERICHE, R.; FONTAINE, R. AND MAITRE, R.: Late results of therapy of leg ulcers by sympathectomy combined with skin grafts; study based on 52 cases. J. de chir. *45:*689–710, May '35
LERICHE, R. AND JUNG, A.: Relation of retraction of palmar aponeurosis to hypocalcemia and parathyroid insufficiency. Presse med. *38:*1641–1642, Dec 3, '30
LERICHE, R. AND JUNG, A.: Tannic acid therapy of burns; case. Lyon chir. *30:*177–179, March–April '33
LERICHE, R.; JUNG, A. AND DE BAKEY, M.: Influence of parathyroid extract on calcification of tissues studies by observation of free transplants (including cartilage). Ann. d'anat. path. *13:*551–555, May '36
LERICHE, R. (see POLICARD, A.) Sept–Oct '22

Leriche Operation
Resection of superior cervical ganglion (Leriche operation) in therapy of peripheral facial paralysis; 3 cases. BERTOLA, V. Prensa med. argent. *23:*2414–2427, Oct 21, '36
Leriche's operation for traumatic peripheral facial paralysis as compared with other operative procedures. JIANU, J. AND BUZOIANU, G. Lyon chir. *25:*10–21, Jan–Feb '28
Postoperative facial paralysis treated with Leriche operation, excision of upper cervical sympathetic ganglion; case. DELLA TORRE, P. L. Cervello *9:*299–312, Nov 15, '30

LERNER, C.: Therapy of common nevi. Urol. and Cutan. Rev. *41:*204–209, March '37
LERNER, C.: Essentials in art of epilation for hypertrichosis (electrolysis). M. Rec. *151:*193–194, March 20, '40
LERNER, C.: Treatment of hypertrichosis by electrocoagulation. New York State J. Med. *42:*879–882, May 1, '42
LERNER, C. (see KARP, F. L. *et al.*) June '39
LEROUX, L.: Hematoma of external ear. Medecine *8:*306–309, Jan '27
LEROUX, R.: Treatment of simple luxations of nasal septum. Ann. d. mal. de l'oreille, du larynx *45:*1064, Nov '26
LEROUX, R.: Surgery of nasal deformities. Vie med. *7:*2499, Dec 3, '26
LEROUX-ROBERT, J. (see MOULONGUET, A.) March '34
LEROY, R.: Massage in burn therapy. Presse med. *49:*535–536, May 14–17, '41
LEROY, R.: Cicatrization of wounds and treatment of cicatrices by massage. Monde med., Paris *56:*11–26, Jan–Feb '46
LERTAS, K. G.: Failures in treatment of melanoma and their causes; study based on recent literature and personal observations. Beitr. z. klin. Chir. *169:*177–213, '39
LESCHTSCHENKO, G. D.: Contractures in peripheral facial paralysis. Ztschr. f. d. ges. Neurol. u. Psychiat. *104:*586–595, '26
LESER, A. J.: Splint for extension and immobilization of digital fractures. Zentralbl. f. Chir. *63:*795–797, April 4, '36
LESEUR, H. H.: Management of hand infections. Am. J. Surg. *2:*38–42, Jan '27
LESHCHINSKIY, Y. L.: Atresia of choana; 3 cases. Zhur. ush., nos. i gorl. bolez. *15:*471–475, '38
LESNÉ, E.; CLÉMENT, R. AND GILBERT-DREYFUS: Dysostosis with acrocephalosyndactylia; case. Bull. Soc. de pediat. de Paris *26:*488–495, Dec '28
LESTER, C. W.: Coaptation splint for immobilization of thumb in abduction. J.A.M.A. *91:*96–97, July 14, '28

LETO, L.: Unusual case of human teratology (complete absence of one nostril). Boll. d. mal. d. orecchio, d. gola, d. naso *50:*129–137, May '32
LEUCUTIA, T. (see EVANS, W. A.) Aug '31

Leukoplakia

Leukoplakia of lip, and its relations to cancer. BROFELDT, S. A. Arb. a. d. path. Inst. *5:*34–109, '27
Study of 80 cases of leukoplakia of mouth. KING, H. AND HAMILTON, C. M. South. M. J. *24:*380–383, May '31
Leukoplakia of mouth and labial and lingual cancer in smokers. HAASE, G. Deutsche Monatschr. f. Zahnh. *49:*881, Sept 15; 929, Oct 1, '31
Leukoplakia buccalis and keratosis labialis (precancerous lesions). STURGIS, S. H. AND LUND, C. C. New England J. Med. *210:*996–1006, May 10, '34
Leukoplakia buccalis and cancer of mouth. STURGIS, S. H. AND LUND, C. C. New England J. Med. *212:*7–9, Jan 3, '35

LEVANDER, G.: Formation of new bone in transplantation. Acta chir. Scandinav. *74:*425–426, '34
LEVANDER, G.: Regeneration of epithelium in grafts. Nord. med. (Hygiea) *10:*1489–1492, May 10, '41
LEVEN: Cleft palate and harelip; familial manifestations. Arch. f. Rassen-u. Gesellsch.-Biol. *20:*71, Dec 20, '27
LEVEN, N. L.: Skin transplantation (including brief historical review). Bull. Minnesota M. Found. *1:*77–79, June '40
LEVEN, N. L.: Burns and reconstructive surgery. Proc. Interst. Postgrad. M. A. North America (1941) pp. 267–269, '42
LEVEN, N. L.: Burn therapy. Minnesota Med. *26:*534–537, June '43
LEVEN, L. N. (see CLARK, W. G. *et al.*) Dec '42
LEVENSON, S. M.: General principles underlying primary local treatment of burns; review. J. Indust. Hyg. and Toxicol. *26:*156–161, May '44
LEVENSON, S. M. *et al.*: Nutrition of patients with thermal burns. Surg. Gynec. and Obst. *80:*449–469, May '45
LEVENSON, S. M.; GREEN, R. W. AND LUND, C. C.: Therapy outline for severe burns. New England J. Med. *235:*76–79, July 18, '46
LEVENSON, S. M. AND LUND, C. C.: Treatment of hand burns with close fitting plaster of paris; cases. J.A.M.A. *123:*272–277, Oct 2, '43
LEVENSON, S. M. AND LUND, C. C.: Dermatome skin grafts in patients prepared with dry dressings and with and without penicillin. New England J. Med. *233:*607–612, Nov 22, '45
LEVENSON, S. M. (see CLOWES, G. H. A. JR. *et al.*) Nov '43
LEVENSON, S. M. (see DAVIDSON, C. S.) June '45
LEVENSON, S. M. (see GREEN, R. W. *et al.*) Aug '45
LEVENSON, S. M. (see TAGNON, H. J. *et al.*) Dec '44
LEVENSON, S. M. (see TAYLOR, F. H. L. *et al.*) March '44
LEVETON, A. L.: Surgical principles of split thickness grafts. J. Bone and Joint Surg. *28:*699–715, Oct '46
LEVEUF, J.: Repair of urethra by temporary joining of penis and scrotum (hypospadias). Bull. et mem. Soc. nat. de chir. *61:*30–31, Jan 19, '35
LEVEUF, J.: Clawhand resulting from mechanical constriction of forearm in plaster casts. Rev. de chir., Paris *80:*79–106, April–Dec '42
LEVEUF, J.: Surgical therapy of hypospadias. J. de chir. *62:*90–98, '46
LEVEUF, J. AND GODARD, H.: Temporary graft of penis to scrotum in therapy of hypospadias; technic and report of cases. J. de chir. *48:*328–341, Sept '36
LEVI, D.: Advance in surgery of cleft palate. Lancet *1:*515–518, March 11, '33
LEVI, D.: Local gigantism involving webbed fingers. Proc. Roy. Soc. Med. *31:*764–765, May '38
LEVI, D.: Operation for penoscrotal hypospadias. Lancet *2:*777, Dec 21, '40
LEVIN, J. J.: Case of successful grafting of ribs into skull for cranial defect. M. J. South Africa *20:*61–63, Oct '24
LEVIN, J. J.: Bone grafting for cranial defect; cases. M. J. S. Africa *21:*283–284, May '26
LEVIN, J. J.: Extroversion of bladder treated by transplantation of ureters. M. J. S. Africa *21:*336–339, July '26
LEVIN, J. J.: Duodenal ulcers following burns, with report of 2 cases. Brit. J. Surg. *17:*110–113, July '29
LEVIN, J. J.: Unusual tendon injuries to fingers; 3 cases. South African M. J. *13:*29–33, Jan 14, '39
LEVIN, W. N. (see WEISENGREEN, H. H.) March '36
LEVINE, B.: Hexenol in burns of limited areas. Am. J. M. Sc. *205:*125–130, Jan '43
LEVINE, J.: Congenital fistula of lacrimal sac. Am. J. Ophth. *12:*745–746, Sept '29
LEVINE, J. M.: Pigmentation of cutaneous scars

in coal miners. Dermat. Ztschr. *73:*135–136, April '36

LEVINE, R.; *et al*: Successful treatment of so-called "irreversible" shock by whole blood supplemented with sodium bicarbonate and glucose. Am. J. Physiol. *141:*209–215, April '44

LEVINGER: Congenital lateral cervical fistula. Munchen. med. Wchnschr. *68:*304, March 11, '21

LEVINSON, L. J. (see DANZIS, M. *et al.*) Aug '38

LEVINSON, S. O.: Use of blood and blood substitutes in shock and hemorrhage. West. J. Surg. *50:*388–391, Aug '42

LEVINSON, S. O.; NEUWELT, F. AND NECHELES, H.: Human serum as blood substitute in treatment of hemorrhage and shock. J.A.M.A. *114:*455–461, Feb 10, '40

LEVINTHAL, D. H.: Tendon transplantation in lower extremity. S. Clin. North America *19:*79–100, Feb '39

LEVITSKIY, M. A.: Blepharoplasty by means of free transplants of skin. Vestnik oftal. *11:*798–802, '37

LEVITT, W. M. AND GILLIES, H.: Radiotherapy in prophylaxis and treatment of keloids. Lancet *1:*440–442, April 11, '42

LEVY, AND MOATTI: Multiple fractures of lower jaw associated with left temporomaxillary luxation; surgical and prosthetic therapy; case. Tunisie med. *32:*175–179, May '38

LÉVY, G.: Harelip in univitelline twins; case. Bull. Soc. d'obst. et de gynec. *17:*661, July '28

LÉVY, G. (see LHERMITTE, J.) April '30

LEVY, J. (see CAHN, L. R.) Jan '22

LEVY, S.: Surgical treatment of atheroma. Munchen. med. Wchnschr. *77:*1030–1031, June 13, '30

Comments by FRANKE, F. AND HALLE, F., Munchen med. Wchnschr., *77:*1277, July 25, '30

LEVY, S.: Reply to Franke and Halle on comments about surgical treatment of atheroma. Munchen. med. Wchnschr. *77:*1845–1846, Oct 24, '30

LEVY, W.: Luxation of tendons of extensor digitorum. Zentralbl. f. Chir. *48:*482, April 9, '21

LEVY, W.: Rupture of thumb tendon (drummer's paralysis). Zentralbl. f. Chir. *49:*15–18, Jan 7, '22

LEVY, W. E. AND MACHECA, H.: Glucose and insulin in treatment of shock. New Orleans M. and S. J. *77:*478–480, May '25

LEVY, W. E. AND MACHECA, H.: Glucose and insulin in shock. Anesth. and Analg. *7:*161–164, May–June '28

LEVY-LENZ: Important errors in plastic surgery of pendulous breasts. Rev. de chir. structive, pp. 233–236, March '36

LÉVY-VALENSI, AND FEIL, A.: Ectrodactylia of last 4 fingers; case. Semaine d. hop. de Paris *6:*61–62, Jan 31, '30

LEWIN, J. M. (see LEVINE, J. M.)

LEWIN, M.: Reconstructive treatment of gunshot wound of face and neck. Arch. Otolaryng. *42:*191–197, Sept '45 also: Tr. Am. Acad. Ophth. (1944) *49:*276–282, May–June '45

LEWIN, M. L. AND PECK, S. M.: Skin graft pigment studies in experimental animals.

LEWIN, P.: Simple splint for baseball finger.

LEWIN, P.: Improved splint for baseball finger. J. A. M. A. *90:*2102, June 30, '28

LEWIN, P.: Preservation of muscle function in Bell's palsy with splint. J.A.M.A. *112:*2273, June 3, '39

LEWIS, D.: Postoperative treatment of tendon injuries. Boston M. and S. J. *194:*913–920, May 20, '26

LEWIS, D.: Reconstructive surgery. Tr. South. S. A. *40:*88–97, '27

LEWIS, D.: Reconstructive surgery (Hodgen lecture). J. Missouri M. A. *25:*185–190, May '28

LEWIS, D.: General principles of plastic surgery; cutaneous graft, sutures; cases. Bull. et mem. Soc. de chir. de Paris *20:*476–487, June 1, '28

LEWIS, E. E. (see PEARSON, R. S. R. *et al*) July '41

LEWIS, E. R.: Transitory conditions contraindicating resection of nasal septum. Tr. Am. Laryng., Rhin. and Otol. Soc. *43:*402–403, '37

LEWIS, F. C. R. (see KENNEDY, R. L.) Jan '45

LEWIS, F. O.: Statistical report on 5 year cures of cancer of larynx. Surg., Gynec. and Obst. *56:*466–467, Feb (No. 2A) '33

LEWIS, G. K.: Skin defects of extremities. Am. Acad. Orthop. Surgeons, Lect., pp. 229–245, '44

LEWIS, J. D.: External nasal deformities; description of operative technic of new method for correction of certain types. Laryngoscope *32:*214–217, March '22 (illus.)

LEWIS, J. D.: Depressed nasal deformities, comparison of prosthetic values of paraffin, bone, cartilage and celluloid, with report of cases corrected with celluloid implants by author's method. Ann. Otol., Rhin. and Laryng. *32:*321–365, June '23 (illus.)

LEWIS, J. D.: New plastic procedure for closure of perforations of nasal septum. Laryngoscope *33:*671–674, Sept '23 (illus.)

LEWIS, J. D.: External nasal deformities of traumatic origin; report of 6 cases. S. Clin. N. America *3:*1409–1420, Oct '23 (illus.)

LEWIS, J. D.: Improved septal punch forceps. Laryngoscope *33:*862–864, Nov '23 (illus.)
LEWIS, J. D.: Correction of congenital deformities of nose.; report of 9 selected cases. Laryngoscope *34:*593–608, Aug '24
LEWIS, L. A. (see PENBERTHY, G. C. *et al.*) Aug '42
LEWIS, L. A. (see PENBERTHY, G. C. *et al.*) May '43
LEWIS, R. S.: Wounds of neck and larynx. Lancet *1:*781–784, June 17, '44
LEWIS, T. W.: Deflection of nasal septum. S. Clin. North America *11:*127–132, Feb '31
LEWIS, W. W.: Disillusionments in nasal surgery. Minnesota Med. *17:*323–329, June '34
LEWISOHN, R.: Postoperative shock following splenectomy for chronic thrombocytopenic purpura. Ann. Surg. *96:*447–450, Sept '32
LEWY, E.: Congenital drumstick fingers. Med. Klin. *17:*845, July 10, '21
LEXER, E.: Fate of bone transplants. Acta chir. Scandinav. *56:*164–180, '23 (illus., in German)
LEXER, E.: Bone transplants and failure to heal. Zentralbl. f. Chir. *51:*258–259, Feb 16, '24
LEXER, E.: Twenty years of transplantation research. Arch. f. klin. Chir. *138:*251–302, '25
LEXER, E.: Treatment of hypertrophic breast; comment on Holländer's article. Deutsche med. Wchnschr. *51:*26, Jan 2, '25
LEXER, E.: Joint transplantations and arthroplasty. Surg., Gynec. and Obst. *40:*782–809, June '25
LEXER, E.: Various methods of treatment of cleft palate. Deutsche Ztschr. f. Chir. *200:*109–128, '27
LEXER, E.: Cosmetic operations of nose. Handb. d. Hals-, Nasen-, Ohrenh. *5:*991–1030, '29
LEXER, E.: Metaplastic formation of bone in transplanted connective tissue. Deutsche Ztschr. f. Chir. *217:*1–32, '29
LEXER, E.: Plastic replacement of flexor tendons of finger. Deutsche Ztschr. f. Chir. *234:*688–698, '31
LEXER, E. W.: Autoplastic covering of cranial defects by transplants from iliac crest. Deutsche Ztschr. f. Chir. *239:*743–749, '33
LEXER, E. W.: Influence of sympathectomy on homoplastic grafts. Deutsche Ztschr. f. Chir. *249:*337–370, '37

Lexer Operation

Lexer operation in eyelid ptosis. BUTLER, R. D. W. Tr. Ophth. Soc. U. Kingdom (pt. 2) *59:*579–585, '39
Lexer operation for ptosis of eyelids. ARMSTRONG, T. M. Tr. Ophth. Soc. Australia (1940) *2:*84–85, '41

Lexer Operation – Cont.
Plastic surgery in therapy of irreparable facial paralyses; Lexer-Rosenthal method. SCHMID, B. Zentralbl. f. Chir. *65:*1296–1297, June 4, '38

LEYRO DIAZ, J.: Total laryngectomy with right hemipharyngectomy; plastic surgery to reconstruct pharynx using laryngeal flap from left vestibular zone. Bol. y trab., Acad. argent. de cir. *30:*815–833, Sept 11, '46
LEYVA PEREIRA, L.: Death resulting from burns on military field. Rev. Fac. de med., Bogota *7:*149–154, Oct '38
LHERMITTE, J. AND LÉVY, G.: Amytrophic mutilating sclerodactylia with vasomotor trophic symptoms due to trauma 30 years previously to hand. Rev. neurol. *1:*622–631, April '30
L'HEUREUX, M.: Repair of large wound of calf by means of graft taken from thigh. Bull. et mem. Soc. nat. de chir. *53:*722, May 28, '27
L'HIRONDEL: Odontoma of jaw complicated by surgical fractures; 2 cases. Rev. de stomatol. *35:*125–139, March '33
L'HIRONDEL, C. AND ARONOWICZ: Surgical resection of upper gingivo-labial frenum and gingivojugal bands. Rev. de stomatol. *37:*436–455, July '35
LIBER, K. E. (see HARBIN, M.) Aug '34
LIBERA, D.: Technic in aesthetic surgery of breast; face. Med. ital. *9:*629–636, Oct '28
LIBERA, DONATO: *Il viso. Igiene cutanea, terapia estetica, chirurgia plastica.* Hoepli, Milan, 1938
LIBERTI, V.: Segmental regeneration of bone due to heteroplastic grafts; experimental study. Ann. ital. di chir. *19:*389–430, May–June '40
LICEAGA, F. J.: Congenital malformation with fingers and toes in flexion; new case. Semana med. *2:*421–425, Aug 13, '36
LICEAGA, F. J.: Complete syndactylia of hands and feet with other deformities in heredosyphilitic; case. Semana med. *2:*1685–1691, Dec 17, '36
LICEAGA, F. J.: Complete syndactylia of hands and feet and other deformities; case. Pediatria prat., Sao Paulo *8:*72–83, March–July '37 also: Monatschr. f. Kinderh. *72:*179–186, '38
LICEAGA, F. J.: Complete syndactylia of hands and feet associated with other deformities; case. Arch. de med. d. enf. *40:*448–452, July '37 Abstr.: Bull. Soc. de pediat. de Paris *35:*141–146, Feb '37
LICHT, S. (see ORNSTEIN, G. G. *et al*) April '39
LICHTENAUER, K.: Formation of artificial vagina from tubular portion of skin; case. Deutsche Ztschr. f. Chir. *232:*375–380, '31

LICHTENSTEIN, M. E.: Common injuries to finger tips and their care. Illinois M. J. *55:*125–127, Feb '29
LICHTENSTEIN, M. E. (see MCNEALY, R. W.) Dec '32
LICHTENSTEIN, M. E. (see MCNEALY, R. W.) March '35
LICHTENSTEIN, M. E. (see MCNEALY, R. W.) Dec '40
LIEBAU, G.: Shock and collapse. Munche. med. Wchnschr. *89:*577, June 26, '42 also: Bull. War Med. *3:*274–275, Jan '43 (abstract)
LIÉBAULT, G.: Resection of nasal septum for obstruction; general discussion. Rev. de laryngol. *47:*677–681, Nov 30, '26
LIEBENAM, L.: Study of family with cleft hands and feet. Ztschr. f. menschl. Vererb.-u. Konstitutionslehre *22:*136–151, '38
LIEBERMAN, S. L.: Sternal transfusions in burns. J.A.M.A. *123:*721, Nov 13, '43
LIEBERMANN, T.: Plastic surgery of nose. Orvosi hetil. *75:*646–649, June 20, '31
LIEBERMANN, T.: Surgical therapy of cleft palate. Orvosi hetil. *75:*1065, Oct 31, '31
LIEBERMANN, T.: Injection anesthesia for submucous resection. Budapesti orvosi ujsag *34:*831–832, Oct 1, '36
LIEBERMANN, T.: Injection anesthesia for submucous resection. Ztschr. f. Hals, Nasen-u. Ohrenh. *41:*290, '37
LIEBERMANN, T. v.: Rare malformation of alae of nose. Klin. Wchnschr. *2:*307, Feb 12, '23
LIEBERMANN, T. v. (see KALÓ, A. v.) March '24
LIEBMANN, E.: Therapy of sudden circulatory failure (collapse and shock). Schweiz. med. Wchnschr. *67:*1086–1089, Nov 13, '37
LIEBMANN, G.: Old and new facts about Chaoul method of close exposure (plesioroentgenotherapy) for cancer of skin and lip; 42 cases. Dermat. Wchnschr. *104:*293–300, March 6, '37
LIEK, E.: Operative treatment of epispadias in the female. Zentralbl. f. Gynak. *47:*604–606, April 14, '23
LIERLE, D. M.: Congenital lymphangiomatous macroglossia with cystic hygroma. Tr. Am. Laryng. A. *66:*194–196, '44
LIERLE, D. M.: Congenital lymphangiomatous macroglossia with cystic hygroma of neck. Ann. Otol., Rhin. and Laryng. *53:*574–575, Sept '44
DE LIETO VOLLARO, A.: Simplified dacryocystorhinostomy, modification of Toti's method. Boll. d'ocul. *8:*561–574, June '29
DE LIETO VOLLARO, A.: Reconstruction of 4 eyelids for ectropion resulting from cicatrix of severe facial burn, by means of free cutaneous grafts; case. Arch. ital. di chir. *51:*588–595, '38
DE LIETO VOLLARO, A.: Simple rapid surgical technic for cure of paralytic ectropion. Boll. d'ocul. *18:*769–780, Oct '39
LIFTON, J. C.: Combined orthodontic and prosthetic treatment of cleft palate. Dental Items Interest *52:*503–513, July '30
LIFTON, J. C.: Orthodontics in treatment of harelip and cleft palate. Am. J. Orthodontics *27:*423–453, Aug '41
LIFTON, J. C. (see WINTER, L. *et al*) Sept '45
LIGAS, A. (see CARDIA, A.) 1934
LIGGETT, H.: Otoplasty for dermatitis congelationis (frost-bite). M. Rec. *142:*278–279, Sept 18, '35
LIGHT, G. (see HYNDMAN, O. R.) Sept '29
LIGHT, G. (see HYNDMAN, O. R.) June '30
LIGHT, R. A. (see JOHNSON, G. S.) Jan '43
LIGHTFOOT, L. H. (see GROSSMAN, M. O.) Aug '45
LIGHTWOOD, R. C. AND SHELDON, W. P. H.: Unilateral hypertelorism, case. Arch. Dis. Childhood *3:*168–172, June '28
LIHOTZKY: Braun's skin grafting after amputations. Med. Klin. *22:*1757–1758, Nov 12, '26
LIISBERG, H. B.: Pedagogic therapy of speech disturbances in congenital palatoschisis. Valsalva *14:*346–351, July '38
LIJÓ PAVÍA, J.: Plastic preparation for prosthesis in extensive symblepharon. Rev. Especialid. *1:*75–82, '26
LILIENTHAL, H.: Epinephrine; method of prolonging its effect in asthma and depression of shock; preliminary note. J.A.M.A. *90:*1192–1193, April 14, '28
LILLIE, H. I.; PASTORE, P. N. AND MOUSEL, L. H.: Methods for producing local anesthesia for intranasal operations. Ann. Otol., Rhin. and Laryng. *49:*38–51, March '40
LILLY, A. J.: Simple technic for simple fractures of mandible. U. S. Nav. M. Bull. *45:*135–139, July '45
LIMA, E.: Medicosurgical anatomy of face. Rev. med.-cir. do Brasil *51:*287–304, April–June '43
LIMA, E. J.; CARDINALE, J. R. AND GREGORINI, H.: Hallomegaly; surgical therapy of case. Semana med. *1:*1098–1102, May 19, '38
LIMA, J.: Physiopathology of phonetic formation and education of cleft palate patients treated surgically. Rev. med. Bahia *9:*74–85, March '41
DE LIMA JUNIOR, B.: Plastic surgery of nose in treatment of rhinophyma; original process of cicatrization. Rev. brasil. de med. e pharm. *4:*243–250, May–June '28
DE LIMA JUNIOR, B.: Plastic surgery of nose in treatment of rhinophyma; original process of cicatrization; cases. Rev. oto-neuro-oft. *4:*80–

87, Feb '29
LIMBERG, A.: Innovations in operative methods for cleft palate. Zentralbl. f. Chir. *54:*1745–1750, July 9, '27
LIMBERG, A. A.: Fasting of protective celluloid plates in uranoplasty. Odont. i stomatol. (no. 11) *6:*5–8, '28
LIMBERG, A. A.: New method of plastic lengthening of mandible in unilateral microgenia and asymmetry of face. J. Am. Dent. A. *15:*851–871, May '28
LIMBERG, A. A.: Formation of end, ala and cutaneous partition of nose by transplanting auricle on round stem. Vestnik khir. (no. 55) *20:*151–159, '30
LIMBERG, A. A.: Reconstruction of nasal tip, wings and septum by T-shaped graft from neck. Novy khir. aekhiv *28:*147–163, '33
LIMBERG, A. A.: Free skin grafts in restoration of defects of conjunctival, oral mucous membranes and cutaneous defects of nasal fossae. Sovet. khir. (nos. 3–4) *6:*462–482, '34
LIMBERG, A. A.: Rhinoplasty with free transplantation from auricle. Sovet. khir., no. 9, pp. 70–90, '35
LIMBERG, A. A.: Apparatus for reducing fractures of zygomatic arch. Vestnik khir. *50:*194–197, '37

Limberg Operation

New surgical technics; Limberg pterygoid displacement in cleft palate. DUFOURMENTEL, L. Bull. et mem. Soc. d. chirurgiens de Paris *27:*130–135, March 1, '35 also: Prat. med. franc. *17:*339–345, June (A–B) '36
Plastic repair of tip of nose, alae and septum with T-shaped round skin flap (Limberg method); case. FALTIN, R. Acta chir. Scandinav. *68:*254–265, '31
Radical uranoplasty (Limberg): new operation (for closure of cleft palate). SCHULTZ, L. J. Am. Dent A. *23:*407–415, March '36

LIMOGES, J. E.: Burn therapy crutique. Ann. med.-chir.de l'Hop. Sainte-Justine, Montreal *4:*69–72, May '44
LIN, C. K.: Restoration of eye socket with Thiersch graft; 6 cases. Chinese M. J. *50:*1335–1344, Oct '36
LINARI, O. T. AND PARODI, L. M.: Elephantiasis; surgical therapy. Rev. de cir. de Buenos Aires *17:*177–180, April '38
LINBERG, B. E.: Plastic surgery of saddle nose (transplantation of toe). Vestnik khir. (no. 52) *18:*70–76, '29
LINDBERG, J. G.: Transplantation of fat in enucleation of eye. Finska lak.-sallsk. handl. *70:*898–902, Nov '28
LINDBERG, L.: Treatment of epithelioma of lips. Arizona Med. *1:*128–130, May–June '44
LINDBERG, L. (see MELAND, O. N.) Sept '36
LINDEMAN, H.: After-examination of patients operated on for sinusitis, especially with regard to results after "broad opening" and Luc-Caldwell operation. Nord. med. *31:*1897–1900, Aug 23, '46
LINDEMANN, AND LEMPKE, H.: Injuries of region of oral cavity by strong electric current. Med. Klin. *37:*155–160, Feb 14, '41

Lindemann Operation

Temporomaxillary arthroplasty (Lindemann operation); results in 2 cases. MARFORT, A.; *et al.* Rev. Asoc. med. argent. *53:*88–90, Feb 15–28, '39
Therapy of progenism by Lindemann method. MARINO, H. Arq. de cir. clin. e exper. *6:*301–306, April–June '42

LINDEMANN, A.: Reconstruction of face. Deutsche Ztschr. f. Chir. *170:*182–208, '22 (illus.) abstr: J.A.M.A. *79:*250, July 15, '22
LINDEMANN, A.: Malignant tumors of jaw; 16 cases. Deutsche Zahnh., Hft. *73:*, pp. 15–56, '28
LINDEMANN, A.: New methods of anesthetizing jaws and face. Narkose u. Anaesth. *1:*3–16, Jan 15, '28
LINDEMANN, A.: Plastic covering of defects of jaws. Chirurg. *1:*817–829, Aug 1, '29
LINDEMANN, A.: New ideas on plastic restoration of congenital and acquired defects. Chirurg *3:*358, April 15, '31; 414, May 1, '31
LINDEMANN, A.: Results of grave inflammations of the jaw and their surgical and orthopedic therapy. Rev. med. german.-ibero-am. *8:*170–176, May–June '35
LINDEMANN, A.: Early diagnosis and therapy of cancer of mouth. Ztschr. f. Stomatol. *35:*145–171, Jan 22, '37
LINDEMANN, A.: New methods of plastic surgery in cleft palate. Deutsche Ztschr. f. Chir. *249:*68–78, '37
LINDEMANN, A.: Surgery and orthopedics of temporomaxillary joint. Rev. de stomatol. *41:*65–77, Feb '39
LINDEN: Treatment of burns and ulcers with Veroform and Epithelan. Deutsche med. Wchnschr. *50:*719–720, May 30, '24
LINDENBAUM, I.: Failures and hazards of Filatov's circular pedicled flap. Beitr. z. klin. Chir. *160:*359–368, '34

LINDENBAUM, I. S.: Errors and dangers of graft with round pedicle flap according to Filatov method. Sovet. khir., no. 3, pp. 126–131, '35
LINDENBAUM, I. S. AND DEPP, M. E.: Blood transfusion in shock therapy. Vestnik khir. *46:*189–198, '36
LINDENBAUM, J.: Failures, hazards and unforeseen complications involved in use of pedicled flap in plastic operations. Arch. f. klin. Chir. *181:*529–547, '35
LINDENBAUM, L. M.: Covering extensive defects of chin and floor of mouth following gunshot wounds. Vrach. delo (nos. 7–8) *26:*469–474, '46
LINDENSTEIN, L.: Spontaneous healing of subcutaneous rupture of tendons in terminal phalanx of finger. Zentralbl. f. Chir. *62:*2961, Dec 14, '35
LINDGREN, S.: Shock. Svenska lak.-tidning. *38:*933–939, April 25, '41
LINDGREN, S. AND WILANDER, O.: Controlled fluid administration in shock. Nord. med. (Hygiea) *12:*3099–3106, Nov 1, '41
LINDNER, K.: Blaskovics operation for eyelid ptosis. Klin. Monatsbl. f. Augenh. *93:*1–12, July '34
LINDQUIST, G.: Healing of skin defects; experimental study on white rat. Acta chir. Scandinav. (supp. 107) *94:*1–163, '46
LINDQVIST, S.: Double fractures of articular processes of lower jaw. Zentralbl. f. Chir. *53:*2777–2778, Oct 30, '26
LINDSAY, H. C. L.: Removal of powder tattoo of face by minor surgery. J.A.M.A. *109:*1530, Nov 6, '37
LINDSAY, H. C. L.: War burns. Urol. and Cutan. Rev. *46:*386–390, June '42
LINDSAY, J. C.: Tannic acid treatment of burns; case report. Canad. Med. and Surg. *61:*9, '27 also: Canad. M. A. J. *17:*86, Jan '27
LINDSTRÖM, E.: Ectopia vesicae; surgical treatment of 3 cases. Acta chir. Scandinav. *72:*134–145, '32
LINDVALL, S. AND WAHLGREN, F.: True hermaphrodite, case. Nord. med. tidskr. *11:*635–641, April 18, '36
LING, W. P.: Ocular neoplasms (orbital hemangiomas) among Chinese; brief clinicopathologic report of 82 cases with discussions. Chinese M. J. *48:*982–986, Sept '34
LINHARES, F.: Correction of saddle nose by inclusion of vitallium. Rev. brasil. de cir. *14:*159–164, March '45
LINK, K. H.: Clinical and experimental study of muscle damage in maxillary fractures. Arch. f. klin. Chir. *181:*24–77, '34
LINK, K. H.: Industrial injuries of jaw. Arch. f. orthop. u. Unfall-Chir. *36:*47–59, '35
LINK, K. H.: Late examination of fractures of upper jaw. Zentralbl. f. Chir. *64:*467–469, Feb 20, '37
LINK, K. H.: Therapy of war injuries to jaws. Zentralbl. f. Chir. *67:*994–998, June 1, '40
LINNARTZ, M.: Technic of suture of divided tendons. Zentralbl. f. Chir. *48:*338, March 12, '21
LINTON, P.: Fracture of lower jaw with bilateral outward dislocation. Acta chir. Scandinav. *81:*304–308, '38
LINTON, P. (see CRAFOORD, C.) Aug '40

Lip, Frenum of

Surgery of labial frenum. CAHN, L. R. Am. J. Surg. *38:*254–255, Oct '24
Surgical resection of upper gingivo-labial frenum and gingivojugal bands. L'HIRONDEL, C. AND ARONOWICZ. Rev. de stomatol. *37:*436–455, July '35
Rational treatment of labial frenum. SCHWARTZ, A. B. AND ABBOTT, T. R. Am. J. Dis. Child. *52:*1061–1064, Nov '36
Synechia of frenum linguae. MAEKAWA, S. AND HASHIMOTO, T. Oto-rhino-laryng. *14:*666, Sept '41
Effect of growth and development on abnormal labial frenum. SCHWARTZ, A. B. AND ABBOTT, T. R. Am. J. Dis. Child. *71:*248–251, March '46
Maxillary labial frenum in School Health Service. FUCHS, E. Brit. Dent. J. *80:*327–329, May 17, '46
Labial adhesions in children. TODD, I. P. Brit. M. J. *2:*13–14, July 6, '46

Lip Pits, Congenital

Three cases of congenital fistulas, mucous membrane pouches on lower lip; nature and cause of malformation, with review of 46 cases on record. HILGENREINER, H. Deutsche Ztschr. f. Chir. *188:*273–309, '24
Congenital labial fistula; case. RUPPE, C. AND MAGDELEINE, J. Rev. de stomatol. *29:*1–8, Jan '27
Congenital fistula of lower lip; embryologic and hereditary factors in pathogenesis of rare congenital abnormalities of face; operative treatment; cases. RUBALTELLI, E. Arch. ital. di otol. *41:*141–154, April '30
Congenital bilateral fistula of lower lip. MEYER, P. Deutsche Ztschr. f. Chir. *229:*391–395, '30
Development of human lower jaw; study of development of fistula of lower lip. SICHER, H. AND POHL, L. Ztschr. f. Stomatol. *32:*552–560, May 25, '34
Congenital fistula of lower lip; etiologic and clinical study. POHL, L. Rev. de chir. plastique, pp. 107–131, Oct '34

Lip Pits, Congenital – Cont.

Congenital fistulas of lower lip; case. BAXTER, H. Am. J. Orthodontics *25:*1002–1007, Oct '39

LIPOWITZ, N. S.: Case of entropion of lower eyelid and case of spastic entropion of upper lid. Klin. Monatsbl. f. Augenh. *80:*353–356, March 23, '28

LIPPMAN, M. C.: Plastic surgical correction of nasal deformities. M. Rec. *152:*399–402, Dec 4, '40

LIPPMANN, O.: Pathogenesis of cleft formation of anterior wall of abdomen (gastroschisis); rare case. Zentralbl. f. Gynak. *61:*516–524, Feb 27, '37

Lips, Cancer

Epithelioma of lip. NASSAU, C. F., S. Clin. N. Amer. *1:*197, Feb '21

Results of surgical treatment of epithelioma of lip. SISTRUNK, W. E. Ann. Surg. *73:*521, May '21

Epithelioma of lower lip; combined surgical and radium treatment. BECK, E. G. Internat. Clinics *1:*31, '21

Epithelioma of lip. TWYMAN, E. D., J.A.M.A. *78:*348–349, Feb 4, '22

Precancer lesion of lip. ANZILOTTI, G. Riforma med. *38:*411–413, May 1, '22

Modern treatment of cancer of lip. PANCOAST, H. K. Surg., Gynec. and Obst. *34:*589–593, May '22

Squamous-cell epithelioma of lip, its surgical indications. SHEPHARD, J. H. Surg., Gynec. and Obst. *35:*107–109, July '22 (illus.)

Cancer of lip. HAMILTON, C. M., J. Tennessee M. A. *15:*190–192, Aug '22

Squamous epithelioma of lower lip. MILIANI, A. Arch. ital. di chir. *6:*105–124, Nov '22 (illus.) abstr: J.A.M.A. *80:*360, Feb 3, '23

Cancer of lip, its treatment by radium and surgery combined. WALL, C. K., J. M. A. Georgia *12:*67–69, Feb '23

Surgical treatment of carcinoma of lower lip. LEIGHTON, W. E., J. Missouri M. A. *20:*90–95, March '23 (illus.)

Cancer of lip. RODRIGUEZ VILLEGAS, R. Semana med. *1:*398–403, March 1 '23 abstr: J.A.M.A. 81:169, July 14, '23

Cancer of lips. PRAT, D. An. de Fac. de med., Montevideo *8:*865–883, Sept '23

Local treatment of cancer of lip. PEÑA NOVO, P. Siglo med. *73:*371–372, April 12, '24

Model of carcinoma of lip reconstructed from serial section. WARWICK, M., J.A.M.A. *82:*1119–1120, April 5, '24

Treatment of cancer of lower lip. NORSWORTHY, O. L. Texas State J. Med. *20:*184–188, July '24

Carcinoma of lower lip. MASON, J. T., S. Clin. N. America *4:*1095–1104, Oct '24

Carcinoma of lip. BROEMAN, C. J., W. Virginia M. J. *20:*27–31, Jan '25

Epithelioma of lip, observations on 150 cases. KENNEDY, W. H. Radiology *4:*319–324, April '25

Cancer of lip, resulting deformity, plastic repair. BOYD, J. E., J. Florida M. A. *12:*27–29, Aug '25

Case report of plastic repair of mutilating operations of lip and cheek following radical removal of carcinoma. COPP, F. A., J. Florida M. A. *12:*29–35, Aug '25

Cancer of lower lip. MCGUFFIN, W. H. Canad. M. A. J. *15:*1046–1049, Oct '25

Treatment of cancer and precancer of lip; clinical and therapeutic study of 191 cases. BUTLER, C. An. de Fac. de med., Montevideo *10:*985–998, Dec '25 abstr: J.A.M.A. *87:*447, Aug 7, '26

Treatment of cancer of lip. WASSINK, W. F. Nederl. Tijdschr. v. Geneesk. *2:*1059–1069, Sept 4, '26 abstr: J.A.M.A. *87:*1524, Oct 30, '26

Cancer of lip, breast and cervix; end result study. WAINWRIGHT, J. M. Bull. Moses Taylor Hosp. *1:*9–14, May '27

Spontaneous cure of cancer of lip. AVRAMOVICI, A. Lyon chir. *24:*257–268, May–June '27

Plastic operation for ulcerative epithelioma of upper lip and cheek. ZAGNI, L. Stomatol. *25:*591–594, July '27

Squamous cell carcinoma of lower lip; case. LANDHAM, J. W. Piedmont Hosp. Bull. *4:*32–35, July–Aug '27

Epithelioma of lip and face. BONDURANT, C. P., J. Oklahoma M. A. *20:*252–256, Sept '27

Leukoplakia of lip, and its relations to cancer. BROFELDT, S. A. Arb. a. d. path. Inst. *5:*34–109, '27

Cancer of upper maxilla and lip; operation; recovery. BONNET-ROY, F. Odontologie *66:*39, Jan '28

Cancer of lips. MCKILLOP, L. M., M. J. Australia *1:*260–263, March 3, '28

Epithelioma of lip; case from Postgraduate Hospital; New York City. ANDERSON, N. P. Physical Therap. *46:*350–352, July '28

Cancer of lower lip; operative technic in plastic repair. FAIRCHILD, F. R. Arch. Surg. *17:*630–640, Oct '28

Cutaneous epithelioma developing rapidly on upper lip after diathermic treatment of supposed verruca carnea; case. HECHT, H.

Lips, Cancer—Cont.
Dermat. Wchnschr. *88:*501-502, April 6, '29
Treatment of cancer of lips. QUICK, D. Am. J. Roentgenol. *21:*322-327, April '29
Cancer of lips. BONÀ, T. Cluj. med. *10:*652-656, Dec 1, '29
Carcinoma of mouth and lip. LELAND, G. A. New England J. Med. *201:*1196-1199, Dec 12, '29
Electrothermic surgery of cancer of lips. STEVENS, J. T. Am. J. Surg. *7:*831-835, Dec '29
Plastic surgery of lip, chin and cheek in man after resection for cancer. CAVINA, C. Arch. ed atti d. Soc. ital. di chir. *35:*526-541, '29
Cancer of lips. JAMES, W. D. Am. J. Surg. *8:*593-597, March '30
Epithelioma developing on site of recurrent herpes simplex of lips. BURGESS, N. Brit. M. J. *2:*249, Aug 16, '30
Early diagnosis and treatment of cancer of lips and mouth. FIGI, F. A. Minnesota Med. *13:*788-792, Nov '30
Rational therapy for cancer of lower lip. FISCHEL, E. Tr. South. S. A. (1929) *42:*306-321, '30
Treatment of uncomplicated primary carcinoma of lips. HAAGENSEN, C. D. Am. J. Cancer *15:*239-245, Jan '31
Differential diagnosis of cancer of lip. NELSON, P. A. Am. J. Cancer *15:*230-238, Jan '31
Special clinic on epithelioma of lips. QUICK, D. Am. J. Cancer *15:*229-270, Jan '31
Treatment of cancer of lips. FISCHEL, E. Colorado Med. *28:*57-61, Feb '31
Etiology of cancer of lips. FRIEDRICH, R. Wien. klin. Wchnschr. *44:*177-179, Feb 6, '31
Epithelioma of lip. FINNERUD, C. W., M. Clin. North America *14:*1148-1150, March '31
Malignancy of lower lip complicated by mouth infections. WILSON, S. J. South M. J. *24:*359-363, April '31
Treatment of cancer of lips. MONTGOMERY, D. W. AND CULVER, G. D., M. J. and Rec. *133:*573-575, June 17, '31
Rational therapy for lower lip cancer. FISCHEL, E. Am. J. Cancer *15:*1321-1337, July '31
Leukoplakia of mouth and labial and lingual cancer in smokers. HAASE, G. Deutsche Monatschr. f. Zahnh. *49:*881, Sept 15; 929, Oct 1, '31
Plastic reconstruction of lower lip in cancer. DALAND, E. M. New England J. Med. *205:*1131-1142, Dec 10, '31

Lips, Cancer—Cont.
Plastic replacement of upper lip in case of epitheliomatous ulcer resulting from x-ray treatment of sycosis barbae. HUTTON, A. J. Glasgow M. J. *117:*225-230, May '32
Coexistence of basal celled epithelioma of temporal region and spinocellular epithelioma of lip; case. MARIN, A. Union med. du Canada *61:*770-772, June '32
Cheiloplasty for advanced carcinoma. MARTIN, H. E. Surg., Gynec. and Obst. *54:*914-922, June '32
Recurring epithelioma of lower lip and chin; diathermy and cautery excision; reconstruction of lower lip. FIGI, F. A., S. Clin. North America *12:*951-954, Aug '32
Surgery for cancer of face and lip. TRUEBLOOD, D. V. West. J. Surg. *40:*401-404, Aug '32
Extensive lupus erythematosus with subsequent carcinoma of lower lip (case). GRAHAM-LITTLE, E. Proc. Roy. Soc. Med. *25:*1741, Oct '32
Diagnosis of cancer of lips. WHITEHILL, N. M. J. Iowa M. Soc. *22:*533-534, Nov '32
Therapy of cancer of lower lip. RUBINROT, S. Nowotwory *7:*240-244, '32
Surgical and radiotherapy of cancer of lips. HARRISON, R. S. Strahlentherapie *46:*401-434, '33 Abstr.: Schweiz. med. Wchnschr. *63:*159-162, Feb 18, '33
Surgical management of cancer of lips. SMITH, F. Surg., Gynec. and Obst. *56:*782-785, April '33
Idiopathic (glandular and exfoliative) cheilitis; relation to epithelioma of lower lip; case. GAY PRIETO, J. AND CAZORLA ROMERO, J. Actas derno-sif. *25:*700-706, May '33
Cancer of lower lip in child 9 years old. ABDANSKI, A. Rev. de chir., Paris *52:*557-559, July '33
Report of results of treatment at Collis P. Huntington Memorial Hospital from 1918-1926. Cancer of lip. LUND, C. C. AND HOLTON, H. M. Am. J. Roentgenol. *30:*59-66, July '33
Operation for epithelioma of lips. WEBSTER, J. P. Am. J. Roentgenol. *30:*82-88, July '33
Surgical therapy of cancer of lips. WIEDHOPF, O. Deutsche Ztschr. f. Chir. *238:*741-744, '33
Early diagnosis of cancer of lips. CURRY, W. A. Canad. M.A.J. *30:*50-53, Jan '34
Abrasive cheilitis; clinical and histologic study of precancerous lesions. MANGANOTTI, G. Arch. ital. di dermat., sif. *10:*25-67, Jan '34

Lips, Cancer–Cont.
Carcinoma of lip and mouth. MARTIN, C. L. Radiology *22:*136-146, Feb '34
Glandular cheilitis, precancerous state of lower lip. TOURAINE, A. AND SOLENTE. Presse med. *42:*191-194, Feb 3, '34
Leukoplakia buccalis and keratosis labialis (precancerous lesions). STURGIS, S. H. AND LUND, C. C. New England J. Med. *210:* 996-1006, May 10, '34
Standard methods of treatment of cancer of lips by surgery and radiation. FISCHEL, E. Surg., Gynec. and Obst. *60:*505-512, Feb (no. 2A) '35
Epithelioma of lips; 385 cases. IACOBOVICI, I. AND ONACA. Rev. de chir., Bucuresti *38:*1-16, March-April '35
Cancer of lip and intra-oral mucous membrane. FRANK, L. W. South. Surgeon *4:*444-456, Dec '35
Surgical therapy of cancer of lips. NARBUTOVSKIY, S. D. Novy khir. arkhiv. *33:*3-14, '35
Treatment of carcinoma of lip. HOLLANDER, L. Arch. Phys. Therapy *17:*17-24, Jan '36
Repair of postoperative defects involving lips and cheeks secondary to removal of malignant tumors. NEW, G. B. AND FIGI, F. A. Surg., Gynec. and Obst. *62:*182-190, Feb '36
Diagnosis and treatment of cancer of lip, mouth and throat. CHRISTIE, A. C. Fortschr. a. d. Geb. d. Rontgenstrahlen *53:*529-534, March '36
General considerations, pathology, clinical picture and diagnosis of cancer of lips. PADGETT, E. C. Internat. J. Orthodontia *22:*387-394, April '36
Cheiloplasty in cancer of lips. PADGETT, E. C. Internat. J. Orthodontia *22:*939-947, Sept '36
Late results of operation for carcinoma of lower lip. KOGON, A. I. Novy khir. arkhiv *37:*227-240, '36
Malignancy and potential malignancy of lower lip. KENNEDY, R. H., S. Clin. North America *17:*297-301, Feb '37
Cancer of lower lip; technic of surgical therapy. MARINO, H. Rev. de cir. de Buenos Aires *16:*53-62, Feb '37
Diagnosis and treatment of cancer of lips. JORSTAD, L. H. Radiol. Rev. and Mississippi Valley M. J. *59:*63-64, March '37
Old and new facts about Chaoul method of close exposure (plesioroentgenotherapy) for cancer of skin and lip; 42 cases. LIEBMANN, G. Dermat. Wchnschr. *104:*293-300, March 6, '37
Treatment of epithelioma of lip by electrodesiccation; technic and preliminary report of results during past 5 years. MORROW, H.; *et al.* Arch. Dermat. and Syph. *35:*821-830, May '37
Cancer of lip and oral cavity and skin. HOLLANDER, L. Pennsylvania M. J. *40:*749-750, June '37
Technic of resection of lower lip in cancer; cases. BREYTFUS, F. F. Khirurgiya, no. 5, pp. 61-62, '37
Radical inferior cheiloplasty for advanced carcinoma of lower lip; 2 cases. WIRTH, J. E. Northwest Med. *37:*109-112, April '38
Cancer of lip and mouth. HAY, A. W. S. Manitoba M. A. Rev. *18:*231-234, Dec '38
Malignant tumors of upper and lower lip treated at Oncologic Institute of Leningrad in past 10 years. SHANIN, A. P. Vestnik khir. *57:*43-62, Jan '39
Treatment of cancer of lips. PADGETT, E. C. J. Missouri M. A. *36:*154-157, April '39
Repair of large defects of lips after removal for cancer. DALAND, E. M. Surg., Gynec. and Obst. *69:*347-357, Sept '39
Superficial cancer of lip. TRUEHEART, M., J. Kansas M. Soc. *40:*419, Oct '39
Treatment of cancer of lips. SHARP, G. S. AND SMITH, H. D. West. J. Surg. *47:*695-705, Dec '39
Reconstruction of lip after cancer. BOYER, B. E., J. Med. *20:*543-544, Feb '40
Prophylaxis, diagnosis and treatment of cancer of lips. HUNT, H. B. Nebraska M. J. *25:*133, April; 187, May '40
Management of cancer of lips. WILSON, H. Memphis M. J. *15:*80-82, May '40
Treatment of large protruding carcinomas of skin and lip by irradiation and surgery. HUNT, H. B. Am. J. Roentgenol. *44:*254-264, Aug '40
Method of therapy of cancer of lower lip. GEKTIN, F. L. Novy khir. arkhiv. *46:*52-59, '40
Cancer of lips and cheeks. FIGI, F. A. Proc. Staff Meet., Mayo Clin. *16:*280-282, April 30, '41
Epidermoid carcinoma of lower lip; case with recovery and survival for 14 years after surgical therapy. MONTEIRO, A. Acta med., Rio de Janeiro *9:*51-58, Feb '42
Cancer of lips. DUNNE, R. E. Connecticut M. J. *6:*175-176, March '42
Extensive plastic repair for restoration of lower lip; report of procedure in case in which lower lip was entirely removed for eradication of epithelioma. FEDERSPIEL, M. N. Am. J. Orthodontics (Oral Surg. Sect.) *28:*163-166, March '42
Repair of extensive loss of substance of lower

Lips, Cancer–Cont.

lip (due to cancer). VIANNA, J. B. Hospital, Rio de Janeiro *23:*69–79, Jan '43

Cancer of upper lip; excision and plastic surgery in case. MARINO, H. Prensa med. argent. *31:*137–140, Jan 19, '44

Cancer of lips. SHARP, G. S. AND FREEMAN, R. G. Eye, Ear, Nose and Throat Monthly *23:*17–26, Jan '44

Cancer of lips. CAZAP, S. Bol. Inst. de med. exper. para el estud. y trat. d. cancer *21:*188–215, April '44

Treatment of epithelioma of lips. LINDBERG, L. Arizona Med. *1:*128–130, May–June '44

Basal cell lesions of nose, cheek and lips. DAVIS, W. B. Ann. Surg. *119:*944–948, June '44

Cancer of lips. DOUGLAS, S. J. Brit. J. Radiol. *17:*185–189, June '44

Cancer of lips. GARLAND, J. G. AND DAVIES, J. A. Marquette M. Rev. *9:*113–118, June '44

Chemosurgical treatment of cancer of lips; microscopically controlled method of excision. MOHS, F. E. Arch. Surg. *48:*478–488, June '44

Cancer of skin, lip and tongue. MARTIN, H. Bull. Am. Soc. Control Cancer *26:*82–83, July '44

Lip carcinoma. ECKERT, C. T. AND PETRY, J. L., S. Clin. North America *24:*1064–1076, Oct '44

Cancer of lips. FREEMAN, D. B. Illinois M. J. *87:*94–96, Feb '45

Acute epithelioma of lip; case. MERCADAL PEYRI, J. AND PEDRAGOSA, R. Actas dermosif. *36:*521–526, Feb '45

Lips, Cancer, Cure Rates

Relationship of cellular differentiation, fibrosis, hyalinization, and lymphocytic infiltration to postoperative longevity of patients with squamous-cell epithelioma of skin and lip. POWELL, L. D., J. Cancer Research *7:*371–378, Oct '22 (illus.)

Results of operations for cancer of lip at Massachusetts General Hospital from 1909 to 1919. SIMMONS, C. C. AND DALAND, E. M. Surg., Gynec. and Obst. *35:*766–771, Dec '22

Carcinoma of lip and cheek; general principles involved in operation and results obtained at Presbyterian, Memorial, and Roosevelt Hospitals. BREWER, G. E. Surg., Gynec. and Obst. *36:*169–184, Feb '23

Carcinoma of jaws, tongue, cheek, and lips; general principles involved in operations and results obtained at Cleveland Clinic.

Lips, Cancer, Cure Rates–Cont.

CRILE, G. W. Surg., Gynec. and Obst. *36:*159–162, Feb '23 (illus.)

Results of surgical treatment of epithelioma of lip from Massachusetts General Hospital and Cancer Commission of Harvard University. SHEDDEN, W. M. Boston M. and S. J. *196:*262–270, Feb 17, '27

Deductions from 191 cases of cancer of lips. FONTS, E. Bol. de la Liga contra el cancer *3:*4–9, Jan 1, '28

End-results of irradiation of cancer of lips; based on study of 173 cases, January 1914 to January 1924. SCHREINER, B. F. AND SIMPSON, B. T. Radiol. Rev. and Chicago M. Rec. *51:*235–245, June '29

Analysis of cases at Pondville Hospital; cancer of lip and mouth. TAYLOR, G. W. Am. J. Cancer (supp.) *15:*2380–2385, July '31

Report of 88 cases of cancer of lips from Steiner Clinic. STEWART, C. B. Surg., Gynec. and Obst. *53:*533–535. Oct '31

Analysis of 137 cases of cancer of lips treated in services of department of laryngology of Instituto del Cancer in Havana. GROS, J. C. Bol. Liga contra el cancer *8:*8–11, Jan '33

Five year cures in cancer of mouth, lip, nose, etc. SMITH, F. Surg., Gynec. and Obst. *56:*470–471, Feb (no. 2A) '33

Five-year end-results obtained by radiation treatment of cancer of lips. SCHREINER, B. F. AND MATTICK, W. L. Am. J. Roentgenol. *30:*67–74, July '33

Treatment and results of cancer of lips; 130 cases. WANGENSTEEN, O. H. AND RANDALL, O. S. Am. J. Roentgenol. *30:*75–81, July '33

Clinicopathologic analysis of 77 cases of cancer of lips and suggestion for rational plan of treatment. HYNDMAN, O. R. Arch. Surg. *27:*250–266, Aug '33

Curability of cancer of lips. JUDD, E. S. AND PHILLIPS, J. R. Proc. Staff Meet., Mayo Clin. *8:*637–640, Oct 18, '33

Results of treatment of cancer of lips by electrocoagulation and irradiation. PFAHLER, G. E. AND VASTINE, J. H. Pennsylvania M. J. *37:*385–389, Feb '34

Epitheliomas of lips; survey of 100 cases. DELREZ, L. AND DESAIVE, P. Liege med. *27:*2057–2085. Oct 7, '34

Epithelioma of lower lip; results of treatment. FIGI, F. A. Surg., Gynec. and Obst. *59:*810–819, Nov '34

Results of therapy in four hundred and twenty-five cases of cancer of lips followed from one to ten years. WILE, U. J. AND HAND, E. A., J.A.M.A. *108:*374–382, Jan

Lips, Cancer, Cure Rates—Cont.
30, '37
Life expectancy and incidence; carcinoma of lip and oral cavity. WELCH, C. E. AND NATHANSON, I. T. Am. J. Cancer *31:*238–252, Oct '37
Five year end-results in treatment of cancer of tongue, lip and cheek. MARTIN, H. E. Surg., Gynec. and Obst. *65:*793–797, Dec '37
Clinical and pathologic study of 390 cases lip cancer, with report of 5 year cures. NEWELL, E. T. JR. Arch. Surg. *38:*1014–1029, June '39
Carcinoma of lower lip; interval statistical survey of end-results in all cases treated at Brooklyn Cancer Institute, 1930 to 1939 inclusive. HOWES, W. E. AND LA ROSA, F. J. Am. J. Roentgenol. *47:*39–49, Jan '42
Study of 56 5-year cases of cancer of lips. WHITCOMB, C. A. Am. J. Surg. *63:*304–315, March '44
Cancer of lips at New Haven Hospital, 1921–1940, inclusive. LAWRENCE, E. A. AND OUGHTERSON, A. W. Connecticut M. J. *8:*353–357, June '44

Lips, Cancer, Distant Metastases

Epithelioma of lip with visceral metastases. WRIGHT-SMITH, R. J., J. Coll. Surgeons, Australasia *2:*421–424, March '30

Lips, Cancer, Neck Metastases

Extirpation of lymphatics with lip cancer. DURANTE, L. Arch. ital. di chir. *8:*201–208, Oct '23
Glandular involvement following cancer of lips, tongue and floor of mouth. REGAUD, C. *et al.* Paris med. *1:*357–372, April 16, '27 also: Strahlentherapie *26:*221–251, '27
Early clinical and therapeutic study of invasion of lymphatic nodes in pavement epitheliomas of lips and tongue; 8 cases. LECÈNE, P. Prat. med. franc. *7:*219–227, May (A) '28
Removal of submaxillary salivary glands in operations for carcinoma of lower lip; responses to questionnaire. BERESOW, E. L. Arch. f. klin. Chir. *151:*767–784, '28
Removal of submaxillary salivary glands and lymph glands in operations for carcinoma of lower lip. BERESOW, E. L. Deutsche Ztschr. f. Chir. *213:*391–415, '29
Neck metastases from lip and mouth cancer. KILGORE, A. R. AND TAUSSIG, L. R., S. Clin. North America *11:*1055–1059, Oct '31
Treatment of epitheliomatous glands of neck following cancer of lips. SCOTT, R. K., M. J.

Lips, Cancer, Neck Metastases—Cont.
Australia *2:*505–512, Oct 24, '31
Radical treatment of cancer of lips. BLAIR, V. P.; *et al.* Am. J. Roentgenol. *29:*229–233, Feb '33
Treatment of neck glands in cancer of lip, tongue and mouth; study of present-day practice (questionnaire report of Cancer Commission of California Medical Association). PFLUEGER, O. H. California and West. Med. *39:*391–397, Dec '33
Epithelioma of lip, with particular reference to lymph node metastases. KENNEDY, R. H. Ann. Surg. *99:*81–93, Jan '34
Surgery as applied to lymph nodes of neck in cancer of lip and buccal cavity; statistical study. FISCHEL, E. Am. J. Surg. *24:*711–731, June '34
Epithelioma of lips; glandular involvement and "wait and see" method of therapy. MYERS, E. S., M. J. Australia *1:*399–400, March 13, '37
Evaluation of neck dissection in cancer of lips. TAYLOR, G. W. AND NATHANSON, I. T. Surg., Gynec. and Obst. *69:*484–492, Oct '39
Treatment of carcinoma of lip (and involved lymph nodes). SMITHERS, D. W. Post-Grad. M. J. *15:*376–381, Nov '39
Current treatment of cancer of lip (and involved lymph nodes); clinical speculation. BLAIR, V. P. AND BYARS, L. T. Surgery *8:*340–352, Aug '40

Lips, Cancer, Radiation Therapy

Radium in treatment of epithelioma of lip. QUICK, D., J. Radiol. *2:*1, Dec '21
Radium treatment of cancer of lip. DUBOIS-ROQUEBERT. Paris med. *12:*110–112, Feb 4, '22
Cancer of lip treated by radiation or combined with electro-coagulation and surgical procedures. PFAHLER, G. E., J. Radiol. *3:*213–218, June '22 (illus.)
Treatment of cancer of lip by radiation. LAIN, E. S. Tr. Sect. Dermat. and Syphilol., A.M.A. pp. 220–233, '22 (illus.) also: Arch. Dermat. and Syph. *6:*434–447, Oct '22
Cancer of lip treated by electrocoagulation and radiation. PFAHLER, G. E. Arch. Dermat. and Syph. *6:*428–433, Oct '22 also: Tr. Sect. Dermat. and Syphilol., A.M.A. pp. 213–219, '22
Radium treatment of carcinoma of lip. TAUSSIG, L. R., S. Clin. N. America *6:*1579–1586. May '23 (illus.)
Contribution to treatment of cancer of lip by irradiation; report on 136 cases. SCHREI-

Lips, Cancer, Radiation Therapy—Cont.
NER, B. F. AND KRESS, L. C., J. Cancer Research *8:*221–233, July '24
Epithelioma of lip treated with radium. MONTGOMERY, D. W. AND CULVER, G. D. California and West. Med. *22:*628–631, Dec '24
Cancer of lip; its treatment by means of electrothermic coagulation, radium and roentgen rays. STEVENS, J. T. Radiology *4:*372–377, May '25
Epithelioma of lip treated by radiation. JACOBS, A. W., M. J. and Rec. *123:*803, June 16, '26
Radio-active substances; their therapeutic uses and applications; radium treatment of carcinoma of lower lip. MUIR, J. Radiology *7:*51–58, July '26
Cancer of lip; report of 25 cases treated with radium. TRUEHEART, M., J. Kansas M. Soc. *26:*311–313, Oct '26
Epidermoid carcinoma (epithelioma) of lip; diagnosis, pathology, and discussion of treatment by non-surgical measures. PENDERGRASS, E. P., S. Clin. N. Amer. *7:*117–163, Feb '27
Radium and radon in treatment of epithelioma of lips. SIMPSON, F. E. AND FLESHER, R. E. Arch. Physical Therapy *9:*207–208, May '28
Radium and radon in treatment of epithelioma of lips. SIMPSON, F. E. AND FLESHER, R. E. Illinois M. J. *54:*48–50, July '28
Cancer of lips; treatment by radium needles. BROWN, R. G., M. J. Australia *1:*421–423, March 30, '29
Epithelioma of lips; radium therapy. LENTH, V. Radiol. Rev. and Chicago M. Rec. *51:*132–135, March '29
Radiotherapy of cancer of lips and mouth. MURPHY, I. J. AND MURPHY, S. L. Radiol. Rev. and Chicago M. Rec. *51:*126–128, March '29
Results of radium treatment of epithelioma of lips; statistics. LACASSAGNE, A. Arch. d'electric. med. *39:*358–366, Oct '29
Radium treatment of early epithelioma of lips. HAILEY, H. South. M. J. *23:*1121–1125, Dec '30
Treatment of bulky lesions of lips by combination of external and interstitial irradiation. DUFFY, J. J. Am. J. Cancer *15:*246–254, Jan '31
Treatment by radiation and gold seed implantation in metastatic nodes in neck from cancer of lips. JOHNSON, S. C. Am. J. Cancer *15:*254–261, Jan '31
Bulky carcinoma of lip treated by irradiation, wide surgical excision and plastic clo-

Lips, Cancer, Radiation Therapy—Cont.
sure. MARTIN, H. E. Am. J. Cancer *15:*261–266, Jan '31
Radiation therapy of cancer of lips and mouth. MARTIN, J. M. Radiology *16:*881–892, June '31
Squamous-celled epithelioma of lower lip; radium therapy. HAILEY, H., J. M. A. Georgia *20:*386–388, Oct '31
Radium treatment of cancer of lips. VAN STUDDIFORD, M. T. New Orleans M. and S. J. *84:*252–259, Oct '31
X-ray therapy as conservative method in cancer of lower lip. MARTIN, J. M. Proc. Internat. Assemb. Inter-State Post-Grad. M. A., North America (1930) *6:*399–403, '31
Radiotherapy of cancer of lips. ARZT, L. AND FUHS, H. Wien. klin. Wchnschr. *45:*15–18, Jan 1, '32
Epithelioma of mucous membrane of lower lip; recovery after radium therapy complicated by partial necrosis of inferior maxilla; case. HOCHE, L. AND ROY. Bull. Assoc. franc. p. l'etude du cancer *21:*381–384, May '32
Radium therapy of cancer of lips, with study of metastasis into regional lymph nodes. COLLIN, E. Acta radiol. *13:*232–237, '32
Radium therapy of cancer of lips, with especial consideration of permanent results. ARTZ, L. AND FUHS, H. Wien. klin. Wchnschr. *46:*706–708, June 9, '33
Cancer of lower lip; efficient treatment by radiation. MUIR, J. Internat. J. Med. and Surg. *46:*590–591, Dec '33
Treatment of early carcinoma of lip, with special reference to use of low kilovoltage x-rays. BELISARIO, J. C., M. J. Australia *1:*91–95, Jan 16, '37
Radiation therapy of cancer of lips. KAPLAN, I. I. Radiology *28:*533–543, May '37
Interstitial radium treatment of cancer of lips; review of 71 cases. DE MONCHAUX, C. M. J. Australia *2:*221–225, Aug 7, '37
Results of irradiation treatment for cancer of lips; analysis of 636 cases from 1926–1936. SCHREINER, B. F. AND CHRISTY, C. J. Radiology *39:*293–297, Sept '42
Clinical study of 778 cases of cancer of lips with particular regard to predisposing factors and radium therapy. EBENIUS, B. Acta radiol., supp. 48, pp. 1–232, '43

Lips, Cross-Lip Flaps (See also Lips, Reconstruction of)
Cheiloplasty; using upper lip to make new lower lip. PÓLYA, E. Zentralbl. f. Chir. *48:*262, Feb 26, '21
Switching of vermilion-bordered lip flaps.

Lips, Cross-Lip Flaps – Cont.
BROWN, J. B. Surg., Gynec. and Obst. *46:*701-704, May '28
Cheiloplasty by Estlander technic. ALFREDO, J. Rev. med. de Pernambuco *5:*233-237, June '35
Split vermilion bordered lip flap in cleft lip. CANNON, B. Surg., Gynec. and Obst. *73:*95-97, July '41
Simplified method of rotating skin and mucous membrane flaps for complete reconstruction of lower lip. OWENS, N. Surgery 15:196-206, Jan '44
Closure of defects with composite vermilion borderlined flaps. MAY, H. Ann. Surg. *120:*214-223, Aug '44

Lips, Deformity of (See also Cleft Lip; Facial Clefts)
Double lip. DORRANCE, G. M. Ann. Surg. *76:*776-777, Dec '22 (illus.)
Treatment of deformities of lips. CATTANI, P. Schweiz. med. Wchnschr. *53:*85-88, Jan 25, '23 (illus.)
Malignant furuncle of lip. ROEDELIUS, E. Klin. Wchnschr. *2:*2348-2353, Dec 24, '23 abstr: J.A.M.A. *82:*506, Feb 9, '24
Treatment of malignant furuncle of lip. ROEDELIUS, E. Dermat. Wchnschr. *78:*37-42, Jan 12, '24
Infections of upper lip. ENGEL, L. P., J. Kansas M. Soc. *24:*44-46, Feb '24
Infections of lip. KAHN, M. J.A.M.A. *82:*1043-1044, March 29, '24
Modification of Estlander's operation for lip defect. TWYMAN, E. D. Surg., Gynec. and Obst. *38:*824-825, June '24
Three cases of congenital fistulas, mucous membrane pouches on lower lip; nature and cause of malformation, with review of 46 cases on record. HILGENREINER, H. Deutsche Ztschr. f. Chir. *188:*273-309, '24
Congenital defects of lips and mouth. FRANK, L. W. Kentucky M. J. *24:*331-335, July '26
Congenital labial fistula; case. RUPPE, C. AND MAGDELEINE, J. Rev. de stomatol. *29:*1-8, Jan '27
Certain fundamental principles of esthetic surgery; with method of plastic reconstruction of lower lip for cicatricial deformity. GIANTURCO, G. Rinasc. med. *4:*507, Nov 1, '27
Abnormally attached frenum labium with surgical interference. PATTON, E. W. Internat. Orthodont. Cong. *1:*701, '27
Deformities of lips from maxillary abnormalities. SCHWARZ, R. Schweiz. Monatschr. f. Zahnh. *39:*331-344, June '29
Congenital fistula of lower lip; embryologic and hereditary factors in pathogenesis of rare congenital abnormalities of face; operative treatment; cases. RUBALTELLI, E. Arch. ital. di otol. *41:*141-154, April '30
Restoration of lower lip by means of Filatov's tubular skin flap. KARTASCHEW, S. Deutsche Ztschr. f. Chir. *229:*395-400, '30
Surgical treatment of double lips. MEYER, H. Deutsche Ztschr. f. Chir. *222:*305-309, '30
Congenital bilateral fistula of lower lip. MEYER, P. Deutsche Ztschr. f. Chir. *229:*391-395, '30
Double lips. EITNER, E. Wien. med. Wchnschr. *83:*429-430, April 8, '33
Therapy of microstomia; case. BUSTAMANTE, S. Ann. Casa de Salud Valdecilla *4:*281-282, '33
Congenital fistula of lower lip; etiologic and clinical study. POHL, L. Rev. de chir. plastique, pp. 107-131, Oct '34
Surgical care of injuries and deformities of nose, lip and premaxilla, with report of cases. FEDERSPIEL, M. N. Internat. J. Orthodontia *22:*1054-1068, Oct '36
Pathology and embryogenesis of deformities of nose and lip. BURIAN, F. Casop. lek. cesk. *76:*101, Jan 29, '37; 138, Feb 5, '37
Double lip; surgical therapy of case. RODRIGUEZ VILLEGAS, R. AND TAULLARD, J. C. Bol. y trab. de la Soc. de cir. de Buenos Aires *21:*45-48, April 14, '37
Surgical consideration of abnormal frena of lip. PARKER, D. B. Internat. J. Orthodontia *23:*1141-1148, Nov '37
Plastic surgery of double lip. ZENO, L. An. de cir. *4:*11-13, March '38
Repair of postoperative defects of lips. NEW, G. B. AND ERICH, J. B. Am. J. Surg. *43:*237-248, Feb '39
Surgical and anatomic aspects of case of double lower lip. MASON, M. L.; *et al.* Surg., Gynec. and Obst. *70:*12-17, Jan '40
Plastic repair of defects of lips and corner of mouth by means of Filatov's tubular flaps. GNILORYBOV, T. E. Vestnik khir. *59:*592-599, June '40
Rare congenital malformation of upper lip. RADCLIFFE, W. Brit. J. Surg. *28:*329-330, Oct '40
Management of nasal deformities in infants and small children and ear, eyelids, lips and palate deform. PEER, L. A. Dis. Eye, Ear, Nose and Throat *2:*166-176, June '42
Ascher syndrome (blepharochalasis, double upper lip and goiter), with report of case. GALLINO, J. A. AND CORA ELISEHT, F. Prensa med. argent. *32:*2423-2426, Dec 7, '45
Macrocheilia. BOUCHER, R. Union med. du Canada *75:*461-462, April '46

Lips, Esthetic Surgery of

Aesthetic correction of lips. DE ASÍS, R. Siglo med. *87:*269–270, March 14, '31
Esthetic surgery of lips. DANTRELLE, A., J. de med. de Paris *56:*57–62, Jan 23, '36
Cheilorthocaliplasty (esthetic surgery of mouth). CODAZZI AGUIRRE, J. A. Rev. med. del Rosario *27:*1111–1131, Nov '37
Plastic correction of lips. EITNER, E. Wien. med. Wchnschr. *89:*89–90, Jan 28, '39
Hypermotility of upper lip, surgery of. DORRANCE, G. M. AND LOUDENSLAGER, P. E. Surg., Gynec. and Obst. *75:*790–791, Dec '42
Plastic operation for lengthening congenitally short upper lip; preliminary report. FORD, J. F., J. Oral Surg. *2:*260–265, July '44
Cosmetic reduction of full, everted lower lip. FIRESTONE, C. Northwest Med. *45:*499–501, July '46

Lips, Infections of

Furuncles of nose and upper lip. DUFOURMENTEL, L. Prat. med. franc. *14:*171–178, March (A) '33
Infections of lip and face. COLLER, F. A. AND YGLESIAS, L. Surg., Gynec. and Obst. *60:*277–290, Feb (no. 2A) '35
Furuncles of upper lip and nose. GAUS, W. Therap. d. Gegenw. *77:*75–76, Feb '36
Furuncle of upper lip; case. FERNANDES, M. Rev. med. de Pernambuco *9:*137–145, May '39
Extensive furunculosis of upper lip treated by roentgenotherapy; case. GRIMAUD, R. AND JACOB, P. Rev. med. de Nancy *67:*701–703, Aug 1, '39
Complications of malignant furuncle of upper lip and their prevention. CALLILAR, N. Turk tip cem mec *12:*44–50, '46

Lips, Lesions of

Differential diagnosis of lesion on lip. STOKES, J. H., S. Clin. N. America *8:*894–898, Nov '24
Diseases of vermillion borders of lips. SHELMIRE, B. Dallas M. J. *14:*82–91, June '28 also: Internat. J. Orthondontia *14:*817–852, Sept '28
Lesions of lower lip. BURFORD, W. N. AND ACKERMAN, L. V. Am. J. Orthodontics (Oral Surg. Sect.) *31:*560–574, Sept '45

Lips, Miscellaneous Procedures

Plastic operations on corner of mouth. FESSLER, J. Deutsche Ztschr. f. Chir. *172:*427–429, '22 (illus.)

Lips, Miscellaneous Procedures—Cont.

Problem of bringing forward retracted upper lip and nose in harelip. BLAIR, V. P. Surg., Gynec. and Obst. *42:*128–132, Jan '26
Lips and teeth and cyclopia and harelips. BOLK, L. Ztschr. f. d. ges. Anat. (Abt. 1) *85:*762–783, May 21, '28
Similarity of reasons for operative failures in congenital harelip and traumatic tear of lip. RENDU, A. Gaz. med. de France, pp. 351–353, May 15, '32
Repair of secondary traumatic defects in mucous membrane of lips. GORDON, S. Canada. M.A.J. *38:*382, April '38
Plastic surgery, with report of original operation for advancement of nasolabial fold. DOUGLAS, B. South. M. J. *31:*1047–1052, Oct '38
Wounds of lips; therapy. ROCHETTE, M. Hopital *27:*195–196, April '39
Problems involving mandibular nerve (ørestheisa of lip). COGSWELL, W. W., J. Am. Dent. A. *29:*964–969, June 1, '42
War wounds of lips and cheek. WEBSTER, G. V., U. S. Nav. M. Bull. *45:*819–826, Nov '45

Lips, Mucosal Grafts from

Exuberance of labial mucosa. FINOCHIETTO, R. Semana med. *1:*1159–1162, May 12, '27
Modification of Lowenstein clamp used in transplantation of lip mucosa. STEIN, R. Klin. Monatsbl. f. Augenh. *88:*370–371, March '32
Lip graft operation for trichiasis of eyelid. ALEXANDER, G. F. Tr. Ophth. Soc. U. Kingdom *52:*162–169, '32
Restoration of vermilion border in certain operation. BALDWIN, J. F. Am. J. Surg. *22:*232, Nov '33
Therapy of trachomatous pannus by transplantation of lip mucosa preserved at low temperature. KIPARISOV, N. M. Vestnik oftal. *17:*227–229, '40
Operation for pterygium using mucous graft from lip. DOZOROVA, N. S. Vestnik oftal. (nos. 1–2) *20:*59–60, '42

Lips, Paralysis of

Operative correction of paralysis of lower lip. SCHMERZ, H. Arch. f. klin. Chir. *131:*353–360, '24 abstr: J.A.M.A. *83:*1464, Nov 1, '24
Permanent enlargement of lips and face, secondary to recurring swellings and associated with facial paralysis; clinical study. NEW, G. B. Tr. Am. Laryng. A. *55:*43–50, '33. Also J.A.M.A. *100:*1230–1233, April 22, '33
Treatment of lip and cheek in cases of facial

Lips, Paralysis of–Cont.
paralysis (by plastic lip cradle). DAHLBERG, A. A., J.A.M.A. *124:*503–504, Feb 19, '44

Lips, Reconstruction of (See also Lips; Cross-Lip Flaps)

Plastic operation on lips. KÖNIG, F. Beitr. z. klin. Chir. *122:*288, '21 abstr: J. A. M. A. *77:*656, Aug 20, '21
Plastic operation on face; and lips. BULLOCK, H., M. J. Australia *2:*220, Sept 17, '21
Reconstruction of lower lip. TZAÏCO, A. Presse med. *29:*723, Sept 10, '21 abstr: J.A.M.A. *77:*1606, Nov 12, '21
Plastic surgery of lip. KAZANJIAN, V. H. J.A.M.A. *77:*1959, Dec 17, '21
Reconstruction of upper lip. DUFOURMENTEL, L. Presse med. *30:*344–346, April 22, '22 (illus.) abstr: J.A.M.A. *78:*1851, June 10, '22
Reconstruction to insure function after plastic operation on lower lip. PICHLER, H. Zentralbl. f. Chir. *49:*1363–1365, Sept 16, '22 (illus.)
Rhinoplasty and cheek, chin, and lip plastics with tubed, temporal-pedicled, forehead flaps. MCWILLIAMS, C. A. AND DUNNING, H. S. Surg., Gynec. and Obst. *36:*1–10, Jan '23 (illus.)
Reconstruction of lower lip. HOFMANN, M. Arch. f. klin. Chir. *131:*338–342, '24
Reconstruction of lower lip according to round pedicle method. WOLOSCHINOW, W. Arch. f. klin. Chir. *135:*770–775, '25
Plastic reconstruction of upper and lower lips. DEMEL, R. Deutsche Ztschr. f. Chir. *196:*210–214, '26
Excision and restoration of upper lip. PICKERILL, H. P. Brit. J. Surg. *14:*536–538, Jan '27
Epithelialized flap from forehead to reconstruction lower lip and cheek. NEW, G. B. S. Clin. N. Amer. *7:*1481–1483, Dec '27
Use of visor flaps from chest in plastic operations upon neck, chin and lip. FREEMAN, L. Ann. Surg. *87:*364–368, March '28
Restoration of upper lip. AXT, E. F. Dental Cosmos *70:*1158–1160, Dec '28
Plastic surgery of lower lip for noma. KOLDAEFF, S. M. Vrach. gaz. *32:*1177–1181, '28
Use of double skin flap in restoration of lip defects. VON CZEYDA-POMMERSHEIM, F. Zentralbl. f. Chir. *56:*2381–2382, Sept 21, '29
Cheiloplastic methods. HAGENTORN, A. Zentralbl. f. Chir. *56:*3031–3032, Nov 30, '29
Cheiloplasty of upper lip. KURTZAHN. Deutsche Ztschr. f. Chir. *218:*378–383, '29

Lips, Reconstruction of–Cont.
Plastic operation for restoration of chin, lower lip, and part of cheeks; method of applying dressing. KRAUSS, F. Zentralbl. f. Chir. *57:*1915–1916, Aug 2, '30
Loss of nasal ala and upper lip reconstruction. FIGI, F. A., S. Clin. North America *11:*834–837, Aug '31
Surgical therapy of ectropion of upper lip; case. MULLER, P. Clinique, Paris *27:*124–125, April (A) '32
Method for cheiloplasty of lower lip. SANCHÍS PERPIÑÁ, V. Actas Soc. de cir. de Madrid *1:*329–352, April–June '32
Destruction of skin of face by irradiation of birthmark in early life; restoration of nose by rhinoplasty, correction of lip by plastic operation, restoration of eyebrow by implantation of narrow flap from hairy scalp, restoration of upper eyelid by full-thickness graft from thigh. BABCOCK, W. W., S. Clin. North America *12:*1409–1410, Dec '32
Extensive cicatrix of face; reconstruction of both eyelids and of both lips by tubular grafts. ROCHER, H. L. Bull. et mem. Soc. de chir. de Bordeaux et du Sud-Ouest, pp. 154–156, '32
Surgery of upper lip to correct loss of tissue due to actinomycosis. DESELAERS, H. Ars med., Barcelona *9:*143–144, April '33
Method for cheiloplasty of lower lip. SANCHÍS PERPIÑÁ, V. Arch. de med., cir. y especialid. *36:*449–458, April 22, '33
Author's cheiloplastic method of surgery of lower lip. SANCHÍS PERPIÑÁ, V. Beitr. z. klin. Chir. *158:*367–380, '33
Preservation of innervation and circulation supply in plastic restoration of upper lip. ESSER, J. F. S. Ann. Surg. *99:*101–111, Jan '34
Frontal flaps of lips; special practice of biological-or artery flaps. ESSER, J. F. S. Rev. de chir. plastique, pp. 288–294, Jan '34
New method of reconstruction of lips. PIERCE, G. W. AND O'CONNOR, G. B. Arch. Surg. *28:*317–334, Feb '34
New method of muscular transplantation applied to cheiloplasty; case. REBELO NETO, J. Rev. de chir. structive, pp. 199–209, March '36
Cheiloplasty of lower lip; case. BROHOVICI, H. Rev. de chir. structive, pp. 210–213, Oct '37
Cicatricial ectropion of upper eyelid and contracture of lower lip following burn; blepharoplasty and labioplasty; case. ROY, J. N. Rev. de chir. structive *8:*85–90, Aug '38
Cheiloplasty for extensive loss of substance of lower lip; 2 cases. LOMBARD, P. Presse med. *47:*525–526, April 8, '39

Lips, Reconstruction of—Cont.
Reconstruction of lower lip. CUNNINGHAM, A. F. Northwest Med. *39:*336–337, Sept '40
One stage operation for closure of large defects of lower lip and chin. MAY, H. Surg., Gynec. and Obst. *73:*236–239, Aug '41
Restoration of subseptum and lower lip by process of tubular autoplasty; case. DA SILVA, G. Arq. de cir. clin. e exper. *6:*287–299, April–June '42
Use of biologic flaps and Esser inlay to form chin and lip. PENHALE, K. W. AND ESSER, J. F. S., J. Am. Dent. A. *29:*1417–1420, Aug 1, '42
Plastic surgery of upper lip with skin flaps from chin. FREY, S. Zentralbl. f. Chir. *70:*539, April 10, '43
Plastic reconstruction of lower lip; French method. IVANISSEVICH, O.; *et al.* Bol. d. Inst. clin. quir. *19:*345–351, June '43
Plastic reconstruction of lower lip (French method). IVANISSEVICH, O.; *et al.* Bol. y trab., Acad. argent. de cir. *27:*353–362, June 23, '43
Simplified method of rotating skin and mucous membrane flaps for complete reconstruction of lower lip. OWENS, N. Am. J. Orthodontics (Oral Surg. Sect.) *30:*340–349, June '44
Cheiloplasties. COVARRUBIAS ZENTENO, R. Rev. med. de Chile *72:*696–698, Aug '44
Plastic reconstruction following gunshot wound of lip; case. CHAMBERS, J. V. U. S. Nav. M. Bull. *46:*588–590, April '46

Lips, Tumors of

Cavernous hemangioma of upper lip. TAVARES, A. Ann. d'anat. path. *3:*147–150, Feb '26
Lymphangioma of lower lip; case. DIEULAFÉ, L. Rev. de stomatol. *29:*193–195, April '27
Angioma of upper lip; case. DIEULAFÉ, L. Rev. de stomatol. *29:*390–392, July '27
Angioma of lower lip reduced by injections of quinine urethane. AUGÉ, A. AND COTSAFTIS, G. G. Arch. Soc. d. sc. med. et biol. de Montpellier *9:*84–86, Feb '28
Neuroma of lower lip; case. DAL POZZO, G. Arch. per le sc. med. *52:*187–190, April '28
Lymphangio-endothelioma of lip and nose. MOOREHEAD, F. B., S. Clin. N. Amer. *9:*329–330, April '29
Lymphangioma of axilla and upper lip. BOYKIN, I. M., S. Clin. N. Amer. *9:*1229–1230, Oct '29
Facial angioma with macrocheilia; case. KIKUCHI, R. AND EBA, M. Oto-rhino-laryng. *12:*1018, Dec '39

Lips, Tumors of—Cont.
Tumors of lips, tongue, gums and alveolar processes. MITTERMAIER, R. Handb. d. Hals-, Nasen-, Ohrenh. *5:*582–618, '29
Voluminous angioma of upper lip; treatment by intratumoral quinine injections followed by extirpation of tumor. SORREL, E. Bull. Soc. de pediat. de Paris *34:*210–215, April '36
Tumors of lip and oral cavity. TRUEBLOOD, D. V. West. J. Surg. *46:*395–411, Aug '38
Tumor of lower lip and right cheek; extirpation followed by pedicled skin graft from head. PORUMBARU, I. Rev. de chir., Bucuresti *41:*714–721, Sept–Oct '38
Pediculate hemangioma of lower lip; case. KABASHIMA, T. Oto-rhino-laryng. *12:*293, April '39
Hemangioma of upper lip; case. COMTOIS, A.; *et al.* Ann. med.-chir. de l'Hop. Sainte-Justine, Montreal *3:*80–88, May '41
Cutaneous horn of upper lip. ARNOLD, A. C. M. J. Australia *1:*662, June 13, '42
Treatment of unusual hemangioma (in Negro) of lip. KAPLAN, I. I. Urol. and Cutan. Rev. *48:*290–291, June '44
Hemangioma of lip. BURFORD, W. N. AND ACKERMAN, L. V. Am. J. Orthodontics (Oral Surg. Sect.) *31:*559–560, Sept '45
Salivary gland tumor of upper lip. CURR, J. F. Brit. M. J. *2:*605, Nov 3, '45
Congenital melanoma of lip with cystic degeneration. REED, H. Brit. J. Surg. *34:*95–96, July '46

LIPSCOMB, P. R. (see GHORMLEY, R. K.) July '44
LIPSCOMB, T. H.: Facial bone fractures as seen in naval service. South. M. J. *36:*665–668, Oct '43
LIPSHUTZ, B.: Fistulae and cysts of neck. Ann. Surg. *79:*499–505, April '24
LISCHER, C. E. AND ELMAN, R.: Experimental burns; effect of elastic pressure applied to burned area (effect on hemoconcentration and mortality). War Med. *3:*482–483, May '43
LISCHER, C. E.; ELMAN, R. AND DAVEY, H. W.: Experimental burns; changes in plasma albumin and globulin. War Med. *5:*43–45, Jan '44
LISCHKOFF, M. A. AND HEINBERG, C. J.: New procedure for closure of nonspecific perforations of nasal septum. Arch. Otolaryng. *4:*342, Oct '26
LISIANSKAIA, V. S. (see BABSKY, A. A.) 1927
LISTER, C. S.: Metal splint for fractures of mandible. U. S. Vet. Bur. M. Bull. *7:*498, May '31
LISTER, W. A.: Natural history of strawberry nevi. Lancet *1:*1429–1434, June 25, '38

Liston, J. J.: Two-stage operation for imperforate anus. Brit. M. J. *1:*852, May 25, '40
Litauer, R. (see Galewska, S.) Jan '36
Litinskiy, A. M.: Transplantation of cartilage from cadaver according to Mikhelson method in correction of nasal deformities. Novy khir. arkhiv. *48:*211–214, '41
Littell, J. J.: Effective method of controlling secondary hemorrhage in nasal surgery. Laryngoscope *42:*207–209, March '32
Little, J. L.: Factor of heredity in harelip. Canad. M.A.J. *40:*482–483, May '39
Little. W. D.: Cutaneous burns. J. Indiana M. A. *24:*415–417, Aug '31
Liu, J. H. and Hsu, Y. H.: Primary Thiersch grafting in radical mastoidectomies, with description of new modified technic. Chinese M. J. *55:*343–356, April '39
Livingston, K. E.: Livingston, W. K. and Davis, E. W.: Technic of suture of peripheral nerves. J. Neurosurg. *3:*270–271, May '46
Livingston, K. E. (see Bradford, F. K.) July '46
Livingston, E. K. (see Livingston, K. E. *et al*) May '46
Llewellyn, J. S. and Biggs, A. D.: Hypoplasia of mandible; report of case, with resume of literature and suggestions for modified form of treatment. Am. J. Dis. Child. *65:*440–444, March '43
Llorens Suque, A.: Radium therapy of giant angiomatous nevi. Strahlentherapie *45:*457–460, '32
Llorens Suque, A.: Radium therapy of giant angiomas of face; 3 cases. J. de radiol. et d'electrol. *16:*211–213, May '32
Lloyd, E. I.: Burns and scalds. Brit. M. J. *2:*177–179, Aug 1, '31
Lloyd, R. S.: Maxillofacial prosthesis. J. Am. Dent. A. *31:*1328–1335, Oct 1, '44
Lloyd, R. S.: Osteotomy for correction of mandibular protrusion. Am. J. Orthodontics (Oral Surg. Sect.) *32:*445–455, Jul '46
Lloyd-Williams, I. H.: Boxer's thumb (dislocation). Brit. M. J. *2:*9, July 5, '30
Lluch Caralps, J. (see Simarro Puig, J. *et al*) July '42
Lluesma Uranga, E.: Palmar contracture of hand as sequel of burn received in infancy; therapy with Gillies tubular graft at age 17 years. Cron. med., Valencia *38:*11–14, Jan 15, '34
Lluesma Uranga, E.: Constructive surgical therapy of syndactylia; case. also: nasal deform. Cron. med. Valencia *41:*201–207, Sept-Oct '37
Loader, G. S.: Trismus in relation to maxillofacial surgery. Brit. Dent. J. *81:*193–196, Sept 20, '46
Lock, N.: Burn therapy. Clin. J. *62:*200–203, May '33
Lockwood, C. D.: Plastic surgery of ear. Surg., Gynec. and Obst. *49:*392–394, Sept '29
Lockwood, C. D.: Plastic surgery of ear. S. Clin. North America *10:*1103–1108, Oct '30
Locy, F. E.: Luetic perforation of hard palate with surgical closure. U. S. Nav. M. Bull. *18:*86–87, Jan '23 (illus.)
Locy, F. E.: Nasal deformities. U. S. Nav. M. Bull. *19:*152–155, Aug '23 (illus.)
Lodge, W. O.: Plastic operation for facial paralysis. Brit. J. Surg. *17:*422–423, Jan '30
Lodge, W. O.: Surgery of eyelids. J. Internat. Coll. Surgeons *9:*383–388, May–June '46
Loeb, C.: Unilateral congenital eyelid ptosis corrected by Hunt-Tansley operation. Am. J. Ophth. *7:*216–217, March '24
Loeb, C.: Bilateral eyelid ptosis cured by Hunt-Tansley operation. Am. J. Ophth. *10:*191–192, March '27
Loeb, H. W.: Fatalities following operations upon nose and throat not dependent upon anesthesia – study of 332 hitherto unreported cases. Ann. Otol. Rhinol. & Laryngol. *31:*273–296, June '22
Loeb, H. W. Further studies of fatalities following operations on nose and throat. Ann. Otol. Rhin. and Laryng. *32:*1103–1107, Dec '23
Loeb, L.: Autotransplantation and homoiotransplantation of cartilage in guinea-pig. Am. J. Path. *2:*111–122, March '26
Loeb, L.: Autotransplantation and homoiotransplantation of cartilage and bone in rat. Am. J. Path. *2:*315–333, July '26
Loeb. L.: Transplantation and individuality. Physiol. Rev. *10:*547–616, Oct '30
Loeb, L. and Harter, J. S.: Heterotransplantation of cartilage and fat tissue and reaction against heterotransplants in general. Am. J. Path. *2:*521–537, Nov '26
Loeb, M. J.: Severe laceration of hand with traumatic amputation of two fingers. J.A.M.A. *86:*1345–1347, May 1, '26
Loeb, M. J.: Glomus tumor of fingers; case. J. Florida M. A. *29:*372–374, Feb '43
Loeb, W. J.: Nasal synechia. M. Bull. North African Theat. Op. *2:*122–123, Nov '44
Loebell, H.: Correction of nasal deformities with use of tricoplast. Ztschr. f. arztl. Fortbild. *29:*329–330, June 1, '32
Loeffler,: Autoplastic and homoplastic implantation of epidermis. Deutsche Ztschr. f. Chir. *236:*169–190, '32
Loeffler, F.: Treatment of weblike dermatogenic contractures of large joints. Zentralbl. f. Chir. *51:*681–683, March 29, '24
Loessl, J.: Nieden's operation for habitual dislocation of lower jaw. Zentralbl f. Chir.

*53:*1749-1751, July 10, '26

LOEWE, O.: Use of pieces of skin in deep plastic operations. Munchen. med. Wchnschr. *76:*2125-2128, Dec 20, '29

LOEWEN, S. L. AND RUPE, L. O.: Exstrophy bladder in pseudohermaphrodite; case. J. Kansas M. Soc. *44:*186-189, June '43

LOFSTROM, J. E. (see WEBSTER, J. E. *et al*) July '46

LOGAN, W. H. G.: Surgery of mouth and face with special reference to cleft palate and cleft lip. Kentucky M. J. *24:*498-505, Oct '26

LOGIE, N. J.: Burn therapy at Tobruk. Lancet *1:*609-611, May 15, '43

LOGIE, N. J.: Burn therapy in warfare. Lancet *2:*138-140, July 29, '44

LOGSDON, C. M.: Fractures of maxillae and mandible. J. Am. Dent. A. *27:*389-392, March '40

LOGSDON, C. M.: Utilization of vitallium appliances to treat edentulous mandible fractures. J. Am. Dent. A. *29:*970-978, June 1, '42

LOGSDON, C. M.: Extraoral utilization of screws or pins in immobilization of mandibular fractures. J. Am. Dent. A. *30:*1529-1540, Oct 1, '43

LOGUE, V. (see LANDAU, E. *et al*) Aug '42

LÖHR, W.: Combination of cod liver oil and plaster bandage in therapy of injuries with tissue losses of fingers. Chirurg. *6:*5-11, Jan 1, '34

LÖHR, W.: Cod liver oil therapy of extensive burns of first, second and third degrees. Chirurg *6:*263-276, April 1, '34

LÖHR, W.: Cod liver oil salve treatment of burns with and without use of plaster of paris cast. Zentralbl. f. Chir. *61:*1686-1695, July 21, '34

LÖHR, W.: Cod liver oil and cod liver oil bandage in therapy of hand injuries. Ztschr. f. arztl. Fortbild. *33:*421-427, Aug 1, '36

LÖHR, W.: Modern burn therapy. Ztschr. f. arztl. Fortbild. *36:*449-453, Aug 1, '39

LÖHR, W. AND ZACHER, K.: Clinical study and pathology of burns of second and third degree (with criticism of tannin therapy). Zentralbl. f. Chir. *66:*5-24, Jan 7, '39

LOIREAU, (see BOURGEOIS, P. *et al*) March '33

LOMAZOV, M. G.: Value of tendon transplantation for rapid restoration of function of wrist following injuries. Vrach. delo *24:*51-54, Dec 1, '44

LOMBARD, P.: Cheiloplasty for extensive loss of substance of lower lip; 2 cases. Presse med. *47:*525-526, April 8, '39

LOMBARD, P.: Failure of intravenous injection of plasma in severe traumatic shock; case. Afrique franc. chir. *1:*17-18, Jan-Feb '43

LOMBARD, P.: Failure of plasma and serum transfusion prolonged during 8 days in extensive burns. Afrique franc. chir. *1:*375-378, Nov-Dec '43

LOMBARD, P.: Another failure of transfusion in severe burns; case. Afrique franc. chir. *2:*77-79, Jan-March '44

LOMBARD, P.: Anesthesia during surgical therapy of cleft palate. Presse med. *54:*566, Aug 31, '46

LOMHOLT, S.: Therapy of facial naevus flammeus with new mercury high pressure lamp (intensol lamp). Dermat. Wchnschr. *109:*898-900, July 29, '39

LONG, C. N. H. (see HARKINS, H. N.) Oct '45

LONG, M. (see HUARD, P.) Aug-Sept '37

LONG, P. H. (see RAVDIN, I. S.) April '42

LONGHI, L.: Congenital malformations of hand; attempted classification and report of cases. Arch. di ortop. *55:*183-212, June 30, '39

LONJUMEAU. (see MILIAN) Dec '27

LOOP, F. A.: Osteotomy and arthroplasty for bony ankylosis of left temporo-mandibular joint of 20 years' duration. J. Indiana M. A. *29:*70-72, Feb '36

Loop Operation

Loop operation for paralysis of adductors of thumb. MAYER, L. Am. J. Surg. *2:*456-458, May '27

LOOPER, E. A.: Surgical treatment of cancer of larynx. South. M. J. *31:*367-374, April '38

LOOPER, E. A.: Use of hyoid bone as graft in laryngeal stenosis. Arch. Otolaryng. *28:*106-111, July '38

LOOPER, E. A.: Diagnosis and surgical treatment of cancer of larynx. South. Surgeon *9:*513-521, July '40

LOOS, J. W.: Burn therapy. Nederl. tijdschr. v. geneesk. *81:*5674-5675, Nov 27, '37

LOPES D'ANDRADE, A.: Plastic surgery of lacrimal organs. Med. contemp. *45:*137-139, May 1, '27

LOPES DE ANDRADE, A.: External dacryocystorhinostomy. Med. contemp. *49:*21-29, Jan 18, '31

LÓPEZ, C. J. (see JIMÉNEZ LÓPEZ, C.)

LOPEZ ESNAURRIZAR, M.: Heterogenous bone grafts. J. Internat. Coll. Surgeons *3:*151-155, April '40

LOPEZ ESNAURRIZAR, M.: Heterogenous bone grafts. Medicina, Mexico *20:*384-392, July 25, '40

LOPEZ-MARTINEZ, (see NOEL, MME.) Feb '28

LÓPEZ VILLORIA, L.: Surgical treatment of harelip. Gac. med. de Caracas *36:*85-88, March 31, '29

LÓPEZ VILLORIA, L.: Facial plastic surgery;

cases. Gac. med. de Caracas *41:*338–344, Nov 30, '34

LORBER, V., KABAT, H. AND WELTE, E. J.: Nervous factor in traumatic shock. Surg., Gynec. and Obst. *71:*469–477, Oct '40

LORD, J. W. JR. (see DINGWALL, J. A. III) Aug '43

LORDY, C.: Female pseudohermaphroditism with hypospadias limited to glans; anomaly due to cessation of development; case. An. brasil. de ginec. *18:*87–93, Aug '44

LORETI, M.: Large cavernous angioma with tumors of thyroid structure in lateral region of neck. Valsalva *3:*353–363, Aug '27

LORETO, C.: Presence of toxic substances in artificial fluid circulating through burned area. Arch. ed atti d. Soc. ital. di chir. *39:*1058–1067, '33

LORETO, C.: Therapy of general manifestations of burns; experimental study; preliminary report. Arch. ed atti d. Soc. ital. di chir. *39:*1068–1072, '33

LORIN, H.: Panaris and phlegmon of hand. Hopital *19:*416–420, June (A) '31

LORING, R. M. (see COTTLE, M. H.) Aug '46

LORTAT-JACOB, E.: Is cryotherapy treatment of choice for angiomas? Monde med., Paris *44:*781–782, July 1, '34

LORTAT-JACOB, E.: Cryotherapy of cutaneous tuberous angioma and injections of sclerosing substances in subcutaneous forms. Gaz. med. de France *45:*1061–1062, Dec 1, '38

LORTAT-JACOB, L.: Results of cryotherapy in angiomas of face in nurslings and in angiomas of eyelids. Bull. et mem. Soc. med. d. hop. de Paris *52:*527–528, March 29, '28

LORTHIOR, P.: Exstrophy of bladder, case. Bruxelles-med. *9:*778–780, May 5, '29

LOSSEN, H.: Hyperphalangism of middle finger with bilateral partial branchydactylia (involving first to third fingers). Fortschr. a. d. Geb. d. Rontgenstrahlen *56:*428–438, Sept '37

LOSSEN, W.: Creation of artificial vagina from intraperitoneal hematocolpos in atresia, with subsequent normal childbirth; case. Zentralbl. f. Gynak. *63:*844–847, April 15, '39

LOSEV, N. A.: Author's modification of van Millingen-Sapejko operation for ectropion and trichiasis. Vestnik oftal. *12:*573–579, '38

LOTIN, A. V.: Reconstruction of orbital cavity for wearing prosthesis long after exenteration of orbit. Sovet. vestnik oftal. *7:*402, '35

LOTIN, A. V.: Successfully operated basalioma of eyelid; case. Vestnik oftal. *10:*891–892, '37

LOTSCH, F.: Correction of exstrophy of bladder. Ztschr. f. Urolog. *17:*385–396, '23 abstr: J.A.M.A. *81:*967, Sept 15, '23

LOTSCH, F.: Pendulous mammae and plastic treatment. Zentralbl. f. Chir. *50:*1241–1244, Aug 11, '23 (illus.)

LOTSCH, F.: Meniscus injuries of temporomaxillary joint resulting in so-called anterior dislocation. Arch. f. klin. Chir. *149:*40–54, '27

LOTSCH, F.: Plastic treatment of pendulous breast. Klin. Wchnschr. *7:*603–606, March 25, '28

LOUBEJAC, A. M.: Mixed tumor of parotid; technic of approach incision. Bol. Soc. cir. d. Uruguay *14:*726–729, '43

LOUDENSLAGER, P. E. (see DORRANCE, G. M.) Feb '35

LOUDENSLAGER, P. E. (see DORRANCE, G. M.) Dec '42

LOUGHRIDGE, J. S.: Shock and its treatment. Ulster M. J. *9:*127–131, Oct '40

LOUNSBERRY, C. R.: Cancer of skin of face and neck. California and West Med. *26:*800–801, June '27

LOUTFALLAH, M. (see BERENS, C.) May '43

LOUYOT, P.: Congenital mutilating lesions of fingers; roentgen and clinical aspects at age of 30; case. Rev. med. de Nancy *66:*822–826, Oct 1, '38

LOVE, J. G.: Compound comminuted depressed fracture of frontal bone and orbit, with recovery. Proc. Staff Meet., Mayo Clin. *10:*291–293, May 8, '35

LOVE, R. J. M.: Simple method of dealing with congenital branchial fistulae. Lancet *2:*122, July 20, '29

LOVE, R. J. M.: Bed-sores and their treatment. Practitioner *138:*277–283, March '37

LOVE, R. J. M.: Minor surgical conditions of hands. Practitioner *142:*261–269, March '39

LOW, M. B.: Tannic acid-silver nitrate burn treatment in children. New England J. Med. *216:*553–556, April 1, '37

LOWELL, H. M.: Thermal burns and their treatment. J. Med. *16:*28–30, March '35

LÖWENSTEIN, A.: Operative treatment for sunken upper lid following enucleation. Klin. Monatsbl. f. Augenh. *80:*233–236, Feb 24, '28

LÖWENSTEIN, A.: Plastic repair of congenital and acquired deformities of palpebral margin by means of cartilage from auricle. Klin. Monatsbl. f. Augenh. *93:*320–323, Sept '34

LÖWENTHAL, K.: Possibility of producing tumors by subcutaneous inoculation of normal, particulary embryonal tissue; experimental study. Med. Klin. *24:*1263–1268, Aug. 17, '28

LOWER, W. E.: Exstrophy of urinary bladder with carcinoma. Ann. Surg. *73:*354, March '21

LOWER, W. E.: Epispadias in women, report of case. J. Urology *10:*149–157, Aug '23 (illus.)

LOWER, W. E.: Ureteral transplantation in

very young (infant 4 months old) with exstrophy of bladder; case. Cleveland Clin. Quart. *4:*23–25, Jan '37

LOWER, W. E.: Transplantation of ureters into rectosigmoid in young children and infants with exstrophy of bladder; preliminary report. J. Mt. Sinai Hosp. *4:*650–653, March-April '38

LOWMAN, C. L.: Use of fascia lata in repair of disability at wrist. J. Bone and Joint Surg. *12:*400–402, April '30

LOWSLEY, O. S.: Medical progress; plastic operations on external genitalia. New York Med. (no. 20) *1:*17, Oct 20, '45

LOWSLEY, O. S. AND BEGG, C. L.: Three-stage operation for hypospadias repair; cases. J.A.M.A. *110:*487–493, Feb 12, '38

LOWSLEY, O. S. AND HUNT, R. W.: Plastic operations of the genitourinary tract. South. M. J. *35:*676–687, July '42

LOWSLEY, O. S.; MORRISSEY, J. H. AND RICCI, J. V.: Use of gum-glucose solution in major urological surgery. J. Urology *6:*381, Nov '21

LÖWY, J.: Heredity in Dupuytren's contracture. Zentralbl. f. inn. Med. *44:*51–52, Jan 27, '23 abstr: J.A.M.A. *80:*1279, April 28, '23

LOZI DIAZ, F. A.: Pseudoankylosis of temporomandibular joint of cicatricial origin; surgical therapy of case. Cir. ortop. y traumatol., Habana *9:*129–136, July–Sept '41

LOZNER, E. L. (see CRONKITE, E. P. *et al*) April '44

LOZNER, E. L. (see NEWHOUSER, L. R.) April '42

LOZNER, E. L. (see RHODE, C. M. *et al*) May '45

LOZOYA SOLIS, J.: Complicated harelip; surgical therapy of case. Bol. med. d. Hosp. inf., Mexico *1:*58–67, July–Aug '44

LUBINEAU, J. (see POMMÉ, B. *et al*) May '31

LUC, J.: Plastic restoration of upper lid and socket. Brit. J. Ophth. *30:*665–668, Nov '46

Luc Operation: See Caldwell-Luc Operation

DE LUCA, R.: Hereditary etiology of syndactylia; remarkable association of polydactylia and syndactylia in case. Minerva med. *2:*324–327, Sept 29, '40

DE LUCCHI, G. (see PALTRINIERI, M.) May–June '38

LUCCIONI, F. (see CHEVALLIER, A. *et al*) Jan '37

LUCHETTI, S. E.: Ganglion of wrist, with special reference to therapy. Semana med. *2:*843–847, Oct 7, '37

DE LUCIA, P.: Angioneuroymomas of tactile region of finger; cases. Arch. ital. di anat. e istol. pat. *7:*106–112, Jan '36

LÜCKER, F. C.: Heredity of malformations, especially harelip and polydactylism. Monatschr. f. Geburtsh. u. Gynak. *66:*327-336, July '24 abstr: J.A.M.A. *83:*882, Sept 13, '24

LUCKSCH, F. (see BUMBA. J.) 1927

LUDWIG, F. E.: Use of saline solution, glycerin, and acetic acid in care of burns; odorless method of treating burns. Surgery *19:*486–491, Apr '46

LUDWIG, F. E.: Use of acetic acid-glycerin-saline solution in skin grafting. Surgery *19:*492–497, Apr '46

LUEKEN, K. G.: Study of family with syndactylia. Ztschr. f. menschl. Vererb.-u. Konstitutionslehre *22:*152–159, '38

LUGONES, C.: Volkmann's contracture. Rev. med. latino-amer. *13:*39–69, Oct '27

LUGONES, L. M. (see MARTINEZ CORDOBA, F. *et al*) Aug '43

LUHMANN, K.: Treatment of protruding intermaxillary bone in case of cleft palate. Beitr. z. klin. Chir. *161:*539–547, '35

LUHMANN, K.: Ankylosis of jaws. Beitr. z. klin. Chir. *162:*449–455, '35

LUHMANN, K.: Surgical therapy of exstrophy of bladder. Beitr. z. klin. Chir. *165:*221–242, '37

LUHMANN, K.: Surgical therapy of epispadias. Beitr. z. klin. Chir. *165:*376–381, '37

LUHMANN, K.: Harelip and cleft palate; age at operation and results in therapy. Therap. d. Gegenw. *79:*300–303, July '38

LUHMANN, K.: New mouth gag for surgery of cleft palate. Zentralbl. f. Chir. *66:*243–244, Feb 4, '39

LUHMANN, K.: New mouth gag for operation of cleft palate. Therap. d. Gegenw. *80:*284–285, June '39

LUHMANN, K.: Question of advisability of surgical closure of traumatic defects of palate. Zentralbl. f. Chir. *68:*460–464, March 8, '41

LÜLSDORF, F.: Late rupture of extensor pollicis longus tendon; case. Ztschr. f. orthop. Chir. *51:*191–199, Jan 11, '29

LUMER, M.: Facial hypertrichosis in female; local therapy by diathermocoagulation, with special reference to technic. Semana med. *2:*891–897, Oct 20, '38

LUMSDEN, R. (see BROWN, D.) Jan '44

LUMSDEN-COOK, J. A. (see COOK, J. A. L.)

LUND, C. C.: Burns. Rhode Island M. J. *26:*197–200, Oct '43

LUND, C. C.: Medical progress; treatment of thermal burns; recent developments. New England J. Med. *229:*868–873, Dec 2, '43

LUND, C. C. *et al:* Collective review of burns. Internat. Abst. Surg. *82:*443–478, '46, in Surg. Gynec. and Obst. June '46

LUND, C. C. AND HOLTON, H. M.: Carcinoma of

buccal mucosa; end results 1918–1926. New England J. Med. *208:*775-780, April 13, '33
LUND, C. C. AND HOLTON, H. M.: Report of results of treatment at Collis P. Huntington Memorial Hospital from 1918–1926 (cancer of lip). Am. J. Roentgenol. *30:*59-66, July '33
LUND, C. C. (see CLOWES, G. H. A. JR. *et al*) Nov '43
LUND, C. C. (see GREEN, R. W. *et al*) Aug '45
LUND, C. C. (see LEVENSON, S. M.) Oct '43
LUND, C. C. (see LEVENSON, S. M.) Nov '45
LUND, C. C. (see LEEVENSON, S. M. *et al*) July '46
LUND, C. C. (see STURGIS, S. H.) May '34
LUND, C. C. (see STURGIS, S. H.) Jan '35
LUND, M.: Clinical connection between Dupuytren's contracture, fibroma plantae, periarthrosis humeri, helodermia, induratio penis plastica and epilepsy, with attempt at pathogenetic valuation. Acta psychiat. et neurol. *16:*465–492, '41
LUNDBLOM, A.: Congenital ulnar deviation of fingers of familial occurrence. Acta orthop. Scandinav. *3:*393–404, '32
LUNDON, A. E.: Rhinoplasty with ivory transplant. Canad. M.A.J. *16:*561-562, May '26
LUNDY, J. S.; ADAMS, R. C. AND SELDON, T. H.: Plasma and blood in treatment of shock in burns. S. Clin. North America *24:*798–807, Aug '44
LUNDY, J. S. (see SELDON, T. H.) Aug '41
LUO, T. H.: Bilateral congenital epicanthus inversus and ptosis; case. Chinese M. J. *48:*814–818, Sept '34
LUONGO, R. A.: Dermoid cyst of bridge of nose. Rinasc. med. *10:*185–186, April 15, '33
LUONGO, R. A.: Dermoid cyst of nasal dorsum. Arch. Otolaryng. *17:*755–759, June '33
LUONGO, R. A.: Typical rhinoplastic operation. Arch. Otolaryng. *40:*68–72, July '44
LUPPI, J. E.: Lymphoepithelial papilliferous cystomas of branchial, thyroglossal and thyropharyngeal origin. Rev. med. de Rosario *33:*608–623, July '43
LUPTON, I. M. (see FENTON, R. A.) June '23

Lupus

Surgical treatment of lupus of face. MOURE, P. Arch. franco-belges de chir. *28:*298–307, April '25
Skin flap transplantation for lupus of neck and chin. SALOMON, A. Deutsche med. Wchnschr. *52:*1821, Oct 22, '26
Spinocellular epithelioma of cheek in patient with old lupus. VIGNE, P. Marseille med. *2:*369–371, Dec 15, '30
Plastic reconstruction of nose destroyed by lupus. KURTZAHN. Chirurg *3:*49–52, Jan 15, '31

Lupus – Cont.

Prosthetic surgery in lupus (Hennig-Zinsser method); DÖRFFEL, J. AND NOSSEN, H. Med. Welt *5:*1172–1174, Aug 15, '31
Use of tubular grafts from scalp in therapy of extensive mutilating lupus. MOURE, P. Bull. Soc. franc. de dermat. et syph. *39:*712–717, June '32
Extensive lupus erythematosus with subsequent carcinoma of lower lip (case). GRAHAM-LITTLE, E. Proc. Roy. Soc. Med. *25:*1741, Oct '32
Surgical treatment of lupus of face (use of tubular cranial flaps and application of Filhos' caustic for destruction of minor facial lesions of lupus). MOURE, P. French M. Rev. *2:*415–419, Oct '32
Combination of Finsen light and plastic surgery in lupus of face. GAUVAIN, H. Strahlentherapie *45:*19–24, '32
Therapy of lupus by transplantation of tubular grafts from scalp. MOURE, P. AND BARRAYA. Bull. Soc. franc. de dermat. et syph. *41:*136–137, Jan '34
Radical surgical therapy of lupus (grafting). SCHMIEDEN, V. Zentralbl. f. Chir. *61:*790–793, April 7, '34
Extensive destruction of eyelids and skin of face caused by lupus and syphillis; surgical therapy. RAUH, W. Ztschr. f. Augenh. *86:*193–199, June '35
Clinically atypical, but histologically typical lupus immediately following burn; case. GOUGEROT, H. AND MEYER, J. Bull. Soc. franc. de dermat. et syph. *44:*269–270, Feb '37
Therapy of certain forms of lupus by free grafts of whole skin; 3 cases. RAPIN, M. Rev. med. de la Suisse Rom. *57:*110–115, Feb 25, '37
Extensive butterfly-shaped lupus of face; surgical excision with immediate implantation of Thiersch graft. JACHIA, A. Boll. e mem. Soc. piemontese di chir. *7:*123–128, '37
Replacement skin grafts in surgical treatment of lupus vulgaris. HOLLANDER, L. AND SHELTON, J. M. Arch. Dermat. and Syph. *40:*263–267, Aug '39
Prosthesis for lupus and other facial defects. STÜMPKE, G. Dermat. Wchnschr. *109:*1058–1061, Sept 2, '39
Surgical treatment of lupus; case. (grafting) MALINIAC, J. W. Am. J. Surg. *55:*123–125, Jan '42
Free full thickness graft in case of lupus erythematosus. MALBEC, E. F. Dia med. *14:*1119–1120, Oct 26, '42

Lupus—Cont.

Free graft of full thickness skin in case of lupus erythematosus of nose. MALBEC, E. F. Semana med. *1:*1232–1235, June 3, '43

Psychosomatic clinical study of case of lupus of nose treated by plastic surgery. ZENO, L. Rev. med. de Rosario *33:*1041–1058, Nov '43 also: An de cir. *9:*125–142, Sept-Dec '43 also: Dia med. *16:*264–268, March 20, '44

Lupus erythematosus of face; free skin graft in case. MALBEC, E. F. Dia med. *16:*160, Feb 21, '44

Replacement skin graft in surgical treatment of lupus vulgaris. HOLLANDER, L. AND SHELTON, J. M. Arch. Dermat. and Syph. *49:*60, Jan '44

LUQUET, G. H.: Digital mutilations. J. de psychol. norm. et path. *35:*548–598, July-Dec '38

LURASCHI, J. C. E. AND PORRINI, E. A.: Paralysis of seventh cranial pair; 2 cases. Dia med. *14:*1214–1216, Nov 16, '42

LURASCHI, J. C. E. AND PORRINI, E. A.: Paralysis of seventh cranial pair; study apropos of 2 cases. Semana med. *1:*218–220, Feb 3, '44

LURIJE, A.: Plastic surgery. Medicina, Kaumas *13:*540–543, Aug '32

LUSCHER, E.: Osteomas of upper jaw. Schweiz. med. Wchnschr. *75:*924–927, Oct 20, '45

LUSENA, G.: Venous cyst of neck. Arch. ital. di chir. *19:*93–108, '27

LUSSIER, E. F.: Laterally displaced mandible; treatment simplified by aid of splint. Internat. J. Orthodontia *22:*139–146, Feb '36

LUSSIER, E. F. AND DAVIS, A. D.: Implantation of bone in chin in severe case of mandibular retraction; case. Am. J. Orthodontics *27:*267–274, May '41

LÜTFÜ, Ö. AND BASTUG, K. Ö.: Linear incision for entropion or trichiasis due to trachoma. Deutsche med. Wchnschr. *62:*2014–2015, Dec 4, '36

LÜTHI, A.: Simple, reliable method for correction of protruding ears. Schweiz. med. Wchnschr. *59:*1268–1269, Dec 7, '29

LUTTENBERGER, A.: Philonin (irradiated cholesterol preparation) in burns. Wien. med. Wchnschr. *83:*88–89, Jan 14, '33

LUTTERLOH, P. W. AND STROUD, H. A.: Detoxification treatment in burns. Internat. J. Med. and Surg. *44:*16–18, Jan '31

LUX, P. (see MCLEOD, J.) June '36

LUXENBERG, L.: Burn treatment (use of rubber sponge bandage). Pennsylvania M. J. *36:*334–335, Feb '33

LUXENBURGER, A.: Contributions to plastic surgery of jaws and palate. Deutsche Ztschr. f. Chir. *172:*384–396, '22 (illus.)

LUZ, F.: Bancroftosis and surgery, with special reference to elephantiasis. Arq. de cir. clin. e esper. *3:*189–201, June '39

LUZHINSKIY, G. F.: Comparative evaluation of marginoplastic operations of eyelids. Sovet. vestnik oftal. *7:*137–142, '35

LVOFF, P. P.: Operation for lengthening palate. Vestnik khir. (nos. 37–38) *13:*212–221, '28

LYAKER, B.: Activate charcoal in therapy of slowly healing ulcers after burns. Sovet. khir., no. 12, pp. 911–913, '36

LYANDE, V. S.: Use of glass for rhinoplastic purposes. Zhur. ush., nos. i gorl. bolez. *16:*322–324, '39

LYERLY, J. G.: Repair of bilateral harelip. Virginia M. Monthly *59:*85–88, May '32

LYFORD, J. III.: Two small wire splints for treatment by traction of fractures and deformities of fingers and metacarpal bones. J. Bone and Joint Surg. *24:*202–203, Jan '42

LYFORD, J. III. (see GRUBER, L. W.) May '42

LYFORD, J. III. (see GRUBER, L. W.) March; '43

LYLE, F. M.: Mangle burn injuries. Am. J. Surg. *61:*148–149, July '43

LYLE, F. M.: Method of treating cystic tumors of neck. Am. J. Surg. *61:*443–444, Sept '43

LYLE, H. H. M.: Disabilities of hand and their physiological treatment. Ann. Surg. *78:*816–845, Dec '23 (illus.)

LYLE, H. H. M.: Skin plastics in treatment of traumatic lesions of hand and forearm. Ann. Surg. *83:*537–542, April '26

LYLE, H. H. M.: Ombredanne's pouch operation in hypospadias. Ann. Surg. *98:*513–519, Oct '33

LYMAN, E. E.: Preanesthetic medication with special consideration of problems in maxillofacial surgery. Mil. Surgeon *88:*57–62, Jan '41

Lyman-Farrell Operation

Experimental and clinical study of cases of exstrophy (technic of Lyman-Farrell operation). KIMBALL, G. H. AND DRUMMOND, N. R., J. Oklahoma M. A. *33:*2–8, Aug '40

Lymph

Flow of lymph from burned tissue, with particular reference to effects of fibrin formation upon lymph drainage and composition. GLENN, W. W. L. *et al.* Surgery *12:*685–693, Nov '42

Lymph Nodes

Lymphangioplastic treatment of elephantiasis of lower extremities. SOKOLOWSKI, M. Zentralbl. f. Chir. *52:*2583–2586, Nov 14, '25

Lymph Nodes—Cont.

Cervical lymph nodes in intra-oral carcinoma. DUFFY, J. J. Radiology *9:*373-379, Nov '27

Removal of submaxillary salivary glands and lymph glands in operations for carcinoma of lower lip. BERESOW, E. L. Deutsche Ztschr. f. Chir. *213:*391-415, '29

Surgical treatment of diseases of lymphatic apparatus. HAYWARD. Med. Klin. *27:*96-97, Jan 16, '31

Conservative procedure in care of cervical lymph nodes in intra-oral carcinoma. DUFFY, J. J. Am. J. Roentgenol. *29:*241-247, Feb '33

Surgical treatment of metastases to cervical lymph nodes from intra-oral cancer. FISCHEL, E. Am. J. Roentgenol. *29:*237-240, Feb '33

Treatment of cancerous or potentially cancerous cervical lymph-nodes (as result of cancers of mouth). BLAIR, V. P. AND BROWN, J. B. Ann. Surg. *98:*650-661, Oct '33

Behavior of lymphatic vessels in autoplastic skin grafts. CAVALLI, M. Sperimentale, Arch. di biol. *89:*504-508, '35

Surgical treatment of lymphatic fields in cancer of mouth. MORRIN, F. J. Irish J. M. Sc., pp. 157-163, April '39

Malignant tumors of rhinopharynx with metastases; 15 cases. SCUDERI, R. Arch. ital. di otol. *54:*273-316, Aug '42

Question of tumor of parotid gland or swelling of preauricular lymph nodes. OESER, H. Monatschr. f. Krebsbekampf. *11:*43, March '43

Neck dissections for metastatic carcinoma. BROWN, J. B. AND McDOWELL, F. Surg., Gynec. and Obst. *79:*115-124, Aug '44

Lymphangiomas (See also Cystic Hygromas; Hemangiomas)

Lymphangioma of neck. THOMPSON, J. E. AND KEILLER, V. H. Ann. Surg. *77:*385-396, April '23 (illus.)

Congenital cystic lymphangioma of neck. TORCHIANA, L. Arch. ital. di chir. *16:*173-192, '26

Lymphangioma of lower lip; case. DIEULAFÉ, L. Rev. de stomatol. *29:*193-195, April '27

Multilocular cystic lymphangioma of neck. DE GAETANO, L. Riforma med. *43:*529-532, June 6, '27

Cystic lymphangioma of chest wall. SAILER, K. Orvosi hetil. *71:*811-813, July 17, '27

Bilateral lymphangioma of neck. VON HEREPEY-CSÁBÁNYI, G. Zentralbl. f. Chir. *54:*1672, July 2, '27

Lymphangioma of nose. HAUTANT, A. AND LANOS. Ann. d. mal. de l'oreille, du larynx *46:*1235, Dec '27

Lymphangioma of neck; case. MILIAN, G. AND LONJUMEAU. Bull. Soc. franc. de dermat. et syph. *34:*859-862, Dec '27

Technic for ideal skin-graft, with report of extensive lymphangioma pigmentosa verrucosa. EMERSON, C. Nebraska M. J. *13:*214-216, June '28

Lymphangio-endothelioma of lip and nose. MOOREHEAD, F. B., S. Clin. N. Amer. *9:*329-330, April '29

Lymphangioma of axilla and upper lip. BOYKIN, I. M., S. Clin. N. Amer. *9:*1229-1230, Oct '29

Cystic tuberous lymphangioma of skin with hypertrichosis. TRÝB, A. Arch. f. Dermat. u. Syph. *158:*468-479, '29

Chylocystic lymphangioma of neck; 3 cases. VOLKMANN, J. Beitr. z. klin. Chir. *146:*654-667, '29

Cystic lymphangioma of neck; case. DELLAMANO, N. Gazz. d. osp. *51:*43-53, Jan 12, '30

Lymphangioma of neck. PLĂCINTIANU, G. Spitalul *51:*51-52, Feb '31

Cystic lymphangioma of neck. BOLINTINEANU, G. AND BĂJEU, G. Spitalul *52:*26-27, Jan '32

Cystic lymphangioma of neck; case. DI CIANNI, E. Rinasc. med. *9:*128-129, March 15, '32

Cavernous lymphangioma of forehead; extirpation and cure. MARTÍNEZ VARGAS, A. Med. de los ninos *33:*89-100, April '32

Recurrent cystic lymphangioma of neck in child; case. GRECO, T. Sperimentale, Arch. di biol. (no. 2) *86:*viii-xii, '32

Congenital recurrent lymphangioma of cheek. FRIEDMAN, M. Eye, Ear, Nose and Throat Monthly *12:*334-335, Sept '33

Therapy of lymphangiomas of neck. CHIARIELLO, A. G. Folia med. *20:*590-594, May 30, '34

Congenital irregular hypertrophy of fingers; case due to lymphangiomas. FEVRE, M. AND BRICAGE, R. Ann. d'anat. path. *13:*337-341, March '36

Diathermy applied to facial lymphangiomas; cases. VAN DEN WILDENBERG, Oto-rhino-laryng. internat. *22:*5-10, Jan '38

Hyperplastic cavernous lymphangioma of forearm; case. GAGLIARDI, P. Arch. ital. di anat. e istol. pat. *8:*608-612, Sept '38

Treatment of lymphangiomas with sclerosing injections of sodium citrate; cases. FONSECA E CASTRO. Arch. de med. d. enf. *41:*798-802, Dec '38

Lymphangiomas – Cont.

Congenital cystic lymphangioma cured by subcutaneous anastomosis (marsupialization); case in infant. CABITZA, A. Riv. di clin. pediat. *38:*681-684, Nov '40

Congenital cystic lymphangioma, with recurrence after surgical therapy; case in newborn infant (neck). VIANA, F. Pediat. prat., Sao Paulo *13:*91-98, March-June '42

Cystic lymphangioma, with report of case (neck). SRIBMAN, I. Dia med. *15:*175-178, March 1, '43

Congenital lymphangiomatous macroglossia with cystic hygroma. LIERLE, D. M. Tr. Am. Laryng. A. 194-196, '44

Lymphedema

Elephantiasis. STROTHER, W. H. Kentucky M. J. *19:*175, April '21

Elephantiasis and the Kondoleon operation. GREEN, T. M. Virginia M. Monthly *48:*196, July '21

Kondoleon operation for elephantiasis. HENRY, A. K. Brit. J. Surg. *9:*111, July '21

Report of end results of Kondoleon operation for elephantiasis. SISTRUNK, W. E. Southern M. J. *14:*619, Aug '21

Elephantiasis chirurgica – its cause and prevention. HALSTED, W. S. Bull. Johns Hopkins Hosp. *32:*309, Oct '21

Elephantiasis. SISTRUNK, W. E., S. Clin. N. Amer. *1:*1525, Oct '21

Kondoleon operation for elephantiasis of leg. PIGNATTI, A. Chir. d. org. di movimento *6:*49-62, Feb '22 (illus.) abstr: J.A.M.A. *78:*1579, May 20, '22

Lymph drainage in elephantiasis. HAUBENREISSER, W. Zentralbl. f. Chir. *49:*474-475, April 8, '22 abstr: J.A.M.A. *79:*511, Aug 5, '22

Elephantiasis treated by Kondoleon operation. HERFF, F. P. Surg., Gynec. and Obst. *34:*758-760, June '22 (illus.)

Mechanism of surgical elephantiasis. HALSTED, W. S. *et al.* Lyon chir. *19:*369-376, July-Aug '22 abstr: J.A.M.A. *79:*1460, Oct 21, '22

Results obtained in elephantiasis through Kondoleon operation. SISTRUNK, W. E. Minnesota Med. *6:*173-177, March '23 (illus.)

Surgical treatment of elephantiasis. LEFEBVRE, C., J. de chir. *21:*434-458, April '23 (illus.) abstr: J.A.M.A. *81:*78, July 7, '23

Elephantiasis; surgical treatment. GIORDANO, D. Riforma med. *39:*889-891, Sept 17, '23 (illus.)

Elephantiasis nostras of genitalia; report of case and operative treatment. ORR, T. G. S. Clin. N. America *3:*1537-1545, Dec '23 (illus.)

Ultimate results of Kondoleon operation for elephantiasic edema. KONDOLEON, E. Arch. franco-belges de chir. *27:*104-110, Feb '24 abstr: J.A.M.A. *82:*2087, June 21, '24

Operative lymph drainage in elephantiasis. TEN HORN, C. Zentralbl. f. Chir. *51:*233, Feb 9, '24

Kondoleon operation and filariasis. STENHOUSE, H. M., U. S. Nav. M. Bull. *20:*715-716, June '24

Surgical treatment of elephantiasis. SAMORINI, G. Policlinico (sez. prat.) *31:*904-908, July 14, '24

Combined operations for elephantiasis of leg. BIRT, E. Deutsche Ztschr. f. Chir. *184:*110-114, '24

Surgical treatment of elephantiasis of lower limbs. GIACINTO, G. Riforma med. *41:*793-795, Aug 24, '25

Treatment of elephantiasis. KIMURA, H. Japan M. World *5:*201-211, Aug '25

Operative treatment of varicose elephantiasis of legs. MELLETTI, M. Policlinico (sez. chir.) *32:*520-536, Oct '25

Lymphangioplastic treatment of elephantiasis of lower extremities. SOKOLOWSKI, M. Zentralbl. f. Chir. *52:*2583-2586, Nov 14, '25

Surgical treatment of elephantiasic conditions in legs by Kondoleon's method. FALCONE, R. Arch. ital. di chir. *13:*662-669, '25

Therapy of elephantiasis of leg. BIRT, E. Tung-chi, Med. Monatschr. *2:*108-113, Dec '26

Surgical treatment of elephantiasis of lower limbs. GOVOROFF, A. P. Vrach. dielo *10:*277-278, Feb 28, '27

Plastic surgery; certain modifications of Kondoleon operation for elephantiasis. SISTRUNK, W. E. Ann. Surg. *85:*190-193, Feb '27

Kondoleon method of treatment of elephantiasis; 2 cases. MIROLLI, A. Minerva med. *7:*637-649, June 20, '27

Operative treatment of elephantiasis of scrotum and penis. NÄGELSBACH, E. Arch. f. Schiffs-u. Tropen-Hyg. *31:*282-291, June '27

Operative treatment in 14 cases of elephantiasis. KEYSSER. Deutsche Ztschr. f. Chir. *203-204:*356-375, '27

Kondoleon operation for elephantiasis. CLUTE, H. M., S. Clin. N. Amer. *8:*119-122, Feb '28

Lymphedema – Cont.
Results in Porto Rico of Kondoleon operations for elephantiasis of extremities. BURKE, G. R. Surg., Gynec. and Obst. *47:*843–847, Dec '28
Surgical treatment of elephantiasis of legs. DE GAETANO, L. Riforma med. *44:*1649–1651, Dec 17, '28
Surgical treatment of elephantiasis of lower extremities. ROMITI, C. Arch. ital. di chir. *20:*607–640, '28
New method for determining of plane of operation in elephantiasis, especially of extremities. ROSENAK, I. Zentralbl. f. Chir. *56:*912–914, April 13, '29
Chronic traumatic edema of dorsum of hand; 7 cases. KLASSEN, P. Monatschr. f. Unfallh. *36:*289–309, July '29
Elephantiasis of lower extremities successfully treated by Kondoleon's operation. WEINSTEIN, M. Am. J. Surg. *7:*704–710, Nov '29
Review of surgical treatment of elephantiasis. KUNTZEN, H. Ergebn. d. Chir. u. Orthop. *22:*431–462, '29
Surgical cure of elephantiasis. BATTISTA, A. Urol. and Cutan. Rev. *34:*431–436, July '30
Surgical treatment of elephantiasis. KUNTZEN, H. Chirurg *2:*667–673, July 15, '30
Surgical treatment of genital elephantiasis in male. DAVIS, D. M. Ann. Surg. *92:*400–404, Sept '30
New operation for elephantiasis. AUCHINCLOSS, H. Porto Rico J. Pub. Health and Trop. Med. *6:*149, Dec '30
Surgery of elephantiasis; clinical, histologic and experimental study. KUNTZEN, H. Arch. f. klin. Chir. *158:*543–583, '30
Surgical treatment of diseases of lymphatic apparatus. HAYWARD. Med. Klin. *27:*96–97, Jan 16, '31
Surgical treatment of chronic lymphedema. PRATT, G. H. AND WRIGHT, I. S. Surg., Gynec. and Obst. *72:*244–248, Feb '41
Non-filarial elephantiasis therapy (Kondoleon operation). SCHOFIELD, J. E. Brit. M. J. *1:*795, May 9, '31
Auchincloss operation in elephantiasis; preliminary report. TORGERSON, W. R. Porto Rico J. Pub. Health and Trop. Med. *6:*411–418, June '31
Case report of 12 Auchincloss or modified Auchincloss operations for filariasis elephantiasis; preliminary report. DEL TORO, J. *et al.* Porto Rico J. Pub. Health and Trop. Med. *7:*3–10, Sept '31
Elephantiasis of right leg. JACKSON, C. AND

Lymphedema – Cont.
BABCOCK, W. W., S. Clin. North America *11:*1243–1244, Dec '31
Surgical therapy of elephantiasis. JIANO, J. Cong. internat. de med. trop. et d'hyg., Compt. rend. (1928) *3:*353–357, '31
Elephantiasis of extremities; surgical therapy. RAGO, G. Gazz. internaz. med.-chir. *40:*747, Dec 15; 783, Dec 30, '32
Elephantiasis of plastic skin graft on thumb. WICHMANN, F. W. Arch. f. klin. Chir. *169:*783–788, '32
Surgical therapy of severe case of elephantiasis of leg. MOENE, I. Med. rev., Bergen *50:*116–121, March '33
Surgical therapy of elephantiasis. MOENE, I. Norsk mag. f. laege-vidensk. *95:*264–275, March '34
Chronic lymphatic edema and its treatment by Kondoleon operation. MAILER, R. Glasgow M.J. *121:*213–217, June '34
Surgical treatment of severe lymphedema of extremities; study of end results. GHORMLEY, R. K. AND OVERTON, L. M. Proc. Staff Meet., Mayo Clin. *9:*564–566, Sept 19, '34
Treatment of lymphedema by plastic operation; preliminary report. GILLIES, H. AND FRASER, F. R. Brit. M. J. *1:*96–98, Jan 19, '35
Chronic edema of arm; recovery of case after surgical therapy. OLIVARES, L. Actas Soc. de cir. de Madrid *4:*223–229, April-June '35
Lymphedema of leg. BIGGS, T. J., M. J. Australia *1:*623–624, May 18, '35
Surgical treatment of lymphedema. MCINDOE, A. H. Proc. Roy. Soc. Med. *28:*1111–1126, June '35
Surgical treatment of severe forms of lymphedema of extremities; end-results. GHORMLEY, R. K. AND OVERTON, L. M. Surg., Gynec. and Obst. *61:*83–89, July '35
Lymphedema of extremities; etiology, classification and treatment; report of 300 cases. ALLEN, E. V. AND GHORMLEY, R. K. Ann. Int. Med. *9:*516–539, Nov '35
Surgical therapy of elephantiasis. FINALY, R. Nederl. tijdschr. v. geneesk. *79:*5298–5301, Nov 16, '35 also: Zentralbl. f. Chir. *63:*389–394, Feb 15, '36
Lymph vessels of human omentum; contribution to treatment of elephantiasis. DICK, W. Beitr. z. klin. Chir. *162:*296–314, '35
Therapy of elephantiasis of extremities by lymphatic drainage by buried tubes (Walther operation); 2 cases. TOURAINE, A. Bull. Soc. franc. de dermat. et syph. *42:*1771–1775, Dec '35
Surgical therapy of elephantiasis. POGGI, J.

Lymphedema – Cont.

Bol. coll. brasil. de cirurgioes *7:*17-30, May '36; in Rev. brasil. de cir., July '36

Elephantiasis of legs; therapy; preliminary report. HOMANS, J. New England J. Med. *215:*1099-1104, Dec 10, '36

Surgical therapy of elephantiasis of lower extremities. GORTER, A. J. Geneesk. tijdschr. v. Nederl.-Indie *77:*1236-1242, May 18, '37

Etiology, pathogenesis and therapy of tropical elephantiasis. LAPEYRE, J. L., J. de chir. *49:*682-717, May '37

Use of muscle pedicle flap for prevention of swelling of arm following radical operation for carcinoma of breast; preliminary report. RIENHOFF, W. F., JR. Bull. Johns Hopkins Hosp. *60:*369-371, May '37

Elephantiasis; lymphangioplasty – fate of silk. HARTLEY, H. AND HARPER, R. A. K. Brit. M. J. *2:*1066-1067, Nov 27, '37

Study of 101 cases of elephantiasis and adenolymphoceles at Negro Hospital, Buta, Belgian Congo, with special reference to surgical technic. DE GREEF, R. Ann. Soc. belge de med. trop. *18:*5-39, March 31, '38

Elephantiasis of legs; unusual case. KOCSARD, E. Dermosifilografo *13:*180-185, March '38

Elephantiasis; surgical therapy. LINARI, O. T. AND PARODI, L. M. Rev. de cir. de Buenos Aires *17:*177-180, April '38

Chronic lymphoedema. TELFORD, E. D. AND SIMMONS, H. T. Brit. J. Surg. *25:*765-772, April '38

Total excision of skin of leg in elephantiasis and closure of defect with Thiersch graft. GERGENREDER, F. A. Vestnik khir. *55:*603-609, May '38

Elephantiasis of legs; surgical therapy. GARAVANO, P. H. Semana med. *2:*1-13, July 7, '38

Hyperplastic cavernous lymphangioma of forearm; case. GAGLIARDI, P. Arch. ital. di anat. e. istol. pat. *8:*608-612, Sept '38

Surgical therapy of elephantiasis. MOLLO, L. Rassegna internaz. di clin. e terap. *19:*699, Aug 31; 765, Sept 15; 809, Sept 30; 857, Oct 15, '38

Surgical and streptococcic vaccine therapy of elephantiasis. MONTEFIORE, L. Tunisie med. *32:*434-435, Dec '38

Therapy of elephantiasis. CONDOLEON, E. Arch. ital. di chir. *51:*464-469, '38

Orthopedic surgical therapy of elephantiasis of leg; case. ZENO, L. AND MAROTTOLI, O. R. Bol. Soc. de cir. de Rosario *6:*10-18, April '39 also: An. de cir. *5:*167-175, June '39

Lymphedema – Cont.

Terminology and therapy of elephantiasis. BIRT, E. Tung-Chi med. Monatschr. *14:*205-214, June '39

Bancroftosis and surgery, with special reference to elephantiasis. LUZ, F. Arq. de cir. clin. e esper. *3:*189-201, June '39

Elephantiasis of vulva and of left leg; results of surgical therapy. ARENAS, N. AND PEPE, A. L. Semana med. *2:*664-673, Sept 21, '39

New surgical procedure for lymphedema of extremities; case. MACEY, H. B. Proc. Staff Meet., Mayo Clin. *15:*49-52, Jan 24, '40

Surgical considerations in treatment of chromic lymphedema. PRATT, G. H. Bull. New York Acad. Med. *16:*381-388, June '40

Edema of arms following radical amputation of breast. JIANU, A. AND POPESCU, C. Rev. de chir., Bucuresti *43:*469-480, July-Aug '40

Nature and cause of swelling of upper limb after radical mastectomy. DEVENISH, E. A. AND JESSOP, W. H. G. Brit. J. Surg. *28:*222-238, Oct '40

Surgical therapy of elephantiasis of legs. JUNGE, W. Arch. f. Schiffs-u. Tropan-Hyg. *44:*549-562, Dec '40

Traumatic edema of hand. SCHÖRCHER, Beitr. z. klin. Chir. *171:*176-194, '40

Surgical treatment of elephantiasis of scrotum and penis. DE SAVITSCH, E., J. Urol. *45:*216-222, Feb '41

Surgical treatment of chronic lymphedema. PRATT, G. H. AND WRIGHT, I. S. Surg., Gynec. and Obst. *72:*244-248, Feb '41

Phagedena (penis); restoration of tissue by pedicle flaps. PASSE, E. R. G. AND BARRY, T., J. Roy. Nav. M. Serv. *27:*185-189, April '41

Operation on huge scrotal elephantiasis performed by Casimiro Saez y Garcia in 1882. MULLER, F. Rev. De med. y cir. Habana *46:*373-383, Aug. 31, '41

Elephantiasis of penis. ROSS, J. C. Brit. J. Surg. *29:*194-196, Oct '41

Kondoleon operation for chronic lymphedema. TELFORD, E. D. AND SIMMONS, H. T. Lancet *2:*667, Nov. 29, '41

Elephantiasis of face cured with rubiazol (sulfonamide); case. MILIAN, G. Ann. de dernat. et syph. (Bull. Soc. dranc. de dermat. et syph) *2:*106-108, Feb '42

Chronic edema of back of hand; simulated sequel of trauma for purpose of collecting insurance. JENNY, F. Praxis *31:*365-367, June 25, '42

Congenital hypertrophy of lower extremity associated with elephantiasis; case. SHU-

Lymphedema—Cont.
MACKER, H. B. JR. Am. J. Surg. *58:*258-263, Nov '42
Lymphedema of arm following radical mastectomy for carcinoma of breast; new operation for its control. STANDARD, S. Ann. Surg. *116:*816-820, Dec '42
Study apropos of 2 cases of elephantiasis with lesions of extraordinary magnitude; therapy. HALTY, M. Rev. argent. dermatol-sif. *26:*991-1000, '42
Elephantiasis of penis and scrotum; study apropos of case treated surgically. FOSSATI, A. Bol. Soc. cir. d. Uruguay *14:*355-364, '43
Elephantiasis of penis and scrotum; clinical study of case treated surgically. FOSSATI, A. Arch. urug. de med., cir. y especialid. *24:*285-294, March '44
Surgical treatment of elephantiasis. BANKOFF, G., J. Trop. Med. *47:*49-53, Oct-Nov '44
Surgical treatment of elephantiasis. YOUNG, H. H. Tr. Am. A. Genito-Urin. Surgeons (1943) *36:*169-173, '44
Surgical treatment of lymphedema (case involving arm after removal of cancer of breast.) RANSOHOFF, J. L. Arch. Surg. *50:*269-270, May '45
Therapy of elephantiasis and lymphangiectasia of lower extremities. VARGAS MOLINARE, R. AND CORREA CASTILLO, H. Arch. Soc. cirujanos hosp. *15:*594-596, June '45 also: Rev. med. de Chile *73:*703-708, Aug '45
Surgical therapy of elephantiasis of extremities; review apropos of case. BERNALDEZ SARMIENTO, P. Rev. espan. cir., traumatol. y ortop. *3:*146-156, Sept '45
Elephantiasis and elephantine conditions; surgical notes, Bahia, 1941. DE SA OLIVEIRA, E. An. Fac. med. Bahia *4:*111-151, '44-'45
Preventation and treatment of postoperative lymphedema of arm (in breast cancer) GUTHRIE, D. AND GAGNON, G. Tr. South. S. A. (1945) *57:*460-471, '46
Postoperative lymphedema of arm (in breast cancer); (Beck operation). GUTHRIE, D. AND GAGNON, G. Ann. Surg. *123:*925-936, May '46

LYONNET, J. H.: Acute hand infections. Dia med. *13:*33-39, Jan 20, '41; 53-55, Jan 27, '41
LYONNET, J. H. AND MOREDA, J. J.: Section of flexor tendons of finger treated by reinsertion; case. Rev. Asoc. med. argent. *48:*260-264, March-April '34
LYONS, B. H.: Traumatic avulsion of penis and scrotum. Canad. M. A. J. *52:*610, June '45
LYONS, C.: Symposium on management of Cocoanut Grove burns at Massachusetts General Hospital; problems of infection and chemotherapy (especially with penicillin and sulfadiazide, sulfonamide). Ann. Surg. *117:*894-902, June '43
LYONS, C. J.: Operative procedure in cleft palate and harelip. J. Am. Dent. A. *14:*1080-1094, June '27
LYONS, C. J.: Etiology of cleft palate and lip; fundamental principles in operative procedure. J. Am. Dent. A. *17:*827-843, May '30
LYONS, C. J.: Malignant and other growths about mouth. J. Am. Dent. A. *20:*3-16, Jan '33
LYONS, D. C.: Jaw injuries. Hygeia *9:*241-244, March '31
LYONS, D. C.: Radical treatment for chronic osteomyelitis of jaws. J. Am. Dent. A. *23:*1092-1095, June '36
LYONS, D. C.: Skeletal anomalies associated with cleft palate and harelip. Am. J. Orthodontics *25:*895-897, Sept '39
LYONS, D. C.: Care of military and civilian injuries; fractures of mandible, maxilla, zygoma and other facial bones; statistical study of 1,149 cases. Am. J. Orthodontics (Oral Surg. Sect.) *29:*67-76, Feb '43
LYONS, S. S.: Vinethene (vinyl ether) burn of face. J.A.M.A. *111:*1284-1285, Oct. 1, '38
LYONS, W. R. (see WOODHALL, B.) June '46
LYTTON, H.: Subcutaneous splitting of eyelid in operative treatment of senile ectropion. Brit. J. Ophth. *29:*378-380, July '45
LYUBARSKAYA, T. E.: Heredofamilial eyelid ptosis. Sovet. nevropat., psikhiat. i psikhogig. (no. 3) *2:*103-104, '33

M

McAFEE, M. F. (see WISER, H. J.) Jan '46
McANENY, J. B. (see POHLE, E. A.) Nov '40
McARTHUR, G. A. D.: Repair of facial nerve lesion by Ballance-Duel graft. M. J. Australia *2:*1123-1124, Dec 31, '38
McARTHUR, G. A. D.: West operation (endonasal dacryocystostomy). M. J. Australia *1:*508-510, April 13, '46
McARTHUR, L. L.: Atypical operations on jaws for malignant growths. J.A.M.A. *79:*1484-1487, Oct 28, '22
MACAULEY, H. F.: Treatment of hare-lip. Brit. M. J. *2:*253-254, Aug 8, '25
MACAULEY, H. F.: Bone transplantation. Irish J. M. Sc., pp. 669-675, Dec '35
McBRIDE, E. D.: Surgical treatment of arthritic joints. Southwestern Med. *17:*321-323, Oct '33
McBRIDE, E. D.: Surgical treatment of arthri-

tis. Southwestern Med. *20:*346-349, Sept '36

McCall, J. W. and Gardiner, F. S.: Facial paralysis following mastoid surgery; 3 cases treated successfully. Laryngoscope *53:*232-239, April '43

McCalla, L. H.: Instrument for obtaining split skin grafts. J. South Carolina M. A. *40:*228, Nov '44

McCarrell, J. D. (see Beecher, H. K.) May '43

McCarroll, H. R.: Regeneration of sensation in transplanted skin. Ann. Surg. *108:*309-320, Aug '38

McCarroll, H. R.: Immediate application of free full-thickness skin graft for traumatic amputation of finger. J. Bone and Joint Surg. *26:*489-494, July '44

McCarter, W. A.: Underdeveloped maxilla and overdeveloped mandible; case report. Internat. Orthodont. Cong. *1:*483, '27 also: Internat. J. Orthodontia *13:*625, July '27

McCarthy, J. F. and Klemperer, P.: Interesting case of exstrophic bladder with neoplastic implant. J. Urology *14:*419-427, Oct '25

McCarthy, M. J. (see Vaughn, A. M.) May '43

McCarthy, W. D. and Burns, S. R.: Preparation of screw lock sectional splint with mechanical retention for fracture of jaw. J. Oral Surg. *4:*343-352, Oct '46

McCaskey, C. H.: Etiology and treatment of facial paralysis. Tr. Am. Laryng., Rhin. and Otol. Soc. *46:*285-295, '40

McCaskey, C. H.: Etiology and treatment of facial paralysis. Ann. Otol., Rhin. and laryng. *49:*199-210, March '40

McClelland, E. S.: Minor plastic surgery (face) and its relation to inferiority complex. M. Rec. *146:*419-424, Nov 17, '37

McClintock, J. A.: Osteomyelitis treated by radical saucerization and early grafting (skin). J. Indiana M. A. *39:*9-14, Jan '46

McClintock, J. A.: Reconstructive surgery following treatment of osteomyelitis by saucerization and early grafting. J. Indiana M. A. *39:*436-439, Sept '46

McClure, R. D.: Burn therapy. J. Connecticut M. Soc. *3:*479-483, Sept '39

McClure, R. D.: Severe burns. J.A.M.A. *113:*1808-1812, Nov 11, '39

McClure, R. D. and Allen, C. I.: Davidson tannic acid treatment of burns; 10 year results. Am. J. Surg. *28:*370-388, May '35

McClure, R. D. and Lam, C. R.: Problems in treatment of burns; liver necrosis as lethal factor. South. Surgeon *9:*223-234, April '40

McClure, R. D. and Lam, C. R.: Burn therapy. Am. J. Nursing *40:*498-501, May '40

McClure, R. D. and Lam, C. R.: Shock factor in burns and its treatment. Univ. Hosp. Bull., Ann Arbor *9:*62-64, July '43

McClure, R. D. and Lam, C. R.: Statistical study of minor industrial burns. J.A.M.A. *122:*909-911, July 31, '43

McClure, R. D.; Lam, C. R. and Romence, H.: Tannic acid in burns; an obsequy.Tr. Am. S. A. *62:*387-405, '44

McClure, R. D.; Lam, C. R. and Romence, H.: Tannic acid in burn therapy; an obsequy. Ann. Surg. *120:*387-398, Sept '44

McClure, R. D.; Warren, K. W. and Fallis, L. S.: Intravenous pectin solution in prophylaxis and treatment of shock. Canad. M.A.J. *51:*206-210, Sept '44

McClure, R. D. (see Harkins, H. N.) Nov '41

McClure, R. D. (see Lam, C. R.) 1944

MacCollum, D. W.: Early and late burn treatment in children. Am. J. Surg. *39:*275-311, Feb '38

MacCollum, D. W.: Wringer arm; report of 26 cases (with special reference to technic of razor skin graft). New England J. Med. *218:*549-554, March 31, '38

MacCollum, D. W.: Lop ear. J.A.M.A. *110:*1427-1430, April 30, '38

MacCollum, D. W.: Webbed fingers. Surg., Gynec. and Obst. *71:*782-789, Dec '40

MacCollum, D. W.: Burns of hand. J.A.M.A. *116:*2371-2377, May 24, '41

MacCollum, D. W.: Elevation of bridge line of nose (use of iliac bone). Surgery *12:*97-108, July '42

MacCollum, D. W.: Practical outline for burn therapy. New England J. Med. *227:*331-336, Aug 27, '42

MacCollum, D. W.: Practical outline for burn therapy. Am. J. Orthodontics (Oral Surg. Sect.) *29:*247-254, May '43

MacConaill, M. A.: Mechanics of synovial joints; hinge-joints and nature of intra-articular displacements. Irish J. M. Sc. pp. 620-626, Sept. '46

McCorkle, H.: Early care of severe thermal injuries. California and West. Med. *53:*72-74, Aug '40

McCorkle, H. J. and Silvani, H.: Selection of time for grafting of skin to extensive defects resulting from deep thermal burns. Ann. Surg. *121:*285-290, March '45

MacCormac, H.: Cancerous and precancerous conditions of the skin. Brit. M. J. *2:*457-460, Sept 13, '24

MacCormack, L. J.; Cauldwell, E. W. and Anson, B. J.: Surgical anatomy of facial nerve with special reference to parotid gland. Surg., Gynec. and Obst. *80:*620-630, June '45

McCown, P. E.: Carcinoma of bladder in exstrophy. J. Urol. *43:*533–542, April '40
McCoy, J.: Physical therapy as aid to surgical procedures on nose. Laryngoscope *37:*756–759, Oct 27
McCoy, J. D.: Factors which control treatment of dwarfed mandible. Am. J. Orthodontics *25:*850–864, Sept '39
McCrackin, R. H.: Cystic hygroma of neck; 2 cases in Bulu children. Am. J. Dis. Child. *51:*349–352, Feb '36
McCrea, L. E.: Congenital absence of penis. J. Urol. *47:*818–823, June '42
McCready, I. A. J.: Two cases of imperforate anus. Brit. M. J. *1:*290, Feb 26, '44
McCready, J. H.: Surgical treatment of laryngeal cancer. Radiology *34:*146–148, Feb '40
McCullough, J. W. S.: Burns in children. Canad. M. A. J. *17:*1176–1177, Oct '27
McCurdy, G. A.: Surgical shock. Bull. Vancouver M. A. *17:*131–138, Feb '41
McCurdy, S. L.: Harelip and cleft palate. Pennsylvania M. J. *25:*560–564, May '22 (illus.)
McCurdy, S. L.: Correction of burn scar deformity by Z-plastic method. J. Bone and Joint Surg. *6:*683–688, July '24
McCutchen, G. T.: Plastic surgical procedures. J. South Carolina M. A. *38:*35–38, Feb '42
MacDermott, E. N.: Implantation method of skin grafting. Irish J. M. Sc., pp. 613–614, Nov '31
MacDonald, A. E.: New treatment of entropion. Tr. Am. Ophth. Soc. *43:*372, '45
McDonald, J. E. and Stuart, F. A.: Stenosing tendovaginitis at radial styloid process (de Quervain's disease). J. Bone and Joint Surg. *21:*1035 Oct '39
McDonald, J. J.; Cadman, E. F. and Scudder, J.: Importance of whole blood transfusions in management of severe burns Ann. Surg. *124:*332–353, Aug '46
McDonald, J. J. and Webster, J. P.: Early covering of extensive traumatic deformities of hand and foot. Plast. and Reconstruct. Surg. *1:*49–57, July '46
McDonough, F. J.: Treatment and complications in fractures of maxillary bones. Am. J. Orthodontics *26:*162–174, Feb '40
McDougall, C.: Parasan and pituitrin in burns. Ugesk. f. Laeger *89:*59, Jan. 20, '27
McDowall, R. J. S.: Experimental shock, with special reference to anesthesia (Arris and Gale lecture). Brit. M. J. *1:*690–693, April 22, '33
McDowall, R. J. S.: Physiologic principles in treatment of traumatic shock. Practitioner *146:*21-26, Jan '41
McDowell, F.: Review of reconstructive surgery of face, 1942–1943. Laryngoscope *53:*433–439, June '43
McDowell, F.: Review of reconstructive surgery, 1943–1945. Laryngoscope *55:*239–276, June '45
McDowell, F.: Deep burns involving bones. J. Indiana M. A. *39:*108–109, Mar '46
McDowell, F., and Brown, J. B.: Syndactylism with absence of the pectoralis major. Surg., *7:*599, April '40
McDowell, F., and Brown, J. B.: Care of severe injuries of the face and jaws. Journal-Lancet (N.S.) *60:*260, June '40
McDowell, F. and Brown, J. B.: Review of reconstructive surgery of face. Laryngoscope *50:*1117–1138, Dec '40
McDowell, F., and Brown, J. B.: Persistence of function of skin grafts through long periods of growth. Surg., Gynec., and Obst., *72:*848, May '41. Also in J. Iowa State Med. Soc., *31:*457, Oct '41
McDowell, F., and Brown, J. B.: Secondary repair of cleft lips and their nasal deformities. Ann. Surg., *114:*101, July '41 also Am. J. Orthodontics and Oral Surg., *27:*712, Dec. '41
McDowell, F., and Brown, J. B.: Internal wire fixation of jaw fractures. Surg., Gynec., and Obst., *74:*227, Feb '42. Also in Am. J. Orthodontics and Oral Surg., *29:*86, Feb '43
McDowell, F., and Brown, J. B.: Massive repairs of burns with thick split skin grafts; emergency dressings with homografts. Ann. Surg., *115:*658, April '42
McDowell, F., and Brown, J. B.: Field-fire and invasive basal cell carcinoma: basal-squamous carcinoma. Surg., Gynec., and Obst., *74:*1128, June '42
McDowell, F., and Brown, J. B.: Epithelial healing and the transplantation of skin. Ann. Surg., *115:*1166, June '42. Also in Trans. American Surgical Assn., *60:*1166, June '42. Also in Digest of Treatment, *6:*481, Jan '43. Also in Anales de Cirugia, pp. 272, '42
McDowell, F., and Brown, J. B.: The plastic repair of burns with free skin grafts. Clinics, *1:*25, June '42
McDowell, F., and Brown, J. B.: Review of reconstructive surgery of the face, 1940–1942. Laryng., *52:*498, June '42. Also in Dentistry, A Digest of Practice, Feb '43. Also in *Rehabilitation of the War Injured*. Philosophical Library, Inc., New York, 1943
McDowell, F., and Brown, J. B.: Internal wire fixation of jaw fractures; second report. Surg., Gynec., and Obst., *75:*361, Sept '42. Also in Dentistry, A Digest of Practice, *3:*6, Feb '43

McDowell, Frank (with J. B. Brown): *Skin Grafting of Burns*. J. B. Lippincott Co., Phila., '43

McDowell, F. and Brown, J. B.: Surgical repair of burns. Wisconsin M. J. *43:*310–315, March '44

McDowell, F., and Brown, J. B.: Treatment of metastatic carcinoma of the neck. Ann. Surg., *119:*543, April '44

McDowell, F., and Brown, J. B.: Neck dissection for metastatic carcinoma. Surg., Gynec., and Obst., *79:*115, Aug '44

McDowell, F., Brown, J. B., Byars, L. T., and Hance, G.: Color matching of skin grafts and flaps with permanent pigment injection. Surg., Gynec., and Obst., *79:*624, Dec '44

McDowell, F., and Brown, J. B.: Simplified design for repair of single cleft lips. Surg., Gynec., and Obst., *80:*12, Jan '45

McDowell, F., and Brown, J. B.: Review of reconstructive surgery, 1943–1945. Laryng., *55:*239, June '45

McDowell, F., and Brown, J. B.: Support of the paralyzed face by fascia. Arch. Surg., *53:*420, Dec '45

McDowell, F., Brown, J. B., and Byars, L. T.: Preoperative and postoperative care in reconstructive surgery. Arch. Surg., *40:*1192, June '40

McDowell, F., Byars, L. T., and Brown, J. B.: Fundamental principles of skin grafting. The Interne, *12:*558, Sept '46

McEachern, A. C. (see de Vidas, J.) Oct '41

McEachern, J. D.: Problems of child with harelip and cleft palate. Canad. M. A. J. *18:*170–174, Feb '28

McEachern, J. S.: Exstrophy of bladder, case. Canad. M. A. J. *25:*324, Sept '31

McElroy, T.: Infections and burns. J. Oklahoma M. A. *29:*443–446, Dec '36

McEvitt, W. G.: Fibrin fixation methods of skin grafting; clinical evaluation. J. Michigan M. Soc. *44:*1347–1351, Dec '45

McEvitt, W. G. (see Straith, C. L.) May '46

McFarland, J.: Ninety tumors of parotid region, in all of which postoperative history was traced. Am. J. M. Sc. *172:*804–848, Dec '26

McFarland, J.: Three hundred mixed tumors of salivary glands, of which sixty-nine recurred. Surg, Gynec. and Obst. *63:*457–468, Oct '36

McFarland, O. W. and Connell, J. H.: Evaluation of various intravenous medications in shock therapy (use of blood serum and plasma). New Orleans M. and S. J. *93:*353–357, Jan '41

MacFee, W. F.: Salivary gland cancer. Ann. Surg. *109:*534–550, April '39

MacFee, W. F.: Full thickness defects of cheek (cancer) involving angle of mouth; method of repair. Surg., Gynec. and Obst. *76:*100–105, Jan '43

MacFee, W. F. and Baldridge, R. R.: Postoperative shock and shock-like conditions; treatment by infusion (physiologic sodium chloride solution with or without dextrose) in large volume. Ann. Surg. *91:*329–341, March '30

MacFee, W. F. and Baldridge, R. R.: Physiological considerations related to infusion treatment of shock. Ann. Surg. *100:*266–278, Aug '34

McFetridge, E. M. (see Veal, J. R.) Jan '34

McGandy, R. F.: Burn therapy. Minnesota Med. *21:*17–23, Jan '38

McGaw, W. H. and Harbin, M.: Role of bone marrow and endosteum in regeneration; experimental study of bone marrow and endosteal transplants. J. Bone and Joint Surg. *16:*816–821, Oct '34

McGivern, C. S.: Suggestions for modification of operative procedure and postoperative treatment of submucous resection. J. M. Soc. New Jersey *27:*28–31, Jan '30

McGivern, C. S.: Simple method for closing septal perforations. M. Rec. *151:*267–268, April 17, '40

McGrail, F. R. and Doherty, J. A.: Roentgenograms of mandibular condyle and zygomatic arch in jaw fractures. Am. J. Roentgenol. *45:*637–639, April '41

McGraw, A. B.: Emergency dressing for burns of extremities. Hosp. Corps Quart. (no. 2) *17:*40–44, March '44

McGraw, J. J. Jr. (see Kendrick, D. B. Jr. *et al*) July '43

MacGregor, A. B.: Simplified method of treatment of maxillary fractures (use of cap splint). Brit. Dent. J. *76:*239–241, May 5, '44

MacGregor, A. B.: Recent advances in treatment of jaw injuries. Proc. Roy. Soc. Med. *38:*201–204, March '45

MacGregor, A. B.: Extraoral pin fixation for fractures of mandible. Lancet *1:*816, June 30, '45

MacGregor, M. W.: Coagulum contact method of skin graft fixation; present status. Permanente Found. M. Bull. *4:*42–46, Feb '46

McGuffin, W. H.: Cancer of lower lip. Canad. M. A. J. *15:*1046–1049, Oct '25

MacGuire, D. P.: Branchiogenetic or bran-

chial fistulae. Am. Med. *41:*324–327, June '35
MacGuire, D. P.: Cystic hygroma of neck. Arch. Surg. *31:*301–307, Aug '35
McGuire, S.: Deformity of neck treated by transplantation of fat. S. Clin. N. America *2:*1259–1261, Oct '22
McGuire, S.: Use of appendix veriformis in formation of urethra in hypospadias. Ann. Surg. *85:*391–399, March '27
McIlroy, J. H.: Hereditary eyelid ptosis with epicanthus; case with pedigree extending over 4 generations. Proc. Roy. Soc. Med. (sect. Ophth.) *23:*17–20, Jan '30
McIndoe, A. H.: Restoration of depressed nose by grafting of cartilage; 6 cases. Proc. Roy. Soc. Med. *27:*1278–1284, July '34
McIndoe, A. H.: Surgical treatment of lymphedema. Proc. Roy. Soc. Med. *28:*1111–1126, June '35
McIndoe, A. H.: Treatment of old traumatic boney lesions of face. Surg., Gynec. and Obst. *64:*376–386, Feb. (no. 2A) '37
McIndoe, A. H.: Operation for cure of adult hypospadias. Brit. M. J. *1:*385–386, Feb 20, '37
McIndoe, A. H.: Applications of cavity grafting with skin. Surgery *1:*535–557, April '37
McIndoe, A. H.: Surgical treatment of hypospadias. Am. J. Surg. *38:*176–185, Oct '37
McIndoe, A. H.: Repair of deformities following surgical removal of malignant tumors of face with grafting. Rev. de chir. structive *8:*181–186, '38
McIndoe, A. H.: Correction of alar deformity in cleft lip. Lancet *1:*607–609, March 12, '38
McIndoe, A. H.: Review of 80 cases of mammaplasty. Rev. de chir. structive *8:*39–47, May '38
McIndoe, A. H.: Surgical and dental treatment of fractures of upper and lower jaws in wartime; review of 119 cases. Proc. Roy. Soc. Med. *34:*267–288, March '41
McIndoe, A. H.: First aid in burns. Lancet *2:*377–378, Sept 27, '41
McIndoe, A. H.: Surgical and dental treatment of jaw fractures in wartime; review based on 119 cases. Rev. san. mil., Habana *6:*178–180, April-June '42
McIndoe, A. H.: Rehabilitation in maxillofacial and plastic center. Post-Grad. M. J. *19:*161–167, July '43
McIndoe, A. H.: Skin grafts in treatment of wounds. Proc. Roy. Soc. Med. *36:*647–656, Oct '43
McIndoe, A. H.: Instrument for manipulation of central middle third of face fractures. Brit. M. J. *1:*14, Jan 1, '44
McIndoe, A. H.: The burned hand. M. Press *211:*57–61, Jan 26, '44
McIndoe, A. H. and Banister, J. B.: Operation for cure of congenital absence of vagina. J. Obst. and Gynaec. Brit. Emp. *45:*490–494, June '38
McIndoe, A. H. (see Banister, J. B.) July '38
McIndoe, A. H. (see Bonney, V.) Feb '44
McIndoe, A. H. (see Gillies, H. D.) March '33
McIndoe, A. H. (see Gillies, H. D.) Dec '33
McIndoe, A. H. (see Gillies, H. D.) April '35
McIndoe, A. H. (see Gillies, H. D.) March '39

McIndoe Operation

Vaginal aplasia (complete absence); formation of new vagina by McIndoe technic. Brea, C. A. and Castro O'Connor, R. Bol. y trab., Acad. argent. de cir. *30:*313–326, June 19, '46

McInturff, D. N. Jr.: Camphorated oil in treatment of minor industrial wounds (burns). U. S. Nav. M. Bull. *34:*70–72, Jan '36
McIntyre, A. D.: Cases of acute oral lesions treated with penicillin. Brit. Dent. J. *78:*262–266, May 4, '45
McIver, M. A.: Extensive cutaneous burns. Ann. Surg. *97:*670–682, May '33
McIver, M. A. and Haggart, W. W.: Traumatic shock; some experimental work on crossed circulation. Surg. Gynec. and Obst. *36:*542–546, April '23 (illus.)
McKay, E. D.: New technic in reconstruction following radical surgery of orbit. Am. J. Ophth. *28:*1017–1018, Sept '45
McKay, H. S.: Plastic operations on nose and forearm. S. Clin. N. America *2:*1597–1608, Dec '22 (illus.)
McKay, J. (see Sinclair, J. G.) Feb '45
McKee, G. K.: Metal anastomosis tubes in suture of tendons. Lancet *1:*659–660, May 26, '45
McKee, S. H.: Plastic repair of right lower eyelid. Canad. M. A. J. *18:*307–308, March '28
McKee, S. H.: Two cases of eyelid repair. Canad. M. A. J. *20:*506–508, May '29
McKee, T. K.: Burn therapy. Virginia M. Monthly *65:*522–523, Sept '38
McKelvey, J. L.: Abnormalities of hind end of body (including hypospadias). J. Coll. Surgeons, Australasia *1:*285–302, March '29
McKelvie, B.: Local anaesthesia in submucous resection of nasal septum. Brit. M. J. *1:*920, May 21, '27
McKenna, C. M.: Surgical correction of hypospadias. J.A.M.A. *113:*2138–2143, Dec 9, '39
McKenna, C. M. and Kiefer, J. H.: Unusual anomaly associated with hypospadias. Urol. and Cutan. Rev. *47:*14–20, Jan '43
McKenney, C. (see Rhodes, G. K.) '30

McKenney, P. W. (see Pollock, W. E. *et al*) Feb '29

MacKenty, J. E.: Surgical treatment of laryngeal cancer with an analysis of 70 cases. New York State J. Med. *22:*456–462, Oct '22

MacKenty, J. E.: Operative treatment of cleft palate; new method. Arch. Otolaryng. *10:*491-512, Nov '29

MacKenzie, A. R.: Roentgen ray therapy in fibrous ankylosis of jaws. South. M. J. *30:*816–819, Aug '37

MacKenzie, C. M.: Facial deformity and change in personality following corrective surgery. Northwest Med. *43:*230–231, Aug '44

MacKenzie, C. M.: Choice of grafts for orbital reconstruction Am. J. Ophth. *29:*867–869, July '46

MacKenzie, C. M. and Sharpless, D. H.: Cosmetic and functional aspects of bone grafting in mandibular fractures. Northwest Med. *40:*372–374, Oct '41

MacKenzie, J. R. (see Mitchell, A) Oct '32

McKenzie, W. R.: Deformity of nasal entrance. South. M. J. *35:*433–443, May '42

McKenzie, W. R.: Surgery of nose. South. M. J. *38:*42–44, Jan '45

McKillop, L. M.: Extensive epitheliomatous ulcer of side of face. M. J. Australia *2:*456, Nov 19, '21

McKillop, L. M.: Cancer of lips. M. J. Australia *1:*260–263, March 3, '28

McKim, L. H.: Hand infections. Canad. M. A. J. *18:*17–22, Jan. '28

McKim, L. H.: Transverse palmar incision. Am. J. Surg. *59:*444–446, Feb '43

McKnight, H. A.: Cancer of parotid in newborn. Am. J. Surg. *45:*128–130, July '39

McLanahan, S. (see Stone, H. B.) July '41

McLaughlin, C. W.: Curling ulcer in burns; study of intestinal ulceration associated with suprarenal damage. Arch. Surg. *27:*490–505, Sept '33

McLaughlin, C. W. Jr.: Corrective surgery. J. Omaha Mid-West. Clin. Soc. *5:*13–20, Jan '44

McLaughlin, C. W. Jr.: Traumatic aneurysm of ulnar artery; case. U. S. Nav. M. Bull. *42:*428–430, Feb '44

McLaughlin, C. W. Jr.: Major burns in naval warfare. Nebraska M. J. *31:*11–19, Jan '46

McLean, D. R. (see Forrester, C. R. G.) Feb '30

McLean, J. M.: Plastic reconstruction of upper eyelid. Am. J. Ophth. *24:*46–48, Jan '41

McLean, J. M.: Some phases of plastic surgery about eye. Mississippi Doctor *19:*335–339, Dec '41

Mac Lean, J. T. and Gerrie, J. W.: Repair of war wounds of bulbous and membranous urethra using split thickness grafts and penicillin. J. Urol. *56:*485–497, Oct '46

McLean, S. and Cannon, A. B.: Treatment of angiomata in infancy and early childhood. Internat. Clinics *3:*40–45, Sept '25

McLean, S. (see Rulison, R. H.) May '23

McLellan, D.: New technique in application of Thiersch skin grafts. Canad. M. A. J. *15:*908–910, Sept '25

MacLennan, A.: Double penis and double vulva. Glasgow M. J. *101:*287–288, May '24

MacLennan, A.: Procedure to fill in medium-sized gap in nostril. Glasgow M. J. *104:*326–327, Dec '25

MacLennan, A.: Burn therapy. Brit. M. J. *2:*590–591, Oct 1, '27

McLeod, A. C. (see Parfitt, G. J. *et al*) Feb '43

McLeod, J. and Lux, P.: Cicatricial ectropion as result of mucocele of frontal sinus; plastic repair. Arch. Ophth. *15:*994–997, June '36

MacLeod, K. M.: Novel method of digital traction in fractures. Brit. M. J. *2:*614, Oct. 26 '46

McMahon, C. G.: Suture of radial nerve, with case report. Nebraska M. J. *17:*28–30, Jan '32

McMahon, J. E.: Simple method of skin grafting. J. Malaya Br., Brit. M. A. *1:*334–335, March '38

McMichael, J.: Circulatory collapse and wound shock (Honyman Gillespie lecture). Edinburgh M. J. *48:*160–172, March '41

McMichael, J.: Treatment of surgical shock. Practitioner *147:*526–530, Aug '41

McMichael, J.: War medicine series; practical management of wound shock. Brit. M. J. *2:*671–673, Dec 5, '42

McMichael, J.: Present status of clinical problem of "shock." Brit. M. Bull. *3:*105–107, '45

McMichael, J. (see Hill, D. K. *et al*) Dec '40

McMillan, W. O.: Surgical shock. Indust. med. *9:*567–569, Nov '40

McMurray, T. P.: Uses and abuses of splints and other instruments in treatment of nerve injuries. Brit. J. Phys. Med. *5:*20–25, Feb '42

McMurtrie, K. F.: Congenital hypertrophy of right hand; case. J. Trop. Med. *35:*343–344, Nov. 15, '32

McNealy, R. W.: Cystic tumors of neck; branchial and thyroglossal cysts. S. Clin. North America *13:*1083–1100, Oct '33

McNealy, R. W.: Cystic tumors; branchial and thyroglossal cysts. J. Am. Dent. A. *29:*1808–1818, Oct 1, '42

McNealy, R. W.: Tumors of neck (other than thyroid). Proc. Interst. Postgrad. M. A., North America (1943) pp. 229–233, '44 also: J. Omaha Mid-West Clin. Soc. *5:*39–45, April '44

McNEALY, R. W. AND LICHTENSTEIN, M. E.: Fractures of metacarpals and phalanges. Surg., Gynec. and Obst. *55:*758–761, Dec '32 Also: West. J. Surg. *43:*156–161, March '35

McNEALY, R. W. AND LICHTENSTEIN, M. E.: Fractures of hand bones. Am. J. Surg. *50:*563–570, Dec '40

McNichol, J. W. (see HARDY, S. B.) April '44

McNICHOLS, W. A.: Treatment of fractures of superior and inferior maxilla. Illinois M. J. *90:*179–185, Sept '46

McNICHOLS, W. A. (see BURKE, H. D. *et al*) Nov-Dec '45

McPHEETERS, H. O.: Skin grafting by seed implantation. Minnesota Med., *17:*360–361, June '34

McPHEETERS, H. C. AND NELSON, H.: Blanket split skin graft for covering large granulating areas. J.A.M.A. *117:*1173–1174, Oct. 4, '41

McQUILLAN, ARTHUR S.: *Surgery of the Head and Neck*. Oxford Press, London, '42

McQUILLAN, A. S. (see WINTER, L. *et al*) Sept '45

MACRAE, A.: Webster's operation for entropion of upper lid. Brit. J. Ophth. *12:*25–30, Jan '28

McRITCHIE, P.: Absence of palpebral fissure of eyelids. Am. J. Ophth. *12:*744–745, Sept '29

McSHANE, J. K. (see DORRANCE, G. M.) Dec '28

McSWAIN, G.: Surgical shock. J. Tennessee M. A. *22:*135–137, Aug '29

McSWAIN, G. H.: Burn therapy. J. Florida M. A. *24:*165–167, Sept '37

MACVICAR, D. N. (see DRIVER, J. R.) Feb '43

McWATTERS, R. C.: Cases of hand surgery. Indian M. Gaz. *65:*276, May '30

McWHORTER, G. L.: Operation on two cases of secondary carcinoma and on one case of primary cystadenoma of parotid gland; relation of lobes of parotid to facial nerve. S. Clin. N. Amer. *7:*489–505, June '27

McWhorter, G. L.: Use of cortical inlay bonegraft in non-union; importance and technic of avoiding encircling bone sutures; clinical and experimental study. S. Clin. N. Amer., *8:*555–560, June, '28

McWHORTER, G. L.: Operative treatment for extensive hypospadias. S. Clin. N. Amer. *10:*275–282, April '30

McWILLIAMS, C. A.: Values of various methods of bone graftings judged by 1,390 reported cases. Ann. Surg. *74:*286, Sept '21

McWILLIAMS, C. A.: Principles of 4 types of skin grafting; with an improved method of treating total avulsion of scalp. J.A.M.A. *83:*183–189, July 19, '24

McWILLIAMS, C. A.: Free, full-thickness skin grafts. Ann. Surg. *84:*237–245, Aug '26

McWILLIAMS, C. A.: Facial disfigurements. Am. J. Surg. *1:*76–79, Aug '26

McWILLIAMS, C. A.: Recent nasal fractures. New Orleans M. and S. J. *85:*336–339, Nov '32

McWILLIAMS, C. A. AND DUNNING, H. S.: Rhinoplasty and cheek, chin, and lip plastics with tubed, temporal-pedicled, forehead flaps. Surg., Gynec. and Obst. *36:*1–10, Jan '23 (illus.)

McWILLIAMS, H. (see DORRANCE, G. M. *et al*) April '24

MACAGGI, D.: True and false Dupuytren contracture in relation to traumatic etiogenesis of condition; interest from medicolegal viewpoint. Policlinico (sez. chir.) *40:*743–759, Dec '33

MACARTNEY, C.: Some minor nasal and aural injuries in recreations. J. Roy. Nav. M. Serv. *26:*139–143, April '40

MACERA, J. M. AND FEIGUES, I.: Craniofacial dysostosis and multiple malformations. Semana med. *2:*793–800, Sept 12, '29

MACEWEN, J. A. C.: Extroversion of bladder treated by vesico-colostomy. Lancet *1:*531, March 18, '22

MACEWEN, J. A. C.: Case of true epispadias. Brit. M. J. *1:*454, March 7, '25

MACEWEN, J. A. C.: Rectal prolapse; treatment by injection. Brit. M. J. *1:*633, April 14, '28

MACEY, H. B.: New surgical procedure for lymphedema of extremities; case. Proc. Staff Meet., Mayo Clin. *15:*49–52, Jan 24, '40

MACEY, H. B.: New instrument for passing portions of tendons and fasciae latae. Am. J. Surg. *47:*686, March '40

MACEY, H. B.: Burn therapy in warfare. Proc. Staff Meet., Mayo Clin. *18:*241–246, July 28, '43

MACEY, H. B.: Practical application of plastic surgery to extremities. S. Clin. North America *23:*1030–1058, Aug '43

MACEY, H. B. (see BLACK, J. R.) Aug '37

MACFARLANE, R. G.: Human fibrin as burn dressing. Brit. M. J. *2:*541–543, Oct 30, '43

MACGREGOR, A. R. (see WILSON, W. C. *et al*) April '38

MACHADO, L. M.: New technic for formation of artificial vagina. Rev. de gynec. e d'obst. *30:*782–789, Oct '36

MACHADO, L. M.: Artificial vagina constructed from Douglas pouch; question of priority. Rev. de gynec. e d'obst. *31:*500–501, Dec '37

MACHADO, R.: Technic in rhinoplasty. Rev. brasil. de med. e pharm. *3:*305–310, July-Aug '27

MACHADO, R.: Plastic surgery of nose. Tribuna med. *33:*239–244, Oct 15, '29

MACHADO, W.: Endometriosis of laparotomy ci-

catrix; case. Bol. San. Sao Lucas *7:*179–184, June '46
MACHAN, V. Y.: Surgical therapy of parotid fistula according to Sapozhkov method. Vestnik khir. *49:*94–95, '37
MACHECA, H. (see LEVY, W. E.) May-June '28
MACHECA, H. (see LEVY, W. E.) May '25

Machek Operation

Machek operation in eyelid ptosis. GIFFORD, S. R. Arch. Ophth. *8:*495-502, Oct '32

MACIEL, H.: Albuminotherapy, plasma therapy and blood transfusion in burns. Rev. brasil. de cir. *12:*375–384, June '43 also: Bol. Col. brasil. de cirurgioes *18:*195–204, July '43
MACINDOE, N. M.: Cure of nasolacrimal obstruction. Tr. Ophth. Soc. Australia (1944) *4:*149, '46
MACINDOE, P. H. Fractures of malar bone. M. J. Australia *1:*317–319, April 10, '43
MACK, C. H. AND CONNELLY, J. H.: Fractures of mandible. U. S. Nav. M. Bull. *32:*31–36, Jan '34
MACKENZIE, D.: Treatment of burns. Brit. M. J. *1:*421–422, March 5, '27
MACKENZIE, G. W.: Syphilis as complicating factor in surgery of nasal septum. Hahneman. Monthly *62:*345–349, May '27
MACKIE, T. J.: Non-specific stimulation of natural antibody in treatment of shock. J. Hygiene *24:*176–188, Oct '25
MACKUTH, E.: Method of restoring function to finger stiffened by venous phlegmon of hand. Arch. f. klin. Chir. *185:*370–372, '36
MACKTA, L.: Acrylic half-splint for jaw injuries. Bull. U. S. Army M. Dept. (no. 72) pp. 81–83, Jan '44
MACLURE, A. F. (see COX, L. B.) July '35
MACLURE, F.: Crush-burns of hand. J. Coll. Surgeons, Australasia *1:*233–235, Nov '28
MACLURE, F.: Diagnosis of depressed zygomatic fracture. Australian and New Zealand J. Surg. *2:*415–416, April '33
MACLURE, F.: Reduction of depressed zygomatic fracture. Australian and New Zealand J. Surg. *2:*420, April '33
MACLURE, F.: Gunshot wounds of face and jaws. M. J. Australia *1:*62–64, Jan 13, '40
MACNAUGHTON, B. F.: Rhinophyma, case. Canad. M. A. J. *24:*271–272, Feb '31
MACOMBER, D. W.: Recent developments in plastic surgery. Rocky Mountain M. J. *35:*532–537, July '38
MACOMBER, D. W.: Ear reconstruction (graft). Rocky Mountain M. J. *36:*37–40, Jan '39
MACOMBER, D. W.: Mastoptosis (with description of surgical reconstruction of case). Rocky Mountain M. J. *38:*50–52, Jan '41
MACOMBER, D. W.: Burn progress. Rocky Mountain M. J. *40:*34–36, Jan '43
MACOMBER, D. W.: Surgical cure of acne rosacea and rhinophyma with skin grafting Rocky Mountain M. J. *43:*466–467, June '46
MACOMBER, D. W.: Reconstruction of bony defects, with special reference to cancellous iliac bone. Surg. Gynec. and Obst. *83:*761–766, Dec '46
MACOMBER, M. H.: Adequate nutrition gains emphasis as vital factor in burn surgery. Hospitals (no. 7) *19:*73–74, July '45
MACOMBER, W. B.: Plastic considerations of burn scars and contractures of hand and forearm. Am. Acad. Orthop. Surgeons, Lect., pp. 174–179, '44
MACPHERSON, N. S.: Skin transplantation. J. Christian M. A. *20:*136–140, Sept '45
MACRAE, D. JR.: Prevention and treatment of wound shock in theatre of army operations. J. Iowa M. Soc. *11:*394, Oct '21
MACY, J. W.: Agranulocytosis associated with surgical infections; case report with comments. S. Clin. North America *14:*1271–1277, Oct '34
MACZEWSKI, S.: Formation of artificial vagina by Kirschner-Wagner operation. Polska gaz. lek. *12:*829–830, Oct 22, '33
MACZEWSKI, S. AND GRUCA, A.: Formation of artificial vagina from epidermis. Ginek. polska *11:*577–579, April–June '32
MADAN, K. E.: Senile blepharospasm. Brit. J. Ophth. *11:*385–386, Aug '27
MADDOCK, W. G.: Use of tannic acid dressing for Ollier-Thiersch graft beds. J.A.M.A. *97:*102, July 11, '31

Madelung's Syndrome

Operative treatment in Madelung deformity of hand; case. TANCREDI, G. Bull. e atti. d. r. Accad. med. di Roma *57:*153–158, June '31
Bilateral congenital dysmorphosis of wrists (Madelung's disease); roentgen study of case. ROUDIL, G. *et al.* J. de radiol. et d'electrol. *20:*241–245, April '36

MADER, J. W. (see ECKERT, G. A.) July '42
MADHOK, G. D.: Ectopia vesicae. Indian M. Gaz. *66:*633, Nov '31
MADIER, J.: Treatment of anterior balanic and penile hypospadias with Beck-von Hacker operation. J. de chir. *18:*234–242, Sept '21 (illus.) J.A.M.A. *78:*688, March 4, '22 (abstr.)
MADLER, N. A.: Burn treatment (use of tannic acid). Colorado Med. *30:*46–49, Feb '33
MADSEN, E.: Extension splint for fingers. Nord. med. (Hospitalstid.) *14:*1650, May 30, '42

MAEKAWA, S. AND HASHIMOTO, T.: Synechia of frenum linguae. Oto-rhino-laryng. *14:*666, Sept. '41
MAES, U.: Curling's ulcer; duodenal ulcer following superficial burns. Ann. Surg. *91:*527-532, April '30
MAES, U.: Curling's ulcer in burns; with report of 2 cases. M. Rec. and Ann. *24:*564-568, June '30
MAES, U. AND RIVES, J. D.: Operation for complete prolapse of rectum. Surg., Gynec. and Obst. *42:*594-599, May '26
MAFFEI, E. (see JACOB, A. C.) Sept-Oct '45
MAGDELEINE, J. (see RUPPE, C.) Jan '27
MAGDELEINE, J. (see FLURIN, H.) Dec '27
MAGGIOROTTI, U.: Congenital fistulas and cysts of neck with report of 17 cases Valsalva *16:*337-365, Sept '40
MAGGIOROTTI, U.: Procaine hydrochloride truncular anesthesia of nerves of nasal lobule; technic. Boll. d. mal. d. orecchio, d. gola, d. naso *59:*17-18, Jan '41
MAGGIOROTTI, U.: New plastic method for correction of velopharyngeal symphysis stricture. Boll. d. mal. d. oreccio, d. gola, d. naso *60:*194-196, May '42
MAGLIULO, A.: Cysts and fistulae of median cervical line. Sperimentale, Arch. di biol *82:*455-504, '28
MAGLIULO, A.: Effect of periarterial sympathectomy on growth of autoplastic skin grafts; experiments. Sperimentale, Arch. di biol. *82:*685-705, '28
MAGNONI, A.: Origin of congenital fistulas of bridge of nose. Acta oto-laryng. *27:*174-180, '39
MAGNUS, J. A.: Correction by 2 strips of fascia lata, eyelid ptosis. Brit. J. Ophth. *20:*460-464, Aug '36
MAGNUSON, P. B.: Finger fractures. Tr. Sect. Surg., General and Abd., A.M.A., pp. 79-84, '28 Also: J.A.M.A. *91:*1339-1340, Nov. 3, '28
MAGNUSSON, R. (see JORDE, A.) Aug '41
MAGUIRE, D. L.: Hand infections. South. Surgeon *9:*11-20, Jan '40
MAGUIRE, D. L. JR.: Extensive second and third degree burns. J. South Carolina M. A. *41:*246-248, Oct '45
MAHAFFEY, H.: Symptoms and control of traumatic shock. Kentucky M. J. *36:*137-142, April '38
MAHAFFEY, H.: Symptoms and control of traumatic shock. Anesth. and Analg. *18:*196-205, July-Aug '39

Maher Operation

Surgical therapy of entropion and trichiasis according to Maher method. GALEWSKA, S.

Maher Operation – Cont.
AND LITAUER, R. Rev. internat. du trachome *13:*41-47, Jan '36
Modification of Maher's operation for entropion. ARKIN, V. Klin. Monatsbl. f. Augenh. *77:*677-680, Nov '26
Modification of Maher's operation (entropion). VON GERNET, R. Klin. Monatsbl. f. Augenh. *78:*73, Jan '27

MAHLSTEDT, H.: Heredity of submucous cleft of palate. Ztschr. f. Laryng., Rhin., Otol. *26:*347-352, '35
MAHONEY, E. B.: Experimental and clinical shock, with special reference to its treatment by intravenous injection of preserved plasma. Ann. Surg. *108:*178-193, Aug '38
MAHONEY, E. B. AND HOWLAND, J. W.: Clinical aspects of shock therapy. Surgery *13:*188-198, Feb '43
MAHONEY, E. B. AND HOWLAND, J. W.: Treatment of severely burned patient, with special reference to controlled protein therapy. New York State J. Med. *43:*1307-1315, July 15, '43
MAHONEY, E. B.; KINGSLEY, H. D. AND HOWLAND, J. W.: Treatment of experimental shock by intravenous injection of dilute, normal and concentrated plasma. Surg., Gynec. and Obst. *74:*319-325, Feb. (no. 2A) '42
MAHONEY, P. L.: Retrobulbar abscess complicating submucous resection. Laryngoscope *42:*199-200, March '32
MAIER, R. L.: Human bite infections of hand. Ann. Surg. *106:*423-427, Sept '37
MAILER, R.: Chronic lymphatic edema and its treatment by Kondoleon operation. Glasgow M. J. *121:*213-217, June '34
MAIR, G.B.: Use of whole skin grafts as substitute for fascial sutures in treatment of hernias; preliminary report. Am. J. Surg. *69:*352-365, Sept '45
MAIR, G. B.: Analysis of series of 454 inguinal hernias, with special reference to morbidity and recurrence after whole skin graft method. Brit. J. Surg. *34:*42-48, July '46
MAIRANO, M. AND VIRANO, G.: Cranioplasty with autografts of elastic cartilage; experiments. Clin. chir. *32:*1687-1705, Dec '29
MAIRE, R. (see ALAJOUANINE, T. *et al*) Dec '30
MAIRE, R. (see WEILL, J.) March '34
MAISONNAVE, R. (see GONZALEZ LOZA, M.) June '43
MAITLAND, A. I. L.: War burns; survey of treatment and results in 100 cases. J. Roy. Nav. M. Serv. *28:*3-17, Jan '42
MAITLAND, G. R.: Treatment of fractures of jaws. J. Michigan M. Soc. *29:*915-917, Dec '30
MAITRE, R. (see LERICHE, R. *et al*) May '35
MAJ, G.: Speed of repair of wounds of mucosa in

mouth. Boll. Soc. ital. biol. sper. *17:*322, May '42

MAJER, E.: Frekasan (tannin preparation) in burns. Munchen. med. Wchnschr. *86:*1433-1435, Sept 22, '39

MAJOR, G.: Kirschner traction in treatment of maxillary fractures. J.A.M.A. *110:*1252-1254, April 16, '38

MAJOR, GLENN: *Fractures of the Jaws and Other Facial Bones.* C. V. Mosby Co., St. Louis, 1943

MAKAI, E.: Local burn therapy. Munchen. med. Wchnschr. *76:*574-575, April 5, '29

MAKAR, N.: Correction of lop-ear; case. J. Egyptian M. A. *13:*299-308, July '30

MAKKAS, M.: Therapy of ectopic bladder. Beitr. z. klin. Chir. *163:*554-570, '36

MAKEL, H. P.: Shock therapy. Mil. Surgeon *80:*436-447, June '37

MAKHLIN, I. M.: Operations for trachomatous eversion of eyelids and trichiasis. Sovet. med. (nos. 1-2) *6:*22-23, '42

Makkas Operation

Makkas operation for exstrophy of bladder in child; case. TAVERNIER. Lyon chir. *29:*587-591, Sept-Oct '32

Modification of Makkas operation in therapy of exstrophy of bladder. MATOLAY, G. Zentralbl. f. Chir. *66:*1130-1133, May 20, '39

Makkas operation in exstrophy of bladder. GORODINSKIY, D. M. Novy khir. arkhiv *33:*290-294, '35

Makkas operation in case of exstrophy of bladder. WALLER, J. B. Zentralbl. f. Chir. *51:*1841-1842, Aug 23, '24

Makkas-Lengemann Operation

Treatment of exstrophy of bladder by Makkas-Lengemann technic. GAZA, W. V. Arch. f. klin. Chir. *126:*515-522, '23

MAKSUD: Autoplastic graft on elbow by Italian method; case. Cong. internat. de med. trop. et d'hyg., Compt. rend (1928) *3:*385, '31

MALAN, R.: Comparison of spinal cord and nerve grafts in repair of loss of peripheral nerve substance; preliminary report. Boll. e mem. Soc. piemontese di chir. *9:*92-99, '39

MALAN, R.: Results of repair of loss of peripheral nerve substance; experimental study. Arch. per le sc. med. *70:*587-605, Dec '40

MALAPLATE. (see ROCHER, H. L.) Feb '29

MALAQUIAS, G.: Results of sulfonamides and penicillin in serious burns. Folha med. *26:*79-80, May 25, '45

MALBEC, E. F.: Cosmetic surgery in correction of protruding pinna, also of nose. Semana med. *1:*170-175, Jan 11, '34

MALBEC, E. F.: Esthetic surgery; cases. Semana med. *1:*31-51, Jan 2, '36

MALBEC, E. F.: Plastic surgery of ears; cases (and face), (and nose). Semana med. *2:*718-728, Sept 10, '36

MALBEC, E. F.: Esthetic surgery (of nose); cases. Semana med. *2:*1632-1643, Dec 10, '36

MALBEC, E. F.: Plastic surgery of ptosis of upper left eyelid; case in child. Semana med. *1:*521-525, Feb 18, '37

MALBEC, E. F.: Plastic surgery of facial wrinkles; case. Semana med. *1:*1225-1227, April 29, '37

MALBEC, E. F.: Esthetic surgery of nose; results in cases. Semana med. *2:*280-289, July 29, '37

MALBEC, E. F.: Plastic surgery. Semana med. *2:*1385-1394, Dec 16, '37

MALBEC, E. F.: Method of obliterating depressions of face; case. Semana med. *1:*600-602, March 17, '38

MALBEC, E. F.: Plastic surgery of ear pavilion. Semana med. *1:*994-1001, May 5, '38

MALBEC, E. F.: Ivory prosthesis in partial rhinoplasty; cases. Semana med. *1:*1374-1382, June 16, '38

MALBEC, E. F.: Plastic surgery of wrinkles. Semana med. *2:*289-294, Aug 4, '38

MALBEC, E. F.: Deformities of ear lobe and their surgical correction. Semana med. *2:*623-631, Sept 15, '38

MALBEC, E. F.: Saddle nose; surgical therapy. Semana med. *2:*860-862, Oct 13, '38

MALBEC, E. F.: Plastic and esthetic surgery of ear; nose and face cases. Semana med. *1:*83-95, Jan 12, '39

MALBEC, E. F.: Corrective surgery of nasal deformities. Semana med. *1:*365-375, Feb 16, '39

MALBEC, E. F.: Mental and psychic condition of certain malformed individuals; value of plastic surgery. Semana med. *1:*716-722, March 30, '39

MALBEC, E. F.: Plastic surgery of nose; case. Dia med. *11:*300-301, April 10, '39

MALBEC, E. F.: Marble prosthesis in correcting saddle nose; 2 cases. Semana med. *1:*1136-1138, May 18, '39

MALBEC, E. F.: Psychic repercussion of facial defects; value of plastic surgery. Semana med. *2:*94-99, July 13, '39

MALBEC, E. F.: Use of marble in correction of nasal deformities. Semana med. *2:*1266-1270, Nov 30, '39

MALBEC, E. F.: Plastic surgery; psychic repercussion and social aspects of deformed ears. Semana med. *2:*1506-1509, Dec 28, '39

MALBEC, E. F.: Esthetic and plastic surgery; historical review. Semana med. *1:*1141-1147,

May 9, '40
MALBEC, E. F.: Function of esthetic sense in plastic surgery of nose. Semana med. *2:*997–1008, Oct 31, '40
MALBEC, E. F.: Partial rhinoplasty using marble prosthesis; cases. Semana med. *2:*1173–1182, Nov 21, '40
MALBEC, E. F.: Plastic surgery of auricle. Semana med. *2:*1479–1482, Dec 26, '40
MALBEC, E. F.: Plastic surgery of auricle; postoperative care and errors committed during surgery. Semana med. *1:*219–221, Jan 23, '41
MALBEC, E. F.: Duraluminum in plastic surgery of nose. Semana med. *1:*1016–1019, May 1, '41
MALBEC, E. F.: Plastic correction of loss of nasal septum. Dia med. *13:*682, July 21, '41
MALBEC, E. F.: Osseous autotransplantations in partial rhinoplasties. Semana med. *2:*350–354, Aug 7, '41
MALBEC, E. F.: Plastic surgery of external ear; case (and nose). Prensa med. argent. *28:*1700–1702, Aug 20, '41
MALBEC, E. F.: Plastic surgery in loss of ear and nose substance. Semana med. *2:*714–716, Sept 18, '41
MALBEC, E. F.: Gynecomastia; surgical therapy of 2 cases. Semana med. *2:*988–989, Oct 23, '41
MALBEC, E. F.: Rhinoplasty by Indian method. Semana med. *2:*1186–1188, Nov 13, '41
MALBEC, E. F.: Plastic surgery of face; 2 cases. Semana med. *2:*1311–1313, Nov 27, '41
MALBEC, E. F.: Bone autografts in partial rhinoplasties. Arq. de cir. clin. e exper. *6:*163–171, April–June '42
MALBEC, E. F.: Plastic surgery of face; 5 cases. Arq. de cir. clin. e exper. *6:*503–512, April–June '42
MALBEC, E. F.: Gynecomastia; surgical therapy of 2 cases. Arq. de cir. clin. e exper. *6:*686–689, April–June '42
MALBEC, E. F.: Plastic surgery of ear and nose. Semana med. *2:*426–431, Aug 20, '42
MALBEC, E. F.: Plastic repair of nostril. Semana med. *2:*625–627, Sept 10, '42
MALBEC, E. F.: Free full thickness graft in case of lupus erythematosus. Dia med. *14:*1119–1120, Oct 26, '42
MALBEC, E. F.: Epithelioma of nose; free graft of whole skin; case. Prensa med. argent. *29:*1763-1765, Nov 4, '42
MALBEC, E. F.: Free full thickness skin graft in nasal cancer; case. Semana med. *2:*1489–1491, Dec 17, '42
MALBEC, E. F.: Free graft of full thickness skin in case of lupus erythematosus of nose. Semana med. *1:*1232–1235, June 3, '43
MALBEC, E. F.: Osteocartilaginous homogenous grafts in partial rhinoplasties. Dia med. *15:*644–645, June 21, '43
MALBEC, E. F.: Free full thickness skin graft; case in cicatrix. Prensa med. argent. *30:*1576–1577, Aug 18, '43
MALBEC, E. F.: Fibrokeloid cicatrix after attempted removal of pilous nevus; free full thickness skin graft; case. Dia med. *15:*1100, Sept 13, '43
MALBEC, E. F.: Dermoid cysts of nasal dorsum; plastic surgery in cases. Semana med. *2:*788–792, Sept 30, '43
MALBEC, E. F.: Esthetic surgery and care of accident cases. Prensa med. argent. *30:*2359–2361, Dec 8, '43
MALBEC, E. F.: Fibrokeloid cicatrix after attempted removal of pilous nevus; free full thickness skin graft; case. Semana med. *2:*1416–1417, Dec 23, '43
MALBEC, E. F.: Lupus erythematosus of face; free skin graft in case. Dia med. *16:*160, Feb 21, '44
MALBEC, E. F.: Rhinophyma. Prensa med. argent. *31:*2274–2284, Nov 8, '44
MALBEC, E. F.: Gynecomastia; new surgical technic. Dia med. *17:*498–500, May 28, '45
MALBEC, E. F.: Gynecomastia; surgical technic. Prensa med. argent. *32:*1759–1763, Sept 7, '45
MALBEC, E. F.: Gynecomastia; surgical technics. Rev. Fac. de med., Bogota *14:*380–391, Dec '45
MALBEC, E. F.: Saddle nose; correction by means of tantalum prosthesis; case Bol. y trab., Soc. argent. de cirujanos *7:*173–177, '46 also: Rev. Asoc. med. argent. *60:*361–363, May 30 '46
MALBEC, E. F.: Technic of plastic surgery hypertrophy breast. Dia med. *18:*375–376, April 15, '46
MALBEC, E. F.: Micrognathia; paladon prosthesis in case. J. Internat. Coll. Surgeons *9:*412–415, May–June '46 Bol. y trab., Acad. argent. de cir. *30:*151–156, May 15 '46
MALBEC, E. F.: Precise technic of local anesthesia in rhinoplasties. J. Internat. Coll. Surgeons *9:*495–505, Jul–Aug '46 also: Prensa med. argent. *33:*1594–1601, Aug 2, '46
MALBEC, E. F.: Gynecomastia; new surgical technic. J. Internat. Coll. Surgeons *9:*652–654, Sept–Oct '46
MALBEC, E. F. (see REBELO NETO, J.) Oct '41

Malbec Operation

Correction of protruding ears; Malbec technic. BEAUX, A. R. Presna med. argent. *32:*2314–2320, Nov 23, '45
Plastic therapy of rhinomegaly and rhinokyphosis using Malbec technics. DEL POZO R.,

Malbec Operation – Cont.
D. D. Bol. y trab., Soc. argent. de cirujanos *6:*522–539, '45
Auriculoplasties in therapy of protruding ears by Malbec technic. DEL POZO, R. D. Bol. y trab. Soc. argent. de cirujanos *7:*205–214, '46 also: Rev. Asoc. med argent. *60:*460–463, June 15, '46

MALBRAN, J.: Surgical correction of eyelid ptosis. Semana med. *2:*1456–1462, Dec 18, '41
MALCOLM, J. D.: Surgical shock. Proc. Roy. Soc. Med. (Sect. Obst. and Gynec.) *15:*71–80, July '22
MALCOLM, R. B. AND BENSON R. E.: Branchial cysts; with report of 2 cases of cyst of cervical sinus. Surgery *7:*187–203, Feb '40
MALEPLATE. (see PONROY, *et al*) July '34
MALINIAC, J. W. (or MALINIAK, J. W.)
MALINIAK, J. W.: Comparative study of ivory and organic transplants in rhinoplasty; endonasal operative technic of some nasal deformities with report of cases. Laryngoscope *34:*882–900, Nov '24
MALINIAK J. W.: Use of ivory in rhinoplasty. Arch. Otolaryng. *1:*599–611, June '25
MALINIAK, J. W.: Causes of failure in corrective rhinoplasty – lantern demonstration. Laryngoscope *35:*832–843, Nov '25 also: Ohio State M. J. *21:*807–814, Nov '25
MALINIAK, J. W.: Prevention and correction of nasal deformities. Eye, Ear, Nose and Throat Month. *5:*689, Jan '27
MALINIAK, J. W.: Facial reconstructive surgery with presentation of cases and lantern slide demonstration. Laryngoscope *37:*157–169, March '27 also: M. Times, New York *55:*57; 72, March '27 also: J. M. Soc. New Jersey *24:*349–355, June '27
MALINIAK, J. W.: Prevention and correction of nasal deformities following submucous resection; presentation of cases. Arch. Otolaryng. *6:*320–329, Oct '27
MALINIAK, J. W.: Correction of facial deformities. M. Rev. of Rev. *33:*571–578, Dec '27
MALINIAK, J. W.: Plastic and reconstructive procedures in rhinology. New York State J. Med. *28:*6–9, Jan 1, '28
MALINIAK, J. W.: Correction of facial deformities. Rhinoplasty, a few statistical data. Eye, Ear, Nose and Throat Monthly *9:*194–198, June '30 also: Laryngoscope *40:*495–501, July '30
MALINIAK, J. W.: Comparative value of surgical procedures in repair of skin defects (including grafts). M. J. and Rec. *133:*82–84, Jan 21, '31
MALINIAK, J. W.: Rhinophyma, treatment and complications. Arch. Otolaryng. *13:*270–274, Feb '31
MALINIAK, J. W.: Plastic surgery; indications and relationship to other specialities. Rev. de chir. plastique, pp. 100–110, July '31 also: J. M. Soc. New Jersey *28:*679–683, Sept '31
MALINIAK, J. W.: Simplified method for correction of dishface. Laryngoscope *41:*715–717, Oct '31
MALINIAK, J. W.: Pendulous breasts. M. Times and Long Island M. J. *59:*355–359, Oct '31
MALINIAK, J. W.: Plastic surgery and specialists. Am. J. Surg. *14:*483–488, Nov '31
MALINIAK, J. W.: Correction of depressions of nose by transposition of lateral cartilages; new method. Arch. Otolaryng. *15:*280–284, Feb '32
MALINIAK, J. W.: Important factors in surgery of common facial deformities. Eye, Ear, Nose and Throat Monthly *11:*95–99, April '32
MALINIAK, J. W.: Important factors in surgery of acquired and congenital facial deformities. J. M. Soc. New Jersey *29:*314–323, April '32
MALINIAK, J. W.: Is surgical restoration of the aged face justified? Indications-method of repair-end results. M. J. and Rec. *135:*321–324, April 6, '32
MALINIAK, J. W.: Plastic repair of pendulous breasts. M. J. and Rec. *136:*312–316, Oct 19, '32
MALINIAK, J. W.: Cartilage and ivory; indications and contraindications for their use as nasal support. Arch. Otolaryng. *17:*649–657, May '33
MALINIAK, J. W.: Problems in plastic surgery. Rev. de chir. plastique, pp. 36–42, May '33 also: J. M. Soc. New Jersey *30:*439–441, June '33
MALINIAK, J. W.: New instruments for use of rib cartilage grafts in rhinoplasty. Arch. Otolaryng. *18:*79–82, July '33
MALINIAK, JACQUES, W.: *Sculpture in the Living*. Lancet Press, New York, 1934
MALINIAK, J. W.: Facts and fallacies of cosmetic surgery (paraffin injections, hair removal, face-lifting, nose-remodeling, etc.). Hygeia *12:*200–202, March '34
MALINIAK, J. W.: Asymmetrical deformities of breast. Ann. Surg. *99:*743–752, May '34
MALINIAK, J. W.: Legal and illegal aspects of plastic surgery. M. Times and Long Island M. J. *62:*165–170, June '34
MALINIAK, J. W.: Aspects of plastic surgery seldom considered. M. Rec. *139:*653–655, June 20, '34
MALINIAK, J. W.: Prevention of necrosis in plastic repair of pendulous breasts. Am. J. Surg. *26:*292–297, Nov '34

MALINIAK, J. W.: Restorative surgery of breast and face. Bull. Assoc. d. med. de lang. franc. de l'Amerique du Nord *1:*199–206, April '35

MALINIAK, J. W.: Your child's face and future. Hygeia *13:*410–413, May '35

MALINIAK, J. W.: Pendulous breast; comparative values of present-day methods of repair and procedure of choice. Arch. Surg. *31:*587–600, Oct '35

MALINIAK, J. W.: Plastic surgeon and crime. J. Crim. Law and Criminol. *26:*594–600, Nov '35

MALINIAK, J. W.: Repair of facial defects with special reference to source of skin grafts. Rev. de chir. structive, pp. 431–439, Dec '36 also: Arch. Surg. *34:*897–908, May '37

MALINIAK, J. W.: Plastic repair of pendulous breast. Vida nueva *39:*327–336, May 15, '37

MALINIAC, J. W.: Breast deformities; anatomic and physiologic considerations in plastic repair. Am. J. Surg. *39:*54–61, Jan '38

MALINIAC, J. W.: Reconstruction of deformed chin in its relationship to rhinoplasty; dermal graft—procedure of choice. Am. J. Surg. *40:*583–587, June '38

MALINIAC, J. W.: Pigmented nevi, with special reference to their surgical therapy. Am. J. Surg. *45:*507–510, Sept '39

MALINIAC, J. W.: Prevention and treatment of late sequelae in corrective rhinoplasty. Am. J. Surg. *50:*84–91, Oct '40

MALINIAC, J. W.: Plastic surgery in war; preparedness of profession at large. M. Rec. *154:*325–326, Nov 5, '41

MALINIAC, J. W.: Surgical treatment of lupus; case (grafting). Am. J. Surg. *55:*123–125, Jan '42

MALINIAC, J. W.: Plastic surgery of nose. Dis. Eye, Ear, Nose and Throat *2:*102–106, April '42

MALINIAC, J. W.: Free skin grafts versus flaps in surface defects of face and neck. Am. J. Surg. *58:*100–109, Oct '42

MALINIAC, J. W.: Early treatment of war wounds, with emphasis on prevention of deformities (grafting). Hebrew M. J. *1:*183, '43

MALINIAC, J. W.: Scope of plastic surgery in war. Bol. d. Hosp. policia mac. *2:*65–68, April 1, '43

MALINIAC, J. W.: 2 cases of pseudogynecomastia in male, with surgical reconstruction. J. Clin. Endocrinol. *3:*364–366, June '43

MALINIAC, J. W.: Arterial supply of breast; revised anatomic data relating to reconstructive surgery. Arch. Surg. *47:*329–343, Oct '43

MALINIAC, J. W.: Critical analysis of mammectomy and free transplantation of nipple. Am. J. Surg. *65:*364–367, Sept '44

MALINIAC, J. W.: Procedure for elevation of nasal dorsum by transposition of lateral cartilages. Arch. Otolaryng. *41:*214–215, March '45

MALINIAC, J. W.: Blood supply of breast in relation to 2-stage mammaplasty. Am. J. Surg. *68:*55–66, April '45

MALINIAC, J. W.: Fracture-dislocations of cartilaginous nose; anatomicopathologic considerations and treatment. Arch. Otolaryng. *42:*131–137, Aug '45

MALINOWSKY, N. N.: Obliteration of orifice of artificial vagina with subsequent suppuration and perforation of blind sac of intestine used in formation of vagina; case. Monatschr. f. Geburtsh. u. Gynak. *83:*77–81, Sept '29

MALIS, S.: Pitfalls in submucous resection. Dis. Eye, Ear, Nose and Throat *2:*343–347, Nov '42

MALKIEL, S. AND BOYD, W. C.: Treatment (with picric acid) of minor burns acquired in laboratory and at home. J. Missouri M. A. *43:*538–539, Aug '46

MALKIN, B.: Treatment of angioma of eyelid by injection of sclerosing solutions. Arch. Ophth. *16:*578–584, Oct '36

MALLARD, R. S.: Reconstruction of urethra and penis following extensive gangrene. J.A.M.A. *95:*332–335, Aug 2, '30

MALLET, L. (see GERNEZ, L. *et al*) Oct '35

MALLET-GUY, P.: Case of permanent constriction of jaws; death, autopsy. Lyon med. *138:*628–631, Nov 28, '26

MALLET-GUY, P.: Phlegmons of 2 carpal sheaths of flexor muscles; excellent function after therapy by disconnected lateral incisions. Lyon chir. *29:*736–740, Nov–Dec '32

MALLET-GUY, P. AND JOUVE, P.: Bilateral temporo-maxillary ankylosis with pleuropneumonia; death; autopsy; case. Ann. d'anat. path. *4:*19–24, Jan '27

MALLET-GUY, P. (see FROMENT, J.) Sept–Oct '38

DE LA T. MALLETT, A. E.: Nerve regeneration; motor and sensory recovery in case of injury to radial nerve. J. Roy. Nav. M. Serv. *32:*61, April; 147, July '46

MALLIK, K. L. B.: Skin-grafting in complete avulsion of scalp. Indian M. Gaz. *66:*86–88, Feb '31

MALLO HUERGO, E. AND QUIRNO LAVALLE, R.: Exposed interphalangeal luxations of hand; cases. Prensa med. argent. *29:*1367–1370, Aug 26, '42

MALMROS, H. AND WILANDER, O.: Question of using preserved whole blood or blood plasma. Svenska lak.-tidning *37:*1026–1029, June 14, '40

MALMSTONE, F. A.: First aid treatment of burns with tannic acid. Internat. J. Med. and Surg. *47:*72–77, Feb '34

MALONE, J. Y.: Suture needle for nasal sur-

gery. Arch. Otolaryng. *17:*562, April '33
MALONE, J. Y.: Simple method of measuring skin for flaps. Ann. Surg. *105:*303-304, Feb '37
MALONE, J. Y. (see SACHS, E.) Sept '22
MALONEY, H. P.: Porcelain faucet handle injuries to hand. J.A.M.A. *103:*1618-1619, Nov 24, '34
MALONY, F. C.: Acute osteomyelitis of mandible. Am. Dent. Surgeon *49:*159-162, April '29
MALTZ, M.: New procedures for tear sac, frontal sinus and endonasal plastic operations. Acta oto-laryng. *9:*144-153, '26 (in English)
MALTZ, M.: New rhinoplastic instruments. Laryngoscope *36:*54-60, Jan '26
MALTZ, MAXWELL: *New Faces—New Futures: Rebuilding Character with Plastic Surgery.* Richard R. Smith, New York, 1936
MALTZ, M.: New method of tube pedicle grafting. Am. J. Surg. *43:*216-222, Feb '39
MALTZ, M.: New method of tube pedicle grafting. J. Internat. Coll. Surgeons. *3:*526-531, Dec '40
MALTZ, M.: Surgical treatment of recent facial wounds. J. Internat. Coll. Surgeons *5:*334-342, July-Aug '42
MALTZ, M.: Reconstruction of thumb; new technic. Am. J. Surg. *58:*429-433, Dec '42
MALTZ, M.: Reconstruction of nasal tip; new technic. Am. J. Surg. *63:*203-205, Feb '44
MALTZ, M.: Surgical treatment of recent wounds of face. Eye, Ear, Nose and Throat Monthly *23:*60-68, Feb '44
MALTZ, MAXWELL: *Evolution of Plastic Surgery.* Froben Press, New York, 1946
MALUCELLI, O.: Atresia, surgical therapy of case of anal. An. paulist. de med. e cir. *51:*193-197, Mar '46
MALUSCHEW, D.: Schubert's method of plastic construction of vagina; 2 cases. Zentralbl. f. Gynak. *53:*428-430, Feb 16, '29
MAMIER (see ROSGEN) 1942
MAMLET, A. M.: Plastic repair of nose as aid in therapeutic surgery. J. M. Soc. New Jersey *34:*664-666, Nov '37

Mammaplasty After Amputation

Plastic covering of defects following breast amputation. KRAFT, R. Deutsche Ztschr. f. Chir. *207:*171-183, '27
Total mammectomy; free autograft of nipple and areola; bilateral aesthetic amputation. DARTIGUES. Bull. et mem. Soc. de chir. de Paris *20:*739-744, Nov 2, '28
Total mastoneoplasty following amputation of breast. REINHARD, W. Deutsche Ztschr. f. Chir. *236:*309-317, '32
Artificial breasts formed by union of 3 flaps following mammectomy for adenofibroma; case. ZORRAQUÍN, G. AND BOIX POU, M. Rev. de cir. de Buenos Aires *13:*244-248, April '34
Attempted plastic surgery in extirpation of breast cancer. ROFFO, A. E. Bol. Inst. de med. exper. para el estud. y trat. d. cancer *21:*163-179, April '44
Free transplant of areola preliminary to amputation of breast for benign tumor; free fat graft; case. ZENO, L. An. de cir. *10:*190-194, Sept-Dec '44

Mammaplasty, Arterial Supply for

Arteries of mammary gland; importance in esthetic surgery; anatomic and roentgenographic study. SALMON, M. Ann. d'anat. path. *16:*477-500, April '39
Blood supply of breast in relation to 2-stage mammaplasty. MALINIAC, J. W. Am. J. Surg. *68:*55-66, April '45

Mammaplasty, Augmentation

Late results of fat transplantation in breast surgery. WREDE, L. Deutsche Ztschr. f. Chir. *203-204:*672-685, '27
Plastic surgery of hypoplasia of breast. HAGENBACH, E. Helvet. med. acta *3:*811-812, Dec '36
Reconstruction of atrophic mammary gland by means of autotransplantation of fat. PASSOT, R. Presse med. *38:*627-628, May 7, '30
Prosthetic restorations of breast; technic using sponge rubber. BROWN, A. M. Arch. Surg. *48:*388-394, May '44

Mammaplasty, Complications

Plastic reconstruction of breast in necrosis following esthetic operation. NOËL, MME. A. Bull. med., Paris *47:*633-634, Oct 7, '33
Prevention of necrosis in plastic repair of pendulous breasts. MALINIAK, J. W. Am. J. Surg. *26:*292-297, Nov '34
Technical mistakes and dangers in plastic surgery of breast. GRODZKI, M. Rev. de chir. structive, pp. 39-57, July '35
Constantly recurring unsatisfactory end results of plastic surgery in hypertrophy of breast. HABERLAND, H. F. O. Zentralbl. f. Chir. *63:*510-511, Feb 29, '36
Important errors in plastic surgery of pendulous breasts. LEVY-LENZ. Rev. de chir. structive, pp. 233-236, March '36
Cicatrix in reparative surgery of breast. CLAOUE, C. AND BERNARD, MME. I., J. de med. de Bordeaux *113:*695-697, Oct 10, '36
Prophylaxis of cicatricial keloid in plastic

Mammaplasty, Complications – Cont.
surgery of breast. SCHWARZMANN, E. AND POLLACZEK, K. F. Wien. med. Wchnschr. *87:*1248–1253, Nov 27, '37
Injury to mammary areola and progressive necrosis after plastic surgery of breast. HABERLAND, H. F. O. Arch. f. klin. Chir. *190:*87–95, '37
Prophylaxis of cicatricial keloid in plastic surgery of pendulous breasts. SCHWARZMANN, E. Rev. de chir. structive *8:*93–98, Aug '38
Problems of plastic surgery and surgery of the breast in particular. BAMES, H. O. Dia med. *10:*907–908, Sept 5, '38
Failures in mammaplastic surgery for hypertrophy of breast. LA ROE, E. K. Am. J. Surg. *66:*339–345, Dec '44

Mammaplasty, Dermal Pedicle

Transplantation of nipple, most complicated form of pedicle graft. BAMES, H. O. Rev. de chir. structive, pp. 93–96, June '37
Avoidance of nipple necrosis by preservation of corium in one-stage plastic surgery of breast. SCHWARZMANN, E. Rev. de chir. structive, pp. 206–209, Oct '37
Twenty-five years' experience with plastic reconstruction of breast and transplantation of nipple. THOREK, M. Am. J. Surg. *67:*445–466, March '45

Mammaplasty, Free Graft of Areola in

Breast surgery with graft of areolar region; 2 cases. DARTIGUES, L. Monde med., Paris *38:*75–85, Feb 1, '28
Total mammectomy; free autograft of nipple and areola; bilateral aesthetic amputation. DARTIGUES, L. Bull. et mem. Soc. de chir. de Paris *20:*739–744, Nov 2, '28
Apparatus for localization of transplanted areolae of breast in plastic surgery. DARTIGUES, L. Bull. et mem. Soc. de chir. de Paris *21:*43, Jan 4, '29
Excision of breast combined with autoplastic areolomammary graft. DARTIGUES, L. Paris chir. *21:*11–19, Jan–Feb '29
Description of new circular incision for breast plastic surgery. DARTIGUES, L. Bull. et mem. Soc. de chir. de Paris *21:*263, March 15, '29
Total bilateral mammectomy with free graft of nipple and areola. DARTIGUES, L. Bull. et mem. Soc. d. chirurgiens de Paris *25:*289–291, May 5, '33
Histological verification of efficacy of free transplantation of nipple. THOREK, M., M. J. and Rec. *134:*474–476, Nov 18, '31

Mammaplasty, Free Graft of Areola in – Cont.
Free transplantation of nipples and areolae in breast hypertrophy. ADAMS, W. M. Surgery *15:*186–195, Jan '44
Critical analysis of mammectomy and free transplantation of nipple. MALINIAC, J. W. Am. J. Surg. *65:*364–367, Sept '44
Plastic reconstruction of breast and free transplantation of nipple (author's one-stage operation; microscopic proof of survival of transplanted nipple). THOREK, M. J. Internat. Coll. Surgeons *9:*194–224, Mar–Apr '46

Mammaplasty for Inverted Nipples

Therapy of inverted nipples. PÖPPELMANN, W. Med. Welt *6:*1317, Sept 10, '32
Plastic reconstruction of nipples. MICHALEK-GRODZKI, S. Bull. et mem. Soc. d. chirurgiens de Paris *28:*387–399, June 19, '36
Plastic reconstruction in deformities of nipples. MICHALEK-GRODSKY. Rev. de chir. structive, pp. 126–136, June '37
Operation to correct crater nipple; contribution to problem of necrosis of nipple and areola. KAST, H. Chirurg. *14:*181–184, March 15, '42

Mammaplasty, Lactation After

Continuation of organic function of female breast after plastic operation; case. REESE, E. Zentralbl. f. Chir. *61:*3011–3012, Dec 29, '34
Ability to nurse child after plastic surgery of pendulous breasts. REESE, E. Zentralbl. f. Chir. *62:*1933–1935, Aug 17, '35
Plastic surgery of breast and preservation of lactating function. GLÄSMER, E. Deutsche med. Wchnschr. *63:*559, April 2, '37
Function of breast following plastic surgery for hypertrophy. VON MATOLCSY, T. Arch. f. klin. Chir. *201:*791–795, '41

Mammaplasty, Local Anesthesia for

Regional anesthesia of breast with procaine hydrochloride in plastic surgery. BRETECHE, *et al.* Bull. med., Paris *49:*685–686, Oct 5, '35

Mammaplasty, Mastopexy (See also Mammaplasty, Reduction)

Pendulous mammae and plastic treatment. LOTSCH, F. Zentralbl. f. Chir. *50:*1241–1244, Aug 11, '23 (illus.)
Low position of right breast. SCHILLING, F. Arch. f. Verdauungskr. *32:*81–82, Sept '23
Plastic correction of sagging breast. PASSOT,

Mammaplasty, Mastopexy—Cont.
R. Presse med. *33:*317–318, March 11, '25 abstr: J.A.M.A. *84:*1308, April 25, '25
Surgical correction of pendulous breasts. DARTIGUES. Arch. franco-belges de chir. *28:*313–328, April '25
Surgery of hypertrophic breast (mastopexy). JOSEPH, J. Deutsche med. Wchnschr. *51:*1103–1105, July 3, '25 abstr: J.A.M.A. *85:*641, Aug 22, '25
Surgical treatment of pendulous breast. DE QUERVAIN, F. Schweiz. med. Wchnschr. *56:*451–453, May 15, '26
Operations for pendulous breast and pendulous abdomen. KÜSTER, H. Monatschr. f. Geburtsh. u. Gynak. *73:*316–341, June '26
Pathology and surgical treatment of pendulous breast. GLAESMER, E. AND AMERSBACH, R. Munchen. med. Wchnschr. *74:*1171–1176, July 15, '27
Plastic operations for pendulous abdomen and pendulous breast; a survey. FRIST, J. Med. Klin. *23:*1269–1271, Aug 19, '27
Operation for pendulous breasts. CESARI, M. Bull. d. sc. med. *5:*373–379, Sept–Oct '27
Plastic surgery of simple and hypertrophied pendulous breasts. JOSEPH, J. Deutsche med. Wchnschr. *53:*1853–1854, Oct 28, '27
Plastic surgery of pendulous breast. EITNER, E. Wein. med. Wchnschr. *77:*1572, Nov 12, '27
Operation for pendulous breast. NOËL, A. Med. Welt *2:*51–53, Jan 14, '28
Operation for pendulous breast. NOËL, MME. AND LOPEZ-MARTINEZ. Arch. franco-belges de chir. *31:*138–153, Feb '28
Plastic treatment of pendulous breast. LOTSCH, F. Klin. Wchnschr. *7:*603–606, March 25, '28
Operative treatment of pendulous breast. WOLFSOHN, G. Med. Welt *2:*477, March 31, '28
Indications for operation to improve shape of female breast. FRISCH, O. Wien. klin. Wchnschr. *41:*640–641, May 3, '28
Operative technic in treatment of prolapsus of breast. SALINAS, F. O. Cultura med. mod. *7:*455–462, July 31, '28
Improved technic for surgical correction of pendulous breast. GLAESMER, E. AND AMERSBACH, R. Munchen. med. Wchnschr. *75:*1547–1549, Sept 7, '28
La chirurgie esthétique—nouveaux procedes de correction du prolpases mammaire. S. NOËL AND L. MARTINEZ. Le Concour Medical, No. 46 (October 27, 1928)
Transpectoral costal mastopexy by peri-areolar route. DARTIGUES, L. Bull. et mem.

Mammaplasty, Mastopexy—Cont.
Soc. de chir. de Paris *21:*287–289, April 19, '29
Operation for pendulous breasts. BAUM, G. Med. Welt *3:*684, May 11, '29
Operation for pendulous breasts. DOWKONTT, C. F., M. J. and Rec. *130:*624–627, Dec 4, '29
Operation for pendulous breast. SCHREIBER, F. Beitr. z. klin. Chir. *147:*56–59, '29
Esthetic surgery of pendulous breast, abdomen and arms in female. THOREK, M. Illinois M. J. *58:*48–57, July '30
Rules and experiences in operative treatment of pendulous breast. AMERSBACH, R. Schweiz. med. Wchnschr. *60:*974–976, Oct 11, '30
Correction of pendulous breasts. BAMES, H. O. Am. J. Surg. *10:*80–83, Oct '30
Simple surgical method for esthetic correction of pendulous breasts. DER BRUCKE, M. G. Am. J. Surg. *11:*324–327, Feb '31
Modification of double circle operation for pendulous breasts. DOWKONTT, C. F. New York State J. Med. *31:*264–266, March 1, '31
Plastic surgery of pendulous breasts. SEBENING, W. Chirurg *3:*510–515, June 1, '31
Plastic surgery of pendulous breasts. MEYER, A. W. Med. Welt *5:*1313, Sept 12, '31
Pendulous breasts. MALINIAK, J. W., M. Times and Long Island M. J. *59:*355–359, Oct '31
Satisfactory operation for pendulous breasts. DUFOURMENTEL, L. Bull. med., Paris *46:*194–195, March 12, '32
Prolapse of breast and its therapy. MICHAŁEK-GRODZKI, S. Ginek. polska *11:*687–698, July–Sept '32
Plastic repair of pendulous breasts. MALINIAK, J. W., M. J. and Rec. *136:*312–316, Oct 19, '32
Bilateral mastopexy and therapy of mammary prolapse of first degree. LAGARDE. Rev. tech. chir. *24:*251–253, Dec '32
Hygienic suspensory operation of breast. OLDAGER, A. Ugesk. f. laeger *95:*202–203, Feb 16, '33
Technic and late results of mastopexy. DUFOURMENTEL, L. Bull. et mem. Soc. d. chirurgiens de Paris *25:*292–295, May 5, '33
Two-stage plastic operation in pendulous breast. NISSEN, R. Zentralbl. f. Chir. *60:*1330–1331, June 10, '33
Improved technic for restoration of pendulous breast. BIDDLE, A. G. Am. J. Surg. *23:*191–193, Jan '34
Plastic surgery for pendulous breast. BJÖRKENHEIM, G. A. Finska lak.-sallsk. handl.

Mammaplasty, Mastopexy—Cont.
*76:*57–77, Jan '34
Plastic correction of pendulous breast. BECK, C. AND BECK, W. C., S. Clin. North America *14:*769–773, Aug '34
New technic for surgical therapy of pendulous breast. ASIS Y GARCÍA DE LA CAMACHA. Actas Soc. de cir. de Madrid *3:*35–42, Oct–Dec '34
Prevention of necrosis in plastic repair of pendulous breasts. MALINIAK, J. W. Am. J. Surg. *26:*292–297, Nov '34
New surgical technic for restoration of pendulous breasts. VERRIER, E. Rev. espan. de med. y cir. *18:*68–70, Feb '35
New points of view in regard to corrective surgery of pendulous breasts, together with description of new method. EHRENFELD, H. Zentralbl. f. Chir. *62:*628–634, March 16, '35
Plastic surgery of pendulous breasts. EITNER, E. Wein. med. Wchnschr. *85:*586, May 18, '35
Pendulous breast; comparative values of present-day methods of repair and procedure of choice. MALINIAK, J. W. Arch. Surg. *31:*587–600, Oct '35
Various technics for plastic surgery of breast; cases. MONTANT. Bull. et mem. Soc. de med. de Paris *139:*566–571, Nov 7, '35
Method of examination of pendulous breasts before reconstructive surgery. DARTIGUES. Bull. et mem. Soc. de med. de Paris *140:*151–160, Feb 29, '36
Important errors in plastic surgery of pendulous breasts. LEVY-LENZ. Rev. de chir. structive, pp. 233–236, March '36
Simplicity versus complicated methods in reconstruction of pendulous breasts. THOREK, M. Illinois M. J. *69:*338–345, April '36
Plastic surgery of pendulous breast. ERCZY, M. Gyogyaszat *77:*324–326, May 23, '37
Pendulous and hypertrophied breasts; operative treatment. DOWKONTT, C. F. New York State J. Med. *37:*643–644, April 1, '37
Surgical therapy of pendulous breast. PALACIO POSSE, R. Semana med. *1:*996–1001, April 8, '37
Plastic surgery of pendulous breast. ERCZY, M. Gyogyaszat *77:*324–326, May 23, '37
Plastic repair of pendulous breast. MALINIAK, J. W. Vida nueva *39:*327–336, May 15, '37
Surgical treatment of pendulous breast. POSSE, P. Am. J. Surg. *38:*293–297, Nov '37
Pendulous breasts; operation limited to one half of breast without cutting all around areola. KAST, H. Chirurg *10:*472–474, July 1, '38

Mammaplasty, Mastopexy—Cont.
One-stage operation for pendulous breasts, using method of peripheral approach in removal of wedge-shaped portion. KAST, H. Zentralbl. f. Chir. *65:*1990–1992, Sept 3, '38
Surgical mastopexy in mastoptosis. GONZALEZ ULLOA, M. Rev. mex. de cir., ginec. y cancer *7:*191–202, May '39
Technic of surgical therapy of pendulous breasts with incision totally encircling nipple. KAST, H. Chirurg *12:*647–649, Nov 1, '40
Mastoptosis (with description of surgical reconstruction of case). MACOMBER, D. W. Rocky Mountain M. J. *38:*50–52, Jan '41
Mammaplasty for pendulous hypertrophied breasts. BERSON, M. I., M. Rec. *153:*89–92, Feb 5, '41
Method of determining correct seat of nipples in plastic surgery for pendulous breasts; new instrument to facilitate it. EHRENFELD, H. J., M. Rec. *154:*92–94, Aug 6, '41
Surgical therapy of pendulous breasts. SCHREIBER, F. An. Fac. de med. de Montevideo *26:*251–271, '41
Surgical treatment of pendulous breast. PALACIO POSSE, R. J. Internat. Coll. Surgeons *6:*361–363, July–Aug '43
Reconstruction of breast deformities (atrophy) (pendulous). MAY, H. Surg., Gynec. & Obst. *77:*523–529, Nov '43
Improved breast lifting operation. BIDDLE, A. G. Am. J. Surg. *67:*488–494, March '45
Plastic surgery in reconstructing enlarged breasts; one-stage mastopexy. LAMONT, E. S. Surgery *17:*379–396, March '45
Operative replacement of mammary prominence. GILLIES, H. Brit. J. Surg. *32:*477–479, April '45
Mammaplasty of pendulous breasts. FRONK, C. E. Hawaii M. J. *5:*23–25, Sept–Oct '45
Two-stage mastopexy in plastic surgery of markedly enlarged breasts. LAMONT, E. S. Ann. Surg. *124:*111–117, July '46

Mammaplasty, Physiology After

Excitation and amelioration of ovarian functions after plastic surgery of breast. MONTANT. Bull. et mem. Soc. de med. de Paris *137:*400–402, May 27, '33
Relations between esthetic surgery of breast and ovarian and mammary glands. NOËL, MME. Bull. med., Paris *48:*611–613, Oct 6, '34
Possible influence of plastic surgery of breast on hypophysio-ovarian function. ROCHAT, R. L. Schweiz. med. Wchnschr. *71:*1307–1308, Oct 25, '41

Mammaplasty, Reduction (See also Mastopexy)
Cosmetic surgery of face, neck and breast. BOOTH, F. A. Northwest Med. *21:*170-172, June '22 (illus.)
Hyperplasia of breast. NITTER, H. Norsk Mag. f. Laegevidensk. *83:*673-677, Sept '22 (illus.) abstr: J. A. M. A. *79:*1730, Nov 11, '22
Operative treatment of hypertrophied mamma. KRASKE, H. Munchen. med. Wchnschr. *70:*672, May 25, '23 (illus.)
Operative treatment of hypertrophied breasts. HÜBENER, A. W. Deutsche Ztschr. f. Chir. *181:*40-47, '23 (illus.) abstr: J. A. M. A. *81:*1566, Nov 3, '23
Mammary plastics. KLEINSCHMIDT, O. Zentralbl. f. Chir. (supp.) *51:*488-493, March 15, '24
Surgical treatment of hypertrophy of breast. HOLLÄNDER, E. Deutsche med. Wchnschr. *50:*1400-1402, Oct 10, '24 abstr: J. A. M. A. *83:*1721, Nov 22, '24
Treatment of hypertrophic breast; reply to Lexer. HOLLÄNDER, E. Deutsche med. Wchnschr. *51:*26, Jan 2, '25
Treatment of hypertrophic breast; comment on Holländer's article. LEXER, E. Deutsche med. Wchnschr. *51:*26, Jan 2, '25
Surgery of hypertrophic breast (mastopexy). JOSEPH, J. Deutsche med. Wchnschr. *51:*1103-1105, July 3, '25 abstr: J. A. M. A. *85:*641, Aug 22, '25
Plastic surgery of breast. AXHAUSEN, G. Med. Klin. *22:*1437-1440, Sept 17, '26
Operative treatment of breast hypertrophy. FOGED, J. Bibliot. f. Laeger *119:*xlvii-lvi, Feb '27
Nasenplastik und sonstige Gesichtsplastik. Nebst einem Anhang über Mammaplastik, by Jacques Joseph. C. Kabitsch, Leipzig, 1928
Chirurgie esthétique; le sein, by M. Virenque. Maloine, Paris, 1928
Indications for operation to improve shape of female breast. FRISCH, O. Wien. klin. Wchnschr. *41:*640-641, May 3, '28
Plastic surgery of breast. LAGARDE. Paris chir. *20:*143-152, July-Aug '28
New method of mammaplasty. BIESENBERGER, H. Zentralbl. f. Chir. *55:*2382-2387, Sept 22, '28
Technic in aesthetic surgery of breast, face. LIBERA, D. Med. ital. *9:*629-636, Oct '28
Description of new circular incision for breast plastic surgery. DARTIGUES, L. Bull. et mem. Soc. de chir. de Paris *21:*263, March 15, '29
Correction of hypertrophy of breasts by cosmetic surgery. HALLA, F. Med. Klin. *25:*1020-1021, June 28, '29

Mammaplasty, Reduction – Cont.
Simplification of plastic method for hypertrophy of breast. HALLA, F. Med. Klin. *25:*1697-1698, Nov 1, '29
Die Förmfehler und die plastischen Operationen der weiblichen Brüst, by Erna Gläsmer. F. Enke, Stuttgart, 1930
Two types of operation for hypertrophy of breast. HALLA, F. Wien. med. Wchnschr. *80:*417, March 15, '30
Cosmetic operations of the breast. GLÄSMER, E. Med. Welt *4:*630, May 3, '30
Surgical treatment of hypertrophic and pendulous breasts. MEYER, A. W. Deutsche med. Wchnschr. *56:*1165, July 11, '30
Method for plastic surgery of hypertrophy of breast. GLÄSMER, E. Zentralbl. f. Gynak. *54:*2202-2204, Aug 30, '30
Technic of plastic operations of breast. SCHWARZMANN, E. Chirurg *2:*932-943, Oct 15, '30
New methods of treatment of hypertrophy of breast by plastic surgery. BIESENBERGER, H. Zentralbl. f. Chir. *57:*2971-2975, Nov 29, '30 (Addendum)
Anisomastia (unilateral hyperplasia) of breast. DE ANGELIS, E. AND ALTSCHUL, R. Deutsche Ztschr. f. Nervenh. *112:*165-176, '30
Operative improvement of form of breasts in women. FRANKENBERG, B. E. Vestnik khir. (no. 61) *21:*67-70, '30
Deformitäten und kosmetische Operationen der weiblichen Brust, by Hermann Biesenberger. Wilhelm Maudrich, Vienna, 1931
Nasenplastik und sonstige Gesichtsplastik. Nebst einem Anhang über Mammaplastik und . . . Körperplastik, by Jacques Joseph. C. Kabitsch, Leipzig, 1931
Technique of complete operation on breast. BARTLETT, E. I. Surg., Gynec. & Obst. *52:*71-78, Jan '31
Cosmetic surgery of breast. KURTZAHN. Chirurg *3:*152-156, Feb 15, '31
Technic of plastic surgery of breasts. PICARD, H. Med. Welt *5:*741-743, May 23, '31
Technic of plastic surgery of breasts. SCHWARZMANN, E. Dia med. *3:*830, May 25, '31
Plastic surgery by Holländer's operation for breasts. SONNTAG, E. Arch. f. klin. Chir. *164:*812-824, '31
Plastic surgery of breast. HABERLAND, H. F. O. Med. Welt *6:*118-120, Jan 23, '32
Satisfactory operation for pendulous breasts. DUFOURMENTEL, L. Bull. med., Paris *46:*194-195, March 12, '32

Mammaplasty, Reduction – Cont.
Unilateral surgical correction of asymmetric breasts. BIESENBERGER, H. Wien. med. Wchnschr. *82:*732–733, June 4, '32
Surgical correction of breast. BIESENBERGER, H. Wien. med. Wchnschr. *82:*734–735, June 4, '32
Plastic surgery of hypertrophy of breast; case. FRAENKEL, L. Zentralbl. f. Gynak. *56:*1506–1510, June 18, '32
Care, preservation and repair of female breasts; review of Erna Glaesmer's "Die Formfehler und die plastischen Operationen de weiblichen Brust," and H. Biesenberger's "Deformitaten und Operationen de weiblichen Brust." SELLHEIM, H. Deutsche med. Wchnschr. *58:*1414–1417, Sept 2, '32
Technic of plastic surgery of breast. NÖE, C. G. N. Zentralbl. f. Gynak. *56:*2721–2723, Nov 5, '32
Importance of dermatogram for plastic operations of breast. GLÄSMER, E. Dermat. Wchnschr. *95:*1713–1718, Nov 26, '32
Chirurgie plastique des seins, by C. Montant and F. Dubois. Maloine, Paris, 1933
New plastic operation of breast. GROSSE, O. Zentralbl. f. Chir. *60:*8–12, Jan 7, '33
Deformities of breast and their correction by plastic surgery. EHRENFELD, H. Gyogyaszat *73:*90–94, Feb 5, '33
Technic of plastic surgery of breast. SCHLESINGER, E. Zentralbl. f. Gynak. *57:*440–442, Feb 18, '33
Plastic operations of face, breast. HABERLAND, H. F. O. Zentralbl. f. Chir. *60:*746–748, March 31, '33
New surgical method in hypertrophy of breast. KAPP, J. F. Med. Welt *7:*631–632, May 6, '33
Cosmetic surgery of breast. TOTIS, B. Gyogyaszat *73:*467–468, July 23–30, '33
Present status of plastic surgery of breast. DARTIGUES, L. Clin. y lab. *23:*737–741, Sept '33
Plastic operation on breast; case. HENNEBERT, P. AND TAISNY, E. Scalpel *86:*1929–1932, Dec 30, '33
Esthetic breast surgery; various technics. BERGERET, A. AND MARTIN, J. Gynec. et obst. *29:*55–70, Jan '34
Plastic surgery of breast. BURIAN. Casop. lek. cesk. *73:*373, April 6; 397, April 13, '34
Plastic surgery of breast hypertrophy. FOGED, J. Nord. med. tidskr. *8:*954–961, July 21, '34
Plastic surgery of breast. GENESIO SALLES. Bahia med. *5:*623–624, Sept '34

Mammaplasty, Reduction – Cont.
Continuation of organic function of female breast after plastic operation; case. REESE, E. Zentralbl. f. Chir. *61:*3011–3012, Dec 29, '34
Marks of alignment in plastic surgery of breast. CLAOUE. Bull. et mem. Soc. de med. de Paris *139:*130–134, Feb 23, '35
Use of skin flaps for cosmetic plastic surgery of breast. EITNER, E. Zentralbl. f. Chir. *62:*625–627, March 16, '35
Routes of access in reparative surgery of breast. CLAOUE. Bull. et mem. Soc. de med. de Paris *139:*205–212, March 23, '35
Restorative surgery of breast and face. MALINIAK, J. W. Bull. Assoc. d. med. de lang. franc. de l'Amerique du Nord *1:*199–206, April '35
Technic of plastic reduction of breast volume. CLAOUE, C. Bull. et mem. Soc. de med. de Paris *139:*454–458, June 29, '35
Technical mistakes and dangers in plastic surgery of breast. GRODZKI, M. Rev. de chir. structive, pp. 39–57, July '35
Esthetic surgery of breasts. KAUFMAN, R. Bull. et mem. Soc. de med. de Paris *139:*484–487, Oct 10, '35
Plastic surgical therapy of dystrophy of breast. MONTANT. Tech. chir. *72:*155–164, Oct '35
Surgical therapy of breast abnormalities. DARTIGUES, L. Bull. et mem. Soc. de med. de Paris *139:*575–569, Nov 7, '35
Various technics for plastic surgery of breast; cases. MONTANT. Bull. et mem. Soc. de med. de Paris *139:*566–571, Nov 7, '35
Plastique mammaire, by Charles Claoué and Irene Bernard. Maloine, Paris, 1936
Chirurgie réparatrice: Plastique et esthétique de la poitrine, des seins, et de l'abdomen, by L. Dartigues. Lépine, Paris, 1936.
Alignment points of nipples in relation to thorax in plastic surgery of breast. DARTIGUES, L. Clin. y lab. *28:*27–37, Jan '36 abstr: Bull. et mem. Soc. de med. de Paris *139:*494–499, Oct 10, '35
Technic of reconstruction of breast. CLAOUE, C. Bull. et mem. Soc. de med. de Paris *140:*33–36, Jan 9, '36
(Comment on article by Claoue on plastic reduction of breast volume). SCHWARZMANN, E. Wien. med. Wchnschr. *86:*100–102, Jan 25, '36
Alignment points of breast in relation to thorax in plastic surgery. DARTIGUES. Spitalul *56:*57–59, Feb '36 also: Rev. de chir. structive, pp. 287–291, June '36
Review of plastic operations of breast.

Mammaplasty, Reduction – Cont.
BAMES, H. O., M. Rec. *143:*273-274, April 1, '36
Plastic reconstruction of breast deformities. BAMES, H. O. Rev. de chir. structive, pp. 293-297, June '36
Special technic for surgical correction of hypertrophy of breast. BOURGUET, J. Bull. et mem. Soc. de med. de Paris *140:*411-417, June 27, '36
Reparative surgery; distribution of skin on neoformed breast. CLAOUE. Bull. et mem. Soc. de med. de Paris *140:*418-423, June 27, '36
Compass for symmetrical measured tracing in plastic surgery of breast. BERTOLA, V. J. Semana med. *2:*197-198, July 16, '36
Surgical treatment of idiopathic breast hypertrophy. FOMON, S. Arch. Surg. *33:*253-266, Aug '36
Restorative surgery of breast in hypertrophy; author's technic. CLAOUE, C. Bull. et mem. Soc. med. et chir. de Bordeaux, pp. 168-182, '36
Reconstruction in hypertrophy of breast. UPDEGRAFF, H. L. California and West. Med. *46:*28-31, Jan '37
Plastic surgery of breast; presentation of colored motion picture. CLAOUE. Arch. f. klin. Chir. *189:*538-547, '37
Alignment points in plastic surgery of breast. CLAOUE, C. Chir. plast. *4:*26-28, Jan-April '38
Breast deformities; anatomic and physiologic considerations in plastic repair. MALINIAC, J. W. Am. J. Surg. *39:*54-61, Jan '38
Plastic operation for correction of breast hypertrophy. SOWLES, H. K. New England J. Med. *218:*253-257, Feb 10, '38
Etiology and therapy of breast hypertrophy. MICHALEK-GRODZKI. Nowiny lek. *50:*113-116, Feb 15, '38
Breast malformations and suggestions for treatment. KAPP, J. F., M. Rec. *147:*252-253, March 16, '38
Plastic operation of breast with flexible adaption. VESTAL, P. W. Am. J. Surg. *39:*614-616, March '38
Plastic surgery of breast hypertrophy; technic. BAMES, H. O. Bol. Soc. de cir. de Rosario *5:*18-20, May '38
Reconstruction for breast hypertrophy. BAMES, H. O. California and West. Med. *48:*341-343, May '38
Experience with mammaplasties. BURIAN, F. Rev. de chir. structive *8:*35-37, May '38
Review of 80 cases of mammaplasty. McINDOE, A. H. Rev. de chir. structive *8:*39-

Mammaplasty, Reduction – Cont.
47, May '38
New corrective method for breast hypertrophy. NEDKOFF, N. Zentralbl. f. chir. *65:*1503-1504, July 2, '38
Corrective operations and development of plastic surgery (including breast). EROZY, M. Gyogyaszat *78:*495-498, Aug 14-21, '38
Plastic surgery of breast hypertrophy during pregnancy; case. DOBRITZ, O. Zentralbl. f. Chir. *65:*1993, Sept 3, '38
Problems of plastic surgery and surgery of the breast in particular. BAMES, H. O. Dia med. *10:*907-908, Sept 5, '38
Technic of plastic surgery of breast. NEUFFER, H. Wien. klin. Wchnschr. *51:*1312-1314, Dec 9, '38
Malformations of mammary glands and their surgical correction. HEIJL, C. Hygiea (Festband) *100:*118-127, '38
Plastic operation for breast hypertrophy. MAY, H. Arch. Surg. *38:*113-117, Jan '39
Plastic reconstruction of female breasts. THOREK, M. Am. J. Surg. *43:*268-278, Feb '39
Technic of mammaplasty (for hypertrophy). GILLIES, H. AND McINDOE, A. H. Surg., Gynec. and Obst. *68:*658-665, March '39
Correction of hypertrophy of breasts by cosmetic surgery. HALLA, F. Med. Klin. *25:*1020-1021, June 28, '29
Hypertrophy of breast corrected by plastic surgery according to Nissen. BUMIN, H. Turk tib cem. mec. *5:*173-183, '39
Results of plastic surgery of breast. MATOLCSY, T. Arch. f. klin. Chir. *195:*666-671, '39
Allgemeine und spezielle Operationslehre. Band III, Die Eingriffe an der Brüst und Brüsthohle, by Otto Kleinschmidt. Edited by Martin Kirschner. Springer-Verlag, Berlin, 1940
Plastic operation for bilateral hypertrophy of breast with asymmetry, ptosis and mastodynia. RIGA, I. T. Rev. de chir., Bucuresti *43:*219-226, March-April '40
Juvenile gigantomastia; surgical therapy of case. BELLOSO, R. A. AND GOLDIE, J. C. Arch. urug. de med., cir. y especialid. *17:*35-52, July '40
Present status of plastic surgery of breast. KRAUSE, W. H. Chirurg *12:*642-647, Nov 1, '40
Surgical therapy of hypertrophy of breast. NORDEN, A. Chirurg *12:*650-655, Nov 1, '40
Correction of abnormally large breasts. BAMES, H. O. Southwestern Med. *25:*10-13, Jan '41
Mammaplasty for pendulous hypertrophied

Mammaplasty, Reduction – Cont.
breasts. BERSON, M. I., M. Rec. *153:*89–92, Feb 5, '41
Operative treatment of hypertrophy of breast; description of new method. ANDREASSEN, M. Ugesk. f. laeger *103:*608–613, May 8, '41
Mastortocaliplasty in hypertrophic ptosis of breasts. CODAZZI AGUIRRE, J. A. Rev. med. de Rosario *31:*564–572, June '41
Plastic Surgery of the Breast and Abdominal Wall, by Max Thorek, C. C. Thomas Co., Springfield, Ill., 1942
Plastic surgery of breast. DOWKONTT, C. F. M. Rec. *155:*132–133, Feb 18, '42
Esthetic surgery for hypertrophy of breast. CODAZZI AGUIRRE, J. A. Rev. med. de Rosario *32:*163–167, March '42
Esthetic breast surgery. CODAZZI AGUIRRE, J. A. Arq. de cir. clin. e exper. *6:*595–597, April–June '42
Unilateral hyperplasia of breast in virgin; study apropos of case treated with plastic surgery. COUTINHO, A. An. brasil. de ginec. *16:*20–27, July '43
Massive hypertrophy breast (approximate weight 35 pounds) in adolescence; notable case. FISHER, G. A.; *et al.* West. J. Surg. *51:*349–355, Sept '43
Plastic surgery; case of hypertrophy of breast. SERTA, S. L. Hospital, Rio de Janeiro *25:*877–887, June '44
Plastic surgery of breast; present status of problems. SORALUCE, J. A. Actas Soc. de cir. de Madrid *5:*137–153, Jan–Mar '46
Technic of plastic surgery hypertrophy breast. MALBEC, E. F. Dia med. *18:*375–376, April 15, '46
Two-stage mastopexy in plastic surgery of markedly enlarged breasts. LAMONT, E. S. Ann. Surg. *124:*111–117, July '46
Plastic surgery of hypertrophy of breast. PICKRELL, K. L. *et al.* S. Clin. North America *26:*1095–1107, Oct '46
Evaluation of common procedures in mammaplasty and new technic. LAROE, E. K. Am. J. Surg. *72:*641–655, Nov '46
Operative correction of hypertrophy and ptosis of female breast; clinical investigation of 300 cases with examination of new method. RAGNELL, A. Acta chir. Scandinav. (supp. 113) *94:*1–149, '46 (abstract) Nord. med. *29:*721–725, Mar 29, '46

MAMOURIAN, M.: Bone graft. Brit. M. J. *2:*934, Dec 3, '21
MAN, I.: Imperforate anus; case. Indian M. Gaz. *43:*81–82, Feb '28
MANABE, K.: Brachyphalangia; rare case. Bull Mav. M. A., Japan (Abstr. Sect.) *27:*37, June 15, '38
MANASSE, P.: Double nerve grafting. Arch. f. klin. Chir. *120:*665–685, '22 (illus.) abstr: J.A.M.A. *80:*515, Feb 17, '23
MANASSE, P.: Plastic correction of defects remaining after original operation. Deutsche med. Wchnschr. *53:*1780, Oct 14, '27
MANCOLL, M. M. (see SEIGALL, H. A.) Oct '31
MANDANAS, A. Y.: Local treatment of burns with use of dusting powders and exposure to air. J. Philippine Islands M. A. *6:*161–162, May '26
MANDE, R. (see COSTE, F. *et al*) May '37
MANDELSHTAM, A. E.: Formation of artificial vagina by Mandelshtam modification of rectal method (Popoff); report of 8 additional cases. Zentralbl. f. Gynak. *58:*222–228, Jan 27, '34
MANDELSTAMM, A.: Popoff's method of formation of artificial vagina; 2 cases. Zentralbl. f. Gynak. *51:*1058–1063, April 23, '27
MANDELSTAMM, A.: Shock in childbirth and sudden death following labor. Arch. f. Gynak. *138:*543–557, '29
MANDELSTAMM, A.: Technic of Popoff method of formation of artificial vagina. Arch. f. Gynak. *138:*739–746, '29

Mandible, Ankylosis: See Jaws, Ankylosis

Mandible, Bone Grafting: See Jaws, Bone Grafting

Mandible, Cancer: See Jaws, Cancer

Mandible, Cysts: See Jaws, Cysts

Mandible, Deformity: See Jaws, Deformity

Mandible, Dislocations (See also Jaws, Dislocations)

Cosmetic incision of soft parts for temporary division of lower jaw. KÖNIG, F. Zentralbl. f. Chir. *49:*362–363, March 18, '22 (illus.)
Reconstruction of mandible after resection. PICHLER, H. Wien. klin. Wchnschr. *36:*465–466, June 28, '23
Method of operative attack for central lesions of lower jaw. BLOODGOOD, J. C. New York State J. Med. *24:*379–385, March 21, '24
Prosthetic restoration of portion of mandible, including temporo-mandibular articulation on one side. MITCHELL, V. E. Am. J. Surg. *38:*274–276, Nov '24
Resection of lower jaw in acromegaly. BLESSING, G. AND ROST, F. Zentralbl. f. Chir. *52:*855–857, April 18, '25
Resection of lower jaw for removal of cancer

Mandible, Dislocations – Cont.
of tongue. KRASSIN, P. M. Zentralbl. f. Chir. *53:*3095–3100, Dec 4, '26
Method of plastic resection of lower jaw. GLUSCHKOV, P. Vestnik khir. (no. 30) *10:*67–70, '27
Dental prosthesis after resection of lower jaw. GREVE, K. Beitr. z. klin. Chir. *142:*747–752, '28
Prosthesis in excision of mandible. LAMÉRIS, H. J. Nederl. Tijdschr. v. Geneesk. *1:*244–246, Jan 12, '29
Restoration of width of lower jaw following loss of both condyles; case. TRAUNER, F. Zentralbl. f. Chir. *56:*1986–1989, Aug 19, '29
Entire resection of lower jaw. VILLARD. Lyon chir. *26:*618–621, Aug–Sept '29
Osteotome for resection of mandible. ROCCIA, B. Minerva med. (pt. 2) *9:*700, Nov 3, '29
Jaw deformity; treatment by orthopedic resection of condyles. DUFOURMENTEL, L. Bull. et mem. Soc. de chir. de Paris *21:*424–431, '29
Extra-oral splinting to support jaw after resection of middle portion of lower jaw. STAHNKE, E. Deutsche Ztschr. f. Chir. *215:*234–239, '29
Operative treatment of losses of substance of mandible, with special reference to fixation of edentulous fragments. IVY, R. H. AND CURTIS, L. Surg., Gynec. and Obst. *52:*849–854, April '31
Maintenance of facial form after removal of right half of mandible. ANDERSON, G. M. Internat. J. Orthodontia *17:*860–864, Sept '31
Plastic surgery after bicondyloid resection of mandible; case. CABROL. Rev. de stomatol. *33:*720–722, Dec '31
Resection and reconstruction of mandible; 2 cases. DOBRZANIECKI, W. Arch. ital. di chir. *35:*207–217, '33
Mandibular resection. HAYNEN, A. S. Am. J. Orthodontics *26:*793–796, Aug '40
Resection of lower jaw by oral route. BERTOLA, V. J. Prensa med. argent. *28:*323–327, Feb 5, '41
Function of lower jaw following partial resection. YOUNG, F. Surgery *11:*966–982, June '42
Function of lower jaw following partial resection. YOUNG, F. Am. J. Orthodontics (Oral Surg. Sect) *28:*581–598, Oct '42
Extensive resections of mandible; collaboration with odontologist in temporary functional therapy. JORGE, J. M. AND VIVONE, R. A. Bol. y trab., Acad. argent. de cir. *28:*134–152, May 3, '44

Mandible, Dislocations – Cont.
Resection of mandible; method that simplifies and overcomes defects of cases reported in the past. PEARSON, W. H. Am. J. Orthodontics *29:*141–147, March '43
Spontaneous regeneration of bone following excision of section of mandible. KAZANJIAN, V. H. Am. J. Orthodontics (Oral Surg. Sect.) *32:*242–248, April '46
Fibrin foam and thrombin as used in surgical removal of large fibromyxoma of mandible. WEINER, L. AND WALD, A. H., J. Am. Dent. A. *33:*731–735, June 1, '46

Mandible, Fractures: See Jaws, Fractures

Mandible, Micrognathia: See Jaws, Micrognathia

Mandible, Prognathism: See Jaws, Prognathism

Mandible, Resection of: See Jaws, Bone Grafting; Jaws, Cancer; Jaws, Surgery, Prostheses in; Jaws, Tumor

MANDI, F.: Typical finger injuries in baseball. Wien. med. Wchnschr. *77:*965, July 16, '27
MANDL, F. AND RABINOVICI, N.: Microscopically verified success of pinch homografting in human case. J. Internat. Coll. Surgeons. *9:*439–446, July–Aug '46
MANDL, F. AND RABINOVICI, N.: Experiments with "cuto-omentopexy" and skin homotransplantation. J. Internat. Coll. Surgeons *9:*525–530, Sept–Oct '46
MANES, A. J.: Dacryocystorhinostomy; radical cure for lacrimation; Semana med. *1:*1020–1027, April 26, '28
MANGABEIRA-ALBERNAZ, P.: Pathogenesis and therapy of rhinophyma. Rev. de laryng. *56:*1199–1214, Dec '35
MANGANO, J. L.: Functioning false joint of finger following severe trauma. Am. J. Surg. *42:*659–661, Dec '38
MANGANOTTI, G.: Abrasive cheilitis; clinical and histologic study of precancerous lesions. Arch. ital. di dermat., sif. *10:*25–67, Jan '34
MANGES, W. F. (see SMITH, R. M.) Nov '37
MANGIARACINA, A.: Congenital atresia of posterior nares. Arch. Otolaryng. *32:*1088–1089, Dec '40
MANGOLD, M. W.: Compound fracture of maxilla. U. S. Nav. M. Bull. *27:*132–133, Jan '29

Mangoldt Technic

Laryngotracheoplasty by Mangoldt technic in therapy of laryngotracheal fistula. LASKIEWICZ, A. Rev. de laryng. *59:*463–471, May '38

MANKEL, W.: Combined developmental abnormalities of outer ear. Hals-, Nasen-u. Ohrenarzt (Teil 1) *27:*354–363, '36

MANN, F. C.: Grafts of organs. Libman Anniv. Vols. *2:*757–771, '32

MANN, I. AND KILNER, T. P.: Deficiency of malar bones with defect of lower eyelids. Brit. J. Ophth. *27:*13–20, Jan '43

MANNA, A.: Surgical treatment of epithelioma of hand. Policlinico (sez. prat.) *29:*753–755, June 5, '22 (illus.) abstr: J.A.M.A. *79:*776, Aug 26, '22

MANNA, A.: Responsibility of surgeon in esthetic surgery; case. Rev. de chir. structive. pp. 149–151, Dec '35

MANNA, A.: Recent progress in plastic surgery. Chir. plast 4:150–170, Oct–Dec '38

MANNHEIM, A. AND ZYPKIN, B.: Free autoplastic cartilage transplantation. Arch. f. klin. Chir. *141:*668–672, '26 abstr: J.A.M.A. *87:*2132, Dec 18, '26

MANNHEIM, A. AND ZYPKIN, B.: Late results of cartilage transplantation. Arch. f. klin. Chir. *149:*31–39, '27

MANNHEIM, H.: Clinical experiences with Braun's epidermal grafts. Arch. f. Klin. Chir. *154:*98–113, '29

MANNHEIM, H.: Homoplastic and heteroplastic transplantation of skin in man. Arch. f. klin. Chir. *162:*551–560, '30

MANNHEIM, H.: Comment on article by Schurch on homoplastic transplantation of epithelium. Zentralbl. f. Chir. *58:*789–790, March 28, '31

DELLA MANO, N.: Cavernous angioma of tendon sheaths; case. Policlinico (sez. chir.) *39:*593–612, Oct '32

MANSFIELD, O. T.: Spontaneous gangrene (Fournier's gangrene). Brit. J. Surg. *33:*275–277, Jan '46

MANSIE, J. W.; MATTHEWS, E. AND ROUND, H.: Symposium on facial restorations (prostheses). Proc. Roy. Soc. Med. *36:*483–487, July '43

DE MARCHI, E.: Congenital median fistula of neck. Arch. ital. di chir. *22:*91–100, '28

MARCHENKO, E.: Artificial vagina formation from large intestine (S. Romanum). Mosk. med. j. (no. 2) *8:*61–65, '28

MARBLE, H. C.; HAMLIN, E. Jr. AND WATKINS, A. L.: Regeneration of radial nerve and ulnar nerve. Am. J. Surg. *55:*274–294, Feb '42

MARBLE, H. C.: Management of hand injuries. J. Indust. Hyg. and Toxicol. *26:*189–192, June '44

MARBLE, H. C.: Purposeful splinting of hand following injuries. J.A.M.A. *116:*1373–1375, March 29, '41

MARAGLIANO, D.: Treatment of extensive subcutaneous angiomas of face by Morestin's method. Arch. ital. di chir. *12:*603–615, '25

MANZANILLA, M. A.: Maggot therapy in infected wound of comminuted jaw fracture; case. Medicina, Mexico *13:*1–7, Jan 10, '33

MANWARING, J. G. R.: Hand infections. J. Michigan M. Soc. *26:*554–555, Sept '27

MANTHEY, P.: Right facial hemiatrophy following thyroidectomy. Ztschr. f. d. ges. Neurol. u. Psychiat. *114:*192–199, '28

MANSON, J. S.: Heredity and Dupuytren's contracture. Brit. M. J. *2:*11, July 4, '31

MANSON, J. S.: Webbing of left arm. Lancet *1:*1182, June 4, '21

MARCHINI, F.: Dermoid cysts of dorsum of nose. Policlinico (sez. prat.) *30:*1422, Oct 29, '23

MARCKS, K. M.: Use of implantation grafts in healing of infected ulcers. Am. J. Surg. *51:*354–361, Feb '41

MARCKS, K. M.: Soft tissue repair in injuries about face and head. Pennsylvania M. J. *45:*801–806, May '42

MARCKS, K. M.: Burn therapy for medical defense unit, with reference to early and late therapy. Am. J. Surg. *58:*174–180, Nov '42

MARCKS, K. M.: Modified calibrated grafting knife. Mil. Surgeon *92:*653–654, June '43

MARCKS, K. M.: Modified calibrated knife in skin grafting; further observations. Surgery *17:*109–115, Jan '45

MARCKS, K. M. AND ZUGSMITH, G. S.: Plastic repair of deformities of socket and minor defects about the orbit. Arch. Ophth. *36:*55–69, July '46

MARCKS, K. M. (see WILLIAMS, P. E.) April '46

MARCOGLOU, A. E.: Therapy of rhinophyma. Presse med. *38:*790, June 7, '30

MARCUS, A. AND GROH, J. A.: X-ray treatment of acute osteomyelitis of fingers; preliminary report. Indust. Med. *9:*551–554, Nov '40

Marcus-Gunn Phenomenon

Synkinesis between third and seventh pairs of cranial nerves (of musculus levator palpebrae superioris and of musculus zygomaticus respectively); similarity to Marcus Gunn phenomenon; case. AZZOLINI, U. Riv. oto-neuro-oftal. *19:*398–412, Nov–Dec '42

MARCY, G. H.: Traumatic shock. Indust. Med. *5:*493–497, Oct '36

Marfan Syndrome

Arachnodactylia, kyphoscoliosis, patent interventricular septum and ectopy of crystalline lens (Marfan syndrome); case. ROCH, M. Presse med. *45:*1429–1430, Oct 9, '37

MARFORT, A. AND BISI, R. H.: Plastic surgery by Axhausen method in cleft palate; case. Rev. Asoc. med. argent. *53:*93–94, Feb 15–28, '39

MARFORT, A.; BISI, R. H. AND VON SOUBIRON, N.: Temporomaxillary arthroplasty (Lindemann operation); results in 2 cases. Rev. Asoc. med. argent. *53:*88–90, Feb 15–28, '39

MARFORT, A. AND EMILIANI, C. M.: Temporomandibular ankylosis. Rev. oto-neuro-oftal. *13:*103–105, April '38

MARFORT, A.; EMILIANI, C. M. AND FARJAT, F. P.: Osteomyelitis of lower jaw; author's surgical therapy of 3 cases. Rev. Asoc. med. argent. *51:*386–387, Oct 15, '37

MARGAROT, J. AND RIMBAUD, P.: Hypertrophic ascending ulnar neuritis following injury; case. Rev. neurol. *65:*134–139, Jan '36

MARGETSON, ELISABETH: *Living Canvas: A Romance of Aesthetic Surgery*. Methuen, London, 1936

MARGOLIN, G. S.: Surgical therapy of injuries of nerve trunks at front. Khirurgiya, no. 5, pp. 68–73, '45

MARIN, A.: Treatment of baso-cellular epithelioma of face. Union med. du Canada *56:*489–500, Sept '27

MARIN, A.: Treatment of rhinophyma; case. Union med. du Canada *57:*641–644, Nov '28

MARIN, A.: Rhinophyma. Canad. M. A. J. *25:*589–591, Nov '31

MARIN, A.: Coexistence of basal celled epithelioma of temporal region and spinocellular epithelioma of lip; case. Union med. du Canada *61:*770–772, June '32

MARIN, A.: Surface angioma of face treated with cryotherapy and radium. Union med. du Canada *65:*446–449, May '36

MARIN, A.: Rhinophyma, case treated and cured. Union med. du Canada *68:*159–160, Feb '39

MARIN, A.: Rhinophyma; therapy by Ollier's surgical decortication. Bull. Soc. franc. de dermat. et syph. *46:*705–709, April '39

MARIN, G. M.: Temporomaxillary ankylosis. Med. espan. *3:*406–428, May '40

MARÍN AMAT, M.: Grave hemorrhage as late complication of dacryocystorhinostomy; 2 cases. Siglo med. *87:*673–675, June 20, '31 also: Arch. d'opht. *48:*632–638, Sept '31

MARÍN-AMAT, M.: Severe hemorrhage as late complication of dacryocystorhinostomy. Bull. et mem. Soc. franc. d'opht. *44:*269–278, '31 also: Arch. de oftal. hispano-am. *31:*629–636, Nov '31

MARÍN AMAT, M.: Comparative results of bipolar electrolysis and radium therapy in angioma of eyelids in infants; 2 cases. Arch. de oftal. hispano-am. *32:*604–613, Nov '32

MARIN GATICA, J.: Dupuytren's contracture. Rev. med. de Chile *67:*1221–1232, Nov '39

MARINESCO, G.; DRAGANESCO, AND VASILIU. Unilateral facial atrophy; 2 cases. Rev. d'oto-neuro-opht. *6:*405–407, May '28

MARINESCO, G.; KREINDLER, A. AND FAÇON, E.: Role of sympathetic nervous system in pathogenesis of facial hemiatrophy with report of case of hemiatrophy of one side of face and other side of body. Paris med. *1:*269–275, March 26, '32 also: Bull. sect. scient. Acad. roumaine (nos. 6–8) *14:*155–166, '31

MARINESCO-SLATINA, D. (see PAULIAN, D. *et al*) March '33

MARINI, J. (see MASI, C.) May '38

MARINO, H.: Cancer of lower lip; technic of surgical therapy. Rev. de cir. de Buenos Aires *16:*53–62, Feb '37

MARINO, H.: Skin grafts. Dia med. *11:*143–146, Feb 20, '39

MARINO, H.: Valgism of third phalanx of finger; therapy of case. Prensa med. argent. *27:*1798–1799. Aug 28, '40

MARINO, H.: Cicatricial ectropion; therapy by free grafts; case. Rev. med.-quir. de pat. fem. *16:*231–236, Sept '40

MARINO, H.: Z-shaped incision in plastic surgery for cicatricial contracture. Rev. Asoc. med. argent. *55:*208–211, March 15–30, '41

MARINO, H.: Therapy of hand infections. Prensa med. argent. *28:*1104–1112, May 21, '41

MARINO, H.: Light aspirator in surgery of palatine fissure and in general surgery. Prensa med. argent. *29:*481–483, March 18, '42

MARINO, H.: Therapy of progenism by Lindemann method. Arq. de cir. clin. e exper. *6:*301–306, April–June '42

MARINO, H.: Cleft palate therapy; Brown operation. Arq. de cir. clin. e exper. *6:*333–336, April–June '42

MARINO, H.: Maxillary osteotomy in extensive palatine fissures of adult. Arq. de cir. clin. e exper. *6:*615–620, April–June '42

MARINO, H.: Dermoepidermal grafts using Padgett dermatome; detail of technic. Dia med. *14:*912–914, Sept 7, '42

MARINO, H.: Congenital fistula of nasal dorsum; radical extirpation; cases. Prensa med. argent. *30:*2297–2299; 2299–2300, Dec 1, '43

MARINO, H.: Plastic surgery in dermatology; large free grafts. Rev. argent. dermatosif. *27:*458–461, '43

MARINO, H.: Plastic surgery of cleft palate. Prensa med. argent. *30:*2350–2352, Dec 8, '43

MARINO, H.: Plastic surgery of cicatrix; case. Prensa med. argent. *30:*2502–2505, Dec 29, '43

MARINO, H.: Cancer of upper lip; excision and plastic surgery in case. Prensa med. argent.

*31:*137–140, Jan 19, '44
MARINO, H.: Work of Jacques Joseph, (1865–1934) especially in plastic surgery. Prensa med. argent. *31:*449–450, March 1, '44
MARINO, H.: Plastic repair of section of flexor tendons of hand and of median nerve; case. Prensa med. argent. *31:*1305–1308, July 12, '44
MARINO, H.: Total pharyngoplasty in cancer. Prensa med. argent. *31:*1509–1516, Aug 9, '44
MARINO, H.: Principles and indications of burn therapy. Bol. y trab., Soc. de cir. de Cordoba *5:*361–375, '44
MARINO, H.: Plastic surgery in present war. Bol. Soc. cir. d. Uruguay *16:*311–321, '45
MARINO, H.: Plastic surgery in war; recent advances in United States and Great Britian. Bol. y trab., Soc. argent. de cirujanos *6:*778–788, '45 also: Rev. Asoc. med. argent. *59:*1373–1376, Dec 15, '45
MARINO, H.: Palatoplasty; procedure for immobilization of mucosa and sutures. Prensa med. argent. *32:*436–438, March 9, '45
MARINO, H.: Extensive infected burns. Gac. med., Lima *1:*177–178, June '45 also: Rev. san. de policia *5:*185–196, July–Aug '45
MARINO, H.: Plastic surgery in second World War. Arch. urug. de med., cir. y especialid. *28:*197–207, Feb '46
MARINO, H.: The asymmetrical face. Prensa med. argent. *33:*1242–1247, June 14, '46
MARINO, H.: Surgical therapy of gigantic nevi. Prensa med. argent. *33:*1321–1325, June 28, '46
MARINO, H.: Free graft in form of cutaneous "bandage"; use in severe burns. Bol. y trab. Acad. argent. de cir. *30:*451–459, July 17 '46
MARINO, H.: Rhinoplasty; importance of microgenia of jaw. Prensa med. argent. *33:*1500–1503, July 19, '46
MARINO, H. AND CRAVIOTTO, M.: Complete harelip; correction of large unilateral fissures of adult. Semana med. *1:*1003–1008, April 25, '40
MARINO, H. AND CRAVIOTTO, M.: Fractures of mandible; Mowlem method of external pin fixation. Prensa med. argent. *33:*1823–1827, Sept 6, '46
MARINO, H. AND ESPERNE, P.: Dermoepidermal grafts; autostabilizing retractor. Rev. med.-quir. de pat. fem. *17:*137–140, Feb '41
MARINO, H. (see FINOCHIETTO, R.) Sept '34
MARINO, H. (see FINOCHIETTO, R.) Oct '35
MARINO, H. (see FINOCHIETTO, R.) June '38
MARINO, H. (see FINOCHIETTO, R. *et al*) Dec '41
MARINO, H. (see FINOCHIETTO, R. *et al*) Nov '42
MARINO, H. (see FINOCHIETTO, R.) Sept–Nov '45
MARINUCCI, C. L.: Muscular (tendinous) avulsion of flexor profundus of middle finger of right hand; case. Riforma med. *48:*1834–1838, Nov 26, '32
MARION, G.: Correction of balanic hypospadias. J. d'urol. *14:*473–478, Dec '22 (illus.) abstr: J.A.M.A. *80:*1032, April 7, '23
MARION, G.: Construction of continent urethra in female; application in exstrophy. J. d'urol. *37:*393–402, May '34

Marion Operation

Hypospadias, correction by plastic surgery of urethra by Marion's operation. SALLERAS, J. Rev. de especialid. *5:*1385–1389, Oct '30 also: Semana med. *1:*10–11, Jan 1, '31

Marion-Heitz-Boyer Operation (See also Heitz-Boyer-Hovelacque Operation)

Exstrophy of bladder, cure by Marion-Heitz-Boyer method (transplantation of ureters into rectum) in man 20 years old. NANDROT. Bull. et mem. Soc. nat. de chir. *61:*1103–1105, Nov 2, '35

MARIQUE: Treatment of pseudohermaphroditism. Arch. franco-belges de chir. *25:*280–281, Dec '21 (illus.)
MARIGUE, P. (see COGNIAUX, P.) July '33
MARIS, A. M.: Jaw fractures. Bull. U. S. Army M. Dept. (no. 75) pp. 81–88, April '44
MARIS, A. M.: Fractures of jaw. Mil. Surgeon *95:*43–47, July '44
MARISCAL, E.: Study of surgical technic in cadaver; hemiresection of lower jaw. Prensa med. mex. *9:*59–61, May 15, '44
MARKOFF, N.: Plastic formation of vagina with bladder. Gynec. et Obst. *19:*182–190, March '29
MARKS, V. O.: Contractures following gunshot wounds; prophylaxis and therapy. Khirurgiya, no. 11, pp. 9–18, '44
MARMASSE, A. (see MAUREL, G.) May '28
MARMELSTEIN, M. (see APPLEBAUM, A.) Feb '43
MARMORSHTEYN, F. F. (see DASHEVSKIY, A. I.) 1940
DE LA MARNIERRE, Primary suture of accidentally sectioned flexor tendons of fingers. Bull. et mem. Soc. nat. de chir. *59:*1314–1317, Nov 18, '33
MARONNEAUD, P. L.: Fractures of lower jaw; indications for new surgical method of pin fixation. J. de med. de Bordeaux *123:*201–205, June '46
MAROTTOLI, O. R.: Results of immediate surgical therapy in grave trauma to face; case. An. de cir. *2:*273–279, Aug '36
MAROTTOLI, O. R.: Tendon transplantation in therapy of permanent radial paralysis; case. Bol. Soc. de cir. de Rosario *5:*434–435, Oct '38

MAROTTOLI, O. R.: Orthopedicosurgical therapy of chronic rheumatism. An. de cir. *5:*137–145, June '39

MAROTTOLI, O. R. AND BRAGAGNOLO, J.: Temporomandibular ankylosis of osteomyelitic origin; case. Bol. Soc. de cir. de Rosario *11:*194–201, July '44

MAROTTOLI, O. R. (see CAMES, O.) Sept '37

MAROTTOLI, O. R. (see ZENO, L.) April '39

MARQUARDT, P.: Burns and their therapy. Fortschr. d. Therap. *18:*27–34, Jan '42

MARQUE, A. M.: Remarks on 1008 cases of facial paralysis. Rev. de especialid. *2:*1195–1199, Dec '27 also: Rev. oto. neuro-oftal. *2:*1–4, Jan '28

MARQUE, A. M.: Peripheral facial paralysis; 1,008 cases. Semana med. *1:*946–949, April 19, '28

MARQUE, A. M. AND LANARI, E.: Electrolysis as cosmetic treatment of keloids and nevus pigmentosus. Semana med. *1:*159–164, Jan 16, '30

MARQUES, A.: Bilateral hypertrophy of breasts. Brazil-med. *35:*129, Sept 17, '21

MARQUES PORTO, E.: Therapy of war burns. Rev. med.-cir. do Brasil *51:*585–608, Nov '43

MARQUEZ, D. E. (see FERNICOLA, C. *et al*) Sept '42

MÁRQUEZ, M.: Argumosa blepharoplastic methods. Arch. de oftal. hispano-am. *33:*1–8, Jan '33

MÁRQUEZ, M.: Cosmetic therapy of mild forms of eyelid ptosis. Arch. de oftal. hispano-am. *33:*363–366, June '33

MÁRQUEZ, M.: Argumosa's 2 methods of blepharoplasty for tumors usually attributed to other authors (especially Dieffenbach). J. Internat. Coll. Surgeons *7:*63–67, Jan–Feb '44

MARQUIS, E.: Treatment of adenopathies which accompany cancer of lower half of face. Bull. et mem. Soc. nat. de chir. *53:*760–767, June 4, '27

MARRE, P.: Burn therapy. Avenir med. *32:*266–269, Nov '35

MARRIQ, AND FAURE, Mme.: Imperforate anus with communication between rectal ampulla and bladder; case. Bull. Soc. med.-chir. de l'Indochine *13:*150–151, Feb–March '35

MARRO, A.: Transcorium tegumental graft; case. Arch. ital. di chir. *52:*897-903, '38

MARRO, A.: Transcorium tegumental graft; value in case. Chir. plast. *4:*49–59, April–June '38

MARRONE, L. V. (see SIEGEL, S. A. *et al*) Sept '45

MARRONEAUD, P. (see LASSERRE, C.) Feb '36

MARSALEK, J.: Artificial vagina construction using fetal membranes. Casop. lek. cesk. *79:*1075–1078, Dec 6, '40

MARSH, F. B.: Plasma protein; physiologic action and therapeutic application in shock. Indust. Med. *10:*352–359, Aug '41

MARSHALL, G.: Circulatory changes in wounded soldiers (shock), with special reference to influence of drugs used for production of anesthesia. Guy's Hosp. Rep. *75:*98–111, Jan '25

MARSHALL, G. D.: Prevention of adhesions to tendons in hand and wrist, with report of 2 cases. J. Bone and Joint Surg. *10:*816–818, Oct '28

MARSHALL, H. K.: Artificial vagina formation; experiences with 3 different corrective procedures. West. J. Surg. *52:*245–255, June '44

MARSHALL, W.: Flap operation for treatment of multiple sebaceous cysts (steatomata). J. Invest. Dermat. *5:*299–302, Dec '42

MARSHALL, W.: Pathogenesis of keloids, with clinical applications in medicine and surgery. Proc. Am. Federation Clin. Research (1943) *1:*25, '44

MARSHALL, W.: Therapy of scars and keloids. New Orleans M. and S. J. *97:*15–17, July '44

MARSHALL, W. AND GREENFIELD, E.: Modified nonadherent gauze pressure treatment of burns. Am. J. Surg. *63:*324–328, March '44

MARSHALL, W. AND ROSENTHAL, S.: Pathogenesis of keloids and similar neoplasms in relation to tissue fluid disturbances (and therapy). Am. J. Surg. *62:*348–357, Dec '43

MARTENS, M.: Artificial vagina made from intestine. Deutsche med. Wchnschr. *47:*1226, Oct 13, '21

MARTENSTEIN, H.: Induratio penis plastica and Dupuytren's contracture. Med. Klin. *17:*44, Jan 9, '21

MARTILLOTTI, F.: Congenital malformation of external ear; 2 cases. Pediatria *45:*337–344, April '37

MARTIN: Repair of urethra with hypospadias by single operation (Duplay's method). Bull. Soc. franc. d'urol. *7:*242–244, Nov 19, '28 also: J. d'urol. *26:*564–567, Dec '28

MARTIN, C. L.: Carcinoma of lip and mouth. Radiology *22:*136–146, Feb '34

MARTIN, C. L. AND MARTIN, J. M.: Cancer in and about mouth, treated with irradiation by European method. Texas State J. Med. *27:*286–291, Aug '31

MARTIN, E. D.: Surgery of injuries and infections of hand. New Orleans M. and S. J. *77:*85–89, Aug '24

MARTIN, E. G.: Plastic use of skin in simple anal stricture; reconstruction of anal lining; pilonidal disease. Clinics *3:*1011–1013, Dec '44

MARTIN, G. E.: Local regional anesthesia in nose and throat operations. J. Laryng. and Otol. *59:*38–43, Jan '44

MARTIN, G. J. (see HUEPER, W. C. et al) June '42

MARTIN, H.: Cancer of skin, lip and tongue. Bull. Am. Soc. Control Cancer *26:*82–83, July '44

MARTIN, H. E.: Bulky carcinoma of lip treated by irradiation, wide surgical excision and plastic closure. Am. J. Cancer *15:*261–266, Jan '31

MARTIN, H. E.: Cheiloplasty for advanced carcinoma. Surg., Gynec. and Obst. *54:*914–922, June '32

MARTIN, H. E.: Carcinoma of mucosa of cheek treated by irradiation only; patient living and free of disease 5 years, 3 months. S. Clin. North America *13:*442–443, April '33

MARTIN, H. E.: Five year end-results in treatment of cancer of tongue, lip and cheek. Surg., Gynec. and Obst. *65:*793–797, Dec '37

MARTIN, H. E.: Benign and malignant tumors of palate. Arch. Surg. *44:*599–635, April '42

MARTIN, J.: Results of roentgen rays, radium diathermocoagulation and surgery in therapy of cutaneous epithelioma (face); 14 cases. Arch. d'electric. med. *44:*444–460, Dec '36

MARTIN, J. (see BERGERET, A.) Jan '34

MARTIN, J. D. JR.: Tannic acid treatment of burns. South. M. J. *26:*321–325, April '33

MARTIN, J. D. JR.: Clinical studies in burn therapy (tannic acid). J. M. A. Georgia *27:*39–46, Feb '38

MARTIN, J. D., JR.: Tannic acid in burns. Internat. Clin. *4:*148–153, Dec '38

MARTIN, J. D. JR.: Burn therapy. Indust. Med. *8:*384–386, Sept '39

MARTIN, J. D. JR.: Congenital preauricular fistula. J. M. A. Georgia *29:*411–413, Aug '40

MARTIN, J. D. JR.: Burn therapy. South. M. J. *35:*513–518, May '42

MARTIN, J. M.: X-ray treatment of epithelioma of face. Proc. Inter-State Post-Grad. M. Assemb., North America (1927) *3:*303–305, '28

MARTIN, J. M.: X-ray therapy as conservative method in cancer of lower lip. Proc. Internat. Assemb. Inter-State Post-Grad. M. A., North American (1930) *6:*399–403, '31

MARTIN, J. M.: Radiation therapy of cancer of lips and mouth. Radiology *16:*881–892, June '31

MARTIN, J. M. (see MARTIN, C. L.) Aug '31

MARTIN, L. AND BONNIOT: Androgynous pseudohermaphroditism; surgical correction of perineal and penile urethra. Bull. Soc. franc. d'urol., pp. 227–235, June 20, '32

MARTIN, L. C. (see WILLIAMS, I. G.) Jan '37

MARTIN, P.: Suture of radial nerve; case with 3 operations; recovery. J. de chir. et ann. Soc. belge de chir. *26:*224–229, Dec '27

MARTIN, R. C.: Toti-Mosher operation (lacrimal ducts) and its end results. Tr. Pacific Coast Oto-Ophth. Soc. *21:*50–58, '33

MARTIN, R. C.: Recent experiences with operation on facial nerve (including 2 cases of paralysis following mastoidectomy). Arch. Otolaryng. *32:*1071–1075, Dec '40

MARTIN, R. C.: Recent experiences with surgery of facial nerve. Tr. Am. Laryng., Rhin. and Otol. Soc. *46:*491–496, '40

MARTIN, R. C.: Repair of peripheral injuries to facial nerve (by anastomosis). J. Nerv. and Ment. Dis. *99:*755–757, May '44

MARTIN, T. M.: Treatment of tumors of parotid; survey of results obtained at Barnard Free Skin and Cancer Hospital. Arch. Surg. *36:*136–143, Jan '38

MARTIN, CALDERIN, A.: Cervicolaryngeal cyst of branchial origin; case. Semana med. espan. *6:*91, Jan 23, '43

MARTIN GROMAZ, L.: Nasal obstruction. An. med. *1:*31–35, July–Sept '40

MARTIN VIVALDI, J.: Scrotal hypospadias treated by Nove-Josserand-Borchers procedure. Rev. clin. espan. *4:*358–359, March 15, '42

MARTINDALE, L.: Plastic surgery and jaw injuries center somewhere in England. M. Woman's J. *49:*299, Oct '42

MARTÍNEZ, E. M.: Analysis of 138 cases of cancer of tongue treated at Instituto del Cancer in Havana. Bol. Liga contra del cancer *8:*12–21, Jan '33

MARTÍNEZ, E. M.: Surgical importance of skin grafts. Rev. med. peruana *5:*964–968, July '33

MARTÍNEZ, E. M.: Surgical therapy of cervical metastases of epithelioma (oral). Bol. Liga contra el cancer *12:*315–320, Sept–Oct '37

MARTÍNEZ, E. M. AND PUENTE DUANY, N.: Infiltrating cancer of nose; acute evolution; treatment by radium; case. Bol. de la Liga contra el cancer *3:*145–149, July 1, '28

MARTÍNEZ CORDOBA, F.; ANSELMO, J. J. AND LUGONES, L. M. Present status of burn therapy. Semana med. *2:*488–493, Aug 26, '43

MARTINEZ, L. (with S. NOËL): La chirurgie esthétique – nouveaux procedes de correction du prolapses mammaire. Le Concour Medical, No. 46 (October 27, 1928)

MARTINEZ SUAREZ, M.: Bone graft of mandible with prosthetic objective. J. Internat. Coll. Surgeons *3:*260–261, June '40

MARTÍNEZ VARGAS, A.: Cavernous lymphangioma of forehead; extirpation and cure. Med. de los ninos *33:*89–100, April '32

DE MARTINI, R.: Congenital choanal atresia; cases. Boll. d. mal. d. orecchio, d. gola, d. naso *57:*14–22, Jan '39

DE MARTINI, R.: Palatine fistula, plastic closure by means of turbinate bone. Boll. d. mal. d.

orecchio, d. gola, d. naso *59:*172–177, May '41
MARTINOTTI, L.: Case of symmetrical bilateral multiple small cysts in neck. Gior. ital. d. ma. ven. *65:*19–25, Feb '24
MARTINOTTI, L.: Superficial epitheliomas of skin. Arch. ital. di chir. *10:*471–556, '24
MARTINS, R.: Decubital eschars. Rev. brasil. de orthop. e traumatol. *1:*147–154, Nov–Dec '39
MARTINY: Harelip and cleft palate in relation to eugenic sterilization, according to German law. Ztschr. f. Stomatol. *36:*947, Aug 26; 1004, Sept 9, '38
MARTMER, E. E.: Talipomanus; three cases in one family. Am. J. Dis. Child. *34:*384–387, Sept '27
MARTON, M. H.: Treatment of hypertichosis by improved apparatus and technic (electrolysis). Arch. Phys. Therapy *21:*678–683, Nov '40
MARVIN, F. W.: Choice of anesthesia for maxillofacial surgery in war and civilian injuries. Am. J. Orthodontics (Oral Surg. Sect) *28:*254–257, May '42
MARX, J.: Problems of congenital origin of lateral fistulas and cysts of neck. Beitr. z. klin. Chir. *168:*435–447, '38 also: Orvosi hetil. *82:*891–895, Sept 10, '38
MARY, A. (see FRUCHAUD, H.) Aug '27
MARZIANI, R.: Indications, technic and results of skin grafting in third degree frostbite of foot. Boll. e mem. Soc. piemontese chir. *12:*277–279, '42
MAS, P. (see EUZIÉRE, J. *et al*) Aug '34
MASCIOTRA, A. A.: Dupuytren's disease from traumatic cause; medicolegal testimony in case. Semana med. *2:*1615–1617, Dec 24, '25
MASCIOTRA, A. A.: Retraction of palmar aponeurosis or Dupuytren's disease due to industrial trauma; medicolegal expertise in case. Semana med. *1:*1063–1066, May 12, '38
MASCIOTTRA, E.: Intra-arterial mercurochrome in hand infections. Rev. med.-quir. de pat. fem. *16:*273–280, Sept '40
MASCIOTTRA, E. L.: Hand infections; intra-arterial mercurochrome. Rev. Asoc. med. argent. *55:*271–273, April 15–30, '41
MASHKARA, K. I. (see MASUROVA, N. A.) Dec '37
MASI, C. AND MARINI, J.: Branchial cyst; case. Semana med. *1:*1061–1062, May 12, '38
MASINI, P.: Burn therapy in sanitary services of army. Hopital *27:*517, Nov; 544, Dec '39
MASLAND, H. C.: Splint for fractures of inferior maxilla. M. Times, New York *58:*75, March '30
MASLAND, H. C.: Implements for hand injuries. Am. J. Surg. *12:*142–143, April '31
MASLOV, I.: Harelip operation by Orlovsky method. Vestnik khir. (no. 33) *11:*146–150, Nov 22, '27
MASMONTEIL, F.: Tannic acid in burns; principles, advantages, method and results of application. Bull. et mem. Soc. d. chirurgiens de Paris *27:*91–96, Feb 1, '35
MASMONTEIL, F.: Sutures or reconstruction (using fascia lata) of sectioned hand tendons; 3 cases. Bull. et mem. Soc. d. chirurgiens de Paris *28:*379–384, June 5, '36
MASMONTEIL, F.: Bone transplantation. Bull. et mem. Soc. de med. de Paris *143:*376–379, June 9, '39
MASON, A.: Hand infections. New Zealand M. J. *38:*304–315, Oct '39
MASON, E. C.: Modern treatment of burns. J. Oklahoma M. A. *24:*273–274, Aug '31
MASON, J. B.: Evaluation of tannic acid treatment of burns. Ann. Surg. *97:*641–647, May '33
MASON, J. T.: Carcinoma of lower lip. S. Clin. N. America *4:*1095–1104, Oct '24
MASON, J. T. AND BAKER, J. W.: Cystic hygroma; 2 cases (neck). S. Clin. North America *11:*1091–1095, Oct '31
MASON, L. W.: Polymastia. Colorado Med. *31:*141–142, April '34
MASON, M.: Immediate treatment of hand injuries. Indust. Med. *6:*536–538, Oct '37
MASON, M. F. (see BLALOCK, A.) May '41
MASON, M. F. (see BLALOCK, A.) June '41
MASON, M. F. (see WOOD, G. O. *et al*) Aug '40
MASON, M. L.: Rupture of tendons with study of extensor tendon insertions in fingers. Surg. Gynec. and Obst. *50:*611–624, March '30
MASON, M. L.: Immediate and delayed tendon repair. Surg., Gynec. and Obst. *62:*449–457, Feb (no. 2A) '36
MASON, M. L.: Tumors of hand. Surg., Gynec. and Obst. *64:*129–148, Feb '37
MASON, M. L.: Surgical principles involved in treatment of open injuries of hand. West. J. Surg. *45:*239–248, May '37
MASON, M. L.: Pitfalls in management of hand infections. Minnesota Med. *20:*485–495, Aug '37
MASON, M. L.: Principles of management of tendon injuries (hand). Physiotherapy Rev. *18:*119–123, May–June '38
MASON, M. L.: Dupuytren's contracture; plastic surgery of hands (grafts). S. Clin. North America *19:*227–248, Feb '39
MASON, M. L.: Immediate treatment of open hand wounds. Mississippi Valley M. J. *61:*136–143, July '39
MASON, M. L.: Primary and secondary suture of tendons; discussion of significance of technic. Surg., Gynec. and Obst. *70:*392–402, Feb (no. 2A) '40

MASON, M. L.: Principles of management of hand infections. Rocky Mountain M. J. *37:*814–824, Nov '40

MASON, M. L.: Significance of function in repair of tendons. Arch. Phys. Therapy *22:*28–34, Jan '41

MASON, M. L.: Plastic surgery and repair of hand, with particular reference to repair of cutaneous defects. Indust. Med. *10:*47–52, Feb '41

MASON, M. L.: Minor surgical conditions of hand. S. Clin. North America *21:*181–195, Feb '41

MASON, M. L.: Injuries to nerves and tendons of hand. J.A.M.A. *116:*1375–1379, March 29, '41

MASON, M. L.: Nerve and tendon injuries of hand. Indust. Med. *11:*61–66, Feb '42

MASON, M. L.: Symposium on surgical infections of hand. S. Clin. North America *22:*455–477, April '42

MASON, M. L.: Treatment of injuries, with particular reference to nerve and tendon repair in hand. Indust. Med. *15:*323–325, May '46

MASON, M. L.: Trauma to hand; with particular reference to indications for primary and secondary nerve and tendon repair J. Oklahoma M. A. *39:*246–251, June '46

MASON, M. L. AND ALLEN, H. S.: Indelible pencil injuries to hands. Ann. Surg. *113:*131–139, Jan '41

MASON, M. L. AND ALLEN, H. S.: Significant factors in development of hand infections. Quart. Bull., Northwestern Univ. M. School *16:*42–56, '42

MASON, M. L.; ANSON, B. J. AND BEATON, L. E.: Surgical and anatomic aspects of case of double lower lip. Surg., Gynec. and Obst. *70:*12–17, Jan '40

MASON, M. L. AND KOCH, S. L.: Human bite infections, with study of route of extension of infection from dorsum of hand. Surg., Gynec. and Obst. *51:*591–625, Nov '30

MASON, M. L. AND QUEEN, F. B.: Grease gun injuries to hand; pathology and treatment of injuries (oleomas) following injection of grease under high pressure. Quart. Bull., Northwestern Univ. M. School *15:*122–132, '41

MASON, M. L. AND SHEARON, C. G.: Process of tendon repair; experimental study of tendon suture and tendon graft. Arch. Surg. *25:*615–692, Oct '32

MASON, M. L. AND WOOLSTON, W. H.: Isolated giant cell xanthomatic tumors of fingers and hand. Arch. Surg. *15:*499–529, Oct Oct '27

MASON, M. L. (see KANAVEL, A. B. *et al*) Feb '29

MASON, M. L. (see KOCH, S. L.) Jan '33

MASON, M. L. (see KOCH, S. L.) Jan '39

MASON, R.: Four generations of harelip. J. Hered. *17:*52, Feb '26

MASON, R. F.: Modern burn treatment. J. Tennessee M. A. *25:*267–271, July '32

MASSA, D. AND TATO, J. M.: External operation for correction of acquired nasal deformity. Rev. de especialid. *4:*129–135, April–May '29

MASSABUAU; GUIBAL, AND DUPONNOIS: Congenital serous cyst of neck; case. Bull. Soc. d. sc. med. et biol. de Montpellier *8:*354–358, Aug '27

MASSABUAU; LAUX, MME. AND GINESTIE, J.: Cause of death of badly burned persons; case of grave icterus. Arch. Soc. d. sc. med. et biol. de Montpellier *16:*213–218, April '35

MASSABUAU, G.: Volkmann contracture. Rev. gen. de clin. et de therap. (no. 42, bis) *45:*691–695, Oct 21, '31

MASSAROTTI, G.: Dupuytren's contracture; case. Gior. di med. mil. *76:*600–602, Nov '28

MASSART, R.: Surgical therapy of articular rheumatism. Bull. et mem. Soc. de med. de Paris *137:*385–395, May 27, '33

MASSART, R.: Surgical therapy of rheumatic arthritis. J. de med. de Paris *53:*644–646, Nov 2, '33

MASSART, R.: Bone graft from mother to child. Bull. et mem. Soc. d. Chirurgiens de Paris *27:*142–144, March 1, '35

MASSART, R.: Transplantation of healthy muscles with their blood vessels and nerves to paralyzed muscles in therapy of sequels of poliomyelitis. Bull. et mem. Soc. d. chirurgiens de Paris *28:*467–472, July 3, '36

MASSART, R. AND VIDAL-NAQUET, G.: Surgical therapy in articular rheumatism. Monde med., Paris *44:*971–977, Nov 1, '34

MASSART, R. AND VIDAL-NAQUET, G.: What to expect of surgical therapy in chronic rheumatism. J. de med. de Paris *55:*69–71, Jan 24, '35

MASSE, (see CHARBONNEL,) March '30

MASSIA, G. (see GATE, J.) Nov '26

MASSIE, F. M.: Skin grafts, use in plastic surgery. Kentucky M. J. *28:*238–246, May '30

MASSIE, G.: Hand deformities. Guy's Hosp. Gaz. *45:*296–298, July 25, '31

MASSIE, J. R. JR. (see RAWLES, B. W. JR.) Dec '44

MASSLOFF, I. D.: Surgical therapy of harelip by Orlowsky's method. Arch. f. klin. Chir. *150:*322–327, '28

MASSLOFF, I. D.: Value of Orloff's method in double harelip. Vestnik khir. (no. 51) *17:*69–73, '29

MASSLOFF, I. D.: Orlowski's method in double harelip. Chirurg *2:*220, March 1, '30

MASSON, J. C.: Congenital absence of vagina

and its treatment. Am. J. Obst. and Gynec. *24:*583–591, Oct '32
MAST, J. R. (see LEE, Q. B.) June '40
MASTEN, M. G.: Facial asymmetry; unilateral atrophy and facial hypertrophy; cases. Arch. Neurol. and Psychiat. *35:*136–145, Jan '36
MASTERS, W. E. (see SMITH, K. D.) March '39

Mastopexy: See Mammaplasty, Mastopexy

MASTROMARINO, A.: Cranial deformites due to premature synosteoses of sutures with particular reference to Crouzon's disease (craniofacial dysostoses) and Apert syndrome (acrocephaly and syndactylia). Arch. di ortop. *51:*233–304, June 30, '35
MASUDA, B. J.: Cancer of oral muscosa and circumoral areas. Am. J. Orthodontics (Oral Surg. Sect.) *31:*730–740, Dec '45
MASUDA, B. J.: Dermoid cyst in floor of mouth. Am. J. Orthodontics (Oral Surg. Sect.) *32:*252–256, Apr '46
MASUMOTO, K.: Processes of regeneration in nerve fibers of transplanted skin. Tr. Jap. Path. Soc. *22:*876–877, '32
MASUMOTO, K.: Regeneration of nerve fibers in transplanted skin; experimental study. Mitt. a. d. med. Akad. zu Kioto *7:*1036–1038, '33
MATA, P.: Dacryocystorhinostomy by modified Gutzeit method. Arch. de oftal. hispano-am. *34:*141–147, March '34
MATERZANINI, A.: Postoperative shock interpreted as secondary hemorrhage following subtotal hysterectomy. Clin. ostet. *4:*593–596, Sept '32
MATHER, K. AND PHILLIP, U.: Harelip inheritance in man. Ann. Eugenics *10:*403–416, Dec '40
MATHEWSON, G. H.: Formation of new lacrimonasal canal after excision of lacrimal sac. Am. J. Ophth. *14:*1252, Dec '31
MATHIEU, C.: Plastic surgery of adherent eyelid; case. J. de l'Hotel-Dieu de Montreal *9:*156–159, May–June '40
MATHIEU, P.: Twelve cases of hypospadias in young boys; operation; immediate and excellent results. Arch. d. mal. d. reins *3:*224–230, Feb '28
MATHIEU, P.: Hypospadias; treatment with cutaneous flap in single operation. Bull. et mem. Soc. nat. de chir. *56:*1314–1316, Nov 29, '30
MATHIEU, P.: Technic of one-stage operation for balanic or juxtabalanic hypospadias. J. de chir. *39:*481–486, April '32
MATHIS, H.: Maxillary injuries in sport. Wien. klin. Wchnschr. *54:*423–427, May 16, '41
MATHYS, A.: Tumors of velum. Bull. Soc. belge d'otol., rhinol., larying., pp. 83–87, '38
MATIS, E. I.: Simple nasal splint. J. Larying. and Otol. *55:*425–426, Sept '40
MATIS, E. I.: Method for suturing of nasal mucous membrane. Acta oto-laryng. *29:*80–82, '41 also: Medicina Kaunas *21:*1031–1034, Dec '40
MATIS, E. T.: Intranasal approach to lacrimal sac (transparent dacryocystotomy). Laryngoscope *53:*357–365, May '43
MATIS, I.: Skin graft in closure of retro-auricular fistulas. Medicina, Kaunas *21:*1027–1031, Dec '40
MATOLAY, G.: Modification of Makkas operation in therapy of exstrohy of bladder. Zentralbl. f. Chir. *66:*1130–1133, May 20, '39
MATOLCSY, T.: Surgical therapy of congenital webbed skin. Arch. f. klin. Chir. *185:*675–681, '36
MATOLCSY, T.: Surgical treatment of congenital webbed skin across joints. Orvosi hetil. *80:*1159–1161, Dec 5, '36
MATOLCSY, T.: Results of plastic surgery of breast. Arch. f. klin. Chir. *195:*666–671, '39
MATSON, D. D.: Tannic acid jelly (tanaburn); use in experimental burns. Surgery *13:*394–400, March '43
MATSON, D. D. (see INGRAHAM, F. D.) June '43
MATSUDA, E.: Congenital angioma of nasal tip; case. Oto-rhino-laryng. *11:*608, July '38
MATSUI, T.: Dacryocystostomy by nasal route. Oto-rhino-laryng. *12:*238–241, March '39 (in Japanese).
MATSUNAGA, T.: Dupuytren's contracture among Polynesians of Truk. Acta dermat. *13:*101, Jan '29
MATTHEWS, D. N.: Modern applications of plastic surgery. M. Press *201:*340–345, April 5, '39
MATTHEWS, D. N.: Skin grafts in casualty department. Lancet *2:*597–598, Sept 9, '39
MATTHEWS, D. N.: Dressing of open wounds and burns with tulle gras. Lancet *1:*43–44, Jan 11, '41
MATTHEWS, D. N.: Value of local chemotherapy (with sulfanilamide and its derivative, sulfathiazole); Hunterian lecture, abridged. (BURNS) Lancet *2:*271–275, Sept 5, '42
MATTHEWS, D. N.: Burn therapy. Practitioner *153:*86–93, Aug '44
MATTHEWS, D. N.: Storage of skin for autogenous grafts (Hunterian lecture, abridged). Lancet *1:*775–778, June 23, '45
MATTHEWS, DAVID N.: *Surgery of Repair, Injuries, and Burns.* CC Thomas Co., Springfield, Ill., 1946
MATTHEWS, E.: Facial prostheses. Brit. M. J. *1:*223, Feb 14, '42

MATTHEWS, E. (see MANSIE, J. W. *et al*) July '43

MATTHEWS, H. B. AND MAZZOLA, V. P.: Intravenous use of hypertonic glucose in gynecology; Experimental and clinical study of surgical shock. Surg., Gynec. and Obst. *62:*781-790, May '36

MATTHEWS, J. L.: Ophthalmic injuries (including burns) of war. War Med. *4:*247-261, Sept '43

MATTI, H.: "Transport" plastic operations of face. Schweiz. med. Wchnschr. *58:*669-673, July 7, '28

MATTI, H.: Osteotomy and transplantation of substantia spongiosa. Schweiz. med. Wchnschr. *59:*1254-1258, Dec 7, '29

MATTI, H.: Free transplantation of substantia spongiosa (bone). Arch. f. klin. Chir. *168:*236-258, '31

Matti Operation: See Reich-Matti Operation

MATTICK, W. L. (see SCHREINER, B. F.) June '29

MATTICK, W. L. (see SCHREINER, B. F.) July '33

MATTISON, J. A.: Discussion of prevention and treatment of shock in combat zone. Mil. Surgeon *88:*114-118, Feb '41

MATTOCKS, A. M. AND LAZIER, W. A.: Hydrophilic acid ointments for debridement of burns. J. Am. Pharm. A. (Scient. Ed.) *35:*275-279, Sept '46

MATTOS, S. O.: Exstrophy of bladder, Coffey-Mayo operations and their results. Rev. de obst. e ginec. de Sao Paulo *4:*107-126, Oct-Dec '39

MATWEJEW, D. N.: Histologic examination of bone transplant after 15 years. Monatschr. f. Ohrenh. *64:*417-422, April '30

MATWEJEW, D. N.: Rule for operation in atresia of nares. Monatschr. f. Ohrenh. *65:*1188-1192, Oct '31

MATWEJEW, F. P.: Formation of vagina by means of modified skin graft method. Zentralbl. f. Gynak. *58:*2727-2736, Nov 17, '34 also: Rev. franc. de gynec. et d'obst. *30:*57-71, Feb '35

MÁTYÁS, M.: Radium therapy of postoperative keloids. Zentralbl. f. Chir. *57:*3039-3040, Dec 6, '30

MATYAS, M.: Accidental skin transplantation in Tschmarke brushing therapy of severe burns. Zentralbl. f. Chir. *67:*2245-2246, Nov 30, '40

MAUCLAIRE, P.: Surgical grafts. Rev. med. franc. *8:*9-30, Jan '27

MAUCLAIRE, P.: Grafts bone and bony implants for repairing large deficiencies in epiphysis and diaphysis; concealed internal prosthesis. Bull. et mem. Soc. nat. de chir. *53:*1363-1373, Dec 17, '27

MAUCLAIRE, P.: Reparation of bone loss by Ollier osteoperiostic grafts, segmentary bone grafts, bone implantations and hidden internal prostheses. Rev. med. franc. *15:*263-273, March '34

MAUCLAIRE, P.: Comparison of various methods of repair of gaps in skull. Maris med. *11:*153, Feb 19, '21 abstr: J.A.M.A. *76:*1049, April 9, '21

MAUCLAIRE, P.: Grafts and implantations of tissue and organs in man and in animals. Medecine (supp.) *13:*1-67, Feb '32

MAULDIN, L. O.: How an eye was saved by plastic surgery. J. South Carolina M. A. *26:*299-300, Dec '30

MAUN, M. E. *et al:* Tissue reactions to medications used in local treatment of burns. Surgery *14:*229-238, Aug '43

MAUN, M. E. (see HIRSHFELD, J. W. *et al*) May '43

MAUN, M. E. (see HIRSHFELD, J. W. *et al*) Oct '43

MAUREL, G.: Surgical correction of cervicofacial scars of dental origin. J. de med. de Paris *46:*577-583, July 21, '27

MAUREL, G.: Autoplastic closure of bucco-nasal and bucco-sinusal communications; illustrations. Rev. de stomatol. *29:*764-781, Nov '27

MAUREL, G.: Maxillofacial surgery; cases. Rev. odont. *50:*377-407, Oct '29

MAUREL, G.: *Chirurgie Maxillofaciale*. Maloine, Paris, 1931. Second Edition, LeFrançois, Paris, 1940

MAUREL, G.: Technic in plastic surgery of upper jaw. Rev. de chir. plastique, pp. 32-62, April '31

MAUREL, G.: Surgical and orthopedic correction of congenital and false (traumatic) prognathism; 3 cases. Rev. de chir. structive, pp. 5-23, March '37

MAUREL, G.: Surgico-orthopedic correction of congenital and of false traumatic prognathism. Chir. plast. *4:*63, April-June; 97, July-Sept; 171, Oct-Dec '38

MAUREL, G. AND MARMASSE, A.: Traumatic infection of lower jaw with fracture; necrosing osteitis; operation; regeneration; case. Rev. odont. *49:*341-357, May '28

MAURER, G.: Dupuytren's contracture of palmar fascia and its treatment. Deutsche Ztschr. f. Chir. *246:*685-692, '36

MAURER, G.: Tetanus after burns. Zentralbl. f. Chir. *65:*2771-2772, Dec 10, '38

MAURER, H.: Development of harelip and cleft palate in embryo 22 mm. in length. Ztschr. f. Anat. u. Entwcklingsgesch. *105:*359-373, '36

MAURER, H.: Healing process in harelip and cleft palate in embryo 23.3 mm. in length.

Ztschr. f. Anat. u. Entwcklngsgesch. *107:*203-211, '37
MAURER, H. (see HOEPKE, H.) 1938
MAURETTE, R. (see GARCIA CASTELLANOS, J. A.) 1943
MAXEINER, S. R.: Case of skin grafting. Minnesota Med. *11:*185, March '28
MAXEINER, S. R. (see TIECK, G. J. E. *et al*) Feb '22

Maxilla, Cancer (See also Jaws, Cancer)

Malignant disease of superior maxillary bone; continued report. DABNEY, S. G. Kentucky M. J. *19:*125, March '21
Epthelioma du Maxillaire Superieur, by Verger. Doin, Paris, 1925
Statistical postoperative prognosis of malignant tumors of upper jaw. OLAISON, F. Hygiea *89:*705-710, Sept 30, '27
Cancer of upper maxilla and lip; operation; recovery. BONNET-ROY, F. Odontologie *66:*39, Jan '28
Combined surgical and radium treatment of carcinoma of superior maxillary; case. JENTZER, A. Schweiz. med. Wchnschr. *58:*659-662, June 30, '28
Management of malignancies of antrum, superior maxilla, pharynx and larynx at Radium Institute of University of Paris. PACK, G. T. Ann. Otol. Rhin. and Laryng. *37:*967-973, Sept '28
Cancer of upper jaw; 4 cases. DUFOURMENTEL, L. Bull. et mem. Soc. de chir. de Paris *22:*745-751, Dec 5, '30
Late results of operations on maxillary bone in cancer of oral cavity; 5 cases. DE-BERNARDI, L. Boll. e mem. Soc. piemontese di chir. *2:*1114-1148, '32
Cancer of maxilla and ethmoid; survey of 50 cases. DAVIS, E. D. D. Brit. M. J. *1:*53-55, Jan 13, '34
Plastic repair of defect following operative treatment of carcinoma of antrum and upper jaw. BECK, J. C. AND GUTMANN, M. R. S. Clin. North America *14:*775-782, Aug '34
Curability of malignant tumors of upper jaw and antrum. NEW, G. B. AND CABOT, C. M. Proc. Staff Meet., Mayo Clin. *9:*684-685, Nov 7, '34
Curability of malignant tumors of upper jaw and antrum. NEW, G. B. AND CABOT, C. M. Surg., Gynec. and Obst. *60:*971-977, May '35
Curability of malignant tumors of upper jaw and antrum. NEW, G. B. AND CABOT, C. M. Tr. Am. Laryng., Rhin. and Otol. Soc. *41:*584-590, '35
Malignant tumors of upper jaw. PORTMANN, G. AND DESPONS, J. Rev. de laryng. *57:*1-44, Jan '36

Maxilla, Cancer—Cont.

Cancer of cheek and neighboring bone. BLAIR, V. P.; *et al.* Internat. J. Orthodontia *22:*183-188, Feb '36
Plastic and prosthetic therapy after resection of upper jaw for cancer; cases. FRENCKNER, P. AND SUNDBERG, S. Acta oto-laryng. *27:*147-158, '39
Malignant tumors of upper jaw; Skinner lecture, 1943. WINDEYER, B. W. Brit. J. Radiol. *16:*362, Dec '43; 17:18, Jan '44
Adenocarcinoma of maxilla. THOMA, K. H. Am. J. Orthodontics (Oral Surg. Sect) *28:*65-85, Feb '42
Malignant tumors of upper jaw. ORSI, J. L. Rev. med. de Rosario *34:*983-1011, Oct '44
Early diagnosis of malignant tumors of upper jaw. KALLENBERGER, K. Schweiz. med. Wchnschr. *75:*990-995, Nov 10, '45
Osteogenic sarcoma of maxilla; case BOIES, L. R.; *et al.* J. Oral Surg. *4:*56-60, Jan '46; correction 4:126, Apr '46

Maxilla, Fractures (See also Jaws, Fractures; War Injuries, Jaws)

Fracture of maxillary sinus plus emphysema of lower eyelid. MOREAU, J. Arch. franco-belges de chir. *25:*421-424, Feb '22 (illus.)
Fracture of condylar region of maxilla; 6 cases. BERCHER, J. Rev. de chir. 61:200-218, '23 (illus.)
Etiology and symptoms of closed temporo-maxillary fractures. DUFOURMENTEL, L. Bull. et mem. Soc. de chir. de Paris *20:*557-565, June 15, '28
Pseudarthrosis of upper jaw after fracture of Guerin type; case. GÓMEZ, O. Bol. y trab. de la Soc. de cir. de Buenos Aires *12:*393-400, Aug 1, '28
Unusual fracture of superior maxilla; appreciation of incapacity for labor. GOMEZ, O. L. Rev. de especialid. *3:*511-519, Sept '28
Compression treatment of fracture of superior maxilla resulting from blow; case. ZARENKO, P. P. Arch. f. klin. Chir. *153:*161-169, '28
Compound fracture of maxilla. MANGOLD, M. W., U. S. Nav. M. Bull. *27:*132-133, Jan '29
Acromioclavicular dislocation; osteosynthesis by kangaroo tendon; fracture of scapula and maxilla. ROCHER, H. L. AND MALAPLATE. J. de med. de Bordeaux *59:*145, Feb 20, '29
Principles of treatment of fractures of superior and inferior maxillae. SCHMUZIGER, P. Schweiz. med. Wchnschr. *60:*101-104, Feb 1, '30
Typical case of Guerin fracture of upper jaw.

Maxilla, Fractures—Cont.

GIOIA, T. Bol. y trab. de la Soc. de cir. de Buenos Aires *14:*976–982, also: Semana med. *2:*1982–1985, Dec 25, '30 Nov 26, '30

Fractures of maxillary zygomatic region and their treatment. STACY, H. S., M. J. Australia *1:*779–780, June 27, '31

Fracture of upper jaw; case. PIERI, G. Valsalva *7:*670–673, Sept '31

Simple treatment of maxillary fracture. ESKES, T. J. Nederl. tijdschr. v. geneesk. *76:*670–674, Feb 13, '32

Fractures of mandible and maxilla; treatment. HUTCHINSON, R. H. Maine M. J. *23:*53–57, March '32

Multiple fractures of upper and lower jaws. HAVENS, F. Z. Proc. Staff Meet., Mayo Clin. *7:*433–434, July 27, '32

Use of splints in complicated maxillary fracture. WUHRMANN, H. Schweiz. med. Wchnschr. *62:*767–769, Aug 20, '32

Horizontal fracture of upper jaw consolidated in defective position and resulting in total malocclusion; functional and esthetic restoration by surgical and prosthetic therapy. DUFOURMENTEL, L.; *et al.* Bull. et mem. Soc. d. chirurgiens de Paris *24:*555–558, Dec 2, '32

Consolidation of horizontal maxillary fracture in vicious position with total loss of dental articulation. DUFOURMENTEL, L.; *et al.* Rev. de stomatol. *35:*339–342, June '33

Fracture of maxilla through left optic foramen; reduction with Kingsley splint, with restoration of vision. LANGDON, H. M. Arch. Ophth. *9:*980–981, June '33

Treatment of fractures of maxillary bones. BERETTA, A. Gior. di med. mil. *81:*952–956, Nov '33

Treatment of fractures of maxilla, mandible and other bones of face. AUFDERHEIDE, P. J., J. Am. Dent. A. *21:*950–961, June '34

Surgical therapy of fractures of upper jaw. JEŽEK, K. Bratisl. lekar. listy *14:*243–246, June '34

Splint for fractures of maxillary bones. MORGAN, W. M., J. Am. Dent. A. *21:*1736–1746, Oct '34

Treatment of maxillary fractures. SIMPSON-SMITH, A. AND GRAVES-MORRIS, W. M. Brit. M. J. *2:*632, Oct 6, '34

Fracture of upper jaw; unusual case. MELCHIOR, M. Ztschr. f. Stomatol. *32:*1331–1335, Nov 23, '34

Clinical and experimental study of muscle damage in maxillary fractures. LINK, K. H. Arch. f. klin. Chir. *181:*24–77, '34

Fractured jaw caused by depression of upper

Maxilla, Fractures—Cont.

jaw; case. DUBECQ, X. J., J. de med. de Bordeaux *112:*43–44, Jan 20, '35

Compound, comminuted fracture of both maxillae and mandible. BRADSHAW, T. L. Internat. J. Orthodontia *21:*260–262, March '35

Fractures of upper jaws. ALONSO, J. M. Ann. d'oto-laryng., pp. 1062–1070, Oct '35

Fractures of mandible and superior maxilla in time of peace. JELINEK, V. J. Voj.-san. glasnik *6:*513–539, '35

Short history of treatment of maxillary fractures. FAIRBANK, L. C. Mil. Surgeon *78:*95–103, Feb '36

Fractures of upper jaw; reduction apparatus with pneumatic cushion. HAMON, J. Rev. de stomatol. *38:*518–521, July '36

Late examination of fractures of upper jaw. LINK, K. H. Zentralbl. f. Chir. *64:*467–469, Feb 20, '37

Treatment of fracture of upper jaw. BLAIR, V. P.; *et al.* Surgery *1:*748–760, May '37

Fractures of upper jaw; treatment. NEUWIRT, F. AND SIMSA, J. Casop. lek. cesk. *76:*1182–1188, July 2, '37

Kirschner traction in treatment of maxillary fractures. MAJOR, G., J.A.M.A. *110:*1252–1254, April 16, '38

Role of sympathetic in maxillary fractures. DECHAUME, M. Presse med. *46:*714–715, May 4, '38

Technic of reduction of fracture of upper jaw; case. THEODORESCO, D. AND CRISTODULO. Rev. de chir., Bucuresti *41:*496–499, July–Aug '38

Fractured maxillae; description of appliance for reduction and fixation with case report. RALPH, H. G. AND MAXWELL, M. M., U. S. Nav. M. Bull. *36:*507–511, Oct '38

Badly consolidated fracture of upper jaw; reduction by osteotomy and elastic traction apparatus. THEODORESCO, D. Rev. de chir., Bucuresti *41:*918–926, Nov–Dec '38

Fracture of upper maxilla associated with extensive trauma of left half of forehead, injury to right optic canal and blindness of right eye; case. SVERDLOV, D. G. AND GOLDIN, L. B. Vestnik oftal. *12:*515–516, '38

Late reduction of fracture of upper jaw. RUSPA, F. Stomatol. ital. *1:*122–130, Feb '39

Treatment of maxillomandibular fractures at aid station and at base hospital. GILKISON, C. C. Mil. Surgeon *84:*441–451, May '39

Diplopia in fracture of upper and lower maxillary and of malar bones; case. PAOLI, M. Rev. de stomatol. *41:*548–552, July '39

Therapy of maxillary fractures. BELTRAMI,

Maxilla, Fractures – Cont.
G. Marseille-med. *1:*32-37, Jan 15, '40
Treatment and complications in fractures of maxillary bones. McDonough, F. J. Am. J. Orthodontics *26:*162-174, Feb '40
Mechanism of temporomaxillary fractures. Beck, H. Ztschr. f. Stomatol. *38:*201-221, March 22, '40
Fractures of maxillae and mandible. Logsdon, C. M., J. Am. Dent. A. *27:*389-392, March '40
Maxillofacial fractures. Hautant, A. Ann. d'oto-laryng., pp. 169-194, March-April '40
Fractures of maxilla. Richison, F. A., J. Am. Dent. A. *27:*558-563, April '40
Management of fractures of maxilla. Davidson, J. B. and Brown, A. M. Mil. Surgeon *87:*26-42, July '40
Incomplete fractures of upper maxilla and their sinusal complications. Dechaume, M. Presse med. *48:*627-628, July 31-Aug 3, '40
New devices for reduction of maxillary fractures. Woodward, C. M. Mil. Surgeon *87:*525-531, Dec '40
Therapy of maxillary fractures according to Ivy. Bakhmutova, E. A. Sovet. med. (no. 4) *4:*38-39, '40
Choice of apparatus for reduction and bandaging in maxillary fractures. Ponroy, and Psaume. Rev. de stomatol. *41:*782-789, '40
Maxillary fractures in relation to dentistry. Frongia, L. Rassegna med. sarda *43:*18-41, Jan-Feb '41
Surgical and dental treatment of fractures of upper and lower jaws in wartime; review of 119 cases. McIndoe, A. H. Proc. Roy. Soc. Med. *34:*267-288, March '41
Fractures of maxillae and mandible; 2 cases (with description of apparatus). Yando, A. H. and Taylor, R. W., U. S. Nav. M. Bull. *40:*155-157, Jan '42
Fractures of maxilla; simplified appliance for craniomaxillary support and fixation. Waldon, C. W. and Balkin, S. G. Surgery *11:*183-194, Feb '42
Treatment of fractures of upper jaw. Erich, J. B., J. Am. Dent. A. *29:*783-793, May '42
Fractures of maxillary bones. Parker, D. B. Laryngoscope *52:*365-370, May '42
Care of military and civilian injuries; fractures of maxilla. Thoma, K. H. Am. J. Orthondontics (Oral Surg. Sect) *28:*275-291, May '42
Compact splints with new fixation method for maxillary fractures. Dimeg, O. Ztschr. f. Stomatol. *40:*485-504, July '42

Maxilla, Fractures – Cont.
New operation for fractures into maxillary sinus and antrum. Warren, E. D. Dis. Eye, Ear, Nose and Throat *2:*304-305, Oct '42
Fractures of upper jaw, malar bone and zygomatic arch. Schildt, E. Nord. med. (Hygiea) *16:*3700-3705, Dec 26, '42
Care of military and civilian injuries; fractures of mandible, maxilla, zygoma and other facial bones; statistical study of 1,149 cases. Lyons, D. C. Am. J. Orthodontics (Oral Surg. Sect.) *29:*67-76, Feb '43
Maxillary fractures. Parker, D. B., J. Oral Surg. *1:*122-130, April '43
Maxillary fractures. Stevenson, W. B. Am. J. Orthodontics *29:*331-332, June '43
Applicances and attachments for treatment of upper jaw fractures. Crawford, M. J. U. S. Nav. M. Bull. *41:*1151-1157, July '43
Review of 215 fractures of maxillae. Hallam, J. W. Brit. Dent. J. *76:*181-182, April 6, '44
Simplified method of treatment of maxillary fractures (use of cap splint). MacGregor, A. B. Brit. Dent. J. *76:*239-241, May 5, '44
Method of fixation in fractures involving maxillary antrum. Scharfe, E. E. Canad. M.A.J. *50:*435-437, May '44
Maxillary forceps in fractures. Gordon, S. Lancet *2:*80, July 15, '44
Maxillary fracture appliance of new principle and design. Johnston, B. and Titze, L. O. Hosp. Corps Quart. (no. 6) *17:*137-139, Nov '44
Alcohol block in delayed consolidation of maxillary fractures. Belskaya, V. M. Khirurgiya, no. 7, pp. 46-49, '44
Modified maxillary fracture splint for jaw. Blausten, S. Bull. U. S. Army M. Dept. (no. 84) pp. 119-121, Jan '45
Appliances for external fixation of mandible and cranial fixation of maxilla. Converse, J. M. Am. J. Orthodontics (Oral Surg. Sect.) *31:*111-112, Feb '45
Fractures of upper jaw; 150 cases in overseas maxillofacial center. Clark, H. B. Jr. J. Oral Surg. *3:*286-303, Oct '45
Reduction of complete transverse fracture of edentulous maxilla. Stevenson, H. N. and Tuoti, F. A., U. S. Nav. M. Bull. *45:*910-913, Nov '45
Fractures of maxilla. Gonzalez Ulloa, M. Vida nueva *56:*175-182, Dec '45
Use of cheek wires in treatment of fractures of maxilla. Holland, N. W. A. Brit. Dent. J. *79:*333-340, Dec 21, '45
Treatment of fractures of superior and inferior maxilla. McNichols, W. A. Illinois M.

Maxilla, Fractures–Cont.
J. *90:*179–185, Sept '46

Maxilla, Infections (See also Jaws, Fractures, Infections: Jaws, Infections)

Diagnosis and treatment of acute and chronic osteomyelitis of mandible and maxilla. MEAD, S. V. Internat. J. Orthodontia *14:*321–340, April '28

Suppurations of maxillary sinus and of orbit with extensive destruction of wall of sinus simulating cancer of upper jaw; case. GUNSETT, *et al.* Bull. et mem. Soc. de radiol. med. de France *24:*170, Feb '36

Gangrenous inflamation of nose and upper jaw of uncertain etiology; 2 cases. JOISTEN, E. Ztschr. f. Hals-, Nasen-u. Ohrenh. *41:*105–128, '36

Spreading osteomyelitis of maxilla (use of surgery and penicillin). HALLBERG, O. E. Minnesota Med. *28:*126–127, Feb '45

Osteomyelitis of superior maxilla; treatment with penicillin. HIRST, O. C. Arch. Otolaryng. *41:*351–352, May '45

Intermaxilloparotid cellular space; abcesses formed there. PONS-TORTELLA, E. AND BROGGI, M. Med. clin., Barcelona *5:*273–277, Oct '45

Total bimaxillary necrobiosis; case with recovery after surgical therapy aided especially by extract of calf jawbone (vaduril). SOLDANO, H. A. O. Prensa med. argent. *30:*1945–1947, Oct 6, '43

Maxilla, Tumors (See also Jaws, Tumors; Maxilla, Cancer)

Congenital tumors of maxilla; report of case with operation. CUTLER, G. D. AND ROCK, J. C. Boston M. and S. J. *192:*1001–1002, May 21, '25

Tumor of upper jaw; surgical therapy with plastic repair; 2 cases. PAVLOVSKY, A. J. AND di PIETRO, A. Bol. y trab. de la Soc. de cir. de Buenos Aires *19:*384–391, June 26, '35

Retromaxillary tonsillar cysts; removal by predigastric incision; case. LERICHE, R. Lyon chir. *35:*574–575, Sept–Oct '38

Plastic surgery of hard palate after excision of huge osteoma of upper jaw; author's technic. PIETRANTONI, L. Valsalva *15:*205–211, May '39

Author's method of plastic reconstruction of palate after removal of huge osteoma of upper jaw. PIERANTONI, L. Plast. chir. *1:*109–112, '40

Tumors of maxilla. ARMBRECHT, E. C. AND APPLE, C. W. Am. J. Orthodontics (Oral Surg. Sect.) *29:*60–64, Jan '43

Maxilla, Tumors–Cont.

Oral and maxillary tumors; experience at First Surgical Clinic of Vienna University during years 1930–1940. TRAUNER, R. Wien. klin. Wchnschr. *57:*192, April 21, '44

Osteomas of upper jaw. LUSCHER, E. Schweiz. med. Wchnschr. *75:*924–927, Oct 20, '45

Maxillary Resection (See also Jaws, Cancer; Maxilla, Cancer)

New method of resection of upper maxillary with lower facial flap. LAUWERS, E. E. Surg., Gynec. and Obst. *39:*499–502, Oct '24

Spontaneous reconstruction of lower maxilla after total surgical removal; case. ALONSO, J. M. AND QUINTELA, U. An. de oto-rino-laring. d. Uruguay *1:*72–76, '31

Apparatus for fixation of skin flap during epithelization of wound cavity after resection of upper jaw. KHARI, A. P. Novy khir. arkhiv *43:*328–330, '39

Maxillofacial Deformities (See also Specific Deformities and Jaws, Deformity)

Duplication of upper jaw. BUMM, E. Arch. f. klin. Chir. *135:*506–519, '25

Maxillofacial dystrophies. MEYER, J. AND NICOLLE. Rev. franc. de pediat. *3:*304–340, July '27

Role of hereditary syphilis in maxillo-facial dystrophies. MEYER, J. Ann. d. mal. ven. *23:*494–505, July '28

Deformities of lips from maxillary abnormalities. SCHWARZ, R. Schweiz. Monatschr. f. Zahnh. *39:*331–344, June '29

Diagnosis of dento-maxillo-facial deformities. MUZII, E. Stomatol. *28:*821–865, Oct '30

Familial aplasia of upper jaw, new type of facial dysostosis. SENDRAIL, M. Prat. med. franc. *15:*127–130, Feb. (B) '34

Therapy and prophylaxis of maxillary deformities by immobilization with monobloc. LASSERRE, C. AND MARRONEAUD, P. Arch. franco-belges de chir. *35:*131–134, Feb '36

Maxillofacial dysmorphism; 5 cases. PEYRUS, J. Rev. de stomatol. *38:*393–409, May '36

Rare congenital malformation of right portion of lower and upper jaw (unilateral micrognathia); case. CASTAY. Bull. et mem. Soc. de radiol. med. de France *25:*125–126, Feb '37

Maxillary deformities and their orthopedic therapy. CAUHEPE, J. Medecine *18:*657–658, Aug '37

Maxillofacial Deformities – Cont.

Complications of dento-maxillo-facial malformations; importance of correction. FAUCONNIER, H. J. AND PATCAS, H. Liege med. *32:*1-9, Jan 1, '39

Unilateral absence of intermaxillary bone without cleft; case. KOZLIK, F. Anat. Anz. *88:*91-100, April 3, '39

Heredity of congenital fossette of lip in conjunction with clefts of upper jaw. TRAUNER, R. Wien. klin. Wchnschr. *54:*427-429, May 16, '41 addendum: *54:*454, May 23, '41

Multiple cleft formations of maxillofacial region and their combination with other malformations. GERKE, J. Munchen. med. Wchnschr. *90:*712, Dec 17, '43

Maxillofacial Injuries (See also Jaws, Fractures; Jaws, Injuries; Maxilla, Fractures; War Injuries, Jaws)

Diagnostic, Traitement, et Expertise des Sequelles des Accidents des Regions Maxillo-faciales, by LÉON DUFOURMENTEL AND LEON FRISON. J. B. Bailliere et fils, Paris, 1922

Fractures of the Jaws, by Robert H. Ivy and Lawrence Curtis. Lea and Febiger, Phila., 1931. Second Edition, 1938. Third Edition, 1945

Relation of traumatic lesions of sense organs to maxillofacial surgery. LACAZE. Rev. odont. *52:*87-99, Feb '31

Fracture of orbit and superior maxilla followed by subcutaneous and deep emphysema from secondary infection. BONNET, P. Lyon chir. *28:*718-719, Nov-Dec '31

Considerations sur les fractures du maxillaire inferieur. Hans Huber, Berne, 1932

Maxillo-facial injuries. GINGRASS, R. P. Wisconsin M. J. *33:*568-571, Aug '34

Maxillo-Facial Injuries, Report of Army Standing Ctte., by War Office of Great Britain. H.M. Stationery Office, London, 1935

Laceration of face with traumatic avulsion of entire maxilla; case. STUMPF, F. W., J. Am. Dent. A. *22:*1206-1208, July '35

Maxillofacial injuries. BOWLER, R. L., J. Missouri M. A. *34:*448-449, Dec '37

Maxillofacial fractures. HAUTANT, A. Ann. d'oto-laryng., pp. 169-194, March-April '40

Feeding and care of patients with maxillofacial wounds. AKS, L. V. Ortop. i. travmatol. (no. 1) *14:*90-96, '40

Maxillofacial injuries; important considerations. IVORY, J., J. Indust. Med. *10:*52-54, Feb '41

Synopsis of Traumatic Injuries of the Face and Jaws, by Douglas B. Parker, C. V. Mosby Co., 1942

Maxillofacial Injuries – Cont.

Traumatic Surgery of the Jaws, Including First-Aid Treatment, by Kurt H. Thoma. C. V. Mosby Co., St. Louis, 1942

Statistics for years 1936-1940 in clinic for dentistry and maxillary injuries at University of Kiel. TILLMANN, G. Ztschr. f. Stomatol. *40:*61-75, Jan 30, '42

Management of recent faciomaxillary and mandibular fractures. WOODWARD, F. D. AND FITZ-HUGH, G. S. Virginia M. Monthly *69:*612-619, Nov '42

Maxillofacial injuries. CHRISTIANSEN, G. W. M. Ann. District of Columbia *14:*76-77, Feb '45

Uses of screw-pin in maxillofacial cases. RUSHTON, M. A. AND WALKER, F. A. Brit. Dent. J. *78:*289-292, May 18, '45

Definitive treatment of maxillofacial injuries. PARKER, D. B., J. Oral Surg. *3:*320-325, Oct '45

Control of bone fragments in maxillofacial surgery. WEISS, L. R., J. Oral Surg. *3:*271-285, Oct '45

Maxillofacial injuries. BLOCKER, T. G. AND WEISS, L. R., J. Indiana M. A. *39:*60-63, Feb '46

Therapy of acute maxillofacial wounds. HENDERSON, J. A. Dia med. *18:*183-184, March 4, '46

Rationale of treatment in maxillofacial injuries, with report of 4 cases. MAXWELL, M. M.; *et al.* J. Oral Surg. *4:*269-303, Oct '46

Aid to prosthetic restorations of maxilla after excision. WALKER, D. G. Lancet *1:*1209-1210, May 27, '39

Buccomaxillofacial prosthesis; artificial nose and palate; case. GRAZIANI, M. Rev. brasil. de oto-rino-laring. *9:*217-221, May-June '41

Maxillofacial prosthesis. NAGLE, R. J. Am. J. Orthodontics (Oral Surg. Sect.) *29:*312-319, June '43

Prosthetic appliance for war injury (maxillofacial injuries). JEFFREYS, F. E., U. S. Nav. M. Bull. *42:*711-714, March '44

Maxillofacial prosthesis. LLOYD, R. S., J. Am. Dent. A. *31:*1328-1335, Oct 1, '44

Maxillofacial prosthesis. DE MONTIGNY, G. Union med. du Canada *74:*1727-1735, Dec '45

Maxillofacial Prostheses (See also Jaws, Prostheses; Prosthesis)

Maxillofacial prosthesis. BODINE, R. L. Internat. J. Orthodontia *14:*998, Nov; 1076, Dec '26; *15:*42, Jan; 163, Feb; 254, March; 371, April '29

Maxillofacial Prostheses – Cont.

Maxillofacial prosthesis. CHENET, H. Odontologie *67:*831-850, Dec '29

Maxillofacial prosthesis of cellulose acetate. LAPIERRE, V. Odontologie *68:*634-653, Sept '30

Immediate maxillary prosthesis. PONT, A. Rev. de chir. plastique, pp. 264-270, Jan '32

La pratique stomatologique. Tome VIII: Restauration et prosthese maxillofaciales. Masson et Cie, Paris, 1935

Maxillofacial Surgery (See also Facial Fractures; Facial Injuries; Facial Surgery; Jaws, Fractures; Jaws, Injuries; Jaws, Surgery of; Maxillofacial Injuries; War Injuries, Jaws)

Plastic surgery, facio-maxillary; case reports. HARTER, J. H. Northwest Med. *25:*404-408, Aug '26

Underdeveloped maxilla and overdeveloped mandible; case report. MCCARTER, W. A. Internat. Orthodont. Cong. *1:*483, '27 also: Internat. J. Orthodontia *13:*625, July '27

Cases illustrating maxillo-facial and plastic surgery. JOHNSON, L. W., U. S. Nav. M. Bull. *26:*843-861, Oct '28

Maxillofacial surgery. BUTOIANU, S. AND STOIAN, C. Rev. san. mil., Bucuresti *28:*344-355, Sept '29

Maxillofacial surgery; cases. MAUREL, G. Rev. odont. *50:*377-407, Oct '29

Plastic repair after operations on upper jaw. WOODMAN, E. M. Proc. Roy. Soc. Med. (Sect. Laryng.) *24:*11-14, Feb '31 also: J. Laryng. and Otol. *46:*405-409, June '31

Technic in plastic surgery of upper jaw. MAUREL, G. Rev. de chir. plastique, pp. 32-62, April '31

Surgical and prosthetic interference for correction of excessive protrusion of maxilla. WOODWARD, C. M. Dental Digest *37:*213-218, April '31

Plastic surgery in loss of substance of alveolar border of incisive region of upper jaw; case. DARCISSAC, M. Bull. et mem. Soc. d. chirurgiens de Paris *23:*507-511, July 3, '31

Simplified method for correction of dishface. MALINIAK, J. W. Laryngoscope *41:*715-717, Oct '31

Tasks and accomplishments of maxillary surgery. AXHAUSEN, G. Deutsche med. Wchnschr. *58:*401-404, March 11, '32

Resection for prognathism of upper jaw; case. An. de cir. *3:*364-368, Dec '37

Corrective osteotomy of maxilla. AXHAUSEN, G. Deutsche Ztschr. f. Chir. *248:*515-522, '37

Surgical Diseases of the Mouth and Jaws, by EARL C. PADGETT. W. B. Saunders Co., Phila., 1938

Significant developments that have contributed to advancement of oral and maxillofacial surgery. CARR, M. W. Ann. Dent. *5:*206-212, Dec '38

Therapy of superior pro-alveolism (superior alveolar prognathism). TSOUCANELIS, A. Stomatol., Athenes *1:*77-90, '38

Chirurgie maxillofaciale, by G. Maurel. Maloine, Paris, 1931. Second Edition, LeFrançois, Paris, 1940

Maxillofacial surgery. IMBERT, L. Marseille-med. *1:*121-124, March 15, '40

Chirurgie de la face et de la région maxillofaciale, by Maurice Aubry and Charles Freidel. Masson et Cie, Paris, 1942

Instruments for maxillofacial and oral surgery. GINESTET, G. Rev. de stomatol. *43:*121-123, July-Aug '42

New ideas in reconstructive maxillofacial surgery. VIRENQUE. Rev. de stomatol. *43:*149-158, Sept-Oct '42

Brenthurst Papers, by JACK PENN (editor). Witwatersrand Univ. Press, Johannesburg, 1944

Lateral osteotomy; anatomic considerations (description of grove on frontal process of maxilla). GALE, C. K. Am. J. Surg. *63:*368-370, March '44

Maxillofacial prognathism; surgical therapy of case. BERTOLA, V. J. AND MOREYRA BERNAN, L. Bol. y trab., Soc. de cir. de Cordoba *6:*59-75, '45

Trismus in relation to maxillofacial surgery. LOADER, G. S. Brit. Dent. J. *81:*193-196, Sept 20, '46

Maxillofacial Surgery, Anesthesia for (See also Jaws, Surgery, Anesthesia for; War Injuries, Jaws)

Ocular complications from local anesthesia in resection of upper jaw. DORON, G. Zentralbl. f. Chir. *54:*2966-2969, Nov 19, '27

Simplified maxillary anesthesia. HARTSTEIN, S. D. Am. Dent. Surgeon *48:*90, Feb '28

Local anesthesia with procaine hydrochloride as anesthesia of choice in operations on upper maxilla. AUBRY, M. Presse med. *43:*592, April 10, '35

Anesthesia for faciomaxillary surgery. MUSHIN, W. W. Post-Grad. M. J. *16:*245-246, July '40

Preanesthetic medication with special consideration of problems in maxillofacial surgery. LYMAN, E. E. Mil. Surgeon *88:*57-62, Jan '41

Maxillofacial Surgery, Anesthesia for—Cont.
Review of local anesthesia in maxillofacial cases. O'HARA, D. M. Mil. Surgeon *89:*652-656, Oct '41
General anesthesia in treatment of maxillofacial cases. FISCHER, T. E. Mil. Surgeon *89:*877-892, Dec '41
Choice of anesthesia for maxillofacial surgery in war and civilian injuries. MARVIN, F. W. Am. J. Orthodontics (Oral Surg. Sect) *28:*254-257, May '42
Practical points in anesthesia at maxillofacial unit. HUNTER, J. T. Anesth. and Analg. *21:*223-228, July-Aug '42
Nitrous oxide-oxygen anesthesia; endotracheal technic in oromaxillofacial surgery. TYLER, E. A. Anesth. and Analg. *22:*177-179, May-June '43

Maxillofacial Surgery, Dental Aspects (See also Jaw Fractures, Teamwork; War Injuries, Jaws)
Surgical correction of maxillary and palatal defects in cooperation with orthodontist and prosthodontist. VAUGHAN, H. S. Dental Cosmos *69:*63-67, Jan '27
Metallic crowns and bridges in maxillofacial orthopedics. FILDERMAN, J. Rev. odont. *52:*5-12, Jan '31
Modern principles in maxillary orthopedics. HÄUPL, K. Wien. klin. Wchnschr. *54:*131-132, Feb 14, '41
Anomalies of maxillary angle; Albrecht's lemurine apophysis. ZENO, L. An. de cir. *8:*48-51, March-June '42
Dental aspect of maxillofacial surgery. GOLDIE, H. South African M. J. *18:*224-225, July 8, '44
Maxillofacial surgical unit mobile dental laboratory. DALLING, E. J. Brit. Dent. J. *78:*10-12, Jan 5, '45
Medical and dental relationship in maxillofacial team. RANKOW, R. M. Ann. Dent. *4:*164-166, Mar '46

MAXWELL, E.: Persistent fistula of lacrimal sac treated by ultraviolet rays; case. Tr. Ophth. Soc. U. Kingson *50:*648, '30
MAXWELL, J. S.: Modification of Hotz operation for entropion due to trachoma. Am. J. Ophth. *24:*298-302, March '41
MAXWELL, M. M.: Treatment of facial fractures of special interest to dental surgeon. U. S. Nav. M. Bull. *36:*501-507, Oct '38
MAXWELL, M. M.: Fractures of interest to dental officer; 3 cases. U. S. Nav. M. Bull. *44:*353-360, Feb '45
MAXWELL, M. M.; SCHORK, C. J. AND HEIDT, E.: Rationale of treatment in maxillofacial injuries, with report of 4 cases. J. Oral Surg. *4:*269-303, Oct '46
MAXWELL, M. M. (see FULCHER, O. H.) May '43
MAXWELL, M. M. (see RALPH, H. G.) Oct '38
MAY, A. (see ROSENBLATT, M. S.) Oct '46
MAY, H.: Vascularization of entire reimplanted radii in dog; relation to regeneration of bone and marrow, to growth and to joint cartilage. Beitr. z. klin. Chir. *160:*30-74, '34
MAY, H.: Regeneration of bone transplants. Ann. Surg. *106:*441-453, Sept '37
MAY, H.: Plastic operation for breast hypertrophy. Arch. Surg. *38:*113-117, Jan '39
MAY, H.: Scope and problems of plastic surgery. Pennsylvania M. J. *42:*1453-1458, Sept '39
MAY, H.: Correction of scars. Am. J. Surg. *50:*754-760, Dec '40
MAY, H.: One stage operation for closure of large defects of lower lip and chin. Surg., Gynec. and Obst. *73:*236-239, Aug '41
MAY, H.: Transplantation and regeneration of tissue. Pennsylvania M. J. *45:*130-135, Nov '41
MAY, H.: Regeneration of joint transplants and intracapsular fragments. Ann. Surg. *116:*297-310, Aug '42
MAY, H.: Reconstruction of breast deformities (atrophy). Surg., Gynec. and Obst. *77:*523-529, Nov '43
MAY, H.: Burn therapy. Am. J. Surg. *63:*34-46, Jan '44
MAY, H.: Closure of defects with composite vermilion borderlined flaps. Ann. Surg. *120:*214-223, Aug '44
MAY, H.: Closure of defects of skin after surgery for cancer. Clinics *4:*53-62, June '45
MAY, H.: Correction of cicatricial contractures of axilla, elbow joint and knee. S. Clin. North America *25:*1229-1241, Oct '45
MAY, H.: Closure of surface defects of hand. Pennsylvania M. J. *49:*116-120, Nov '45
MAY, H.: Tendon transplantation in hand. Surg. Gynec. and Obst. *83:*631-638, Nov '46
MAY, J.: Orientation in etiology of permanent retraction of fingers. An. Fac. de med. de Montevideo *28:*675-685, '43
MAY, R. M.: Repercussions of nerve grafts. Encephale *27:*885-902, Dec '32
MAY, R. M.: New studies on brephoplastic grafts. Arch. d'anat. micr. *35:*147-199, '40
MAYANTS, I. A.: New plastic operation for avulsion of skin of thumb; utilization of scrotal skin. Arch. f. klin. Chir. *181:*303-310, '34 abstr.: Novy khir. arkhiv. *32:*180-184, '34
MAYCOCK, W. D'A. AND WHITBY, L. E. H.: As-

pects of wound shock with experiences in treatment. J. Roy. Army M. Corps *77:*173-187, Oct '41

MAYCOCK, W. D'A. AND WHITBY, L. E. H.: Wound shock with experiences in treatment. J. Roy. Nav. M. Serv. *27:*358-371, Oct '41

Maydl Operation (See also Borelius-Maydl Operation)

Remote results of Maydl's operation for exstrophy of bladder. MUGNIÉRY, E. Lyon chir. *18:*481, July-Aug '21 abstr: J.A.M.A. *77:*1606, Nov 12, '21

Case operated according to method of Maydl-Borelius (exstrophy of bladder). BRATTSTRÖM, E. Acta chir. Scandinav. *55:*33-37, '22 (illus.; in English) abstr: J.A.M.A. *79:*1562, Oct 28, '22

Maydl-Borelius operation for exstrophy of bladder. BRATTSTRÖM, E. Beitr. z. klin. Chir. *127:*419-421, '22 Abstr: J.A.M.A. *80:*364, Feb 3, '23

Remote results of Maydl's operation for exstrophy. ROLOFF, F. Zentralbl. f. Chir. *57:*1977-1979, Aug 9, '30

Late results of Maydl operation for congenital ectopy of bladder. GRAUBNER, E. Zentralbl. f. Chir. *63:*2657-2658, Nov 7, '36

Maydl operation in child 1½ years old for exstrophy. HEYN, W. Zentralbl. f. Gynak. *64:*194-198, Feb 3, '40

Pregnancy in woman 25 years old after Maydl operation in childhood for exstrophy of bladder and cleft pelvis; review of clinical aspects of exstrophy. SCHUMANN, H. Geburtsh. u. Frauenh. *4:*318-333, Aug '42

Surgical therapy of exstrophy of bladder, with special reference to Maydl and Coffey operations. TILK, G. U. Deutsche Ztschr. f. Chir. *257:*287, '43

MAYEDA, T.: Treatment of head scars in Japan. Ztschr. d. japan. chirurg. Gesellsch. *35:*59-60, '34

MAYER, A.: Operative treatment of exstrophy of bladder. Zentralbl. f. Gynak. *51:*1887-1898, July 23, '27

MAYER, F. J.: Two instruments for modelling transplanted cartilage in closure of laryngeal and tracheal defects. Monatschr. f. Ohrenh. *69:*1193-1196, Oct '35

MAYER, F. J.: Nasal furuncle. Monatschr. f. Ohrenh. *74:*167-182, April '40

MAYER, F. O.: Hand injuries during boxing. Arch. f. orthop. u. Unfall-Chir. *32:*245-246, '32

MAYER, L.: Free transplantation of tendons. Am. J. Surg. *35:*271, Sept '21

MAYER, L.: Physiological method of tendon transplantation. Surg., Gynec. and Obst. *33:*528, Nov '21

MAYER, L.: Tendon transplantations for division of extensor tendon of fingers. J. Bone and Joint Surg. *8:*383-394, April '26

MAYER, L.: Loop operation for paralysis of adductors of thumb. Am. J. Surg. *2:*456-458, May '27

MAYER, L.: Interesting case of hand infection and injury. Am. J. Surg. *8:*1087-1088, May '30

MAYER, L.: Recurrent dislocation of jaws. J. Bone and Joint Surg. *15:*889-896, Oct '33

MAYER, L.: Repair of severed tendons in hand. Am. J. Surg. *42:*714-722, Dec '38

MAYER, L.: Celloidin tube reconstruction of extensor digitorum communis sheath. Bull. Hosp. Joint Dis. *1:*39-45, July '40

MAYER, L.: Generalities and fundamentals of tendon surgery. Medicina, Mexico *25:*468-474, Nov 10, '45

MAYER, F. X. AND PESTA, H.: Spectral analysis of eschars. Wien. klin. Wchnschr. *53:*397-399, May 17, '40

MAYER, L. AND RANSOHOFF N. S.: Physiological method of repair of damaged finger tendons; preliminary report on reconstruction of destroyed tendon sheath. Am. J. Surg. *31:*56-58, Jan '36

MAYER, L. AND RANSOHOFF, N. S.: Reconstruction of digital tendon sheath; contribution to physiological method of repair of damaged finger tendons. J. Bone and Joint Surg. *18:*607-616, July '36

MAYER, O.: Payment epithelial cancer of nasal cavity cured by roentgen treatment; case. Wien. med. Wchnschr. *78:*587, April 28, '28

MAYER, O.: Medical care of injuries of external nasal surface. Wien. klin. Wchnschr. *47:*109-110, Jan 26, '34

MAYET, H.: Late results of cranioplasty by hinging method of bone grafts. Bull. et mem. Soc. d. chirurgiens de Paris *24:*138-140, Feb 19, '32

MAYET, H.: Von Hacker's operation for hypospadias. Bull. et mem. Soc. de chir. de Paris *21:*394-403, May 17, '29 also: Paris chir. *21:*149-154, July-Aug '29

MAYFIELD, F. H.: New elastic splint for wrist drop. Bull. U. S. Army M. Dept. (no. 73) pp. 96-97, Feb '44

MAYFIELD, F. H.: Peripheral nerve injuries. J. Michigan M. Soc. *44:*269-275, March '45

MAYNARD, A. DE L.: Technic of skin grafting. Am. J. Surg. *37:*92-105, July '37

MAYNE, W.: Present day treatment of cancer of mouth. Am. J. M. Sc. *210:*548-554, Oct '45

MAYO, C. H.: Formation of cloaca in treatment of exstrophy of bladder. S. Clin. N. Amer. *1:*1257, Oct '21

MAYO, C. H.: Exstrophy of bladder. Proc. Staff

Meet., Mayo Clin. *3:*289, Oct 3, '28

MAYO, C. H.: Ureterosigmoidal transplantation for exstrophy of bladder. Sovet. khir. (nos. 1–3) *5:*308–313, '33

MAYO, C. H. AND DIXON, C. F.: Ureteral transplantation for exstrophy of bladder. S. Clin. N. Amer. *10:*1–6, Feb '30

MAYO, C. H. AND HENDRICKS, W. A.: Exstrophy of bladder. Surg., Gynec. and Obst. *43:*129–134, Aug '26

MAYO, C. H. AND WALTERS, W.: Transplantation of ureters into rectum, end-results in 35 cases of exstrophy of bladder. J.A.M.A. *82:*624–626, Feb 23, '24

Mayo Operation: See Coffey's Operation

Mayo-Walters Operation

Technic of Mayo-Walters operation in exstrophy of bladder. KRABBEL, M. Zentralbl. f. Chir. *64:*693–696, March 20, '37

MAYORAL, J.: Classification of dentofacial anomalies. Am.J. Orothodontics *31:*429–439, Sept '45

MAZEL, Z. A.: Burn therapy with high frequency currents; preliminary report. Vrach. delo *22:*269–274, '40

MAZEL, Z. A.; YUDILEVICH, S. L. AND VARSHAVSKAYA, A. D.: Radiant energy from artificial light in burns. Vrach. delo *18:*913–916, '35

MAZUROVA, N. A. AND MASHKARA, K. I.: Primary treatment of wounds of hand and fingers. Sovet. vrach. zhur. *41:*1809–1814, Dec 15, '37

MAZZI, L.: Bilateral facial colobomas, with oculopalpebral adhesions and eye complications. Arch. di ottal. *41:*148–157, March '34

MAZZI, L.: Plastic and esthetic reparative surgery of eyelid. Chir. plast. *4:*138–141, July-Sept '38

MAZZINI, O. F.: Black grain mycetoma of hand; case. Bol. y trab. de la Soc. de cir. de Buenos Aires *18:*943–946, Sept 19, '34

MAZZINI, O. F.: Fatal tetanus following burns; case. Bol. y trab. de la Soc. de cir. de Buenos Aires *21:*651–654, Aug 25, '37

MAZZINI, O. F.: Fatal tetanus in burn; case. Prensa med. argent. *25:*554–556, March 16, '38

MAZZINI, O. F.: Total avulsion of skin of male genital organs; therapy of case. Bol. y trab., Acad. argent. de cir. *30:*591–594, July 31, '46

MAZZOLA, V. P. (see MATTHEWS, H. B.) May '36

MAZZONI, E.: Three cases of Dupuytren's contracture. Gazz. d. osp. *55:*1323–1329, Oct 28, '34

MEAD, S. V.: Diagnosis and treatment of acute and chronic osteomyelitis of mandible and maxilla. Internat. J. Orthodontia *14:*321–340, April '28

MEAD, S. V.: Surgical treatment of case of acute osteomyelitis of mandible. Internat. J. Orthodontia *14:*416–424, May '28

MEAD, S. V.: Diagnosis and treatment of chronic osteomyelitis of jaws. J. Am. Dent. A. *15:*2272–2286, Dec '28

MEAD, STERLING V.: *Oral Surgery*. C. V. Mosby Co., St. Louis, 1933. Second Edition, 1940. Third Edition, 1946

MEADE, H. S.: Volkmann's ischaemic contracture treated by transplantation of internal condyle. Clin. J. *59:*8, Jan 1, '30

MEADE, H. S.: New method for treatment of fracture of lower jaw. Irish J. M. Sc., pp. 318–319, July '35

MEADE, H. S.: Fracture-dislocation of mandible. Irish J. M. Sc. pp. 98–99, March '46

MEADOFF, N. (see WIESENFELD, I. H.) March '44

MEAKINS, J. C.: Present views of shock therapy; address in medicine before Royal College of Physicians and Surgeons of Canada. Canad. M.A.J. *49:*21–29, July '43

MEAKINS, J. C.: Shock therapy. Canad. M.A.J. *43:*201–205, Sept '40

MEAKINS, J. C. (see WEIL, P. G.) June '42

MEALLA, E. S. (see JORGE, J. M.) April-June '42

MEALLA, E. S. (see JORGE, J. M.) April '43

MECCA, G.: Methods of burn therapy. Prat. pediat. *10:*61–65, Feb '32

MECHTENBERG, W. R.: Types of skin grafts and indications. Nebraska M. J. *13:*454–457, Dec '28

MEDAWAR, P. B.: Chemical coagulants in burn therapy. Lancet *1:*350–352, March 21, '42

MEDAWAR, P. B.: Problem of skin homografts. Bull. War Med. *4:*1–4, Sept '43

MEDAWAR, P. B.: Experimental study of skin transplantation. Brit. M. Bull. *3:*79–81, '45

MEDAWAR, P. B.: Immunity to homologous grafted skin; suppression of cell division in grafts transplanted to immunized animals. Brit. J. Exper. Path. *27:*9–14, Feb '46

MEDAWAR, P. B.: Immunity to homologous grafted skin; relationship between antigens of blood and skin. Brit. J. Exper. Path. *27:*15–24, Feb '46

MEDAWAR, P. B.: Relationship between antigens of blood and skin (grafts). Nature, London *157:*161–162, Feb 9, '46

MEDAWAR, P. B. (see GIBSON, T.) July '43

MEDAWAR, P. B. (see SEDDON, H. J.) July '42

MEDAWAR, P. B. (see SEDDON, H. J. *et al*) Sept '43

MEDINA AGUILAR, R.: Symptomology and general therapy of extensive burns. Medicina, Mexico *24:*323–340, Aug 25, '44

MEDVEDEV, N. I.: Therapy of trachomatous entropion. Sovet. vestnik oftal. *3:*36–42, '33
MEEK, R. E.: Operation for spastic entropion. Arch. Ophth. *24:*547–551, Sept '40
MEEK, R. E.: Ptosis; applied anatomy of eye; relation to ophthalmic surgery. Arch. Ophth. *26:*494–513, Sept '41
MEEK, W. J.: Present day conception of therapy of shock. Northwest. Med. *35:*325–334, Sept '36
MEEKER, L. H.: Relation of tonsil to branchiogenetic cysts. Laryngoscope *47:*164–183, March '37
MEEKISON, D. M.: Instrument for insertion of Kirschner wire in phalanges for skeletal traction. J. Bone and Joint Surg. *19:*234, Jan '37
MEHERIN, J. M. AND GREELEY, P. W.: Symposium on war surgery; rehabilitation of burned hand. S. Clin. North America *23:*1651–1665, Dec '43
MEHERIN, J. M. AND SCHOMAKER, T. P.: Cement burn; etiology, pathology and treatment. J.A.M.A. *112:*1322–1326, April 8, '39
MEHN, W. H. (see GLASER, K. *et al*) June '46
MEHTA, K. B. AND MODI, N. J. Syndactyly. Indian J. Pediat. *3:*241–243, Oct'36
MEIGNANT. (see CAUSSADE, L. *et al*) July '37
MEIGS, J. V. (see BENEDICT, E. B.) Nov '30
MEILLÈRE, J. (see DEPLAS, B.) March '32
MEILLIÈRE, J. (see DESPLAS, B.) Aug '32
MEISSNER, A.: Lengthening of velum and shortening of pharynx for amelioration of voice after uranoplasty. Rev. de stomatol. *35:*405–411, July '33
MEISSNER, K.: Diseases of ear in patients with cleft palate. Hals-, Nasen-u. Ohrenarzt (Teil 1) *30:*6–20, Jan '39
MEIXNER, K.: Operations on hermaphrodites. (Comment on Moszkowicz's article). Med. Klin. *25:*986, June 21, '29. Comment by Moszkowicz, L. Med. Klin. *25:*986, June 21, '29
MEKIE, D. E. C.: Anatomy of subhyoid region with reference to diagnosis of mid-line swellings of neck. Malayan M. J. *11:*178–179, Sept '36
MELA, B.: Progressive hypertrophy of half of mandible; case. Boll. e mem. Soc. piemontese di chir. *6:*1070–1087, '36
MELA, B.: Pathogenesis and surgical therapy of ankylosis of temporomandibular joint. Minerva med. *1:*553–556, May 26, '38
MELA, B. AND SEGRE, R.: Experiences with new obturator in cleft palate. Stomatol. *30:*854–869, Sept '32
MELAND, O. N.: Treatment of extensive injuries of scalp. Minnesota Med. *8:*116–120, Feb '25
MELAND, O. N.: Treatment of metastasic involvement of neck secondary to intraoral cancer. Am. J. Roentgenol. *26:*20–22, July '31
MELAND, O. N.: Treatment of epitheliomas of nasolabial fold. Am. J. Roentgenol. *38:*730–739, Nov '37
MELAND, O. N. AND LINDBERG, L.: Malignant melanoma; course and treatment. Southwestern Med. *20:*336–346, Sept '36
MELAND, O. N. (see SOILAND, A.) Aug '30

Melanomas

Research on melanomas of skin. HALKIN, H. Ann. de med. *12:*189–225, Sept '22 (illus.) abstr: J.A.M.A. *79:*1722, Nov 11, '22
Treatment of nevocarcinoma by diathermocoagulation. RAVAUT, P. AND FERRAND, M. Bull. Soc. franc. de dermat. et syph. *34:*96–105, Feb '27
Prognosis in malignant melanoma; 40 consecutive cases. GLEAVE, H. H. Lancet *2:*658–659, Sept 28, '29
Differential diagnosis of subungual melanomas; 4 cases. ADAIR, F. E. *et al*. Bull. Assoc. franc. p. l'etude du cancer *19:*549–566, July '30
Treatment of pigmented moles and malignant melanomas. EVANS, W. A. AND LEUCUTIA, T. Am. J. Roentgenol. *26:*236–259, Aug '31
Present opinion about malignant melanotic tumors of skin and their most suitable treatment. FRANKENTHAL, L. Arch. f. klin. Chir. *166:*678–693, '31
Cutaneous melanomas with special reference to prognosis. FARRELL, H. J. Arch. Dermat. and Syph. *26:*110–124, July '32
Electrocoagulation of melanomas and its dangers. AMADON, P. D. Surg., Gynec. and Obst. *56:*943–946, May '33
Malignant melanomas arising in moles; report of 50 cases. BUTTERWORTH, T. AND KLAUDER, J. V. J.A.M.A. *102:*739–745, March 10, '34
Melanoma of skin. BECKER, S. W. Am. J. Cancer *22:*17–40, Sept '34
Melonomas; 5 year cures. SCOTT, A. C. JR. Surg., Gynec. and Obst. *60:*465–466, Feb (no. 2A) '35
Technic for covering defects after extirpation of malignant melanoma of skin (grafts). ORBACH, E. Wien. med. Wchnschr. *85:*1112–1113, Oct 5, '35
Use of cobra venom in generalized nevocarcinoma; case. PRUD'HOMME, E., J. de l'Hotel-Dieu de Montreal *4:*372–378, Dec '35
Diathermocoagulation as only therapy for nevocarcinoma. JOLY, M. Bull. et mem. Soc. de med. de Paris *140:*70–71, Jan 25, '36

Melanomas – Cont.
Melanoma treatment; 400 cases. ADAIR, F. E. Surg., Gynec. and Obst. *62:*406–409, Feb (no. 2A) '36
Benign nevus: malignant melanoma; problem of borderline case. GREENBLATT, R. B. *et al.* South. M. J. *29:*122–129, Feb '36
Malignant melanoma; course and treatment. MELAND, O. N. AND LINDBERG, L. Southwestern Med. *20:*336–346, Sept '36
Nevocarcinoma of skin and mucous membranes. WILLIAMS, I. G. AND MARTIN, L. C. Lancet *1:*135–138, Jan 16, '37
Cutaneous melanoma; 2 cases alive 30 and 38 years after operation. PRINGLE, J. H. Lancet *1:*508–509, Feb 27, '37
Nevocarcinoma of cheek in child 3 years old. PERIN, L. AND BLAIRE, G. Rev. franc. de dermat. et de venereol. *13:*491–499, Dec '37
Patient operated on for melanoma of thigh 30 years ago still without obvious recurrence. PRINGLE, J. H. Tr. Roy. Med.-Chir. Soc. Glasgow, pp. 52–53, '36–'37; in Glasgow M. J. March '37
Malignant melanomas, with particular reference to subungual type. NEWELL, C. E. South. M. J. *31:*541–547, May '38
Subungual melanoma; differential diagnosis of tumors of nail bed. PACK, G. T. AND ADAIR, F. E. Surgery *5:*47–72, Jan '39
Failures in treatment of melanoma and their causes; study based on recent literature and personal observations. LERTAS, K. G. Beitr. z. klin. Chir. *169:*177–213, '39
Malignant melanoma; statistical and pathological review of 35 cases. TAUSSIG, L. R. AND TORREY, F. A. California and West. Med. *52:*15–18, Jan '40
Clinical discussion of malignant melanoma. LEE, Q. B. AND MAST, J. R. South. Surgeon *9:*437–441, June '40
Malignant melanomas, with report of 4 and 7 year cures. BROWN, J. B. AND BYARS, L. T. Surg., Gynec. and Obst. *71:*409–415, Oct '40
Malignant melanomas with report of 4- and 7-year cures. BROWN, J. B. AND BYARS, L. T. Am. J. Orthodontics (Oral Surg. Sect) *27:*90–100, Feb '41
Malignant melanoma; clinical study of 117 cases. DE CHOLNOKY, T. Ann. Surg. *113:*392–410, March '41
Malignant melanoma cutis. PELLER, S. Cancer Research *1:*538–542, July '41
Conservative autoplasty for malignant melanoma of upper eyelid; case. BADEAUX, F. AND PERRON, L. Union med. du Canada *70:*1065–1066, Oct '41
Malignant melanoma of nose. KAPLAN, I. I. Arch. Otolaryng. *35:*85–90, Jan '42

Melanomas – Cont.
Melanomas of skin; clinical study of 60 cases. DRIVER, J. R. AND MACVICAR, D. N. J.A.M.A. *121:*413–420, Feb 6, '43
Melanoepithelioma (melanosarcoma, melanocarcinoma, malignant melanoma) of extremities. BICKEL, W. H. *et al.* Surg., Gynec. and Obst. *76:*570–576, May '43
Malignant melanoma of skin. ABERNATHY, S. Memphis M. J. *19:*54–58, April '44
Malignant degeneration of gigantic pigmented nevus of shoulder; case. FUSTE, R. AND MORA MORALES, L. Rev. med. cubana *55:*307–314, April '44
Symposium on reparative surgery; treatment of malignant melanomas. WEBSTER, J. B. *et al.* S. Clin. North America *24:*319–339, April '44
Tragedy of malignant melanoma. TOD, M. C. Lancet *2:*532–534, Oct 21, '44
Principle of excision and dissection in continuity for primary and metastatic melanoma. PACK, G. T. *et al.* Surgery *17:*849–866, June '45
Melanoma of skin. CORREA ITURRASPE, M. Dia med. *17:*1449–1454, Dec 10, '45
Malignant melanomas; clinical study based on 20 cases. SANCHEZ DORDERO, R. Rev. med. d. Hosp. gen. *8:*332–339, Jan '46
Principles of excision and continuous dissection for malignant melanoma, both primary and metastatic; cases. PACK, G. T. AND NUNEZ, R. A. Arch. cubanos cancerol. *5:*20–51, Jan–Mar '46
Principle of excision and dissection in continuity for primary and metastatic malignant melanoma. PACK, G. T. AND NUNEZ, R. A. Rev. med. cubana *57:*106–137, Feb '46
Melanoma of skin. SCHARNAGEL, I. M., J. Am. M. Women's A. *1:*76–83, June '46
Melanoma of vulva with pregnancy. CLAYTON, S. G. Proc. Roy. Soc. Med. *39:*578–579, July '46
Inappropriate treatment of moles predisposing to melanotic malignancies. PUTZKI, P. S. AND SCULLY, J. H., M. Ann. District of Columbia *15:*320–324, July '46
Congenital melanoma of lip with cystic degeneration. REED, H. Brit. J. Surg. *34:*95–96, July '46

MELCHOIR, E.: New operation for total epispadia. Zentralbl. f. Chir. *48:*220, Feb 19, '21
MELCHIOR, E.: Treatment of furuncles of face. Beitr. z. klin. Chir. *135:*681–695, '26
MELCHIOR, E.: Biology of skin transplants. Beitr. z. klin. Chir. *147:*45–52, '29
MELCHER, K.: Internal treatment of extensive

second degree burns. Orvosi hetil. *83:*878–879, Sept 9, '39
MELCHIOR, M.: Alveolar fractures of jaw. Ztschr. f. Stomatol. *30:*251–268, '32
MELCHIOR, M.: Unusual case of fractured jaw. Hospitalstid. *76:*829–835, Aug 10, '33
MELCHIOR, M.: Fracture of upper jaw; unusual case. Ztschr. f. Stomatol. *32:*1331–1335, Nov 23, '34
MELENEY, F. L.: Chemotherapy in prevention and treatment of infection in burns; panel discussion; introduction. Am. Acad. Orthop. Surgeons, Lect., pp. 314–316, '43
MELENEY, F. L.: Prevention of infection in contaminated accidental wounds, compound fractures and burns (report on 1500 cases, especially evaluation of sulfonamides). Ann. Surg. *118:*171–186, Aug '43
MELENEY, F. L.: Prevention of infection in wounds, fractures and burns (report on 1500 cases, especially evaluation of sulfonamides). Bull. U. S. Army M. Dept. (no. 72) pp. 41–46, Jan '44
MELENEY, F. L. AND WHIPPLE, A. O.: Statistical analysis of study of prevention of infection in burns, with special reference to sulfonamides. Surg. Gynec. and Obst. *80:*263–296, March '45
MELESHKO, E. R.: Dupuytren's contracture and its therapy. Khirurgiya, no. 12, pp. 78–85, '39
MELLETTI, M.: Operative treatment of varicose elephantiasis of legs. Policlinico (sez. chir.) *32:*520–536, Oct '25
MELLICK, A.: Secondary oblique facial cleft; case. Brit. J. Ophth. *30:*221–224, Apr '46
MELLINGER, WILLIAM J. (with JOHN F. BARNHILL): *Surgical Anatomy of the Head and Neck,* Second Edition. Wm. Wood and Co., New York, 1940
DE MELLO, C.: Operative method in cleft palate. Beitr. z. Anat., Physiol., Path. u. Therap. d. Ohres *28:*120–123, May '30
MELLON, R. R.: New sulfhydryl solution (hydrosulphosol) in burns. Indust. Med. *11:*14–18, Jan '42
MELNIK, D. A. (see KOTELNIKOV, F. S.) 1941
DE MELO, C.: Esthetic operations on crooked noses. Med. contemp. *50:*153–154, May 1, '32
MELO, N. L.: Macromastia in girl of 17; case. Rev. med. veracruzana *11:*238–240, Feb 1, '31

Meloplasty: See Rhytidectomy

MELOY, T. M. JR. AND GUNTER, J. H.: Skeletal fixation of pathologic fractures of mandible with extensive loss of substance; 2 cases. Am. J. Orthodontics (Oral Surg. Sect.) *30:*567–571, Sept '44
MELTZER, H.: Treatment of new injuries of fingers. Munchen. med. Wchnschr. *77:*498–503, March 21, '30
MELTZER, H.: Therapy of fractures of fingers and middle hand. Chirurg. *4:*58–64, Jan 15, '32
MELTZER, H.: Wire extension treatment of fractures of fingers. Surg., Gynec. and Obst. *55:*87–89, July '32
MELTZER, H. AND FILLINGER, F.: Permanent results of plastic surgery of finger tips. Chirurg *8:*397–404, May 15, '36
MELTZER, H. (see STOLZE, M.) Oct '29
MELZNER, E.: Comment on Heyer's article about formation of vagina. Zentralbl. f. Gynak. *54:*2072–2075, Aug 16, '30
MENDELSOHN, S. N. (see RANSOHOFF, J. L.) Feb '32
MENDIZÁBAL, P.: Simple surgical therapy of cleft palate. Gac. med. de Mexico *63:*327–332, June '32
MENDIZÁBAL, P.: Stomatoplasty in loss of cheek due to gangrene. Cir. y cirujanos *12:*427–431, Oct–Nov '44
MENDIZÁBAL, P.: Procedure for closing cleft palate (uranoplasty for uranoschisis). Cir. y cirujanos *12:*432–435, Oct–Nov '44
MÉNÉGAUX, G. (see BELOT, J.) Feb '31
MENESES, J. G. J.: Multilocular serous cyst in neck, probably of congenital origin. Arch. espan. de pediat. *9:*91–95, Feb '25
MENESTRINA, G.: Plastic surgery of eyelid. Boll. d'ocul. *8:*667–685, July '29
MENGELE, J.: Studies on family groups with harelip and clefts of jaw and palate. Ztschr. f. menschl. Vererb.-u. Konstitutionslehre *23:*17–42, '39
MENGER, L. C.: Otological sepsis following submucous resection. Laryngoscope *42:*371–375, May '32
MENNE, F. R. (see JOYCE, T. M. *et al*) Feb '41
MENNELL, J.: Massage, movements and exercises in treatment of suture and repair of nerves. Brit. J. Phys. Med. *5:*40–47, March '42
MENNINGER, K. A. (see UPDEGRAFF, H. L.) Sept '34
MENSING, E. H. (see FISHER, D.) April '25
MENYHÁRD, I.: Peculiar malformation of nose. Jahrb. f. Kinderh. *106:*128–129, June '24
MENZEL, K. M.: Congenital absence of vomer and causes of septal deformities. Wien. med. Wchnschr. *77:*1081–1083, Aug 13, '27
MENZEL, K. M.: Development of saddle nose and formation of small multiple hemangiomas of mucous membrane of nose and pharynx complicating diffuse sclerode ma; case. Monatschr. f. Ohrenh. *70:*1409–1418, Dec '36

MERCADAL PEYRI, J.: Disseminated keloid acne; case. Actas dermo-sif. *35:*839–849, May '44
MERCADAL PEYRI, J. AND PEDRAGOSA, R.: Acute epithelioma of lip; case. Actas dermo-sif. *36:*521–526, Feb '45
MERCANDINO, C. P. (see GAMES, F.) March '32
MERCANDINO, C. P. (see JUST TISCORNIA, B.) July '35
MERCIER, O.: Surgical therapy of epispadias in women. Union med. du Canada *61:*1004–1009, Sept '32
MERCIER, O.: Epispadias, personal technic for cure in women. Brit. J. Urol. *6:*313–319, Dec '34
MERCIER, O.: Author's technic for cure of female epispadias. J. de l'Hotel-Dieu de Montreal *4:*84–90, March–April '35
MEREDITH, D. T. AND LEE, C. O.: Antiseptic compounds (especially trinitrophenolate of ethyl aminobenzoate) in burns. J. Am. Pharm. A. *28:*369–373, June '39
MERELLO, M. (see KENNY, T. B.) May '29
MERENLENDER, J. (see HERMAN, E.) Oct '35
MERIC, A. J. L.: Thermocauterization in therapy of facial cancer. Rev. de laryng. *57:*768–802, July–Aug '36
MERINO EUGERCIOS, E. AND GONZALEZ CALVO, S.: Primary keloids with spontaneous remission. Actas dermo-sif. *37:*616–622, Feb '46
MERKLIN, L.: Aural fistula; retropharyngeal abscess with fistulization into external auditory canal; report of 2 cases. Arch. Pediat. *55:*395–399, July '38
MERLE-BERAL. (see ROBERT) Oct–Dec '35
MERLE-BERAL, J.: Malformations of profile due to malposition of teeth and deformities of jaws; importance of complete lesional diagnosis. J. de med. de Bordeaux *115:*113–137, Aug 6–13, '38
MERLE D'AUBIGNE, R. AND LANCE, P.: Tendon transplant in treatment of post-traumatic radial paralysis. Semaine d. hop. Paris *22:*1666–1671, Sept 21, '46
MERLE D'AUBIGNE, R.; LANCE, P. AND ZIMMER, M.: Treatment of diaphysial pseudarthrosis, including grafts, in repair of soft parts. Semaine d. hop. Paris *22:*1644–1652, Sept 21, '46
MERLE D'AUBIGNE, R. AND ZIMMER, M.: Peripheral nerves; treatment of war wounds. Semaine d. hop. Paris *22:*1652–1657, Sept 21, '46
MERMINGAS, K.: Exposure of articulation of jaw. Zentralbl. f. Chir. *53:*1510–1511, June 12, '26
MERRIFIELD, F. W.: Management of fractured jaws. Radiology *41:*539–542, Dec '43
MERRILL, W. J.: Tendon substitution to restore function of extensor muscles of fingers and thumb. J.A.M.A. *78:*425–426, Feb 11, '22 (illus.)
MERRIMAN, B.: Complete repair of "mallet finger." Brit. M. J. *2:*760, Oct 17, '36
MERRITT, K. K.; FABER, H. K. AND BRUCH, H.: Progressive facial hemiatrophy; 2 cases with cerebral calcification. J. Pediat. *10:*374–395, March '37
MERRY, C. R.: Recent advances in burn therapy. J. Nat. M. A. *37:*117–120, July '45
MERSHON, H. F.: Ulcerating epithelioma of cheek; case treated with 500,000 volt therapy. South. Surgeon *7:*262, June '38
MERTENS, G.: Case of bilateral harelip. Zentralbl. f. Chir. *48:*1794–1795, Dec 10, '21
MESA, C.: Ankylosis of lower jaw; case. Bol. y trab. de la Soc. de cir. de Buenos Aires *12:*317–326, July 18, '28
MESA, C.: Ankylosis of jaws, case. Semana med. *2:*1178–1181, Nov 1, '28
MESHCHANINOV, A. I.: Classification, prophylaxis and rational treatment of hand infections. Novy khir. arkhiv *31:*388–394, '34
DE MESQUITA SAMPAIO, J. A. AND DA ROCHA AZEVEDO, L. G.: Physiopathology of extensive burns and their therapy in light of endocrinology. Sao Paulo med. *1:*25–55, Jan '44
MESSINA, P. (see MOORE, W. G.) Jan '36
MESTSCHANINOV, A.: Inborn crook-hands; case. Vrach. dielo *10:*1000, July 15, '27
METZ, W. R.: Multiple carpo-metacarpal dislocations, with report of case. New Orleans M. and S. J. *79:*327–330, Nov '26
METZ, W. R.: Cartilaginous and osteo-cartilaginous rib grafts in correction of nasal deformities. New Orleans M. and S. J. *82:*831–840, June '30
METZ, W. R.: Nasal septum; – twisted nose. New Orleans M. and S. J. *92:*180–185, Oct '39
METZ, W. R.: Fundamentals of plastic repair. South. Surgeon *11:*502–513, July '42
METZENBAUM, M. F.: Deformities of nose of developmental type. Ohio State M. J. *17:*382, June '21
METZENBAUM, M. F.: Replacement of lower end of dislocated septal cartilage versus submucous resection of dislocated end of septal cartilage. Tr. Sect. Laryng., Otol. and Rhin., A.M.A., pp. 236–251, '28 also: Arch. Otolaryng. *9:*282–296, March '29
METZENBAUM, M. F.: Nasal reconstruction by means of auto and iso-grafts. Ohio State M. J. *24:*196–200, March '28 also: Laryngoscope *38:*197–205, March '28
METZENBAUM, M. F.: Nasal reconstruction by means of bone and cartilage existing within

old traumatized nose; illustrated by plaster models and lantern slides of preoperative and postoperative cases. Laryngoscope *40:*488–494, July '30

METZENBAUM, M. F.: Asymmetry of nares; positive diagnostic sign or entity establishing anatomic displacement of lower end of cartilaginous nasal septum. Arch. Otolaryng. *16:*690–697, Nov '32

METZENBAUM, M. F.: Dislocations of lower end of nasal septal cartilage in new-born (injury sustained at birth), in infants and in young children and with their anatomic replacement by orthopedic procedures. Arch. Otolaryng. *24:*78–88, July '36

METZENBAUM, M. F.: Oblique-angled knife for resetting lower end of dislocated septal cartilage and operations on harelip and cleft palate. Arch. Otolaryng. *24:*199, Aug '36

METZENBAUM, M. F.: Photographic record of case of unusual congenital nasal deformity. Rev. de chir. structive *8:*20–21, May '38

METZENBAUM, M. F.: Recent fracture of nasal base lines of both outer nasal walls, with divergent displacement; orthopedic procedures for obtaining anatomic reduction of osseous and cartilaginous nasal framework. Arch. Otolaryng. *34:*723–735, Oct '41

METZENBAUM, M. F.: Submucous elevator. Arch. oto-laryng. *34:*847, Oct '41

Metzenbaum Operation

Metzenbaum operation for correction of deflected nasal septum. RIDPATH, R. F., S. Clin. North America *15:*231–237, Feb '35

METZGER, J. (see PICKRELL, K. L. *et al*) Oct '46

METZLER, F.: Experimental study of surgical shock. Deutsche Ztschr. f. Chir. *228:*340–348, '30

MEURMAN, Y.: New knife for dacryocystorhinostomy. Acta otolaryng. *21:*343–345, '34

MEYER, A. W.: Surgical treatment of hypertrophic and pendulous breasts. Deutsche med. Wchnschr. *56:*1165, July 11, '30

MEYER, A. W.: Plastic surgery of pendulous breasts. Med. Welt *5:*1313, Sept 12, '31

MEYER, G. E.: Maxillofacial injuries produced by gunshot wounds in modern warfare. J. Am. Dent. A. *30:*1576–1583, Oct 1, '43

MEYER, H.: Correction of nose deformities at operations for harelip. Zentralbl. f. Chir. *49:*220, Feb 18, '22 (illus.)

MEYER, H.: Treatment of harelip. Beitr. z. klin. Chir. *135:*136–149, '25

MEYER, H.: New plastic operation for hypospadias. Arch. f. klin. Chir. *155:*588–596, '29

MEYER, H.: Phalloplasty after traumatic loss of skin of penis. Arch. f. Orthop. *27:*437–442, July 18, '29

MEYER, H.: Surgical treatment of double lips. Deutsche Ztschr. f. Chir. *222:*305–309, '30

MEYER, H. E.: Facial hemiatrophy. Med. Klin. *32:*352–354, March 13, '36

MEYER, H. W.: Case of epithelioma of outer canthus of eye. S. Clin. N. Amer. *1:*1643, Dec '21

MEYER, H. W.: Case for Thiersch skin-grafting. S. Clin. N. Amer. *1:*1650, Dec '21

MEYER, H. W.: Congenital complete branchiogenetic cyst and duct. Am. J. Surg. *40:*121, May '26

MEYER, H. W.: Cancer of face. Am. J. Surg. *5:*352–357, Oct '28

MEYER, H. W.: Congenital cysts and fistulas of neck. Ann. Surg. *95:*1, Jan; 226, Feb '32

MEYER, H. W.: Neglected and recurrent basal cell epitheliomas of face. Surg., Gynec. and Obst. *64:*675–683, March '37

MEYER, H. W.: True branchiogenic cyst and fistula of neck. Arch. Surg. *35:*766–771, Oct '37

MEYER, H. W.: Hypospadias. Surgery *8:*781–790, Nov '40

MEYER, J.: Role of hereditary syphilis in maxillo-facial dystrophies. Ann. d. mal. ven. *23:*494–505, July '28

MEYER, J. AND NICOLLE: Maxillofacial dystrophies. Rev. franc. de pediat. *3:*304–340, July '27

MEYER, J. (see GOUGEROT, H.) Feb '37

MEYER, K. A. AND GRADMAN, R.: Sulfadiazine (sulfonamide) treatment of burns; comparative study (bismuth tribromophenate pressure dressings.) Surg., Gynec. and Obst. *76:*584–586, May '43

MEYER, K. A.; KOZOLL, D. D.; POPPER, H. AND STEIGMANN, F.: Pectin solutions in treatment of shock. Surg., Gynec. and Obst. *78:*327–332, March '44

MEYER, K. A. AND WILKEY, J. L.: Modern burn treatment; evaluation of various methods used in 968 cases in Cook County Hospital. Minnesota Med. *21:*644–649, Sept '38

MEYER, M. F.: Fractures of malar bone and zygoma with eye, ear, nose and throat complications. New Orleans M. and S. J. *92:*90–94, Aug '39

MEYER, N. C.: Guillotine amputation modified to preserve skin flaps. U. S. Nav. Bull. *46:*1844–1847, Dec '46

MEYER, O.: Pressure ointment method of burn therapy. Indust. Med. *12:*727–728, Nov '43

MEYER, O.: Phlebitis and burns (role of pressure bandages). Indust. Med. *14:*440, May '45

MEYER, P.: Congenital bilateral fistula of lower lip. Deutsche Ztschr. f. Chir. *229:*391–395, '30

MEYER, R.: Experimental studies in skin grafting. Wien. klin. Wchnschr. *50:*1424–1425, Oct 15, '37

MEYER, W. C.: Changes in gluteal muscles and their significance in development of bedsores. Virchows Arch. f. path. Anat. *294:* 159–170, '34

MEYER-BURGDORFF, H.: Simple method of plastic surgery in syndactylia. Zentralbl. f. Chir. *58:*998–1000; April 18, '31

MEYER-BURGDORFF, H.: Plastic repair of avulsion of scalp. Zentralbl. f. Chir. *59:*1209–1211, May 14, '32

MEYER-WILDISEN, R.: Plastic surgery to restore function after loss of thumb. Helvet. med. acta *6:*872–873, March '40

MEYERDING, H. W.: Volkmann's ischemic contracture. S. Clin. N. Amer. *10:*49–52, Feb '30

MEYERDING, H. W.: Volkmann's ischemic contracture. J.A.M.A. *94:*394–400, Feb 8, '30 abstr: Gazz. d. osp. *51:*338–343, March 16, '30

MEYERDING, H. W.: Surgical treatment of chronic arthritis. J.A.M.A. *97:*751–757, Sept 12, '31

MEYERDING, H. W.: Volkmann's contracture. Physiotherapy Rev. *12:*96–97, March–April '32

MEYERDING, H. W.: Dupuytren's contracture. Proc. Staff Meet., Mayo Clin. *10:*694–696, Oct 30, '35

MEYERDING, H. W.: Dupuytren's contracture. Arch. Surg. *32:*320–333, Feb '36

MEYERDING, H. W.: Volkmann's ischemic contracture associated with supracondylar fracture of humerus. J.A.M.A. *106:*1139–1144, April 4, '36

MEYERDING, H. W.: Treatment of Dupuytren's contracture. Am. J. Surg. *49:*94–103, July '40

MEYERDING, H. W.; BLACK, J. R. AND BORDERS, A. C.: Etiology and pathology of Dupuytren's contracture. Surg., Gynec. and Obst. *72:*582–590, March '41

MEYERDING, H. W. AND DICKSON, D. D.: Correction of congenital hand deformations. Am. J. Surg. *44:*218–231, April '39

MEYERDING, H. W. AND KRUSEN, F. H.: Physical therapy for Dupuytren's contracture. Physiotherapy Rev. *16:*42–45, March–April '36

MEYERDING, H. W. AND OVERTON, L. M.: Bilateral Dupuytren's contracture. Proc. Staff Meet., Mayo Clin. *10:*801–803, Dec 18, '35

MEYERDING, H. W. (see BICKEL, W. H. *et al*) May '43

MEYERS, E. S.: Epithelioma of lips; glandular involvement and "wait and see" method of therapy. M. J. Australia *1:*399–400, March 13, '37

MEYSSONNIER. (see LAROYENNE) March '29

MEZEI, K.: New electrical epilation apparatus. Dermat. Wchnschr. *85:*1107, Aug 6, '27

MEZEI, K.: Multiple epilation with diathermy by simultaneous use of several needles. Dermat. Wchnschr. *88:*720, May 16, '29

MEZZATESTA, F.: Hemiatrophy of face with visual disturbances. Riv. oto-neuro-oftal. *4:*315–327, March–June '27

MICHAEL, H.: Formation of artificial vagina. Zentralbl. f. Gynak. *45:*1665-1667, Nov 19, '21

MICHAËL, P. R.: Traumatic shock. Nederl. tijdschr. v. geneesk. *2:*5415–5426, Nov 16, '29

MICHAËL, P. R.: Surgical therapy of cleft palate. Beitr. z. klin. Chir. *161:*468–475, '35

MICHAËL, P. R.: Burns and frostbite. Geneesk. gids *18:*476, May 31, '40; 494, June 7, '40

MICHAEL, P. AND ABBOTT, W. D.: Sutures, use of human fibrinogen in reconstructive surgery. J.A.M.A. *123:*279, Oct 2, '43

MICHAËLIS, L.: Fractures of zygoma as result of collision with device on automobile which gives signal for turning; case. Beitr. z. klin. Chir. *154:*252–253, '31

MICHAELSON, I. C.: Device for fixation of Wolfe graft. Brit. M. J. *2:*49, July 14, '45

MICHAELSON, N. M.: Jaw fractures. Sovet. khir. *1:*287–290, '31

MICHAELSON, N. M.: Tongue wounds. Am. Rev. Soviet Med. *1:*216–219, Feb '44 also: Sovet. med., no. 1, pp. 6–7, '43

MICHAŁEK-GRODZKI, S.: Prolapse of breast and its therapy. Ginek. polska *11:*687–698, July–Sept '32

MICHAŁEK-GRODZKI, S.: Plastic reconstruction of nipples. Bull. et mem. Soc. d. chirurgiens de Paris *28:*387–399, June 19, '36

MICHAŁEK-GRODSKY, S.: Plastic reconstruction in deformities of nipples. Rev. de chir. structive, pp. 126–136, June '37

MICHAŁEK-GRODZKI, S.: Nasal deformities in harelip; surgical therapy. Rev. de chir. structive *8:*205–210, '38

MICHAŁEK-GRODZKI, S.: Etiology and therapy of breast hypertrophy. Nowiny lek. *50:*113–116, Feb 15, '38

MICHALOWSKI, E.: Electrocoagulation therapy of hemangiomas. Munchen. med. Wchnschr. *84:*101, Jan 15, '37

MICHALOWSKI, E.: Rhinoplasty; 2 cases. Rev. de chir. structive, pp. 214–222, Oct '37

MICHAUX, J.; LAMACHE, A. AND PICARD, J.: Four cases of contraction of palmar fascia in lead-poisoning. Bull. et mem. Soc. med. d. hop. de Par. *49:*782–786, May 22, '25 abstr: J.A.M.A. *85:*308, July 25, '25

MICHANS, J. R. AND GARCIA FRUGONI, A.: Subcutaneous rupture of tendon of extensor pollicis longus after fracture of inferior epiphysis of radius; case. Prensa med. argent. *30:*1221–1235, July 7, '43 also: Bol. y trab., Acad. argent. de cir. *27:*288–298, June 9, '43 (abstr)

MICHEL, L.: Tourniquet method in retractile cicatrices caused by burns in articular regions. J. de med. de Bordeaux *113:*184–185, March 10, '36

MICHEL, P. J. (see GATÉ, J. *et al*) Dec '32

MICHELI, E.: Reconstruction of crucial ligaments of knee with kangaroo tendons; late results. Boll. e mem. Soc. piemontese di chir. *3:*874–883, '33

MICHELSON, H. E.: Fissure of lip; a simple and efficient method of treatment. Arch. Dermat. and Syph. *10:*332, Sept '24

MICHELSON, J. M.: Treatment of hypospadias by method of Nové-Josserand. Arch. d. mal. d. reins *2:*513–517, April 1, '27

MICHELTHWAITE, G. R.: Newer method in treatment of burns with report of cases. Ohio State M. J. *18:*198–200, March '22

MICHON, L.: Transplantation of bone in hand. J. de chir. *20:*260–273, Sept '22 (illus.) abstr: J.A.M.A. *79:*1884, Nov 25, '22

MICHON, L. (see BONNET, P.) Nov–Dec '29

Micrognathia: See Jaws, Micrognathia of

Microtia: See Otoplasty

MIEREMET, C. W. G.: Electric burns of skin. Klin. Wchnschr. *2:*1362–1364, July 16, '23

MIESCHER, G.: Precancerous conditions of skin and adjacent mucosa. Schweiz. med. Wchnschr. *73:*1072, Sept 4, '43

MIGRAY, J.: Plastic surgery of nose. Orvos. koz. *2:*167–172, May 31, '41

MIHĂILESCU, S. P.: New operative technic for facial salivary cyst of traumatic nature. Rev. de chir., Bucuresti *37:*713–715, Sept–Dec '34

MIKHELSON, N. M.: Malunited fractures of jaw. Novy khir. arkhiv *38:*549–550, '37

MIKHELSON, N. M.: Surgical therapy of cicatricial contracture of neck after burns. Ortop. i travmatol. (no. 1) *12:*74–82, '38

MIKHELSON, N. M.: Treatment of wounds of face. Khirurgiya, no. 1, pp. 33–40, '39

MIKHELSON, N. M.: Cadaver cartilage as material for free transplantation. Khirurgiya, no. 10, pp. 29–34, '39

MIKHELSON, N. M.: Tongue wounds. Sovet. med. (no. 1) *7:*6–7, '43

Mikhelson Operation

Transplantation of cartilage from cadaver according to Mikhelson method in correction of nasal deformities. LITINSKIY, A. M. Novy khir. arkhiv. *48:*211–214, '41

MIKHLIN, E. G.: Electric injury to ear. Sovet. med. (no. 23) *4:*29–30, '40

MIKI, Y.: Cleft hand; 2 cases. Okayama-Igakkai-Zasshi *44:*2295–2296, Aug '32

MIKKELSEN, O.: Post-traumatic arteriospasms in fingers. Hospitalstid. *80:*177–184, Feb 16, '37

MIKKELSEN, O.: New type of finger splints (for fractures). Ugesk. f. laeger *99:*790–791, July 22, '37

MILÄNDER, J.: Advantages of Kirschner-Wagner operation for artificial vagina. Zentralbl. f. Gynak. *55:*2746–2749, Sept 12, '31

MILCH, H.: Thomas finger splint for fractures. M. J. and Rec. *128:*473, Nov 7, '28

MILCH, H.: Recurrent dislocations of thumb; capsulorrhaphy. Am. J. Surg. *6:*237–239, Feb '29

MILCH, H.: Button-hole rupture of extensor tendon of finger. Am. J. Surg. *13:*244–245, Aug '31

MILCH, H.: Bayonet incision for temporomandibular arthrotomy. Am. J. Orthodontics *24:*287–288, March '38

MILCH, H.: Anterior closed space infections of finger (surgical treatment). M. Rec. *152:*361–362, Nov 20, '40

MILCH, H.: Excision of ankylosed sesamoid of thumb. M. Rec. *156:*541–542, Sept '43

MILES, A. A. (see WILLIAMS, R. E. O.) Jan '45

MILES, A. E. W.: Unilateral gigantism of face and teeth; case. Brit. Dent. J. *77:*197–199, Oct 6, '44

MILHIET, H.: Therapy of salivary fistulae. Progres med., p. 742, May 4, '35

MILIAN, G.: Elephantiasis of face cured with rubiazol (sulfonamide); case. Ann. de dermat. et syph. (Bull. Soc. dranc. de dermat. et syph) *2:*106–108, Feb '42

MILIAN, G. AND DELARUE, J.: Ulcerating angioma of face; case. Bull. Soc. franc. de dermat. et syph. *34:*189–192, March '27

MILIAN, G. AND GARNIER, G.: Professional epithelioma of lower eyelid following burn by hot tar; case. Bull. Soc. franc. de dermat. et syph. *35:*793, Nov '28

MILIAN, G. AND LONJUMEAU: Lymphangioma of neck; case. Bull. Soc. franc. de dermat. et syph. *34:*859–862, Dec '27

MILIANI, A.: Squamous epithelioma of lower lip. Arch. ital. di chir. *6:*105–124, Nov '22 (illus.) abstr: J.A.M.A. *80:*360, Feb 3, '23

Military Surgery: See War Injuries

MILLANT. (see BRETECHE, *et al*) Oct '35

MILLARD, J. J.: Orthodontia and its uses in preliminary treatment of extreme cases of harelip and cleft palate. Internat. Orthodont. Cong. *1:*493–496, '27 also: Internat. J. Ortho-

dontia *13:*621–624, July '27
MILLER, A.: Knife for submucous resection. Lancet *1:*1395, June 30, '34
MILLER, CHARLES C.: *Cosmetic Surgery: The Correction of Featural Imperfections.* F. A. Davis Co., Phila., 1924
MILLER, C. C.: Excision of tattoo marks. Am. J. Surg. *39:*121, May '25
MILLER, C. C.: Fascial bands as supports to relaxed facial tissue. Ann. Surg. *82:*603–608, Oct '25
MILLER, CHARLES C.: *Cannula Implants and Review of Implantation Technics in Esthetic Surgery.* Oak Printing and Pub. Co., Chicago, 1926
MILLER, C. C.: Surgery of skin of face. Am. Med. *23:*345–350, May '28
MILLER, C. J.: Construction of an artificial vagina, with report of case. Am. J. Obst. and Gynec. *8:*333–334, Sept '24
MILLER, E. M.: Congenital ankylosis of joints of hands and feet. J. Bone and Joint Surg. *4:*560–569, July '22 (illus.)
MILLER, F. M.: Injured hand. Internat. J. Med. and Surg. *47:*18, Jan '34
MILLER, H.: Repair of severed tendons of hand and wrist; statistical analysis of 300 cases. Surg., Gynec. and Obst. *75:*693–698, Dec '42
MILLER, H. AND WINFIELD, J. M.: Human bites of hand. Surg., Gynec. and Obst. *74:*153–160, Feb '42
MILLER, H. A. (see IVY, R. H.) May '38
MILLER, H. A. (see IVY, R. H.) July '39
MILLER, H. A. (see IVY, R. H.) July '40
MILLER, H. A. (see IVY, R. H.) July '41
MILLER, H. A. (see IVY, R. H.) July '42
MILLER, H. E. (see MORROW, H. *et al*) May '37
MILLER, I. D.: Causation and treatment of surgical shock. M. J. Australia *1:*522–523, April 27, '35
MILLER, I. D.: Ankylosis of temporomandibular joints; cure by Esmarch operation. Australian and New Zealand J. Surg. *8:*406–407, April '39
MILLER, J. F.: Postoperative considerations in oral surgery. J. Am. Dent. A. *31:*1627-1631, Dec 1, '44
MILLER, J. M. (see SHEARER, T. P. *et al*) July '45
MILLER, J. W.: Intranasal operations with special reference to post-operative packing. New York M. J. *113:*456, March 16, '21
MILLER, J. W.: Pollex varus; 2 cases. Univ. Hosp. Bull., Ann Arbor *10:*10–11, Feb '44
MILLER, L. I.: Branchial fistulae; with report of surgical case. Colorado Med. *18:*110, May '21
MILLER, L. M.: New skin for burns. Hygeia *19:*884–885, Nov '41
MILLER, N. F.; WILLSON, J. R. AND COLLINS, J.: Surgical correction of congenital aplasia of vagina; evaluation of operative procedures, end result and functional activity of transplanted epithelium. Am. J. Obst. and Gynec. *50:*735–747, Dec '45
MILLER, O. L.: Treatment of contracture deformities secondary to burns. Southern M. J. *17:*522–526, July '24
MILLER, O. L.: Massive bone grafts; cases. South. M. J. *25:*211–218, March '32
MILLER, O. L. AND ROBERTS, W. M.: Treatment (with skin grafts) of deformities from burns. South. Surgeon *4:*52–62, March '35
MILLER, O. L.: Plastic operation of flat foot. Am. Acad. Orthop. Surgeons, Lect., pp. 224–225, '43
MILLER, O. R.: Wry-neck following burns, relieved by skin flaps; case report. Kentucky M. J. *26:*190–192, April '28
MILLER, S. J. C.: Harelip and cleft palate. Univ. West. Ontario M. J. *11:*14–19, Nov '40
MILLER, T. AND RUBENSTEIN, B.: Curling ulcer in burns. Dallas M. J. *18:*8–9, Jan '32
MILLER, T. AND RUBENSTEIN, B.: Unusual case of burn complication (development of Curling ulcer; recovery). Texas State J. Med. *27:*873, April '32
MILLET. (see DESJACQUES, R.) Aug '33
MILLHON, J. A. AND PARKHILL, E. M.: Myxomatous tumor simulating dentigerous cyst of jaw. J. Oral Surg. *4:*129–132, April '46
MILLHON, J. A. AND STAFNE, E. C.: Incidence of supernumerary and congenitally missing lateral incisor teeth in 81 cases of harelip and cleft palate. Am. J. Orthodontics (Oral Surg. Sect) *27:*599–604, Nov '41

Millingen-Sapezhko Operation
Modification of Millingen-Sapezhko operation (eyelids). MINEEV, P. Vestnik oftal. (no. 2) *15:*40–42, '39
Technic of Millingen-Sapezhko operation (eyelid). MITSKEVICH, L. D. Vestnik oftal. *13:*848–849, '38
Comparison of immediate and late results of Panas, Snellen and Millingen-Sapezhko eyelid operations. AVGUSHEVICH, P. L. Vestnik oftal. *11:*557–563, '37
Transplantation of mucous membrane from lips of cadavers in Millingen-Sapezhko operation. ALEKSEEV, S. A. Vestnik oftal. (no. 6) *15:*77–79, '39
Modification of Millingen-Sapezhko operation for trachomatous entropion. SERGIEVA, M. Sovet. vestnik oftal. *8:*244–245, '36

MILLS, H. P.: Cause of death in burns. Southwestern Med. *9:*111, March '25
MILLS, J. T. (see KIRKHAM, H. L. D. *et al*) Dec

'43
MILNE, G. R. (see CLARK, A. M. *et al*) April '45
MILNER, R.: Operation for harelip and cleft palate. Zentralbl. f. Chir. *49:*80–81, Jan 21, '22 (illus.)
MILONE, S.: Reaction of skin in homoplastic grafts studied by means of phenol red (phenol sulphon-phthalein). Gior. d. r. Accad. di med. di Torino *33:*147–150, March '27
MILONE, S. (see MORPURGO, B.) May '27
MILONE, S. (see MORPURGO, B.) July '27
MILONE, S. (see MORPURGO, B.) Nov '27
MILONE, S. (see MORPURGO, B.) 1928
MILOVIDOVA, A. N. (see KURLOV, I. N.) 1939
MILTNER, L. J. AND WOLFE, J. J.: Treatment of suppurative osteomyelitis of mandible. Surg., Gynec. and Obst. *59:*226–235, Aug '34
MILTON, W. T.: Self-retaining anaesthetic and post-anaesthetic gag and tongue tractor. Indian M. Gaz. *66:*298, May '31
MILTON, R. F. (see CAMERON, G. R. *et al*) Aug '43
MIMS, A. T. (see HOLMES, R. L. JR.) Nov '45
MINCHEW, B. H.: Transplantation flap repair of lower eyelid following removal of epithelioma. J. M. A. Georgia *11:*110–111, March '22
MINDER, W. (see RUEDI, J.) 1944
MINEÀ, I.: Grafting with dead tissue; conserved nerves. Cluj. med. *11:*53–57, Feb 1, '30
MINEEV, P.: Modification of Millingen-Sapezhko operation (eyelids). Vestnik oftal. (no. 2) *15:*40–42, '39
MINKEWITSCH, I.: Epidemiology and prophylaxis of scarlet fever after burns. Med. Welt *4:*1397, Sept 27, '30
MINOT, A. S. AND BLALOCK, A.: Plasma loss in severe dehydration, shock and other conditions as affected by therapy. Ann. Surg. *112:*557–567, Oct '40
MINSKY, H.: Surgical repair of recent lacerations of eyelids; intramarginal splinting suture. Surg., Gynec. and Obst. *75:*449–456, Oct '42

Mirault Operation

Mirault operation for single harelip. BLAIR, V. P. AND BROWN, J. B. Surg., Gynec. and Obst. *51:*81–98, July '30
Mirault operation for single harelip. BLAIR, V. P. AND BROWN, J. B. Internat. J. Orthodontia *17:*370–396, April '31
Vilray P. Blair's modification of Mirault operation for cleft lip. BROWN, R. G., M. J. Australia *1:*499–503, April 11, '36
Blair-Brown modification of Mirault method of treating unilateral harelip; results in cases. CHIATELLINO, A. Gior. med. d. Alto Adige *11:*131–145, March '39

MIRIC, B.: Simple surgical method in post-trachomatous entropion and trichiasis. Klin. Monatsbl. f. Augenh. *101:*381–386, Sept '38
MIRIZZI, P. L.: Burns on both forearms and back of hand; treatment by graft from thigh. Bull. et mem. Soc. nat. de chir. *55:*780–785, June 8, '29
MIRIZZI, P. L.: Plastic surgery in retractile cicatrices or extensive loss of skin; cases. Rev. de cir. *8:*337–348, Aug '29
MIRIZZI, P. L.: General principles of plastic surgery of face. Schweiz. med. Wchnschr. *59:*1011–1019, Oct 5, '29
MIRIZZI, P. L.: Surgical aspect of therapy in hand infections. Semana med. *1:*1052–1068, March 30, '33
MIRIZZI, P. L.: Extensive burns on both forearms and back of hand; remote results of resection of retractile scar and pedicled graft from thigh. Bull. et mem. Soc. nat. de chir. *59:*694–695, May 6, '33
MIRIZZI, P. L. AND URRUTIA, J. M.: Malignant tumor of parotid gland treated by Duval operation, with transplantation of digastric muscle to relieve resulting paralysis (Cadenat operation); case. Bol. y trab., Soc. de cir. de Cordoba (no. 4) *1:*52–55, '40
MIROLLI, A.: Kondoleon method of treatment of elephantiasis; 2 cases. Minerva med. *7:*637–649, June 20, '27

Mirotvortzeff Operation

Transplantation of ureters into rectum by Mirotvortzeff's method in exstrophy of bladder. SHILOVTZEFF, S. P. Lancet *2:*412–415, Aug 19, '39

MISCALL, L. AND JOYNER, A.: Hemostatic globulin and plasma clot dressing in local treatment of burns. Surgery *16:*419–421, Sept '44
MISRA, B.: Treatment of burns. Antiseptic *42:*488–491, Sept '45
MISRACHI: Postoperative shock. Presse med. *31:*565–567, June 23, '23
MISSET. (see VEAU, V. *et al*) May '37
MITCHELL, A. AND MACKENZIE, J. R.: Cleft palate repair, with notes on administration of anesthetics. Brit. J. Surg. *20:*214–219, Oct '32
MITCHELL, G. F.: Total avulsion of scalp; new method of restoration. Brit. M. J. *1:*13–14, Jan 7, '33
MITCHELL, V. E.: Prosthetic restoration of portion of mandible, including temporo-mandibular articulation on one side. Am. J. Surg. *38:*274–276, Nov '24
MITCHELL, V. E.: Treatment of cleft palate. Dental Cosmos *71:*230–235, March '29
MITCHINER, P. H.: Treatment of burns and scalds, with especial reference to use of tannic acid (Hunterian lecture). Lancet

*1:*233–239, Feb 4, '33 also: Brit. M. J. *1:*447-452, March 18, '33
MITCHINER, P. H.: Treatment of burns and scalds (with special reference to use of tannic acid). St. Thomas's Hosp. Gaz. *34:*71–78, June '33
MITCHINER, P. H.: Practical hints on use of tannic acid for burns and scalds. Clin. J. *63:*221–224, June '34
MITCHINER, P. H.: Hints on prophylaxis, diagnosis and treatment of deep hand infections. St. Thomas's Hosp. Gaz. *35:*10–13, Feb '35
MITCHINER, P. H.: Burns and scalds; therapy. Brit. M. J. *1:*27–30, Jan 1, '38
MITCHINER, P. H.: Burn therapy under war conditions. M. Press. *202:*26–31, July 12, '39
MITCHINER, P. H. AND COWELL, E. M.: Air raids; wound shock, hemorrhage and blood transfusion. Lancet *1:*228–231, Jan 28, '39
MITCHINER, P. H. AND COWELL, E. M.: Air-raid injuries to face. Lancet *1:*601–602, March 11, '39
MITERSTEIN, B. AND KORNBLUETH, W.: Transplantation of mucous membrane (Denig operation) in severe burns of eyes. Harefuah *29:*152, Oct 1, '45
MITSKEVICH, L. D.: Homotransplantation of mucous membrane in ophthalmic surgery. Sovet. vestnik oftal. *3:*299–302, '33
MITSKEVICH, L. D.: Technic of Millingen-Sapezhko operation (eyelid). Vestnik oftal. *13:*848–849, '38
MITTELSTAEDT: Tannin in burns. Kinderarztl. Praxis *5:*152–153, April '34
MITTERMAIER, R.: Tumors of lips, tongue, gums and alveolar processes. Handb. d. Hals-, Nasen-, Ohrenh. *5:*582–618, '29
MIXTER, C. G.: Contractures of neck following burns (treatment by use of tubular skin graft). New England J. Med. *208:*190–196, Jan 26, '33
MIXTER, W. J. AND GRANT, F. C.: Relief of pain of facial cancer. Tr. Am. S. A. *45:*473–482, '27 also: Ann. Surg. *87:*179–185, Feb '28
MIYATA, R. (see TAKAHASHI, N.) 1922
MIYATA, S. AND KAYASHIMA, K.: Clinical observations on patients (sailors) with scalding burns. Far East. Sc. Bull. *3:*12, March '43 (abstract)
MOATTI. (see LEVY) May '38
MOATTI, L.: Pathogenesis of lateral fistulae and cysts of neck. Ann. d'oto-laryng., pp. 11–41, Jan '31
MOATTI, L.: Anatomy, pathogenesis and clinical aspects of congenital fistulas of neck. Rev. med. franc. *12:*39–57, Jan '31
MOBERG, E.: Tendon surgery of hand. Nord. med. (Hygiea) *25:*535–539, March 23, '45
MOBLEY, H. E.: Hand infections. J. Arkansas M. Soc. *34:*269–270, May '38
MOCCIA, G.: Author's experience with orthopedicosurgical therapy of chronic primary polyarthritis. Arch. ital. di chir. *53:*124–134, '38
MOCHALOV, S. P.: Burn therapy. Vestnik khir. *55:*531–536, May '38
MOCK, H. E.: Fractures of fingers and toes. Am. J. Surg. *35:*109, May '21
MOCK, H. E.: Reconstructive surgery. Minnesota Med. *4:*343, June '21
MOCK, H. E.: Reconstructive surgery; case of congenital absence of arms. J.A.M.A. *86:*541–544, Feb 20, '26
MOCK, H. E. AND ELLIS, J. D.: Treatment of fractures of fingers and metacarpals with description of authors' finger caliper. Surg., Gynec. and Obst. *45:*551–556, Oct '27
MOCK, A. E. AND WEBB, C. C.: Hand infections. J. Florida M. A. *27:*296–298, Dec '40
MOCK, J.: Renal abscess following panaris of sheath of flexor tendon developing from cut of palm; case. Bull. et mem. Soc. d. chirurgiens de Paris *24:*295–298, May 20, '32
MÓCZÁR, L.: New operative method in habitual temporomaxillary dislocations; case. Rev. de stomatol. *32:*129–143, March '30
MÓCZÁR, L.: Treatment of habitual dislocation of mandible. Orvosi hetil. *74:*1081–1084, Oct 25, '30
MODI, N. J. (see MEHTA, K. B.) Oct '36
MOE, R.: Treatment of nasal fractures of long standing. Nord. med. (Norsk mag. f. laegevidensk.) *27:*1907–1917, Sept 21, '45
MOE, R.: Plastic surgery of nose according to Gillies. Nord. med. (Norsk mag. f. laegevidensk.) *28:*2329–2332, Nov 2, '45
MOFFETT, A. J.: Postural instillation (for induction of local anesthesia); added note (nose). J. Laryng. and Otol. *59:*151–153, April '44
MOENE, I.: Surgical therapy of severe case of elephantiasis of leg. Med. rev., Bergen *50:*116–121, March '33
MOENE, I.: Surgical therapy of elephantiasis. Norsk mag. f. laege-vidensk. *95:*264–275, March '34
MOERS: Skin grafting after enucleation of eye; case. Rev. de chir. structive, pp. 119–120, June '37
MOERS: Cartilage autograft in therapy of saddle nose; case. Bull. Soc. belge d'oto., rhinol., laryng., pp. 23–24, '38
MOFFETT, A. J.: Results of operative treatment of nasal infections and deformities. Birmingham M. Rev. *14:*161–169, Sept '39
MOFFETT, A. J.: Postural instillation; method of inducing local anesthesia. J. Laryng. and Otol. *56:*429–436, Dec '41
MOFFETT, A. J.: Postural instillation (for induction of local anesthesia); added note. J. Laryng. and Otol. *59:*151–153, April '44
MOHS, F. E.: Chemosurgical treatment of can-

cer of lips; microscopically controlled method of excision. Arch. Surg. *48:*478–488, June '44
MOLESWORTH, E. H.: Treatment of vascular naevi. M. J. Australia *1:*576–578, May 27, '22
MOLIN DE TEYSSIEU, AND PONS: Post-traumatic ptosis and atrophic myopathies of eyelid. Rev. d'oto-neuro-ocul. *5:*284–287, April '27
MOLINIÉ, J.: Technic for reconstruction of face. Paris med. *11:*89, July 30, '21 abstr: J.A.M.A. *77:*1053, Sept 24, '21
MOLLÁ, V. M.: Branchiogenic tumors; surgical therapy. Cron. med., Valencia *38:*501–509, July 15, '34
MOLLARET, P.: Clinical and etiologic study of progressive facial hemiatrophy; case in woman with dental focus of infection; regression after therapy of infection. Rev. neurol. *2:*463–474, Nov '32
MOLLO, L.: Surgical therapy of elephantiasis. Rassegna internaz. di clin. e terap. *19:*699, Aug 31; 765, Sept 15; 809, Sept 30; 857, Oct 15, '38

Mommsen Procedure

Prevention of decubitus ulcers during therapy of contracture by Mommsen cast method. VERESHCHAKOVSKIY, I. I. Ortop. i travmatol. (no. 1) *9:*100, '35
Mommsen's bloodless treatment of Volkmann's contracture. TANCREDI, G. Arch. di ortop. *43:*362–377, '27

MONA, C.: Fractures of lower jaw; therapy by Böhler method. Policlinico (sez. prat.) *48:*659–666, April 14, '41
MONACO, U.: Bone grafts. Policlinico (sez. chir.) *30:*203–220, April '23 abstr: J.A.M.A. *81:*341, July 28, '23
MONAGHAN, J. F. (see STRUMIA, M. M. *et al*) April '40
MONASTERIO ODENA, R.: Present status of burn therapy in United States. Dia med. (sup) *3:*1–12, April 15, '46
MONBERG, A.: Snapping finger and its treatment. Hospitalstid. *68:*295–300, April 2, '25
DE MONCHAUX, C.: Interstitial radium treatment of cancer of lips; review of 71 cases. M. J. Australia *2:*221–225, Aug 7, '37
MONCORPS, C.: Cosmetic operations. Zentralbl. f. Haut-u. Geschlechtskr. *28:*1–14, Oct 5, '28
MONCORPS, C.: Subcutaneous division of sebaceous glands in treatment of acne vulgaris. Munchen. med. Wchnschr. *76:*997–998, June 14, '29
MONCORPS, C.: Surgical correction of unusual type of syphilitic deformity of nostril. Dermat. Wchnschr. *94:*383–386, March 12, '32
MONCORPS, C. (see SCHMID, R.) Nov '38
MONCORPS, C. (see SIEMENS, H. W.) Dec '38
MONDADORI, E. C. F.: Problem of anesthesia in surgery of temporomaxillary joint. An. paulist. de med. e cir. *42:*227–230, Sept '41
MONDRY, F.: Surgical therapy of post-traumatic functional disturbance of proximal joint of thumb. Zentralbl. f. Chir. *67:*1532–1535, Aug 17, '40
MONEY, R. A.: Osteoplastic restoration of skull. M. J. Australia *2:*269–270, Aug 27, '32
MONEY, R. A.: Plastic surgery for deformity and contractures after nitric acid burns to face (case). M. J. Australia *2:*848–853, Dec 19, '36
MONEY, R. A.: Ear reconstruction. M. J. Australia *1:*819–820, May 7, '38
MONEY, R. A.: Repair of defects by bone grafting (especially from ilium) in cranium. Surgery *19:*627–650, May '46
MONNIER, E.: Cleft palate operations. Schweiz. med. Wchnschr. *51:*970, Oct 20, '21
MONNIER, E.: Remote results of cleft palate operations. Jahrb. f. Kinderh. *105:*200–211, '24
MONNIER, E.: Technic of cleft palate operation. Schweiz. med. Wchnschr. *59:*595, June 8, '29
MONNIER, E.: Surgical therapy of cleft palate; 150 cases. Schweiz. med. Wchnschr. *61:*1207, Dec 12, '31
MONNIER, E.: Surgical therapy of exstrophy of bladder in young children. Schweiz. med. Wchnschr. *64:*202–203, March 10, '34
MONNIER, E.: Progress in plastic operations performed during childhood (for exstrophy of bladder and harelip) (cleft palate). Schweiz. med. Wchnschr. *68:*613–614, May 21, '38
MONOD, O. (see HAUTANT, A. *et al*) Sept '26
MONOD, O. (see HAUTANT, A.) April '30
MONOD, O. (see ROUX-BERGER, J. L.) May '27
MONOD, R. AND ISELIN, M.: Colpoplasty for congenital absence of vagina by modified method of Thiersch grafts mounted on rigid supports. Mem. Acad. de chir. *62:*997–1002, June 24, '36
MONSARRAT, K. W.: High or third-degree prolapse of rectum. Brit. J. Surg. *14:*89–93, July '26
MONSERRATE, D. N.: Hand and fingers infections. M. Bull. Vet. Admin. *13:*321–326, April '37
MONT-REID. (see HALSTED, W. S. *et al*) July–Aug '22
MONTANARI-REGGIANI, M.: Isolated fractures of zygomatic arch. Arch. ortop. *57:*431–450, Dec '42
MONTANARO, J. C. AND PIERINI, L. E.: Progressive facial hemiatrophy; case. Semana med. *1:*704–710, March 31, '38

MONTANT: Reactions of soft parts and periosteum after fractures without displacement and contusion of fingers. Bull. et mem. Soc. d. chirurgiens de Paris *25:*60–67, Jan 20, '33
MONTANT: Excitation and amelioration of ovarian functions after plastic surgery of breast. Bull. et mem. Soc. de med. de Paris *137:*400–402, May 27, '33
MONTANT: Plastic surgical therapy of dystrophy of breast. Tech. chir. *27:*155–164, Oct '35
MONTANT, C., AND DUBOIS, F.: *Chirurgie plastique des seins.* Maloine, Paris, 1933
MONTANT: Various technics for plastic surgery of breast; cases. Bull. et mem. Soc. de med. de Paris *139:*566–571, Nov 7, '35
MONTANT, R.: Personal restorative technic of section of flexor tendons of fingers. J. de chir. *53:*768–774, June '39
MONTANT, R. AND BAUMANN, A.: Rupture and luxation of dorsal (extensor) tendons of fingers at first interphalangeal articulation; physiologic and clinical study. Rev. d'orthop. *25:*5–22, Jan '38
MONTEFIORE, L.: Surgical and streptococcic vaccine therapy of elephantiasis. Tunisie med. *32:*434–435, Dec '38
MONTEIRO, A.: Epidermoid carcinoma of lower lip; case with recovery and survival for 14 years after surgical therapy. Acta med., Rio de Janeiro *9:*51–58, Feb '42
MONTEIRO, J. (see CORA ELISEHT, F. *et al*) Aug '44
MONTEIRO, J. (see CORREIA NETO, A.) Sept-Oct '45
MONTEIRO, O.: Serious burns. Hospital, Rio de Janeiro *19:*929–935, June '41
MONTEIRO FILHO, A.: Etiopathogenesis and therapy of shock. Rev. med. brasil. *17:*489–500, Oct '44
MONTEITH, S. R.: Horse serum in burns; cases. Gazz. d. osp. *50:*550–554, April 28, '29
MONTEITH, S. R. AND CLOCK, R. O.: Normal horse serum in burns; cases. J.A.M.A. *92:*1173–1177, April 6, '29
MONTEMARTINI, G.: Advantages and method of surgical therapy in Volkmann contracture; case. Policlinico (sez. chir.) *44:*12–19, Jan '37
MONTENEGRO, J. (see FERRAZ ALVIM, J. *et al*) Feb '34
MONTFORD, T. M.: Hereditary hypertelorism without mental deficiency. Arch. Dis. Childhood *4:*381–384, Dec '29
MONTGOMERY, A. H.: Splint for overcoming contractures of fingers. Surg., Gynec. and Obst. *44:*404–405, March '27
MONTGOMERY, A. H.: Tannic acid treatment of burns in children. Surg., Gynec. and Obst. *48:*277–280, Feb '29
MONTGOMERY, A. H.: Treatment of burns (tannic acid and silver nitrate). Indust. Med. *6:*639–642, Dec '37
MONTGOMERY, D. W.: Epitheliomata; clinical notes. California and West. Med. *45:*134–137, Aug '36
MONTGOMERY, D. W. AND CULVER, G. D.: Epithelioma of auricle. Arch. Dermat. and Syph. *7:*472–478, April '23
MONTGOMERY, D. W. AND CULVER, G. D.: Epithelioma of back of hand. New York M. J. *118:*674–676, Dec 5, '23 (illus.)
MONTGOMERY, D. W. AND CULVER, G. D.: Epithelioma of lip treated with radium. California and West. Med. *22:*628–631, Dec '24
MONTGOMERY, D. W. AND CULVER, G. D.: Treatment of cancer of lips. M. J. and Rec. *133:*573–575, June 17, '31
MONTGOMERY, H.: Benign and malignant moles; differentiation and treatment. M. Clin. North America *28:*968–977, July '44
MONTGOMERY, M. L.: Congenital auricular fistula; 3 cases in same family. S. Clin. North America *11:*141–148, Feb '31
DE MONTIGNY, G.: Maxillofacial prosthesis. Union med. du Canada *74:*1727–1735, Dec '45
MOON, V. H.: Shock syndrome in surgery. Ann. Int. Med. *8:*1633–1648, June '35
MOON, V. H.: Early recognition and management of shock. Urol. and Cutan. Rev. *44:*5–12, Jan '40
MOON, V. H.: Shock—circulatory failure of capillary origin. J.A.M.A. *114:*1312–1318, April 6, '40
MOON, V. H.; MORGAN, D. R.; LIEBER, M. M. AND MCGREW, D.: Similarities and distinctions between shock and effects of hemorrhage. J.A.M.A. *117:*2024–2030, Dec 13, '41
MOORE, A. T. AND COOK, W. C.: Reconstruction of lower jaw; case. J. South Carolina M. A. *40:*73–75, April '44
MOORE, B. H.: Macrodactyly and associated peripheral nerve changes. J. Bone and Joint Surg. *24:*617–631, July '42
MOORE, F. D.: Symposium on management of Cocoanut Grove burns at Massachusetts General Hospital; note on thrombophlebitis encountered. Ann. Surg. *117:*931–936, June '43
MOORE, F. D.; PEACOCK, W. C.; BLAKELY, E. AND COPE, O.: Anemia of thermal burns. Ann. Surg. *124:*811–839, Nov '46
MOORE, F. T.: Discussion on treatment of hand injury. Brit. J. Surg. *34:*70–74, July '46
MOORE, J. R. A.: Plea for co-operation in congenital cleft palate treatment. S. African M. Record *24:*335–338, Aug 14, '26
MOORE, P. M.: Indications and technic for sub-

mucous resection. S. Clin. North America *17:*1437–1448, Oct '37

MOORE, P. M.: Skin grafting in case of chronic laryngeal stenosis. Cleveland Clin. Quart. *11:*5–8, Jan '44

MOORE, P. M. JR. AND HARRIS, H. E.: Nasal fractures. Am. J. Surg. *50:*668–671, Dec '40

MOORE, S. (see BLAIR, V. P. *et al*) April '30

MOORE, S. (see BLAIR, V. P. *et al*) Feb '31

MOORE, S. (see BLAIR, V. P.) 1941

MOORE, T.: Spontaneous rupture of extensor pollicis longus tendon associated with Colles fracture. Brit. J. Surg. *23:*721–726, April '36

MOORE, T.: Unusual finger accident. Brit. J. Surg. *26:*198–199, July '38

MOORE, W. G. AND MESSINA, P.: Camptodactylism and its variable expression. J. Hered. *27:*27–30, Jan '36

MOOREHEAD, F. B.: Correction of congenital cleft palate and harelip, surgical principles involved. J.A.M.A. *77:*1951, Dec 17, '21

MOOREHEAD, F. B.: Congenital cleft lip and palate; some personal observations. J. Am. Dent. A. *14:*1098–1107, June '27

MOOREHEAD, F. B.: Correction of secondary palate defects. J.A.M.A. *90:*1614–1615, May 19, '28

MOOREHEAD, F. B.: Bone graft to jaw. S. Clin. N. Amer. *9:*321–323, April '29

MOOREHEAD, F. B.: Cartilage graft to nose. S. Clin. N. Amer. *9:*327–328, April '29

MOOREHEAD, F. B.: Lymphangio-endothelioma of lip and nose. S. Clin. N. Amer. *9:*329–330, April '29

MOOREHEAD, F. B.: Cartilage graft to malar bone. S. Clin. N. Amer. *9:*331–332, April '29

MOOREHEAD, F. B.: Lesions of jaw, nose and cheek; cleft lip and palate; cartilage transplant; tube graft. S. Clin. North America *12:*57–66, Feb '32

MOOREHEAD, F. B.: Better method of treating jaw fractures. J.A.M.A. *102:*1655–1657, May 19, '34

MOOREHEAD. F. B.: Two cases illustrating elastic traction in plastic surgery; pedicle flap to close large opening in hard palate. S. Clin. North America *14:*745–749, Aug '34

MOOREHEAD, F. B.: Management of jaw fractures. S. Clin. North America *16:*197–213, Feb '36

MOOREHEAD, F. B.: Jaw fractures and their management. Am. J. Surg. *38:*474–479, Dec '37

MOORHEAD, J. J.: Laceration of tendons of thumb. S. Clin. N. America *5:*170–173, Feb '25

MOORHEAD, J. J.: Symposium on reparative surgery after amputation. S. Clin. North America *24:*435–452, April '44

MOORHEAD, J. J. AND UNGER, L. J.: Human red cell concentrate for surgical dressings for burns. Am. J. Surg. *59:*104–105, Jan '43

MOORHEAD, S. W.: Drainage after uretero-intestinal anastomosis for exstrophy of bladder. Am. J. Surg. *22:*215–216, Nov '33

MOORHOUSE, M. S. (see TAYLOR, N. B.) Oct '43

MOOSE, S. M.: Correction of abnormal mandibular protrusion by intraoral operation. J. Oral Surg. *3:*304–310, Oct '45

MOOTNICK, M. W.: Plastic surgery of saddle nose. Laryngoscope *42:*376–384, May '32

MOOTNICK, M. W.: Lengthening septum nobile nasi; new plastic procedure. New York State J. Med. *37:*1509–1510, Sept 1, '37

MOOTNICK, M. W.: Lowering glabella in rhinoplasty. Laryngoscope *55:*28–29, Jan '45

MORA MORALES, L. (see FUSTE, R.) April '44

DE MORAES, A.: Modern treatment of burns (paraffin). Brasil-med. *1:*242–244, May 13, '22 abstr: J.A.M.A. *79:*858, Sept 2, '22

DE MORAES, A.: Supernumerary breasts; surgical therapy of case. Obst. y ginec. latino-am. *4:*1–6, Jan '46

MORAES BARROS FILHO, N.: Surgery of peripheral nerves; basis and technic. Rev. de cir. de Sao Paulo *7:*93–135, Sept–Oct '41

DE MORAES LEME, J.: Plaster casts in burns. Rev. paulista de Med. *28:*109–125, Feb '46

DE MORAIS LEME, J. B.: Uncomplicated unilateral harelip; general review. Arq. de cir. clin. e exper. *6:*359–457, April–June '42

MORAL, H. AND SCHLAMPP, H.: Causes and treatment of jaw fractures. Fortschr. d. Zahnheilk. *5:*1055–1076, Nov '29

MORAL, H. AND SCHLAMPP, H.: Dental aspect of jaw fractures. Fortschr. d. Zahnh. *6:*973–994, Nov '30

MORAL, H. AND SCHLAMPP, H.: Diagnosis and therapy of jaw fractures. Fortschr. d. Zahnh. *7:*1017–1038, Nov '31

MORALES, A.: Hypospadias. Siglo med. *71:*549–550, June 9, '23

MORALES, L. (see ESTELLA, J.) July '30

MORALES, M. F. (see RHODE, C. M. *et al*) May '45

MORAN, H. M.: Radium therapy of cancer of nose. M. J. Australia *2:*814–817, Dec 20, '30

MORANI, A. D.: Burn therapy in industry. Am. J. Surg. *64:*361–372, June '44

MORANI, A. D.: Indications for plastic surgery. M. Woman's J. (no. 2) *52:*21–27, Feb '45

MORANDI, G.: Anterior transposition of ulnar nerve. Bull. War Med. *4:*513–514, May '44 (abstract)

MORANDI, G.: Reconstruction of thumb; indications and results of 15 cases. Chir. d. org. di movimento *30:*41-51, Jan-Mar '46

MORAX, V.: Plastic repair of eyelid after excision of tumor. Bull. Soc. d'opht. de Paris, pp. 411, Oct '26

MORAX, V.: Skin grafting in 2 cases of epithelioma of eyelids. Ann. d'ocul. *164:*6-15, Jan '27

Morax Operation

Morax operation in correction of symblepharon orbitale. CHISTYAKOV, P. I. Vestnik oftal. *11:*795-797, '37

MORAYTA, M.: Maxillofacial traumatology in military medicine. An. med. d. Ateneo Ramon y Cajal (no. 4) *2:*45-46, Dec '44

MORAZA, M.: Hypertrophy of ear; case. and fingers. Med. ibera *2:*630-633, Dec 6, '30

MOREAU, J.: "Dovetail" bone graft. Arch. franco-belges de chir. *25:*256-267, Dec '21 (illus.) abstr: J.A.M.A. *78:*618, Feb 25, '22

MOREAU, J.: Fracture of maxillary sinus plus emphysema of lower eyelid. Arch. francobelges de chir. *25:*421-424, Feb '22 (illus.)

MOREAU, L.: Two cases of hand deformity. Ann. d'anat. path. *6:*1132-1133, Nov '29

MOREDA, J. J. (see LYONNET, J. H.) March-April '34

MOREHEAD, R. P.: Angiomatoid formations in genital organs with tumor formation. Arch. Path. *42:*56-63, July '46

MOREIRA, E.: Perforating ulcer of septum (Hajek's ulcer), with report of case. Rev. brasil. de oto-rino-laring. *8:*265-267, July-Aug '40

MOREMEN, C. W.: Fractures of upper and lower jaw and their correction with dental splint. J. Florida M. A. *15:*207-209, Oct '28

MORENO, J.: Therapy of decubitus ulcers. Rev. clin. espan. *3:*243-244, Sept 1, '41

Morestin Operation

Treatment of extensive subcutaneous angiomas of face by Morestin's method. MARGLIANO, D. Arch. ital. di chir. *12:*603-615, '25

Surgical treatment of large contraction scars of burns according to Morestin's plastic operations. STEGEMANN, H. Zentralbl. f. Chir. *53:*1880-1884, July 24, '26

Morestin operation in dermatogenous contractures after burns. PRISELNOFF, P. V. Vestnik khir. (no. 64) *22:*111-114, '30

Clawhand; Morestin plastic surgery with free full-thickness skin graft. ZENO, L. Bol. Soc. de cir. de Rosario *7:*308-315, Aug '40 also: An. de cir. *6:*315-321, Sept '40

MOREU, A.: Dacryocystorhinostomy and its clinical results. Arch. de oftal. hispano-am. *35:*127-139, March '35

MOREYRA BERNAN, L. (see BERTOLA, V. J.) 1945

MORFIT, M. (see PACK, G. T. *et al*) June '45

MORGAN, A. L.: Plastic repair of deformities of eyelids. Canad. M.A.J. *44:*560-562, June '41

MORGAN, E. K. (see SENGER, F. L.) Dec '42

MORGAN, E. M. (see ERB, I. H. *et al*) Feb '43

MORGAN, J. R. E. (see MURRAY, D. W. G.) April '35

MORGAN, O. G.: Treatment of epiphora, with special reference to some cases treated by dacryocystorhinostomy. Tr. Ophth. Soc. U. Kingdom (pt. 1) *58:*163-172, '38

MORGAN, W. M.: Splint for fractures of maxillary bones. J. Am. Dent. A. *21:*1736-1746, Oct '34

MORGANTI, R.: Surgical repair of extensive tendon loss by tendon transplantation; 7 cases. Chir. d. org. di movimento *25:*182-188, Dec '39

MORGENSTERN, D. J.: Congenital atresia of postnasal orifices; simple, effective office technic for treatment by electrocoagulation. Arch. Otolaryng. *31:*653-662, April '40

MORGENTHALER, C. F.: Gentle means for reducing fracture of jaw. J. Am. Dent. A. *23:*1736-1738, Sept '36

MORHARDT, P. E.: Accidents with electricity; burns of mouth. Presse med. *48:*480, May 8-11, '40

MORHARDT, P. E.: Tannin and gentian violet in burn therapy. Presse med. *48:*660, Aug 14-17, '40

MORI, A.: Conservative surgery and its limitations in industrial injuries to hands. Rassegna d. previd. sociale *23:*12-30, March '36

MORI, M.: Artificial vagina; comment on Paunz's article. Zentralbl. f. Gynak. *48:*859, April 19, '24 abstr: J.A.M.A. *83:*77, July 5, '24

MORI, S.: Experimental studies on transplantation of cartilage (ear) to cover tracheal defect. Okayama-Igakkai-Zasshi *48:*516, March '36

Mori Operation

Revision of vagina formed according to Mori after 3 years. PARSAMOW, O. S. Zentralbl. f. Gynak. *50:*55-551, Feb 27, '26

MORIAN, R.: Furuncles on face and their treatment. Deutsche Ztschr. f. Chir. *193:*45-58, '25 abstr: J.A.M.A. *85:*1437, Oct 31, '25

MORIKAWA, G.: Extensive cleft of hard palate; case. Oto-rhino-laryng. *14:*574, Aug '41

MORIN, E.: Traumatic shock in war wounded; blood transfusion therapy. Union med. du Canada *75:*400-404, April '46

MORIOKA, K.: Zygoma fractures; five cases. Taiwan Igakkai Zasshi (Abstr. Sect.) *33:*108, July '34

MORISON, A. E.: Principles of bone graft surgery. Tr. Medico-Chir. Soc., Edinburgh, pp. 65–80, '22–'23; in Edinburgh M. J., April '23

MORISON, J. E.: Extroversion of primitive hind gut. Arch. Dis. Childhood *15:*105–114, June '40

MORISON, J. H. S.: Burn therapy. M. Bull. Vet. Admin. *16:*146–148, Oct '39

MORISON, R.: "Bipp" method of treatment of bone cavities and bone grafts. Surg., Gynec. and Obst. *34:*642–666, May '22 (illus.)

MORITZ, A. R. (see HARBIN, M.) June '30

MORLEY, G. H.: Plastic surgery cooperation with orthopedic surgery. Proc. Roy. Soc. Med. *35:*762–763, Oct '42

MORLEY, G. H. AND BENTLEY, J. P.: Propamidine in burns. Lancet *1:*138–139, Jan 30, '43

MORLEY, MURIEL E: *Cleft Palate and Speech*. E. and S. Livingstone Ltd., Edinburgh, 1945.

MORNARD, P.: Technic and results of plastic surgery of nasal deformities. Rev. franc. de dermat. et de venereol. *3:*386–405, July–Aug '27

MORONE, G.: Atypical craniofacial dysostosis associated with atrophy of optic nerve. Arch. ottal. *50:*45–74, Mar–Apr '46

MORONEY, P. B.: Conservation of metacarpus by skin and bone grafting in 3 patients. Brit. J. Surg. *32:*464–466, April '45

MORPURGO, B.: Influence of inanition on homeoplastic transplantations. Centralbl. f. allg. Path. u. path. Anat. *40:*1–3, July 1, '27

MORPURGO, B. AND MILONE, S.: Deep homoplastic grafts and successive superficial grafts. Arch. per le sc. med. *49:*306–309, May '27

MORPURGO, B. AND MILONE, S.: Influence of inanition on homoplastic skin-grafts. Boll. d. Soc. ital. di biol. sper. *2:*709–712, July '27

MORPURGO, B. AND MILONE, S.: Influence of insufficient nutrition on taking of skin-grafts. Arch. per le sc. med. *49:*648–664, Nov '27

MORPURGO, B. AND MILONE, S.: Comparative effects on skin of homo- and heteroplastic grafts. Arch. ed atti d. Soc. ital. di chir (1927) *34:*lxxxiv, '28

MORPURGO, B. AND MILONE, S.: Effect of insufficient nutrition on growth of homoplastic skin grafts. Arch. ed atti d. Soc. ital. di chir. (1927) *34:*lxxxv, '28

MORRIN, F. J.: Surgical treatment of lymphatic fields in cancer of mouth. Irish J. M. Sc., pp. 157–163, April '39

MORRIS, C. J. O. R. (see CROOKE, A. C. *et al*) Nov '44

MORRIS, F. (see HALL, C.) Dec '41

MORRIS, H. D.: Metacarpal defects due to gunshot wounds; tenon and mortise grafts. Surgery *20:*364–372, Sept '46

MORRIS, J. H.: Chronic temporomaxillary subluxation. Am. J. Surg. *1:*288, Nov '26

MORRIS, J. H.: Chronic recurring temporomaxillary subluxation; surgical consideration of "snapping jaw" with report of successful operative result. Surg., Gynec. and Obst. *50:*483–491, Feb '30

MORRIS, K. A.: Free tendon grafts in fingers; case. J. Florida M. A. *17:*161–164, Oct '30

MORRIS, M. H. (see COBEY, M. C. *et al*) July '43

MORRIS, M. H. (see COBEY, M. C. *et al*) June '44

MORRIS, S. L. JR.: Practical treatment of extensive burns, with report of case. South. Surgeon *11:*210–217, March '42

MORRIS, W. M.: Surgical treatment of facial paralysis; review of 46 cases (nerve transplant). Lancet *2:*558–561, Sept 2, '39

MORRIS, W. M.: Surgical treatment of facial paralysis (with nerve grafting). Lancet *2:*1172–1174, Nov 14, '36

MORRIS, W. M.: Surgical treatment of Bell's palsy. Lancet *1:*429–431, Feb 19, '38

MORRISON, G. M. (see COTTON, F. J. *et al*) July '38

MORRISON, O. C.: Traumatic removal of entire scalp. Surg. J. *33:*93–96, March–April '27

MORRISSEY, J. H. (see LOWSLEY, O. S. *et al*) Nov '21

MORROW, H.; MILLER, H. E. AND TAUSSIG, L. R.: Treatment of epithelioma of lip by electrodesiccation; technic and preliminary report of results during past 5 years. Arch. Dermat. and Syph. *35:*821–830, May '37

MORROW, H. AND TAUSSING, L.: Epitheliomas of face and their treatment with radium. Arch. Dermat. and Syph. *5:*73–87, Jan '22 (illus.)

MORROW, H. AND TAUSSIG, L. R.: Statistics and technic in treatment of malignant disease of skin by radiation. Am. J. Roentgenol. *10:*212–218, March '23; *10:*867–871, Nov '23

MORROW, H. AND TAUSSIG, L. R.: Radium therapy of vascular nevi. Am. J. Roentgenol. *10:*867–871, Nov '23

MORROW, J.: Burn therapy. Minnesota Med. *17:*330–332, June '34

MORSE, J. L.: Moles, warts and keloids. Am. J. Surg. *36:*137–144, April '37

MORTON, A. M.: Cutaneous burns. M. Times, New York *58:*73, March '30

MORTON, C. B. AND JORDAN, H. E.: Median cleft of lower lip and mandible, cleft sternum and absence of basihyoid (inferior gnathoschisis); case. Arch. Surg. *30:*647-656, April '35

MORTON, H. M.: Treatment of eyelid ptosis. Eye, Ear, Nose and Throat Monthly *8:*155-158, May '29

MORTON, H. S.: Fractures of hand. Canad. M. A. J. *51:*430-434, Nov '44

MORVAN. (see SOLCARD) May '31

MOSCARIELLO, T.: Keloid and its radium therapy, with report of cases. Arch. di radiol. *13:*317-337, July-Aug '37

MÓSCISKER, E.: Submucous bone defect of palate. Wien. med. Wchnschr. *78:*961, July 14, '28

DE MOSCOSO, A.: Operative treatment of keloids. Rev. brasil. de med. e pharm. *6:*209-218, July-Sept '30

MOSCOSO, A.: Blood transfusion in shock. Rev. med.-cir. do Brasil *43:*125-139, April '35

MOSENTHAL: Development of stiffness of fingers (congenital and hereditary). Verhandl. d. deutsch. orthop. Gesellsch. (1931) Kong. 26, pp. 66-68, '32

MOSER, E.: Tendon sutures. Zentralbl. f. Chir. *54:*1606, June 25, '27

MOSER, E.: Dupuytren's contracture of finger. Zentralbl. f. Chir. *63:*149-151, Jan 18, '36

MOSHER, H. P.: Mosher-Toti operation on lacrimal sac. Laryngoscope *31:*284, May '21

MOSHER, H. P.: Re-establishing intranasal drainage of lacrimal sac. Laryngoscope *31:*492, July '21

Mosher-Toti Operation

- Dacryocystorhinostomy (Mosher-Toti operation). HOOVER, W. B., S. Clin. North America *16:*1695-1699, Dec '36
- Mosher-Toti operation on lacrimal sac. MOSHER, H. P. Laryngoscope *31:*284, May '21
- Dacryocystorhinoplasty, Mosher's modification of Toti method. COWEN, S. B. Ohio State M. J. *21:*902-905, Dec '25
- Mosher-Toti dacryocystorhinostomy. SPAETH, E. B. Arch. Ophth. *4:*487-496, Oct '30

MOSIMAN, R. E.: Significance of subcutaneous scar tissue. West. J. Surg. *47:*397-401, July '39

MOSKOFF, G.: Skin graft use in reparation of tendinous lesions with loss of substance. J. de chir. *50:*607-620, Nov '37

Moskovits Operation

- Rectal prolapse treated by Moskovits technic. ETZEL, E. Rev. de cir. de Sao Paulo *3:*333-347, Dec '37

MOSOTEGUY, C. AND SAMMARTINO, E. S.: Traumatic irreducible posterior luxation of metacarpophalangeal articulation of thumb. Dia med. *10:*462-464, May 30, '38

MOSS, O. W.: Chemical burns to eyes. New Orleans M. and S. J. *89:*302-306, Dec '36

MOSZKOWICZ, L.: Plastic construction of artificial vagina. Zentralbl. f. Gynak. *45:*80, Jan 15, '21

MOSZKOWICZ, L.: Gersuny's pedunculated flaps for reconstruction of face. Arch. f. klin. Chir. *130:*796-798, '24

MOSZKOWICZ, L.: Fasciaplasty in treatment of facial paralysis. Wien. klin. Wchnschr. *41:*1151-1153, Aug 9, '28

MOSZKOWICZ, L.: Operations on hermaphrodites. Med. Klin. *25:*517-519, March 28, '29 (comment on Moszkowicz's article). MEIXNER, K. Med. Klin. *25:*986, June 21, '29

MOSZKOWICZ, L.: Reply to Meixner's comments article about operations on hermaphrodites. Med. Klin. *25:*986, June 21, '29

MOSZKOWICZ, L.: Treatment of facial hemiatrophy by means of transplantation of fat tissues. Med. Klin. *26:*1478, Oct 3, '30

MOSZKOWICZ, L.: Surgical therapy of x-ray injuries of skin. Wien. klin. Wchnschr. *45:*885, July 8, '32

MOSZKOWICZ, L.: Question of surgical therapy of hypospadias. Chirurg *6:*401-402, June 1, '34

Motais Operation

- Motais operation for eyelid ptosis, report of 6 cases. O'CONNOR, R. California State J. Med. *19:*409, Oct '21
- Modification of Motais' operation for ptosis of eyelid. TAGGART, H. J. Tr. Ophth. Soc. U. Kingdom *53:*417-421, '33
- Modified Motais operation for eyelid ptosis. KIRBY, D. B. Arch. Ophth. *57:*327-331, July '28
- Technique of Motais operation for ptosis. WEEKS, W. W. Am. J. Ophth. *11:*879-883, Nov '28
- On permanence of results of Motais' operation for eyelid ptosis. BRUNS, H. D. Am. J. Ophth. *5:*269-270, April '22 (illus.)
- Modification of Motais operation for eyelid ptosis. DE SAINT-MARTIN, R. Bull. Soc. d'opht. de Paris *50:*100-102, Feb '38
- Modified Motais operation for eyelid ptosis. DE SAINT-MARTIN, R. Ann. d'ocul. *175:*589-596, Aug '38

MOUCHET, A.: Volkmann's disease. J. de med. et chir. prat. *98:*229-238, April 10, '27

MOUCHET, A.: Traumatic avulsion of ungual phalanx of thumb and of its flexor tendon.

Bull. et mem. Soc. nat. de chir. *59:*1244–1247, Oct 28, '33

Mouchet, A.: Late rupture of tendon of extensor pollicis longus 10 years after fracture of lower end of radius; case. Presse med. *48:*1007–1008, Dec 11–14, '40

Mouchet, A.: Traumatic luxation of extensor tendon of middle finger. Presse med. *50:*455, July 11, '42

Mouchet, A. and Desfosses, P.: Fracture of base of first phalanx of thumb resulting in fragment resembling sesamoid bone; difficulty in interpreting radiograph. J. de radiol. et d'electrol. *12:*331–333, July '28

Moulages

Use of negocoll and hominit in making moulages of face as aid in plastic surgery. Iglauer, S. Laryngoscope *42:*774–778, Oct '32

Life-masks in conjunction with models of mouth in cleft palate. Broderick, R. A. Proc. Roy. Soc. Med. *28:*1667–1672, Oct '35

Simple and practical technic for making facial casts. Bulbulian, A. H., J. Am. Dent. A. *26:*347–354, March '39

Technic for producing facial masks and models. West, B. S. Ann. Surg. *109:*474–478, March '39

Moulage prosthesis for face. Clarke, C. D. J. Lab. and Clin. Med. *26:*901–912, Feb '41 also: Am. J. Orthodontics (Oral Surg. Sect) *27:*214–225, April '41

Facial masks; new technic using newly deviced matrix for impression. Kaufman, J. L., J. Am. Dent. A. *28:*64–66, Jan '41

Moulages as aid to maxillofacial restorations. Jacobsen, H. H. and Barron, J. B. Mil. Surgeon *92:*511–520, May '43

Moulonguet: Use of free grafts in surgical therapy of frontal sinusitis. Ann. d'oto-laryng. *12:*501–503, Oct–Dec '45

Moulonguet, A. and Leroux-Robert, J.: Rectal anesthesia with tribrom-ethanol in cervicofacial surgery; indications, technic, results and experimental studies. Ann. d'oto-laryng., pp. 283–304, March '34

Moulonguet, P.: Therapy of anorectal cancers exteriorized to perineum by diathermocoagulation; subsequent plastic operation. Mem. Acad. de chir. *71:*298–300, June 13–20, '45

Moulonguet, P. (see Gernez, L. *et al.*) Oct '35

Mounier-Kuhn: Vascular changes in eye just after endonasal operations. Rev. d'oto-neuro-opht. *6:*679–685, Nov '28

Mount, L. A.: Cranioplasty with tantalum, case. Rev. argent. de neurol. y psiquiat. *10:*127–131, June '45

Mourad, A.: A case of clubhand. Lancet *2:*1222, Dec 9, '22 (illus.)

Moure, P.: Scalp flaps in reconstruction of face. Presse med. *29:*1021–1022, Dec 4, '21 (illus.) Abstr: J.A.M.A. *78:*470, Feb 11, '22

Moure, P.: Reconstruction of face. J. de chir. *21:*414–422, April '23 (illus.) abstr: J.A.M.A. *81:*78, July 7, '23

Moure, P.: Surgical treatment of lupus of face. Arch. franco-belges de chir. *28:*298–307, April '25

Moure, P.: Avulsion of scalp; treatment by dermo-epidermic grafts; case. Bull. et mem. Soc. nat. de chir. *53:*1040–1043, July 16, '27

Moure, P.: Phlegmon of tendon sheaths; operation. Bull. et mem. Soc. nat. de chir. *54:*572–576, April 28, '28

Moure, P.: Autotransplantation of fascia by cutaneous flaps with tubulate pedicles. Rev. odont. *51:*5–10, Jan '30

Moure, P.: Treatment of harelip. Bull. et mem. Soc. nat. de chir. *57:*899–901, June 27, '31

Moure, P.: Total rhinoplasty. Am. J. Surg. *14:*298–308, Oct '31

Moure, P.: Use of tubular grafts from scalp in therapy of extensive mutilating lupus. Bull. Soc. franc. de dermat. et syph. *39:*712–717, June '32

Moure, P.: Surgical treatment of lupus of face (use of tubular cranial flaps and application of Filhos' caustic for destruction of minor facial lesions of lupus). French M. Rev. *2:*415–419, Oct '32

Moure, P. and Barraya: Therapy of lupus by transplantation of tubular grafts from scalp. Bull. Soc. franc. de dermat. et syph. *41:*136–137, Jan '34

Mourgeon, A.: Superior incisive prognathism; prevention and therapy. Presse med. *41:*1353–1354, Aug 30, '33

Mourgue-Molines, E.: Tannic acid in burns. Montpellier med. *53:*45, Feb 1; 79, Feb 15, '31

Mourgue-Molines, E.: Prognosis and therapy of severe burns. Gaz. d. hop. *106:*1013, July 8, '33; 1045, July 15, '33

Mourgue-Molines, E.: Recent extensive cutaneous burns. Montpellier med. *12:*201–212, Dec '37

Mourgue-Molines, E. (see Duval, P.) Oct '37

Mourgue-Molines, E. (see Riche, V. *et al*) Jan '32

Mourgues, (see Roudil, G. *et al*) April '36

Mourot, A. J.: Burn therapy. Virginia M. Monthly *71:*25–28, Jan '44

Mourot, A. J. (see Strange, W. W.) July '43

MOUSEL, L. H.: Regional anesthesia of head and neck. Anesthesiology *2:*61-73, Jan '41
MOUSEL, L. H. (see LILLIE, H. I. *et al*) March '40

Mouth, Cancer

Prophylaxis of malignant growths of mouth, face and jaws. EASTMAN, J. R., J.A.M.A. *79:*118-120, July 8, '22
Carcinoma of floor of mouth. QUICK, D. Am. J. Roentgenol. *10:*461-470, June '23 (illus.)
Cancer of mouth. GRANT, W. W. Colorado Med. *20:*248-251, Sept '23 (illus.)
Treatment of precancerous and cancerous lesions in mouth. SCHMIDT, W. H. New York M. J. *118:*732-737, Dec 19, '23 (illus.)
Surgery in cancer of mouth and throat. HEIDRICH, L. Beitr. z. klin. Chir. *128:*310-347, '23 abstr: J.A.M.A. *80:*1348, May 5, '23
Malignancies of oral cavity. PETTIT, J. A. Northwest Med. *23:*153-157, April '24
Suggestion for relief of pain from carcinoma of mouth and cheek. GRANT, F. C. Ann. Surg. *81:*494-498, Feb '25
Radium emanation in treatment of intra-oral cancer; with report of 141 cases. SIMPSON, F. E. AND FLESHER, R. E. Tr. Sect. Dermat. and Syphil., A.M.A., pp. 120-129, '25
Epithelioma of face and buccal cavity. WETZEL, J. O. New York State J. Med. *26:*634-639, July 15, '26
Cancer of skin and mouth. KING, J. M., J. Tennessee M. A. *19:*115-121, Sept '26
Technique of operations for carcinoma of buccal mucous membranes. PÓLYA, E. Surg., Gynec. and Obst. *43:*343-354, Sept '26
Cancer of mouth; results of treatment by operation and radiation; 376 cases observed at Massachusetts General and Collis P. Huntington Memorial Hospitals in three-year period, 1918-1920. SIMMONS, C. C. Surg., Gynec. and Obst. *43:*377-382, Sept '26
Repair of defects caused by surgery and radium in cancer of hand, mouth and cheek. BLAIR, V. P. Am. J. Roentgenol. *17:*99-100, Jan '27
Glandular involvement following cancer of lips, tongue and floor of mouth. REGAUD, C. *et al*. Paris med. *1:*357-372, April 16, '27 also: Strahlentherapie *26:*221-251, '27
Precancerous lesions of oral cavity and their treatment. BASS, H. H. Internat. J. Med. and Surg. *40:*321-323, Aug '27
Cervical lymph nodes in intra-oral carcinoma. DUFFY, J., J. Radiology *9:*373-379, Nov '27
Cancer of nose and mouth, with special reference to treatment by irradiation. EWING. J. Radiology *9:*359-365, Nov '27
Surgery of cancer of mouth. JUDD, E. S. AND NEW, G. B., J. Radiology *9:*380-383, Nov '27
Carcinoma of mucosa of cheek treated surgically; 10 cases. SERAFINI, G. AND ANTONIOLI, G. M. Gior. d. r. Accad. di med. di Torino *91:*51-56, Jan-March '28 also: Minerva med. (pt. 2) *8:*599-610, Sept 15, '28
Treatment of epithelioma about face, mouth and jaws. PADGETT, E. C., J. Missouri M. A. *25:*190-194, May '28
Cancer in and about mouth; 211 cases. BLAIR, V. P. *et al*. Ann. Surg. *88:*705-724, Oct '28
Cancer of tongue and floor of mouth. DORRANCE, G. M. AND MCSHANE, J. K. Ann. Surg. *88:*1007-1021, Dec '28
Cancer in and about mouth; study of 211 cases. BLAIR, V. P. *et al*. Tr. Am. S. A. *46:*395-414, '28
Statistics on 1,323 operations on mouth, pharynx and esophagus for cancer. SIMEONI, V. Valsalva *5:*86-89, Feb '29
Electrodesiccation and electro-coagulation in neoplastic and allied diseases of oral cavity and adjacent parts; clinical, physical, historical and photographic studies based upon 20 years' experience. CLARK, W. L. Am. J. Surg. *6:*257-275, March '29
Radiotherapy of cancer of lips and mouth. MURPHY, I. J. AND MURPHY, S. L. Radiol. Rev. and Chicago M. Rec. *51:*126-128, March '29
Management of intra-oral cancers at Radium Institute of University of Paris. PACK, G. T. Ann. Surg. *90:*15-25, July '29
Five year end-results of radiation treatment of cancer of oral cavity, nasopharynx and pharynx, based on study of 309 cases, 1912-1923. SCHREINER, B. F. AND SIMPSON, B. T. Radiol. Rev. and Chicago M. Rec. *51:*327-332, Aug '29
Carcinoma of mouth and lip. LELAND, G. A. New England J. Med. *201:*1196-1199, Dec 12, '29
Plastic surgery of floor of mouth after excision of malignant tumors. GAIDUKOFF, M. F. Odessky M. J. *4:*332-334, '29
Cancer in and about mouth; study of 211 cases. BLAIR, V. P. *et al*. Internat. J. Orthodontia *16:*188-209, Feb '30
Necessity of early diagnosis and early treatment of cancer of mouth for effective therapy; 202 cases treated in hospitals of Eastern Switzerland from 1919-1928. SCHÜRCH, O. Schweiz. med. Wchnschr. *60:*96-101, Feb 1, '30

Mouth, Cancer—Cont.

Treatment of malignant tumors of mouth and throat. FIGI, F. A. Am. J. Roentgenol. *23:*648–653, June '30

Intraoral cancer and its treatment. SOILAND, A. AND MELAND, O. N. California and West. Med. *33:*559–562, Aug '30

Early diagnosis and treatment of cancer of lips. and mouth. FIGI, F. A. Minnesota Med. *13:*788–792, Nov '30

Principles of and results in radium treatment of buccal carcinoma. BIRKETT, G. E. Canad. M.A.J. *23:*780–784, Dec '30

Results of treatment of cancer of mouth in 82 cases. SEGALE, G. C. Arch. ed atti d. Soc. ital. di chir. *36:*770, '30

Position of surgery and radium in treatment of cancer of mouth. PADGETT, E. C., J. Kansas M. Soc. *32:*167–172, May '31

Radiation therapy of cancer of lips and mouth. MARTIN, J. M. Radiology *16:*881–892, June '31

Treatment of metastasic involvement of neck secondary to intraoral cancer. MELAND, O. N. Am. J. Roentgenol. *26:*20–22, July '31

Analysis of cases at Pondville Hospital; cancer of lip and mouth. TAYLOR, G. W. Am. J. Cancer (supp.) *15:*2380–2385, July '31

Cancer in and about mouth treated with irradiation by European method. MARTIN, C. L. AND MARTIN, J. M. Texas State J. Med. *27:*286–291, Aug '31

Leukoplakia of mouth and labial and lingual cancer in smokers. HAASE, G. Deutsche Monatschr. f. Zahnh. *49:*881, Sept 15; 929, Oct 1, '31

Neck metastases from lip and mouth cancer. KILGORE, A. R. AND TAUSSIG, L. R., S. Clin. North America *11:*1055–1059, Oct '31

Late results of operations on maxillary bone in cancer of oral cavity; 5 cases. DEBERNARDI, L. Boll. e mem. Soc. piemontese di chir. *2:*1114–1148, '32

Malignant and other growths about mouth. LYONS, C. J., J. Am. Dent. A. *20:*3–16, Jan '33

Summary of 65 "cures" of cancer about mouth. BLAIR, V. P. Surg., Gynec. and Obst. *56:*469, Feb (No. 2A) '33

Conservative procedure in care of cervical lymph nodes in intra-oral carcinoma. DUFFY, J. J. Am. J. Roentgenol. *29:*241–247, Feb '33

Surgical treatment of metastases to cervical lymph nodes from intra-oral cancer. FISCHEL, E. Am. J. Roentgenol. *29:*237–240, Feb '33

Five year cures in cancer of mouth, lip, nose, etc. SMITH, F. Surg., Gynec. and Obst. *56:*470–471, Feb (no. 2A) '33

Care of cervical glands in intra-oral carcinoma. STEWART, C. B. Am. J. Roentgenol. *29:*234–236, Feb '33

Carcinoma of buccal mucosa; end results 1918–1926. LUND, C. C. AND HOLTON, H. M. New England J. Med. *208:*775–780, April 13, '33

Carcinoma of mouth and its treatment. STACY, H. S., M. J. Australia *1:*549–550, May 6, '33

Management of facial teguments in extensive exeresis for cancers of inferior maxilla, of floor of mouth, of tonsils and of pharynx. BERNARD, R. Presse med. *41:*748–751, May 10, '33

Treatment of cancerous or potentially cancerous cervical lymph-nodes (as result of cancers of mouth). BLAIR, V. P. AND BROWN, J. B. Ann. Surg. *98:*650–661, Oct '33

Treatment of neck glands in cancer of lip, tongue and mouth; study of present-day practice (questionnaire report of Cancer Commission of California Medical Association). PFLUEGER, O. H. California and West. Med. *39:*391–397, Dec '33

Carcinoma of lip and mouth. MARTIN, C. L. Radiology *22:*136–146, Feb '34

Cancer of mouth. BROWN, J. B. South. Surgeon *3:*47–52, March '34

Leukoplakia buccalis and keratosis labialis (precancerous lesions). STURGIS, S. H. AND LUND, C. C. New England J. Med. *210:*996–1006, May 10, '34

Carcinoma of buccal mucosa; analysis of cases observed at Massachusetts General Hospital in 3 year period 1924–1926. TAYLOR, G. W. Surg., Gynec. and Obst. *58:*914–916, May '34

Surgery as applied to lymph nodes of neck in cancer of lip and buccal cavity; statistical study. FISCHEL, E. Am. J. Surg. *24:*711–731, June '34

Role of surgery in carcinoma of buccal cavity. STACY, H. S., M. J. Australia *1:*712–717, June 2, '34

Leukoplakia buccalis and cancer of mouth. STURGIS, S. H. AND LUND, C. C. New England J. Med. *212:*7–9, Jan 3, '35

Five year cures of cancer of larynx and mouth and pharynx. NEW, G. B. AND FIGI, F. A. Surg., Gynec. and Obst. *60:*483–484, Feb (no. 2A) '35

Surgical therapy of secondary adenopathies of neck in buccopharyngeal cancer. DUCUING, J. Ars med., Barcelona *11:*353–359, Sept '35

Mouth, Cancer–Cont.

Cancer of mouth. FIGI, F. A., S. Clin. North America *15:*1233–1240, Oct '35

Malignant disease of mouth and accessory structures. NEW, G. B. Am. J. Surg. *30:*46–52, Oct '35

Cancer of lip and intra-oral mucous membrane. FRANK, L. W. South. Surgeon *4:*444–456, Dec '35

Treatment of carcinoma of mouth and buccopharynx, nose and nasal sinus, with some remarks on diagnosis. PATTERSON, N. Tr. Am. Laryng., Rhin. and Otol. Soc. *41:*1–34, '35

Cancer of mouth. FIGI, F. A., J. Am. Dent. A. *23:*216–224, Feb '36

Diagnosis and treatment of cancer of lip, mouth and throat. CHRISTIE, A. C. Fortschr. a. d. Geb. d. Rontgenstrahlen *53:*529–534, March '36

Epidermoid carcinoma of mouth; general considerations and etiologic factors. PADGETT, E. C. Internat. J. Orthodontia *22:*283–293, March '36

Pathology, clinical features and diagnosis of cancer of mouth. PADGETT, E. C. Internat. J. Orthodontia *22:*504–515, May '36

Results and prognosis of cancer in and about oral cavity. PADGETT, E. C. Internat. J. Orthodontia *22:*1255–1267, Dec '36

Early diagnosis and therapy of cancer of mouth. LINDEMANN, A. Ztschr. f. Stomatol. *35:*145–171, Jan 22, '37

Management of cancer in and about oral cavity. PADGETT, E. C. Internat. J. Orthodontia *23:*73–82, Jan '37

Diagnosis and treatment of malignancy of mouth. FITZGERALD, L. M., J. Am. Dent. A. *24:*763–770, May '37

Cancer of lip and oral cavity and skin. HOLLANDER, L. Pennsylvania M. J. *40:*749–750, June '37

Surgical therapy of cervical metastases of epithelioma (oral). MARTINEZ, E. M. Bol. Liga contra el cancer *12:*315–320, Sept–Oct '37

Our responsibility toward oral cancer. BLAIR, V. P. *et al.* Ann. Surg. *106:*568–576, Oct '37

Life expectancy and incidence; carcinoma of lip and oral cavity. WELCH, C. E. AND NATHANSON, I. T. Am. J. Cancer *31:*238–252, Oct '37

Results of surgical therapy and radiotherapy of epitheliomas of mouth, tongue and larynx. CHRYSSICOS, J. AND LAMBADARIDIS, A. Ztschr. f. Hals-, Nasen-u. Ohrenh. *40:*410–413, '37

Indications for and limits of surgical therapy in extensive cancers of buccofacial region; 3 cases. BERARD, L. *et al.* Lyon chir. *35:*318–327, May–June '38

Cancer of lip and mouth. HAY, A. W. S. Manitoba M. A. Rev. *18:*231–234, Dec '38

Surgical treatment of lymphatic fields in cancer of mouth. MORRIN, F. J. Irish J. M. Sc., pp. 157–163, April '39

Surgical therapy of metastases in cervical lymph nodes from cancer of mouth. SCHÜRCH, O. AND FEHR, A. Deutsche Ztschr. f. Chir. *251:*641–672, '39

Malignant disease of face, buccal cavity, pharynx and larynx in first three decades of life. HERTZ, C. S. Proc. Staff Meet., Mayo Clin. *15:*152–156, March 6, '40

Extirpation of cervical lymph nodes in cancer of mouth with metastases. PRUDENTE, A. Bol. y trab., Acad. argent. de cir. *26:*1030–1031, Oct 28, '42

Full thickness defects of cheek (cancer) involving angle of mouth; method of repair. MACFEE, W. F. Surg., Gynec. and Obst. *76:*100–105, Jan '43

Cancer of mouth. (and face) BLAIR, V. P. AND BYARS, L. T. Texas State J. Med. *38:*641–645, March '43

Cancer of floor of mouth. KAPLAN, I. I., J. Am. Dent. A. *30:*737–740, May 1, '43

Cancer of mouth and jaws (with emphasis on therapy). SOMERVELL, T. H. Indian J. Surg. (no. 2) *5:*5–28, June '43

Symposium on 20 cases of benign and malignant lesions of oral cavity, from Ellis Fischel State Cancer Hospital, Columbia, Missouri. BURFORD, W. N.; *et al.* Am. J. Orthodontics (Oral Surg. Sect.) *30:*353–398, July '44

Surgical treatment of pain; malignant lesions of face, nose and mouth. ROBERTSON, J. S. Tr. Roy. Med.-Chir. Soc. Glasgow, pp. 29–31, '43–'44; in Glasgow M. J. May '44

Therapy of malignant tumors of mouth at Bern. RUEDI, J. AND MINDER, W. Pract. oto-rhino-laryng. *6:*113–144, '44

Carcinoma of oral cavity; 10 year survey in general hospital. LAWRENCE, E. A. AND BREZINA, P. S., J.A.M.A. *128:*1012–1016, Aug 4, '45

Carcinoma of buccal mucosa. BURFORD, W. N. AND ACKERMAN, L. V. Am. J. Orthodontics (Oral Surg. Sect) *31:*547–551, Sept '45

Present day treatment of cancer of mouth. MAYNE, W. Am. J. M. Sc. *210:*548–554, Oct '45

Cancer of oral mucosa and circumoral areas. MASUDA, B. J. Am. J. Orthodontics (Oral Surg. Sect.) *31:*730–740, Dec '45

Mouth Deformities (See also Jaws, Deformity; Maxillofacial Deformities)

Some mouth and jaw conditions responsible for defects in speech. GREENE, J. S. Med. Rec. *100:*8, July 2, '21
Congenital deformities of mouth and face. VON WEDEL, C., J. Oklahoma M. A. *15:*46–49, Feb '22 (illus.)
Accessory mouth. BAYLEY DE CASTRO, A. Indian M. Gaz. *58:*162–163, April '23 (illus.)
Congenital defects of lips and mouth. FRANK, L. W. Kentucky M. J. *24:*331–335, July '26
Bucco-facial prosthesis in case of grave mutilation. BRUSOTTI, A. Stomatol. *25:*649–658, Aug '27
Restoration of buccal sulcus by intraoral skin grafting. PICKERILL, H. P., M. J. and Rec. *126:*671–674, Dec 7, '27
Case of nearly complete cicatrizing of mouth. RICHTER, G. Klin. Med. *5:*700–702, '27
Plastic surgery of jaw deformities and mouth. WASSMUND, M. Med. Welt *4:*327, March 8, '30
Diagnosis and treatment of lesions preventing normal opening of mouth; 6 illustrative cases. BROWN, J. B. AND HAMM, W. G. Internat. J. Orthodontia *18:*353–362, April '32
Therapy of microstomia; case. BUSTAMANTE, S. Ann. Casa de Salud Valdecilla *4:*281–282, '33
Plastic method of correcting microstomia, particularly of type following Estlander cheiloplastic operation. TUOMIKOSKI, V. Acta chir. Scandinav. *70:*353–362, '33
Congenital deformities of mouth (including cleft lip and palate). BROWNE, D. Practitioner *132:*658–670, June '34
Free skin grafts in restoration of defects of conjunctival, oral mucous membranes and cutaneous defects of nasal fossae. LIMBERG, A. A. Sovet. khir. (nos. 3–4) *6:*462–482, '34
Surgical prosthetics of oral and facial defects. OLINGER, N. A. AND AXT, E. F. Am. J. Surg. *31:*24–37, Jan '36
Abnormally large mouth with ear abnormality on same side; case. EITNER, E. Monatschr. f. Ohrenh. *70:*714–717, June '36
Harelip, cleft palate; congenital deformities of mouth and face. KIMBALL, G. H., J. Oklahoma M. A. *31:*85–89, March '38
Plastic repair of defects of lips and corner of mouth by means of Filatov's tubular flaps. GNILORYBOV, T. E. Vestnik khir. *59:*592–599, June '40
Speech defects in relation to oral defects. OLINGER, N. A. Am. J. Orthodontics (Oral Surg. Sect.) *32:*469–471, July '46

Mouth, Infections (See also Jaws, Infections; Maxilla, Infections)

Malignancy of lower lip complicated by mouth infections. WILSON, S. J. South. M. J. *24:*359–363, April '31
Rare complications in osteomyelitis of lower jaw; Filatov's grafts in defects of oral cavity. STEPANOFF, N. M. Vestnik khir. (nos. 70–71) *24:*233–236, '31
Types of chronic infection about mouth. BROWN, J. B. Internat. J. Orthodontia *18:*1311, Dec '32; *19:*59, Jan '33
Oral and genital aphthae of mutilating character; case. DEGAUDENZI, C. Dermosifilografo *17:*520–526, Sept '42
Osteomyelitis of jaw; mandibular operation; buccal operation. TURCO, N. B. Prensa Med. argent. *30:*2209–2210, Nov 17, '43
Penicillin in oral and maxillofacial surgery. CHRISTIANSEN, G. W. Mil. Surgeon *96:*51–54, Jan '45
Cases of acute oral lesions treated with penicillin. MCINTYRE, A. D. Brit. Dent. J. *78:*262–266, May 4, '45
Recurrent aphthous ulceration of oral mucous membrane and genitals associated with recurrent hypopyon iritis (Behcet syndrome); 3 cases. KATZENELLENBOGEN, I. Brit. J. Dermat. *58:*161–172, Jul–Aug '46

Mouth, Injuries of (See also Burns, Chemical; Burns, Electrical; Maxillofacial Injuries)

Surgical treatment of accidental wounds of mouth and face, with special reference to those complicated by bone injury. IVY, R. H., J. Am. Dent. A. *17:*967–974, June '30
Burns of oral cavity. NADOLECZNY, M. Arch. f. Ohren-, Nasen-u. Kehlkopfh. *133:*283–287, '32
Clinical cases in stomatology (including fractures). BOISSON, R. Rev. de stomatol. *38:*625–662, Sept '36
Chemical burns of mouth. DELPH, J. F., S. Clin. North America *17:*585–592, April '37
Electrical injuries of oral cavity. OPPIKOFER, E. Schweiz. med. Wchnschr. *69:*1197–1198, Nov 25, '39
Accidents with electricity; burns of mouth. MORHARDT, P. E. Presse med. *48:*480, May 8–11, '40
Oral and pharyngeal injuries from pointed objects. KLIMPEL, W. Ztschr. f. Hals-, Nasen-u. Ohrenh. *45:*328–338, '40
Injuries of region of oral cavity by strong electric current. LINDEMANN, AND LEMPKE, H., Med. Klin. *37:*155–160, Feb 14, '41
Speed of repair of wounds of mucosa in mouth. MAJ, G. Boll. Soc. ital. biol. sper. *17:*322, May '42

Mouth, Injuries of—Cont.

Symposium on industrial surgery; fractures of jaws and injuries of face, mouth and teeth. THOMAS, E. H., S. Clin. North America *22:*1029–1048, Aug '42

Injuries to nose, paranasal sinuses, mouth and ears. CANFIELD, N. Connecticut M. J. *6:*796–798, Oct '42

Care of military and civilian injuries; use of remote flaps in repairing defects of face and mouth. CANNON, B. Am. J. Orthodontics (Oral Surg. Sect.) *29:*77–85, Feb '43

Burns of ear, nose, mouth and adjacent tissues (with special reference to therapy with hydrosulphosol, sulfhydryl solution). CRUTHIRDS, A. E. Laryngoscope *53:*478–494, July '43

Burns of ear, nose, mouth and adjacent tissues (including use of hydrosulphosol, sulfhydryl solution). CRUTHIRDS, A. E. Tr. Am. Laryng., Rhin. and Otol. Soc., pp. 219–235, '43

Use of stents in skin grafting in mouth. BEDER, O. E., J. Oral Surg. *2:*32–38, Jan '44

Covering extensive defects of chin and floor of mouth following gunshot wounds. LINDENBAUM, L. M. Vrach. delo (nos. 7–8) *26:*469–474, '46

Mouth, Miscellaneous

Permanent fistula of floor of mouth; case. COELST. Rev. de chir. structive *8:*128–130, Aug '38

Brief review of anatomy, blood and nerve supply of mouth, jaws and teeth. GREEN, R. M. Am. J. Orthodontics (Oral Surg. Sect.) *27:*469–471, Sept '41

Differential diagnosis of lesions of mouth. DE OLIVEIRA, L. C. Hora med., Rio de Janeiro *2:*9–16, July '43

Postoperative considerations in oral surgery. MILLER, J. F., J. Am. Dent. A. *31:*1627–1631, Dec 1, '44

Orofacial cripple. BEDER, O. E. AND SAPORITO, L. A. Am. J. Orthodontics (Oral Surg. Sect.) *32:*351–358, Jun '46

Mouth, Prostheses (See also Jaws, Prostheses; Prostheses)

Prosthesis of mouth and face. KAZANJIAN, V. H. *et al.* J. Dent. Research *12:*651–693, Oct '32

Progressive facial hemiatrophy treated by means of expansion prosthesis of oral cavity; case. BØE, H. W. Med. rev., Bergen *50:*212–225, May '33

Oral prosthesis in repair of war injuries. POUND, E. Am. J. Orthodontics (Oral Surg. Sect.) *32:*435–439, Aug '46

Mouth, Surgery of (See also Jaws, Surgery of; Maxillofacial Surgery)

Skin-grafting in buccal cavity. KILNER, T. P. AND JACKSON, T. Brit. J. Surg. *9:*148, July '21

Surgical principles of mouth. DAVIS, A. D. Nebraska M. J. *7:*27–29, Jan '22

Plastic operations on corner of mouth. FESSLER, J. Deutsche Ztschr. f. Chir. *172:*427–429, '22 (illus.)

Some diseases of mouth, jaws, and face surgically treated. FEDERSPIEL, M. N. Journal-Lancet *43:*267–275, June 1; 297–301, June 15, '23

Restoration of function of mouth. BLAIR, V. P. Ann. Clin. Med. *3:*242–244, Sept '24

Surgical restoration of lining of mouth. BLAIR, V. P. Surg., Gynec. and Obst. *40:*165–174, Feb '25

Case of contracture of mouth. NARASIMHAN, N. S. Indian M. Gaz. *60:*72, Feb '25

Case of skin plastic operation for mucous membrane replacement in mouth. SMYTHE, G. J. C., S. African M. Rec. *24:*408–409, Sept 25, '26

Surgery of mouth and face with special reference to cleft palate and cleft lip. LOGAN, W. H. G. Kentucky M. J. *24:*498–505, Oct '26

Rhinoplasty and stomatoplasty. Arch. f. klin. Chir. *142:*572–589, '26

Bucco-antral fistula; plastic operation. VOORHEES, I. W. Internat. J. Surg. *40:*19, Jan '27

Case of nearly complete cicatrizing of mouth. RICHTER, G. Klin. Med. *5:*700–702, '27

Plastic surgery of chin and mouth mucosa; case. SMITAL, W. Zentralbl. f. Chir. *55:*142–145, Jan 21, '28

Endoral plastic correction of results of paralysis of facial nerve. BRUNNER, H. Wien. klin. Wchnschr. *41:*876–877, June 21, '28

Simple method for raising corner of mouth in facial paralysis. BLUME, AND SCHOLZ. Deutsche med. Wchnschr. *55:*272, Feb 15, '29

Operative treatment of trachomatous pannus by transplantation of buccal mucosa. VEJDOVSKÝ, V. Casop. lek. cesk. *69:*1561–1565, Nov 14, '30

Ankylosis of mandible due to scarring of cheek; restoration of cheek lining with skin graft. KIRCH, W. Proc. Staff Meet., Mayo Clin. *5:*339–341, Nov 26, '30

Study of 80 cases of leukoplakia of mouth. KING, H. AND HAMILTON, C. M. South. M. J. *24:*380–383, May '31

Autoplastic graft of flap by Italian method in reconstructive surgery of mouth; case. RE-

Mouth, Surgery of–Cont.

BELO NETO, J. Bol. Soc. de med. e cir. de Sao Paulo *16:*94–108, Nov '32

Technic of plastic surgery for correction of microstomia resulting from Estlander cheiloplasty. TUOMIKOSKI, V. Duodecim *48:*691–698, '32

Plastic surgery of corner of mouth (Rehn operation). VON BRANDIS, H. J. Deutsche Ztschr. f. Chir. *241:*479–482, '33

Skin grafting in mouth; 2 cases. FIGI, F. A. Proc. Staff Meet., Mayo Clin. *9:*740–742, Dec 5, '34

Reconstructive plastic and oral surgery. SMITH, A. E., J. Am. Dent. A. *21:*2190–2200, Dec '34

Reconstructive plastic and oral surgery. SMITH, A. E. California and West. Med. *42:*432–438, June '35

Transplantation of skin into oral cavity. ZHAKOV, M. P. Novy khir. arkhiv. *35:*573–577, '36

Role of intra-oral and intranasal grafts in contour restoration of face. KILNER, T. P. Rev. de chir. structive, pp. 1–3, March '37

Reconstructive plastic and oral surgery. SMITH, A. E. AND JOHNSON, J. B., J. Am. Dent. A. *24:*1142–1153, July '37

Cheilorthocaliplasty (esthetic surgery of mouth). CODAZZI AGUIRRE, J. A. Rev. med. del Rosario *27:*1111–1131, Nov '37

Surgical Diseases of the Mouth and Jaws, by EARL C. PADGETT. W. B. Saunders Co., Phila., 1938

Treatment of complications of surgical diseases of the mouth. IVY, R. H. West. J. Surg. *46:*202–208, April '38

Plastic surgery of alveolar process as preparation for artificial plates. JAKABHAZY, I. Orvosi hetil. *82:*338–340, April 9, '38

Skin grafts and suspension of labial commissure by skin sutures for facial paralysis. ZENO, L. An. de cir. *4:*187–189, Sept '38 Also: Bol. Soc. de cir. de Rosario *5:*412–414, Oct '38

Surgical therapy of facial paralysis by intraoral neurotization. DOROSCHENKO, I. T. Acta oto-laryng. *26:*702–709, '38

Vestibulo-alveolar adhesions; destruction by plastic reconstruction of gingivo-jugo-labial groove. CLAOUE, C. Oto-rhino-laryng. internat. *24:*41–45, Feb '40 also: Rev. gen. de clin. et de therap. *54:*95–96, Feb 24, '40

Oral and plastic surgery. SCHAEFER, J. E. J. Indiana M. A. *33:*60–66, Feb '40

Plastic surgery of mouth. DUNNING, H. S. Laryngoscope *50:*532–534, June '40

Resection of lower jaw by oral route. BERTOLA, V. J. Prensa med. argent. *28:*323–

Mouth, Surgery of–Cont.

327, Feb 5, '41

Use of vermillion bordered flaps in surgery about mouth. CANNON, B. Surg., Gynec. and Obst. *74:*458–462, Feb. (no. 2A) '42

Use of vermillion bordered flaps in surgery about mouth. CANNON, B. Am. J. Orthodontics (Oral Surg. Sect.) *28:*423–430, July '42

Surgery of face, mouth and jaws, 30 years ago and now. IVY, R. H., J. Oral Surg. *1:*95–99, April '43

Counterstroke electrocoagulation of buccal mucosa during treatment of facial lesions. BARMAN, J. M. Rev. argent. dermatosif. *28:*191–192, June '44

Stomatoplasty in loss of cheek due to gangrene. MENDIZABAL, P. Cir. y cirujanos *12:*427–431, Oct–Nov '44

Buccal mucosal grafts in therapy of total symblepharon. BERTOTTO, E. V. Rev. med. de Rosario *35:*317–322, April '45

New technic for correction of macrostomia. HARRIS, H. I., J. Oral Surg. *3:*156–163, April '45

Correction of case of cicatricial oral atresia. BERGER, A., J. Am. Dent. A. *32:*1427–1430, Nov 1–Dec 1, '45

Oral surgery case reports. SAGHIRIAN, L. M. Am. J. Orthodontics (Oral Surg. Sect.) *32:*472–492, July '46

Orbicularis oris muscle in double harelip. LEE, F. C. Arch. Surg. *53:*407–413, Oct '46

Mouth Surgery, Anesthesia for (See also Jaws, Surgery, Anesthesia for; Maxillofacial Surgery, Anesthesia for; War Injuries, Jaws)

Nitrous oxide-oxygen anesthesia; endotracheal technic in oromaxillofacial surgery. TYLER, E. A. Anesth. and Analg. *22:*177–179, May–June '43

Anesthesia (topical anesthesia and administration of pentothal sodium, barbital derivative, before intratracheal use of nitrous oxide and oxygen) for oral surgery in presence of cautery and diathermy. ELLIOT, H. L. AND ARROWOOD, J. G. Anesthesiology *6:*32–39, Jan '45

Anesthesia for oropharyngeal surgery. PERNWORTH, P. H. Anesth. and Analg. *25:*200–203, Sept–Oct '46

Mouth Surgery, Instruments for

Mouth gag and tongue depressor combination. WOLF, G. D. Tr. Sect. Laryng. Otol. and Rhin., A.M.A. p. 287, 1921

Combined gag and tongue retractor. BOYLE, H. E. G. Lancet *2:*1130, Nov 25, '22 (illus.)

Mouth, Surgery, Instruments for—Cont.

Automatic gag and tongue holder. SAMENGO, L. Semana med. *1:*734–738, April 19, '23 (illus.)

Modification of Davis Boyle gag. BROWN, R. G. Lancet *2:*756, Oct 11, '24

Dangers of Whitehead mouth-gag used on young children. TRENDTEL. Klin. Wchnschr. *6:*2436–2437, Dec 17, '27

Adjustable mouthgag tongue depressor. LEWIS, E. R. Arch. Otolaryng. *7:*636, June '28

Self-retaining anesthetic and post-anaesthetic gag and tongue tractor. MILTON, W. T. Indian M. Gaz. *66:*298, May '31

Improved gag. WADE, R. Lancet *2:*1220, Dec 3, '32

Retractor for intra-oral operations. JOHNSON, B. Lancet *2:*1052, Nov 10, '34

Life-masks in conjunction with models of mouth in cleft palate. BRODERICK, R. A. Proc. Roy. Soc. Med. *28:*1667–1672, Oct '35

Rubber plate as support for mouth following cleft palate operation. JANTZEN, J. Deutsche Ztschr. f. Chir. *249:*651–656, '38

New mouth retractor for oral surgery. BALOGH, K. Ztschr. f. Stomatol. *40:*669–671, Sept 11, '42

Instruments for maxillofacial and oral surgery. GINESTET, G. Rev. de stomatol. *43:*121–123, July–Aug '42

Mouth, Tumors (See also Jaws, Tumors; Maxilla, Tumors)

Tumors of jaws. and mouth. KAZANJIAN, V. H. New England J. Med. *201:*1200–1201, Dec 12, '29

Tumors of lips, tongue, gums and alveolar processes. MITTERMAIER, R. Handb. d. Hals-, Nasen-, Ohrenh. *5:*582–618, '29

Angiomas of face and mouth. CLARK, C. M. Ohio State M. J. *30:*438–441, July '34

Tumors and cysts of mouth and jaws of interest to otolaryngologist. IVY, R. H. Tr. Am. Acad. Ophth. *41:*163–185, '36

Congenital branchial cyst of floor of mouth; case. CHAVES, D. A. Rev. med.-cir. do Brasil *46:*620–626, May '38

Tumors of the jaws. (and mouth) IVY, R. H. Delaware State M. J. *10:*147–152, July '38

Tumors of lip and oral cavity. TRUEBLOOD, D. V. West. J. Surg. *46:*395–411, Aug '38

Mixed tumors of submaxillary gland; extirpation by buccal route. IVANISSEVICH, O. AND FERRARI, R. C. Bol. y trab., Acad. argent. de cir. *24:*1051–1054, Oct 30, '40

Cysts of floor of mouth. JOHNSTON, W. H. Tr. Am. Laryng., Rhin. and Otol. Soc. *48:*83–96, '42

Mouth, Tumors—Cont.

Blood and lymph vessel tumors involving mouth. BELLINGER, D. H., J. Oral Surg. *2:*141–151, April '44

Oral and maxillary tumors; experience at First Surgical Clinic of Vienna University during years 1930–1940. TRAUNER, R. Wien. klin. Wchnschr. *57:*192, April 21, '44

Dermoid cyst in floor of mouth. MASUDA, B. J. Am. J. Orthodontics (Oral Surg. Sect.) *32:*252–256, Apr '46

MOWLEM, R.: Use and behavior of iliac bone grafts in restoration of nasal contour; clinical and radiographic observations. Rev. de chir. structive *8:*23–29, May '38

MOWLEM, R.: Modern treatment of soft tissue injuries (skin grafts). Clin. J. *68:*271–276, July '39

MOWLEM, R.: Burn therapy. Proc. Roy. Soc. Med. *34:*221–224, Feb '41

MOWLEM, R.: Symposium on sequelae to war wounds; scarring and contracture. M. Press *205:*384–387, May 7, '41

MOWLEM, R.: Bone (iliac) and cartilage transplants to ear and nose; use and behavior. Brit. J. Surg. *29:*182–193, Oct '41

MOWLEM, R.: Experiences with various methods of skeletal fixation in jaw fractures. Proc. Roy. Soc. Med. *35:*415–426, April '42

MOWLEM, R.: Surgical treatment of congenital defects. Proc. Roy. Soc. Med. *35:*683–684, Aug '42

MOWLEM, R.: Surgery and penicillin in mandibular infection. Brit. M. J. *1:*517–519, April 15, '44

MOWLEM, R.: Relation of transport speed to type and treatment of facial injuries. M. Press. *212:*310–312, Nov 15, '44

MOWLEM, R. *et al*: Fixation of mandibular fractures by means of extraoral apparatus based on pins. Rev. san. mil., Buenos Aires *43:*1055–1058, July '44

MOWLEM, R. *et al*: Discussion on modern methods of skin grafting. Proc. Roy. Soc. Med. *37:*215–225, March '44

MOWLEM, R. *et al*: External pin fixation for mandible fractures. Lancet *2:*391–393, Oct 4, '41

MOWLEM, R. (see GILLIES, H. D.) Dec '36

Mowlem Operation

Fractures of mandible; Mowlem method of external pin fixation. MARINO, H. AND CRAVIOTTO, M. Prensa med. argent. *33:*1823–1827, Sept 6, '46

MOYER, C. A. *et al*: Interrelationship of salt solutions, serum and defibrinated blood in treatment of severely scalded, anesthetized dogs. Ann. Surg. *120:*367-376, Sept '44

MUCCI, D.: Isolated fracture of coronoid apophysis of jaw from direct violence; case. Gazz. internaz. med.-chir. *32:*403-407, Nov 30, '27

Mucosal Grafts

Technique of transplanting mucous membrane in intercostal region. PILLMAN, N. Vrach. Gaz. *31:*370-372, March 15, '27

Transplantation of oral mucosa in diseases of cornea and burns of eyes. DENIG. R. Arch. f. Ophth. *118:*729-737, '27

Wedge-shaped implantation of oral mucosa into intermarginal border of eyelid in trichiasis. KREIKER, A. Klin. Monatsbl. f. Augenh. *80:*386-389, March 23, '28

Circumcorneal transplantation of oral mucosa as curative measure in diseases of eye. DENIG, R. Arch. Ophth. *1:*351-357, March '29

Denig operation in trachomatous pannus (grafting). DERKAČ, V. Klin. Monatsbl. f. Augenh. *85:*409-411, Sept 26, '30

Operative treatment of trachomatous pannus by transplantation of buccal mucosa. VEJDOVSKÝ, V. Casop. lek. cesk. *69:*1561-1565, Nov 14, '30

Transplantation of lip mucosa by Denig method in treatment of trachoma. KAMINSKI, D. S. Klin. Monatsbl. f. Augenh. *87:*60-70, July '31

Histologic changes in membrane transplanted from lip to trachomatous eye (Denig's method). TOWBIN, B. G. Arch. f. Ophth. *125:*643-651, '31

Modification of Lowenstein clamp used in transplantation of lip mucosa. STEIN, R. Klin. Monatsbl. f. Augenh. *88:*370-371, March '32

Technic of transplanting mucosa. DANTRELLE. Rev. de chir. plastique, pp. 274-287, Oct '32

Homotransplantation of mucous membrane in ophthalmic surgery. MITSKEVICH, L. D. Sovet. vestnik oftal. *3:*299-302, '33

Transplantation of oral mucosa in recurrent pterygium. GREEN, J. Am. J. Ophth. *20:*942-943, Sept '37

Free autoplastic graft of gastric mucosa to replace urinary bladder tissue loss. STEFANINI, P. Arch. ed atti d. Soc. ital. di chir. *43:*951-967, '37

Therapeutic homoplastic transplantation of conserved mucous membrane. FILATOV, V. P. Vestnik oftal. *12:*307-310, '38

Therapy of trachomatous pannus by transplantation of mucous membrane from cadaver conserved in cold. KOSTENKO, F. M. Med. zhur. *8:*533-542, '38

New technic for mucous graft in ophthalmology. KOLEN, A. A. Vestnik oftal. (nos. 3-4) *15:*100-102, '39

Mucosal graft in therapy of corneoconjunctival burns. VON GROLMAN, G. Arch. de oftal. de Buenos Aires *15:*429-434, Sept '40 also: Rev. med. y cien. afines *2:*629-632, Sept 30, '40

Application of mucous membrane grafts to congenital and acquired states. SHEEHAN, J. E., M. Rec. *152:*404-408, Dec 4, '40

Biomicroscopic picture of healing of "normal" Denig transplant (lip mucosa). ROSHCHIN, V. P. Vestnik oftal. *16:*333-336, '40

Recidivating symblepharon in leper treated with conjunctival transplant; case. BEAUJON, O. Arch. venezol. Soc. de oto-rino-laring., oftal., neurol. *2:*23-27, March '41

Therapy of trachomatous pannus by transplantation of mucous (lip) preserved at low temperature. KOTELNIKOV, F. S. AND BELOUSOVA, N. M. Vestnik oftal. *18:*620-623, '41

Operation for pterygium using mucous graft from lip. DOZOROVA, N. S. Vestnik oftal. (nos. 1-2) *20:*59-60, '42

Preliminary graft of buccal mucosa in closure of extensive perforations of hard palate. REBELO NETO, J. Rev. brasil. de oto-rino-laring. *12:*297-301, July-Oct '44

Buccal mucous membrane grafts in treatment of burns of eye. SIEGEL, R. Arch. Ophth. *32:*104-108, Aug '44

Early transplantation of buccal mucosa and conjunctiva in chemical burns of eyes. PAVISIC, Z. Ophthalmologica *108:*297-304, Dec '44

Buccal mucosal grafts in therapy of total symblepharon. BERTOTTO, E. V. Rev. med. de Rosario *35:*317-322, April '45

Transplantation of mucous membrane (Denig operation) in severe burns of eyes. MITERSTEIN, B. AND KORNBLUETH, W. Harefuah *29:*152, Oct 1, '45

Mucous Membrane

Idiopathic perforation of nasal septum; autoplasty with peduncluated flap of mucous membrane; cure. ROY, J. N. Ann. Otol., Rhin. and Laryng. *32:*554-560, June '23

Surgical restoration of lining of mouth. BLAIR, V. P. Surg., Gynec. and Obst. *40:*165-174, Feb '25

Early plastic operation (transplantation of

Mucous Membrane – Cont.
oral mucosa) in caustic injuries of eye. THIES, O. Arch. f. Ophth. *123:*165-170, '29
Lip-graft operation for trichiasis of eyelid. ALEXANDER, G. F. Tr. Ophth. Soc. U. Kingdom *52:*162-169, '32
Early grafting of mucous membrane in burns of eye. O'CONNOR, G. B. Arch. Ophth. *9:*48-51, Jan '33
Modification of operation for trachomatous entropion (trichiasis) by means of free transplant. BURSUK, G. G. Sovet. vestnik oftal. *2:*251-252, '33
Plastic replacement of extensive mucosal defects of cheek. HOFER, O. Wien. klin. Wchnschr. *49:*990-992, July 31, '36
Restoration of orbit and repair of conjunctival defects, with grafts from prepuce and labia minora. CLAY, G. E. AND BAIRD, J. M. Tr. Sect. Ophth., A.M.A., pp. 252-259, '36
Use of mucosa of lips in Toti operation on lacrimal ducts. JANCKE, G. Ber. u. d. Versamml. d. deutsch. ophth. Gesellsch. *51:*478-479, '36
Transplantation of oral mucosa in recurrent pterygium. GREEN, J. Am. J. Ophth. *20:*942-943, Sept '37
Use of mucous membrane in ophthalmic surgery. SPAETH, E. B. Am. J. Ophth. *20:*897-907, Sept '37
Method of maintaining apposition of mucosal flaps after submucous resection. KEARNEY, H. L. Tr. Am. Laryng., Rhin. and Otol. Soc. *43:*109-110, '37
Free autoplastic graft of gastric mucosa to replace urinary bladder tissue loss. STEFANINI, P. Arch. ed atti d. Soc. ital. di chir. *43:*951-967, '37
Repair of secondary traumatic defects in mucous membrane of lips. GORDON, S. Canad. M.A.J. *38:*382, April '38
Therapeutic homoplastic transplantation of conserved mucous membrane. FILATOV, V. P. Vestnik oftal. *12:*307-310, '38
Therapy of trachomatous pannus by transplantation of mucous membranes of cadaver conserved at low temperature. KOSTENKO, F. M. Vestnik oftal. *13:*500-506, '38
Abstr: Gaz. clin. *36:*453-454, Dec '38
Transplantation of conjunctiva in surgical therapy of trichiasis. KLAUBER, E. Ann. d'ocul. *176:*476-477, June '39
Transplantation of mucous membrane from lips of cadavers in Millingen-Sapezhko operation. ALEKSEEV, S. A. Vestnik oftal. (no. 6) *15:*77-79, '39
Possibility of repairing loss of bony substance of cranium by means of graft of bladder

Mucous Membrane – Cont.
mucosa. BEZZA, P. Arch. ital. di chir. *55:*405-429, '39
Transplantation of conjunctiva from cadaver. ROZENTSVEYG, M. G. Vestnik oftal. (nos. 2-3) *14:*26-36, '39
Mucosal graft in therapy of corneoconjunctival burns. VON GROLMAN, G. Arch. de oftal. de Buenos Aires *15:*429-434, Sept '40
also: Rev. med. y cien. afines *2:*629-632, Sept 30, '40
Application of mucous membrane grafts to congenital and acquired states. SHEEHAN, J. E., M. Rec. *152:*404-408, Dec 4, '40
Double-edged knife for removing mucous membrane and skin grafts. BERENS, C. Tr. Sect. Ophth., A.M.A., p. 291, '40
Therapy of trachomatous pannus by transplantation of lip mucosa preserved at low temperature. KIPARISOV, N. M. Vestnik oftal. *17:*227-229, '40
Biomicroscopic picture of healing of "normal" Denig transplant (lip mucosa). ROSHCHIN, V. P. Vestnik oftal. *16:*333-336, '40
Recidivating symblepharon in leper treated with conjunctival transplant; case. BEAUJON, O. Arch. venezol. Soc. de oto-rino-laring., oftal., neurol. *2:*23-27, March '41
Conjunctival burn due to ammonia treated by Denig method (excision of tissue and graft of buccal mucosa); case. VON GROLMAN, G. Prensa med. argent. *28:*839-840, April 16, '41
Transplantation of conjunctiva of cadaver; clinical and histologic aspects. SIE BOEN LIAN. Geneesk. tijdschr. v. Nederl.-Indie *81:*2097-2101, Sept 30, '41
Therapy of trachomatous pannus by transplantation of mucous (lip) preserved at low temperature. KOTELNIKOV, F. S. AND BELOUSOVA, N. M. Vestnik oftal. *18:*620-623, '41
Speed of repair of wounds of mucosa in mouth. MAJ, G. Boll. Soc. ital. biol. sper. *17:*322, May '42
Use of palpebral conjunctiva in reconstruction of inferior fornix. PUGA, R. Amatus *2:*207-211, Mar '43
Buccal mucosal grafts in therapy of total symblepharon. BERTOTTO, E. V. Rev. med. de Rosario *35:*317-322, April '45
Precancerous condistions of skin and adjacent mucosa. MIESCHER, G. Schweiz. med. Wchnschr. *73:*1072, Sept 4, '43
Simplified method of rotating skin and mucous membrane flaps for complete reconstruction of lower lip. OWENS, N. Surgery *15:*196-206, Jan '44

Mucous Membrane – Cont.
Sulfonamide-impregnated membranes; further experience. ANDRUS, W. DEW. AND DINGWALL, J. A. III. Ann. Surg. *119:*694–699, May '44
Preliminary graft of buccal mucosa in closure of extensive perforations of hard palate. REBELO NETO, J. Rev. brasil. de oto-rino-laring. *12:*297-301, July-Oct '44
Buccal mucous membrane grafts in treatment of burns of eye. SIEGEL, R. Arch. Ophth. *32:*104–108, Aug '44
Carcinoma of buccal mucosa. BURFORD, W. N. AND ACKERMAN, L. V. Am. J. Orthodontics (Oral Surg. Sect.) *31:*547-551, Sept '45
Autoplastic dacryorhinostomy; new process for reconstructing lacrimal organs by means of labial mucosal graft. NIEMEYER, W. Arq. brasil. de oftal. *8:*181- 185, Dec '45
Conjunctival palpebral autoplasty. BELFORT MATTOS, W. Arq. brasil. de oftal. *8:*103–109, '45

Mucous Membranes, Tumors
Nevocarcinoma of skin and mucous membranes. WILLIAMS, I. G. AND MARTIN, L. C. Lancet *1:*135–138, Jan 16, '37

MUDD, S. AND FLOSDORF, E. W.: Military symposium; blood and blood substitutes in burn treatment. New England J. Med. *225:*868–870, Nov 27, '41

MUECKE, F. F. AND SOUTTAR, H. S.: Case of double nose. Proc. Roy. Soc. Med. (sect. Laryng.). *17:*8-9, Jan '24

MUELLER, R. F.: Management of compound injuries of hand. Minnesota Med. *27:*110–114, Feb '44

MÜHLPFORDT, H.: Simultaneous appearance of acuminate condylomata and warts on face with keloid. Dermat. Wchnschr. *84:*463-466, April 2, '27

MÜHSAM, E.: Plastic surgery of fingers. Zentralbl. f. Chir. *53:*585–588, March 6, '26

MÜLLER. G.: Formation of artificial vagina by skin flap (Ostrčil method); case. Rozhl. v chir. a gynaek. (cast gynaek.) *11:*55–59, '32

MÜLLER, G.: Artificial vagina obtained by section of urethro-vesico-rectal septum. Casop. lek. cesk. *75:*1393–1399, Nov 6, '36

MÜLLER, G.: Construction of artificial vagina from vesico-urethro-rectal septum; late results. Casop. lek. cesk. *78:*169–171, Feb 17, '39

MÜLLER, H.: Granugenol in burns. Deutsche med. Wchnschr. *58:*1759-1760, Nov 4, '32

MÜLLER, H. K.: Congenital entropion due to epiblepharon. Klin. Monatsbl. f. Augenh. *87:*184–190, Aug '31

MÜLLER, O.: Suture of tendons; technic and outcome in 101 cases. Beitr. z. klin. Chir. *128:*754–765, '23

MÜLLER, P.: New procedure for formation of artificial vagina. (Comment on Kirschner and Wagner's article). Zentralbl. f. Gynak. *55:*201-203, Jan 24, '31

MÜLLER, P.: Formation of artificial vagina with use of skin flaps. Vereinsbl. d. pfalz. Aerzte *44:*21, Jan 15; 42, Feb 1, '32

MÜLLER, P.: Formation of artificial vagina from epidermis. Chirurg. *4:*527-533, July 1, '32

MÜLLER, P.: Elimination of cicatricial ectropion by free Thiersch graft. Schweiz. med. Wchnschr. *71:*5–6, Jan 4, '41

MÜLLER, R.: Five years' experience with radium therapy of hemangiomas. Munchen. med. Wchnschr. *87:*538–541, May 17, '40

MÜLLER, S.: Case of lateral fistulas in neck. Deutsche Ztschr. f. Chir. *193:*401–408, '25

MÜLLER, S.: Exstrophy of bladder; operation by Borelius-Maydl method. Hospitalstid. (Dansk kir. selsk. forh.) *73:*23, Aug 14, '30

MÜLLER, W.: Triphalangeal thumb. Arch. f. klin. Chir. *185:*377–386, '36

MUGNIÉRY, E.: Remote results of Maydl's operation for exstrophy of bladder. Lyon chir. *18:*481, July–Aug '21 abstr: J.A.M.A. *77:*1606, Nov 12, '21

MUGRAGE, R. (see GOOD, R. W. *et al*) July '34

MUIR, D. C.: Case of hypertelorism. Brit. J. Child. Dis. *22:*102–109, April–June '25

MUIR, E.: Treatment of perforating ulcer of foot. Leprosy Rev. *14:*49, July '43

MUIR, J.: Radio-active substances; their therapeutic uses and applications; radium treatment of carcinoma of lower lip. Radiology *7:*51–58, July '26

MUIR, J.: Radio-active substances; their therapeutic uses and applications; radiation of cancer of cheek. Radiology *7:*131–136, Aug '26

MUIR, J.: Cancer of lower lip; efficient treatment by radiation. Internat. J. Med. and Surg. *46:*590–591, Dec '33

MUIRHEAD, E. E. AND HILL, J. M.: Advantages and clinical uses of desiccated plasma in shock prepared by adtevac process. Ann. Int. Med. *16:*286–302, Feb '42

MUIRHEAD, E. E. AND HILL, J. M.: Intrasternal administration of plasma in burns; sulfadiazine (sulfonamide) complications. Dallas M. J. *28:*156-161, Dec '42

MUIRHEAD, E. E.; HILL, J. M. AND ASHWORTH, C. T.: Use of human plasma protein solutions in shock. South. Surgeon *11:*414–431, June '42

MUIRHEAD, E. E.; HILL, J. M. AND ASHWORTH,

C. T.: Rationale of use of concentrated plasma protein solutions in treatment of hematogenic shock. Texas State J. Med. *38:*199–207, July '42

MUIRHEAD, E. E. (see HILL, J. M.) Dec '42

MUKASA, H.: Postoperative psychosis; dementia praecox following operation on nasal septum; case. Oto-rhino-laryng. *12:*139, Feb '39

MUKASA, H.: Hypertrophic angioma of cheek; case. Oto-rhino-laryng. *14:*487, July '41

MUKERJI, A.: Burn therapy in general practice. J. Indian M. A. *13:*146–; 48, Feb '44

MUKERJI, S. N.: Case of stiff jaw after cancrum oris; surgical interference; cure. Indian M. Gaz. *62:*387, July '27

MUKERJI, S. N.: Imperforate anus; case. Indian M. Gazz. *62:*521–522, Sept '27

MUKHERJI, M.: Club hands; case. Brit. J. Radiol *4:*507–508, Oct '31

MUKHIN, M. V.: Rare case of tetanus following burn. Sovet. vrach. zhur., pp. 1820–1821, Dec 15, '36

MULDOON, W. E.: Restoration of patency of nasolacrimal duct by means of vitallium tube; preliminary report. Am. J. Ophth. *28:*1340–1345, Dec '45

MULHOLLAND, J. H. *et al*: Protein metabolism and bed sores. Ann. Surg. *118:*1015–1023, Dec '43

MULLEN, T. F.: Epispadias in male. Northwest Med. *24:*63–67, Feb '25

MULLEN, T. F.: Treatment of congenital cleft lip. M. J. and Rec. (supp.) *122:*402–407, Oct 7, '25

MULLEN, T. F.: Plastic repair of facial defects. Northwest Med. *25:*408–416, Aug '26

MULLEN, T. F.: Early treatment of facial wounds. S. Clin. North America *23:*1458–1464, Oct '43

MULLER, F.: Operation on huge scrotal elephantiasis performed by Casimiro Saez y Garcia in 1882. Rev. de med. y cir. Habana *46:*373–383, Aug 31, '41

MULLER, G. P.: Surgical treatment of exstrophy of bladder. S. Clin. North America *15:*275–283, Feb '35

MULLER, H. K. AND LANGGUTH, H.: Measuring force of elevation of upper eyelid and its clinical significance; description of apparatus. Arch. f. Ophth. *144:*234–246, '41

MULLER, P.: Surgical therapy of ectropion of upper lip; case. Clinique, Paris *27:*124–125, April (A) '32

MULLER, P. (see IRRMANN, E.) April '35

MULLER, VALENTIN: *Frühe Plastik in Griechenland und Vorderasien* (rund 3000 bis 600 v. Christ). B. Filser, Augsburg, 1929

MULLER-MEERNACH, O.: Simple instrument for cutting Thiersch flaps. Munchen. med. Wchnschr. *89:*591, June 26, '42

MULLIGAN, R. M.: Metastasis of mixed tumors of salivary glands. Arch. Path. *35:*357–365, March '43

MULLIN, W. V. AND DARSIE, L. L.: Study of 133 cases of laryngeal cancer. S. Clin. North America *15:*851–858, Aug '35

MULVIHILL, D. A.: Kineplastic surgery for amputated arms. S. Clin. North America *18:*467–481, April '38

MUNGER, I. C. JR.: Burns and their treatment. Nebraska M. J. *18:*300–306, Aug '33

MUNOZ ARENOS, J. M.: Fundamental principles of esthetic surgery. Arch. de med., cir. y especialid. *38:*756–760, Nov 30, '35

MUNOZ ARENOS, J. M.: Nondiffused infections of hand in daily practice. Semana med. espan. *3:*636–642, May 18, '40

MUNOZ ARENOS, J. M.: Burn of cranium due to electric current; rare case. Semana med. espan. *3:*1070–1073, Aug 31, '40

MUNOZ ARENOS, J. M.: Diffuse phlegmons of hand and forearm. Semana med. espan. *4:*167–171, Feb 15, '41

MUNRO, D.: Care of back following spinal cord injuries; consideration of bed sores. New England J. Med. *223:*391–398, Sept 12, '40

MUNRO, D.: Treatment of patients with injuries of spinal cord and cauda equina preliminary to making them ambulatory. Clinics *4:*448–474, Aug '45

MUNROE, A. R.: Rational treatment of surgical shock based on proven physiological data. Canad. M.A.J. *12:*136–138, March '22

MUNROE, A. R.: Operation of cartilage-cranioplasty. Canad. M.A.J. *14:*47–49, Jan '24

MUNSON, F. T. AND HERON, D. F.: Facial reconstruction with acrylic resin. Am. J. Surg. *53:*291–295, Aug '41

DE MUNTER, L. AND BARAKIN, M.: Mechanism and therapy of facial paralysis. Liege med. *30:*415–434, April 4, '37

MURARD, J. (see COMBIER, V.) Nov '27

MURAT, J. (see ISELIN, M.) July '37

MURATA, M. (see FUZII, M.) 1931

MURDOCH, R. L.: Tunnel skin grafts into stricture of rectum. Tr. Am. Proct. Soc. *33:*156–158, '32

MURDOCH, R. L.: New operation for atresia ani vaginalis. Tr. Am. Proct. Soc. (1941) *42:*274–285, '42

MURESANU, J.: Therapy of inoperable cysts of neck. Zentralbl. f. Chir. *65:*1453–1455, June 25, '38

MURDY, W. F.: Treatment of fracture of mandible in child. U. S. Nav. M. Bull. *33:*114–115, Jan '35

MURLESS, B. C.: Treatment (especially tannic acid) of infected burns. Brit. M. J. *1:*51–53, Jan 13, '40

MURPHY, D. R. JR.: Brachial plexus block anesthesia; improved technic. Ann. Surg. *119:*935–943, June '44

MURPHY, A. B.: Jaw fractures. Northwest Med. *38:*44–46, Feb '39

MURPHY, D. L. (see BURKE, H. D. *et al*) Nov–Dec '45

MURPHY, D. P.: Exstrophy with cancer of bladder and absence of umbilicus; report of case. J.A.M.A. *82:*784–785, March 8, '24

MURPHY, D. P.: Congenital familial finger contracture and associated familial knee-joint subluxation. J.A.M.A. *86:*395–397, Feb 6, '26

MURPHY, F. G.: Technic in using trichloroacetic acid for removal of moles from eyelids. J. Iowa M. Soc. *26:*147–148, March '36

MURPHY, F. G.: Repair of laceration of flexor pollicis longus tendon (by faucet handle). J. Bone and Joint Surg. *19:*1121–1123, Oct '37

MURPHY, F. G.: Italian method of plastic repair of denuded areas followed by mermaid cast immobilization. Surgery *12:*294–301, Aug '42

MURPHY, I. J. AND MURPHY, S. L.: Radiotherapy of cancer of lips and mouth. Radiol. Rev. and Chicago M. Rec. *51:*126–128, March '29

MURPHY, S. L. (see MURPHY, I. J.) March '29

Murphy's Operation

Jaw ankylosis; treatment by Murphy's arthroplastic operation; case. FERNÁNDEZ SARALEGUI, A.: Bol. y trab. de la Soc. de cir. de Buenos Aires *13:*165–171, May 29, '29

MURRAY, C. R.: Fractures of bones of hand. New York State J. Med. *36:*1749–1761, Nov 15, '36

MURRAY, D. W. G. AND MORGAN, J. R. E.: Gonococcal tenosynovitis of hand. Canad. M.A.J. *32:*374–375, April '35

MURRAY, G.: Small bone grafts of extremities. Canad. M.A.J. *48:*137–139, Feb '43

MURRAY, J. J. AND BOOKHALTER, S.: Complete hypospadias; case. Brit. M. J. *2:*659–660, Sept 24, '38

MURRAY, R. A. (see KELLY, R. P. *et al*) 1946

MURRAY, R. A. (see KELLY, R. P. *et al*) April '46

Murray-Nelson-Hulsman Operation

Priority of Murray-Nelson-Hulsman original method for avoiding perforation in submucous resection. NELSON, R. M., J. M. A. Georgia *32:*338–339, Oct '43

MUSCHAT, M.: Case of complete epispadias associated with incontinence of urine cured by operation; 4 additional cases. J. Urol. *18:*177–185, Aug '27

MUSCHAT, M.: Experiences with Ombredanne operation for hypospadias. J. Urol. *51:*437–438, April '44

Muscles

Reconstruction of muscles and tendons. CHARBONNEL. J. de med. de Bordeaux *92:*437, Aug 10, '21 abstr: J.A.M.A. *77:*1210, Oct 8, '21

Muscles and nerves in total bilateral harelip. CADENAT, M. E. Ann. d'anat. path. *8:*353–358, April '31

Surgery of muscles and tendons for contracture. GILL, A. B., S. Clin. North America *15:*203–212, Feb '35

New aspect of muscle reinnervation; preliminary report. BILLIG, H. E. JR. AND VAN HARREVELD, A., U. S. Nav. M. Bull. *41:*410–414, March '43

Myotomy in repair of divided flexor tendons. BLUM, L., U. S. Nav. M. Bull. *42:*1317–1322, June '44

Shock associated with deep muscle burns. ANTOS, R. J.; *et al*. Proc. Soc. Exper. Biol. and Med. *57:*11–13, Oct '44

Problem of central nervous reorganization after nerve regeneration and muscle transposition. SPERRY, R. W. Quart. Rev. Biol. *20:*311–369, Dec '45

Muscle Grafts, Free

Experiments with free transplantation of entire muscle. SERRA, A. Arch. ital. di chir. *12:*355–370, '25

Experimental researches on homoplastic transplantation of striated muscle preserved in vitro. BERTOCCHI, A. AND BIANCHETTI, C. F. Arch. per le sc. med. *51:*347–363, '27

Fate of free muscular transplants. SICILIANI, G. Morgagni *70:*329–353, Feb 19, '28

Influence of nervous system on transplantation of homoplastic grafts of striated muscular tissue. BARTOLI, O. Policlinico (sez. chir.) *37:*361–370, Aug '30

Neurotization of homoplastic grafts of striated muscle. BARTOLI, O. Arch. ed atti d. Soc. ital. di chir. *36:*1170, '30

Neurotization of muscular tissue transplanted into striated muscles. COMOLLI, A. Arch. ed atti d. Soc. ital. di chir. *36:*967, '30

Attachment of autoplastic grafts of striated muscles in relation to their nervous connections. COMOLLI, A. Chir. d. orig. di movimento *16:*151–180, June '31

Muscle Grafts, Free—Cont.

Muscular autotransplants and nerve connections; experimental study. Iovino, F. Ann. ital. di chir. *12:*1521-1546, Dec 31, '33

Muscle-nerve graft. Sheehan, J. E., S. Clin. North America *15:*471-482, April '35

Muscle-nerve graft in paralysis of facial nerve. Yaritsyn, A. A. Vestnik-khir. *39:*132-134, '35

Transplantation of healthy muscles with their blood vessels and nerves to paralyzed muscles in therapy of sequels to poliomyelitis. Massart, R. Bull. et mem. Soc. d. chirurgiens de Paris *28:*467-472, July 3, '36

Transplantation of motor nerves and muscles in forelimb of rat. Sperry, R. W., J. Comp. Neurol. *76:*283-321, April '42

Free muscle transplantation in restoration of lips and cheeks. Prudente, A. Rev. paulista de med. *23:*344-345, Dec '43 J. Internat. Coll. Surgeons *7:*312-313, July-Aug '44

Muscles, Transposition of

Restoration of cheek and temporal region by pedicled and sliding grafts of skin and muscle. Whitham, J. D., J.A.M.A. *76:*448, Feb 12, '21

Case of epispadias associated with complete incontinence treated by rectus transplantation. Thompson, A. R. Brit. J. Child. Dis. *20:*146-151, July-Sept '23

Nerve grafting versus musculoplasty in paralysis of facial nerve. Perthes, G. Zentralbl. f. Chir. *51:*2073-2076, Sept 20, '24

Muscle transplantation. Petta, G. Policlinico (sez. chir.) *32:*303-320, June '25

Muscle transplantation. Scheel, P. F. Deutsche Ztschr. f. Chir. *192:*136-142, '25

Epispadias in female, transplantation of gracilis muscle for incontinence. Deming, C. L., J.A.M.A. *86:*822-825, March 20, '26

Muscle transplantation, method for cure of urinary incontinence in male. Player, L. P. and Callander, C. L., J.A.M.A. *88:*989-991, March 26, '27

Use of muscle grafts in mastoid operations. Kisch, H. Post-Grad. M. J. *8:*270-271, July '32

Formation of artificial vagina by transplantation of muscular flap. Soler Juliá, J. Rev. de cir. de Barcelona *7:*194-198, March '34

Treatment of persistent bronchial fistula by use of pedicled muscle flap. Garlock, J. H. S. Clin. North America *14:*307-313, April '34

Plastic surgery of muscular paralysis; formation of muscular loops. König, F. Zentralbl. f. Chir. *62:*2531-2536, Oct 26, '35

Muscles, Transposition of—Cont.

New method of muscular transplantation applied to cheiloplasty; case. Rebelo Neto, J. Rev. de chir. structive, pp. 199-209, March '36

Extirpation of benign parotid tumors; use of digastric muscle as guide during operation and in correction of facial paralysis. Cadenat, F. M., J. de chir. *48:*625-629, Nov '36

Use of muscle pedicle flap for prevention of swelling of arm following radical operation for carcinoma of breast; preliminary report. Rienhoff, W. F., Jr. Bull. Johns Hopkins Hosp. *60:*369-371, May '37

Plastic surgery of anus; using fatty flap of bulbocavernosus muscle, in therapy of incontinence of feces, following transplantation of vestibular anus; case. Holterman, C. Zentralbl. f. Gynak. *63:*60-66, Jan 7, '39

Utilization of temporal muscle and fascia for facial paralysis. Brown, J. B. Ann. Surg. *109:*1016-1023, June '39

Use of pedicled muscular flaps in surgical therapy of residual empyema and indirect bronchial fistula. Zschau, H. Zentralbl. f. Chir. *66:*2529-2534, Dec 2, '39

Utilization of temporal muscle and fascia in facial paralysis. Brown, J. B. Am. J. Orthodontics *26:*80-87, Jan '40

Pedicled muscle flap in treatment of bronchial fistulas; 16 cases. Crafoord, C. and Linton, P. J. Thoracic Surg. *9:*606-611, Aug '40

Correction of facial paralysis. (muscle transplant.) Alexander, R. J. Rocky Mountain M. J. *38:*713-716, Sept '41

Use of muscular flap to fill bone cavities in osteomyelitis due to gunshot wounds. Stotz, W. Zentralbl. f. Chir. *69:*427, March 14, '42

Muscle transplants; opposition of thumb. Bunnell, S. Am. Acad. Orthop. Surgeons, Lect., pp. 283-288, '44

Transplantation of muscles in paralysis of radial nerve following gunshot wounds. Tikhonovich, A. V. Khirurgiya, no. 3, pp. 72-73, '44

Muscle flap closure of cavity resulting from lung abcess. Prioleau, W. H. Ann. Surg. *123:*664-672, April '46

Muscle transplant for paralysis of radial nerve. Altman, H. and Trott, R. H. J. Bone and Joint Surg. *28:*440-446, July '46

Mushin, W. W.: Anesthesia for faciomaxillary surgery. Post-Grad. M. J. *16:*245-246, July '40

MUSHKATIN, V. I.: Burn therapy; fumigation with iodine vapors. Novy khir. arkhiv. *39:*485–503, '37

MUSITZ, G.: Congenital fistula of lacrimal sac; case. Budapesti orvosi ujsag *31:*28–30, Jan 12, '33

MUSKAT, G.: Fracture of fingers during baseball game. Deutsche med. Wchnschr. *58:*2032–2033, Dec 23, '32

MUSSER, J. H.: Symphalangism. New Orleans M. and S. J. *83:*325–326, Nov '30

MUSSO, A. (see REBAUDI, F.) Jan '40

MUYLE, G. AND BATSELAERE, R.: Syndrome of "forked hands and feet" and oligophrenia; 2 cases. J. belge de neurol. et de psychiat. *36:*441–455, July '36

MUZII, E.: Prevention of postoperative recurrence of ankylosis of jaws; case. Stomatol. *27:*136–147, Feb '29

MUZII, E.: Diagnosis of dento-maxillo-facial deformities. Stomatol. *28:*821–865, Oct '30

MYERS, B. L.: Peripheral burns. J. Missouri M. A. *30:*25–29, Jan '33

MYERS, D.: War injuries to mastoid and facial nerve. Arch. Otolaryng. *44:*392–405. Oct '46

MYERS, D. (see ERSNER, M. S.) April '36

MYERS, S. A.: Early care of facial wounds. U. S. Nav. M. Bull. *42:*1019–1020, May '44

MYERS, T.: New finger splint. Minnesota Med. *13:*840, Nov '30

MYERSON, M. C.: New elevator for submucous resection. Laryngoscope *34:*660, Aug '24

N

NACHLAS, I. W.: Splint for correction of extension contractures of metacarpophalangeal joints. J. Bone and Joint Surg. *27:*507–512, July '45

NADOLECZNY, M.: Burns of oral cavity. Arch. f. Ohren-, Nasen-u. Kehlkopfh. *133:*283–287, '32

NAEGELI, T.: A new method of operation for congenital cleft palate. Schweiz. med. Wchnschr. *54:*62–63, Jan 10, '24

NAFFZIGER, H. C.: Methods to secure end-to-end suture of peripheral nerves. Surg., Gynec. and Obst. *32:*193, March '21

NAFFZIGER, H. C. AND JONES, O. W., JR.: Surgical treatment of progressive exophthalmos following thyroidectomy. J.A.M.A. *99:*638–642, Aug 20, '32

NAFTZGER, J. B.: Fractures involving nasal accessory sinuses. Ann. Otol. Rhin. and Laryng. *37:*486–499, June '28

NAFTZGER, J. B.: Fractures of facial bones involving nasal accessory sinuses. Tr. Am. Laryng., Rhin. and Otol. Soc. *34:*383–394, '28

NAFTZGER, J. B.: Facial fractures involving nasal accessory sinuses. Ann. Otol., Rhin. and Laryng. *51:*414–423, June '42

NAFTZGER, J. B.: Fractures involving nasal accessory sinuses. Tr. Am. Laryng., Rhin. and Otol. Soc. *48:*333–341, '42

NAGEL, Z.: "New operation for hypospadias." Zentralbl. f. Chir. *49:*982–984, July 8, '22

Nagel

Reply to Nagel's remarks on my article, "Operation for hypospadias." FISCHER, A. Zentralbl. f. Chir. *49:*1748, Nov 25, '22

NÄGELSBACH, E.: Operative treatment of elephantiasis of scrotum and penis. Arch. f. Schiffs-u. Tropen-Hyg. *31:*282–291, June '27

NAGEOTTE, J.: Grafts of fresh tendon unite with tissue of host later than grafts of devitalized tendon. Compt. rend. Soc. de biol. *95:*669–672, Sept 21, '26

NAGEOTTE, J.: Remote effects of grafting of dead tissue (tendon injury). Compt. rend. Soc. de biol. *95:*1552–1554, Dec 31, '26

NAGEOTTE, J.: Transplantation of dead connective tissue. Virchow's Arch. f. path. Anat. *263:*69–88, '27

NAGEOTTE, J.: Use of grafts of devitalized connective tissue (tendon and nerve) in reparative surgery. Presse med. *47:*1365–1366, Sept 27, '39

Nageotte Operation

Histologic document on fate of heterotransplantation of nerves of Nageotte type. POLICARD, A. AND LERICHE, R. Lyon chir. *19:*544–549, Sept–Oct '22 (illus.) abstr: J.A.M.A. *80:*1182, April 21, '23

Repair of radialis through grafting of dead calf nerve according to Nageotte's method. SOLÉ, R. Semana med. *2:*452–454, Aug 19, '26

NAGER, F. R. AND RÜEDI, L.: Ear injuries due to electricity. Rassegna ital. di oto-rino-laring. *5:*129–140, Jan–Dec '31

NAGLE, P.: Use of antiseptic anesthetic agent locally in extensive burn. J. Oklahoma M. A. *33:*14–16, Jan '40

NAGLE, P. S.: Hyperthermic epidermal destruction. J. Oklahoma M. A. *32:*7–14, Jan '39

NAGLE, R. J.: Maxillofacial prosthesis. Am. J. Orthodontics (Oral Surg. Sect.) *29:*312–319, June '43

NAGY, B.: Cosmetic correction of long nose. Med. Klin. *24:*1310–1311, Aug 24, '28

NAKAJIMA, K. (see TAKEZAWA, N.) May '38

NAKONOVA, E. I.: New method of burn treatment. Sovet. vrach. zhur., pp. 1262–1263, Aug 30, '36

NALIVKIN, P. A.: Burn therapy. Novy khir. arkhiv. *38:*436–447, '37

NANDROT: Exstrophy of bladder, cure by Marion-Heitz-Boyer method (transplantation of ureters into rectum) in man 20 years old. Bull. et mem. Soc. nat. de chir. *61:*1103–1105, Nov 2, '35

NAPALKOV, N.: Contracture of fingers due to cicatrices on back of hand. Ortop. i. travmatol. (no. 6) *9:*43–47, '35

NAPIER, J. R.: Corrective splint for paralysis of thenar muscles. Brit. M. J. *1:*15, Jan 5, '46

NARASIMHAN, N. S.: Case of contracture of mouth. Indian M. Gaz. *60:*72, Feb '25

NARAT, J. K.: Brilliant green in burns. Am. J. Surg. *36:*54–56, April '37

NARBUTOVSKIY, S. D.: Surgical therapy of cancer of lips. Novy khir. arkhiv. *33:*3–14, '35

NARDUCCI, F.: Multiple gigantic keloids; case. Dermosifilografo *5:*145–156, March '30

NARIO, C. V.: Volkmann's disease and syndromes of arterial obliteration in extremities. An. de Fac. de med., Montevideo *14:*422–589, May–June '29

NÄRVI, E. J.: Regeneration of tendons and treatment of ruptures of tendons, especially in region of synovial sheaths. Acta chir. Scandinav. *60:*1–54, '26 abstr: J.A.M.A. *86:*1670, May 22, '26

NASAROW, N. N. AND KUSCHEWA, M. N.: Osteoplastic partial resection of lower jaw by Krassin's method for removal of lingual cancer; 5 cases. Deutsche Ztschr. f. Chir. *215:*145–146, '29

NASE, H.: Hairy polyps of soft palate as cause of cleft formation; case. Zentralbl. f. Chir. *66:*29–32, Jan 7, '39

NASON, L. H.: Keloids and their treatment. New England J. Med. *226:*883–886, May 28, '42

Nasopharynx, Cancer

Treatment of malignant tumors of pharynx and nasopharynx. NEW, G. B. Surg., Gynec. and Obst. *40:*177–182, Feb '25

Nasopharynx, Tumors

Treatment of fibromas of nasopharynx; report of 32 cases. NEW, G. B. AND FIGI, F. A. Am. J. Roentgenol. *12:*340–343, Oct '24

Treatment of fibromas of naso-pharynx; report of 32 cases. NEW, G. B. AND FIGI, F. A. Ann. Otol., Rhin. and Laryng. *34:*191–196, March '25

Therapy of nasopharyngeal tumors. PORDES, J. M. Acta oto-laryng. orient. *1:*45–49, '45

NASSAU, C. F.: Epithelioma of lip. S. Clin. N. Amer. *1:*197, Feb '21

NASSAU, C. F.: Tubed pedicle flap for scar contracture. S. Clin. North America *14:*13–18, Feb '34

NASTA, T.; BÂLCU, S. AND VLĂDESCU, V.: Phalangization of first metacarpal bone in surgical therapy of thumb injuries. Rev. de chir., Bucuresti *37:*234–237, March–April '34

Nataf-Saunders Operation

Cuénod and Nataf modification of Saunders' operation for trichiasis and entropion. CUNNINGHAM, E. R. Chinese M. J. *48:*819–829, Sept '34

NATALE, A. M. AND BARBERIS, J. C.: Plastic surgery of nose by Italian method under general ether anesthesia by peritoneal route with J. B. Abalos' technic; case. Rev. med. del Rosaro *20:*487–489, Oct '30

NATALE, A. M. (see ABALOS, J. B.) Dec '28

NATANZON, A. M.: Rhinoplastic operations following gunshot wounds. Vrach. delo (nos. 1–2) *25:*61–66, '45

NATHAN, P. W.: Biology of bone development in its relation to bone transplantation. New York M. J. *114:*454, Oct 19, '21

NATHAN, P. W. AND RENNIE, A. M.: Value of Tinel sign (in relation to regeneration of peripheral nerve lesions). Lancet *1:*610–611, April 27, '46

NATHANSON, G.: Therapy of fractures of cranial base involving nasal sinuses. Acta oto-laryng. *25:*430–439, '37

NATHANSON, I. T.: Large carcinoma of cheek. Am. J. Orthodontics (Oral Surg. Sect.) *31:*284–286, April '45

NATHANSON, I. T. (see TAYLOR, G. W.) Oct '39

NATHANSON, I. T. (see WELCH, C. E.) Oct '37

NATIONAL RESEARCH COUNCIL: Medical progress; treatment of thermal burns; general outline. New England J. Med. *229:*817–823, Nov 25, '43

NATTINGER, J. K.: Total reconstruction of external ear. Northwest Med. *36:*172–174, May '37

NAUJOKS: Surgical and hormonal therapy of true hermaphroditism. Arch. f. Gynak. *156:*93–96, '33

NAVA, V.: Experimental skin grafting. Boll. d. Soc. ital. di biol. sper. *2:*858–860, July '27

NAVA, V.: Grafting of fixed skin. Boll. d. Soc. med. chir. di Pavia *2:*369–372, '27

NAVA VERA: Transplantation of skin preserved in fluids. Arch. per le sc. med. *52:*236–242, May '28

DE NAVASQUEZ, S.: Metastasizing basal cell carcinoma of face. J. Path. and Bact. *53:*437–

439, Nov '41

NEBLETT, H. C.: Late complications and sequels following blunt trauma to eye and orbital wall. South. Med. and Surg. *106:*436–437, Nov '44

NECHELES, H. AND OLSON, W. H.: Experimental investigation of gastrointestinal secretions and motility following burns and their relation to ulcer. Surgery *11:*751–765, May '42

NECHELES, H. (see LEVINSON, S. O. *et al*) Feb '40

NECHELES, H. (see OLSON, W. H.) Aug '43

Neck

Surgical conditions of neck other than goiter. LAHEY, F. H. Proc. Internat. Assemb. Inter-State Post-Grad. M. A., North America (1929) *5:*388–392, '30

Hemorrhagic cyst on side of neck. IWATÔ, Y. Okayama-Igakkai-Zasshi *44:*1727–1728, June '32

Anatomy of subhyoid region with reference to diagnosis of mid-line swellings of neck. MEKIE, D. E. C. Malayan M. J. *11:*178–179, Sept '36

Deep infections of neck; collective review. NEW, G. B. AND ERICH, J. B. Internat. Abstr. Surg. *68:*555–567, '39; in Surg. Gynec. and Obst., June '39

Differential diagnosis of swellings of face and neck. WINTER, L. Am. J. Orthodontics *25:*1087–1116, Nov '39

Anomalies and complex abnormalities of region of first pharyngeal arch. GÜNTHER, H. Ztschr. f. menschl. Vererb.-u. Konstitutionslehre *23:*43–52, '39

Cervicofacial arc, apparatus for isolating surgical field. BERTOLA, V. J. Prensa med. argent. *27:*997–998, May 8, '40

Pseudolaryngocele (aerocele) of neck; case. KILPATRICK, F. R. Guy's Hosp. Rep. *90:*15–20, '40–'41

Concepts of anatomy of head and neck. BUCHANAN, A. R. Am. J. Orthodontics *28:*152–166, March '42

Retractor for use in neck surgery. BEATTY, H. G. Arch. Otolaryng. *35:*651–652, April '42

Neck lesions; therapy. BRITTO, R. Imprensa med., Rio de Janeiro *19:*59–70, Sept '43

Placement of neck incisions. HOLMAN, E. Surg., Gynec. and Obst. *78:*533–534, May '44

Diagnosis and management of surgical conditions of neck. LAHEY, F. H. Proc. Interst. Postgrad. M. A. North America (1944) pp. 102–106, '45

Neck, Cancer of (See also Neck Dissections)

Surgical relief of pain in deep carcinoma of face and neck. FAY, T. Am. J. Roentgenol. *14:*1–5, July '25

Cervical lymph nodes in intra-oral carcinoma. DUFFY, J. J. Radiology *9:*373–379, Nov '27

Cancer of skin of face and neck. LOUNSBERRY, C. R. California and West Med. *26:*800–801, June '27

Glandular involvement following cancer of lips, tongue and floor of mouth. REGAUD, C. *et al*. Paris med. *1:*357–372, April 16, '27 also: Strahlentherapie *26:*221–251, '27

Early clinical and therapeutic study of invasion of lymphatic nodes in pavement epitheliomas of lips and tongue; 8 cases. LECÈNE, P. Prat. med. franc. *7:*219–227, May (A) '28

Aberrant thyroid glands in neck. LEECH, J. V. *et al*. Am. J. Path. *4:*481–492, Sept '28

Cancer and malignant tumors of neck; with special reference to incidence, pathology and prognosis. SILVERMAN, I. Long Island M. J. *22:*651–656, Nov '28

Treatment by radiation and gold seed implantation in metastatic nodes in neck from cancer of lips. JOHNSON, S. C. Am. J. Cancer *15:*254–261, Jan '31

Treatment of metastatic involvement of neck secondary to intraoral cancer. MELAND, O. N. Am. J. Roentgenol. *26:*20–22, July '31

Neck metastases from lip and mouth cancer. KILGORE, A. R. AND TAUSSIG, L. R., S. Clin. North America *11:*1055–1059, Oct '31

Radium therapy of cancer of lips, with study of metastasis into regional lymph nodes. COLLIN, E. Acta radiol. *13:*232–237, '32

Conservative procedure in care of cervical lymph nodes in intra-oral carcinoma. DUFFY, J. J. Am. J. Roentgenol. *29:*241–247, Feb '33

Care of cervical glands in intra-oral carcinoma. STEWART, C. B. Am. J. Roentgenol. *29:*234–236, Feb '33

Papillary tumors of lateral aberrant thyroid origin; discussion and report of 4 cases. STRODE, J. E. Proc. Staff Meet. Clin., Honolulu *9:*103–113, Nov '43

Treatment of neck glands in cancer of lip, tongue and mouth; study of present-day practice (questionnaire report of Cancer Commission of California Medical Association). PFLUEGER, O. H. California and West. Med. *39:*391–397, Dec '33

Neck, Cystic Hygroma (See also Cystic Hygroma)

Lymphangioma of neck. THOMPSON, J. E. AND KEILLER, V. H. Ann. Surg. *77:*385-396, April '23 (illus.)

Hygroma cystica treated with radium. NEW, G. B., S. Clin. N. America *4:*527-529, April '24

Multilocular serous cyst in neck, probably of congenital origin. MENESES, J. G. J. Arch. espan. de pediat. *9:*91-95, Feb '25

Lymphatic cysts of neck with report of case. WAFFLE, E. B. AND FOWLER, F. E. Northwest Med. *25:*142-144, March '26

Congenital cystic lymphangioma of neck. TORCHIANA, L. Arch. ital. di chir. *16:*173-192, '26

Multilocular cystic lymphangioma of neck. DE GAETANO, L. Riforma med. *43:*529-532, June 6, '27

Bilateral lymphangioma of neck. VON HEREPEY-CSÁBÁNYI, G. Zentralbl. f. Chir. *54:*1672, July 2, '27

Lymphangioma of neck; case. MILIAN, G. AND LONJUMEAU. Bull. Soc. franc. de dermat. et syph. *34:*859-862, Dec '27

Radium in treatment of multilocular lymph cysts (cystic hygromas) of neck in children. FIGI, F. A. Am. J. Roentgenol. *21:*473-480, May '29

Chylocystic lymphangioma of neck; 3 cases. VOLKMANN, J. Beitr. z. klin. Chir. *146:*654-667, '29

Cystic lymphangioma of neck; case. DELLAMANO, N. Gazz. d. osp. *51:*43-53, Jan 12, '30

Lymphangioma of neck. PLĂCINTIANU, G. Spitalul *51:*51-52, Feb '31

Cystic hygroma of neck. NEW, G. B., S. Clin. North America *11:*771-773, Aug '31

Cystic hygroma; 2 cases. (neck) MASON, J. T. AND BAKER, J. W., S. Clin. North America *11:*1091-1095, Oct '31

Cystic lymphangioma of neck. BOLINTINEANU, G. AND BĂJEU, G. Spitalul *52:*26-27, Jan '32

Cystic lymphangioma of neck; case. DI CIANNI, E. Rinasc. med. *9:*128-129, March 15, '32

Pseudo-unilocular serous cyst of neck in infant; case. TERCERO, M. Arch. espan. de pediat. *16:*306-309, July '32

Hygroma cysticum colli; case report with review of literature. HYATT, C. N., J. Iowa M. Soc. *22:*406-408, Aug '32

Recurrent cystic lymphangioma of neck in child; case. GRECO, T. Sperimentale, Arch. di biol. (no. 2) *86:*viii-xii, '32

Neck, Cystic Hygroma — Cont.

Therapy of lymphangiomas of neck. CHIARIELLO, A. G. Folia med. *20:*590-594, May 30, '34

Cystic hygroma of neck; report of case and review of literature. VAUGHN, A. M. Am. J. Dis. Child. *48:*149-158, July '34

Cystic hygroma of neck. MACGUIRE, D. P. Arch. Surg. *31:*301-307, Aug '35

Cystic lymphangioma associated with grave congenital malformations; study of cervical hygromas. QUADRI, S. Clin. pediat. *17:*755-777, Oct '35

Therapy of serous cysts of neck. BELLONE, G. Riv. san. siciliana *23:*1717-1724, Dec 1, '35

Cystic hygroma of neck; 2 cases in Bulu children. MCCRACKIN, R. H. Am. J. Dis. Child. *51:*349-352, Feb '36

Cystic hygroma. BAILEY, H. Clin. J. *66:*242-244, June '37

Hygroma colli cysticum and hygroma axillare; pathologic and clinical study and report of 12 cases. GOETSCH, E. Arch. Surg. *36:*394-479, March '38

Cystic hygroma of neck. FLEMING, B. L., J.A.M.A. *110:*1899-1900, June 4, '38

Therapy of inoperable cysts of neck. MURESANU, J. Zentralbl. f. Chir. *65:*1453-1455, June 25, '38

Cystic hygroma (of neck). BAILEY, H., J. Internat. Coll. Surgeons *2:*31-33, Jan-April '39

Cystic hygroma of neck; 27 cases. GROSS, R. E. AND GOERINGER, C. F. Surg., Gynec. and Obst. *69:*48-60, July '39

Congenital cystic lymphangioma, with recurrence after surgical therapy; case in newborn infant (neck). VIANA, F. Pediat. prat., Sao Paulo *13:*91-98, March-June '42

Cystic lymphangioma, with report of case. (neck) SRIBMAN, I. Dia med. *15:*175-178, March 1, '43

Cervicomediastinal lymphangioma (cystic hygroma); 2 cases in infants. ARNHEIM, E. E. J. Mt. Sinai Hosp. *10:*404-410, Sept-Oct '43

Congenital lymphangiomatous macroglossia with cystic hygroma of neck. LIERLE, D. M. Ann. Otol., Rhin. and Laryng. *53:*574-575, Sept '44

Neck Dissections

Extirpation of lymphatics with lip cancer. DURANTE, L. Arch. ital. di chir. *8:*201-208, Oct '23

Injuries to nerves from surgical treatment of

Neck Dissections – Cont.

diseases of face and neck. BABCOCK, W. W. J.A.M.A. *84:*187-192, Jan 17, '25

Experience in treatment of epitheliomata of tongue with glandular involvement. ROUX-BERGER, J. L. AND MONOD, O. Bull. et mem. Soc. nat. de chir. *53:*648-659, May 14, '27

Treatment of adenopathies which accompany cancer of lower half of face. MARQUIS, E. Bull. et mem. Soc. nat. de chir. *53:*760-767, June 4, '27

Surgical treatment of invasion of cervical glands in lingual cancer. ROUX-BERGER, J. L. Presse med. *35:*881, July 13, '27

Removal of submaxillary salivary glands in operations for carcinoma of lower lip; responses to questionnaire. BERESOW, E. L. Arch. f. klin. Chir. *151:*767-784, '28

Treatment of epitheliomatous glands of neck following cancer of lips. SCOTT, R. K., M. J. Australia *2:*505-512, Oct 24, '31

Neck metastases from lip and mouth cancer. KILGORE, A. R. AND TAUSSIG, L. R., S. Clin. North America *11:*1055-1059, Oct '31

Surgical treatment of metastases to cervical lymph nodes from intra-oral cancer. FISCHEL, E. Am. J. Roentgenol. *29:*237-240, Feb '33

Treatment of cancerous or potentially cancerous cervical lymph-nodes (as result of cancers of mouth). BLAIR, V. P. AND BROWN, J. B. Ann. Surg. *98:*650-661, Oct '33

Epithelioma of lip, with particular reference to lymph node metastases. KENNEDY, R. H. Ann. Surg. *99:*81-93, Jan '34

Surgery as applied to lymph nodes of neck in cancer of lip and buccal cavity; statistical study. FISCHEL, E. Am. J. Surg. *24:*711-731, June '34

Surgical therapy of secondary adenopathies of neck in buccopharyngeal cancer. DUCUING, J. Ars med., Barcelona *11:*353-359, Sept '35

Present day status of irradiation and surgery of cancer of neck. BECK, J. C. AND GUTTMAN, M. R. South. M. J. *29:*606-609, June '36

Epithelioma of lips; glandular involvement and "wait and see" method of therapy. MEYERS, E. S., M. J. Australia *1:*399-400, March 13, '37

Surgical therapy of cervical metastases of epithelioma (oral). MARTINEZ, E. M. Bol. Liga contra el cancer *12:*315-320, Sept-Oct '37

Surgical treatment of lymphatic fields in cancer of mouth. MORRIN, F. J. Irish J. M. Sc., pp. 157-163, April '39

Cancer of head and neck; management of lesions with borderline operability and curability. KIME, E. N. Arch. Phys. Therapy *20:*282-287, May '39

Evaluation of neck dissection in cancer of lips. TAYLOR, G. W. AND NATHANSON, I. T. Surg., Gynec. and Obst. *69:*484-492, Oct '39

Treatment of carcinoma of lip (and involved lymph nodes). SMITHERS, D. W. Post-Grad. M. J. *15:*376-381, Nov '39

Surgical therapy of metastases in cervical lymph nodes from cancer of mouth. SCHÜRCH, O. AND FEHR, A. Deutsche Ztschr. f. Chir. *251:*641-672, '39

Current treatment of cancer of lip (and involved lymph nodes); clinical speculation. BLAIR, V. P. AND BYARS, L. T. Surgery *8:*340-352, Aug '40

Extirpation of cervical lymph nodes in cancer of mouth with metastases. PRUDENTE, A. Bol. y trab., Acad. argent. de cir. *26:*1030-1031, Oct 28, '42

Treatment of metastatic carcinoma of neck. BROWN, J. B. AND McDOWELL, F. Ann. Surg. *119:*543-555, April '44

Neck dissections for metastic carcinoma. BROWN, J. B. AND McDOWELL, F. Surg., Gynec. and Obst. *79:*115-124, Aug '44

Treatment of metastatic carcinoma of neck. BROWN, J. B. AND McDOWELL, F. Tr. South. S. A. (1943) *55:*254-266, '44

Neck Surgery

Serous cysts of neck. CEVARIO, L. Gazz. d. osp. *42:*200, Feb 27, '21

Plastic and cosmetic surgery of head, face and neck; correction of nasal deformities. TIECK, G. J. E. AND HUNT, H. L. Am. J. Surg. *35:*234, Aug '21

Plastic and cosmetic surgery of head, neck and face. (including keloids). TIECK, G. J. E. AND HUNT, H. L. Am. J. Surg. *35:*173, June '21; 355, Nov '21

Cosmetic surgery of face, neck and breast. BOOTH, F. A. Northwest. Med. *21:*170-172, June '22 (illus.)

Deformity of neck treated by transplantation of fat. McGUIRE, S., S. Clin. N. America *2:*1259-1261, Oct '22

Plastic surgery of head and neck. RISDON, F. Canad. M.A.J. *12:*797-798, Nov '22

Delayed pedicle flap in plastic surgery of face and neck. NEW, G. B. Minnesota Med. *6:*721-724, Dec '22 (illus.)

Plastic surgery of face and neck. SHEEHAN, J. E. New York M. J. *118:*676-678, Dec 5, '23 (illus.)

Case of extensive plastic repair of face and

Neck Surgery – Cont.
neck with "visor flap". GOLDSCHMIDT, T. Zentralbl. f. Chir. *52:*688-691, March 28, '25
Plastic surgery about face, head and neck. BECK, J. C., J. Indiana M. A. *18:*167-184, May '25
Principles in plastic surgery about head and neck (and nose) BECK, J. C. Illinois M. J. *48:*194-202, Sept '25
Combined satchel handle or tubed pedicle and large delayed whole skin pedicle flaps in case of plastic surgery of face, neck and chest. ALDEN, B. F. Surg., Gynec. and Obst. *41:*493-496, Oct '25
Contractures due to burns of face, neck and body. BEHREND, M., S. Clin. N. America *6:*237-243, Feb '26
New procedures and method in plastic surgery of face and neck. NEW, G. B. South M. J. *19:*138-140, Feb '26
Details in repair of cicatricial contractures of neck. DOWD, C. N. Surg., Gynec. and Obst. *44:*396-399, March '27
Surgical correction of cervicofacial scars of dental origin. MAUREL, G., J. de med. de Paris *46:*577-583, July 21, '27
Plastic surgery of face, neck and chest skin losses. BLAIR, V. P. Tr. Am. S. A. *45:*190-199, '27
Use of visor flaps from chest in plastic operations upon neck, chin and lip. FREEMAN, L. Ann. Surg. *87:*364-368, March '28
Wry-neck following burns, relieved by skin flaps; case report. MILLER, O. R. Kentucky M. J. *26:*190-192, April '28
Treatment of acne-keloid of nape of neck by diathermocoagulation; cases. RAVAUT, P. AND FILLIOL, L. Bull. Soc. franc. de dermat. et syph. *35:*942-946, Dec '28
Free transplants of skin in plastic surgery of face and neck. SANVENERO-ROSSELLI, G. Arch. ital. di chir. *21:*245-265, '28
Plastic surgery of face and neck to remove cicatricial adhesions caused by burns; case. VASCONCELLOS ALVARENGA, E. Rev. brasil. de med. e pharm. *7:*334-337, '31
Use of pedicled flaps and skin grafts in reconstructive surgery of (face) head and neck. FIGI, F. A. Nebraska M. J. *17:*361-365, Sept '32
Contracted dense scar of neck despite use of many Thiersch grafts. BABCOCK, W. W. S. Clin. North America *12:*1405-1407, Dec '32
Contractures of neck following burns (treatment by use of tubular skin graft). MIXTER, C. G. New England J. Med. *208:*190-196, Jan 26, '33
Developments in plastic surgery of face and

Neck Surgery – Cont.
neck. NEW, G. B. Wisconsin M. J. *32:*243-246, April '33
Cicatricial contraction of neck. NEW, G. B. S. Clin. North America *13:*868-869, Aug '33
Tubular skin graft in therapy of extensive contracture of neck. KARTASHEV, Z. I. Sovet. khir., no. 11, pp. 22-30, '35
Plastic surgery of head, face and neck; psychic reactions. BLAIR, V. P., J. Am. Dent. A. *23:*236-240, Feb '36
Repair of loss of substance of throat due to extensive burns. PRUDENTE, A. Rev. Assoc. paulista de med. *11:*43-51, July '37
Extensive loss of substance in subhyoid region; recovery after fat transplantation. STEPLEANU-HORBATZKY. Rev. de chir., Bucuresti *41:*512-515, July-Aug '38
Surgical therapy of cicatricial contracture of neck after burns. MIKHELSON, N. M. Ortop. i travmatol. (no. 1) *12:*74-82, '38
Fibrous contracture of head and neck after extensive burns. GJANKOVIC, H. Lijecn. vjes. *61:*279-284, May '39
Epithelial inlay for scars in neck dragging lower jaw downwards. ESSER, J. F. S. Am. J. Surg. *45:*148-149, July '39
Modern changes in plastic and reconstructive surgery of face and neck. GUTTMAN, M. R. Illinois M. J. *76:*349-351, Oct '39
Brachiothoracic adhesions. BURTON, J. F. Surg., Gynec. and Obst. *70:*938-944, May '40
Labiomentothoracic synechia due to burn; plastic repair of case. JOHOW, A. AND URZUA, R. Rev. med. de Chile *68:*1482-1487, Nov '40
Retractile scars of cervicofacial region; biologic fundamentals for plastic reconstruction. ZENO, L. Bol. Soc. de cir. de Rosario *7:*446-454, Nov '40 also: An. de cir. *6:*341-349, Dec '40 also: Dia med. *13:*264-266, April 14, '41
Use of abdominal skin to correct cervical defect due to burn. GABARRO, P. Rev. Fac. de med., Bogota *10:*339-342, Oct '41
Free full-thickness skin graft for relief of burn contracture of neck. BLOCKER, T. G., JR. South. Surgeon *10:*849-857, Dec '41
Axillary-iliac tubed flap in neck surgery. HAVENS, F. Z. AND DIX, C. R. Proc. Staff Meet., Mayo Clin. *17:*167-169, March 18, '42
Free skin grafts versus flaps in surface defects of face and neck. MALINIAC, J. W. Am. J. Surg. *58:*100-109, Oct '42
Thoracofacial synechia following burn; case. COVARRUBIAS ZENTENO, R. Rev. med. de Chile *71:*899-901, Sept '43
Evaluation of pedicle flaps versus skin grafts

Neck Surgery–Cont.

in reconstruction of surface defects and scar contractures of chin, cheeks and neck. AUFRICHT, G. Surgery *15:*75–84, Jan '44

Full-thickness skin grafts from neck for function and color in eyelid. BROWN, J. B. AND CANNON, B. Ann. Surg. *121:*639–643, May '45

Reconstructive treatment of gunshot wound of face and neck. LEWIN, M. Arch. Otolaryng. *42:*191–197, Sept '45 also: Tr. Am. Acad. Ophth. (1944) *49:*276–282, May–June '45

Full-thickness skin grafts from neck for function and color in eyelid. BROWN, J. B. AND CANNON, B. Tr. South. S. A. (1944) *56:*255–259, '45

Neck Surgery, Anesthesia for

Anesthesia in operations on face and neck. Ann. d. mal. de l'oreille, du larynx *49:*516–524, May '30

Rectal anesthesia with tribrom-ethanol in cervicofacial surgery; indications, technic, results and experimental studies. MOULONGUET, A. AND LEROUX-ROBERT, J. Ann. d'oto-laryng., pp. 283–304, March '34

Rectal anesthesia with mixture of ether, tribromethanol and oil in cervicofacial surgery. JACOD, M. Lyon chir. *32:*35–42, Jan–Feb '35

Regional anesthesia of head and neck. MOUSEL, L. H. Anesthesiology *2:*61–73, Jan '41

Regional anesthesia for operations about neck. ADAMS, R. C. Anesthesiology *2:*515–529, Sept '41

Anesthesia by procaine hydrochloride block of cervical plexus in neck surgery. FINOCHIETTO, R. Prensa med. argent. *31:*1757–1760, Sept 6, '44

Neck Tumors (See also Cystic Hygroma; Neck, Cysts and Fistulae)

Swellings of submaxillary regions. IVY, R. H. Ann. Surg. *81:*605–610, March '25

Diagnosis of tumors of neck. TRUFFERT, P. Bull. med., Paris *41:*726–731, June 18, '27

Lipoma of cheek and neck. DALEPPA, K. Indian M. Gaz. *62:*385–386, July '27

Large cavernous angioma with tumors of thyroid structure in lateral region of neck. LORETI, M. Valsalva *3:*353–363, Aug '27

Tumors of neck. SEARBY, H., M. J. Australia *2:*406–408, Sept 20, '30

Tumors of hyo-thyro-pharyngeal region; laryngocele and branchial cyst. VAN DEN WILDENBERG, L. Scalpel *85:*265–271, Feb 27, '32

Massive congenital cervicofacial cavernous hemangioma; case. GIUSTINIAN, V. AND ESTIÚ, M. D. Semana med. *2:*245–246, July 28, '32

Tumors of head and neck. JORSTAD, L. H. J. Missouri M. A. *34:*82–84, March '37

Tumors of neck; diagnosis and treatment, cervical cysts and fistulas. HICKEN, N. F. AND POPMA, A. M. Nebraska M. J. *23:*209–212, June '38

Differential diagnosis of swellings of face and neck. WINTER, L. Am. J. Orthodontics *25:*1087–1116, Nov '39

Tumors and cysts of neck. BOYD, W. Tr. West. S. A. (1938) *48:*172–182, '39

Unusual tumors of cervical region. JOYCE, T. M. *et al*. Arch. Surg. *42:*338–370, Feb '41

Deep cavernous hemangioma of neck; case. LAIRD, E. G. Am. J. Surg. *53:*158–162, July '41

Benign lesions of neck. DINSMORE, R. S. Proc. Interst. Postgrad. M. A. North America (1940) pp. 322–324, '41

Tumors of head, face and neck. WOLFER, J. A. Indust. Med. *11:*528–529, Nov '42

Treatment of pigmented nevi of neck. FIGI, F. A., S. Clin. North America *23:*1059–1075, Aug '43

Method of treating cystic tumors of neck. LYLE, F. M. Am. J. Surg. *61:*443–444, Sept '43

Tumors of neck. PETERSON, E. W. Am. J. Surg. *61:*350–359, Sept '43

Differential diagnosis of neck tumors. DORE, R. Union med. du Canada *73:*269–271, March '44

Tumors of neck (other than thyroid). McNEALY, R. W. Proc. Interst. Postgrad. M. A., North America (1943) pp. 229–233, '44 also: J. Omaha Mid-West Clin. Soc. *5:*39–45, April '44

Surgical management of large tumors of neck; unusual case (mixed tumor). DIXON, C. F. AND BENSON, R. E. Am. J. Surg. *69:*384–390, Sept '45

Neck Wounds

Tracheotomy for grave subcutaneous emphysema following cervicofacial trauma; cases. CASTELNAU, M. Oto-rhino-Laryng. internat. *22:*195–196, April '38

Treatment of facial wounds and cut throat. TAYLOR, J. Brit. M. J. *1:*792–795, April 9, '38

Wounds of neck and lesions of larynx, trachea and esophagus in war surgery. DE ANDRADE MEDICIS, J. Arq. brasil. de cir. e ortop. *10:*155–179, '42

Neck Wounds—Cont.

Wounds of the neck. AGUILERA V., M. Arch. Soc. cirujanos hosp. *13:*3-11, June '43

Early treatment of facial wounds. (and neck) NEW, G. B. Minnesota Med. *26:*619-622, July '43

Wounds of neck and larynx. LEWIS, R. S. Lancet *1:*781-784, June 17, '44

DE NECKER, J.: Ideas of Dr. Crile on operative shock and their clinical application. Arch. franco-belges de chir. *27:*411-421, May '24

NEDKOFF, N.: New corrective method for breast hypertrophy. Zentralbl. f. Chir. *65:*1503-1504, July 2, '38

NEDVED, M. (see VONDRACEK, V.) Feb '41

NEEL, H. B. AND PEMBERTON, J. DEJ.: Lateral cervical (branchial) cysts and fistulas; clinical and pathologic study. Surgery *18:*267-286, Sept '45

NEFF, E. AND DIMOND, W. B.: Novocain (procaine hydrochloride) applied topically as local anesthetic in nasal surgery; preliminary report. Ann. Otol., Rhin. and Laryng. *39:*593-594, June '30

NEFF, J. M.: Arthoplasty of jaw, with some general remarks on focal infection and on formation of new joints. Surg., Gynec. and Obst. *33:*8, July '21

NEFROTTI, G. M.: Double fracture of lower jaw. Riforma med. *37:*438, May 7, '21

NEGLO, L. G. AND SPEKTOR, I. Z.: Orbital fractures; case with air embolism. Vestnik oftal. (nos. 1-2) *20:*60-63, '42

NEGUS, V. E.: Treatment of chronic laryngeal stenosis, with special reference to skin grafting. Ann. Otol., Rhin. and Laryng. *47:*891-901, Dec '38

NEGUS, V. E.: Treatment of chronic laryngeal stenosis, with special reference to skin grafting. Tr. Am. Laryng. A. *60:*82-92, '38

NEGUS, V. E. AND KILNER, T. P.: Discussion of nasal injury. Proc. Roy. Soc. Med. *35:*513-518, June '42 also: J. Laryng. and Otol. *57:*270-279, May '42

NEIDELMAN, M. L.: Fibrosarcoma protuberans arising on old burn scar. Ann. Surg. *123:*311-314, Feb '46

NEIL, J. F.: Apparatus for treating bedsores. Brit. M. J. *2:*390, Sept 22, '45

NEILL, C. L. (see SMITH, B. *et al*) Oct '45

NEILL, W. JR.: Mixed tumors of parotid gland; 71 cases. M. J. and Rec. *136:*187-189, Sept 7, '32

NEJROTTI, G. M.: Fracture of jaw. Riforma med. *37:*891, Sept 17, '21 abstr: J.A.M.A. *77:*1689, Nov 19, '21

NEKULA, R.: Surgical therapy of severe burns. Casop. lek. cesk. *72:*1487-1491, Nov 24, '33

NELSON, H.: Ganglia of tendon sheaths (bursae). Minnesota Med. *26:*734-737, Aug '43

NELSON, H. F. (see LAHEY, F. H.) April '41

NELSON, H. (see MCPHEETERS, H. O.) Oct '41

NELSON, L. S.: Opera-glass hand in chronic arthritis; "la main en lorgnette" of Marie and Leri. J. Bone and Joint Surg. *20:*1045-1049, Oct '38

NELSON, L. S.: Treatment of commoner injuries of hand. J. Kansas M. Soc. *41:*236-239, June '40

NELSON, O. G.: Local treatment of burns. J. Tennessee M. A. *37:*159-161, May '44

NELSON, P. A.: Differential diagnosis of cancer of lip. Am. J. Cancer *15:*230-238, Jan '31

NELSON, R. M.: Priority of Murray-Nelson-Hulsman original method for avoiding perforation in submucous resection. J. M. A. Georgia *32:*338-339, Oct '43

Nelson Operation: See Murray-Nelson-Hulsman Operation

NEMES, A.: Formation of vagina from rectum. Zentralbl. f. Gynak. *45:*787, June 4, '21

NERTNEY, E. G.: Fractures of mandible. U. S. Vet. Bur. M. Bull. *4:*360-362, April '28

Nerves, Dupuytren's Contracture and

Nervous etiology of Dupuytren's contracture; cases. GUBERN-SALISACHS, L. Rev. de cir. de Barcelona *6:*81-115, Sept '33

Association of retraction of palmar aponeurosis and scleroderma; relation to diseases of endocrine glands and of sympathetic nervous system. WEILL, J. AND MAIRE, R. Paris med. *1:*263-268, March 24, '34

Traumatic Claude Bernard-Horner syndrome associated with Dupuytren's contracture and paroxysmal anxiety (precordial pain) caused by aerophagy; case. LAIGNEL-LAVASTINE *et al.* Rev. neurol. *2:*784-787, Dec '34

Bilateral Dupuytren's contracture due to injury of cubital nerve in lower third of forearm. NOICA, D. *et al.* Romania med. *15:*261-262, Oct 15. '37

Nerves, Effects of Sympathectomy on Skin Grafts

Action of periarterial sympathectomy on skin grafts. DALGER, J. Lyon chir. *23:*451-452, July-Aug '26

Skin grafts; effect of cervical sympathectomy; experiments. TINOZZI, F. P. Rassegna internaz. di clin. e terap. *7:*585-604, Nov 10, '26

Periarterial decortication as aid to skin graft-

Nerves, Effects of Sympathectomy on Skin Grafts – Cont.

ing. BERTOCCHI, A. Gior. d. r. Accad. di med. di Torino *33:*129-134, March '27

Good results of combined periarterial sympathectomy and skin grafts on leg; 24 cases. LERICHE, R. AND FONTAINE, R. Strasbourgh-med. (pt. 2) *86:*101-105, April 20,'28

Influence of ablation of sympathetic ganglions on evolution of different forms of skin grafts; experimental study. DOBRZANIECKI, W. Lyon chir. *27:*537-578, Sept-Oct '30

Effect of removal of sympathetic ganglia on cutaneous autoplastic and homoplastic transplants (skin). DOBRZANIECKI, W. Polska gaz. lek. *10:*262, April 5; 287, April 12, '31

Periarterial decortication by Leriche method and autoplastic and homoplastic grafts. BERTOCCHI, A. Arch. ital. di chir. *29:*1-36, '31

Effect of removal of cervical ganglion of sympathetic nerve on growth of autoplastic and homoplastic skin transplants. VASILEV, A. A. AND ZHOLONDZ, A. M. Arch. f. klin. Chir. *178:*148-169, '33 also: Novy khir. arkhiv *29:*3-20, '33

Late results of therapy of leg ulcers by sympathectomy combined with skin grafts; study based on 52 cases. LERICHE, R. *et al.* J. de chir. *45:*689-710, May '35

Periarterial sympathectomy and Thiersch graft in therapy of varicose veins. AREL, F. Turk tib cem. mec. *3:*394-395, '37

Nerves, Facial Hemiatrophy and

Trophic disorders of central origin; report of case of progressive facial hemiatrophy, associated with lipodystrophy and other metabolic derangements. WOLFF, H. G. AND EHRENCLOU, A. H., J.A.M.A. *88:*991-994, March 26, '27

Progressive facial hemiatrophy; case with other signs of disease of central nervous system. WOLFF, H. G. Arch. Otolaryng. *7:*580-582, June '28

Role of sympathetic nervous system in pathogenesis of facial hemiatrophy with report of case of hemiatrophy of one side of face and other side of body. MARINESCO, G. *et al.* Paris med. *1:*269-275, March 26, '32 also: Bull. sect. scient. Acad. roumaine (nos. 6-8) *14:*155-166, '31

Atypical facial hemiatrophy of sympathetic origin. WORMS, G. Rev. d'oto-neuro-opht. *11:*99-103, Feb '33

Congenital hemiatrophy of face with Claude Bernard-Horner syndrome; case. VELASCO BLANCO, L. AND WAISBEIN, S. Arch. am. de med. *14:*74-76, '38

Nerves, Facial

Successful grafting of hypoglossal on facial nerve. SCHMIDT, W. T. Munchen. med. Wchnschr. *69:*708-709, May 12, '22 (illus.)

Facial paralysis and surgical repair of facial nerve. NEY, K. W. Laryngoscope *32:*327-347, May '22 (illus.)

Surgical treatment of facial paralysis. COLEMAN, C. C. Virginia M. Monthly *49:*180-188, July '22 (illus.)

Case of facio-hypoglossal anastomosis for facial palsy. STONEY, R. A. Irish J. M. Soc. pp. 404-408, Nov '22

Preservation of facial nerve in radical treatment of parotid tumors. ADSON, A. W. AND OTT, W. O. Arch. Surg. *6:*739-746, May '23 (illus.)

Anastomosis of facial nerve to correct contracture. ALURRALDE, M. AND ALLENDE, C. T. Rev. Asoc. med. argent. *36:*259-266, May-June '23 (illus.) abstr: J.A.M.A. *81:*1730, Nov 17, '23

Anastomosis of seventh and eleventh cranial nerves to correct facial paralysis. NIX, J. T. New Orleans M. and S. J. *77:*123-126, Sept '24

Spinofacial anastomosis; result after 16 years. LECOUTURIER. Arch. franco-belges de chir. *28:*308-312, April '25

Operative correction of facial paralysis. BLAIR, V. P. South. M. J. *19:*116-120, Feb '26

Results of hypoglossofacial anastomosis for facial paralysis in 2 cases. BROWN, A. Surg., Gynec. and Obst. *42:*608-613, May '26

Immediate results of operations for facial paralysis. TAVERNIER, L. Bull. et mem. Soc. nat. de chir. *52:*992-994, Nov 20, '26

Plastic operations for paralysis of facial nerve. BRUNNER, H. Arch. f. klin. Chir. *140:*85-100, '26

Hypoglossal-facial nerve anastomosis. CANESTRO, C. AND CAMPORA, G. Riv. otoneuro-oftal. *4:*81-90, Jan-Feb '27

Facial paralysis treated by spino-facial anastomosis; 2 cases. ANTONIOLI, G. M. Gior. d. r. Accad. di med. di Torino *33:*80-88, Feb '27

Peripheral facial paralysis and progressive facial hemiatrophy as sequels of teeth extraction. BÖNHEIM, E. Deutsche Monatschr. f. Zahnh. *45:*353-366, April 15, '27

Operation on two cases of secondary carcinoma and on one case of primary cystadenoma of parotid gland; relation of lobes of parotid to facial nerve. MCWHORTER, G. L. S. Clin. N. Amer. *7:*489-505, June '27

Suture of facial nerve within temporal bone, with report of first successful case. BUN-

Nerves, Facial – Cont.
NELL, S. Surg., Gynec. and Obst. *45:*7-12, July '27
Glossopharyngeal-facial nerve anastomosis. WATSON-WILLIAMS, E. Proc. Roy. Soc. Med. (Sect. Otol.) *20:*59-63, July '27 also: J. Laryng. and Otol. *42:*516-519, Aug '27
Facial paralysis; causes, symptoms and treatment. SIEMERLING, E. Deutsche med. Wchnschr. *53:*1467-1470, Aug 26, '27
Treatment of facial paralysis due to exposure. BERTWISTLE, A. P. Brit. M. J. *2:*494, Sept 17, '27
Remarks on 1008 cases of facial paralysis. MARQUE, A. M. Rev. de especialid. *2:*1195-1199, Dec '27 also: Rev. oto. neuro-oftal. *2:*1-4, Jan '28
Leriche's operation for traumatic peripheral facial paralysis as compared with other operative procedures. JIANU, J. AND BUZOIANU, G. Lyon chir. *25:*10-21, Jan-Feb '28
Surgery of traumatic facial paralysis. ANTONIOLI, G. M. Clin. chir. *31:*81-104, Feb '28
Rational treatment of facial paralysis; with special reference to Bell's palsy. FELDMAN, L. Am. J. Phys. Therapy *4:*539-544, March '28
Peripheral facial paralysis; 1,008 cases. MARQUE, A. M. Semana med. *1:*946-949, April 19, '28
Preservation of facial nerve in excision of parotid tumors; 2 cases. SHAAR, C. M., U. S. Nav. M. Bull. *27:*351-360, April '29
Facial nerve anastomosis in paralysis. BALLANCE, C., J. Egyptian M. A. *12:*63-68, May '29
Classification of peripheral facial paralyses. ZIMMERN, A. AND CHAVANY, J. A. Medecine *11:*453-457, June '30
Experiments in which central endo of divided cervical sympathetic nerve was anastomosed to peripheral end of divided facial nerve and to peripheral end of divided hypoglossal nerve. BALLANCE, C. Arch. Neurol. and Psychiat. *25:*1-28, Jan '31
Surgical therapy of facial paralysis. WERTHEIMER, P. Lyon chir. *28:*111-113, Jan-Feb '31
Facial nerve anastomosis for relief of paralysis. BROWN, A. Illinois M. J. *59:*130, Feb '31
Freezing of facial nerve in treatment of harelip. GOETZE, O. Zentralbl. f. Chir. *58:*927-930, April 11, '31
Neurolysis of facial nerve after 10 years inclusion within scar tissue; operation, with returning function. BUNTEN, W. A. Nebraska M. J. *16:*169-173, May '31
Surgical therapy of peripheral facial paralysis. WERTHEIMER, P. AND CARCASSONNE,

Nerves, Facial – Cont.
F. Lyon chir. *28:*560-570, Sept-Oct '31
Operative treatment of facial palsy by introduction of nerve grafts into fallopian canal and by other intratemporal methods. BALLANCE, C. AND DUEL, A. B. Tr. Am. Otol. Soc. *21:*288-295, '31
Suture of facial nerve trunk. NEUGEBAUER, F. Beitr. z. klin. Chir. *152:*625-628, '31
Treatment of clonic facial spasm; alcohol injection; nerve anastomosis. (with hypoglossal). HARRIS, W. AND WRIGHT, A. D. Lancet *1:*657-662, March 26, '32
Successful treatment of postoperative facial paralysis. ARWINE, J. T., M. Bull., Vet. Admin. *8:*404, May '32
Technic of total or subtotal extirpation of parotid gland with conservation of superior branch of facial nerve in so-called mixed tumors; clinical results. DUVAL, P. AND REDON, H. J. de chir. *39:*801-808, June '32
Anastomosis of hypoglossal and facial nerves 10 months after operation; presentation of case. LEARMONTH, J. R. Proc. Staff Meet., Mayo Clin. *7:*389-390, July 6, '32
Correction of unilateral facial paralysis. SHEEHAN, J. E., J. M. Soc. New Jersey *29:*556-560, July '32
Peripheral facial nerve injuries. POLLOCK, L. J. AND DAVIS, L. Am. J. Surg. *18:*553-595, Dec '32
Therapy of peripheral facial paralysis by resection of superior cervical sympathetic ganglion. WERTHEIMER, P. Bull. et mem. Soc. nat. de chir. *59:*4-7, Jan 14, '33
Fascia lata grafts in facial paralysis. WARDILL, W. E. M. Newcastle N. J. *13:*35-38, Jan '33
Facial nerve damage; repair. GRAHAM, H. B. California and West. Med. *40:*174-177, March '34
Plastic use of fascia in treatment of facial paralysis. DEMEL, R. Zentralbl. f. Chir. *61:*1445-1448, June 23, '34
Clinical presentation of improvement in surgical repair of facial nerve (transplant). DUEL, A. B. Laryngoscope *44:*599-611, Aug '34
Experience with fascia lata grafts in operative treatment of facial paralysis. GILLIES, H. Proc. Roy. Soc. Med. *27:*1372-1378, Aug '34 also: J. Laryng. and Otol. *49:*743-756, Nov '34
Buccal-facial anastomosis in facial nerve injury. PONS TORTELLA, E. Rev. de cir. de Barcelona *8:*82-89, Sept-Dec '34
Surgical treatment of facial paralysis by autoplastic nerve graft. SULLIVAN, J. A. Canad. M.A.J. *31:*474-479, Nov '34
Results of resection of superior cervical gan-

Nerves, Facial—Cont.
glion and of part of trunk of cervical sympathicus in peripheral facial paralysis of long standing; case. ROASENDA, G. AND DOGLIOTTI, A. M. Boll. e mem. Soc. piemontese di chir. *4:*980–990, '34
Results of stellectomy in facial paralysis due to section of facial nerve involved in parotid tumor; case. CAEIRO, J. A. Semana med. *1:*572–579, Feb 20, '36
Total removal of parotid gland with preservation of facial nerve. SALTZSTEIN, H. C. Ann. Surg. *103:*635–638, April '36
Method for correcting paralysis of lower part of face due to nerve injury in extirpation of benign parotid tumors. CADENAT, F. M. Mem. Acad. de chir. *62:*961–962, June 17, '36
Resection of superior cervical ganglion in therapy of peripheral facial paralysis caused by injury to cranium; case. HUARD, P. Bull. Soc. med.-chir. de l'Indochine *14:*1289–1293, Nov '36
Extirpation of tumors of parotid gland; technic to avoid injury to facial nerve. DUFOURMENTEL, L. Oto-rhino-laryng. internat. *21:*75–76, Feb '37
Surgery of facial nerve. DOGLIOTTI, A. M. Arch. ed atti d. Soc. ital. di chir. *43:*537–691, '37
Follow-up report on facial nerve repair. ELLIS, B. E. Tr. Indiana Acad. Ophth. and Otolaryng. *21:*22–27, '37
Treatment of clonic facial spasm by nerve anastomosis. PHILLIPS, G., M. J. Australia *1:*624–626, April 2, '38
Cutaneous femoris lateralis nerve, direct implantation of free nerve grafts between facial musculature and facial trunk; first case to be reported. CARDWELL, E. P. Arch. Otolaryng. *27:*469–471, April '38
Plastic surgery in therapy of postoperative facial paralysis; case. COELST. Rev. de chir. structive *8:*107–109, Aug '38
Repair of facial nerve lesion by Ballance-Duel graft. MCARTHUR, G. A. D. M. J. Australia *2:*1123–1124, Dec 31, '38
Transplantation of nerves in facial palsy. BAUER, G. Acta chir. Scandinav. *81:*130–138, '38
Spinofacial anastomosis for bilateral traumatic facial paralysis; late results. COSTANTINI, H. AND CURTILLET, E. Lyon chir. *36:*50–53, Jan–Feb '39
Surgical treatment of facial paralysis; review of 46 cases (nerve transplant). MORRIS, W. M. Lancet *2:*588–561, Sept 2, '39

Nerves, Facial—Cont.
Facial paralysis treated by incision of sheath of facial nerve. HORGAN, J. B. Brit. M. J. *2:*768, Oct 14, '39
Parotidectomy with conservation of superior facial nerve (Duval operation); 2 cases. COGNIAUX, P. J. de chir. et ann. Soc. belge de chir. *38–36:*370–372, Dec '39
Intratemporal repair of facial nerve for facial paralysis (Ballance-Duel operation). CASSIDY, W. A. Nebraska M. J. *25:*47–50, Feb '40
Etiology and treatment of facial paralysis. MCCASKEY, C. H. Ann. Otol., Rhin. and Laryng. *49:*199–210, March '40
Surgical repair of seventh cranial nerve. HOOVER, W. B. AND POPPEN, J. L., S. Clin. North America *20:*685–695, June '40
Possible new operation for therapy of definitive paralysis; anastomosis of facial and sympathetic nerves. LERICHE, R. Presse med. *48:*721–722, Sept 17, '40
Recent experiences with operation on facial nerve (including 2 cases of paralysis following mastoidectomy). MARTIN, R. C. Arch. Otolaryng. *32:*1071–1075, Dec '40
Recent experiences with surgery of facial nerve. MARTIN, R. C. Tr. Am. Laryng., Rhin. and Otol. Soc. *46:*491–496, '40
Surgical intervention on second and third portions of seventh cranial nerves in therapy; preliminary report. VAQUERO, L. An. Soc. mex. de oftal. y oto-rino-laring. *16:*264–272, Sept–Oct '41
Late result of hypoglossofacial anastomosis: inadaptation of centers. BOURGUIGON, G. Rev. neurol. *73:*601–603, Nov–Dec '41
Extirpation of parotid gland with complete conservation of facial nerve. FINOCHIETTO, R. *et al.* Rev. med. munic. *2:*790–803, Dec '41
Unusual possible injuries of facial nerves. TATRALLYAY, Z. Monatschr. f. Ohrenh. *76:*30–37, Jan '42
Treatment of facial paralysis. ELLIS, B. E. North Carolina M. J. *3:*130–132, March '42
Treatment facial paralysis. LATHROP, F. D. Lahey Clin. Bull. *3:*20–27, July '42
Paralysis of seventh cranial pair; 2 cases. LURASCHI, J. C. E. AND PORRINI, E. A. Dia med. *14:*1214–1216, Nov. 16, '42
Facial nerve repair. JUERS, A. L. Kentucky M. J. *40:*453–455, Nov. '42
Anastomosis between hypoglossal and facial nerves; case. THOMAS, A. AND DE AJURIAGUERRA. Rev. neurol. *74:*308–310, Nov–Dec '42

Nerves, Facial—Cont.

Combined plastic surgery on facial and facial-hypoglossal nerves for facial paralysis. BERGGREN, S. AND FROSTE, N. Acta oto-laryng. *30:*325-327, '42

Peripheral facial paralysis, based upon 50 observations. ADLER, E. Acta med. orient. *2:*1-9, Dec '42-Jan '43

Facial palsy of otitic origin, with special regard to its prognosis under conservative treatment and possibilities of improving results by active surgical intervention; account of 264 cases subjected to reexamination. KETTEL, K. Arch. Otolaryng. *37:*303-348, March '43

Cervical sympathectomy in therapy of facial paralysis. ALBANESE, A. R. Prensa med. argent. *31:*415-417, March 1, '44

Procedure to correct facial paralysis (by spinofacial anastomosis and fascial strips). HANRAHAN, E. M. AND DANDY, W. E. J.A.M.A. *124:*1051-1053, April 8, '44

Surgical lesions of facial nerve, with comments on anatomy. COLEMAN, C. C. Ann. Surg. *119:*641-655, May '44

Repair of peripheral injuries to facial nerve (by anastomosis). MARTIN, R. C., J. Nerv. and Ment. Dis. *99:*755-757, May '44

Successful suture of facial nerve trunk. STARR, K. W. Australian and New Zealand J. Surg. *14:*53-57, July '44

Total parotidectomy with conservation of facial nerve; 3 cases. GONI MORENO, I. AND RUSSO, A. G. Bol. y trab., Acad. argent. de cir. *28:*722-739, Sept 6, '44

Facial nerve; experiences in surgery. VIOLE, P. Laryngoscope *54:*455-466, Sept. '44

Surgical lesions of facial nerve, with comments on anatomy. COLEMAN, C. C. Tr. South. S. A. (1943) *55:*318-332, '44

Reconstruction of facial nerve (especially in operations on parotid gland). FURSTENBERG, A. C. Arch. Otolaryng. *41:*42-47, Jan '45

Facial nerve surgery in 300 cases. TICKLE, T. G. Laryngoscope *55:*191-195, May '45

Facial nerve lesions due to war injuries and their repair. LATHROP, F. D. J. Laryng. and Otol. *60:*257-266, June '45

Surgical anatomy of facial nerve with special reference to parotid gland. MCCORMACK, L. J. *et al.* Surg., Gynec. and Obst. *80:*620-630, June '45

Facial nerve lesions due to war injuries and their repair. LATHROP, F. D. Proc. Roy. Soc. Med. *38:*629-634, Sept '45

Technic of total parotidectomy with conservation of facial nerve. REDON, H. J. de chir. *61:*14-20, '45

Facial nerve; repair of traumatic lesions secondary to war wounds LATHROP, F. D. S. Clin. North America *26:*763-773, June '46

Anatomic findings concerning morphology and relations of intraparotid facial nerve. DARGENT, M. AND DUROUX, P. E. Presse med. *54:*523-524, Aug 10, '46

War injuries to mastoid and facial nerve. MYERS, D. Arch. Otolaryng. *44:*392-405, Oct '46

Nerves, Grafts

Nerve transplants to bridge nerve defects. CASSIRER, R. AND UNGER, E. Deutsche med. Wchnschr. *47:*586, May 26, '21

Spinofacial anastomosis for facial paralysis. TITONE, M. Lyon chir. *18:*601-605, Sept-Oct '21 (illus.) abstr: J.A.M.A. *78:*249, Jan 21, '22

Changes in nerve implants. ALBANESE, A. Arch. ital. di chir. *4:*215-228, Nov '21 (illus.) abstr: J.A.M.A. *78:*250, Jan 21, '22

Experimental artificial neurotization of paralyzed muscle. JINNAKA, S. Mitt. a. d. med. Fakult. d. k. Univ. zu Tokyo *25:*367-441, '21

Facial palsy and its treatment by nerve anastomosis. DE PAIVA MEIRA, S. Internat. Clinics *2:*241, '21

Fate of nerve grafts. GOSSET, A. AND CHARRIER, J. J. de chir. *19:*1-14, Jan '22 abstr: J.A.M.A. *78:*848, March 18, '22

Successful grafting of hypoglossal on facial nerve. SCHMIDT, W. T. Munchen. med. Wchnschr. *69:*708-709, May 12, '22 (illus.)

Histologic document on fate of heterotransplantation of nerves of Nageotte type. POLICARD, A. AND LERICHE, R. Lyon chir. *19:*544-549, Sept-Oct '22 (illus.) abstr: J.A.M.A. *80:*1182, April 21, '23

Experimental study of method for bridging nerve defects; with description of new method of autotransplant (auto-autotransplant). SACHS, E. AND MALONE, J. Y. Arch. Surg. *5:*314-333, Sept. '22 (illus.)

Experimental results of cable grafts and tubes of fascia lata in repair of peripheral nerve defects. OTT, W. O. Minnesota Med. *5:*581-588, Oct '22 (illus.)

Case of facio-hypoglossal anastomosis for facial palsy. STONEY, R. A. Irish J. M. Soc. pp. 404-408, Nov '22

Double nerve grafting. MANASSE, P. Arch. f. klin. Chir. *120:*665-685, '22 (illus.) abstr:

Nerves, Grafts – Cont.
J.A.M.A. *80:*515, Feb 17, '23
Anastomosis of facial nerve to correct contracture. ALURRALDE, M. AND ALLENDE, C. T. Rev. Asoc. med. argent. *36:*259–266, May–June '23 (illus.) abstr: J.A.M.A. *81:*1730, Nov 17, '23
Results of nerve anastomosis; preliminary remarks: lateral implantation of 2 ends of divided nerve into neighbouring uninjured nerve. BALLANCE, C. Brit. J. Surg. *11:*327–346, Oct '23 (illus.).
Free grafts of nerves. CHIASSERINI, A. Policlinico (sez. chir.) *30:*489–497, Oct '23 (illus.)
Nerve grafting versus musculoplasty in paralysis of facial nerve. PERTHES, G. Zentralbl. f. Chir. *51:*2073–2076, Sept 20, '24
Spinofacial anastomosis; result after 16 years. LECOUTURIER. Arch. franco-belges de chir. *28:*308–312, April '25
Grafting of nerve preserved in alcohol. SALCADO, L. V. Presse med. *33:*558–559, April 29, '25 abstr: J.A.M.A. *84:*1966, June 20, '25
Experimental study of transplantation of nerve supply of muscles, STEWART, J. E., J. Bone & Joint Surg. *7:*948–956, Oct '25
Results of hypoglossofacial anastomosis for facial paralysis in 2 cases. BROWN, A. Surg., Gynec. and Obst. *42:*608–613, May '26
Repair of radialis through grafting of dead calf nerve according to Nageotte's method. SOLÉ, R. Semana med. *2:*452–454, Aug 19, '26
Hypoglossal-facial nerve anastomosis. CANESTRO, C. AND CAMPORA, G. Riv. otoneuro-oftal. *4:*81–90, Jan–Feb '27
Study of nerve grafts with case of heterografts of sciatic. JIANU, J. AND BUZOIANU, G. Lyon chir. *24:*625–641, Nov–Dec '27
Alcoholized nerve graft; experimental study. SWEET, P. W. Ann. Surg. *89:*191–198, Feb '29
Facial nerve anastomosis in paralysis. BALLANCE, C., J. Egyptian M. A. *12:*63–68, May '29
Transplantation of skin, fat, blood vessels, nerves, etc. EISELSBERG, A. Wien. med. Wchnschr. *80:*50–55, Jan 4, '30
Sensory-motor restoration after section of nerves of arm; suture of radial nerve with subsequent graft of median and ulnar nerves. THOMAS, A. AND PETIT-DUTAILLIS. Rev. neurol. *1:*56–60, Jan '30
Grafting with dead tissue; conserved nerves. MINEÀ, I. Cluj. med. *11:*53–57, Feb 1, '30

Nerves, Grafts – Cont.
Neurotization of paralyzed muscles in nerve transplant. FELIX, W. Arch. f. klin. Chir. *162:*681–692, '30
Facial paralysis; causes; treatment by neurosurgery (muscular neurotization). ROSENTHAL, W. Deutsche Ztschr. f. Chir. *223:*261–270, '30
Experiments in which central end of divided cervical sympathetic nerve was anastomosed to peripheral end of divided facial nerve and to peripheral end of divided hypoglossal nerve. BALLANCE, C. Arch. Neurol. and Psychiat. *25:*1–28, Jan '31
Section of radial nerve and heterograft of dog's fresh nerve into man; case. THALHEIMER, M. AND BLONDIN-WALTHER, M. Bull. et mem. Soc. nat. de chir. *57:*535–543, April 25, '31
Operative treatment of facial palsy by introduction of nerve grafts into fallopian canal and by other intratemporal methods. BALLANCE, C. AND DUEL, A. B. Tr. Am. Otol. Soc. *21:*288–295, '31
Neurotization of nerve transplants. FINKEL, Z. I. J. nevropat. i psikhiat. (no. 8) *24:*24–31, '31
Operative treatment of facial palsy by introduction of nerve grafts into fallopian canal and by other intratemporal methods. BALLANCE, C. AND DUEL, A. B. Arch. Otolaryng. *15:*1–70, Jan '32
Technic of grafting living nervous tissue. DUROUX, E. Rev. tech. chir. *24:*21–26, Jan–Feb '32
Paralysis of branchial plexus; rupture of superior roots in supraclavicular fossa; nerve graft; beginning of functional restoration 3 years later. TAVERNIER, L. Lyon chir. *29:*110–112, Jan–Feb '32
Treatment of clonic facial spasm; alcohol injection; nerve anastomosis (with hypoglossal). HARRIS, W. AND WRIGHT, A. D. Lancet *1:*657–662, March 26, '32
Therapy of trophic disturbances (ulcer) following injury of limb by resection of neuroma of posterior tibial nerve and by autotransplantation of nervous tissue. LASSERRE, C. Bull. et mem. Soc. nat. de chir. *58:*500–502, April 16, '32
Anastomosis of hypoglossal and facial nerves 10 months after operation; presentation of case. LEARMONTH, J. R. Proc. Staff Meet., Mayo Clin. *7:*389–390, July 6, '32
Clinical experiences in surgical treatment of facial palsy by autoplastic grafts; Ballance-Duel method. DUEL, A. B. Arch. Otolaryng. *16:*767–788, Dec '32

Nerves, Grafts – Cont.

Repercussions of nerve grafts. May, R. M. Encephale *27:*885-902, Dec '32

History and development of surgical treatment of facial palsy (including grafts). Duel, A. B. Surg., Gynec. and Obst. *56:*382-390, Feb (No. 2A) '33

Muscular autotransplants and nerve connections; experimental study. Iovino, F. Ann. ital. di chir. *12:*1521-1546, Dec 31, '33

Experimental studies in nerve transplantation. Davis, L. and Cleveland, D. A. Ann. Surg. *99:*271-283, Feb '34

Advanced methods in surgical treatment of facial paralysis (Mütter lecture) (nerve transplants). Duel, A. B. Ann. Otol., Rhin. and Laryng. *43:*76-88, March '34

Operative treatment of facial palsy, with observations on prepared nerve graft. Ballance, C. Proc. Roy. Soc. Med. *27:*1367-1372, Aug '34 also: J. Laryng. and Otol. *49:*709-718, Nov '34

Clinical presentation of improvement in surgical repair of facial nerve (transplant). Duel, A. B. Laryngoscope *44:*599-611, Aug '34

Buccal-facial anastomosis in facial nerve injury. Pons Tortella, E. Rev. de cir. de Barcelona *8:*82-89, Sept-Dec '34

Surgical treatment of facial paralysis by autoplastic nerve graft. Sullivan, J. A. Canad. M. A. J. *31:*474-479, Nov '34

Operative treatment of facial palsy (transplant). Duel, A. B. Brit. M. J. *2:*1027-1031, Dec 8, '34

Muscle-nerve graft. Sheehan, J. E., S. Clin. North America *15:*471-482, April '35

Bilateral spinofacial anastomosis and resection of superior cervical ganglion for bilateral facial paralysis; case. Costantini, H. and Curtillet, E. Lyon chir. *32:*291-305, May-June '35

Wounds of median nerve with surgical therapy in 5 cases; interest of external route of access; anatomic possiblility of anastomosis of anterior branch of radial with peripheral end of median in extended loss of nerve substance. Huard, P. and Boutareau. Bull. Soc. med.-chir. de l'Indochine *13:*1856-1873, Dec '35

Muscle-nerve graft in paralysis of facial nerve. Yaritsyn, A. A. Vestnik-khir. *39:*132-134, '35

Nerve grafting. Bentley, F. H. and Hill, M. Brit. J. Surg. *24:*368-387, Oct '36

Surgical treatment of facial paralysis (with nerve grafting). Morris, W. M. Lancet *2:*1172-1174, Nov 14, '36

Nerves, Grafts – Cont.

Recent work in anatomy bearing on surgical practice (transplantation of nerves). Gowland, W. P. Australian and New Zealand J. Surg. *6:*339-349, April '37

Nerve transplantation in facial paralysis. Cawthorne, T. Tr. M. Soc. London *60:*171-177, '37

Treatment of clonic facial spasm by nerve anastomosis. Philips, G., M. J. Australia *1:*624-626, April 2, '38

Cutaneous femoris lateralis nerve, direct implantation of free nerve grafts between facial musculature and facial trunk; first case to be reported. Cardwell, E. P. Arch. Otolaryng. *27:*469-471, April '38

Anesthesia of inferior maxillary nerve by way of zygoma in jaw surgery. Popescu, G. and Pricoriu, S. Rev. san. mil., Bucuresti *37:*873-875, Oct '38

Repair of facial nerve lesion by Ballance-Duel graft. McArthur, G. A. D., M. J. Australia *2:*1123-1124, Dec 31, '38

Transplantation of nerves in facial palsy. Bauer, G. Acta chir. Scandinav. *81:*130-138, '38

Spinofacial anastomosis for bilateral traumatic facial paralysis; late results. Costantini, H. and Curtillet, E. Lyon chir. *36:*50-53, Jan-Feb '39

Nerve (hypoglossal-facial) anastomosis in treatment of facial paralysis. Trumble, H. C., M. J. Australia *1:*300-302, Feb 25, '39

Nerve grafts. Bunnell, S. and Boyes, J. H. Am. J. Surg. *44:*64-75, April '39

Nerve transplant for facial paralysis. Tickle, T. G. Laryngoscope *49:*475-481, June '39

Facial paralysis; recent treatment with case report (nerve graft). Juers, A. L. Kentucky M. J. *37:*368-371, Aug '39

Surgical treatment of facial paralysis; review of 46 cases (nerve transplant). Morris, W. M. Lancet *2:*558-561, Sept 2, '39

Use of grafts of devitalized connective tissue (tendon and nerve) in reparative surgery. Nageotte, J. Presse med. *47:*1365-1366, Sept 27, '39

Wrist-drop; graft of 15 cm of rabbit's spinal cord and infiltration of stellate ganglion followed by rapid recovery; case. Soubiran. J. de med. de Bordeaux *116:*353-354, Nov 4-25, '39

Comparative study of repair of loss of peripheral nerve substance by interposition of fixed spinal cord or nerve. Gianotti, M. and Ferrando, M. Boll. e mem. Soc. piemontese di chir. *9:*100-128, '39

Comparison of spinal cord and nerve grafts in

Nerves, Grafts – Cont.

repair of loss of peripheral nerve substance; preliminary report. MALAN, R. Boll. e mem. Soc. piemontese di chir. *9:*92–99, '39

Results of facio-hypoglossal anastomosis in treatment of facial paralysis. COLEMAN, C. C. Ann. Surg. *111:*958–970, June '40

Nerve regeneration; importance of peripheral stump and value of nerve grafts. YOUNG, J. Z. *et al.* Lancet *2:*128–130, Aug 3, '40

Possibilities of nerve transplantation. BENTLEY, F. H. AND HILL, M. Brit. M. J. *2:*352–353, Sept 14, '40

Duel-Ballance nerve graft for cure of complete traumatic facial paralysis; case. HORGAN, J. B. Irish J. M. Sc., pp. 196–198, May '41

Nerve repair in man; studies on 2 cases, 10 weeks and 6 months after operation; evaluations of grafts and tubular prosthesis. VERNE, J. AND ISELIN, M. Presse med. *49:*789–791, July 22, '41

Late result of hypoglossofacial anastomosis; inadaptation of centers. BOURGUIGNON, G. Rev. neurol. *73:*601–603, Nov–Dec '41

Transplantation of motor nerves and muscle in forelimb of rat. SPERRY, R. W. J. Comp. Neurol. *76:*283–321, April '42

Repair of large gaps in peripheral nerves (including use of grafts). SANDERS, F. K. Brain *65:*281–337, Sept '42

Experiments on cadaver nerve graft and "glue" suture of divided nerves. DE REZENDE, N. New York State J. Med. *42:*2124–2128, Nov 15, '42

Anastomosis between hypoglossal and facial nerves; case. THOMAS, A. AND DE AJURIAGUERRA. Rev. neurol. *74:*308–310, Nov–Dec '42

Technic for transplanting ulnar nerve. LEARMONTH, J. R. Surg., Gynec. and Obst. *75:*792–793, Dec '42

Degeneration and re-innervation of grafted nerves. SANDERS, F. K. AND YOUNG, J. Z. J. Anat. *76:*143–166, Jan '42

Histologic condition of autograft of nerve in man. SEDDON, H. J. *et al.* Brit. J. Surg. *29:*378–384, April '42

Combined plastic surgery on facial and facial-hypoglossal nerves for facial paralysis. BERGGREN, S., AND FROSTE, N. Acta otolaryng. *30:*325–327, '42

Peripheral nerve injuries in war; transplantation of nerves. GRASHCHENKOV, N. I. P. Sovet. med. (no. 9) *6:*8–10, '42

Instructions for transplantation of formalized

Nerves, Grafts – Cont.

nerve to replace defect of injured nerve. GRASHCHENKOV, N. I. P. AND ANOKHIN, P. K. Nevropat. i psikhiat. (nos. 1–2) *11:*44–45, '42

New aspect of muscle reinnervation; preliminary report. BILLIG, H. E. JR. AND VAN HARREVELD, A. U. S. Nav. M. Bull. *41:*410–414, March '43

Peripheral nerve repair by grafts of frozen-dried nerve. WEISS, P. AND TAYLOR, A. C. Proc. Soc. Exper. Biol. and Med. *52:*326–328, April '43

Nerve transplantation in mastoid surgery. SULLIVAN, J. A. Arch. Otolaryng. *37:*845–851, June '43

Degeneration and reinnervation of nerve transplants. SANDERS, F. K. AND YOUNG, J. Z. Rev. oto-neuro-oftal. *18:*117–119, July–Aug '43

Nerve graft from cadaver to repair sectioned nerve; case. JARA ROBLES, R. Arch. Soc. cirujanos hosp. *13:*214–215, Sept '43

Autopsy nerve grafts in peripheral nerve surgery; clinical application; "glue" suture technic. KLEMME, R. M. *et al.* J.A.M.A. *123:*393–396, Oct 16, '43

Nerve transplantation. GRASHCHENKOV, N. I. P. Am. Rev. Soviet Med. *1:*28–31, Oct '43 also: Sovet. med (no. 9) *6:*8–10, '42

Amputated limbs as source for nerve graft. LAM, C. R., J.A.M.A. *123:*1067, Dec 18, '43

Preserved transplants in repair of defects of peripheral nerves; disadvantages of this method. ORLOV, G. A. Sovet. med. (nos. 11–12) *7:*7–9, '43

Principles of and method for compensating for nerve deficiency by grafting prepared nervous tissue. SCHABADASCH, A. Compt. rend. Acad. d. sc. URSS *43:*40–42, April 10, '44

Transplantation of nerves from cadavers in human surgery. DE REZENDE, N. Rev. brasil. de cir. *13:*245–258, May '44

Late condition of nerve homografts in man. SEDDON, H. J. AND HOLMES, W. Surg., Gynec. and Obst. *79:*342–351, Oct '44

Preparation and storage of autopsy nerve grafts. SACCOMANNO, G. *et al.* Science *100:*436, Nov 10, '44

Nerve regeneration in end to end sutures, grafts and gunshot nerve injuries. DAVIS, L. AND HILLER, F. Tr. Am. Neurol. A. *70:*178–179, '44

Transplantation of nerves treated with formalin (solution of formaldehyde). FIRER, S. L. Sovet. med. (nos. 4–5) *8:*19, '44

Peripheral nerve injuries; experimental

Nerves, Grafts – Cont.
study of recovery of function following repair by end to end sutures and nerve grafts. DAVIS, L. *et al.* Surg., Gynec. and Obst. *80:*35–59, Jan '45
Importance of adequate blood supply in nerve transplantation. TARLOV, I. M. AND EPSTEIN, J., J. Neurosurg. *2:*49–71, Jan '45
Failure of whole fresh homogenous nerve grafts in man. SPURLING, R. G. *et al.* J. Neurosurg. *2:*79–101, March '45
Peripheral nerve injuries; surgical principles underlying use of grafts in repair. DAVIS, L. *et al.* Ann. Surg. *121:*686–699, May '45
Histologic study of predegenerated autograft (ulnar). BARNES, R. *et al.* Brit. J. Surg. *33:*130–135, Oct '45
Peripheral nerve injuries; surgical principles underlying use of grafts in repair. DAVIS, L. *et al.* Tr. South S. A. (1944) *56:*302–315, '45
Surgical principles underlying use of peripheral nerve grafts in repair of injuries. DAVIS, L. *et al.* Tr. West. S. A. (1944) *52:*526–537, '45
Restoration of sectioned or destroyed nerves, with special reference to grafting. ROUHIER, G. Mem. Acad. de chir *72:*170–174, Mar 20–Apr 3, '46
Fate of peripheral nerve homografts in man. BARNES, R. *et al.* Brit. J. Surg. *34:*34–41, July '46
Cross nerve anastomosis in man. SADR, A. R. Ann. Surg. *124:*599–603, Sept '46
Source of autografts in clinical surgery; technic for their suture. TARLOV, I. M. *et al.* Am. J. Surg. *72:*700–710, Nov '46

Nerves, Injuries (See also Nerves, Grafts; Nerves, Injuries, Hand; War Injuries, Nerve)
Methods to secure end-to-end suture of peripheral nerves. NAFFZIGER, H. C. Surg., Gynec. and Obst. *32:*193, March '21
Results of 98 cases of nerve suture. DANE, P. G. Brit. M. J. *1:*885, June 18, '21
Possibilities of suture after extensive nerve injury. FORRESTER-BROWN, M. F., J. Orthop. Surg. *3:*277, June '21
Treatment of nerve injuries. NEY, K. W. Mil Surgeon *49:*277, Sept '21
Technic for suturing nerves. LANGEMAK, O. Zentralbl. f. Chir. *49:*1253–1255, Aug 26, '22 (illus.)
Ultimate outcome of suture of nerves. DIETERICH. Med. Klinik *19:*237–238, Feb 25, '23 abstr: J.A.M.A. *80:*1742, June 9, '23
Essential in technic of nerve suture; with

Nerves, Injuries – Cont.
report of 2 cases. LACROIX, P. G. Am. J. Surg. *37:*282–283, Nov '23
Remote results of operations for injuries of peripheral nerves. PLATT, H. AND BRISTOW, W. R. Brit. J. Surg. *11:*535–567, Jan '24
Further results of nerve anastomosis. BALLANCE, C. *et al.* Brit. J. Surg. *13:*535–558, Jan '26
Primary repair of lacerated tendons and nerves. EISBERG, H. B. AND SONNENSCHEIN, H. D. Am. J. Surg. *3:*582–587, Dec '27
Use of rubber in plastic operations on tendons and nerves, in repairing defects in abdominal wall, in hernia and in fractures with loss of substance. DELBET, P. Rev. de chir. *66:*181–213, '28
Neurotization of nerve transplants. FINKEL, Z. I., J. nevropat. i psikhiat. (no. 8) *24:*24–31, '31
Finger injuries with injury of peripheral nerves. TURNER, G. I. Vestnik khir. (nos. 65–66) *22:*49–55, '31
Results of suturing divided nerves (particularly in horses). BALLANCE, C. *et al.* Proc. Roy. Soc. Med. *27:*1207–1210, July '34
Nerve and tendon suture: illustrative case. WHELAN, H. M. J. Roy. Nav. M. Serv. *22:*234–237, July '36
Successful primary suture of nerves in seriously infected wounds. SEIFFERT, L. Zentralbl. f. Chir. *63:*1890–1892, Aug 8, '36
Late results of surgical therapy of traumatic lesions of peripheral nerves. THÉVENARD. Bull. et mem. Soc. de chirurgiens de Paris *28:*479–485, Nov 6, '36
Surgical treatment of peripheral nerve injuries. ADSON, A. W., J. Kansas M. Soc. *37:*497, Dec '36
Repair of peripheral nerve injuries. TINKER, M. B. AND TINKER, M. B. JR. Ann. Surg. *106:*943–951, Nov '37
Experimental study upon prevention of adhesions about repaired nerves and tendons (especially by use of allantoic and amniotic membranes). DAVIS, L. AND ARIES, L. J. Surgery 2:877–888, Dec '37
Late results of surgical therapy of nerves. HERBIG, B. Beitr. z. klin. Chir. *166:*414–436, '37
Restorative surgery of peripheral nerves. CHRISTOPHE, L., J. de chir. et ann. Soc. belge de chir., Seances extraord., pp. 122–154, June 25–26, '38
Surgery of peripheral nerves, including therapy of neurinoma. JENTZER, A. Schweiz.

Nerves, Injuries – Cont.
med. Wchnschr. *68:*1162–1164, Oct 15, '38
Injuries of nerves of upper extremities. GINZBURG, R. L. Ortop. i travmatol. (no. 3) *12:*105–119, '38
Comparative study of repair of loss of peripheral nerve substance by interposition of fixed spinal cord or nerve. GIANOTTI, M. AND FERRANDO, M. Boll. e mem. Soc. piemontese di chir. *9:*100–128, '39
Comparison of spinal cord and nerve grafts in repair of loss of peripheral nerve substance; preliminary report. MALAN, R. Boll. e mem. Soc. piemontese di chir. *9:*92–99, '39
New modification of technic of laterolateral anastomosis. (nerves) POZZAN, A. Arch. ital. di chir. *57:*363–376, '39
Technic of laterolateral anastomosis (nerve). POZZAN, A. Arch. ital. di chir. *57:*458–482, '39
Peripheral nerve injuries, with results of early and delayed suture. FORRESTER, C. R. G. Am. J. Surg. *47:*555–572, March '40
Results of repair of loss of peripheral nerve substance; experimental study. MALAN, R. Arch. per le sc. med. *70:*587–605, Dec '40
Surgical principles in repair of divided nerves and tendons. KOCH, S. L. Quart. Bull., Northwestern Univ. M. School *14:*1–8, '40
Surgery of peripheral nerves; basis and technic. MORAES BARROS FILHO, N. Rev. de cir. de Sao Paulo *7:*93–135, Sept–Oct '41
Uses and abuses of splints and other instruments in treatment of nerve injuries. MCMURRAY, T. P. Brit. J. Phys. Med. *5:*20–25, Feb '42
Autologous plasma clot suture of nerves. TARLOV, I. M. AND BENJAMIN, B. Science *95:*258, March 6, '42
Massage, movements and exercises in treatment of suture and repair of nerves. MENNELL, J. Brit. J. Phys. Med. *5:*40–47, March '42
Splintage of peripheral nerve injuries. HIGHET, W. B. Lancet *1:*555–558, May 9, '42
Fibrin suture of human nerves. SEDDON, H. J. AND MEDAWAR, P. B. Lancet *2:*87–88, July 25, '42
Tendon and nerve injuries. KOCH, S. L. New York State J. Med. *42:*1819–1823, Oct 1, '42
Effects of immobilization and activity on neuromuscular regeneration (after injury). HINES, H. M., J.A.M.A. *120:*515–517, Oct 17, '42
Nerve regeneration after immediate and delayed suture. HOLMES, W. AND YOUNG, J. Z., J. Anat. *77:*63–96, Oct '42

Nerves, Injuries – Cont.
Peripheral nerve suture; 13 cases. SORREL, E. AND MME SORREL-DEJERINE. Mem. Acad. de chir. *68:*448–452, Dec 9–16, '42
Peripheral nerve injuries; basic methods of surgical therapy. IGNATOV, M. G. Nevropat. i psikhiat. (no. 4) *11:*73, '42
Peripheral nerve injuries; early therapy. SEPP, E. K. Klin. med. (no. 8–9) *20:*7–11, '42
Peripheral nerve traction injuries after suture. HIGHET, W. B. AND HOLMES, W. Brit. J. Surg. *30:*212–233, Jan '43
Plastic problems in surgery of peripheral nerves. LEARMONTH, J. R. AND WALLACE, A. B. Surg., Gynec. and Obst. *76:*106–109, Jan '43
Repair of traumatic gaps in peripheral nerves. BODIAN, D., J.A.M.A. *121:*662–664, Feb 27, '43
Peripheral nerve injuries (John Burns Trust lecture). SEDDON, H. J. Glasgow M. J. *139:*61–75, March '43
Plasma clot and silk suture of nerves; experimental study of comparative tissue reaction. TARLOV, I. M. AND BENJAMIN, B. Surg., Gynec. and Obst. *76:*366–374, March '43
Experimental study on nerve suture with various suture materials. CUTTMANN, L. Brit. J. Surg. *30:*370–375, April '43
Effects of stretching nerves after suture. HIGHET, W. B. AND SANDERS, F. K. Brit. J. Surg. *30:*355–369, April '43
Nerve and tendon injuries. KOCH, S. L. Bull. Am. Coll. Surgeons *28:*125–126, June '43
Physical therapy following suture of nerves. DUBE, P., M. Clin. North America *27:*1091–1096, July '43
Peripheral nerve injuries; physical medicine in treatment. KINNEMAN, R. E., M. Clin. North America *27:*1097–1108, July '43
Peripheral nerve lesions; diagnosis and treatment. PORTUGAL, J. R. Imprensa med., Rio de Janeiro *19:*71–82, July '43
Plasma clot suture of peripheral nerves; experimental technic. TARLOV, I. M. *et al.* Arch. Surg. *47:*44–58, July '43
Peripheral nerve injuries; physical therapy. KOVACS, R. New York State J. Med. *43:*1403–1408, Aug 1, '43
Injury and repair of peripheral nerves (importance of blood supply as shown by transparent chamber technic). ESSEX, H. E. AND DE REZENDE, N. T. Am. J. Physiol. *140:*107–114, Oct '43
Peripheral nerve lesions; time element in restorative surgery. LEBEDENKO, V. V. Am. Rev. Soviet Med. *1:*23–27, Oct '43 also:

Nerves, Injuries – Cont.
Khirurgiya, no. 10, pp. 48–52, '42
Nerve reunion with sleeves of frozen-dried artery in rabbits, cats and monkeys. WEISS, P. Proc. Soc. Exper. Biol. & Med. *54:*274–277, Dec '43
Experiments on repair of peripheral nerves. WEISS, P. Tr. Am. Neurol. A. *69:*42–45, '43
Peripheral nerve injuries; review of recent literature. BRENNER, C. War Med. *5:*21–35, Jan '44
Peripheral nerve injuries; principles of treatment. SCHNITKER, M. T. Northwest Med. *43:*5–9, Jan '44 also: Bull. U. S. Army M. Dept. (no. 73) pp. 53–61, Feb '44
Peripheral nerve injuries; surgical treatment. COLEMAN, C. C. Surg., Gynec. and Obst. *78:*113–124, Feb '44 abstr: Tr. Am. Neurol. A. *69:*51–55, '43
Peripheral nerve injuries; early management. SEDDON, H. J. Practitioner *152:*101–107, Feb '44
Plasma clot suture of peripheral nerves; illustrated technic. TARLOV, I. M. Surgery *15:*257–269, Feb '44
Peripheral nerve suture; forty years' experience. STONEY, R. A. Irish J. M. Sc. pp. 85–92, March '44
Peripheral nerve injuries; treatment. WRIGHT, H. W. S., M. Press *211:*228–230, April 12, '44
Sutureless reunion of severed nerves with elastic cuffs of tantalum. WEISS, P., J. Neurosurg. *1:*219–225, May '44
Personal experience of exploration and reexploration of injured nerves. LEARMONTH, J. R. Proc. Roy. Soc. Med. *37:*553–556, Aug '44
Effect of delay on success of suture of peripheral nerves. YOUNG, J. Z. Proc. Roy. Soc. Med. *37:*551–552, Aug '44
Autologous plasma clot suture of nerves; use in clinical surgery. TARLOV, I. M. J.A.M.A. *126:*741–748, Nov 18, '44
Technology of regeneration; review; sutureless tubulation and related methods of nerve repair. WEISS, P., J. Neurosurg. *1:*400–450, Nov '44
Preliminary and substitution operations in treatment of lesions; peripheral nerves. KÖSTLER, J. Deutsche Ztschr. f. Chir. *259:*1, '44
Plastic reconstruction of peripheral nerves. OVNATANYAN, K. T. Sovet. med. (no. 9) *8:*27–29, '44
Peripheral nerve surgery; technical considerations. SPURLING, R. G. Am. Acad. Orthop. Surgeons, Lect. pp. 259–269, '44
Manual of Diagnosis and Management of Peripheral Nerve Injuries, by ROBERT A. GROFF AND SARA J. HOUTZ. J. B. Lippincott Co., Phila., 1945
Peripheral nerve injuries; therapy. JULLIARD, C. Praxis *34:*147–148, March 1, '45
Peripheral nerve injuries. MAYFIELD, F. H., J. Michigan M. Soc. *44:*269–275, March '45
New uses of tantalum in suture and control of neuroma formation; illustration of technical procedures. WHITE, J. C. AND HAMLIN, H., J. Neurosurg. *2:*402–413, Sept '45
Surgical treatment of injuries of brain, spinal cord and peripheral nerves. SCARFF, J. E. Surg., Gynec. and Obst. *81:*405–424, Oct '45
Prevention of formation of end-bulb neuromata. POTH, E. J. *et al.* Proc. Soc. Exper. Biol. and Med *60:*200–207, Nov '45
Early nerve and bone repair in war wounds. SCHWARTZ, H. G. AND PARKER, J. M., J. Neurosurg. *2:*510–515, Nov '45
Nerve injuries; management in late stages. TURNBULL, F. Canad. M. A. J. *53:*438–443, Nov '45
Peripheral nerve injuries; therapy. BOROVSKIY, M. L. Khirurgiya, no. 5, pp. 50–52, '45
Peripheral nerve injuries; surgical principles underlying use of grafts in repair. DAVIS, L. *et al.* Tr. South. S. A. (1944) *56:*302–315, '45
Surgical therapy of combined injuries of peripheral nerves and bones. FETISOVA, E. V. Khirurgiya, No. 2, pp. 55–58, '45
Suture of peripheral nerves. JENTZER, A. Confinia neurol. *6:*257–269, '45
Peripheral nerve surgery; review of incisions for operative exposure; preliminary report. SELETZ, E., J. Neurosurg. *3:*135–147, March '46
Regeneration and reconstitution of severed nerves. WEBER, A. Lyon chir. *41:*129–137, Mar–Apr '46
Peripheral nerve injuries; treatment. PRUCE, A. M. South. M. J. *39:*289–291, April '46
Suture of posterior tibial nerve below knee, with follow-up study of clinical results. FAHLUND, G. T. R., J. Neurosurg. *3:*223–233, May '46
Technic of suture of peripheral nerves. LIVINGSTON, K. E. *et al.* J. Neurosurg. *3:*270–271, May '46
Peripheral nerve injuries; experience with early nerve surgery. SPURLING, R. G. AND WOODHALL, B. Ann. Surg. *123:*731–748, May '46
Peripheral nerve injuries; results of "early" nerve suture; preliminary report. WOODHALL, B. AND LYONS, W. R. Surgery *19:*757–789, June '46

Nerves, Injuries – Cont.

Metallic tube for nerve suture. SICARD, A. AND FAUREL. Mem. Acad. de chir. *72:*393, July 3-10, '46

Removal suture method of repair peripheral nerves. POTTER, S. E., J. Neurosurg. *3:*354-357, July '46

Surgery of peripheral nerve injury. AIRD, I. Post-Grad. M. J. *22:*225-254, Sept '46

Peripheral nerve lesions; repair. HOEN, T. I. Am. J. Surg. *72:*489-495, Sept '46

Cross-nerve anastomosis in man. SADR, A. R. Ann. Surg. *124:*599-603, Sept '46

Guides for regeneration of peripheral nerves across gaps. WEISS, P. AND TAYLOR, A. C. J. Neurosurg. *3:*375-389, Sept '46

Separation at suture site as cause of failure in regeneration of peripheral nerves. WHITCOMB, B. B., J. Neurosurg. *3:*399-406, Sept '46

Painful injuries of nerves and their surgical treatment. WHITE, J. C. Am. J. Surg. *72:*468-488 Sept '46

Peripheral nerve surgery. SILBER, W. South African M. J. *20:*601, Oct 12, '46; 634, Oct 26, '46

Peripheral nerve injuries; early surgery. SPURLING, R. G. AND WOODHALL, B. Tr. South S. A. (1945) *57:*269-286, '46

Nerves, Injuries, Hand (See also Nerves, Median; Nerves, Radial; Nerves, Ulnar)

Peripheral nerve lesions of the hand. ALLISON, W. L. Texas State J. Med. *20:*46-51, May '24

Surgery of nerves of hand. BUNNELL, S. Surg., Gynec. and Obst. *44:*145-152, Feb '27

Repair of nerves and tendons of hand and grafting. BUNNELL, S., J. Bone & Joint Surg. *10:*1-26, Jan '28 abstr: Arch. franco-belges de chir. *30:*93-97, Feb '27

Abnormalities of nerves in palmar region of man. CAPONNETTO, A. Monitore zool. ital. *41:*180-183, '30

Plastic surgery of tendons and nerves of hand. CHIARIELLO, A. G. Policlinico (sez. prat.) *39:*520-525, April 4, '32

Division of nerves and tendons of hand, with discussion of surgical treatment and its results. KOCH, S. L. AND MASON, M. L. Surg., Gynec. and Obst. *56:*1-39, Jan '33

Injuries of nerves and tendons of hand (surgical therapy). KOCH, S. L., J. Oklahoma M. A. *26:*323-327, Sept '33

Injuries to nerves and tendons of hand.

Nerves, Injuries, Hand – Cont.

KOCH, S. L. Pennsylvania M. J. *37:*555-557, April '34; Wisconsin M. J., *33:*655-661, Sept '34

Late results of secondary plastic operations on tendons and nerves of hand. KALALOVA-DI LOTTIOVA, V. Bratisl. lekar. listy *16:*162-174, April '36

Industrial accidents; management of injuries of tendons and nerve of hand. GARLOCK, J. H. New York State J. Med. *36:*1740-1748, Nov 15, '36

Severed tendons and nerves of hand and forearm. O'SHEA, M. C. Ann. Surg. *105:*228-242, Feb '37

Treatment and results of 870 severed tendons and 57 severed nerves of hand and forearm (in 362 patients). O'SHEA, M. C. Am. J. Surg. *43:*346-366, Feb '39

Extensive primary nerve and tendon suture at wrist; 2 cases. HOWARD, R. N., M. J. Australia *2:*322-323, Aug 26, '39

Traumatic lesions of nerves of wrist and hand. HARMER, T. W. Am. J. Surg. *47:*517-541, Feb '40

"Dead hand"; lesion produced by rapid vibration. CUMMINS, R. C., Irish J. M. Sc., pp. 171-175, April '40

Injuries to nerves and tendons of hand. MASON, M. L., J.A.M.A. *116:*1375-1379, March 29, '41

Ascending neuropathy due to injury of hand; predominance and unusual nature of trophic phenomena. COUTO, DEOLINDO. Cultura med. *3:*355-370, Feb '42

Nerve and tendon injuries of hand. MASON, M. L. Indust. Med. *11:*61-66, Feb '42

Post-traumatic neuralgia as serious complication of section of tendons of hand in cultivators of sugar cane. OLIVERAS GUERRA, A. Bol. Asoc. med. de Puerto Rico *35:*47-51, Feb '43

Repair of lacerated nerves at wrist. SONNENSCHEIN, H. D., S. Clin. North America *23:*487-496, April '43

Trauma to hand; with particular reference to indications for primary and secondary nerve and tendon repair. MASON, M. L., J. Oklahoma M. A. *39:*246-251, June '46

Treatment of injuries, with particular reference to nerve and tendon repair in hand. MASON, M. L. Indust. Med. *15:*323-325, May '46

Injuries of nerves and tendons of hand. KOCH, S. L. Cincinnati J. Med. *27:*515-521, Aug '46

Nerves, Median

Remote results of suture of ulnar and median nerves. CAEIRO, J. A. Semana med. *2:*495-497, Aug 27, '25

Sensory-motor restoration after section of nerves of arm; suture of radial nerve with subsequent graft of median and ulnar nerves. THOMAS, A. AND PETIT-DUTAILLIS. Rev. neurol. *1:*56-60, Jan '30

Incised wound of palm; severance of median nerve; immediate nerve suture. COHN, I. Internat. Clin. *2:*104-106, June '31

Results of suture of median and radial nerves in therapy of fracture of left radius. CHENUT, A. Bordeaux chir. *3:*136-138, April '32

Surgical therapy of paralysis of median nerve caused by section following wound with resultant neuroma formation. GODOY MOREIRA, F. E. Sao Paulo med. *1:*211-215, Jan '33

Wounds of median nerve with surgical therapy in 5 cases; interest of external route of access; anatomic possibility of anastomosis of anterior branch of radial with peripheral end of median in extended loss of nerve substance. HUARD, P. AND BOUTAREAU. Bull. Soc. med.-chir. de l'Indochine *13:*1856-1873, Dec '35

Neuritis of median nerve due to compression by luxated semilunar bone; case in workman. BRUNI, A. Rassegna d. previd. sociale *24:*42-43, Nov-Dec '37

Flexion of distal phalanx of thumb in lesions of median nerve. SUNDERLAND, S. Australian and New Zealand J. Surg. *13:*157-159, Jan '44

Plastic repair of section of flexor tendons of hand and of median nerve; case. MARINO, H. Prensa med. argent. *31:*1305-1308, July 12, '44

Nerves, Miscellaneous Items

Injuries to nerves from surgical treatment of diseases of face and neck. BABCOCK, W. W. J.A.M.A. *84:*187-192, Jan. 17, '25

Accidents in conduction anesthesia of sphenopalatine ganglion; 4 cases. ULLMANN, S. Ztschr. f. Hals-, Nasen-u. Ohrenh. *21:*587-595, May 10, '28

Neurogenic tumors of nose. TOBECK, A. Ztschr. f. Hals-, Nasen-u. Ohrenh. *23:*329-339, Sept 10, '29

Peripheral neurectomy in blepharospasm. FRIEDE, R. Ztschr. f. Augenh. *72:*299-303, Oct '30

Neurotization of muscular tissue transplanted into striated muscles. COMOLLI, A. Arch. ed atti d. Soc. ital. di chir. *36:*967, '30

Deep block anesthesia of second and third divisions of fifth nerve. BROWN, J. B. Surg., Gynec. and Obst. *53:*832-835, Dec '31

Clinical sequelae of injury to inferior alveolar nerve following fractures of mandible. STEIDL, H. Deutsche Ztschr. f. Chir. *230:*129-146, '31

Dystrophic disorders due to lesions of nerves in spinomedullary trauma; clinical and therapeutic study. DRAGONETTI, M. Gazz. internaz. med.-chir. *47:*416-421, July 15, '37

Role of sympathetic in maxillary fractures. DECHAUME, M. Presse med. *46:*714-715, May 4, '38

Elective traumatism of extensor digitorum and flexor digitorum profundus in injury to forearm; reflex inhibition of extension; infiltration of stellate ganglion; Volkmann contracture; tendinous transmutation. FROMENT, J. AND MALLET-GUY, P. Lyon chir. *35:*623-629, Sept-Oct '38

Nervous factor in traumatic shock. LORBER, V. *et al.* Surg., Gynec. and Obst. *71:*469-477, Oct '40

Procaine hydrochloride blocking of stellate ganglion in therapy of traumatic hard edema of hand. LÄWEN, A. Arch. f. klin. Chir. *201:*687-691, '41

Transplantation of motor nerves and muscles in forelimb of rat. SPERRY, R. W., J. Comp. Neurol. *76:*283-321, April '42

Problems involving mandibular nerve (paresthesia of lip). COGSWELL, W. W., J. Am. Dent. A. *29:*964-969, June 1, '42

Macrodactyly and associated peripheral nerve changes. MOORE, B. H., J. Bone and Joint Surg. *24:*617-631, July '42

Synkinesis between third and seventh pairs of cranial nerves (of musculus levator palpebrae superioris and of musculus zygomaticus respectively); similarity to Marcus Gunn phenomenon; case. AZZOLINI, U. Riv. oto-neuro-oftal. *19:*398-412, Nov-Dec '42

Inferior alveolar nerve and fractured mandible. HALLAM, J. W. Guy's Hosp. Gaz. *57:*22, Jan 23, '43

Innervation and function of thenar muscles. HIGHET, W. B. Lancet *1:*227-230, Feb 20, '43

New aspect of muscle reinnervation; preliminary report. BILLIG, H. E. JR. AND VAN HARREVELD, A., U.S. Nav. M. Bull. *41:*

Nerves, Miscellaneous Items–Cont.

410–414, March '43

Rate of peripheral nerve regeneration in man. SEDDON, H. J. *et al.* J. Physiol. *102:*191–215, Sept 30, '43

Partial gigantism of face with neurologic complications. KARNOSH, L. J. AND GARDNER, W. J. Cleveland Clin. Quart. *12:*43–47, April '45

Problem of central nervous reorganization after nerve regeneration and muscle transposition. SPERRY, R. W. Quart. Rev. Biol. *20:*311–369, Dec '45

Value of Tinel sign (in relation to regeneration of peripheral nerve lesions). NATHAN, P. W. AND RENNIE, A. M. Lancet *1:*610–611, April 27, '46

Restorative operations in reflex disorders caused by nerve trauma. CHIBUKMAKHER, N. B. Vrach. delo (nos. 7-8) *26:*435–440, '46

Nerves, Neuromas

Preventing formation of painful neuromas after amputations by direct implantation of nerves into muscle (neurotization). TOMOFF, W. Ztschr. f. d. ges. exper. Med. *84:*287–300, '32

Method of restoring nerves requiring resection (by removing neuroma, shortening bone and suturing nerve). DANDY, W. E. J.A.M.A. *122:*35–36, May 1, '43

Role of neuroma in evolution of wounds. WEISS, A. C. AND WARTER, J. Bull. War Med. *3:*607, July '43 (abstract)

Surgical treatment of pain in peripheral nervous system (following amputations of fingers). PARKES, A. R. Tr. Roy. Med.-Chir. Soc. Glasgow, pp. 23–25, '43–'44; in Glasgow M. J. May '44

Prevention of neuroma formation by encasement of severed nerve end in rigid tubes. POTH, E. J. AND BRAVO-FERNANDEZ, E. Proc. Soc. Exper. Biol. and Med. *56:*7–8, May '44

Method of treating nerve ends in amputations. BATE, J. T. Am. J. Surg. *64:*373–374, June '44

Ligature of nerve in prevention of neuroma of amputation-stump. EGOROV, M. A. Khirurgiya, no. 4, pp. 38–42, '44

Ligature for prevention of terminal neuromas. TROITSKIY, V. V. Khirurgiya, no. 2, pp. 61–65, '45

Traumatic and amputation neuromas. CIESLAK, A. K. AND STOUT, A. P. Arch Surg. *53:*646–651, Dec '46

Nerves, Radial

Tendon transplantation for radial paralysis. RIOSALIDO. Arch. espan. de pediat. *5:*210, April '21 abstr: J.A.M.A. *77:*497, Aug 6, '21

Tendon transplantation for musculospiral (radial) nerve injury. BILLINGTON, R. W. J. Bone and Joint Surg. *4:*538–547, July '22 (illus.)

Tendon transplantations for musculo-spiral paralysis. STEVENSON, G. H. Glasgow M. J. *99:*225–230, April '23

Repair of radialis through grafting of dead calf nerve according to Nageotte's method. SOLE, R. Semana med. *2:*452–454, Aug 19, '26

Tendon transplantation for radial paralysis. COMBAULT, A. Clinique, Paris *21:*315–320, Nov '26

Treatment of radial paralysis by tendon anastomosis. DUPUY DE FRENELLE. Paris chir. *19:*20–27, Jan '27

Suture of radial nerve; case with 3 operations; recovery. MARTIN, P., J. de chir. et ann. Soc. belge de chir. *26:*224–229, Dec '27

Transplantation of tendons in paralysis of radial nerve. HASS, J. Wien. klin. Wchnschr. *42:*642–644, May 9, '29

Tendon transplantation for irreparable musculo-spiral injury (radial nerve). KRIDA, A. Am. J. Surg. *9:*331–332, Aug '30

Section of radial nerve and heterograft of dog's fresh nerve into man; case. THALHEIMER, M. AND BLONDIN-WALTHER, M. Bull. et mem. Soc. nat. de chir. *57:*535–543, April 25, '31

Suture of radial nerve, with case report. MCMAHON, C. G. Nebraska M. J. *17:*28–30, Jan '32

Results of suture of median and radial nerves in therapy of fracture of left radius. CHENUT, A. Bordeaux chir. *3:*136–138, April '32

Remote results in radial paralysis after tendon transplantation; 4 cases. SOLCARD. Bull. et mem. Soc. nat. de chir. *58:*677–682, May 7, '32

Subcutaneous rupture of extensor pollicis longus simulating partial radial paralysis; case. CROUZON, O. *et al.* Bull. et mem. Soc. med. d. hop. de Paris *48:*1043–1046, June 27, '32

Radial nerve injuries. POLLOCK, L. J. AND DAVIS, L. Am. J. Surg. *16:*549–600, June '32

Results of suture of radial nerve in therapy of fracture of radius. CHENUT, A. Bull. et mem. Soc. de chir. de Bordeaux et du Sud-Ouest, pp. 254–257, '32

Nerves, Radial – Cont.
Wounds of median nerve with surgical therapy in 5 cases; interest of external route of access; anatomic possibility of anastomosis of anterior branch of radial with peripheral end of median in extended loss of nerve substance. HUARD, P. AND BOUTAREAU. Bull. Soc. med.-chir. de l'Indochine *13:*1856–1873, Dec '35
Tendon transplantation in therapy of inveterate radial paralysis; physiologic aims, technic and results. BONOLA, A. Chir. d. org. di movimento *22:*239–254, Aug '36
Tendon transplantation in therapy of complete paralysis of radial nerve; case. GIULIANI, G. M. Arch. ital. di chir. *42:*613–626, '36
Peripheral radial paralysis following burns. BAHLS, G. Med. Welt *11:*857–858, June 19, '37
Tendon transplantation in therapy of inveterate radial paralysis. (Comment on Bonola's article). GIULIANI, G. M. Chir. d. org. di movimento *23:*102, Oct '37
Tendon transplants in surgical therapy of radial paralysis; case. VEZINA, C. *et al.* Laval med. *3:*181–186, June '38
Tendon transplantation in therapy of permanent radial paralysis; case. MAROTTOLI, O. R. Bol. Soc. de cir. de Rosario *5:*434–435, Oct '38
Complete traumatic section of radial nerve in young girl; rapid regeneration following immediate suture; case. DE GIRARDIER, J. Lyon med. *163:*13–15, Jan 1, '39
Recurrent pseudoarthrosis of humerus complicated by irreparable paralysis of radial nerve; curative osteoplasty and functional reconstruction of hand by means of tendon transplants. INCLAN, A. Cir. ortop. y traumatol., Habana *7:*43–53, April–June '39
Tendon transplantation for radial nerve paralysis. YOUNG, H. H. Proc. Staff Meet., Mayo Clin. *15:*26–28, Jan 10, '40
Tendon transplantation for paralysis of radial nerve. GHORMLEY, R. K. AND CAMERON, D. M. Proc. Staff Meet., Mayo Clin. *15:*537–539, Aug 21, '40
Tendon transplantation in radial paralysis. SPISIC, B. Lijecn. vjes. *63:*12–13, Jan '41
Tendon transplantation, in therapy of inveterate radial paralysis. ARGUELLES LOPEZ, R. Rev. clin. espan. *2:*319–323, April 1, '41
Block of branches of trigeminal nerve for surgery. PLAZA, F. L. Jorn. neuro-psiquiat. panam., actas (1939) *2:*104–112, '41
Regeneration of radial nerve; and ulnar nerve. MARBLE, H. C. *et al.* Am. J. Surg.

Nerves, Radial – Cont.
*55:*274–294, Feb '42
Erosion of ala nasi following trigeminal denervation. SCHORSTEIN, J., J. Neurol. and Psychiat. *6:*46–51, Jan-April '43
Subtitute tenoplasties in therapy of radial paralysis. D'HARCOURT, J. Pasteur *1:*121–127, June 15, '43
Substitute tenoplasties according to Perthes in therapy of radial paralysis. STUMPFEGGER, L. Chirurg *15:*430, July 15, '43
Plastic surgery in radial paralysis. SUDECK, P. Chirurg *15:*665, Nov 15, '43
War injuries to radial nerve; treatment. SOUTTAR, H. S., M. Press *210:*345–347, Dec 1, '43
Radial nerve injuries. KOCH, S. L. Quart. Bull., Northwestern Univ. M. School *17:* 1–6, '43
Tendon transplant for complete radial paralysis; case. CHARBONNEL AND BARROUX, R. Bordeaux chir. *1-2:*55, Jan–Apr '44
Reconstructive orthopedic surgery (tendon transplantation and arthrodesis of wrist) for disabilities resulting from irreparable injuries to radial nerve. ABBOTT, L. C., J. Nerv. and Ment. Dis. *99:*466–474, May '44
Plastic operations in radial nerve paralysis. SUDECK, P. Bull. War Med. *4:*627–628, July '44 (abstract)
Splint for radial (musculospiral) nerve palsy. THOMAS, F. B., J. Bone and Joint Surg. *26:*602–605, July '44
Splint for radial nerve palsies. HERZOG, E. G. Lancet *2:*754, Dec 9, '44
Transplantation of muscles in paralysis of radial nerve following gunshot wounds. TIKHONOVICH, A. V. Khirurgiya, no. 3, pp. 72–73, '44
Peripheral nerve injuries; simple compression injuries of radial nerve. SUNDERLAND, S. Brain *68:*56–72, March '45
Radial paralysis; tenoplasty of extensors. POINOT, J. Bordeaux chir. *3-4:*148–149, July-Oct, '45
Surgical repair of deep branch of radial nerve. ALLBRITTEN, F. F. JR. Surg., Gynec. and Obst. *82:*305–310, March '46
Tendon transplant for radial paralysis. ZACHARY, R. B. Brit. J. Surg. *33:*358–364, April '46
Muscle transplant for paralysis of radial nerve. ALTMAN, H. AND TROTT, R. H. J. Bone and Joint Surg *28:*440–446, July '46
Nerve regeneration; motor and sensory recovery in case of injury to radial nerve. DE LA T. MALLETT, A. E., J. Roy. Nav. M. Serv. *32:*61, April; 147, July '46

Nerves, Radial – Cont.

Radial nerve lesions; course and rate of regeneration of motor fibers. SUNDERLAND, S. Arch. Neurol. and Psychiat. *56:*133–157, Aug '46

Tendon transplant in treatment of post-traumatic radial paralysis. MERLE D'AUBIGNE, R. AND LANCE, P. Semaine d. hop. Paris *22:*1666–1671, Sept. 21, '46

Nerves, Recovery of Sensation in Skin Grafts and Flaps

Sensibility of flap in remote plastic operations. LEHMANN, W. AND JUNGERMANN, E. Mitt. a. d. Grenzgeb. d. Med. u. Chir. *32:*653–658, '20

Histologic observations on regeneration of sensory nerve fibres in skin transplantations. KADANOFF, D. Klin. Wchnschr. *4:*1266, June 25, '25

Recuperation of innervation in skin transplants. POLISSADOWA, X. Zentralbl. f. Chir. *52:*2166–2168, Sept 26, '25

Processes of regeneration in nerve fibers of transplanted skin. MASUMOTO, K. Tr. Jap. Path. Soc. *22:*876–877, '32

Regeneration of nerves in grafts and flaps. DAVIS, J. S. AND KITLOWSKI, E. A. Am. J. Surg. *24:*501–545, May '34

Return of sensation to transplanted skin. DAVIS, L. Surg., Gynec. and Obst. *59:*533–543, Sept '34

Changes in cutaneous localization in pedicle flap. DOUGLAS, B. AND LANIER, L. H. Arch. Neurol. and Psychiat. *32:*756–762, Oct '34

General sensations in pedunculated skin flaps. DAVIS, J. S. AND KITLOWSKI, E. A. Arch. Surg. *29:*982–1000, Dec '34

Influence of sympathectomy on homoplastic grafts. LEXER, E. W. Deutsche Ztschr. f. Chir. *249:*337–370, '37

Regeneration of sensation in transplanted skin. MCCARROLL, H. R. Ann. Surg. *108:*309–320, Aug '38

Recovery of sympathetic nerve function in skin transplants. KREDEL, F. E. AND PHEMISTER, D. B. Arch. Neurol. and Psychiat. *42:*403–412, Sept '39

Nerves, Sympathectomy for Facial Paralysis

Mechanism involved in return of contractility of facial muscles when cervical sympathectomy is performed for facial paralysis. LERICHE, R. AND FONTAINE, R. Compt. rend. Soc. de biol. *99:*858–860, Sept 18, '28

Treatment of facial paralysis by excision of cervical sympathetic ganglion; case. ALBERT, F. Liege med. *22:*592–599, April 28, '29

Nerves, Sympathectomy for Facial Paralysis – Cont.

Postoperative facial paralysis treated with Leriche operation, excision of upper cervical sympathetic ganglion; case. DELLA TORRE, P. L. Cervello *9:*299–312, Nov 15, '30

Old-standing facial paralysis treated by removal of inferior cervical ganglion of sympathetic (case). WAKELEY, C. P. G. Proc. Roy. Soc. Med. *25:*795, April '32

Therapy of peripheral facial paralysis by resection of superior cervical sympathetic ganglion. WERTHEIMER, P. Bull. et mem. Soc. nat. de chir. *59:*4–7, Jan 14, '33

Facial paralysis from gunshot wound caused by attempted suicide; therapy by resection of superior cervical sympathetic ganglion and suspension of corners of mouth. ROQUES, P. Bull. et mem. Soc. nat. de chir. *60:*981–984, July 21, '34

Results of resection of superior cervical ganglion and of part of trunk of cervical sympathicus in peripheral facial paralysis of long standing; case. ROASENDA, G. AND DOGLIOTTI, A. M. Boll. e mem. Soc. piemontese di chir. *4:*980–990, '34

Results of stellectomy in facial paralysis due to section of nerve involved in parotid tumor; case. CAEIRO, J. A. Bol. y trab. de la Soc. de cir. de Buenos Aires *19:*392–403, June 26, '35

Resection of superior cervical ganglion in therapy of peripheral facial paralysis caused by injury to cranium; case. HUARD, P. Bull. Soc. med.-chir. de l'Indochine *14:*1289–1293, Nov '36

Excision of superior cervical ganglion in therapy of peripheral paralysis (facial). PLACINTEANU, G. AND DOBRESCU, D. Zentralbl. f. Chir. *69:*323, Feb 21, '42

Stellectomy in therapy of case of facial paralysis. DIEZ, J. Bol. y trab., Acad. argent. de cir. *27:*564–566, July 21, '43

Cervical sympathectomy in therapy of facial paralysis. ALBANESE, A. R. Prensa med. argent. *31:*415–417, March 1, '44

Nerves, Ulnar

Remote results of suture of ulnar and median nerves. CAEIRO, J. A. Semana med. *2:*495–497, Aug 27, '25

Tenoplasty for ulnar paralysis. SILFVERSKIÖLD, N. Acta chir. Scandinav. *64:*300–302, '28

Sensory-motor restoration after section of nerves of arm; suture of radial nerve with subsequent graft of median and ulnar nerves. THOMAS, A. AND PETIT-DUTAILLIS. Rev. neurol. *1:*56–60, Jan '30

Nerves, Ulnar–Cont.

Section of flexor tendons and ulnar nerve in injury to wrist; good results from secondary tendon and nerve sutures. POUZET, F. Lyon chir. *28:*203-206, March-April '31

Suture of ulnar nerve. HEYMAN, J. A. AND CONNER, P. K. Texas State J. med. *26:*861-864, April '31

Nerve suture and muscle repair; primary suture of ulnar nerve and secondary reconstruction of extensor tendons of forearm. HORGAN, E. Ann. Surg. *95:*93-100, Jan '32

Suture of ulnar nerve and reconstruction of brachial triceps tendon by grafting. ROCHER, H. L. Bordeaux chir. *3:*133-136, April '32

Peripheral ulnar nerve injuries. POLLOCK, L. J. AND DAVIS, L. Am. J. Surg. *17:*299-343, Aug '32

Technic and results of suture of ulnar nerve in gunshot injury; case. TANAKAYA, K. Okayama-Igakkai-Zasshi *45:*2677, Nov '33

Suture of ulnar nerve and reconstruction of brachial triceps tendon by grafting. ROCHER, H. L. Bull. et mem. Soc. de chir. de Bordeaux et du Sud-Ouest, pp. 247-254, '32

Gunshot wound of upper third of arm with complete section of ulnar nerve and compression of median nerve; late suture of ulnar nerve. FERRAZ ALVIM, J. *et al.* Rev. oto-neuro-oftal. *9:*44-52, Feb '34

Hypertrophic ascending ulnar neuritis following injury; case. MARGAROT, J. AND RIMBAUD, P. Rev. neurol. *65:*134-139, Jan '36

Clinical forms of ulnar paralysis. CARRIERE, G. AND PARIS, J. Gaz. d. hop. *113:*5, Jan 3-6; 21, Jan 10-13, '40

Ulnar paralysis due to holding of tool handle. LANG, H. Zentralbl. f. Chir. *67:*301-302, Feb 17,'40

Hemiatrophy of face coexisting with diffuse cutaneous neurofibromatosis; case. GUILLAIN, G. *et al.* Rev. neurol. *74:*87-88, Jan-Feb '42

Regeneration of radial nerve, and ulnar nerve. MARBLE, H. C. *et al.* Am. J. Surg. *55:*274-294, Feb '42

Technic for transplanting ulnar nerve. LEARMONTH, J. R. Surg., Gynec. and Obst. *75:*792-793, Dec '42

Simple splint in treatment of ulnar paralysis. RAFFLER, K. Zentralbl. f. Chir. *70:*764, May 22, '43

Operative position for transposition of ulnar nerve. DOBELLE, M. AND PROCTOR, S. E. Am. J. Surg. *64:*254-256, May '44

Anterior transposition of ulnar nerve. MORANDI, G. Bull. War Med. *4:*513-514, May '44 (abstract)

Splint to correct deformity (clawhand) resulting from injury to ulnar nerve. PRUCE, A. M., J. Bone and Joint Surg. *28:*397, Apr '46

NESBIT, R. M.: Plastic procedure for correction of hypospadias. J. Urol. *45:*699-702, May '41

NESBITT, B. E. AND LEEDS, C. R. D.: Fractures of zygoma. Brit. M. J. *1:*512-513, April 14, '45

NEUFELD, A. J. (see TAYLOR, G. M.) April '38

NEUFFER, H.: Technic of plastic surgery of breast. Wien. klin. Wchnschr. *51:*1312-1314, Dec 9, '38

NEUFFER, H. (see LAPP, F. W.) June '31

NEUGEBAUER, F. Construction of vagina from small intestine. Zentralbl. f. Gynak. *46:*381-384, March 11, '22

NEUGEBAUER, F:. Suture of facial nerve trunk. Beitr. z. klin. Chir. *152:*625-628, '31

NEUHÄUSER, H.: Comment on article by Kohn on skin grafting. Zentralbl. f. Chir. *59:*2532, Oct 15, '32

NEUHOF, H.: Transplantation of toe for missing finger; end-result. Ann. Surg. *112:*291-293, Aug '40

NEUHOF, H.: Free transplantation of fat for bronchopulmonary cavity; case. Ann. Surg. *113:*153-155, Jan '41

NEUMANN, A. G.: Plastic repair of penis by autografts. Rev. med. del Rosario *22:*292-299, May '32

NEUMANN, B.: Shock, collapse and hemorrhage. Harefuah *20:*71, June 1, '41

NEUMANN, B. I.: Treatment of hypertrophic cicatrices. Vestnik khir. (no. 47) *16:*65-76, '29

NEUMANN, C. (see FOSTER, A. D. JR. *et al*) May '45

NEUMANN, H.: Mucous-periostal covering and its consideration in surgical therapy of nasal septal deviations. Monatschr. f. Ohrenh. *65:*1399-1405, Nov '31

NEUMANN, H.: Burns and their therapy. Med. Klin. *40:*245, April 28, '44

NEUMANN, H. O.: Congenital scalp defects. Zentralbl. f. Gynak. *48:*628-634, March 15, '24

NEUSCHULER, I.: New instrument for detachment of sac in dacryocystectomy. Arch. d'opht. *48:*829-831, Dec '31

NEUWELT, F. (see LEVINSON, S. O. *et al*) Feb '40

NEUWIRT, F. AND SIMSA, J.: Fractures of upper jaw; treatment. Casop. lek. cesk. *76:*1182-1188, July 2, '37

NEVE, E. F.: Method of skin grafting. Brit. M. J. *2:*987, Dec 10, '21

NEVEU, J. (with J. AUDOUIN): *Technique de la*

parotidectomie totale avec conservation du nerf faciale. Maloine, Paris, 1941

Nevi, Giant

Extensive nevus covering nearly whole body. HELLE. Deutsche med. Wchnschr. *48:*1316, Sept 26, '22 (illus.)

Bathing trunk nevus. CONWAY, H. Surgery *6:*585–597, Oct '39

Plastic surgery of giant pigmented nevus; case. REBELO NETO, J. Rev. med. brasil. *8:*607–611, May '40

Giant nevus with malignant degeneration; case. PINHEIRO, J. AND BARRETO NETO, M. Arq. Serv. nac. doen. ment., pte. 1, pp. 173–205, '43

Malignant degeneration of gigantic pigmented nevus of shoulder; case. FUSTE, R. AND MORA MORALES, L. Rev. med. cubana *55:*307–314, April '44

Giant nevus of thigh successfully treated by complete excision and primary grafting. PICKRELL, K. L. AND CLAY, R. C. Arch. Surg. *48:*319–324, April '44

Surgical therapy of gigantic nevi. MARINO, H. Prensa med. argent. *33:*1321–1325, June 28, '46

Nevi, Pigmented

Nevi in children and their treatment. FITZWILLIAMS, D. C. L. Practitioner *107:*153, Sept '21

Treatment of naevi. STEVENS, R. H., J. Radiol. *2:*33, Nov '21

Treatment of hairy nevi. DU BOIS, C. Rev. med. de la Suisse Rom. *41:*769–772, Dec '21 (illus.) abstr: J.A.M.A. *78:*690, March 4, '22

Treatment of warts and moles. SEMON, H. C. Lancet *1:*1359–1360, June 27, '25

Cosmetic treatment of small nevus. EITNER, E. Wien. med. Wchnschr. *78:*366, March 10, '28

Treatment of nevi, with particular reference to high frequency current. KLAUDER, J. V. J.A.M.A. *90:*1763–1768, June 2, '28

Birthmarks. KLAUDER, J. V. Hygeia *7:*351–352, April '29

Pigmented growths of skin; their significance and treatment. CANNON, A. B. New York State J. Med. *29:*857–864, July 15, '29

Electrolysis as cosmetic treatment of keloids and nevus pigmentosus. MARQUE, A. M. AND LANARI, E. Semana med. *1:*159–164, Jan 16, '30

Multiple pigmented papillary nevi of face (pigmented mole). FIGI, F. A., S. Clin. N. Amer. *10:*101–103, Feb '30

Nevi, Pigmented—Cont.

Injection treatment of nevi. PORRITT, A. E. Proc. Roy. Soc. Med. (sect. Surg.) *24:*81–85, May '31

Removal of large scars or blemishes (nevi) by graduated partial removal. PACKARD, G. B. JR. Colorado Med. *28:*289–292, July '31

Cutaneous epithelioma developed on pigmented nevi. HALKIN, H. Cancer, Bruxelles *9:*241–247, '32

Sebaceous nevus of face; case. REDAELLI, E. Gior. ital. di dermat. e sif. *74:*122–129, Feb '33

Treatment of pigmented moles. REID, M. R. Internat. Clin. *4:*222–232, Dec '33

Therapy of birthmarks. CASKEY, C. R. California and West. Med. *41:*385–388, Dec '34

Technic in using trichloroacetic acid for removal of moles from eyelids. MURPHY, F. G., J. Iowa M. Soc. *26:*147–148, March '36

Therapy of birthmarks. FOX, E. C. Urol. and Cutan. Rev. *40:*820–823, Nov '36

Unusual case of congenital naevus of forefinger and thumb. BRAITHWAITE, L. R. Brit. J. Surg. *14:*538–540, Jan '27

Therapy of common nevi. LERNER, C. Urol. and Cutan. Rev. *41:*204–209, March '37

Moles, warts and keloids. MORSE, J. L. Am. J. Surg. *36:*137–144, April '37

Pilous verrucous pigmentary nevus of nose; autoplasty using Thiersch graft. ROY, J. N. Union med. du Canada *66:*945–948, Sept '37

Pigmentary verrucous pilose nasal nevus; autoplasty by means of Thiersch graft; case. ROY, J. N. Rev. de chir. structive, pp. 180–184, Oct '37

Pilous verrucous pigmented nevus of nose; autoplasty using Thiersch graft; case. ROY, J. N. Rev. argent. de oto-rhino-laring. *7:*53–57, March–April '38

Prognosis and therapy of blue nevi. SCHUERMANN, H. Med. Welt *12:*1102–1104, July 30, '38

Nevi, review of literature. WENDLBERGER, J. Dermat. Ztschr. *78:*95–111, July '38

Therapy of nevi. REUTER, M. J. Wisconsin M. J. *38:*207–208, March '39

Pigmented nevi, with special reference to their surgical therapy. MALINIAC, J. W. Am. J. Surg. *45:*507–510, Sept '39

Dermatologic esthetics; pigmentation, freckles, etc. of exposed parts; means of preventing, improving and curing them. SAINZ DE AJA, E. A. Actas dermo-sif. *32:*145–151, Nov '40

Extensive mole of face and scalp; excision and full thickness skin graft. FIGI, F. A. Proc. Staff Meet., Mayo Clin. *16:*280 282, April 30, '41

Nevi, Pigmented—Cont.

Pigmented nevi. Pires de Lima, J. A. Coimbra med. *9:*5–14, April '42 also: Arq. trab. Fac. med. do Porto Jan–April '42

Error in diagnosis and treatment of nevus; case. Culla, E. Bol. d. Inst. clin. quir. *18:*643–645, Sept '42

Plastic correction of superficial pigmented nevi. Greeley, P. W. Tr. West. S. A. (1941) *51:*398–414, '42

Therapy of nevi; relationship to skin malignancies. Traub, E. F., J. Michigan M. Soc. *42:*297–300, April '43

Verrucous hairy nevus of interciliary region; extirpation and free skin graft; case with recovery. Ivanissevich, O. and Ferrari, R. C. Bol. y trab., Acad. argent. de cir. *27:*422–424, June 30, '43

Treatment of pigmented nevi of neck. Figi, F. A., S. Clin. North America *23:*1059–1075, Aug '43

Fibrokeloid cicatrix after attempted removal of pilous nevus; free full thickness skin graft; case. Malbec, E. F. Dia med. *15:*1100, Sept 13, '43

Treatment of birthmarks. Bailey, W. and Kiskadden, W. California and West. Med. *59:*265–268, Nov '43

Treatment of nevi. Traub, E. F. Clinics *3:*974–981, Dec '44

Fibrokeloid cicatrix after attempted removal of pilous nevus; free full thickness skin graft; case. Malbec, E. F. Semana med. *2:*1416–1417, Dec 23, '43

Pigmented mole of hand. Stout, A. P. Texas State J. Med. *41:*579–580, Mar '46

Plastic correction of superficial pigmented nevi. Greeley, P. W. Surgery *19:*467–481, April '46

Removal of adjacent nevi of eyelids. Callahan, A. Am. J. Ophth. *29:*563–565, May '46

Nevi, Pigmented, Malignancy in (*See also Nevi, Giant*)

Moles, pigmented and nonpigmented, and other skin defects in precancerous stage. Bloodgood, J. C. Northwest Med. *28:*543–547, Dec '29

Treatment of nevi; hazard of insufficient destruction of pigmented nevi. Klauder, J. V. Pennsylvania M. J. *33:*472–477, April '30

Treatment of pigmented moles and malignant melanomas. Evans, W. A. and Leucutia, T. Am. J. Roentgenol. *26:*236–259, Aug '31

Malignant melanomas arising in moles; report of 50 cases. Butterworth, T. and Klauder, J. V. J.A.M.A. *102:*739–745, March 10, '34

Nevi, Pigmented Malignancy in—Cont.

Use of cobra venom in generalized nevocarcinoma; case, Prud'Homme, E., J. de l'Hotel-Dieu de Montreal *4:*372–378, Dec '35

Benign nevus: malignant melanoma; problem of borderline case. Greenblatt, R. B. *et al.* South. M. J. *29:*122–129, Feb '36

Epitheliomas developing on pigmented nevi and pigmented epitheliomas; cases. Halkin, H. Paris med. *1:*241–249, March 20, '37

Nevocarcinoma of cheek in child 3 years old. Perin, L. and Blaire, G. Rev. franc. de dermat. et de venereol. *13:*491–499, Dec '37

Question of relationship between nevus and carcinoma. Beek, C. H. Nederl. tijdschr. v. geneesk. *82:*1199–1203, March 12, '38

"Common mole"; clinicopathologic relations and question of malignant degeneration. Traub, E. F. and Keil. H. Arch. Dermat. and Syph. *41:*214–252, Feb '40

Birth-marks; relationship to skin cancer. Traub, E. F. Hygeia *18:*513, June '40

Benign and malignant moles; differentiation and treatment. Montgomery, H., M. Clin. North America *28:*968–977, July '44

Inappropriate treatment of moles predisposing to melanotic malignancies. Putzki, P. S. and Scully, J. H., M. Ann. District of Columbia *15:*320–324, July '46

Nevi, Vascular

Radium treatment of vascular nevi. Laborde, S. Medecine *2:*696, June '21 abstr: J.A.M.A. *77:*409, July 30, '21

Radium treatment of vascular nevi. Laborde, S. Progres med. *36:*531–532, Nov 12, '21

Treatment of vascular naevi. Molesworth, E. H., M. J. Australia *1:*576–578, May 27, '22

Treatment of vascular nevi with radium. Rulison, R. H. and McLean, S. Am. J. Dis. Child. *25:*359–370, May '23 (illus.)

Radium therapy of vascular nevi. Morrow, H. and Taussig, L. R. Am. J. Roentgenol. *10:*867–871, Nov '23

Case of cavernous angioma (facial nevus). Dreyer. Munchen. med. Wchnschr. *74:*563, April 1, '27

Radium in removal of "birthmarks." Simpson, F. E. and Flesher, R. E. Clin. Med. and Surg. *34:*605–607, Aug '27

Cosmetic applications of carbon dioxide snow to nevi. Kren, O. Wien. klin. Wchnschr. *40:*1329–1331, Oct 20, '27

Radium treatment of haemangiomata, lymphangiomata and naevi pigmentosi. Experiences from "Radium-hemmet," 1909–1924. Andren, G. Acta radiol *8:*1–45, '27

Nevi, Vascular–Cont.

Radium treatment of vascular nevi in infants. STRYKER, G. V., J. Missouri M. A. *25:*417–421, Sept '28

Treatment of vascular nevi in children with roentgen and radium therapy. COTTENOT, P. Med. inf. *37:*72–83, March '30 also: J. de med. de Paris *50:*376–378, May 1, '30

Treatment of vascular nevi by injection of sclerosing solutions. ANDREWS, G. C. AND KELLY, R. J. Arch. Dermat. and Syph. *26:*92–94, July '32

Irradiation treatment of red birth-marks; experiences in over 200 cases. KROMAYER, E. Deutsche med. Wchnschr. *58:*1199–1201, July 29, '32 also: Urol. and Cutan. Rev. *36:*524–527, Aug '32

Radium therapy of giant angiomatous nevi. LLORENS SUQUE, A. Strahlentherapie *45:*457–460, '32

Should vascular nevi be treated? TRAUB, E. F. Arch. Pediat. *50:*272–278, April '33

Therapy of vascular nevus in children. FRIEDJUNG, J. K. Wien. klin. Wchnschr. *46:*1520, Dec 15, '33

Pediculated vascular tumor developed on large nevus of face; case. NICOLAS, J. AND ROUSSET, J. Bull. Soc. franc. de dermat. et syph. (Reunion dermat., Lyon) *42:*1050–1051, July '35

Vascular nevi and their treatment. BLAISDELL, J. H. New England J. Med. *215:*485–488, Sept 10, '36

Natural history of strawberry nevi. LISTER, W. A. Lancet *1:*1429–1434, June 25, '38

Therapy of nevi with thorium X; case. WENDT, H. Dermat. Wchnschr. *108:*10–14, Jan 7, '39

Radium therapy in birth-marks. FEUERSTEIN, B. L. Mississippi Valley M. J. *62:*77, May '40

Radium treatment of vascular nevi; analysis of 152 cases seen during 1928–1938. POHLE, E. A. AND MCANENY, J. B. Am. J. Roentgenol. *44:*747–755, Nov '40

Angiomatous nevus; cases in infants. RUEDA, P. Rev. Soc. pediat. d. litoral *9:*139–142, May-Aug '44

Discussion of angiomata and pigmented nevi. BIVINGS, L. South. M. J. *38:*241–244, April '45

NEVIASER, J. S.: Splint for correction of clawhand. J. Bone and Joint Surg. *12:*440–443, April '30

NEW, G. B.: Rhinophyma. S. Clin. N. Amer. *1:*1393, Oct '21

NEW, G. B.: Delayed pedicle flap in plastic surgery of face and neck. Minnesota Med. *6:*721–724, Dec '22 (illus.)

NEW, G. B.: Use of delayed flap in secondary operations on palate and antrum. Minnesota Med. *6:*214–220, April '23 (illus.)

NEW, G. B.: Hygroma cystica treated with radium. S. Clin. N. America *4:*527–528, April '24

NEW, G. B.: Nasal deformities. Minnesota Med. *7:*629–633, Oct '24

NEW, G. B.: Treatment of malignant tumors of pharynx and nasopharynx. Surg., Gynec. and Obst. *40:*177–182, Feb '25

NEW, G. B.: Tumors of nose, throat and ear; review of literature. Arch. Otolaryng. *1:*545–552, May '25

NEW, G. B.: Plastic surgery of nose. S. Clin. N. America *5:*721–728, June '25

NEW, G. B.: New procedures and method in plastic surgery of face and neck. South. M. J. *19:*138–140, Feb '26

NEW, G. B.: Tumors of nose and throat. Arch. Otolaryng. *3:*461–465, May '26

NEW, G. B.: Carcinoma of larynx. Minnesota Med. *9:*365–368, July '26

NEW, G. B.: Tumors of nose and throat; review of literature. Arch. Otolaryng. *5:*352–356, April '27

NEW, G. B.: Removal of tumor of cheek and temporal region with secondary plastic operation. S. Clin. N. Amer. *7:*1479–1481, Dec '27

NEW, G. B.: Epithelialized flap from forehead to reconstruct lower lip and cheek. S. Clin. N. Amer. *7:*1481–1483, Dec '27

NEW, G. B.: Bone transplantation from crest of ilium for reconstruction of ascending ramus and two-thirds of body of lower jaw-bone. S. Clin. N. America *7:*1483–1486, Dec '27

NEW, G. B.: Two stage laryngectomy. Proc. Staff Meet., Mayo Clin. *3:*221, July 25, '28 also: Surg., Gynec. and Obst. *47:*826–830, Dec '28

NEW, G. B.: Total rhinoplasty. J.A.M.A. *91:*380–381, Aug 11, '28

NEW, G. B.: Reconstruction of upper lip and portion of nose. S. Clin. N. Amer. *9:*75–78, Feb '29

NEW, G. B.: Cavernous hemangioma in adult. S. Clin. N. Amer. *9:*78–80, Feb '29

NEW, G. B.: Adamantinoma of lower jaw treated with surgical diathermy. S. Clin. N. Amer. *9:*80–82, Feb '29

NEW, G. B.: Extrinsic epithelioma of larynx. S. Clin. N. Amer. *9:*84–87, Feb '29

NEW, G. B.: Two-stage thyrotomy in cases considered bad risks. Arch. Otolaryng. *9:*538–542, May '29

NEW, G. B.: Scarring and ulceration of neck

following roentgen therapy. S. Clin. N. Amer. *10:*89-92, Feb '30
NEW, G. B.: Reconstruction of upper lip and cheek. S. Clin. N. Amer. *10:*92-94, Feb '30
NEW, G. B.: Keloid of neck. S. Clin. N. Amer. *10:*95-96, Feb '30
NEW, G. B.: Osteomyelitis of jaws. S. Clin. N. Amer. *10:*96-98, Feb '30
NEW, G. B.: Problems in plastic surgery of nose. Minnesota Med. *13:*242-246, April '30
NEW, G. B.: Reconstruction of ear; case. Proc. Staff Meet., Mayo Clin. *6:*97, Feb 18, '31
NEW, G. B.: Harelip, and cleft palate. S. Clin. North America. *11:*761-765, Aug '31
NEW, G. B.: Cystic hygroma of neck. S. Clin. North America *11:*771-773, Aug '31
NEW, G. B.: Highly malignant tumors of pharynx and nasopharynx. Tr. Am. Acad. Ophth. *36:*39-44, '31
NEW, G. B.: Status of thyrotomy in cancer of larynx. Tr. Am. Laryng., Rhin. and Otol Soc. *37:*241-247, '31
NEW, G. B.: Use of pedicled flaps in reconstructive surgery of face. Tr. Am. Laryng., Rhin. and Otol. Soc. *37:*485-491, '31
NEW, G. B.: Tumors of tonsil and pharynx; 357 cases. Tr. Am. Laryng. A. *53:*277-309, '31
NEW, G. B.: Lymphosarcoma of antrum treated 12 years ago; no recurrence. Proc. Staff Meet., Mayo Clin. *7:*317-318, June 1, '32
NEW, G. B.: Developments in plastic surgery of face and neck. Wisconsin M. J. *32:*243-246, April '33
NEW, G. B.: Postoperative double harelip deformity. S. Clin. North Amea *13:*867-868, Aug '33
NEW, G. B.: Cicatricial contraction of neck. S. Clin. North America *13:*868-869, Aug '33
NEW, G. B.: Permanent enlargement of lips and face, secondary to recurring swellings and associated with facial paralysis; clinical study. Tr. Am. Laryng. A. *55:*43-50, '33
NEW, G. B.: Laryngectomy for carcinoma in aged patient; case. Proc. Staff Meet., Mayo Clin. *10:*186-187, March 20, '35
NEW, G. B.: Scarring of face and neck with keloid from burn treated with radium and plastic operation; case. Proc. Staff Meet., Mayo Clin. *10:*283-285, May 1, '35
NEW, G. B.: Correction of deformities of forehead and nose; presentation of 2 patients. Proc. Staff Meet., Mayo Clin. *10:*519-521, Aug 14, '35
NEW, G. B.: Malignant disease of mouth and accessory structures. Am. J. Surg. *30:*46-52, Oct '35
NEW, G. B.: Fractures of nasal and malar bones. S. Clin. North America *15:*1241-1250, Oct '35
New, G. B. Cancer of tongue and lower jaw. Tr. Am. Laryng., Rhin. and Otol. Soc. *41:*610-613, '35
NEW, G. B.: Skin, cartilage and bone grafts to face. Proc. Staff Meet., Mayo Clin. *11:*791-794, Dec 9, '36
NEW, G. B.: Traumatic deformites of nose and other bones of face. Surg., Gynec. and Obst. *64:*532-537, Feb (no. 2A) '37
NEW, G. B.: Surgical treatment of cancer of larynx. Surg., Gynec. and Obst. *68:*462-466, Feb (no. 2A) '39
NEW, G. B.: Immediate care of automobile injuries to face at scene of accident. Proc. Staff Meet., Mayo Clin. *15:*728-729, Nov 13, '40
NEW, G. B.: Cancer of face. Proc. Staff Meet., Mayo Clin. *16:*71-72, Jan 29, '41
NEW, G. B. Treatment of cancer of face, including reconstructive surgery. S. Clin. North America *21:*969-978, Aug '41
NEW, G. B.: Immediate and later care of facial injuries. Tr. Pacific Coast Oto-Ophth. Soc. *27:*14-16, '42
NEW, G. B.: Early treatment of facial wounds (and neck). Minnesota Med. *26:*619-622, July '43
NEW, G. B.: Sickle flap for nasal reconstruction. Surg., Gynec. and Obst. *80:*497-499, May '45
NEW, G. B.: Sickle flap for reconstruction of nose. Proc. Staff Meet., Mayo Clin. *20:*353-356, Oct 3, '45
NEW, G. B.; BRODERS, A. C. AND CHILDREY, J. H.: Highly malignant tumors of pharynx and base of tongue; identification and treatment. Surg., Gynec. and Obst. *54:*164-174, Feb '32
NEW, G. B. AND CABOT, C. M.: Curability of malignant tumors of upper jaw and antrum. Proc. Staff Meet., Mayo Clin. *9:*684-685, Nov 7, '34
NEW, G. B. AND CABOT, C. M.: Curability of malignant tumors of upper jaw and antrum. Surg., Gynec. and Obst. *60:*971-977, May '35
NEW, G. B. AND CABOT, C. M.: Curability of malignant tumors of upper jaw and antrum. Tr. Am. Laryng., Rhin. and Otol. Soc. *41:*584-590, '35
NEW, G. B. AND DEVINE, K. D.: Methods and indications for skin transplantation S. Clin. North America *26:*890-905, Aug '46
NEW, G. B. AND DIX, C. R.: Repair of defects of frontal bone. Surg., Gynec. and Obst. *70:*698-701, March '40
NEW, G. B. AND ERICH, J. B.: Dermoid cysts of neck and head. Surg., Gynec. and Obst. *65:*48-55, July '37
NEW, G. B. AND ERICH, J. B.: Benign tumors of larynx; 722 cases. Arch. Otolaryng. *28:*841-910, Dec '38

New, G. B. and Erich, J. B.: Benign tumors of larynx; study of 722 cases. Tr. Sect. Laryng., Otol. and Rhin., A.M.A., pp. 17–96, '38

New, G. B. and Erich, J. B.: Repair of postoperative defects of lips. Am. J. Surg. *43:*237–248, Feb '39

New, G. B. and Erich, J. B.: Deep infections of neck; collective review. Internat. Abstr. Surg. *68:*555–567, '39; in Surg., Gynec. and Obst., June '39

New, G. B. and Erich, J. B.: Care of automobile injuries to face. Minnesota Med. *23:*1–8, Jan '40

New, G. B. and Erich, J. B.: Protruding ears; method of plastic correction. Am. J. Surg. *48:*385–390, May '40

New, G. B. and Erich, J. B.: Retruded chins; correction by plastic operation. J.A.M.A. *115:*186–191, July 20, '40

New, G. B. and Erich, J. B.: Method to prevent fresh costal cartilage grafts from warping. Proc. Staff Meet., Mayo Clin. *16:*199–200, March 26, '41

New, G. B. and Erich, J. B.: Surgical correction of mandibular prognathism. Am. J. Surg. *53:*2–12, July '41

New, G. B. and Erich, J. B.: Method to prevent fresh cartilage grafts from warping (facial surgery). Am. J. Surg. *54:*435–438, Nov '41

New, G. B. and Erich, J. B.: Bone grafts to mandible. Am. J. Surg. *63:*153–167, Feb '44

New, G. B. and Erich, J. B.: Hair-bearing scalp flap for repair of unilateral scalp defects. S. Clin. North America *24:*741–750, Aug '44

New, G. B. and Figi, F. A.: Treatment of fibromas of nasopharynx; report of 32 cases. Am. J. Roentgenol. *12:*340–343, Oct '24

New, G. B. and Figi, F. A.: Use of full thickness skin grafts. Minnesota Med. *7:*714–716, Nov '24

New, G. B. and Figi, F. A.: Treatment of fibromas of naso-pharynx; report of 32 cases. Ann.Otol., Rhin. and Laryng. *34:*191–196, March '25

New, G. B. and Figi, F. A.: Treatment of secondary deformity in cases of harelip (nose). Minnesota Med. *14:*514–516, June '31

New, G. B. and Figi, F. A.: Use of pedicled flaps in reconstruction of nose. Surg., Gynec. and Obst. *53:*780–787, Dec '31

New, G. B. and Figi, F. A.: Use of reconstructive surgery in certain types of facial deformities; and nasal. J.A.M.A. *103:*1434–1438, Nov 10, '34

New, G. B. and Figi, F. A.: Use of reconstructive surgery in certain types of deformities (face, nose). Tr. Sect. Laryng., Otol. and Rhin., A.M.A., pp. 52–63, '34

New, G. B., and Figi, F. A.: Five year cures of cancer of larynx and mouth and pharynx. Surg., Gynec. and Obst. *60:*483–484, Feb (no. 2A) '35

New, G. B. and Figi, F. A.: Repair of postoperative defects involving lips and cheeks secondary to removal of malignant tumors. Surg., Gynec. and Obst. *62:*182–190, Feb '36

New, G. B. and Figi, F. A.: Treatment of carcinoma of larynx. Surg., Gynec. and Obst. *62:*420–423, Feb (no. 2A) '36

New, G. B.; Figi, F. A. and Havens, F. Z.: Replacement of tissues of forehead and scalp. S. Clin. North America *14:*607–613, June '34

New, G. B. and Fletcher, E.: Selection of treatment for cancer of larynx. J.A.M.A. *99:*1754–1758, Nov 19, '32

New, G. B. and Fletcher, E. M.: Selection of treatment of cancer of larynx. Tr. Sect. Laryng., Otol. and Rhin., A.M.A., pp. 27–42, '32

New, G. B. and Harper, F. R.: Osteitis deformans affecting bones of face. Proc. Staff Meet., Mayo Clin. *8:*465–466, Aug 2, '33

New, G. B. and Havens, F. Z.: Epithelioma of face; treatment and subsequent surgical reconstruction. J.A.M.A. *97:*687-690, Sept 5, '31

New, G. B. and Havens, F. Z.: Epithelioma of face; treatment and subsequent surgical reconstruction. Tr. Sect. Surg., Gen. and Abd., A.M.A., pp. 166–176, '31

New, G. B. and Kirch, W.: Tumors of nasopharynx; review of literature. Arch. Otolaryng. *8:*600–607, Nov '28

New, G. B. and Kirch, W.: Nasal tumors. Arch. Otolaryng. *9:*445–450, April '29

New, G. B. and Kirch, W.: Review of literature of nasal tumors. Arch. Otolaryng. *11:*657–668, May '30

New, G. B. and Kirch, W.: Tumors of nose and throat; summary of bibliographic material available in field of otolaryngology. Arch. Otolaryng. *15:*623–633, April '32

New, G. B. and Kirch, W.: Tumors of nose. Arch. Otolaryng. *29:*457–467, March '39

New, G. B. and Kirch, W.: Permanent enlargement of lips and face secondary to recurring swellings and associated with facial paralysis; clinical entity. J.A.M.A. *100:*1230–1233, April 22, '33

New, G. B.; Kirch, W. and Erich, J. B.: Tumors of nose and throat; summaries of bibliographic material available in field of otolaryngology. Arch. Otolaryng. *30:*283–297, Aug '39

New, G. B. and Waugh, J. M.: Curability of

cancer of larynx. Surg., Gynec. and Obst. *58:*841–844, May '34
NEW, G. B. (see JUDD, E. S.) Feb '23
NEW, G. B. (see JUDD, E. S.) Nov '27
NEW, G. B. (see FIGI, F. A.) April '29
NEW, G. B. (see FIGI, F. A.) 1929
NEW, G. B. (see FIGI, F. A. *et al*) Sept '43

New-Erich Operation

Projecting auricle (lop ear); case corrected by surgery (New-Erich method). AUSTIN, E. R. Proc. Staff Meet. Clin., Honolulu *9:*45–48, May '43

NEWELL, C. E.: Malignant melanomas, with particular reference to subungual types. South. M. J. *31:*541–547, May '38
NEWELL, E. T., JR.: Clinical and pathologic study of 390 cases lip cancer, with report of 5 year cures. Arch. Surg. *38:*1014–1029, June '39
NEWHOUSER, L. R. AND LOZNER, E. L.: Human serum albumin (concentrated); clinical indications and dosage (shock). U. S. Nav. M. Bull. *40:*277–279, April '42
NEWIRK, H. D.: New mouth gag for cleft palate operation. Laryngoscope *44:*587, July '34
NEWLAND, H. S.: Whole thickness dermo-epidermal grafts. J. Coll. Surgeons, Australasia *1:*62–64, July '28
NEWLAND, H. S. (see LENDON, A. A.) July '21
NEWMAN, J.: Reconstruction of external ear. Surg., Gynec. and Obst. *73:*234–235, Aug '41
NEWMAN, J. Repair of prognathic and retruded jaws. Am. J. Surg. *58:*35–39, Oct '42
NEWMAN, J. (see WEISS, B. *et al*) Jan '41
NEWMAN, L. I. (see GOTTLIEB, A.) Sept '21
NEWSOM, R. A.: Treatment of septic hands and feet on shipboard. Brit. M. J. *1:*809–810, May 4, '29
NEWTON, K.: Nursing responsibilities in plastic surgery. Am. J. Nursing *43:*155–162, Feb '43
NEWTON, M. E.: Pressure areas; practical suggestions on how to prevent bed sores. Am. J. Nursing *38:*888–892, Aug '38
NEY, K. W.: Treatment of nerve injuries. Mil. Surgeon *49:*277, Sept '21
NEY, K. W.: Tendon transplant for intrinsic hand muscle paralysis. Surg., Gynec. and Obst. *33:*342, Oct '21
NEY, K. W.: Facial paralysis and surgical repair of facial nerve. Laryngoscope *32:*327–347, May '22 (illus.)
NEY, K. W.: Repair of cranial defects with celluloid. Am. J. Surg. *44:*394–399, May '39

Ney Operation

Results of tendon transplantation for intrinsic hand paralysis (Ney's operation). JOHNSTON, J. G., J. Bone and Joint Surg. *5:*278–283, April '23 (illus.)

NEYMAN, V. N.: Use of ocular prosthesis during plastic reconstruction of conjunctival sac with free cutaneous or mucous graft. Vestnik oftal. (no. 5) *14:*45–46, '39
NI, T. G.: Use of ah-chiao (donkey skin glue) for circulatory failure encountered in severe hemorrhage and shock. Chinese J. Physiol. *10:*125–132, Feb 15, '36
NICHOLSON, M. E. (see ADAIR, F. E. *et al*) July '30
NICITA, A.: Congenital syndactylia; study of 3 generations. Minerva med. *1:*346–352, April 14, '36
NICKEL, W. F. (see ANDRUS, W. DEW. *et al*) Jan '43
DE NICOLA, C. P. AND VILAFANE, A. R.: Clinical aspect of severe burns. An. Cong. brasil. e am. cir. *3:*364–374, '42

Nicoladoni Operation

Transplantation of toe to replace thumb; Nicoladoni method. DZBANOVSKIY, V. P. Vestnik khir. *55:*626–629, May '38
Transplantation of toe according to method of Nicoladoni; case. KUSLIK, M. I. Arch. Surg. *32:*123–130, Jan '36

NICOLAS. (see CAUSSADE, L.) Nov '29
NICOLAS, J. AND ROUSSET, J.: Pediculated vascular tumor developed on large nevus of face; case. Bull. Soc. franc. de dermat. et syph. (Reunion dermat., Lyon) *42:*1050–1051, July '35
NICOLATO, A.: Results of reconstruction of eyelids following loss of substance due to grave trauma. Ann. di ottal. e clin. ocul. *67:*81–92, Feb '39
NICOLAU, S. AND POINCLOUX, P.: Skin grafts in herpes recurrens. Compt. rend. Soc. de biol. *98:*360–363, Feb 10, '28
NICOLLE. (see MEYER, J.) July '27
NICOLLE, A.: Peripheral facial paralysis; electrologic, diagnostic and therapeutic technic. Rev. d'actinol. *8:*510–524, Nov–Dec '32
NIDA, X.: Cancer in right eye; unsuccessful radium therapy; extended exeresis and graft of medio-frontal, pediculated flap; 2 photographs. Bull. Soc. d'opht. de Paris, no. 9, pp. 532–536, '27
NIDA, M.: Ptosis of eyelid; case operated by new method. Ann. d'ocul. *166:*639–645, Aug '29

Nida Operation

Surgical therapy of eyelid ptosis with special reference to Nida technic; results in cases. VALERIO, M. Rassegna ital. d'ottal. *8:*62–83, Jan–Feb '39

Nida method of correcting ptosis of upper eyelid. BARDANZELLU, T. Rassegna ital. d'ottal. *8:*449–453, July–Aug '39

NIEDELMAN, M. L.: Epilation; fifteen year comparative evaluation of electrolysis and electrocoagulation. Arch. Phys. Med. *26:*290–296, May '45

NIEDEN, H.: Operative treatment of habitual dislocation of jaw. Deutsche Ztschr. f. Chir. *183:*358–363, '24

NIEDEN, H. AND ASBECK, C.: Congenital cartilaginous remains in neck; relation to lateral cervical fistulas. Beitr. z. klin. Chir. *153:*47–59, '31

Nieden's Operation

Nieden's operation for habitual dislocation of lower jaw. LOESSL, J. Zentralbl. f. Chir. *53:*1749–1751, July 10, '26

NIEDERLAND, W.: Dupuytren's contracture; relation to occupation. Arch. f. Gewerbepath. u. Gewerbehyg. *3:*23–43, '32

NIEDERLAND, W.: Dupuytren's contracture; relation to occupation. Med. Welt *7:*126–127, Jan 28, '33

NIEDERLAND, W.: Dupuytren's contracture of fingers as result of injury; case. Med. Klin. *29:*614–615, April 28, '33

NIEDERLAND, W.: Dupuytren's contracture. Zentralbl. f. Chir. *62:*2238–2243, Sept 21, '35

NIEDERLAND, W.: Dupuytren's contracture as industrial injury. Jahresk. f. arztl. Fortbild. *27:*60–65, Sept '36

NIEDERMAYR, R.: Plastic treatment of hypospadias. Munchen. med. Wchnschr. *68:*773, June 24, '21

NIEHUES, X.: Traumatic origin of Dupuytren's contracture. Aerztl. Sachverst.-Ztg. *33:*250–255, Sept 15, '27

NIELSEN, M.: Plastic operation for vaginal defect ad modum Kirschner-Wagner. Acta obst. et gynec. Scandinav. *14:*314–320, '34

NIELSEN, M.: Plastic formation of artificial vagina by Kirschner-Wagner operation; case. Acta obst. et gynec. Scandinav. *16:*179–188, '36

NIEMAN, H. A. (see KARP, F. L. *et al*) June '39

NIEMEYER, W.: Autoplastic dacryorhinostomy; new process for reconstructing lacrimal organs by means of labial mucosal graft. Arq. brasil. de oftal. *8:*181–185, Dec '45

NIENHUIS, J. H.: So-called congenital fistulae of neck. Geneesk. Gids *6:*625–633, July 6, '28

NIENY, K.: Surgical treatment of arthritis. Zentralbl. f. Chir. *54:*3218–3219, Dec 10, '27

NIGRISOLI, P.: Experimental implantation of cartilage into kidney and transplantation of cartilage into bone defects. Arch. per le sc. med. *49:*689–703, Dec '27

NIGRISOLI, P.: Experiments to improve survival of homoplastic transplants. Arch. per sc. med. *52:*65–75, Feb '28

NIJKERK, M.: Iontophoresis in treatment of Dupuytren's contracture and keloids. Nederl. tijdschr. v. geneesk. *83:*5135–5140, Oct 28, '39

NIKANOROV, A. M.: Flat skin graft in restoration of extensive facial defects. Novy khir. arkhiv *40:*255–258, '38

NIKIFOROVA, E. K.: Reconstruction of tendons of fingers. Vestnik khir. *58:*255–260, Sept '39

NIKIFOROVA, E. K.: Bandage for Perthes operation (tendon transplant). Khirurgiya, no. 6, p. 94, '45

NIKITIN, A. A.: Transformation of osseous tissue used for filling bone defects. Ortop. i travmatol. (no. 6) *11:*64–65, '37

NIKOLAEV, G. F.: Experimental data on plastic surgery of tendons according to Bunnell. Ortop. i travmatol. (no. 6) *11:*3–11, '37

NIKOLAEV, G. F.: Restoration of function of injured tendons of upper extremities. Ortop. i travmatol. (no. 2) *12:*3–17, '38

NIKOLAEV, G. F.: Use of various materials for isolation of suture to prevent adhesion in tendon surgery; experimental study. Ortop. i travmatol. (no. 4) *14:*18–26, '40

NIKOLAEV, G. F.: Significance of early resumption of function following plastic repair of tendons according to Bunnell. Novy khir. arkhiv. *45:*327–331, '40

NIKOLSKY, A. M.: Osteoplastic resection of both alveolar processes according to Kocher. Ann. Otol., Rhin. and Laryng. *39:*701–719, Sept '30

NIRENBERG, B. B. AND FUKS, B. I.: Preparation of splint for extra-oral extension in jaw fractures. Sovet. khir. (no. 4) *7:*732–734, '34

NISHIMURA, I.: Branchiogenic cysts of neck; 2 cases. Okayama-Igakkai-Zasshi *47:*235, Jan '35

NISHIYAMA, A.: War injuries of nose and nasal sinuses; 5 cases. Oto-rhino-laryng. *12:*476–477, June '39

NISSEL, W.: Normet's citrated solution in shock. Chirurg *4:*363–369, May 1, '32

NISSEN, R.: Transplantation of leg; Sauerbruch's plastic operation. Umschau *31:*526, June 25, '27

NISSEN, R.: Urethroplasty for scrotal hypospadias. Zentralbl. f. Chir. *56:*962–964, April 20, '29

NISSEN, R.: Bone transplantation by Axhausen's method in case of pseudoarthrosis of lower jaw resulting from defective healing. Deutsche Ztschr. f. Chir. *229:*140–142, '30

NISSEN, R.: Two-stage plastic operation in pendulous breast. Zentralbl. f. Chir. *60:*1330–1331, June 10, '33

Nissen Operation

Hypertrophy of breast corrected by plastic surgery according to Nissen. BUMIN, H. Turk tib cem. mec. *5:*173–183, '39

Modification of Nissen's operation in hypospadias. KAÏRIS, Z. Zentralbl. f. Chir. *57:*3047–3048, Dec 6, '30

NITTER, H.: Hyperplasia of breast. Norsk. Mag. f. Laegevidensk. *83:*673–677, Sept '22 (illus.) abstr. J.A.M.A. *79:*1730, Nov 11, '22

NIVEN, R. B. (see PEARSON, R. S. R. *et al*) July '41

NIX, J. T.: Anastomosis of seventh and eleventh cranial nerves to correct facial paralysis. New Orleans M. and S. J. *77:*123–126, Sept '24

NIŽETIĆ, Z.: Construction of lacrimal passages. Klin. Monatsbl. f. Augenh. *102:*67–71, Jan '39

NIŽETIĆ, Z.: Two-stage dacryocystorhinostomy. Klin. Monatsbl. f. Augenh. *102:*71–76, Jan '39

NIŽETIĆ, Z.: Inversion of tarsus as surgical procedure in correction of granulous entropion. Ann. d'ocul. *177:*211–217, June '40

NIŽETIĆ, Z.: Technic of operation for correction of trachomatous entropion. Klin. Monatsbl. f. Augenh. *105:*641–647, Dec '40

NOBL, G.: Treatment of xanthoma of eyelid. Med. Klinik *19:*1631–1633, Dec 16, '23 abstr: J.A.M.A. *82:*344, Jan 26, '24

NOBL, G.: Cosmetic depilation of hair. Med. Klinik *20:*369–371, March 23, '24 abstr: J.A.M.A. *82:*1575, May 10, '24

NOBLE, R. P. AND GREGERSEN, M. I.: Extent and cause of blood volume reduction in traumatic, hemorrhagic and burn shock. J. Clin. Investigation *25:*172–183, Mar '46

NOBLE, T. B. JR.: Rationalization of treatment of cellulitis of hand. J. Indiana M. A. *25:*12–16, Jan '32

NOCITO, J. P.: Surgical technic in therapy of eyelid ptosis. Semana med. *2:*496–497, Aug 14, '30

NOË, C. G. N.: Technic of plastic surgery of breast. Zentralbl. f. Gynak. *56:*2721–2723, Nov 5, '32

NOE, M.: Musculotendinous surgery in treatment of sequels of poliomyelitis. Rev. chilena de pediat. *17:*20–22, Jan '46

NÖEL: Therapy of cavernous angioma of face; cases. Rev. de chir. structive *8:*199–203, '38

NOËL, A.: Relations between esthetic surgery of breast and ovarian and mammary glands. Bull. med., Paris *48:*611–613, Oct 6, '34

NOËL, A.: Operation for pendulous breast. Med. Welt *2:*51–53, Jan 14, '28

NÖEL, A. AND LOPEZ-MARTINEZ: Operation for pendulous breast. Arch. franco-belges de chir. *31:*138–153, Feb '28

NOËL, A.: Plastic surgery of ear; 2 cases. Ann. d. mal. de l'oreille, du larynx *47:*478–482, May '28

NOËL, A.: Plastic reconstruction of breast in necrosis following esthetic operation. Bull. med., Paris *47:*633–634, Oct 7, '33

NOËL, A.: *La chirurgie esthétique, son role social.* Masson et Cie, Paris, 1926. (German translation by A. Hardt published by Barth, Leipzig, 1932)

NOËL, A.: Correction esthétique veineuses des mains. Bull. Medical, 14 octobre, 1933

NOËL, A. (see BRETECHE *et al*) Oct '35

Noël Operation

Noël technic in plastic surgery of nipple. VENETIANER, P. Gyogyaszat *73:*553–555, Sept 3, '33

NOËL, S. AND MARTINEZ, L.: La chirurgie esthétique—nouveaux procedes de correction du prolapses mammaire. Le Concour Medical, No. 46 (October 27, 1928)

NØRVIG, J.: Acrocephalosyndactylia in brother and sister. Hospitalstid. *72:*165–178, Feb 14, '29

NOGUCHI, M. AND KOTAKE, Y.: Pouch ear; case. Oto-rhino-laryng. *9:*820, Sept '36

NOGUEIRA, A. JR.: Peripheral circulatory insufficiency with shock; present status of theories on physiopathogenesis and treatment. Med. cir. farm., pp. 242–276, May '46

NOGUEIRA, N. G.: Veritol therapy of shock. Ann. brasil. de gynec. *6:*123–126, Aug '38

NOGUEIRA, P.: Thyroglossal fistula in children; surgical therapy; 2 cases. Rev. Assoc. paulista de med. *2:*206–212, April '33

NOGUERA, A. M.: Burn therapy with special reference to use of tannic acid (Davidson method). Gac. med. de Caracas *42:*223–224, July 31, '35

NOGUERA, A. M.: Burn therapy, with special

reference to use of tannic acid (Davidson method). Gac. med. de Caracas *42:*226–240, Aug 15, '35

NOICA, D.; ARAMA, O.; LUPULESCU, I. AND STROESCU, G.: Bilateral Dupuytren's contracture due to injury of cubital nerve in lower third of forearm. Romania med. *15:*261–262, Oct 15, '37

NOICA, D.; ARAMA, O.; PARVULESCU, N. AND LUPULESCU, I.: New data on pathogenesis of Dupuytren's contracture. Rev. san. mil., Bucuresti *35:*513–518, May '36

NOICA, D. AND PARVULESCU: Nervous etiology of Dupuytren's contracture. Rev. neurol. *1:*703–708, April '32

NOICA, I. AND PÂRVULESCU, N.: Pathogenesis of Dupuytren's contracture. Rev. san. mil., Bucuresti *31:*3–9, Jan–Feb '32

NOLAND, L. AND Wilson, C. H.: More recent ideas on burn therapy. J. M. A. Alabama *10:*157–162, Nov '40

NOLTENIUS, F.: Technic of intranasal operation for humpnose. Arch. f. Ohren-, Nasen-u. Kehlkopfh. *128:*355, May 11, '31

Noma

- Plastic operations for defects of face due to noma. HORSLEY, J. S. Southern M. J. *15:*557–561, July '22 (illus.)
- Case of stiff jaw after cancrum oris; surgical interference; cure. MUKERJI, S. N. Indian M. Gaz. *62:*387, July '27
- Plastic surgery of lower lip for noma. KOLDAEFF, S. M. Vrach. gaz. *32:*1177–1181, '28
- Cancrum oris with recovery; subsequent repair of defect by plastic operation. GOODALL, E. W. Brit. J. Child. Dis. *27:*204–208, July–Sept '30
- Plastic operation of face following noma. SMYRNOFF, S. S., M. Rec. *143:*186–188, March 4, '36
- Reparative operation for maxillary ankylosis and labiofacial destruction due to noma. KANKAT, C. T. Turk tip cem. mec. *12:*163–168, '46

NOMLAND, R.: Treatment of acne vulgaris with comedos by monoterminal electrodesiccation. Arch. Dermat. and Syph. *48:*302–304, Sept '43

NOMLAND, R. AND WALLACE, E. G.: Penicillin for ulcers of leg treated by pinch grafts. J.A.M.A. *130:*563-564, March 2, '46

NORCROSS, N. C.: Operative experiences on wounds of peripheral nerves from Pacific combat area; preliminary report based on 50 cases. Bull. Am. Coll. Surgeons *28:*127–128, June '43

NORD, C. F. L.: Hemihypertrophy of jaw. Tijdschr. v. tandheelk. *35:*811–814, Dec 15, '28

NORDEN, A.: Surgical therapy of hypertrophy of breast. Chirurg *12:*650–655, Nov 1, '40

NORDMANN, O.: Therapy of neuropathic ulcers of foot (mal perforant) by implantation of sensory nerves. Chirurg *14:*116–122, Feb 15, '42

NORENBERG, A. E.: Comparative evaluation of Bettmann-Davidson method in burns. Vestnik khir. *60:*9–17, July–Aug '40

NORES, A. JR.: Surgical shock, review of literature. Rev. med. de Cordoba *29:*474, Aug; 545–553, Sept; 585–560, Oct '41

NORES, A. JR.: Review of literature on shock. Rev. med. de Cordoba *29:*629–643, Nov '41

NORMET: Normet's citrated solution in shock; cases. Bull. et mem. Soc. nat. de chir. *55:*848–853, June 22, '29

NORMET, L.: Therapy of hemorrhages and states of traumatic shock in armies in wartime. Bruxelles-med. *19:*1474–1482, Oct 8, '39

NORSA, G.: Retraction of palmar aponeuroses and scleroderma. Gazz. d. osp. *55:*1285–1287, Oct 21, '34

NORSWORTHY, O. L.: Treatment of cancer of lower lip. Texas State J. Med. *20:*184–188, July '24

NORTH, J. P. (see OWEN, H. R.) Dec '39

NORTHCUTT, E. W.: Hand fractures. Kentucky M. J. *35:*8–10, Jan '37

NORTHCUTT, J. D.: Avulsion of scalp; skin grafting; with report of unusual case. Kentucky M. J. *23:*493–497, Oct '25

NORTHFIELD, D. W. C. (see ALLEN, A. G.) Aug '44

NORTHFIELD, D. W. C. (see ALLEN, A. G.) Oct '45

NORTHROP, H. L.: Keloid of forehead. S. Clin. N. Amer. *5:*1671, Dec '25

NORTHROP, H. L.: Transplantation of ureters into sigmoid in exstrophy of bladder. J. Am. Inst. Homeop. *26:*33–34, Jan '33

NORVOLD, R. W. (see RUDOLPH, C. E.) April '44

Nose, Anterior Atresia (See also Nose, Choanal Atresia)

- Operative treatment of congenital nasal atresia. KAFEMANN, A. W. AND BESELIN, O. Arch. f. Ohren-, Nasen-u. Kehlkopfh. *116:*116–118, Dec '26
- New operative method in anterior nasal atresia. BOCKSTEIN, F. Ztschr. f. Hals-, Nasen-u. Ohrenh. *17:*180–187, Jan 31, '27
- Rule for operation in atresia of nares. MATWEJEW, D. N. Monatschr. f. Ohrenh. *65:*1188–1192, Oct '31

Nose, Anterior Atresia–Cont.

Cicatricial atresia of nasal fossa; 5 cases. CORDEIRO LOBATO, J. Lisboa med. *9:*155-163, Feb '32

Congenital atresia or obstruction of air passages. BLAIR, V. P. Ann. Otol., Rhin. and Laryng. *40:*1021-1035, Dec '31 also: Tr. Am. Laryng. A. *53:*229-246, '31 also: Internat. J. Orthodontia *18:*516-526, May '32

Congenital atresia of anterior nares; 2 cases in sisters. WASHBURNE, A. C. Arch. Otolaryng. *16:*789-790, Dec '32

Plastic surgery for atresia of anterior portion of nose, case. ARAI, A. Oto-rhino-laryng. *9:*605, July '36

Operation for correction of atresia or stenosis of anterior nares. O'CONNOR, G. B. Arch. Otolaryng. *25:*208-210, Feb '37

Bilateral anterior nasal atresia; cure; case. HOSOMI, E. Oto-rhino-laryng. *10:*329, April '37

Plastic surgery in atresia of nostrils; cases. REBELO NETO, J. Rev. oto-laring. de Sao Paulo *5:*259-265, May-June '37

Treatment of functional and organic stenosis of entrance to nose. RETHI, A. Rev. de chir. structive, pp. 137-147, June '37

Congenital atresia of pyriform orifice as cause of respiratory insufficiency; surgical correction. ESCAT, M. Oto-rhino-laryng. internat. *22:*65-74, Feb '38

Reconstruction of anterior nares following stenosis. O'CONNOR, G. B. Rev. de chir. structive *8:*77-83, Aug '38

Congenital bilateral imperforation of nostril; case. PRUDENTE DE AQUINO, F. Rev. brasil. de oto-rino-laring *7:*255-262, May-June '39

Nasal atresia; surgical critique. CINELLI, A. A., Ann. Otol., Rhin. and Laryng. *49:*912-923, Dec '40

Congenital closure of anterior nasal aperture and of nasal cavities; 2 cases. KANZAKI, T. AND KAMIO, T. Oto-rhino-laryng. (Abst. Sect.) *14:*5, Feb '41

Surgical therapy of cicatricial stenosis and atresia of vestibule and interior of nose. ESCH, A. Ztschr. f. Hals-, Nasen-u. Ohrenh. *48:*41-46, '41

Nose, Atrophic Rhinitis of

Ivory implant in atrophic rhinitis. BERNHEIMER, L. B. Illinois M. J. *55:*420-422, June '29

Treatment (with ivory implants) of atrophic rhinitis. BERNSTIEN, J., J. Laryng. and Otol. *48:*603-607, Sept '33

Correction of saddle nose with ozena by endonasal inclusions of costal grafts; case. PERI, M. Rev. de chir. structive, pp. 299-302, June '36

Nose, Atrophic Rhinitis of–Cont.

Atrophic rhinitis in plastic surgery. KOPP, M. M. Laryngoscope *50:*510-519, June '40

Cartilage implants in therapy of ozena; first cases in Venezuela. CELIS PEREZ, A. Gac. med. de Caracas 54:14-16, Jan-Mar '46

Nose, Bone and Cartilage Autografts to

Treatment of a "saddle nose" by costal cartilage graft. CAMERER, C. B., U. S. Nav. M. Bull. *15:*397, April '21

Correction of nasal deformities with autogenous transplants. STOTTER, J. AND STOTTER, A. L. Ohio State M. J. *17:*384, June '21

Transplantation for correction of depressed deformities of nose. CARTER, W. W. New York M. J. *117:*59-60, Jan 3, '23

Value and ultimate fate of bone and cartilage transplants in correction of nasal deformities. CARTER, W. W. Laryngoscope *33:*196-202, March '23 (illus.)

Free cartilage grafts (nasal deformities). RUEF, H. Med. Klinik *20:*1428-1429, Oct 12, '24 abstr: J.A.M.A. *83:*1722, Nov 22, '24

Plastic repair of "saddle nose" deformity by autogeneous cartilaginous graft. CAMERER, C. B., U. S. Nav. M. Bull. *22:*186, Feb '25

Rib implant for depressed bridge of nose. EADIE, C. M., M. J. Australia *2:*137-139, Aug 1, '25

How soon should nasal deformities, due to abscess of septum be corrected by transplantation of bone. CARTER, W. W., M. J. and Rec. *122:*247-248, Sept 2, '25

Method of nasal plastic repair by cartilage graft. WATSON-WILLIAMS, E. Brit. M. J. *2:*987-988, Nov 28, '25

Case of developmental deformity of nose corrected by bone and cartilage transplants. CARTER, W. W. Laryngoscope *36:*664-666, Sept '26

Reconstruction of nasal bridge by means of autogenous rib cartilage grafts. GARRETSON, W. T., J. Michigan M. Soc. *26:*36-41, Jan '27

Rhinoplasty by cartilaginous grafts. LECLERC, G. Bull. et mem. Soc. nat. de chir. *53:*671-678, May 21, '27

Correction of pronounced types of saddle nose with mixed implants of bone and cartilage. COHEN, L. Ann. Otol., Rhin. and Laryng. *36:*639-647, Sept '27

Correction of pronounced types of saddle nose with mixed implants of bone and cartilage. COHEN, L. Tr. Am. Laryng., Rhin. and Otol. Soc. *33:*233-242, '27

Use of autogenous transplants vs. foreign

Nose, Bone and Cartilage Autografts to – Cont.
bodies in correction of nasal deformities. Carter, W. W. Am. Med. *23:*363–366, May '28
Resector for removing shaped piece of rib cartilage for nasal transplant. Fornell, C. H. Laryngoscope *38:*733–734, Nov '28
Cartilage graft to nose. Moorehead, F. B., S. Clin. N. Amer. *9:*327–328, April '29
Plastic operation with costal cartilage in concave nose; cases. Roy, J. N. Union med. du Canada *58:*408–414, July '29
Cartilaginous and osteo-cartilagenous rib grafts in correction of nasal deformities. Metz, W. R. New Orleans M. and S. J. *82:*831–840, June '30
Narrowing of wide alae of nose by reimplantation of cartilage from tip of nose. Érczy, N. Ztschr. f. Hals-, Nasen-u. Ohrenh. *26:*194–197, July 3, '30
Transposition of section from auricle for correction of nasal defect; case. Carter, W. W. Arch. Otolaryng. *12:*178–183, Aug '30
Ultimate fate of bone when transplanted into nose for purpose of correcting deformity. Carter, W. W. Arch. Otolaryng. *15:*563–573, April '32
Cartilage and ivory; indications and contraindications for their use as nasal support. Maliniak, J. W. Arch. Otolaryng. *17:*649–657, May '33
Restoration of shape of nose by cartilaginous autograft after old fracture. Dantlo, R. Strasbourg med. *93:*485–487, July 15, '33
Correction of nasal deformities by plastic methods and by transplantation of bone and cartilage (from rib). Carter, W. W. Internat. J. Orthodontia *19:*1012–1016, Oct '33
Value of bone and cartilage grafts in rhinoplasty. Carter, W. W. Laryngoscope *43:*905–910, Nov '33
Plastic correction of nasal deformities after operation for harelip. Eitner, E. Deutsche Ztschr. f. Chir. *238:*644–646, '33
Correction of posttraumatic saddle nose by costal graft. Peri. Rev. de chir. plastique, pp. 334–338, Jan '34
Restoration of depressed nose by grafting of cartilage; 6 cases. McIndoe, A. H. Proc. Roy. Soc. Med. *27:*1278–1284, July '34
Correction of saddle nose by autograft from costal cartilage. Tetu, I. and Dumitrescu, J. Spitalul *55:*65–66, Feb '35
Rhinoplasty with free transplantation from auricle. Limberg, A. A. Sovet. khir., no. 9, pp. 70–90, '35
Correction of saddle nose with ozena by endonasal inclusions of costal grafts; case. Peri,

Nose, Bone and Cartilage Autografts to – Cont.
M. Rev. de chir. structive, pp. 299–302, June '36
Costal graft and ivory inclusions in reconstruction of saddle nose by transsupraciliary route. Alves, O. Rev. oto-laring. de Sao Paulo (no. 5, bis) *4:*843–863, Sept–Oct '36
Chrondral autoplasty in correction of saddle nose. Prisant, M. Folia oto-laryng. orient. *3:*205–211, '36
Use of costal cartilage in restorative surgery of saddle nose; 3 cases. Peri, M. Rev. de chir. structive, pp. 103–107, June '37
Correction of depressed deformities of external nose with rib graft. Cohen, L. South. M. J. *30:*680–685, July '37
Free transplantation of cartilage in rhinoplasty. Dujardin, E. Ugesk. f. laeger *99:*1292, Dec 2, '37
Implantation of costal cartilage for correction of nasal deformities. Gill, E. G. Virginia M. Monthly *65:*279–281, May '38
Use and behavior of iliac bone grafts in restoration of nasal contour; clinical and radiographic observations. Mowlem, R. Rev. de chir. structive *8:*23–29, May '38
Principle to be considered in transplanting costal cartilage for repairing deficiencies of nasal skeleton. Young, F. Ann. Surg. *108:*1113–1117, Dec '38
Cartilage autograft in therapy of saddle nose; case. Moers. Bull. Soc. belge d'oto., rhinol., laryng., pp. 23–24, '38
Correction of saddleback deformities of nose by specially cut cartilage from ear. Harbert, F. Arch. Otolaryng. *31:*339–341, Feb '40
Plastic surgery with cartilage for saddle nose. Rehn, E. Zentralbl. f. Chir. *67:*548–550, March 30, '40
Advantage of mixed bone and cartilage grafts in correction of saddle nose and other depressed deformities of dorsum. Cohen, L. Ann. Otol., Rhin. and Laryng. *49:*410–417, June '40
Graft of costal cartilage in therapy of saddle nose; case. Pedemonte, P. V. Arch. urug. de med., cir. y especialid. *17:*65–67, July '40
Prevention and correction of dorsal depressions by septal implants (nose). Goldman, I. B. Arch. Otolaryng. *32:*524–529, Sept '40
Advantage of mixed bone and cartilage grafts in correction of saddle nose and other depressed deformities of dorsum. Cohen, L. Tr. Am. Laryng., Rhin. and Otol. Soc. *46:*370–376, '40
Osseous autotransplantations in partial rhinoplasties. Malbec, E. F. Semana med.

Nose, Bone and Cartilage Autografts to—Cont.
2:350-354, Aug 7, '41
Bone (iliac) and cartilage transplants to ear and nose; use and behavior. MOWLEM, R. Brit. J. Surg. *29:*182-193, Oct '41
Bone autografts in partial rhinoplasties. MALBEC, E. F. Arq. de cir. clin. e exper. *6:*163-171, April-June '42
Elevation of bridge line of nose (use of iliac bone). MACCOLLUM, D. W. Surgery *12:*97-108, July '42
Cancellous bone transplants for correction of saddle nose. FOMON, S. *et al.* Ann. Otol., Rhin. and Laryng. *54:*518-533, Sept '45

Nose, Bone and Cartilage Heterografts to

Nasal reconstruction by means of auto and iso-grafts. METZENBAUM, M. Ohio State M. J. *24:*196-200, March '28 also: Laryngoscope *38:*197-205, March '28
Bovine cartilage in correction of nasal deformities. STOUT, P. S. Laryngoscope *43:*976-979, Dec '33
Use of bone from cattle in restoration of saddle nose. GONZALEZ ULLOA, M. Rev. mex. de cir., ginec. y cancer *9:*321-329, Aug '41
Use of bone from cattle in restoration of saddle nose. GONZALEZ ULLOA, M. Arq. de cir. clin. e exper. *6:*535-538, April-June '42

Nose, Cancer

Caustic treatment of superficial cancer of ear, nose. CITELLI, AND CALICETI. Tumori *8:*165, Aug '21 abstr: J.A.M.A. *77:*1139, Oct 1, '21
Surgical treatment of saddle nose and malignancies. SMITH, F., J. Michigan M. Soc. *20:*413, Oct '21
Clinical study of carcinoma of nose. SUTTON, R. L., J.A.M.A. *77:*1561, Nov 12, '21
Electrocoagulation and radiation therapy in malignant disease of ear, nose and throat. PFAHLER, G. E., J.A.M.A. *85:*344-347, Aug 1, '25
Basocellular epithelioma of nose. GATÉ, J. AND MASSIA, G. Bull. Soc. franc. de dermat. et syph. *33:*668-673, Nov '26
Epithelioma of nose in girl of 15. FOLLMANN, E. Dermat. Wchnschr. *85:*940-943, July 2, '27
Cancer of nose, and mouth with special reference to treatment by irradiation. EWING, J. Radiology *9:*359-365, Nov '27
Payment epithelial cancer of nasal cavity cured by roentgen treatment; case. MAYER, O. Wien. med. Wchnschr. *78:*587, April 28, '28
Sarcoma of nasal bones; subtotal removal of nose and its reconstruction. COUGHLIN, W. T. Arch. Otolaryng. *7:*588-600, June '28
Inflitrating cancer of nose; acute evolution; treatment by radium; case. MARTÍNEZ, E. AND PUENTE DUANY, N. Bol. de la Liga contra el cancer *3:*145-149, July 1, '28
Cure of epithelioma of nose with Bucky's border rays (grenz rays). BUCKY, G. Arch. f. Dermat. u. Syph. *155:*109-111, '28
One stage plastic surgery after removal of epithelioma of nose and contiguous areas. KURTZAHN, H. Beitr. z. klin. Chir. *144:*50-57, '28
Multiple dermal cancer in face and on neck; case. ODQVIST, H. Acta radiol. *9:*302-304, '28
Operative treatment of radium resistant epitheliomata; cases (of nose). HAUTANT, A. AND MONOD, O. Ann. d. mal. de l'oreille, du larynx *49:*394-410, April '30
Surgical diathermy of cancer of nose. HESSE, W. Deutsche med. Wchnschr. *56:*1479-1481, Aug 29, '30
Rhinophyma with carcinomatous degeneration; case. NOVY, F. G. JR. Arch. Dermat. and Syph. *22:*270-273, Aug '30
Radium therapy of cancer of nose. MORAN, H. M., M. J. Australia *2:*814-817, Dec 20, '30
Plastic operations on cheeks and nose for cancer. WOLF, H. Arch. f. klin. Chir. *160:*105-117, '30
Operation followed by radium therapy in epithelioma of nasal septum; 2 cases. SAKON, H. Ann. d'oto-laryng., pp. 55-60, Jan '31
Naso-orbital epitheliomas; 10 cases. ABOULKER, H. AND GOZLAN, A. Ann. d'oto-laryng., pp. 381-398, April '31
Epithelioma on bridge of nose; case. DERR, J. S. Radiology *16:*955-956, June '31
Case of carcinomatous degeneration of rhinophyma, with remarks on treatment of rhinophyma. EISENKLAM, D. Wien. klin. Wchnschr. *44:*1407-1408, Nov 6, '31
Plastic surgery of face following electrocoagulation treatment of malignant tumors of nose and accessory sinuses. ÖHNGREN, G. Acta oto-laryng. *16:*292-305, '31
Destruction of nose and part of face by squamous-celled carcinoma of rodent ulcer type. RIDOUT, C. A. S. Proc. Roy. Soc. Med. *25:*1767, Oct '32
Five year cures in cancer of mouth, lip, nose, etc. SMITH, F. Surg., Gynec. and Obst. *56:*470-471, Feb (no. 2A) '33
Curability of carcinoma of skin of nose. ERICKSEN, L. G., J. Iowa M. Soc. *25:*309-311, June '35

Nose, Cancer – Cont.

Treatment of carcinoma of mouth and buccopharynx, nose and nasal sinus, with some remarks on diagnosis. PATTERSON, N. Tr. Am. Laryng., Rhin. and Otol. Soc. *41:*1–34, '35

Reparation of loss of substance due to electrosurgical therapy of nasofacial cancer. PRUDENTE, A. Rev. oto-laring. de Sao Paulo (no. 5, bis) *4:*749–810, Sept–Oct '36

Diagnosis and therapy of malignant tumors of nasopharynx. GERLINGS, P. G. AND DEN HOED, D. Nederl. tijdschr. v. geneesk. *81:*581–589, Feb 6, '37

Therapy of epitheliomas of septum of nose. GROS, J. C. Bol. Liga contra el cancer *12:*148–154, May '37

Treatment of epitheliomas of nasolabial fold. MELAND, O. N. Am. J. Roentgenol. *38:*730–739, Nov '37

Gonzalez Loza operation for removing tip of nose. CORA ELISEHT, F. AND BERRI, C. Rev. Asoc. med. argent. *53:*214–215, April 15, '39

Malignant tumors of nasopharynx; anatomicopathologic study. VILLATA, I. Oto-rino-laring. ital. *10:*106–151, March '40

Treatment of cancer of nose. KING, E. Ohio State M. J. *36:*627–628, June '40

Early diagnosis and therapy of cancer of nose. GROS, J. C. Bol. Liga contra el cancer *15:*305–311, Nov '40

Malignant melanoma of nose. KAPLAN, I. I. Arch. Otolaryng. *35:*85–90, Jan '42

Plastic surgery in exeresis of epitheliomas of dorsum of nose. SILVEIRA, L. M. Arq. de cir. clin. e exper. *6:*573–577, April–June '42

Malignant tumors of rhinopharynx with metastases; 15 cases. SCUDERI, R. Arch. ital. di otol. *54:*273–316, Aug '42

Epithelioma of nose; free graft of whole skin; case. MALBEC, E. F. Prensa med. argent. *29:*1763–1765, Nov 4, '42

Free full thickness skin graft in nasal cancer; case. MALBEC, E. F. Semana med. *2:*1489–1491, Dec 17, '42

Basal cell lesions of nose, cheek and lips. DAVIS, W. B. Ann. Surg. *119:*944–948, June '44

Restoration of ala nasi following its excision for cancer. AUBRY, M. AND DUCOURTIOUX, M. Ann. d'oto-laryng., pp. 89–92, July–Sept, '44

Surgical treatment of pain; malignant lesions of face, nose and mouth. ROBERTSON, J. S. Tr. Roy. Med.-Chir. Soc. Glasgow, pp. 29–31, '43- '44; in Glasgow M. J. May -44

Nose, Cartilage Homografts to

Transplantation of cartilage from cadaver according to Mikhelson method in correction of nasal deformities. LITINSKIY, A. M. Novy khir. arkhiv. *48:*211–214, '41

Osteocartilaginous homogenous grafts in partial rhinoplasties. MALBEC, E. F. Dia med. *15:*644–645, June 21, '43

Nose, Choanal Atresia (See also Nose, Anterior Atresia)

Stenosis of nasopharynx. FIGI, F. A. Arch. Otolaryng. *10:*480–490, Nov '29

Choanal atresia; case. FISHBEIN, J. N. Rhode Island M. J. *14:*180–182, Nov '31

Cicatricial stenosis of choanae narium. TORTOLONE, V. Arch. ital. di otol. *43:*265–276, May '32

Congenital atresia of right posterior naris. GROVE, R. C. Virginia M. Monthly *60:*682–684, Feb '34

Permanent results of von Eicken operation for choanal atresia. LABHARDT, E. Schweiz. med. Wchnschr. *66:*1153–1154, Nov 21, '36

Relation between nasal occlusion and development of paranasal sinuses, with special reference to 2 cases of congenital occlusion of choanae. BARBERA, S. Oto-rino-laring. ital. *6:*563–576, Dec '36

Surgery of choanal atresia; roentgenography with iodipin (iodized oil). UFFENORDE, W. Hals-, Nasen-u. Ohrenarzt (Teil 1) *28:*174–175, May '37

Congenital choanal atresia; 2 cases of complete bilateral obstruction. COLVER, B. N. Ann. Otol., Rhin. and Laryng. *46:*358–375, June '37

Congenital occlusion of choana. ANDERSON, C. M., J.A.M.A. *109:*1788–1792, Nov 27, '37

Diathermocoagulation in therapy of congenital imperforation of choanae; 2 cases. GIGNOUX, A. Lyon med. *160:*652–654, Dec 12, '37

Congenital occlusion of choana. ANDERSON, C. M. Tr. Sect. Laryng., Otol. and Rhin., A.M.A., pp. 83–97, '37

Technic of surgical therapy of osseous choanal diaphragm. BORGHESAN, E. Valsalva *14:*73–75, Feb '38

New method of operation for congenital atresia of posterior nares. DONNELLY, J. C. Arch. Otolaryng. *28:*112–125, July '38

Unilateral choanal imperforation, with report of case. VIALE DEL CARRIL, A. Rev. Asoc. med. argent. *52:*977–979, Sept 30, '38

Nose, Choanal Atresia – Cont.

Atresia of choana; 3 cases. LESHCHINSKIY, Y. L. Zhur. ush., nos. i gorl. bolez. *15:*471–475, '38

Congenital occlusion of posterior nasal choanae. KELLY, D. B. Brit. M. J. *1:*157–158 Jan 28, '39

Congenital choanal atresia; cases. DE MARTINI, R. Boll. d. mal. d. orecchio, d. gola, d. naso *57:*14–22, Jan '39

Unilateral congenital imperforation of choana; case with slight surgical correction. OLIVE LEITE, A. Rev. brasil. de oto-rino-laring. *7:*49–58, Jan–Feb '39

Nasopharyngeal atresia; description of operation. GOODYEAR, H. M. Arch. Otolaryng. *29:*974–976, June '39

Congenital atresia of posterior choana of nose. BROWNELL, D. H. Univ. Bull. Ann Arbor *5:*68, Sept '39

Congenital occlusion of choanae; brief review of 12 cases. PASTORE, P. N. AND WILLIAMS, H. L. Proc. Staff Meet., Mayo Clin. *14:*625–627, Oct 4, '39

Choanal imperforation of nose. PADILLA Y CESPEDES, V. M. Rev. san. mil., Habana *4:*292–294, Oct–Dec '40

Congenital bilateral diaphragm of choana; case. DAL LAGO, E. Boll. d. mal. d. orecchio, d. gola, d. naso *58:*450–458, Dec '40

Congenital atresia of posterior nares. MANGIARACINA, A. Arch. Otolaryng. *32:*1088–1089, Dec '40

Congenital atresia of posterior choanae. COOK, J. A. L. South African M. J. *15:*498–499, Dec 27, '41

Congenital atresia of posterior nares; 2 cases. SCHWARTZ, A. A. AND ISAACS, H. J. Arch. Otolaryng. *35:*603–612, April '42

Transpalatine route in therapy of bilateral congenital inperforation of choanae, with report of cases. REBELO NETO, J. Rev. brasil. de oto-rino-laring. *10:*431–441, July–Aug '42

Treatment of congenital atresia of choanae. KAZANJIAN, V. H. Ann. Otol., Rhin. and Laryng. *51:*704–711, Sept '42

Congenital choanal atresia. ROBERTS, G. J. U. S. Nav. M. Bull. *43:*1216–1219, Dec '44

Congenital atresia of posterior nares; descriptions of technics used in meeting operative difficulties and report of case. BOYD, H. M. E. Arch. Otolaryng. *41:*261–271, April '45

Bilateral congenital atresia of choanae. KLAFF, D. D. Arch. Otolaryng. *41:*298–299, April '45

Transpalatine operation for congenital atresia of choanae in small child or infant. RUDDY, L. W. Arch. Otolaryng. *41:*432–438, June '45

Postoperative results in 2 cases of congenital choanal occlusion. BONHAM, W. L. Eye, Ear, Nose and Throat Monthly *25:*387–393, Aug '46

Nasopharyngeal stenosis and its correction. KAZANJIAN, V. H. AND HOLMES, E. M. Arch. Otolaryng. *44:*261–273, Sept '46

Nose, Cleft Lip Deformities of

Reconstruction of nostril in simple hare-lip. OMBRÉDANNE, L. Presse med. *29:*703, Sept 3, '21

Nasal relation of harelip operations. BROWN, G. V. I., J.A.M.A. *77:*1954, Dec 17, '21

Correction of nose deformities at operations for harelip. MEYER, H. Zentralbl. f. Chir. *49:*220, Feb 18, '22 (illus.)

Recommended procedure for relief of ala deformity in certain cases in adult associated with harelip and its mechanical counterpart. SHEEHAN, J. E., M. J. and Rec. *120:*72–73, July 16, '24

Treatment of unilateral harelip with special reference to associated deformity of nose. COLEMAN, C. C. Virginia M. Monthly *51:*393–399, Oct '24

Nasal deformities associated with congenital cleft of lip. BLAIR, V. P., J.A.M.A. *84:*185–187, Jan 17, '25

Problem of bringing forward retracted upper lip and nose in harelip. BLAIR, V. P. Surg., Gynec. and Obst. *42:*128–132, Jan '26

Role of median nasal process in development of face; study of hare-lip. VEAU, V. Ann. d'anat. path. *3:*305–348, April '26 abstr: J.A.M.A. *87:*1160, Oct 2, '26

Transplantation of strip of cheek and naris in harelip therapy. EHRENFELD, H. Arch. f. klin. Chir. *144:*486–488, '27

Plastic surgery of face and harelip and nose, and cleft palate. JOBSON, G. B. Atlantic M. J. *31:*716–723, July '28

Flat nose, consequent to harelip operations; operative treatment. OMBRÉDANNE, L. AND OMBRÉDANNE, M. Ann. d. mal. de l'oreille, du larynx *47:*1090–1111, Dec '28

Repair of harelip and accompanying nasal deformity. PADGETT, E. C., J. Kansas M. Soc. *30:*143–147, May '29

Treatment of secondary deformity in cases of harelip (nose). NEW, G. B. AND FIGI, F. A. Minnesota Med. *14:*514–516, June '31

Correction of losses and deformities of exter-

Nose, Cleft Lip Deformities of–Cont.
nal nose, including those associated with harelip. BLAIR, V. P. California and West. Med. *36:*308–313, May '32
Plastic correction of nasal deformities after operation for harelip. EITNER, E. Deutsche Ztschr. f. Chir. *238:*644–646, '33
Correction of alar deformity in cleft lip. MCINDOE, A. H. Lancet *1:*607–609, March 12, '38
Cases of cheiloplasty; description of apparatus for feeding infants with harelip and cleft palate. Also: rhinoplasty. BRISOTTO, P. Boll. d. mal. d. oreccio, d. gola, d. naso *56:*89–99, March '38
Nostril in secondary harelip. HUMBY, G. Lancet *1:*1275, June 4, '38
Practical problems in surgical correction of harelip; and nose, palate defects. CALLISTER, A. C. Rocky Mountain M. J. *35:*698–701, Sept '38
Nasal deformities in harelip; surgical therapy. MICHALEK-GRODZKI. Rev. de chir. structive *8:*205–210, '38
Nasal deformity in harelip; technic of plastic correction. ZENO, L. Bol. Soc. de cir. de Rosario *7:*408–414, Oct '40 also: An. de cir. *6:*388–394, Dec '40
Secondary repair of cleft lips and their nasal deformities. BROWN, J. B. AND MC5-DOWELL, F. Ann. Surg. *114:*101–117, July '41
Secondary nasal deformities following correction of cleft lip. CINELLI, A. A. Laryngoscope *51:*1053–1058, Nov '41
Secondary repair of cleft lips and their nasal deformities. BROWN, J. B. AND MCDOWELL, F. Am. J. Orthodontics (Oral Surg. Sect) *27:*712–727, Dec '41
Nasal deformity in harelip; anatomic study. APOLO, E. Arq. de cir. clin. e exper. *6:*339–343, April–June '42
Nasal deformity in harelip; surgical problem. APOLO, E. Arq. de cir. clin. e exper. *6:*645–651, April–June '42
Wide nostril in unilateral cleft lip. VAUGHAN, H. S. Tr. Am. Soc. Plastic and Reconstructive Surg. *12:*117–123, '43

Nose, Deformity
Gillies new method in giving support to depressed nasal bridge and columella. SHEEHAN, J. E. New York M. J. *113:*448, March 16, '21
Deformities of nose of developmental type. METZENBAUM, M. Ohio State M. J. *17:*382, June '21
Surgery of nasal deformities. GUTHRIE, D. Edinburgh M. J. *27:*365, Dec '21

Nose, Deformity–Cont.
Bifid nose. WILKINSON, G., J. Laryngol. and Otol. *37:*560–563, Nov '22 (illus.)
Rare malformation of alae of nose. LIEBERMANN, T. V. Klin. Wchnschr. *2:*307, Feb 12, '23
Malformations of nose and their correction. PRECECHTĚL, A. Cas. lek. cesk. *62:*305–308, March 24, '23 (illus.)
Correction of deformities of nose and about orbit bz plastic surgery. DE RIVER, J. P. Southwestern Med. *7:*226–232, July '23
Correction of nasal deformities. SHEEHAN, J. E. Brit. M. J. *2:*981–982, Nov. 24, '23
Case of double nose. MUECKE, F. F. AND SOUTTAR, H. S. Proc. Roy. Soc. Med. (sect. Laryng.). *17:*8–9, Jan '24
Nasal deformities and their correction. WILSON, A. K., J. Florida M. A. *10:*270–273, April '24
Martyrdom of the nose. PULLEINE, R. H., M. J. Australian (supp.) *1:*385–386, June 7, '24
Peculiar malformation of nose. MENYHÁRD, I. Jahrb. f. Kinderh. *106:*128–129, June '24
Correction of congenital deformities of nose; report of 9 selected cases. LEWIS, J. D. Laryngoscope *34:*593–608, Aug '24
Congenital defect of left ala of nose. REDER, F., S. Clin. N. America *5:*1313–1320, Oct '25
Absence of one nostril. JUARISTI, V. Arch. espan. de pediat. *10:*299–300, May '26
Rare congenital malformations of nose; case histories, and treatment: (1) fibrolipoma of septum, harelip; (2) bull-dog nose, fibrolipoma of dorsum of nose. FEYGIN, N. Zentralbl. f. Chir. *53:*1686, July 3, '26
Surgery of nasal deformities. LEROUX, R. Vie med. *7:*2499, Dec 3, '26
Congenital anomaly of external nose. BENJAMINS, C. E. AND STIBBE, F. H. Nederl. Tijdschr. v. Geneesk. *2:*2543–2549, Dec 4, '26
Particular form of congenital median fissure of nose; independence of pars lacrimalis of nasal process. SCHWOERER, M. Frankfurt. Ztschr. f. Path. *34:*48–64, '26
New operative method in anterior nasal atresia. BOCKSTEIN, F. Ztschr. f. Hals-, Nasen- u. Ohrenh. *17:*180–187, Jan 31, '27
Nasal deformities plastic repair; cases. BRUSOTTI, A. Stomatol. *25:*161–181, March '27
Aspiration of ala nasi and its operative treatment. Bosviel J. J. de med. de Paris *46:*417, May 26, '27
Surgery of nasal deformities. SANVENERO-ROSSELLI, G. Ann. di laring., otol. *28:*193–216, July '27
Surgical correction of congenital and acquired deformities of nasal pyramid. SEBI-

Nose, Deformity–Cont.

LEAU, P. AND DUFOURMENTEL, L. Ann. d. mal. de l'oreille, du larynx *46:*753, Aug; 853, Sept '27

Technic of correction of nasal deformity by adjustment of proper tissues. SANVENERO-ROSSELLI, G. Rassegna ital. di oto-rino-laring. *1:*223–231, Sept-Oct '27

Congenital deformity of nasal bones. BENJAMINS, C. E. AND STIBBE, F. H. Acta oto-laryng. *11:*274–284, '27

Case of bulldog nose. BUMBA, J. AND LUCKSCH, F. Virchow's Arch. f. path. Anat. *264:*554–562, '27

Congenital choanal imperforation; operation. BEYNES, E. Arch. internat. de laryng. *34:*179–183, Feb '28

Best method of correction of snub-nose. ROY, J. N. Arch. internat. de laryng. *34:*166–178, Feb '28

Congenital malformation of nose; case. DI VESTEA, D. Valsalva *5:*214–219, April '29

Sincipital hydro-encephalocele with deformity of nose. BENDER, E. Arch. f. klin. Chir. *161:*625–632, '30

Meningo-encephaloma of right nasofrontal region with malformation of nose and forehead; case. ROCHER, H. L., J. de med. de Bordeaux *107:*571–573, July 20, '30

Loss of nasal ala and upper lip reconstruction. FIGI, F. A., S. Clin. North America *11:*834–837, Aug '31

Rule for operation in atresia of nares. MATWEJEW, D. N. Monatschr. f. Ohrenh. *65:*1188–1192, Oct '31

Defects of tip of nose; surgical correction. (Comment on Wodak's article.) HALLA, F. Med. Klin. *28:*50, Jan 8, '32

Osseous atresia of posterior choanae. STINSON, W. D. Arch. Otolaryng. *15:*101–103, Jan '32

Surgical correction of unusual type of syphilitic deformity of nostril. MONCORPS, C. Dermat. Wchnschr. *94:*383–386, March 12, '32

Unusual case of human teratology (complete absence of one nostril). LETO, L. Boll. d. mal. d. orecchio, d. gola, d. naso *50:*129–137, May '32

Noseless man. KHANDEKAR, K. G. Indian M. Gaz. *67:*267–268, May '32

Plastic surgery of nasal deformities. WODAK, E. Rev. de chir. plastique, pp. 157–169, July '32

Surgical therapy of nasal deformities; 2 cases. LARROUDÉ, C. Rev. de chir. plastique, pp. 246–250, Oct '33

Histology and pathogenesis of some marked abnormalities of nose. STUPKA, W. Acta oto-laryng. *19:*1–5, '33

Nose, Deformity–Cont.

Arrhinencephalia with incomplete development of nose; case. HENZE, K. Beitr. z. prakt. u. theoret. Hals-, Nasen-u. Ohrenh. *31:*241–247, '34

Correction of deformities of forehead and nose; presentation of 2 patients. NEW, G. B. Proc. Staff Meet., Mayo Clin. *10:*519–521, Aug 14, '35

Hypertelorism, case with unusual congenital malformation of external portion of nose, double overlapping external parts. VAN VOORTHUYSEN, D. G. W. Acta oto-laryng. *22:*540–544, '35

Surgical correction of bull-dog nose; case. DOBRZANIECKI, W., J. de chir. *48:*191–196, Aug '36

Rare congenital malformation of nose (transverse duplication of fossa); case. SIMONETTA, B. Boll. d. mal. d. orecchio, d. gola. d. naso *54:*361–366, Oct '36

Pathology and embryogenesis of deformities of nose and lip. BURIAN, F. Casop. lek. cesk. *76:*101, Jan 29, '37; 138, Feb 5, '37

Persistent bucconasal membrane in newborn. LEMERE, H. B., J.A.M.A. *109:*347–348, July 31, '37

Rare congenital malformation of nose and lower eyelid. GRITTI, P. Boll. d. mal. d. orecchio, d. gola, d. naso *55:*321–334, Sept '37

Plastic repair of deformities about lower part of nose resulting from loss of tissue. KAZANJIAN, V. H. Tr. Am. Acad. Ophth. *42:*338–366, '37

Transpalatinal therapy of congenital choanal atresia. SCHWECKENDIEK, H. Ztschr. f. Hals-, Nasen-u. Ohrenh. *42:*367–373, '37

Atresia of choana of nose; case. CHILDREY, J. H. Laryngoscope *48:*51–53, Jan '38

Photographic record of case of unusual congenital nasal deformity. METZENBAUM, M. Rev. de chir. structive *8:*20–21, May '38

Congenital eyelid ptosis with rhinomalacia (lack of ossification of nasal bones); case. REBELO NETO, J. Rev. Assoc. paulista de med. *12:*455–464, May '38

Rare malformation of nose; case. SCHMIDT, B. Monatschr. f. Ohrenh. *72:*880–893, Sept '38

Crooked nose. CINELLI, A. A. Laryngoscope 48:760–764, Oct '38

Rhinocele; case. CORA ELISEHT, F. Rev. Asoc. med. argent. *53:*18–19, Jan 15–30, '39

Joseph operation in plastic repair of bulldog nose; case. OHNO, T. Oto-rhino-laryng. *12:*10, Jan '39

Blocking and forming of nose in child aged 4. DUJARDIN, E. Ugesk. f. laeger *101:*211–212, Feb 16, '39

Two congenital deformities; bifid nose and

Nose, Deformity – Cont.

bulldog nose. KOPP, M. M. Laryngoscope *49:*1128–1133, Nov '39

Gibbous nose; plastic surgery. RODRIGUEZ DIAZ, A. Rev. de cien. med. *2:*79–82, March '39

Correction of cleft nose. EITNER, E. Deutsche Ztschr. f. Chir. *252:*507–510, '39

Median fissure of nose; surgical therapy of cases. ESSER, E. Plast. chir. *1:*40–50, '39

Deformities of nose due to septal abnormalities. KOPP, M. M., M. Rec. *151:*111–116, Feb 21, '40

Congenital atresia of postnasal orifices; simple, effective office technic for treatment by electrocoagulation. MORGENSTERN, D. J. Arch. Otolaryng. *31:*653–662, April '40

Plastic correction of cartilaginous crooked nose. KLICPERA, L. Arch. f. Ohren-, Nasen-u. Kehlkopfh. *147:*170–172, '40

Rare congenital malformation of face; median harelip with dissociation without deformation of 2 halves of nose (double nose); case. STEFANI, F. Plast. chir. *1:*162–166, '40

Nasal deformities. SCHER, S. L. Arch. Otolaryng. *34:*307–320, Aug '41

Method of plastic surgery in correction of unilateral arrhinia; case. RUDERT, H. Arch. f. Ohren-, Nasen-u. Kehlkopfh. *150:*168–174, '41

Congenital choanal occlusion. BONHAM, W. L. South. M. J. *35:*252–257, March '42

Hypertelorism; case with median nasal fissure. ZENO, L. An. de cir. *8:*37–39, March–June '42 also: Bol. Soc. de cir. de Rosario *9:*59–62, May '42

Nasal defects in students; psychologic aspects and plastic correction. CODAZZI AGUIRRE, J. A. Arq. de cir. clin. e exper. *6:*194–197, April–June '42

Nasal deformity of syphilitic type due to injury; loss of mucosa and of supporting bone and cartilage; modified Gillies operation in therapy of case. DELLEPIANE RAWSON, R. AND PEREZ FERNANDEZ, M. Arq. de cir. clin. e exper. *6:*492–503, April–June '42

Deformity of nasal entrance. MCKENZIE, W. R. South. M. J. *35:*433–443, May '42

Management of nasal deformities in infants and small children; and ear, eyelids, lips and palate deform. PEER, L. A. Dis. Eye, Ear, Nose and Throat *2:*166–176, June '42

Hypertelorism associated with median nasal cleft; case. ZENO, L. An. argent. de oftal. *4:*3–5, Jan–March '43

New technic for surgical therapy of congenital coloboma of ala nasi. REBELO NETO, J. Rev. brasil. de oto-rino-laring. *11:*159–165, March–April '43

Nose, Deformity – Cont.

Treatment of nasal deformities. DE RYNCK, G., M. Press *210:*154–157, Sept 8, '43

Case showing partial deficient fusion of maxillary process with lateral nasal process on one side. DODDS, G. E. Brit. J. Ophth. *27:*414–415, Sept '43

Congenital occlusion of both anterior nares. JERVEY, J. W. JR. Ann. Otol., Rhin. and Laryng. *53:*182–184, March '44

Median harelip and bifid nose; case. LAGOS GARCIA, A. Semana med. *2:*237–241, Aug 3, '44

Correction of multiple deformities of nose. GATEWOOD, W. L. Eye, Ear, Nose and Throat Monthly *24:*134–138, March '45

Postoperative results in 2 cases of congenital choanal occlusion. BONHAM, W. L. Eye, Ear, Nose and Throat Monthly *25:*387–393, Aug '46

Bifid nose associated with midline cleft of upper lip. WEAVER, D. F. AND BELLINGER, D. H. Arch. Otolaryng. *44:*480–482, Oct '46

Nose, Dermoid Cyst

Dermoid cysts of dorsum of nose. MARCHINI, F. Policlinico (sez. prat.) *30:*1422, Oct 29, '23

Dermoid cyst of dorsum of nose; citation of case. HART, V. K. Laryngoscope *37:*760–763, Oct '27

Congenital fistulae and dermoid cysts on dorsum of nose. VERMEULEN, B. S. Geneesk. gids *7:*1117–1126, Dec 6, '29

Cystic tumors of anterior nares due to embryonal maldevelopment; 3 cases. ARNOLDI, W. Ztschr. f. Laryng., Rhin. *18:*58–69, '29

Dermoid cyst of nose; case. TRAMPNAU. Ztschr. f. Hals-, Nasen-u. Ohrenh. *28:*163–165, March 3, '31

Etiology and operation of congenital dermoid on dorsum of nose. BESELIN, O. Arch. f. Ohren-, Nasen-u. Kehlkopfh. *129:*47–49, June 6, '31

Dermoid cysts of dorsum of nose; 3 cases. HACQUEBORD, P. Geneesk. gids *9:*721–728, July 31, '31

Congenital fistulae and dermoid cysts on dorsum of nose. VERMEULEN, B. S. Acta oto-laryng. *16:*48–56, '31

Dermoid cyst of bridge of nose. LUONGO, R. Rinasc. med. *10:*185–186, April 15, '33

Dermoid cyst of nasal dorsum. LUONGO, R. A. Arch. Otolaryng. *17:*755–759, June '33

Origin of congenital fistula of dorsum of nose. SIMONETTA, B. Boll. d. mal. d. orecchio, d. gola, d. naso *51:*503–512, Dec '33

Nose, Dermoid Cyst—Cont.

Medial nasal fistula. KHARCHAK, E. Acta oto-laryng. *19:*73-76, '33

Dermoid cyst of nasal dorsum. POWELL, L. S. Arch. Otolaryng. *19:*67-68, Jan '34

Congenital epithelial ducts and cysts of bridge of nose. BENJAMINS, C. E. Nederl. tijdschr. v. geneesk. *80:*1886-1890, May 2, 36 also: Acta oto-laryng. *24:*284-297, '36

Congenital fistula and dermoid cyst of nasal dorsum; surgical therapy of 2 cases. PORTO, G. Rev. oto-laring. de Sao Paulo *5:*275-278, May-June '37 also: Arq. Inst. Penido Burnier *4:*320-323, June '37

Congenital fistula and dermoid cyst of nasal dorsum. JAROS, Z. Casop. lek. cesk. *77:*540-541, April 29, '38

Congenital dermoid cyst and fistula of dorsum of nose; case. HAGENS, E. W. Arch. Otolaryng. *28:*399-403, Sept '38

Origin of congenital fistulas of bridge of nose. MAGNONI, A. Acta oto-laryng. *27:*174-180, '39

Dermoid cysts of nasal dorsum; plastic surgery in cases. MALBEC, E. F. Semana med. *2:*788-792, Sept 30, '43

Congenital fistula of nasal dorsum; radical extirpation; cases. MARINO, H. Prensa med. argent. *30:*2297-2300, Dec 1, '43

Fissural cyst of nose (facial cleft). ROSENBERGER, H. C. Arch. Otolaryng. *40:*288-290, Oct '44

Nose, Fractures

Reduction of old fractures of nose. WHITHAM, J. D. Laryngoscope *31:*620, Aug '21

Fracture of nose and its treatment. JACQUES. Paris med. *11:*199, Sept 3, '21 abstr: J.A.M.A. *77:*1289, Oct 15, '21

Management of recent fractures of nose. COHEN, L. Ann. Otol. Rhinol. and Laryng. *30:*690, Sept '21

Recent fractures of nose; how to diagnose and treat them. CARTER, W. W. Med. Rec. *101:*237-239, Feb 11, '22

Recent nasal fractures. FRANK, I. Ann. Otol., Rhin. and Laryng. *32:*768-779, Sept '23

Immediate and late treatment of nasal fractures. COHEN, L. Laryngoscope *33:*847-853, Nov '23 (illus.)

Nasal fractures; treatment of same by new adjustable splint. SALINGER, S. Ann. Otol., Rhin. and Laryng. *33:*413-416, June '24

Fractures of nose. GILE, B. C. Atlantic M. J. *28:*512-515, May '25

Adjustable splint for fractures of nose. SALINGER, S. Illinois M. J. *48:*304-306, Oct '25

Treatment of old and recent nasal fractures. SARGNON, A. Arch. internat. de laryngol.

Nose, Fractures—Cont.

*33:*129-148, Feb '27

Aims of early treatment of nasal fractures. HUET, P. C. Medecine *9:*317-318, Jan '28

Early treatment of nasal fractures. HUET, P. C., J. de chir. *31:*649-658, May '28

Esthetic reduction of nasal fractures with new apparatus; case. PROBY, H. Arch. internat. de laryng. *34:*866-868, July-Aug '28

Pathogenesis and treatment of nasal fractures. HUET, P. C. Ann. d. mal. de l'oreille, du larynx *47:*797-833, Sept '28

Treatment of nasal fractures. GILLES, H. D. AND KILNER, T. P. Lancet *1:*147-149, Jan 19, '29

Importance of early treatment of recent nasal fractures. CARTER, W. W. Am. J. Surg. *6:*51-55, Jan '29

Treatment of nasal fractures. JESSAMAN, L. W. New England J. Med. *200:*753-756, April 11, '29

Nasal fractures and their treatments. FUCHS, V. H. New Orleans M. and S. J. *81:*802-806, May '29

Treatment of nasal deformities and fractures. RISDON, F. Canad. M. A. J. *20:*631-633, June '29

New instrument for reduction of nasal fractures. SALINGER, S. Arch. Otolaryng. *9:*657-658, June '29

Nasal fractures. BECK, C. K. Kentucky M. J. *27:*387-390, Sept '29

Prevention of nasal deformities (fractures). CARTER, W. W. Ann. Otol., Rhin. and Laryng. *39:*696-700, Sept '30

Plea for early treatment of nasal fractures. WHITE, F. W. Laryngoscope *41:*253-256, April '31

Recent nasal fractures. ATKINSON, D. T. Eye, Ear, Nose and Throat Monthly *10:*147-148, May '31

Treatment of recent nasal fractures. SARGNON, A. Rev. de chir. plastique, pp. 111-130, July '31

Treatment of fresh nasal fractures and nasal sinuses. KLESTADT, W. Med. Klin. *27:* 1235-1237, Aug 21, '31

Fractures involving nasal bones. SEIGALL, H. A. AND MANCOLL, M. M., M. J. and Rec. *134:*328-329, Oct 7, '31

Nasal fractures. WATSON-WILLIAMS, E. Brit. M. J. *2:*791-794, Oct 31, '31

Management of nasal fractures. RISDON, E. F. Ann. Otol., Rhin. and Laryng. *40:*1094-1098, Dec '31

Fracture of inferior turbinate bone of nose. RICHTER, E. Deutsche Ztschr. f. Chir. *232:*380-381, '31

Nose, Fractures – Cont.

Management of nasal fractures. RISDON, E. F. Tr. Am. Acad. Ophth. *36:*193–198, '31

Straightening of recently fractured nose. SARGNON, AND EUVRARD. Lyon med. *149:*353–355, March 20, '32

Plastic surgery of nasal fractures. COELST. Rev. de chir. plastique, pp. 54–68, April '32

Therapy of nasal fractures. GONZÁLEZ LOZA, M. Rev. med. del Rosario *22:*514–529, July '32

Scarless reconstruction of nose broken in childhood. HEINEMANN, O. Med. Klin. *28:*1427–1428, Oct 7, '32

Recent nasal fractures. MCWILLIAMS, C. A. New Orleans M. and S. J. *85:*336–339, Nov '32

Restoration of shape of nose by cartilaginous autograft after old fracture. DANTLO, R. Strasbourg med. *93:*485–487, July 15, '33

Treatment of severer cases of nasal fractures (splint). WATKINS, A. B. K. Brit. M. J. *2:*917–918, Nov 18, '33

Unsuspected chronic bronchiectasis from inhalation of fragment of bone – unusual sequel to comminuted fracture of nasal bones. CRAN, B. S., J. Laryng. and Otol. *48:*821–823, Dec '33

Treatment of nasal fractures. COX, G. H., M. Times and Long Island M. J. *62:*171–175, June '34

Nasal fractures in connection with fracture of facial cranium. CSILLAG, S. Monatschr. f. Ohrenh. *68:*663–669, June '34 also: Orvosi hetil. *78:*586–588, June 30, '34

Nasal fractures. BERMAN, H. L., M. Rec. *140:*17, July 4, '34

Nasal fractures. DUFOURMENTEL, L. Bull. med., Paris *48:*811–814, Dec 29, '34

Depression fracture of root of nose. VOGEL, K. Ztschr. f. Laryng., Rhin. Otol. *25:*426–428, '34

Simple rules for management of recent nasal fractures in general practice. SCHWARTZ, V. J. Minnesota Med. *18:*101–106, Feb '35

Correction of recent and old nasal fractures. COX, G. H. Laryngoscope *45:*188–197, March '35

Management of recent fractures of nose and sinuses. WOODWARD, F. D. Ann. Otol., Rhin. and Laryng. *44:*264–273, March '35

Nasal fractures in clinical practice. FELDSTEIN, E. Rev. gen. de clin. et de therap. *49:*388–390, June 15, '35

Therapy of nasal fractures. POULT, J. Schweiz. med. Wchnschr. *65:*638–639, July 13, '35

Fractures of nasal and malar bones. NEW, G. B., S. Clin. North America *15:*1241–1250, Oct '35

Nose, Fractures – Cont.

Treatment of old unreduced nasal fractures. FOMON, S. Ann. Surg. *104:*107–117, July '36

Late complications of nasal fractures. DUFOURMENTEL, L. Paris med. *2:*152–155, Sept 5, '36

Cranial prosthesis and restoration of nose in fractures of nose and frontal part of cranium. PONT, A. Rev. de chir. structive, pp. 34–37, March '37

New type of plaster of paris protector for use in therapy of nasal fractures. GAUS, W. Hals-, Nasen-u. Ohrenarzt (Teil 1) *28:*94–97, April '37

Nasal fractures. KELLY, J. D. Am. J. Surg. *36:*77–82, April '37

Therapy of old nasal fractures; 3 cases. EITNER, E. Zentralbl. f. Chir. *64:*1096–1101, May 8, '37

Endonasal free graft in therapy of old fractures of nose. SARGNON, A. Rev. de chir. structive, pp. 185–204, Oct '37

Modern management of nasal fractures; collective review. STRAITH, C. L. AND DE KLEINE, E. H. Internat. Abstr. Surg. *66:*9–15, '38; in Surg., Gynec. and Obst. Jan '38

Lateral pressure splint in nasal fractures. KAZANJIAN, V. H. Arch. Otolaryng. *27:*474–475, April '38

Treatment of nasal fractures. IBBOTSON, W. M. Press *197:*8–12, July 6, '38

Favorable time for reposition of nasal fractures. HOGEWIND, F. Geneesk. gids *16:*781, July 15, '38

Plaster cast in therapy of nasal fractures. ZENO, L. An. de cir. *4:*124–127, June '38 also: Bol. Soc. de cir. de Rosario *5:*269–272, July '38

Traumatic fracture of nasal septum and its therapy. ALVES, O. Rev. oto-laring. de Sao Paulo *6:*373–378, Sept–Oct '38

One hundred broken noses. GERRIE, J. W. Canad. M. A. J. *39:*433–436, Nov '38

Fractures of nose and their otorhinolaryngologic complications. COELST. Bull. Soc. belge d'oto., rhinol., laryng., pp. 69–71, '38

Technic of making plaster of paris cast for nasal fractures and deformities. RODE, B. Ztschr. f. Hals-, Nasen-u. Ohrenh. *43:*294–295, '38

Recent nasal fractures; surgical therapy. GOT, A. Rev. de laryng. *60:*166–171, Feb '39

Therapy of nasal fractures. IVANISSEVICH, O. *et al.* Bol. y trab. de la Soc. de cir. de Buenos Aires *23:*9–14, April 12, '39

Treatment of facial fractures and nose. WHITHAM, J. D. Laryngoscope *49:*394–400, May '39

Nasal fractures and their therapy. ROSTOCK,

Nose, Fractures – Cont.

P. Med. Welt *13:*953-954, July 8, '39

Maneuvers for reducing fractures of nasal pyramid with luxation or simple luxations of bones. VERNAZA, F. Colombia med. *2:*70-73, March-April '40

Nasal fractures. MOORE, P. M. JR. AND HARRIS, H. E. Am. J. Surg. *50:*668-671, Dec '40

Treatment of nasal fractures. HUME, E. C. Am. J. Orthodontics (Oral Surg. Sect) *27:*105, Feb '41

Recent fracture of nasal base lines of both outer nasal walls, with divergent displacement; orthopedic procedures for obtaining anatomic reduction of osseous and cartilaginous nasal framework. METZENBAUM, M. F. Arch. Otolaryng. *34:*723-735, Oct '41

Nasal fractures in children; diagnosis and treatment. SALINGER, S. Arch. Otolaryng. *34:*936-951, Nov '41

New traction and fixation apparatus for fractured nose. GONZALEZ ULLOA, M. Rev. mex. de cir., ginec. y cancer *10:*65-74, Feb '42 also: Rev. brasil. de cir. *11:*215-218, May '42

Nasal fractures. WALDRON, C. W. Minnesota Med. *25:*258-267, April '42

Plaster splint for fractured noses. PARSONS, H. H. Mil. Surgeon *91:*212, Aug '42

Fractures involving nasal accessory sinuses. NAFTZGER, J. B. Tr. Am. Laryng., Rhin. and Otol. Soc. *48:*333-341, '42

Nasal fracture device. WOMACK, D. R., U. S. Nav. M. Bull. *41:*852-856, May '43

Early care of nasal fractures. CURDIN, M. U. S. Nav. M. Bull. *41:*1706-1712, Nov '43

Nasal fractures and their treatment. WODAK, E. Harefuah *25:*211, Dec 1, '43

Dental arch of upper jaw as support for apparatus during surgical interventions on head in cases of nasal fractures and corrections, skin grafts of face and mobilization of maxillary ankylosis. KUNZENDORF, W. Deutsche Ztschr. f. Chir. *258:*348, '43

Nasal fractures; cases. DUARTE CARDOSO, A. Rev. brasil. de oto-rino-laring. *12:*284-296, July-Oct '44

Prosthetic appliance for comminuted fracture of nose; case. SCHORK, C. J., J. Oral Surg. *2:*324-328, Oct '44

Nasal fractures. FOX, S. L. Eye, Ear, Nose and Throat Monthly *24:*286-287, June '45

Plastic surgery of nasal fractures. LAMONT, E. S. Am. J. Surg. *69:*144-154, Aug '45

Fracture-dislocations of cartilaginous nose; anatomico-pathologic considerations and treatment. MALINIAC, J. W. Arch. Otolaryng. *42:*131-137, Aug '45

Management of fractures of bony vault of nose. HERSH, J. H. Ann. Otol., Rhin. and Laryng. *54:*534-553, Sept '45

Treatment of nasal fractures of long standing. MOE, R. Nord. med. (Norsk mag. f. laegevidensk.) *27:*1907-1917, Sept 21, '45

Fracture of frontal and nasal bones. GONZALEZ ULLOA, M. Vida nueva *56:*195-201, Dec '45

Fractures of nose. WATSON, O. A., J. Oklahoma M. A. *39:*337-340, Aug '46

Nose, Infections of

Abscesses of nasal septum, their etiology and treatment with reference to resulting deformities. CARTER, W. W., M. J. and Rec. *119:*11-13, Feb 6, '24

Furuncles of nose and upper lip. DUFOURMENTEL, L. Prat. med. franc. *14:*171-178, March (A) '33

Furuncles of upper lip and nose. GAUS, W. Therap. d. Gegenw. *77:*75-76, Feb '36

Gangrenous inflammation of nose and upper jaw of uncertain etiology; 2 cases. JOISTEN, E. Ztschr. f. Hals-, Nasen-u. Ohrenh. *41:*105-128, '36

Results of operative treatment of nasal infections and deformities. MOFFETT, A. J. Birmingham M. Rev. *14:*161-169, Sept '39

Nasal furuncle. MAYER, F. J. Monatschr. f. Ohrenh. *74:*167-182, April '40

Intranasal granuloma of sporothrix type producing marked deformity. ORTMAYER, M. AND HUMPHREYS, E. M. Ann. Surg. *113:*118-122, Jan '41

Microaerophilic hemolytic streptococcus infection causing destruction of nose. COSTELLO, M. J., J.A.M.A. *121:*36-38, Jan 2, '43

Nasal septal abscess. LAUB, G. R. South. Med. and Surg. *106:*374, Oct '44

Nose, Injuries of

External nasal deformities of traumatic origin; report of 6 cases. LEWIS, J. D., S. Clin. N. America *3:*1409-1420, Oct '23 (illus.)

Relation of minor injuries of nose during childhood to subsequent deformities of organ. CARTER, W. W. Ann. Otol., Rhin. and Laryng. *35:*825-833, Sept '26

External, traumatic deformity of nose with total destruction of both fossae; surgical treatment. ZUBIZARRETA, H. Rev. de cir. *7:*380-384, Aug '28 also: Rev. de especialid. *3:*646-652, Nov '28

Treatment of crushing injuries to nose and adjacent structures. POTTS, J. B. Surg. J. *34:*196-198, Nov-Dec '28

Nasal injuries. KARÁSEK, M. Casop. lek. cesk. *69:*92-94, Jan 10, '30

Nose, Injuries of–Cont.

Nasal reconstruction by means of bone and cartilage existing within old traumatized nose; illustrated by plaster models and lantern slides of preoperative and postoperative cases. METZENBAUM, M. Laryngoscope *40:*488–494, July '30

Development of nose; dynamic relation to traumatic injuries and to submucous resection. CARTER, W. W. Laryngoscope *42:*189–194, March '32

Treatment of automobile accidents in cases where nose and face are involved. CARTER, W. W. Ann. Otol., Rhin. and Laryng. *41:*571–575, June '32

Injuries to nose in automobile accidents; importance of early treatment. CARTER, W. W. Eye, Ear, Nose and Throat Monthly *12:*150–152, May '33

Immediate transplantation on defects of ear and nose due to accident; 2 cases. AUFRICHT, G. Arch. Otolaryng. *17:*769–773, June '33

Medical care of injuries of external nasal surface. MAYER, O. Wein. klin. Wchnschr. *47:*109–110, Jan 26, '34

Nasal injuries and their cosmetic therapy. EITNER, E. Wein. med. Wchnschr. *84:*307–309, March 10, '34

Treatment of traumatic injuries to nose in automobile accidents. CARTER, W. W. Arch. Otolaryng. *20:*513–517, Oct '34

Importance of correct technic in primary treatment of nasal injuries. CARTER, W. W., M. Rec. *140:*465–466, Nov 7, '34

Birth injuries to nose of new-born. BIRKE, L. Monatschr. F. Geburtsh. u. Gynak. *98:*144–152, Nov '34

External injuries of nose. DUBOV, M. D. Sovet. khir. (no. 4) *7:*670–680, '34

Tattooing of nose and face following automobile injuries. CARTER, W. W. New York State J. Med. *35:*573–575, June 1, '35

Tip of nose completely sectioned and sutured 3 hours after accident; recovery. ROY, J. N. Rev. de chir. structive, pp. 211–217, March '36

Surgical care of injuries and deformities of nose, lip and premaxilla, with report of cases. FEDERSPIEL, M. N. Internat. J. Orthodontia *22:*1054–1068, Oct '36

Plastic surgery of nasal injuries. DOROSCHENKO, I. T. Arch. f. Ohren-, Nasen-u. Kehlkopfh. *141:*5–11, '36

Traumatic origin of late angioneurotic condition in region of nose and cheek; 3 cases. SEMRAU, J. Hals-, Nasen-u. Ohrenarzt (Teil 1) *27:*363–370, '36

Nose, Injuries of–Cont.

Traumatic deformities of nose and other bones of face. NEW, G. B. Surg., Gynec. and Obst. *64:*532–537, Feb (no. 2A) '37

Management of nasal injuries. RENIE, R. O. S. Clin. North America *19:*467–473, April '39

Traumatic tear of ala nasi and of tip; surgical repair in case. ZENO, L. An. de cir. *5:*15–16, March '39 also: Bol. Soc. de cir. de Rosario *6:*8–9, April '39

Fractures of malar bone and zygoma with eye, ear, nose and throat complications. MEYER, M. F. New Orleans M. and S. J. *92:*90–94, Aug '39

Trauma of nasal pyramid. RIVAS, C. I. Rev. med. de Chile *68:*306–320, March '40

Traumatic affections of nose. KIMBALL, G. H. AND DRUMMOND, N. R., J. Oklahoma M. A. *33:*1–3, April '40

Some minor nasal and aural injuries in recreations. MACARTNEY, C., J. Roy. Nav. M. Serv. *26:*139–143, April '40

Plastic surgery for enlarged and small nose resulting from accidents. PEARLMAN, R. C. M. Rec. *152:*402–404, Dec 4, '40

Trauma of nasal pyramid. RIVAS, C. I. Acta med., Rio de Janeiro *7:*187–202, May '41

Nasal injury. BLACK, J. I. M., Clin. J. *70:*177–183, July '41

Plastic surgery in loss of ear and nose substance. MALBEC, E. F. Semana med. *2:*714–716, Sept 18, '41

Abrasions and accidental tattoos, scars, keloids and scar contractures and nasal deformities. GREELEY, P. W., S. Clin. North America *22:*253–276, Feb '42

Discussion of nasal injury. NEGUS, V. E. AND KILNER, T. P. Proc. Roy. Soc. Med. *35:*513–518, June '42 also: J. Laryng. and Otol. *57:*270–279, May '42

Nose and sinus injuries; necessity of early surgical intervention. BERENDES, J. Deut. Militararzt *7:*579–581, Sept '42

Injuries to nose, paranasal sinuses, mouth and ears. CANFIELD, N. Connecticut M. J. *6:*796–798, Oct '42

Injury to nose. STRAITH, C. L. Tr. Indiana Acad. Ophth. and Otolaryng. *26:*88–99, '42

Burns of ear, nose, mouth and adjacent tissues (with special reference to therapy with hydrosulphosol, sulfhydryl solution). CRUTHIRDS, A. E. Laryngoscope *53:*478–494, July '43

Burns of ear, nose, mouth and adjacent tissues (including use of hydrosulphosol, sulfhydryl solution). CRUTHIRDS, A. E. Tr. Am. Laryng., Rhin. and Otol. Soc., pp.

Nose, Injuries of–Cont.

219–235, '43

Traumatic deformities to nose. SALINGER, S. Ann. Otol., Rhin. and Laryng. *53:*274–285, June '44

Wounds and injuries of nose and their implications. ERSNER, M. S. Pennsylvania M. J. *49:*840–844, May '46

Nose, Leishmaniasis of

Total rhinoplasty following destruction of leishmaniasis; case. DUARTE CARDOSO, A. Rev. med. e cir. de Sao Paulo *5:*271–277, Sept–Dec '45

Nose, Leprosy of

Development of saddle nose and formation of small multiple hemangiomas of mucous membrane of nose and pharynx complicating diffuse scleroderma; case. MENZEL, K. M. Monatschr. f. Ohrenh. *70:*1409–1418, Dec '36

Surgical correction of deformities due to leprosy in nose. PRUDENTE, A. Presse med. *48:*156–158, Feb 6, '40

Problem of nasal deformity in leprosy. SILVEIRA, L. M. Arq. de cir. clin. e exper. *6:*531–535, April–June '42

Nose, Lupus of

Nasal prosthesis in lupus treated with ultraviolet rays. DAUBRESSE-MORELLE, E. Ann. de l'Inst. chir. de Bruxelles *29:*161–165, Nov 15, '28

Prosthetic surgery in lupus (Hennig-Zinsser method); total rhinoneoplasty. DÖRFFEL, J. AND NOSSEN, H. Med. Welt *5:*1172–1174, Aug 15, '31

Plastic reconstruction of nose destroyed by lupus. KURTZAHN. Chirurg *3:*49–52, Jan 15, '31

Free graft of full thickness skin in case of lupus erythematosus of nose. MALBEC, E. F. Semana med. *1:*1232–1235, June 3, '43

Psychosomatic clinical study of case of lupus of nose treated by plastic surgery. ZENO, L. Rev. med. de Rosario *33:*1041–1058, Nov '43 also: An. de cir. *9:*125–142, Sept–Dec '43 also: Dia med. *16:*264–268, March 20, '44

Nose, Miscellaneous

Trophic postencephalitic ulcerations of outer nose and of cheek. SCHLITTLER, E. Schweiz. med. Wchnschr. *59:*1121–1122, Nov 9, '29

Fistulas of nasal entrance. SZENDE, B. Orvosi hetil. *83:*112, Feb 4, '39

Nose, Polyps of

Deforming and recurring polyps of nose of youth. LAFF, H. I. Arch. Otolaryng. *30:*795–799, Nov '39

Deforming recidivating polyposis of nose, with report of case. RIESCO MAC-CLURE, J. S. Rev. otorrinolaring. *1:*61–64, Dec '41

Deforming polyposis of nose, with report of case. RIVAS, J. J. Arch. venezol. Soc. de oto-rino-laring., oftal., neurol. *2:*194–199, Dec '41

Nose, Prostheses

Treatment of nasal deformities, with special reference to nasal prosthesis. KAZANJIAN, V. H., J.A.M.A. *84:*177–181, Jan 17, '25

Replacement of nose and ear by gelatin prosthesis. STRAUSS. Schweiz. med. Wchnschr. *56:*464–465, May 15, '26

Prosthetic aids in reconstructive surgery about head; presentation of new methods (including ear), nose. LEDERER, F. L. Arch. Otolaryng. *8:*531–554, Nov '28

New nasal prosthesis (celluloid). ALEKSIEWICZ, J. Polska gaz. lek. *9:*214–216, March 16, '30

Prosthetic nose and face. CSERNYEI, G. Schweiz. med. Wchnschr. *62:*116, Jan 30, '32

Nasal prosthesis. WHYTE, D. Australian and New Zealand J. Surg. *3:*74–75, July '33

Prosthesis covering orbital region, nose and upper lip. PONT, AND LAPIERRE, V. Bull. Soc. franc. de dermat. et syph. (Reunion dermat., Lyon) *43:*908–910, May '36

Nasal prosthesis to hide deformity; case. ALVES, O. Rev. oto-laring. de Sao Paulo (no. 5, bis) *4:*873–877, Sept–Oct '36

Cranial prosthesis and restoration of nose in fractures of nose and frontal part of cranium. PONT, A. Rev. de chir. structive, pp. 34–37, March '37

Articulated prosthesis of eye, nose and upper lip; case. PONT, A. AND LAPIERRE, V. Rev. de chir. structive, pp. 38–41, March '37

Technic of making artificial noses. SIMONS, R. D. G. P. Nederl. tijdschr. v. geneesk. *81:*1421–1425, April 3, '37

Useful prostheses for nasal and facial defects due to destructive lesions. SCHMID, R. Munchen. med. Wchnschr. *85:*1784–1786, Nov 18, '38 comment by Moncorps *86:*252–253, Feb 17, '39

Elastic prosthesis for nasal defects. SIEMENS, H. W. Munchen. med. Wchnschr. *85:*1987–1988, Dec 23, '38 comment by Zinsser

Nose, Prostheses – Cont.

*86:*252, Feb 17, '39 comment by Moncorps *86:*252–253, Feb 17, '39 comment by Bering *86:*253–254, Feb 17, '39 reply by Siemens *86:*254, Feb 17, '39

Construction of nose by prosthesis (case). CLAFLIN, R. S. Am. J. Orthodontics *25:*92–93, Jan '39

Artificial ear and nose. BULBULIAN, A. H. Hygeia *18:*980–982, Nov '40

Prosthetic reconstruction of nose and ear with latex compound. BULBULIAN, A. H. J.A.M.A. *116:*1504–1506, April 5, '41

Buccomaxillofacial prosthesis; artificial nose and palate; case. GRAZIANI, M. Rev. brasil. de oto-rino-laring. *9:*217–221, May–June '41

Psychology of lupus patients with nasal prostheses. KALKOFF, K. W. Dermat. Wchnschr. *113:*597–601, July 12, '41

Adjustable, non-solid appliance for nasal restoration, attached to upper denture. ASHWORTH, H. S. Brit. Dent. J. *80:*157–160, March 1, '46

Nose, Rat Bite of

Rhinoplasty to replace nose bitten off by a rat. BEHREND, M., J.A.M.A. *76:*1752, June 18, '21

Nose, Septal Abscess of

Abscesses of nasal septum, their etiology and treatment with reference to resulting deformities. CARTER, W. W., M. J. and Rec. *119:*11–13, Feb 6, '24

Management of abscess of nasal septum. VOORHEES, I. W. Laryngoscope *39:*652–654, Oct '29

Abscess (traumatic) of nasal septum in children; importance of early diagnosis and treatment. CARTER, W. W. Eye, Ear, Nose and Throat Monthly *11:*352–354, Oct '32

Use of T tube for drainage of septal abscess in nose. WEILLE, F. L. AND DE BLOIS, E. Arch. Otolaryng. *39:*85–86, Jan '44

Nasal septal abscess. LAUB, G. R. South. Med. and Surg. *106:*374, Oct '44

Nose, Septal Obstruction in Children

Submucous resection in children. WHITE, F. W. Ann. Otol., Rhin. and Laryng. *33:*526–533, June '24

Submucous resection in children. WINDHAM, R. E. Eye, Ear, Nose and Throat Monthly *7:*307–311, July '28 Also: Northwest Med. *27:*392–396, Aug '28

Deviated nasal septums and their correction

Nose, Septal Obstruction in Children – Cont.

in young children. ALEXANDER, G. J. J. Ophth., Otol. and Laryng. *32:*325–337, Oct '28

Relief of obstruction in children without subsequent deformity of nose. CARTER, W. W. Laryngoscope *40:*55–58, Jan '30

Relief of obstruction of nose in children due to deviation of septum. CARTER, W. W. Ann. Otol., Rhin. and Laryng. *39:*199–203, March '30

Submucous resection in children. YEARSLEY, M. Practitioner *129:*581–583, Nov '32

Nasal obstruction in children due to septal abnormalities; what shall we do for them? CARTER, W. W. Laryngoscope *43:*377–382, May '33

Dislocations of lower end of nasal septal cartilage in new-born (injury sustained at birth), in infants and in young children and with their anatomic replacement by orthopedic procedures. METZENBAUM, M. Arch. Otolaryng. *24:*78–88, July '36

After-effects of nasal septal operation on children. BARTON, J. F. Tr. Pacific Coast Oto-Ophth. Soc. *23:*172–177, '38

Nasal septal surgery in children. COTTLE, M. H. Illinois M. J. *75:*161–163, Feb '39

Anatomic and functional results of 50 operations for marked deviations of traumatic origin in young children (nasal septum). OMBREDANNE. Ann. d'oto-laryng., pp. 145–150, July–Sept '42

Nose, Septal Perforations

Idiopathic perforation of nasal septum; autoplasty with pedunculated flap of mucous membrane; cure. ROY, J. N. Ann. Otol., Rhin. and Laryng. *32:*554–560, June '23

New plastic procedure for closure of perforations of nasal septum. LEWIS, J. D. Laryngoscope *33:*671–674, Sept '23 (illus.)

Postoperative perforations of nasal septum. ŠERCER, A. Cas. lek. cesk. *63:*842–845, May 31, '24 abstr: J.A.M.A. *83:*161, July 12, '24

Technic for autoplastic repair of septum of nose. FRÓES, H. Brazil-med. *1:*349–352, June 21, '24

New procedure for closure of nonspecific perforations of nasal septum. LISCHKOFF, M. A. AND HEINBERG, C. J. Arch. Otolaryng. *4:*342, Oct '26

Case report of repair of nasal septal perforation. HOMPES, J. J. Tr. Am. Laryng., Rhin. and Otol. Soc. *33:*565–568, '27

Perforation of nasal septum occurring in manufacture of calcium arsenate. STINSON, W. D., J. Tennessee M. A. *24:*65, Feb '31

Nose, Septal Perforations – Cont.

Autoplasty of nasal septal perforations. SEKULIĆ, B. Otolaryng. slavica. *4:*40, Jan '32

Nasal septal perforation. BROWNE, H. S. J. Oklahoma M. A. *25:*382–383, Sept '32

Nasal septal autoplasty in therapy of perforation; cases. TORRES LUQUIN, P. An. Soc. mex. de oftal. y oto-rino-laring. *10:*47–54, March–June '33

Nasal septal perforation in workers with arsenic. DRESCHKE. Med. Klin. *29:*1378, Oct 6, '33

New plastic method of repairing nasal septal perforation. DOROSCHENKO, J. T. Acta oto-laryng. *23:*553–554, '36

Immediate therapy of surgical perforations of nasal septum. AUBONE, J. C. Rev. Asoc. med. argent. *50:*669–671, May–June '37

Plastic surgery in complete loss of lobules and subpartition of nose; case. COELST. Rev. de chir. structive *8:*103–105, Aug '38

New method of plastic surgery for septal defects; case. SASAKI, M. AND SUEMITSU, S. Oto-rhino-laryng. *12:*834, Oct '39

Simple method for closing septal perforations. MCGIVERN, C. S., M. Rec. *151:*267–268, April 17, '40

New surgical technic for correcting septal perforation in nose. AUBONE, J. C. Rev. Asoc. med. argent. *55:*288–290, April 15–30, '41

Plastic correction of loss of nasal septum. MALBEC, E. F. Dia med. *13:*682, July 21, '41

Reconstruction of nasal septum by tubular skin graft; cases. ZENO, L. AND RECALDE, J. F. Arq. de cir. clin. e exper. *6:*185–194, April–June '42

Nasal perforation; free transplantation; experiments with fascia lata. BEHRMAN, W. Acta oto-laryng. *34:*78–81, '46

Nose, Septal Resection

Submucous resection of nasal septum. DUNNING, W. M. Am. J. Surg. *35:*1, Jan '21

Observations upon operation for deflection of nasal septum. DONALD, J. Practitioner *106:*250, April '21

Use of hollow tube following submucous resection of nasal septum. GOODYEAR, H. M. J.A.M.A. *77:*1103, Oct 1, '21

Submucous resection of nasal septum. BROWN, K. T., J. Indiana M. A. *14:*339, Oct '21

Modification of submucous resection operation. NOTHENBERG, O. J. Illinois M. J. *40:*385, Nov '21

Intranasal reconstruction. PRATT, F. J. AND

Nose, Septal Resection – Cont.

PRATT, J. A. Laryng. Otol. and Rhin., A.M.A. p. 95, 1921

Intranasal reconstruction. PRATT, F. J. AND PRATT, J. A. Ann. Otol. Rhinol. and Laryngol. *31:*46–105, March '22 (illus.)

After treatment of submucous resection. JONES, D. H. New York M. J. *115:*494, April 19, '22

Submucous resection of nasal septum. NOTTAGE, H. P. China M. J. *36:*469–473, Nov '22

Indications and contraindications for submucous resection of nasal septum. HOFFMANN, J. N. Laryngoscope *33:*13–15, Jan '23

Symptoms and treatment of deviations of nasal septum. EDMONDSON, E. E. Illinois M. J. *43:*208–210, March '23

Few notes of Halle's Clinic; with special reference to his endonasal surgery. COHN, R. D. California State J. Med. *22:*6–8, Jan '24

Method of holding septal membranes in apposition after a submucous resection without use of packing, description and demonstration of instruments and method of use. SIMPSON, H. L., J. Michigan M. Soc. *23:*64–67, Feb '24

Submucous resection of nasal septum; simple flap suture. WILSON, W. F. Brit. M. J. *2:*814, Nov 1, '24

Correction of nasal deformities following septum operations. SAFIAN, J. Laryngoscope *34:*957–960, Dec '24

Technic for submucous resection, with presentation of membrane elevator. JONES, M. J. Laryngoscope *35:*406–408, May '25

Endonasal plastic surgery. BASAVILBASO, J. Prensa med. argent. *13:*23–25, June 10, '26

Submucous resection of nasal septum. WAHRER, F. L., J. Iowa M. Soc. *16:*371–372, Aug '26

What septa demand operation? PRATT, F. J. Ann. Otol. Rhin. and Laryng. *35:*940–943, Sept '26

New nasal septum operation. WOJATSCHEK, W. I. Monatschr. f. Ohrenh. *60:*910–914, Oct '26

Resection of nasal septum for obstruction; general discussion. LIÉBAULT, G. Rev. de laryngol. *47:*677–681, Nov 30, '26

Evolution of submucous resection with new technic. ATKINSON, D. T. Laryngoscope *37:*132–136, Feb '27

Deviated nasal septum. LAWWILL, S., J. Tennessee M. A. *19:*284–286, Feb '27

Local anesthesia in submucous resection of nasal septum. STURM, F. P. Brit. M. J. *1:*720, April 16, '27

Nose, Septal Resection – Cont.

Local anaesthesia in submucous resection of nasal septum. McKelvie, B. Brit. M. J. *1:*920, May 21, '27

Syphilis as complicating factor in surgery of nasal septum. Mackenzie, G. W. Hahneman. Monthly *62:*345-349, May '27

Prevention and correction of nasal deformities following submucous resection; presentation of cases. Maliniak, J. W. Arch. Otolaryng. *6:*320-329, Oct '27

Treatment of minor degrees of nasal obstruction; deflections of septum. Jory, P. Lancet *1:*147-148, Jan 21, '28

Essentials of nasal septal operations. Yearsley, M. Practitioner *121:*178-182, Sept '28

Modified nasal septal resection. Roost, F. H. J. Iowa M. Soc. *18:*432-434, Nov '28

Endonasal surgery with aid of new instrument; simplified technic. Wachsberger, A. Arch. Otolaryng. *8:*712-714, Dec '28

Limitations of septum operation. Curtin, L. J., J. Laryng. and Otol. *44:*24-26, Jan '29

Causes and operative treatment of deformities of nasal septum. Weleminsky, J. Monatschr. f. Ohrenh. *63:*530-535, May '29

Submucous resection of nasal castration symbol. Oberndorf, C. P. Internat. J. Psycho-Analysis *10:*228-241, April-July '29

Correction of deviation of nasal septum; case. Duerto, J. Rev. espan. de med. y cir. *12:*600-603, Oct '29

Modification of present radical operation for deflection of nasal septum. Burkhardt, C. F. Illinois M. J. *56:*353-355, Nov '29

High submucous excision of nasal septum. Takahashi, K. Ztschr. f. Laryng., Rhin. *19:*22-40, Nov '29

Method of correcting lax, boggy septa following submucous resection. Pratt, J. A. Ann. Otol., Rhin. and Laryng. *38:*1156-1157, Dec '29

Submucous resection in children. White, F. W. Tr. Sect. Laryng., Otol. and Rhin., A. M. A., pp. 123-134, '29 also: Arch. Otolaryng. *11:*415-425, April '30

Suggestions for modification of operative procedure and postoperative treatment of submucous resection. McGivern, C. S., J. M. Soc. New Jersey *27:*28-31, Jan '30

Diathermo-surgical treatment of septal malformations. Jouffray. Rev. d'actinol. *6:*35-39, Jan-Feb '30

Indications for resection of nasal septum. Richter, H. Ztschr. f. Laryng., Rhin. *19:*399-402, July '30 also: Munchen. med. Wchnschr. *77:*1354-1356, Aug 8, '30

Nose, Septal Resection – Cont.

Septal deformities and their correction. Salmon, D. L. Kentucky M. J. *28:*485-488, Oct '30

Submucous resection. Baldenweck, L. Medecine *12:*75-79, Jan '31

Deflection of nasal septum. Lewis, T. W. S. Clin. North America *11:*127-132, Feb '31

Submucous resection from technical, respiratory and esthetic viewpoints. Tempea, V. Spitalul. *51:*98-99, March '31

Technic of resection of nasal septum. Zambrini, A. R. Semana med. *1:*1153-1155, April 30, '31

Local anesthesia in nasal septal surgery. Sonntag, A. Ztschr. f. Laryng., Rhin. *21:*32-36, June '31

Mucous-periostal covering and its consideration in surgical therapy of nasal septal deviations. Neumann, H. Monatschr. f. Ohrenh. *65:*1399-1405, Nov '31

New method for removal of vomerine ridge in septal obstruction. Ridpath, R. F. Tr. Am. Laryng., Rhin. and Otol. Soc. *37:*339-343, '31

Endonasal surgery and terrain. Aubriot, P. Rev. med. de l'est *60:*269-277, April 15, '32

Submucous resection in children. Windham, R. E. Texas State J. Med. *27:*859-862, April '32

Technic of submucous resection. Hutter, F. Monatschr. f. Ohrenh. *66:*584-585, May '32

Indications for operations and operations most commonly performed on nasal septum. Silveira, R. Rev. de med. y cir. de la Habana *38:*428-436, June 30, '33

Nasal septal deformities. Adkins, G. E. New Orleans M. and S. J. *86:*102-105, Aug '33

Ways of treating most anterior portions during submucous resection. Behrman, W. Acta oto-laryng. *21:*248-255, '34

Metzenbaum operation for correction of deflected nasal septum. Ridpath, R. F. S. Clin. North America *15:*231-237, Feb '35

Submucous resection. Berman, H. L. Laryngoscope *45:*184-187, March '35

External nasal deformities corrected and removal of existing intranasal obstruction advantageously accomplished at same operation. Cohen, L. Ann. Otol., Rhin. and Laryng. *44:*233-241, March '35

Late results of operations on septum in cases of obstruction of nasal respiration. Ipolyi, F. Monatschr. f. Ohrenh. *69:*685-689, June '35

Behavior of cartilage in submucous resection; histopathologic study. Gianni, O. Arch. ital. di otol. *47:*487-498, July '35

Nose, Septal Resection – Cont.

Direct incision in submucous resection; modification of Killian operation. TEMPEA, V. Rev. san. mil., Bucuresti *35:*1077–1079, Oct '36

Practical points on submucous resection; pitfalls and corrections. LASZLO, A. F. Laryngoscope *46:*840–847, Nov '36

Nasal spine as stenosing factor; surgical therapy. DELLEPIANE RAWSON, R. Rev. otoneurol-oftal. *11:*343–344, Dec '36

New postoperative pack for submucous resection. DIXON, O. J. Ann. Otol., Rhin. and Laryng. *45:*1184–1185, Dec '36

Submucous resection in relation to nasal plastic surgery. WOLFE, M. M. Laryngoscope *47:*281–285, April '37

Indications and technic for submucous resection. MOORE, P. M., S. Clin. North America *17:*1437–1448, Oct '37

Evaluation of submucous resection; points as to technic. FRANK, P., M. Rec. *146:*469–470, Dec 1, '37

Deviation of septum with insufficient nasal respiration as indication for submucous resection; preliminary report. AMERSBACH, K. Arch. f. Ohren-, Nasen-u. Kehlkopf. *143:*241–245, '37

Method for maintaining apposition of mucosal flaps after submucous resection. KEARNEY, H. L. Tr. Am. Laryng., Rhin. and Otol. Soc. *43:*109–110, '37

Transitory conditions contraindicating resection of nasal septum. LEWIS, E. R. Tr. Am. Laryng., Rhin. and Otol. Soc. *43:*402–403, '37

Injection anesthesia for submucous resection. LIEBERMANN, T. Ztschr. f. Hals, Nasen-u. Ohrenh. *41:*290, '37

Direct incision in submucous resection; modification of Killian operation. TEMPEA, V. Ztschr. f. Hals-, Nasen-u. Ohrenh. *40:*548–552, '37

New splint for nasal septum. SOLO, A. Arch. Otolaryng. *27:*343–346, March '38

Deflection of nasal septum. SYME, W. S. Brit. M. J. *2:*656–657, Sept 24, '38

Nasal septal deviations and their results. VALDES, G. Rev. mex. de cir., ginec. y cancer *6:*559–569, Oct '38

Essential points in submucous resection. YEARSLEY, M., M. Press *197:*518–520, Dec 7, '38

Submucous resection; methods of preventing post-operative fluttering and perforation. DÖDERLEIN, W. Hals-, Nasen-u. Ohrenarzt (Teil 1) *30:*273–285, July '39

Improved surgical technic for subperichondrial nasal septum resection used in Colonial Hospital of National Railroads of Mexico, Federal District. SCIANDRA, A. Cir. y cirujanos *7:*389–394, Sept 30–Oct 31, '39

Septal structural changes; sequels and therapy. HAYMANN, L. Med. Klin. *35:*1365–1368, Oct 20, '39

Prevention of hematoma after submucous resection. CHAMBERLIN, W. B. Tr. Am. Laryng. A. *61:*21–28, '39

Nasal obstruction. MARTIN GROMAZ, L. An. med. *1:*31–35, July–Sept '40

Surgical establishment of nasal ventilation. PARKINSON, S. N. Ann. Otol., Rhin. and Laryng. *49:*1023–1029, Dec '40

Nasal obstruction and impairment of hearing; 46 cases of submucous resection with audiometric studies. JOHNSON, M. R. Arch. Otolaryng. *33:*536–549, April '41

Treatment of nasal obstruction in adults. ROSS, A. M., M. Press *207:*112–114, Feb 18, '42

Submucous resection of septum of nose. SNYDER, W. S. JR. Kentucky M. J. *40:*59–62, Feb '42

Dressings after submucous resection of septum. PRUVOT, M. Rev. de laryng. *63:*196–199, June–July '42

Pitfalls in submucous resection. MALIS, S. Dis. Eye, Ear, Nose and Throat *2:*343–347, Nov '42

Nasal septal operation; technic to avoid postoperative tamponade. LANZA CASTELLI, R. A. Rev. otorrinolaring. d. litoral *2:*112–128, Dec '42

Use of diathermy in submucous resection. JONES, A. C. Tr. Am. Laryng., Rhin. and Otol. Soc. *48:*331–332, '42

Priority of Murray-Nelson-Hulsman original method for avoiding perforation in submucous resection. NELSON, R. M., J. M. A. Georgia *32:*338–339, Oct '43

Use of diathermy in submucous resection. JONES, A. C. Arch. Otolaryng. *38:*445–446, Nov '43

Nasal septum operation; successes and failures. DE PAULA PINTO HARTUNG, F. Rev. brasil. de oto-rino-laring. *12:*112–121, March–April '44

Technic of secondary resection of nasal septum demonstrating regeneration of cartilage. EISENSTODT, L. W. Laryngoscope *54:*190–197, April '44

Surgical treatment of nasal obstruction; indications for plastic approach to septal deformity; details of plastic procedures. BOLOTOW, N. A. Arch. Otolaryng. *40:*198–202,

Nose, Septal Resection – Cont.
Sept '44
Operation of nasal septum; successes and failures. DE PAULA PINTO HARTUNG, F. Rev. paulista de med. *25:*197–207, Sept '44
Relation of deflections of nasal septum to rhinoplasty. BERSON, M. I., M. Rec. *158:*734–736, Dec '45
Cartilaginous septum in reconstruction of nose; modified procedure. EISBACH, E. J. Arch. Otolaryng. *44:*207–211, Aug '46
Plastic repair of deflected septum of nose. FOMON, S.; *et al.* Arch. Otolaryng. *44:*141–156, Aug '46

Nose, Septal Resection, Complications of

Fatal meningitis following submucous resection of nasal septum, post-mortem discovery of latent sphenoidal sinusitis. POWELL, W. E., J. Laryngol. and Otol. *37:*39–40, Jan '22
Post-operative complications of submucous resection and their treatment. SCHWARTZ, A. A. Am. J. Surg. *36:*133–136, June '22
Submucous resection; complications and after-results. WEINBERGER, N. S. Ann. Otol., Rhin. and Laryng. *32:*387–393, June '23
Submucous resection followed by complications of acute otitis, mastoiditis and sinus thrombosis. HOUSER, K. M. Arch. Otolaryng. *7:*631–634, June '28
Vulnerability of sphenopalatine artery in deep endonasal surgery. VIÉLA, A. AND ESCAT, M. Ann. d. mal. de l'oreille, du larynx *47:*980–985, Nov '28
Delayed healing of septal resections due to Vincent's infection; 3 cases. HOLLENDER, A. R. Arch. Otolaryng. *9:*422–424, April '29
Complications following resections of submucous septum. CLAUS, G. Ztschr. f. Hals-, Nasen-u. Ohrenh. *23:*444–449, Sept 10, '29
Embolic infarction of lung after excision of septum of nose. KELEMEN, G. Ztschr. f. Hals-, Nasen-u. Ohrenh. *26:*139–142, July 3, '30
Acute pulmonary edema in course of local anesthesia for deviation of nasal septum; case. VAN DEN BOSSCHE, P. Ann. d. mal. de l'oreille, du larynx. *49:*983–995, Oct '30
Necrosis of septum after correction in latent syphilis; 2 cases. BURGDORF, K. Arch. f. Ohren-, Nasen-u. Kehlhopfh. *129:*175–180, July 21, '31
Retrobulbar abscess complicating submucous resection. MAHONEY, P. L. Laryngoscope *42:*199–200, March '32
Otological sepsis following submucous resection. MENGER, L. C. Laryngoscope *42:*371–375, May '32

Nose, Septal Resection, Complications of – Cont.
Complications of local anesthesia in surgery of nasal septum. ZIEGLER, E. Ztschr. f. Hals-, Nasen-u. Ohrenh. *32:*476–479, '33
Septal hematomas and their complications. COMBECHER, W. Ztschr. f. Laryng., Rhin., Otol. *26:*156–171, '35
Death of patient after Killian operation for deformed septum. ERRECART, P. L. Rev. Asoc. med. argent. *50:*974–977, June '36
Complications of submucosal resection (Killian operation). CARANDO, V.; *et al.* Semana med. *1:*225–227, Jan 21, '37
Septicemia due to Micrococcus catarrhalis after resection of nasal septum; case. HERCOG, P. Gior. di clin. med. *19:*315–318, April 10, '38
Hemorrhage in nasal septal resection. HARTUNG, F. Rev. oto-laring. de Sao Paulo *6:*379–382, Sept–Oct '38
Therapy of postoperative hematoma of nasal septum by means of laminaria. DE CERQUEIRA FALCAO, E. Rev. oto-laring. de Sao Paulo *6:*471–477, Nov–Dec '38 also: Brasil-med. (no. 5) *53:*143–145, '39
Postoperative psychosis; dementia praecox following operation on nasal septum; case. MUKASA, H. Oto-rhino-laryng. *12:*139, Feb '39
Accidents to septum in anesthesia with novocain (procaine hydrochloride) in nose. LEDERER, L. Arch. f. Ohren-, Nasen-u. Kehlkopfh. *150:*162–167, '41
Complications of plastic surgery of nasal septum. COHEN, S. Dis. Eye, Ear, Nose and Throat *2:*235–243, Aug '42
Hematoma, abscess and necrosis of septum (especially following injury). BIRDSALL, S. E. St. Barth. Hosp. J. *47:*68–70, Feb '43

Nose, Septal Resection Instruments

New perichondrium elevator for resection of nasal septum. CAMPBELL, C. A. Laryngoscope *31:*973, Dec '21 (illus.)
Nasal septum splint. VERDIER, R. A. Am. J. Surg. *36:*44, Feb '22 (illus.)
New nasal septal chisel. BARKER, C. J.A.M.A. *79:*216, July 15, '22 (illus.)
New nasal septal chisel. OLSHO, S. L. Laryngoscope *33:*308, April '23 (illus.)
Nasal drill for removal of septal spur. YOUNG, H. H., J.A.M.A. *80:*1216, April 28, '23 (illus.)
Improved septal punch forceps. LEWIS, J. D. Laryngoscope *33:*862–864, Nov '23 (illus.)
Guarded septum chisel. RUSKIN, S. L. Laryngoscope *34:*288–289, April '24
New elevator for submucous resection.

Nose, Septal Resection Instruments—Cont.
MYERSON, M. C. Laryngoscope *34:*660, Aug '24
Submucosa dissector. GRAHAM, A. J. Surg., Gynec. and Obst. *40:*709, May '25 also: M. J. and Rec. *122:*527, Nov 4, '25
Two new instruments; septum needle and thread-holder for ear surgery. POLLAK, E. Monatschr. f. Ohrenh. *61:*1252, Nov '27
Modified nasal septal forceps. TAKAHASHI, K. Ztschr. f. Hals-, Nasen-u. Ohrenh. *22:*130, June 16, '28
New combined submucous dissector and suction cannula. HAMRICK, D. W. Arch. Otolaryng. *9:*655-656, June '29
Submucous septum punch. REAVES, R. G. Tr. Am. Acad. Ophth. *35:*475, '30
Submucous flap punch for nasal septal surgery. REAVES, R. G. Arch. Otolaryng. *15:*754, May '32
New instruments for submucous resection of nasal septum. GAMMAGE, F. V. Arch. Otolaryng. *16:*573-574, Oct '32
Knife for submucous resection. MILLER, A. Lancet *1:*1395, June 30, '34
Nasal septum trephine. BOILER, W. F. Laryngoscope *40:*438-439, June '40
Submucous elevator. METZENBAUM, M. F. Arch. oto-laryng. *34:*847, Oct '41

Nose, Septum, Dislocation of

Treatment of simple luxations of nasal septum. LEROUX, R. Ann. D. mal. de l'oreille, du larynx *45:*1064, Nov '26
Replacement of lower end of dislocated septal cartilage versus submucous resection of dislocated end of septal cartilage. METZENBAUM, M. Tr. Sect. Laryng., Otol. and Rhin., A.M.A., pp. 236-251, '28 also: Arch. Otolaryng. *9:*282-296, March '29
Correction of dislocation of nasal subseptum from functional and esthetic points of view. GONZÁLEZ LOZA, M. Rev. med. del Rosario *22:*929-941, Nov '32
Asymmetry of nares; positive diagnostic sign or entity establishing anatomic displacement of lower end of cartilaginous nasal septum. METZENBAUM, M. Arch. Otolaryng. *16:*690-697, Nov '32
Oblique-angled knife for resetting lower end of dislocated septal cartilage and operations on harelip and cleft palate. METZENBAUM, M. Arch. Otolaryng. *24:*199, Aug '36
Correction of displaced nasal cartilage, especially in children. COHEN, S. Pennsylvania M. J. *40:*925-930, Aug '37
Operation to repair lateral displacement of lower border of septal cartilage. PEER, L. A. Arch. Otolaryng. *25:*475-477, April '37

Nose, Septum, Dislocation of—Cont.
Nasal septum; —twisted nose. METZ, W. R. New Orleans M. and S. J. *92:*180-185, Oct '39
New instrument for conservative operations on nasal septum. TSYPIN, M. Y. Zhur. ush., nos. i gorl. bolez *16:*141-145, '39
Correction of lateral displacement of free border of nasal septal cartilage. HARBERT, F. Arch. Otolaryng. *31:*341-343, Feb '40
Reconstruction of deformed septum; critical evaluation of orthodox submucous resection from anatomophysiologic standpoint. ERSNER, M. S. Arch. Otolaryng. *39:*476-484, June '44
Plastic repair of deviated septum associated with deflected nasal tip. SELTZER, A. P. Arch. Otolaryng. *40:*433-444, Dec '44
Corrective surgery of external pyramid and septum for restoration of normal physiology. COTTLE, M. H. AND LORING, R. M. Illinois M. J. *90:*119-131, Aug '46
Plastic repair of deflected septum of nose. FOMON, S.; *et al.* Arch. Otolaryng. *44:*141-156, Aug '46
New operation for dislocated nasal cartilage. KAYSER, R. Am. J. Surg. *72:*248-251, Aug '46

Nose, Septum, Excision of

Indications for excision of nasal septum. RICHTER, H. Prakt. Arzt. *16:*5-11, Jan 5, '31
Removal of nasal septum. SMITH, C. Arch. Otolaryng. *20:*709-710, Nov '34

Nose, Septum, Miscellaneous

Correction of nasal deformities following septum operations. SAFIAN, J. Laryngoscope *34:*957-960, Dec '24
How soon should nasal deformities, due to abscess of septum be corrected by transplantation of bone? CARTER, W. W., M. J. and Rec. *122:*247-248, Sept 2, '25
Depressed nose following submucous resection. BABCOCK, W. W., S. Clin. N. Amer. *6:*48-52, Feb '26
Use of septal flap in closure of unilateral clefts of palate. THOMPSON, J. E., J.A.M.A. *87:*1384-1388, Oct 23, '26
Partial rhinoplasty; restoration of nasal tip, alae and septum. GOLKIN, M. Deutsche Ztschr. f. Chir. *199:*354-359, '26
Closure of defects of palate by flaps of mucosa from nasal septum. PERWITZSCHKY, R. Arch. f. Ohren-, Nasen-u. Kehlkopfh. *116:*196-203, March '27
Congenital absence of vomer and causes of septal deformities. MENZEL, K. M. Wien. med. Wchnschr. *77:*1081-1083, Aug 13, '27

Nose, Septum, Miscellaneous—Cont.

Prevention and correction of nasal deformities following submucous resection; presentation of cases. MALINIAK, J. W. Arch. Otolaryng. *6:*320–329, Oct '27

Saddle nose; unfortunate result of too thorough operation for deflected septum. SCHAEFFER, G. C. Ohio State M. J. *23:*989, Dec '27

Prevention of nasal deformity following submucous resection. CARTER, W. W. Arch. Otolaryng. *8:*555–563, Nov '28

Origin of nasal septal deflections. IVINS, H. M., J. Iowa M. Soc. *18:*428–432, Nov '28

Prevention of deformities following submucous resection. CARTER, W. W. Tr. Am. Laryng., Rhin. and Otol. Soc. *34:*123–131, '28 also: Laryngoscope *39:*52–57, Jan '29

Causes of deformities of middle portion of nose. KLESTADT, W. Ztschr. f. Laryng., Rhin. *17:*326–334, Jan '29

Congenital tendency of nasal septum and intermaxillary bone to abnormal longitudinal growth. PICHLER, H. Ztschr. f. Stomatol. *27:*21–26, Jan '29

Restoration of subseptal portion of nose. DOBRZANIECKI, W. Ann. Surg. *90:*974–977, Dec '29

Plastic surgery of septum on account of saddle nose. HEINEMANN, O. Med. Klin. *26:*1188, Aug 8, '30

Surgical therapy of ozena by transplantation of bone into septum. OLIVARES, M. G. An. Soc. mex. de oftal. y oto-rino-laring. *9:*28–32, July–Sept '31

Development of nose; dynamic relation to traumatic injuries and to submucous resection. CARTER, W. W. Laryngoscope *42:*189–194, March '32

Sinking of nasal bone following submucous resection. DUFOURMENTEL, L. Oto-rhino-laryng. internat. *16:*233–234, May '32

Development, structure and changes of form of human nasal septum in fetal life. HILLENBRAND, K. Arch. f. Ohren-, Nasen-u. Kehlkopfh. *135:*1–24, '33

Reconstruction of nasal tip, wings and septum by T-shaped graft from neck. LIMBERG, A. A. Novy khir. arkhiv *28:*147–163, '33

Cosmetic corrections of abnormalities of septal cartilage. EITNER, E. Ztschr. f. Laryng., Rhin., Otol. *25:*40–45, '34

Clinical observations on influence of septum on development of nose and palatal arch. CARTER, W. W. Laryngoscope *45:*355–365, May '35

Typical method for reconstruction of nasal tip, septum and median portion of alae nasi. FALTIN, R. Acta chir. Scandinav. *78:*492–511, '36

Etiology of congenital deformities of nasal septum. RICHTER, H. Hals-, Nasen-u. Ohrenarzt (Teil 1) *27:*53–55, '36

Submucous resection in relation to nasal plastic surgery. WOLFE, M. M. Laryngoscope *47:*281–285, April '37

Lengthening septum mobile nasi; new plastic procedure. MOOTNICK, M. W. New York State J. Med. *37:*1509–1510, Sept 1, '37

Traumatic fracture of nasal septum and its therapy. ALVES, O. Rev. oto-laring. de Sao Paulo *6:*373–378, Sept–Oct '38

Deviation of septum in relation to twisted nose. SALINGER, S. Arch. Otolaryng. *29:*520–532, March '39

Role of septum in surgery of nasal contour. COHEN, S. Arch. Otolaryng. *30:*12–20, July '39

Deformities of nose due to septal abnormalities. KOPP, M. M., M. Rec. *151:*111–116, Feb 21, '40

Positive method for ablation of septoturbinal synechiae. FIRESTONE, C. Arch. Otolaryng. *31:*976–978, June '40

Perforating ulcer of septum (Hajek's ulcer), with report of case. MOREIRA, E. Rev. brasil. de oto-rino-laring. *8:*265–267, July–Aug '40

Prevention and correction of dorsal depressions by septal implants (nose). GOLDMAN, I. B. Arch. Otolaryng. *32:*524–529, Sept '40

Complementary turbinotomy in submucosal resection of septum. RESENDE, E. Acta med., Rio de Janeiro *6:*166–167, Sept '40

Histologic study of development of septal deformities. SERCER, A. Acta oto-laryng. *28:*529–547, '40

Nasal obstruction and impairment of hearing; 46 cases of submucous resection with audiometric studies. JOHNSON, M. R. Arch. Otolaryng. *33:*536–549, April '41

Reconstruction of nasal tip and subseptum by means of tubular graft; case. ZENO, L. Bol. y trab., Acad. argent. de cir. *25:*1028–1033, Sept 10, '41

Reconstruction of nasal tip and subseptum by means of tubular graft. ZENO, L. An. de cir. *7:*183–190, Sept '41

High cartilaginous septal trauma. CINELLI, A. A. Dis. Eye, Ear, Nose and Throat *2:*6–9, Jan '42

Cavernous hemangioma of nose, nasal septum and forehead. SALINGER, S. Ann. Otol., Rhin. and Laryng. *51:*268–272, March '42

Nasal synechia. LOEB, W. J., M. Bull. North

Nose, Septum, Miscellaneous–Cont.

African Theat. Op. *2:*122–123, Nov '44
Traumatic deformities of nasal septum. SALINGER, S. Tr. Am. Laryng. A. *66:*46–58, '44

Nose, Sinuses

Fracture of maxillary sinus plus emphysema of lower eyelid. MOREAU, J. Arch. franco-belges de chir. *25:*421–424, Feb '22 (illus.)
Thiersch graft in radical cure of frontal sinus and maxillary antrum diseases; its further application to tonsil and gingival sulci. SHEEHAN, J. E. Surg., Gynec. and Obst. *35:*358–360, Sept '22 (illus.)
Use of delayed flap in secondary operations on palate and antrum. NEW, G. B. Minnesota Med. *6:*214–220, April '23 (illus.)
New procedures for tear sac, frontal sinus and endonasal plastic operations. MALTZ, M. Acta oto-laryng. *9:*144–153, '26 (in English)
Bucco-antral fistula; plastic operation. VOORHEES, I. W. Internat. J. Surg. *40:*19, Jan '27
Fractures involving nasal accessory sinuses. NAFTZGER, J. B. Ann. Otol. Rhin. and Laryng. *37:*486–499, June '28
Fractures of facial bones involving nasal accessory sinuses. NAFTZGER, J. B. Tr. Am. Laryng., Rhin. and Otol. Soc. *34:*383–394, '28
Fracture of frontal sinus and ethmoid through dura, orbit and maxillary sinus; case; phenomenal recovery. SEIBERLING, J. D. Laryngoscope *41:*93–96, Feb '31
Three new instruments for fronto-ethmo-sphenoid operation. SMITH, F. Ann. Otol., Rhin. and Laryng. *40:*198–200, March '31
Treatment of fresh nasal fractures and nasal sinuses. KLESTADT, W. Med. Klin. *27:*1235–1237, Aug 21, '31
Fractures involving orbit and paranasal sinuses, with special reference to diagnosis and treatment. GILL, W. D. Texas State J. Med. *27:*351–358, Sept '31
Plastic surgery of face following electrocoagulation treatment of malignant tumors of nose and accessory sinuses. ÖHNGREN, G. Acta oto-laryng. *16:*292–305, '31
Prognosis of fractures of frontal sinus. BONNET, P. Bull. Soc. d'opht. de Paris, pp. 327–328, May '32
Chronic maxillary sinusitis; fatal complications of traumatic fracture of wall of sinus in patient with sinusitis. FEUZ, J. Rev. med. de la Suisse Rom. *52:*347–354, May 25, '32
Lymphosarcoma of antrum treated 12 years

Nose, Sinuses–Cont.

ago; no recurrence. NEW, G. B. Proc. Staff Meet., Mayo Clin. *7:*317–318, June 1, '32
Posttraumatic frontal sinusitis; recovery after replacement of bone segment of frontal bone displaced by accident; case. ARÁUZ, S. AND GAMES, F. Rev. Asoc. med. argent. *46:*509–510, July '32
Sequestra and suppurative mucocele in frontal sinus following fracture; operation; case. ZAMBRINI, A. R. AND CASTERÁN, E. Rev. Asoc. med. argent. *46:*788–789, Aug '32
Technic of plastic surgery after opening of antrum. KLESTADT, W. Ztschr. f. Laryng., Rhin., Otol. *23:*80–84, '32
Chondrosarcoma of ethmoid; surgical therapy; radiotherapy and autoplasty with tubular flap. LARROUDÉ, C. Rev. de chir. plastique, pp. 239–245, Oct '33
Cancer of maxilla and ethmoid; survey of 50 cases. DAVIS, E. D. D. Brit. M. J. *1:*53–55, Jan 13, '34
Facial bone fractures, especially orbits and sinuses. GILL, W. D. South. M. J. *27:*197–205, March '34
Plastic repair of defect following operative treatment of carcinoma of antrum and upper jaw. BECK, J. C. AND GUTTMAN, M. R. S. Clin. North America *14:*775–782, Aug '34
Curability of malignant tumors of upper jaw and antrum. NEW, G. B. AND CABOT, C. M. Proc. Staff Meet., Mayo Clin. *9:*684–685, Nov 7, '34
Celluloid prosthesis in cosmetic correction after disfiguring surgery of frontal sinus. STUPKA, W. Arch. f. Ohren-Nasen-u. Kehlkopfh. *138:*79–86, '34
Management of recent fractures of nose and sinuses. WOODWARD, F. D. Ann. Otol., Rhin. and Laryng. *44:*264–273, March '35
Treatment of carcinoma of mouth and buccopharynx, nose and nasal sinus, with some remarks on diagnosis. PATTERSON, N. Tr. Am. Laryng., Rhin. and Otol. Soc. *41:*1–34, '35
Suppurations of maxillary sinus and of orbit with extensive destruction of wall of sinus simulating cancer of upper jaw; case. GUNSETT, *et al.* Bull. et mem. Soc. de radiol. med. de France *24:*170, Feb '36
Transplantation of parotid (Stensen's) duct in cancer of antrum. FIGI, F. A. Proc. Staff Meet., Mayo Clin. *11:*241–243, April 15, '36
Observations on sinus abnormalities in congenital total and hemi-absence of nose. BLAIR, V. P.; *et al.* Ann. Otol., Rhin. and Laryng. *46:*592–599, Sept '37
Unusual complication (facial hemi-atrophy)

Nose, Sinuses – Cont.
following Caldwell-Luc operation. J. Arkansas M. Soc. *34:*94, Oct '37
Fracture of skull involving paranasal sinuses. COLEMAN, C. C. J.A.M.A. *109:*1613–1616, Nov 13, '37
Sinus abnormalities in congenital total and hemi-absence of nose. BLAIR, V. P. Tr. Am. Laryng. A. *59:*223–229, '37
Fracture of skull involving paranasal sinuses and mastoids. COLEMAN, C. C. Tr. Sect. Laryng., Otol. and Rhin., A.M.A., pp. 58–67, '37
Therapy of fractures of cranial base involving nasal sinuses. NATHANSON, G. Acta otolaryng. *25:*430–439, '37
Contour reconstruction after external frontal sinus operation. O'CONNOR, G. B. Ann. Otol., Rhin. and Laryng. *47:*183–188, March '38
Paradental cyst of upper maxillary sinus with fistulization into lower eyelid; case. (Palpebral fistula.) PIQUET, J. AND DETROY, L. Echo med. du Nord *9:*337–339, June 30, '38
Plastic repair after removal of extensive malignant tumors of antrum. FIGI, F. A. Arch. Otolaryng. *28:*29–41, July '38
Unusual complication of radical antrum operation (hemiatrophy of face following Caldwell-Luc operation). FULLER, T. E. South. M. J. *31:*1094–1095, Oct '38
Fractures involving frontal sinus; 2 cases. BONNET, P. Bull. Soc. d'opht. de Paris *51:*83–84, Jan '39
War injuries of nose and nasal sinuses; 5 cases. NISHIYAMA, A. Oto-rhino-laryng. *12:*476–477, June '39
Sinusofacial wounds in war surgery with report of cases. ESCAT, M. Oto-rhino-laryng. internat. *24:*241–252, Sept '40
Orbital prosthesis after Riedel operation in frontal sinusitis; case. ALVES, O. Arq. de cir. clin. e exper. *6:*322–323, April–June '42
Facial fractures involving nasal accessory sinuses. NAFTZGER, J. B. Ann. Otol., Rhin. and Laryng. *51:*414–423, June '42
Nose and sinus injuries; necessity of early surgical intervention. BERENDES, J. Deut. Militararzt *7:*579–581, Sept '42
Discussion on injuries of frontal and ethmoidal sinuses. CALVERT, C. A. AND CAIRNS, H. Proc. Roy. Soc. Med. *35:*805–810, Oct '42 also: J. Laryng. and Otol. *57:*499–508, Nov '42
Injuries to nose, paranasal sinuses, mouth and ears. CANFIELD, N. Connecticut M. J. *6:*796–798, Oct '42

Nose, Sinuses – Cont.
New operation for fractures into maxillary sinus and antrum. WARREN, E. D. Dis. Eye, Ear, Nose and Throat *2:*304–305, Oct '42
Management of facial fractures involving paranasal sinuses. SHEA, J. J., J.A.M.A. *120:*745–749, Nov 7, '42
Surgical treatment of war injuries of nasal accessory sinuses. ESCHER, F. Schweiz. med. Wchnschr. *73:*715, May 29, '43 abstr. Bull. War Med. *4:*278, Jan '44
Surgical importance of abnormalities of frontal sinus; result of postoperative plastic correction using vitallium inclusion. GONZALEZ LOZA, M. AND MAISONNAVE, R. Rev. otorrinolaring. d. litoral *2:*298–306, June '43
Skin grafting in operations of the frontal sinus. BRADBEER, W. H., J. Laryng. and Otol. *59:*36–37, Jan '44
Lesions associated with fistula of frontal sinus. HICKEY, H. L. Ann. Otol., Rhin. and Laryng. *54:*143–158, March '45
Nose and sinuses; primary war injuries. CANFIELD, N. Proc. Roy. Soc. Med. *38:*627–628, Sept '45
Use of free grafts in surgical therapy of frontal sinusitis. MOULONGUET. Ann. d'oto-laryng. *12:*501–503, Oct–Dec '45
Primary war injuries involving nose and sinuses. CANFIELD, N., J. Laryng. and Otol. *60:*458–460, Nov '45
Management of fractures into nasal sinuses. SHEA, J. J. Laryngoscope *56:*22–25, Jan '46
Fractures involving frontal air sinuses, due to localized violence; 30 cases. SARTORIUS, K. South African M. J. *20:*202–208, April 27, '46
Fractures involving frontal air sinuses due to localized violence; 30 cases. SARTORIUS, K. South African M. J. *20:*234–237, May 11, '46
After-examination of 131 patients who had been operated on according to Caldwell-Luc procedure. HAASE, E. B. Acta oto-laryng. *34:*23–30, '46

Nose Surgery, Complications: See Rhinoplasty, Complications

Nose, Syphylitic Deformity of

Plastic repair of syphilitic nose. SHEEHAN, J. E. Laryngoscope *35:*22, Jan '25
Repair of spyhilitic nose. SHEEHAN, J. E. M. J. and Rec. (supp.) *120:*81–84, Sept 17, '24
Deformities of syphilitic nose. GILLIES, H. D. Brit. M. J. *2:*977–979, Nov 24, '23 (illus.)

Nose, Syphilitic Deformity of—Cont.

Plastic and reconstructive surgery; total rhinoplasty for syphilitic defect. IVY, R. H., S. Clin. N. Amer. *6:*248–251, Feb '26

Repair of syphilitic nasal deformity. JACQUES, P. Rev. med. de l'est *55:*81–84, Feb 15, '27

Plastic surgery in malignant syphilis of face and nasal fossae; case. PORTMANN, G. Rev. de laryng. *52:*199–208, March 31, '31

Late syphilis with destructive gummatous manifestations in nasal bones and first cervical vertebrae; cleft palate; case. RADAELI, A. Gior. ital. di dermat. e sif. *73:*531, Feb '32

Surgical correction of unusual type of syphilitic deformity of nostril. MONCORPS, C. Dermat. Wchnschr. *94:*383–386, March 12, '32

Method for repair of syphilitic nose. STRAATSMA, C. R. Arch. Otolaryng. *15:*906–909, June '32

Surgical correction of syphilitic saddle nose by Joseph operation and Filatov graft; case. REBELO NETO, J. Bol. Soc. de med. e cir. de Sao Paulo *16:*123–130, Dec '32

Syphilitic origin of perforation of palate and destruction of nose; uranoplasty; reconstruction of nose by tubular grafts with cartilaginous support of costal origin. ROCHER, H. L. Bull. et mem. Soc. de chir. de Bordeaux et du Sud-Ouest, pp. 150–152, '32

Syphilitic deformities of nose. FABIAN, A. Bratisl. lekar. listy *15:*749–768, June '35

Partial rhinoplasty after destruction of nose by syphilis; case. ALVES, O. Rev. oto-laring. de Sao Paulo (no. 5, bis) *4:*865–871, Sept–Oct '36

Etiology of saddle nose; preliminary report (syphilis). WOLFE, M. M. Ann. Otol., Rhin. and Laryng. *46:*504–509, June '37

Syphilitic saddle nose. GILLIES, H. Deutsche Ztschr. f. Chir. *250:*379–401, '38

Nose, Toe Transplants to

Transplantation of fleshy tip of toe to tip of nose. KURTZAHN, H. Deutsche Ztschr. f. Chir. *209:*401–402, '28

Plastic surgery of saddle nose (transplantation of toe). LINBERG, B. E. Vestnik khir. (no. 52) *18:*70–76, '29

Nose, Tumors

Treatment of fibromas of nasopharynx; report of 32 cases. NEW, G. B. AND FIGI, F. A. Am. J. Roentgenol. *12:*340–343, Oct '24

Hemangioma of nose. ROSENTHAL, M. Laryngoscope *35:*54, Jan '25

Nose, Tumors—Cont.

Tumors of nose, throat and ear; review of literature. NEW, G. B. Arch. Otolaryng. *1:*545–552, May '25

Tumors of nose and throat. NEW, G. B. Arch. Otolaryng. *3:*461–465, May '26

Giant hemangiofibroma of nose; case. BAYMA, F. Ann. paulist. de med. e cir. *18:*1–10, Jan '27

Tumors of nose and throat; review of literature. NEW, G. B. Arch. Otolaryng. *5:*352–356, April '27

Lymphangioma of nose. HAUTANT, A. AND LANOS. Ann. d. mal. de l'oreille, du larynx *46:*1235, Dec '27

Angioma of nose following erysipelas; radium therapy proposed; case. WALLON, E. Bull. Soc. franc. de dermat. et syph. *35:*406–408, May '28

Tumors of nasopharynx; review of literature. NEW, G. B. AND KIRCH, W. Arch. Otolaryng. *8:*600–607, Nov '28

Lymphangio-endothelioma of lip and nose. MOOREHEAD, F. B., S. Clin. N. Amer. *9:*329–330, April '29

Nasal tumors. NEW, G. B. AND KIRCH, W. Arch. Otolaryng. *9:*445–450, April '29

Fibroglioma of nose; case. DELLEPIANE RAWSON, J. AND VIVOLI, D. Rev. med. latino-am. *14:*860–868, May '29

Encephaloma or so-called nasal glioma. BROWDER, J. Ann. Otol. Rhin. and Laryng. *38:*395–403, June '29

Neurogenic tumors of nose. TOBECK, A. Ztschr. f. Hals-, Nasen-u. Ohrenh. *23:*329–339, Sept 10, '29

Cystic tumors of anterior nares due to embryonal maldevelopment; 3 cases. ARNOLDI, W. Ztschr. f. Laryng., Rhin. *18:*58–69, '29

Review of literature of nasal tumors. NEW, G. B. AND KIRCH, W. Arch. Otolaryng. *11:*657–668, May '30

Personal and practical experiences with neoplasms about head and neck, with special reference to ear, nose and throat. BECK, J. C. Pennsylvania M. J. *34:*467–469, April '31

Angioma of nose; case. PLEWKA. Ztschr. f. Hals-, Nasen-u. Ohrenh. *28:*560–564, Aug 20, '31

Tumors of nose and throat; summary of bibliographic material available in field of otolaryngology. NEW, G. B. AND KIRCH, W. Arch. Otolaryng. *15:*623–633, April '32

Hemangioma of nose; late results of radiotherapy. PANNETON, J. E. Union med. du Canada *61:*940–944, Aug '32

Nose, Tumors—Cont.

Congenital angiomas with nasofacial localization; case. FRANCHINI, Y. AND RICCITELLI, E. An. de oto-rino-laring. d. Uruguay *3:*193–203, '33

Angiomatous tumor of nasal fossae; ligature of external carotid and Rouge-Denker operation; case. PIQUET, J. AND BECUWE. Ann. d'oto-laryng., pp. 393–397, May '37

Pilous verrucous pigmentary nevus of nose; autoplasty using Thiersch graft. ROY, J. N. Union med. du Canada *66:*945–948, Sept '37

Pilous verrucous pigmented nevus of nose; autoplasty using Thiersch graft; case. ROY, J. N. Rev. argent. de oto-rhino-laring. *7:*53–57, March–April '38

Congenital angioma of nasal tip; case. MATSUDA, E. Oto-rhino-laryng. *11:*608, July '38

Tumors of nose. NEW, G. B. AND KIRCH, W. Arch. Otolaryng. *29:*457–467, March '39

Tumors of nose and throat; summaries of bibliographic material available in field of otolaryngology. NEW, G. B.; *et al.* Arch. Otolaryng. *30:*283–297, Aug '39

Deforming and recurring polyps of nose of youth. LAFF, H. I. Arch. Otolaryng. *30:*795–799, Nov '39

Paraffinoma of nose; surgical therapy of case. ZENO, L. Bol. Soc. de cir. de Rosario *7:*415–418, Oct '40

Paraffinoma of nose; surgical therapy; cases. ZENO, L. An. de cir. *7:*41–45, March–June '41

Deforming recidivating polyposis of nose, with report of case. RIESCO MAC-CLURE, J. S. Rev. otorrinolaring. *1:*61–64, Dec '41

Deforming polyposis of nose, with report of case. RIVAS, J. J. Arch. venezol. Soc. de oto-rino-laring., oftal., neurol. *2:*194–199, Dec '41

Cavernous hemangioma of nose, nasal septum and forehead. SALINGER, S. Ann. Otol., Rhin. and Laryng. *51:*268–272, March '42

Nasal tumors. EGGSTON, A. A. New York State J. Med. *43:*2403–2412, Dec 15, '43

Therapy of nasopharyngeal tumors. PORDES, J. M. Acta oto-laryng. orient. *1:*45–49, '45

NOSSEN, H. (see DÖRFFEL, J.) Aug '31

NOTHENBERG, O. J.: Modification of submucous resection operation. Illinois M. J. *40:*385, Nov '21

NOTTAGE, H. P.: Submucous resection of nasal septum. China M. J. *36:*469–473, Nov '22

NOVA, P. L. (see SHAAR, C. M. *et al*) Oct '42

NOVACHENKO, N. P.: Sources of regeneration of transplanted bone; experimental study. Ortop. i travmatol. (no. 1) *15:*5–13, '41

NOVACHENKO, N. P.: Present status of reconstructive surgery of organs of support and locomotion. Vrach. delo (nos. 11–12) *25:*587–592, '45

NOVAK, E.: Gastrointestinal ulceration following cutaneous burns; with report of case. Am. J. M. Sc. *169:*119–125, Jan '25

NOVAK, F. V.: Therapy of ulcerations and dermatoses of hands of roentgenologists and radiologists. Casop. lek. cesk. *74:*434–436, April 19, '35

NOVAK, J.: Plastic formation of artificial vagina by Schubert operation; 4 cases. Zentralbl. f. Gynak. *53:*2902–2908, Nov 16, '29

NOVAK, M.: Prevention of pain and treatment of burns. Munchen. med. Wchnschr. *77:*1669–1670, Sept 26, '30

NOVAK, V.: Consequences of hand injuries. Rozhl. v chir. a gynaek. (cast chir.) *14:*20–24, '35

Nové-Josserand Operation

Treatment of hypospadias by method of Nové-Josserand. MICHELSON, J. M. Arch. d. mal. d. reins *2:*513–517, April 1, '27

Nové-Josserand-Borchers Operation

Scrotal hypospadias treated by Nové-Josserand-Borchers procedure. MARTIN VIVALDI, J. Rev. clin. espan. *4:*358–359, March 15, '42

NOVELLA MONLEON, F.: Evolution of burn treatment. Med. clin., Barcelona *2:*505–509, June '44

NOVIS FILHO, A.: Acrocephalosyndactylia (Apert syndrome); case. Brasil-med. *49:*28–32, Jan 12, '35

NOVITSKIY, S. T.: Total transplantation of large toe to replace thumb. Vestnik khir. *57:*352–361, Feb–March '39

NOVOSHINOVA, E. N.: Use of tubular flap for transplantation of cartilage (ear) in surgical restoration of alae nasi. Zhur. ush., nos. i gorl. bolez. *15:*164–168, '38

NOVY, F. G. JR.: Rhinophyma with carcinomatous degeneration; case. Arch. Dermat. and Syph. *22:*270–273, Aug '30

NOWAK, H.: Familial ankylosis of finger joints (camptodactylia). Deutsche med. Wchnschr. *63:*937–938, June 11, '37

NOYA BENITEZ, J.: Burns. Bol. Asoc. med. de Puerto Rico *34:*90–95, March '42

NUBOER, J. F.: Rupture of subcutaneous tendon

of thumb; case. Nederl. tijdschr. v. geneesk. *2:*5645-5649, Nov 30, '29

NUBOER, J. F.: Treatment of ectopy of bladder. Deutsche Ztschr. f. Chir. *240:*390-393, '33

NUNEZ, R. A. (see PACK, G. T.) Jan-Mar '46

NUNEZ, R. A. (see PACK, G. T.) Feb '46

NUNN, L. L.: Cadaver cartilage banks. Bull. U. S. Army M. Dept. (no. 74) pp. 99-101, March '44

NUNZIATA, A.: Metacarpophalangeal luxation of index finger. Prensa med. argent. *31:*1760-1762, Sept 6, '44

NUNZIATA, A.: Clawhand; capsulotomies. Prensa med. argent. *31:*2169-2171, Oct 25, '44

NURI, M. K.: Exstrophy of bladder with abnormal symphysis pubis. J. de radiol. et d'electrol. *15:*254, May '31

Nursing

Nursing responsibilities in plastic surgery. NEWTON, K. Am. J. Nursing *43:*155-162, Feb '43

NUTINI, L. G. (see WALSH, T. F. P.) Aug '43

Nutrition

Malnutrition in infants with cleft palate, with description of new external obturator. FOOTE, J. A. Am. J. Dis. Child. *30:*343-346, Sept '25

Influence of inanition on homeoplastic transplantations. MORPURGO, B. Zentralbl. f. allg. Path. u. path. Anat. *40:*1-3, July 1, '27

Influence of inanition on homeoplastic skin-grafts. MORPURGO, B. AND MILONE, S. Boll. d. Soc. ital. di biol. sper. *2:*709-712, July '27

Influence of insufficient nutrition on taking of skin-grafts. MORPURGO, B. AND MILONE, S. Arch. per le sc. med. *49:*648-664, Nov '27

Feeding of liquid diet in jaw fractures. BROWN, J. B. Internat. J. Orthodontia *18:*614-617, June '32

Cleft palate associated with congenital and hypo-alimentary debility and pulmonary tuberculosis; case. PÉREZ MORENO, B. Siglo med. *93:*325-328, March 24, '34

Cases of cheiloplasty; description of apparatus for feeding infants with harelip and cleft palate. also: rhinoplasty. BRISOTTO, P. Boll. d. mal. d. oreccio, d. gola, d. naso *56:*89-99, March '38

Feeding and care of patients with maxillofacial wounds. AKS, L. V. Ortop. i. travmatol. (no. 1) *14:*90-96, '40

Organizational problem of nutrition in maxillofacial trauma. PYATNITSKIY, F. A. Klin. med. (nos. 3-4) *20:*22-28, '42

Nutrition – Cont.

Problems of protein nutrition in burn patients. TAYLOR, F. H. L. *et al.* Ann. Surg. *118:*215-224, Aug '43

Congenital cleft palate and harelip in infants; mode of nutrition in preoperative period. TAYLOR, H. P. Brit. Dent. J. *78:*1-7, Jan 5, '45

Alterations following thermal burns; effect of variations in food intake on nitrogen balance of burned patients. HIRSHFELD, J. W. *et al.* Arch. Surg. *50:*194-200, April '45

Nutrition of patients with thermal burns. LEVENSON, S. M. *et al.* Surg. Gynec. and Obst. *80:*449-469, May '45

Fluid and nutritional therapy in burns. HARKINS, H. N. *et al.* J.A.M.A. *128:*475-479, June 16, '45

Adequate nutrition gains emphasis as vital factor in burn surgery. MACOMBER, M. H. Hospitals (no. 7) *19:*73-74, July '45

NUTTING, R. J.: Plastic surgery in and about eyelids. California State J. Med. *20:*15-16, Jan '22

NUYTTEN, J.: Epitheliomas and their therapy. Echo med. du Nord. *6:*544-563, Sept 27, '36

NUZUM, T. W.: Avulsion of scalp; with report of 3 cases. Surg. J. *33:*117-119, May-June '27

NUZZI, O.: Correction of deformity of hand. Riforma med. *37:*248, March 12, '21 abstr: J.A.M.A. *76:*1435, May 21, '21

NYI, P. C.: Cleft lip repair under bilateral infra-orbital nerve block at infra-orbital foramina. Chinese M. J. *48:*373-374, April '34

NYKA, W. AND LAVEDAN, J.: Therapy of cancer by means of transplantation of normal organs; review. Paris med. *1:*229-240, March 18, '33

NYLANDER, P. E. A.: Congenital cervical fistulae and cysts. Arb. a. d. path. Inst. *5:*114-231, '27

NYLANDER, P. E. A.: Parathyroidal cyst of neck; case. Acta chir. Scandinav. *64:*539-547, '29

NYLANDER, P. E. A.: Genesis of congenital lateral cervical fistulas and cysts. Deutsche Ztschr. f. Chir. *215:*139-145, '29

NYLANDER, P. E. A.: Therapy of congenital branchial fistulas. Zentralbl. f. Chir. *65:*1095-1097, May 7, '38

NYST, P. M. E. P.: Intrapharyngeal nitrous oxide insufflation in staphylorrhaphy. Nederl. tijdschr. v. geneesk. *75:*2059-2061, April 18, '31

O

OAKS, L. W.: Improved treatment for chemical burns of eye. Am. J. Ophth. *28:*370–373, April '45

OBERDORFER, A. Z.: Primary skin graft for repair of traumatic skin loss of face; case. U. S. Nav. M. Bull. *42:*695–696, March '44

OBERHOFF, K.: Measures to protect eye in facial paralysis. Munchen. med. Wchnschr. *87:*33, Jan 12, '40

OBERNDORF, C. P.: Submucous resection of nasal castration symbol. Internat. J. Psycho-Analysis *10:*228–241, April–July '29

OBERNIEDERMAYR, A.: Surgical therapy of harelip and cleft palate. Chirurg. *9:*641–645, Sept 1, '37

OBERNIEDERMAYR, A.: Therapy of congenital bladder ectopia. Med. Klin. *36:*971–973, Aug 30, '40

OBRAZTSOV, G. D.: Experimental and clinical contributions to question of alcohol therapy of traumatic shock. Vestnik khir. *53:*123–129, '37

OBSTÄNDER, E. (see BRÜCKNER, S.) Sept '32

OČENÁŠEK, M.: Progressive hemiatrophy of face. Cas. lek. cesk. *61:*378–382, April 29, '22

OCHSNER, A. J.: Treatment of cancer of jaws; observations continued since 1918, covering 26 additional cases. Ann. Surg. *76:*328–332, Sept '22

OCHSNER, C. G.: Branchial cysts. Minnesota Med. *20:*31–33, Jan '37

OCHSNER, E. H.: Treatment of extensive burns and scalds (with special reference to Unna's paste, zinc oxide preparation). New Zealand M. J. *38:*180–187, June '39 also: M. Rec. *150:*193–196, Sept 20, '39

OCHSNER, E. W. A. (see DEUCHER, W. G.) 1924

Free homeoplastic skin grafting; comment on Deucher and Ochsner's article. ASCHER, K. W. Arch. f. klin. Chir. *137:*198, '25

O'CONNELL, R. J. JR. (see BEEKMAN, F.) Sept '33

O'CONNOR, D. C.: Surgical shock. Journal-Lancet *41:*287, May 15, '21

O'CONNOR, G. B.: Early grafting of mucous membrane in burns of eye. Arch. Ophth. *9:*48–51, Jan '33

O'CONNOR, G. B.: Application of grafts early in burns of eye. Rev. de chir. structive, pp. 273–277, June '36

O'CONNOR, G. B.: Glove flap method of dorsal repair in hand surgery. Am. J. Surg. *32:*445–447, June '36

O'CONNOR, G. B.: Glove flap method of dorsal hand repair. Rev. de chir. structive, pp. 384–389, Dec '36

O'CONNOR, G. B.: Operation for correction of atresia or stenosis of anterior nares. Arch. Otolaryng. *25:*208–210, Feb '37

O'CONNOR, G. B.: Pharyngeal reconstruction in stenosis; new operative procedure. Ann. Otol., Rhin. and Laryng. *46:*376–386, June '37

O'CONNOR, G. B.: Contour reconstruction after external frontal sinus operation. Ann. Otol., Rhin. and Laryng. *47:*183–188, March '38

O'CONNOR, G. B.: Reconstruction of anterior nares following stenosis. Rev. de chir. structive *8:*77–83, Aug '38

O'CONNOR, G. B.: Merthiolate (mercury compound): tissue preservative and antiseptic (for "refrigerated cartilage isografts"). Am. J. Surg. *45:*563–565, Sept '39

O'CONNOR, G. B.: Refrigerated cartilage isografts; source, storage and use. California and West. Med. *52:*21–23, Jan '40

O'CONNOR, G. B.: Plastic repair of scrotum following gangrene; case. U. S. Nav. M. Bull. *44:*1060–1062, May '45

O'CONNOR, G. B.: Reconstruction of penis after traumatic fracture. U. S. Nav. M. Bull. *45:*147–149, July '45

O'CONNOR, G. B. AND KESSLER, H. H.: Symposium on amputation from Naval Amputation Center, U. S. Naval Hospital, Mare Island, California; plastic surgery of stumps. U. S. Nav. M. Bull. *44:*1167–1180, June '45

O'CONNOR, G. B. AND PIERCE, G. W.: Dermo-subcutaneous flaps; management in reconstructive surgery. California and West. Med. *40:*151–156, March '34

O'CONNOR, G. B. AND PIERCE, G. W.: Repair and restoration of orbit. Arch. Ophth. *12:*493–499, Oct '34

O'CONNOR, G. B. AND PIERCE, G. W.: Refrigerated cartilage isografts in facial surgery. Surg., Gynec. and Obst. *67:*796–798, Dec '38

O'CONNOR, G. B. (see PIERCE, G. W.) Aug '31

O'CONNOR, G. B. (see PIERCE, G. W.) Feb '34

O'CONNOR, G. B. (see PIERCE, G. W.) June '37

O'CONNOR, G. B. (see PIERCE, G. W.) June '38

O'CONNOR, R.: Motias operation for eyelid ptosis, report of 6 cases. California State J. Med. *19:*409, Oct '21

ODELBERG, A.: Therapy of contracture of underarm. (Comment on Kappis' article). Zentralbl. f. Chir. *59:*2915–2918, Dec 3, '32

ODEN, L. H. JR. (see HARBISON, S. P.) July '46

ODQVIST, H.: Multiple dermal cancer in face and on neck; case. Acta radiol. *9:*302–304, '28

OERTEL, T. E.: Submucous replacement for external deviation of nose. Ann. Otol. Rhinol.

and Laryng. *30:*147, March '21

OESER, H.: Question of tumor of parotid gland or swelling of preauricular lymph nodes. Monatschr. f. Krebsbekampf. *11:*43, March '43

OEHLECKER, F.: Transplants in fingers, fate of joint transplants. Beitr. z. klin. Chir. *126:*135–181, '22 (illus.) abstr: J.A.M.A. *79:*778, Aug 26, '22

OEHLECKER, F.: Contracture of fingers (ischemic myositis). Beitr. z. klin. Chir. *149:*333–364, '30

OEHLECKER, F.: Late results of transplantation of large toe to replace lost thumb. Arch. f. klin. Chir. *189:*674–680, '37

O'FARRELL. (see SIBBALD) 1926

O'FARRELL, G. (see SIBBALD, D.) 1925

O'FERRALL, J. T.: Surgical treatment of arthritis. New Orleans M. and S. J. *81:*899–902, June '29

D'OFFAY, T. M. J.: Rehabilitation of injured hand. M. Press. *211:*76–79, Feb 2, '44

OFFRET, G. (see WELTI, H.) Oct–Nov '42

OGHI, A. (see PAVLOWSKY, A. J. *et al*) Feb '46

OGILVIE, A. G. AND POSEL, M. M.: Scaphocephaly, oxycephaly and hypertelorism, with reports of cases. Arch. Dis. Childhood *2:*146–154, June '27

OGILVIE, W. H.: Hand infections. Guy's Hosp. Gaz. *44:*314–321, Aug 23, '30

OGILVIE, W. H.: Hand infections. J. Roy. Army M. Corps *56:*261–274, April '31

OGILVIE, W. H.: Hand infections. Guy's Hosp. Gaz. *51:*114, March 13, '37; *51:*177–184, April 24, '37

OGILVIE, W. H.: Burn therapy. East Africa M. J. *18:*131–139, Aug '41

OGLE, M. W.: Chemotherapy (with sulfanilamide and its derivatives) in gunshot wounds of face, neck and jaws. Mil. Surgeon *90:*650–655, June '42

OGLE, M. W.: Chemotherapy (with sulfonamides) in gunshot wounds of face, neck and jaws. Rev. san. mil., Habana *6:*312–317, Oct–Dec ('42)

OGNEFF, B. V.: New principle in formation of artificial vagina. Vestnik khir. (no. 64) *22:*105–110, '30

OGNEV, B. V.: Method of reduction of luxation of temporomaxillary joint. Sovet. med. (no. 4) *4:*17–18, '40

O'HARA, D. M.: Review of local anesthesia in maxillofacial cases. Mil. Surgeon *89:*652–656, Oct '41

OHM, J.: Historical observation on improvement of Toti's operation (dacryocystorhinostomy). Klin. Monatsbl. f. Augenh. *77:*825–832, Dec '26

ÖHNGREN, G.: Plastic surgery of face following electrocoagulation treatment of malignant tumors of nose and accessory sinuses. Acta oto-laryng. *16:*292–305, '31

ÖHNGREN, G.: Cosmesis and surgery. Nord. med. tidskr. *4:*342–345, May 21, '32

OHNO, T.: Cavernous angioma of face with homolateral glaucoma; case. Jap. J. Dermat. and Urol. *29:*33, May '29

OHNO, T.: Joseph operation in plastic repair of bulldog nose; case. Oto-rhino-laryng. *12:*10, Jan '39

OKUDA, S.: Clinical and experimental studies on transplantation of living hairs. Jap. J. Dermat. and Urol. *46:*135–138, Dec 20, '39

OKUMA, M.: Mechanism of development of epithelial cysts; behavior of autogenous skin particle implanted subcutaneously. Nagasaki Igakkwai Zasshi *14:*94–96, Jan 25, '36

OLÁH, E.: Operative procedure in trachomatous entropion of upper lid. Klin. Monatsbl. f. Augenh. *79:*388, Sept 30, '27

OLÁH, E.: Therapy of epicanthus tarsalis. Klin. Monatsbl. f. Augenh. *90:*233–234, Feb '33

OLAISON, F.: Statistical postoperative prognosis of malignant tumors of upper jaw. Hygiea *89:*705–710, Sept 30, '27

OLDAGER, A.: Hygienic suspensory operation of breast. Ugesk. f. laeger *95:*202–203, Feb 16, '33

OLDENSTAM, R. A.: Entire restoration of auricle after complete traumatic separation; case. Nederl. Tijdschr. v. Geneesk. *1:*1097, March 2, '29

OLDFIELD, MICHAEL C.: *Speech Training for Cases of Cleft Palate.* H. K. Lewis and Co., London, 1938

OLDFIELD, M. C.: Encephalocele associated with hypertelorism and cleft palate. Brit. J. Surg. *25:*757–764, April '38

OLDFIELD, M. C.: Burn therapy in wartime. J. Roy. Army M. Corps *77:*1–13, July '41

OLDFIELD, M. C.: Cleft palate and mechanism of speech. (Arris and Gale lecture). Brit. J. Surg. *29:*197–227, Oct '41

OLDFIELD, M. C.: Early treatment of war wounds of upper part of face. Brit. M. J. *2:*163–165, Aug 7, '43

OLDFIELD, M. C.: Early treatment of war wounds of upper part of face. Rev. san. mil., Buenos Aires. *43:*11–17, Jan '44

OLDFIELD, M. C.: Reparative surgery of face in Middle East, with short review of 1,200 cases treated during last 2 years. Brit. J. Surg. *32:*237–246, Oct '44

OLDFIELD, M. C. AND KING, C. J.: Finger exerciser for burned hands. Lancet *2:*109, July 22, '44

Oldham, J. B.: War wounds of fingers. M. Press *204:*476-480, Dec 18, '40

Olesen, M.: Skin grafts with film bandage. Ugesk. f. laeger *101:*144-147, Feb 2, '39

Olinger, N. A.: Care of military and civilian facial injuries; surgical prosthesis. Am. J. Orthodontics (Oral Surg. Sect.) *28:*222-238, April '42

Olinger, N. A.: Eugenic aspect of cleft palate and other facial deformities. J. Am. Dent. A. *31:*1431-1434, Nov 1, '44

Olinger, N. A.: Prosthetic restoration of congenital cleft palate. Am. J. Orthodontics (Oral Surg. Sect.) *32:*456-468, July '46

Olinger, N. A.: Speech defects in relation to oral defects. Am. J. Orthodontics (Oral Surg. Sect.) *32:*469-471, July '46

Olinger, N. A. and Axt, E. F.: Surgical prosthetics of oral and facial defects. Am. J. Surg. *31:*24-37, Jan '36

Olivares, L.: Etiology, pathogenesis, semeiology, surgical and nonsurgical treatment of Volkmann's contracture. Med. ibera *1:*313-319, March 24, '28

Olivares, L.: Chronic edema of arm; recovery of case after surgical therapy. Actas Soc. de cir. de Madrid *4:*223-229, April-June '35

Olivares, L.: Irreducible luxation of lower jaw; surgical therapy of case. Actas Soc. de cir. de Madrid *4:*279-284, April-June '35

Olivares, M. G.: Surgical therapy of ozena by transplantation of bone into septum. An. Soc. mex. de oftal. y oto-rino-laring. *9:*28-32, July-Sept '31

Olive Leite, A.: Unilateral congenital imperforation of choana; case with slight surgical correction. Rev. brasil. de oto-rino-laring. *7:*49-58, Jan-Feb '39

de Oliveira, L. C.: Differential diagnosis of lesions of mouth. Hora med., Rio de Janeiro *2:*9-16, July '43

de Oliveira Matos, J.: Braun graft in therapy of varicose ulcers; histopathologic evolution of graft. Arq. de cir. clin. e exper. *6:*653-669, April-June '42

Oliveras Guerra, A.: Primary tenorrhaphy in therapy of section of tendons during cane cutting. Bol. Asoc. med. de Puerto Rico *28:*114-118, June '36

Oliveras Guerra, A.: Post-traumatic neuralgia as serious complication of section of tendons of hand in cultivators of sugar cane. Bol. Asoc. med. de Puerto Rico *35:*47-51, Feb '43

Olivier, E.; Piedelievre, R. and Desoille, H.: Evaluation of degree of invalidity in amputation of various segments of fingers. Ann. de med. leg. *17:*883-888, Oct '37

Olivier, G. and Barasch: Generalized keloids treated by parathyroidectomy; case. Progr. med., Paris *7:*292-293, July 10, '46

Oller, A.: Rare traumatic lesions of wrist and hand. Arch. de med., cir. y espec. *26:*465-469, April 9, '27

Oller, A.: Examples of restorative surgery and functional adaptation of hand and feet. Siglo med. *83:*77-82, Jan 5, '29

Oller, A.: Dupuytren's contracture as result of industrial accident. Arch. de med., cir. y espec. *30:*333-335, March 16, '29

Ollerenshaw, R.: Tendon transplantation. Brit. M. J. *2:*77-78, July 15, '22

Ollier, A.: Dupuytren's contracture not occupational accident; case. Ars med. *5:*96-98, March '29

Ollier Operation

Rhinophyma; therapy by Ollier's surgical decortication. Marin, A. Bull. Soc. franc. de dermat. et syph. *46:*705-709, April '39

Reparation of bone loss by Ollier osteoperiostic grafts, segmentary bone grafts, bone implantations and hidden internal prostheses. Mauclaire. Rev. med. franc. *15:*263-273, March '34

Olsho, S. L.: New nasal septal chisel. Laryngoscope *33:*308, April '23 (illus.)

Olsho, S. L.: Use of prisms in bilateral eyelid ptosis; case. Am. J. Ophth. *16:*141-142, Feb '33

Olson, C. T.: Tantalum in plastic surgery; glimpse of surgical future. Indust. Med. *13:*738, Sept '44

Olson, W. H. and Necheles, H.: Vasopressor effect of thermal trauma. Am. J. Physiol. *139:*574-582, Aug '43

Olson, W. H. (see Necheles, H.) May '42

Oltramare, H. (see Oltramare, J. H.) May '24

Oltramare, H. (see Oltramare, J. H.) Oct '24

Oltramare, J. H. and Oltramare, H.: Traumatic shock. Schweiz. med. Wchnschr. *54:*420, May 1, '24 abstr: J.A.M.A. *82:*1997, June 14, '24

Oltramare, J. H. and Oltramare, H.: Traumatic shock and inspissation of blood. Schweiz. med. Wchnschr. *54:*912-914, Oct 2, '24 abstr: J.A.M.A. *83:*1625, Nov 15, '24

O'Malley, T. S.: Full thickness skin grafts in finger amputations. Wisconsin M. J. *33:*337-340, May '34

Omar Bey, T.: Clinical note on burns. J. Egyptian M. A. *17:*653, July '34

Omar Bey, T.: Thiersch method of skin grafting. J. Egyptian M. A. *17:*654, July '34

Ombrédanne: Cleft palate treatment in children. Rev. odont. *50:*230-237, June '29

OMBRÉDANNE: Anatomic and functional results of 50 operations for marked deviations of traumatic origin in young children (nasal septum). Ann. d'oto-laryng., pp. 145–150, July–Sept '42

OMBRÉDANNE, L.: Correction of facial paralysis. Presse med. *29:*636, Aug 10, '21 abstr: J.A.M.A. *77:*1053, Sept 24, '21

OMBRÉDANNE, L.: Reconstruction of nostril in simple hare-lip. Presse med. *29:*703, Sept 3, '21

OMBRÉDANNE, L.: Treatment of harelip. Medecine *4:*21–27, Oct '22 abstr: J.A.M.A. *79:*1962, Dec 2, '22

OMBRÉDANNE, L.: *Les hermaphrodites et la chirurgie*. Masson et Cie, Paris, 1923

OMBRÉDANNE, L.: Autoplastic surgery of ear. Presse med. *39:*982–983, July 4, '31

OMBRÉDANNE, L.: Surgical correction of hermaphroditism. Clinics *1:*615–630, Oct '42

OMBRÉDANNE, L. AND OMBRÉDANNE, M.: Flat nose, consequent to harelip operations; operative treatment. Ann. d. mal. de l'oreille, du larynx *47:*1090–1111, Dec '28

OMBRÉDANNE, M. (see OMBRÉDANNE, L.) Dec '28

OMBRÉDANNE, M.: Autoplasty in rhinologic surgery (face). Semaine d. hop. de Paris *7:*44–48, Jan 31, '31

OMBRÉDANNE, M.: Protruding ears and their surgical correction. Semaine d. hop. de Paris *15:*404–411, Nov '39

OMBRÉDANNE, M.: Imperforate auditory canal in connection with congenital malformations of auricle. Ann. d'oto-laryng., pp. 1–5, Jan–March '44

OMBRÉDANNE, M.: Imperforation of external auditory canal with aplasia of auricle; results of operation. Arch. franc. pediat. *2:*73–74, '44

Ombredanne Operation

Therapy of penal and penoscrotal hypospadias; supplementary notes on Ombredanne operation. BARCAT, J. R., J. de chir. *58:*418–426, '41–'42

Posterior hypospadias cured by Ombredanne operation; case. BIANCALANA, L. Boll. e mem. Soc. piemontese di chir. *7:*325–327, '37

Ombredanne's pouch operation in hypospadias. LYLE, H. H. M. Ann. Surg. *98:*513–519, Oct '33

Experiences with Ombredanne operation for hypospadias. MUSCHAT, M. J. Urol. *51:*437–438, April '44

Hypospadias treated by Ombredanne technic. FLYNN, R., M. J. Australia *2:*479, Sept 18, '37

Ombredanne-Lyle operation for hypospadias; case. WALTERS, W. Proc. Staff Meet., Mayo Clin. *8:*467–469, Aug 2, '33

Ombredanne operation in hypospadias; case. BIANCALANA, L. Boll. e mem. Soc. piemontese di chir. *6:*18–25, '36

Ombredanne's method for grave hypospadias. RIVAROLA, R. A. Rev. Asoc. med. argent. *35:*634, Aug '21

Plastic surgery (modified Ombredanne operation) in therapy of epispadias with urinary incontinence; case. DE BRUIN, T. R. Nederl. tijdschr. v. geneesk. *90:*1127–1129, Sept 7, '46

ONACA. (See IACOBOVICI, I.) March–April '35

O'NEILL, C. P. (see VESEEN, L. L.) Sept '33

O'NEILL, J. F.; TOCANTINS, L. M. AND PRICE, A. H.: Technic of administering blood and other fluids via bone marrow; further experiences (shock). North Carolina M. J. *3:*495–500, Sept '42

O'NEILL, J. F. (see TOCANTINS, L. M. *et al*) Dec '41

O'NEILL, T.: Congenital absence of vagina treated successfully by Baldwin technic. Brit. M. J. *2:*746–747, Dec 11, '43

ONGJOCO, J. S. (see SANTILLAN, J. S. *et al*) Jan '41

ONKEN, T.: Therapy of positional abnormalities of eyelids. Klin. Monatsbl. f. Augenh. *90:*78–79, Jan '33

OPIZZI, J.: Traumatic shock; review. Rev. san. mil., Buenos Aires *40:*76–78, Jan '41

OPPEGAARD, M. O.: Treatment of hand infections and injuries. Minnesota Med. *9:*373–375, July '26

OPPENHEIM, A.: Prognathism from anthropological and orthodontic viewpoint. Ztschr. f. Stomatol. *25:*518–573, June '27

OPPENHEIM, A.: Prognathism from anthropological and orthodontic viewpoints. Dental Cosmos *70:*1092–1110, Nov '28

OPPENHEIM, A.: Prognathism from anthropological and orthodontic viewpoints. Ztschr. f. Stomatol. *28:*313–339, April '30 also: Dental Cosmos *72:*645, June; 736, July '30

OPPIKOFER, E.: Electrical injuries of oral cavity. Schweiz. med. Wchnschr. *69:*1197–1198, Nov 25, '39

OPPENHEIMER, E. D.: Splint for correction of finger contracture. J. Bone and Joint Surg. *19:*247–248, Jan '37

Oral Surgery (See also Maxillofacial Surgery, Mouth, etc)

Principles and Technique of Oral Surgery, by ADOLPH BERGER. Dental Items of Interest Publishing Co., Brooklyn, 1923

Oral Surgery—Cont.

Essentials of Oral Surgery, by VILRAY P. BLAIR AND ROBERT H. IVY AND (in the Second and Third Edition) J. B. BROWN. C. V. Mosby Co., St. Louis, 1923. Second Edition, 1936. Third Edition, 1944

Principles and Practice of Oral Surgery, by S. L. SILVERMAN. Blakiston Co., Phila., 1926

Oral Surgery, by STERLING V. MEAD. C. V. Mosby Co., St. Louis, 1933. Second Edition, 1940. Third Edition, 1946

Surgical Diseases of the Mouth and Jaws, by EARL C. PADGETT. W. B. Saunders Co., Phila., 1938

Operative Oral Surgery, by LEO WINTER. C. V. Mosby Co., St. Louis, 1941

ORBACH, E.: Division of palmar fascia in therapy of Dupuytren's contracture. Med. Welt *6:*955–956, July 2, '32

ORBACH, E.: Functional therapy of finger contractures. Arch. f. orthop. u. Unfall-Chir. *34:*572–579, '34

ORBACH, E.: Technic for covering defects after extirpation of malignant melanoma of skin (grafts). Wien. med. Wchnschr. *85:*1112–1113, Oct 5, '35

ORBELI, L. A.: Physiologic bases of traumatic shock. Voen.-med. sborn. *1:*5–13, '44

Orbit

Orbital phlegmons as sequels of endonasal operations. BACHMANN, R. Med. Klin. *17:*192, Feb 13, '21

Plastic surgery of eyelids and orbit. WALDRON, C. W. Minnesota Med. *4:*504, Aug '21

Reconstruction of orbit. TERRIEN, F. Paris med. *12:*157–159, Feb 25, '22

Correction of deformities of nose and about orbit by plastic surgery. DE RIVER, J. P. Southwestern Med. 7:226–232, July '23

Hypertelorism; a hitherto undifferentiated congenital cranio-facial deformity. GREIG, D. M. Edinburgh M. J. *31:*560–593, Oct '24

Newer Methods of Ophthalmic Plastic Surgery, by EDMUND B. SPAETH. Blakiston Co., Phila., 1925

Hypertelorism. COMBY, J. Arch. de med. d. enf. *28:*570–573, Sept '25

Present day advances in plastic surgery, with special reference to correction of deformities of nose and about orbit. DE RIVER, J. P. Ann. Otol., Rhin. and Laryng. *34:*904–916, Sept '25

Hypertelorism. COCKAYNE, E. A. Brit. J. Child. Dis. *22:*265–274, Oct–Dec '25

Orbit—Cont.

Present day advance in plastic surgery, with special reference to correction of deformities of nose and about orbit. DE RIVER, J. P. California and West. Med. *24:*64–68, Jan '26

Plastic surgery of supra-orbital region. JOHNSON, L. W., J.A.M.A. *86:*14–16, Jan 2, '26

Plastic Surgery of the Orbit, by J. EASTMAN SHEEHAN. Macmillan Co., New York, 1927

Scaphocephaly, oxycephaly and hypertelorism, with reports of cases. OGILVIE, A. G. AND POSEL, M. M. Arch. Dis. Childhood *2:*146–154, June '27

Hypertelorism in several generations. ABERNETHY, D. A. Arch. Dis. Childhood *2:*361–365, Dec '27

Eyelid surgery for partial contraction of socket. GREEVES, R. A. Tr. Ophth. Soc. U. Kingdom *47:*101–106, '27

Four cases of unusual eye injuries; eyelash in iris; horsehair in lens; ink pencil injury; traumatic enophthalmos. HORAY, G. Klin. Monatsbl. f. Augenh. *80:*202–208, Feb 24, '28

Hypertelorism. REUBEN, M. S. AND FOX, H. R. Arch. Pediat. *45:*105–115, Feb '28

Congenital craniofacial deformity (hypertelorism); case. BABONNEIX, L. *et al.* Bull. Soc. de pediat. de Paris *26:*118, March '28

Lips and teeth and cyclopia and harelips. BOLK, L. Ztschr. f. d. ges. Anat. (Abt. 1) *85:*762–783, May 21, '28

Unilateral hypertelorism, case. LIGHTWOOD, R. C. AND SHELDON, W. P. H. Arch. Dis. Childhood *3:*168–172, June '28

Plastic surgery of orbit. WILDE, A. G. Texas State J. Med. *24:*336–344, Sept '28

Orbital grafting of cartilage from nasal ala; technic. DANTRELLE AND SHEEHAN. Ann. d'ocul. *165:*902–909, Dec '28

Repair of roof of orbit by means of cartilaginous graft. RHÉAUME, P. Z. AND BABEAUX, F. Presse med. *36:*1604, Dec 15, '28

Hereditary hypertelorism without mental deficiency. MONTFORD, T. M. Arch. Dis. Childhood *4:*381–384, Dec '29

Ocular hypertelorism. REGNAULT, F. AND CROUZON, O. Ann. d'anat. path. *7:*571–576, May '30

Congenital ocular hypertelorism; case. DELLEPIANE RAWSON, R. AND GONZÁLEZ AVILA, E. Rev. de especialid. *5:*1090–1096, Aug '30 also: Semana med. *2:*1206–1209, Oct 16, '30

Plastic surgery of orbit. WILDE, A. G. New Orleans M. and S. J. *83:*239–244, Oct '30

Naso-orbital epitheliomas; 10 cases.

Orbit—Cont.
ABOULKER, H. AND GOZLAN, A. Ann. d'oto-laryng., pp. 381–398, April '31
Hypertelorism, four cases. REILLY, W. A. J.A.M.A. *96:*1929–1933, June 6, '31
Plastic surgery of orbit. CSAPODY, I. Gyogyaszat *72:*65–67, Jan 31, '32
Plastic surgery of orbital cavity with dermo-epidermal grafts. WORMS, G. Bull. Soc. d'opht. de Paris, pp. 358–361, June '32
Unusual familial developmental disturbance of face, (acrocephalosyndactylia, craniofacial dystosis and hypertelorism). CHOTZEN, F. Monatschr. f. Kinderh. *55:*97–122, '32
Types of reconstructive surgery of orbital region. BLAIR, V. P.; *et al.* South. Surgeon *1:*293–300, Jan '33
Hypertelorism, case. TOZER, F. H. W. Roy. Berkshire Hosp. Rep., pp. 17–21, '33
Anomalies of eye and orbit in acrocephalosyndactylia (Apert syndrome). WAARDENBURG, P. J. Maandschr. v. kindergeneesk. *3:*196–212, Feb '34
Repair and restoration of orbit. O'CONNOR, G. B. AND PIERCE, G. W. Arch. Ophth. *12:*493–499, Oct '34
Reconstruction of orbital cavity for wearing prosthesis long after exenteration of orbit. LOTIN, A. V. Sovet. vestnik oftal. *7:*402, '35
Ocular hypertelorism. SLO-BODKIN, S. G. Arch. Pediat. *53:*191–196, March '36
Potassium bromide as anesthetic in facial orbital surgery. KHRAMELASHVILI, N. G. Sovet. vrach. zhur., pp. 677–678, May 15, '36
Prosthesis covering orbital region, nose and upper lip. PONT AND LAPIERRE, V. Bull. Soc. franc. de dermat. et syph. (Reunion dermat., Lyon) *43:*908–910, May '36
Restoration of orbit and repair of conjunctival defects, with grafts from prepuce and labia minora. CLAY, G. E. AND BAIRD, J. M. J.A.M.A. *107:*1122–1125, Oct 3, '36
Restoration of eye socket with Thiersch graft; 6 cases. LIN, C. K. Chinese M. J. *50:*1335–1344, Oct '36
Plastic surgery of orbit. FOLK, M. L. Illinois M. J. *70:*419–424, Nov '36
Restoration of orbit and repair of conjunctival defects, with grafts from prepuce and labia minora. CLAY, G. E. AND BAIRD, J. M. Tr. Sect. Ophth., A.M.A., pp. 252–259, '36
Cavernous hemangioma of orbit successfully removed by Krönlein's operation. STALLARD, H. B. Lancet *1:*131–133, Jan 15, '38
Buried grafts used to repair depressions in brow, eye socket, skull and nose. PEER, L. A., J. M. Soc. New Jersey *35:*601–605, Oct '38

Orbit—Cont.
Notes on 3 cases of hypertelorism. PICKERILL, H. P. Brit. J. Surg. *26:*588–592, Jan '39
Epithelial inlay with Kerr-material to form eye socket. CZUKRASZ, I. Brit. J. Ophth. *23:*343–347, May '39
Total plastic reconstruction of orbit. GANZER, H. Plast. chir. *1:*72–76, '39
Plastic surgery about eye and orbit. SPAETH, E. B. Tr. Indiana Acad. Ophth. and Otolaryng. *23:*81–83, '39
Plastic restoration of deformity caused by complete exenteration of orbit. HAGEDOORN, A. Surg., Gynec. and Obst. *70:*193–195, Feb '40
Method of dealing with fractures through infraorbital margin. LAW, T. B., M. J. Australia *1:*666–667, May 31, '41
Eye socket reconstruction; new form and method of handling skin graft. HUGHES, W. L. Arch. Ophth. *26:*965–968, Dec '41
Roentgen diagnosis of blunt and gunshot injuries to orbit. BALTIN, M. M. AND SVYADOSHCH, B. I. Vestnik oftal. *18:*306–311, '41
Prosthesis of orbit and surrounding parts of face. RUMYANTSEVA, A. F. Vestnik oftal (nos. 3–4) *19:*153–154, '41
Hypertelorism; case with median nasal fissure. ZENO, L. An. de cir. *8:*37–39, March–June '42 also: Bol. Soc. de cir. de Rosario *9:*59–62, May '42
Orbital prosthesis after Riedel operation in frontal sinusitis; case. ALVES, O. Arq. de cir. clin. e exper. *6:*322–323, April–June '42
Wounds and deformities of orbital region. HAYNES, L. K. Mil. Surgeon *91:*83-90, July '42
Hypertelorism associated with median nasal cleft; case. ZENO, L. An. argent. de oftal. *4:*3–5, Jan–March '43
Lagrange's law of indirect ocular war injuries (facial fractures). SOUDAKOFF, P. S. Am. J. Ophth. *26:*293–296, March '43
Hypertelorism. BERKOVE, A. B. Arch. Otolaryng. *38:*587–589, Dec '43
Reconstruction of contracted eye socket. HUGHES, W. L. Tr. Am. Soc. Plastic and Reconstructive Surg. *12:*25–28, '43
Plastic reconstruction of eye socket. GOLDMANN, H. Ophthalmologica *107:*60–63, Jan–Feb '44
Gunshot wounds of fronto-orbital region. SCHORSTEIN, J. Lancet *1:*44–47, Jan 8, '44
Two plastic operations for repair of orbit following severe trauma and extensive comminuted fracture. CONVERSE, J. M. Arch. Ophth. *31:*323–325, April '44

Orbit – Cont.

Prostheses for eye and orbit. BROWN, A. M. Arch. Ophth. *32:*208-212, Sept '44

Recuperation of war wounded with orbital-ocular injuries. PAIVA GONCALVES. Hospital, Rio de Janeiro *26:*429-444, Sept '44

Late complications and sequels following blunt trauma to eye and orbital wall. NEBLETT, H. C. South. Med. and Surg. *106:*436-437, Nov '44

New method and appliance for grafting eye sockets. PICKERILL, H. P. Brit. M. J. *1:*596, April 28, '45

Plastic operations of orbit. RISDON, F. Bull. Acad. Med., Toronto *18:*139-141, April '45

Reconstruction of orbit by Esser-Wheeler technic. SVERDLICK, J. AND FERNANDEZ, L. L. Semana med. *2:*142-144, July 26, '45

New technic in reconstruction following radical surgery of orbit. McKAY, E. D. Am. J. Ophth. *28:*1017-1018, Sept '45

Orbitotemporal osteoma with exorbitism in syphilitics, with report of cases. CHAVANY, J. A. Presse med. *53:*702, Dec 22, '45

Plastic surgery of eye cavity. LECH, JR. Arq. Inst. Penido Burnier *7:*30-56, Dec '45

Cavernous hemangioma of orbit successfully removed by Shugrue operation. PAUL, M. Brit. J. Ophth. *30:*35-41, Jan '46

Choice of grafts for orbital reconstruction. MACKENZIE, C. M. Am. J. Ophth. *29:*867-869, July '46

Plastic repair of deformities of socket and minor defects about the orbit. MARCKS, K. M. AND ZUGSMITH, G. S. Arch. Ophth. *36:*55-69, July '46

Management of orbitocranial wounds. WEBSTER, J. E.; *et al.* J. Neurosurg. *3:*329-336, July '46

Reconstruction of floor of orbit; case. GIVNER, I. Am. J. Ophth. *29:*1010-1012, Aug '46

Plastic restoration of upper lid and socket. LUC, J. Brit. J. Ophth. *30:*665-668, Nov '46

Repair of eyelids and periorbital structures. RANK, B. K. Tr. Ophth. Soc. Australia (1944) *4:*84-97, '46

Orbit, Fracture

Signs of fracture of orbit. KEHL, H. Beitr. z. klin. Chir. *123:*203, '21 abstr: J.A.M.A. *77:*1292, Oct 15, '21

Plastic repair of depressed fracture of lower orbital rim. GOLDTHWAITE, R. H., J.A.M.A. *82:*628-629, Feb 23, '24

Fracture of 3 orbital walls with suppurative ethmoiditis case. BERTEIN. Lyon med. *142:*79, July 15, '28

Orbit, Fracture – Cont.

Fractures about orbit. GILL, W. D. South. M. J. *21:*527-534, July '28

Fracture of frontal sinus and ethmoid through dura, orbit and maxillary sinus; case; phenomenal recovery. SEIBERLING, J. D. Laryngoscope *41:*93-96, Feb '31

Fractures involving orbit and paranasal sinuses, with special reference to diagnosis and treatment. GILL, W. D. Texas State J. Med. *27:*351-358, Sept '31

Fracture of orbit and superior maxilla followed by subcutaneous and deep emphysema from secondary infection. BONNET, P. Lyon chir. *28:*718-719, Nov-Dec '31

Traumatic scarring and depressed fracture of right malar bone and orbital border; cartilage implant. FIGI, F.A., S. Clin. North America *12:*949-951, Aug '32

Fractures about orbit. EVANS, S. S. South. M. J. *26:*548-549, June '33

Facial bone fractures, especially orbits and sinuses. GILL, W. D. South. M. J. *27:*197-205, March '34

Compound comminuted depressed fracture of frontal bone and orbit, with recovery. LOVE, J. G. Proc. Staff Meet., Mayo Clin. *10:*291-293, May 8, '35

Fractures of lower margin of orbit; reduction and visualization by X-ray. EITZEN, A. C. J. Kansas M. Soc. *39:*15, Jan '38

Orbital fractures; case with air embolism. NEGLO, L. G. AND SPEKTOR, I. Z. Vestnik oftal. (nos. 1-2) *20:*60-63, '42

Two plastic operations for repair of orbit following severe trauma and extensive comminuted fracture. CONVERSE, J. M. Arch. Ophth. *31:*323-325, April '44

Symposium on reparative surgery; depressed fracture of orbital rim, with report of case treated by reduction through Caldwell-Luc approach, with maintenance of position of fragment by water-filled balloon. JOHNSON, M. R., S. Clin. North America *24:*340-347, April '44

Late complications and sequels following blunt trauma to eye and orbital wall. NEBLETT, H. C. South. Med. and Surg. *106:*436-437, Nov '44

Orbit, Infections

Suppurations of maxillary sinus and of orbit with extensive destruction of wall of sinus simulating cancer of upper jaw; case. GUNSETT, *et al.* Bull. et mem. Soc. de radiol. med. de France *24:*170, Feb '36

Orbit, Tumors

Ocular neoplasms (orbital hemangiomas) among Chinese; brief clinicopathologic report of 82 cases with discussions. LING, W. P. Chinese M. J. *48:*982–986, Sept '34

O'REAGAN, R. (see WHYTE, D.) Feb '37
O'REAGAN, R. (see WHYTE, D.) Dec '37
OREGGIA, J. C.: Temporomandibular ankylosis; surgical therapy of case in child following otitis with mastoiditis. Arch. de pediat. d. Uruguay *15:*223–234, April '44
ORELL, S.: Experimental studies and application of bone transplantation in practical surgery; preliminary report. Deutsche Ztschr. f. Chir. *232:*701–713, '31
ORELL, S.: Interposition of os purum in osteosynthesis after osteotomy, resections of bones and joints, etc. (interposition-osteosynthesis). Surg., Gynec. and Obst. *59:*638–643, Oct '34
ORELL, S.: Bone implantation and new growth; implantation of "os purum" and transplantation of "os novum." Acta chir. Scandinav. (supp. 31) *74:*1–274, '34
ORELL, S.: Bone transplantation. Acta chir. Scandinav. *74:*424–425, '34
ORELL, S.: Surgical implantation of pure bone, new bone and boiled bone. Mem. Acad. de chir. *61:*1376–1378, Dec 21, '35
ORELL, S.: Surgical grafting with "os purum," "os novum" and "boiled bone." J. Bone and Joint Surg. *19:*873–885, Oct '37 also: J. de chir. *49:*857–870, June '37
ORELL, S.: Use of os purum in implantations (bone). Surg., Gynec and Obst. *66:*23–26, Jan '38
ORELL, S.: Finger prosthesis made from hard and soft rubber joined by vulcanizing. Nord. med. (Hygiea) *4:*3346–3348, Nov 11, '39
ORELL, S.: Surgical bone transplantation; review. Zentralbl. f. Chir. *68:*1398–1403, July 26, '41
ORELL, S.: Ankylosis of jaw and its treatment in connection with case. Nord. med. (Hygiea) *29:*83–88, Jan 11, '46

Orell Operation

Orell method of bone transplantation; cases. RISINGER, W. Acta orthop. Scandinav. *9:*152–180, '38
Transplantation of dead heterologus bone in surgery; present status of problem; preparation of Orell's os purum. CASANUEVA DEL C., M. AND VELASCO S., A. Rev. med. de Chile *70:*424–428, June '42

ORIENTE, L. AND DE ALMEIDA MOURA, J. C.: Burn therapy. Arq. de cir. clin e exper. (supp.) *6:*1–56, April–June '42
ORLOV, G. A.: Preserved transplants in repair of defects of peripheral nerves; disadvantages of this method. Sovet. med. (nos. 11–12) *7:*7–9, '43
ORLOVA, G. N. (see BRAUN, A. A.) April '45
ORNSTEIN, G. G.; LICHT, S. AND HERMAN, M.: Method of raising venous pressure (stimulation of voluntary muscles by faradic current), to be used in surgical and traumatic shock (preliminary report). Quart. Bull., Sea View Hosp. *4:*333–338, April '39

Oroantral Fistula

Bucco-antral fistula; plastic operation. VOORHEES, I. W. Internat. J. Surg. *40:*19, Jan '27
Autoplastic closure of bucco-nasal and bucco-sinusal communications; illustrations. MAUREL, G. Rev. de stomatol. *29:*764–781, Nov '27
Perforation of palate due to suction attachment of dental plate. AXHAUSEN, G. Deutsche Zahn-, Mund-u. Kieferh. *1:*343–348, '34
Palatine fistula, plastic closure by means of turbinate bone. DE MARTINI, R. Boll. d. mal. d. orecchio, d. gola, d. naso *59:*172–177, May '41
Closure of alveolosinusal communications by pedicled palatine strip. RAMADIER, J. A. Ann. d'oto-laryng. *12:*315–316, April–June '45
Traumatic palatine fistula. WIBLE, L. E. AND HOWARD, J. C. JR. Arch. Otolaryng. *44:*159–165, Aug '46

ORR, H. W.: History of transplantation in general and orthopedic surgery. Am. J. Surg. *43:*547–553, Feb '39
ORR, T. G.: Elephantiasis nostras of genitalia; report of case and operative treatment. S. Clin. N. America *3:*1537–1545, Dec '23 (illus.)
ORR, T. G. (see PADGETT, E. C.) June '28
ORR, T. G. (see SCHNEDORF, J. G.) July '41
ORR, T. G. (see SCHNEDORF, J. G.) Oct '41
ORRIN, H. C.: *Fascial Grafting in Principle and Practice*. Oliver and Boyd, Ltd., London, 1928
ORSI, J. L.: Fracture of lower edentulous jaw; surgical therapy of case. Bol. Soc. de cir. de Rosario *10:*230–235, July '43
ORSI, J. L.: Malignant tumors of upper jaw. Rev. med. de Rosario *34:*983–1011, Oct '44
ORSÓS, J. (see KREIKER, A.) 1923
ORSOS, J. I.: Rational treatment of burns. Gyo-

gyaszat *79:*613, Nov 26; 626, Dec 3, '39 also: Munchen. med. Wchnschr. *87:*297-299, March 15, '40

ORTH, O.: Surgical therapy of exstrophy of bladder with intestinal transplantation of ureters. Ztschr. f. Urol. *36:*214-216, '42

ORTHNER, F.: Therapy of large ulcers of leg with Thiersch grafts. Wien. klin. Wchnschr. *47:*1047-1048, Aug 24, '34

ORTIGA, S. JR. (see SANTOS, H. A. *et al*) Nov '40

Orthodontia

Role of orthodontia following cleft lip and palate surgery. DAVIS, A. D. Pacific Dent. Gaz. *39:*571-580, Aug '31

Role of plastic surgery in relation to orthodontia. DAVIS, A. D. Internat. J. Orthodontia *19:*1214-1222, Dec '33

Surgical correction of jaw deformities and their relationship to orthodontia. KAZANJIAN, V. H. Internat. J. Orthodontia *22:*259-282, March '36

Orthodontic treatment of jaw fractures and cleft palate. CARTWRIGHT, F. S. Internat. J. Orthodontia *23:*159-163, Feb '37

Orthodontics as aid in repairing congenital cleft palate. ABELSON, J. M. Am. J. Orthodontics *25:*154-158, Feb '39

Responsibility of orthodontist in treatment of traumatic injuries of face and jaws. FAIRBANK, L. C. Am. J. Orthodontics *27:*414-422, Aug '41

Orthodontics in treatment of harelip and cleft palate. LIFTON, J. C. Am. J. Orthodontics *27:*423-453, Aug '41

Orthopedics

Plastic surgery in orthopedics. CAMPBELL, H. H. Tr. Roy. Med.-Chir. Soc. Glasgow, pp. 7-12, '42-'43; in Glasgow M. J. Dec '42

ORTIZ, C. (see BERTOLA, V. J. *et al*) April '45

ORTIZ TIRADO, A.: Bone tissue as filling material in loss of substances. Cir. y cirujanos *10:*65-70, Feb 28, '42

ORTMAYER, M. AND HUMPHREYS, E. M.: Intranasal granuloma of sporothrix type producing marked deformity. Ann. Surg. *113:*118-122, Jan '41

ORTNER, A. B.: Skin transplantation. Kentucky M. J. *41:*176-178, May '43

ORTON, H. B.: Surgical treatment of cancer of larynx; results. Mississippi Doctor *17:*128-135, Aug '39

ORY, M.: Value of lateral incisions in hand phlegmons. Liege med. *26:*404-411, March 26, '33

ORY, M.: Lateral incisions in phlegmons of tendon sheaths of hand. Ann. Soc. med.-chir. de Liege, no. 1, pp. 30-35, '33 abstr: Liege med. *27:*384-387, March 18, '34

ORZALESI, F.: Good esthetic and functional results in correction of cicatricial ectropion by means of plastic graft operation. Boll. d'ocul. *12:*906-931, Sept '33

OSACAR, E. M. (see TORRES, G. A.) 1946

OSBORN, C. H.: Management of fractures of bones of face (and wounds). M. J. Australia *2:*41-49, July 9, '38

OSBORNE, E. D.: Morphea associated with hemiatrophy of face. Arch. Dermat. and Syph. *6:*27-34, July '22 (illus.)

OSBORNE, R. P.: Treatment of burns and wounds with skin loss by envelope method (using electrolytic sodium hypochlorite solution). Brit. J. Surg. *32:*24-32, July '44

OSBORNE, R. P.: Modern methods of burn therapy. J. Roy. Inst. Pub. Health and Hyg. *9:*169-177, June '46

OSGOOD, R. B. (see WILSON, P. D.) July '33

O'SHEA, M. C.: Severed tendons and nerves of hand and forearm. Ann. Surg. *105:*228-242, Feb '37

O'SHEA, M. C.: Treatment and results of 870 severed tendons and 57 severed nerves of hand and forearm (in 362 patients). Am. J. Surg. *43:*346-366, Feb '39

OSIPOVSKIY, V. M. (see KRASIN, P. M.) 1933

OSORIO, L. A.: Crouzon's disease (craniofacial dysostosis); case. An. Fac. de med. de Porto Alegre (fasc. 2) *5:*98-99, July-Dec '44

OSTENFELD, J.: Blood cysts of neck. Nord. med. (Hospitalstid.) *22:*758-759, April 21, '44

OSTERBERG, A. E.: Symposium on acute burns; biochemical studies. Proc. Staff Meet., Mayo Clin. *8:*121-123, Feb 22, '33

OSTERHAGEN, H. F. (see LEECH, C. H. *et al*) Oct '46

OSTERMANN, F. A.: Nerve gunshot wounds; surgical therapy. Deut. Militararzt *9:*42, Jan '44

Ostrčil

Formation of artificial vagina by skin flap (Ostrčil method); case. MÜLLER, G. Rozhl. v. chir. a gynaek. (cast gynaek.) *11:*55-59, '32

OSTRČIL, A.: Operative methods in formation of artificial vagina. Casop. lek. cesk. *70:*596-599, April 24, '31

OSTRČIL, A.: Colpopoiesis by means of transplantation according to Thiersch method. Zentralbl. f. Gynak. *55:*1900-1901, June 13, '31

O'SULLIVAN, T. J.: Plastic surgery of face; interesting cases. Maine M. J. *26:*167–173, Nov '35

OTERO SANCHEZ, A. (see SIMARRO PUIG, J. *et al*) July '42

O'TOOLE, J. B. JR.: Celluloid splint in traumatic amputation of distal phalanges. U. S. Nav. M. Bull. *42:*460–461, Feb '44

Otoplasty

Otoplasty. PÓLYA, E. Zentralbl. f. Chir. *48:*219, Feb 19, '21

Reconstruction of ears. DAY, H. F. Boston M. and S. J. *185:*146, Aug 4, '21

Total reconstruction of external ear. ESSER, J. F. S. Munchen. med. Wchnschr. *68:*1150, Sept 9, '21

Correction of flaring ears. EITNER, E. Med. Klinik *18:*1117–1118, Aug 27, '22

Reconstruction of ear. ESSER, J. F. S. AND AUFRICHT, G. Arch. f. klin. Chir. *120:*518–525, '22 (illus.) abstr: J.A.M.A. *79:*1887, Nov 25, '22

Surgical treatment of abnormal flaring of ears. HOULIÉ. Progres med. *38:*85–86, Feb 24, '23 (illus.)

Technic for correcting deformities of ears among natives of Dutch East Indies acquired from wearing heavy things in ear lobes. WAAR, C. A. H. Nederlandsch Tijdschr. v. Geneesk. *2:*32–35, July 7, '23 (illus.)

Case of microtia, with occlusion of left external auditory canal; operated with satisfactory results. SHEMELEY, W. G. Laryngoscope *33:*841–844, Nov '23 (illus.)

Plastic operation on protruding ears (Gersuny). BIESENBERGER, H. Zentralbl. f. Chir. *51:*1126–1127, May 24, '24

Cosmetic surgery of nose and ear. SOLONCOV, N. Cas. lek. cesk. *63:*833–839, May 31, '24

Cosmetic surgery of nose and ear. WODAK, E. Med. Klinik *20:*1042–1044, July 27, '24

Plastic reconstruction of ear with pedunculated tube flap. VAN DIJK, J. A. Nederl. Tijdschr. v. Geneesk. *1:*895–900, Feb 21, '25

Anatomy, psychology, diagnosis and treatment of congenital malformation and absence of ear. BECK, J. C. Laryngoscope *35:*813–831, Nov '25

Surgical treatment of flopping ear. EITNER, E. Wien. klin. Wchnschr. *39:*868, July 22, '26

Making lobule of ear smaller. EITNER, E. Wien. klin. Wchnschr. *39:*1423–1424, Dec 2, '26

Experimental transplantation of cartilage and skin for repair of concha. GUSSIO, S. Valsalva *3:*58–77, Feb '27

Otoplasty—Cont.

Restoration of auricle. DE RIVER, J. P. California and West. Med. *26:*654–656, May '27

Treatment for acute traumatic hematoma of external ear. BRITTON, H. A. J.A.M.A. *89:*111–112, July 9, '27

Plastic surgery of protruding ears. KOSCH, W. Deutsche med. Wchnschr. *54:*569, April 6, '28

Technic of plastic operations on ear. ALEXANDER, G. Ztschr. f. Hals-, Nasen-u. Ohrenh. *21:*6–10, May 10, '28

Treatment of protruding ears. IVANISSEVICH, O. AND FERRARI, R. C. Semana med. *1:*1161–1170, May 10, '28

Plastic surgery of ear; 2 cases. NOEL, MME. A. Ann. d. mal. de l'oreille, du larynx *47:*478–482, May '28

Plastic correction of protruding ears. ALEXANDER, G. Wien. klin. Wchnschr. *41:*1217–1218, Aug 23, '28

Projecting or lop ear; case corrected by operation. WAGERS, A. J., M. J. and Rec. *128:*623–624, Dec 19, '28

Entire restoration of auricle after complete traumatic separation; case. OLDENSTAM, R. A. Nederl. Tijdschr. v. Geneesk. *1:*1097, March 2, '29

Surgical correction of protruding ears. KLICPERA, L. Wien. klin. Wchnschr. *52:*536–538, June 2, '39

Plastic operation on auditory canal after complete opening of middle ear with chisel. UFFENORDE, W. Ztschr. f. Hals-, Nasen-u, Ohrenh. *23:*317, Sept 10, '29

Window operation for hematoma auris and perichondritis, with effusion. HOWARD, R. C. Laryngoscope *39:*590–594, Sept '29

Plastic surgery of ear. LOCKWOOD, C. D. Surg., Gynec. and Obst. *49:*392–394, Sept '29

Operative treatment of ear deformities. DOBRZANIECKI, W. Ann. d. mal. de l'oreille, du larynx *48:*998–1003, Oct '29

Simple, reliable method for correction of protruding ears. LÜTHI, A. Schweiz. med. Wchnschr. *59:*1268–1269, Dec 7, '29

Plastic surgery of nose, ear, face. DAVIS, A. D. Arch. Otolaryng. *10:*575–584, Dec '29

Reconstruction of external ear. PIERCE, G. W. Surg., Gynec. and Obst. *50:*601–605, March '30

Plastic surgery of ear. HEERMANN, H. Ztschr. f. Hals-, Nasen-u. Ohrenh. *26:*35–41, May 6, '30

Correction of lop-ear; case. MAKAR, N. J. Egyptian M. A. *13:*299–308, July '30

Surgical correction of abnormally protruding

Otoplasty – Cont.
ears. SCHLANDER, E. Chirurg *2:*699–704, Aug 1, '30
Plastic surgery for large and protruding ears. EISENKLAM, J. Wien. klin. Wchnschr. *43:*1176, Sept 18, '30
Plastic surgery of ear. LOCKWOOD, C. D., S. Clin. North America *10:*1103–1108, Oct '30
Reply to Eitner's comments on article on plastic surgery for large and protruding ears. EISENKLAM, I. Wien. klin. Wchnschr. *43:*1377, Nov 6, '30
Plastic surgery for large and protruding ears. (Comment on Eisenklam's article). EITNER, E. Wien. klin. Wchnschr. *43:*1377, Nov 6, '30
Surgical treatment of protruding ears. ZAAIJER, J. H. Nederl. tijdschr. v. geneesk. *74:*5572–5575, Nov 15, '30
Reconstruction of ear; case. NEW, G. B. Proc. Staff Meet., Mayo Clin. *6:*97, Feb 18, '31
Plastic surgery in abnormalities of direction, convolution and flexion of external ear. BOURGUET, J. Monde med., Paris *41:*483–492, April 1, '31
Surgical correction of protruding ears. DEMEL, R. AND FEIGL, E. Deutsche Ztschr. f. Chir. *233:*453–459, '31
Korrektiv-cosmetische Chirurgie der Näse, der Ohren, und den Gesichts, by VICTOR FRÜHWALD. Wilhelm Maudrich, Vienna, 1932. (Also English edition, translated by Geoffrey Morey.)
Artificial ear, replacement of entire auricle. GULEKE. Chirurg *4:*274–278, April 1, '32
Plastic surgery of ear. SANVENERO-ROSSELLI, G. Rev. de chir. plastique, pp. 27–52, April '32
Plastic surgery of ear deformities. FERRARI, R. C. AND FIORINI, J. M. Rev. de chir. plastique, pp. 150–156, July '32
Technic of plastic correction of external ear; 3 cases. GONZÁLEZ LOZA, M. Rev. med. del Rosario *22:*833–837, Oct '32
Cosmetic correction of pinna which turns forward in abnormal fashion. EITNER, E. Wien. klin. Wchnschr. *45:*1537–1538, Dec 9, '32
Plastic replacement of upper rim of ear. EITNER, E. Monatschr. f. Ohrenh. *67:*222–225, Feb '33
Surgical therapy of abnormalities of external ear. BOURGUET, J. Bull. Acad. de med., Paris *109:*602–604, April 25, '33
Plastic surgery in correction of ear deformities. EHRENFELD, H. Gyogyaszat *73:*374, June 11, '33
Auricular dyschondrogenesis; technic of surgical correction. TORELLÓ CENDRA, M. But. Soc. catalana de pediat. *6:*193–198, July–Aug '33
Abnormalities of external ear and their surgical correction. EITNER, E. Chirurg *5:*618–625, Aug 15, '33
Esthetic surgery in correction of abnormally protruding pinna. BOURGUET, J. Clinique, Paris *28:*318–320, Oct (B) '33
Plastic operation for protruding ears. GOODYEAR, H. M. Arch. Otolaryng. *18:*527–530, Oct '33 also: J. Med. *14:*479–480, Nov '33
Surgical correction of deformed external ear and nose; case. REBELLO NETO, J. Rev. med. de Pernambuco *3:*285–290, Oct '33
Surgical therapy of congenital abnormalities of external ear. PIERI, G. Valsalva *9:*842–846, Nov '33
Surgical correction of deformities of external ear; 3 cases. BOURGUET, J. Bull. et mem. Soc. de med. de Paris *137:*656–659, Dec 8, '33
Cosmetic correction of Darwin's ear. EITNER, E. Ztschr. f. Hals-, Nasen-u. Ohrenh. *33:*564–567, '33
Congenital malformation of region of pinna; case. GESCHELIN, A. I. Arch. f. Ohren-, Nasen-u. Kehlkopfh. *136:*332–334, '33
Cosmetic surgery in correction of protruding pinna. also of nose. MALBEC, E. F. Semana med. *1:*170–175, Jan 11, '34
Technic of radical operation in plastic surgery of ear. POGÁNY, O. Gyogyaszat *74:*38, Jan 21, '34
Reconstruction of nasal ala; case. JULLIARD, C. Rev. med. de la Suisse Rom. *54:*463–467, April (25), '34
Total reconstruction of ear; original technic. BETTMAN, A. G. Rev. de chir. plastique, pp. 3–13, May '34
Cosmetic corrections of form of external ear. EITNER, E. Wien. med. Wchnschr. *84:*810–811, July 14, '34
Otoneoplasty. PRUDENTE, A. Rev. oto-laring. de Sao Paulo *2:*388–391, Sept–Oct '34
Plastic reconstruction of auricle. EITNER, E. Deutsche Ztschr. f. Chir. *242:*797–801, '34
New and simple method for plastic surgery in congenital or accidental absence of ear. ESSER, J. F. S. Presse med. *43:*325–326, Feb 27, '35
Window operation for hematoma and perichondritis with effusion of ear. HOWARD, R. C. Laryngoscope *45:*81–105, Feb '35
Microtia with meatal atresia, with description of operation for its correction; 2 cases. HUME, J. R. AND OWENS, N. Ann. Otol., Rhin. and Laryng. *44:*213–219, March '35

Otoplasty – Cont.

Otoplasty for dermatitis congelationis (frostbite). LIGGETT, H., M. Rec. *142:*278–279, Sept 18, '35

Results of treatment of protruding ears. DEMEL, R. Wien. klin. Wchnschr. *48:*1185, Sept 27, '35

Complete atresia of auditory canal due to trauma; plastic repair; case. SAES, P. Rev. oto-laring. de Sao Paulo *4:*83–86, March-April '36

Plastic reconstruction of large portion of pavilion of ear by new method. GUCCIARDELLO, S. Riv. san. siciliana *24:*640–642, June 15, '36

New method of plastic surgery in complicated deformities of pinna; cat's ear and coloboma in 2 cases. DOROSCHENKO, J. T. Monatschr. f. Ohrenh. *70:*718–721, June '36

Plastic repair of mutilated ear. ESSER, J. F. S. Rev. de chir. structive, pp. 269–271, June '36

Plastic surgery of ear. GRAHAM, H. B. West. J. Surg. *44:*478–480, Aug '36

Plastic surgery of ears; cases (and face and nose). MALBEC, E. F. Semana med. *2:*718–728, Sept 10, '36

Protruding ears; psychological effect and plastic correction. WOLFE, M. M., M. Rec. *144:*306–307, Oct 7, '36

Technic of reparation of ear lobe by tubular skin grafts. GONZALEZ ULLOA, M. Rev. mex. de cir., ginec. y cancer *5:*33–41, Jan '37

Total reconstruction of external ear. NATTINGER, J. K. Northwest Med. *36:*172–174, May '37

Simple method for correction of protruding ears. EITNER, E. Wien. klin. Wchnschr. *50:*1206, Aug 20, '37

Reconstruction of external ear with special reference to use of maternal ear cartilage as supporting structure (cases). GILLIES, H. Rev. de chir. structive, pp. 169–179, Oct '37

Abnormal prominence of ear; method of readjustment. DAVIS, J. S. AND KITLOWSKI, E. A. Surgery *2:*835–848, Dec '37

Plastic correction of boxer's ears and nose. DUJARDIN, E. Ugesk. f. laeger *100:*115, Feb 3, '38

Esthetic and psychologic principles of plastic surgery (ear), (face), (nose). WODAK, E. Monatschr. f. Ohrenh. *72:*288–303, March '38

Lop ear. MACCOLLUM, D. W. J.A.M.A. *110:*1427–1430, April 30, '38

Repair for partial loss of auricle. THOMAS, C. H., J. Laryng. and Otol. *53:*259–260, April '38

Esthetic and psychologic principles of plastic surgery of nose, ears and face. WODAK, E. Monatschr. f. Ohrenh. *72:*424, April; 490, May '38

Plastic surgery of ear pavilion. MALBEC, E. F. Semana med. *1:*994–1001, May 5, '38

Ear reconstruction. MONEY, R. A., M. J. Australia *1:*819–820, May 7, '38

Cosmetic operation for protruding ears. EHRENFELD, H. Zentralbl. f. Chir. *65:*1236–1239, May 28, '38

Reconstruction of pavilion using skin grafts (ear); case. DUFOURMENTEL, L. Rev. de laryng. *59:*517–518, May '38 also: Oto-rhino-laryng. internat. *22:*395–396, July '38

Plastic surgery of ear lobule. EITNER, E. Wien. med. Wchnschr. *88:*774–775, July 11, '38

Treatment of ear deformities. HINDMARSH, J. Nord. med. tidskr. *16:*1178–1181, July 23, '38

Deformities of ear lobe and their surgical correction. MALBEC, E. F. Semana med. *2:*623–631, Sept 15, '38

Lop ear; psychologic importance of early surgical correction. ZENO, L. An. de cir. *4:*190–192, Sept '38 also: Bol. Soc. de cir. de Rosario *5:*429–431, Oct '38

Deformation of auricular pavilion and its surgical corrections. CORA ELISEHT, F. AND AUBONE, J. Rev. argent. de oto-rino-laring. *7:*411–421, Nov-Dec '38

Total reconstruction of auricle. PADGETT, E. C. Surg., Gynec. and Obst. *67:*761–768, Dec '38

Repair of permanent cavity behind left ear, following petromastoid evident; excision of concha of ear; case. COELST. Rev. de chir. structive *8:*113–115, Aug '38

Use of full thickness free grafts in surgical therapy of microtia; case. COELST, M. Rev. de chir. structive *8:*155–159, '38

New operation for radical treatment of winged, projecting and distorted ears. SAMY, M. Rev. de chir. structive *8:*192–194, '38

Surgical correction of too large auricles. VOGEL, K. Ztschr. f. Hals-, Nasen-u. Ohrenh. *44:*366–367, '38

Plastic and esthetic surgery of ear, nose and face; cases. MALBEC, E. F. Semana med. *1:*83–95, Jan 12, '39

Restoration of partial defect of auricle by free transplantation. ERCZY, M. Gyogyaszat *79:*319–320, May 21, '39

Otoplasty—Cont.
Surgical correction of protruding ears. KLICPERA, L. Wien. klin. Wchnschr. *52:*536-538, June 2, '39
Psychology of plastic surgery of ear. BERNDORFER, A. Gyogyaszat *79:*349-351, June 4, '39
Plastic repair with cartilagoperiosteal bridge in drooping (or dog) ear. RIGG, J. P. AND WALDAPFEL, R. J.A.M.A. *113:*125-126, July 8, '39
Surgical correction of protruding ear. PRUDENTE, A. Rev. de cir. de Sao Paulo *5:*17-26, July-Aug '39
Deformities of ear and nose treated by plastic surgery. COX, G. H. New York State J. Med. *39:*1956-1961, Oct 15, '39
Protruding ears and their surgical correction. OMBREDANNE, M. Semaine d. hop. de Paris *15:*404-411, Nov '39
Plastic surgery; psychic repercussion and social aspects of deformed ears. MALBEC, E. F. Semana med. *2:*1506-1509, Dec 28, '39
Plastic reconstruction of auricle. GNILORYBOV, T. E. Novy khir. arkhiv. *45:*148-156, '39
Correction of abnormally protruding ears. KLICPERA, L. Ztschr. f. Hals-, Nasen-u. Ohrenh. *46:*367-368, '39
Protruding ears; surgical therapy. IVANISSEVICH, O.; *et al.* Bol. d. Inst. clin. quir. *16:*33-47, Jan-March '40
Surgical correction of hypertrophy of auricular lobe in leprosy. SILVEIRA, L. M. Rev. brasil. de leprol. *8:*1-3, March '40
Use of preserved cartilage in ear reconstruction. KIRKHAM, H. L. D. Ann. Surg. *111:*896-902, May '40
Protruding ears; method of plastic correction. NEW, G. B. AND ERICH, J. B. Am. J. Surg. *48:*385-390, May '40
Protruding ears; technical detail of surgical correction. FERNANDEZ, L. L. Semana med. *2:*89-90, July 11, '40
Congenital abnormalities (with surgical therapy of prominent ear). FOUCAR, H. O. Canad. M.A.J. *43:*26-27, July '40
Protruding ear; psychologic effect, morphologic classification and surgical therapy. PEDEMONTE, P. V. Arch. urug. de med., cir. y especialid. *17:*458-472, Oct '40
Autoplastic methods for surgical restoration of congenital agenesis of ear. VEINTEMILLAS, F. Rev. brasil. de oto-rino-laring. *8:*413-418, Nov-Dec '40
Plastic surgery of auricle. MALBEC, E. F. Semana med. *2:*1479-1482, Dec 26, '40
Argyrosis of auricles with certain practical observations on plastic operations. KESSEL, O. Hals-, Nasen-u. Ohrenarzt (Teil 1) *31:*250-252, Dec '40

Otoplasty—Cont.
Plastic surgery of auricle; postoperative care and errors committed during surgery. MALBEC, E. F. Semana med. *1:*219-221, Jan 23, '41
Harmful effects of malformed ears in school; plastic surgery of protruding ears. CODAZZI AGUIRRE, J. A. Semana med. *1:*456-462, Feb 20, '41
Plastic surgery for positional anomalies of ear. EITNER, E. Wien. med. Wchnschr. *91:*140-142, Feb 22, '41
Protruding ear; psychologic effect, morphologic classification and surgical therapy. PEDEMONTE, P. V. An. d. ateneo clin. quir. *7:*73-87, Feb '41
Surgery of auricle, including total reconstruction and protuberant ears. COX, G. H. Laryngoscope *51:*791-797, Aug '41
Reconstruction of external ear. NEWMAN, J. Surg., Gynec. and Obst. *73:*234-235, Aug '41
Plastic correction of protruding ears in children. BAXTER, H. Canad. M.A.J. *45:*217-220, Sept '41
Reconstructive otoplasty (by transplantation of cartilage). GREELEY, P. W. Surgery *10:*457-461, Sept '41
Technic in construction of auricle. GILLIES, H. Tr. Am. Acad. Ophth. (1941) *46:*119-121, Jan-Feb '42
Plastic reconstruction of ear lobe with circular pedicled flap from neck. SCHUCHARDT, K. Zentralbl. f. Chir. *69:*345, Feb 28, '42
Use of meniscus of knee in plastic surgery (ear). DELLEPIANE RAWSON, R. Prensa med. argent. *29:*654-658, April 22, '42
Correction of lop ears. COE, H. E. Northwest Med. *41:*126, April '42
Surgical therapy of protruding ears. ALVES, O. Arq. de cir. clin. e exper. *6:*517-519, April-June '42
New surgical therapy of protruding ears without resection of cartilage. PALACIO POSSE, R. Arq. de cir. clin. e exper. *6:*489-492, April-June '42
Plastic correction of deformities of ear lobe in leprosy. SILVEIRA, L. M. Arq. de cir. clin. e exper. *6:*485-488, April-June '42
Plastic surgery of ear and nose. MALBEC, E. F. Semana med. *2:*426-431, Aug 20, '42
Auriculoplasty for hypoplasia of pavilion using tubular skin graft; case. ZENO, L. Bol. y trab., Acad. argent. de cir. *26:*807-812, Sept 16, '42

Otoplasty – Cont.

Plastic method to correct occlusions of meatus and auditory canal. CITELLI, S. Oto-rino-laring. ital. *12:*300-305, '42

Complete reconstruction of auricle. BERSON, M. I. Am. J. Surg. *60:*101-104, April '43

Projecting auricle (lop ear); case corrected by surgery (New-Erich method). AUSTIN, E. R. Proc. Staff Meet. Clin., Honolulu *9:*45-48, May '43

Protruding ears; original technic of surgical therapy. FERNANDEZ, J. C. Bol. y trab., Soc. argent. de cirujanos *4:*768-772, '43 also: Rev. Asoc. med. argent. *57:*1019-1020, Nov 30, '43

Present status of complete reconstruction of external ear. PEER, L. A. Tr. Am. Soc. Plastic and Reconstructive Surg. *12:*11-16, '43

Reconstructive plastic surgery of absent ear with necrocartilage; original method. LAMONT, E. S. Arch. Surg. *48:*53-72, Jan '44

Correction of abnormally prominent ears. YOUNG, F. Surg., Gynec. and Obst. *78:*541-550, May '44

Microtia; therapeutic problem. CORA ELISEHT, F.; *et al.* Prensa med. argent. *31:*1671-1673, Aug 23, '44

Plastic surgery of ear; case. HERNANDEZ, A. Prensa med. argent. *31:*2367-2373, Nov 22, '44

Plastic reconstruction of acquired defects of external ear, with case reports. SURACI, A. J. Am. J. Surg. *66:*196-202, Nov '44 (no. 1) *1:*13-14, Jan '44

Imperforation of external auditory canal with aplasia of auricle; results of operation. OMBREDANNE, M. Arch. franc. pediat. *2:*73-74, '44

Surgical correction of protruding ears. BECKER, O. J. Eye, Ear, Nose and Throat Monthly *24:*177-181, April '45

External agenesis of ear treated surgically by Humberto and Ricardo Bisi. IVANISSEVICH, O. Bol. y trab., Acad. argent. de cir. *29:*666-668, Aug 1, '45

Plastic repair for protruding ears. BERSON, M. I. Eye, Ear, Nose and Throat Monthly *24:*423-426, Sept '45

Correction of protruding ears; Malbec technic. BEAUX, A. R. Prensa med. argent. *32:*2314-2320, Nov 23, '45

Total loss of pavilion of ear and its plastic repair; technic in case. ASIS, R. Actas Soc. de cir. de Madrid *5:*131-136, Jan-Mar '46

Protruding ear and its surgical treatment. ABBOTT, A. C. Manitoba M. Rev. *26:*335-339, June '46

Otoplasty – Cont.

Plastic surgery for outstanding ears; simple surgical procedure. FISHMAN, L. Z. AND FISHMAN, V. P. Bull. Pract. Ophth. *16:*19-21, July '46

Reconstructive otoplasty; further observations; utilization of tantalum wire mesh support. GREELEY, P. W. Arch. Surg. *53:*24-31, July '46

Correction of congenital protruding ear; new surgical concept. SEELEY, R. C. Am. J. Surg. *72:*12-15, July '46

Protruding ears; author's technic of correction. FERNANDEZ, J. C. Dia med. *18:*1052-1053, Aug 5, '46

Auriculoplasties in therapy of protruding ears by Malbec technic. DEL POZO, R. D. Bol. y trab. Soc. argent. de cirujanos *7:*205-214, '46 also: Rev. Asoc. med. argent. *60:*460-463, June 15, '46

Otorhinolaryngology

Plastic methods in otorhinolaryngology. SANVENERO-ROSSELLI, G. Rassegna ital. di oto-rino-laring. *2:*241-257, Nov-Dec '28

Plastic surgery, summary of material available in field of otolaryngology. SHEEHAN, J. E. Arch. Otolaryng. *12:*527-530, Oct '30

Plastic surgery; summary of bibliographic material available in field of otolaryngology. SHEEHAN, J. E. Arch. Otolaryng. *16:*867-870, Dec '32

Results of plastic operations at R. Clinica Otorinolaringoiatrica in Turin. SANVENERO-ROSSELLI, G. Arch. ital. di laring. (supp.) *51:*301-324, '32

Plastic surgery; summary of bibliographic material available in field of otolaryngology. SHEEHAN, J. E. Arch. Otolaryng. *18:*531-533, Oct '33

Reconstructive surgery in ophthalmology and otolaryngology. GILL, W. D. Texas State J. Med. *29:*616-622, Feb '34

Postoperative cicatrices in otorhinolaryngologic surgery. DUFOURMENTEL, L. Prat. med. franc. *15:*243-247, April (B) '34

Plastic surgery; summary of bibliographic material available in field of otolaryngology. SHEEHAN, J. E. Arch. Otolaryng. *20:*577-582, Oct '34

Correction during infancy of congenital and acquired deformities in otorhinolaryngology to prevent later increased disfigurement, with special reference to plastic surgery. REBELO NETO, J. Rev. oto-laring. de Sao Paulo *3:*11-24, Jan-Feb '35

Relationship between otolaryngologist and plastic surgeon. HAYS, H. Am. J. Surg. *31:*38-47, Jan '36

Otorhinolaryngology – Cont.
The different application of free grafts in oto-rhino-laryngology. DUFOURMENTEL, L. Prat. med. franc. *18:*187–195, June '37
Congenital anomalies in otorhinolaryngology. VAN DEN WILDENBERG, Bull. Soc. belge d'otol., rhinol., laryng., pp. 282–292, '37
Plastic surgery; summaries of bibliographic material available in field of otolaryngology, 1936–1938. IVY, R. H. AND MILLER, H. A. Arch. Otolaryng. *27:*622–642, May '38
New suction elevator for otorhinolaryngologic operations. YOSHIDA, S. Oto-rhino-laryng. *11:*651, July '38
Plastic surgery, 1938; summaries of bibliographic material available in field of otolaryngology. IVY, R. H. AND MILLER, H. A. Arch. Otolaryng. *30:*99–114, July '39
Tumors of nose and throat; summaries of bibliographic material available in field of otolaryngology. NEW, G. B.; *et al.* Arch. Otolaryng. *30:*283–297, Aug '39
Plastic surgery; summaries of bibliographic material available in field of otolaryngology. IVY, R. H. AND MILLER, H. A. Arch. Otolaryng. *36:*135–148, July '42
Plastic surgery for 1942; summaries of bibliographic material available in field of otolaryngology. PEER, L. A. Arch. Otolaryng. *38:*171–189, Aug '43
Anesthesia in otorhinolaryngology. CULLEN, S. C. Tr. Am. Acad. Ophth. (1943) *48:*240–247, March–April '44
Role of plastic surgery in field of otolaryngology. FOMON, S. Arch. Otolaryng. *39:*518–520, June '44
Contribution to plastic surgery during 1943; summaries of bibliographic material available in field of otolaryngology. PEER, L. A. Arch. Otolaryng. *39:*537–555, June '44
Contributions to plastic surgery during 1944; summaries of bibliographic material available in field of otolaryngology. PEER, L. A. Arch. Otolaryng. *42:*56–79, July '45
Contributions to plastic surgery during 1945; summaries of bibliographic material available in field of otolaryngology. PEER, L. A. Arch. Otolaryng. *44:*715–758, Dec '46

OTSUKA, H.: Pouch ear; case. Oto-rhino-laryng. *9:*813, Sept '36
OTT, W. O.: Experimental results of cable grafts and tubes of fascia lata in repair of peripheral nerve defects. Minnesota Med. *5:*581–588, Oct '22 (illus.)
OTT, W. O. (see ADSON, A. W.) May '23
OTTENDORF: Treatment of snapping thumb. Zentralbl. f. Chir. *57:*1273, May 24, '30
OTTO, T. O.: Avulsion of scalp treated without grafting. Ann. Surg. *102:*315–317, Aug '35
OTTOBRINI COSTA, M. AND LABATE, F.: Thyroglossal fistulas and cysts. Pediatria prat., Sao Paulo *10:*287–300, July–Aug '39
OTTOLENGHI, C. E. AND SPINELLI, C. A.: Stenosing tenosynovitis; surgical therapy of 2 cases. Rev. ortop. y traumatol. *6:*196–202, Oct '36
OTTOW, B.: Congenital polyps of urethra with peni-scrotal hypospadias. Ztschr. f. urol. Chir. *32:*64–68, '31
OUGHTERSON, A. W. AND TENNANT, R.: Angiomas of hands and feet. Surgery *5:*73–100, Jan '39
OUGHTERSON, A. W. (see LAWRENCE, E. A.) June '44
OUSAROFF, V. M.: Blood supply of hard palate in connection with plastic operations. Vestnik khir. (nos. 37–38) *13:*222–229, '28
OVENS, J. M.: Management of cleft lip. Arizona Med. *2:*298–303, Sept '45
OVERTON, L. M. (see GHORMELY, R. K.) Sept '34
OVERTON, L. M. (see GHORMELY, R. K.) July '35
OVERTON, L. M. (see MEYERDING, H. W.) Dec '35
OVNATANYAN, K. T.: Osteomyelitis of ungual phalanges of fingers. Sovet. med. (no. 4) *4:*18–20, '40
OVNATANYAN, K. T.: Plastic reconstruction of peripheral nerves. Sovet med. (no. 9) *8:*27–29, '44
OVNBOL, A.: Severe burns treated by blood transfusion, adrenal cortical hormone and ascorbic acid. Ugesk. f. laeger *105:*1331, Dec 30, '43
OWEN, H. R.: Fractures of bones of hand. Surg., Gynec. and Obst. *66:*500–505, Feb (no. 2A) '38
OWEN, H. R. AND NORTH, J. P.: Present status of treatment of burn patient. S. Clin. North America *19:*1489–1511, Dec '39
OWEN, M. (see HYDE, T. L. *et al*) Feb '44
OWENS, N.: Indications, limitations and uses of various types of skin grafts. New Orleans M. and S. J. *87:*158–165, Sept '34
OWENS, N.: Skin grafting in relation to general surgery. J. M. A. Alabama *5:*41–46, Aug '35
OWENS, N.: Plastic repair of defects resulting from radical extirpation of facial cancer. South. M. J. *29:*654–664, July '36
OWENS, N.: Treatment of chronic varicose ulcers of lower extremities (grafting). New Orleans M. and S. J. *89:*483–491, March '37
OWENS, N.: Plastic surgery as allied with treatment of cancer (grafts). New Orleans M. and S. J. *90:*417–424, Jan '38

OWENS, N.: Harelip repair (cleft palate). South. M. J. *31:*959–968, Sept '38

OWENS, N.: Reconstruction for traumatic denudation of penis and scrotum; case. Surgery *12:*88–96, July '42

OWENS, N.: Simplified method for formation of artificial vagina by split graft; case. Surgery *12:*139–150, July '42

OWENS, N.: Pressure dressings in burns. S. Clin. North America *23:*1354–1366, Oct '43

OWENS, N.: Simplified method of rotating skin and mucous membrane flaps for complete reconstruction of lower lip. Surgery *15:*196–206, Jan '44

OWENS, N.: Simplified method of rotating skin and mucous membrane flaps for complete reconstruction of lower lip. Am. J. Orthodontics (Oral Surg. Sect.) *30:*340–349, June '44

OWENS, N.: Rayon, ideal surgical dressing for surface wounds. Surgery *19:*482–485, April '46

OWENS, N. AND VINCENT, R. W.: Management of facial injuries. New Orleans M. and S. J. *94:*221–232, Nov '41

OWENS, N. (see HUME, J. R.) March '35

OWENS, R. W. (see BONAR, B. E.) Dec '29

P

PACAUD, H. E. L. AND BERGERET, P. M.: Osteomyelitis of lower jaw with spontaneous fracture in hereditary syphilitic; case. Rev. de stomatol. *32:*785–790, Oct '30

PACHER, W.: Plastic surgery of flexor tendon of hand, with special reference to paralysis of opponens pollicis. Arch. f. orthop. u. Unfall-Chir. *40:*93–101, '39

PACHNER, E.: Autoplastic operations on thumb. Arch. di ortop. *48:*817–828, Dec 31, '32

PACHNER, F.: Various methods for construction of artificial vagina in correction with 7 cases. Gynaekologie *18:*142–150, '39

PACIFICO, A.: Dupuytren's contracture; importance of morbid processes of cervical spine in pathogenesis. Rassegna di neurol. veget. *1:*34–80, '38

PACK, G. T.: Management of malignancies of antrum, superior maxilla, pharynx and larynx at Radium Institute of University of Paris. Ann. Otol. Rhin. and Laryng. *37:*967–973, Sept '28

PACK, G. T.: Management of intra-oral cancers at Radium Institute of University of Paris. Ann. Surg. *90:*15–25, July '29

PACK, GEORGE T.: *Tumors of the Hands and Feet.* C. V. Mosby Co., St. Louis, 1939

PACK, G. T. AND ADAIR, F. E.: Subungual melanoma; differential diagnosis of tumors of nail bed. Surgery *5:*47–72, Jan '39

PACK, G. T. AND NUNEZ, R. A.: Principles of excision and continuous dissection for malignant melanoma, both primary and metastatic; cases. Arch. cubanos cancerol. *5:*20–51, Jan–Mar '46

PACK, G. T. AND NUNEZ, R. A.: Principle of excision and dissection in continuity for primary and metastatic malignant melanoma. Rev. med. cubana *57:*106–137, Feb '46

PACK, G. T. AND PARSONS, J. L.: Unusual deformity sequential to a burn of hand. Am. J. Surg. *38:*159, June '24

PACK, G. T.; SCHARNAGEL, I. AND MORFIT, M.: Principle of excision and dissection in continuity for primary and metastatic melanoma. Surgery *17:*849–866, June '45

PACK, G. T. (see ADAIR, F. E. *et al*) July '30

PACKARD, G. B. JR.: Tannic acid in burns. Colorado Med. *26:*173–176, June '29

PACKARD, G. B. JR.: Removal of large scars or blemishes (nevi) by graduated partial removal. Colorado Med. *28:*289–292, July '31

PACKARD, J. W. JR.: Metal finger splint. U. S. Nav. M. Bull. *45:*769–770, Oct '45

PADDOCK, R. (see PEER, L. A.) Feb '37

PADGETT, E. C.: Cleft palate. J. Kansas M. Soc. *27:*50–51, Feb '27

PADGETT, E. C.: Free full-thickness skin transplantation. J. Kansas M. Soc. *27:*145–148, May '27

PADGETT, E. C.: Treatment of epithelioma about face, mouth and jaws. J. Missouri M. A. *25:*190–194, May '28

PADGETT, E. C.: Repair of harelip and accompanying nasal deformity. J. Kansas M. Soc. *30:*143–147, May '29

PADGETT, E. C.: Plastic surgery. Kansas City Southwest Clin. Soc. Monthly Bull. *5:*19–24, July '29

PADGETT, E. C.: Cleft palate repair after unsuccessful operations, with special reference to cases with extensive loss of palatal tissue. Tr. Sect. Surg., General and Abd., A.M.A., pp. 336–358, '29 also: Arch. Surg. *20:*453–472, March '30

PADGETT, E. C.: Repair of cleft palates after unsuccessful operations, with special reference to cases with extensive loss of palatal tissue. Internat. J. Orthodontia *16:*1299–1316, Dec '30

PADGETT, E. C.: Position of surgery and radium in treatment of cancer of mouth. J. Kansas M. Soc. *32:*167–172, May '31

PADGETT, E. C.: Full-thickness skin graft in correction of soft tissue deformities (cicatrices). Tr. Sect. Surg., Gen. and Abd., A.M.A., pp. 304–319, '31 also: J.A.M.A. *98:*18–23, Jan 2, '32

PADGETT, E. C.: Is iso-skin grafting practicable? South. M. J. *25:*895–900, Sept '32

PADGETT, E. C.: Is grafting with isografts or homografts practicable? West. J. Surg. *41:*205–212, April '33

PADGETT, E. C.: Early and late treatment of burns. J. Kansas M. Soc. *34:*184–188, May '33

PADGETT, E. C.: Epidermoid carcinoma of mouth; general considerations and etiologic factors. Internat. J. Orthodontia *22:*283–293, March '36

PADGETT, E. C.: General considerations, pathology, clinical picture and diagnosis of cancer of lips. Internat. J. Orthodontia *22:*387–394, April '36

PADGETT, E. C.: Pathology, clinical features and diagnosis of cancer of mouth. Internat. J. Orthodontia *22:*504–515, May '36

PADGETT, E. C.: Cheiloplasty in cancer of lips. Internat. J. Orthodontia *22:*939–947, Sept '36

PADGETT, E. C.: Repair of palates primarily unsuccessfully operated upon. Surg., Gynec. and Obst. *63:*483–496, Oct '36

PADGETT, E. C.: Results and prognosis of cancer in and about oral cavity. Internat. J. Orthodontia *22:*1255–1267, Dec '36

PADGETT, E. C.: Management of cancer in and about oral cavity. Internat. J. Orthodontia *23:*73–82, Jan '37

PADGETT, E. C.: Management of injuries of face and jaws, with special reference to common automobile injury. J. Kansas M. Soc. *38:*240–248, June '37

PADGETT, E. C.: Care of severely burned, with special reference to skin grafting. Arch. Surg. *35:*64–86, July '37

PADGETT, EARL C.: *Surgical Diseases of the Mouth and Jaws.* W. B. Saunders Co., Phila., 1938

PADGETT, E. C.: Total reconstruction of auricle. Surg., Gynec. and Obst. *67:*761–768, Dec '38

PADGETT, E. C.: Skin grafting in severe burns. Am. J. Surg. *43:*626–636, Feb '39

PADGETT, E. C.: Treatment of cancer of lips. J. Missouri M. A. *36:*154–157, April '39

PADGETT, E. C.: Calibrated intermediate skin grafts. Surg., Gynec. and Obst. *69:*779–793, Dec '39

PADGETT, E. C.: Late care of severe facial injuries and jaw. Surg., Gynec. and Obst. *72:*437–452, Feb (no. 2A) '41 also: Am. J. Orthodontics (Oral Surg. Sect) *27:*190–207, April '41

PADGETT, E. C.: Severe facial injuries and jaws. Am. J. Surg. *51:*829–846, March '41

PADGETT, E. C.: Skin grafting and "three quarter" thickness skin graft for prevention and correcton of cicatricial formation. Ann. Surg. *113:*1034–1049, June '41

PADGETT, EARL C.: *Skin Grafting from a Personal and Experimental Viewpoint.* C C Thomas Co., Springfield, Ill., 1942

PADGETT, E. C.: Care of military and civilian injuries of face and jaws. Am. J. Orthodontics (Oral Surg. Sect.) *28:*213–221, April '42

PADGETT, E. C.: Improved methods of skin grafting. Proc. Interst. Postgrad. M. A. North America (1942) pp. 32–34, '43

PADGETT, E.: How to use dermatome. Am. Acad. Orthop. Surgeons, Lect., pp. 216–224, '44

PADGETT, E. C.: Indications for determination of thickness for split grafts. Am. J. Surg. *72:*683–693, Nov '46

PADGETT, E. C. AND GASKINS, J. H.: Use of skin flaps in repair of scarred defects over bone and tendons. Surgery *18:*287–298, Sept '45

PADGETT, E. C. AND GASKINS, J. H.: Use of skin flaps in repair of scarred or ulcerative defects over bone and tendons. Tr. West. S. A. (1944) *52:*195–211, '45

PADGETT, E. C. AND ORR, T. G.: Insulin-glucose treatment of traumatic shock; discussion with experimental report. Surg., Gynec. and Obst. *46:*783–788, June '28

PADGETT, E. C. AND SODERBERG, N. B.: Three-fourths graft and other thicknesses cut with dermatome. Dia med. *14:*8–11, Jan 5, '42

PADGETT, E. C. (see ROBINSON, D. W. *et al*) July '46

PADILLA Y CESPEDES, V. M.: Choanal imperforation of nose. Rev. san. mil., Habana *4:*292–294, Oct–Dec '40

PAGANELLI, T. R.: Paganelli's modification of operation for entropion. Dis. Eye, Ear, Nose and Throat *2:*347–349, Nov '42

DE PAGANETTO, M. J. T.: Hypertrichosis in women and its therapy, with special reference to diathermocoagulation. Semana med. *1:*1792–1794, May 25, '33

PAGANI, M.: Skin grafting method favoring epidermic and dermo-epidermic growth. Boll. d'ocul. *7:*442–444, May '28

PAGE: Burn therapy. M. Bull. Bombay *12:*261–264, July 8, '44

PAGE, C. M.: Operation for relief of flexion-contracture in forearm. J. Bone and Joint Surg. *5:*233–234, April '23

PAGE, C. M.: Scope of surgery in treatment of chronic rheumatoid and osteo-arthritis. Brit. M. J. *1:*343–345, March 3, '28

PAGE, C. M.: Apparatus for treatment of finger fractures by skeletal traction. Lancet *1:*986, May 7, '32

PAGE, C. M. AND PERKINS, G.: Some observations on bone-grafting; with special reference to bridge-grafts. Brit. J. Surg. *9:*540–552, April '22 (illus.)

PAGE, I. H.: Occurence of vasoconstrictor substance in blood during shock induced by trauma, hemorrhage and burns. Am. J. Physiol. *139:*386–398, July '43

PAGE, I. H. (see KOHLSTAEDT, K. G.) Aug '43

PAGE, J. R.: Angioma of auricle; case. Ann. Otol. Rhin. and Laryng. *37:*358–360, March '28

PAGEL, W.: Role of allergy in degeneration of tissues transplanted into peritoneal cavity. Krankheits-forschung *6:*337–377, Aug '28

PAGENSTECHER, G. A.: Burn therapy. J.A.M.A. *84:*1917, June 20, '25

PAGENSTECHER, G. A.: Congenital anomalies of the neck. Texas State J. Med. *25:*786–789, April '30

PAGENSTECHER, G. A.: Rhinoplasty. Am. J. Surg. *25:*491–493, Sept '34

PAGLIANI, F.: Lateral cyst of neck; surgical removal followed by development of malignant branchioma; clinical and pathologic study. Bull. d. sc. med., Bologna *105:*405–428, Sept–Oct '33

PAGLIOLI, E.: Bilateral ankylosis of temporomaxillary joint; technic of surgical therapy; case. Rev. radiol. clin. *2:*613–620, April '33

PAGNAMENTA, E.: Late anatomic and functional results of cleft palate operation; 150 cases. Deutsche Ztschr. f. Chir. *235:*214–233, '32

PAIS, C.: Isolated fracture of zygomatic arch; case. Gior. veneto di sc. med. *12:*685–690, Nov '38

PAISLEY, J. C.: Stretcher head support in cases of smashed jaw. Brit. M. J. *1:*16, Jan 3, '42

PAITRE, F.: Treatment of synovial and lymphangitic phlegmonata; practical importance of anatomic data on cellular spaces of hand and fingers. Bull. med., Paris *43:*1171–1177, Nov 2, '29

PAIVA GONCALVES: Recuperation of war wounded with orbital-ocular injuries. Hospital, Rio de Janeiro *26:*429–444, Sept '44

DE PAIVA MEIRA, S.: Facial palsy and its treatment by nerve anastomosis. Internat. Clinics *2:*241, '21

PALACIO POSSE, R.: Plastic surgery in correction of nasal hypertrophy; intranasal route. Rev. de especialid. *5:*1856–1866, Nov '30

PALACIO POSSE, R.: Social role of esthetic surgery. Semana med. *1:*330–335, Jan 26, '33

PALACIO POSSE, R.: Surgical therapy of pendulous breast. Semana med. *1:*996–1001, April 8, '37

PALACIO POSSE, R.: Use of osteocartilaginous hump of nose for correction of underdeveloped chin. Arq. de cir. clin. e exper. *6:*299–301, April–June '42

PALACIO POSSE, R.: New surgical therapy of protruding ears without resection of cartilage. Arq. de cir. clin. e exper. *6:*489–492, April–June '42

PALACIO POSSE, R.: Surgical treatment of pendulous breast. J. Internat. Coll. Surgeons *6:*361–363, July–Aug '43

PALACIO POSSE, RAMON: *Cirugia estética.* El Ateñeo Press, Buenos Aires, 1946

Palate (See also Cleft Palate)

Reconstruction of hard palate. BURIAN, F. Rev. de chir. *59:*49, '21

Two rare congenital anomalies; 1. hydro-encephalocele; 2. intra-uterine adhesion of tip of tongue to hard palate. ESAU, P. Arch. f. klin. Chir. *118:*817–820, '21

Reconstruction of palate after injury. BIEDERMANN, H. Beitr. z. klin. Chir. *125:*444–450, '22 (illus.) abstr: J.A.M.A. *79:*84, July 1, '22

Surgical anatomy of palate. VEAU, V. AND RUPPE, C., J. de chir. *20:*1–30, July '22 (illus.) abstr: J.A.M.A. *79:*687, Aug 19, '22

Contributions to plastic surgery of jaws and palate. LUXENBURGER, A. Deutsche Ztschr. f. Chir. *172:*384–396, '22 (illus.)

Luetic perforation of hard palate with surgical closure. LOCY, F. E., U. S. Nav. M. Bull. *18:*86–87, Jan '23 (illus.)

Use of delayed flap in secondary operations on palate. NEW, G. B. Minnesota Med. *6:*214–220, April '23 (illus.)

Staphylorrhaphy. VEAU, V. Medecine *5:*21–25, Oct '23

Plastic operations on hard palate. ROSENTHAL, W. Zentralbl. f. Chir. *51:*1621–1627, July 26, '24

Plastic operations on hard palate; comment on Rosenthal's article. ERNST, F. Zentralbl. f. Chir. *52:*464–470, Feb 28, '25

Plastic operation to reconstruct syphilitic defect in palate. CAVINA, C. Gior. ital. di dermat. e sifil. *66:*678–679, April '25

Speech complications involved in certain types of inadequate palate, especially congenital short palate, with exhibition of patients. KENYON, E. L. Ann. Otol., Rhin. and Laryng. *34:*887–900, Sept '25

Treatment of perforations and fissures in hard and soft palates. CRESPI, R. A. Semana med. *1:*666–683, April 1, '26; *1:*710–723, April 8; *1:*755–776, April 15, '26

Technic of uranostaphylorrhaphy. PIZZAGALLI, L. Boll. d. spec. med.-chir. *1:*7–16, Jan–March '27

Surgical correction of maxillary and palatal defects in cooperation with orthodontist

Palate—Cont.
and prosthodontist. VAUGHAN, H. S. Dental Cosmos *69:*63–67, Jan '27
Velo-palatine prosthesis. RUPPE, L. AND RUPPE, C. Odontologie *65:*69–86, Feb 28, '27
Prolongation of palate by retrotransposition of pterygoid processes in cleft palate. PŘECHECHTĚL, A. Casop. lek. cesk. *66:*541-543, March 28, '27
Treatment of perforations and fissures of palate and soft palate. CRESPI, R. A. Semana med. *1:*666; 710; 755, '27
Operation for lengthening palate. LVOFF, P. P. Vestnik khir. (nos. 37–38) *13:*212–221, '28
Blood supply of hard palate in connection with plastic operations. OUSAROFF, V. M. Vestnik khir. (nos. 37–38) *13:*222–229, '28
Old and new methods of palate surgery. CAMPOS, J. Ars med. *5:*229–238, July '29
Suture technic of palate. SCHOEMAKER, J. Chirurg. *1:*1012, Oct 1, '29
Uranostaphylorrhaphy. GATTI, G. Surg., Gynec. and Obst. *51:*224–226, Aug '30
Bifid uvula. DUCUING, L. Rev. de laryng. *52:*76–80, Jan 31, '31
Intrapharyngeal nitrous oxide insufflation in staphylorrhaphy. NYST, P. M. E. P. Nederl. tijdschr. v. geneesk. *75:*2059–2061, April 18, '31
Uranoplasty at several sittings. EICHHOFF, E. Chirurg *3:*595–599, July 1, '31
Rhinolalia clausa palatina functionalis. DAITÔ, T. Fukuoka-Ikwadaigaku-Zasshi *24:*87–90, Sept '31
Correction of short palate. PŘECECHTĚL, A. Casop. lek. cesk. *70:*1544–1548, Nov 13, '31 also: Otolaryng. slavica *4:*23–24, Jan '32
Schönborn operation (velopharyngorrhaphy) for correction of defective speech. SEEMANN, M. Casop. lek. cesk. *70:*1570–1574, Nov 20, '31 also: Otolaryng. slavica *4:*24–25, Jan '32
Simple plastic method of covering palatal defects. SPANIER, F. Deutsche Ztschr. f. Chir. *231:*284–293, '31
New treatment of palatopharyngeal synechiae of traumatic origin. LEMOINE, J. Ann. d'oto-laryng., pp. 404–410, April '32
Congenital functional defect of soft palate and uvula with other malformations of first and second branchial arches in unshortened palate. BERNFELD, K. Monatschr. f. Ohrenh. *66:*916–921, Aug '32
Syphilitic origin of perforation of palate and destruction of nose; uranoplasty; reconstruction of nose by tubular grafts with

Palate—Cont.
cartilaginous support of costal origin. ROCHER, H. L. Bull. et mem. Soc. de chir. de Bordeaux et du Sud-Ouest, pp. 150–152, '32
Treatment of adherent and deficient palates following injury. DENEHY, W. J. AND AMIES, A., M. J. Australia *1:*150–154, Feb 4, '33
Therapy of malformations and acquired lesions of palate. HECKER, I. W. Rev. de stomatol. *35:*412–420, July '33
Lengthening of velum and shortening of pharynx for amelioration of voice after uranoplasty. MEISSNER, A. Rev. de stomatol. *35:*405–411, July '33
Closure of defect in hard palate by pedicled tube graft. BURNELL, G. H., M. J. Australia *2:*484, Oct 7, '33
Functional results of 200 staphylorrhaphies. VEAU, V. AND BOREL-MAISONNY, MME. Bull. et mem. Soc. nat. de chir. *59:*1372–1382, Nov 25, '33
Plastic closure of defective hard palate by means of round pedicled flap (Filatov). FRANKENBERG, B. E. Sovet khir. *4:*591–595, '33
Palatoplasty using extra-oral tissues. DAVIS, A. D. Ann. Surg. *99:*94–100, Jan '34
Two cases illustrating elastic traction in plastic surgery; pedicle flap to close large opening in hard palate. MOOREHEAD, F. B., S. Clin. North America *14:*745–749, Aug '34
Rhinolalia aperta caused by velopalatine insufficiency; case. VARGA, V. Cluj. med. *15:*576–578, Oct 1, '34
Correcting deformities of velum and mesopharynx to insure better speech following cleft palate surgery. BOYNE, H. N. Nebraska M. J. *19:*407–409, Nov '34
Perforation of palate due to suction attachment of dental plate. AXHAUSEN, G. Deutsche Zahn-, Mund-u. Kieferh. *1:*343–348, '34
"Push-back operation" of palate. DORRANCE, G. M. Ann. Surg. *101:*445–459, Jan '35
Therapeutic technic for staphylolalia (so-called short palate speech). VOELKER, C. H. Arch. Otolaryng. *21:*94–96, Jan '35
Therapeutic methods in palatopharyngeal adhesion in connection with 2 successfully treated cases. PESTI, L. Monatschr. f. Ohrenh. *69:*330–335, March '35
Clinical observations on influence of septum on development of nose and palatal arch. CARTER, W. W. Laryngoscope *45:*355–365, May '35
Roentgenologic studies of closure of orophar-

Palate—Cont.
ynx against nasopharynx and position of tongue during blowing up of cheeks in persons with cleft palate; function tests of soft palate. SEIFERTH, L. B. Klin. Wchnschr. *14:*897–899, June 22, '35
Technic of therapy (palatopharyngorrhaphy) of rhinolalia aperta due to too short palate. SERCER, A. Rev. de chir. structive, pp. 5–18, July '35
Technic and results of plastic surgery of the palate. AXHAUSEN, G. Zentralbl. f. Chir. *62:*2211–2215, Sept 14, '35
Protective prosthesis for plastic operation on palate. HOTTA, H. Ztschr. d. japan, chirurg. Gesellsch. *36:*100–101, '35
Phonation and staphylorraphy. VEAU, V. AND BOREL-MAISONNY, S. Rev. franc. de phoniatrie *4:*133–141, July '36
Prosthetic appliance for atresia palati in edentulous patient. AMIES, A. AND BAGHEL, D., M. J. Australia *2:*600–601, Oct 31, '36
Repair of palates primarily unsuccessfully operated upon. PADGETT, E. C. Surg., Gynec. and Obst. *63:*483–496, Oct '36
Tumors and ulcers of palate and fauces (Semon lecture, abstract). HOWARTH, W. Lancet *2:*1139–1142, Nov 14, '36
Protective prosthesis for plastic operations of palate. HOTTA, H. Nagoya J. M. Sc. *10:*280–284, Dec '36
Combined congenital malformation of tongue and hard palate; case. KOLESOV, G. G. Sovet. khir., no. 9, pp. 524–526, '36
Pharyngo-staphylo-uranoplasty, operation in older children and adults. TROELL, A. Svenska lak.-tidning. *34:*521–524, April 9, '37
Results of bridge plastic (Axhausen) operation for cleft palate in 45 cases. IMMENKAMP, A. Deutsche Ztschr. f. Chir. *249:*326–336, '37
Prosthetic therapy of acquired palatal defects. EHRICKE, A. Med. Welt *12:*775–776, May 28, '38
Uranostaphylorrhaphy with Donati suture. SCHOEMAKER, J. Arch. ital. di chir. *54:*513–515, '38
Hairy polyus of soft palate as cause of cleft formation; case. NASE, H. Zentralbl. f. Chir. *66:*29–32, Jan 7, '39
Plastic surgery of hard palate after excision of huge osteoma of upper jaw; author's technic. PIETRANTONI, L. Valsalva *15:*205–211, May '39
Injuries to tongue and palate; therapy. ROCHETTE, M. Hôpital *27:*281–282, May '39
New periosteotome for hard palate. BERTOLA, V. J. Prensa med. argent. *26:*1853–1854, Sept 20, '39
Double elongations of partially cleft palates and elongations of palates with complete clefts. BROWN, J. B. Surg., Gynec. and Obst. *70:*815–818, April '40
Unusual case of submucosal cleft palate in conjunction with deformity of soft palate and nasal speech. ARNOLD, G. E. Arch. f. Ohren-, Nasen-u. Kehlkopfh. *147:*173–176, '40
Author's method of plastic reconstruction of palate after removal of huge osteoma of upper jaw. PIERANTONI, L. Plast. chir. *1:*109–112, '40
Question of advisability of surgical closure of traumatic defects of palate. LUHMANN, K. Zentralbl. f. Chir. *68:*460–464, March 8, '41
Palatine fistula, plastic closure by means of turbinate bone. DE MARTINI, R. Boll. d. mal. d. orecchio, d. gola, d. naso *59:*172–177, May '41
Buccomaxillofacial prosthesis; artificial nose and palate; case. GRAZIANI, M. Rev. brasil. de oto-rino-laring. *9:*217–221, May–June '41
Intramural tumors of soft palate. UTRATA-BANYAI, J. Ztschr. f. Hals-, Nasen-u. Ohrenh. *48:*113–116, '41
Self-retaining illuminating palate retractor. DALTON, S. E. Tr. Am. Acad. Ophth. (1941) *46:*151, Jan–Feb '42
New method of elongating short palates. BAXTER, H. Canad. M.A.J. *46:*322–325, April '42
New plastic method for correction of velopharyngeal symphysis stricture. MAGGIOROTTI, U. Boll. d. mal. d. oreccio, d. gola, d. naso *60:*194–196, May '42
Management of nasal deformities in infants and small children and ear, eyelids, lips and palate deform. PEER, L. A. Dis. Eye, Ear, Nose and Throat *2:*166–176, June '42
Serious mutilation of palate due to tonsillectomy. ARNOLD, G. Monatschr. f. Ohrenh. *76:*377–381, Aug '42
Method of keeping palatal mucoperiosteum against bony structures following surgery. GROSS, P. P. Am. J. Orthodontics (Oral Surg. Sect) *28:*522–524, Sept '42
Vincent's ulceration of soft palate. HOUSER, K. M. Tr. Am. Laryng. A. *64:*141–143, '42
Injury of hard palate by indelible pencil. KUNG, H. Arch. f. Ohren-, Nasen-u. Kehlkopfh. *151:*272–274, '42
Fissural cysts of median palatine suture. COHEN, M. M. Am. J. Orthodontics (Oral Surg. Sect.) *29:*442–451, Aug '43

Palate – Cont.

Attempt to correct congenital rhinolalia aperta by plastic operation. WODAK, E. Harefuah *27:*8, July 2, '44

Congenital anteflexion accompanied by swelling of soft palate; correction by plastic methods. WODAK, E. Ann. Otol., Rhin. and Laryng. *53:*581-582, Sept '44

Palatoplasty; procedure for immobilization of mucosa and sutures. MARINO, H. Prensa med. argent. *32:*436-438, March 9, '45

Closure of alveolosinusal communications by pedicled palatine strip. RAMADIER, J. A. Ann. d'oto-laryng. *12:*315-316, April–June '45

Prosthesis for palate; treatment of case with hollow-ball obturator. CANTOR, B. B. Am. J. Orthodontics (Oral Surg. Sect.) *31:*740–743, Dec '45

Traumatic palatine fistula. WIBLE, L. E. AND HOWARD, J. C. JR. Arch. Otolaryng. *44:*159-165, Aug '46

Responsibility of surgeon in treating palatal and related defects. KEMPER, J. W. Am. J. Orthodontics (Oral Surg. Sect.) *32:*667–670, Nov '46

Palate, Cancer (See also Jaws, Cancer; Mouth, Cancer)

Tumors and ulcers of palate and fauces (Semon lecture, abstract). HOWARTH, W. Lancet *2:*1139-1142, Nov 14, '36

Benign and malignant tumors of palate. MARTIN, H. E. Arch. Surg. *44:*599-635, April '42

Palate, Tumors

Tumors of velum. MATHYS, A. Bull. Soc. belge d'oto., rhinol., laryng., pp. 83-87, '38

Intramural tumors of soft palate. UTRATA-BANYAI, J. Ztschr. f. Hals-, Nasen-u. Ohrenh. *48:*113-116, '41

Benign and malignant tumors of palate. MARTIN, H. E. Arch. Surg. *44:*599-635, April '42

PALAZZI, S.: Fractured jaw; case. Stomatol. *32:*662-665, July '34

PALAZZI, S.: Mandibular fracture treated by emergency methods; preliminary report. Stomatol. *33:*1076-1079, Dec '35

PALAZZI, S.: Therapy of jaw fractures by simple stomatologic means obtainable by general practitioner. Gior. di med. mil. *85:*833-837, Aug '37

PALAZZI, S.: Naphthalene in therapy of gangrene following grave trauma of face due to bullet wounds. Gior. di med. mil. *85:*944-952, Sept '37

PALAZZI, S.: Care and therapeutic provisions for maxillofacial wounds on battlefield; limits and possibilities of aid in dressing stations of troops, battalions and regiments and in advanced posts of sanitary service. Gior. di med. mil. *88:*500-508, July '40

PALAZZO, O. R.: Artificial vagina, plastic formation in uterovaginal aplasia, with report of case. Semana med. *2:*189-200, July 22, '37

PALAZZO, O. R.: Artificial vagina covered with dermoepidermal graft. Bol. Soc. de obst. y ginec. de Buenos Aires *24:*183-192, June 21, '45

PALAZZO, R. (see FERNICOLA, C. *et al*) Sept '42

PALCHEVSKIY, E. I. AND POLYAK, S. O.: Fate of flap in esophagoplasty after circular resection of cervical part of esophagus. Vestnik khir. *53:*113-115, '37

PALLARÉS MACHÍ, V.: Therapy of acute hand infections following industrial accidents. Cron. med., Valencia *37:*31-48, Jan 15, '33

PALMA, R.: Operative treatment of rhinophyma; 3 cases. Rev. sud-am. de med. et de chir. *2:*49-57, Jan '31

PALMA, R.: Modifications of Zeller operation in therapy of syndactylia. Ann. ital. di chir. *13:*1068-1074, Sept 30, '34

PALMÉN, A. J.: Serrated plastic surgery; one of several beneficial methods of treating syndactylia and Dupuytren's. Zentralbl. f. Chir. *59:*1377-1379, May 28, '32

PALMÉN, A. J.: Technic of autoplastic grafts. Duodecim *48:*36-39, '32

PALMÉN, A. J.: Improvised finger splint. Nord. med. *27:*1960, Sept 28, '45

PALMER, A.: Rhinoplasty; past and present. Eye, Ear, Nose and Throat Monthly *11:*58–62, March '32

PALMER, A.: Complications following rhinoplasty. Arch. Otolaryng. *28:*538-545, Oct '38

PALMER, A.: Plastic surgery training; visual aids. Plast. and Reconstruct. Surg. *1:*113–117, July '46

PALMER, B. M. (see COUNSELLER, V. S.) Aug '29

PALMER, D. H.: Plastic surgery. Northwest Med. *27:*296-298, June '28

PALMER, D. H.: Problems in plastic surgery. Northwest Med. *38:*136-138, April '39

PALMER, E. P. AND PALMER, E. P. JR.: War burns. Southwestern Med. *26:*251-255, Aug '42

PALMER, E. P. JR. (see PALMER, E. P.) Aug '42

PALMER, F. E. AND REIFSNEIDER, J. S.: Plastic reconstruction of external auditory meatus. Laryngoscope *43:*618-621, Aug '33

PALMER, L. A. AND SOUTHWORTH, J. L.: Bridge operation for Dupuytren's contracture. Am. J. Surg. *68:*351–354, June '45
PALMER, R. G.: Retraction of palmar aponeurotic fascia. Gaz. d. hop. *106:*1369–1375, Sept 23, '33
PALMSTIERNA, K.: Plastic surgery of thumb. Nord. med. (Hygiea) *1:*243–244, Jan 28, '39
PALOMO MARTINEZ, J.: Conservative and restorative surgery in accidents. Rev. med. veracruzana *18:*2539–2546, May 1, '38
PALTRINIERI, M. AND DE LUCCHI, G.: Hereditary transmission of rare deformity of thumb. Bull. d. sc. med., Bologna *110:*158–167, May–June '38

Panas Operation

Surgical treatment of entropion by method of Panas. CANGE, A. Medecine *4:*261–262, Jan '23 abstr: J.A.M.A. *80:*1183, April 21, '23
Modification of Panas operation for cicatricial ectropion. PARADOKSOV, L. F. Sovet. vestnik oftal. *7:*381–383, '35
Comparison of immediate and late results of Panas, Snellen and Millingen-Sapezhko eyelid operations. AVGUSHEVICH, P. L. Vestnik oftal. *11:*557–563, '37

PANCOAST, H. K.: Modern treatment of cancer of lip. Surg., Gynec. and Obst. *34:*589–593, May '22
PANGLOSS: Limits of esthetic surgery. Policlinico (sez. prat.) *36:*1087, July 29, '29
PANKRATIEV, B. E.: Dead bone grafts to repair skull defects. Ann. Surg. *97:*321–326, March '33
PANNELLA, P.: Influence of epinephrine on shock caused by removal of hemostatic bandage; clinical and experimental study. Ann. ital. di chir. *14:*1–14, Jan '35
PANNETON, J. E.: Hemangioma of nose; late results of radiotherapy. Union med. du Canada *61:*940–944, Aug '32
PANNETON, P.: Facial wounds and their plastic repair. Union med. du Canada. *72:*392–397, April '43
PANNETON, P.: New technic for correcting symblepharon. Union med. du Canada *73:*42–44, Jan '44
PAOLI, M.: Therapy of complicated jaw fracture in patient with no upper teeth. Rev. de stomatol. *41:*398–402, May '39
PAOLI, M.: Diplopia in fracture of upper and lower maxillary and of malar bones; case. Rev. de stomatol. *41:*548–552, July '39
PAOLINI LANDA, J. AND FARINA, R. C.: Dupuytren's contracture; with report of case. Semana med. *2:*1607–1612, Dec 31, '42
PAOLUCCI, F.: Lack of taking of autoplastic skin-grafts. Ann. ital. di chir. *7:*41–64, Jan '28
PAOLUCCI, R.: Therapy of extensive burns, with special reference to use of tannic acid. Ann. di med. nav. e colon. *46:*501–504, Nov–Dec '40
PAPE: Surgical therapy of nasal deformities. Ztschr. f. Laryng., Rhin., Otol. *24:*73–74, '33
PAPPER, E. M.: Anesthesia for patient in burn therapy. Surgery *17:*116–121, Jan '45
PAPPER, E. M. AND ROVENSTINE, E. A.: Anesthetic management in reconstructive surgery of mandible. Am. J. Orthodontics (Oral Surg. Sect.) *32:*433–438, Jul '46
PARADIS, B. (see HUDON, F.) Feb '45
PARADOKSOV, L. F.: Modification of Panas operation for cicatricial ectropion. Sovet. vestnik oftal. *7:*381–383, '35
PARADOKSOV, L. F.: Surgical therapy of cicatricial entropion of lower eyelid. Vestnik oftal. *13:*550–551, '38
PARAMONOV, V. A.: Combined open method of burn therapy. Khirurgiya, no. 10, pp. 37–39, '37
PARANAGUA, C.: War burns; traumatologic study on action of flame throwers and explosives. Imprensa med., Rio de Janeiro *19:*57–72, Aug '43
PARAVICINI: Extensive burns. Schweiz. med. Wchnschr. *57:*22, Jan 1, '27
PARCE, A. D.: An improved method of skin grafting. Ann. Surg. *75:*658–662, June '22 (illus.)
PARDO-CASTELLO, V.: Contracture of palmar aponeurosis. Acta dermat.-venereol. *13:*649–654, Dec '32
PARDO DE TAVERA, V.: Complete fracture of horizontal branch of inferior maxillary bone. Semana med. *2:*539–540, Aug 14, '30
PARDO DE TAVERA, V.: Exposed comminuted fracture of inferior maxilla caused by bullet; case. Semana med. *2:*598–599, Aug 21, '30

Pare, Ambroise

Ambroise Pare's onion treatment of burns. SIGERIST, H. E. Bull. Hist. Med. *15:*143–149, Feb '44

PAREDAS, J.: Clinical aspects and treatment of hand infections. Med. contemp. *46:*269–274, Aug 19, '28
PARFITT, G. J.; MCLEOD, A. C. AND SHEPHERD, P. R.: Teeth in fracture line. Bull. War Med. *3:*328, Feb '43 (abstract)
PARIN, B.: Technic of Filatov's tubular pedicle. Sovet. khir. *1:*141–144, '31
PARIN, B.: Transplantation of large pieces of skin with aid of Filatov cutaneous pedicle. Arch. f. klin. Chir. *168:*191–198, '31

PARIN, B. V.: Method of shortening healing process in Filatov graft. Vestnik khir. (no. 67) *23:*90–95, '31
PARIN, B. V.:Restoration of lost fingers. Trudy Molotovsk. gos. med. Inst. *21:*125–142, '42
PARIN, B. V.: *Reconstruction of the Fingers*. U.S.S.R. "Medgiz" Press, Moscow, 1944
PARIN, B. V.: Skin grafts in war wounded. Sovet. med. (nos. 7–8) *8:*4–8, '44
PARIN, B. V.: Immediate and late results of free transplantation in form of perforated flap; preliminary report. Khirurgiya, no. 12, pp. 21–29, '44
PARIN, B. V.: Mobilization of hand following loss of all fingers. Khirurgiya no. 3, p. 89, '45 (comment on Geymanovich's article)
PARIN, B. V.: Reconstruction of fingers. Bull. War Med. *6:*524, Aug '46 (Abstract)
PARIN, V. N.: Grafting of hairy skin with aid of pedunculated flap for formation of eyebrows, mustache and beard. Vestnik khir. (nos. 73–74) *24:*10–12, '31
PARINA, G. A.: Local anesthesia with nupercaine in reconstructive surgery. Khirurgiya, no. 1, pp. 25–27, '45
PARIS, J. (see CARRIERE, G.) Jan '40
PARIS, M.: Streptococcic inflammation of 2 large tendon sheaths of right hand; case. Liege med. *23:*137–142, Feb 2, '30
PARISEAU, L.: Branchial fistula; case. J. de l'Hotel-Dieu de Montreal *4:*276–283, Nov '35
PARISH, B. B. AND WHITAKER, L. W.: Multiple facial fractures. U. S. Vet. Bur. M. Bull. *7:*162–163, Feb '31
PARK, W. D.: Treatment of wounds of fingers. M. Press *216:*26–262, Oct 9, '46
PARKER, D. B.: Surgical treatment of clefts of palate and lip. Am. J. Surg. *4:*385–389, April '28
PARKER, D. B.: Surgical consideration of abnormal frena of lip. Internat. J. Orthodontia *23:*1141–1148, Nov '37
PARKER, DOUGLAS B.: *Synopsis of Traumatic Injuries of the Face and Jaws*. C. V. Mosby Co., St. Louis, 1942
PARKER, D. B.: Fractures of maxillary bones. Laryngoscope *52:*365–370, May '42
PARKER, D. B.: Maxillary fractures. J. Oral Surg. *1:*122–130, April '43
PARKER, D. B.: Skeletal fixation in treatment of fractures of mandible. S. Clin. North America *24:*381–391, April '44
PARKER, D. B.: Definitive treatment of maxillofacial injuries. J. Oral Surg. *3:*320–325, Oct '45
PARKER, E. F.: Present concept of surgical shock. J. South Carolina M. A. *38:*12–15, Jan '42
PARKER, W. R.: Ophthalmic plastic surgery; clinical procedure in certain cases. Am. J. Ophth. *10:*109–113, Feb '27
PARKER, W. S.: Surgical emphysema of hand due to use of pneumatic tools (case). J. Roy. Nav. M. Serv. *23:*347–348, Oct '37
PARKES, A. R.: Surgical treatment of pain in peripheral nervous system (following amputations of fingers). Tr. Roy. Med.-Chir. Soc. Glasgow, pp. 23–25, '43–'44; in Glasgow M. J. May '44
PARKHILL, E. M. (see MILLHON, J. A.) April '46
PARKINS, W. M. *et al*: Gelatin as plasma substitute, with particular reference to burn shock. Ann. Surg. *118:*193–214, Aug '43
PARKINS, W. M.; *et al*: Desoxycorticosterone (adrenal preparation) as prophylactic foretreatment for prevention of circulatory failure following hemorrhage and surgical trauma in adrenalectomized dog. Am. J. Physiol. *134:*426–435, Sept '41
PARKINSON, S. N.: Surgical establishment of nasal ventilation. Ann. Otol., Rhin. and Laryng. *49:*1023–1029, Dec '40
PARNELL, H. S. (see COX, F. J. *et al*) Dec '44
PARODI, L.: Sequestrectomy and autoplasty with skin flaps in therapy of subacute and chronic nonspecific osteomyelitis. Ann. ital. di chir. *21:*307–314, May '42
PARODI, L. M. (see LINARI, O. T.) April '38

Parotid, Cancer

Parotid gland cancer, surgical therapy, recurrence and cure by radiotherapy. BELOT, J. AND MÉNÉGAUX, G. J. de radiol. et d'electrol. *15:*90–91, Feb '31
Cancer of parotid in new-born. MCKNIGHT, H. A., Am. J. Surg. *45:*128–130, July '39
Malignant tumor of parotid gland treated by Duval operation, with transplantation of digastric muscle to relieve resulting paralysis (Cadenat operation); case. MIRIZZI, P. L. AND URRUTIA, J. M. Bol. y trab., Soc. de cir. de Cordoba (no. 4) *1:*52–55, '40

Parotid Gland

Primary repair of injuries to parotid duct. TEES, F. J. Canad. M.A.J. *16:*145–146, Feb '26
Operation on two cases of secondary carcinoma and on one case of primary cystadenoma of parotid gland; relation of lobes of parotid to facial nerve. MCWHORTER, G. L. S. Clin. N. Amer. *7:*489–505, June '27
Preservation of facial nerve in excision of parotid tumors; 2 cases. SHAAR, C. M. U. S. Nav. M. Bull. *27:*351–360, April '29

Parotid Gland—Cont.
Branchial cysts of parotid gland. CUNNINGHAM, W. F. Ann. Surg. *90:*114–117, July '29
Cancer of parotid gland, indications and technic for total removal; 2 cases. SANTOS, M. Bol. do coll. brasil. de cir. *3:*10–20, April–July '32
Technic of total or subtotal extirpation of parotid gland with conservation of superior branch of facial nerve in so-called mixed tumors; clinical results. DUVAL, P. AND REDON, H., J. de chir. *39:*801–808, June '32
Questions of malignancy of parotid tumors, diagnosis and therapy. FRENYÓ, L. Deutsche Ztschr. f. Chir. *235:*130–139, '32
Treatment of persistent parotid fistulas; 2 cases. KONJETZNY, G. E. Zentralbl. f. Chir. *61:*243–247, Feb 3, '34
Extirpation of parotid gland by Duval method. FIORILLO, J. F. Prensa med. argent. *22:*150–152, Jan 16, '35
Primary repair of severed parotid duct; method of fixation of inlying dowel. BROHM, C. G. AND BIRD, C. E., J.A.M.A. *104:*733–734, March 2, '35
Technic of local anesthesia for total extirpation of parotid gland. FINOCHIETTO, R. AND DICKMANN, G. H. Semana med. *2:*1349–1352, Nov 7, '35
Results of stellectomy in facial paralysis due to section of facial nerve involved in parotid tumor; case. CAEIRO, J. A. Semana med. *1:*572–579, Feb 20, '36
Transplantation of parotid (Stensen's) duct in cancer of antrum. FIGI, F. A. Proc. Staff Meet., Mayo Clin. *11:*241–243, April 15, '36
Total removal of parotid gland with preservation of facial nerve. SALTZSTEIN, H. C. Ann. Surg. *103:*635–638, April '36
Treatment of parotid fistula. COOK, J. Lancet *1:*1239, May 30, '36
Local anesthesia in total excision of parotid. GUTIERREZ, A. Rev. de cir. de Buenos Aires *15:*288–292, May '36
Method for correcting paralysis of lower part of face due to nerve injury in extirpation of benign parotid tumors. CADENAT, F. M. Mem. Acad. de chir. *62:*961–962, June 17, '36
Branchioma of right parotid in young girl; extracapsular extirpation and closure of resulting defect by Thiersch graft. GOUFAS, G. Ann. d'oto-laryng., pp. 677–685, July '36
Modern trends in therapy of parotid tumors. COGNIAUX, P. AND SIMON, S. J. de chir. et ann. Soc., belge de chir. (no. 4) *36–34:*152–163, May '37

Parotid Gland—Cont.
Repair of traumatic fistulas of Stenson's duct (parotid). GLASCOCK, H. AND GLASCOCK, H. JR. Surg., Gynec. and Obst. *65:*355–356, Sept '37
Acute purulent parotitis caused by facial trauma; case. YAMASAKI, Y. Oto-rhino-laryng. *10:*1027, Nov '37
Surgical therapy of parotid fistula according to Sapozhkov method. MACHAN, V. Y. Vestnik khir. *49:*94–95, '37
Treatment of tumors of parotid; survey of results obtained at Barnard Free Skin and Cancer Hospital. MARTIN, T. M. Arch. Surg. *36:*136–143, Jan '38
Parotidectomy with conservation of superior facial nerve (Duval operation); 2 cases. COGNIAUX, P. J. de chir. et ann. Soc. belge de chir. *38–36:*370–372, Dec '39
Diagnosis and surgical therapy of parotid tumors. ZAVALETA, D. E. Rev. med. y cien afines *2:*422–424, June 30, '40
Treatment of mixed tumors of parotid. PATEY, D. H. Brit. J. Surg. *28:*29–38, July '40
Treatment of parotid tumors with special reference to total parotidectomy. BAILEY, H. Brit. J. Surg. *28:*337–346, Jan '41
Extirpation of parotid gland with complete conservation of facial nerve. FINOCHIETTO, R.; *et al.* Rev. med. munic. *2:*790–803, Dec '41
Mixed tumor of parotid; technic of approach incision. LOUBEJAC, A. M. Bol. Soc. cir. d. Uruguay *14:*726–729, '43
Total parotidectomy with conservation of facial nerve; 3 cases. GONI MORENO, I. AND RUSSO, A. G. Bol. y trab., Acad. argent. de cir. *28:*722–739, Sept 6, '44
Reconstruction of facial nerve (especially in operations on parotid gland). FURSTENBERG, A. C. Arch. Otolaryng. *41:*42–47, Jan '45
Temporary external salivary drainage (from Stenson's duct) following arthroplasty. GOODSELL, J. O., J. Oral Surg. *3:*174–176, April '45
New method of treatment of parotid fistula; cauterization and silence cure. COSTANTINI, H. Afrique franc. chir., nos. 3–4, pp. 65–68, May–Aug '45
Surgical anatomy of facial nerve with special reference to parotid gland. MCCORMACK, L. J.; *et al.* Surg., Gynec. and Obst. *80:*620–630, June '45
Total parotidectomy; cases. SIBILLA, C. E. AND CATALANO, F. E. Bol. y trab., Soc. argent. de cirujanos *6:*142–150, '45 also: Rev. Asoc. med. argent. *59:*698–700, Jun 30, '45

Parotid Gland—Cont.

Sistrunk operation (parotid); case. ZAVALETA, E. E. Prensa med. argent. *32:*1331–1334, July 13, '45

Intermaxilloparotid cellular space; abscesses formed there. PONS-TORTELLA, E. AND BROGGI, M. Med. clin., Barcelona *5:*273–277, Oct '45

Primary repair of parotid duct. WALLACE, F. T. Am. J. Surg. *70:*412–413, Dec '45

Technic of total parotidectomy with conservation of facial nerve. REDON, H. J. de chir. *61:*14–20, '45

Anatomic findings concerning morphology and relations of intraparotid facial nerve. DARGENT, M. AND DUROUX, P. E. Presse med. *54:*523–524, Aug 10, '46

Parotid Tumors

Mixed tumors of parotid. SISTRUNK, W. E. Minnesota Med. *4:*155, March '21

Preservation of facial nerve in radical treatment of parotid tumors. ADSON, A. W. AND OTT, W. O. Arch. Surg. *6:*739–746, May '23 (illus.)

Ninety tumors of parotid region, in all of which postoperative history was traced. MCFARLAND, J. Am. J. M. Sc. *172:*804–848, Dec '26

Study of 225 cases of parotid tumors with complete end-results in 80 cases. BENEDICT, E. B. AND MEIGS, J. V. Surg., Gynec. and Obst. *51:*626–647, Nov '30

Mixed tumors of parotid gland; 71 cases. NEILL, W. JR. M. J. and Rec. *136:*187–189, Sept 7, '32

Results of stellectomy in facial paralysis due to section of nerve involved in parotid tumor; case. CAEIRO, J. A. Bol. y trab. de la Soc. de cir. de Buenos Aires *19:*392–403, June 26, '35

Management of tumors of the parotid. STEWART, C. B. Am. J. Surg. *30:*18–20, Oct '35

Branchioma of right parotid in young girl; extracapsular extirpation and closure of resulting defect by Thiersch graft. GOUFAS, G. Ann. d'oto-laryng., pp. 677–685, July '36

Extirpation of benign parotid tumors; use of digastric muscle as guide during operation and in correction of facial paralysis. CADENAT, F. M., J. de chir. *48:*625–629, Nov '36

Extirpation of tumors of parotid gland; technic to avoid injury to facial nerve. DUFOURMENTEL, L. Oto-rhino-laryng. internat. *21:*75–76, Feb '37

Modern trends in therapy of parotid tumors. COGNIAUX, P. AND SIMON, S., J. de chir. et ann. Soc., belge de chir. (no. 4) *36-34:*152–

Parotid Tumors—Cont.

163, May '37

Treatment of tumors of parotid; survey of results obtained at Barnard Free Skin and Cancer Hospital. MARTIN, T. M. Arch. Surg. *36:*136–143, Jan '38

Diagnosis and surgical therapy of parotid tumors. ZAVALETA, D. E. Rev. med. y cien. afines *2:*422–424, June 30, '40

Treatment of mixed tumors of parotid. PATEY, D. H. Brit. J. Surg. *28:*29–38, July '40

Branchiogenous cysts and cystadenolymphomas. BIANCHI, A. E. AND PAVLOVSKY, A. An. Inst. modelo de clin. med. *21:*436–452, '40

Technique de la parotidectomie totale avec conservation du nerf faciale, by J. AUDOUIN AND J. NEVEU. Maloine, Paris, 1941

Treatment of parotid tumors with special reference to total parotidectomy. BAILEY, H. Brit. J. Surg. *28:*337–346, Jan '41

Question of tumor of parotid gland or swelling of preauricular lymph nodes. OESER, H. Monatschr. f. Krebsbekampf. *11:*43, March '43

Parotid tumors; clinical observations and surgical experiences. TRUEBLOOD, D. V. West. J. Surg. *52:*109–118, March '44

Mixed tumors of parotid, with report of cases. CATALANO, F. E. AND SIBILLA, C. E. Rev. Asoc. med. argent. *59:*507–510, May 15, '45

The problem of tumors of the parotid gland. BURCH, J. C. AND FISHER, H. C., S. Clin. North America *26:*489–494, April '46

Early recurrence of mixed tumor of parotid in cicatrix of total parotidectomy; case. SANTY, P. AND DARGENT, M. Mem. Acad. de chir. *72:*225–232, April 10–May 15, '46

Congenital hemangioma of parotid gland. GLASER, K.; *et al.* J. Pediat. *28:*729–732, June '46

PARROTT, A. H.: Fractures of bones of face in war-time; president's address. Proc. Roy. Soc. Med. *32:*53–58, Nov '38

PARSAMOW, O. S.: Revision of vagina formed according to Mori after 3 years. Zentralbl. f. Gynak. *50:*55–551, Feb 27, '26

PARSONS, F.: Speech training for cleft palate patients. Proc. Roy. Soc. Med. *27:*1301–1303, July '34

PARSONS, H. H.: Plaster splint for fractured noses. Mil. Surgeon *91:*212, Aug '42

PARSONS, J. G.: Block anesthesia in nasal surgery. Northwest Med. *24:*223–227, May '25

PARSONS, J. L. (see PACK, G. T.) June '24

PARSONS, L. (see BORNEMEIER, W. C.) Mar '46

PARSONS, W. B. JR.: Thyroglossal fistula with

submental opening (case). Ann. Surg. *97:*143, Jan '33
PARSONS, W. H.: Clinical aspects of acute shock. Mississippi Doctor *21:*70–74, Aug '43
PARTHIOT (see REBATTU) Dec '28
PARTRIDGE, G. T.: Value of skin grafts in traumatic lesions. M. Press. *196:*132–135, Feb 16, '38
PARVULESCO (see NOICA, D.) April '32
PÂRVULESCU, N. (see NOICA, I.) Jan–Feb '32
PASCALIS, G.: Closure of cranial openings by cartilaginous autotransplantation. Gaz. d. hop. *100:*1314–1316, Oct 5, '27
PASCALIS, G.: Creation of artificial vagina by perineal autoplasty in case of congenital aplasia. Rev. de chir., Paris *77:*304–306, April '39
PASCAU, I.: Plastic repair of talipes calcaneovalgus due to cicatricial adhesions following burns; case. Cir. ortop. y traumatol. *3:*185–189, July–Sept '35
PASCHOUD, H.: Cervical cysts and fistulas; 3 cases. Rev. med. de la Suisse Rom. *54:*300–319, March 25, '34
PASQUALINO, G.: Complete thyroglossal fistula; case. Riv. san. siciliana *25:*586–593, May 15, '37

Passaggi-Galliera Operation

Urethroplasty in penoscrotal hypospadias using Passaggi-Galliera technic. TORRE, D. Ann. ital. di chir. *16:*841–854, Oct '37

PASSALACQUA, L. A.: Wartime burns. Bol. Asoc. med. de Puerto Rico *34:*140–146, April '42
PASSALACQUA, L. A.: Surgical therapy of simple and complicated harelip. Bol. Asoc. med. de Puerto Rico *36:*56–61, Feb '44
PASSALACQUA, L. A.: Autoplastic grafts in cicatricial deformities due to burns. Bol. Asoc. med. de Puerto Rico *37:*285–295, Aug '45
PASSALACQUA, L. A.: Cicatrix prevention and treatment; general considerations. Bol. Asoc. med. de Puerto Rico *37:*355–360, Sept '45
PASSE, E. R. G.: Immediate treatment of facial injuries preparatory to plastic repair. J. Roy. Nav. M. Serv. *26:*273–275, July '40
PASSE, E. R. G. AND BARRY, T.: Phagedena (penis); restoration of tissue by pedicle flaps. J. Roy. Nav. M. Serv. *27:*185–189, April '41
PASSEBOIS. (see ETIENNE, *et al*) June '39
PASSOT, R.: Plastic correction of sagging breast. Presse med. *33:*317–318, March 11, '25 abstr: J.A.M.A. *84:*1308, April 25, '25
PASSOT, R.: Two corrective operations; good results. Hopital *16:*246, April (A, bis) '28
PASSOT, RAYMOND: *Chirurgie esthétique pure.* GASTON Doin et Cie, Paris, 1930
PASSOT, R.: Reconstruction of atrophic mammary gland by means of autotransplantation of fat. Presse med. *38:*627–628, May 7, '30
PASSOT, R.: Keloids, esthetic therapy, surgical ablation followed immediately by radium irradiation. Presse med. *41:*544–546, April 5, '33
PASSOT, R.: Technic of corrective surgery of wrinkles of face. Rev. de chir. plastique, pp. 23–33, May '33
PASTEUR. (see JAUSION, *et al*) Nov '26
PASTORE, P. N. AND ERICH, J. B.: Congenital preauricular cysts and fistulas. Arch. Otolaryng. *36:*120–125, July '42
PASTORE, P. N. AND WILLIAMS, H. L.: Congenital occlusion of choanae; brief review of 12 cases. Proc. Staff Meet., Mayo Clin. *14:*625–627, Oct 4, '39
PASTORE, P. N. (see LILLIE, H. I. *et al*) March '40
PATARO, V. F.: Chronic ulcer of leg; perifemoral sympathectomy and skin graft. Prensa med. argent. *31:*2376–2379, Nov 22, '44
PATCAS, H. (see FAUCONNIER, H. J.) Jan '39
PATEL: Extensive burns treated by exposure to air. Lyon chir. *28:*617–618, Sept–Oct '31
PATEL: Results of exposure to air and use of tannic acid in burns. Lyon chir. *36:*474–476, July–Aug '39
PATEL, M. AND PONTHUS, P.: Early treatment of severe, extensive burns, without dressing. Progres med., pp. 497–501, March 22, '30
PATERSON, R. AND TOD, M. C.: Radium treatment of angiomas in children. Am. J. Roentgenol. *42:*726–730, Nov '39
PATEY, D. H.: Treatment of mixed tumors of parotid. Brit. J. Surg. *28:*29–38, July '40
PATEY, D. H.: Treatment of hand infections; necessity for new approach. Practitioner *152:*329–330, May '44
PATEY, D. H. AND RICHES, E. W.: Emergency treatment of smashed-in face; value of tracheotomy and laryngotomy. Lancet *2:*161–162, Aug 7, '43
PATEY, D. H. AND SCARFF, R. W.: Diagnosis of depth of skin destruction in burns and its bearing on treatment. Brit. J. Surg. *32:*32–35, July '44
PATEY, D. H. AND SCARFF, R. W.: Burns with partial skin destruction; illustrative case. Lancet *1:*146, Feb 3, '45
PATHAN, H. A. H.: Transgrafting operation for trichiasis and entropion of upper eyelid. Indian M. Gaz. *77:*204–206, April '42
PATRICK, J.: Branchial plexus block anesthesia (procaine hydrochloride) in operations on upper extremity. Tr. Roy. Med.-Chir. Soc. Glas-

gow, pp. 39–45, '40–'41; in Glasgow M. J. Nov '41

PATRIGNANI, F.: Aqueous solution of tannic acid in burns. Riv. osp. *21:*257–264, Aug '31

PATRIKALAKIS, M. (see TAMMANN, H.) 1927

PATTERSON, D. C.: de Quervain's disease; stenosing tendovaginitis at radial styloid. New England J. Med. *214:*101–103, Jan 16, '36

PATTERSON, N.: New method of treating carcinoma of cheek. Lancet *2:*703, Oct 1, '27

PATTERSON, N.: Treatment of carcinoma of mouth and buccopharynx, nose and nasal sinus, with some remarks on diagnosis. Tr. Am. Laryng., Rhin. and Otol. Soc. *41:*1–34, '35

PATTERSON, N.: Carcinoma of cheek; original method of treatment, with reports on 10 cases. Brit. J. Surg. *25:*330–336, Oct '37

PATTERSON, R.: Carpometarcarpal arthroplasty of thumb. J. Bone and Joint Surg. *15:*240–241, Jan '33

PATTERSON, R.: Treatment of facial fractures. J. Tennessee M. A. *30:*273–279, Aug '37

PATTERSON, R. F.: Treatment of depressed fractures of zygomatic (malar) bone and zygomatic arch. J. Bone and Joint Surg. *17:*1069–1071, Oct '35

PATTON, C. L.: Burn therapy. Illinois M. J. *76:*141–144, Aug '39

PATTON, E. W.: Abnormally attached frenum labium with surgical interference. Internat. Orthodont. Cong. *1:*701, '27

PATTON, H. S. (see STRAITH, C. L.) Nov '43

PAUCHET, V.; ROSENTHAL, P. AND BERTREUX, H.: Fresh embryonal juices in shock after surgical therapy of peptic ulcers; 2 cases. Compt. rend. Acad. d. sc. *197:*1470–1472, Dec 4, '33

PAUFIQUE. (see BONNET, P. *et al*) March '34

PAUL, M.: Cavernous hemangioma of orbit successfully removed by Shugrue operation. Brit. J. Ophth. *30:*35–41, Jan '46

DE PAULA PINTO HARTUNG, F.: Nasal septum operation; successes and failures. Rev. brasil. de oto-rino-laring. *12:*112–121, March–April '44

DE PAULA PINTO HARTUNG, F.: Operation of nasal septum; successes and failures. Rev. paulista de med. *25:*197–207, Sept '44

PAULIAN, D. E.; POPESCU, S. AND MARINESCO-SLATINA, D.: Subungual glomus tumor causing hemihyperthermia; complete cure after surgical removal; case. Ann. d'anat. path. *10:*271–276, March '33

PAULIAN, E. D.: Automatic pseudocorrection in ocular ptosis and strabismus. Encephale *19:*506–508, Sept–Oct '24 abstr: J.A.M.A. *83:*1623, Nov 15, '24

PAUNZ, A.: Formation of an artificial vagina to remedy congenital defect. Zentralbl. f. Gynak. *47:*883–888, June 2, '23. Comment by MORI, M. Zentralbl. f. Gynak. *48:*859, April 19, '24 abstr: J.A.M.A. *83:*77. July 5, '24

PAUTIENIS, K.: Surgical and medical therapy of third degree burns. Medicina, Kaunas *20:*869–874, Oct–Nov '39

PAUTRIER, L. M. AND ROEDERER, J.: Massive angioma of scalp; rapid growth; case. Bull. Soc. franc. de dermat. et syph. (Reunion dermat., Strasbourg) *45:*692–694, May '38

PAVIA, J. L.: Burn of cornea and conjunctiva; how to prevent symblepharon. Rev. oto-neuro-oftal. *19:*159–171, Nov–Dec '44 also: Semana med. *2:*1117–1122, Dec 7, '44

PAVISIC, Z.: Early transplantation of buccal mucosa and conjunctiva in chemical burns of eyes. Ophthalmologica *108:*297–304, Dec '44

PAVLENKO, S. M.: Pantocrine in thermal and chemical burns. Khirurgiya, no. 5, pp. 19–22, '44

PAVLOVSKY, A. (see BIANCHI, A. E.) 1940

PAVLOVSKY, A. J.: Congenital absence of vagina; creation of artificial vagina by autoplastic graft. Bol. y trab. de la Soc. de cir. de Buenos Aires *21:*307–328, June 9, '37 also: Rev. de cir. de Buenos Aires *16:*344–362, July '37

PAVLOVSKY, A. J.: Congenital absence of vagina; creation of artificial vagina by author's autoplastic procedure. Bol. Soc. de cir. de Rosario *6:*453–458, Nov '39

PAVLOVSKY, A. J.: Angioma arteriale racemosum of face and tongue; surgical therapy; case. Bol. y trab., Acad. argent. de cir. *26:*670–672, Aug 19, '42

PAVLOVSKY, A. J. AND HARRIS, M. M.: Free grafts (called intermediate or transchorionic) using Padgett dermatome. Semana med. *2:*709–713, Sept 24, '42

PAVLOVSKY, A. J.; OGHI, A. AND HARRIS, M. M.: Burns and their sequels; therapy with free skin grafts. Rev. Asoc. med. Argent. *60:*78–83, Feb 15–28, '46

PAVLOVSKY, A. J. AND DI PIETRO, A.: Tumor of upper jaw; surgical therapy with plastic repair; 2 cases. Bol. y trab. de la Soc. de cir. de Buenos Aires *19:*384–391, June 26, '35

PAVLOVSKY, A. J. AND SAVAGE, R.: Exstrophy of bladder, case with abnormalities of genitals. Bol. Soc. de obst. y ginec. *8:*64–74, June 5, '29 also: Semana med. *2:*615–620, Aug 29, '29

PAWLONSKY, J. M.: Attempt at nephropexy by means of pedicled cutaneous-subcutaneous flap. (Sokolow method). Zentralbl. f. Chir. *58:*1306–1312, May 23, '31

PAYNE, J. L.: Artificial velum for congenital cleft palate. Proc. Roy. Soc. Med. (Sect. Odontology) *14*:36, Feb '21

PAYNE, J. L.: Fracture of mandible. Clin. J. *58:*77–84, Feb 13, '29

PAYNE, R. L.: Congenital cysts of neck in children. Am. J. Surg. *3:*1–5, July '27

PAYNE, R. L. JR. (see SHAW, D. T.) May '46

PAYNE, R. L., JR. (see SHAW, D. T.) Aug '46

PAYNE, R. L., JR. (see SHAW, D. T.) 1946

PAYR, E.: Plastic restoration of all 4 eyelids, with use of skin from arm in 3 cases. Arch. f. klin. Chir. *152:*532–540, '28

PAYR, E.: Treatment and restoration of totally crippled hands. Arch. f klin. Chir. *200:*527–545, '40

PAZ, J. C.: Prontosil (sulfonamide); indications for use in burns. Dia med. *16:*354–357, April 10, '44

PEABODY, C. W.: Tendon transplantation, end-result study. J. Bone and Joint Surg. *20:*193–205, Jan '38

PEACHER, G. M. (see PEACHER, W. G.) May '46

PEACHER, W. G. AND PEACHER, G. M.: Methods of examination of dysarthria and dyslalia in World War. II. J. Nerv. and Ment. Dis. *103:*484–493, May '46

PEAKE, J.: Ultra-violet light for burns, with special reference to technique used by C. B. Heald. M. D., M. R. C. P. Brit. J. Actinotherapy *4:*96–97, Aug '29

PEARCE, E. C.: Nursing and care of bedridden patient (especially prevention of bed-sores). Practitioner *139:*55–62, July '37

PEARLMAN, A. C.: Plastic surgeon looks at a nose. Kentucky M. J. *34:*467–469, Oct '36

PEARLMAN, L. M.: Surgical relationship between inner and outer nose. M. Rec. *149:*329–332, May 17, '39

PEARLMAN, L. M.: Improved instruments and postoperative splint for nasal plastic operations; combined chisel and periosteal elevator. Arch. Otolaryng. *32:*338–340, Aug '40

PEARLMAN, R. C.: New developments in application of plastic surgery to accident cases involving the face. Kentucky M. J. *36:*30–34, Jan '38

PEARLMAN, R. C.: Plastic surgeon and surgery of today. Rev. med.-cir. do Brasil *46:*689–691, June '38

PEARLMAN, R. C.: Plastic surgery for enlarged and small nose resulting from accidents. M. Rec. *152:*402–404, Dec 4, '40

PEARLMAN, R. C.: Use of tantalum in tendon reconstruction of hand. U. S. Nav. M. Bull *46:*1647–1650, Nov '46

PEARMAN, R. O. AND THOMPSON, F. G. JR.: Modern concepts of burn therapy. J. Missouri M. A. *39:*342–346, Nov '42

PEARSE, H. E.: Burns. J. Missouri M. A. *18:*323, Sept '21

PEARSON, R. S. R.; LEWIS, E. E. AND NIVEN, R. B.: Local treatment of burns (using tulle gras with sulfanilamide powder or envelope irrigation with electrolytic sodium hypochlorite solution). Brit. M. J. *2:*41–45, July 12, '41

PECK, S. M. (see LEWIN, M. L.) Dec '41

PECK, W. S.: Application of physical therapy measures in burns. Arch. Phys. Therapy *12:*327–333, June '31 Abstr. Brit. J. Phys. Med. *6:*175, Nov '31

PECK, W. S. (see POTTER, E. B.) Nov '31

Pectoralis Muscle, Absence of

Syndactylism with absence of the pectoralis major. BROWN, J. B. AND MCDOWELL, F. Surgery, *7:*599, April '40

PEDEMONTE, P. V.: Rhinomegaly and rhinokyphosis; corrective therapy. Arch. urug. de med., cir. y especialid. *16:*601–616, June '40

PEDEMONTE, P. V.: Graft of costal cartilage in therapy of saddle nose; case. Arch. urug. de med., cir. y especialid. *17:*65–67, July '40

PEDEMONTE, P. V.: Protruding ear; psychologic effect, morphologic classification and surgical therapy. Arch. urug. de med., cir. y especialid. *17:*458–472, Oct '40

PEDEMONTE, P. V.: Rhinomegaly and rhinokyphosis; corrective therapy. An. d. ateneo clin. quir. *7:*40–48, Jan '41

PEDEMONTE, P. V.: Protruding ear, psychologic effect, morphologic classification and surgical therapy. An. d. ateneo clin. quir. *7:*73–87, Feb '41

PEDEMONTE, P. V.: Total loss of skin and subcutaneous cellular tissue of heel; monopedicled graft; case. Arch. urug. de med., cir. y especialid. *23:*154–157, Aug '43

PEDEMONTE, P. V.: Total loss of skin and of subcutaneous cellular tissue of heel; monopedicled graft; case. Bol. Soc. cir. d. Uruguay *14:*57–60, '43

PEDEMONTE, P. V.: Tubed pedicle graft in therapy of burn cicatrix; resulting keloids. Bol. Soc. cir. d. Uruguay *14:*106–108, '43 also: Arch. urug. de med., cir. y especialid. *23:*296–298, Sept '43

PEDEMONTE, P. V.: Plastic surgery; advantages and inconveniences of tubular transplants in grave cicatrices of hand. Bol. Soc. cir. d. Uruguay *14:*114–122, '43 also: Arch. urug. de med., cir. y especialid. *23:*453–461, Nov '43

PEDEMONTE, P. V.: Plastic surgery of flexed fingers; semeiologic and therapeutic study.

Bol. Soc. cir. d. Uruguay *14:*318–344, '43
PEDEMONTE, P. V.: Plastic surgery of hand; fingers in flexion contracture; semeiologic and therapeutic study. Arch. urug. de med., cir. y especialid. *24:*249–274, Mar '44
PEDLOW, W. L.: Surgical shock. West. J. Surg. *51:*81–84, Feb '43
PEDOTTI, F.: Therapy of lesions of extensor tendons of fingers. Helvet. med. acta *3:*161–165, May '36
PEDOTTI, F.: Severe burns. Helvet. med. acta *5:*914–915, Dec '38
PEDOTTI, F.: Burn therapy. Arch. ital. di chir. *53:*499–500, '38
PEDRAGOSA, R. (see MERCADAL PEYRI, J.) Feb '45
PEARSON, W. H.: Resection of mandible; method that simplified and overcomes defects of cases reported in the past. Am. J. Orthodontics *29:*141–147, March '43
PEEPLES, D. L.: Keloid removal by electro-coagulation. Am. J. Phys. Therapy *4:*160, July '27
PEER, L. A.: Tube flaps in reconstructive surgery of face. J. M. Soc. New Jersey *28:*86–89, Feb '31
PEER, L. A.: Plastic surgery of nose. Arch. Otolaryng. *14:*462–466, Oct '31
PEER, L. A.: Plastic surgery of nasal deformities. J. M. Soc. New Jersey *30:*123–130, Feb '33
PEER, L. A.: Repair of coloboma of upper eyelid. Arch. Ophth. *11:*1028–1031, June '34
PEER, L. A.: Skin grafts. J. M. Soc. New Jersey *32:*484–487, Aug '35
PEER, L. A.: Presentation of cases requiring plastic repair (grafts). J. M. Soc. New Jersey *34:*15–20, Jan '37
PEER, L. A.: Operation to repair lateral displacement of lower border of septal cartilage. Arch. Otolaryng. *25:*475–477, April '37
PEER, L. A.: Cartilage transplanted beneath skin of chest in man; experimental studies with sections of cartilage preserved in alcohol and buried from 7 days to 14 months. Arch. Otolaryng. *27:*42–58, Jan '38
PEER, L. A.: Buried grafts used to repair depressions in brow, eye socket, skull and nose. J. M. Soc. New Jersey *35:*601–605, Oct '38
PEER, L. A.: Fate of living and dead cartilage transplanted in humans. Surg., Gynec. and Obst. *68:*603–610, March '39
PEER, L. A.: Cysts; fate of buried skin grafts in man. Arch. Surg. *39:*131–144, July '39
PEER, L. A.: Types of buried grafts used to repair deep depressions of cranium. J.A.M.A. *115:*357–360, Aug 3, '40
PEER, L. A.: Fate of autogenous cartilage after transplantation in human tissues. Arch. Otolaryng. *34:*696–709, Oct '41
PEER, L. A.: Management of nasal deformities in infants and small children, and ear, eyelids, lips and palate deform. Dis. Eye, Ear, Nose and Throat *2:*166–176, June '42
PEER, L. A.: Diced cartilage grafts; new method for repair of skull defects. Arch. Otolaryng. *38:*156–165, Aug '43
PEER, L. A.: Plastic surgery for 1942; summaries of bibliographic material available in field of otolaryngology. Arch. Otolaryng. *38:*171–189, Aug '43
PEER, L. A.: Present status of complete reconstruction of external ear. Tr. Am. Soc. Plastic and Reconstructive Surg. *12:*11–16, '43
PEER, L. A.: Cartilage transplantation. S. Clin. North America *24:*404–419, April '44
PEER, L. A.: Contribution to plastic surgery during 1943; summaries of bibiliographic material available in field of otolaryngology. Arch. Otolaryng. *39:*537–555, June '44
PEER, L. A.: Contributions to plastic surgery during 1944; summaries of bibliographic material available in field of otolaryngology. Arch. Otolaryng. *42:*56–79, July '45
PEER, L. A.: Experimental observations on growth of human cartilage grafts. Arch. Otolaryng. *42:*384–396, Nov–Dec '45
PEER, L. A.: Contributions to plastic surgery during 1945; summaries of bibliographic material available in field of otolaryngology. Arch. Otolaryng. *44:*715–758, Dec '46
PEER, L. A. AND PADDOCK, R.: Histologic studies on fate of deeply implanted skin grafts; observations on sections of implants buried from one week to one year. Arch. Surg. *34:*268–290, Feb '37
PEER, L. A. (see STRAATSMA, C. R.) April '32
PEIPER, H.: Snapping finger. Arch. f. klin. Chir. *150:*496–505, '28
PEIRIS, M.V.P.: Use of tea in burn therapy. Indian M. Gaz. *72:*718–720, Dec '37
PELAGATTI, V.: Pathogenesis of death due to burns; role of acidosis. Ateneo parmense *9:*209–227, July–Aug '37
PELKONEN, E.: Results and indications for Kirschner-Wagner operation in connection with 2 cases of vaginal aplasia. Duodecim *53:*1003–1017, '37
PELLER, S.: Malignant melanoma cutis. Cancer Research *1:*538–542, July '41
PELLERAT, J. (see RICARD, A. *et al*) Jan–Feb '45
PELLERIN, R. (see BADEAUX, F.) Oct '41
PELLINI, M.: Infra-red irradiation as therapy in serious burns of children; cases. Pediatria *49:*507–516, Sept '41

PELNER, L. (see RABINOWITZ, H. M.) April '44
PEMBERTON, F. A.: Formation of an artificial vagina. Am. J. Obst. and Gynec. *10:*294–303, Aug '25
PEMBERTON, J. DE J. AND STALKER, L. K.: Thyroglossal cysts, sinuses and fistulae; results in 293 surgical cases. Ann. Surg. *111:*950–957, June '40
PEMBERTON, J. DEJ. (see NEEL, H. B.) Sept '45
PEMBERTON, P. A.: Infection of fascial spaces of palm. Am. J. Surg. *50:*512–515, Dec '40
PEÑA NOVO, P.: Local treatment of cancer of lip. Siglo med. *73:*371–372, April 12, '24
PENALVER, R.: Trauma to jaw and its sequel. Cir. ortop. y traumatol., Habana *11:*73–83, July–Dec '43
PENBERTHY, G. C.: Tannic acid in burns. J. Michigan M. Soc. *34:*1–4, Jan '35
PENBERTHY, G. C.: Burn therapy. New England J. Med. *214:*306–310, Feb 13, '36
PENBERTHY, G. C.: Burn therapy. Indust. Med. *11:*277–280, June '42
PENBERTHY, G. C.: Trends in burn therapy. Surgery *12:*345–348, Sept '42
PENBERTHY, G. C. AND WELLER, C. N.: Complications associated with treatment of burns. Am. J. Surg. *26:*124–132, Oct '34
PENBERTHY, G. C. AND WELLER, C. N.: Burn therapy. Am. J. Surg. *46:*468–476, Dec '39
PENBERTHY, G. C. AND WELLER, C. N.: Burn therapy. Surg., Gynec. and Obst. *74:*428–432, Feb (no. 2A) '42
PENBERTHY, G. C. AND WELLER, C. N.: Treatment of burns (including shock). Am. Acad. Orthop. Surgeons, Lect., pp. 188–198, '43
PENBERTHY, G. C.; WELLER, C. N. AND LEWIS, L. A.: Symposium on industrial surgery; burn therapy. S. Clin. North America *22:*1215–1233, Aug '42
PENBERTHY, G. C.; WELLER, C. N. AND LEWIS, L. A.: Burn therapy. Dia med. *15:*518–522, May 24, '43
PENBERTHY, G. C. (see DAVIDSON, E. C.) 1930
PENDERGRASS, E. P.: Epidermoid carcinoma (epithelioma) of lip; diagnosis, pathology, and discussion of treatment by non-surgical measures. S. Clin. N. Amer. *7:*117–163, Feb '27
PENDLETON, R. C.: Paraffin wax open air treatment of burns. J.A.M.A. *122:*414–417, June 12, '43
PENDLETON, R. C.: Paraffin wax open air treatment of burns. Am. Acad. Orthop. Surgeons, Lect., pp. 198–202, '43
PENDLETON, R. C.: Paraffin wax open air treatment of burns. Semana med. *1:*1344–1346, June 29, '44
PENHALE, K. W.: Acrylic resin as implant for correction of facial deformities. Arch. Surg. *50:*233–239, May '45
PENHALE, K. W. AND ESSER, J. F. S.: Use of biologic flaps and Esser inlay to form chin and lip. J. Am. Dent. A. *29:*1417–1420, Aug 1, '42
PENICK, R. M. JR.: Burn therapy with especial reference to use of gentian violet. Internat. Clin. *1:*31–42, March '33
PENICK, R. M. JR.: Preauricular sinuses; diagnosis and treatment. South. M. J. *38:*103–105, Feb '45
PENIDO BURNIER, E. M.: Procaine hydrochloride block of phrenic nerve in therapy of postoperative complications, with report of case of autoplastic repair of face. Rev. med.-cir. do Brasil *49:*53–68, Feb '41

Penis

Induratio penis plastica and Dupuytren's contracture. MARTENSTEIN, H. Med. Klin. *17:*44, Jan 9, '21
Avulsion of scrotum, left testicle and sheath of penis. COTTLE, G. F., U. S. Nav. M. Bull. *20:*457–460, April '24
Double penis and double vulva. MACLENNAN, A. Glasgow M. J. *101:*287–288, May '24
Keloid of penis. SMITH, E. O., J. Urology *11:*515–524, May '24
Strangulation of finger and penis by long hair. GROSSE. Munchen. med. Wchnschr. *72:*1887–1888, Oct 30, '25
Hypospadias, relation to abnormalities of penis. SIEVERS, R. Deutsche Ztschr. f. Chir. *199:*286–306, '26
Operative treatment of elephantiasis of scrotum and penis. NÄGELSBACH, E. Arch. f. Schiffs-u. Tropen-Hyg. *31:*282–291, June '27
Plastic surgery of penis; case. and scrotum. CORNEJO SARAVIA, E. Rev. de cir. *6:*662–670, Dec '27
Treatment of case of male hypospadias. CECIL, A. B., S. Clin. N. Amer. *8:*1343–1350, Dec '28
Plastic surgery of penis. HOLDEN, W. B., S. Clin. N. Amer. *8:*1409–1410, Dec '28
Epispadias; operation. DANZIGER, F. Ztschr. f. urol. Chir. *25:*21–24, '28
Plastic operation of penis; case. BUZZI, A. AND CORNEJO SARAVIA, E. Bol. y trab. de la Soc. de cir. de Buenos Aires *13:*143, May 22, '29
Genitoplasty; restitution of skin of penis and of scrotum by autograft; restitution of function after trauma. KENNY, T. B. AND MER-

Penis – Cont.
ELLO, M. Prensa med. argent. *15:*1549-1560, May 30, '29
Phalloplasty after traumatic loss of skin of penis. MEYER, H. Arch. f. Orthop. *27:*437-442, July 18, '29
Avulsion of skin of penis and scrotum. COUNSELLER, V. S. AND PALMER, B. M., S. Clin. N. Amer. *9:*993-996, Aug '29
Plastic operation; avulsion of skin of penis; good functional results of graft of scrotum. VADI, E. Bol. Asoc. med. de Puerto Rico *22:*25-26, Sept-Oct '29
Cases of diphallus. BÓKAY, J. Orvosi hetil. *73:*1138-1141, Nov 16, '29 also: Jahrb. f. Kinderh. *127:*127-136, April '30
Reconstruction of urethra and penis following extensive gangrene. MALLARD, R. S. J.A.M.A. *95:*332-335, Aug 2, '30
Surgical treatment of genital elephantiasis in male. DAVIS, D. M. Ann. Surg. *92:*400-404, Sept '30
Plastic surgery of urethra and prepuce in surgical treatment of perineal hypospadias. KURTZAHN, H. Zentralbl. f. Chir. *58:*1945-1948, Aug 1, '31
Ureterosigmoidal transplantation and plastic operations on penis in exstrophy of bladder. WALTERS, W. *et al.* S. Clin. North America *11:*823-828, Aug '31
Double penis and scrotum (diphallus); case. HARRENSTEIN, R. J. Beitr. z. klin. Chir. *154:*308-314, '31
New method for staightening penis in hypospadias. HAGNER, F. R. Tr. South S. A. *44:*245-246, '31 also: J.A.M.A. *99:*116, July 9, '32
Diphallism; case. TSCHMARKE, G. Beitr. z. klin. Chir. *151:*631-637, '31
Phalloplasty; case. RIHMER, B. Budapesti orvosi ujsag *30:*73-75, Jan 21, '32
Plastic repair of penis by autografts. NEUMANN, A. G. Rev. med. del Rosario *22:*292-299, May '32
Traumatic avulsion of skin of penis and scrotum. TÜRSCHMID, W. Polska gaz. lek. *11:*373-374, May 15, '32
Partial biphallism (double penis) associated with exstrophy of bladder and multiple abnormalities of hands and feet; case. BAUZÁ, J. A. Arch. de pediat. d. Uruguay *3:*353-355, Aug '32
Denudation of penis and scrotum; case. DEXELMANN, J. Zentralbl. f. Chir. *59:*2760-2761, Nov 12, '32
Traumatic removal of entire external cutaneous covering of penis with subsequent partial necrosis of urethra; plastic repair;

Penis – Cont.
case. VON RIHMER, B. Ztschr. f. Urol. *26:*369-373, '32
Hypospadias of penis in uniovular twins. VOÛTE, P. A. Nederl. tijdschr. v. geneesk. *77:*2431-2433, May 27, '33
Plastic operation of penis; case. VESEEN, L. L. AND O'NEILL, C. P., J. Urol. *30:*375-377, Sept '33
Operative treatment of complete epispadias. DE QUERVAIN, F. Ztschr. f. urol. Chir. *36:*237-242, '33
Repair of urethra by temporary joining of penis and scrotum (hypospadias). LEVEUF, J. Bull. et mem. Soc. nat. de chir. *61:*30-31, Jan 19, '35
Congenital absence of penis. DRURY, R. B. AND SCHWARZELL, H. H. Arch. Surg. *30:*236-242, Feb '35
Congenital implantation of penis with hypospadias in perineum between scrotum and anus; case. SISTO HONTAN, E. Pediatria espan. *24:*344-347, Sept '35
Complete removal of foreskin by factory machine; plastic replacement; case. TAKASHIMA, R. AND KUSANO, M. Zentralbl. f. Chir. *63:*84-86, Jan 11, '36
Plastic construction of penis capable of accomplishing coitus; case. BOGORAZ, N. Zentralbl. f. Chir. *63:*1271-1276, May 30, '36
Traumatic rupture of penis; case. FETTER, T. R. AND GARTMAN, E. Am. J. Surg. *32:*371-372, May '36
Urethroplasty for congenital strictures; method of temporary graft of penis to scrotum; case. GODARD, H. Rev. de chir., Paris *74:*374-386, May '36
Temporary graft of penis to scrotum in therapy of hypospadias; technic and report of cases. LEVEUF, J. AND GODARD, H., J. de chir. *48:*328-341, Sept '36
Traumatic loss of skin; "skinning" of genitals. KANTOR, A. Chirurg *8:*972-974, Dec 15, '36
Plastic restoration of penis. BOGORAZ, N. A. Sovet. khir., no. 8, pp. 303-309, '36
Plastic induration of penis with retraction of palmar aponeurosis; case. POLICARO, R. D. Gior. med. d. Alto Adige *9:*13-16, Jan '37
Foreskins as skin grafts. ASHLEY, F. Ann. Surg. *106:*252-256, Aug '37
Restoration of entire skin of penis. BROWN, J. B. Surg., Gynec. and Obst. *65:*362-365, Sept '37
Traumatic loss of skin of penis. DUNE, M. V. Vestnik khir. *53:*51, '37
Plastic operations of penis. ILINSKIY, V. P. Khirurgiya, no 1, pp. 142-143, '37

Penis – Cont.

Use of prepuce to epithelialize tract in treatment of imperforate anus. DAVISON, T. C. South. Surgeon *7:*68–70, Feb '38

Plastic restoration of penis; case. BLUM, V., J. Mt. Sinai Hosp. *4:*506–511, March–April '38

Total loss of skin of external male genitals due to unusual industrial trauma; plastic repair; case. PLACITELLI, G. Arch. ital. di urol. *15:*423–428, Aug '38

Phalloplasty; technic of skin grafting in avulsion of skin of penis and scrotum; review of literature and report of case. AGOSTINELLI, E. Policlinico (sez. prat). *46:*1303–1306, July 17, '39

Association of hypospadias with gonococcal infections in male. LAMBERSON, H. H. Rocky Mountain M. J. *37:*668–671, Sept '40

Straightening hypospadiac penis. CREEVY, C. D. Surgery *8:*777–780, Nov '40

Fistula of penile urethra after gunshot wound. TURNER, G. G. Lancet *2:*649, Nov 23, '40

Plastic surgery of urethra and penis in total epispadias. VOZNESENSKIY, V. P. Novy khir. arkhiv *47:*281–283, '40

Surgical treatment of elephantiasis of scrotum and penis. DE SAVITSCH, E., J. Urol. *45:*216–222, Feb '41

Phagedena (penis); restoration of tissue by pedicle flaps. PASSE, E. R. G. AND BARRY, T., J. Roy. Nav. M. Serv. *27:*185–189, April '41

Plastic induration of penis and Dupuytren's disease with negative Frei reaction; case. CONEJO MIR, J. Actas dermo-sif. *32:*834–836, June '41

Congenital ventral curvature of penis and its surgical correction. WEHRBEIN, H. L. Urol. and Cutan. Rev. *45:*359–360, June '41

Elephantiasis of penis. ROSS, J. C. Brit. J. Surg. *29:*194–196, Oct '41

Dupuytren's contracture, relation to plastic induration of penis. VOLAVSEK, W. Ztschr. f. Urol. *35:*173–178, '41

Plastic induration of penis and Dupuytren's contracture; cases. LANA MARTINEZ, F. AND LANA SALARRULLANA, F. Med. espan. *7:*450–456, May '42

Congenital absence of penis. MCCREA, L. E. J. Urol. *47:*818–823, June '42

Reconstruction for traumatic denudation of penis and scrotum; case. OWENS, N. Surgery *12:*88–96, July '42

Cavernous hemangioma of penis; case. GORODNER, J. Rev. argent. de urol. *11:*413–418, Nov–Dec '42

Penis – Cont.

Dislocation (luxation) of penis; case. PERRUELO, N. N. Semana med. *2:*1371–1376, Dec 3, '42

Congenital absence of penis; case. LAL, K. M. Indian M. Gaz. *78:*152, March '43

Foreskin isografts. SACHS, A. E. AND GOLDBERG, S. L. Am. J. Surg. *60:*255–259, May '43

Avulsion of scrotum and skin of penis; technic of delayed and immediate repair (using skin grafts). BYARS, L. T. Surg., Gynec. and Obst. *77:*326–329, Sept '43

Traumatic avulsion of skin of penis and scrotum. JUDD, E. S. JR. AND HAVENS, F. Z. Am. J. Surg. *62:*246–252, Nov '43

Reconstruction following complete avulsion of skin of penis and scrotum; case. SUTTON, L. E. New York State J. Med. *43:*2279–2282, Dec 1, '43

Elephantiasis of penis and scrotum; study apropos of case treated surgically. FOSSATI, A. Bol. Soc. cir. d. Uruguay *14:*355–364, '43

Elephantiasis of penis and scrotum; clinical study of case treated surgically. FOSSATI, A. Arch. urug. de med., cir. y especialid. *24:*285–294, March '44

Traumatic avulsion of entire penis (both corpora cavernosa and urethra). DELPRAT, G. D., J.A.M.A. *125:*274–275, May 27, '44

Traumatic avulsion of skin of penis and scrotum. ROTH, R. B. AND WARREN, K. W., J. Urol. *52:*162–168, Aug '44

New operation for midscrotal hypospadias DAVIS, D. M., J. Urol. *52:*340–345, Oct '44

Reconstruction of male genitals. FRUMKIN, A. P. Am. Rev. Soviet Med. *2:*14–21, Oct '44

Use of preputial skin in "structive" surgery. ESSER, J. F. S., J. Internat. Coll. Surgeons *7:*469–470, Nov–Dec '44

Artificial penis. BRAKE, B. S. West Virginia M. J. *41:*45–47, Feb '45

Fracture of penis; surgical therapy of case. BERTOLA, V. J.; *et al.* Prensa med. argent. *32:*703–707, April 20, '45

Chemical burn of penis. HOOPES, B. F., U. S. Nav. M. Bull. *44:*846–847, April '45

Traumatic avulsion of penis and scrotum. LYONS, B. H. Canad. M. A. J. *52:*610, June '45

Reconstruction of penis after traumatic fracture. O'CONNOR, G. B., U. S. Nav. M. Bull. *45:*147–149, July '45

Medical progress; plastic operations on external genitalia. LOWSLEY, O. S. New York Med. (no. 20) *1:*17, Oct 20, '45

Therapy of shortness of frenum of penis.

Penis – Cont.
Yoel, J. Prensa med. argent. *32:*2539–2540, Dec 21, '45
Fistula of penile urethra; method of repair utilizing stainless steel "pull-out" sutures. Cordonnier, J. J., J. Urol. *55:*278–286, Mar '46
Strangulation of penis; 3 cases. Hermans, A. G. J. Nederl. tijdschr. v. geneesk. *90:*810–816, July 13, '46
Total avulsion of skin of male genital organs; therapy of case. Mazzini, O. F. Bol. y trab., Acad. argent. de cir. *30:*591–594, July 31 '46
Angiomatoid formations in genital organs with tumor formation. Morehead, R. P. Arch. Path. *42:*56–63, July '46
Avulsion of skin of penis and scrotum; reparative genitoplasty. Torres, G. A. and Osacar, E. M. Bol. y trab. Soc, de cir. de Cordoba *7:*225–237, '46

Penn, J.: Harelip treatment (and cleft palate). South African M. J. *12:*425–429, June 25, '38
Penn, J.: Aspects of civilian plastic surgery. South African M. J. *14:*335–338, Sept 14, '40
Penn, J.: Plastic surgery, historical background. Leech *13:*23, June '42
Penn, Jack (editor): *Brenthurst Papers*. Witwatersrand Univ. Press, Johannesburg, 1944
Penn, J. and Rand, W. W.: Modern treatment of jaw fractures. Clin. Proc. *3:*455–460, Dec '44
Pennacchietti, M.: Contracture of hands with arthropathies in postencephalitic parkinsonism; clinical and anatomicopathologic study of cases. Minerva med. *1:*423–431, May 5, '36
Pennisi, A.: Transplants of fat tissue. Policlinico (sez. chir.) *28:*62, Feb '21 abstr: J.A.M.A. *76:*1202, April 23, '21
Pepe, A. L. (see Arenas, N.) Sept '39
Perazzo, G.: Factors of resistance and receptivity in skin transplanted in epitheliomatous regions. Arch. ital. di dermat., sif. *7:*573–584, Dec '31
Percival, R. T.: Surgical treatment for dysfunction of temporomandibular joint. New York State J. Med. *45:*186–189, Jan 15, '45
Pereira, A.: Surgical adaptation of female pseudohermaphrodite to true sex; case. Rev. urol. de S. Paulo *4:*169–177, May–June '37
Pereira, R. F.: Dacryocystorhinostomy; author's experience. Arch. de oftal. de Buenos Aires *15:*603–613, Dec '40
Pereira, R. F.: Hess operation; new bandage substitute (eyelid ptosis). Arch. de oftal. de Buenos Aires *16:*241–242, May '41
Pereira de Queiroz, R.: Luxations of lower jaw; surgical pathology and therapy. Ann. paulist. de med. e cir. *33:*521–527, June '37
Peremans, G.: Volkmann's ischemic contracture. Arch. franco-belges de chir. *27:*1076–1086, Dec '24
Perez Dueño, F.: Modern methods of burn therapy, especially tannic acid. Arch. de med., cir. y espec. *32:*593–597, June 7, '30
Perez Dueño, F.: Modern methods of burn therapy. Cron. med. mex. *29:*511–516, Nov 1, '30
Perez Fernandez, M. (see Dellepiane Rawson, R.) April–June '42
Pérez Moreno, B.: Cleft palate associated with congenital and hypo-alimentary debility and pulmonary tuberculosis; case. Siglo med. *93:*325–328, March 24, '34
Pérez Olivares, C.: Total and partial absence of vagina; 2 cases. Bol. an. clin. ginec. *2:*124–136, '32
Pergola, A.: Congenital eyelid ptosis associated with ocular abnormalities; 3 cases. Rassegna ital. d'ottal. *4:*371–384, May–June '35
Péri, M.: Diathermy in treatment of rhinophyma. Practicien du Nord de l'Afrique *5:*150–151, March 15, '32
Péri, M.: Therapy of humpnose. Oto-rhino-laryng. internat. *16:*174–175, April '32
Péri, M.: Correction of posttraumatic saddle nose by costal graft. Rev. de chir. plastique, pp. 334–338, Jan '34
Péri, M.: Correction of saddle nose with ozena by endonasal inclusions of costal grafts; case. Rev. de chir. structive, pp. 299–302, June '36
Péri, M.: Use of costal cartilage in restorative surgery of saddle nose; 3 cases. Rev. de chir. structive, pp. 103–107, June '37
Péri, M.: Rhinoplasty by frontal flap; case. Rev. de chir. structive *8:*216–217, '38
Périn, L.: Angiomas of skin; therapy. Rev. franc. de dermat. et de venereol. *10:*27–39, Jan '34
Périn, L. and Blaire, G.: Nevocarcinoma of cheek in child 3 years old. Rev. franc. de dermat. et de venereol. *13:*491–499, Dec '37
Perkins, G. (see Page, C. M.) April '22
Perkins, H. W. and Silver, E. I.: Rehabilitation of children with cleft palate, harelip or both. Am. J. Orthodontics *28:*567–575, Sept '42
Perkins, P. A.: Traumatic shock. J. Tennessee M. A. *28:*461–464, Nov '35
Perkoff, D.: Syndactylism in 4 generations. Brit. M. J. *2:*341–342, Aug 25, '28
Perla, D. *et al*: Prevention of shock by cortical hormone (desoxycorticosterone acetate and cortin) and saline. Proc. Soc. Exper. Biol. and Med. *43:*397–404, Feb '40
Perles, L. (see Weissenbach, R. J. *et al*) April '35

PERLOW, S. (see KATZ, L. N. *et al*) May '43
PERMAN, E.: Treatment of acute septic tendovagnitis. Hygiea *93:*197–199, March 15, '31
PERMAN, E.: Aluminum splints for fractures of forearm and hand. Svenska lak.-tidning. *29:*769–784, July 15, '32
PERMAN, E.: Aluminum splints in hand fractures. Acta chir. Scandinav. *72:*331–343, '32
PERMAN, E.: Surgical therapy of cleft palate from social-medical point of view. Svenska lak.-tidning. *35:*2025–2029, Dec 9, '38
PERMAN, E.: Experiences in surgical therapy of cleft palate. Acta chir. Scandinav. *83:*83–89, '39
PERNWORTH, P. H.: Anesthesia for oropharyngeal surgery. Anesth. and Analg. *25:*200–203, Sept–Oct. '46
PERNYÉSZ, S.: Gas phlegmon in connection with accidental hand injury. Gyogyaszat *74:*534–536, Sept 16, '34
PERREAU, E. H.: Lawful character of plastic surgery; medicolegal aspects. Paris med. (annexe) *2:*iv-vii, Sept 18, '37
PERRET, C. A.: Treatment of furuncles on face by "chemical incision" with phenol. Schweiz. med. Wchnschr. *55:*469–470, May 28, '25 abstr: J.A.M.A. *85:*393, Aug 1, '25
PERRET, G. (see DAVIS, L. *et al*) May '45
PERRET, G. (see DAVIS, L. *et al*) 1945
PERRIN, E.: Technic, indications and results of cervicocystopexy (for orthostatic incontinence of urine in women). Lyon chir. *41:*270–278, May–June '46
PERRON, L. (see BADEAUX, F.) Oct '41
PERRONCITO, A.: Regeneration and grafts. Tratt. di anat. patol., no. 5, pp. 3–148, '27
PERRONCITO, A.: Grafting or transplantation of tissues. Tratt. di anat. patol. no. 5, pp. 79–155, '27
PERROT. (see ROUSSY, *et al*) June '27
PERRUELO, N. N.: Grave burns during pregnancy; case. Semana med. *1:*452–456, Feb 20, '41
PERRUELO, N. N.: Dislocation (luxation) of penis; case. Semana med. *2:*1371–1376, Dec 3, '42
PERRY, K. M. A. (see BUTLER, E. C. B. *et al*) Jan '45
PERSCHL, A.: Fractures of ungual phalanx of fingers. Munchen. med. Wchnschr. *84:*810, May 21, '37
PERSCHL, A.: Volar dislocation of semilunar bone as distinguished from perilunar dorsal dislocation of hand; case. Arch. f. orthop. u. Unfall-Chir. *38:*657–661, '38
PERTHES, G.: Visor scalp flap reconstruction of face. Arch. f. klin. Chir. *127:*165–177, '23 (illus.) abstr: J.A.M.A. *81:*2155, Dec 22, '23
PERTHES, G.: Nerve grafting versus musculoplasty in paralysis of facial nerve. Zentralbl. f. Chir. *51:*2073–2076, Sept 20, '24
PERTHES, G.: Fractures and dislocation fractures of condyle of lower jaw and its operative treatment. Arch. f. klin. Chir. *133:*418–433, '24
PERTHES, G.: Rhinoplasty and stomatoplasty. Arch. f. klin. Chir. *142:*572–589, '26

Perthes Operation

Bandage for Perthes operation (tendon transplant). NIKIFOROVA, E. K. Khirurgiya, no. 6, p. 94, '45
Substitute tenoplasties according to Perthes in therapy of radial paralysis. STUMPFEGGER, L. Chirurg *15:*430, July 15, '43

PERUSSIA, F.: Cavernous angiomas of face in children; late results of radium therapy. Strahlentherapie *57:*109–120, '36
PERVÈS, J.: Congenital ankylosis and osseous fusion of phalanges; familial disease. Rev. d'orthop. *19:*628–632, Nov–Dec '32
PERWITZSCHKY, R.: Closure of defects of palate by flaps of mucosa from nasal septum. Arch. f. Ohren-, Nasen-u. Kehlkopfh. *116:*196–203, March '27
PERWITZSCHKY, R.: Use of buttons with wire suture in gunshot wounds of face and jaw. Ztschr. f. Hals-, Nasen-u. Ohrenh. *48:*270; 458, '42
PESME, P. (see ROCHER, H. L.) Oct '30
PESME, P. (see ROCHER, H. L.) Oct '45
PESSANO, J. E. AND GOÑI MORENO, I.: Plastic surgery of traumatic cleft of hard palate in adult; case. Semana med. *1:*1678–1679, May 31, '34
PESTA, H. (see MAYER, F. X.) May '40
PESTI, L.: Therapeutic methods in palatopharyngeal adhesion in connection with 2 successfully treated cases. Monatschr. f. Ohrenh. *69:*330–335, March '35
PETEL, R.: Development and therapy of phlegmons of hand. Progres med., pp. 1873–1881, Nov 5, '32
PETER, K.: Genesis of facial clefts. Kinderarztl. Praxis *4:*335–339, July '33
PETER, K. L.: Fractures of lower jaw in children. Ztschr. f. Stomatol. *35:*1371–1377, Oct 22, '37
PETERS, A.: Covering of recurrent crural ulcers by means of plastic use of skin flap from thigh of other leg. Deutsche med. Wchnschr. *55:*1458–1461, Aug 30, '29
PETERS, R. A. (see CROFT, P. B.) Feb '45
PETERS, R. A. (see ROSSITER, R. J.) Jan '44

Peters Operation

Complete exstrophy of bladder with split pelvis; Peters operation in 1912 with subsequent complication of pregnancy; caesarean section and recovery in 1926. GREEN-ARMYTAGE, V. B., J. Obst. and Gynec. Brit. Emp. *33:*436–438, '26

Late results of Peters operation for exstrophy. FOULDS, G. S. AND ROBINSON, T. A. Brit. J. Urol. *4:*20-26, March '32

Historical data on ureteral transplantation in exstrophy; Peters operation. FOULDS, G. S. Am. J. Surg. *22:*217-219, Nov '33

Case of ureteral transplantation (Peters operation) for exstrophy of bladder surviving 22 years. FISHER, J. H. Brit. J. Urol. *10:*241-244, Sept '38

PETERSEN, N.: Plastic reconstruction of thumb. South African M. J. *17:*137-138, May 8, '43

PETERSEN, N.: Surgical repair of harelip. South African M. J. *19:*132-134, April 28, '45

PETERSEN, O. H.: Skin grafts in military surgery. Zentralbl. f. Chir. *70:*1624, Nov 6, '43

PETERSON, D. K. (see GLENN, W. W. L. *et al*) Nov '42

PETERSON, E. W.: Tumors of neck. Am. J. Surg. *61:*350-359, Sept '43

PETERSON, L. (see BERMAN, J. K. *et al*) April '44

PETERSON, L. W. (see BELLINGER, D. H. *et al*) Jan '43

PETERSON, L. W. (see BROWN, J. B.) July '46

PETERSON, R. G.: Tie-loop wiring of fractured jaws. J. Oral Surg. *1:*246-249, July '43

PETERSON, R. G.: Bilateral osteotomy of mandibular rami for correction of prognathism in edentulous mouth; case. J. Oral Surg. *4:*203-206, July '46

PETERSON, R. G.; FREEMAN, J. T. AND WALDRON, C. W.: Method of facilitating insertion of pins in skeletal fixation of jaw fractures. J. Oral Surg. *3:*258-262, July '45

PETERSON, R. G. (see WALDRON, C. W. *et al*) July '43

PETERSON, R. G. (see WALDRON, C. W. *et al*) Jan '46

PETGES, AND WANGERMEZ: Short wave therapy of alopecia; cases. Bull. et mem. Soc. de radiol. med. de France *24:*477-478, May '36

PETHEÖ, J.: Congenital synosteosis of maxilla and mandible; case. Ztschr. f. Kinderh. *47:*447-448, '29

PETIT, A. M.: Brief panoramic study of nasal surgery. Vida nueva *51:*138-145, April '43

PETIT, P.: Therapy of imperforate anus in newborn infants. Semaine d. hop. de Paris *16:*38-42, Feb '40

PETIT, R.: Plastic repair of vagina by graft of 2 prepuces; case. Rev. franc. de gynec. et d'obst. *26:*605-607, Nov '31

PETIT-DUTALILLIS (see THOMAS, A.) Jan '30

PETIT ODDO: Most recent advances in burn therapy; question of therapy used in present war. Publ. med., Sao Paulo *14:*43-56, March–April '43

PETIT DE LA VILLÉON: Treatment of phlegmons of hand with bacteriophage, minimizing surgery. Bull. et mem. Soc. d. chirurgiens de Paris *23:*430-434, June 19, '31 also: Cron. med. mex. *30:*435-438, Oct '31

PETITPIERRE, M.: Avulsion injuries to extremities in skiing. Helvet. med. acta *6:*968-973, March '40

PETRIDIS, P. A.: Congenital bilateral club hand with absence of thumbs; case. Rev. d'orthop. *14:*419-421, Sept '27

PETRIK, L.: Orthopedic correction of congenital fissures of jaws. Ztschr f. Stomatol. *37:*1235-1252, Sept '39

PETROFF, N. N.: Plastic operation for saddlenose. Zentralbl. f. Chir. *55:*2755-2757, Nov. 3 '28

PETROFF, N. N.: Rhinoplasty. Vestnik khir. (nos. 48-49) *16-17:*37-41, '29

Petroff Operation: See Darcissac-Bruhn-Petroff Operation

PETROV, I. R.: Pathogenesis of functional disturbances in traumatic shock and significance of blood transfusion in therapy. Vestnik khir. *60:*119-126, Sept '40

PETROV, I. R.: Therapy of traumatic shock. Klin. med. (no. 10) *20:*3-9, '42

PETROV, I. R.: Traumatic shock and its therapy, Voen.-med. sborn, *2:*61-97, '45

PETROV, N. Late results of Subbotin's operation for complete epispadias with urinary incontinence; 2 cases. Arch. f. klin. Chir. *149:*762-768, '28

PETROVA, A. A.: Conservative therapy of crushing injuries of fingers. Ortop. i travmatol. (nos. 3-4) *6:*53-58, '32

PETROVITCH, G. AND YOVANOVITCH, I.: Traumatic shock; mechanism, symptomatology and treatment. Voj. san. glasnik *1:*192-206, July–Dec '30

PETROW, N.: Twenty-five year old bone transplant. Arch. f. klin. Chir. *175:*176-180, '33

PETROW, N. N.: Russian method of rhinoplasty. Zentralb. f. Chir. *51:*36-39, Jan 12, '24

PETRY, J. L. (see ECKERT, C. T.) Oct '44

PETTA, G.: Muscle transplantation. Policlinico (sez. chir.) *32:*303-320, June '25

PETTAVEL, C. A.: Burn therapy. Rev. med. de la Suisse Rom. *62:* 769-798, Oct 25, '42

PETTERINO PATRIARCA, A. AND DUC, C.: Dacryocystorhinostomy by nasal route. Rassegna ital. d'ottal. *5:*205–224, March–April 36

PETTERSSON, G.: Temporomandibular ankylosis. Nord. med. (Hygiea) *23:*1521–1523, Aug 18, '44

PETTINARI, V.: Surgical therapy of hypospadias. Arch. ital. di urol. *10:*555–588, Oct '33

PETTIT, J. A.: Mandibular tumors. J.A.M.A. *77:*1881, Dec 10, '21

PETTIT, J. A.: Some consideration of cleft palate surgical technic. Northwest Med. *21:*52–55, Feb '22 (illus.).

PETTIT, J. A.: Underlying principles of plastic surgery. California State J. Med. *20:*398–401, Nov '22 (illus.)

PETTIT, J. A.: Malignancies of oral cavity. Northwest Med. *23:*153–157, April '24

PETTIT, J. A.: Surgical correction of prognathism. J. Am. Dent. A. *24:*1837–1842, Nov '37

PETTIT, J. A. AND WALRATH, C. H.: New surgical procedure for correction of prognathism. J.A.M.A. *99:*1917–1919, Dec 3, '32

PETTIT, J. A. AND WALRATH, C. H.: Prognathism and its surgical correction by new procedure. J. Am. Dent. A. *21:* 125–129, Jan '34

PETTIT, R. T.: Use of small amounts of radium at distance in treatment of cancer of face. Radiology *14:*55–59, Jan '30

PETZAL, E.: Injuries of ear by electricity. Internat. Zentralbl. f. Ohrenh. *34:*65–76, July '31

PEUGNIEZ: Surgical correction of facial deformities. Bull. et mem. Soc. d. chirurgiens de Paris *25:*315–318, May 19, '33

PEYRET, J. A.: Stricturotomy and injections of iodized oil in therapy of dacryocystitis; results in recent cases. Arch. de oftal. de Buenos Aires *11:*429–435, July '36

PEYRI, J.: Skin grafts in extirpation of cancer due to roentgen irradiation. Actas dermo-sif. *32:*736–738, May '41

PEYRUS, J.: Maxillofacial dysmorphism; 5 cases. Rev. de stomatol. *38:*393–409, May '36

PEYRUS, J. J.: War wounds of face and jaws. Rev. serv. de san. mil. *111:*1017–1030, Dec '39

PEYTEL, A.: Medicolegal aspects of plastic surgery. Paris med. (annexe) *1:*viii-x, May 9, '31

PEYTEL, A.: Plastic surgery from medicolegal point of view. Paris med. (annexe) *1:*ix, May 16; vi, May 30; xiv, June 6, '31

PEYTON, W. T.: Dimensions and growth of palate in infant with gross maldevelopment of upper lip and palate; quantitative study. Arch. Surg. *22:*704–737, May '31

PEYTON, W. T.: Dimensions and growth of palate in infants with gross maldevelopment of upper lip and palate; further investigations (including cleft lip and palate). Am. J. Dis. Child. *47:*1265–1268, June '34

PEYTON, W. T.: Hemangioma and its treatment. Minnesota Med. *21:*590–593, Aug '38

PEYTON, W. T. AND RITCHIE, H. P.: Quantitative studies on congenital clefts. Arch. Surg. *33:*1046–1053, Dec '36

PEZCOLLER, A.: Congenital cyst of thymic origin in neck. Clin. chir. *32:*272–284, March '29

PFAB, B.: Medical and surgical treatment of hand injuries. Monatschr. f. Unfallh. *35:*148–160, Mary '28

PFAB, B.: Silver foil in burn therapy. Munchen. med Wchnschr. *77:*857–858, May 16, '30

PFAHLER, G. E.: Cancer of lip treated by radiation or combined with electro-coagulation and surgical procedures. J. Radiol. *3:*213–218, June '22 (illus.)

PFAHLER, G. E.: Cancer of lip treated by electrocoagulation and radiation. Arch. Dermat. and Syph. *6:*428–433, Oct '22 also: Tr. Sect. Dermat. and Syphilol., A.M.A. pp. 213–219, '22

PFAHLER, G. E.: Treatment of skin cancer. New York M. J. *116:*553–555, Nov 15, '22

PFAHLER, G. E.: Electrocoagulation of desiccation in treatment of keratoses and malignant degeneration which follow radiodermatitis. Am. J. Roentgenol. *13:*41–48, Jan '25

PFAHLER, G. E.: Electrocoagulation and radiation therapy in malignant disease of ear, nose and throat. J.A.M.A. *85:*344–347, Aug 1, '25

PFAHLER, G. E. AND VASTINE, J. H.: Results of treatment of cancer of lips by electrocoagulation and irradiation. Pennsylvania M. J. *37:*385–389, Feb '34

PFEFFER, M. (see FUCHS, A.) Oct '24

PFEIFFER, C.: Plastic correction of defects in larynx and trachea. Zentralbl. f. Chir. *48:*965, July 9, '21

PFEIFFER, C. C.; HALLMAN, L. F. AND GERSH, I.: Boric acid ointment in burn therapy; study of possible intoxication. J.A.M.A. *128:*266–274, May 26, '45

PFEIFFER, R. L.: Traumatic enophthalmos. Arch. Ophth. *30:*718–726, Dec '43

PFLAUMER, E.: Successful treatment of exstrophy of bladder. Beitr. z. klin. Chir. *122:*346, '21

PFLUEGER, O. H.: Treatment of neck glands in cancer of lip, tongue and mouth; study of present-day practice (questionnaire report of Cancer Commission of California Medical Association). California and West. Med. *39:*391–397, Dec '33

PFOHL, A. C.: Review of modern burn problem. J. Iowa M. Soc. *26:*100–103, Feb '36

Pharynx

Nasopharyngeal cyst of branchial origin; case. GUISSANI, M. Ann. di laring., otol. *29:*213-226, July '28

Management of malignancies of antrum, superior maxilla, pharynx and larynx at Radium Institute of University of Paris. PACK, G. T. Ann. Otol. Rhin. and Laryng. *37:*967-973, Sept '28

Cleft palate and rhinopharyngeal functions; case. SEGRÈ, R. Arch. ital. di otol. *40:*633-643, Oct '29

Stenosis of nasopharynx. FIGI, F. A. Arch. Otolaryng. *10:*480-490, Nov '29

Plastic operation in pharygostoma following laryngectomy; case. GROS, J. C. Rev. de med. y cir. de la Habana *36:*65-70, Jan 13, '31

New treatment of palotopharyngeal synechiae of traumatic origin. LEMOINE, J. Ann. d'oto-laryng., pp. 404-410, April '32

Two atypical methods for plastic closure of pharynx. WESSELY, E. Monatschr. f. Ohrenh. *66:*423-430, April '32

Surgical contraction of pharynx in therapy of rhinolalia aperta. RÉTHI, A. Monatschr. f. Ohrenh. *66:*842-848, July '32

Lengthening of velum and shortening of pharynx for amelioration of voice after uranoplasty. MEISSNER, A. Rev. de stomatol. *35:*405-411, July '33

Pharyngolaryngeal burns and scalds; prognosis, complications and therapy. AGUERRE, J. A. JR. Arch. de pediat. d. Uruguay *5:*181-190, May '34

Correcting deformities of velum and mesopharynx to insure better speech following cleft palate surgery. BOYNE, H. N. Nebraska M. J. *19:*407-409, Nov '34

Therapeutic methods in palatopharyngeal adhesion in connection with 2 successfully treated cases. PESTI, L. Monatschr. f. Ohrenh. *69:*330-335, March '35

Method of treating atresia of pharynx. BECK, K. Chirurg *8:*957-958, Dec 15, '36

Development of saddle nose and formation of small multiple hemangiomas of mucous membrane of nose and pharynx complicating diffuse scleroderma; case. MENZEL, K. M. Monatschr. f. Ohrenh. *70:*1409-1418, Dec '36

Pharyngeal reconstruction in stenosis; new operative procedure. O'CONNOR, G. B. Ann. Otol., Rhin. and Laryng. *46:*376-386, June '37

Scalds of pharynx in small children. IDEMITSU, K. Oto-rhino-laryng. *10:*1047, Nov '37

Nasopharyngeal atresia; description of operation. GOODYEAR, H. M. Arch. Otolaryng. *29:*974-976, June '39

Death due to shock after scalding of pharynx and larynx. TANAKA, H. Oto-rhino-laryng. (Abstr. Sect.) *13:*45-46, Oct '40

Oral and pharyngeal injuries from pointed objects. KLIMPEL, W. Ztschr. f. Hals-, Nasen-u. Ohrenh. *45:*328-338, '40

New plastic method for correction of velopharyngeal symphysis stricture. MAGGIOROTTI, U. Boll. d. mal. d. oreccio, d. gola, d. naso *60:*194-196, May '42

Nasopharyngeal stenosis and its correction. KAZANJIAN, V. H. AND HOLMES, E. M. Arch. Otolaryng. *44:*261-273, Sept '46

Total laryngectomy with right hemipharyngectomy; plastic surgery to reconstruct pharynx using laryngeal flap from left vestibular zone. LEYRO DIAZ J. Bol. y trab., Acad. argent. de cir. *30:*815-833, Sept 11, '46

Pharynx, Cancer

Treatment of malignant tumors of pharynx and nasopharynx. NEW, G. B. Surg., Gynec. and Obst. *40:*177-182, Feb '25

Statistics on 1,323 operations on mouth, pharynx and esophagus for cancer. SIMEONI, V. Valsalva *5:*86-89, Feb '29

Five year end-results of radiation treatment of cancer of oral cavity, nasopharynx and pharynx, based on study of 309 cases, 1912-1923. SCHREINER, B. F. AND SIMPSON, B. T. Radiol. Rev. and Chicago M. Rec. *51:*327-332, Aug '29

Repair of defects after operation on pharynx for removal of malignant tumours. COLLEDGE, L. Proc. Roy. Soc. Med. (Sect. Laryng.) *24:*14-17, Feb '31 also: J. Laryng. and Otol. *46:*409-413, June '31

Highly malignant tumors of pharynx and nasopharynx. NEW, G. B. Tr. Am. Acad. Ophth. *36:*39-44, '31

Highly malignant tumors of pharynx and base of tongue; identification and treatment. NEW, G. B. *et al.* Surg., Gynec. and Obst. *54:*164-174, Feb '32

Five year cures of cancer of larynx and mouth and pharynx. NEW, G. B. AND FIGI, F. A. Surg., Gynec. and Obst. *60:*483-484, Feb (no. 2A) '35

Treatment of carcinoma of mouth and buccopharynx, nose and nasal sinus, with some remarks on diagnosis. PATTERSON, N. Tr. Am. Laryng., Rhin. and Otol. Soc. *41:*1-34, '35

Selection of treatment of cancer of pharynx.

Pharynx, Cancer – Cont.

FIGI, F. A. Radiol. Rev. and Mississippi Valley M. J. *58:*13-19, Jan '36

Diagnosis and therapy of malignant tumors of nasopharynx. GERLINGS, P. G. AND DEN HOED, D. Nederl. tijdschr. v. geneesk. *81:*581-589, Feb 6, '37

Cancer of pharynx, treatment and its results. COLLEDGE, L. Brit. M. J. *2:*167-168, July 23, '38

Surgical therapy of laryngopharyngeal cancer. AUBRY, M. Ann. d'oto-laryng., pp. 905-908, Nov-Dec '39

Malignant disease of face, buccal cavity, pharynx and larynx in first three decades of life. HERTZ, C. S. Proc. Staff Meet., Mayo Clin. *15:*152-156, March 6, '40

Malignant tumors of nasopharynx; anatomicopathologic study. VILLATA, I. Oto-rino-laring. ital. *10:*106-151, March '40

Results of treatment of malignant tumors of larynx and hypopharynx. WOODWARD, F. D. AND ARCHER, V. W. Virginia M. Monthly *67:*751-755, Dec '40

Malignant tumors of rhinopharynx with metastases; 15 cases. SCUDERI, R. Arch. ital. di otol. *54:*273-316, Aug '42

Surgical therapy of cancer of hypopharynx. ALONSO, J. M. An. Fac. de med. de Montevideo *28:*812-818, '43

Total pharyngoplasty in cancer. MARINO, H. Prensa med. argent. *31:*1509-1516, Aug 9, '44

Pharynx, Tumors

Treatment of fibromas of nasopharynx; report of 32 cases. NEW, G. B. AND FIGI, F. A. Am. J. Roentgenol. *12:*340-343, Oct '24

Tumors of nasopharynx; review of literature. NEW, G. B. AND KIRCH, W. Arch. Otolaryng. *8:*600-607, Nov '28

Tumors of tonsil and pharynx; 357 cases. NEW, G. B. Tr. Am. Laryng. A. *53:* 277-309, '31

Therapy of nasopharyngeal tumors. PORDES, J. M. Acta oto-laryng. orient. *1:*45-49, '45

PHEMISTER, D. B.: Repair of fractures by bone transplantation. Proc. Interst. Postgrad. M. A. North America (1942) pp. 105-108, '43

PHEMISTER, D. B.: Mechanism and management of shock. J.A.M.A. *127:*1109-1112, April 28, '45

PHEMISTER, D. B. (see KREDEL, F. E.) Sept '39

PHILIP, U. (see MATHER, K.) Dec '40

PHILIPPIDES, D.: Present status of surgical therapy of cleft palate. Ergebn. d. Chir. u. Orthop. *30:*316-371, '37

PHILIPS, W. P.: Facial lacerations. Dallas M. J. *24:*41-43, March '38

PHILLIPS, G.: Treatment of clonic facial spasm by nerve anastomosis. M. J. Australia *1:*624-626, April 2, '38

PHILLIPS, J. R.: Funnel chest; case successfully treated by chondrosternal resection. Dis. of Chest *10:*422-426, Sept-Oct '44

PHILLIPS, J. R. (see: JUDD, E. S.) Oct '33

PHILLIPS, M. H.: Obstetric shock. Brit. M. J. *1:*833-837, May 16, '31

PHILLIPS, R. B. (see DEAVER, J. M. *et al*) May '44

PHILLIPS, W. H.: Anatomic considerations in local anesthesia of jaws. J. Oral Surg. *1:*112-121, April '43

Photography

Functional restoration in repair of facial injuries; value of color photography in this work. SHEEHAN, J. E., J. M. Soc. New Jersey *24:*618-621, Nov '27

Photographic records in plastic surgery, with special reference to textual aspects of facial portrayal. BUTLER, E., M. Press *209:*109-112, Feb 17, '43

Physical Therapy

Exercise after burns. SCHWARTZ, A. Paris med. *2:*175-176, Aug. 30, '24

Physical therapy as aid to surgical procedures on nose. MCCOY, J. Laryngoscope *37:*756-759, Oct '27

Surgical and physical therapy of contractures. SAXL, A. Wien. klin. Wchnschr. *42:*1266-1267, Sept. 26, '29

Application of physical therapy measures in burns. PECK, W. S. Arch. Phys. Therapy *12:*327-333, June '31 Abstr. Brit. J. Phys. Med. *6:*175, Nov '31

Physiotherapy of keloids. BELOT, J. Bull. Soc. franc. de dermat. et syph. (Reunion dermat., Strasbourg) *38:*965-976, July '31

Treatment of extensive granulating areas, with special reference to use of physical therapy measures in burns. and skin grafts. POTTER, E. B. AND PECK, W. S. Am. J. Surg. *14:*472-476, Nov '31

New light on cause and possibility of physiotherapy (Dupuytren's contracture). POWERS, H. Am. J. Phys. Therapy *8:*239-241, Dec '31

Table for gymnastic after-treatment of hand injuries. KOTILAINEN, T. Duodecim *56:* 333-335, '40

Massage in burn therapy. LEROY, R. Presse med. *49:*535-536, May 14-17, '41

Massage, movements and exercises in treatment of suture and repair of nerves. MEN-

Physical Therapy—Cont.
NELL, J. Brit. J. Phys. Med. *5:*40–47, March '42
Physical therapy following suture of nerves. DUBE, P., M. Clin. North America *27:*1091-1096, July '43
Peripheral nerve injuries; physical therapy. KOVACS, R. New York State J. Med. *43:*1403-1408, Aug. 1, '43
Physical medicine in maxillofacial injuries. WEISENGREEN, H. H. Mil. Surgeon *93:*294–298, Sept '43
Physical therapy in plastic surgery unit. WILSON, H. C. Physiotherapy Rev. *25:*3–21, Jan–Feb, '45

PIATT, A. D. (see POSNER, I.) July '40
PIAZZA DE ROSENFELD, A.: Rational surgical conduct in osteomyelitis of lower jaw; cases. Semana med. *1:*248–249, Feb 3, '38
PIAZZA DE ROSENFELD, A. (see JORGE, J. M.) April '38
PIAZZA DE ROSENFELD, A. (see JORGE, J. M.) June '39
PICARD, H.: Technic of plastic surgery of breasts. Med. Welt *5:*741–743, May 23, '31
PICARD, J.: Dupuytren's contraction. Vie med. *8:*225–228, Feb. 4, '27
PICARD, J. (see MICHAUX, J. *et al*) May '25
PICCARDI, G.: Multiple malignant skin epitheliomas in the young. Gior. ital. d. mal. ven. *65:*338–343, April '24
PICARD, MAX: *The Human Face* (translated from the German by G. Endore). Cassell and Co., London, 1931
PICENA, J. P. (see SYLVESTRE BEGNIS, C.) May '46
PICHLER, H.: Reconstruction to insure function after plastic operation on lower lip. Zentralbl. f. Chir. *49:*1363–1365, Sept 16, '22 (illus.)
PICHLER, H.: Reconstruction of mandible after resection. Wien. klin. Wchnschr. *36:*465–466, June 28, '23
PICHLER, H.: Operation for double cleft palate and harelip. Deutsche Ztschr. f. Chir. *195:*104–107, '26
PICHLER, H.: Surgical correction of prognathism of lower jaw. Wien. klin. Wchnschr. *41:*1333–1334, Sept 20, '28
PICHLER, H.: Congenital tendency of nasal septum and intermaxillary bone to abnormal longitudinal growth. Ztschr. f. Stomatol. *27:*21–26, Jan '29
PICHLER, H.: Resection, plastic surgery and prosthesis of jaw. Fortschr. d. Zahnheilk. *5:*1027–1043, Nov '29
PICHLER, H.: Operations on congenital harelip and cleft of both hard and soft palates. Wien. klin. Wchnschr. *47:*70–72, Jan 19, '34
PICHLER, H.: Therapy of bullet wounds of jaw at Vienna Surgical Clinic. Wien. klin. Wchnschr. *53:*22–24, Jan 5, '40
PICHLER, H. (see EISELSBERG, A.) 1922
PICHLER, K.: Typical cicatricial bridges between fingers of dairymaids. Wien. klin. Wchnschr. *36:*850–851, Nov 29, '23 (illus.)
PICHON, E. AND WIRZ, S.: Multiple congenital malformations including hand with 5 fingers and no thumb. Bull. Soc. de pediat. de Paris *34:*310–311, June '36
PICK, F. AND BARTON, D.: Viacutan (silver dianphthylmethane disulfonate) in burn therapy. (hand) Lancet *2:*408–410, Oct 2, '43
PICK, J. F.: Present status of plastic surgery. Illinois M. J. *72:*177–182, Aug '37
PICK, J. F.: Dermoplasty of healed burned dorsum of hand. J. Internat. Coll. Surgeons *8:*217–223, May–June '45
PICK, J. F.: Dermoplasty of war wounds of lower leg. Am. J. Surg. *69:*25–38, July '45
PICK, J. F.: Critique of free graft. South. M. J. *38:*827–831, Dec '45
PICKELL, F. W.: Burns (fundamentals of tannic acid therapy). J.M.A. Alabama *8:*203–208, Dec '38
PICKEN, L. E. R. (see HARRISON, G. A.) May '41
PICKERILL, C. M.: Harelip and cleft palate; 70 consecutive cases. New Zealand M. J. *41:*121–129, June '42
PICKERILL, C. M. (see PICKERILL, H. P.) Feb '45
PICKERILL, C. M. (see PICKERILL, H. P.) Oct '45
PICKERILL, H. P.: *Facial Surgery*. Wm. Wood and Co., New York, 1924
PICKERILL, H. P.: Excision and restoration of upper lip. Brit. J. Surg. *14:*536–538, Jan '27
PICKERILL, H. P.: Restoration of buccal sulcus by intraoral skin grafting. M. J. and Rec. *126:*671–674, Dec 7, '27
PICKERILL, H. P.: Facial hemiatrophy. Australian and New Zealand J. Surg. *4:*404–406, April '35
PICKERILL, H. P.: Optimum time for operation in plastic surgery. New Zealand M. J. *34:*154–159, June '35
PICKERILL, H. P.: *Speech Training for Cleft Palate Patients*. Whitcombe and Tombs, Ltd., London, 1937
PICKERILL, H. P.: Eyelid ptosis. New Zealand M. J. *36:*308–309, Oct '37
PICKERILL, H. P.: Notes on 3 cases of hypertelorism. Brit. J. Surg. *26:*588–592, Jan '39
PICKERILL, H. P.: Plastic reconstruction of scars

after burns, with report of 6 cases. New Zealand M. J. *39:*327–329, Dec '40
PICKERILL, H. P.: Cartilage graft restoration of jaw ankylosis; new operation. Australian and New Zealand J. Surg. *11:*197–206, Jan '42
PICKERILL, H. P.: Reorientation in burn therapy. New Zealand M. J. *41:*70–78, April '42
PICKERILL, H. P.: Skin graft restoration after excision for malignant disease. Australian and New Zealand J. Surg. *13:*147–154, Jan '44
PICKERILL, H. P.: Construction of artificial vagina. New Zealand M. J. *44:*37–40, Feb '45
PICKERILL, H. P.: New method and appliance for grafting eye sockets. Brit. M. J. *1:*596, April 28, '45
PICKERILL, H. P.: Advantages of early skin grafting. New Zealand M. J. *45:*45–49, Feb '46
PICKERILL, H. P. AND PICKERILL, C. M.: Elimination of cross-infection; experimental (special hospital for infants undergoing plastic surgery). Brit. M. J. *1:*159–160, Feb 3, '45
PICKERILL, H. P. AND PICKERILL, C. M.: Early treatment of Bell's palsy. Brit. M. J. *2:*457–459, Oct. 6, '45
PICKERILL, H. P. AND WHITE, J. R.: Plastic surgery, tube skin-flap in plastic surgery of face. Brit. J. Surg. *9:*321–333, Jan '22 (illus.)
PICKERILL, P.: Reconstruction of smaller defects and lesions of face. M. J. Australia *2:*605–610, Oct 29, '27
PICKERILL, P.: Hypospadias; case. M. J. Australia *1:*527–528, April 28, '28
PICKERILL, P.: Facial paralysis, palatal repair and some other plastic operations. M. J. Australia *1:*543–548, May 5, '28
PICKERILL, P.: Plastic restorations after specific lesions of face. M. J. Australia *1:*414–417, March 29, '30
PICKRELL, K. L.: New burn treatment (spraying solution of sulfadiazine, sulfanilamide derivative); preliminary report. Bull. Johns Hopkins Hosp. *69:*217–221, Aug '41
PICKRELL, K. L. AND CLAY, R. C.: Giant nevus of thigh successfully treated by complete excision and primary grafting. Arch. Surg. *48:*319–324, April '44
PICKRELL, K. L.; METZGER, J.; AND HOLLOWAY, J. B. JR.: Plastic surgery of hypertrophy of breast. S. Clin. North America *26:*1095–1107, Oct '46
PIEDELIEVRE, R. (see OLIVIER, E. *et al*) Oct '37
PIERANTONI, L.: Author's method of plastic reconstruction of palate after removal of huge osteoma of upper jaw. Plast. chir. *1:*109–112, '40
PIERCE, G. S. (see BERMAN, J. K. *et al*) Nov '46
PIERCE, G. W.: Problems in plastic surgery. California State J. Med. *19:*231, June '21
PIERCE, G. W.: Surgical treatment of burn scars. S. Clin. N. America *3:*841–855, June '23 (illus.)
PIERCE, G. W.: Plastic surgery of nose. Surg., Gynec. and Obst. *40:*469–475, April '25
PIERCE, G. W.: Reconstruction of thumb after total loss. Surg., Gynec. and Obst. *45:*825–826, Dec '27
PIERCE, G. W.: Reconstruction of external ear. Surg., Gynec. and Obst. *50:*601–605, March '30
PIERCE, G. W.: Advantages of Padgett dermatome. California and West. Med. *57:*16–18, July '42
PIERCE, G. W.: Useful plastic procedures of eyes. Tr. Am. Acad. Ophth. (1943) *48:*309–322, May–June '44
PIERCE, G. W.; KLABUNDE, E. H. AND EMERSON, D.: Repair of burned hand. Surgery *15:*153–172, Jan '44
PIERCE, G. W. AND O'CONNOR, G. B.: Tubed pedicle flap in reconstructive surgery; cases. California and West. Med. *35:*94–97, Aug '31
PIERCE, G. W. AND O'CONNOR, G. B.: New method of reconstruction of lips. Arch. Surg. *28:*317–334, Feb '34
PIERCE, G. W. AND O'CONNOR, G. B.: Pedicle flap patterns for reconstruction of hand. Rev. de chir. structive, pp. 85–90, June '37 also: Surg., Gynec. and Obst. *65:*523–527, Oct '37
PIERCE, G. W. AND O'CONNOR, G. B.: Reconstructive surgery of nose. Ann. Otol., Rhin. and Laryng. *47:*437–452, June '38
PIERCE, G. W. (see O'CONNOR, G. B.) March '34
PIERCE, G. W. (see O'CONNOR, G. B.) Oct '34
PIERCE, G. W. (see O'CONNOR, G. B.) Dec '38
PIERCE, G. W. (see EBERBACH, C. W.) Oct '28
PIERCE, W. F.: Sulfhydryl solution (hydrosulphosol) in burns; preliminary report. Am. J. Surg. *53:*434–439, Sept '41
PIERI, G.: Plastic reconstruction of thumb. Chir. d. org. di movimento *11:*89–93, Sept '26
PIERI, G.: Skin grafts on extremities. Arch. ital. di chir. *18:*607–621, '27
PIERI, G.: Fracture of upper jaw; case. Valsalva *7:*670–673, Sept '31
PIERI, G.: Surgical therapy of congenital abnormalities of external ear. Valsalva *9:*842–846, Nov '33
PIERI, G.: Surgical therapy of penoscrotal hypospadias. Urologia *1:*140–143, Sept 1, '34
PIERI, P. F.: New instrument for correction of hump nose. Boll. d. mal. d. orecchio, d. gola, d. naso *54:*180–187, May '36
PIERINI, L. E. (see MONTANARO, J. C.) March '38

PIERITZ, G.: Therapy of wounds of maxillofacial region; later experiences with war wounded who were first treated at field hospitals. Deut. Militararzt *8:*693, Dec '43

Pierre Robin Syndrome (See also Cleft Palate; Micrognathia)

Glossoptosis in micrognathia; 2 cases. ULLRICH, G. Deutsche med. Wchnschr. *61:*1033–1036, June 28, '35

Hypoplasia of mandible (micrognathy) with cleft palate; treatment in early infancy by skeletal traction. CALLISTER, A. C. Am. J. Dis. Child. *53:*1057-1059, April '37

PIETRANTONI, L.: Harelip with cleft palate; 2 cases. Sperimentale Arch. di biol. *80:*651–664, Jan 25, '27

PIETRANTONI, L.: Plastic surgery of hard palate after excision of huge osteoma of upper jaw; author's technic. Valsalva *15:*205–211, May '39

DI PIETRO, A. (see PAVLOVSKY, A. J.) June '35

PIFFAULT, C. (see PONTHUS, P. *et al*) April '42

PIGNATELLI, G.: Modern therapy of burns; review of literature Progr. med. Napoli *2:*307–310, May 15 '46

PIGNATTI, A.: Kondoleon operation for elephantiasis of leg. Chir. d. org. di movimento *6:*49–62, Feb '22 (illus.) abstr: J.A.M.A. *78:*1579, May 20, '22

PIGNOT, M.: Eyebrow alopecias and their therapy. Presse med. *46:*843–844, May 25, '38

PIKIN, K. I.: Therapy of fresh wounds by transplantation of chemically treated tissues (skin and fetal membranes). Sovet. med. (no. 9) *6:*15–16, '42

PILLING, M. A. (see HIRSHFELD, J. W. *et al*) May '43

PILLING, M. A. (see HIRSHFELD, J. W. *et al*) Oct '43

PILLMAN, N.: Technique of transplanting mucous membrane in intercostal region. Vrach. Gaz. *31:*370–372, March 15, '27

PILON, A.: Dupuytren's contracture, two cases. J. de l'Hotel-Dieu de Montreal *5:*75–81, '36

PINCOCK, D. F.: Horizontal pin fixation for fractures of mandible using pin guide. Surg., Gynec. and Obst. *77:*493–496, Nov '43

PINCOCK, D. F.: Horizontal pin fixation for fractures of mandible using pin guide. Am. J. Orthodontics (Oral Surg. Sect.) *30:*67–72, Feb '44

PINEDA, E. V. (see YAP, S. E.) Jan '22

PINEDA, J. C.: Necessity for transplantation of living bone and cartilage; cases. Rev. de med. y cir. de la Habana *33:*862, Dec. 31, '28

PINEIRO SORONDO, J. AND FERRE, R. L.: Dupuytren's contracture; with special reference to therapy. Dia med. *16:*487–490, May 15, '44

PINHEIRO, J. AND BARRETO NETO, M.: Giant nevus with malignant degeneration; case. Arq. Serv. nac. doen. ment., pte. 1, pp. 173–205, '43

PINHEIRO CAMPOS, O.: Skin grafting for spina bifida with meningocele or myelomeningocele. J. Internat. Coll. Surgeons *3:*438–440, Oct '40

PINHEIRO GUIMARAES, U.: Shock in war surgery. Rev. med.-cir. do Brasil *50:*1043–1078, Dec '42

PINHEIRO GUIMARAES, U.: Shock in war traumatology. Imprensa med., Rio de Janeiro *19:*73–92, Aug '43

PINI, R. AND ZERBINI, C.: Urethropubic fistula; surgical therapy of case. Semana med. *2:*639–641, Aug 31, '33

PINSONNEAULT, G.: Obstetric shock, case. Union med. du Canada *59:*477–482, Aug '30

PINTO DE SOUZA, O.: Habitual temporomaxillary luxation. Arq. de cir. clin. e exper. *2:*351–366, Oct '38

PINTO DE SOUZA, O.: Wounds with loss of distal phalangeal substance of fingers. Rev. Assoc. paulista de med. *14:*219–226, April '39

PIQUE, J. A. (see SAMMARTINO, E. S.) March '40

PIQUET, J.: Sulfonamides in prophylaxis of postoperative meningitis in nasal surgery. Monatschr. f. Ohrenh. *76:*68–75, Feb '42

PIQUET, J. AND BECUWE: Angiomatous tumor of nasal fossae; ligature of external carotid and Rouge-Denker operation; case. Ann. d'oto-laryng., pp. 393–397, May '37

PIQUET, J. AND DETROY, L.: Paradental cyst of upper maxillary sinus with fistulization into lower eyelid; case (palpebral fistula). Echo med. du Nord *9:*337–339, June 30, '38

PIRES: Cosmetic surgery of wrinkles (face). Fortschr. d. Med. *52:*576, June 25, '34 also: Marseille-med. *1:*635–638, May 15, '34 also: Rev. de med. y cir. de la Habana *39:*409–412, June 30, '34 also: Strasbourg med. *94:*393–394, July 5, '34 also: Rev. med. de l'est *62:*554–557, Aug 15, '34

PIRES: Cosmetic surgery of facial wrinkles. Rev. med. peruana *6:*1997-2000, Sept '34

PIRES DE LIMA, J. A.: Congenital atrophy of fingers; 19 cases. Arq. de anat. *10:*401–429, '27

PIRES DE LIMA, J. A.: Anomalies of outer ear. Ann. d'anat. path. *7:*377–378, March '30

PIRES, DE LIMA, J. A.: Hypospadias as cause of error in determining sex. J. de sif. e urol. *10:*35–39, Feb '39

PIRES DE LIMA, J. A.: Pigmented nevi. Coimbra

med. *9:*5-14, April '42 also: Arq. trab. Fac. med. do Porto Jan-April '42
PITKIN, H. C. (see WATKINS, J. T.) Feb '30
PITTS, A. T.: Treatment of fractures of jaws. Lancet *2:*1336-1337, Dec 25, '26
PITTS, H. C.: Reconstruction of vagina from portion of sigmoid; case. Tr. New England S. Soc. *18:*273-275, '35
PITTS, H. C.: Reconstruction of vagina from portion of sigmoid; case. New England J. Med. *213:*1136-1137, Dec 5, '35
PITZEN, P.: Plastic operations on great toe and thumb. Ztschr. f. Orthop. *70:*93-98, '39
PIULACHS, P.: Procaine hydrochloride anesthesia of carotid sinus in treatment of shock; experimental study. Med. clin., Barcelona *3:*223-236, Sept '44
PIULACHS, P. AND ARANDES, R.: Post-traumatic hematoma of tendon sheaths. Rev. clin. espan. *8:*435-436, March 30, '43
PIULACHS, P. AND PLANAS-GUASCH, J.: Recidivation of vulvar cancer in arm, due to graft to prevent local recurrence; case. Med. clin., Barcelona *6:*334-336, May '46
PIZARRO CRESPO, E. (see ZENO, L.) March '40
PIZZAGALLI, L.: Technic of uranostaphylorrhaphy. Boll. d. spec. med.-chir. *1:*7-16, Jan-March '27
PIZZAGALLI, L.: Exstrophy of bladder; case. Boll. d. spec. med.-chir. *4:*321-328, '30
PIZZAGALLI, L.: Surgical therapy of congenital cleft palate. Boll. d. spec. med.-chir. *5:*129-266, '31
PLACINTEANU, G. AND DOBRESCU, D.: Excision of superior cervical ganglion in therapy of peripheral paralysis (facial). Zentralbl. f. Chir. *69:*323, Feb. 21, '42
PLACINTIANU, G.: Lymphangioma of neck. Spitalul *51:*51-52, Feb '31
PLACITELLI, G.: Total loss of skin of external male genitals due to unusual industrial trauma; plastic repair; case. Arch. ital. di urol. *15:*423-428, Aug '38
PLANAS-GUASCH, J. (see PIULACHS, P.) May '46
PLANK, T. H.: Electrocoagulation and desiccation of surface malignancies. Physical Therap. *44:*363-367, July '26

Plastic Surgery

Reconstruction surgery and its application to civilian practice. STARR, C. L. Surg., Gynec. and Obst. *32:*311, April '21
Plastic procedures for obliteration of cavities with non-collapsible walls. KANAVEL, A. B. Surg., Gynec. and Obst. *32:*453, May '21
Reconstructive surgery. MOCK, H. E. Minnesota Med. *4:*343, June '21

Plastic Surgery—Cont.

Problems in plastic surgery. PIERCE, G. W. California State J. Med. *19:*231, June '21
Plastic surgery, tube skin-flap in plastic surgery of face. PICKERILL, H. P. AND WHITE, J. R. Brit. J. Surg. *9:*321-333, Jan '22 (illus.)
Plastic operations. ELOESSER, L. Surg., Gynec. and Obst. *34:*532-537, April '22 (illus.)
Constructive surgery. ESSER, J. F. S. Munchen. med. Wchnschr. *69:*502-503, April 7, '22 (illus.)
Constructive surgery. ESSER, J. F. S. Med. Klinik *18:*793-796, June 18, '22 abstr: J.A.M.A. *79:*2043, Dec 9, '22
Foundation in plastic surgery. ESSER, J. F. S. Munchen. med. Wchnschr. *69:*966-967, June 30, '22
Incisions in plastic surgery. ESSER, J. F. S. Munchen. med. Wchnschr. *69:*818-819, June 2, '22
Source of material for plastic operations. ESSER, J. F. S. Munchen. med. Wchnschr. *69:*888, June 16, '22
Use of tissues for various plastic purposes. ESSER, J. F. S. Munchen. med. Wchnschr. *69:*1186-1187, Aug 11, '22
Underlying principles of plastic surgery. PETTIT, J. A. California State J. Med. *20:*398-401, Nov '22 (illus.)
Possibilities in reconstruction of human form. THOREK, M. New York M. J. *116:*572-575, Nov 15, '22 (illus.)
Some points in reconstructive surgery. GIRDLESTONE, G. R. Practitioner *109:*456-459, Dec '22
Notes on plastic surgery. JOHNSON, L. W., U. S. Nav. M. Bull. *18:*214-219, Feb '23 (illus.)
General plastic surgery. DAVIS, J. S. Ann. Surg. *77:*257-262, March '23
"Eternal (plastic) triangle," simple cure. GILLIES, H. D. Lancet *2:*930-931, Oct 27, '23 (illus.)
Priority in plastic surgery. FILATOFF, W. Presse med. *31:*1061-1062, Dec 19, '23
Recent advances in plastic surgery. BROWN, G. V. I. Wisconsin M. J. *22:*427-428, Feb '24
Destructive and constructive surgery of malignancy. RITCHIE, H. P. Minnesota Med. *8:*4-7, Jan '25
Plastic surgery, its relation to general surgery. SCHAEFFER, G. C. Ohio State M. J. *21:*11-14, Jan '25
Plastic surgery. SHEEHAN, J. E. Am. J. Surg. *39:*88-90, April '25
Remote results of plastic operations. JUARISTI, V. Arch. espan. de pediat. *9:*385-391,

Plastic Surgery—Cont.
July '25 abstr: J.A.M.A. *85:*1262, Oct 17, '25
Principles in plastic surgery about head and neck (and nose). BECK, J. C. Illinois M. J. *48:*194-202, Sept '25
General review of field of plastic surgery SHEEHAN, J. E., J. M. Soc. New Jersey *22:*338-341, Sept '25
Problems in reconstructive surgery. JOHNSON, C. C. Nebraska M. J. *10:*435-438, Nov '25
Principles in plastic surgery. KILNER, T. P. Irish J. M. Sc., pp. 77-81, Feb '26
Art and science of plastic surgery. DAVIS, J. S. Ann. Surg. *84:*203-210, Aug '26
Plastic operation on chest. SHIPLEY, A. M. Ann. Surg. *84:*246-250, Aug '26
Plastic surgery. SHEEHAN, J. E. Arch. Otolaryng. *4:*427-429, Nov '26
Cutaneous plastics; their scientific basis. URKOV, J. Illinois M. J. *51:*469-471, June '27
Problems in plastic surgery. BASTOS ANSART, M. Rev. med. de Barcelona *8:*18-35, July '27 also: Arch. de med., cir. y espec. *27:*356-365, Sept 24, '27
Plastic surgery. SHEEHAN, J. E. Arch. Otolaryng. *6:*385-389, Oct '27
Reconstructive surgery. LEWIS, D. Tr. South. S. A. *40:*88-97, '27
Progress in plastic surgery. DUFOURMENTEL, L. Arch. franco-belges de chir. *31:*126-132, Feb '28
Plastic surgery. KIRKHAM, H. L. D. Texas State J. Med. *23:*725-727, March '28
Two corrective operations; good results. PASSOT, R. Hopital *16:*246, April (A, bis) '28
Plastic surgery. SHEEHAN, J. E. Arch. Otolaryng. *7:*299-311, April '28
Reconstructive surgery (Hodgen lecture). LEWIS, D. J. Missouri M. A. *25:*185-190, May '28
General principles of plastic surgery; cutaneous graft, sutures; cases. LEWIS, D., Bull. et mem. Soc. de chir. de Paris *20:*476-487, June 1, '28
Plastic surgery. PALMER, D. H. Northwest Med. *27:*296-298, June '28
Cases illustrating maxillo-facial and plastic surgery. JOHNSON, L. W., U. S. Nav. M. Bull. *26:*843-861, Oct '28
Plastic surgery. SHEEHAN, J. E. Arch. Otolaryng. *8:*448-451, Oct '28
Plastic methods in otorhinolaryngology. SANVENERO-ROSSELLI, G. Rassegna ital. di oto-rino-laring. *2:*241-257, Nov-Dev '28
Freedom in plastic surgery. ABRAJANOFF, A. A. Vestnik khir. (no. 35-36) *12:*10-19, '28

Plastic Surgery—Cont.
Examples of restorative surgery and functional adaptation of hand and feet. OLLER, A. Siglo med. *83:*77-82, Jan 5, '29
Reconstructive surgery in relation to cancer defects. SHEEHAN, J. E. Internat. J. Med. and Surg. *42:*177-180, April '29
Technic in plastic surgery. DE QUERVAIN, F. Zentralbl. f. Chir. *56:*1218-1219, May 18, '29
Plastic surgery. PADGETT, E. C. Kansas City Southwest Clin. Soc. Monthly Bull. *5:*19-24, July '29
Plastic surgery. WILKINSON, D. E. Vet. Rec. *9:*579-588, July 13, '29
General principles of plastic surgery of face. MIRIZZI, P. L. Schweiz. med. Wchnschr. *59:*1011-1019, Oct 5, '29
Plastic surgery. SHEEHAN, J. E. Arch. Otolaryng. *10:*426-428, Oct '29
Principles of plastic surgery of importance to general practitioners (for face.) BROWN, G. V. I. Proc. Internat. Assemb. Inter-State Post-Grad. M. A., North America (1928), pp. 542-547, '29
Plastic surgery cases. DESELAERS, H. Rev. espan. de med. y cir. *13:*2-11, Jan '30
Rights and duties of surgeon in plastic surgery. SEBILEAU, P. Ann. d. mal. de l'oreille, du larynx *49:*1-9, Jan '30
Plastic surgery in industry (industrial surgery). COHEN, I. New Orleans M. and S. J. *83:*623-631, March '31
Newer methods in plastic surgery. VON WEDEL, C., J. Oklahoma M. A. *24:*75-76, March '31
New ideas on plastic restoration of congenital and acquired defects. LINDEMANN, A. Chirurg *3:*358, April 15, '31
Formation and work of Société Scientifique Française de Chirurgie Réparatrice, Plastique et Esthétique. JÁUREGUI, P. Semana med. *2:*396-398, July 30, '31
Plastic surgery; indications and relationship to other specialities. MALINIAK, J. W. Rev. de chir. plastique, pp. 100-110, July '31 also: J. M. Soc. New Jersey *28:*679-683, Sept '31
Plastic surgery; practice and biology. LEOZ ORTIN, G. Med. ibera *2:*213-223, Aug. 22, '31
Plastic surgery. SHEEHAN, J. E. Arch. Otolaryng. *14:*377-379, Sept '31
Variety in plastic surgery. SHEEHAN, J. E. Rev. de chir. plastique, pp. 161-181, Oct '31
Technic and biology of plastic surgery. LEOZ ORTÍN, G. Arch. de oftal. hispano-am. *31:*593-617, Nov '31

Plastic Surgery – Cont.

Plastic surgery and specialists. MALINIAK, J. W. Am. J. Surg. *14:*483–488, Nov '31

Plastic surgery methods. HENRY, A. K. Cong. internat. de med. trop. et d'hyg., Compt. rend. (1928) *2:*293–301, '31

Plastic surgery (of keloids). ALHAIQUE, A. Rinasc. med. *9:* 25–27, Jan 15, '32

Uses and limitations of plastic surgery. STRAATSMA, C. R. New York State J. Med. *32:*253–257, March 1, '32

Legal responsibility in plastic surgery; advisability of establishing regulations protecting both physician and patient. RIBEIRO, L. Folha med. *13:*175–178, May 25, '32

Types of contour repair in plastic surgery. BLAIR, V. P. South. Surgeon *1:*162–166, July '32

Plastic surgery. LURIJE, A. Medicina, Kaumas *13:*540–543, Aug '32

Plastic surgery (skin grafts). VON WEDEL, C. Southwestern Med. *16:*409–411, Oct '32

Division of plastic surgery; its needs; its field of usefulness. DAVIS, J. S. Tr. West. S. A. *42:*209–225, '32

Results of plastic operations at R. Clinica Otorinolaringoiatrica in Turin. SANVENERO-ROSSELLI, G. Arch. ital. di laring. (supp.) *51:*301-324, '32

Plastic operations developed by Dr. Mackenty in field of otorhinolaryngology. FAULKNER, E. R. Laryngoscope *43:*103–105, Feb '33

Developments in plastic surgery of face and neck. NEW, G. B. Wisconsin M. J. *32:*243–246, April '33

Division of plastic surgery; organization, needs and field of usefulness. DAVIS, J. S. South. Surgeon *2:*136–142, June '33

Problems in plastic surgery. MALINIAK, J. W. Rev. de chir. plastique, pp. 36–42, May '33 also: J. M. Soc. New Jersey *30:*439–441, June '33

Progress in plastic and reconstructive surgery. SHEEHAN, J. E. Union med. du Canada *62:*639-643, July '33

Technic of incisions and sutures in plastic surgery (face). DANTRELLE. Rev. de chir. plastique, pp. 75–108, Aug '33

Healing of surface wounds for prevention of deformities. BEEKMAN, F. AND O'CONNELL, R. J. JR. Ann. Surg. *98:*394–407, Sept '33

Problems of plastic and reconstructive surgery. SHEEHAN, J. E. Bruxelles-med. *14:*39–48, Nov 12, '33

Role of plastic surgery in relation to orthodontia. DAVIS, A. D. Internat. J. Orthodontia *19:*1214–1222, Dec '33

Plastic Surgery – Cont.

Plastic surgery (grafts) in pathology and in clinical conditions. BERDICHEVSKIY, G. A. Novy khir. arkhiv *28:*79–87, '33

Data on plastic surgical operations. GINZBERG, M. M. Sovet. klin. *19:*447–452, '33

Aspects of plastic surgery seldom considered. MALINIAK, J. W., M. Rec. *139:*653–655, June 20, '34

Reparative surgery. SHEEHAN, J. E., M. Rec. *139:*647–653, June 20, '34

Task of plastic surgeon. HUNT, H. L. Am. Med. *40:*361-362, Sept '34

Mission to U.S.S.R. to study plastic surgery. DUFOURMENTEL, L. Bull. et mem. Soc. d. chirurgiens de Paris *26:*571–590, Nov 2, '34

Reconstructive plastic and oral surgery. SMITH, A. E., J. Am. Dent. A. *21:*2190–2200, Dec '34

Development and scope of plastic surgery (Charles H. Mayo lecture). GILLIES, H. D. Northwestern Univ. Bull., Med. School *35:*1–32, Jan 28, '35

Correction during infancy of congenital and acquired deformities in otorhinolaryngology to prevent later increased disfigurement, with special reference to plastic surgery. REBELO NETO, J. Rev. oto-laring. de Sao Paulo *3:*11–24, Jan–Feb '35

Reconstructive surgery; repair of superficial injuries. GILLIES, H. Surg., Gynec. and Obst. *60:*559-567, Feb (no. 2A) '35

Recent advances in plastic surgery with special reference to vascularization of implants (face). GOLDEN, H. M. Illinois M. J. *67:*175–181, Feb '35

Conclusive remarks from personal experience in plastic surgery. BECK, J. C. Ann. Otol., Rhin. and Laryng. *44:*90-93, March '35

Use of medicated gauze dressing (tulle gras) in plastic and esthetic surgery. CODAZZI AGUIRRE, J. A. Rev. med. del Rosario *25:*441-446, April '35

Optimum time for operation in plastic surgery. PICKERILL, H. P. New Zealand M. J. *34:*154–159, June '35

Reconstructive plastic and oral surgery. SMITH, A. E. California and West. Med. *42:*432–438, June '35

Institute of Plastic and Esthetic Surgery in Czechoslovakia. KUBERTOVA, E. Rev. de chir. structive, pp. 19–33, July '35

Reparative and reconstructive surgery. SHEEHAN, J. E. Guy's Hosp. Gaz. *49:*327–336, Aug 31, '35

Relationship between otolaryngologist and plastic surgeon. HAYS, H. Am. J. Surg. *31:*38–47, Jan '36

Plastic Surgery—Cont.

Modern plastic surgery (face). ALFREDO, J. Rev. med. de Pernambuco *6:*109–118, April '36

Abnormalities and plastic surgery of lower urogenital tract (Ramon Guiteras lecture). YOUNG, H. H., J. Urol. *35:*417–480, April '36

Treatment of disfiguring scars (keloids), defects and malformations. DUJARDIN, E. Hospitalstid. *79:*524–533, May 19, '36

Plastic surgery, what to expect. SARNOFF, J. M. Rec. *144:*58–62, July 15, '36

Medical responsibility in plastic surgery; possible precautions for protection of practitioner; how much should patient know of risks. DARTIGUES, L. Vie med. *17:*893–899, Dec 10, '36

Prognosis in plastic surgery. GILLIES, H. D. AND MOWLEM, T. Lancet *2:*1346–1347, Dec 5, '36

Prognosis in plastic surgery. GILLIES, H. D. AND MOWLEM, R. Lancet *2:*1411–1412, Dec 12, '36

Contribution of stomatology to esthetic or reconstructive surgery. POHL, L. Rev. de chir. structive, pp. 426–429, Dec '36

Value of reparative surgery, inclusive of free transplantations. REHN, E. Arch. f. klin. Chir. *186:*244–266, '36

Reparative plastic surgery; loss of thumb and methods of substitution. SORALUCE, J. Cir. ortop. y tramatol., Madrid *1:*247–254, '36

Plastic surgery for general practitioner (grafts). BARSKY, A. J. Radiol. Rev. & Mississippi Valley M. J. *59:*13–15, Jan '37

Presentation of cases requiring plastic repair (grafts). PEER, L. A., J. M. Soc. New Jersey *34:*15–20, Jan '37

Nomenclature in plastic surgery. FINESILVER, E. M. Am. J. Surg. *35:*549–553, March '37

Indications and limitations of plastic surgery. BARSKY, A. J. Radiol. Rev. and Mississippi Valley M. J. *59:*95–98, May '37

Restorative surgery following surgical or pathologic loss of substance in cancer and leprosy. PRUDENTE, A. Rev. de chir. structive, pp. 148–154, June '37

Reconstructive plastic and oral surgery. SMITH, A. E. AND JOHNSON, J. B., J. Am. Dent. A. *24:*1142–1153, July '37

Present status of plastic surgery. PICK, J. F. Illinois M. J. *72:*177–182, Aug '37

Modern surgery (plastic); achievements and possibilities. AUFRICHT, G., M. Rec. *146:*310–313, Oct 6, '37

Plastic surgery. ECKHOFF, N. Guy's Hosp. Gaz. *51:*440–448, Oct 23, '37

Plastic Surgery—Cont.

Variety in reparative surgery. SHEEHAN, J. E., M. Rec. *146:*307–310, Oct 6, '37

Plastic surgery. MALBEC, E. F. Semana med. *2:*1385–1394, Dec 16, '37

Reparative surgery. DEMEL, R. Arch. f. klin. Chir. *188:*207–214, '37

Results achieved with plastic surgery. ADAMS, W. M. Memphis M. J. *13:*3–6, Jan '38

Role of plastic surgery in general practice. DAVIS, A. D. Urol. and Cutaneous Rev. *42:*40–45, Jan '38

Plastic surgery; use of rubber (nuova carne); results in various cases after 25 years. FIESCHI, D. Rev. de chir., Paris *76:*1–36, Jan '38

New developments in application of plastic surgery to accident cases involving the face. PEARLMAN, R. C. Kentucky M. J. *36:*30–34, Jan '38

Reconstructive surgery (face). ADAMS, W. M. Mississippi Doctor *15:*23–28, Feb '38

Emergency plastic surgery. UPDEGRAFF, H. L. Mil. Surgeon *82:*315–321, April '38

Plastic surgery. BAMES, O. Rev. med. peruana *10:*249–256, May '38

Conservative and restorative surgery in accidents. PALOMO MARTINEZ, J. Rev. med. veracruzana *18:*2539–2546, May 1, '38

Plastic surgeon and surgery of today. PEARLMAN, R. C. Rev. med.-cir. do Brasil *46:*689–691, June '38

Plastic surgery. ZENO, L. An. de cir. *4:*65–74, June '38

Corrective operations and development of plastic surgery. ERCZY, M. Gyogyaszat *78:*454–456, July 17–24, '38

Recent developments in plastic surgery. MACOMBER, D. W. Rocky Mountain M. J. *35:*532–537, July '38

Corrective operations and development of plastic surgery (including breast). ERCZY, M. Gyogyaszat *78:*495–498, Aug 14–21, '38

Problems of plastic surgery and surgery of the breast in particular. BAMES, H. O. Dia med. *10:*907–908, Sept 5, '38

Plastic surgery (face, nose). KING, E. D. J. Med. *19:*348–354, Sept '38

Plastic surgery in relation to automobile accidents (face). LANGE, W. A., J. Michigan M. Soc. *37:*787–792, Sept '38

Reconstructive surgery. ALBEE, F. H. Cir. ortop. y traumatol., Habana *6:*153–155, Oct–Dec '38

Recent progress in plastic surgery. MANNA, A. Chir. plast. *4:*150–170, Oct–Dec '38

Regenerative-reconstructive operations and late results of bone and tissue transplanta-

Plastic Surgery—Cont.
tions. Ertl, J. Budapesti orvosi ujsag *36:*949–953, Nov 3, '38
Significant developments that have contributed to advancement of oral and maxillofacial surgery. Carr, M. W. Ann. Dent. *5:*206–212, Dec '38
Recent advances in plastic and reconstructive surgery. Guttman, M. R. Am. J. M. Sc. *196:*875–882, Dec '38
General principles and application of plastic surgery. von Seemen, H. Jahresk. f. arztl. Fortbild. *29:*31–42, Dec '38
Fall and rise of plastic surgery. Updegraff, H. L. Am. J. Surg. *43:*637–656, Feb '39
Plastic surgery; progress in Argentina. Zeno, L. An. de cir. *5:*82–84, March '39
Value and limitations of plastic surgical procedures. Davis, A. D., M. Times, New York *67:*158–163, April '39
Plastic surgery in Prague, Czechoslovakia; recent experiences. Guttman, M. R. Laryngoscope *49:*291–296, April '39
Modern applications of plastic surgery. Matthews, D. N., M. Press *201:*340–345, April 5, '39
Problems in plastic surgery. Palmer, D. H. Northwest Med. *38:*136–138, April '39
Plastic surgery. Urzua, R. Dia med. *11:*556–558, June 26, '39 also: Arq. de cir. clin. e exper. *3:*103–105, April '39
Concept of plastic surgery. Urzua, R. Rev. med. brasil. *4:*41–44, June '39
Scope and problems of plastic surgery. May, H. Pennsylvania M. J. *42:*1453–1458, Sept '39
Plastic surgery in Italy. Zeno, L. Bol Soc. de cir. de Rosario *6:*430–438, Nov '39
Plastic surgery at 72. Gerrie, J. W. Canad. M. A. J. *41:*548–549, Dec '39
Problems in plastic and reconstructive surgery. Greeley, P. W., J. Am. Dent. A. *26:*1954–1965, Dec '39
Recent developments in plastic surgery. La Dage, L. H., J. Iowa M. Soc. *29:*609–611, Dec '39
Plastic surgery and transplantations in dermatology. Tappeiner, S. Wien. klin. Wchnschr. *52:*1140–1143, Dec 22, '39
Plastic surgery in Italy. Zeno, L. An. de cir. *5:*311–319, Dec '39
Science and art of plastic surgery; present and future. Sanvenero-Rosselli, G. Plast. chir. *1:*3–28, '39
Reparative surgery. Updegraff, H. L. Australian and New Zealand J. Surg. *9:*237–258, Jan '40
Oral and plastic surgery. Schaefer, J. E. J. Indiana M. A. *33:*60–66, Feb '40

Plastic Surgery—Cont.
Year's work in plastic surgery. Covarrubias Zenteno, R. Rev. med. de Chile *68:*227–237, March '40
Preoperative and postoperative care in reconstructive surgery. Brown, J. B., Byars, L. T., and McDowell, F. Arch. Surg., *40:*1192, June '40
Plastic surgery in service of dermatology. Ragnell, A. Nord. med. (Hygiea) *7:*1259–1264, July 20, '40
Aspects of civilian plastic surgery. Penn, J. South African M. J. *14:*335–338, Sept 14, '40
Skin grafting and reconstructive surgery. Thuss, C. J. J.M.A. Alabama *10:*77–83, Sept '40
Importance of department for plastic surgery and advisory center for disfigurations at dermatologic clinic. Hartmann, M. Dermat. Wchnschr. *111:*1089–1091, Dec 21, '40
Medical responsibility in plastic surgery. Zeno, L. Rev. med. leg. y jurisp. med. *5:*17–24, Jan–June '41
Plastic surgery; medical responsibility. Zeno, L. An. de cir. *7:*57–62, March–June '41
American Board of Plastic Surgery, Inc. J.A.M.A. *117:*752–753, Aug 30, '41
Plastic surgery; conception and tendencies in North America. Adler, D. Hospital, Rio de Janeiro *20:*643–650, Oct '41
Plastic orientation in treatment of wounds. Zeno, L. Arq. de cir. clin. e exper. *5:*97–123, Oct '41
Local supracutaneous serotherapy used in skin diseases and surgery for esthetic results. de Campos, A. Rev. paulista de med. *20:*12–19, Jan '42
Plastic surgical procedures. McCutchen, G. T., J. South Carolina M. A. *38:*35–38, Feb '42
Plastic surgery field. Cronin, T. D., M. Rec. and Ann. *36:*260–264, March '42
Emergency plastic surgery. Adler, D. Arq. de cir. clin. e exper. *6:*651–653, April–June '42
Plastic surgery, concept and tendencies in North America. Adler, D. Arq. de cir. clin. e exper. *6:*695–702, April–June '42
Plastic surgery, human aspects. Campos, F. Arq. de cir. clin. e exper. *6:*280–286, April–June '42
Histophilic asepsis (in plastic surgery). Tiscornia, A. Minerva med. *1:*481–485, June 16, '42
Fundamentals of plastic repair. Metz, W. R. South. Surgeon *11:*502–513, July '42
Surgical treatment of congenital defects.

Plastic Surgery – Cont.
MOWLEM, R. Proc. Roy. Soc. Med. *35:*683–684, Aug '42
Plastic surgery for general practitioner. WOLFRAM, S. Wien. klin. Wchnschr. *55:*878–879, Oct 30, '42
Plastic surgery cooperation with orthopedic surgery. MORLEY, G. H. Proc. Roy. Soc. Med. *35:*762–763, Oct '42
Burns and reconstructive surgery. LEVEN, N. L. Proc. Interst. Postgrad. M. A. North America (1941) pp. 267–269, '42
Structive surgery as carried on in North Dakota. FOSTER, G. C. Journal-Lancet *63:*62–66, March '43
Plastic surgery. ZENO, L. An. de cir. *9:*52–57, March–June '43
Plastic surgical advances in Latin America. BAMES, H. O. Tr. Am. Soc. Plastic and Reconstructive Surg. *12:*43–45, '43
Strategy in solution of problems in reconstructive surgery. BAMES, H. O. Tr. Am. Soc. Plastic and Reconstructive Surg. *12:*17–21, '43
Plastic procedures in burn therapy. KIRKHAM, H. L. D. Am. Acad. Orthop. Surgeons, Lect., pp. 202–208, '43
Plastic surgery in dermatology; large free grafts. MARINO, H. Rev. argent. dermatosif. *27:*458–461, '43
Corrective surgery. MCLAUGHLIN, C. W. JR. J. Omaha Mid-West. Clin. Soc. *5:*13–20, Jan '44
Plastic surgery, possibilities and limitations. BYARS, L. T. AND KAUNE, M. M. Am. J. Nursing *44:*334–342, April '44
Symposium on reparative surgery; cineplastic amputations. KESSLER, H. H., S. Clin. North America *24:*453–466, April '44
Symposium on reparative surgery after amputation. MOORHEAD, J. J., S. Clin. North America *24:*435–452, April '44
Plastic surgical contribution to emergency surgery. ARESPACOCHAGA, F. E. Dia med. *16:*626–630, June 12, '44
Plastic principles in common surgical procedures. RANK, B. K. Australian and New Zealand J. Surg. *14:*14–36, July '44
Plastic surgical principles. KILNER, T. P. Practitioner *153:*65–72, Aug '44
Elementary theories on therapy of hand from point of view of plastic surgery. REBELO NETO, J. An. paulist. de med. e cir. *48:*97–118, Aug '44
Paladon in plastic surgery. RECALDE, J. F. JR. Rev. med. d. Paraguay *7:*40–42, Oct–Dec '44
Relation of physiotherapy to plastic surgery.

Plastic Surgery – Cont.
REIDY, J. P. Proc. Roy. Soc. Med. *37:*705–708, Oct '44
Amputation surgery and plastic repair. THOMPSON, T. C. AND ALLDREDGE, R. H. J. Bone and Joint Surg. *26:*639–644, Oct '44
Indications for plastic surgery. MORANI, A. D., M. Woman's J. (no. 2) *52:*21–27, Feb '45
Case of serious burns; problem of reconstructive surgery, SMITH, P. E. Mississippi Doctor *22:*258–262, March '45
Plastic surgery of harelip. Science and art of plastic surgery; present and future status. SANVENERO-ROSSELLI, G. Salud y belleza *1:*8–9, April–May '45
Indications for plastic surgery. SAMMIS, G. F. M. Times, New York *73:*160–162, June '45
Plastic repair of hereditary and developmental anomalies. SELTZER, A. P. Arch. Pediat. *62:*248–254, June '45
Plastic surgery in past and future. GONZALEZ ULLOA, M. Salud y belleza (no. 4) *1:*18–21, Aug–Sept '45
Specialized surgery (plastic surgery). CURTILLET, E. Afrique franc. chir., nos. 5–6, pp. 201–213, Sept–Dec '45
Plastic surgery in congenital deformities about face. LAMONT, E. S. Eye, Ear, Nose and Throat Monthly *24:*571, Dec '45; *25:*25, Jan; 85, Feb '46
Surgical impressions from England; burns and plastic surgery. TEN KATE, J. Geneesk. gids. *24:*25, Jan 31, '46; 52, Feb 28, '46
Plastic aspects of neurosurgery, with special reference to use of tantalum. CONTRERAS, M. V. AND ROCCA, E. D. Arch. Soc. cirujanos hosp. *16:*353–358, Mar '46
Rehabilitation; plastic and reconstructive surgery of stumps. DUPERTUIS, S. M. AND HENDERSON, J. A., U.S. Nav. M. Bull. (supp.) pp. 65–77, Mar '46
Medical progress; recent developments in plastic surgery. AUFRICHT, G. New York Med. (no. 8) *2:*17–20, April 20, '46
Principles in reparative plastic surgery; experiences in general hospital in tropics. CONWAY, H. AND COLDWATER, K. B. Surgery *19:*437–459, April '46
Plastic surgery in Great Britian. GALTIER, M. Presse med. *54:*329–330, May 18, '46
Plastic surgery tour of United States centers. CLARKSON, P. Guy's Hosp. Gaz. *60:*141, May 25, '46; 165, June 22, '46; 193, July 20, '46
Anesthesia in Plastic Surgery Unit Canadian Army Overseas. GORDON, R. A. Bull. Acad. Med., Toronto *19:*233–237, Aug '46

Plastic Surgery—Cont.

Use of plastic materials in plastic surgery. BLAINE, G., M. Press *216:*223–224, Sept 25, '46 also: Lancet *2:*525–528, Oct 12, '46

Common errors in plastic surgery and how to avoid them. BEINFIELD, H. H. Eye, Ear, Nose and Throat Monthly *25:*491–495, Oct '46

Plastic Surgery Articles, Reviews of

Plastic surgery, summary of material available in field of otolaryngology. SHEEHAN, J. E. Arch. Otolaryng. *12:*527–530, Oct '30

Plastic surgery; summary of bibliographic material available in field of otolaryngology. SHEEHAN, J. E. Arch. Otolaryng. *16:*867–870, Dec '32

Plastic surgery; summary of bibliographic material available in field of otolaryngology. SHEEHAN, J. E. Arch. Otolaryng. *18:*531–533, Oct '33

Plastic surgery; summary of bibliographic material available in field of otolaryngology. SHEEHAN, J. E. Arch. Otolaryng. *20:*577–582, Oct '34

Plastic surgery; summaries of bibliographic material available in field of otolaryngology, 1936–1938. IVY, R. H. AND MILLER, H. A. Arch. Otolaryng. *27:*622–642, May '38

Plastic surgery, 1938; summaries of bibliographic material available in field of otolaryngology. IVY, R. H. AND MILLER, H. A. Arch. Ololaryng. *30:*99–114, July '39

Review of reconstructive surgery of the face, 1938–1940. BROWN, J. B. AND MCDOWELL, F. Laryng., *50:* 1117, Dec '40

Progress of plastic surgery of head (including ears, mouth, jaws, nose, etc.); review of literature for 1939. REBELO NETO, J. Rev. brasil. de oto-rino-laring. *8:*111–120, March-April '40

Plastic surgery, 1940; summaries of bibliographic material available in field of otolaryngology. IVY, R. H. AND MILLER, H. A. Arch. Otolaryng. *34:*179–192, July '41

Plastic surgery; summaries of bibliographic material available in field of otolaryngology. IVY, R. H. AND MILLER, H. A. Arch. Otolaryng. *36:*135–148, July '42

Review of reconstructive surgery of the face, 1940–1942. MCDOWELL, F. AND BROWN, J. B. Laryng., *52:*498, June '42. Also in Dentistry, A Digest of Practice, Feb '43. Also in *Rehabilitation of the War Injured,* Philosophical Library, Inc., New York, '43

Surgery of head, progress of plastic surgery; review of literature for 1942. REBELO NETO, J. Rev. brasil. de oto-rino-laring. *11:*173–185, March–April '43

Plastic Surgery Articles, Reviews of—Cont.

Review of reconstructive surgery of the face, 1942–1943. MCDOWELL, F. AND BROWN, J. B. Laryng., *53:*433, June '43

Plastic surgery for 1942; summaries of bibliographic material available in field of otolaryngology. PEER, L. A. Arch. Otolaryng. *38:*171–189, Aug '43

Progress of plastic surgery; review of literature for 1943. REBELO NETO, J. Rev. brasil. de oto-rino-laring. *12:*140–150, Mar-Apr '44

Contribution to plastic surgery during 1943; summaries of bibliographic material available in field of otolaryngology. PEER, L. A. Arch. Otolaryng. *39:*537–555, June '44

Progress of plastic surgery; review of literature for 1944 and notes of trip to United States. REBELO NETO, J. Rev. brasil. de oto-rino-laring. *13:*158–166, Mar-Apr '45

Review of reconstructive surgery, 1943–1945. MCDOWELL, F. AND BROWN, J. B. Laryng., *55:*239, June '45

Contributions to plastic surgery during 1944; summaries of bibliographic material available in field of otolaryngology. PEER, L. A. Arch. Otolaryng. *42:*56–79, July '45

Contributions to plastic surgery during 1945; summaries of bibliographic material available in field of otolaryngology PEER, L. A. Arch. Otolaryng. *44:*715–758, Dec '46

Plastic Surgery Books: See Books

Plastic Surgery, History: See History of Plastic Surgery

Plastic Surgery, Medicolegal Aspects

French law and aesthetic surgery. DARTIGUES. Vie med. *10:*289–298, March 25, '29

Medicolegal aspects of plastic surgery. PEYTEL, A. Paris med. (annexe) *1:*viii–x, May 9, '31

Plastic surgery from medicolegal point of view. PEYTEL, A. Paris med. (annexe) *1:*ix, May 16; vi, May 30; xiv, June 6, '31

Cosmetic surgery in relation to legal liability. REBELO NETO, J. Rev. oto-laryng. de Sao Paulo *1:*23–45, Jan–Feb '33

Legal responsibility in plastic surgery. REBELLO NETO, J. Rev. med. de Pernambuco *3:*204, July; 244, Aug; 271, Sept '33

Medicolegal aspects of esthetic surgery. FAURE, J. L. Presse med. *41:*1677–1678, Oct 28, '33

Authorization of physician to perform plastic,

Plastic Surgery, Medicolegal Aspects—Cont.
and particularly cosmetic operations. WULLE, H. Med. Welt *8:*132, Jan 27; 171, Feb 3, '34
Legal and illegal aspects of plastic surgery. MALINIAK, J. W., M. Times and Long Island M. J. *62:*165–170, June '34
Legal responsibility of plastic surgeons. REBELLO NETO, J. Arch. Soc. de med. leg. e criminol. de S. Paulo *4:*81–109, '34
Plastic surgery and criminals; surgeon's responsibility. HOOVER, J. E. Am. J. Surg. *28:*156, April '35
Practitioner's responsibility when fugitives attempt to conceal identity by means of surgery. HOOVER, J. E., J.A.M.A. *104:*1663–1664, May 4, '35
Medicolegal responsibility for failures in plastic surgery; case. WARNEYER, Chirurg *7:*294–298, May 1, '35
Plastic surgeon and crime. MALINIAK, J. W. J. Crim. Law and Criminol. *26:*594–600, Nov '35
Lawful character of plastic surgery; medicolegal aspects. PERREAU, E. H. Paris med. (annexe) *2:*iv–vii, Sept 18, '37
Medicolegal aspects in plastic surgery. SCHNEIDER, P. Wien. klin. Wchnschr. *52:*1029–1031, Nov 17, '39
Medicolegal aspects of plastic surgery. ALFREDO, J. Rev. med. de Pernambuco *14:*173–180, Aug '44

Plastic Surgery, Military (See also War Injuries)
Maxillo-facial centers. LEMAITRE, F. Mil. Surgeon *57:*242–255, Sept '25
Plastic surgery in relation to armed forces; past, present and future (Kober lecture). JOHNSON, L. W. Mil. Surgeon *79:*90–120, Aug '36
Centers for restorative surgery and prosthesis after war wounds. LEMAITRE. Mem. Acad. de chir. *65:*1143–1147, Oct 25–Nov 8, '39
Principles of reconstructive surgery in war wounds. REHN, E. Beitr. z. klin. Chir. *171:*1–24, '40
Plastic surgery in war; preparedness of profession at large. MALINIAC, J. W., M. Rec. *154:*325–326, Nov 5, '41
Symposium on military surgery; plastic and maxillofacial surgery. IVY, R. H., S. Clin. North America *21:*1583–1592, Dec '41
Plastic surgery and jaw injuries center somewhere in England. MARTINDALE, L., M. Woman's J. *49:*299, Oct '42
Scope of plastic surgery in war. MALINIAC, J. W. Bol. d. Hosp. policia mac. *2:*65–68, April 1, '43

Plastic Surgery, Military—Cont.
Corrective surgery in war; progress, advantages and possibilities. HERNANDEZ RAMIREZ, S. Pasteur *2:*15–18, July 15, '43
Rehabilitation in maxillofacial and plastic center. MCINDOE, A. H. Post-Grad. M. J. *19:*161–167, July '43
Plastic surgery and war. PRUDENTE, A. Imprensa med., Rio de Janeiro *19:*39–58, Sept '43
Plastic surgery as related to war surgery. KIRKHAM, H. L. D. *et al.* S. Clin. North America *23:*1603–1611, Dec '43
Plastic surgery in wartime; how to manage head and neck wounds. REBELO NETO, J. Rev. paulista de med. *23:*345–346, Dec '43
Reconstruction in times of war and peace. BROWN, G. V. I. Proc. Interst. Postgrad. M. A. North America (1942) pp. 63–66, '43
(Plastic) surgery heals scars of war. BROWN, D. AND LUMSDEN, R. Hygeia *22:*26, Jan '44
Plastic surgery in combat and civilian casualities. IVY, R. H., M. Ann. District of Columbia *13:*45–49, Feb '44
Symposium on war medicine; plastic and reconstruction surgery. IVY, R. H. *et al.* Symposium on war medicine; plastic and reconstruction surgery. Clinics *2:*1165–1193, Feb '44
Plastic surgery of war wounds. ASCHAN, P. E. Deut. Militararzt *9:*142, March '44
Reparative surgery in the war. COVARRUBIAS ZENTENO, R. Arch. Soc. cirujanos hosp. *14:*49–56, March '44
Initial care of wounds from reconstructive viewpoint. GALLAGHER, J. L. Mil. Surgeon *94:*212–216, April '44
Plastic surgery and its association with orthopedic surgery. BROWN, J. B. AND CANNON, B. Am. Acad. Orthop. Surgeons, Lect. pp. 212–216, '44
Reconstruction surgery of Imperial and Union Defense Force. FOUCHE, F. P. Am. Acad. Orthop. Surgeons, Lect. pp. 542–546, '44
Physical therapy in plastic surgery unit. WILSON, H. C. Physiotherapy Rev. *25:*3–21, Jan–Feb, '45
Plastic and reconstructive surgery in military. STRAATSMA, C. R. Mil. Surgeon *96:*255–257, March '45
Reconstructive surgery of war wounded. WILSON, P. D. Rocky Mountain M. J. *42:*267–274, April '45
Reconstructive surgery of war wounded. WILSON, P. D. New England J. Med. *233:*492–497, Oct 25, '45

Plastic Surgery, Military–Cont.

Military plastic surgery. SHAW, M. H. M. Press *214:*312-317, Nov 14, '45

Reconstructive surgery of war wounds. WILSON, P. D. Medicina, Mexico *25:*475-491, Nov 25, '45

Plastic surgery in war; recent advances in United States and Great Britian. MARINO, H. Bol. y trab., Soc. argent. de cirujanos *6:*778-788, '45 also: Rev. Asoc. med. argent. *59:*1373-1376, Dec 15, '45

Plastic surgery in present war. MARINO, H. Bol. Soc. cir. d. Uruguay *16:*311-321, '45

Plastic surgery in second World war. MARINO, H. Arch. urug. de med., cir. y especialid. *28:*197-207, Feb '46

Advances in England; impressions gained during trip in October 1945. RAGNELL, A. Nord. med. *29:*261-263, Feb 8, '46

Plastic surgery in World War I and in World War II. DAVIS, J. S. Ann. Surg. *123:*610-621, April '46

Plastic surgery in World War I and in World War II. DAVIS, J. S. Tr. South. S. A. (1945) *57:*141-152, '46

Plastic Surgery, Psychology of

Treatment of facial scars, with remarks on their psychological aspects. HUNT, H. L. Am. J. Surg. *4:*313-320, March '28

Plastic surgery; psychology of appearances. BETTMAN, A. G. Northwest Med. *28:*182-185, April '29

Congenital deformities of external ear; their mental effect. STRAATSMA, C. R. Arch. Otolaryng. *11:*609-613, May '30

Defects of nose–fancied and real; reaction of patient; attempted correction. BLAIR, V. P. AND BROWN, J. B. Surg., Gynec. & Obst. *53:*797-819, Dec '31

Psychological aspects of plastic surgery. STRAITH, C. L., J. Michigan M. Soc. *31:*13-18, Jan '32

Nasal abnormalities, fancied and real; reaction of patient; attempted correction. BLAIR, V. P. AND BROWN, J. B. Internat. J. Orthodontia *18:*363-401, April '32

Psychoanalytic aspects of plastic surgery. UPDEGRAFF, H. L. AND MENNINGER, K. A. Am. J. Surg. *25:*554-558, Sept '34

Plastic surgery of head, face and neck; psychic reactions. BLAIR, V. P., J. Am. Dent. A. *23:*236-240, Feb '36

Plastic surgery from point of view of mental hygiene (face). ROY, J. N. Rev. san. mil., Bucuresti *35:*1070-1076, Oct '36

Protruding ears; psychological effect and plastic correction. WOLFE, M. M., M. Rec. *144:*306-307, Oct 7, '36

Plastic Surgery, Psychology of –Cont.

Importance of plastic surgery for relieving mental condition of deformed individuals (psychocosmeticopathy). CODAZZI AGUIRRE, J. A. Semana med. *1:*675-680, March 4, '37

Psychologic aspects of relationship between surgeon and patient (plastic surgery). WODAK, E. Med. Klin. *33:*833-835, June 18, '37

Minor plastic surgery (face) and its relation to inferiority complex. MCCLELLAND, E. S. M. Rec. *146:*419-424, Nov 17, '37

Esthetic and psychologic principles of plastic surgery (ear), (face), (nose). WODAK, E. Monatschr. f. Ohrenh. *72:*288-303, March '38

Esthetic and psychologic principles of plastic surgery of nose, ears and face. WODAK, E. Monatschr. f. Ohrenh. *72:*424, April; 490, May '38

Lop ear; psychologic importance of early surgical correction. ZENO, L. An. de cir. *4:*190-192, Sept '38 also: Bol. Soc. de cir. de Rosario *5:*429-431, Oct '38

Plastic surgery in children; medical and psychologic aspects of deformity. STRAITH, C. L. AND DE KLEINE, E. H. J.A.M.A. *111:*2364-2370, Dec 24, '38

Postoperative psychosis; dementia praecox following operation on nasal septum; case. MUKASA, H. Oto-rhino-laryng. *12:*139, Feb '39

Mental and psychic condition of certain malformed individuals; value of plastic surgery. MALBEC, E. F. Semana med. *1:*716-722, March 30, '39

Psychology of plastic surgery of ear. BERNDORFER, A. Gyogyaszat *79:*349-351, June 4, '39

Psychic repercussion of facial defects; value of plastic surgery. MALBEC, E. F. Semana med. *2:*94-99, July 13, '39

Plastic surgery; psychic repercussion and social aspects of deformed ears. MALBEC, E. F. Semana med. *2:*1506-1509, Dec 28, '39

Plastic surgery and psychology. ZENO, L. AND PIZARRO CRESPO, E. An. de cir. *6:*1-22, March '40 also: Semana med. *2:*231-244, Aug 1, '40

Protruding ear; psychologic effect, morphologic classification and surgical therapy. PEDEMONTE, P. V. Arch. urug. de med., cir. y especialid. *17:*458-472, Oct '40

Harmful effects of malformed ears in school; plastic surgery of protruding ears. CODAZZI AGUIRRE, J. A. Semana med. *1:*456-462, Feb 20, '41

Protruding ear; psychologic effect, morphologic classification and surgical therapy.

Plastic Surgery, Psychology of –Cont.
PEDEMONTE, P. V. An. d. ateneo clin. quir. *7:*73–87, Feb '41
Improving mental attitude by means of plastic surgery of face. RICHISON, F. A., J. Am. Dent. A. *28:*437-441, March '41
Psychology of lupus patients with nasal prostheses. KALKOFF, K. W. Dermat. Wchnschr. *113:*597-601, July 12, '41
Nasal defects in students; psychologic aspects and plastic correction. CODAZZI AGUIRRE, J. A. Arq. de cir. clin. e exper. *6:*194–197, April–June '42
Nasal deformities in students; psychologic aspects and plastic correction. CODAZZI AGUIRRE, J. A. Semana med. *1:*981-988, May 14, '42
Symposium on neuropsychiatry; changing character through corrective surgery. EHRENFELD, H. J., M. Rec. *155:*531–533, Dec '42
Psychosomatic clinical study of case of lupus of nose treated by plastic surgery. ZENO, L. Rev. med. de Rosario *33:*1041–1058, Nov '43 also: An. de cir. *9:*125–142, Sept–Dec '43 also: Dia med. *16:*264-268, March 20, '44
Psychology of patient undergoing plastic surgery. BARSKY, A. J. Am. J. Surg. *65:*238–243, Aug '44

PLATT, H. AND BRISTOW, W. R.: Remote results of operations for injuries of peripheral nerves. Brit. J. Surg. *11:*535-567, Jan '24
PLAYER, L. P., AND CALLANDER, C. L.: Muscle transplantation, method for cure of urinary incontinence in male. J.A.M.A. *88:*989-991, March 26, '27
PLAZA, F. L.: Block of branches of trigeminal nerve for surgery. Jorn. neuro-psiquiat. panam., actas (1939) *2:*104-112, '41
PLESSIER, P. (see VEAU, V.) June '31
PLESSIER, P. (see VEAU, V.) Sept '32
PLEWKA: Angioma of nose; case. Ztschr. f. Hals-Nasen-u. Ohrenh. *28:*560-564, Aug 20, '31
PLOMAN, K. G.: Contribution to knowledge of fistula interna sacci lacrymalis. Acta opth. *5:*277–284, '27
PLOUSSARD, C. N.: Hand infections. Southwestern Med. *14:*319-322, July '30
PLUCIŃSKI, K.: Acrocephalosyndactylia (Apert syndrome). Ginek. polska *11:*661-676, July-Sept '32
PLUMMER, S. C. AND BUMP, W. S.: Massive hypertrophy of breasts. Ann. Surg. *85:*61–66, Jan '27
POATE, H. R. G.: Bone grafts. M. J. Australia *1:*209–215, Feb 25, '22 (illus.)
POCHISSOFF, N.: New marginoplastic method of operation in trichiasis of eyelids. Klin. Monatsbl. f. Augenh. *86:*213–218, Feb '31
POCHY-RIANO, R.: Question of electrolysis or diathermocoagulation in therapy of vascular tumors of face; experimental study. Arch. di radiol. *12:*121-133, March–April '36
PODGAETSKIY, G. B.: Unilateral gigantic development of auricle; case. Zhur. ush., nos. i gorl. bolez. *15:*551-552, '38
PODLAHA, J.: Crossed dislocation of lower jaw; anatomic and physiologic conception of dislocations of jaw. Zentralbl. f. Chir. *53:*2199–2202, Aug 28, '26
PODVINEC, J.: Artificial vagina construction from fetal membranes; 2 cases. Casop. lek. cesk. *76:*48–49, Jan 15, '37
POE, D. L.: Rhinolalia aperta; further studies. Arch. Pediat. *50:*147–157, March '33
POE, J. G.: General anesthesia in submucous and other nasal operations. Am. J. Surg. (Anesthesia supp.) *37:*56-57, April '23
POENARU-CAPLESCU: Burn therapy. Romania med. *10:*239–242, Oct 15, '32
POER, D. H. (see BARKER, D. E.) Apr '46
POER, D. H. (see BARKER, D. E. *et al*) 1946
POGÁNY, O.: Technic of radical operation in plastic surgery of ear. Gyogyaszat *74:*38, Jan 21, '34
POGGI, J.: Treatment of partial loss of right side of nose; case. Folha med. *9:*413–415, Dec 15, '28
POGGI, J.: Bone autoplasty; 3 cases. Folha med. *10:*13–17, Jan 15, '29
POGGI, J.: History and development of plastic surgery. Folha med. *10:*241–243, July 25, '29
POGGI, J.: Free and pediculated skin grafts. Folha med. *10:*403-406, Nov 25, '29
POGGI, J.: Plastic surgery of face. Bol. do coll. brasil. de cir. *2:*91–99, April-Nov '31
POGGI, J.: Surgical therapy of elephantiasis. Bol. coll. brasil. de cirurgioes *7:*17–30, May '36; in Rev. brasil. de cir., July '36
POHL, H.: Tendovaginitis stenosans of extensor pollicis longus sinister. Med. Klin. *32:*1596–1597, Nov 20, '36
POHL, L.: Facial deformities caused by abnormalities of jaw; operative and dental treatment; cases. Rev. odont. *50:*134–150, April '29
POHL, LEANDER (editor): *Chirurgische und konservative Kosmetik der Gesichtes*. Urban and Schwarzenberg, München, 1931
POHL, L.: Congenital fistula of lower lip; etiologic and clinical study. Rev. de chir. plastique, pp. 107–131, Oct '34
POHL, L.: Contribution of stomatology to esthetic or reconstructive surgery. Rev. de chir. structive, pp. 426–429, Dec '36

POHL, L.: Extra-oral splinting of edentulous mandible in fractures. Lancet *2:*389-391, Oct 4, '41

POHL, L. (see SICHER, H.) May '34

POHLE, E. A.: Treatment (radium) of infected hemangiomata. Am. J. Roentgenol. *43:*408-415, March '40

POHLE, E. A. AND MCANENY, J. B.: Radium treatment of vascular nevi; analysis of 152 cases seen during 1928-1938. Am. J. Roentgenol. *44:*747-755, Nov '40

PÖHLMANN, G.: Burn therapy at surgical clinic in Munich. Arch. f. klin. Chir. *197:*666-722, '40

POILLEUX, F.: Surgical indications in rheumatoid arthritis. Gaz. med. de France *44:*923-925, Nov 1, '37

POINCLOUX, P. (see NICOLAU, S.) Feb '28

POINOT, J.: Radial paralysis; tenoplasty of extensors. Bordeaux chir. *3-4:*148-149, July-Oct, '45

POINSO, R.; RECORDIER, M. AND SARRADON, P.: Hemithoracic pain following zona, with disturbances of cutaneous pigmentation; bilateral contracture of palmar aponeuroses; case. Marseille-med. *1:*20-29, Jan 5, '35

POIRIER, B. (see DAMAYE, H.) Aug '30

POKA, L.: Unusual hand injuries and face. Orvosi hetil. *85:*105-107, March 1, '41

POKHISOV, N. Y.: Operation for spastic entropion. Sovet. vestnik oftal. *6:*131-135, '35

POKHISOV, N. Y.: New technic in therapy of eversion of lacrimal point and ectropion of lower lid; preliminary report. Vestnik oftal. *11:*218-222, '37

POKHISOV, N. Y.: Surgical therapy of obstruction of lacrimal ducts. Vestnik oftal. *16:*356-360, '40

POKOTILO, V. L. AND KOZDOBA, A. Z.: Fate of bone transplanted into soft tissue; experimental study. Sovet. khir., no. 1, pp. 73-82, '36

POKOTILO, W. L.: Two modifications of technic in making use of skin flaps in esophagoplasty. Zentralbl. f. Chir. *57:*2295-2300, Sept 13, '30

POKOTILO, W. L. AND KOZDOBA, A. Z.: Fate of bone explants grafted into soft tissue; experimental studies. Mitt. a. d. Grenzgeb. d. Med. u. Chir. *44:*390-400, '36

POLACCO, E.: Comparative study of bony new growth in auto- and homo-plastic grafts of periosteum and young bones. Arch. per le sc. med. *53:*476-480, Aug '29 also: Gior. d. r. Accad. di med. di Torino *92:*153-157, April-June '29

POLANO, H.: Clinical aspects of plastic use of skin, especially for repair of postoperative hernia. Beitr. z. klin. Chir. *154:*551-562, '32

POLETTI, G. B.: Ankylosis of temporomandibular articulation. Stomatol. *31:*392-429, April '33

POLETTINI, B.: Experimental growth of bone and cartilage. Arch. ital. di chir. *6:*179-191, Nov '22 (illus.) abstr: J.A.M.A. *80:*360, Feb 3, '23

POLICARD, A. AND LERICHE, R.: Histologic document on fate of heterotransplantation of nerves of Nageotte type. Lyon chir. *19:*544-549, Sept-Oct '22 (illus.) abstr: J.A.M.A. *80:*1182, April 21, '23

POLICARO, R. D.: Plastic induration of penis with retraction of palmar aponeurosis; case. Gior. med. d. Alto Adige *9:*13-16, Jan '37

POLISADOVA, K. I. AND SINITSKIY, A. A.: Application of cultures of Bacillus bulgaricus in treatment of purulent wounds after burns. Sovet. khir. (no. 6) *6:*786-794, '34

POLISSADOWA, X.: Recuperation of innervation in skin transplants. Zentralbl. f. Chir. *52:*2166-2168, Sept 26, '25

POLISSADOWA, X. AND BJELOSOR, I.: Atypical epithelial proliferation of transplanted mammary tissue. Virchows Arch. f. path. Anat. *272:*759-762, '29

POLITZER, G.: Origin of facial cleft, harelip and cleft palate. Monatschr. f. Ohrenh. *71:*63-73, Jan '37

POLITZER, G. (see VEAU, V.) March '36

POLJAK, G. D.: Modification of Toti's dacryocystorhinostomy. Klin. Monatsbl. f. Augenh. *83:*510-515, Oct-Nov '29

POLLACZEK, K. F. (see SCHWARZMANN, E.) Nov '37

POLLAK, E.: Two new instruments; septum needle and thread-holder for ear surgery. Monatschr. f. Ohrenh. *61:*1252, Nov '27

POLLOCK, B.: Dried plasma sheets in burn therapy; preliminary reports. U.S. Nav. M. Bull. *42:*1171-1173, May '44

POLLOCK, G. A.: Conservative operation for severe injury to hand. Brit. J. Surg. *32:*535-536, April '45

POLLOCK, G. A. AND HENDERSON, M. S. Value of periosteum in grafting operation. Proc. Staff Meet., Mayo Clin. *15:*443-448, July 10, '40

POLLOCK, H. L.: Use of foreign bodies in ear, nose and throat surgery. Ann. Otol., Rhin. and Laryng. *36:*463-471, June '27

POLLOCK, H. L.: Implants in nasal deformities; history and uses. Ann. Otol., Rhin. and Laryng. *41:*1103-1107, Dec '32

POLLOCK, L. J. AND DAVIS, L.: Radial nerve injuries. Am. J. Surg. *16:*549-600, June '32

POLLOCK, L. J. AND DAVIS, L.: Peripheral ulnar nerve injuries. Am. J. Surg. *17:*299-343, Aug '32

POLLOCK, L. J. AND DAVIS, L.: Peripheral facial nerve injuries. Am. J. Surg. *18:*553–595, Dec '32

POLLOCK, W. E.; MC KENNEY, P. W. AND BLAISDELL, F. E.: Viability of bone grafts; experimental study. Arch. Surg. *18:*607–623, Feb '29

POLLOSSON, AND DE ROUGEMONT: Diagnosis and treatment of joint injuries in wounds of dorsal surface of fingers. Lyon chir. *28:*227–230, March–April '31

POLLOSSON, E. AND FREIDEL: Recurrent temporomaxillary luxation; osteoplastic abutment (Elbim method); case. Lyon chir. *35:*460–463, July–Aug '38

PÓLYA, E.: Otoplasty. Zentralbl. f. Chir. *48:*219, Feb 19, '21

PÓLYA, E.: New technic for rhinoplasty. Zentralbl. f. Chir. *48:*257, Feb 26, '21

PÓLYA, E.: Meloplasty. Zentralbl. f. Chir. *48:*261, Feb 26, '21

PÓLYA, E.: Cheiloplasty; using upper lip to make new lower lip. Zentralbl. f. Chir. *48:*262, Feb 26, '21

PÓLYA, E.: Technique of operations for carcinoma of buccal mucous membranes. Surg., Gynec. and Obst. *43:*343–354, Sept '26

PÓLYA, E.: Simple apparatus for relief of palsies of upper extremities. Surgery *8:*1023, Dec '40

POLYA, E. see POLYA, J.

POLYA, J.: Surgical therapy of syndactylia; case. Riv. di chir. *1:*469–472, Aug '35

POLYA, J.: Surgical therapy of syndactylia. Orvosi hetil. *80:*38–40, Jan 11, '36

POLYACK, G. D.: Dacryocystorhinostomy; 2 cases. Ann. d'ocul. *164:*942–951, Dec '27

POLYAK, B. L.: Extirpation of lacrimal sac. (Comment on Strakhov's article.) Strakhov's reply. Vestnik oftal. *10:*450–451, '37 Vestnik oftal. *10:*448–450, '37

POLYAK, S. O. (see PALCHEVSKIY, E. I.) 1937

POLYAKOV, K. L.: Effect of experimental sleep on healing of skin defects in man. Voen.-med. sborn. *2:*223–233, '45

POMMÉ, B.; TRICAULT, G. AND LUBINEAU, J.: Etiology of Dupuytren's contracture. Rev. neurol. *1:*633–638, May '31

POMMRICH, W.: Congenital salivary fistula in cleft cheek. Deutsche Ztschr. f. Chir. *191:*136–142, '25

POMOSOV, V. N.: Effect of procaine hydrochloride block of nerve trunks in traumatic shock. Novy khir. arkhiv. *35:*109–113, '35

PONCHER, H. G. (see PUESTOW, C. B. *et al*) March '38

PONROY, AND CABROL: Care after surgical therapy in prognathism of lower jaw. Rev. de stomatol. *35:*89–95, Feb '33

PONROY; DECHAUME, M. AND MALEPLATE: Complex fracture (craniofacial disjunction and vertical fractures) of upper jaw and double fracture of lower jaw; simplified therapy of case. Rev. de stomatol. *36:*470–471, July '34

PONROY, AND PSAUME: Choice of apparatus for reduction and bandaging in maxillary fractures. Rev. de stomatol. *41:*782–789, '40

PONROY; PSAUME, AND BOUTROUX: Permanent reduction of jaw fractures; 7 cases. Rev. de stomatol. *29:*795–814, Nov '27

PONROY; PSAUME, AND BOUTROUX: Emergency treatment of fractures of mandible. Paris med. *2:*195–199, Sept 1, '28

PONROY (see BOURGUET *et al*) Dec '31

PONROY (see LEMAÎTRE, F.) Dec '28

PONS (see MOLIN DE TEYSSIEU) April '27

PONS, J. A. (see DEL TORO, J. *et al*) Sept '31

PONS TORTELLA, E.: Buccal-facial anastomosis in facial nerve injury. Rev. de cir. de Barcelona (8):82–89, Sept–Dec '34

PONS-TORTELLA, E. AND BROGGI, M.: Intermaxilloparotid cellular space; abscesses formed there. Med. clin., Barcelona *5:*273–277, Oct '45

PONT, A.: Immediate maxillary prosthesis. Rev. de chir. plastique, pp. 264–270, Jan '32

PONT, A.: Cranial prosthesis and restoration of nose in fractures of nose and frontal part of cranium. Rev. de chir. structive. pp. 34–37, March '37

PONT, A. AND LAPIERRE, V.: Prosthesis covering orbital region, nose and upper lip. Bull. Soc. franc. de dermat. et syph. (Reunion dermat., Lyon) *43:*908–910, May '36

PONT, A. AND LAPIERRE, V.: Articulated prosthesis of eye, nose and upper lip; case. Rev. de chir. structive, pp. 38–41, March '37

PONT, A. (see SANTY, P.) Nov–Dec '38

PONTES, A.: Branchial cysts; 2 cases. Brasil-med. *55:*610–614, Sept 6, '41

PONTHUS, P.; PIFFAULT, C. AND DARGENT, M. Relation between sympathetic phenomena and contracture in facial paralysis; therapeutic conclusions. Presse med. *50:*308–309, April 20, '42

PONTHUS, P. (see PATEL, M.) March '30

Pontoppidan Operation

Transplantation of epidermal flaps by Pontoppidan method in radical surgery in otitis media. VON MAGNUS, R. Ztschr. f. Laryng., Rhin., Otol. *25:*48–52, '34

POOL, F. L.: Genesis of genopathic syndrome (Bardet-Biedl acrocephalosyndactylia). Wien. Arch. f. inn. Med. *31:*187–200, '37

POOL, H. H.: Interlocking finger bandage which

needs no anchor. J. Michigan M. Soc. *43:*406, May '44

Popenoe, P.: Split-hand deformity. J. Hered. *28:*174–176, May '37

Popescu, A. and Vlad, V.: Powdered tannin in burns. Romania med. *19:*73–74, March 15, '41

Popescu, C. (see Jianu, A.) July–Aug '40

Popescu, G. and Pricoriu, S.: Anesthesia of inferior maxillary nerve by way of zygoma in jaw surgery. Rev. san. mil., Bucuresti *37:*873–875, Oct '38

Popescu, S. and Buzoianu, G. V.: Actual surgery in digitopalmar infections. Romania med. *7:*51–52, March 1, '29

Popescu, S. (see Paulian, D. E. *et al*) March '33

Popma, A. M. (see Hicken, N. F.) June '38

Poppe, J. K.: Use of cold air blast on precancerous skin lesions and hemangiomas. Surgery *11:*460–465, March '42

Pöppelmann, W.: Therapy of inverted nipples. Med. Welt *6:*1317, Sept 10, '32

Poppen, J. L.: Intractable and non-intractable exophthalmos; causes and surgical treatment. Proc. Interst. Postgrad. M. A. North America (1942) pp. 266–269, '43

Poppen, J. L.: Diagnosis and surgical treatment of intractable cases of exophthalmos. Am. J. Surg. *64:*64–79, April '44

Poppen, J. L. (see Hoover, W. B.) June '40

Popper, H. *et al*: Evaluation of gelatin and pectin solutions as substitutes for plasma; histologic changes produced in human beings. Arch. Surg. *50:*34–45, Jan '45 also: abst., Proc. Central Soc. Clin. Research *17:*9–10, '44 abstr., J. Lab. & Clin. Med. *30:*352–354, April '45

Popoff, D.: Technic in creation of artificial vagina from rectum. Rev. franc. de gynec. et d'obst. *37:*225–236, Oct '42

Popoff Operation

Popoff's method of formation of artificial vagina; 2 cases. Mandelstamm, A. Zentralbl. f. Gynak. *51:*1058–1063, April 23, '27

Artificial vagina formation by Popoff's method and its remote results. Zdravomysloff, V. I., J. akush. i zhensk. boliez. *39:*333–344, '28

Technic and results of Popoff's method of formation of artificial vagina; 7 cases. Sdrawomyslow, W. I. Monatschr. f. Geburtsh. u. Gynak. *82:*182–204, June '29

Technic of Popoff method of formation of artificial vagina. Mandelstamm, A. Arch. f. Gynak. *138:*739–746, '29

Popoff method of formation of artificial vagina. Tchernigovsky, N. N. Vrach. gaz. *34:*216–218, Feb 15, '30

Popoff Operation – Cont.

Formation of artificial vagina by Mandelshtam modification of rectal method (Popoff); report of 8 additional cases. Mandelshtam, A. E. Zentralbl. f. Gynak. *58:*222–228, Jan 27, '34

Popovici, V. M.: New incision for ligature of palmar arch. Lyon chir. *26:*686–693, Sept–Oct '29 also: Rev. de chir., Bucuresti *21:*437–443, July '29

Porcu-Maccioni, G.: Wounds of hand, particularly of thumb in miners; statistics. Rassegna d. previd. soc. *16:*8–17, Feb '29

Pordes, J. M.: Therapy of nasopharyngeal tumors. Acta oto-laryng. orient. *1:*45–49, '45

Porges, H.: Technic of primary suture of tendons. Wien. klin. Wchnschr. *37:*285–286, March 20, '24 abstr: J.A.M.A. *82:*1486, May 3, '24

Porosz, A.: Operative treatment of rhinophyma. Dermat. Wchnschr. *84:*776, June 4, '27

Porosz, A.: Successful treatment of rhinophyma. Urol. and Cutan. Rev. *32:*519, Aug '28

Porrini, E. A. (see Luraschi, J. C. E.) Nov '42

Porrini, E. A. (see Luraschi, J. C. E.) Feb '44

Porritt, A. E.: Injection treatment of nevi. Proc. Roy. Soc. Med. (sect. Surg.) *24:*81–85, May '31

Porritt, A. E.: New methods of burn therapy. Mil. Surgeon *94:*227–228, April '44

Porritt, A. E. and Barbieri, P.: Modern methods of burn therapy. Rev. san. mil., Buenos Aires *43:*1366–1368, Oct '44

Port, K.: Unfortunate results of tendon transplantation. Deutsche Ztschr. f. Chir. *232:*12–18, '31

Porter, C. A.: Surgical treatment of roentgenray lesions. Am. J. Roentgenol. *13:*31–37, Jan '25

Porter, C. A. and Shedden, W. M.: Avulsion of scalp; review of literature and report of a case. Boston M. and S. J. *186:*727–730, June 1, '22 (illus.)

Porter, C. P.: Bilateral syndactylism, case. Brit. M. J. *1:*502, March 16, '29

Porter, M. F.: Shall we wait for shock to pass before operating? J. Indiana M. A. *19:*401–402, Oct '26

Portmann, G.: Plastic surgery in malignant syphilis of face and nasal fossae; case. Rev. de laryng. *52:*199–208, March 31, '31

Portmann, G. and Despons, J.: Technic of closure of esophageal fistula; significance in

surgical treatment of laryngo-esophageal cancer. Bordeaux chir. *3:*252–261, July '32
PORTMANN, G. AND DESPONS, J.: Malignant tumors of upper jaw. Rev. de laryng. *57:*1–44, Jan '36
PORTMANN, U. V.: Diathermia for prevention and treatment of shock. Arch. Physical Therapy *9:*385–388, Sept '28
PORTMANN, U. V.: Cystic hygroma; 3 cases. Cleveland Clin. Quart. *12:*98–104, July '45
PORTO, G.: Congenital fistula and dermoid cyst of nasal dorsum; surgical therapy of 2 cases. Rev. oto-laring. de Sao Paulo *5:*275–278, May–June '37 also: Arq. Inst. Penido Burnier *4:*320–323, June '37
PORTUGAL, J. R.: Peripheral nerve lesions; diagnosis and treatment. Imprensa med., Rio de Janeiro *19:*71–82, July '43
PORTUGAL, J. R. (see AUSTREGESILO, A. *et al*) Nov-Dec '43
PORTUGALOV, S. O.: Formation of artificial vagina. Vestnik khir. *44:*261–270, '36

Port-Wine Stains (See also Hemangiomas; Nevi)

Cure of nevus flammeus by freezing with ethyl chloride; case. KOSSACK, G. Med. Klin. *23:*2003, Dec 30, '27
Technic of treating naevus flammeus with infraroentgen (grenz) rays. KALZ, F. Strahlentherapie *57:*510–515, '36
Therapy of facial naevus flammeus with new mercury high pressure lamp (intensol lamp). LOMHOLT, S. Dermat. Wchnschr. *109:*898–900, July 29, '39
Treatment of portwine birthmarks (nevus flammeus) by grenz (infra-roentgen) rays. WHITE, C. Illinois M. J. *76:*449–451, Nov '39

PORUMBARU, I.: Tumor of lower lip and right cheek; extirpation followed by pedicled skin graft from head. Rev. de chir., Bucuresti *41:*714–721, Sept-Oct '38
PORZELT, W.: Adamantinoma of jaw recurs after 45 years. Arch. f. klin. Chir. *130:*142–150, '24
PORZELT, W.: Soft parts in finger amputations. Zentralbl. f. Chir. *51:*1343–1345, June 21, '24
PORZELT, W.: Successful thumb plasty from big toe from opposite side 4½ years after unsuccessful transplantation. Arch. f. klin. Chir. *135:*340–355, '25
PORZELT, W.: Method of placing dressing in order to relieve tension of suture after operation for harelip. Zentralbl. f. Chir. *59:*2165–2167, Sept 3, '32
PORZELT, W.: Reconstruction of thumb from mutilated index finger with preservation and extension of skin fold from thumb to middle finger. Chirurg *5:*61–65, Jan 15, '33
PORZELT, W.: Transplantation of forefinger as substitute for lost thumb; preservation of fold dividing forefinger from middle finger and new formation of ball of thumb by transplantation of pedicled flap of abdominal skin. Zentralbl. f. Chir. *62:*2248–2253, Sept 21, '35
PORZELT, W.: Usefulness of single finger; justifiability of using uninjured index finger to replace lost thumb. Zentralbl. f. Chir. *64:*550–551, March 6, '37
POSEL, M. M. (see OGILVIE, A. G.) June '27
POSER, E. AND HAAS, E.: Phosphates in therapy of chemical burns. J.A.M.A. *123:*630–631, Nov 6, '43
POSKA-TEISS, L. (see KLEITSMAN, R.) March '35
POSNER, I. AND PIATT, A. D.: Ocular hypertelorism with cleft palate and giant-cell tumor. Radiology *35:*79–81, July '40
POSSE, R.: Surgical treatment of pendulous breast. Am. J. Surg. *38:*293–297, Nov '37
POST, K.: Therapy of dislocation fracture of head of mandible. Zentralbl. f. Chir. *60:*2118–2121, Sept 9, '33
POSTNIKOV, B. N.: Chalk dressing in ambulant burn therapy. Khirurgiya, no. 1, pp. 28–33, '37
POSTNIKOV, B. N. (see BELYAEVA, V. I.) 1934
POTEL, G.: Treatment of epispadias in women. Gynec. et Obst. *10:*94–101, Aug '24
POTEL, G.: Operative treatment of balanic hypospadias. J. d'urol. *19:*236–239, March '25
POTH, E. J.: New technic for cutting skin grafts, including description of new instruments. Surgery *6:*935–939, Dec '39
POTH, E. J.: Skin graft technic. Surg., Gynec. and Obst. *75:*779–784, Dec '42
POTH, E. J.: Free graft; special technic. Texas State J. Med. *40:*290–294, Sept '44
POTH, E. J.: Technical aspects of skin transplantation. M. Rec. and Ann. *39:*1081–1088, July '45
POTH, E. J. AND BRAVO-FERNANDEZ, E.: Prevention of neuroma formation by encasement of severed nerve end in rigid tubes. Proc. Soc. Exper. Biol. and Med. *56:*7–8, May '44
POTH, E. J.; FERNANDEZ, E. B. AND DRAGER, G. A.: Prevention of formation of end-bulb neuromata. Proc. Soc. Exper. Biol. and Med. *60:*200–207, Nov '45
POTIQUET, H.: Dacryocystorhinostomy by method of Dupuy-Dutemps and Bourguet. Ann. d'ocul. *166:*470–487, June '29
POTOTSCHNIG, G.: Reconstruction of cheek. Arch. ital. di chir. *8:*209–224, Oct '23

POTTER, A. H.: Ectopia vesicae, imperforate rectum and anus, true hermaphroditism and other anomalies. Am. J. Surg. *31:*172–178, Jan '36

POTTER, E. B.: Free transplantation of skin. Univ.Hosp. Bull., Ann Arbor *1:*5–6, April '35

POTTER, E. B.: Free transplantation of skin: evaluation of methods. Surg., Gynec. and Obst. *61:*713–720, Dec '35

POTTER, E. B. AND PECK, W. S.: Treatment of extensive granulating areas, with special reference to use of physical therapy measures in burns and skin grafts. Am. J. Surg. *14:*472–476, Nov '31

POTTER, L. E. (see KIRKHAM, H. L. D. *et al*) Dec '43

POTTER, P. C.: Diagnosis and treatment of more common infections of hand. S. Clin. North America *16:*763–769, June '36

POTTER, S. E.: Removal suture method of repair peripheral nerves. J. Neurosurg. *3:*354–357, July '46

POTTER, W. B.: Bilateral congenital coloboma of upper eyelids; case. Am. J. Ophth. *26:*1087–1089, Oct '43

POTTER, W. W.: Conservatism in nasal surgery. Southern M. J. *16:*560–563, July '23

POTTS, J. B.: Treatment of crushing injuries to nose and adjacent structures. Surg. J. *34:*196–198, Nov–Dec '28

POULARD, A.: Surgical therapy of entropion of external angular origin. Ann. d'ocul. *172:*97–105, Feb '35

POULSEN, V.: Burn therapy. Ugesk. f. laeger *102:*578–579, May 30, '40

POULT, J.: Therapy of nasal fractures. Schweiz. med. Wchnschr. *65:*638–639, July 13, '35

POUND, A. E. (see GREELEY, P. W.) May '46

POUND, E.: Oral prosthesis in repair of war injuries. Am. J. Orthodontics (Oral Surg. Sect) *32:*435–439, Aug '46

POUYANNE, L. (see ROCHER, H. L.) March '36

POUYANNE, L. (see ROCHER, H. L.) Aug '38

POUZET, F.: Section of flexor tendons and ulnar nerve in injury to wrist; good results from secondary tendon and nerve sutures. Lyon chir. *28:*203–206, March–April '31

POUZET, F.: Partial resection of wrist for Volkmann contracture; case. Lyon chir. *30:*581–584, Sept–Oct '33

POUZET, F. AND LECLERC, G.: Volkmann paralysis; appearance of lesions 70 hours after beginning circulatory disturbances; case. Lyon chir. *34:*187–190, March–April '37

POUZET, F. (see TAVERNIER) May–June '38

POUZET, F. (see TAVERNIER, L. *et al*) Dec '36

POWELL, L. D.: Relationship of cellular differentiation, fibrosis, hyalinization, and lymphocytic infiltration to postoperative longevity of patients with squamous-cell epithelioma of skin and lip. J. Cancer Research *7:*371–378, Oct '22 (illus.)

POWELL, L. S.: Dermoid cyst of nasal dorsum. Arch. Otolaryng. *19:*67–68, Jan '34

POWELL, W. E.: Fatal meningitis following submucous resection of nasal septum, post-mortem discovery of latent sphenoidal sinusitis. J. Laryngol. & Otol. *37:*39–40, Jan '22

POWER, D. A.: Bygone operations in surgery; removal of sebaceous cyst from King George IV. Brit. J. Surg. *20:*361–365, Jan '33

POWERS, H.: New light on cause and possibility of physiotherapy (Dupuytren's contracture). Am J. Phys. Therapy *8:*239–241, Dec '31

POWERS, H.: One hundred years after Dupuytren; interpretation. J. Nerv. & Ment. Dis. *80:*386–409, Oct '34

POWERS, J. H. (see BECK, C. S.) July '26

POYNER, H.: Analysis of 235 cases burn therapy. Texas State J. Med. *32:*274–279, Aug '36

POYNER, H.: Treatment of industrial burns, with report of 350 cases. Am. J. Surg. *42:*744–749, Dec '38

DEL POZO, R. D.: Auriculoplasties in therapy of protruding ears by Malbec technic. Bol. y trab. Soc. argent. de cirujanos *7:*205–214, '46 also: Rev. Asoc. med. argent. *60:*460–463, June 15, '46

DEL POZO, R., D. D.: Plastic therapy of rhinomegaly and rhinokyphosis using Malbec technics. Bol. y trab., Soc. argent. de cirujanos *6:*522–539, '45

POZZAN, A.: New modification of technic of laterolateral anastomosis (nerves). Arch. ital. di chir. *57:*363–376, '39

POZZAN, A.: Technic of laterolateral anastomosis (nerve). Arch. ital. di chir. *57:*458–482, '39

DAL POZZO, G.: Neuroma of lower lip; case. Arch. per le sc. med. *52:*187–190, April '28

PRACY, J. P.: Facial splint for treatment of Bell's palsy. Brit. M. J. *1:*528, April 6, '46

PRADHAN, K. N.: Electric-ionisation and nose operations. Indian M. Gas. *57:*137–138, April '22

PRASOL, F. I.: Pathogenesis, therapy and prophylaxis of spontaneous fractures of lower jaw. Novy khir. arkhiv *40:*414–425, '38

PRAT, D.: Cancer of lips. An. de Fac. de med., Montevideo *8:*865–883, Sept '23

PRATI, M.: Importance of tendinous union in lesion of extensor tendons of fingers. Arch. ital. di chir. *17:*597–610, '27

PRATT, D. R.: Suggestions on immobilization of hand. Bull. U. S. Army M. Dept. (no. 86) pp. 105–108, March '45

PRATT, D. R.: Suggestions on immobilization of

hand injuries. Arch. Phys. Med. *26:*649–653, Oct '45

PRATT, D. R. (see SLOCUM, D. B.) July '44

PRATT, F. J.: What septa demand operation? Ann. Otol., Rhin. & Laryng. *35:*940–943, Sept '26

PRATT, F. J. AND PRATT, J. A.: Intranasal reconstruction. Laryng. Otol. & Rhin., A.M.A. p. 95, 1921

PRATT, F. J. AND PRATT, J. A.: Intranasal reconstruction. Ann. Otol., Rhin. & Laryng. *31:*46–105, March '22 (illus.)

PRATT, G. H.: Surgical considerations in treatment of chronic lymphedema. Bull. New York Acad. Med. *16:*381–388, June '40

PRATT, G. H. AND WRIGHT, I. S.: Surgical treatment of chronic lymphedema. Surg., Gynec. & Obst. *72:*244–248, Feb '41

PRATT, J. A.: Method of correcting lax, boggy septa following submucous resection. Ann. Otol., Rhin. & Laryng. *38:*1156–1157 Dec '29

PRATT, J. A. (see: PRATT, F. J.) 1921

PRATT, J. A. (see: PRATT, F. J.) March '22

Preauricular Cysts and Sinuses

Pre-auricular fistulae. STAMMERS, F. A. R. Brit. J. Surg. *14:*359–363, Oct '26

Congenital preauricular fistula. FISCHER, H. J. de med. de Bordeaux *59:*711–714, Sept 10, '29

Bilateral congenital preauricular fistula, with report of case in congenital syphilitic. BERGARA, R. A. AND BERGARA, C. Rev. Asoc. med. argent. *48:*44–50, Jan '34

Sinus preauricularis (fistula preauricularis congenita). BECKER, S. W. AND BRUNSCHWIG, A. Am. J. Surg. *24:*174–177, April '34

Preauricular fistula; development of external ear. JONES, F. W. AND WEN, I. C., J. Anat. *68:*525–533, July '34

Pringle's disease with hemifacial hyperplasia (of cheeks, lips, conjunctiva and concha of ear), but without any psychoneurologic symptoms. HERMAN, E. AND MERENLENDER, J. Acta dermat.-venereol. *16:*276–291, Oct '35

Preauricular fistulae; two cases. KLABER, R. Proc. Roy. Soc. Med. *28:*1553–1554, Oct '35

Congenital preauricular sinus. DINGMAN, R. O. Arch. Otolaryng. *29:*982–984, June '39

Congenital preauricular sinus; treatment. HAVENS, F. Z. Arch. Otolaryng. *29:*985–986, June '39

Congenital preauricular fistula. MARTIN, J. D. JR. J.M.A.Georgia *29:*411–413, Aug '40

Preauricular fistula. KHANNA, M. N. Indian M. Gaz. *76:*72–75, Feb '41

Preauricular Cysts and Sinuses—Cont.

Congenital preauricular sinus. HARDING, R. L. Am. J. Orthodontics (Oral Surg. Sect.) *28:*399–401, July '42

Congenital preauricular cysts and fistulas. PASTORE, P. N. AND ERICH, J. B. Arch. Otolaryng. *36:*120–125, July '42

Preauricular sinuses; diagnosis and treatment. PENICK, R. M. JR. South. M. J. *38:*103–105, Feb '45

Ear-pit (congenital aural and preauricular fistula). AIRD, I. Edinburgh M. J. *53:*498–507, Sept '46

Preauricular congenital sinuses. WEAVER, D. F. Laryngoscope *56:*246–251, May '46

PRECECHTĚL, A.: Malformations of nose and their correction. Cas. lek. cesk. *62:*305–308, March 24, '23 (illus.)

PŘECECHTĚL, A.: Pedigree of anomalies in first and second branchial cleft, inherited according to laws of Mendel, and contribution to technique of extirpation of congenital lateral fistulae coli. Acta oto-laryng. *11:*23–30, '27

PŘECECHTĚL, A.: Prolongation of palate by retrotransposition of pterygoid processes in cleft palate. Casop. lek. cesk. *66:*541–543, March 28, '27

PŘECECHTĚL, A.: Developmental abnormalities of second branchial slit. Otolaryng. slavica *3:*437–449, Oct '31

PŘECECHTĚL, A.: Correction of short palate. Casop. lek. cesk. *70:*1544–1548, Nov 13, '31 also: Otolaryng. slavica *4:*23–24, Jan '32

PREOBRASCHENSKI, B. S.: Modified technic in plastic surgery for correction of atresia and stenosis of external ear developing after otitis media. Otolaryng. slavica *4:*249–255, Aug '33

PREOBRAZHENSKIY, V. V.: External dacryocystorhinostomy. Sovet. vrach. gaz., pp. 388–390, March 15, '34

PRESMAN, D. L. *et al*: Intensive human serum treatment of burn shock; modified formula for calculating amount of infusion. J.A.M.A. *122:*924–928, July 31, '43

PRESNO ALBARRAN, J. A.: Modern concept of shock therapy. Rev. de med. y cir. Habana *48:*295–313, July 31, '43

Pressure Sores

Prevention and treatment of bed-sores. BONNE. Med. Klinik *20:*784–785, June 8, '24

Treatment of decubitus. HAYWARD. Med. Klin. *25:*1328–1329, Aug 23, '29

Treatment of decubitus ulcers with epithelin. SELLEI, J. Dermat. Wchnschr. *89:*1911–1916, Nov 30, '29

Pressure Sores – Cont.
Therapy of trophic disturbances (ulcer) following injury of limb by resection of neuroma of posterior tibial nerve and by autotransplantation of nervous tissue. LASSERRE, C. Bull. et mem. Soc. nat. de chir. *58:*500–502, April 16, '32
Mummification of skin (decubitus). FREUDENTHAL, P. Ugesk. f. laeger *95:*1095–1096, Oct 5, '33
Sacral eschar occurring early in puerperium; case. FERRARI, R. A. AND BRUZZONE, I. A. Semana med. *2:*1977–1979, Dec 21, '33
Treatment of decubitus ulcers with tannic acid. LATIMER, E. O., J.A.M.A. *102:*751–752, March 10, '34
Changes in gluteal muscles and their significance in development of bed-sores. MEYER, W. C. Virchows Arch. f. path. Anat. *294:*159–170, '34
Decubitus ulcer, treatment with elastic adhesive plaster. CARTY, T. J. A. Brit. M. J. *1:*105–106, Jan 19, '35
Decubitus ulcer, therapy of Cook County Hospital. FANTUS, B., J.A.M.A. *104:*46–48, Jan 5, '35
Trophic lesions in multiple sclerosis (decubitus). BYRNES, C. M. JR. J. Nerv. & Ment. Dis. *82:*373–380, Oct '35
Tannic acid therapy of decubitus ulcers. COWLEY CAMPODONICO, R. Rev. de med. y cir. de la Habana *40:*555–557, Oct 31, '35
Prevention of decubitus ulcers during therapy of contracture by Mommsen cast method. VERESHCHAKOVSKIY, I. I. Ortop. i travmatol. (no. 1) *9:*100, '35
Use of alveolate rubber in preventive and curative therapy of sacral eschar. THEVENET, V. Lyon med. *157:*709–711, June 14, '36
Hospital therapy of skin defects (decubitus ulcers). REINSTEIN, H. Psychiat.-neurol. Wchnschr. *38:*454–455, Sept 5, '36
Unguentolan (cod liver oil ointment) in therapy of decubitus and postoperative fistula and wound infection; 15 cases. WEBER, H. Wien. med. Wchnschr. *87:*219–221, Feb 20, '37
Bed-sores and their treatment. LOVE, R. J. M., Practitioner *138:*277–283, March '37
Decubitus. SPIESMAN, M. G. Am. J. Surg. *36:*17–21, April '37
Dystrophic disorders due to lesions of nerves in spinomedullary trauma; clinical and therapeutic study. DRAGONETTI, M. Gazz. internaz. med.-chir. *47:*416–421, July 15, '37
Nursing and care of bedridden patient (especially prevention of bed-sores). PEARCE, E. C. Practitioner *139:*55–62, July '37
Therapy of decubitus ulcers. EWALD, C. Med. Klin. *33:*1202–1205, Sept 3, '37
Underwater douche for decubitus ulcers. HORSCH, K. Balneologe *4:*512–517, Nov '37
Therapy of decubitus ulcer. SELETSKIY, V. V. Klin. med. *15:*241–246, '37
Decubitus ulcers; operative treatment of scars following bedsores. DAVIS, J. S. Surgery *3:*1–7, Jan '38
Cricoid perichondritis due to decubitus ulcer; case. VON SOUBIRON, N. *et al.* Rev. Asoc. med. argent. *52:*529–530, June 15, '38
Pressure areas; practical suggestions on how to prevent bed sores. NEWTON, M. E. Am. J. Nursing *38:*888–892, Aug '38
Prevention and treatment of bed-sores. COPE, V. Z. Brit. M. J. *1:*737–738, April 8, '39
Protection of heels of bedridden patients with half-shells of oranges, lemons or grapefruit. HENSCHEN, C. Zentralbl. f. Chir. *66:*782–785, April 8, '39
Decubital eschars. MARTINS, R. Rev. brasil. de orthop. e traumatol. *1:*147–154, Nov-Dec '39
Bed frame for severe decubitus and sacral wounds. HELLER, E. Zentralbl. f. Chir. *67:*1530–1532, Aug 17, '40
Care of back following spinal cord injuries; consideration of bed sores. MUNRO, D. New England J. Med. *223:*391–398, Sept 12, '40
Prevention of decubitus ulcers in fractures. FOX, T. A. AND APFELBACH, G. L., J.A.M.A. *115:*1438–1439, Oct 26, '40
Therapy of decubitus ulcers. ASTLEY, G. M. Am. J. Surg. *50:*734–737, Dec '40
Sawdust beds – summary of 7 years' experience (measure for prevention and treatment of bedsores). HOFMANN, H. M. Mod. Hosp. *56:*49–50, March '41
Therapy of decubitus ulcers. MORENO, J. Rev. clin. espan. *3:*243–244, Sept 1, '41
Topical use of sulfathiazole (sulfanilamide derivative) in decubitus ulcers; preliminary report. GOODMAN, J. I. AND CORSARO, J. F. Ohio State M. J. *37:*956–958, Oct '41
Trophic ulcers and their surgical therapy in injuries of sciatic nerve. TRAKHTENBERG, K. I. Vopr. neyrokhir. (no. 4) *5:*61, '41
Experimental studies in decubitus ulcer. GROTH, K. E. Nord. med. (Hygiea) *15:*2423–2428, Aug 29, '42
Half suspension of pelvis (to prevent bedsores). WESTHUES, H. Chirurg. *14:*489–493, Aug 15, '42
Decubitus ulcers. STUBINGER, K. Med. Klin. *38:*913–916, Sept 25, '42

Pressure Sores—Cont.

Pregnancy and labor complicated by ascending myelitis and bedsore of unusual size. DAWSON, J. B., J. Obst. & Gynaec. Brit. Emp. *50:*63, Feb '43

Decubitus ulcers. FUHS, H. Wien. klin. Wchnschr. *56:*145, Feb 26, '43

Clinical experiments with riboflavin (in decubital ulcer). VORHAUS, M. G. *et al.* Am. J. Digest. Dis. *10:*45–48, Feb '43

Half suspension of pelvis (to prevent bedsores). WESTHUES, H. Bull. War Med. *3:*440–441, April '43 (abstract)

Protein metabolism and bed sores. MULHOLLAND, J. H. *et al.* Ann. Surg. *118:*1015–1023, Dec '43

Acute postoperative decubitus following gynecologic and obstetric interventions. CLERC, J. P. Monatschr. f. Geburtsh. u. Gynak. *115:*128–137, '43

Blood transfusion in treatment of decubitus. SHAPIRO, S. E. Klin. med. (nos. 4-5) *21:*66, '43

Abdominal surgery in old age; mechanism of development of "bedsores." WANGENSTEEN, O. H. Journal-Lancet *64:*178–183, June '44

Therapy of decubitus. GROSSMAN, M. O. AND LIGHTFOOT, L. H. Hospital, *1:*35–36, Aug '45

War wounds of spinal cord; surgical treatment of decubitus ulcers. BARKER, D. E. J.A.M.A. *129:*160, Sept 8, '45

Apparatus for treating bedsores. NEIL, J. F. Brit. M. J. *2:*390, Sept 22, '45

Treatment of bedsores by total excision with plastic closure. WHITE, J. C. *et al.* U. S. Nav. M. Bull. *45:*454–463, Sept '45

Vitamin B complex therapy of decubital eschars. JACOB, A. C. AND MAFFEI, E. Rev. med. Rio Grande do Sul *2:*47–49, Sept-Oct '45

Operative treatment of decubitus ulcer. CROCE, E. J. *et al.* Ann. Surg. *123:*53–69, Jan '46

New hope for spinal cord sufferers (with decubitus). GUTTMANN, L., M. Times, New York *73:*318–326, Nov '45 also: South African M.J. *20:*141–144, March 23, '46

Methods of closure of decubitus ulcers in paralyzed patient. BARKER, D. E. *et al.* Ann. Surg. *123:*523–530, Apr '46

Methods of closure of decubitus ulcers in paralyzed patient. BARKER, D. E. *et al.* Tr. South. S. A. (1945) *57:*54–61, '46

PREVITALI, G. AND JACOBZINER, H.: Progressive facial and crossed hemiatrophy complicated by transient hypoglycemia. Am. J. Dis. Child. *60:*116–129, July '40

PREVITERA, A.: Failure of parathyroid extract in Dupuytren's contracture; 4 cases. Arch. ed atti d. Soc. ital. di chir. *40:*578–583, '34

PREVOT, M.: Hypertrophic fibrous cicatrix following esthetic operation on nose by endonasal route. Rev. de chir. structive, pp. 43–44, March '37

PREVOT, M.: Fissures of face, apropos of case of unusual labiogenal malformation. Rev. de chir. structive *8:*196–198, '38

PŘÍBRSKÝ, J.: Surgical technic for formation of artificial vagina. Zentralbl. f. Gynak. *59:*403–406, Feb 16, '35

PRICE, A. H. (see O'NEILL, J. F. *et al*) Sept '42

PRICE, A. H. (see TOCANTINS, L. M. *et al*) Dec '41

PRICE, P. B.: Transplantation of ureters into sigmoid in exstrophy; 3 operations on 2 cases. China M. J. *45:*634–643, July '31

PRICE, P. B.: Shock; prevention and treatment. S. Clin. North America *22:*1297–1310, Oct '42

PRICE, P. B. (see BLALOCK, A.) April '42

PRICORIU, S. (see POPESCU, G.) Oct '38

PRIESTLEY, J. B. (see WALTERS, W. *et al*) Aug '31

PRIESTLEY, J. T. (see RANKIN, F. W.) Dec '33

PRIMA, C.: Therapy of extensive burns. Zentralbl. f. Chir. *68:*243–245, Feb 8, '41

PRIMLANI, C. H.: Burns and their treatment. Sind M. J. *7:*1–7, Jun '34

Prince, D.

Plastic surgery in Mississippi Valley; David Prince. BLACK, C. E. Tr. West. S.A. (1937) *47:*287–309, '38

PRINGLE, J. H.: Cutaneous melanoma; 2 cases alive 30 and 38 years after operation. Lancet *1:*508–509, Feb 27, '37

PRINGLE, J. H.: Patient operated on for melanoma of thigh 30 years ago still without obvious recurrence. Tr. Roy. Med.-Chir. Soc. Glasgow, pp. 52–53, '36–'37; in Glasgow M. J. March '37

PRINGLE, J. H.: Treatment of acquired defects of skull (especially use of celluloid plates). Brit. M. J. *2:*1105–1107, Dec 4, '37

PRINZMETAL, M. AND BERGMAN, H. C.: The heart in experimental shock. J. Mt. Sinai Hosp. *12:*579–583, May–June '45

PRINZMETAL, M. AND BERGMAN, H. C.: Nature of circulatory changes in burn shock. Clin. Sc. *5:*205–227, Dec '45

PRINZMETAL, M.; BERGMAN, H. C. AND HECHTER, O.: Demonstration of 2 types of shock in burns. Surgery *16:*906–913, Dec '44

PRINZMETAL, M.; FREED, S. C. AND KRUGER, H. E.: Pathogenesis and treatment of shock resulting from crushing of muscle. War Med. *5:*74–79, Feb '44
PRINZMETAL, M. *et al*: Principle from liver effective against shock due to burns; preliminary report. J.A.M.A. *122:*720–723, July 10, '43. Also: J. Clin. Investigation *23:*795–806, Sept '44
PRINZMETAL, M. (see BERGMAN, H. C.) April '45
PRINZMETAL, M. (see BERGMAN, H. C. *et al*) April '45
PRINZMETAL, M. (see BERGMAN, H. C.) June '46
PRINZMETAL, M. (see HECHTER, O. *et al*) April '45
PRIOLEA, W. H.: Common hand infections; etiology and treatment. J. South Carolina M. A. *28:*276–278, Nov '32
PRIOLEAU, W. H.: Local treatment of surface burns. South. Med. & Surg. *106:*201–202, June '44
PRIOLEAU, W. H.: Harelip and cleft palate; plan of management. J. South Carolina M. A. *41:*129–130, June '45
PRIOLEAU, W. H.: Full thickness flap closure of large thoracotomy due to chemical destruction of chest wall (by injection of nitric acid). J. Thoracic Surg. *14:*433–437, Dec '45
PRIOLEAU, W. H.: Muscle flap closure of cavity resulting from lung abscess. Ann. Surg. *123:*664–672, April '46
PRISANT, M.: Chrondral autoplasty in correction of saddle nose. Folia oto-laryng. orient. *3:*205–211, '36
PRISSELKOFF, P. V.: Cork as prosthesis in correction of nasal defects. Vrach. gaz. *34:* 534–536, April 15, '30
PRISSELKOFF, P. V.: Morestin operation in dermatogenous contractures after burns. Vestnik khir. (no. 64) *22:*111–114, '30
PRITCHARD, J. E.: Biopsy as accurate guide to decision of early skin grafting. Ann. Surg. *121:*164–171, Feb '45
PRIWES, M. G. (see RUBASCHEWA, A.) 1932
PROBSTEIN, J. G.: Treatment of hand infections. S. Clin. North America *20:*1457–1472, Oct '40
PROBSTEIN, J. G. AND BROOKES, H. S. JR.: Treatment of infections of the terminal phalanges of hand. J. Missouri M. A. *21:*307–309, Sept '24
PROBY, H.: Esthetic reduction of nasal fractures with new apparatus; case. Arch. internat. de laryng. *34:*866–868, July-Aug '28
PROCHAZKA, A.: Making of arm and hand splints. Physiotherapy Rev. *18:*59–64, March-April '38
PROCTOR, S. E. (see DOBELLE, M.) May '44
PROELL, F.: First aid in jaw fractures. Deutsche med. Wchnschr. *65:*1538–1543, Oct 13, '39
PROETZ, A. W.: Planning surgery of nose. Tr. Am. Laryng., Rhin. & Otol. Soc. *48:*33–39, '42
PROETZ, A. W.: Planning nasal surgery. Arch. Otolaryng. *37:*502–506, April '43
PROETZ, A. W.: Nasal physiology from standpoint of plastic surgeon. Arch. Otolaryng. *39:*514–517, June '44
PRONK, K. J.: Flexor contracture of little finger, typical late tertiary symptom of tropical frambesia. Geneesk. tijdschr. v. Nederl.-Indie *81:*1403–1407, July 1, '41
PROPPE, A. AND GAHLEN, W.: Late sequels of roentgen depilation of scalp. Arch. f. Dermat. u. Syph. *108:*155–164, '40

Propper-Grashchenkov, N. I.: See Grashchenkov, N. I. P.

PROSKE, R.: Dorsal dislocation of proximal phalanx of second to fifth fingers. Beitr. z. klin. Chir. *136:*528–536, '26

Prostheses

Artificial velum for congenital cleft palate. PAYNE, J. L. Proc. Roy. Soc. Med. (Sect. Odontology) *14:*36, Feb '21
Prosthesis to correct facial paralysis. SICARD, J. A. Bull. et mem. Soc. med. d. hop. de Paris *45:*612, May 6, '21 abstr: J.A.M.A. *76:*1862, June 25, '21
Present status of prostheses, etc., for jaws. SCHROEDER, H. Arch. f. klin. Chir. *118:*275–297, '21 (illus.)
Prosthesis after removal of auricle for carcinoma. FENTON, R. A. AND LUPTON, I. M. Northwest Med. *22:*212, June '23 (illus.)
Treatment of nasal deformities, with special reference to nasal prosthesis. KAZANJIAN, V. H., J.A.M.A. *84:*177–181, Jan 17, '25
Appliance for pendulous breasts. GLASS, E. Deutsche med. Wchnschr. *51:*660, April 17, '25 abstr: J.A.M.A. *84:*1881, June 13, '25
Malnutrition in infants with cleft palate, with description of new external obturator. FOTTE, J. A. Am. J. Dis. Child. *30:*343–346, Sept '25
Replacement of nose and ear by gelatin prosthesis. STRAUSS. Schweiz. med. Wchnschr. *56:*464–465, May 15, '26
Prosthetic appliance in jaw surgery. EISELSBERG, A. Internat. Clin. *4:*220, Dec '26
Prosthetic treatment of harelip and cleft palate complications. RUPPE, L. AND RUPPE, C. Odontologie *64:*831–845, Dec 30, '26
Plastic preparation for prosthesis in extensive symblepharon. LIJÓ PAVÍA, J. Rev. Especialid. *1:*75–82, '26

Prostheses – Cont.
Velo-palatine prosthesis. RUPPE, L. AND RUPPE, C. Odontologie *65:*69–86, Feb 28, '27
Aids to palatal sufficiency after cleft palate operations. WOODS, R. Brit. M. J. *1:*371–372, Feb 26, '27
Prosthesis for cleft palate. RUPPE, L. AND RUPPE, C. Odontologie *65:*276–302, April '27
Case of surgical prosthesis of ear. AXT, E. F. Dental Cosmos *69:*828–830, Aug '27
Bucco-facial prosthesis in case of grave mutilation. BRUSOTTI, A. Stomatol. *25:*649–658, Aug '27
Grafts and bony implants for repairing large deficiencies in epiphysis and diaphysis; concealed internal prosthesis. MAUCLAIRE. Bull. et mem. Soc. nat. de chir. *53:*1363–1373, Dec 17, '27
Enucleation of eye-ball and cartilage transplantation as basis for prosthesis. FABER, A. Beitr. z. klin. Chir. *141:*524–527, '27
De la prosthèse immédiate des maxillaires. LeGrand, Paris, 1928
Obturators in treatment of rhinolalia aperta. FRÖSCHELS, E. AND SCHALIT, H. Wien. med. Wchnschr. *78:*840, June 23, '28
Nasal voice; treatment by obturator. SCHALIT, A. Wien. med. Wchnschr. *78:*964–966, July 14, '28
Form of new obturator (meatus obturator) for preventing nasal speech in cleft palate. FRÖSCHELS, E. Ztschr. f. Stomatol. *26:*882–888, Sept '28
Interdental fixation appliance for jaw fractures. WILLETT, R. C. Dental Items Interest *50:*788–799, Oct '28
Maxillofacial prosthesis. BODINE, R. L. Internat. J. Orthodontia *14:*998, Nov; 1076, Dec '28; *15:*42, Jan; 163, Feb; 254, March; 371, April '29
Nasal prosthesis in lupus treated with ultraviolet rays. DAUBRESSE-MORELLE, E. Ann. de l'Inst. chir. de Bruxelles *29:*161–165, Nov 15, '28
Prosthetic aids in reconstructive surgery about head; presentation of new methods (including ear, nose). LEDERER, F. L. Arch. Otolaryng. *8:*531–554, Nov '28
Dental prosthesis after resection of lower jaw. GREVE, K. Beitr. z. klin. Chir. *142:*747–752, '28
Simple wooden appliance for righting horizontal dislocations in treatment of jaw fractures. KUBASSOFF, M. N. Odont. i. stomatol. (no. 11) *6:*36–37, '28
Fastening of protective celluloid plates in

Prostheses – Cont.
uranoplasty. LIMBERG, A. A. Odont. i. stomatol. (no. 11) *6:*5–8, '28
Prosthesis in excision of mandible. LAMÉRIS, H. J. Nederl. Tijdschr. v. Geneesk. *1:*244–246, Jan 12, '29
Principles of prosthetic treatment in cleft palate. FISCHER, A. Ugesk. f. Laeger *91:*108–110, Feb 7, '29
Fracture of lower jaw; prosthetic treatment. ALEMAN. Cluj. med. *10:*378–395, Aug 1, '29
New obturator to combat nasalization in patients with cleft of hard palate. FRÖSCHELS, E. AND SCHALIT, A. Wien. klin. Wchnschr. *42:*1442–1444, Nov 7, '29
Resection, plastic surgery and prosthesis of jaw. PICHLER, H. Fortschr. d. Zahnheilk. *5:*1027–1043, Nov '29
Maxillofacial prosthesis. CHENET, H. Odontologie *67:*831–850, Dec '29
Prosthetic treatment of defects of mandible following unilateral exarticulation of mandible for adamantinoma; case. BERGENFELDT, E. Acta chir. Schandinav. *64:*473–492, '29
Prosthetic treatment of congenital gnathopalatoschisis; case. BAGGER, H. Ugesk. f. laeger *92:*66–69, Jan 16, '30
New nasal prosthesis (celluloid). ALEKSIEWICZ, J. Polska gaz. lek. *9:*214–216, March 16, '30
Correction of congenital cleft-palate speech by appliances. FITZ-GIBBON, J. J. Dental Cosmos *72:*231–238, March '30
Combined orthodontic and prosthetic treatment of cleft palate. LIFTON, J. C. Dental Items Interest *52:*503–513, July '30
Maxillofacial prosthesis of cellulose acetate. LAPIERRE, V. Odontologie *68:*634–653, Sept '30
Jaw resection; plastic and prosthetic surgery. AXHAUSEN, G. Fortschr. d. Zahnh. *6:*917–952, Nov '30
Preparation and adjustment of prosthesis in loss of auricular substance. CHENET, H. Odontologie *68:*861–870, Dec '30 also: Ann. d'oto-laryng., pp. 1–9, Jan '31
Correction of nasal speech from congenital defects of palate by obturators. REICHENBACH, E. Vrtljsschr. f. Zahnh. *46:*418–434, '30
Metallic crowns and bridges in maxillofacial orthopedics. FILDERMAN, J. Rev. odont. *52:*5–12, Jan '31
Fitz-Gibbon's prosthesis for correcting phonetic troubles in congenital cleft palate. FITZ-GIBBON, J. J. Odontologie *69:*760–767, Nov '31

Prostheses – Cont.
Facial prosthesis. ALESSANDRINI, I. *et al.* Bol. Soc. de cir., Chile *9:*450–451, Dec 23, '31
Substitute for implantation prosthesis and for osteoplasty in resection of jaw. SPANIER, F. Deutsche Ztschr. f. chir. *231:*456–469, '31
Prosthetic nose and face. CZERNYEI, G. Schweiz. med. Wchnschr. *62:*116, Jan 30, '32
Immediate maxillary prosthesis. PONT, A. Rev. de chir. plastique, pp. 264–270, Jan '32
Artificial ear, replacement of entire auricle. GULEKE. Chirurg *4:*274–278, April 1, '32
Experiences with new obturator in cleft palate. MELA, B. AND SEGRE, R. Stomatol. *30:*854–869, Sept '32
Use of negocoll and hominit in making moulages of face as aid in plastic surgery. IGLAUER, S. Laryngoscope *42:*774–778, Oct '32
Prosthesis of mouth and face. KAZANJIAN, V. H. *et al.* J. Dent. Research *12:*651–693, Oct '32
"Open bite"; surgical and prosthetic treatment. SCHMIDT, G. AND REICHENBACH, E. Deutsche Ztschr. f. Chir. *237:*167–176, '32
Progressive facial hemiatrophy treated by means of expansion prosthesis of oral cavity; case. BØE, H. W. Med. rev., Bergen *50:*212–225, May '33
Chenet technic in prosthesis of ear deformities. GRIMAUD, *et al.* Rev. med. de l'est. *61:*485–486, July 1, '33
Nasal prosthesis. WHYTE, D. Australian & New Zealand J. Surg. *3:*74–75, July '33
Facial prosthesis with cellulose acetate, technic. LAPIERRE, V. Rev. de chir. plastique, pp. 168–217, Oct '33
New obturator for use in case of unsuccessful uranoplasty, with reference to surgical and prosthetic therapeutic methods in palatine defects. KAHN, W. Ztschr. f. Stomatol. *32:*18–27, Jan 12, '34
Reparation of bone loss by Ollier osteoperiostic grafts, segmentary bone grafts, bone implantations and hidden internal prostheses. MAUCLAIRE. Rev. med. franc. *15:*263–273, March '34
Surgical and orthopedic prosthetic correction of depression of middle portion of face due to automobile accidents; cases. DUFOURMENTEL, L. AND DARCISSAC, M. Rev. de stomatol. *36:*447–457, July '34
Dental prosthesis in relation to reparative surgery of face. KAZANJIAN, V. H. Surg., Gynec. & Obst. *59:*70–80, July '34
Fractures of lower jaw; prosthetic therapy.

Prostheses – Cont.
CITOLER SESÉ, R. Clin. y lab. *25:*129–132, Aug '34
Facial hemiatrophia progressiva treated with expansion prosthesis in mouth; case. BØE, H. W. Acta psychiat. et neurol. *9:*1–27, '34
Celluloid prosthesis in cosmetic correction after disfiguring surgery of frontal sinus. STUPKA, W. Arch. f. Ohren-Nasen-u. Kehlkopfh. *138:*79–86, '34
La pratique stomatologique. Tome VIII: Restauration et prosthese maxillofaciales. Ed. by Chompret. Masson et Cie, Paris, 1935
Use of moulages in application of skin grafts; 2 cases. ESSER, J. F. S. Presse med. *43:*1286–1288, Aug 14, '35
Use of gelatin prosthesis in restoration of face. BATSON, O. V. Tr. Am. Acad. Ophth. *40:*317–326, '35
Protective prosthesis for plastic operation on palate. HOTTA, H. Ztschr. d. japan, chirurg. Gesellsch. *36:*100–101, '35
Reconstruction of orbital cavity for wearing prosthesis long after exenteration of orbit. LOTIN, A. V. Sovet. vestnik oftal. *7:*402, '35
Surgical prosthetics of oral and facial defects. OLINGER, N. A. AND AXT, E. F. Am. J. Surg. *31:*24–37, Jan '36
Loss of external ear and its artificial replacement. HARTMANN, E. Nord. med. tidskr. *11:*728–729, May 2, '36
Prosthesis covering orbital region, nose and upper lip. PONT, AND LAPIERRE, V. Bull. Soc. franc. de dermat. et syph. (Reunion dermat., Lyon) *43:*908–910, May '36
Preoperative and postoperative prosthesis in application of skin, cutaneomucosal, cartilage and bone grafts and in improvement of cicatrix of face. DARCISSAC, M. Bull. et mem. Soc. d. chirurgiens de Paris *28:*424–433, June 19, '36
Prosthetic therapy for cleft palate. SEGRE, R. Monatschr. f. Ohrenh. *70:*865–884, July '36
Nasal prosthesis to hide deformity; case. ALVES, D. Rev. oto-laring. de Sao Paulo (no. 5 bis) *4:*873–877, Sept–Oct '36
Prosthetic appliance for atresia palati in edentulous patient. AMIES, A. AND BAGHEL, D., M. J. Australia *2:*600–601, Oct 31, '36
Surgical therapy of temporomaxillary ankylosis followed by prosthesis of dental arches. VARGAS SALCEDO, L. AND ILABACA L., L. Bol. y trab. de la Soc. de cir. de Buenos Aires *20:*1071–1082, Oct 21, '36
Prosthesis in restorative surgery of face. DARCISSAC, M. Rev. de chir. structive, pp. 420–424, Dec '36

Prostheses – Cont.

Protective prosthesis for plastic operations of palate. HOTTA, H. Nagoya J. M. Sc. *10:*280–284, Dec '36

Claims of various obturators, from standpoint of correction of speech defects in cleft palate. REICHENBACH, E. Hals-, Nasen-. u. Ohrenarzt (Teil 1) *28:*29–33, Feb '37

Apparatus for immediate treatment and prosthesis in jaw fractures. DI GIUSEPPE, F. Gior. ital. di clin. trop. *1:*81, March 31, '37

Articulated prosthesis of eye, nose and upper lip; case. PONT, A. AND LAPIERRE, V. Rev. de chir. structive, pp. 38–41, March '37

Technic of making artificial noses. SIMONS, R. D. G. P. Nederl. tijdschr. v. geneesk. *81:*1421–1425, April 3, '37

Personal reminiscences of men and methods in field of prosthesis in jaw surgery. STOPPANY, G. A. Ztschr. f. Stomatol. *35:*525–531, April 23, '37

Prosthetic treatment of cleft palate. BAGGER, H. Nord. med. tidskr. *13:*685–689, May 1, '37

Nasal prosthesis with heavy paraffin. FRIEDMANN, L. Romania med. *15:*186–187, July 1–15, '37

Orthopedic plate in therapy of jaw deformities. JARDENI, J. AND AUERBACH, H. Ztschr. f. Stomatol. *35:*1019–1028, Aug 13, '37

Use of rubber sponge (new flesh) over period of 25 years. FIESCHI, D. Arch. ital. di chir. *46:*221–251, '37

Formation of artificial hand. FUKS, B. I. Novy khir. arkhiv *39:*125–129, '37

Cleft palate operation supplemented by obturator in treatment. FITZGERALD, R. R. Brit. J. Surg. *25:*816–825, April '38

Plastic surgery of alveolar process as preparation for artificial plates. JAKABHAZY, I. Orvosi hetil. *82:*338–340, April 9, '38

Prosthetic therapy of acquired palatal defects. EHRICKE, A. Med. Welt *12:*775–776, May 28, '38

Ivory prosthesis in partial rhinoplasty; cases. MALBEC, E. Semana med. *1:*1374–1382, June 16, '38

Construction of the amputated shoulder in order to fit a prosthesis with a mechanical arm. COELST. Rev. de chir. structive *8:*117–122, Aug '38

Useful prostheses for nasal and facial defects due to destructive lesions. SCHMID, R. Munchen. med. Wchnschr. *85:*1784–1786, Nov 18, '38 comment by Moncorps *86:*252–253, Feb 17, '39

Feeding infant with cleft palate with aid of dental plate; 5 cases. SILLMAN, J. H. Am. J. Dis. Child. *56:*1055–1058, Nov '38

Deformation of lower jaw corrected by surgical intervention and prosthesis. THEODORESCO, D. Rev. de chir., Bucuresti *41:*926–930, Nov–Dec '38

Elastic prosthesis for nasal defects. SIEMENS, H. W. Munchen. med. Wchnschr. *85:*1987–1988, Dec 23, '38 comment by Zinsser *86:*252, Feb 17, '39 comment by Moncorps *86:*252–253, Feb 17, '39 comment by Bering *86:*253–254, Feb 17, '39 reply by Siemens *86:*254, Feb 17, '39

Rubber plate as support for mouth following cleft palate operation. JANTZEN, J. Deutsche Ztschr. f. Chir. *249:*651–656, '38

Dental prosthesis in relation to plastic and reconstructive surgery of face. JOACHIM. Rev. de chir. structive *8:*212–215, '38

Construction of nose by prosthesis (case). CLAFLIN, R. S. Am. J. Orthodontics *25:*92–93, Jan '39

Simple and practical technic for making facial cases. BULBULIAN, A. H., J. Am. Dent. A. *26:*347–354, March '39

Technic for producing facial masks and models. WEST, B. S. Ann. Surg. *109:*474–478, March '39

Os purum as biologic element of internal prosthesis. DE ROMANA, J. Dia med. (Ed. espec.), no. 2, pp. 19–20, April '39

Aid to prosthetic restorations of maxilla after excision. WALKER, D. G. Lancet *1:*1209–1210, May 27, '39

Improved technic for prosthetic restoration of defects of face by use of latex compound. BULBULIAN, A. H. Proc. Staff Meet., Mayo Clin. *14:*433–439, July 12, '39

Prosthesis for lupus and other facial defects. STÜMPKE, G. Dermat. Wchnschr. *109:*1058–1061, Sept 2, '39

Centers for restorative surgery and prosthesis after war wounds. LEMAITRE. Mem. Acad. de chir. *65:*1143–1147, Oct 25–Nov 8, '39

Prosthetic restorations of defects of face by use of latex compound; further detailed description of technic used. BULBULIAN, A. H. Proc. Staff Meet., Mayo Clin. *14:*721–727, Nov 15, '39

Finger prosthesis made from hard and soft rubber joined by vulcanizing. ORELL, S. Nord. med. (Hygiea) *4:*3346–3348, Nov 11, '39

Psychologic aspects of problem of artificial ear, with critical comment on rigid permanent prosthesis and elastic temporary pros-

Prostheses – Cont.
thesis. FUNK, F. Dermat. Wchnschr. *109:*1402-1407, Dec 30, '39
Use of ocular prosthesis during plastic reconstruction of conjunctival sac with free cutaneous or mucous graft. NEYMAN, V. N. Vestnik oftal. (no. 5) *14:*45-46 '39
Silver-plated vaginal prosthesis for construction of artificial vagina. WORD, B. Am. J. Obst. & Gynec. *39:*1071, June '40
Artificial ear and nose. BULBULIAN, A. H. Hygeia *18:*980-982, Nov '40
Facial masks; new technic using newly devised matrix for impression. KAUFMAN, J. L., J. Am. Dent. A. *28:*64-66, Jan '41
Repair of facial defects with prosthesis using latex compound. BULBULIAN, A. H., J. Am. Dent. A. *28:*559-571, April '41 abstr., Mil. Surgeon *88:*179-182, Feb '41
Moulage prosthesis for face. CLARKE, C. D., J. Lab. and Clin. Med. *26:*901-912, Feb '41 also: Am. J. Orthodontics (Oral Surg. Sect) *27:*214-225, April '41
Rhinoplastic surgery combined with paraffin prosthesis in correction of saddle nose. DUJARDIN, E. Ugesk. f. laeger *103:*404-405, March 27, '41
Prosthetic reconstruction of nose and ear with latex compound. BULBULIAN, A. H. J.A.M.A. *116:*1504-1506, April 5, '41
Repair of facial defects with prosthesis using latex compound. BULBULIAN, A. H., J. Am. Dent. A. *28:*559-571, April '41 abstr., Mil. Surgeon *88:*179-182, Feb '41
Buccomaxillofacial prosthesis; artificial nose and palate; case. GRAZIANI, M. Rev. brasil. de oto-rino-laring. *9:*217-221, May-June '41
Prosthetic inclusions. ZENO, L. Bol. Soc. de cir. de Rosario *8:*158-169, June '41
Psychology of lupus patients with nasal prostheses. KALKOFF, K. W. Dermat. Wchnschr. *113:*597-601, July 12, '41
Facial reconstruction with acrylic resin. MUNSON, F. T. AND HERON, D. F. Am. J. Surg. *53:*291-295, Aug '41
Prosthetic inclusions in plastic surgery. ZENO, L. An. de cir. *7:*108-118, Sept '41
Application and wearing of facial prostheses. CLARKE, C. D., J. Lab. and Clin. Med. *27:*123-126, Oct '41
Facial prosthesis. CARNEY, H. J. Am. J. Orthodontics (Oral Surg. Sect.) *27:*689-697, Dec '41
Prosthesis of orbit and surrounding parts of face. RUMYANTSEVA, A. F. Vestnik oftal. (nos. 3-4) *19:*153-154, '41
Facial prostheses. MATTHEWS, E. Brit. M. J. *1:*223, Feb. 14, '42

Prostheses – Cont.
Latex prosthesis for cosmetic restoration of amputated breast. BROWN, A. M. South. Surgeon *11:*181-188, March '42
Extraoral device for immobilization of mandibular fractures. ALESSANDRINI, I. Rev. med. de Chile *70:*298-299, April '42
Orbital prosthesis after Riedel operation in frontal sinusitis; case. ALVES, O. Arq. de cir. clin. e exper. *6:*322-323, April-June '42
Internal prosthesis with autotransplant of bone or cartilage. JORGE, J. M. AND MEALLA, E. S. Arq. de cir. clin. e exper. *6:*539-540, April-June '42
Care of military and civilian facial injuries; surgical prosthesis. OLINGER, N. A., Am. J. Orthodontics (Oral Surg. Sect) *28:*222-238, April '42
Osteoplasty of mandibular arch and complementary surgical prosthesis. SOUZA CUNHA, A. Arq. de cir. clin. e exper. *6:*587-593, April-June '42
Prosthetic inclusions in plastic surgery. ZENO, L. Arq. de cir. clin. e exper. *6:*523-531, April-June '42
Correction of facial defects with latex prostheses; technic. BROWN, A. M. Arch. Otolaryng. *35:*720-731, May '42
Utilization of vitallium appliances to treat edentulous mandible fractures. LOGSDON, C. M., J. Am. Dent. A. *29:*970-978, June 1, '42
Congenital and postoperative loss of ear; reconstruction by prosthetic method. BULBULIAN, A. H., J. Am. Dent. A. *29:*1161-1168, July 1, '42
Simple device for temporary support of fractured mandible. ROMMEL, R. W., U. S. Nav. M. Bull. *40:*977, Oct '42
Extensive mutilating defect of face; cosmetic correction with latex mask. BROWN, A. M. Surgery *12:*957-961, Dec '42
Submucous cleft palate; traumatic perforation by denture. GINGRASS, R. P. Am. J. Orthodontics (Oral Surg. Sect) *28:*113-114, Feb '42
Artist's approach to restorative prosthetics. EDWARDS, B. Mil. Surgeon *92:*197-201, Feb '43
Appliance for use in conservative treatment of collum fractures of mandible, in maintaining vertical dimension of jaw, and for overcoming spasm of elevator muscles of mandible. GRUBER, L. W. AND LYFORD, J. III. Am. J. Orthodontics (Oral Surg. Sect.) *29:*160-162, March '43
Facial restorations. BIGELOW, H. M., J. Am. Dent. A. *30:*509-512, April 1, '43
Simple procedure for relief of entropion (de-

Prostheses—Cont.
vice attached to spectacle frame). WIENER, A. Arch. Ophth. *29:*634, April '43
Orthopedic-prosthetic therapy of fractures of condyloid process of mandible. HED, H. Nord. med. (Hygiea) *18:*789–793, May 8, '43
Moulages as aid to maxillofacial restorations. JACOBSEN, H. H. AND BARRON, J. B. Mil. Surgeon *92:*511-520, May '43
Nasal fracture device. WOMACK, D. R., U. S. Nav. M. Bull. *41:*852–856, May '43
Maxillofacial prosthesis. NAGLE, R. J. Am. J. Orthodontics (Oral Surg. Sect.) *29:*312–319, June '43
Appliances and attachments for treatment of upper jaw fractures. CRAWFORD, M. J., U. S. Nav. M. Bull. *41:*1151-1157, July '43
Plastic as substitute for metal in fracture appliances in facial fractures. FREEMAN, J. J. Oral Surg. *1:*241-245, July '43
Symposium on facial restorations (prostheses). MANSIE, J. W. *et al.* Proc. Roy. Soc. Med. *36:*483-487, July '43
Coloring and applying prosthesis to face. CLARKE, C. D., J. Lab. and Clin. Med. *28:*1517-1534, Sept '43
Severe retrusion of mandible treated by buccal inlay and dental prosthesis. FICKLING, B. W. Proc. Roy. Soc. Med. *37:*7-10, Nov '43
Use of acrylic and elastic resin prosthesis for deformities of face. SWEEZEY, E. *et al.* Canad. M. A. J. *50:*16–21, Jan '44
Construction of simple obturator in cleft palate. GEMMELL, J. A. M. Brit. Dent. J. *76:*69–70, Feb 4, '44
Prosthetic reconstruction of face. GERRIE, J. W., Canad. M. A. J. *50:*104-109, Feb '44
Extraoral facial prosthesis; elastic vinyl (vinylite resin) plastic method. GURDIN, M. M. *et al.* U. S. Nav. M. Bull. *42:*644–650, March '44
Prosthetic appliance for war injury (maxillofacial injuries). JEFFREYS, F. E., U. S. Nav. M. Bull. *42:*711-714, March '44
Practical elastic permanent prosthesis for facial defects. SCHMID, R. Munchen. med. Wchnschr. *91:*183, April 7, '44
Prosthesis in relation to war wounds of face. CLARKE, C. D., M. Bull. North African Theat. Op. (no. 1) *1:*17–24, Jan '44 also: J. Lab. and Clin. Med. *29:*667-672, June '44
Use of acrylic resin for prostheses of face. COFFIN, F. Brit. Dent. J. *77:*36–39, July 21, '44
Prostheses for eye and orbit. BROWN, A. M. Arch. Ophth. *32:*208–212, Sept '44
Obturators for palate; review. BEDER, O. E. J. Oral Surg. *2:*356–368, Oct '44

Prostheses—Cont.
Maxillofacial prosthesis. LLOYD, R. S., J. Am. Dent. A. *31:*1328–1335, Oct 1, '44
Prosthetic appliance for comminuted fracture of nose; case. SCHORK, C. J., J. Oral Surg. *2:*324-328, Oct '44
Hemiresection of lower jaw; immediate prosthesis with later iliac bone graft. FINOCHIETTO, R. *et al.* Semana med. (tomo cincuent., fasc. 1) pp. 65–71, '44
Facial and Body Prosthesis, by CARL D. CLARKE. C. V. Mosby Co., St. Louis, 1945
Facial Prosthesis, by ARTHUR H. BULBULIAN. W. B. Saunders Co., Phila., 1945
Cleft palate prosthesis. SCHOLE, M. L. AND KATZ, T. Bull. U. S. Army M. Dept. (no.84) pp. 90–93, Jan '45
Adamantinoma of lower jaw; surgical therapy with immediate prosthesis; case. RONCORONI, E. J. AND CICCHETTI, J. N. Bol. Soc. de cir. de Rosario *12:*27–40, May '45
Correction of cleft palate using stress-breaker type partial appliance with obturator attached. BEDER, O. E. *et al.* Am. J. Orthodontics (Oral Surg. Sect.) *31:*377–380, June '45
Fracture of mandible at angle; appliance to depress posterior fragment. HARRIS, L. W. AND CHRISTIANSEN, G. W., J. Oral Surg. *3:*212–214, July '45
Prosthetic device for support of eyelids. KOHOUT, J. J. Bull. U. S. Army M. Dept. *4:*117–118, July '45
Obturator (acrylic) for newborn infant with cleft palate. SCHAPIRO, I. E. *et al.* J. Pediat. *27:*288–290, Sept '45
Embedment of vitallium mandibular prosthesis as integral part of operation for removal of adamantinoma. WINTER, L. *et al.* Am. J. Surg. *69:*318–324, Sept '45
Prosthesis for palate; treatment of case with hollow-ball obturator. CANTOR, B. B. Am. J. Orthodontics (Oral Surg. Sect.) *31:*740–743, Dec '45
Maxillofacial prosthesis. DE MONTIGNY, G. Union med. du Canada *74:*1727–1735, Dec '45
Adjustable, non-solid appliance for nasal restoration, attached to upper denture. ASHWORTH, H. S. Brit. Dent. J. *80:*157-160, March 1, '46
Technic for taking imprint for construction of prosthesis for cleft palate. CABROL. Rev. de stomatol. *47:*157–159, May–June '46
Plastic and dental prosthetic repair of jaw injuries. GREELEY, P. W. AND POUND, A. E. Illinois M. J. *89:*216–221, May '46
Micrognathia; paladon prosthesis in case. MALBEC, E. F. J. Internat. Coll. Surgeons

Prostheses – Cont.
*9:*412–415, May–June '46 Bol. y trab., Acad. argent. de cir. *30:*151–156, May 15 '46
Saddle nose; correction by means of tantalum prosthesis; case. MALBEC, E. F. Bol. y trab., Soc. argent. de cirujanos *7:*173–177, '46 also: Rev. Asoc. med. argent. *60:*361–363, May 30, '46
Prosthetic restoration of congenital cleft palate. OLINGER, N. A. Am. J. Orthodontics (Oral Surg. Sect.) *32:*456–468, July '46
Temporary prosthesis as aid in treatment of war injuries of face. EMORY, L. Mil. Surgeon *99:*105–109, Aug '46
Oral prosthesis in repair of war injuries. POUND, E. Am. J. Orthodontics (Oral Surg. Sect) *32:*435–439, Aug '46
Cineplastic forearm amputations and prostheses. RANK, B. K. AND HENDERSON, G. D. Surg. Gynec. and Obst. *83:*373–386, Sept '46
Present status of speech training of patients who wear speech correction appliances. BAKES, F. P. Am. J. Orthodontics (Oral Surg. Sect.) *32:*718–723, Nov '46
Responsibility of prosthodontist in treatment of cleft palate. HARKINS, C. S. Am. J. Orthodontics (Oral Surg. Sect.) *32:*684–687, Nov '46
Responsibility of speech correctionist in treatment of patient who has received surgical or prosthetic treatment. KOEPP-BAKER, H. Am. J. Orthodontics (Oral Surg. Sect.) *32:*714–717, Nov '46
Obturator of choice for congenital cleft palate. SCHALIT, A. Am. J. Orthodontics (Oral Surg. Sect.) *32:*688–713, Nov '46
Modern Plastic Surgical Prosthetics, by ADOLPH M. BROWN. Grune and Stratton Co., New York, 1947

PROWSE, C. B.: Acute nephritis following acute cellulitis of hand and forearm; case. St. Barth. Hosp. J. *39:*191–193, July '32
PRUCE, A. M.: Splint to correct deformity (claw-hand) resulting from injury to ulnar nerve. J. Bone and Joint Surg. *28:*397, Apr '46
PRUCE, A. M.: Peripheral nerve injuries; treatment. South. M. J. *39:*289–291, April '46
PRUDENTE, A.: Surgical correction of uncomplicated saddle nose by partial inclusion of ivory. Rev. Assoc. paulista de med. *5:*75–78, Aug '34
PRUDENTE, A.: Otoneoplasty. Rev. oto-laring. de Sao Paulo *2:*388–391, Sept–Oct '34
PRUDENTE, A.: Reparation of loss of substance due to electrosurgical therapy of nasofacial cancer. Rev. oto-laring. de Sao Paulo (no. 5, bis) *4:*749–810, Sept–Oct '36
PRUDENTE, A.: Reconstruction following ablation of cancer of face. Bull. et mem. Soc. d. chirurgiens de Paris *28:*485–496, Nov 6, '36
PRUDENTE, A.: Restorative surgery following surgical or pathologic loss of substance in cancer and leprosy. Rev. de chir. structive, pp. 148–154, June '37
PRUDENTE, A.: Repair of loss of substance of throat due to extensive burns. Rev. Assoc. paulista de med. *11:*43–51, July '37
PRUDENTE, A.: Hemiresection of lower jaw with immediate osteoperiosteal graft in multilocular cancer; technical study. Rev. de cir. de Sao Paulo *3:*245–258, Aug '37
PRUDENTE, A.: Skin grafts in protection of exposed area after extirpation of cancer. Arch. urug. de med., cir. y especialid. *12:*196–209, Feb '38
PRUDENTE, A.: Surgical correction of protruding ear. Rev. de cir. de Sao Paulo *5:*17–26, July–Aug '39
PRUDENTE, A.: Surgical correction of deformities due to leprosy, in nose. Presse med. *48:*156–158, Feb 6, '40
PRUDENTE, A.: Plastic repair of total loss of nose; 8 cases. Arq. de cir. clin. e exper. *6:*174–183, April–June '42
PRUDENTE, A.: Regeneration technic in plastic surgery of buttocks, using blood as "nutritive bed"; illustrative case. Arq. de cir. clin. e exper. *6:*272–280, April–June '42
PRUDENTE, A.: Keysser's work and plastic surgery of cancer. Arq. de cir. clin. e exper. *6:*316–320, April–June '42
PRUDENTE, A.: Extirpation of cervical lymph nodes in cancer of mouth with metastases. Bol. y trab., Acad. argent. de cir. *26:*1030–1031, Oct 28, '42
PRUDENTE, A.: Musculocutaneous graft and its importance in war surgery. Rev. paulista de med. *22:*435–436, June '43
PRUDENTE, A.: Skin grafting in plastic surgery. Rev. paulista de med. *22:*439–441, June '43
PRUDENTE, A.: Plastic surgery and war. Imprensa med., Rio de Janeiro *19:*39–58, Sept '43
PRUDENTE, A.: Biologic recovery of skin grafts doomed to necrosis, by means of histamine; preliminary report. Rev. paulista de med. *23:*262–265, Nov '43
PRUDENTE, A.: Free muscle transplantation in restoration of lips and cheeks. Rev. paulista de med. *23:*344–345, Dec '43 J. Internat. Coll. Surgeons *7:*312–313, July–Aug '44
PRUDENTE, A. AND ARIE, G.: Physiologic integration of skin grafts. Arq. de cir. clin. e exper. *6:*577–586, April–June '42

PRUDENTE DE AQUINO, F.: Congenital bilateral imperforation of nostril; case. Rev. brasil. de oto-rino-laring *7:*255-262, May-June '39

PRUD'HOMME, E.: Use of cobra venom in generalized nevocarcinoma; case. J. de l'Hotel-Dieu de Montreal *4:*372-378, Dec '35

PRUVOT, M.: Dressings after submucous resection of septum. Rev. de laryng. *63:*196-199, June-July '42

PSAUME. (see PONROY) 1940

PSAUME. (see PONROY, *et al*) Nov '27

PSAUME. (see PONROY, *et al*) Sept '28

Psychology: See Plastic Surgery, Psychology of

PTIC, D.: Congenital anomalies of fingers. Polski przegl. radjol. *10-11:*65-70, '36

PUDENZ, R. H. (see WEBSTER, G. V. *et al*) July '45

PUENTE DUANY, N.: Branchial dermoepidermic cysts, with report of cases. Arch. cubanos cancerol. *3:*133-156, April-June '44

PUENTE DUANY, N.: Dermoepidermal branchial cysts. Rev. med. cubana *55:*398, May; 449, June '44

PUENTE, DUANY, N. (see MARTÍNEZ, E.) July '28

PUESTOW, C. B.; PONCHER, H. G. AND HAMMATT, H.: Vitamin oils in burns; experimental study. Surg., Gynec. and Obst. *66:*622-627, March '38

PUHL, H.: Anuria and symptoms of uremia in clinical picture of postoperative shock. Deutsche Ztschr. f. Chir. *235:*393-413, '32

PUGA, R.: Use of palpebral conjunctiva in reconstruction of inferior fornix. Amatus *2:*207-211, Mar '43

PUIG, J. (see BERCHER, J. *et al*) Oct '27

PULFORD, D. S. AND ADSON, A. W.: Surgical removal and pathological study of massive squamous cell epithelioma associated with angioma of scalp. Surg., Gynec. and Obst. *42:*846-848, June '26

PULFORD, D. S. (see LARSON, E. E.) 1929

PULIDO, A. (see GIMENO Y RODRÍGUEZ JAÉN, V.) May-June '23

PULLEINE, R. H.: Martyrdom of the nose. M. J. Australia (supp.) *1:*385-386, June 7, '24

PUND, E. R. (see GREENBLATT, R. B. *et al*) Feb '36

PUNTENNEY, I.: Plastic procedures of eyelids. Illinois M. J. *88:*238-242, Nov '45

PUNTENNEY, I. (see GIFFORD, S. R.) Nov '42

PUPPENDAHL, M. (see LAM, C. R.) June '45

PUSITZ, M. E.: Burn therapy. J. Kansas M. Soc. *36:*148, April '35

PUTSCHKOWSKY, A.: Pedicled grafts in therapy of defects of hard palate. Ztschr. f. Laryng., Rhin., Otol. *22:*98-102, '31

Putti-Krukenberg Operation

Phalangization of stumps of forearm amputations (Putti-Krukenberg operation); 13 cases. BIRCKEL, A. Strasbourg-med. (pt. 2) *85:*437-447, Dec 20, '27

PÜTZ, T.: Deformities of ventral line of abdominal closure; umbilical hernia and gastroschisis. Geburtsh. u. Frauenh. *1:*663-671, Oct '39

PUTZKI, P. S. AND SCULLY, J. H.: Inappropriate treatment of moles predisposing to melanotic malignancies. M. Ann. District of Columbia *15:*320-324, July '46

PUTZU DONEDDU, F.: Monolateral amastia; case. Arch. di ostet. e ginec. *41:*1-13, Jan '34

PUYO VILLAFANE, E.: Application of Wolff's law to bone transplants. Semana med. *2:*840-843, Oct 8, '42

PYATNITSKIY, F. A.: Organizational problem of nutrition in maxillofacial trauma. Klin. med. (nos. 3-4) *20:*22-28, '42

Q

QUADRI, S.: Cystic lymphangioma associated with grave congenital malformations; study of cervical hygromas. Clin. pediat. *17:*755-777, Oct '35

QUARTERO: Cavernous angioma of cheek; case. Nederl. Tijdschr. v. Geneesk. *1:*1997, April 21, '28

QUEEN, F. B. (see MASON, M. L.) 1941

QUELPRUD, T.: Ear pit and its inheritance; fistula auris congenita, described in 1864, still genetic and embryologic puzzle. J. Hered. *31:*379-384, Sept '40

QUEMADURAS: Burn review. Semana med. *2:*33-37, July 1, '43

QUÉNU: Research of Fenton B. Turck on traumatic shock. Bull. Acad. de med., Par. *87:*92-97, Jan 24, '22

DE QUERVAIN, F.: Surgical treatment of pendulous breast. Schweiz. med. Wchnschr. *56:*451-453, May 15, '26

DE QUERVAIN, F.: Technic in plastic surgery. Zentralbl. f. Chir. *56:*1218-1219, May 18, '29

DE QUERVAIN, F.: Electrocoagulation therapy of subcutaneous angiomas. Schweiz. med. Wchnschr. *61:*1169-1170, Dec 5, '31

DE QUERVAIN, F.: Operative treatment of complete epispadias. Ztschr. f. urol. Chir. *36:*237-242, '33

DE QUERVAIN, F.: Surgical therapy of prognathism. Chirurg *10:*256-260, April 15, '38

QUESADA, F.: Rhinoplasty; 3 cases. Dia med. *4:*16, Aug 3, '31

QUICK, B.: Gillies tubed pedicle flap in cleft

palate. J. Coll. Surgeons, Australasia *2:*395-400, March '30
QUICK, B.: Treatment of bone cavities (including use of molds for grafts). Australian and New Zealand J. Surg. *13:*3-10, July '43
QUICK, D.: Radium in treatment of epithelioma of lip. J. Radiol. *2:*1, Dec '21
QUICK, D.: Carcinoma of floor of mouth. Am. J. Roentgenol. *10:*461-470, June '23 (illus.)
QUICK, D.: Treatment of cancer of lips. Am. J. Roentgenol. *21:*322-327, April '29
QUICK, D.: Special clinic on epithelioma of lips. Am. J. Cancer *15:*229-270, Jan '31
QUICK, D. A. AND JOHNSON, F. M.: Statistics and technique in treatment of malignant neoplasms of larynx. Am. J. Roentgenol. *9:*599-606, Sept '22
QUIGLEY, R. A.: Intestinal obstruction simulated by segregated closed loop of bowel; case following Baldwin operation for artificial vagina. Northwest Med. *28:*122-123, March '29
QUINTARELLI, L.: Necrotic ulcer from cocaine-epinephrine injections; 2 cases (palatal vault). Ann. di med. nav. *1:*67-75, Jan-Feb '27
QUINTELA, U. (see ALONSO, J. M.) 1931
QUIRNO LAVALLE, R. (see MALLO HUERGO, E.) Aug '42
QUIROGA, P.: Rural esthetic surgery. Semana med. *2:*1454-1456, Dec 30, '43
QUIROZ, F.: Complete lateral alternate bisexual hermaphroditism; surgical therapy of case. Cir. y cirujanos *5:*299-307, July '37

R

DE RAAD, H.: Operation for aplasia of vagina. Nederl. tijdschr. v. verlosk. en gynaec. *40:*153-158, '37
RABINOVICI, N. (see MANDL, F.) July-Aug '46
RABINOVICI, N. (see MANDL, F.) Sept-Oct '46
RABINOVITCH, C. N.: Formation of artificial vagina; contribution to 25th anniversary of Baldwin operation. Am. J. Surg. *13:*480-483, Sept '31
RABINOVITCH, P.: Homio transplantation of skin flaps. Proc. Soc. Exper. Biol. and Med. *25:*798-799, June '28
RABINOWITCH, I. M.: Treatment of phosphorus burns (with note on acute phosphorus poisoning). Canad. M. A. J. *48:*291-296, April '43
RABINOWITSCH, K. N.: Artificial vagina made by Baldwin's method for congenital defect in vagina. Zentralbl. f. Gynak *50:*1851-1864, July 10, '26 abstr: J.A.M.A. *87:*1081, Sept 25, '26
RABINOWITZ, H. M. AND PELNER, L.: Topical application of horse serum in extensive burns. Am. J. Surg. *64:*55-63, April '44
RABL, R. AND SCHULZ, F.: Congenital cardiac defects and harelip with clefts of jaw and palate in twins. Virchows Arch. f. path. Anat. *305:*505-520, '39
RABUT, R.: Various methods of treating keloids. Hopital *21:*763-765, Dec (B) '33
RABUT, R.: Traumatic alopecias of scalp; different types. Presse med. *46:*379-380, March 9, '38
RACOVEANU, V.: Plastic surgery of nose. Spitalul *52:*402-414, Oct '32
RACZ, B.: Tannic acid in burns. Orvosi hetil. *80:*756-757, Aug 8, '36
RADAELI, A.: Late syphilis with destructive gummatous manifestations in nasal bones and first cervical vertebrae; cleft palate; case. Gior. ital. di dermat. e sif. *73:*531, Feb '32
RADCLIFFE, F. (see LEE, W. D.) Jan '40
RADCLIFFE, W.: Rare congenital malformation of upper lip. Brit. J. Surg. *28:*329-330, Oct '40

Radial Nerve: See Nerves, Radial

Radiation Injuries

X-ray burn of third degree followed by rapid healing. BLAINE, E. S. Am. J. Roentgenol. *8:*183, April '21
X-ray burns. BEVAN, A. D., S. Clin. N. Amer. *1:*935, Aug '21
Surgical treatment of X-ray burns. BLAIR, E. G., J. Radiol. *5:*149-152, May '24
Treatment of grave roentgen burns of hands with radium and Doramad ointment. FABRY, J. Med. Klinik *21:*1498, Oct 2, '25
Treatment of X-ray burn. BARROW, S. C. Radiology *4:*54, Jan '25
Electrocoagulation of desiccation in treatment of keratoses and malignant degeneration which follow radiodermatitis. PFAHLER, G. E. Am. J. Roentgenol. *13:*41-48, Jan '25
Surgical treatment of roentgen-ray lesions. PORTER, C. A. Am. J. Roentgenol. *13:*31-37, Jan '25
Treatment of deep roentgen-ray burns by excision and tissue shifting. DAVIS, J. S. J.A.M.A. *86:*1432-1435, May 8, '26
Treatment of burns by actinotherapy. KESSLER, E. B. Arch. Physical Therapy *7:*347-354, June '26
Lesions of fingers and hands secondary to roentgen rays. JUARISTI, V. AND ARRAIZA, D. Progresos de la clinica *35:*301-304, April '27
Carbon dioxide snow in injuries of skin due to X-ray. EISNER. Zentralbl. f. Haut-u. Geschlechtskr. *24:*580, Oct 5, '27
Cancer of hand in radiologist, cured by dia-

Radiation Injuries – Cont.

thermo-coagulation; case. BORDIER, H. Cancer, Bruxelles *4:*328-330, '27

Treatment of X-ray and radium burns. SHEEHAN, J. E. Laryngoscope *38:*612-617, Sept '28

Treatment of cutaneous ulcer due to roentgen ray burn. ISELIN, H. Schweiz. med. Wchnschr. *59:*629-630, June 15, '29

Surgical treatment of roentgen ray burns. HAYWARD. Med. Klin. *25:*1548-1550, Oct 4, '29

Plastic repair of severe radium burns and angioma of face. STRAATSMA, C. R. New York J. Med. *30:*9-10, Jan 1, '30

Treatment of roentgen ulcerations of skin. BRUNER, E. Strahlentherapie *36:*373-384, '30

Serious case of roentgen necrosis of face and mandible. ESSER, J. F. S. Rev. de chir. structive *8:*1-3, May '38

Treatment of roentgen ray ulcers. STÜHMER, A. AND WUCHERPFENNIG, V. Ztschr. f. arztl. Fortbild. *27:*689-695, Nov 1, '30

Late injuries of roentgen rays. KUSS, H. Rontgenpraxis *2:*1133-1136, Dec 15, '30

Treatment of roentgen ulcerations of skin. BRUNER, E. Strahlentherapie *36:*373-384, '30

Extensive X-ray burns; repeated blood transfusions. ZALEWSKI, F. Rev. de chir., Paris *68:*75-79, '30

Burns of roentgenologists; therapy. HOLZKNECHT, G. Fortschr. a. d. Geb. d. Rontgenstrahlen *44:*78-81, July '31

Treatment of injuries with rays of long wave length. BRÖCKER, W. Strahlentherapie *42:*551-570, '31

Deep roentgen-ray burns. DAVIS, J. S. Am. J. Roentgenol. *26:*890-893, Dec '31

Deep X-ray burns. DAVIS, J. S. Tr. South. S. A. *44:*227-236, '31

Filatov grafts in large ulcers due to X-ray burns. SOKOLOFF, A. P. Vestnik khir. (nos. 70-71) *24:*237-241, '31

Therapy of late injuries of skin with ointment containing radium emanations. ROST, G. A. AND UHLMANN, E. Deutsche med. Wchnschr. *58:*655-656, April 22, '32

Surgical therapy of X-ray injuries of skin. MOSZKOWICZ, L. Wien. klin. Wchnschr. *45:*885, July 8, '32

Actinodermatitis (roentgen-ray burn) of entire neck; replacement with tubed flap from thorax. FIGI, F. A., S. Clin. North America *12:*947-949, Aug '32

Destruction of skin of face by irradiation of birthmark in early life; restoration of nose

Radiation Injuries – Cont.

by rhinoplasty, correction of lip by plastic operation, restoration of eyebrow by implantation of narrow flap from hairy scalp, restoration of upper eyelid by full-thickness graft from thigh. BABCOCK, W. W., S. Clin. North America *12:*1409-1410, Dec '32

Surgical therapy of post-radiation keratosis. BLAIR, V. P. *et al.* Radiology *19:*337-344, Dec '32

Ulcerous radiodermatitis of 16 years' duration cured by periarterial sympathectomy and skin grafts; case. LERICHE, R. AND FONTAINE, R. Lyon chir. *30:*107-108, Jan-Feb '33

Plastic surgery in chronic radiodermatitis and radionecrosis. GILLIES, H. D. AND McINDOE, A. H. Brit. J. Radiol. *6:*132-147, March '33

Treatment of roentgen burn of elbow with salicyclic acid solution and skin graft. THOMASSEN, C. Nederl. tijdschr. v. geneesk. *78:*1621-1624, April 14, '34

Roentgen burns, with report of 9 cases from University Hospital, Philadelphia, 1907-1933. ZUGSMITH, G. S. Radiology *23:*36-44, July '34

Role of plastic surgery in burns due to roentgen rays and radium. GILLIES, H. D. AND McINDOE, A. H. Ann. Surg. *101:*979-996, April '35

Therapy of ulcerations and dermatoses of hands of roentgenologists and radiologists. NOVAK, F. V. Casop. lek. cesk. *74:*434-436, April 19, '35

Ulcerated radiodermatitis of hand cured by perihumeral sympathectomy; case. BAUDET, G. Bull. et mem. Soc. nat. de chir. *61:*991-994, July 20, '35

Successful therapy of injuries of skin from roentgen and radium rays. UHLMANN, E. AND SCHAMBYE, G. Strahlentherapie *52:*282-298, '35

Dangers of roentgenotherapy of hypertrichosis of chin; 2 cases. ESSER, J. F. S. An. de cir. *4:*260-262, Sept '38

Serious case of roentgen necrosis of face and mandible. ESSER, J. F. S. Rev. de chir. structive *8:*1-3, May '38

Dangers of roentgenotherapy of hypertrichosis of chin; 2 cases. ESSER, J. F. S. An. de cir. *4:*260-262, Sept '38

Perianal actinodermatitis; treatment by excision and pedicle graft. SMITH, N. D. Proc. Staff Meet., Mayo Clin. *14:*113-115, Feb 22, '39

Treatment of injuries produced by roentgen rays and radioactive substances. UHL-

Radiation Injuries – Cont.

MANN, E. Am. J. Roentgenol. *41:*80-90, Jan '39

Treatment of X-ray burns and other superficial disfigurements of skin (and keloids). CANNON, A. B. New York State J. Med. *40:*391-399, March 15, '40

Surgical treatment of roentgen and radium dermatitis. GHORMLEY, R. K. AND FAIRCHILD, R. D. Surgery *7:*737-752, May '40

Late sequels of roentgen depilation of scalp. PROPPE, A. AND GAHLEN, W. Arch. f. Dermat. u. Syph. *108:*155-164, '40

Surgical treatment of roentgen and radium dermatitis. GHORMLEY, R. K. Proc. Staff Meet., Mayo Clin. *16:*69, Jan 29, '41

Skin grafts in extirpation of cancer due to roentgen irradiation. PEYRI, J. Actas dermo-sif. *32:*736-738, May '41

Treatment of X-ray and radium burns by radical excision and grafting. DOUGLAS, B., J. Tennessee M. A. *34:*220-224, June '41

Surgical management of postradiation scars and ulcers. CONWAY, H. Surgery *10:*64-84, July '41

Surgical treatment of radiation damage to tissue. KIMBALL, G. H., J. Oklahoma M. A. *34:*285-289, July '41

Glycerin-gelatin base for irradiation dermatitis and burns. COLE, P. P. AND LEDERMAN, M. Lancet *2:*329, Sept 13, '41

X-ray or radium burn. FICHARDT, T. South African M. J. *15:*403-405, Oct 25, '41

Surgical management of radiation ulceration (grafting). ADAMS, H. D. Lahey Clin. Bull. *2:*203-206, Jan '42

Skin grafts in therapy of late reactions to roentgen or radium therapy; cases. CAMPOS MARTIN, R. *et al.* Actas dermo-sif. *34:*564-575, April '43

Radiodermatitis of head and neck, with discussion of its surgical treatment (skin grafting). FIGI, F. A. *et al.* Surg., Gynec. and Obst. *77:*284-294, Sept '43

Chronic radiodermatitis and plastic surgery. ZWANCK, T. Semana med. *1:*471-476, March 15, '45

Plastic repair of radiation ulcers of sole. GREELEY, P. W., U.S. Nav. M. Bull. *45:*827-830, Nov '45

Subtotal replacement of skin of face for actinodermatitis due to roentgenotherapy with multiple areas of squamous cell carcinoma. JENKINS, H. P. Ann. Surg. *122:*1042-1048, Dec '45

Radiation Treatment of Benign Conditions

Radium treatment of vascular nevi. LABORDE, S. Medecine *2:*696, June '21 abstr: J.A.M.A. *77:*409, July 30, '21

Radium treatment of vascular nevi. LABORDE, S. Progres med. *36:*531-532, Nov 12, '21

Contracture of aponeurosis of palms and soles plus neuralgia treated with X-ray. SPECKLIN, P. AND STOEBER, R. Presse med. *30:*743-745, Aug 30, '22 abstr: J.A.M.A. *79:*1368, Oct 14, '22

Epithelization of skin grafts with roentgen rays. HABERLAND, H. F. O. Klin. Wchnschr. *2:*353-354, Feb 19, '23

Treatment of vascular nevi with radium. RULISON, R. H. AND MCLEAN, S. Am. J. Dis. Child. *25:*359-370, May '23 (illus.)

Radium therapy of vascular nevi. MORROW, H. AND TAUSSIG, L. R. Am. J. Roentgenol. *10:*867-871, Nov '23

Hygroma cystica treated with radium. NEW, G. B., S. Clin. N. America *4:*527-528, April '24

Rhinophyma; report of 6 cases cured by radical operations followed by X-ray and acid treatments to relieve associated hypertrophy of skin and to reduce operative scars to state of invisibility. GRATTAN, J. F. Surg., Gynec. and Obst. *41:*99-102, July '25

Angioma cavernosum; report of case of face treated with radium. FRAZIER, C. N. Arch. Dermat. and Syph. *12:*506-508, Oct '25

Hereditary contracture of palmar fascia; efficiency of radium emanation. APERT, E. Bull. et mem. Soc. med. d. hop. de Paris *49:*1502-1505, Nov 27, '25 abstr: J.A.M.A. *86:*380, Jan 30, '26

Roentgen ray in treatment of skin disease, with special reference to acne vulgaris. FISHER, J. E. Ohio State M. J. *23:*374-378, May '27

Radium in removal of "birthmarks." SIMPSON, F. E. AND FLESHER, R. E. Clin. Med. and Surg. *34:*605-607, Aug '27

Radium treatment of haemangiomata, lymphangiomata and naevi pigmentosi. Experiences from "Radium-hemmet," 1909-1924. ANDREN, G. Acta radiol *8:*1-45, '27

Angioma of nose following erysipelas; radium therapy proposed; case. WALLON, E. Bull. Soc. franc. de dermat. et syph. *35:*406-408, May '28

Radium treatment of vascular nevi in infants. STRYKER, G. V., J. Missouri M. A. *25:*417-421, Sept '28

Rhinophyma; case cured by radiotherapy. HARET. Bull. et mem. Soc. de radiol. med. de France *16:*236, Nov '28

Radiation Treatment of Benign Conditions—Cont.

Radium in treatment of multilocular lymph cysts (cystic hygromas) of neck in children. FIGI, F. A. Am. J. Roentgenol. *21:*473–480, May '29

Effect of radium rays on transplanted tissues. KRONTOVSKY, A. A. Vrach. dielo *12:*669–671, May 31, '29

Indications for technic of radium treatment of cutaneous angiomas. WALLON, E. Presse med. *37:*803–804, June 19, '29

Roentgen treatment of thermal and chemical burns of skin. TAMIYA, C. AND KOYAMA, M. Strahlentherapie *34:*808–812, '29

Treatment of vascular nevi in children with roentgen and radium therapy. COTTENOT, P. Med. inf. *37:*72–83, March '30 also: J. de med. de Paris *50:*376–378, May 1, '30

Treatment of late injuries of skin with radium ointment; 3 cases. UHLMANN, E. Dermat. Wchnschr. *91:*1825–1828, Dec 13, '30

Radium treatment of angioma of external ear in infant. DHALLUIN, M. Gaz. med. de France (supp. radiol.) no.6, pp. 136–138, Oct 1, '31

Treatment of injuries with rays of long wave length. BRÖCKER, W. Strahlentherapie *42:*551–570, '31

Bilateral hypertrophy of breasts treated by x-rays. LAIRD, A. H. Brit. J. Radiol. *5:*249, March '32

Radium therapy of giant angiomas of face; 3 cases. LLORENS SUQUE, A., J. de radiol. et d'electrol. *16:*211–213, May '32

Irradiation treatment of red birth-marks; experiences in over 200 cases. KROMAYER, E. Deutsche med. Wchnschr. *58:*1199–1201, July 29, '32 also: Urol. and Cutan. Rev. *36:*524–527, Aug '32

Hemangioma of nose; late results of radiotherapy. PANNETON, J. E. Union med. du Canada *61:*940–944, Aug '32

Cavernous hemangioma of skin; radium therapy in infants. RATTI, A. Gior. ital. di dermat. e sif. *73:*1430–1436, Aug '32

Comparative results of bipolar electrolysis and radium therapy in angioma of eyelids in infants; 2 cases. MARÍN AMAT, M. Arch. de oftal. hispano-am. *32:*604–613, Nov '32

Radium therapy of giant angiomatous nevi. LLORENS SUQUE, A. Strahlentherapie *45:*457–460, '32

Radium therapy of cutaneous angiomas. LABORDE, S. Presse med. *41:*103–104, Jan 18, '33

Radium treatment of angiomas. TYLER, A. F. Radiol. Rev. and Chicago M. Rec. *55:*51–54, March '33

Radiation Treatment of Benign Conditions—Cont.

Use of radium in traumatic and postoperative scars. KEITH, D. Y. Radiol. Rev. and Chicago M. Rec. *56:*61–63, March '34

Radium therapy of Dupuytren's contracture. TOMÁNEK, F. Casop. lek. cesk. *74:*46–47, Jan 11, '35

Short wave therapy of alopecia; cases. PETGES, AND WANGERMEZ. Bull. et mem. Soc. de radiol. med. de France *24:*477–478, May '36

Radium therapy in Dupuytren's contracture. FEURSTEIN, J. G. Wien. klin. Wchnschr. *49:*1090–1092, Sept 4, '36

Technic of treating naevus flammeus with infraroentgen (grenz) rays. KALZ, F. Strahlentherapie *57:*510–515, '36

Cavernous angiomas of face in children; late results of radium therapy. PERUSSIA, F. Strahlentherapie *57:*109–120, '36

Injuries following epilation by electrolysis or roentgen rays. (Further comment on Nobl's article.) KARPELIS, E. Wien. med. Wchnschr. *87:*685, June 19, '37

Roentgen ray therapy in fibrous ankylosis of jaws. MACKENZIE, A. R. South. M. J. *30:*816–819, Aug '37

Roentgen treatment of infection from human bite of hand. SMITH, R. M. AND MANGES, W. F. Am. J. Roentgenol. *38:*720–725, Nov '37

Interstitial radiation treatment of hemangiomata. BROWN, J. B. AND BYARS, L. T. Am. J. Surg. *39:*452–457, Feb '38

Roentgen therapy of Dupuytren's contracture. BEATTY, S. R. Radiology *30:*610–612, May '38

Cavernous angioma; radium and roentgen therapy; cases. GARDINI, G. F. Bull. d. sc. med., Bologna *110:*293–314, Sept–Oct '38

Radium therapy of hemangiomas. BAENSCH, W. Strahlentherapie *63:*496–505, '38

Roentgen epilation. ARONSTEIN, E. Radiology *32:*95–96, Jan '39

Extensive furunculosis of upper lip treated by roentgenotherapy; case. GRIMAUD, R. AND JACOB, P. Rev. med. de Nancy *67:*701–703, Aug 1, '39

Radium treatment of angiomas in children. PATERSON, R. AND TOD, M. C. Am. J. Roentgenol. *42:*726–730, Nov '39

Treatment of portwine birthmarks (nevus flammeus) by grenz (infra-roentgen) rays. WHITE, C. Illinois M. J. *76:*449–451, Nov '39

Radium treatment of cutaneous cavernous haemangiomas, using surface application of radium tubes in glass capsules.

Radiation Treatment of Benign Conditions—Cont.

STRANDQVIST, M. Acta radiol. *20:*185–211, '39

Treatment (radium) of infected hemangiomata. POHLE, E. A. Am. J. Roentgenol. *43:*408–415, March '40

Radium treatment of hemangiomata. HARWELL, W. R. New Orleans M. and S. J. *92:*576–580, April '40

Radium therapy in birth-marks. FEUERSTEIN, B. L. Mississippi Valley M. J. *62:*77, May '40

Five years' experience with radium therapy of hemangiomas. MÜLLER, R. Munchen. med. Wchnschr. *87:*538–541, May 17, '40

X-ray treatment of acute osteomyelitis of fingers; preliminary report. MARCUS, A. AND GROH, J. A. Indust. Med. *9:*551–554, Nov '40

Radium treatment of vascular nevi; analysis of 152 cases seen during 1928–1938. POHLE, E. A. AND MCANENY, J. B. Am. J. Roentgenol. *44:*747–755, Nov '40

Experiences with thorium-x needles in therapy of hemangiomas. HOEDE, K. AND SCHAEFER, F. Strahlentherapie *67:*23–38, '40

Radiation treatment of hemangioma of skin. SPENCER, J. Am. J. Roentgenol. *46:*220–223, Aug '41

Roentgen therapy of hypertrophic scars and keloids. HUNTER, A. F. Rev. radiol. y fisioterap. *10:*101–109, May–June '43

Cavernous hemangioma of face in infant treated with radium; case. JACOBS, A. W. Am. J. Roentgenol. *49:*816–818, June '43

Use of X-rays in treatment of indurations due to scars and chronic inflammation. RHYS-LEWIS, R. D. S. Proc. Roy. Soc. Med. *39:*150–151, Feb '46

Radiation Treatment of Cancer

Carcinoma of eyelids treated with radium. WITHERS, S. Am. J. Ophth. *4:*8, Jan '21

Radium in treatment of epithelioma of lip. QUICK, D., J. Radiol. *2:*1, Dec '21

Carcinoma of external ear; combined surgical and radium treatment. BECK, E. G. Internat. Clinics *1:*29, '21

Epitheliomas of face and their treatment with radium. MORROW, H. AND TAUSSIG, L. Arch. Dermat. and Syph. *5:*73–87, Jan '22 (illus.)

Radium treatment of cancer of lip. DUBOIS-ROQUEBERT. Paris med. *12:*110–112, Feb 4, '22

Cancer of lip treated by radiation or combined with electro-coagulation and surgical procedures. PFAHLER, G. E., J. Radiol. *3:*213–218, June '22 (illus.)

Treatment of cancer of lip by radiation. LAIN, E. S. Tr. Sect. Dermat. and Syphilol., A. M. A. pp 220–233, '22 (illus.) also: Arch. Dermat. and Syph. *6:*434–447, Oct '22

Cancer of lip, its treatment by radium and surgery combined. WALL, C. K., J. M. A. Georgia *12:*67–69, Feb '23

Statistic and technique in treatment of malignant disease of skin by radiation. MORROW, H. AND TAUSSIG, L. R. Am. J. Roentgenol. *10:*212–218, March '23; *10:*867–871, Nov '23

Radium treatment of carcinoma of lip. TAUSSIG, L. R., M. Clin. N. America *6:*1579–1586, May '23 (illus.)

Radiotherapy in treatment of superficial malignant disease of face. JOSSELYN, R. B., J. Maine M. A. *13:*279–284, June '23 (illus.)

Contribution to treatment of cancer of lip by irradiation; report on 136 cases. SCHREINER, B. F. AND KRESS, L. C., J. Cancer Research *8:*221–233, July '24

Epithelioma of lip treated with radium. MONTGOMERY, D. W. AND CULVER, G. D. California and West. Med. *22:*628–631, Dec '24

Radium treatment of epithelioma of face. KENNEDY, W. H., J. Radiol. *6:*52–55, Feb '25

Radium treatment of cancer of face. TRUEHART, M., J. Kansas M. Soc. *25:*70–73, March '25

Cancer of lip; its treatment by means of electrothermic coagulation, radium and roentgen rays. STEVENS, J. T. Radiology *4:*372–377, May '25

Radium emanation in treatment of intra-oral cancer; with report of 141 cases. SIMPSON, F. E. AND FLESHER R. E. Tr. Sect. Dermat. and Syphil., A. M. A., pp. 120–129, '25

Epithelioma of lip treated by radiation. JACOBS, A. W., M. J. and Rec. *123:*803, June 16, '26

Radio-active substances; their therapeutic uses and applications; radium treatment of carcinoma of lower lip. MUIR, J. Radiology *7:*51–58, July '26

Carcinoma of larynx and laryngopharynx treated with radium; analysis of 30 cases. IMPERATORI, C. J. Arch Otolaryng. *4:*151–159, Aug '26

Radio-active substances; their therapeutic uses and applications; radiation of cancer of cheek. MUIR, J. Radiology *7:*131–136, Aug '26

Surgery associated with radium in treatment

Radiation Treatment of Cancer—Cont.
of epitheliomas of upper jaw. HAUTANT, A. *et al.* J. de chir. *28:*257–274, Sept '26
Radium treatment of epithelioma of ear. KENNEDY, W. H. Radiology *7:*249-252, Sept '26
Cancer of mouth; results of treatment by operation and radiation; 376 cases observed at Massachusetts General and Collis P. Huntington Memorial Hospitals in three-year period, 1918–1920. SIMMONS, C. C. Surg., Gynec. and Obst. *43:*377–382, Sept '26
Cancer of lip; report of 25 cases treated with radium. TRUEHEART, M., J. Kansas M. Soc. *26:*311–313, Oct '26
Ten years' experience with radium therapy of cancer of larynx. SARGNON, A., J. de radiol. et d'electrol. *10:*553–555, Dec '26
Repair of defects caused by surgery and radium in cancer of hand, mouth and cheek. BLAIR, V. P. Am. J. Roentgenol. *17:*99–100, Jan '27
Treatment of advanced carcinoma of skin of face with radium. BRADLEY, R. A. AND SNOKE, P. O., S. Clin. N. Amer. *7:*165–168, Feb '27
Radium treatment in 13 cases of cancer of face. FRUCHAUD, H. AND MARY, A. Gazettes med., Paris, pp. 465–471, Aug 15, '27
Radium therapy of cancer of tongue; 143 cases. CAPIZZANO, N. Rev. med. latino-am. *13:*464–470, Dec '27
Cancer of eyelid; radium therapy; case. CAPIZZANO, N. Bol. Inst. de med. exper. para el estud. y trat. del cancer *4:*139, April '28
Payment epithelial cancer of nasal cavity cured by roentgen treatment; case. MAYER, O. Wien. med. Wchnschr. *78:*587, April 28, '28
Treatment of facial cancer by irradiation. KAPLAN, I. I. Am. J. Roentgenol. *19:*437–439, May '28
Radium and radon in treatment of epithelioma of lips. SIMPSON, F. E. AND FLESHER, R. E. Arch. Physical Therapy *9:*207–208, May '28
Combined surgical and radium treatment of carcioma of superior maxillary; case. JENTZER, A. Schweiz. med. Wchnschr. *58:*659–662, June 30, '28
Infiltrating cancer of nose; acute evolution; treatment by radium; case. MARTÍNEZ, E. AND PUENTE DUANY, N. Bol. de la Liga contra el cancer *3:*145–149, July 1, '28
Radium and radon in treatment of epithelioma of lips. SIMPSON, F. E. AND FLESHER, R. E. Illinois M. J. *54:*48–50, July '28

Radiation Treatment of Cancer—Cont.
Value and dangers of radium therapy of tumors of jaws; osteonecrosis; cases. VALLEBONA, A. Minerva med. (pt.2) *8:*422–440, Aug 25, '28
Epithelioma of face treated by grattage and radiotherapy. BELOT, J. AND LEPENNETIER, F. Bull. et mem. Soc. de radiol. med. de France *16:*227, Nov '28
Cure of epithelioma of nose with Bucky's border rays (grenz rays). BUCKY, G. Arch. f. Dermat. u. Syph. *155:*109–111, '28
X-ray treatment of epithelioma of face. MARTIN, J. M. Proc. Inter-State Post-Grad. M. Assemb., North America (1927) *3:*303–305, '28
Roentgenotherapy in inoperable epithelioma of face. SCADUTO, G. Urol. and Cutan. Rev. *33:*28–35, Jan '29
Cancer of lips; treatment by radium needles. BROWN, R. G., M. J. Australia *1:*421–423, March 30, '29
Epithelioma of lips; radium therapy. LENTH, V. Radiol. Rev. and Chicago M. Rec. *51:*132–135, March '29
Radiotherapy of cancer of lips and mouth. MURPHY, I. J. AND MURPHY, S. L. Radiol. Rev. and Chicago M. Rec. *51:*126–128, March '29
Effect of radium rays on transplanted tissues. KRONTOVSKY, A. A. Vrach. dielo *12:*669–671, May 31, '29
Five year end-results of radiation treatment of cancer of oral cavity, nasopharynx and pharynx, based on study of 309 cases, 1912–1923. SCHREINER, B. F. AND SIMPSON, B. T. Radiol. Rev. and Chicago M. Rec. *51:*327–332, Aug '29
Results of radium treatment of epithelioma of lips; statistics. LACASSAGNE, A. Arch. d'electric. med. *39:*358–366, Oct '29
Value of radium in treatment of cancer of face. LARKIN, A. J. Am. J. Surg. *8:*164–165, Jan '30
Use of small amounts of radium at distance in treatment of cancer of face. PETTIT, R. T. Radiology *14:*55–59, Jan '30
Epithelioma of eyelids; indications for radium treatment and surgical intervention. VILLARD, H. Medecine *11:*19–23, Jan '30
Treatment of surface cancers of face with scraping and roentgen therapy; value in relation to other methods. BELOT, J. AND BUHLER, Y. E. Rev. d'actinol. *6:*91–107, March-April '30
Results of treatment of cancer of jaws by operation and radiation. SIMMONS, C. C. Ann. Surg. *92:*681–693, Oct '30

Radiation Treatment of Cancer—Cont.
Radium treatment of epitheliomas of eyelids. APPELMANS, M. Rev. belge sc. med. *2:*829-840, Dec '30
Principles of and results in radium treatment of buccal carcinoma. BIRKETT, G. E. Canad. M. A. J. *23:*780-784, Dec '30
Radium treatment of early epithelioma of lips. HAILEY, H. South. M. J. *23:*1121-1125, Dec '30
Radium therapy of cancer of nose. MORAN, H. M., M. J. Australia *2:*814-817, Dec 20, '30
Results of radium therapy in cancer of larynx; 150 cases. ESCAT, *et al.* Cancer, Bruxelles *7:*121-126, '30
Treatment by radiation and gold seed implantation in metastatic nodes in neck from cancer of lips. JOHNSON, S. C. Am. J. Cancer *15:*254-261, Jan '31
Operation followed by radium therapy in epithelioma of nasal septum; 2 cases. SAKON, H. Ann. d'oto-laryng., pp. 55-60, Jan '31
Parotid gland cancer, surgical therapy, recurrence and cure by radiotherapy. BELOT, J. AND MÉNÉGAUX, G., J. de radiol. et d'electrol. *15:*90-91, Feb '31
Recurrence after roentgenotherapy and then after excision of epithelioma of internal angle and of upper right eyelid; case. COSTE, J. Bull. Soc. franc. de dermat. et syph. (Reunion dermat., Lyon) *38:*501-504, April '31
Position of surgery and radium in treatment of cancer of mouth. PADGETT, E. C., J. Kansas M. Soc. *32:*167-172, May '31
Cancer in and about mouth, treated with irradiation by European method. MARTIN, C. L. AND MARTIN, J. M. Texas State J. Med. *27:*286-291, Aug '31
Squamous-celled epithelioma of lower lip; radium therapy. HAILEY, H., J.M.A. Georgia *20:*386-388, Oct '31
Radium treatment of cancer of lips. VAN STUDDIFORD, M. T. New Orleans M. and S. J. *84:*252-259, Oct '31
X-ray therapy as conservative method in cancer of lower lip. MARTIN, J. M. Proc. Internat. Assemb. Inter-State Post-Grad. M. A., North America (1930) *6:*399-403, '31
Radiotherapy of cancer of lips. ARZT, L. AND FUHS, H. Wien. klin. Wchnschr. *45:*15-18, Jan. 1, '32
Radiotherapy of epithelioma of eyelids; aesthetic results. ARCELIN, F. Lyon med. *149:*289-292, March 6, '32
Late results of fractional roentgenotherapy of intrinsic cancer of larynx; results of 5 years' experience. GUNSETT, A. Gaz. med.

Radiation Treatment of Cancer—Cont.
de France (supp. radiol.), pp. 173-177, May 1, '32
Epithelioma of mucous membrane of lower lip; recovery after radium therapy complicated by partial necrosis of inferior maxilla; case. HOCHE, L. AND ROY. Bull. Assoc. franc. p. l'etude du cancer *21:*381-384, May '32
Plastic replacement of upper lip in case of epitheliomatous ulcer resulting from X-ray treatment of sycosis barbae. HUTTON, A. J. Glasgow M. J. *117:*225-230, May '32
Radium therapy of cancer of lips, with study of metastasis into regional lymph nodes. COLLIN, E. Acta radiol. *13:*232-237, '32
Surgical and radiotherapy of cancer of lips. HARRISON, R. S. Strahlentherapie *46:*401-434, '33 Abstr.: Schweiz. med. Wchnschr. *63:*159-162, Feb. 18, '33
Carcinoma of mucosa of cheek treated by irradiation only; patient living and free of disease 5 years, 3 months. MARTIN, H. E. S. Clin. North America *13:*442-443, April '33
Radium therapy of cancer of lips, with especial consideration of permanent results. ARTZ, L. AND FUHS, H. Wien. klin. Wchnschr. *46:*706-708, June 9, '33
Five-year end-results obtained by radiation treatment of cancer of lips. SCHREINER, B. F. AND MATTICK, W. L. Am. J. Roentgenol. *30:*67-74, July '33
Radium therapy of cancer of larynx; results in 150 cases. CAPIZZANO, N. Bol. Inst. de med. exper. para el estud. y trat. del cancer *10:*575-579, Oct '33
Chondrosarcoma of ethmoid; surgical therapy, radiotherapy and autoplasty with tubular flap. LARROUDÉ, C. Rev. de chir. plastique, pp. 239-245, Oct '33
Cancer of lower lip; efficient treatment by radiation. MUIR, J. Internat. J. Med. and Surg. *46:*590-591, Dec '33
Standard methods of treatment of cancer of lips by surgery and radiation. FISCHEL, E. Surg., Gynec. and Obst. *60:*505-512, Feb (no. 2A) '35
Present day status of irradiation and surgery of cancer of neck. BECK, J.C. AND GUTTMAN, M. R. South. M. J. *29:*606-609, June '36
Results of roentgen rays, radium, diathermocoagulation and surgery in therapy of cutaneous epithelioma (face); 14 cases. MARTIN, J. Arch. d'electric. med. *44:*444-460, Dec '36
Radiation therapy of cancer of lips. KAPLAN, I. I. Radiology *28:*533-543, May '37

Radiation Treatment of Cancer—Cont.

Results of roentgenotherapy of cancer of larynx after 5 and 10 years of control. Coutard, H., J. de radiol. et d'electrol. *21:*402-409, Sept '37

Results of surgical therapy and radiotherapy of epitheliomas of mouth, tongue and larynx. Chryssicos, J. and Lambadaridis, A. Ztschr. f. Hals-, Nasen-u. Ohrenh. *40:*410-413, '37

Ulcerating epithelioma of cheek; case treated with 500,000 volt therapy. Mershon, H. F. South. Surgeon *7:*262, June '38

Plastic surgery of eyelid following removal of epithelioma caused by irradiation. Lauber, H. Ophthalmologica *97:*312-316, July '39

Comparison of results obtained by surgery and radiation therapy in cancer of larynx. Arbuckle, M. F. South. M. J. *32:*1008-1014, Oct '39

Treatment of large protruding carcinomas of skin and lip by irradiation and surgery. Hunt, H. B. Am. J. Roentgenol. *44:*254-264, Aug '40

Symposium on cancer: radiation damage to tissue and its repair. Daland, E. M. Surg., Gynec. and Obst. *72:*372-383, Feb (no. 2A) '41

Results of irradiation treatment for cancer of lips; analysis of 636 cases from 1926-1936. Schreiner, B. F. and Christy, C. J. Radiology *39:*293-297, Sept '42

Giant epithelioma of lower extremity; roentgenotherapy and Reverdin grafts; case. Campos Martin, R. and Usua Marine, J. Actas dermo-sif. *34:*747-750, June '43

Clinical study of 778 cases of cancer of lips with particular regard to predisposing factors and radium therapy. Ebenius, B. Acta radiol., supp. 48, pp. 1-232, '43

Radiation Treatment of Keloids

Mixed surgical and radium treatment of prominent keloids. Sáinz de Aja. Siglo med. *72:*1185-1187, Dec 8, '23

Treatment of keloids with radium. Taussig, L. R. California State J. Med. *21:*520-522, Dec '23

Roentgen-ray treatment of keloids. Hazen, H. H. Am. J. Roentgenol. *11:*547-549, June '24

Successful radiotherapy of cicatrices and keloids with case report. Du Bois, C. Rev. med. de la Suisse Rom. *44:*705-713, Nov '24

Roentgen-ray treatment of keloid. Grier, G. W., Am. J. Roentgenol. *16:*22-26, July '26

Deep, cicatricial keloid treated by radium;

Radiation Treatment of Keloids—Cont.

case. Guilera, L. G. An. Hosp. de Santa Cruz y San Pablo *2:*234, July 15, '28

Radium therapy of keloids. Rieti, E. Arch. di radiol. *4:*941-955, Sept-Dec '28

Roentgenotherapy and electrotherapy of keloids. Lepennetier, F. Rev. d'actinol. *5:*69, Jan-Feb '29

Therapy of keloids by filtered roentgen rays. Kilbane, C. V. New England J. Med. *203:*1238-1241, Dec 18, '30

Radium therapy of postoperative keloids. Mátyás, M. Zentralbl. f. Chir. *57:*3039-3040, Dec 6, '30

Treatment of keloids and hypertrophic scars by introduction of radio-active substances into tissue. Simons, A. Strahlentherapie *37:*89-123, '30

Prevention of keloid formation by prophylactic irradiation of fresh operative wound. Bab, M. Deutsche med. Wchnschr. *57:*319-320, Feb. 20, '31

Radium in therapy of cicatrices and keloids. Degrais, P. and Bellot, A. Bull. med., Paris *46:*196-198, March 12, '32

X-ray treatment of keloidal and hypertrophic scars. Sherman, B. H. Radiology *18:*754-757, April '32

Keloids, radium therapy; case, with suggestions of other physiotherapeutic methods (electrolysis, electropuncture, ionization, cryotherapy, electrocoagulation and roentgenotherapy). Trépagne, D. Ann. de med. phys. *25:*291-297, '32

Keloids, esthetic therapy, surgical ablation followed immediately by radium irradiation. Passot, R. Presse med. *41:*544-546, April 5, '33

Surgical removal followed by radiotherapy of cicatricial keloids. Vialle, P. Arch. med. -chir. de Province *23:*429-432, Dec '33

Radium treatment of cicatricial keloids. Fuhs, H. Med. Klin. *30:*160-161, Feb. 2, '34

Radiation therapy of keloid and keloidal scars. Hodges, F. M. Am. J. Roentgenol. *31:*238-243, Feb '34

Surgical and radium therapy of keloids. Weill, R. Bull. et mem. Soc. de med. de Paris *139:*340-343, May 10, '35

Keloid tumor and its cure by radiotherapy. Hintze, A. Strahlentherapie *57:*224-240, '36

Roentgen and radium treatment in prevention and therapy of keloids. Deplaen, P. Rev. de chir. structive, pp. 99-102, June '37

Keloid and its radium therapy, with report of cases. Moscariello, T. Arch. di radiol. *13:*317-337, July-Aug '37

Radiation Treatment of Keloids – Cont.

Radium treatment of keloids. Davis, A. H. and Brown, W. L. Radiol. Rev. and Mississippi Valley M. J. *60:*67-69, March '38

Radiotherapy in prophylaxis and treatment of keloids. Levitt, W. M. and Gillies, H. Lancet *1:*440-442, April 11, '42

Roentgen therapy of hypertrophic scars and keloids. Hunter, A. F. Radiology *39:*400-409, Oct '42

Radice, J. C. (see Finochietto, R. *et al*) Nov '42

Rado, T.: Cosmetic surgery in Dutch East Indies. Geneesk. tijdschr. v. Nederl. -Indie *73:*291-295, Feb 28, '33

Radusch, D. F. (see Worman, H. G. *et al*) Jan '46

Radulesco, A. D.: *Greffes et Transplants Osseux chez l'Homme*. Romaneasca, Bucharest, 1924

Radushkevich, V. P.: Intra-arterial blood transfusion in irreversible form of shock and hemorrhage. Khirurgiya, no. 8, pp. 38-40, '44

Rae, S. L. and Wilkinson, A. W.: Liver function after burns in childhood; changes in levulose tolerance (especially in relation to tannic acid therapy). Lancet *1:*332-334, March 11, '44

Rafal, H. S. (see Evans, E. I.) 1945

Rafal, H. S. (see Evans, E. I.) April '45

Raffler, K.: Simple splint in treatment of ulnar paralysis. Zentralbl. f. Chir. *70:*764, May 22, '43

Raffo, J. M. and Arcone, R.: Complete tearing of ungual phalanx of ring finger and of its extensor tendon; case. Rev. ortop. y traumatol. *7:*29-31, July '37

Ragnell, A.: Operative treatment of progeni in Sweden. Rev. de chir. structive *8:*187-191, '38

Ragnell, A.: Field of activity and methods of modern plastic surgery including cosmetic surgery. Nord. med. tidskr. *15:*361-370, March 5, '38

Ragnell, A.: Plastic surgery in service of dermatology. Nord. med. (Hygiea) *7:*1259-1264, July 20, '40

Ragnell, A.: Correction of jaw deformities. Acta chir., Scandinav. *88:*344-352, '43

Ragnell, A.: Operative correction of hypertrophy and ptosis of female breast; clinical investigation of 300 cases with examination of new method. Acta chir. Scandinav. (supp. 113) *94:*1-149, '46 (abstract) Nord. med. *29:*721-725, Mar 29, '46

Ragnell, A.: Advances in England; impressions gained during trip in October 1945. Nord. med. *29:*261-263, Feb 8, '46

Ragnell, A.: Treatment of secondary deformity of harelip. M. Press. *216:*281-286, Oct. 16, '46

Rago, G.: Elephantiasis of extremities; surgical therapy. Gazz. internaz. med.-chir. *40:*747, Dec. 15; 783, Dec 30, '32

Rahm, H.: Plastic operation on contracted finger. Beitr. z. klin. Chir. *127:*214-217, '22 (illus.) abstr: J.A.M.A. *79:*1726, Nov 11, '22

Raia, A.: Solutions of acacia in shock. Rev. de cir. de Sao Paulo *5:*463-476, May-June '40

Raiga, A.: d'Herelle's bacteriophage in paronychia and wounds of hand; cases. Progres med. *44:*415-429, Mar 9, '29

Raison, C. A.: Hand infections. Am. J. Surg. *6:*530-534, April '29

Rajasingham, A. S.: Brief survey of burn therapy, with account of new method adopted by author. J. Ceylon Br., Brit. M. A. *40:*136-146, April '44

Rakhmanov, V. A.: First aid in chemical burns. Sovet. khir., no. 8, pp. 10-15, '35

Rakonitz, J.: Secretion of sweat in Romberg's progressive facial hemiatrophy. Orvosi hetil. *79:*1369-1372, Dec 28, '35

Rallo, A.: Hypertrophied thumb; case. Ann. di. med. nav. *1:*257-273, May-June '28

Ralph, H. G. and Maxwell, M. M.: Fractured maxillae; description of appliance for reduction and fixation with case report. U. S. Nav. M. Bull. *36:*507-511, Oct '38

Ramadier, J. A.: Closure of alveolosinusal communications by pedicled palatine strip. Ann. d'oto-laryng. *12:*315-316, April-June '45

Rambo, V. C.: Surgical treatment of trachoma (complicated by entropion). Am. J. Ophth. *21:*277-285, March '38

Rameev, R. S.: Chemical burns to eyes. Vestnik oftal. *16:*381-383, '40

Ramirez, V.: Carbon dioxide snow in treatment of keloids. Gac. med. de Mexico *57:*318-320, May-June '26

Ramírez Olivella, J.: Diffuse hypertrophy of breast during pregnancy; case. Rev. med. cubana *41:*131-137, Feb '30

Ramiro Moreno, A.: Burn therapy. Rev. mex. de cir., ginec. y cancer *2:*28-45, Jan '34

Ramiš, V.: Ichtoxyl (sulphoichthyolate preparation) in burns. Ceska dermat. (supp.) *12:*517-522, '31

Ramond, L.: Diagnosis of cutaneous cancer of face. Presse med. *37:*951-952, July 20, '29

Ramsay, A. (see Waud, R. A.) Feb '43

Ramsey, E. M. (see Choisser, R. M.) June '38

Ramstedt, C.: Operation for complex harelip. Zentralbl. f. Chir. *49:*1556-1558, Oct. 21, '22

RANCKEN, D.: Prognosis and treatment of Volkmann's ischemic paralysis. Finska lak. -salsk. handl. *71:*22-28, Jan '29
RAND, W. W. (see PENN, J.) Dec '44
RANDALL, H. E.: Therapy of traumatic shock (insulin and dextrose). J. Michigan M. Soc. *26:*19-20, Jan '27
RANDALL, L. M.: Obstetric shock; treatment with intravenous injections of acacia. Tr. Sect. Obst., Gynec. and Abd. Surg., A. M. A., pp. 141-148, '29
RANDALL, L. M.: Treatment of obstetric shock with intravenous injections of acacia. J.A.M.A. *93:*845-847, Sept 14, '29
RANDALL, L. M. AND HARDWICK, R. S.: Pregnancy and parturition following bilateral ureteral transplantation for congenital exstrophy of bladder. Surg., Gynec. and Obst. *58:*1018-1020, June '34
RANDALL, O. S. (see WANGENSTEEN, O. H.) July '33
RANFT, G.: Bandaging after harelip operation. Zentralbl. f. Chir. *50:*598-600, April 14, '23 (illus.)
RANGANATHAN, K. S.: Role of transfusion and infusion in treatment of wound shock. Antiseptic *39:*646-654, Oct '42
RANGANI, S.: Treatment of simple fractures of lower jaw. Sind M. J. *7:*64-68, Sept '34
RANK, B. K.: Use of Thiersch graft. Brit. M. J. *1:*846-849, May 25, '40
RANK, B. K.: Base hospital management of soft tissue injuries (including skin grafts). Australian and New Zealand J. Surg. *11:*171-184, Jan '42
RANK, B. K.: Therapy of burns (coagulation therapy; saline regime; skin grafting). Australian and New Zealand J. Surg. *12:*103-110, Oct '42
RANK, B. K.: Scar disabilities in hand. Australian and New Zealand J. Surg. *12:*191-206, Jan '43
RANK, B. K.: Facial bone fractures. Australian and New Zealand J. Surg. *13:*184-198, Jan '44
RANK, B. K.: Hand retraction piece for hand surgery. Brit. M. J. *1:*496, April 8, '44
RANK, B. K.: Plastic principles in common surgical procedures. Australian and New Zealand J. Surg. *14:*14-36, July '44
RANK, B. K.: Repair of eyelids and periorbital structures. Tr. Ophth. Soc. Australia (1944) *4:*84-97, '46
RANK, B. K. AND HENDERSON, G. D.: Cineplastic forearm amputations and prostheses. Surg. Gynec. and Obst. *83:*373-386, Sept '46
RANKIN, C. A.: Factor in repair of wounds of eyelids. Pennsylvania M. J. *49:*258-259, Dec '45
RANKIN, F. W. *et al*: Therapy of war burns. Clinics *2:*1194-1218, Feb '44
RANKIN, J. O.: Bone transplantation. W. Virginia M. J. *24:*18-24, Jan '28
RANKIN, W.: Hare-lip and other developmental lesions of face. Glasgow M. J. *106:*350-358, Dec '26
RANKOW, R. M.: Medical and dental relationship in maxillofacial team. Ann. Dent. *4:*164-166, Mar '46
RANSCHBURG, P. (see ESSER, J. F. S.) April '40
RANSOHOFF, J. L.: Surgical treatment of lymphedema (case involving arm after removal of cancer of breast). Arch. Surg. *50:*269-270, May '45
RANSOHOFF, J. L. AND MENDELSOHN, S. N.: Treatment of surgical shock (blood transfusion and intravenous drip). J. Med. *12:*637-641, Feb '32
RANSOHOFF, N. S. (see MAYER, L.) Jan '36
RANSOHOFF, N. S. (see MAYER, L.) July '36
RANSON, J. R. (see WITHERS, S.) April '24

Ranula

Cysts of floor of mouth. JOHNSTON, W. H. Tr. Am. Laryng., Rhin. and Otol. Soc. *48:*83-96, '42

RAOUL. (see ESSER, J. F. S.) May '34
RAPIN, M.: Therapy of certain forms of lupus by free grafts of whole skin; 3 cases. Rev. med. de la Suisse Rom. *57:*110-115, Feb 25, '37
RAPIN, M.: Plastic surgery of nose; 5 cases. Rev. med. de la Suisse Rom. *57:*405-412, June 10, '37
RAPIN, M.: Prethoracic esophagoplasty by new esthetic method with enclosed epithelial graft. Helvet. med. acta *8:*429-435, Aug '41
RAPIN, M.: Plastic procedure in correction of laryngotracheostenosis with dermoepidermic skin grafts. Pract. oto-rhino-laryng. *4:*88-91, '42
RAPIN, M.: Materials for corrective plastic surgery of nose. Pract. oto-rhino-laryng. *4:*133-141, '42
RAPIN, M.: Use of tubular flaps in repair of defects of face. Helvet. med. acta *9:*787-792, Dec '42
RAPIN, M.: Plastic reconstruction of lower and upper eyelids. Ophthalmologica *105:*233-239, May '43
RAPIN, M.: New plastic procedures for covering stumps. Mem. Acad. de chir. *71:*488, Nov 28-Dec 19, '45
RAPOPORT, D. M.: Methyl violet in burns. Sovet. med. (nos. 13-14) *4:*15-16, '40
RAPOPORT, D. M.: Methyl violet in burns.

Sovet. vrach. zhur. *44:*843–846, Dec '40

RAPPORT, D.: Studies in experimental traumatic shock; liberation of epinephrine in traumatic shock. Am. J. Physiol. *60:*461–475, May '22

RASTELLI, E.: Medial cervical fistula due to persistence of thyroglossal tract; case. Gior. med. d. Alto Adige *11:*3–14, Jan '39

RATTI, A.: Cavernous hemangioma of skin; radium therapy in infants. Gior. ital. di dermat. e sif. *73:*1430–1436, Aug '32

RAU, U. M.: War burns and their treatment. Antiseptic *39:*655–665, Oct '42

RAUER, A. E.: Present status of therapy of maxillofacial war wounds. Sovet. med. (nos. 7–8) *7:*22–24, '43

RAUH, W.: Extensive destruction of eyelids and skin of face caused by lupus and syphillis; surgical therapy. Ztschr. f. Augenh. *86:*193–199, June '35

RAVAUT, P. AND FERRAND, M.: Treatment of nevocarcinoma by diathermocoagulation. Bull. Soc. franc. de dermat. et syph. *34:*96–105, Feb '27

RAVAUT, P. AND FILLIOL, L.: Treatment of acne-keloid of nape of neck by diathermocoagulation; cases. Bull. Soc. franc. de dermat. et syph. *35:*942–946, Dec '28

RAVDIN, I. S.: Treatment of superficial burns. S. Clin. N. America *5:*1579–1583, Dec '25

RAVDIN, I. S.: Superficial burns. Atlantic M. J. *30:*679–683, Aug '27

RAVDIN, I. S.: General considerations of burn problem. Clinics *1:*1–5, June '42

RAVDIN, I. S.: Burn problem. Am. J. Surg. *59:*330–340, Feb '43

RAVDIN, I. S. AND FERGUSON, L. K.: Early treatment of superficial burns. Ann. Surg. *81:*439–456, Feb '25

RAVDIN, I. S. AND LONG, P. H.: Burn casualties at Pearl Harbor. U. S. Nav. M. Bull. *40:*353–358, April '42

RAVDIN, I. S. AND RHOADS, J. E.: Problems illustrating importance of knowledge of biochemistry by surgeon (including shock). S. Clin. North America *15:*85–100, Feb '35

RAVEN, R. W.: Syndrome of traumatic shock. Post-Grad. M. J. *16:*118–124, April '40

RAVEN, R. W.: Proflavine (acridine dye) powder in burn wounds. Lancet *2:*73–75, July 15, '44

RAVEN, R. W.: Treatment of patient (burns), with reference to proflavine (acridine dye) powder technic. Brit. M. J. *1:*261–262, Feb. 24, '45

RAVERDINO, E.: Turbinotome for "ab externo" dacryocystorhinostomy. Rassegna ital. d'ottal. *7:*499–503, July–Aug '38

RAVN, J. (see KEMP, T.) 1932

RAWLES, B. W. JR.: Routine for early skin grafting of deep burns. Surgery *18:*696–706, Dec '45

RAWLES, B. W. JR. AND MASSIE, J. R. JR.: Review of burn cases treated in overseas general hospital. Virginia M. Monthly *71:*605–609, Dec '44

RAY, V.: Two cases of cavernous angioma of eyelid and case of lymphangioma of bulbar conjunctiva. Ohio State M. J. *21:*720–722, Oct '25

RAYNER, H. H.: Operative treatment of cleft-palate, record of results in 125 consecutive cases. Lancet *1:*816–817, April 18, '25

RAZEMON. (see BIZARD, G. *et al*) July '32

RAZEMON, P.: Traumatic dislocation of extensor tendon of second finger. Ann. d'anat. path. *7:*238–241, Feb '30

RAZEMON, P.: Traumatic dislocation of extensor tendons of fingers; case. Echo m. du nord *34:*213–216, May 3, '30

REA, C. E.: Shock therapy. Minnesota Med. *26:*531–534, June '43

REA, R. L.: Bilateral eyelid ptosis operation; Blaskovics method. Proc. Roy. Soc. Med. *31:*667–669, April '38

READ, C. D.: Surgical treatment of congenital (stricture) absence of vagina. Irish J. M. Sc., pp. 52–57, Feb '44

READ, F. L. AND HASLAM, E. T.: Immediate skin grafts on finger injuries. U. S. Nav. M. Bull. *42:*183–186, Jan '44

REAVES, R. G.: Submucous septum punch. Tr. Am. Acad. Ophth. *35:*475, '30

REAVES, R. G.: Submucous flap punch for nasal septal surgery. Arch. Otolaryng. *15:*754, May '32

REAVES, R. G.: Preserving physiologic functions in nasal surgery. J. Tennessee M. A. *34:*403–406, Oct '41

REAVES, R. G.: Importance of preserving physiologic functions of nose in intranasal surgery. South. Surgeon *11:*574–580, Aug '42

REBATTU, J. AND PARTHIOT: Amygdaloid cyst of neck; case. Rev. de laryng. *49:*771–773, Dec 31, '28

REBAUDI, F. AND JANNUZZI, V.: Surgical correction of harelip; 26 cases. Boll. Soc. ital. di med. e ig. trop. (nos.5–6) *5:*253–264, '45

REBAUDI, F. AND MUSSO, A.: Therapy of deformities of extremities due to burn cicatrices. Gior. di med. mil. *88:*46–55, Jan '40

REBAUDI, L.: Paraffin spray in burns. Munchen. med. Wchnschr. *70:*179, Feb 9, '23

REBELO NETO, J.: Cirugia plastica de las cavidades retro-auriculares posoperatorias. Semana med. *1:*1286–1291, June 18, '42

REBELO NETO, J.: Autoplastic graft of flap by

Italian method in reconstructive surgery of mouth; case. Bol. Soc. de med. e cir. de Sao Paulo *16:*94–108, Nov '32

Rebelo Neto, J.: Surgical correction of syphilitic saddle nose by Joseph operation and Filatov graft; case. Bol. Soc. de med. e cir. de Sao Paulo *16:*123–130, Dec '32

Rebelo Neto, J.: Cosmetic surgery in relation to legal liability. Rev. oto-laryng. de Sao Paulo *1:*23–45, Jan–Feb '33

Rebelo Neto, J.: Legal responsibility in plastic surgery. Rev. med. de Pernambuco *3:*204, July; 244, Aug; 271, Sept '33

Rebelo Neto, J.: Surgical correction of deformed external ear and nose; case. Rev. med. de Pernambuco *3:*285–290, Oct '33

Rebelo Neto, J.: Legal responsibility of plastic surgeons. Arch. Soc. de med. leg. e criminol. de S. Paulo *4:*81–109, '34

Rebelo Neto, J.: Plastic surgery of face in relation to identification. Arq. de med. leg. e indent. (no. 10) *4:*87–93, '34

Rebelo Neto, J.: Surgical correction of aquiline nose; technic and results. Rev. oto-laring. de Sao Paulo *2:*97–99, March–April '34

Rebelo Neto, J.: Correction during infancy of congenital and acquired deformities in otorhinolaryngology to prevent later increased disfigurement, with special reference to plastic surgery. Rev. oto-laring. de Sao Paulo *3:*11–24, Jan–Feb '35

Rebelo Neto, J.: New method of muscular transplantation applied to cheiloplasty; case. Rev. de chir. structive, pp. 199–209, March '36

Rebelo Neto, J.: Rhinophyma; with special reference to surgical therapy. Rev. oto-laring. de Sao Paulo (no.5, bis) *4:*811–840, Sept–Oct '36

Rebelo Neto, J.: Plastic surgery in atresia of nostrils; cases. Rev. oto-laring. de Sao Paulo *5:*259–265, May–June '37

Rebelo Neto, J.: Congenital eyelid ptosis with rhinomalacia (lack of ossification of nasal bones); case. Rev. Assoc. paulista de med. *12:*455–464, May '38

Rebelo Neto, J.: Progress of plastic surgery of head (including ears, mouth, jaws, nose, etc.); review of literature for 1939. Rev. brasil. de oto-rino-laring. *8:*111–120, March–April '40

Rebelo Neto, J.: Plastic surgery of giant pigmented nevus; case. Rev. med. brasil. *8:*607–611, May '40

Rebelo Neto, J.: Surgical therapy of harelip should be at birth. Rev. brasil. de oto-rino-laring. *8:*601–608, Nov–Dec '40

Rebelo Neto, J.: Progress of surgery of head (including face, ears, nose, mouth, etc.) and throat (esophagus and larynx); review of literature for 1940. Rev. brasil. de oto-rino-laring. *9:*37–46, Jan–Feb '41

Rebelo Neto, J.: Technical devices in surgical therapy of harelip and velopalatine fissures, with report of cases. Arq. de cir. clin. e exper. *6:*343–358, April–June '42

Rebelo Neto, J.: Protection of surgeon against anesthetic gases while performing plastic surgery on cleft palate. Arq. de cir. clin. e exper. *6:*641–645, April–June '42

Rebelo Neto, J.: Plastic surgery, Latin American bibliography. Arq. de cir. clin. e exper. *6:*721–776, April–June '42

Rebelo Neto, J.: Surgical progress; head and throat; review of literature for 1941. Rev. brasil. de oto-rino-laring. *10:*347–357, May–June '42

Rebelo Neto, J.: Transpalatine route in therapy of bilateral congenital imperforation of choanae, with report of cases. Rev. brasil. de oto-rino-laring. *10:*431–441, July–Aug '42

Rebelo Neto, J.: New technic for surgical therapy of congenital coloboma of ala nasi. Rev. brasil. de oto-rino-laring. *11:*159–165, March–April '43

Rebelo Neto, J.: Surgery of head, progress of plastic surgery; review of literature for 1942. Rev. brasil. de oto-rino-laring. *11:*173–185, March–April '43

Rebelo Neto, J.: Plastic surgery in wartime; how to manage head and neck wounds. Rev. paulista de med. *23:*345–346, Dec '43

Rebelo Neto, J.: Progress of plastic surgery; review of literature for 1943. Rev. brasil. de oto-rino-laring. *12:*140–150, Mar–Apr '44

Rebelo Neto, J.: Preliminary graft of buccal mucosa in closure of extensive perforations of hard palate. Rev. brasil. de oto-rino-laring. *12:*297–301, July–Oct '44

Rebelo Neto, J.: Elementary theories on therapy of hand from point of view of plastic surgery. An. paulist. de med. e cir. *48:*97–118, Aug '44

Rebelo Neto, J.: Schema of surgical technic in congenital fissures (palate). Rev. brasil. de oto-rino-laring. *12:*393–400, Nov–Dec '44

Rebelo Neto, J.: Importance of keloids to plastic surgeons. Hospital, Rio de Janeiro *27:*33–43, Jan '45

Rebelo Neto, J.: Progress of plastic surgery; review of literature for 1944 and notes of trip to United States. Rev. brasil. de oto-rino-laring. *13:*158–166, Mar–Apr '45

Rebelo Neto, J. and Malbec, E. F.: Implants in plastic surgery. Arq. de cir. clin. e exper. *5:*245–314, Oct '41

Rebhorn, E. H.: Tannic acid in burns. Bull. Moses Taylor Hosp. *1:*21–23, May '27

RECALDE, J. F. JR.: Plastic surgery of nasal deformities. Rev. med. d. Paraguay *5:*32–37, Jan–March '42

RECALDE, J. F. JR.: Physiology of free full thickness skin graft. Arq. de cir. clin. e exper. *6:*547–549, April–June '42

RÉCAMIER, JACQUES (with Victor Veau): *Bec-de-lièvre*. Masson et Cie, Paris, 1938

RECALDE, J. F. JR.: Tubed pedicle graft. Rev. med. d. Paraguay *5:*24–28, April–June '42

RECALDE, J. F. JR.: Paladon in plastic surgery. Rev. med. d. Paraguay (7):40–42, Oct–Dec '44

RECALDE, J. F. (see ZENO, L.) April–June '42

RECORDIER, M. (see POINSO, R. *et al*) Jan '35

Rectum

Formation of vagina from rectum. NEMES, A. Zentralbl. f. Gynak. *45:*787, June 4, '21

Artificial vagina made from rectum (Schubert's method). HARTTUNG, H. Zentralbl. f. Gynak. *46:*1610–1612, Oct 7, '22

Exstrophy of bladder with successful transplantation of ureters into rectum, report of 2 cases. HUTCHINS, E. H. AND HUTCHINS, A. F. Surg., Gynec. and Obst. *36:*731–741, June '23 (illus.)

Transplantation of ureters into rectum, end-results in 35 cases of exstrophy of bladder. MAYO, C. H. AND WALTERS, W. J.A.M.A. *82:*624–626, Feb 23, '24

Rectal incontinence relieved by plastic operation. FERRARINI, G. Arch. ital. di chir. *10:*85–107, '24 abstr: J.A.M.A. *83:*1544, Nov 8, '24

Artificial vagina made from rectum. KAKUSCHKIN, N. Zentralbl. f. Gynak. *48:*2702–2704, Dec 6, '24

Remote sequelae of rectal implantation of ureters for exstrophy; findings at necropsy 14 years after Bergenhem operation. RICHEY, DEW. G., Arch. Surg. *11:*408–416, Sept '25

Construction of artificial vagina from rectum, with presence of uterus. SCHUBERT, G., Beitr. z. klin. Chir. *134:*421–425, '25 abstr: J.A.M.A. *85:*1844, Dec 5, '25

Formation of artificial vagina from rectum in deficiency of vagina. FRANZ, R. Zentralbl. f. Gynak. *50:*545–547, Feb 27, '26

Exstrophy of bladder; junction of ureters with upper part of rectum; results 24 years after operation. ESTOR, E., J. d'urol. *22:*242–243, Sept '26

Artificial vagina formed from rectum; 2 cases. SCHMELEW, W. Med. Welt *2:*403–405, March 17, '28

Treatment of persistent tubular urogenital sinus by formation of vagina from rectum; case. SCHUBERT, G. Arch. f. Gynak. *141:*228–236, '30

Rectum – Cont.

Transplantation of ureters into rectum in exstrophy. HIGGINS, C. C. Ohio State M. J. *27:*705–708, Sept '31

Tunnel skin grafts into stricture of rectum. MURDOCH, R. L. Tr. Am. Proct. Soc. *33:*156–158, '32

Ectopia vesicae; full report of case treated by transplantation of ureters into recto-sigmoid and complete cystectomy. EL-KATIB, A., J. Egyptian M. A. *16:*3–16, Jan '33

Annular stricture of rectum and anus; treatment by tunnel skin graft; preliminary report. KELLER, W. L. Am. J. Surg. *20:*28–32, April '33

Question of advantages of use of loop of small intestine, of segment of rectum or Thiersch grafts in colpoplasty for congenital absence of vagina. FORGUE, E. Paris med. *2:*479–486, Dec 15, '34

Exstrophy of bladder, cure by Marion-Heitz-Boyer method (transplantation of ureters into rectum) in man 20 years old. NANDROT. Bull. et mem. Soc. nat. de chir. *61:*1103–1105, Nov 2, '35

Transplantation of ureter to rectum in exstrophy of bladder. COLOMBINO, S. Boll. e mem. Soc. piemontese di chir. *5:*333–341, '35

Technic in creation of artificial vagina from rectum. POPOFF, D. Rev. franc. de gynec. et d'obst. *37:*225–236, Oct '42

Rectal stricture (method for surgical relief). BODKIN, L. G. Am. J. Surg. *61:*277–279, Aug '43

Transplantation of ureters into rectosigmoid in infants with exstrophy of bladder; review of 19 cases. HIGGINS, C. C., J. Urol. *50:*657–666, Dec '43

Restoration of rectum after injury. HARTZELL, J. B., U.S. Nav. M. Bull. *42:*1151–1155, May '44

Rectal herniation with intrasphincteric repair. ALLEN, V. K. Clinics *3:*1014–1022, Dec '44

REDAELLI, E.: Sebaceous nevus of face; case. Gior. ital. di dermat. e sif. *74:*122–129, Feb '33

REDER, F.: Angioma of left temporal and malar regions. S. Clin. N. America *5:*1303–1311, Oct '25

REDER, F.: Congenital defect of left ala of nose. S. Clin. N. America *5:*1313–1320, Oct '25

REDON, H.: Technic of total parotidectomy with conservation of facial nerve. J. de chir. *61:*14–20, '45

REDON, H. (see DUVAL, P.) June '32

REED, E. N.: Pin and stirrup for finger and toe traction. J. Bone and Joint Surg. *20:*786, July '38

REED, F. R.: Acute adrenal cortex exhaustion and its relationship to shock. Am. J. Surg. *40:*514–528, June '38

REED, H.: Congenital melanoma of lip with cystic degeneration. Brit. J. Surg. *34:*95–96, July '46

REED, J. V. AND HARCOURT, A. K.: Immediate full thickness grafts to finger tips. Surg., Gynec. and Obst. *68:*925-929, May '39

REED, T. G.: Traumatic shock. West Virginia M. J. *26:*205-207, April '30

REEL, P. J.: Artificial vagina in congenital absence. Ohio State M. J. *39:*1117-1119, Dec '43

REES, C. E.: Penetration of tissue by fuel oil under high pressure from Diesel engine (hand). J.A.M.A. *109:*866–867, Sept 11, '37

REES, C. E.: Repair of severed tendons; new tendon suture. Arizona Med. *1:*12–15, Jan–Feb '44

REESE, A. B.: Partial resection of eyelid and plastic repair for epithelioma involving margin of lid. Arch. Ophth. *32:*173-178, Sept '44

REESE, E.: Continuation of organic function of female breast after plastic operation; case. Zentralbl. f. Chir. *61:*3011-3012, Dec 29, '34

REESE, E.: Ability to nurse child after plastic surgery of pendulous breasts. Zentralbl. f. Chir. *62:*1933-1935, Aug 17, '35

REESE, E. C.: Local treatment of burns with pressure dressings and films containing sulfonamide. Am. J. Surg. *67:*524-529, March '45

REESE, J. D.: Dermatape; new method for management of split grafts. Plast. and Reconstruct. Surg. *1:*98–105, July '46

REESE, R. G.: Operation for blepharoptosis with formation of a fold in eyelid. Arch. Ophth. *53:*26–30, Jan '24

REEVE, B. B.: Burn management. Illinois M. J. *83:*26–31, Jan '43

REGARD, G. L.: Surgiology and survival of bone grafts. Paris med. *11:*292, Oct 8, '21 abstr: J.A.M.A. *77:*1847, Dec 3, '21

REGARD, G. L.: Treatment of paralysis by dead tendon grafting. Rev. med. de la Suisse Rom. *43:*364–374, June '23

REGAUD, C.; LACASSAGNE, A. *et al*: Glandular involvement following cancer of lips, tongue and floor of mouth. Paris med. *1:*357–372, April 16, '27 also; Strahlentherapie *26:*221–251, '27

REGNAULT, F. AND CROUZON, O.: Ocular hypertelorism. Ann. d'anat. path. *7:*571–576, May '30

REGNAULT, F. (see APERT) July '29

REGELE, H.: Congenital bilateral flexion contracture of thumb (spring finger) in children. Munchen. med. Wchnschr. *83:*391–392, March 6, '36

REGGI, J. P.: Fractures of malar bone and of zygomatic arch. Bol. y trab., Soc. argent. de cirujanos *4:*905–914, '43 also: Rev. Asoc. med. argent. *58:*21–24, Jan–Feb '44

REGGI, J. P.: Burns. Dia med. *15:*1424-1427, Dec 20, '43

REGNART, R. L. F.: Social sequels of maxillofacial wounds received in war. Rev. odont. *51:*372-378, Sept-Oct '30

REGNER. (see BAILLEUL) July '35

REGO, G.: Plastic correction of depressed deformities of facial bones, especially by means of traction apparatus. Arq. de cir. clin. e exper. *6:*200–234, April–June '42

REGOLI, G.: Experiments on implantation of dead preserved tissue. Policlinico (sez. chir.) *29:*559–574, Oct '22 (illus.)

REH, H.: Congenital fistulas of lacrimal sac combined with congenital aural fistulas and anosmia. Klin. Monatsbl. f. Augenh. *104:*55–59, Jan '40

REHN, E.: Surgical shock. Arch. f. klin. Chir. *177:*360–370, '33 also: Internat. Clin. *2:*57–65, June '34 abstr: Ztschr. f. Urol. *27:*709–710, '33

REHN, E.: Value of reparative surgery, inclusive of free transplantations. Arch. f. klin. Chir. *186:*244–266, '36

REHN, E.: Shock and surgical collapse in war wounded. Deutsche med. Wchnschr. *65:*1594–1598, Oct 27, '39

REHN, E.: Principles of reconstructive surgery in war wounds. Beitr. z. klin. Chir. *171:*1-24, '40

REHN, E.: Plastic surgery with cartilage for saddle nose. Zentralbl. f. Chir. *67:*548–550, March 30, '40

Rehn's Operation

Plastic surgery by Rehn's method of shifting soft parts to cover defect of face. FOHL, T. AND KILLIAN, H. Deutsche Ztschr. f. Chir. *222:*309–320, '30

Plastic surgery of corner of mouth (Rehn operation). VON BRANDIS, H. J., Deutsche Ztschr. f. Chir. *241:*479–482, '33

REICH, W.: Flexion contracture of fingers. Zentralbl. f. Chir. *53:*1503-1504, June 12, '26

Reich-Matti Operation

Reich-Matti operation for double harelip. FRÜND, H. Munchen. med. Wchnschr. *75:*1067-1070, June 22, '28

REICHEL: Etiology of finger contracture (Dupuytren's). Deutsche Ztschr. f. Chir. *230:*291-295, '31
REICHEL, J. JR. (see KENDRICK, D. B. JR. *et al*) July '43
REICHEL, J. JR. (see KENDRICK, D. B. JR.) Sept '43
REICHENBACH, E.: Present status of treatment of jaw fractures. Munchen. med. Wchnschr. *76:*530-532, March 29, '29
REICHENBACH, E.: Correction of nasal speech from congenital defects of palate by obturators. Vrtljsschr. f. Zahnh. *46:*418-434, '30
REICHENBACH, E.: Nonsurgical treatment of habitual dislocation of lower jaw especially when accompanied by prognathism. Deutsche Ztschr. f. Chir. *231:*470-476, '31
REICHENBACH, E.: Rare forms of fractures of mandible. Ztschr. f. Stomatol. *29:*719-728, June '31
REICHENBACH, E.: Claims of various obturators, from standpoint of correction of speech defects in cleft palate. Hals-, Nasen-. u. Ohrenarzt (Teil 1) *28:*29-33, Feb '37
REICHENBACH, E.: Wire reposition in linear fractures of lower jaw. Ztschr. f. Stomatol. *38:*347-357, May 24, '40
REICHENBACH, E.: Results of front line plastic surgery of face; experiences with the Army at Eastern Front. I. Zentralbl. f. Chir. *69:*1333-1350, Aug 15, '42
REICHENBACH, E. (see SCHMIDT, G.) 1932
REICHERT, E. L. (see HALSTED, W. S. *et al*) July-Aug '22
REICHL, E.: Surgical therapy of Dupuytren's contracture. Zentralbl. f. Chir. *64:*1570-1573, July 3, '37
REICHL, E.: Dupuytren's contracture; etiology. Wien. klin. Wchnschr. *52:*315-316, March 31, '39
REID, M. R.: Treatment of pigmented moles. Internat. Clin. *4:*222-232, Dec '33
REID, M. R. (see SILER, V. E.) June '42
REID, W. L.: Traumatic slow intraperitoneal hemorrhage with delayed shock; 3 cases. Southwestern Med. *19:*160-162, May '35
REIDY, J. P.: Relation of physiotherapy to plastic surgery. Proc. Roy. Soc. Med. *37:*705-708, Oct '44
REIFFERSCHEID, K.: Operative cure of incontinence of urine in epispadias by Goebell-Stoeckel operation. Zentralbl. f. Gynak. *45:*97, Jan 22, '21
REIFSNEIDER, J. S. (see PALMER, F. E.) Aug '33
REILLY, W. A.: Hypertelorism; four cases. J.A.M.A. *96:*1929-1933, June 6, '31
REIMERS, C.: Treatment of air raid burn casualties at base hospital; experiences in Chinese war. Chirurg *12:*145-152, March 15, '40
REINBERG, H.: Extensive facial reconstructive surgery; 2 cases. Zentralbl. f. Chir. *56:*530-534, March 2, '29
REINECKE, R.: Cysts and fistulas of lateral branchial canal. Arch. f. klin. Chir. *136:*99-108, '25
REINER, J.: Surgical correction of marked prognathism of the mandible. Internat. J. Orthodontia. *18:*271-281, March '32
REINHARD, W.: Total mastoneoplasty following amputation of breast. Deutsche Ztschr. f. Chir. *236:*309-317, '32
REINHARD, W.: Restorative surgery of lower jaw. Deutsche Ztschr. f. Chir. *257:*407, '43
REINHARD, W. AND LAUER, A.: Dangers in pedicled graft in homeoplasty; case of serious blood changes in patient and donor. Deutsche Ztschr. f. Chir. *254:*661-668, '41
REINSTEIN, H.: Hospital therapy of skin defects (decubitus ulcers). Psychiat.-neurol. Wchnschr. *38:*454-455, Sept 5, '36
REISNER, A.: Therapy of keloids and angiomas. Med. Klin. *34:*1233-1235, Sept 16, '38
REITER, E.: Fractures of mandible. Dental Cosmos *70:*772-782, Aug '28
REITZ, G. B.: Trauma to sesamoid bones of thumb. Am. J. Surg. *72:*284-285, Aug '46
REMZI, T.: New method of surgical therapy of acquired vaginal stenosis. J. Egyptian M. A. *19:*137-139, March '36
RENAUD, MME. A. (see BOIDE) May '38
RENAULT, P. (see TOURAINE, A.) Feb '33
RENAUX, R.: Keloids, with special reference to curative therapy and prevention. Monde med., Paris *45:*702-706, May 15, '35
RENDU, A.: Similarity of reasons for operative failures in congenital harelip and traumatic tear of lip. Gaz. med. de France, pp. 351-353, May 15, '32
RENEDO: Operative treatment of eyelid ptosis; case. Arch. de med., cir. y espec. *30:*628-631, May 25, '29
RENIE, R. O.: Management of nasal injuries. S. Clin. North America *19:*467-473, April '39
RENIE, R. O.: Economic considerations of cosmetic surgery. Am. J. Surg. *55:*126-130, Jan '42
RENNIE, A. M. (see NATHAN, P. W.) April '46
RENNIE, J. G.: Burn therapy with special reference to use of sulfadiazine (sulfonamide). Virginia M. Monthly *70:*24-30, Jan '43
RENNIE, S. W.: Therapy of thermal burns. Delaware State M. J. *17:*111-113, June '45

Replantation

Transplantation of leg; Sauerbruch's plastic operation. NISSEN, R. Umschau *31:*526, June 25, '27

Replantation – Cont.
Application to study of human constitution, of biological laws discovered by transplantation of extremities. BRANDT. Verhandl. d. anat. Gesellsch. *37:*38–41, '28
Tip of nose completely severed and sutured 3 hours after accident. ROY, J. N., J. Laryng. and Otol. *50:*518-520, July '35 also: Union med. du Canada *64:*847–852, Aug '35 also: Ann. Otol., Rhin. and Laryng. *44:*893–898, Sept '35
Tip of nose completely sectioned and sutured 3 hours after accident; recovery. ROY, J. N. Rev. de chir. structive, pp. 211–217, March '36
Autograft of amputated digit; suggested operation. GILLIES, H. Lancet *1:*1002–1003, June 1, '40
Whole upper extremity transplant for human beings; general plans of procedure and operative technic. HALL, R. H. Ann. Surg. *120:*12–23, July '44
Autograft of amputated thumb. GORDON, S. Lancet *2:*823, Dec 23, '44
Refrigeration in treatment of trauma (lacerated and almost detached thumb). KANAAR, A. G. Anesth. and Analg. *25:*177–190, Sept–Oct '46 *25:*228, Nov–Dec '46

REQUARTH, W.H.: Care of injured hand. U. S. Nav. M. Bull. *41:*1329–1335, Sept '43
REQUE, P. G.: Hypertrichosis with particular reference to electrolysis. South. Med. and Surg. *103:*376–379, July '41
RESCHKE, K.: Tschmarke's antiseptic treatment of burns. Arch. f. klin. Chir. *146:*763–776, '27
RESCHKE, K.: Transplantation of pedicled cartilaginous symphysis. Beitr. z. klin. Chir. *146:*713–720, '29
RESCHKE, K.: Treatment of ischemic contracture of wrist. Beitr. z. klin. Chir. *147:*302–307, '29
RESCHKE, K.: Surgical treatment of acquired club-hand. Deutsche Ztschr. f. Chir. *232:*458–462, '31
RESCHKE, K.: Tschmarke method of burn therapy. Med. Welt *5:*444, March 28, '31
RESENDE, E.: Complementary turbinotomy in submucosal resection of septum. Acta med., Rio de Janeiro *6:*166–167, Sept '40
RESNICK, E.: Congenital unilateral absence of pectoral muscles often associated with syndactylism. J. Bone and Joint Surg. *24:*925–928, Oct '42
RETEZEANU, MME. (see URECHIA, C. I.) March '36
RÉTHI, A.: Tamponing after operations on nose. Wien. klin. Wchnschr. *35:*637–638, July 20, '22
RÉTHI, A.: Operative treatment for saddle-nose. Zentralbl. f. Chir. *50:*1393–1397, Sept 8, '23 (illus.)
RÉTHI, A.: Enfolding flap in correction of nasal deformities. Acta oto-laryng. *11:*443–452, '27
RÉTHI, A.: Plastic operations on nasal cartilages. Ztschr. f. Hals-, Nasen-u. Ohrenh. *18:*515–517, '27–'28
RÉTHI, A.: Operative treatment of cicatricial stenosis of larynx; case. Ztschr. f. Laryng., Rhin. *16:*215–224, Nov '27
RÉTHI, A.: Plastic formation of tip of nose. Chirurg *1:*539–545, May 1, '29
RÉTHI, A.: Operation for hump-nose. Chirurg *1:*1103–1113, Nov 1, '29
RÉTHI, A.: Operative depilation in plastic surgery. Chirurg *1:*695–698, June 15, '29
RÉTHI, A.: Surgical contraction of pharynx in therapy of rhinolalia aperta. Monatschr. f. Ohrenh. *66:*842–848, July '32
RÉTHI, A.: Plastic surgery in destruction of tip of nose. Rev. de chir. plastique, pp. 327–349, Jan '33
RÉTHI, A.: Corrective operations; lowering of protruding nasal bridge and point. Chirurg *5:*503–511, July 1, '33
RÉTHI, A.: Shortening of nose. Rev. de chir. plastique, pp. 85–106, Oct '34
RÉTHI, A.: Treatment of functional and organic stenosis of entrance to nose. Rev. de chir. structive, pp. 137–147, June '37
RETTERER, E.: Plant and animal grafts. Progres med., pp. 1041–1050, June 11, '32
REUBEN, M. S. AND FOX, H. R.: Hypertelorism. Arch. Pediat. *45:*105–115, Feb '28
REUSS, A.: Acrocephalosyndactylia; 2 cases. Wien. med. Wchnschr. *77:*1208, Sept 3, '27
REUTER, M. J.: Therapy of nevi. Wisconsin M. J. *38:*207–208, March '39
REY, J.: Orthopedic treatment of hand and finger contractures. Ztschr. f. orthop. Chir. *48:*21–31, Feb 11, '27
REYNBERG, G. A.: Replacement of almost entire skin of upper extremity by skin graft; case. Khirurgiya, no.12, pp. 144–145, '37
REYNOLDS, T. E. (see HITCHCOCK, H. H.) Feb '36
DE REZENDE, N.: Experiments on cadaver nerve graft and "glue" suture of divided nerves. New York State J. Med. *42:*2124–2128, Nov 15, '42
DE REZENDE, N.: Transplantation of nerves from cadavers in human surgery. Rev. brasil. de cir. *13:*245–258, May '44
DE REZENDE, N. T. (see ESSEX, H. E.) Oct '43
DE REZENDE, N. T. (see KLEMME, R. M. *et al*) Oct '43
RHEA, B. S.: Facial injuries and scalp. J. Ten-

nessee M. A. *24:*41-42, Feb '31

RHÉAUME, P. Z. AND BABEAUX, F.: Repair of roof of orbit by means of cartilaginous graft. Presse med. *36:*1604, Dec 15, '28

RHINELANDER, F. W. (see COPE, O.) June '43

Rhinolalia (See also: Cleft Palate)

Rhino-laryngologic phases of harelip and cleft palate work. DAVIS, W. B. Internat. Clinics *2:*258-266, '22 (illus.)

Rhinolalia aperta. STREPOWSKA, A. Polaska gaz. lek. *8:*183-185, March 10, '29

Pathology and treatment of rhinolalia. STEIN, L. Wien. klin. Wchnschr. *43:*1068-1069, Aug 21, '30

Rhinolalia aperta; further studies. POE, D. L. Arch. Pediat. *50:*147-157, March '33

Rhinophyma

Surgical treatment of rhinophyma, with report of case. HANRAHAN, E. M. JR. Bull. Johns Hopkins Hosp. *32:*49, Feb '21

Rhinophyma. NEW, G. B., S. Clin. N. Amer. *1:*1393, Oct '21

Rhinophyma, report of case. ISRAEL, S. Laryngoscope *32:*218-219, March '22 (illus.)

Case of rhinophyma and its cure. SHEEHAN, J. E., M. J. and Rec. *119:*94-95, Jan 16, '24

Rhinophyma; report of 6 cases cured by radical operations followed by X-ray and acid treatments to relieve associated hypertrophy of skin and to reduce operative scars to state of invisibility. GRATTAN, J. F. Surg., Gynec. and Obst. *41:*99-102, July '25

Rhinophyma. SEELIG, M. G., S. Clin. N. America *5:*1381-1386, Oct '25

Operative treatment of rhinophyma. POROSZ, A. Dermat. Wchnschr. *84:*776, June 4, '27

Operative treatment of rhinophyma. RIVAS JORDAN, R. Rev. med. del Rosario *18:*68, Feb '28

Plastic surgery of nose in treatment of rhinophyma; original process of cicatrization. DE LIMA JUNIOR, B. Rev. brasil. de med. e pharm. *4:*243-250, May-June '28

Operative treatment of rhinophyma. SANVENERO-ROSSELLI, G. Rassegna ital. di otorino-laring. *2:*149-159, July-Aug '28

Successful treatment of rhinophyma. POROSZ, A. Urol. and Cutan. Rev. *32:*519, Aug '28

Rhinophyma; case cured by radiotherapy. HARET. Bull. et mem. Soc. de radiol. med. de France *16:*236, Nov '28

Treatment of rhinophyma; case. MARIN, A. Union med. du Canada *57:*641-644, Nov '28

Diathermic treatment of rhinophyma; 2 cases. BEHDJET, H. Dermat. Wchnschr. *88:*129-130, Jan 26, '29

Rhinophyma—Cont.

Plastic surgery of nose in treatment of rhinophyma; original process of cicatrization; cases. DE LIMA JUNIOR, B. Rev. oto-neuro-oft. *4:*80-87, Feb '29

Use of ferric chloride solution as hemostatic during operative treatment of rhinophyma; 2 cases. WETSCHTOMOW, A. A. Zentralbl. f. Chir. *57:*333-335, Feb 8, '30

Rhinophyma, with report of case. FEDERSPIEL, M. N. Wisconsin M. J. *29:*75-79, Feb '30

Operative treatment in case of gigantic rhinophyma. CAPRIOLI, N. Rinasc. med. *7:*144, March 15, '30

Effective use of electric coagulation in rhinophyma. BORDIER, H. Presse med. *38:*538-539, April 19, '30

Rhinophyma. SALINGER, S. Arch. Otolaryng. *11:*620-621, May '30

Therapy of rhinophyma. MARCOGLOU, A. E. Presse med. *38:*790, June 7, '30

Rhinophyma with carcinomatous degeneration; case. NOVY, F. G. JR. Arch. Dermat. & Syph. *22:*270-273, Aug '30

Treatment of rhinophyma. COLDREY, R. S. Brit. M. J. *2:*518, Sept. 27, '30

Operative treatment of rhinophyma; 3 cases. PALMA, R. Rev. sud-am. de med. et de chir. *2:*49-57, Jan '31

Rhinophyma, case. MACNAUGHTON, B. F. Canad. M. A. J. *24:*271-272, Feb '31

Rhinophyma, treatment and complications. MALINIAK, J. W. Arch. Otolaryng. *13:*270-274, Feb '31

Rhinophyma; representations in art and literature. DIECKMANN, F. Dermat. Ztschr. *62:*20-31, Sept '31

Case of carcinomatous degeneration of rhinophyma, with remarks on treatment of rhinophyma. EISENKLAM, D. Wien. klin. Wchnschr. *44:*1407-1408, Nov 6, '31

Surgical therapy of rhinophyma; case. ALBERTI, V. Rassegna internaz. di clin. e terap. *12:*1050-1060, Nov 15, '31

Rhinophyma. MARIN, A. Canad. M. A. J. *25:*589-591, Nov '31

Rhinophyma, with report of case. FEDERSPIEL, M. N. Internat. J. Orthodontia *18:*92-98, Jan '32

Rhinophyma. GLATT, M. A. Illinois M. J. *61:*174-175, Feb '32

Diathermy in treatment of rhinophyma. PÉRI, M. Practicien du Nord de l'Afrique *5:*150-151, March 15, '32

Rhinophyma, case with unusual involvement of chin. SAMS, W. M. Arch. Dermat. & Syph. *26:*834-837, Nov '32

Rhinophyma—Cont.
Rhinophyma, case. HUNT, H. L. Laryngoscope *43:*282, April '33
Simple procedure for cure of rhinophyma. ELLER, J. J. New York State J. Med. *33:*741–743, June 15, '33
Technic of surgical therapy of rhinophyma. DESGOUTTES, L. Tech. chir. *25:*177–188, Oct '33
Roentgenotherapy of rhinophyma. BLASI, R. Gior. ital. di mal. esot. e trop. *7:*16–22, Jan 31, '34
Diathermocoagulation in rhinophyma; case. FIUMICELLI, F. Dermosifilografo *9:*35–38, Jan '34 also: Minerva med. *1:*228–229, Feb 17, '34
Surgical therapy of rhinophyma; case. SPILIMANN, L.; *et al.* Bull. Soc. franc. de dermat. et syph. (Reunion dermat., Nancy) *41:*813–815, June '34
Technic of plastic surgery for rhinophyma. LEDO, E. Actas dermo-sif. *27:*249–254, Nov '34
Rhinophyma in woman. GINSBURG, L. Arch. Dermat. and Syph. *32:*468, Sept '35
Pathogenesis and therapy of rhinophyma. MANGABEIRA-ALBERNAZ, P. Rev. de laryng. *56:*1199–1214, Dec '35
Combined use of surgery and radium in treatment of rhinophyma. CAMPOS, R. Ars med., Barcelona *12:*85–91, Feb '36
Treatment of rhinophyma by electrodesiccation. KLAUDER, J. V. Arch. Dermat. and Syph. *33:*885, May '36
Results of nasal decortication performed 20 years ago for rhinophyma; case. JORGE, J. M., Bol. y trab. de la Soc. de cir. de Buenos Aires *20:*472–475, July 1, '36
Rhinophyma; with special reference to surgical therapy. REBELO NETO, J. Rev. otolaring. de Sao Paulo (no. 5, bis) *4:*811–840, Sept–Oct '36
Rhinophyma. CRABTREE, W. C. California and West. Med. *45:*485–487, Dec '36
Use of electric bistoury for removing rhinophyma; case. DORIGO, L. Bollettino *11:*62–72, '37
Rhinophyma, case treated and cured. MARIN, A. Union med. du Canada *68:*159–160, Feb '39
Rhinophyma; cosmetic surgery in primary stage. EITNER, E. Wien. med. Wchnschr. *89:*442–443, April 29, '39
Rhinophyma; therapy by Ollier's surgical decortication. MARIN, A. Bull. Soc. franc. de dermat. et syph. *46:*705–709, April '39
Rhinophyma and its treatment. DUCOURTIOUX, M. Presse med. *47:*799–800, May 24, '39
Rhinophyma. CINELLI, J. A. New York State J. Med. *40:*1672–1674, Nov 15, '40
Plasty surgery of nose; case of rhinophyma. SODRE FILHO, L. Arq. de cir. clin. e exper. *6:*692–695, April–June '42
Rhinophyma with new etiologic and therapeutic considerations (case with ascorbic acid deficiency). WOLFE, M. M. Laryngoscope *53:*172–180, March '43
Rhinophyma and hypertrophic acne; treatment by means of cold (high frequency) knife. IBARRA PEREZ, R. Vida nueva *52:*231–236, Nov '43
Rhinophyma. MALBEC, E. F. Prensa med. argent. *31:*2274–2284, Nov 8, '44
Surgical cure of acne rosacea and rhinophyma with skin grafting. MACOMBER, D. W. Rocky Mountain M. J. *43:*466–467, June '46

Rhinoplasty (See Nose, Various Categories)

Rhinoplasty, Alar Collapse

Lobulation of ala nasi. KALÓ, A. V. AND LIEBERMANN, T. V. Klin. Wchnschr. *3:*452, March 11, '24
Fascia implant to correct respiratory sinking in of nasal wings. BOECKER, W. Zentralbl. f. Chir. *48:*1796–1797, Dec 10, '21
Aspiration of ala nasi and its operative treatment. BOSVIEL, J., J. de med. de Paris *46:*417, May 26, '27
Treatment of alar collapse of nose. BROWN, E., J. Laryng. and Otol. *46:*545–546, Aug '31
Inversion of ala nasi. DESELAERS. Rev. espan. de med. y cir. *15:*9–10, Jan '32
Correction of collapse of ala nasi; 2 cases. ALFREDO, J. Rev. oto-laring. de Sao Paulo *2:*207–210, May–June '34
Therapy of collapse of nostril. ALFREDO, J. Rev. med. de Pernambuco *5:*22–26, Jan '35
Surgical correction of collapsed alar cartilages; case. GURNEY, C. E. Arch. Otolaryng. *33:*199–203, Feb '41
Collapse of nares. CINELLI, A. A. Arch. Otolaryng. *33:*683–693, May '41

Rhinoplasty, Anesthesia for

General versus local anesthesia in operations on nose and throat. WATSON, W. R. New York M. J. *113:*444, March 16, '21
A new local anesthetic for nose and throat work. BULSON, A. E. JR. Ann. Otol. Rhinol. and Laryngol. *31:*131–136, March '22
General anesthesia in submucous and other nasal operations. POE, J. G. Am. J. Surg. (Anesthesia supp.) *37:*56–57, April '23

Rhinoplasty, Anesthesia for—Cont.

Block anesthesia in nasal surgery. PARSONS, J. G. Northwest Med. *24:*223-227, May '25

Essential facts in connection with use of local anesthesia in nose and throat surgery. GATEWOOD, W. L. Virginia M. Monthly *54:*163-166, June '27

Topical application of cocaine in nose. HOWARD, E. F. New Orleans M. and S. J. *80:*162-167, Sept '27

Resection under local anesthesia of lower part of jaw, with integrity of nasal membrane; case. HEYNINX, A. Ann. d. mal. de l'oreille, du larynx *47:*996, Nov '28

Morphine-scopolamine narco-anaesthesia in nasal surgery. THACKER NEVILLE, W. S. Proc. Roy. Soc. Med. (Sect. Laryng.) *22:*61-64, Sept '29

Depth of action of percaine solution by application to mucous membrane of nose in surgical anesthesia. BIRKHOLZ. Klin. Wchnschr. *9:*72, Jan 11, '30

General anesthesia for nasal surgery. FORBES, S. B. South. M. J. *23:*305-308, April '30

Novocain (procaine hydrochloride) applied topically as local anesthetic in nasal surgery; preliminary report. NEFF, E. AND DIMOND, W. B. Ann. Otol., Rhin. and Laryng. *39:*593-594, June '30

Local anesthesia in nasal septal surgery. SONNTAG, A. Ztschr. f. Laryng., Rhin. *21:*32-36, June '31

Plastic preparation of nose; preliminary report on new local anesthetic. STRAATSMA, C. R., M. J. and Rec. *135:*399-400, April 20, '32

Method of local anesthesia for intranasal operations. LANE, F. F., U.S. Nav. M. Bull. *33:*55-59, Jan '35

Anesthesia in plastic surgery of nose. ERCZY, M. Orvosi hetil. *79:*641-643, June 8, '35

Injection anesthesia for submucous resection. LIEBERMANN, T. Budapesti orvosi ujsag *34:*831-832, Oct 1, '36

Discussion on choice and technic of anesthetics for nasal surgery. LAYTON, T. B. *et al.* J. Laryng. and Otol. *52:*501-512, July '37

Intranasal procaine anesthesia in nasal surgery. LEAMER, B. V., U.S. Nav. M. Bull. *36:*498-499, Oct '38

Nerve trunk anesthesia of nasal cavity. GATTI-MANACINI. Arch. ital. di otol. *51:*495-512, Oct '39

Methods for producing local anesthesia for intranasal operations. LILLIE, H. I. *et al.* Ann. Otol., Rhin. and Laryng. *49:*38-51, March '40

Procaine hydrochloride truncular anesthesia of nerves of nasal lobule; technic. MAGGIOROTTI, U. Boll. d. mal. d. orecchio, d. gola, d. naso *59:*17-18, Jan '41

Postural instillation; method of inducing local anesthesia. MOFFETT, A. J., J. Laryng. and Otol. *56:*429-436, Dec '41

Nasal surgery—local anesthesia; technic and practical considerations. HOOVER, W. B., S. Clin. North America *22:*661-673, June '42

Local regional anesthesia in nose and throat operations. MARTIN, G. E., J. Laryng. and Otol. *59:*38-43, Jan '44

Regional anesthesia of nose. DALE, H. W. L. Lancet *1:*562-563, April 29, '44

Postural instillation (for induction of local anesthesia); added note (nose). MOFFETT, A. J., J. Laryng. and Otol. *59:*151-153, April '44

Monocaine hydrochloride; clinical experiences and technic of administration in rhinoplasty. BERSON, M. I. Anesth. and Analg. *23:*189-195, Sept-Oct '44

Precise technic of local anesthesia in rhinoplasties. MALBEC, E. F., J. Internat. Coll. Surgeons *9:*495-505, Jul-Aug '46 also: Prensa med. argent. *33:*1594-1601, Aug 2, '46

Rhinoplasty, Chin Corrections with

Combined nasal plastic and chin plastic; correction of microgenia by osteocartilaginous transplant from large hump nose. AUFRICHT, G. Am. J. Surg. *25:*292-296, Aug '34

Reconstruction of deformed chin in its relationship to rhinoplasty; dermal graft—procedure of choice. MALINIAC, J. W. Am. J. Surg. *40:*583-587, June '38

Use of osteocartilaginous hump of nose for correction of underdeveloped chin. PALACIO POSSE, R. Arq. de cir. clin. e exper. *6:*299-301, April-June '42

Rhinoplasty; importance of microgenia of jaw. MARINO, H. Prensa med. argent. *33:*1500-1503, July 19, '46

Rhinoplasty, Complications

Orbital phlegmons as sequels of endonasal operations. BACHMANN, R. Med. Klin. *17:*192, Feb 13, '21

Pulmonary complications following nose and throat operations. BORDEN, C. R. C. Laryngoscope *31:*851, Nov '21

Fatalities following operations upon nose and throat not dependent upon anesthesia—study of 332 hitherto unreported cases. LOEB, H. W. Ann. Otol. Rhinol. and Laryngol. *31:*273-296, June '22

Rhinoplasty, Complications—Cont.

Fatalities after operations on nose. BURGER, H. Nederlandsch. Tijdschr. v. Geneesk. *1:*2356–2366, June 2, '23 abstr: J.A.M.A. *81:*1061, Sept 22, '23

Further studies of fatalities following operations on nose and throat. LOEB, H. W. Ann. Otol. Rhin. and Laryng. *32:*1103–1107, Dec '23

Corrective rhinoplasty, some reasons for faulty results. COHEN, L. Tr. Sect. Laryng., Otol. and Rhin., A. M. A., pp. 122–133, '23 (illus)

Causes of failure in corrective rhinoplasty—lantern demonstration. MALINIAK, J. Laryngoscope *35:*832–843, Nov '25 also: Ohio State M. J. *21:*807–814, Nov '25

Prevention of angina after nasal operations. HAARDT, W. Wien. klin. Wchnschr. *40:*320, March 10, '27

Peroral endoscopy; its use in complications following operations on nose and throat. TUCKER, G. Arch. Otolaryng. *5:*321–333, April '27

Reflections on hazards of nasal surgery in person with senile changes. HILL, F. T. Ann. Otol. Rhin. and Laryng. *36:*503–510, June '27

Saddle nose; unfortunate result of too thorough operation for deflected septum. SCHAEFFER, G. C. Ohio State M. J. *23:*989, Dec '27

Vascular changes in eye just after endonasal operations. MOUNIER-KUHN. Rev. d'oto-neuro-opht. *6:*679–685, Nov '28

Delayed healing of septal resections due to Vincent's infection; 3 cases. HOLLENDER, A. R. Arch. Otolaryng. *9:*422–424, April '29

Cerebrospinal rhinorrhea following nasal surgery. BULSON, A. E. AND BULSON, E. L. J.A.M.A. *93:*1969–1970, Dec 21, '29

Tetany following use of cocaine and epinephrine in nasal surgery; observations and treatment; preliminary report. ROBERTS, S. E. Tr. Sect. Laryng., Otol. and Rhin., A. M. A., pp. 22–30, '29

Rhinoplasty; facts and fiction. WOLF, G. D. Tr. Sect. Laryng., Otol. and Rhin., A. M. A. , pp.174–189, '29 also: Arch. Otolaryng. *11:*322–335, March '30

Etiology of postoperative anginas in nasal surgery. VON ZWEHL, W. Beitr. z. Anat., Physiol., Path. u. Therap. d. Ohres *28:*311–325, Oct '30

Rhinophyma, treatment and complications. MALINIAK, J. W. Arch. Otolaryng. *13:*270–274, Feb '31

Necrosis of septum after correction in latent

Rhinoplasty, Complications—Cont.

syphilis; 2 cases. BURGDORF, K. Arch. f. Ohren-, Nasen-u. Kehlhopfh. *129:*175–180, July 21, '31

Complications of minor endo-nasal operations. DUFOURMENTEL, L. Paris med. *2:*203–206, Sept 5, '31

Near-fatal postoperative secondary hemorrhage in nasal surgery. EFFLER, L. R. Laryngoscope *42:*201–206, March '32

Effective method of controlling secondary hemorrhage in nasal surgery. LITTELL, J. J., Laryngoscope *42:*207–209, March '32

Complications of minor nasal operations. DUFOURMENTEL, L. Rev. de laryng. *53:*447–474, April '32

Postoperative hemorrhage in nose and throat operations; treatment with clauden. THACKER NEVILLE, W. S. Lancet *2:*624–625, Sept 17, '32

Complications following nasal surgery. WALDAPFEL, R. Wien. med. Wchnschr. *83:*1431–1433, Dec 16, '33

Postoperative disturbances in nasal surgery. TOBECK, A. Med. Klin. *30:*629–631, May 11, '34

Keloid of nose; case. TAVANI, E. Boll. d. mal. d. orecchio, d. gola, d. naso *52:*281–288, June '34

Death of patient after Killian operation for deformed septum. ERRECART, P. L. Rev. Asoc. med. argent. *50:*974–977, June '36

Late complications of nasal fractures. DUFOURMENTEL, L. Paris med. *2:*152–155, Sept 5, '36

Hypertrophic fibrous cicatrix following esthetic operation on nose by endonasal route. PREVOT, M. Rev. de chir. structive, pp. 43–44, March '37

Precaution against hemorrhage and infections following intranasal operations. BOEHS, C. J., Texas State J. Med. *32:*824–827, April '37

Complications following rhinoplasty. PALMER, A. Arch. Otolaryng. *28:*538–545, Oct '38

Postoperative psychosis; dementia praecox following operation on nasal septum; case. MUKASA, H. Oto-rhino-laryng. *12:*139, Feb '39

Discussion on complications of intranasal surgery. HOWARTH, W. AND DAVIS, E. D. D. Proc. Roy. Soc. Med. *32:*1238–1246, Aug '39 also: J. Laryng. and Otol. *54:*627–640, Oct '39

Complications of rhinoplastic surgery. KOPP, M. M., J. Internat. Coll. Surgeons *2:*346–350, Oct '39

Rhinoplasty, Complications – Cont.
Atrophic rhinitis in plastic surgery. Kopp, M. M. Laryngoscope *50:*510–519, June '40
Prevention and treatment of late sequelae in corrective rhinoplasty. Maliniac, J. W. Am. J. Surg. *50:*84–91, Oct '40
Failures in rhinoplastic surgery; causes and prevention. Safian, J. Am. J. Surg. *50:*274–280, Nov '40
Arterial vascularization of nose; relation to certain plastic reactions after corrective interventions. Thevenin, J. Plast. chir. *1:*155–161, '40
Fallacious views and factors influencing more successful results in nasal surgery. Hollender, A. R., J. Florida M. A. *28:*27–29, July '41
Sulfonamides in prophylaxis of postoperative meningitis in nasal surgery. Piquet, J. Monatschr. F. Ohrenh. *76:*68–75, Feb '42
Critical review of causes of unsuccessful end results of nasal surgery. Hollender, A. R. South. M. J. *35:*363–372, April '42
Complications of plastic surgery of nasal septum. Cohen, S. Dis. Eye, Ear, Nose and Throat *2:*235–243, Aug '42
Nasal septal operation; technic to avoid postoperative tamponade. Lanza Castelli, R. A., Rev. otorrinolaring. d. litoral *2:*112–128, Dec '42
Critical review of causes of unsuccessful end results in nasal surgery. Hollender, A. R. Eye, Ear, Nose and Throat Monthly *22:*21–26, Jan '43
Do corrective operations of nose cause pathologic disorders? Hernandez Ramirez, S. Pasteur *2:*35–37, Aug 15, '43
Fixity of facial expression following undermining of skin over nose; modified method by which it is avoided. Seltzer, A. P. Am. J. Surg. *68:*326–335, June '45

Rhinoplasty, Corrective
Cosmetic surgery of nose. Selfridge, G. Laryngoscope *31:*337, June '21
Corrective rhinoplasty, with presentation of case. Weil, A. I. New Orleans M. and S. J. *73:*507, June '21
Operation on nose without skin incision. Esser, J. F. S. Deutsche Ztschr. f. Chir. *164:*211, June '21 abstr: J.A.M.A. *77:*898, Sept 10, '21
Plastic and cosmetic surgery of head, face and neck; correction of nasal deformities. Tieck, G. J. E. and Hunt, H. L. Am. J. Surg. *35:*234, Aug '21
An invisible scar method in cosmetic nasal surgery. Frank, I. and Strauss, J. S.

Rhinoplasty, Corrective – Cont.
Ann. Otol. Rhinol. and Laryng. *30:*670, Sept '21
Further observations in correction of external deformities of nose by intranasal route. Israel, S. Texas State J. Med. *17:*302, Oct '21
Surgery of nasal deformities. Guthrie, D. Edinburgh M. J. *27:*365, Dec '21
External nasal deformities; description of operative technic of new method for correction of certain types. Lewis, J. D. Laryngoscope *32:*214–217, March '22 (illus.)
Intranasal reconstruction. Pratt, F. J. and Pratt, J. A. Ann. Otol. Rhinol. and Laryngol. *31:*46–105, March '22 (illus.)
Cosmetic operations on nose. Gallusser, E. Schweiz. med. Wchnschr. *52:*381–383, April 20, '22 (illus.) abstr: J.A.M.A. *78:*1931, June 17, '22
External deformities of nose and their correction by intra-nasal route. Israel, S. Southern M. J. *15:*324–327, April '22 (illus.)
Bone surgery of nose. Carter, W. W. Surg., Gynec. and Obst. *34:*800–803, June '22 (illus.)
Corrective rhinoplasty, some anatomicosurgical considerations. Cohen, L. Surg., Gynec. and Obst. *34:*794–799, June '22 (illus.)
Plastic repair of nasal displacement and deformity. Goldthwaite, R. H. Mil. Surgeon *51:*42–43, July '22
Correction of external deformities of nose. Israel, S. Tr. Sect. Laryng. Otol. and Rhin., A. M. A., pp. 111–119, '22 (illus.)
Clinical observations on correction of external deformities of nose by intranasal route, with lantern demonstration. Blackwell, H. B. Laryngoscope *33:*21–26, Jan '23 (illus.)
Plastic correction for nose deformities. Eitner, E. Med. Klinik *19:*238–239, Feb 25, '23
Corrective rhinoplasty. Aud, G. Kentucky M. J. *21:*105–110, Feb '23
Nasal disfigurement and its correction. Guthrie, D. J. Laryng. and Otol. *38:*300–303, June '23 (illus.)
Correction of external deformities of nose. Israel, S. Ann. Otol., Rhin. and Laryng. *32:*504–517, June '23 (illus.)
Conservatism in nasal surgery. Potter, W. W. Southern M. J. *16:*560–563, July '23
Correction of deformities of nose and about orbit by plastic surgery. de River, J. P. Southwestern Med. *7:*226–232, July '23
Nasal deformities. Locy, F. E., U.S. Nav. M. Bull. *19:*152–155, Aug '23 (illus.)
Correction of nasal deformities. Sheehan, J.

Rhinoplasty, Corrective—Cont.
E. Brit. M. J. *2:*981-982, Nov 24, '23
Nasal deformities and their correction. WILSON, A. K., J. Florida M. A. *10:*270-273, April '24
Cosmetic surgery of nose and ear. SOLONCOV, N. Cas. lek. cesk. *63:*833-839, May 31, '24
Correction of external nasal deformities. DE RIVER, J. P. California and West. Med. *22:*214-216, May '24
New Method for rhinoplasty. IVANISSEVICH, O. Surg., Gynec. and Obst. *38:*828-829, June '24
Cosmetic surgery of nose and ear. WODAK, E. Med. Klinik *20:*1042-1044, July 27, '24
Nasal deformities. NEW, G. B. Minnesota Med. *7:*629-633, Oct '24
Correction of nasal deformities following septum operations. SAFIAN, J. Laryngoscope *34:*957-960, Dec '24
Plastic Surgery of the Nose, by J. EASTMAN SHEEHAN. Paul Hoeber Co., New York, 1925. Second Edition, 1936
Surgery of deformities of nose. DUFOURMENTEL, L. Arch. franco-belges de chir. *28:*273-292, April '25
Corrective plastic operations on nose. WODAK, E. Med. Klinik *21:*1573-1575, Oct 16, '25
Correction of nasal deformities. CARTER, W. W., New York State J. Med. *25:*1070-1073, Dec 1, '25
Correction of nasal deformities by external route. GILL, E. G. Virginia M. Monthly *52:*578-581, Dec '25
Plastic surgery of nose. BETTMAN, A. G., M. J. and Rec. *123:*417-421, April 7; 499-501, April 21, '26
Endonasal plastic surgery. BASAVILBASO, J. Prensa med. argent. *13:*23-25, June 10, '26
New method for plastic operations in bony frame of nose. SOUZA MENDES, J. Brazil-med. *2:*100-102, Aug 21, '26
Corrective rhinoplasty. BLANCHARD, H. E. Rhode Island M. J. *9:*161-165, Oct '26
Surgery of nasal deformities. LEROUX-ROBERT. Vie med. *7:*2499, Dec 3, '26
Example of Joseph nose improvement. DANELIUS, B. Acta oto-laryng. *9:*49-52, '26 (in English)
Rhinoplasty and stomatoplasty. PERTHES, G. Arch. f. klin. Chir. *142:*572-589, '26
Correction chirurgicales des difformités congenitales et acquises de la pyramide nasale, by PIERRE SEBILEAU AND LÉON DUFOURMENTEL. Arnette, Paris, 1927
Eine Nasenplastik, ausgeführt in Lokalanesthesie. Kinegrammata medica. (In German, English, French, Italian, Russian,

Rhinoplasty, Corrective—Cont.
and Spanish test) P. 14. G. Stilke, Berlin, 1927
Outline of methods of nasal plastic surgery. BOSVIEL, J., J. de med. de Paris *46:*87, Jan 31, '27
Prevention and correction of nasal deformities. MALINIAK, J. Eye, Ear, Nose and Throat Month. *5:*689, Jan '27
Plastics of external nose. VON WEDEL, C., J. Oklahoma M. A. *20:*44-45, Feb '27
Correction of nasal disfigurements by readjustment of nasal tissues. SHEEHAN, J. E. M. J. and Rec. *125:*585, May 4; 664, May 18, '27
Technic of plastic surgery of face and nose. VAN DEN BRANDEN, J. Bruxelles-med. *7:*917-920, May 15, '27
Experiences with corrective plastic surgery of nose. GRIESSMANN, B. Klin. Wchnschr. *6:*1045, May 28, '27
Plastic surgery of face (including nose). IVY, R. H. Atlantic M. J. *30:*572-575, June '27
Plastic surgery of nose. IVY, R. H. Laryngoscope *37:*486-497, July '27
Surgery of nasal deformities. SANVENERO-ROSSELLI, G. Ann. di laring., otol. *28:*193-216, July '27
Technic and results of plastic surgery of nasal deformities. MORNARD, P. Rev. franc. de dermat. et de venereol. *3:*386-405, July-Aug '27
Surgical correction of congenital and acquired deformities of nasal pyramid; with 105 illustrations. SEBILEAU, P. AND DUFOURMENTEL, L. Ann. d. mal. de l'oreille, du larynx *46:*753, Aug '27
Surgical correction of congenital and acquired deformities of nasal pyramid. SEBILEAU, P. AND DUFOURMENTEL, L. Ann. d. mal. de l'oreille, du larynx *46:*753, Aug; 853, Sept '27
Technic of correction of nasal deformity by adjustment of proper tissues. SANVENERO-ROSSELLI, G. Rassegna ital. di oto-rino-laring. *1:*223-231, Sept-Oct '27
Plastic operations on nasal cartilages. RÉTHI, A. Ztschr. f. Hals-, Nasen-u. Ohrenh. *18:*515-517, '27-'28
Nasenplastik und sonstige Gesichtsplastik, etc., by JACQUES JOSEPH. C. Kabitsch, Leipzig, 1928
Plastic and reconstructive procedures in rhinology. MALINIAK, J. W. New York State J. Med. *28:*6-9, Jan 1, '28
Best method of correction of snub-nose. ROY, J. N. Arch. internat. de laryng. *34:*166-178, Feb '28
Corrective surgery of eyelids and nose. AT-

Rhinoplasty, Corrective—Cont.
KINSON, D. T., J. Ophth., Otol. and Laryng. *32:*73-82, March '28
Results obtained in corrective rhinoplasty. COHEN, L., M. J. and Rec. *127:*354-357, April 4, '28
Nasal plastic surgery; 7 cases. DE FLINES, E. W., Nederl. Tijdschr. v. Geneesk. *1:*1984, April 21, '28
New technic for plastic operations of nose. KELLY, J. D. Arch. Otolaryng. *8:*433-445, Oct '28
Nasal deformities. BLAIR, V. P. Tr. Am. Laryng. A. *50:*36-40, '28
Rhinoplasty; 3 cases. SCHREIBER, F. Beitr. z. klin. Chir. *144:*307, '28
Chirurgie correctrice du nez, by LÉON DUFOURMENTEL. University Press of France, Paris, 1929.
Recent results in rhinoplasty. COHEN, L. Virginia M. Monthly *55:*781-788, Feb '29
Plastic surgery of nose. INGEBRIGTSEN, R. Norsk Mag. f. Laegevidensk. *90:*169-175, Feb '29
Plastic surgery of nose. BIANCULLI, H. Semana med. *1:*741-748, March 28, '29
Plastic operation for saddle nose. SIMONT, D. Zentralbl. f. Chir. *56:*910-912, April 13, '29
External operation for correction of acquired nasal deformity. MASSA, D. AND TATO, J. M. Rev. de especialid. *4:*129-135, April-May '29
Treatment of nasal deformities and fractures. RISDON, F. Canad. M. A. J. *20:*631-633, June '29
Corrective plastic surgery of nose. TZUKERMANN, M. A. Vrach. dielo *12:*1020-1023, Aug 31, '29
Technic of cosmetic surgery of nose. FORERO, A. Semana med. *2:*1461-1474, Nov 21, '29
Plastic surgery of nose. COHEN, S. Pennsylvania M. J. *33:*50-52, Nov '29
Plastic surgery of nose, ear, face. DAVIS, A. D. Arch. Otolaryng. *10:*575-584, Dec '29
Problem of rhinoplasty. UPDEGRAFF, H. L. Ann. Surg. *90:*961-973, Dec '29
Cosmetic operations of nose. LEXER, E. Handb. d. Hals-, Nasen-, Ohrenh. *5:*991-1030, '29
Technic of rhinoplasty. HAGENTORN, A. Zentralbl. f. Chir. *57:*600-603, March 8, '30
Rhinoplasty. IVANISSEVICH, O. AND FERRARI, R. C. Semana med. *1:*967-974, April 17, '30
Problems in plastic surgery of nose. NEW, G. B. Minnesota Med. *13:*242-246, April '30
Sheehan's method of plastic surgery of nose. DELLEPIANE RAWSON, R. Rev. med. latino-am. *15:*1055-1090, May '30

Rhinoplasty, Corrective—Cont.
Technic of cosmetic operations of nose. WOJATSCHEK, W. Monatschr. f. Ohrenh. *64:*1066-1070, Sept '30
Nasal surgery. DELLEPIANE RAWSON, R. AND GONZÁLEZ AVILA, E. Semana med. *2:*1351-1357, Oct 30, '30
Nasenplastik und sonstige Gesichtsplastik. Nebst einem Anhang über Mammaplastik und . . . Körperplastik, by JACQUES JOSEPH. C. Kabitsch, Leipzig, 1931
Chirurgia plastica del naso, by GUSTAVO SANVENERO-ROSSELLI. Luigi Pozzi, Rome, 1931
Plastic surgery of nose. FORERO, A. Semana med. *1:*187-191, Jan 15, '31
Plastic surgery of nose; 2 cases. GONZÁLEZ LOZA, M. Rev. med. del Rosario *21:*701-706, Jan '31
Autoplasty in rhinologic surgery (face). OMBRÉDANNE, M. Semaine d. hop. de Paris *7:*44-48, Jan 31, '31
End results in nasal surgery. WOLF, G. D., M. J. and Rec. *133:*178-182, Feb 18, '31
Correction of disfigurements of nose by readjustment of frame-work and tissues. SHEEHAN, J. E. Arch. Otolaryng. *13:*584-596, April '31
Plastic surgery of nose. LIEBERMANN, T. Orvosi hetil. *75:*646-649, June 20, '31
Rhinoplasty; 3 cases. QUESADA, F. Dia med. *4:*16, Aug 3, '31
Technic of correcting nasal deformities. KING, E. Arch. Otolaryng. *14:*483-488, Oct '31
Plastic surgery of nose. PEER, L. A. Arch. Otolaryng. *14:*462-466, Oct '31
Experiences in rhinoplasty. ŠERCER, A. Otolaryng. slavica *3:*415-435, Oct '31
Plastic surgery of nose. KING, E. D., J. Med. *12:*518-524, Dec '31
Plastic surgery of nose. SMIRNOV, A. A. Russk. oto-laring. *24:*356-358, '31
Korrektiv-cosmetische Chirurgie der Näse, der Ohren, und des Gesichts, by VICTOR FRÜHWALD. Wilhelm Maudrich, Vienna, 1932. (Also English edition, translated by Geoffrey Morey.)
Plastic surgery of nose. COHEN, S. Eye, Ear, Nose and Throat Monthly *10:*493-498, Jan '32
Plastic surgery of nose. GAMES, F. AND MERCANDINO, C. Semana med. *1:*727-736, March 3, '32
Rhinoplasty; past and present. PALMER, A. Eye, Ear, Nose and Throat Monthly *11:*58-62, March '32
Plastic surgery in nasal reconstruction; classification of deformities. GONZÁLEZ LOZA,

Rhinoplasty, Corrective – Cont.
M. Rev. med. del Rosario *22:*268–282, May '32
Simplification of nasal plastic surgery. STRAATSMA, C. R. New York State J. Med. *32:*871–872, July 15, '32
Plastic surgery of nasal deformities. WODAK, E. Rev. de chir. plastique, pp. 157–169, July '32
External nasal deformities and their correction. ISRAEL, S. South. M. J. *25:*916–919, Sept '32
Scarless reconstruction of nose broken in childhood. HEINEMANN, O. Med. Klin. *28:*1427–1428, Oct 7, '32
Nasal deformities and their correction. SALINGER, S. Arch. Otolaryng. *16:*510–525, Oct '32
Conservatism in surgery as applied to nasal mucosa. GROSS, W. A. Am. J. Phys. Therapy *9:*199–200, Nov '32 also: Eye, Ear, Nose and Throat Monthly *11:*392–393, Nov '32
New method of surgical correction of nasal deformities. VON LIEBERMANN, T. Ztschr. f. Hals, Nasen-u. Ohrenh. *30:*560–566, '32
Plastic surgery of nasal deformities. PEER, L. A., J. M. Soc. New Jersey *30:*123–130, Feb '33
Cosmetic surgery of nose. WEISS, J. Semana med. *1:*1779–1783, May 25, '33
Method of rhinoplasty. STRAITH, C. L. Rev. de chir., Plastique, pp. 109–115, Aug '33
Surgical therapy of nasal deformities; 2 cases. LARROUDÉ, C. Rev. de chir. plastique, pp. 246–250, Oct '33
Surgical correction of deformed external ear and nose; case. REBELLO NETO, J. Rev. med. de Pernambuco *3:*285–290, Oct '33
Nasal deformities and their repair. KAZANJIAN, V. H. Laryngoscope *43:*955–975, Dec '33
Plastic surgery of nose. WATKINS, A. B. K. J. Laryng. and Otol. *48:*809–820, Dec '33
Surgical therapy of nasal deformities. PAPE. Ztschr. f. Laryng., Rhin., Otol. *24:*73–74, '33
Cosmetic surgery in correction of protruding pinna, also of nose. MALBEC, E. F. Semana med. *1:*170–175, Jan 11, '34
Facial and nasal plastic surgery from esthetic point of view. VILARDOSA LLUBES, E. Rev. de cir. de Barcelona *8:*1, July–Aug; 99, Sept–Dec '34
Rhinoplasty. PAGENSTECHER, G. A. Am. J. Surg. *25:*491–493, Sept '34
Plastic surgery of nasal deformities. COHEN, S., M. Rec. *140:*536–539, Nov 21, '34
Cosmetic corrections of abnormalities of septal cartilage. EITNER, E. Ztschr. f. Laryng., Rhin., Otol. *25:*40–45, '34

Rhinoplasty, Corrective – Cont.
Corrective Rhinoplastic Surgery, by JOSEPH SAFIAN. Paul Hoeber Co., New York, 1935
External nasal deformities corrected and removal of existing intranasal obstruction advantageously accomplished at same operation. COHEN, L. Ann. Otol., Rhin. and Laryng. *44:*233–241, March '35
Plastic surgery of nose; 6 cases. IVANISSEVICH, O. AND FERRARI, R. C. Semana med. *1:*973–989, April 4, '35
Shortening and lengthening of nose. EITNER, E. Wien. klin. Wchnschr. *48:*799–800, June 7, '35
Cases of rhinoplasty. ROY, J. N. Union med. du Canada *64:*644–658, June '35 also: Canad. M. A. J. *33:*158–160, Aug '35
External nasal deformities and their correction. ISRAEL, S. Texas State J. Med. *31:*281–284, Aug '35
Esthetic surgery of nose. DANTRELLE, A. J. de med. de Paris *55:*865–870, Oct 3, '35
Plastic surgery of ears; cases (and face and nose). MALBEC, E. F. Semana med. *2:*718–728, Sept 10, '36
Esthetic surgery (of nose); cases. MALBEC, E. F. Semana med. *2:*1632–1643, Dec 10, '36
Problems in cosmetic surgery of nose. KOVACS, A. Laryngoscope *47:*92–96, Feb '37
Correction of nasal deformities. CINELLI, J. A. New York State J. Med. *37:*1018–1024, June 1, '37
Plastic surgery of nose; 5 cases. RAPIN, M. Rev. med. de la Suisse Rom. *57:*405–412, June 10, '37
Esthetic surgery of nose; results in cases. MALBEC, E. F. Semana med. *2:*280–289, July 29, '37
Operative procedures for cosmetic purposes (nose). VON WEIDEL, C., J. Oklahoma M. A. *30:*249–252, July '37
Correction of displaced nasal cartilage, especially in children. COHEN, S. Pennsylvania M. J. *40:*925–930, Aug '37
Rhinoplasty; 2 cases. MICHALOWSKI, E. Rev. de chir. structive, pp. 214–222, Oct '37
Plastic repair of nose as aid in therapeutic surgery. MAMLET, A. M., J. M. Soc. New Jersey *34:*664–666, Nov '37
Corrective rhinoplasty. ZENO, L. An. de cir. *3:*357–363, Dec '37
Plastic surgery of nose; technic and instruments. CLAOUE. Ztschr. f. Hals-, Nasen-u. Ohrenh. *40:*660–662, '37
Plastic surgery of nose. KULAKCI, N. Anadolu klin. *5:*199–200, '37
Plastic correction of boxer's ears and nose. DUJARDIN, E. Ugesk. f. laeger *100:*115, Feb 3, '38
Corrective operations of nose and develop-

Rhinoplasty, Corrective—Cont.
ment of plastic surgery. ERCZY, M. Gyogyaszat *78:*272–276, April 24, '38
Esthetic and psychologic principles of plastic surgery of nose, ears and face. WODAK, E. Monatschr. f. Ohrenh. *72:*424, April; 490, May '38
Evaluation of rhinoplasty. SAFIAN, J. Rev. de chir. structive *8:*14–18, May '38
Combined nasal reconstruction and submucous resection. TAMERIN, J. A. New York State J. Med. *38:*1129–1133, Aug 15, '38
Cosmetic rhinoplasty; 150 cases. ISHII, T. Oto-rhino-laryng. *11:*722, Aug '38
Technic of surgical correction of nasal deformities. ZENO, L. Bol. Soc. de cir. de Rosario *5:*345–348, Aug '38
Plastic surgery (nose). ZENO, L. Rev. Asoc. med. argent. *52:*902–907, Sept 15, '38
Plastic surgery (face) (nose). KING, E. D. J. Med. *19:*348–354, Sept '38
New technic for plastic operations of nose. KELLY, J. D. Arch. Otolaryng. *8:*433–445, Oct '28
Plastic surgery of nose. ZERO, L. An. de otorino-laring. d. Uruguay *8:*225–235, '38
Plastic and esthetic surgery of ear, nose and face; cases. MALBEC, E. F. Semana med. *1:*83–95, Jan 12, '39
Esthetic surgery; criteria or artistic precepts (nose). SCAVUZZO, R. Semana med. *1:*144–146, Jan 19, '39
Corrective surgery of nasal deformities. MALBEC, E. F. Semana med. *1:*365–375, Feb 16, '39
Plastic surgery of nose. ADLER, D. Rev. med. brasil. *2:*67–82, Feb '39
Plastic surgery of nose; case. MALBEC, E. F. Dia med. *11:*300–301, April 10, '39
Rhinoplasty. COMORA, H. C. Laryngoscope *49:*484–488, June '39
Rhinoplasty. INGEBRIGTSEN, R. Lyon chir. *26:*548–553, Aug–Sept '29
Deformities of ear and nose treated by plastic surgery. COX, G. H. New York State J. Med. *39:*1956–1961, Oct 15, '39
Plastic surgery of nose. SORALUCE, J. A. Semana med. espan. *2:*782–789, Dec 30, '39
Nasal surgery in women. COELST. Bull. Soc. belge d'otol., rhinol., laryng., pp. 316–318, '39
Plastic operations of nose. ENGLAND, M. C. J. Oklahoma M. A. *33:*10–12, Jan '40
Plastic surgery of nose. DE VILLIERS, R. Rev. san. mil., Habana *4:*27–40, Jan–March '40
Possibilities and principles of plastic surgery of nose. WEICHHERZ, I. Budapesti orvosi ujsag *38:*134–136, March 21, '40
Two-stage plastic operation for nasal deformities. KLICPERA, L. Monatschr. f. Ohrenh. *74:*183–186, April '40
Problems in plastic surgery of nose. STRAATSMA, C. R. Laryngoscope *50:*1092–1099, Nov '40
Plastic surgical correction of nasal deformities. LIPPMAN, M. C., M. Rec. *152:*399–402, Dec 4, '40
Plastic surgery for enlarged and small nose resulting from accidents. PEARLMAN, R. C. M. Rec. *152:*402–404, Dec 4, '40
Plastic surgery of nose. COHEN, S. Laryngoscope *51:*363–377, April '41
Plastic surgery of nose. MIGRAY, J. Orvos. koz. *2:*167–172, May 31, '41
Plastic surgery of face and nose. KING, E. D. West Virginia M. J. *37:*293–297, July '41
Plastic surgery of external ear, case (and nose). MALBEC, E. F. Prensa med. argent. *28:*1700–1702, Aug 20, '41
Plastic surgery of nasal deformities. RECALDE, J. F. JR. Rev. med. d. Paraguay *5:*32–37, Jan–March '42
Plastic surgery of nose; cases. WEAVER, D. F. J. Michigan M. Soc. *41:*229–232, March '42
Plastic surgery of nose. MALINIAC, J. W. Dis. Eye, Ear, Nose and Throat *2:*102–106, April '42
Plastic surgery of nasal deformities. ALVES, O. Arq. de cir. clin. e exper. *6:*320–322, April–June '42
Plastic surgery of nose. DE SANSON, R. D. Arq. de cir. clin. e exper. *6:*144, April–June '42
Rhinoplasty from cosmetic point of view. SALINGER, S., J. Iowa M. Soc. *32:*199–202, May '42
Plastic surgery of nose. KING, E. Kentucky M. J. *40:*264–266, July '42
Plastic surgery of ear and nose. MALBEC, E. F. Semana med. *2:*426–431, Aug 20, '42
External deformities of nose and methods used in their repair. DAVIS, W. B. Arch. Otolaryng. *36:*619–628, Nov '42
External nasal deformities and methods used in their repair. DAVIS, W. B. Tr. A. Laryng. A. *64:*80–90, '42
Materials for corrective plastic surgery of nose. RAPIN, M. Pract. oto-rhino-laryng. *4:*133–141, '42
Hints and surgical details in rhinoplasty. AUFRICHT, G. Laryngoscope *53:*317–335, May '43
Improved method of narrowing the nose. SELTZER, A. P. Ann. Otol., Rhin. and Laryng. *52:*460–472, June '43
Treatment of nasal deformities. DE RYNCK, G., M. Press *210:*154–157, Sept 8, '43
Principles of rhinoplasty. FELDERMAN, L. Pennsylvania M. J. *47:*13–20, Oct '43

Rhinoplasty, Corrective—Cont.

Important considerations in rhinoplastic procedures. BERSON, M. I. Eye, Ear, Nose and Throat Monthly *22:*424–430, Nov '43

Lateral osteotomy; anatomic considerations (description of grove on frontal process of maxilla). GALE, C. K. Am. J. Surg. *63:*368–370, March '44

Retaining correct septolabial angle in rhinoplasty. DALEY, J. Arch. Otolaryng. *39:*348–349, April '44

Muscles and cartilages of nose from standpoint of typical rhinoplasty. GRIESMAN, B. L. Arch. Otolaryng. *39:*334–341, April '44

Correction of multiple deformities of nose. GATEWOOD, W. L. Virginia M. Monthly *71:*227–231, May '44

Typical rhinoplastic operation. LUONGO, R. A. Arch. Otolaryng. *40:*68–72, July '44

Rhinology and plastic surgery of nasal pyramid. ALCAINO, Q. A. Rev. otorrinolaring. *4:*73–123, Sept '44

Correction of multiple deformities of nose. GATEWOOD, W. L. Eye, Ear, Nose and Throat Monthly *24:*134–138, March '45

Fixity of facial expression following undermining of skin over nose; modified method by which it is avoided. SELTZER, A. P. Am. J. Surg. *68:*326–335, June '45

Cosmetic surgery of nose. FIRESTONE, C. Northwest Med. *44:*213–216, July '45

Plastic surgery of nasal fractures. LAMONT, E. S. Am. J. Surg. *69:*144–154, Aug '45

Anatomic and physiologic principles underlying plastic surgery of nasal deformities. ROSEDALE, R. S. Ohio State M. J. *41:*724–728, Aug '45

Rhinoplastic correction of common deformities. BARRETT, J. H. Texas State J. Med. *41:*315–318, Oct '45

Corrective surgery of external pyramid and septum for restoration of normal physiology. COTTLE, M. H. AND LORING, R. M. Illinois M. J. *90:*119–131, Aug '46

Cartilaginous septum in reconstruction of nose; modified procedure. EISBACH, E. J. Arch. Otolaryng. *44:*207–211, Aug '46

New operation for dislocated nasal cartilage. KAYSER, R. Am. J. Surg. *72:*248–251, Aug '46

Problem of rhinoplastic surgery. COATES, G. M. Tr. Am. Acad. Ophth. *51:*11–17, Sept-Oct '46

Rhinoplasty, Deviated Nose

Submucous replacement for external deviation of nose. OERTEL, T. E. Ann. Otol. Rhinol. and Laryng. *30:*147, March '21

Rhinoplasty, Deviated Nose—Cont.

Operation to correct crooked nose. BOSERUP, O. AND KRAGH, J. Ugesk. f. Laeger *85:*808, Nov 15; 830, Nov 22, '23

Lower nasal deflection; new operation for its correction. COHEN, S. Arch. Otolaryng. *8:*399–404, Oct '28

Surgical correction of crooked nose. SALINGER, S. Illinois M. J. *54:*368–373, Nov '28

Operation for bony wry-nose. LAUTENSCHLÄGER, A. Chirurg *1:*260–263, Feb 1, '29

Plastic operations for wry-nose. EITNER, E. Med. Klin. *25:*600, April 12, '29

Correction of bony wry and flat nose. HEERMANN, H. Ztschr. f. Hals-, Nasen-u. Ohrenh. *23:*133–136, June 10, '29

Nasal reconstruction by means of bone and cartilage existing within old traumatized nose; illustrated by plaster models and lantern slides of preoperative and postoperative cases. METZENBAUM, M. Laryngoscope *40:*488–494, July '30

Cosmetic correction of deviations of tip of nose. EITNER, E. Wien. klin. Wchnschr. *43:*1260, Oct 9, '30

Esthetic operations on crooked noses. DE MELO, C. Med. contemp. *50:*153–154, May 1, '32

Asymmetry of nares; positive diagnostic sign of entity establishing anatomic displacement of lower end of cartilaginous nasal septum. METZENBAUM, M. Arch. Otolaryng. *16:*690–697, Nov '32

Plastic surgery in correction of crooked noses; technic and report of cases. FORERO, A. Semana med. *2:*1631–1637, Dec 1, '32

Cosmetic correction of wry-nose. EITNER, E. Wien. med. Wchnschr. *83:*739–740, June 24, '33

Metzenbaum operation for correction of deflected nasal septum. RIDPATH, R. F. S. Clin. North America *15:*231–237, Feb '35

Operation to repair lateral displacement of lower border of septal cartilage. PEER, L. A. Arch. Otolaryng. *25:*475–477, April '37

New operations for correction of external deviations of lower end of nose. TAMERIN, J. A. Ann. Otol., Rhin. and Laryng. *47:*235–239, March '38

Crooked nose. CINELLI, A. A. Laryngoscope *48:*760–764, Oct '38

Deviation of septum in relation to twisted nose. SALINGER S. Arch. Otolaryng. *29:*520–532, March '39

Nasal septum; —twisted nose. METZ, W. R. New Orleans M. and S. J. *92:*180–185, Oct '39

Plastic correction of cartilaginous crooked

Rhinoplasty, Deviated Nose—Cont.

nose. KLICPERA, L. Arch. f. Ohren-, Nasen- u. Kehlkopfh. *147:*170–172, '40

Simplified method of removing triangular wedge of nasal bone in plastic correction of lateral deviation. SPARER, W. Arch. Otolaryng. *33:*666–667, April '41

One-stage rhinoplasty for deflected bony nose, with sequelae. FRIEDMAN, G. A., M. Rec. *155:*123–124, Feb 18, '42

Plastic repair of deviated septum associated with deflected nasal tip. SELTZER, A. P. Arch. Otolaryng. *40:*433–444, Dec '44

Rhinoplasty, Function in

Rhinoplastic surgeon versus rhinologist. BERNE, L. P. Tr. Sect. Laryng., Otol. and Rhin., A.M.A., pp. 118–121, '23

Plastic and reconstructive procedures in rhinology. MALINIAK, J. W. New York State J. Med. *28:*6–9, Jan 1, '28

Dangers of permitting anyone except rhinologist to operate on nose. BÜHR, R. Deutsche med. Wchnschr. *55:*1554, Sept 13, '29

Surgical relationship between inner and outer nose. PEARLMAN, L. M., M. Rec. *149:*329–332, May 17, '39

Preserving physiologic functions in nasal surgery. REAVES, R. G., J. Tennessee M. A. *34:*403–406, Oct '41

Rhinoplasty and its relation to rhinology. WOLF, G. D. Tr. Sect. Laryng., Otol. and Rhin., A.M.A., pp. 81–95F, '41

Importance of preserving physiologic functions of nose in intranasal surgery. REAVES, R. G. South. Surgeon *11:*574–580, Aug '42

Rhinoplasty and its relation to rhinology. WOLF, G. D. Am. J. Surg. *62:*216–224, Nov '43

Nasal physiology from standpoint of plastic surgeon. PROETZ, A. W. Arch. Otolaryng. *39:*514–517, June '44

Rhinology and plastic surgery of nasal pyramid. ALCAINO Q., A. Rev. otorrinolaring. *4:*73–123, Sept '44

Anatomic and physiologic principles underlying plastic surgery of nasal deformities. ROSEDALE, R. S. Ohio State M. J. *41:*724–728, Aug '45

Corrective surgery of external pyramid and septum for restoration of normal physiology. COTTLE, M. H. AND LORING, R. M. Illinois M. J. *90:*119–131, Aug '46

Physiology of nose and its relation to plastic surgery LAMONT, E. S. Am. J. Surg. *72:*238–245, Aug '46

Rhinoplasty, History of (See also History of Plastic Surgery)

Restoration of nose by transplantation of skin from forehead in year 1881. TEALE, T. P. Brit. J. Surg. *9:*449, Jan '22 (illus.)

Rhinoplastic surgery through ages. CLERY, A. B. Irish J. M. Sc., pp. 170–176, April '32

Joseph Constantine Carpue and revival of rhinoplasty. Internat. Abstract Surg., pp. 275–280, Oct '30

References to nasal and auricular esthetic surgery in work of Hippocrates. CODAZZI AGUIRRE, J. A. Semana med. *1:*445–449, Feb 25, '43

Rhinoplasty, Implants in

Use of paraffin and wax in ear and nose surgery. STAHLMAN, T. M. Pennsylvania M. J. *24:*875, Sept '21

Inlays in plastic nasal operations. ESSER, J. F. S. Munchen. med. Wchnschr. *69:*1154–1155, Aug 4, '22

Depressed nasal deformities, comparison of prosthetic values of paraffin, bone, cartilage and celluloid, with report of cases corrected with celluloid implants by author's method. LEWIS, J. D. Ann. Otol., Rhin. and Laryng. *32:*321–365, June '23 (illus.)

Comparative study of ivory and organic transplants in rhinoplasty; endo-nasal operative technic of some nasal deformities with report of cases. MALINIAK, J. Laryngoscope *34:*882–900, Nov '24

Use of ivory in rhinoplasty. MALINIAK, J. Arch. Otolaryng. *1:*599–611, June '25

Rhinoplasty over silver frame. BOGORODIZKY, W. A. Zentralbl. f. Chir. *52:*2830–2835, Dec 12, '25

Rhinoplasty with ivory transplant. LUNDON, A. E. Canad. M. A. J. *16:*561–562, May '26

Ivory in alloplasty of nasal fossae. BASAVILBASO, J. Prensa med. argent. *13:*597–598, Nov 30, '26 also: Rev. de especialid. *1:*564–567, '26

Use of foreign bodies in ear, nose and throat surgery. POLLOCK, H. L. Ann. Otol., Rhin. and Laryng. *36:*463–471, June '27

Cosmetic operations of nose; paraffin injections. BLEGVAD, N. R. Ugesk. f. Laeger *89:*1141–1144, Dec 8, '27

Cartilage and ivory in plastic surgery of nose. SALINGER, S. Arch. Otolaryng. *6:*552–558, Dec '27

Cosmetic operations on nose and paraffin injections; 6 cases. BLEGVAD, N. R. Ugesk. f. Laeger *90:*286–290, March 29, '28

Plastic surgery of nose with bone graft and

Rhinoplasty, Implants in—Cont.
paraffin. CHÉRIDJIAN, Z. Rev. med. de la Suisse Rom. *49:*751-753, Oct 25, '29
Cork as prosthesis in correction of nasal defects. PRISSELKOFF, P. V. Vrach. gaz. *34:*534-536, April 15, '30
Ivory in cosmetic operations of nose. EITNER, E. Med. Welt *4:*1615, Nov 8, '30
Cork as plastic material for correction of saddle noses. DAHMANN, H. Ztschr. f. Laryng., Rhin. *20:*451-457, March '31
Implantation of ivory in ozena of nose; approved technic; further observations. KEMLER, J. I. Arch. Otolaryng. *13:*726-731, May '31
Ivory implants for saddle nose; results in 50 cases. SALINGER, S. Ann. Otol., Rhin. and Laryng. *40:*801-808, Sept '31
Correction of nasal deformities with use of tricoplast. LOEBELL, H. Ztschr. f. arztl. Fortbild. *29:*329-330, June 1, '32
Implants in nasal deformities; history and uses. POLLOCK, H. L. Ann. Otol., Rhin. and Laryng. *41:*1103-1107, Dec '32
Results of implantations of porous gold in plastic surgery of nose. THIELEMANN. Ztschr. f. Laryng., Rhin., Otol. *24:*175-180, '33
Facts and fallacies of cosmetic surgery (paraffin injections, hair removal, face-lifting, nose-remodeling, etc.). MALINIAK, J. W. Hygeia *12:*200-202, March '34
Surgical correction of uncomplicated saddle nose by partial inclusion of ivory. PRUDENTE, A. Rev. Assoc. paulista de med. *5:*75-78, Aug '34
Problem of inclusions in surgical therapy of saddle nose; answers to questionnaire (le probleme des inclusions). VARIOUS AUTHORS. Rev. de chir. plastique, pp. 132-141, Oct '34
Correction of saddle nose, with special reference to implantation of ivory. CLAUS, G. Ztschr. f. Hals-, Nasen-u. Ohrenh. *35:*198-211, '34
Problem of inclusions in surgical therapy of saddle nose; answers to questionnaire (le probleme des inclusions). VARIOUS AUTHORS Rev. de chir. structive, pp. 59-64, July '35
Nasal prosthesis with heavy paraffin. FRIEDMANN, L. Romania med. *15:*186-187, July 1-15, '37
Saddle nose; ivory and cartilage implants. SALINGER, S. Illinois M. J. *72:*412-417, Nov '37
Ivory prosthesis in partial rhinoplasty; cases. MALBEC, E. Semana med. *1:*1374-1382, June 16, '38

Rhinoplasty, Implants in—Cont.
Technic of ivory implant for correction of saddle nose. WOLFE, M. M. Arch. Surg. *37:*800-807, Nov '38
New approach for nasal implants. COHEN, S. Ann. Otol., Rhin. and Laryng. *47:*1101-1106, Dec '38
Marble prosthesis in correcting saddle nose; 2 cases. MALBEC, E. F. Semana med. *1:*1136-1138, May 18, '39
Marble prosthesis in correction of saddle nose. ZENO, L. Bol. y trab. de la Soc. de cir. de Buenos Aires *23:*332-338, June 21, '39 also: An. de cir. *5:*111-122, June '39
Marble implantation by transsupracilliary route in saddle nose; case. ALVES, O. Rev. brasil. de oto-rino-laring. *7:*347-350, July-Aug '39
Use of marble in correction of nasal deformities. MALBEC, E. F. Semana med. *2:*1266-1270, Nov 30, '39
Marble prosthesis in correction of saddle nose. ZENO, L. Dia med. (Ed. espec., no. 9), pp. 170-171, Nov '39
Use of glass for rhinoplastic purposes. LYANDE, V. S. Zhur. ush., nos. i gorl. bolez. *16:*322-324, '39
Partial rhinoplasty using marble prosthesis; cases. MALBEC, E. F. Semana med. *2:*1173-1182, Nov 21, '40
Vitallium for skeleton support of nose. KIMBALL, G. H. AND DRUMMOND, N. R., J. Oklahoma M. A. *34:*9-12, Jan '41
Rhinoplastic surgery combined with paraffin prosthesis in correction of saddle nose. DUJARDIN, E. Ugesk. f. laeger *103:*404-405, March 27, '41
Paraffinoma of nose; surgical therapy; cases. ZENO, L. An. de cir. *7:*41-45, March-June '41
Duraluminum in plastic surgery of nose. MALBEC, E. F. Semana med. *1:*1016-1019, May 1, '41
Marble inclusion by trans-supraciliary route in saddle nose. ALVES, O. Arq. de cir. clin. e exper. *6:*512-517, April-June '42
Correction of saddle nose by inclusion of vitallium. LINHARES, F. Rev. brasil. de cir. *14:*159-164, March '45
Correction of deformities of tip of nose with implantations of paladon. RIVAS, C. I. AND IZURIETA, F. A. Bol. y trab., Acad. argent. de cir. *29:*240-247, May 9, '45
Saddle nose; correction by means of tantalum prosthesis; case. MALBEC, E. F. Bol. y trab., Soc. argent. de cirujanos *7:*173-177, '46 also: Rev. Asoc. med. argent. *60:*361-363, May 30, '46

Rhinoplasty, Instruments for

New intra-nasal suture set. ISRAEL, S. Laryngoscope *31:*633, Aug '21

New instruments used in nose and throat and plastic surgery. SHEEHAN, J. E. New York M. J. *115:*493–494, April 19, '22 (illus.)

Apparatus for restoring shape to sunken nose. FREUND. Deutsche med. Wchnschr. *48:*1422, Oct 20, '22

An instrument (drill) to facilitate correction of certain types of external deformities of nose. ISRAEL, S., J.A.M.A. *80:*690, March 10, '23 (illus.)

Simple knot for intranasal sutures. JOHNSTON, W. Ann. Otol., Rhin. and Laryng. *32:*201–209, March '23 (illus.)

New nasal septal chisel. OLSHO, S. L. Laryngoscope *33:*308, April '23 (illus.)

Electrically driven nasal saw and rasp. IGLAUER, S. Laryngoscope *35:*78, Jan '25

New nasal splint. WHITE, F. W. Laryngoscope *35:*76, Jan '25

New rhinoplastic instruments. MALTZ, M. Laryngoscope *36:*54–60, Jan '26

Splint for treatment of wide depressed nasal bridges. WATKINS, A. B. K., M. J. Australia *2:*556–557, Oct 23, '26

Forceps for inserting grafts in corrective operations of nose. EITNER, E. Munchen. med. Wchnschr. *74:*1876, Nov 4, '27

Double-end arrow elevator for nasal plastic operations and submucous resections. FISHBEIN, J. N. Laryngoscope *38:*97, Feb '28

New rhinoplastic instrument. SAFIAN, J. Arch. Otolaryng. *8:*78, July '28

New instrument for intranasal suture. TAKAHASHI, K. Ztschr. f. Laryng., Rhin. *17:*211–216, Sept '28

New nasal brace. SAFIAN, J. Arch. Otolaryng. *8:*566–568, Nov '28

Nasal suturing instrument. CAMPBELL, C. A. Arch. Otolaryng. *11:*95–96, Jan '30

Improved nasofrontal rasp. SPRATT, C. N. Arch. Otolaryng. *11:*783, June '30

Cutting hook and inverse hammer for nasal surgery. VAN DER HOEVEN LEONHARD, J. Oto-rhino-laryng. internat. *17:*27–31, Jan '33

Suture needle for nasal surgery. MALONE, J. Y. Arch. Otolaryng. *17:*562, April '33

New instruments for use of rib cartilage grafts in rhinoplasty. MALINIAK, J. W. Arch. Otolaryng. *18:*79–82, July '33

Adjustable nasal elevator. HOMME, O. H. Arch. Otolaryng. *20:*711, Nov '34

New instruments for nasal reconstructive surgery. BARSKY, A. J. Arch. Otolaryng. *22:*487–490, Oct '35

New type nasal rasp in plastic surgery. ISRAEL, S. Laryngoscope *46:*388–389, May '36

New instrument for correction of hump nose. PIERI, P. F. Boll. d. mal. d. orecchio, d. gola, d. naso *54:*180–187, May '36

Simplified intranasal suture. CHILDREY, J. H. Arch. Otolaryng. *27:*618, May '38

Two improved instruments for use in plastic surgery of nose. FIRESTONE, C. Laryngoscope *48:*356–357, May '38

Nasal splint. SCHLESSELMAN, J. T. Arch. Otolaryng. *29:*988–989, June '39

Use of knitting needle for suture of conjunctiva in rhinostomy. KURLOV, I. N. AND MILOVIDOVA, A. N. Vestnik oftal. (no. 2) *15:*38–39, '39

Improved instruments and postoperative splint for nasal plastic operations; combined chisel and periosteal elevator. PEARLMAN, L. M. Arch. Otolaryng. *32:*338–340, Aug '40

Simple nasal splint. MATIS, E. I., J. Laryng. and Otol. *55:*425–426, Sept '40

New instruments for use in rhinoplastic surgery. CINELLI, J. A. Arch. Otolaryng. *32:*1102–1106, Dec '40

New set of automatic retractors for nasal surgery. VELLOSO VIANNA, E. Rev. brasil. de oto-rino-laring. *10:*533–550, Sept–Oct '42

Needle and needle holder for intranasal use. SIMPSON, R. K. Am. J. Ophth. *25:*1368–1369, Nov '42

Angled bistoury with retrograde uniform cutting edge for use in plastic surgery of nose. DELLEPIANE RAWSON, R. AND JAROLAVSKY, N. N. Dia med. *14:*1280, Dec 7, '42

New instrument for use in rhinoplastic surgery. KAYSER, R. Arch. Otolaryng. *39:*186–188, Feb '44

New nasal tissue clamp used in new method of narrowing columella. SELTZER, A. P. J. Internat. Coll. Surgeons *8:*154–159, March–April '45

New instruments in rhinoplastic surgery. SUNSHINE, L. Am. J. Surg. *71:*434–435, March '46

Aids in rhinoplastic procedures. BECKER, O. J. Ann. Otol., Rhin. and Laryng. *55:*562–571, Sept '46

Rhinoplasty, Miscellaneous

Electric-ionisation and nose operations. PRADHAN, K. N. Indian M. Gaz. *57:*137–138, April '22

Surgery of throat, nose and ear. DUNDAS-GRANT, J. Practitioner *110:*11–25, Jan '23

Rhinoplasty, Miscellaneous—Cont.

Simple knot for intranasal sutures. JOHNSTON, W. Ann. Otol., Rhin. and Laryng. *32:*201–209, March '23 (illus.)

Use of gold-wire splints in intranasal plastic surgery. CARTER, W. W. Laryngoscope *35:*942–943, Dec '25

New procedures for tear sac, frontal sinus and endonasal plastic operations. MALTZ, M. Acta oto-laryng. *9:*144–153, '26 (in English)

Physical therapy as aid to surgical procedures on nose. McCOY, J. Laryngoscope *37:*756–759, Oct '27

Influence of nasal bacteria on healing process of surgical wounds. LAKOS, T. Z. Ztschr. f. Hals-, Nasen-u. Ohrenh. *23:*426–435, Sept 10, '29

Cleft palate and rhinopharyngeal functions; case. SEGRÈ, R. Arch. ital. di otol. *40:*633–643, Oct '29

Plastic surgery of nose, ear, face. DAVIS, A. D. Arch. Otolaryng. *10:*575–584, Dec '29

Surgical method of nasal surgery which does not cause shock. WOJATSCHEK. Acta oto-laryng. *15:*327–341, '31

Endonasal surgery and terrain. AUBRIOT, P. Rev. med. de l'est *60:*269–277, April 15, '32

Conservatism in surgery as applied to nasal mucosa. GROSS, W. A. Am. J. Phys. Therapy *9:*199–200, Nov '32 also: Eye, Ear, Nose and Throat Monthly *11:*392–393, Nov '32

Correction of deformities of forehead and nose; presentation of 2 patients. NEW, G. B. Proc. Staff Meet., Mayo Clin. *10:*519–521, Aug 14, '35

Simplified intranasal suture. CHILDREY, J. H. Arch. Otolaryng. *27:*618, May '38

Technical improvements on Glatzel's mirror for examination of width of nose. JOCHIMS, J. Ztschr. f. Kinderh. *60:*147–153, '38

Development of bridge of nose. GOLDSTEIN, M. S. Am. J. Phys. Anthropol. *25:*101–117, April–June '39

Indications for nasal surgery. SAUVAIN, Y. Paris med. *2:*434–436, Sept 21–28, '40

Method for suturing of nasal mucous membrane. MATIS, E. I. Acta oto-laryng. *29:*80–82, '41 also: Medicina Kaumas *21:*1031–1034, Dec '40

Minor surgery of nose and throat. SHAMBAUGH, G. JR. S. Clin. North America *21:*21–36, Feb '41

Minor nasal surgery. DAVIS, E. D. D. Practitioner *148:*244–249, April '42

Planning surgery of nose. PROETZ, A. W. Tr. Am. Laryng. Rhin. and Otol. Soc. *48:*33–39, '42

Deficient respiration due to malformation of lobe of nose; surgical therapy of case. CORA ELISEHT, F. Prensa med. argent. *30:*175–179, Jan 27, '43

Erosion of ala nasi following trigeminal denervation. SCHORSTEIN, J., J. Neurol. and Psychiat. *6:*46–51, Jan–April '43

Brief panoramic study of nasal surgery. PETIT, A. M. Vida nueva *51:*138–145, April '43

Planning nasal surgery. PROETZ, A. W. Arch. Otolaryng. *37:*502–506, April '43

Structure of external nose; study from point of view of plastic surgery. GRIESMAN, B. L. Arch. Otolaryng. *42:*117–122, Aug '45

Rhinoplasty, Planning

Corrective rhinoplasty, some anatomicosurgical considerations. COHEN, L. Surg., Gynec. and Obst. *34:*794–799, June '22 (illus.)

Corrective rhinoplasty, some reasons for faulty results. COHEN, L. Tr. Sect. Laryng., Otol. and Rhin., A.M.A., pp. 122–133, '23 (illus.)

Rhinoplasty from an artist's standpoint. BERNE, L. P., J. M. Soc. New Jersey *21:*121–123, April '24

Corrective rhinoplasty; some reasons for faulty results. COHEN, L. Ann. Otol., Rhin. and Laryng. *33:*342–350, June '24

Causes of failure in corrective rhinoplasty—lantern demonstration. MALINIAK, J. Laryngoscope *35:*832–843, Nov '25 also: Ohio State M. J. *21:*807–814, Nov '25

Rhinoplasty; facts and fiction. WOLF, G. D. Tr. Sect. Laryng., Otol. and Rhin., A.M.A., pp. 174–189, '29 also: Arch. Otolaryng. *11:*322–335, March '30

Importance of plastic surgery of nose. CARTER, W. W. Laryngoscope *40:*502–506, July '30

Surgery of nose in relation to orthodontia and facial harmony. IVY, R. H. Internat. J. Orthodontia *19:*888–898, Sept '33

Facial and nasal plastic surgery from esthetic point of view. VILARDOSA LLUBES, E. Rev. de cir. de Barcelona *8:*1, July–Aug; 99, Sept–Dec '34

Ideals in rhinoplastic surgery. CARTER, W. W. Am. J. Surg. *26:*524–527, Dec '34

Plastic surgeon looks at a nose. PEARLMAN, A. C. Kentucky M. J. *34:*467–469, Oct '36

New profilometer (instrument for plastic surgery of nasal deformities). STRAITH, C. L. Rev. de chir. structive, pp. 156–157, June '37

Technic of making plaster of paris cast for nasal fractures and deformities. RODE, B. Ztschr. f. Hals-, Nasen-u. Ohrenh. *43:*294–295, '38

Rhinoplasty, Planning—Cont.

Esthetic surgery; criteria or artistic precepts (nose). SCAVUZZO, R. Semana med. *1:*144-146, Jan 19, '39

Construction of ideal nose with aid of masks and measurements. BERSON, M. I., M. Rec. *149:*80-82, Feb 1, '39

Role of septum in surgery of nasal contour. COHEN, S. Arch. Otolaryng. *30:*12-20, July '39

Nasal surgery in women. COELST. Bull. Soc. belge d'otol., rhinol., laryng., pp. 316-318, '39

Possibilities and principles of plastic surgery of nose. WEICHHERZ, I. Budapesti orvosi ujsag *38:*134-136, March 21' 40

Indications for nasal surgery. SAUVAIN, Y. Paris med. *2:*434-436, Sept 21-28, '40

Function of esthetic sense in plastic surgery of nose. MALBEC, E. F. Semana med. *2:*997-1008, Oct 31, '40

Prevention and treatment of late sequelae in corrective rhinoplasty. MALINIAC, J. W. Am. J. Surg. *50:*84-91, Oct '40

Failures in rhinoplastic surgery; causes and prevention. SAFIAN, J. Am. J. Surg. *50:*274-280, Nov '40

Fallacious views and factors influencing more successful results in nasal surgery. HOLLENDER, A. R., J. Florida M. A. *28:*27-29, July '41

Ideal nose. CINELLI, A. A. New York State J. Med. *42:*64-66, Jan 1, '42

Modification of facial characteristics through remodeling of nose. EHRENFELD, H. J., M. Rec. *155:*5-8, Jan 7, '42

Critical review of causes of unsuccessful and results of nasal surgery. HOLLENDER, A. R. South. M. J. *35:*363-372, April '42

Prevention of nasal deformity in corrective rhinoplasty (description of rhinometer). BERSON, M. I. Laryngoscope *53:*276-287, April '43

Planning nasal surgery. PROETZ, A. W. Arch. Otolaryng. *37:*502-506, April '43

Important considerations in rhinoplastic procedures. BERSON, M. I. Eye, Ear, Nose and Throat Monthly *22:*424-430, Nov '43

New rhinometer. BERSON, M. I. Am. J. Surg. *63:*148-149, Jan '44

Muscles and cartilages of nose from standpoint of typical rhinoplasty. GRIESMAN, B. L. Arch. Otolaryng. *39:*334-341, April '44

Rhinoplastic analysis. FOMON, S. *et al.* Eye, Ear, Nose and Throat Monthly *24:*19-24, Jan '45

Introduction of artistic point of view in regard to rhinoplastic diagnosis. DALEY, J. Arch. Otolaryng. *42:*33-41, July '45

Structure of external nose; study from point of view of plastic surgery. GRIESMAN, B. L. Arch. Otolaryng. *42:*117-122, Aug '45

Planning rhinoplasty. COHEN, S. Arch. Otolaryng. *43:*283-292, Mar '46

Rhinoplasty, Postoperative Care

Adhesive plaster bandage for plastic operations of nose. FISHBEIN, J. N. Laryngoscope *38:*128, Feb '28

Fixative bandage in corrective nasal plastic surgery. ERCZY, M. Orvosi hetil. *76:*657-658, July 23, '32

Copper molded nasal splint; new method of application. SALINGER, S. Arch. Otolaryng. *20:*211-214, Aug '34

Dental molding compound cast and adhesive strapping in rhinoplastic procedure. AUFRICHT, G. Arch. Otolaryng. *32:*333-338, Aug '40

Postoperative care in plastic surgery of nose. RIUS, M. Arq. de cir. clin. e exper. *6:*171-174, April-June '42

Materials for corrective plastic surgery of nose. RAPIN, M. Pract. oto-rhino-laryng. *4:*133-141, '42

Aids in rhinoplastic procedures. BECKER, O. J. Ann. Otol., Rhin. and Laryng. *55:*562-571, Sept '46

Rhinoplasty, Postoperative Packing

Intranasal operations with special reference to postoperative packing. MILLER, J. W. New York M. J. *113:*456, March 16, '21

Tamponing nose (after surgery). SCHMIDT, C. Schweiz. med. Wchnschr. *52:*540-541, May 25, '22 (illus.)

Tamponing after operations on nose. RÉTHI, L. Wien. klin. Wchnschr. *35:*637-638, July 20, '22

Post-operative endo-nasal tamponade with cotton sachets (in nasal surgery). LAVAL, F. Ann. d. mal. de l'oreille, du larynx *46:*377-379, April '27

Use of packing in postoperative treatment in nasal surgery. WOODBURN, J. J., M. J. Australia *2:*390-392, Sept 26, '31

Question of tamponade after nasal operations. (Comment on von Liebermann's article.) KREBS, G. Ztschr. f. Hals-, Nasen-u. Ohrenh. *30:*684-685, '32

Use of sulfanilamide and gauze packing following intranasal operation. KERN, E. C. Arch. Otolaryng. *36:*134, July '42

Elimination of intranasal pack by topical use of thrombin. STEVENSON, H. N. Ann. Otol., Rhin. and Laryng. *53:*159-162, March '44

New medicated gauze for use in nasal operations. SELTZER, A. P. Eye, Ear, Nose and Throat Monthly *24:*189, April '45

Rhinoplasty, Psychology of

Martyrdom of the nose. PULLEINE, R. H., M. J. Australia (supp.) *1:*385-386, June 7, '24

Plastic surgery of nose; patient's viewpoint. BLAIR, V. P. Tr. Am. Acad. Ophth. *33:*436-444, '28

Facial abnormalities, fancied and real; reaction of patient; attempted correction (including nose). BLAIR, V. P. Proc. Inst. Med., Chicago *8:*217-223, April 15, '31

What plastic surgery is doing for deformed and badly proportioned noses. WOLF, G. D. Hygeia *9:*1005-1006, Nov '31

Defects of nose – fancied and real; reaction of patient; attempted correction. BLAIR, V. P. AND BROWN, J. B. Surg., Gynec. and Obst. *53:*797-819, Dec '31

Nasal abnormalities, fancied and real; reaction of patient; attempted correction. BLAIR, V. P. AND BROWN, J. B. Internat. J. Orthodontia *18:*363-401, April '32

Disillusionments in nasal surgery. LEWIS, W. W. Minnesota Med. *17:*323-329, June '34

Esthetic and psychologic principles of plastic surgery (ear), (face), (nose). WUDAK, E. Monatschr. f. Ohrenh. *72:*288-303, March '38

Nasal defects in students; psychologic aspects and plastic correction. CODAZZI AGUIRRE, J. A. Arq. de cir. clin. e exper. *6:*194-197, April-June '42 also: Semana med. *1:*981-988, May 14, '42

Rhinoplasty, Reconstructive

New technic for rhinoplasty. PÓLYA, E. Zentralbl. f. Chir. *48:*257, Feb 26, '21

Gillies new method in giving support to depressed nasal bridge and columella. SHEEHAN, J. E. New York M. J. *113:*448, March 16, '21

Partial and total rhinoneoplasty. JOSEPH, J. Klin. Wchnschr. *1:*678-680, April 1, '22 (illus.)

Five years of surgery of ear and nose. HAAG, H. Schweiz. med. Wchnschr. *52:*498-504, May 25, '22

Inlays in plastic nasal operations. ESSER, J. F. S. Munchen. med. Wchnschr. *69:*1154-1155, Aug 4, '22

Plastic operations on nose and forearm. McKAY, H. S., S. Clin. N. America *2:*1597-1608, Dec '22 (illus.)

Rhinoplasty and cheek, chin, and lip plasties with tubed, temporal-pedicled, forehead flaps. MCWILLIAMS, C. A. AND DUNNING, H. S. Surg., Gynec. and Obst. *36:*1-10, Jan '23 (illus.)

Rhinoplasty, Reconstructive – Cont.

Rhinoplasty with flap from patient's chest. STEINTHAL, K. Zentralbl. f. Chir. *50:*508-509, March 31, '23 (illus.)

Reconstructive surgery of nose. IVANISSEVICH, O. Rev. Asoc. med. argent. *36:*197-202, May-June '23

Conservatism in nasal surgery POTTER, W. W. Southern M. J. *16:*560-563, July '23

Russian method of rhinoplasty. PETROW, N. N. Zentralbl. f. Chir. *51:*36-39, Jan 12, '24

New method for rhinoplasty. IVANISSEVICH, O. Surg., Gynec. and Obst. *38:*828-829, June '24

Surgical reconstruction of nose. BRANSFIELD, J. W. Atlantic M. J. *27:*637-640, July '24

Repair of acquired defects of face (and nose). IVY, R. H., J.A.M.A. *84:*181-185, Jan 17, '25

Plastic surgery of nose. PIERCE, G. W. Surg., Gynec. and Obst. *40:*469-475, April '25

Plastic surgery of nose. NEW, G. B., S. Clin. N. America *5:*721-728, June '25

Principles in plastic surgery about head and neck (and nose). BECK, J. C. Illinois M. J. *48:*194-202, Sept '25

Total and subtotal restoration of nose. BLAIR, V. P., J.A.M.A. *85:*1931-1935, Dec 19, '25

Procedure of fill in medium-sized gap in nostril. MACLENNAN, A. Glasgow M. J. *104:*326-327, Dec '25

Rhinoplasty by rotation of flaps from cheek. D'AGATA, G. Policlinico (sez. prat). *34:*168, Jan 31, '26

Plastic and reconstructive surgery; total rhinoplasty for syphilitic defect. IVY, R. H. S. Clin. N. Amer. *6:*248-251, Feb '26

Plastic surgery of nose. BETTMAN, A. G., M. J. and Rec. *123:*417-421, April 7; 499-501, April 21, '26

New method for plastic operations in bony frame of nose. SOUZA MENDES, J. Brazil-med. *2:*100-102, Aug 21, '26

Partial rhinoplasty; restoration of nasal tip, alae and septum. GOLKIN, M. Deutsche Ztschr. f. Chir. *199:*354-359, '26

Rhinoplasty and stomatoplasty. PERTHES, G. Arch. f. klin. Chir. *142:*572-589, '26

Outline of methods of nasal plastic surgery. BOSVIEL, J., J. de med. de Paris *46:*87, Jan 31, '27

Plastics of external nose. VON WEDEL, C. J. Oklahoma M. A. *20:*44-45, Feb '27

Nasal deformities plastic repair; cases. BRUSOTTI, A. Stomatol. *25:*161-181, March '27

Technic of plastic surgery of face and nose. VAN DEN BRANDEN, J. Bruxelles-med. *7:*917-920, May 15, '27

Correction of nasal deformities (including

Rhinoplasty, Reconstructive—Cont.
skin grafts). SHEEHAN, J. E. Virginia M. Monthly *54:*138–141, June '27
Technic in rhinoplasty. MACHADO, R. Rev. brasil. de med. e pharm. *3:*305–310, July-Aug '27
Argentine method of rhinoplasty; 3 cases. IVANISSEVICH, O. AND FERRARI, R. C. Bol. Inst. de clin. quir. *3:*103–106, '27
Enfolding flap in correction of nasal deformities. RÉTHI, A. Acta oto-laryng. *11:*443–452, '27
Total rhinoplasty. SMITH, F. Warthin Ann. Vol., pp. 601–612, '27
Nasal reconstruction by means of auto and iso-grafts. METZENBAUM, M. Ohio State M. J. *24:*196–200, March '28 also: Laryngoscope *38:*197–205, March '28
Nasal plastic surgery; 7 cases. DE FLINES, E. W. Nederl. Tijdschr. v. Geneesk. *1:*1984, April 21, '28
New method of partial rhinoplasty. DUJARDIN, E. Ugesk. f. Laeger *90:*384–386, April 26, '28 also: Lancet *1:*1280–1281, June 23, '28
Problem of rhinoplasty. SHATKINSKY, M. P. Klin. j. saratov. Univ. *5:*463–471, April '28
Sarcoma of nasal bones; subtotal removal of nose and its reconstruction. COUGHLIN, W. T. Arch. Otolaryng. *7:*588–600, June '28
Loss of substance in nostril; rhinoplasty with skin graft; case. ROY, J. N. Ann. d. mal. de l'oreille, du larynx *47:*571–576, June '28 also: Union med. du Canada *57:*505–510, Sept '28
Traumatic loss of substance of nostril; rhinoplasty with dermo-epidermic graft. ROY, J. N. Arch. Otolaryng. *7:*601–605, June '28 also: J. Laryng. and Otol. *43:*490–495, July '28
Total rhinoplasty. NEW G. B., J.A.M.A. *91:*380–381, Aug 11, '28
Treatment of partial loss of right side of nose; case. POGGI, J. Folha med. *9:*413–415, Dec 15, '28
Die frühindische Plastik. K. Wolff, Munich, 1929
Plastic surgery of nose. INGEBRIGTSEN, R. Norsk Mag. f. Laegevidensk. *90:*169–175, Feb '29
Reconstruction of upper lip and portion of nose. NEW, G. B., S. Clin. N. Amer. *9:*75–78, Feb '29
Plastic surgery of nose. BIANCULLI, H. Semana med. *1:*741–748, March 28, '29
Plastic formation of tip of nose. RÉTHI, A. Chirurg *1:*539–545, May 1, '29
Partial reconstruction of nose. FIGI, F. A. S. Clin. N. Amer. *9:*923–928, Aug '29

Rhinoplasty, Reconstructive—Cont.
Rhinoplasty. INGEBRIGTSEN, R. Lyon chir. *26:*548–553, Aug-Sept '29
Plastic surgery of nose. MACHADO, R. Tribuna med. *33:*239–244, Oct 15, '29
Partial rhinomyoplasty. ALFREDO, J. Brasil-med. *43:*1564–1567, Dec 21, '29
Restoration of subseptal portion of nose. DOBRZANIECKI, W. Ann. Surg. *90:*974–977, Dec '29
Rhinoplasty. PETROFF, N. N. Vestnik khir. (nos. 48–49) *16–17:*37–41, '29
Further observations on rhinoplasty. SHATKINSKY, M. P. Vestnik khir. (no. 52) *18:*77–84, '29
Technic of rhinoplasty. HAGENTORN, A. Zentralbl. f. Chir. *57:*600–603, March 8, '30
Total rhinoplasty; cases. HAZEN, S. F. Proc. Staff Meet., Mayo Clin. *5:*69–71, March 12, '30
Rhinoplasty. IVANISSEVICH, O. AND FERRARI, R. C. Semana med. *1:*967–974, April 17, '30
Problems in plastic surgery of nose. NEW, G. B. Minnesota Med. *13:*242–246, April '30
Plastic repair of partial losses of nasal tip. STRAATSMA, C. R. Ann. Surg. *91:*792–794, May '30
Nasal surgery. DELLEPIANE RAWSON, R. AND GONZÁLEZ AVILA, E. Semana med. *2:*1351–1357, Oct 30, '30
Closure of large nasal breach by grafts of frontal and cervicothoracic flaps placed side by side; case. DUPUY-DUTEMPS, L. AND BOURGUET. Bull. Soc. d'opht. de Paris, pp. 435–442, Oct '30
Plastic surgery of nose by Italian method under general ether anesthesia by peritoneal route with J. B. Abalos' technic; case. NATALE, A. M. AND BARBERIS, J. C. Rev. med. del Rosario *20:*487–489, Oct '30
Reconstruction of nasal ala by Argentine method; cases. IVANISSEVICH, O., AND FERRARI, R. C. Bol. Inst. de clin. quir. *6:*279–294, '30
Formation of end, ala and cutaneous partition of nose by transplanting auricle on round stem. LIMBERG, A. A. Vestnik. khir. (no. 55) *20:*151–159, '30
Use of tubular stem in transplantation from ear to defect of ala. VETCHTOMOFF, A. A. Vestnik khir. (no. 55) *20:*143–150, '30
Plastic surgery of nose. BIANCULLI, H. Semana med. *1:*292–297, Jan 29, '31
Plastic surgery of nose. FORERO, A. Semana med. *1:*187–191, Jan 15, '31
Plastic surgery of nose; 2 cases. GONZÁLEZ LOZA, M. Rev. med. del Rosario *21:*701–706, Jan '31
Autoplasty in rhinologic surgery (face). OM-

Rhinoplasty, Reconstructive—Cont.
BRÉDANNE, M. Semaine d. hop. de Paris *7:*44–48, Jan 31, '31
Plastic surgery of nose. LIEBERMANN, T. Orvosi hetil. *75:*646–649, June 20, '31
Loss of nasal ala and upper lip reconstruction. FIGI, F. A., S. Clin. North America *11:*834–837, Aug. '31
Rhinoplasty; 3 cases. QUESADA, F. Dia med. *4:*16, Aug 3, '31
Plastic surgery of nose by Italian method using tubular grafts. BURIAN, F. Presse med. *39:*1418–1420, Sept 26, '31
Total rhinoplasty. MOURE, P. Am. J. Surg. *14:*298–308, Oct '31
Plastic surgery of nose. PEER, L. A. Arch. Otolaryng. *14:*462–466, Oct '31
Experiences in rhinoplasty. ŠERCER, A. Otolaryng. slavica *3:*415–435, Oct '31
Defects of tip of nose; surgical correction. WODAK, E. Med. Klin. *27:*1606–1608, Oct 30, '31
Plastic surgery of nose. KING, E. D., J. Med. *12:*518–524, Dec '31
Use of pedicled flaps in reconstruction of nose. NEW, G. B. AND FIGI, F. A. Surg., Gynec. and Obst. *53:*780–787, Dec '31
Plastic repair of tip of nose, alae and septum with T-shaped round skin flap (Limberg method); case. FALTIN, R. Acta chir. Scandinav. *68:*254–265, '31
Plastic surgery of nose. SMIRNOV, A. A. Russk. oto-laring. *24:*356–358, '31
Technic of total rhinoplasty in which portions of abdominal skin are used. TROFIMOW, A. M. Arch. f. klin. Chir. *163:*681–692, '31
Surgical method of nasal surgery which does not cause shock. WOJATSCHEK. Acta otolaryng. *15:*327–341, '31
Defects of tip of nose; surgical correction. (Comment on Wodak's article.) EITNER, E. Med. Klin. *28:*49–50, Jan 8, '32
Defects of tip of nose; surgical correction. (Comment on Wodak's article.) HALLA, F. Med. Klin. *28:*50, Jan 8, '32
Plastic operation for denudation of nasolacrimal region. FAVALORO, G. Rassegna ital. d'ottal. *1:*197–209, March–April '32
Plastic surgery of nose. GAMES, F. AND MERCANDINO, G. Semana med. *1:*727–736, March 3, '32
Correction of losses and deformities of external nose, including those associated with harelip. BLAIR, V. P. California and West. Med. *36:*308–313, May '32
Plastic surgery in nasal reconstruction; classification of deformities. GONZÁLEZ LOZA, M. Rev. med. del Roasario *22:*268–282, May '32
Forced method of total rhinoplasty. TOPROWER, G. S. Wien. klin. Wchnschr. *45:*1015–1017, Aug 12, '32
Technic of autoplastic operation to restore whole nose. CAFORIO, L. Rinasc. med. *9:*467–469, Oct 15, '32
Plastic surgery of nose. RACOVEANU, V. Spitalul *52:*402–414, Oct '32
Use of dermal graft in repair of small saddle defects (nose). STRAATSMA, C. R. Arch. Otolaryng. *16:*506–509, Oct '32
Plastic surgery in destruction of tip of nose. RETHI, A. Rev. de chir. plastique, pp. 327–349, Jan '33
Plastic replacement of tip of nose. EITNER, E. Med. Klin. *29:*358, March 10, '33
Restoration of protein of nostril. GONZÁLEZ LOZA, M. Rev. med. del Rosario *23:*217–219, March '33
Plastic surgery of nose. WATKINS, A. B. K. J. Laryng. and Otol. *48:*809–820, Dec '33
Reconstruction of nasal tip, wings and septum by T-shaped graft from neck. LIMBERG, A. A. Novy khir. arkhiv *28:*147–163, '33
Reconstruction of nasal ala; case. JULLIARD, C. Rev. med. de la Suisse Rom. *54:*463–467, April 25, '34
Rhinoplasty. PAGENSTECHER, G. A. Am. J. Surg. *25:*491–493, Sept '34
Use of reconstructive surgery in certain types of facial and nasal deformities. NEW, G. B. AND FIGI, F. A., J.A.M.A. *103:*1434–1438, Nov 10, '34
Free skin grafts in restoration of defects of conjunctival, oral mucous membranes and cutaneous defects of nasal fossae. LIMBERG, A. A. Sovet. khir. (nos. 3–4) *6:*462–482, '34
Use of reconstructive surgery in certain types of deformities (face) (nose). NEW, G. B. AND FIGI, F. A. Tr. Sect. Laryng., Otol. and Rhin., A. M. A., pp. 52–63, '34
Plastic surgery of nose; 6 cases. IVANISSEVICH, O. AND FERRARI, R. C. Semana med. *1:*973–989, April 4, '35
Cases of rhinoplasty. ROY, J. N. Union med. du Canada *64:*644–658, June '35 also: Canad. M. A. J. *33:*158–160, Aug '35
Reconstruction of columella nasi. UPDEGRAFF, H. L. Am. J. Surg. *29:*29–31, July '35
Rhinoplasty using cutaneous flap from abdomen via forearm. CLAOUE. Bull. et mem.

Rhinoplasty, Reconstructive – Cont.
Soc. de med. de Paris *140:*208-209, March 28, '36
Surgical correction of bull-dog nose; case. DOBRZANIECKI, W., J. de chir. *48:*191-196, Aug '36
Technic of rhinoplasty by tubular grafts. CLAOUE, C., J. de med. de Bordeaux *113:*633-635, Sept 10-30, '36
Plastic surgery of ears; cases (and face and nose). MALBEC, E. F. Semana med. *2:*718-728, Sept 10, '36
Typical method for reconstruction of nasal tip, septum and median portion of alae nasi. FALTIN, R. Acta chir. Scandinav. *78:*492-511, '36
Partial rhinoplasty using tissue from auricle on round Filatov pedicle. KHRIZMAN, I. A. Sovet. Khir., no. 6, pp. 975-980, '36
Plastic repair of frontal deformity using hump from nose. STRAATSMA, C. R. Tr. Am. Acad. Ophth. *41:*625-626, '36
Autoplasty of alae nasi (nose). DOROCHENKO, I. T. Acta otolaryng. *25:*147-149, March-April '37
Role of intra-oral and intranasal grafts in contour restoration of face. KILNER, T. P. Rev. de chir. structive, pp. 1-3, March '37
Rhinoplasty using cutaneous flap from abdomen via forearm. CLAOUE. Bull. et mem. Soc. de med. de Paris *14:*278-280, April 24, '37
Plastic surgery of nose; 5 cases. RAPIN, M. Rev. med. de la Suisse Rom. *57:*405-412, June 10, '37
Constructive surgical therapy of syndactylia; case. Also: nasal deform. LLUESMA URANGA, E. Cron. med., Valencia *41:*201-207, Sept-Oct '37
Reconstruction of upper and middle portions of nose by author's technic; case. STEFANI, F. Riv. di chir. *3:*433-439, Sept '37
Plastic repair of nose as aid in therapeutic surgery. MAMLET, A. M., J. M. Soc. New Jersey *34:*664-666, Nov '37
Plastic repair of deformities about lower part of nose resulting from loss of tissue. KAZANJIAN, V. H. Tr. Am. Acad. Ophth. *42:*338-366, '37
Plastic surgery of nose. KULAKCI, N. Anadolu klin. *5:*199-200, '37
Rhinoplasty; result 25 years after operation. FINOCHIETTO, E. Prensa med. argent. *25:*897-901, May 11, '38
Plastic replacement of tip of nose. HELLENTHAL, Chirurg *10:*359-361, May 15, '38
Reconstructive surgery of nose. PIERCE, G.

Rhinoplasty, Reconstructive – Cont.
W. AND O'CONNOR, G. B. Ann. Otol., Rhin. and Laryng. *47:*437-452, June '38
Plastic surgery in complete loss of lobules and subpartition of nose; case. COELST. Rev. de chir. structive *8:*103-105, Aug '38
Reconstruction of nasal lobule, using skin graft. BAMES, H. O. An. de cir. *4:*224-229, Sept '38
Rhinoplasty. CORA ELISEHT, F. Rev. argent. de oto-rino-laring. *7:*301-341, Sept-Oct. '38
Buried grafts used to repair depressions in brow, eye socket, skull and nose. PEER, L. A., J. M. Soc. New Jersey *35:*601-605, Oct '38
Use of tubular flap for transplantation of cartilage (ear) in surgical restoration of alae nasi. NOVOSHINOVA, E. N. Zhur. ush., nos. i. gorl. bolez. *15:*164-168, '38
Rhinoplasty by frontal flap; case. PERI. Rev. de chir. structive *8:*216-217, '38
Joseph operation in plastic repair of bulldog nose; case. OHNO, T. Oto-rhino-laryng. *12:*10, Jan '39
Gibbous nose; plastic surgery. RODRIGUEZ DIAZ, A. Rev. de cien. med. *2:*79-82, March '39
Gonzalez Loza operation for removing tip of nose. CORA ELISEHT, F. AND BERRI, C. Rev. Asoc. med. argent. *53:*214-215, April 15, '39
Plastic surgery of nose. SORALUCE, J. A. Semana med. espan. *2:*782-789, Dec 30, '39
Partial nasal defects; new modification of "French" method of restoration with sliding flaps of adjoining tissue. TWYMAN, E. D. West. J. Surg. *48:*106-109, Feb '40
Loss of cutaneous substance of nasal pyramid; skin grafts in therapy. RIVAS, C. I. Rev. Asoc. med. argent. *54:*167-169, March 15-30, '40
Rhinoplasty; Argentine method. IVANISSEVICH, O. AND FERRARI, R. C. Surg., Gynec. and Obst. *71:*187-190, Aug '40
Rhinoplasties by Italian and Hindu methods. COVARRUBIAS ZENTENO, R. Rev. med. de Chile *68:*1331-1346, Oct '40
Grafts and inclusions in nasal surgery. ADLER, D. Rev. brasil. de oto-rino-laring. *8:*679-682, Nov-Dec '40
Modern surgical therapy of total loss of nose. COELST. Bull. Soc. belge d'otol., rhinol., laryng., pp. 103-106, '40
Primary rhinoplasty. KHASKELEVICH, M. G. Zhur. ush., nos. i gorl. bolez. *17:*108-112, '40
Facial autoplasty in nasal surgery; cases.

Rhinoplasty, Reconstructive – Cont.

KROEFF, M. Hospital, Rio de Janeiro *19:*773–781, May '41; *20:*11, July '41

Plastic surgery in loss of ear and nose substance. MALBEC, E. F. Semana med. *2:*714–716, Sept 18, '41

Reconstruction of nasal tip and subseptum by means of tubular graft. ZENO, L. An. de cir. *7:*183–190, Sept '41 also: Bol. y trab., Acad. argent. de cir. *25:*1028–1033, Sept 10, '41

Free graft of closely sutured skin in small rhinoplasties. ZENO, L. Bol. Soc. de cir. de Rosario *8:*361–365, Oct '41 also: An. de cir. *7:*295–299, Dec '41

Rhinoplasty by Indian method. MALBEC, E. F. Semana med. *2:*1186–1188, Nov 13, '41

Method of plastic surgery in correction of unilateral arrhinia; case. RUDERT, H. Arch. f. Ohren-, Nasen-u. Kehlkopfh. *150:*168–174, '41

Restoration of subseptum and lower lip by process of tubular autoplasty; case. DA SILVA, G. Arq. de cir. clin. e exper. *6:*287–299, April–June '42

Nasal deformity of syphilitic type due to injury; loss of mucosa and of supporting bone and cartilage; modified Gillies operation in therapy of case. DELLEPIANE RAWSON, R. AND PEREZ FERNANDEZ, M. Arq. de cir. clin. e exper. *6:*492–503, April–June '42

Plastic repair of total loss of nose; 8 cases. PRUDENTE, A. Arq. de cir. clin. e exper. *6:*174–183, April–June '42

Plastic repair of nostril. MALBEC, E. F. Semana med. *2:*625–627, Sept 10, '42

New forehead flap for nasal reconstruction. CONVERSE, J. M. Proc. Roy. Soc. Med. *35:*811–812, Oct '42 also: J. Laryng. and Otol. *57:*508–509, Nov '42

Nasal mutilation in India and new rhinoplasty. TAUBER-HRADSKY, H. T., J. Internat. Coll. Surgeons *6:*27–34, Jan–Feb '43

New technic for surgical therapy of congenital coloboma of ala nasi. REBELO NETO, J. Rev. brasil. de oto-rino-laring. *11:*159–165, March–April '43

New free graft (of skin and ear cartilage) applied to reconstruction of nostril. GILLIES, H. Brit. J. Surg. *30:*305–307, April '43

Uses of transplanted pedicle flaps for restoration or correction of nose. BLAIR, V. P. Tr. Am. Soc. Plastic and Reconstructive Surg. *12:*23–24, '43

New method for repair of small loss of alar rim. BARSKY, A. J. Arch. Otolaryng. *39:*325–326, April '44

Technic of total rhinoplasty by method of double frontal flap. VIRENQUE, M. Ann. d'oto-laryng., pp. 45–57, April–June '44

Restoration of ala nasi following its excision for cancer. AUBRY, M. AND DUCOURTIOUX, M. Ann. d'oto-laryng., pp. 89–92, July–Sept, '44

Reconstructive surgery in congenital deformity, injury and disease of nose. LAMONT, E. S. Am. J. Surg. *65:*17–45, July '44

Typical rhinoplastic operation. LUONGO, R. A. Arch. Otolaryng. *40:*68–72, July '44

Plastic surgery in reconstructing partially absent nose; original technic. LAMONT, E. S. Ann. Otol., Rhin. and Laryng. *53:*561–568, Sept '44

Surgery of nose. MCKENZIE, W. R. South. M. J. *38:*42–44, Jan '45

Treatment of partial loss of substance of ala nasi. GALTIER. Semaine d. hop. Paris *21:*491–493, May 14, '45

Sickle flap for nasal reconstruction. NEW, G. B. Surg., Gynec. and Obst. *80:*497–499, May '45

Reconstruction of columella nasi; method advantageous for female patient. HAVENS, F. Z., S. Clin. North America *25:*877–879, Aug '45

Sickle flap for reconstruction of nose. NEW, G. B. Proc. Staff Meet., Mayo Clin. *20:*353–356, Oct 3, '45

Plastic surgery of nose according to Gillies. MOE, R. Nord. med. (Norsk mag. f. laegevidensk.) *28:*2329–2332, Nov 2, '45

"Hits, strikes and outs" in use of pedicle flaps for restoration or correction of nose. BLAIR, V. P. AND BYARS, L. T. Surg. Gynec. and Obst. *82:*367–385, April '46

Repair of nasal defects with median forehead flap; primary closure of forehead wound. KAZANJIAN, V. H. Surg. Gynec. and Obst. *83:*37–49, July '46

Repair of nasal losses. YOUNG, F. Surgery *20:*670–683, Nov '46

Nasal perforation; free transplantation; experiments with fascia lata. BEHRMAN, W. Acta oto-laryng. *34:*78–81, '46

Rhinoplasty, Reduction

Operations to reduce size of nose. EITNER, E. Med. Klin. *17:*908, July 24, '21 abstr: J. A. M. A. *77:*1215, Oct 8, '21

Intranasal correction of hump and hooked noses. BALSINGER, W. E. Am. J. Surg. *36:*184–186, Aug '22 (illus.)

Operation for correction of elongated and humped noses. WHITHAM, J. D. Laryngoscope *34:*271–273, April '24

Rhinoplasty, Reduction – Cont.

Nasal hump; simplified external operation. ROBERTS, S. E. Ann. Otol., Rhin. and Laryng. *33:*1251–1253, Dec '24

Correction of hump or saddle bridge nose. JOBSON, G. B. Arch. Otolaryng. *2:*45–49, July '25

Shortening the nose. EITNER, E. Med. Klin. *22:*999, June 25, '26

Example of Joseph nose improvement. DANELIUS, B. Acta oto-laryng. *9:*49–52, '26 (in English).

Cosmetic surgery of pendulous humped nose. COELST, M. Brux.-med. *7:*530–532, Feb 20, '27

Subcutaneous plastic correction of rhinokyphosis. EITNER, E. Wien. klin. Wchnschr. *40:*1449–1450, Nov 17, '27

Cosmetic correction of long nose. NAGY, B. Med. Klin. *24:*1310–1311, Aug 24, '28

Operation for hump-nose. RÉTHI, A. Chirurg *1:*1103–1113, Nov 1, '29

Method of choice for correction of hump nose. ROY, J. N. Canad. M. A. J. *22:*803–807, June '30 also J. Laryng. and Otol. *45:*398–408, June '30 also: Union med. du Canada *59:*329–339, June '30 also: Bull. med. de Quebec *31:*207–219, June '30 also: Arch. Otolaryng. *12:*484–492, Oct '30

Plastic surgery in correction of nasal hypertrophy; intranasal route. PALACIO POSSE, R. Rev. de especialid. *5:*1856–1866, Nov '30

Cosmetic correction of convex nasal profile. EITNER, E. Med. Klin. *26:*1924, Dec 24, '30

Plastic surgery; convex nose in women. HARTER, J. H. Northwest Med. *30:*74–77, Feb '31

Choice of operative technic for convex nose; case. ROY, J. N. Ann. d'oto-laryng., pp. 155–162, Feb '31

Technic of intranasal operation for hump-nose. NOLTENIUS, F. Arch. f. Ohren-, Nasen-u. Kehlkopfh. *128:*355, May 11, '31

Therapy of humpnose. PÉRI, M. Oto-rhino-laryng. internat. *16:*174–175, April '32

Corrective operations; lowering of protruding nasal bridge and point. RÉTHI, A. Chirurg *5:*503–511, July 1, '33

Humped nose; cosmetic and plastic correction. KAHN, K., M. Times and Long Island M. J. *62:*42–44, Feb '34

Surgical correction of aquiline nose; technic and results. REBELLO NETO, J. Rev. otolaring. de Sao Paulo *2:*97–99, March–April '34

Shortening of nose. RETHI, A. Rev. de chir. plastique, pp. 85–106, Oct '34

Extreme hypertrophy of nasal pyramid (exclusively osseous); plastic surgery of case. CODAZZI AGUIRRE, J. A. Rev. med. del Rosario *26:*654–660, July '36

Cosmetic correction of convex nasal profile. EITNER, E. Chirurg *8:*528–532, July 1, '36

Cosmetic shortening of broad nose bridge. EITNER, E. Monatschr. f. Ohrenh. *71:*313–315, March '37

Technic for correcting rhinomegaly and rhinokyphosis. IVANISSEVICH, O. AND RIVAS, C. I. Bol. y. trab. de la Soc. de cir. de Buenos Aires *23:*442–451, July 12, '39

Plastic operations for hump nose; notes on artistic anatomy. BROWN, A. M. Arch. Otolaryng. *31:*827–837, May '40

Rhinomegaly and rhinokyphosis; corrective therapy. PEDEMONTE, P. V. Arch. urug. de med., cir. y especialid. *16:*601–616, June '40

Simplified plastic operation for hump, hook and twist of nose. SARNOFF, J. Surgery *7:*908–909, June '40

Rhinomegaly and rhinokyphosis; corrective therapy. PEDEMONTE, P. V. An. d. ateneo clin. quir. *7:*40–48, Jan '41

Plastic operation to correct large hump with deviation of nasal axis; modified technic. SPARER, W., M. Rec. *153:*92–94, Feb 5, '41

Correction of extreme rhinomegaly. RIVAS, C. I. Bol. y trab., Soc. argent. de cirujanos *2:*794–811, '41

Improved method of narrowing the nose. SELTZER, A. P. Ann. Otol., Rhin. and Laryng. *52:*460–472, June '43

Localized rhinomegalias; treatment of nose with pendulous tip. RIVAS, C. I. Bol. y trab., Soc. argent. de cirujanos *4:*812–817, '43 also: Rev. Asoc. med. argent. *57:*1075–1076, Dec 15, '43

Lowering glabella in rhinoplasty. MOOTNICK, M. W. Laryngoscope *55:*28–29, Jan '45

Precise technic for correcting rhinomegaly and rhinokyphosis. IVANISSEVICH, O. *et al.* Salud y belleza (no. 5) *1:*12–16, Oct-Dec '45

Plastic therapy of rhinomegaly and rhinokyphosis using Malbec technics. DEL POZO R., D. D. Bol. y trab., Soc. argent. de cirujanos *6:*522–539, '45

Rhinoplasty, Results

Correction of facial deformities. Rhinoplasty, a few statistical data. MALINIAK, J. W. Eye, Ear, Nose and Throat Monthly *9:*194–198, June '30 also: Laryngoscope *40:*495–501, July '30

End results in nasal surgery. WOLF, G. D. M. J. and Rec. *133:*178–182, Feb 18, '31

Rhinoplasty; result 25 years after operation.

Rhinoplasty, Results—Cont.

FINOCHIETTO, E. Prensa med. argent. *25:*897-901, May 11, '38

Rhinoplasty, Reviews of

Review of 25 years' observation in plastic surgery, with special reference to rhinoplasty. BECK, J. C. Laryngoscope *31:*487, July '21

Five years of surgery of ear and nose. HAAG, H. Schweiz. med. Wchnschr. *52:*498–504, May 25, '22

Present status of plastic surgery of nose and face. DA SILVA, S. C. Brazil-med. *2:*96–97, Aug 12, '22

Present day advance in plastic surgery, with special reference to correction of deformities of nose and about orbit. DE RIVER, J. P. Ann. Otol., Rhin. and Laryng. *34:*904–916, Sept '25

Present day advance in plastic surgery, with special reference to correction of deformities of nose and about orbit. DE RIVER, J. P. California and West. Med. *24:*64–68, Jan '26

Rhinoplasty; past and present. PALMER, A. Eye, Ear, Nose and Throat Monthly *11:*58–62, March '32

Progress in plastic surgery of ear and nose. FRUEHWALD, V. Rev. de chir. plastique, pp. 155–167, Oct '33

Recent advances in plastic and reconstructive surgery (of ears, nose and throat). GUTTMAN, M. R. Am. J. M. Sc. *196:*875–882, Dec '38

Progress of plastic surgery of head (including ears, mouth, jaws, nose, etc.); review of literature for 1939. REBELO NETO, J. Rev. brasil. de oto-rino-laring. *8:*111–120, March–April '40

Progress of surgery of head (including face, ears, nose, mouth, etc.) and throat (esophagus and larynx); review of literature for 1940. REBELO NETO, J. Rev. brasil. de oto-rino-laring. *9:*37-46, Jan–Feb '41

Brief panoramic study of nasal surgery. PETIT, A. M. Vida nueva *51:*138–145, April '43

Rhinoplasty, Saddle Nose

Surgical treatment of saddle nose and malignancies. SMITH, F., J. Michigan M. Soc. *20:*413, Oct '21

Rhinoplasty, with special reference to saddle nose. BLAIR, V. P., J.A.M.A. *77:*1479, Nov 5, '21

New surgical procedure for relief of depression of nasal bridge and columella; its further application for relief of hump and deflected noses; plastic treatment of syphilitic nose. SHEEHAN, J. E. Laryngoscope *32:*709–718, Sept '22 (illus.)

Restoration of sunken nose. BURROWS, H. Brit. M. J. *2:*688–689, Oct 14, '22 (illus.)

Apparatus for restoring shape to sunken nose. FREUND. Deutsche med. Wchnschr. *48:*1422, Oct 20, '22

Operative treatment for saddle-nose. RÉTHI, A. Zentralbl. f. Chir. *50:*1393–1397, Sept 8, '23 (illus.)

Correction of sunken noses. EITNER, E. Med. Klinik *20:*1000–1001, July 20, '24

Plastic surgery of nose; with special reference to correction of "saddle nose" deformities. BAUM, H. L. Colorado Med. *22:*140–144, April '25.

Correction of hump or saddle bridge nose. JOBSON, G. B. Arch. Otolaryng. *2:*45–49, July '25

Plastic operation for correction of saddle nose. SHIMOZUMA, T. Sei-I-Kwai M. J. *44:*13–24, Oct '25

Plastic and reconstructive surgery; repair of traumatic saddle nose. IVY, R. H., S. Clin. N. Amer. *6:*245–247, Feb '26

Method of choice for correction of saddle nose. ROY, J. N. Arch. Otolaryng. *5:*258–268, March '27 also: Union med. du Canada *56:*156–169, March '27 Surg. Gynec. and Obst. *45:*88–92, July '27

"Saddle-nose" deformity in children. STRACHAN, J. G. Canad. M. A. J. *17:*324–326, March '27

Saddle nose; unfortunate result of too thorough operation for deflected septum. SCHAEFFER, G. C. Ohio State M. J. *23:*989, Dec '27

Plastic operation for saddle-nose. PETROFF, N. N. Zentralbl. f. Chir. *55:*2755–2757, Nov 3, '28

Plastic operation for saddle nose. SIMONT, D. Zentralbl. f. Chir. *56:*910–912, April 13, '29

Plastic surgery of septum on account of saddle nose. HEINEMANN, O. Med. Klin. *26:*1188, Aug 8, '30

Technic of plastic operation for saddle nose. ADLER, H. Arch. f. klin. Chir. *160:*780–781, '30

Correction of depressions of nose by transposition of lateral cartilages; new method. MALINIAK, J. W. Arch. Otolaryng. *15:*280–284, Feb '32

Plastic surgery of saddle nose. MOOTNICK, M. W. Laryngoscope *42:*376–384, May '32

Use of dermal graft in repair of small saddle defects (nose) STRAATSMA, C. R. Arch. Otolaryng. *16:*506–509, Oct '32

Rhinoplasty, Saddle Nose—Cont.
Esthetic surgery of saddle nose. BELLELLI, F. Riforma med. *49:*442–448, March 25, '33
Correction of saddle nose. GONZÁLEZ LOZA, M. Rev. med. del Rosario *23:*220–225, March '33
Cosmetic sugery in correction of saddle nose deformity; case. GARCIA SIERRA, S. Clin. y lab. *23:*673–675, Aug '33
Correction of saddle nose; 3 cases. FEUZ, J. Rev. med. de la Suisse Rom. *53:*801–819, Nov. 25, '33
Plastic surgery of saddle nose. WOLFE, M. M. Laryngoscope *43:*897–904, Nov '33
Plastic correction of saddle nose. WALDE, I. Monatschr. f. Ohrenh. *69:*850–863, July '35
Correction of saddle nose. WOLF, G. D. Arch. Otolaryng. *22:*304–311, Sept '35
Plastic correction of saddle nose. KEYZER, A. F. Sovet. khir., no. 7, pp. 44–54, '35
Multiple stage operation for difficult saddle nose, avoidance of scar. ESSER, J. F. S. Surg., Gynec. and Obst. *64:*102, Jan '37
Surgical correction of saddle nose. ROLLIN, H. Hals-, Nasen-u. Ohrenarzt (Teil 1) *28:*97-100, April '37
Correction of flattened nose without graft; author's technic. GONZALEZ LOZA, M. Rev. argent. de oto-rino-laring. *6:*147–160, May-June '37
Correction of flattened nose without graft; author's technic. GONZALEZ LOZA, M. Rev. med. de Rosario *28:*388–400, April '38 also: Bol. Soc. de cir. de Rosario *5:*21–32, May '38
Saddle nose, flattened nose and lateral deviation; surgical therapy. ZENO, L. An. de cir. *4:*128–133, June '38
Saddle nose. CINELLI, A. A. AND CINELLI, J. A. New York State J. Med. *38:*977–981, July 1, '38
Saddle nose; surgical therapy. MALBEC, E. Semana med. *2:*860–862, Oct 13, '38
Depression of bridge of nose (case following abscess of septum) and its plastic treatment. HU, M. L. Chinese M. J. *54:*563–567, Dec '38
Procedure of choice in correction of saddle nose. SARNOFF, J., M. Rec. *151:*155–156, March 6, '40
Prevention and correction of dorsal depressions by septal implants (nose). GOLDMAN, I. B. Arch. Otolaryng. *32:*524–529, Sept '40
Partial saddle nose; simplified technic without use of implant or transplant. WOLFE, M. M. Ann. Otol., Rhin. and Laryng. *49:*700–708, Sept '40
Correction of flattened nose without graft, according to Gonzalez Loza procedure; author's experience. BERGAGLIO, E. O. Rev. otorrinolaring. d. litoral *1:*373–377, March '42
Correction of flat nose without graft. GONZALEZ LOZA, M. Arq. de cir. clin. e exper. *6:*145–148, April–June '42
Saddle nose deformity. FLEMMING, P. N. Dis. Eye, Ear, Nose and Throat *2:*244–245, Aug '42
Procedure for elevation of nasal dorsum by transposition of lateral cartilages. MALINIAC, J. W. Arch. Otolaryng. *41:*214–215, March '45
Fracture-dislocations of cartilaginous nose; anatomicopathologic considerations and treatment. MALINIAC, J. W. Arch. Otolaryng. *42:*131–137, Aug '45
Repair of depressed nasal bridge. SUGGIT, S. J. Laryng. and Otol. *40:*501–503, Dec '45
Saddle nose; correction by means of tantalum prosthesis; case. MALBEC, E. F. Bol. y trab., Soc. argent. de cirujanos *7:*173–177, '46 also: Rev. Asoc. med. argent. *60:*361–363, May 30 '46

Rhinoplasty, Tip Corrections
Endonasal plastic operation on alar cartilages of nose. TSCHIASSNY, K. Wien. klin. Wchnschr. *34:*120, March 17, '21
Intranasal plastic operation of deformed end of nose. ADLER, H. J. Acta oto-laryng. *10:*130–134, '26
Subcutaneous plastic operation of deformed end of nose. EITNER, E. Wien. klin. Wchnschr. *40:*916, July 14, '27
Plastic operations on nasal cartilages. RÉTHI, A. Ztschr. f. Hals-, Nasen-u. Ohrenh. *18:*515–517, '27–'28
Plastic formation of tip of nose. RÉTHI, A. Chirurg *1:*539–545, May 1, '29
Narrowing of wide alae of nose by reimplantation of cartilage from tip of nose. ÉRCZY, N. Ztschr. f. Hals-, Nasen-u. Ohrenh. *26:*194–197, July 3, '30
Cosmetic correction of deviations of tip of nose. EITNER, E. Wien. klin. Wchnschr. *43:*1260, Oct 9, '30
Reply to Eitner's comments on article about nasal tip defects, and Halla's comments. WODAK, E. Med. Klin. *28:*50, Jan 8, '32
Cosmetic correction of defects of tip of nose. EITNER, E. Ztschr. f. Laryng., Rhin. Otol. *26:*46–53, '35
Simple method for reducing abnormally protruding nasal tip. WAHL, S. Rev. de chir. structive, pp. 315–318, June '36
New method of rhinoplasty for sinking tip of nose. ROY, J. N. Rev. de chir. structive, pp. 441–446, Dec '36 also: Ann. Otol., Rhin. and

Rhinoplasty, Tip Corrections—Cont.
Laryng. *46:*203-207, March '37 also: Union med. du Canada *66:*266-270, March '37 also: Canad. M. A. J. *36:*603-605, June '37
Reconstructions about nasal tip. STRAITH, C. L. Am. J. Surg. *43:*223-236, Feb '39
Corrective plastic surgery of nasal lobe. ZENO, L. An. de cir. *5:*3-14, March '39
Corrective surgery of nasal tip. CONVERSE, J. M. Ann. Otol., Rhin. and Laryng. *49:*895-911, Dec '40
Reconstruction of nasal tip; case. FREYTES, M. V. AND SUAREZ, A. R. Bol. y trab., Soc. de cir. de Cordoba *2:*193-205, '41
Plastic correction of prominent nasal tip. RIUS, M. Arq. de cir. clin. e exper. *6:*639-641, April-June '42
Depressions of nasal tip; plastic surgery. SANTA MARINA IRAOLA, J. A. Semana med. *2:*726-729, Sept 23, '43
Corrections of depressions of nasal tip. RIVAS, C. I. Bol. y trab., Acad. argent. de cir. *27:*936-941, Oct 6, '43
Reconstruction of nasal tip; new technic. MALTZ, M. Am. J. Surg. *63:*203-205, Feb '44
Corrections of depressions of nasal tip. RIVAS, C. I. Bol. d. Inst. clin. quir. *20:*573-580, April '44

RHOADS, J. E.; WOLFF, W. A. AND LEE, W. E.: Use of adrenal cortical extract in treatment of traumatic shock. of burns. Ann. Surg. *113:*955-968, June '41
RHOADS, J. E.; WOLFF, W. A. AND LEE, W. E.: Sulfonamides (sulfanilamide and its derivatives) in local treatment of burns. Pennsylvania M. J. *46:*13-16, Oct '42
RHOADS, J. E. *et al*: Use of plasma in treatment of burn shock. Clinics *1:*37-42, June '42
RHOADS, J. E. *et al*: Adrenal cortical extract in burn shock; further experiences. Ann. Surg. *118:*982-987, Dec '43
RHOADS, J. E. (see LEE, W. E.) July '44
RHOADS, J. E. (see RAVDIN, I. S.) Feb '35
RHOADS, J. E. (see WOLFF, W. A. *et al*) Nov '42
RHODE, C. M.; MORALES, M. F. AND LOZNER, E. L.: Quantitative evaluation of certain treatments in healing of experimental third degree burns. J. Clin. Investigation *24:*372-379, May '45
RHODE, J.: Dacryocystorhinostomy in Venezuela. Arch. venezol. Soc. de oto-rino-laring., oftal., neurol. *3:*1-56, March '42
RHODE, J.: Dacryocystorhinostomy in Venezuela. Gac. med. de Caracas *50:*231, Nov 30, '43; 241, Dec 15, '43; 251, Dec 31, '43 *51:*261, Jan 15, '44 comment by Lopez Villoria *51:*264, Jan 15, '44; 11, Jan 31, '44
RHODES, G. K. AND MCKENNEY, C.: Traumatic shock; newer aspects and treatment. California and West. Med. *33:*665-670, Sept '30
RHODES, J. E.: Newer aspects of burn therapy. Clinics *3:*1618-1622, April '45
RHYS-LEWIS, R. D. S.: Use of X-rays in treatment of indurations due to scars and chronic inflammation. Proc. Roy. Soc. Med. *39:*150-151, Feb '46

Rhytidectomy

Meloplasty. PÓLYA, E. Zentralbl. f. Chir. *48:*261, Feb 26, '21
Esthetic surgery of face. BOURGUET. Arch. franco-belges de chir. *28:*293-297, April '25
Fascial bands as supports to relaxed facial tissue. MILLER, C. C. Ann. Surg. *82:*603-608, Oct '25
Truth and fallacies of face peeling and face lifting. BAMES, H. O., M. J. and Rec. *126:*86-87, July 20, '27
Operative removal of skin folds for cosmetic purposes. EITNER, E. Wien. med. Wchnschr. *77:*1006, July 23, '27
Improved technique for removal of wrinkles of face and neck. LAGARDE, M. Am. J. Surg. *3:*132-138, Aug '27 also: Cron. med., Lima *44:*33-42, Feb '27
Removal of folds and wrinkles of face; indications and technic. STEIN, R. O. Wien. klin. Wchnschr. *40:*1168-1172, Sept 15, '27
Cosmetic results of treatment of facial wrinkles. (Wie sind die kosmetischen Erfolge bei operativer Behandlung der Runzein?) Various Authors. Wien. med. Wchnschr. *77:*1320, Sept 24, '27
Treatment of facial wrinkles; 17 photographs. BOURGUET, J. Monde med., Paris *38:*41-51, Jan 15, '28
Surgical treatment of facial and neck wrinkles; new technics. LAGARDE, M. Arch. franco-belges de chir. *31:*154-163, Feb '28
Joseph's improvement of his technic for plastic surgery of pendulous cheeks (meloplasty). JOSEPH, J. Deutsche med. Wchnschr. *54:*567-568, April 6, '28
Surgery of skin of face. MILLER, C. C. Am. Med. *23:*345-350, May '28
Indications and technic of cosmetic correction of facial wrinkles. EITNER, E. Wien. klin. Wchnschr. *41:*1281-1283, Sept 6, '28
Indications and technic of cosmetic correction of facial wrinkles (comment on Eitner's article). HALLA. Wien. klin. Wchnschr. *41:*1442, Oct 11, '28
Reply to comment by Halla on cosmetic correction of facial wrinkles. EITNER. Wien. klin. Wchnschr. *41:*1530, Nov 1, '28

Rhytidectomy—Cont.
Excision of oval pieces of skin in treatment of facial wrinkles. STEIN, R. O. Arch. f. Dermat. u. Syph. *155:*304–307, '28
Removal of facial wrinkles; healing of wound without suture. KROMAYER. Deutsche med. Wchnschr. *55:*912–914, May 31, '29
Comment on Kromayer's article on facial wrinkle removal. HALLA, F. Deutsche med. Wchnschr. *55:*1262–1263, July 26, '29
Comment on Kromayer's article on removal of facial wrinkles. SCHLESINGER. Deutsche med. Wchnschr. *55:*1512–1513, Sept 6, '29
Excision of unsightly skin folds. GUMPERT, M. Med. Welt. *4:*219, Feb 15, '30
Cosmetic surgery of face. HOFFMANN, K. F. Med. Welt. *4:*185–187, Feb 8, '30
Cosmetic facial surgery. BROEMAN, C. J. Urol. and Cutan. Rev. *34:*319–323, May '30
Making of a Beautiful Face, or Face-Lifting Unveiled, by J. HOWARD CRUM. Walton Book Co., New York, 1931
Plastic or esthetic surgery of face. CUCCO, A. Ann. di ottal. e clin. ocul. *59:*253–271, March '31
Korrektiv-cosmetische Chirurgie der Näse, der Ohren, und den Gesichts, by VICTOR FRÜHWALD. Wilhelm Maudrich, Vienna, 1932. (Also English edition, translated by Geoffrey Morey.)
Is surgical restoration of the aged face justified? Indications-method of repair-end results. MALINIAK, J. W., M. J. and Rec. *135:*321–324, April 6, '32
Technic of surgical restoration of aged face. CLAOUÉ, C. Bull. Acad. de med., Paris *109:*257–265, Feb 28, '33
Esthetic surgery (face). BOURGUET, J. Bull. et mem. Soc. d. chirurgiens de Paris *25:*282–288, May 5, '33
Technic of corrective surgery of wrinkles of face. PASSOT, R. Rev. de chir. plastique, pp. 23–33, May '33
Facts and fallacies of cosmetic surgery (paraffin injections, hair removal, face-lifting, nose-remodeling, etc.). MALINIAK, J. W. Hygeia *12:*200–202, March '34
Cosmetic surgery of wrinkles (face). PIRES. Fortschr. d. Med. *52:*576, June 25, '34 also: Marseille-med. *1:*635–638, May 15, '34 also: Rev. de med. y cir. de la Habana *39:*409–412, June 30, '34 also: Strasbourg med. *94:*393–394, July 5, '34 also: Rev. med. de l'est *62:*554–557, Aug 15, '34
Cosmetic surgery of facial wrinkles. PIRES. Rev. med. peruana *6:*1997–2000, Sept '34
Cosmetic surgery of facial wrinkles. EITNER, E. Wien. med. Wchnschr. *85:*244, Feb 23, '35

Rhytidectomy—Cont.
Technic of increasing tone of skin of skin and removing wrinkles. BURIAN, F. Med. Welt *10:*930–931, June 27, '36
New ideas with regard to plastic surgery of pendulous cheeks with description of new method. EHRENFELD, H. Zentralbl. f. Chir. *64:*202–205, Jan 23, '37
Plastic surgery of facial wrinkles; case. MALBEC, E. F. Semana med. *1:*1225–1227, April 29, '37
Plastic surgery of wrinkles. MALBEC, E. F. Semana med. *2:*289–294, Aug 4, '38
Esthetics of plastic surgery (face). BERNDORFER, A. Gyogyaszat *78:*638–641, Oct 30, '38
Cosmetic surgery of face. RIUS, M. Arq. de cir. clin. e exper. *6:*586, April–June '42

RIBAS, G.: Congenital absence of vagina; surgical therapy. Ann. de Hosp. de Santa Creu i Sant Pau *9:*66–83, Jan 15, '35
RIBAS Y RIBAS, E.: Shock therapy. Arch. de med., cir. y espec. *29:*393–398, Oct 6, '28
RIBEIRO, E. B.: Practical method of burn treatment; preliminary report. Bol. San. Sao Lucas *7:*93–95, Dec '45
RIBEIRO, L.: Legal responsibility in plastic surgery; advisability of establishing regulations protecting both physician and patient. Folha med. *13:*175–178, May 25, '32
RIBÓN, V. (see JIMÉNEZ LÓPEZ, C.) Oct '22

Rib Grafts (See also Bone Grafts; Cranioplasty; Jaws, Bone Grafts to)

Case of successful grafting of ribs into skull for cranial defect. LEVIN, J. J., M. J. South Africa *20:*61–63, Oct '24
Cranioplasty by split rib method. BROWN, R. C., J. Coll. Surgeons, Australiasia *1:*238–246, Nov '28
Correction of depressed deformities of external nose with rib graft. COHEN, L. South. M. J. *30:*680–685, July '37

RICARD AND FANJEAUX: Resuscitation and transfusion service during offensives in Italy from May 11 to July 27, 1944. Bull. internat. serv. san. *19:*7–22, Jan '46
RICARD, A.: Conservative hand surgery. Lyon chir. *26:*596–599, Aug–Sept '29
RICARD, A.; FRANCILLON, J. AND PELLERAT, J.: Use of polyvinyl pyrrolidine as blood substitute in therapy of postoperative shock. Lyon chir. *40:*110–113, Jan–Feb '45
RICCI, B.: Third grade hypoplasia of right auricle, absence of auditory canal and malformation of tympanic cavity. Boll. d. mal. d. orecchio, d. gola, d. naso *52:*57–70, Feb '34

RICCI, J. V. (see: LOWSLEY, O. S. *et al*) Nov '21
RICCIARDI, M.: Senile form of ectropion. Ann. di ottal. e clin. ocul. *55:*51-57, Jan-Feb '27
RICCITELLI, E. (see: FRANCHINI, Y.) 1933
RICE, E. R.: Conservation of fingers in injuries and infections. Internat. J. Med. and Surg. *46:*105-108, March '33
RICHARDS, D. W. JR.: Circulation in traumatic shock in man. Harvey Lect. (1943-1944) *39:*217-253, '44
RICHARDS, D. W. JR.: Blood circulation in traumatic shock in man. Nord. med. *26:*1069-1080, May 25, '45
RICHARDS, R. L.: Methods of immobilization of fractured mandible. Am. J. Orthodontics *24:*973-979, Oct '38
RICHARDS, R. L.: Vasomotor disturbances in hand after injuries. Edinburgh M. J. *50:*449-468, Aug '43
RICHARDS, R. T.: Burn therapy. Rocky Mountain M. J. *38:*521-525, July '41
RICHARDS, R. T.: Burns. Rocky Mountain M. J. *40:*810-815, Dec '43
RICHARDSON, F. M.: Modern burn treatment (with special reference to physiologic changes). M. J. Australia *2:*337-339, Oct 10, '42
RICHE, V.; MOURGUE-MOLINES, E. AND CADÉRAS, J.: Burn therapy without bandaging; continuous exposure to hot air and electric light. Arch. Soc. d. sc. med. et biol. de Montpellier *13:*36-45, Jan '32
RICHER, V.: Urethroplasty; general review of technics using free or pedicled grafts in restoration of hypospadias or of loss of substance of masculine urethra. (Comment on Godard's article.) J. d'urol. *42:*339-340, Oct '36
RICHERI, S.: Palatographic researches on phonation in cleft palate. Arch. ital. di otol. *45:*487-509, July '34
RICHES, E. W. (see PATEY, D. H.) Aug '43
RICHEY, DEW. G.: Remote sequelae of rectal implantation of ureters for exstrophy; findings at necropsy 14 years after Bergenhem operation. Arch. Surg. *11:*408-416, Sept '25
RICHISON, F. A.: Treatment of malar and zygomatic fractures. U. S. Nav. M. Bull. *37:*566-571, Oct '39
RICHISON, F. A.: Fractures of maxilla. J. Am. Dent. A. *27:*558-563, April '40
RICHISON, F. A.: Improving mental attitude by means of plastic surgery of face. J. Am. Dent. A. *28:*437-441, March '41
RICHISON, F. A.: Multiple facial fractures; case. J. Am. Dent. A. *29:*3-6, Jan '42
RICHISON, F. A. AND KENNEDY, J. T.: Skeletal fixation splint in mandibular fractures as aid to early denture construction. J. Am. Dent. A. *31:*646-648, May 1, '44
RICHLIN, P. (see GLASSER, B. F.) April '44
RICHON, KISSEL, AND SIMONIN, J.: Dupuytren's contracture and nervous disturbances. Rev. med. de l'est *61:*231-237, March 15, '33
RICHTER, E.: Fracture of inferior turbinate bone of nose. Deutsche Ztschr. f. Chir. *232:*380-381, '31
RICHTER, G.: Case of nearly complete cicatrizing of mouth. Klin. Med. *5:*700-702, '27
RICHTER, H.: Indications for resection of nasal septum. Ztschr. f. Laryng., Rhin. *19:*339-402, July '30 also: Munchen. med. Wchnschr. *77:*1354-1356, Aug 8, '30
RICHTER, H.: Indications for excision of nasal septum. Prakt. Arzt *16:*5-11, Jan 5, '31
RICHTER, H.: Etiology of congenital deformities of nasal septum. Hals-, Nasen-u. Ohrenarzt (Teil 1) *27:*53-55, '36
RIDARD, L.: Osteosynthesis of lower jaw after fracture; cases. Rev. de stomatol. *31:*883-888, Dec '29
RIDARD, L.: Methods of immobilization with mouth open and closed in fracture of lower jaw. Rev. gen. de clin. et de therap. *44:*454-456, July 12, '30
RIDDOCH, J. W.: Surgical shock. Birmingham M. Rev. *11:*131-143, June '36
RIDER, D. L.: Finger fractures. Am. J. Surg. *38:*549-559, Dec '37
RIDER, D. L. (see SMITH, F. L.) Jan '35
RIDOUT, C. A. S.: Destruction of nose and part of face by squamous-celled carcinoma of rodent ulcer type. Proc. Roy. Soc. Med. *25:*1767, Oct '32
RIDPATH, R. F.: New method for removal of vomerine ridge in septal obstruction. Tr. Am. Laryng., Rhin. & Otol. Soc. *37:*339-343, '31
RIDPATH, R. F.: Metzenbaum operation for correction of deflected nasal septum. S. Clin. North America *15:*231-237. Feb '35
RIEHL, G. JR.: Twenty-eight cases of grave burns treated by blood transfusion. Arch. f. Dermat. u. Syph. *153:*41-65, '27
RIEHL, G. JR.: Peptic ulcer following burns of skin; 5 cases. Acta dermat.-venereol. *11:*277-294, Sept '30
RIEHL, G. JR.: Prognosis, therapy and complications in burns. Arch. f. Dermat. u. Syph. *164:*409-471, '31
RIEHL, G. JR: Burns causing death; review of past and recent literature. Zentralbl. f. Haut-u. Geschlechtskr. *38:*289-296, Sept 5, '31
RIEHL, G. JR.: Pathology and therapy of burns. Wien. klin. Wchnschr. *46:*1041-1043, Aug 25, '33
RIEHL, G. JR.: Burns in very young children. Wien. klin. Wchnschr. *46:*1147-1150, Sept 22, '33
RIEMKE, V.: Cleft palate operations. Hospital-

stid. *78:*741, July 9; 753, July 16, '35

RIENHOFF, W. F., JR.: Use of muscle pedicle flap for prevention of swelling of arm following radical operation for carcinoma of breast; preliminary report. Bull. Johns Hopkins Hosp. *60:*369–371, May '37

RIESCO MAC-CLURE, J. S.: Deforming recidivating polyposis of nose, with report of case. Rev. otorrinolaring. *1:*61–64, Dec '41

RIETI, E.: Radium therapy of keloids. Arch. di radiol. *4:*941–955, Sept–Dec '28

RIFE, C. S.: Shock and hemorrhage; management in evacuation hospital. M. Bull. North African Theat. Op. (no. 6) *1:*3–4, June '44

RIECKE, H. G.: Wounds of larynx due to burns during childhood. Hals-, Nasen-u. Ohrenarzt (Teil 1) *30:*111–118, March '39

Riedel Operation

Orbital prosthesis after Riedel operation in frontal sinusitis; case. ALVES, O. Arq. de cir. clin. e exper. *6:*322–323, April–June '42

RIEDER, W.: Progressive furuncle of face. Zentralbl. f. Chir. *50:*1024–1025, June 30, '23 abstr: J.A.M.A. *81:*1155, Sept 29, '23

RIEDER, W. (see SUDECK, P.) 1929

RIEDL, L.: Report of 30 cases of Dupuytren's contracture observed in 1932–1938. Zentralbl. f. Chir. *66:*1093–1096, May 13, '39

RIEDL, L.: Bilateral Dupuytren's contracture in three children of one family; case. Casop. lek. cesk. *78:*1114–1115, Oct 6, '39

RIEHL, G. JR.: Live-wire injuries of skin. Munchen. med. Wchnschr. *70:*1119–1120, Aug 31, '23

RIEHL, G. JR.: Treatment of severe burns by blood transfusion. Wien. klin. Wchnschr. *38:*833–834, July '23, '25 abstr: J.A.M.A. *85:*860, Sept 12, '25

RIFE, C. S. (see TURNER, J. W.) May '38

RIGA, I. T.: Plastic operation for bilateral hypertrophy of breast with asymmetry, ptosis and mastodynia. Rev. de chir., Bucuresti *43:*219–226, March–April '40

RIGA, I. T. (see SARRU, P. *et al*) May '40

RIGANO-IRRERA, D. AND SACERDOTE, G.: Behavior of autoplastic and homoplastic grafts placed in subcutaneous tissue; experiments on rabbits. Arch. ital. di chir. *20:*190–198, '27

RIGAUD. (see ESCAT, *et al*) 1930

RIGG, J. P. AND WALDAPFEL, R.: Plastic repair with cartilagoperiosteal bridge in drooping (or dog) ear. J.A.M.A. *113:*125–126, July 8, '39

RIGNEY, P.: Utilization of autoplastic bone grafts in orthopedic and plastic surgery. Southwestern Med. *12:*564–565, Dec '28

RIHMER, B.: Phalloplasty; case. Budapesti orvosi ujsag *30:*73–75, Jan 21, '32

RIKHTER, G. A.: Extensive plastic reconstruction of shoulder joint following gunshot wound. Khirurgiya, no. 8, pp. 79–80, '44

RILEY, J. G.: Present conception of cause and treatment of shock. Lahey Clin. Bull. *2:*154–160, July '41

RIMBAUD, P. (see MARGAROT, J.) Jan '36

RIN, K.: Progressive facial hemiatrophy; case. Taiwan Igakkai Zasshi *35:*1156, May '36

RING, H. J.: Management and treatment of burns. California and West. Med. *23:*1296–1297, Oct '25

RINGROSE, E. J.: Treatment of large stasis ulcers by pinch grafts. J. Iowa M. Soc. *33:*175–178, April '43

RIOSALIDO: Tendon transplantation for radial paralysis. Arch. espan. de pediat. *5:*210, April '21 abstr: J.A.M.A. *77:*497, Aug 6, '21

RIOU, M.: New technic of bandaging of epidermic grafts; application in therapy of ulcers of leg. Bull. Soc. path. exot. *26:*1296–1301, '33

RISAK, E.: Ankylosis of fingers; pathologic study. Deutsche Ztschr. f. Chir. *211:*86–115, '28

RISDON, E. F.: Management of nasal fractures. Ann. Otol., Rhin. and Laryng. *40:*1094–1098, Dec '31

RISDON, E. F.: Management of nasal fractures. Tr. Am. Acad. Ophth. *36:*193–198, '31

RISDON, E. F.: Surgical repair of facial injuries and harelip and cleft palate deformities. Canad. M. A. J. *32:*51–54, Jan '35

RISDON, F.: Treatment of nonunion of fractures of mandible by free autogenous bone-grafts. J.A.M.A. *79:*297–299, July 22, '22

RISDON, F.: Plastic surgery of head and neck, Canad. M. A. J. *12:*797–798, Nov '22

RISDON, F.: Arthroplasty of temporomaxillary joint. J.A.M.A. *85:*2011–2013, Dec 26, '25

RISDON, F. Treatment of harelip and cleft palate. J. Am. Dent. A. *15:*2017–2020, Nov '28

RISDON, F.: Treatment of jaw fractures. Canad. M. A. J. *20:*260–262, March '29

RISDON, F.: Treatment of nasal deformities and fractures. Canad. M. A. J. *20:*631–633, June '29

RISDON, F.: Surgical treatment of harelip and cleft palate in children. Canad. M. A. J. *25:*563–565, Nov '31

RISDON, F.: Ankylosis of jaws. J. Am. Dent. A. *21:*1933–1937, Nov '34

RISDON, F.: Jaw fractures. J. Am. Dent. A. *23:*1639–1641, Sept '36

RISDON, F.: Surgical treatment of fractures of bones of face. Canad. M. A. J. *38:*33–36, Jan '38

RISDON, F.: Jaw fractures. Canad. M. A. J. *39:*572–573, Dec '38

RISDON, F.: Plastic operations of orbit. Bull. Acad. Med., Toronto *18:*139–141, April '45

RISINGER, W.: Orell method of bone transplantation; cases. Acta orthop. Scandinav. *9:*152-180, '38

RISK, P. A.: Role of orthodontist and general practitioner in treatment of jaw fractures. J. Am. Dent. A. *28:*884-894, June '41

RISK, R. (see SMITH, S. *et al*) Oct '39

RISMONDO, P.: Neoplasty of vagina by Wagner-Thiersch method (grafts). Lijecn. vjes. *56:*312-313, '34

RITCHIE, H. P.: Repair of harelip and cleft palate deformity. Minnesota Med. *4:*15, Jan '21

RITCHIE, H. P.: Uses of dermal graft and delayed flap. S. Clin. N. America *3:*1371-1387, Oct '23 (illus.)

RITCHIE, H. P.: Destructive and constructive surgery of malignancy. Minnesota Med. *8:*4-7, Jan '25

RITCHIE, H. P.: Congenital cleft lip and palate; muscle theory repair of cleft lip. Ann. Surg. *84:*211-222, Aug '26

RITCHIE, H. P.: Congenital cleft lip and palate; series of congenital clefts. Minnesota Med. *9:*664-666, Dec '26

RITCHIE, H. P.: Congenital cleft lip and palate; embryology of upper jaw interpreted in terms of surgical repair of process and palate of clefts. Tr. Am. S. A. *45:*170-178, '27

RITCHIE, H. P.: Congenital clefts of face and jaw; survey of 350 operated cases. Tr. West. S. A. *42:*37-98, '32

RITCHIE, H. P.: Congenital clefts of face and jaws; 350 cases in which operation was performed. Arch. Surg. *28:*617-658, April '34

RITCHIE, H. P.: Discussion of subject of hypospadias from viewpoint of reconstructive surgery and report of use of depilated scrotal flap. Surgery *5:*911-931, June '39

RITCHIE, H. P.: Congenital clefts of face and jaws; report of operations used and discussion of results. Surg., Gynec. and Obst. *73:*654-670, Nov '41

RITCHIE, H. P. (see DAVIS, J. S.) Oct '22

RITCHIE, H. P. (see PEYTON, W. T.) Dec '36

RITCHIE, R. N.: Primary carcinoma of vagina following Baldwin reconstruction operation for congenital absence of vagina. Am. J. Obst. and Gynec. *18:*794-799, Dec '29

RITCHIE, W. P.: Correlation of anatomic and functional results following operation for cleft palate. Arch. Surg. *35:*548-570, Sept '37

RITT, A. E.: New method for cutting full thickness or split thickness grafts. Minnesota Med. *29:*437, May '46

RITTER, C.: End results of covering amputation stumps with free fascia transplants. Zentralbl. f. Chir. *56:*2565-2566, Oct 12, '29

RITTER, C.: Surgical treatment of Dupuytren's contracture. Deutsche Ztschr. f. Chir. *227:*544-546, '30

RITTER, H. H.: Burn therapy (skin grafts). Am. J. Surg. *31:*48-55, Jan '36

RITTER H. H.: Treatment of shock and fresh wounds. Am. J. Surg. *60:*112-114, April '43

RITTER, R. (see LEHMANN, W.) 1939

RITTERSKAMP, P.: Family with camptodactylia. Munchen. med. Wchnschr. *83:*724-725, May 1, '36

RIUS, M.: Postoperative care in plastic surgery of nose. Arq. de cir. clin. e exper. *6:*171-174, April-June '42

RIUS, M.: Cosmetic surgery of face. Arq. de cir. clin. e exper. *6:*586, April-June '42

RIUS, M.: Plastic correction of prominent nasal tip. Arq. de cir. clin. e exper. *6:*639-641, April-June '42

RIVARD, J. H.: Suture of tendon of flexor digitorum profundus; case. Union med. du Canada *59:*28-30, Jan '30

RIVAROLA, R. A.: Ombredanne's method for grave hypospadias. Rev. Asoc. med. argent. *35:*634, Aug '21

RIVAROLA, R. A.: Exstrophy of bladder, treatment by Heitz-Boyer-Hovelacque operation; 9 cases. Semana med. *2:*1023-1027, Oct 20, '27

RIVAS, C. I.: Trauma of nasal pyramid. Rev. med. de Chile *68:*306-320, March '40

RIVAS, C. I.: Loss of cutaneous substance of nasal pyramid; skin grafts in therapy. Rev. Asoc. med. argent. *54:*167-169, March 15-30, '40

RIVAS, C. I.: Trauma of nasal pyramid. Acta med., Rio de Janeiro *7:*187-202, May '41

RIVAS, C. I.: Correction of extreme rhinomegaly. Bol. y trab., Soc. argent. de cirujanos *2:*794-811, '41

RIVAS, C. I.: Surgical infections of hand. Bol. d. Inst. clin. quir. *18:*917-1382, Dec '42

RIVAS, C. I.: Corrections of depressions of nasal tip. Bol. y trab., Acad. argent. de cir. *27:*936-941, Oct 6, '43

RIVAS, C. I.: Localized rhinomegalias; treatment of nose with pendulous tip. Bol. y trab., Soc. argent. de cirujanos *4:*812-817, '43 also: Rev. Asoc. med. argent. *57:*1075-1076, Dec 15, '43

RIVAS, C. I.: Corrections of depressions of nasal tip. Bol. d. Inst. clin. quir. *20:*573-580, April '44

RIVAS, C. I.: Acute hand infections; surgical concept. Dia med. *17:*63-66, Jan 22, '45

RIVAS, C. I.: Therapy of war trauma of facial region. Bol. d. Inst. clin. quir. *21:*90-95, Feb '45

RIVAS, C. I.: Use of flaps. Dia med. *18:*946-955, July 15, '46

RIVAS, C. I. AND IZURIETA, F. A.: Correction of deformities of tip of nose with implantations of paladon. Bol. y trab., Acad. argent. de cir. *29:*240–247, May 9, '45

RIVAS, C. I.; URZUA C, C. R., AND GOBICH, E.: Use of implants in plastic surgery of face. Arq. de cir. clin. e exper. *6:*621–638, April-June '42

RIVAS, C. I. (see IVANISSEVICH, O. *et al*) April '39

RIVAS, C. I. (see IVANISSEVICH, O.) July '39

RIVAS, C. I. (see IVANISSEVICH, O. *et al*) Jan-March '40

RIVAS, C. I. (see IVANISSEVICH, O. *et al*) June '41

RIVAS, C. I. (see IVANISSEVICH, O.) Sept '42

RIVAS, C. I. (see IVANISSEVICH, O.) July '43

RIVAS, C. I. (see IVANISSEVICH, O. *et al*) Oct-Dec '45

RIVAS, J. J.: Deforming polyposis of nose, with report of case. Arch. venezol. Soc. de oto-rino-laring., oftal., neurol. *2:*194–199, Dec '41

RIVAS DIEZ, B. AND DELRIO, J. M. A.: Trophoanesthetic treatment of burns; preliminary report. Dia med. *16:*209, March 6, '44

RIVAS DIEZ, B. AND DELRIO, J. M. A.: Local anesthesia in burn therapy. Bol. y trab., Acad. argent. de cir. *28:*1182–1192, Nov 22, '44

RIVAS JORDAN, R.: Operative treatment of rhinophyma. Rev. med. del Rosario *18:*68, Feb '28

DERIVER, J. P.: Correction of deformities of nose and about orbit by plastic surgery. Southwestern Med. *7:*226–232, July '23

DE RIVER, J. P.: Correction of external nasal deformities. California and West. Med. *22:*214–216, May '24

DE RIVER, J. P.: Use of dental stent in skin grafts of middle ear and mastoid cavities. M. J. and Rec. *122:*63–64, July 15, '25

DE RIVER, J. P.: Present day advance in plastic surgery, with special reference to correction of deformities of nose and about orbit. Ann. Otol., Rhin. and Laryng. *34:*904–916, Sept '25

DE RIVER, J. P.: Present day advance in plastic surgery, with special reference to correction of deformities of nose and about orbit. California and West. Med. *24:*64–68, Jan '26

DE RIVER, J. P.: Jump method or interrupted tube flap; new technic in fashioning tube flaps for skin grafts. J.A.M.A. *87:*662–663, Aug 28, '26

DE RIVER, J. P.: Restoration of auricle. California and West. Med. *26:*654–656, May '27

DE RIVER, J. P.: Plastic surgery of face. California and West. Med. *28:*651–655, May '28

RIVEROS, M.: Cutaneous burns. An. Cong. brasil. e am. cir. *3:*174–278, '42

RIVEROS, M.: Burn therapy with report of cases. An. Fac. de cien. med., Asuncion (no. 18) *11:*7–68, '43

RIVES, J. D. (see MAES, U.) May '26

RIVIERE, M.: Phenomena of shock in obstetrics. Arch. franco-belges de chir. *29:*106–109, Feb '26

RIVIÈRE, M.: Case of obstetric shock. Bull. Soc. d'obst. et de gynec. *16:*225–228, March '27

RIVIERE, M. (see LAFARGUE, P.) April '37

ROA, R. L.: Sulfonamides in burn therapy. Dia med. *15:*608, June 14, '43

ROA, R. L.: Successful repair of severely wounded hand; case. Rev. med.-quir. de pat. fem. *22:*456–457, Dec '43

ROASENDA, G. AND DOGLIOTTI, A. M.: Results of resection of superior cervical ganglion and of part of trunk of cervical sympathicus in peripheral facial paralysis of long standing; case. Boll. e mem. Soc. piemontese di chir. *4:*980–990, '34

ROBACK, R. A. AND IVY, A. C.: Comparative experimental study including medicated (with potassium iodide and sulfathiazole, sulfonamide) pliable gelatin film (sulfagel) in burns; effect of firm dressings on rate of healing. Surg., Gynec. and Obst. *79:*469–477, Nov '44

ROBB, J. J.: Burn therapy. Brit. M. J. *1:*466–467, March 9, '35

ROBB-SMITH, A. H. T. (see CONVERSE, J. M.) Dec '44

ROBBINS, A. R.: Treatment of spastic entropion. Arch. Ophth. *25:*475–476, March '41

ROBBINS, B. H. (see LAMSON, P. D. *et al*) March '45

ROBBIO CAMPOS, J. (see CARANDO, V. *et al*) Jan '37

ROBERT, AND MEARLE-BERAL: Fractures of lower jaw; 2 methods of therapy; 2 cases. Arch. de med. et pharm. nav. *125:*703–715, Oct-Dec '35

ROBERT, P.: Medical therapy of burns. Union med. du Canada *71:*262–268, March '42

ROBERTS, C.: Operation for treatment of ectopia vesicae. Lancet *1:*1125, May 28, '21

ROBERTS, F. W.: Review of cases of squamous cell carcinoma at New Haven Hospital from January 1, 1920, to November 1, 1931. Yale J. Biol. and Med. *4:*187–198, Dec '31

ROBERTS, G. J.: Congenital choanal atresia. U.S. Nav. M. Bull. *43:*1216–1219, Dec '44

ROBERTS, L. B. (see ASHE, W. F. JR.) Feb '45

ROBERTS, M. A. W. (see ANDERSON, T. F.) June '32

ROBERTS, N.: Fractures of phalanges of hand and metacarpals. Proc. Roy. Soc. Med. *31:*793–798, May '38

ROBERTS, R. E. (see JONES, H. W.) Jan '26
ROBERTS, S. E.: Nasal hump; simplified external operation. Ann. Otol., Rhin. and Laryng. *33:*1251-1253, Dec '24
ROBERTS, S. E.: Fracture of malar zygomatic arch; review of literature; simplified operative technic; case reports. Ann. Otol., Rhin. and Laryng. *37:*826-838, Sept '28
ROBERTS, S. E.: Tetany following use of cocaine and epinephrine in nasal surgery; observations and treatment; preliminary report. Tr. Sect. Laryng., Otol. and Rhin., A. M. A., pp. 22-30, '29
ROBERTS, W. M. AND SCHAUBEL, H. J.: Vaseline gauze contact fixation of split thickness (Padgett) skin grafts. Am. J. Surg. *67:*16-22, Jan '45
ROBERTS, W. M. (see MILLER, O. L.) March '35
ROBERTS, W. R.: Control of mandibular fragments by external fixation. Brit. Dent. J. *80:*257, April 18, '46; 291, May 3, '46
ROBERTS, W. S.: Tendon transplantation. Southern M. J. *16:*545-550, July '23
ROBERTSON, B.: Blood transfusion in severe burns in infants and young children. Canad. M. A. J. *11:*744, Oct '21
ROBERTSON, B. AND BOYD, G. L.: Toxemia of severe superficial burns in children. Am. J. Dis. Child. *25:*163-167, Feb '23
ROBERTSON, B. AND BOYD, G. L.: Toxemia of severe superficial burns. J. Lab. and Clin. Med. *9:*1-14, Oct '23
ROBERTSON, F.: Symptoms, recognition and treatment of severe shock. Newcastle M. J. *21:*67-77, July '42
ROBERTSON, J. F.: Avulsion of skin of scrotum and reconstruction. South. Med. and Surg. *93:*527-528, July '31
ROBERTSON, J. S.: Surgical treatment of pain; malignant lesions of face, nose and mouth. Tr. Roy. Med.-Chir. Soc. Glasgow, pp. 29-31, '43-'44; in Glasgow M. J. May '44
ROBERTSON, R. C.; CAWLEY, J. J. JR. AND FARIS, A. M.: Treatment of fracture-dislocation of interphalangeal joints of hand. J. Bone and Joint Surg. *28:*68-70, Jan '46
ROBERTSON, T. S.: Exstrophy of bladder. Illinois M. J. *58:*66-69, July '30
ROBIN, P.: Dangers and treatment of hypotrophy of lower jaw in infants. Odontologie *69:*499-505, July '31
ROBINSON, C. C.: Present status of burn therapy. J. Indiana M. A. *24:*652-656, Dec '31
ROBINSON, C. N.: Triple-dye-soap mixture in burn therapy. Lancet *2:*351-353, Sept 18, '43
ROBINSON, H. B. G. (see BURFORD, W. N. *et al*) July '44
ROBINSON, R. L. (see SKINNER, H. L.) April '43
ROBINSON, T. A. AND FOULDS, G. S.: Late results after operation for exstrophy of bladder. Brit. J. Surg. *14:*529-530, Jan '27
ROBINSON, T. A. (see FOULDS, G. S.) March '32
ROBINSON, W. H.: Simplified method of traction for finger fractures. Am. J. Surg. *8:*791-792, April '30
ROBISON, J. T.: Radical mastoid graft. Texas State J. Med. *29:*525-528, Dec '33
ROBITSHEK, E. C.: Tannic acid treatment of cutaneous burns. Journal-Lancet *50:*470-472, Oct 1, '30
ROBITSHEK, E. C.: Branchial fistulas; treatment with sclerosing fluids; case presentation and report. Minnesota Med. *16:*760-762, Dec '33
ROBSON, J. M. AND WALLACE, A. B.: Glycerinsulfonamide paste (euglamide, acetylsulfanilamide preparation) in burns. Brit. M. J. *1:*469-472, March 29, '41
ROBSON, L. C.: Perforated esophagus with burns. Brit. M. J. *1:*414, April 3, '43
ROCCA, E. D. (see CONTRERAS, M. V.) Mar '46
ROCCIA, B.: Spontaneous fractures of lower jaw; cases. Minerva med. (pt. 1) *9:*701-708, May 12, '29
ROCCIA, B.: Osteotome for resection of mandible. Minerva med. (pt. 2) *9:*700, Nov 3, '29
ROCCIA, B.: Therapy of temporomandibular ankylosis. Boll. e mem. Soc. piemontese di chir. *2:*502-518, April 30, '32
ROCCIA, B.: Therapy of mandibular fractures. Boll. e mem. Soc. piemontese di chir. *5:*1161-1176, '35
ROCCIA, B.: Hemiatrophy of face complicated by spontaneous fracture of jaw; case. Stomatol. *35:*448-458, July '37
ROCCIA, B.: Late surgical reduction of badly consolidated fracture of mandible by means of osteotomy. Boll. e mem. Soc. piemontese di chir. *8:*643-655, '38
ROCCIA, B.: Late surgical therapy of badly consolidated mandibular fracture by means of osteotomy. Stomatol. ital. *1:*197-204, March '39
ROCH: Acrocephalosyndactylia (Apert syndrome) in congenital syphilitic; case. Bull. et mem. Soc. med. d. hop. de Paris *49:*513-518, April 17, '33
ROCH, M.: Arachnodactylia, kyphoscoliosis, patent interventricular septum and ectopy of crystalline lens (Marfan syndrome); case. Presse med. *45:*1429-1430, Oct 9, '37
DA ROCHA, J.: New device for suturing skin. Dia med. *17:*77, Jan 22, '45
ROCHA AZEVEDO, L. G.: Burn therapy. An.

Cong. brasil. e am. cir. *3:*384–395, '42
DA ROCHA AZEVEDO, L. G.: Modern theories on burns. An. paulist. de med. e cir. *44:*277–297, Oct '42
DA ROCHA AZEVEDO, L. G.: Burn therapy in infants. Rev. paulista de med. *24:*87–91, Feb '44
DA ROCHA AZEVEDO, L. G.: New acquisitions in burn therapy. Rev. paulista de med. *25:*227–232, Oct '44
DA ROCHA AZEVEDO, L. G. (see DE MESQUITA SAMPAIO, J. A.) Jan '44
ROCHAT, G. F.: Formation of new upper eyelid from auricle. Nederl. Tijdschr. v. Geneesk. *2:*709, Aug 6, '27
ROCHAT, R. L.: Urethral fistula. Helvet. med. acta *4:*67–69, Feb '37
ROCHAT, R. L.: Possible influence of plastic surgery of breast on hypophysio-ovarian function. Schweiz. med. Wchnschr. *71:*1307–1308, Oct 25, '41
ROCHE, G. K. T.: Maxillofacial anesthesia at base hospital. Brit. J. Anaesth. *19:*141–160, July '45
ROCHE, G. K. T.: Anesthesia of recent injuries of jaw and face. Anesthesiology *7:*233–254, May '46
ROCHER: Perfect phonetic results of uranostaphylorrhaphy (Langenbeck-Trelat method). J. de med. de Bordeaux *109:*402–403, May 20, '32
ROCHER, C. (see ROCHER, H. L.) Nov '35
ROCHER, H. L.: Volkmann syndrome in obstetric fractures of humerus. Arch. franco-belges de chir. *32:*625–627, July '30
ROCHER, H. L.: Meningo-encephaloma of right nasofrontal region with malformation of nose and forehead; case. J. de med. de Bordeaux *107:*571–573, July 20, '30
ROCHER, H. L.: Atrophy of external ear with hemiatrophy of face and paresis of lower facial nerve; case. J. de med. de Bordeaux *108:*231, March 20, '31
ROCHER, H. L.: Syphilitic origin of perforation of palate and destruction of nose; uranoplasty; reconstruction of nose by tubular grafts with cartilaginous support of costal origin. Bull. et mem. Soc. de chir. de Bordeaux et du Sud-Ouest, pp. 150–152, '32
ROCHER, H. L.: Extensive cicatrix of face; reconstruction of both eyelids and of both lips by tubular grafts. Bull. et mem. Soc. de chir. de Bordeaux et du Sud-Ouest, pp. 154–156, '32
ROCHER, H. L.: Suture of ulnar nerve and reconstruction of brachial triceps tendon by grafting. Bull. et mem. Soc. de chir. de Bordeaux et du Sud-Ouest, pp. 247–254, '32
ROCHER, H. L.: Postpuerperal ankylosing polyarthritis; subluxation of atlas and axis; temporomaxillary and articulatory ankylosis; radiologic and etiologic study. Bull. et mem. Soc. med. et chir. de Bordeaux, pp 279–293, '32
ROCHER, H. L.: Suture of ulnar nerve and reconstruction of brachial triceps tendon by grafting. Bordeaux chir. *3:*133–136, April '32
ROCHER, H. L.: Reconstruction of lower jaw with tibial grafts. Bordeaux chir. *3:*272–277, July '32
ROCHER, H. L.: Extensive cicatrices of legs and feet due to burns; cicatricial pes talus; autoplasty and disarticulation of Chopart's joint of left foot; case. Rev. de chir. structive, pp. 111–114, June '37
ROCHER, H. L.: Absence of hand, two cases. J. de med. de Bordeaux *116:*115–117, July 22–29, '39
ROCHER, H.L.: Esthetic repair of face (after burn) by free grafts of skin; case. Bordeaux chir. *3–4:*98–100, July-Oct '44
ROCHER, H. L. AND FISCHER, H.: Unilateral and congenital agenesis of jaws; cases. J. de med. de Bordeaux *59:*611–621, July 30, '29
ROCHER, H. L. AND MALAPLATE: Acromioclavicular dislocation; osteosynthesis by kangaroo tendon; fracture of scapula and maxilla. J. de med. de Bordeaux *59:*145, Feb 20, '29
ROCHER, H. L. AND PESME, P.: Facial coloboma with complete, unilateral velopalatine fissure; case. J. de med. de Bordeaux *107:*763, Oct 10, '30
ROCHER, H. L. AND PESME, P.: Bilateral complicated harelip with bilateral palpebral coloboma and left iridic coloboma; total ectromelia of right upper extremity J. de med. de Bordeaux *121–122:*493–494, Oct '45
ROCHER, H. L. AND POUYANNE, L.: Avulsion of last 2 phalanges of forefinger and 15 cm. of 2 flexor tendons in child 7 years old; case. J. de med. de Bordeaux *115:*175–176, Aug 20–27, '38
ROCHER, H. L. AND ROCHER, C.: Bilateral congenital radial clubhand complicated in one case by luxation of elbow, in other by luxation of shoulder. J. de med. de Bordeaux *112:*880–882, Nov 30, '35
ROCHER, H. L. *et al:* Coloboma (Morian's second type) with extensive facial malformations; anatomic study of case in infant 6 months old. Ann. d'anat. path. *9:*487–498, May '32
ROCHETTE, M.: Wounds of lips; therapy. Hopital *27:*195–196, April '39
ROCHETTE, M.: Injuries to tongue and palate; therapy. Hopital *27:*281–282, May '39
ROCHETTE, M.: Therapy of wounds of face and

jaws at battalion or regiment first aid stations, in army corps field hospital and in evacuation hospital. Hopital *27:*521–527, Nov '39

Rochlin, D. G. and Simonson, S. G.: Congenital stiffness of digital joints. Fortschr. a. d. Geb. d. Rontgenstrahlen *46:*193–204, Aug '32

Rock, J. C. (see Cutler, G. C.) May '25

Rockey, E. W.: Repair of epispadias and exstrophy of bladder. S. Clin. N. Amer. *8:*1503–1509, Dec '28

Rockey, E. W.: Repair of severed tendons. S. Clin. North America *14:*1497–1499, Dec '34

Roddis, L. H.: Treatment of burns incident to war; Wellcome prize essay. Mil. Surgeon *94:*65–75, Feb '44

Rode, B.: Technic of making plaster of paris cast for nasal fractures and deformities. Ztschr. f. Hals-, Nasen-u. Ohrenh. *43:*294–295, '38

Roden, S.: Nonmalignant pharyngopalatal tumors and their surgical treatment. Acta chir. Scandinav. *91:*369–385, '44

Röden, S. H.: Tannic acid in burns; results from Maria Hospital and description of simplified quick method. Nord. med. tidskr. *16:*1188–1191, July 23, '38

Rodin, F. H.: Pedigree of four generations of hereditary congenital ptosis affecting only one eye and pedigree of one generation of congenital ptosis with epicanthus. Am. J. Ophth. *19:*597–599, July '36

Rodin, F. H. and Barkan, H.: Hereditary congenital eyelid ptosis; report of pedigree and review of literature. Am. J. Ophth. *18:*213–225, March '35

Rodino, D.: Modern therapy of burns. Riforma med. *60:*273–282, June 15 '46

Rodionov, F. I.: Artificial vagina formation by grafting tissue from small intestine. Vestnik khir. (nos. 37–38) *13:*342–345, '28

Rodriguez, R. (see Inclan, A.) July–Sept '38

Rodríguez, D. M. (see Alcaino, A.) Feb '31

Rodriguez Baz, L.: Shock in war medicine. Rev. med.-social san. y benef. munic. *2:*272–281, Oct-Dec '42

Rodríguez Berceruelo, S.: Development and present status of cosmetic surgery. Siglo med. *92:*436, Oct 21, '33

Rodrigues da Costa Doria, J.: Partial amputation as barbarous unusual crime; case. Brasil med. *60:*264–266, Aug 3–10, '46

Rodriguez Diaz, A.: Gibbous nose; plastic surgery. Rev. de cien. med. *2:*79–82, March '39

Rodriguez Lopez, M. B.: Construction of artificial vagina by Palazzo technic. Arch. ginec. y obst. *5:*7–18, Feb '46

Rodríguez de Mata: Ulcer of leg, resistant to therapy, cured by cutaneous autotransplant; case. Actas Soc. de cir. de Madrid *3:*53–56, Oct-Dec '33

Rodríguez de Mata: Traumatic ulcer of leg resisting all therapy, finally cured by autoplastic skin graft; case. Rev. espan. de cir. *16:*105–108, March-April '34

Rodriguez Molina, R. (see del Toro, J. *et al*) Sept '31

Rodriguez Segade: Emergency therapy of gunshot wounds of lower jaw. Med. espan. *6:*59–69, July '41

Rodríguez Villegas, R. and Brachetto-Brian, D.: Retraction of superficial palmar aponeurosis; case. Bol. y trab. de la Soc. de cir. de Buenos Aires *14:*809–821, Oct 29, '30

Rodriguez Villegas, R.: Cancer of lip. Semana med. *1:*398–403, March 1, '23 abstr: J.A.M.A. *81:*169, July 14, '23

Rodriguez Villegas, R. and Taullard, J. C.: Double lip; surgical therapy of case. Bol. y trab. de la Soc. de cir. de Buenos Aires *21:*45–48, April 14, '37

Rodriguez Villegas, R. and Taullard, J. C.: Recidivating temporomaxillary subluxation; surgical therapy of case. Bol. y trab. de la Soc. de cir. de Buenos Aires *21:*484–492, July 21, '37

Roedelius, E.: Malignant furuncle of lip. Klin. Wchnschr. *2:*2348–2353, Dec 24, '23 abstr: J.A.M.A. *82:*506, Feb 9, '24

Roedelius, E.: Treatment of malignant furuncle of lip. Dermat. Wchnschr. *78:*37–42, Jan 12, '24

Roedelius, E.: Gangrene of fingers after operation for Dupuytren's contracture. Zentralbl. f. Chir. *57:*936–939, April 12, '30

Roeder, C. A.: Virulent hand infections; treatment by prophylactic chemical and traumatic inflammation. J.A.M.A. *90:*1371–1373, April 28, '28

Roederer, C.: Arachnodactylia; case. Bull. Soc. de pediat. de Paris *35:*225–231, April '37

Roederer, J. (see: Pautrier, L. M.) May '38

Roffo, A. E.: Attempted plastic surgery in extirpation of breast cancer. Bol. Inst. de med. exper. para el estud. y trat. d. cancer *21:*163–179, April '44

Rogachevskiy, S. L.: New apparatus (heat tent) in burn therapy. Klin. med. (no. 7) *20:*91–92, '42

Roger, H.: Volkmann contracture; clinical and pathogenetic study. Marseille-med. *1:*213–228, Feb 15, '34

Roger, H.; Siméon, and Coulange: Friedreich's disease with club-hand in hereditary syphilitic; case. Gaz. d. hop. *101:*501–504, April 4, '28

Rogers, C. S. (see Bancroft, F. W.) July '26

Rogers, C. S. (see Bancroft, F. W.) 1927

Rogers, C. S. (see Bancroft F. W.) May '28

Rogers, L.: Maldevelopment of wrist and hand.

Edinburgh M. J. *32:*407-409, Aug '25
ROGERS, L.: Hand infections. and injuries. J. Roy. Nav. M. Serv. *22:*2-6, Jan '36
ROGERS, L.: Amputation of fingers. J. Roy. Nav. M. Serv. *27:*137-141, April '41
ROGERS, L.; HALL, C. T. AND SHACKELFORD, J. H.: Fractures and incomplete dislocations of jaws. Radiology *18:*28-40, Jan '32
ROGERS, S. P. AND ESPINOSA ROBLEDO, M.: Therapy of section of tendons of hand in industrial accidents; 50 cases. Cir. ortop. y traumatol. *3:*177-181, July-Sept '35
ROGERS, W. L.; COHEN, T. M. AND GOLDBERG, R. R.: Value of sulfonated oils (for cleansing) in treatment of burns and other denuded surfaces. U. S. Nav. M. Bull. *42:*1125-1128, May '44
ROHDE, C.: Attempts to overcome difficulties in healing of homoplastic transplants. Beitr. z. klin. Chir. *134:*111-127, '25
ROHLICH, K.: Formation of blood cells in devitalized bone transplants. Ztschr. f. mikr.-anat. Forsch. *49:*616-625, '41
RÖHLICH, K.: Formation of new bone substance in devitalized bone transplants. Ztschr. f. mikr.-anat. Forsch. *50:*132-145, '41
ROIG, A. (see JACQUES, P.) April '28
ROJAS, N.: Medical responsibility in practice of cosmetic surgery. Rev. de especialid. *4:*520-527, July '29
ROJO, J. J. (see CORNILLON, A.) Dec '42
ROLLIN, H.: Surgical correction of saddle nose. Hals-, Nasen-u. Ohrenarzt (Teil 1) *28:*97-100, April '37
ROLLO, S.: Homotransplantation and heterotransplantation in man with reference to blood groups. Riforma med. *47:*1190-1192, Aug 3, '31
ROLOFF, F.: Operation for exstrophy of bladder. Zentralbl. f. Chir. *51:*2432-2433, Nov 1, '24
ROLOFF, F.: Remote results of Maydl's operation for exstrophy. Zentralbl. f. Chir. *57:*1977-1979, Aug 9, '30
ROMAGNA MANOIA, A.: Acrocephalosyndactylia; case. Riv. di antropol. *28:*165-188, '28-'29
ROMAN, C. L.: Severe industrial injuries to fingers and their treatment. Canad. M. A. J. *13:*633-635, Sept '23
DE ROMANA, J.: Os purum as biologic element of internal prosthesis. Dia med. (Ed. espec.), no. 2, pp. 19-20, April '39
ROMANI, A.: Traumatic lesions of hand. Arch. ital. di chir. *22:*1-39, '28

Romanum, S.

Artificial vagina formation from large intestine (S. Romanum). MARCHENKO, E. Mosk. med. j. (no. 2) *8:*61-65, '28

ROMBACH, K. A.: Subcutaneous rupture of tendon in finger injuries. Nederl. tijdschr. v. geneesk. *77:*2938-2939, June 24, '33
ROMBACH, K. A.: Treatment of fractures of fingers. Nederl. tijdschr. v. geneesk. *79:*1112-1113, March 16, '35
ROMENCE, H. (see HARKINS, H. N. *et al*) Oct '42
ROMENCE, H. (see MC CLURE, R. D. *et al*) 1944
ROMENCE, H. (see MC CLURE, R. D. *et al*) Sept '44
ROMENCE, H. L. (see HARTMAN, F. W.) Sept '43
RÖMER, H.: Web fingers. Deutsche Ztschr. f. Chir. *174:*1-9, '22 (illus.) abstr: J.A.M.A. *79:*2124, Dec 16, '22
ROMERO ALVAREZ, A. M.: Plasma therapy in burns. Semana med. *1:*1117-1129, June 1, '44
ROMERO ALVAREZ, A. M.: Early massive plasma therapy in burns of children; preliminary report. Dia med. *17:*309-313, April 9, '45
ROMITI, C.: Surgical treatment of elephantiasis of lower extremities. Arch. ital. di chir. *20:*607-640, '28
ROMITI, C.: Surgical treatment of trophic ulcers of leg and foot; autoplastic operation by Italian method, periarterial sympathectomy, lumbar sympathetic ganglionectomy and ramisection. Tr. Roy. Soc. Trop. Med. and Hyg. *27:*185-194, July '33
ROMMEL, R. W.: Simple device for temporary support of fractured mandible. U. S. Nav. M. Bull. *40:*977, Oct '42
RONCHESE, F.: Duodenal ulcers in case of grave burns. Riforma med. *40:*753-755, Aug 11, '24 abstr: J.A.M.A. *83:*1038, Sept 27, '24
RONCORONI, E. J. AND CICCHETTI, J. N.: Adamantinoma of lower jaw; surgical therapy with immediate prosthesis; case. Bol. Soc. de cir. de Rosario *12:*27-40, May '45
RONKA, E. K. F.: Solid double rudimentary uterus with absence of cervix and vagina. New England J. Med. *207:*945-946, Nov 24, '32
RONNEAUX, G. AND BRUNEL: Congenital variations in number of fingers. Bull. et mem. Soc. de radiol. med. de France *21:*712-718, Nov '33
ROOF, C. S.: Surgical shock. Rocky Mountain M. J. *41:*100-103, Feb '44
ROOKE, C. J. (see BROOKE, R.) Dec '39
ROOME, N. W. (see HARKINS, H. N.) July '37
ROOME, N. W. (see WILSON, H.) Nov '33
ROONEY, J. C.: Symposium on industrial medicine in wartime – widening field of industrial medicine; treatment of burns. California and West. Med. *62:*23-24, Jan '45
ROOS, J.: Liquefaction of fatty tissue and softening of scars; experimental studies on action of pepsin. Zentralbl. f. Chir. *53:*2136-2144, Aug 21, '26

ROOS, W.: Wire grating chin cap in military surgery of jaw fractures. Schweiz. med. Wchnschr. *70:*770, Aug 10, '40

ROOS, W.: Wire screen chin cap; suggestion for first aid for jaw injuries in field. Schweiz. med. Wchnschr. *71:*719–720, June 7, '41

ROOST, F. H.: Modified nasal septal resection. J. Iowa M. Soc. *18:*432–434, Nov '28

ROOT, G. T.: Brief review of etiology of shock. Proc. Staff Meet., Mayo Clin. *17:*218–221, April 8, '42

ROOT, H. F.: Thermal burns in diabetes mellitus. New England J. Med. *232:*279, March 8, '45

RÖPER, W.: Use of small skin grafts for treating recent injuries of nail bed. Zentralbl. f. Chir. *64:*2679–2681, Nov 20, '37

ROQUES, P.: Facial paralysis from gunshot wound caused by attempted suicide; therapy by resection of superior cervical sympathetic ganglion and suspension of corners of mouth. Bull. et mem. Soc. nat. de chir. *60:*981–984, July 21, '34

ROQUES, P. AND SOHIER, H.: Subcutaneous rupture of tendon of extensor pollicis longus; case. Rev. d'orthop. *26:*230–235, May '39

ROQUES-SATIVO, R.: Dysplasias of external ear. Rev. de laryng. *57:*304–371, March '36

DE ROSA, G.: Surgical treatment of senile ectropion. Arch. di ottal. *34:*15–19, Jan '27

ROSATI, L. M. (see KELLY, R. P. *et al*) 1946

ROSATI, L. M. (see KELLY, R. P. *et al*) April '46

ROSE, B.; WEIL, P. G. AND BROWNE, J. S. L.: Use of concentrated pooled human serum and pooled lyophile serum in shock therapy. Canad. M. A. J. *44:*442–448, May '41

ROSE, B. (see WEIL, P. G. *et al*) July '40

ROSE, H. W.: Initial cold water treatment of burns. Northwest Med. *35:*267–270, July '36

ROSE, H. W.: Severe burns complicated by appendicitis. Northwest Med. *36:*113–114, April '37

ROSE, J. E.: Differential diagnosis of certain types of facial deformities and their treatment (including jaws). Internat. J. Orthodontia *20:*222–228, March '34

ROSE, T. F.: Bilateral trigger thumb in infants. M. J. Australia *1:*18–20, Jan 5, '46

ROSENDALE, R. S.: Anatomic and physiologic principles underlying plastic surgery of nasal deformities. Ohio State M. J. *41:*724–728, Aug '45

ROSEDALE, R. S. (see STREICHER, C. J.) Jan '44

ROSENAK, I.: New method for determining plane of operation in elephantiasis, especially of extremities. Zentralbl. f. Chir. *56:*912–914, April 13, '29

ROSENAK, I.: Imperforate anus, plastic repair. Zentralbl. f. Chir. *63:*2235–2238, Sept 19, '36

ROSENÁK, STEFON (ISTVON) see ROSENAK, I.

ROSENAK, STEPHAN (ISTVAN) see ROSENAK, I.

ROSENAUER, F.: Branchiogenic anomalies (cysts and fistulas) associated with larynx. Deutsche Ztschr. f. Chir. *226:*304–307, '30

ROSENBAUM, W.: Sclerosing treatment (using sylnasol, fatty acid solution) for subluxation of temporomandibular joint. Am. J. Orthodontics *32:*551–571, Oct '46

ROSENBERG, N.: Detergents; use in cleansing and local treatment of burns. Surgery *13:*385–393, March '43

ROSENBERG, W. A. AND SMITH, E. M. JR.: Removal of superfluous hair with cutting current. Arch. Phys. Therapy *24:*277–279, May '43

ROSENBERGER, H. C.: Fissural cyst of nose (facial cleft). Arch. Otolaryng. *40:*288–290, Oct '44

ROSENBLATT, M. S. AND MAY, A.: Malformation of anus and rectum. Surg., Gynec. and Obst. *83:*499–506, Oct '46

ROSENBLATT, S.: Gynecomastia; pathogenesis and therapy. Dia med. *15:*1147–1149, Oct 4, '43

ROSENBURG, S.: Fascia lata transplant in eyelid ptosis. Am. J. Surg. *47:*142–148, Jan '40

ROSENHECK, C.: Facial palsies and their management. M. J. and Rec. *129:*266–269, March 6, '29

ROSENQVIST, H.: Organization for treatment of burns; important aspect of preparedness. Nord. med. *25:*419–423, March 9, '45

ROSENSTEIN: Artificial vagina from intestine; 2 cases. Monatschr. f. Geburtsh. u. Gynak. *58:*176–183, July '22 abstr: J.A.M.A. *79:*1372, Oct 14, '22

ROSENSTEIN, P.: Method for plastic construction of a urethra in penoscrotal hypospadias by means of flap of mucosa of bladder. Ztschr. f. Urol. *23:*627–637, '29

ROSENSTEIN, P.: Hypospadias, cure by transplantation of bladder mucosa; 2 cases. Zentralbl. f. Chir. *58:*1874–1880, July 25, '31

Rosenthal

Plastic operations on hard palate; comment on Rosenthal's article. ERNST, F. Zentralbl. f. chir. *52:*464–470, Feb 28, '25

ROSENTHAL: Artificial vagina made from small intestine. Zentralbl. f. Gynak. *46:*1102–1104, July 8, '22

ROSENTHAL. (see GRIMAUD, *et al*) July '33

ROSENTHAL, M.: Hemangioma of nose. Laryngoscope *35:*54, Jan '25

ROSENTHAL, P. (see PAUCHET, V. *et al*) Dec '33
ROSENTHAL, S. (see MARSHALL, W.) Dec '43
ROSENTHAL, S. M.: Experimental chemotherapy of burns; effects of local therapy upon mortality from shock. Pub. Health Rep. *57:*1923–1935, Dec 18, '42
ROSENTHAL, S. M.: Experimental chemotherapy of burns and shock; effects of systemic therapy on early mortality. Pub. Health Rep. *58:*513–522, March 26, '43
ROSENTHAL, S. M. AND TABOR, H.: Electrolyte changes and chemotherapy in experimental burn and traumatic shock and hemorrhage (use of isotonic sodium chloride solution). Arch. Surg. *51:*244–252, Nov-Dec, '45
ROSENTHAL, W.: Plastic operations on hard palate. Zentralbl. f. Chir. *51:*1621–1627, July 26, '24
ROSENTHAL, W.: New plastic operation for chronic cases of contracture of jaws. Vrtljschr. f. Zahnh. *42:*499–507, '26
ROSENTHAL, W.: Reconstructive surgery of jaw necrosis, and after excision. Arch. f. klin. Chir. *147:*248–284, '27
ROSENTHAL, W.: Pathology and therapy of cleft palate. Fortschr. d. Zahnheilk. *5:*1044–1054, Nov '29
ROSENTHAL, W.: Pathology and therapy of cleft palate and harelip. Fortschr. d. Zahnh. *6:*953–972, Nov '30
ROSENTHAL, W.: Facial paralysis; causes; treatment by neurosurgery (muscular neurotization). Deutsche Ztschr. f. Chir. *223:*261–270, '30
ROSENTHAL, W.: Pathology and therapy of cleft palates. Fortschr. d. Zahnh. *7:*989–1016, Nov '31
ROSENTHAL, W.: Modern therapy of cleft palate. Ztschr. f. Stomatol. *30:*530–540, '32
ROSENTHAL, W.: Surgery of fetal clefts (harelip, cleft palate, etc.); review of literature. Zentralbl. f. Chir. *59:*2345–2379, Sept 24, '32

Rosenthal Operation (See also Lexer-Rosenthal Operation; Schonborn-Rosenthal Operation)

Staphylopharyngoplasty by Rosenthal's method. HARBITZ, H. F. Norsk. Mag. f. Laegevidensk. *90:*13–16, Jan '29

ROSGEN AND MAMIER: Question of physical deformities, especially clubhand; special case of amniotic stricture. Ztschr. f. Orthop. *74:*45–52, '42
ROSHCHIN, V. P.: Biomicroscopic picture of healing of "normal" Denig transplant (lip mucosa). Vestnik oftal. *16:*333–336, '40
ROSITO, E. (see SANTAS, A. A. *et al*) Aug '42
ROSNER, S.: Results of therapy of keloids obtained at Instituto de Medicina Experimental in Buenos Aires. Bol. Inst. de med. exper. para el estud. y trat. del cancer *7:*1375–1381, Dec '30
ROSS, A. M. Treatment of nasal obstruction in adults. M. Press. *207:*112–114, Feb 18, '42
ROSS, F. P. (see BRANCH, C.D. *et al*) Apr '46
ROSS, J. A. AND HULBERT, K. F.: Silver nitrate, tannic acid and gentian violet in burn therapy. Brit. M. J. *2:*702–703, Nov 23, '40
ROSS, J. A. AND HULBERT, K. F.: Treatment of 100 war wounds and burns. Brit. M. J. *1:*618–621, April 26, '41
ROSS, J. C.: Elephantiasis of penis. Brit. J. Surg. *29:*194–196, Oct '41
ROSS, J. P.: Prognosis of hand infections. St. Barth. Hosp. J. *45:*269–270, Aug '38
ROSS, N.: Congenital epicanthus and ptosis of eyelid transmitted through 4 generations. Brit. M. J. *1:*378–379, Feb 27, '32
ROSS, R. A.: Hand infections. M. J. South Africa *20:*84–96, Nov '24 also: South African M. Rec. *23:*245–257, June 27, '25
ROSSANO, I.: Origin of cysts, fistulas and tumors of lateral region of neck. Rev. de path. comparee *32:*951, Sept; 1127, Oct '32
ROSSANO, I.: Origin of cysts, fistulas and tumors of lateral region of neck. Rev. de path. comparee *32:*1269–1307, Nov '32
ROSSELLI, D. Skin transplantation with tubular flap. Pathologica *34:*209–225, July '42
ROSSELLO, H. J. AND BENATTI, D.: Traumatic abdominal shock. An. de Fac. de med., Montevideo *11:*295–302, May '26 abstr: J.A.M.A. *87:*2131, Dec 18, '26
ROSSI, D.: Cysts of skin graft into rectovaginal septum; case. Clin. ostet. *38:*464–470, Sept '36
ROSSITER, R. J.: Plasma loss in burns (review of literature, prepared on behalf of Burns Sub-Committee, M. R. C. War Wounds Committee). Bull. War Med. *4:*181–189, Dec '43
ROSSITER, R. J. AND PETERS, R. A.: Controlled external pressure and edema formation in burns. Lancet *1:*9–11, Jan 1, '44
ROSSITER, R. J. (see BARNES, J. M.) Aug '43
ROSSITER, R. J. (see CLARK, E. J.) March '44
ROST, F. (see BLESSING, G.) April '25
ROST, G. A. AND UHLMANN, E.: Therapy of late injuries of skin with ointment containing radium emanations. Deutsche med. Wchnschr. *58:*655–656, April 22, '32
ROSTA, G.: Otitis media and cerebellar abscess developing after burns. Budapesti orvosi ujsag *36:*902–904, Oct 20, '38
ROSTENBERG, A.: Epilation with diathermy; preliminary report. M. J. and Rec. *121:*751, June 17, '25

ROSTOCK, P.: Burn therapy. Fortschr. d. Therap. *4:*386–388, June 25, '28

ROSTOCK, P.: Nasal fractures and their therapy. Med. Welt *13:*953–954, July 8, '39

ROTH, E.: Method of nasal packing following submucous resection which allows free nasal respiration. Arch. Otolaryng. *13:*732, May '31

ROTH, R. B. AND WARREN, K. W.: Traumatic avulsion of skin of penis and scrotum. J. Urol. *52:*162–168, Aug '44

ROTHMAN, M.; TAMERIN, J. AND BULLOWA, J. G. M.: Burn therapy with 2.5 per cent sulfadiazine (sulfanilamide derivative) in 8 per cent triethanolamine solution. J.A.M.A. *120:*803–805, Nov 14, '42

ROUDIL, G. AND ASSALI, J.: Velopalatine fissure; result of staphylorrhaphy in case. Marseille-med. *1:*37–38, Jan 5, '35

ROUDIL, G.; DREVON, AND MOURGUES: Bilateral congenital dysmorphosis of wrists (Madelung's disease); roentgen study of case. J. de radiol. et d'electrol. *20:*241–245, April '36

ROUDINESCO, MME.: Acrocephalosyndactyly; case. Bull. et mem. Soc. med. d. hop. de Paris *56:*624–627, Nov 25, '40

Rouge-Denker operation

Angiomatous tumor of nasal fossae; ligature of external carotid and Rouge-Denker operation; case. PIQUET, J. AND BECUWE. Ann. d'oto-laryng., pp. 393–397, May '37

DE ROUGEMONT, J.: Treatment of hand infections. Presse med. *39:*1088, July 18, '31

DE ROUGEMONT, J.: Lateral luxation of portion of extensor tendon of finger. Presse med. *47:*1197, Aug 2, '39

DE ROUGEMONT, J. AND CARCASSONNE, F.: Regional anesthesia with solution of procaine hydrochloride and epinephrine in surgery of fingers. Presse med. *41:*218–220, Feb 8, '33

DE ROUGEMONT, J. (see POLLOSSON) March-April '31

DE ROUGEMONT, J. (see TIXIER, L. *et al*) Nov-Dec '31

ROUHIER, G.: Restoration of sectioned or destroyed nerves, with special reference to grafting. Mem. Acad. de chir *72:*170–174, Mar 20–Apr 3, '46

ROULHAC, G. E. (see SCHWARTZ, H. G.) Jan '46

ROULSTON, T. J.: Closed-plaster burn treatment. Brit. M. J. *2:*611–613, Nov 1, '41

ROUND, H. (see BILLINGTON, W.) Jan '26

ROUND, H. (see BILLINGTON, W.) March '30

ROUND, H. (see BILLINGTON, W.) May '30

ROUND, H. (see MANSIE, J. W. *et al*) July '43

ROUNTREE, C. R.: Luxated and severed tendons. Am. J. Surg. *50:*516–518, Dec '40

ROUS, P.: Relative reaction within mammalian tissues; factors determining reaction of skin grafts; study by indicator method of conditions within ischemic tissue. J. Exper. Med. *44:*815–834, Dec '26

ROUS, P.: Activation of skin grafts. J. Exper. Med. *83:*383–400, May '46

ROUSSEAU-DECELLE, L.: Osteomyelitis of jaws; cure; case. Rev. de stomatol. *33:*86–94, Feb '31

ROUSSEL, J. M. (see CAUSSADE, L. *et al*) March '38

ROUSSET, J. (see LACASSAGNE, J.) July '35

ROUSSET, J. (see NICOLAS, J.) July '35

ROUSSY, SORTON, AND PERROT: Epithelioma of forearm developed upon scar of ancient burn. Bull. de l'Assoc. franc. p. l'etude du cancer *16:*504–509, June '27

ROUSSY, G.; HUGUENIN, R. AND SARACINO, R.: Clinical problems of tumors of skin. Presse med. *50:*193–196, Feb 24, '42

ROUTIER: Retraction of palmar aponeurosis; therapy; case. Bull. et mem. Soc. nat. de chir. *57:*1467, Dec 5, '31

ROUVILLOIS, H.: Treatment of traumatic deformity of hand. Bull. Acad. de med., Par. *92:*1094–1097, Nov 4, '24 abstr: J.A.M.A. *83:*2050, Dec 20, '24

ROUVILLOIS, H.: Bone grafting in pseudoarthrosis of lower jaw. Paris med. *2:*237–245, Sept 26, '25 abstr: J.A.M.A. *85:*1433, Oct 31, '25

ROUVILLOIS, H.: Therapy of pseudoarthrosis with loss of substance of inferior maxilla. Arch. ital. di chir. *54:*351–356, '38

ROUX, C.: Ectopia vesicae. Beitr. z. klin. Chir. *142:*482–489, '28

ROUX-BERGER, J. L.: Surgical treatment of invasion of cervical glands in lingual cancer. Presse med. *35:*881, July 13, '27

ROUX-BERGER, J. L.: Whole skin grafted on dura mater in case of cancer of parietal bone. Bull. et mem. Soc. nat. de chir. *53:*1305–1308, Dec 3, '27

ROUX-BERGER, J. L. AND MONOD, O.: Experience in treatment of epitheliomata of tongue with glandular involvement. Bull. et mem. Soc. nat. de chir. *53:*648–659, May 14, '27

ROUZAUD, M. (see GUILLAIN, G. *et al*) Jan-Feb '42

ROVENSTINE, E. A. (see FOSTER, A. D. JR. *et al*) May '45

ROVENSTINE, E. A. (see PAPPER, E. M.) July '46

ROVIDA, F.: Roentgen ray findings in case of acrocephaly with syndactylia. Gazz. med. lomb. *87:*49–56, April 10, '28

ROVIRALTA, E.: Surgical therapy of cleft palate must be performed before child begins to talk. Ars med., Barcelona *7:*395–398, Dec '31

ROVIRALTA, E.: New apparatus for wire skeletal traction used in therapy of fractures, burns and traumas. But. Soc. catalana de pediat. *6:*233–237, July-Aug '33

ROVIRALTA, E.: Correction of phonetic disorders in cleft palate lacking timely surgical therapy. Rev. clin. espan. *4:*48–49, Jan 15, '42

ROWBOTHAM, S. (see THORNTON, H. L.) Nov '45

ROWBOTHAM, S. E. (see COLE, P. P. *et al*) May '30

ROWE, A. T. (see KAZANJIAN, V. H. *et al*) Oct '32

ROWHANAVONGSE, S. (see CONGDON, E. D. *et al*) Nov '32

ROWLAND, W. D. (see WEBSTER, G. V.) Aug '46

ROWLANDS, J. S.: New method of obtaining autogenous fascial grafts without extensive incision. Practitioner *119:*321–326, Nov '27

ROWLETTE, A. P. (see WEINER, D. O. *et al*) May '36

ROY (see GINESTET, G. *et al*) July '39

ROY (see HOCHE, L.) May '32

ROY, F.: Therapy of harelip and cleft palate. Laval med. *5:*197–201, May '40

ROY, J. N.: Plastic operations on face by means of fat grafts. Laryngoscope *31:*65, Feb '21

ROY, J. N.: Idiopathic perforation of nasal septum; autoplasty with pedunculated flap of mucous membrane; cure. Ann. Otol., Rhin. and Laryng. *32:*554–560, June '23

ROY, J. N.: Method of choice for correction of saddle nose. Arch. Otolaryng. *5:*258–268, March '27

ROY, J. N.: Method of choice for correction of saddle nose. Union med. du Canada *56:*156–169, March '27 also: Surg., Gynec. and Obst. *45:*88–92, July '27

ROY, J. N.: Best method of correction of snubnose. Arch. internat. de laryng. *34:*166–178, Feb '28

ROY, J. N.: Loss of substance in nostril; rhinoplasty with skin graft; case. Ann. d. mal. de l'oreille, du larynx *47:*571–576, June '28 also: Union med. du Canada *57:*505–510, Sept '28

ROY, J. N.: Traumatic loss of substance of nostril; rhinoplasty with dermo-epidermic graft. Arch. Otolaryng. *7:*601–605, June '28 also: J. Laryng. and Otol. *43:*490–495, July '28

ROY, J. N.: Plastic operation with costal cartilage in concave nose; cases. Union med du Canada *58:*408–414, July '29

ROY, J. N.: Method of choice for correction of hump nose. Canad. M. A. J. *22:*803–807, June '30

ROY, J. N.: Method of choice for correction of hump nose. J. Laryng. and Otol. *45:*398–408, June '30 also: Union med. du Canada *59:*329–339, June '30 also: Bull. med. de Quebec *31:*207–219, June '30 also: Arch. Otolaryng. *12:*484–492, Oct '30

ROY, J. N.: Choice of operative technic for convex nose; case. Ann. d'oto-laryng., pp. 155–162, Feb '31

ROY, J. N.: Peripheral facial paralysis following frostbite; case. Union med. du Canada *60:*223–229, April '31

ROY, J. N.: Plastic surgery in cicatrices of eyelid caused by burn; case. Bull. med. de Quebec *32:*322–328, Oct '31

ROY, J. N.: Cases of rhinoplasty. Union med. du Canada *64:*644–658, June '35 also: Canad. M. A. J. *33:*158–160, Aug '35

ROY, J. N.: Tip of nose completely severed and sutured 3 hours after accident. J. Laryng. and Otol. *50:*518–520, July '35 also: Union med. du Canada *64:*847–852, Aug '35 also: Ann. Otol., Rhin. and Laryng. *44:*893–898, Sept '35

ROY, J. N.: Tip of nose completely sectioned and sutured 3 hours after accident; recovery. Rev. de chir. structive, pp. 211–217, March '36

ROY, J. N.: Plastic surgery from point of view of mental hygiene (face). Rev. san. mil., Bucuresti *35:*1070–1076, Oct '36

ROY, J. N.: New method of rhinoplasty for sinking tip of nose. Rev. de chir. structive, pp. 441–446, Dec '36 also: Ann. Otol., Rhin. and Laryng. *46:*203–207, March '37 also: Union med. du Canada *66:*266–270, March '37 also: Canad. M. A. J. *36:*603–605, June '37

ROY, J. N.: Pilous verrucous pigmentary nevus of nose; autoplasty using Thiersch graft. Union med. du Canada *66:*945–948, Sept '37

ROY, J. N.: Pigmentary verrucous pilose nasal nevus; autoplasty by means of Thiersch graft; case. Rev. de chir. structive, pp. 180–184, Oct '37

ROY, J. N.: Pilous verrucous pigmented nevus of nose; autoplasty using Thiersch graft; case. Rev. argent. de oto-rhino-laring. *7:*53–57, March-April '38

ROY, J. N.: Cicatricial ectropion of upper eyelid and contracture of lower lip following burn; blepharoplasty and labioplasty; case. Rev. de chir. structive *8:*85–90, Aug '38

ROY, L. P. (see VEZINA, C. *et al*) June '38

ROYER AND BARBIZET: Shock; medical treatment and surgical intervention in war wounded. Mem. Acad. de chir. *71:*334–335, July 4–11, '45

Royer, A. (see Bisson, C.) 1946

Royle, N. D.: Living suture in tendon transplantation. M. J. Australia *1:*333–334, April 5, '24

Royle, N. D.: Original technique in transplantation of tendons. J. Coll. Surgeons, Australasia *1:*115–119, July '28

Royle, N. D.: Operation for thenar paralysis. M. J. Australia *2:*155–156, Aug 1, '36

Royle, N. D.: Operation for paralysis of intrinsic muscles of thumb. J.A.M.A. *111:*612–613, Aug 13, '38

Royster, H. P. (see Cook, T. J. *et al*) Oct '45

Rozentsveyg, M. G.: Experimental studies on transplantation of conjunctiva from eye of cadaver; preliminary report. Vestnik oftal. *11:*311-316, '37

Rozentsveyg, M. G.: Transplantation of conjunctiva from cadaver. Vestnik oftal. (nos. 2–3) *14:*26–36, '39

Rozhanskiy, V. I.: Treatment of minor hand injuries. Khirurgiya, no. 3, pp. 53–59, '37

Rozov, V. I.: Instruments for restoration of severed flexor tendons of fingers according to Bunnell method. Sovet. khir. (nos. 3–4) *6:*458–461, '34

Rozov, V. I.: Open fractures of fingers and their treatment. Sovet. khir., no. 7, pp. 119–122, '36

Rozov, V. I.: Injuries of extensor tendons of fingers and their therapy. Vestnik khir. *54:*95–105, '37

Rozov, V. I.: Splint for therapy of lesions of extension tendons of fingers. Ortop. i. travmatol. (no. 2) *11:*98–100, '37

Rozov, V. I.: Primary and secondary suture of flexor tendons of wrist and fingers. Novy khir. arkhiv *41:*490–504, '38

Rua, L. and Venturino, H.: Local and general therapy of grave burns; authors' experience. Dia med. *15:*356–363, April 19, '43

Ruata, G.: Coagulant medications in burns. Rassegna di med. indust. *11:*213–220, April '40

Rubaltelli, E.: Congenital fistula of lower lip; embryologic and hereditary factors in pathogenesis of rare congenital abnormalities of face; operative treatment; cases. Arch. ital. di otol. *41:*141–154, April '30

Rubaschewa, A. and Priwes, M. G.: Vascularization of long bones by autotransplantation. Beitr. z. klin. Chir. *156:*299–312, '32

Rubashev, S. M.: Treatment of traumatic avulsion of skin. Vestnik khir. *47:*87–88, '36

Rubashev, S. M.: History of burns in connection with Fabricius Hildanus' book published in 1610. Vestnik khir. *56:*876–880, Dec '38

Rubbreciit, R.: Technic and indications of dacryocystorhinostomy. Bull. Soc. belge d'opht., no. 57, pp. 94–106, '28

Rubens, E.: Hereditary cleidocranial dysostosis with features of ocular hypertelorism; 2 cases. Arch. Pediat. *56:*771–780, Dec '39

Rubenstein, A. D.; Tabershaw, I. R. and Daniels, J.: Pseudo-gas gangrene of hand (role of magnesium). J.A.M.A. *129:*659-662, Nov 3, '45

Rubenstein, B. (see Miller, T.) Jan '32

Rubenstein, B. (see Miller, T.) April '32

Ruberg, G. (see Derra, E.) June '38

Rubi, R. A. (see Grimaldi, F. E.) June '34

Rubin, L. R.: Simplification of split skin grafts; gum acacia technic. M. Bull. North African Theat. Op. (no. 6) *1:*14–15, June '44

Rubin, L. R.: Simplification of split grafting; gum acacia technic. Am. J. Surg. *70:*302–307, Dec '45

Rubin, L. R.: Contiguous skin flaps for wounds of extremities. Am. J. Surg. *71:*36–54, Jan '46

Rubin, L. R.: Repair of avulsion wounds by flap graft technic. Am. J. Surg. *72:*373–384, Sept '46

Rubinrot, S.: Therapy of cancer of lower lip. Nowotwory *7:*240–244, '32

Rubinshteyn, A. Y.: Structure of carpal bones in connection with problem of reconstructive operations. Khirurgiya, no. 6, pp. 68–72, '44

Rubritius, H.: When should hypospadias be operated on? Chirurg *6:*402–403, June 1, '34

Ruckensteiner, E.: Roentgenographic examination of midcervical fistula. Fortschr. a. d. Geb. d. Rontgenstrahlen *54:*321-325, Sept '36

Rudanovskaya, V. A. and Struchkov, V. I.: Chemical burns. Novy khir. arkhiv *38:*471–475, '37

Rudaux, P. (see Garcin, R. *et al*) Nov '32

Rudaux, P. (see Garcin, R. *et al*) June '33

Ruddy, L. W.: Transpalatine operation for congenital atresia of choanae in small child or infant. Arch. Otolaryng. *41:*432–438, June '45

Rudert, H.: Method of plastic surgery in correction of unilateral arrhynia; case. Arch. f. Ohren-, Nasen-u. Kehlkopfh. *150:*168–174, '41

Rudler, J. C.: Modern therapy of superficial burns in medical practice. Bull med., Paris *49:*343-347, May 18, '35

Rudler, J. C.: Mechanism of death following burns. Bull. med., Paris *52:*765-767, Oct 22, '38

Rudler, J. C.: General accidents and treatment (burns). Presse med. *47:*1366–1368, Sept 27, '39

Rudofsky, F.: Treatment of chronically recurring paronychias and related ungual diseases by excision and by Thiersch grafts. Med. Klin. *30:*198, Feb 9, '34

Rudolf, A.: Formation of artificial vagina and bladder from sigmoid. Beitr. z. klin. Chir. *153:*103-109, '31

RUDOLPH, C. E. AND NORVOLD, R. W.: Congenital partial hemihypertrophy involving marked malocclusion. J. Dent. Research *23:*133–139, April '44

RUEDA, P.: Angiomatous nevus; cases in infants. Rev. Soc. pediat. d. litoral *9:*139–142, May-Aug '44

RUEDA MAGRO, G.: Congenital anorectal imperforation; case. Rev. med. veracruzana *15:*1544–1546, July 1, '35

RUEDEMANN, A. D.: Immediate treatment of eye injuries including burns. S. Clin. North America *16:*979–989, Aug '36

RUEDEMANN, A. D.: Surgical treatment of eyelid ptosis. S. Clin. North America *17:*1503–1509, Oct '37

RÜEDI, G.: Fracture of condyle of mandible. Schweiz. Monatschr. f. Zahnh. *38:*727, Nov; 805, Dec '28

RUEDI, J. AND MINDER, W.: Therapy of malignant tumors of mouth at Bern. Pract. oto-rhino-laryng. *6:*113–114, '44

RUEDI, L.: Restorative surgery of the larynx. Pract. oto-rhino-laryng. *7:*186–197, '45

RÜEDI, L. (see NAGER, F.R.) Jan-Dec '31

RUEF, H.: Subcutaneous skin transplants. Arch. f. klin. Chir. *125:*366–377, '23 (illus.) abstr: J.A.M.A. *81:*1322, Oct 13, '23

RUEF, H.: To improve outcome of suture of tendon in hand. Arch. f. klin. Chir. *130:*757–762, '24 abstr: J.A.M.A. *83:*1379, Oct 25, '24

RUEF, H.: Free cartilage grafts. (Nasal deformities.) Med. Klinik *20:*1428–1429, Oct 12, '24 abstr: J.A.M.A. *83:*1722, Nov 22, '24

RUGE, E.: Construction of artificial vagina from sigmoid flexure in case of congenital aplasia. Monatschr. f. Geburtsh. u. Gynak. *78:*313–326, March '28

RUGE, E.: Artificial vagina formation from sigmoid flexure. Zentralbl. f. Chir. *56:*2958, Nov 23, '29

Ruge Operation

Plastic replacement of vagina with portion of sigmoid flexure (Ruge operation) after Wertheim operation for total extirpation; case. BALKOW, E. Deutsche med. Wchnschr. *62:*586–588, April 10, '36

RUGH, J. T.: Tenotomy; indications and technic. Am. J. Surg. *44:*272–278, April '39

RÜHL, A.: Cystic tumors of neck; struma papillomatosa cystica lateralis. Deutsche Ztschr. f. Chir. *198:*90–98, '26

RUIZ MORENO, A.: Spring finger and Dupuytren's contracture; case in woman. Semana med. *1:*939–946, March 19, '36

RUIZ MORENO, V.: Free full thickness skin grafts in children; cases. Semana med. *1:*1089–1097, June 28, '45

RUIZ RUBIO, M.: Crushing injury of hand; conservative reparative surgery; case. Arch. Soc. cirujanos hosp. *16:*398–400, June '46

RULISON, E. T.: Postoperative care of Ollier-Thiersch skin grafts; advisability of daily surgical dressings. Surg., Gynec. and Obst. *45:*708–710, Nov '27

RULISON, R. H. AND MC LEAN, S.: Treatment of vascular nevi with radium. Am. J. Dis. Child. *25:*359–370, May '23 (illus.)

RUMOLD, M. J. (see WEAVER, J. B.) April '43

RUMSEY, H. ST. J.: Speech reeducation in cleft palate. Guy's Hosp. Gaz. *58:*6–8, Jan 8, '44

RUMYANTSEVA, A. F.: Prosthesis of orbit and surrounding parts of face. Vestnik oftal. (nos. 3–4) *19:*153–154, '41

RUPE, L. O. (see LOEWEN, S. L.) June '43

RUPPE, C.: Relations of osseous fragments in total cleft palates. Rev. de stomatol. *30:*670–681, Nov '28

RUPPE, C.: Veau operation for cleft palate. Ann. d'oto-laryng., pp.1029–1043, Oct '31

RUPPE, C.: Uranostaphylorrhaphy according to method of Victor Veau. French M. Rev. *2:*259–275, May '32

RUPPE, C.: War wounds of face. Presse med. *47:*1334–1336, Sept 13, '39

RUPPE, C. AND MAGDELEINE, J.: Congenital labial fistula; case. Rev. de stomatol. *29:*1–8, Jan '27

RUPPE, C. (see LAMAITRE, F.) July-Aug '29

RUPPE, C. (see LEMAITRE, F.) March '29

RUPPE, C. (see RUPPE, L.) Jan '23

RUPPE, C. (see RUPPE, L.) Dec '26

RUPPE, C. (see RUPPE, L.) Feb '27

RUPPE, C. (see RUPPE, L.) April '27

RUPPE, C. (see VEAU, V.) April '21

RUPPE, C. (see VEAU, V.) 1922

RUPPE, C. (see VEAU, V.) July '22

RUPPE, C. (see VEAU, V.) Aug '22

RUPPE, L. AND RUPPE, C.: Training of speech in children with cleft palate. Arch. de med. d. enf. *26:*19–35, Jan '23 (illus.)

RUPPE, L. AND RUPPE, C.: Prosthetic treatment of harelip; and cleft palate complications. Odontologie *64:*831–845, Dec 30, '26

RUPPE, L. AND RUPPE, C.: Velo-palatine prosthesis. Odontologie *65:*69–86, Feb 28, '27

RUPPE, L. AND RUPPE, C.: Prosthesis for cleft palate. Odontologie *65:*276–302 April '27

RUSCHENBERG, E.: Flexion contracture of thumb in small children, typical phenomenon. Ztschr. f. Orthop. *68:*172–178, '38

RUSH, H. L. AND RUSH, L. V.: Planning plastic operation of face. New Orleans M. and S. J. *84:*948–953, June '32

RUSH, H. L. (see RUSH, L. V. *et al*) Dec '29
RUSH, H. L. (see RUSH, L. V.) July '42
RUSH, J. H. (see RUSH, L. V. *et al*) Dec '29
RUSH, L. V.; RUSH, J. H. AND RUSH, H. L.: Bridging of osseous defects of forehead, using metal models as guides for shaping cartilage transplants. Am. J. Surg. *7:*805–807, Dec '29
RUSH, L. V. (see RUSH, H. L.) June '32
RUSHMORE, S.: Formation of artificial vagina. Am. J. Obst. and Gynec. *18:*427–429, Sept '29
RUSHTON, M. A. AND WALKER, F. A.: Unilateral secondary facial cleft with excess tooth and bone formation. Proc. Roy. Soc. Med. *30:*79–82, Nov '36
RUSHTON, M. A. AND WALKER, F. A.: Care of military and civilian injuries; mandibular fractures treated by pin fixation; 21 cases. Am. J. Orthodontics (Oral Surg. Sect) *28:*307–315, May '42
RUSHTON, M. A. AND WALKER, F. A.: Uses of screw-pin in maxillofacial cases. Brit. Dent. J. *78:*289–292, May 18, '45
RUSKIN, S. L.: Guarded septum chisel. Laryngoscope *34:*288–289, April '24
RUSPA, F.: Surgical and orthopedic treatment of jaw ankylosis. Boll.e mem.Soc.piemontese di chir. *4:*130–141, '34
RUSPA, F.: Late reduction of fracture of upper jaw. Stomatol. ital. *1:*122–130, Feb '39
RUSSELL, A. Y.: Method for treating fracture of neck of condyle of mandible. Internat. J. Orthodontia *16:*84–86, Jan '30
RUSSELL, C. V.: New method of skin grafting. J. Michigan M. Soc. *31:*804, Dec '32
RUSSELL, E. P.: Deep infections of hand. J. Iowa M. Soc. *26:*689, Dec '36
RUSSELL, K. F.: Exstrophy of bladder, case presenting many unusual features. Brit. J. Urol. *11:*31–47, March '39
RUSSELL, R. D.: Cysts and fistulae of neck. Ann. Otol., Rhin. and Laryng. *44:*532–543, June '35
RUSSI, J. C. (see GARCIA CAPURRO, R.) 1943
RUSSI, J. C. (see GARCIA CAPURRO, R.) Aug '43
RUSSO, A. G. (see GONI MORENO, I.) Sept '44
RUSSOLILLO, M.: Cure of salivary fistula following wound of Stensen's duct; case. Riforma med. *53:*139–140, Jan 23, '37
RUTH, V. A.: Injuries to hand. J. Iowa M. Soc. *26:*90–92, Feb '36
RUTHERFORD, A. G.: Shock and its treatment. W. Virginia M. J. *18:*298–302, Dec '23
RUTHERFORD, A. G.: Injuries to hand. W. Virginia M. J. *23:*83–86, Feb '27
RUTHERFORD, A. G.: Significance and management of shock. West Virginia M. J. *26:*26–28, Jan '30
RUTHERFORD, R.: Hand infection and its treatment. Clin. J. *67:*444–452, Nov '38
RUTTEN, E.: Surgery of ankylosis of jaws. Beitr. z. klin. Chir. *163:*414–415, '36
RUTTIN, E.: Congenital aural fistula; case. Wien. med. Wchnschr. *77:*1019, July 30, '27
RUTTIN, E.: Clinical and pathologic aspects of branchiogenic cysts. Monatschr. f. Ohrenh. *66:*1111–1114, Sept '32
RYBNIKOVA, O. I.: Fate of implanted tissue in eyelid after Schneller operation. Sovet. vestnik oftal. *9:*324–325, '36
RYCHENER, R. O.: Present status of surgery of lacrimal sac. Surg., Gynec. and Obst. *68:*414–418, Feb (no. 2A) '39
RYLANDER, C. M. AND KISNER, W. H.: Avulsion of scalp; case. Am. J. Surg. *58:*150–151, Oct '42
RYLL-NARDZEWSKA, J.: Cleft palate and bilateral lack of development of upper extremities; case. Ginek. polska *11:*678–683, July-Sept '32
DE RYNCK, G.: Treatment of nasal deformities. M. Press *210:*154–157, Sept 8, '43
RYSKINA, Z. B. (see KAGANOVICH-DVORKIN, A. L.) 1945
RYZHIKH, A. N.: Plaster of paris bandage in therapy of gunshot wounds of fingers. Khirurgiya, no. 4, pp. 65–69, '44

S

SABATUCCI, F.: Drumstick fingers from freezing. Policlinico (sez. med.) *28:*233, June '21 abstr: J.A.M.A. *77:*580, Aug 13, '21
SACCOMANNO, G. *et al*: Preparation and storage of autopsy nerve grafts. Science *100:*436, Nov 10, '44
SACERDOTE, G. (see RIGANO-IRRERA, D.) 1927
SACHARIEW, G.: "Transplantation microtome" new apparatus for obtaining uniformly thick epidermal and cutaneous grafts. Chirurg. *15:*94, Feb 1, '43
SACHS, A. E. AND GOLDBERG, S. L.: Foreskin isografts. Am. J. Surg. *60:*255–259, May '43
SACHS, E. AND MALONE, J. Y.: Experimental study of method for bridging nerve defects; with description of new method of autotransplant (auto-autotransplant). Arch. Surg. *5:*314–333, Sept '22 (illus.)
SACHS, M.: Surgery of blepharospasm. Wien. klin. Wchnschr. *38:*215, Feb 19, '25 abstr: J.A.M.A. *84:*1161, April 11, '25
SACKS, S.: Congenital defect of lower jaw associated with cleft palate (case). South African M. J. *15:*34, Jan 25, '41
SADLER, L.: Management of congenital absence of vagina. J. Oklahoma M. A. *34:*382–385, Sept '41

SADR, A. R.: Cross nerve anastomosis in man. Ann. Surg. *124:*599–603, Sept '46
SAEGESSER, M.: Tannic acid in burns. Schweiz. med. Wchnschr. *62:*117–118, Jan 30, '32
SAEGESSER, M.: Treatment of ganglion. Schweiz. med. Wchnschr. *66:*663–664, July 11, '36
SAEGESSER, M.: Burn therapy. Chirurg *12:*708–711, Dec 1, '40
SAES, P.: Complete atresia of auditory canal due to trauma; plastic repair; case. Rev. otolaring. de Sao Paulo *4:*83–86, March–April '36
SAFAR, K.: Alcohol injection in blepharospasm and spastic entropion. Ztschr. f. Augenh. *71:*135–141, May '30
SAFFORD, F. K. JR. (see ALLEN, F. M. *et al*) May '43
SAFFORD, F. K. JR. (see CROSSMAN, L. W.) Feb '45
SAFIAN, J.: Correction of nasal deformities following septum operations. Laryngoscope *34:*957–960, Dec '24
SAFIAN, J.: New rhinoplastic instrument. Arch. Otolaryng. *8:*78, July '28
SAFIAN, J.: New nasal brace. Arch. Otolaryng. *8:*566–568, Nov '28
SAFIAN, J.: *Corrective Rhinoplastic Surgery.* Paul Hoeber Co., New York, 1935
SAFIAN, J.: Evaluation of rhinoplasty. Rev. de chir. structive *8:*14–18, May '38
SAFIAN, J.: Receding chin; plastic reconstruction. New York State J. Med. *38:*1331–1335, Oct 15, '38
SAFIAN, J.: Failures in rhinoplastic surgery; causes and prevention. Am. J. Surg. *50:*274–280, Nov '40
SÀFTA, E.: Congenital cysts of neck. Cluj. med. *12:*595–598, Nov 1, '31
SAGE, E. C.: Unusual example of exstrophy of bladder with marked separation of pubic bones. Am. J. Obst. and Gynec. *8:*497–500, Oct '24
SAGHER, F. (see DOSTROVSKY, A.) April '43
SAGHIRIAN, L. M.: Oral surgery case reports. Am. J. Orthodontics (Oral Surg. Sect) *32:*472–492, July '46
SAGRERA, J. M. (see SALLERAS LLINARES, V.) July '46
SAILER, K.: Cystic lymphangioma of chest wall. Orvosi hetil. *71:*811–813, July 17, '27
DE SAINT-MARTIN: Plastic surgery in ectropion or loss of substance, with special reference to Hungarian method. Rev. med. de Nancy *64:*879–903, Dec 1, '36 also: Bull. Soc. d'opht. de Paris, pp. 648–671, Oct '36
DE SAINT-MARTIN: Excision of cancer of eyelids and autoplastic surgery according to Imre technic. Bull. Soc. d'opht. de Paris *49:*36–40, Jan '37
DE SAINT-MARTIN, R.: Modification of Motais operation for eyelid ptosis. Bull. Soc. d'opht. de Paris *50:*100–102, Feb '38
DE SAINT-MARTIN, R.: Modified Motais operation for eyelid ptosis. Ann. d'ocul. *175:*589–596, Aug '38
SAINT-ONGE, G.: Tannic acids in burns; useful and dangerous fixative. J. de l'Hotel-Dieu de Montreal *13:*270–282, Sept–Oct '44
SÁINZ DE AJA: Mixed surgical and radium treatment of prominent keloids. Siglo med. *72:*1185–1187, Dec 8, '23
SAITO, R.: Studies of scalding. Mitt. d. med. Gessellsch. zu Tokio *46:*2137–2138, Dec '32
SAJDOVÁ, V.: Dupuytren's contracture; etiology, with report of case. Rev. v neurol. a psychiat. *29:*188–194, Sept '32
SAKAGUSHI, S. (see SCHAEFFER, A. A.) May '45
SAKLER, B. R.: Plastic repair of eyelid hernia with fascia lata. Am. J. Ophth. *20:*936–938, Sept '37
SAKON, H.: Operation followed by radium therapy in epithelioma of nasal septum; 2 cases. Ann. d'oto-laryng., pp 55–60, Jan '31
SALA, F. (see BERTOLA, V. *et al*) Oct '36
SALA, F. (see BERTOLA, V. J. *et al*) April '45
SALAS, N. E. (see VILLARAN, C.) May '39
SALAS GONZÁLEZ, J.: Digitalis therapy of cardiac insufficiency in primary and secondary traumatic shock. Rev. espan. de med. y cir. *17:*489–490, Oct '34
SALAZAR DE SOUSA, C.: Unusual types of congenital abnormalities of hand. Arq. de anat. *13:*119–128, '29–'30
SALCADO, L. V.: Grafting of nerve preserved in alcohol. Presse med. *33:*558–559, April 29, '25 abstr: J.A.M.A. *84:*1966, June 20, '25
SALEZ. (see DEBEYRE, A.) Nov '29
SALINAS, F. O.: Operative technic in treatment of prolapsus of breast. Cultura med. mod. *7:*455–462, July 31, '28
SALINGER, S.: Nasal fractures; treatment of same by new adjustable splint. Ann. Otol., Rhin. and Laryng. *33:*413–416, June '24
SALINGER, S.: Adjustable splint for fractures of nose. Illinois M. J. *48:*304–306, Oct '25
SALINGER, S.: Cartilage and ivory in plastic surgery of nose. Arch. Otolaryng. *6:*552–558, Dec '27
SALINGER, S.: Surgical correction of crooked nose. Illinois M. J. *54:*368–373, Nov '28
SALINGER, S.: New instrument for reduction of nasal fractures. Arch. Otolaryng. *9:*657–658, June '29
SALINGER, S.: Rhinophyma. Arch. Otolaryng. *11:*620–621, May '30
SALINGER, S.: Ivory implants for saddle nose; results in 50 cases. Ann. Otol., Rhin. and

Laryng. *40:*801-808, Sept '31
SALINGER, S.: Nasal deformities and their correction. Arch. Otolaryng. *16:*510-525, Oct '32
SALINGER, S.: Copper molded nasal splint; new method of application. Arch. Otolaryng. *20:*211-214, Aug '34
SALINGER, S.: Saddle nose; ivory and cartilage implants. Illinois M. J. *72:*412-417, Nov '37
SALINGER, S.: Deviation of septum in relation to twisted nose. Arch. Otolaryng. *29:*520-532, March '39
SALINGER, S.: Nasal fractures in children; diagnosis and treatment. Arch. Otolaryng. *34:*936-951, Nov '41
SALINGER, S.: Cavernous hemangioma of nose, nasal septum and forehead. Ann. Otol., Rhin. and Laryng. *51:*268-272, March '42
SALINGER, S.: Rhinoplasty from cosmetic point of view. J. Iowa M. Soc. *32:*199-202, May '42
SALINGER, S.: Traumatic deformities of nasal septum. Tr. Am. Laryng. A. *66:*46-58, '44
SALINGER, S.: Traumatic deformities to nose. Ann. Otol., Rhin. and Laryng. *53:*274-285, June '44

Salivary Fistula

Case of facial fistula due to submaxillary sialolithiasis. CAHN, L. R. AND LEVY, J. Am. J. Surg. *36:*11, Jan '22 (illus.).
Salivary fistula; case report. DABNEY, S. G. Kentucky M. J. *20:* 589, Sept '22
Treatment of salivary fistulas. KLEINSCHMIDT, K. Munchen. med. Wchnschr. *70:* 809, June 22, '23 abstr: J.A.M.A. *81:*1245, Oct 6, '23
Salivary fistula behind ear; 2 cases. KAUSCH, W. Zentralbl. f. Chir. *52:*914-917, April 25, '25
Congenital salivary fistula of neck. SMITH, R. R. AND TORGERSON, W. R. Surg., Gynec. and Obst. *41:*318-319, Sept '25
Congenital salivary fistula in cleft cheek. POMMRICH, W. Deutsche Ztschr. f. Chir. *191:*136-142, '25
Case of abnormal salivary fistula. CHAWLA, G. S. Indian M. Gaz. *61:*233, May '26
Simple operation for closing salivary fistula. SAPOSCHKOFF, K. Zentralbl. f. Chir. *53:*2905-2909, Nov 13, '26
Inflammations and fistulae of salivary glands and their treatment. WAKELEY, C. P. G. Lancet *2:*7-10, July 7, '28
Salivary fistula communicating with external auditory meatus. ABERCROMBIE, P. H. J. Laryng. and Otol. *45:*474-476, July '30
Retro-auricular salivary fistula; therapy. BORKOWSKI, J. Warszawskie czasop. lek. *9:*653, July 14, '32

Salivary Fistula – Cont.
Treatment of persistent parotid fistulas; 2 cases. KONJETZNY, G. E. Zentralbl. f. Chir. *61:*243-247, Feb 3, '34
New operative technic for facial salivary cyst of traumatic nature. MIHĂILESCU, S. P. Rev. de chir., Bucuresti *37:*713-715, Sept-Dec '34
Primary repair of severed parotid duct; method of fixation of inlying dowel. BROHM, C. G. AND BIRD, C. E., J.A.M.A. *104:*733-734, March 2, '35
Therapy of salivary fistulae. MILHIET. Progres med., p. 742, May 4, '35
Treatment of parotid fistula. COOK, J. Lancet *1:*1239, May 30, '36
Cure of salivary fistula following wound of Stensen's duct; case. RUSSOLILLO, M. Riforma med. *53:*139-140, Jan 23, '37
Repair of traumatic fistulas of Stenson's duct (parotid). GLASCOCK, H. AND GLASCOCK, H. JR. Surg., Gynec. and Obst. *65:*355-356, Sept '37
Surgical therapy of parotid fistula according to Sapozhkov method. MACHAN, V. Y. Vestnik khir. *49:*94-95, '37
Salivary fistulas following gunshot wounds to face, and their therapy. GUTNER, Y. I. Khirurgiya, no. 7, pp. 54-58, '44
New method of treatment of parotid fistula; cauterization and silence cure. COSTANTINI, H. Afrique franc. chir., nos. 3-4, pp. 65-68, May-Aug '45
Salivary fistula of submaxillary gland following excision of thyroglossal cyst. JENKINS, H. B. Am. J. Surg. *70:*118-120, Oct '45
Plastic closure of salivary fistula with transposed skin flaps. AMELIN. Khirurgiya, no. 6, pp. 43-44, '45

Salivary Glands, Cancer (See also Cancer, Jaws; Neck; Parotid, Cancer)

Removal of submaxillary salivary glands in operations for carcinoma of lower lip; responses to questionnaire. BERESOW, E. L. Arch. f. klin. Chir. *151:*767-784, '28
Salivary gland cancer. MACFEE, W. F. Ann. Surg. *109:*534-550, April '39
Metastasis of mixed tumors of salivary glands. MULLIGAN, R. M. Arch. Path. *35:*357-365, March '43

Salivary Glands, Stone

Calculi of salivary glands. IVY, R. H. AND CURTIS, L. Ann. Surg. *96:*979-986, Dec '32

Salivary Glands, Tumors

Swellings of submaxillary regions. IVY, R. H. Ann. Surg. *81:*605-610, March '25

Tumors of salivary glands. WAKELEY, C. P. G. Surg., Gynec. and Obst. *48:*635-638, May '29

Study of 66 cases of salivary gland tumors. SCHREINER, B. F. AND MATTICK, W. L. Am. J. Roentgenol. *21:*541-546, June '29

Three hundred mixed tumors of salivary glands, of which sixty-nine recurred. MCFARLAND, J., Surg., Gynec. and Obst. *63:*457-468, Oct '36

Salivary gland tumors. SWINTON, N. W. AND WARREN, S. Surg., Gynec. and Obst. *67:*424-435, Oct '38

Salivary gland tumors. SNYDER, C. D., J. Kansas M. Soc. *41:*389-390, Sept '40

Mixed tumors of submaxillary gland; extirpation by buccal route. IVANISSEVICH, O. AND FERRARI, R. C. Bol. y trab., Acad. argent. de cir. *24:*1051-1054, Oct 30, '40

Treatment of salivary gland tumors by radical excision. JANES, R. M. Canad. M. A. J. *43:*554-559, Dec '40

Salivary gland tumors. SINGLETON, A. O. AND DUREN, N. Texas State J. Med. *36:*784-792, April '41

Surgical treatment of salivary gland tumors. JANES, R. M., S. Clin. North America *23:*1429-1439, Oct '43

Mixed tumor of salivary gland type on left hand. HIGHMAN, B. Arch. Path. *37:*387-388, June '44

Salivary gland tumor of upper lip. CURR, J. F. Brit. M. J. *2:*605, Nov 3, '45

SALLERAS, J.: Hypospadias, correction by plastic surgery of urethra by Marion's operation. Rev. de especialid *5:*1385-1389, Oct '30 also: Semana med. *1:*10-11, Jan 1, '31

SALLERAS, J.: Penoscrotal hypospadias; satisfactory results of Duplay operation with hypogastric derivation of urine; case. Rev. Asoc. med. argent. *46:*988-990, Sept '32

SALLERAS, J. see SALLERAS PAGÉS, J.

SALLERAS LLINAERS, V. AND SAGRERA, J. M.: Therapy of furunculosis of face. Med. clin. Barcelona *7:*36-44, July '46

SALLERAS PAGÉS, J.: Treatment of fistulas into male urethra by inversion of skin. Semana med. *28:*602, May 26, '21 abstr: J.A.M.A. *77:*580, Aug 13, '21

SALLERAS PAGÉS, J.: Correction of balanic hypospadias. Semana med. *1:*797-798, May 18, '22 (illus.) abstr: J.A.M.A. *79:*924, Sept 9, '22

SALLFELD, U.: Therapy of keloids. Therap. d. Gegenw. *72:*410-412, Sept '31

SALMAN, I.: Sclerosing agent in treatment of subluxation of mandible and hemangiomas. U.S. Nav. M. Bull. *44:*361-369, Feb '45

SALMON, D. D.: Complete compound dislocation, without fracture, of distal joint of ring finger. Radiology *40:*79-80, Jan '43

SALMON, D. L.: Septal deformities and their correction. Kentucky M. J. *28:*485-488, Oct '30

SALMON, M.: Arteries of mammary gland; importance in esthetic surgery; anatomic and roentgenographic study. Ann. d'anat. path. *16:*477-500, April '39

SALOJ, C. D. AND CID, J. M.: Lympho-epithelial cysts of neck; cases. An. de cir. *1:*48-60, June '35

SALOMON, A.: Fate of sutured tendons. Zentralbl. f. Chir. *49:*74-76, Jan 21, '22 abstr: J.A.M.A. *78:*1769, June 3, '22

SALOMON, A.: Skin flap transplantation for lupus of neck and chin. Deutsche med. Wchnschr. *52:*1821, Oct 22, '26

SALOMON, A.: Treatment of open tendon injuries. Ztschr. f. arztl. Fortbild. *28:*559-562, Sept 1, '31

SALSBURY, C. R.: Practical points in hand surgery. J. Oklahoma M. A. *26:*315-319, Sept '33

SALSBURY, C. R.: Tendons in hand injuries. Am. J. Surg. *21:*354-357, Sept '33

SALTONSTALL, H. AND LEE, W. E.: Modified technic in skin grafting of extensive deep burns. Ann. Surg. *119:*690-693, May '44

SALTZSTEIN, H. C.: Total removal of parotid gland with preservation of facial nerve. Ann. Surg. *103:*635-638, April '36

SALVATI, G.: Repair of conjunctival fornix by Reverdin-Thiersch graft. Gior. di ocul. *9:*56, May '28

SALVATI, G.: New method in correction of cicatricial entropion. Ann. d'ocul. *167:*311-314, April, '30

SALVIN, A. A.: Skin-grafting of arm wound; successful outcome despite unusual difficulties. Am. J. Surg. *26:*572-574, Dec '34

SAMENGO, L.: Automatic gag and tongue holder. Semana med. *1:*734-738, April 19, '23 (illus.)

SAMENGO, L. AND ERRECART, P. L.: Treatment and diagnostic considerations in cleft palate. Semana med. *2:*913-914, Oct 4, '28

SAMENGO, L. AND ERRECART, P. L.: Cause and treatment of cleft palate. Rev. de especialid. *3:*658-662, Nov '28

SAMMARTINO, E. S. AND PIQUE, J. A.: Splitting of thenar eminence with protrusion of muscles due to crushing of hand in industrial accident; therapy of case. Rev. Asoc. med. argent. *54:*178-180, March 15-30, '40

SAMMARTINO, E. S. (see MOSOTEGUY, C.) May '38

SAMMIS, G. F.: New method of transfer of full-thickness skin; grille graft. Am. J. Surg. *36:*46–49, April '37

SAMMIS, G. F.: Indications for plastic surgery. M. Times, New York *73:*160–162, June '45

SAMORINI, G.: Surgical treatment of elephantiasis. Policlinico (sez. prat.) *31:*904–908, July 14, '24

SAMPAIO DORIA, A. (see ALVARO, M. E.) Nov '37

SAMPAIO, DORIA, A. (see ALVARO, M. E.) 1938

SAMPSON, W. C.: The burned patient. J. Nat. M. A. *36:*143–151, Sept '44

SAMS, W. M.: Rhinophyma, case with unusual involvement of chin. Arch. Dermat. and Syph. *26:*834–837, Nov '32

SAMSONOVA, Z. P.: Burn therapy, open method as practiced at Traumatologic Clinic of Sklifasovskiy Institute. Novy khir. arkhiv *38:*476–479, '37

SAMSONOVA, Z. P. (see GORINEVSKAYA, V. V.) 1935

SAMUEL, S.: Method of skin-grafting. Brit. M. J. *2:*632, Oct 22, '21

SAMUELS, L.: Hare-lip surgery; a suggestion. Lancet *2:*860, Oct 22, '21

SAMY, M.: New operation for radical treatment of winged, projecting and distorted ears. Rev. de chir. structive *8:*192–194, '38

SANCHEZ-ARBIDE, A.: Free skin grafts; classification. Rev. de chir. structive, pp. 270–272, Dec '37

SANCHEZ ARBIDE, A.: Skin grafts for plastic surgery of face. Semana med. *2:*1281–1286, Dec 2, '37

SANCHEZ BULNES, L.: Surgical technic for correction of spastic entropion and senile ectropion. Arch. Assoc. para evit. ceguera Mexico *2:*125–135, '44

SANCHEZ BULNES, L. AND SILVA, D.: New instruments for dacryocystorhinostomy. Arch. Asoc. para evit. ceguera Mexico *3:*249–255, '45

SANCHEZ CORDERO, R.: Malignant melanomas; clinical study based on 20 cases. Rev. med. d. Hosp. gen. *8:*332–339, Jan '46

SANCHEZ-COVISA, I.: Treatment of hypospadias and epispadias. Arch. espan. de pediat. *6:*577–613, Oct '22 (illus.) abstr: J.A.M.A. *80:*285, Jan 27, '23

SANCHEZ GALINDO, J.: Therapy of loss of substance of lower jaw by auto-plastic bone graft. Med. espan. *4:*35–45, July '40

SÁNCHEZ TOLEDO, P.: Volkmann contracture of hand; therapy by Henle operation; case. Cir. ortop. y traumatol. *1:*113–118, April '33

SANCHÍS PERPIÑÁ, V.: Plastic surgery of penobalanic and penoscrotal hypospadias. Actas Soc. de cir. de Madrid *1:*197–229, Jan–March '32

SANCHÍS PERPIÑÁ, V.: Method for cheiloplasty of lower lip. Actas Soc. de cir. de Madrid *1:*329–352, April–June '32

SANCHÍS PERPIÑÁ, V.: Author's cheiloplastic method of surgery of lower lip. Beitr. z. klin. Chir. *158:*367–380, '33

SANCHÍS PERPIÑÁ, V.: Method for cheiloplasty of lower lip. Arch. de med., cir. y especialid. *36:*449–458, April 22, '33

SANCHÍS PERPIÑÁ, V.: Plastic surgery of penobalanic and penoscrotal hypospadias. Arch. de med., cir. y especialid. *36:*989–1002, Sept 2, '33

SANCHÍS PERPIÑÁ, V.: Plastic methods for surgical correction of penobalanic and penoscrotal hypospadias. Zentralbl. f. Chir. *61:*209–216, Jan 27, '34

SANDBERG, I. R.: Snapping fingers due to tendosynovitis; case. Nord. med. (Hygiea) *9:*707–709, March 8, '41

SANDER, P.: Congenital eyelid coloboma; case. Ztschr. f. Augenh. *61:*180–183, Feb '27

SANDERS, F. K.: Repair of large gaps in peripheral nerves (including use of grafts). Brain *65:*281–337, Sept '42

SANDERS, F. K. AND YOUNG, J. Z.: Degeneration and re-innervation of grafted nerves. J. Anat. *76:*143–166, Jan '42

SANDERS, F. K. AND YOUNG, J. Z.: Degeneration and reinnervation of nerve transplants. Rev. oto-neuro-oftal. *18:*117–119, July–Aug '43

SANDERS, F. K. (see HIGHET, W. B.) April '43

SANDERS, F. K. (see YOUNG, J. Z. *et al*) Aug '40

SANDERS, J.: Inheritance of harelip and cleft palate. Genetica *15:*433–510, '34

SANDES, T. L.: Tendon transplantation. M. J. South Africa *17:*217–220, June '22

SANGVICHIEN, S.: Thoracopagus, one with harelip and cleft palate. Anat. Rec. *67:*157–158, Jan 25, '37

SAINT-GIRONS, F. (see BRODIN, P.) Nov '39

SAINZ DE AJA, E. A.: Dermatologic esthetics; pigmentation, freckles, etc. of exposed parts; means of preventing, improving and curing them. Actas dermo-sif. *32:*145–151, Nov '40

SAINZ DE AJA, E. A.: Substances promoting formation of skin. Actas dermo-sif. *32:*229–233, Dec '40

SANO, M. E.: New method of skin grafting based on principles of tissue culture. Am. J. Surg. *61:*105–106, July '43

SANO, M. E.: Coagulum-contact method as applied to human grafts. Surg., Gynec. & Obst. *77:*510–513, Nov '43

SANO, M. E.: Possibilities and advantages of gluing grafts in place (coagulum-contact method). Am. Acad. Orthop. Surgeons, Lect. pp. 224–225, '44

SANO, M. E.: New method of skin grafting (coagulum-contact method). Delaware State M. J. *16:*51–52, April '44

SANO, M. E.: New coagulum-contact method of skin grafting; further simplications in technic. Am. J. Surg. *64:*359–360, June '44

SANO, M. E.; HOLLAND, C. A. AND BABCOCK, W. W.: Use of coagulum-contact method in surgery for grafting. S. Clin. North America *23:*1673–1695, Dec '43

DE SANSON, R. D.: Braun's skin grafts. Brazil-med. *35:*299, June 11, '21 abstr: J.A.M.A. *77:*977, Sept 17, '21

DE SANSON, R. D.: Cancer of larynx and its therapy. Rev. oto-laring. de Sao Paulo *3:*197–214, May–June '35 also: Rev. de laryng. *56:*964–985, Sept–Oct '35

DE SANSON, R. D.: Surgical therapy of cleft palate by Veau technic. Rev. oto-laring de Sao Paulo *4:*349–364, July–Aug '36

DE SANSON, R. D.: Osteomyelitis of mandible; surgical therapy. Rev. oto-laring. de Sao Paulo *4:*1297–1318, Nov–Dec '36

DE SANSON, R. D.: Plastic surgery of nose. Arq. de cir. clin. e exper. *6:*144, April–June '42

DE SANSON, R. D.: Harelip and cleft palate: results of plastic surgery. Arq. de cir. clin. e exper. *6:*336–339, April–June '42

DE SANSON, R. D. AND AMARANTE, R. C. L.: Labiovelopalatine fissure; surgical therapy with report of cases. Rev. brasil. de cir. *12:*215–246, March '43

SANTA MARINA IRAOLA, J. A.: Depressions of nasal tip; plastic surgery. Semana med. *2:*726–729, Sept 23, '43

SANTAS, A. A.: Biologic (plasma) and chemical therapy of burns. Rev. Asoc. med. argent. *57:*850–854, Oct 30, '43 also: Bol. d. Inst. clin. quir. *19:*690–697, Dec '43

SANTAS, A. A.: Shock in war surgery. Bol. d. Inst. clin. quir. *21:*55–61, Feb '45

SANTAS, A. A.; ROSITO, E. AND JURADO, P.: Plan for grave burns. Bol. d. Inst. clin. quir. *18:*549–553, Aug '42

SANTAS, A. A.; ROSITO, E. AND JURADO, P.: Plan for grave burns. Semana med. *2:*424–426, Aug 20, '42

SANTI, E.: Effect of periarterial sympathectomy on autoplastic grafts (including bone); experimental study. Arch. ital. de chir. *31:*209–227, '32

SANTI, E.: Formation of artificial vagina by use of labial tissue. Clin. obstet. *34:*517–520, Aug '32

SANTIAGO RIESCO MAC-CLURE, J. (see RIESCO MAC-CLURE, J. S.)

SANTILLAN, J. S.; ONGJOCO, J. S. AND SORIANO, F. S.: Avulsion of scalp; case. Rev. filipina de med. y farm. *32:*1–5; 10, Jan '41

SANTORO, E.: Lateral, congenital, cervical fistula; clinical aspects, histogenesis, operative technic; case. Ann. ital. di chir. *8:*59–71, Jan '29

DOS SANTOS, F.: Facial war surgery. Arq. brasil. de cir. e ortop. *11:*24–35, '43

SANTOS, H. A.; CRUZ, A. AND ORTIGA, S. JR.: Human ascitic fluid and starch-Ringer solution in shock therapy. U.S. T. J. Med. *1:*75–85, Nov '40

SANTOS, M.: Cancer of parotid gland, indications and technic for total removal; 2 cases. Bol. do coll. brasil. de cir. *3:*10–20, April–July '32

SANTY, P.: Extensive chronic ulceration on leg; successful treatment by autoplastic skin grafts. Lyon chir. *26:*456–457, May–June '29

SANTY, P. AND BERARD, M.: Recurrent dislocation of jaw; bilateral ablation of temporomaxillary menisci; case. Lyon chir. *33:*75–76, Jan–Feb '36

SANTY, P. AND DARGENT, M.: Early recurrence of mixed tumor of parotid in cicatrix of total parotidectomy; case. Mem. Acad. de chir. *72:*225–232, April 10–May 15, '46

SANTY, P. AND PONT, A.: Mandibular "obtusism"; surgical therapy; case. Lyon chir. *35:*727–728, Nov–Dec '38

SANVENERO-ROSSELLI, G.: Surgery of nasal deformities. Ann. di laring., otol. *28:*193–216, July '27

SANVENERO-ROSSELLI, G.: Technic of correction of nasal deformity by adjustment of proper tissues. Rassegna ital. di oto-rino-laring. *1:*223–231, Sept–Oct '27

SANVENERO-ROSSELLI, G.: Free transplants of skin in plastic surgery of face and neck. Arch. ital. di chir. *21:*245–265, '28

SANVENERO-ROSSELLI, G.: Operative treatment of rhinophyma. Rassegna ital. di oto-rino-laring. *2:*149–159, July–Aug '28

SANVENERO-ROSSELLI, G.: Plastic methods in otorhinolaryngology. Rassegna ital. di oto-rino-laring. *2:*241–257, Nov–Dec '28

SANVENERO-ROSSELLI, G.: Methods and results of plastic surgery of face. Bruxelles-med. *9:*476–482, Feb 24, '29 abstr: Bruxelles med. (supp.) *9:*63, '28

SANVENERO-ROSSELLI, G.: Plastic surgery of cicatrices. Igiene e vita *12:*406–410, Oct '29

SANVENERO-ROSSELLI, GUSTAVO: *Chirurgia plastica del naso*. Luigi Pozzi, Rome, 1931

SANVENERO-ROSSELLI, G.: Results of plastic operations at R. Clinica Otorinolaringoiatrica in Turin. Arch. ital. di laring. (suppl) *51:*301–324, '32

SANVENERO-ROSSELLI, G.: Methods and results of plastic surgery of face. Boll. e mem. Soc piemontese di chir. *2:*1024–1050, '32

SANVENERO-ROSSELLI, G.: Plastic surgery of ear. Rev. de chir. plastique, pp. 27–52, April '32

SANVENERO-ROSSELLI, G.: Surgical restoration by means of grafts in severe burns of face with cicatrix. Bull. et mem. Soc. d. chirurgiens de Paris *27:*391–403, July 5, '35

SANVENERO-ROSSELLI, G.: Surgical therapy of congenital cleft palate. Rev. de chir. structive, pp. 413–418, Dec '36

SANVENERO-ROSSELLI, G.: Plastic surgery for mutilations of face resulting from exeresis of malignant tumors from soft parts. Arch. ital. di chir. *54:*491–501, '38

SANVENERO-ROSSELLI, G.: Science and art of plastic surgery; present and future. Plast. chir. *1:*3–28, '39

SANVENERO-ROSSELLI, G.: Plastic surgery of harelip. Science and art of plastic surgery; present and future status. Salud y belleza *1:*8–9, April–May '45

SANVENERO-ROSSELLI, G. (see COLOMBINO, C.) Sept–Oct '39

SANYAL, S. N.: Crude vegetable oil (Calophyllum oil) for local burn treatment. Calcutta M. J. *38:*255–258, May '41

SANZ DE FRUTOS, F.: Therapy of acute hand infections. Medicina, Madrid *3:*509–548, Oct '32

DE SA OLIVEIRA, E.: Elephantiasis and elephantine conditions; surgical notes, Bahia, 1941. An. Fac. med. Bahia *4:*111–151, '44–'45

Sapejko Operation: See Van Millingen Operation

Sapezhko Operation: See Millingen-Sapezhko Operation

SAPORITO, L. A. (see BEDER, O. E.) June '46

SAPOSCHKOFF, K.: Simple operation for closing salivary fistula. Zentralbl. f. Chir. *53:*2905–2909, Nov 13, '26

Sapozhkov Operation

Surgical therapy of parotid fistula according to Sapozhkov method. MACHAN, V. Y. Vestnik khir. *49:*94–95, '37

SARACINO, R. (see ROUSSY, G. *et al*) Feb '42

SARAVAL, U.: Therapy of fractures of lower jaw. Riforma med. *46:*675–678, May 5, '30

SARAZIN, A.: Rare case of exstrophy of bladder. Bull. et mem. Soc. de radiol. med. de France *24:*324–327, April '36

SARGNON, AND EUVRARD: Straightening of recently fractured nose. Lyon med. *149:*353–355, March 20, '32

SARGNON. (see BÉRARD, *et al*) May '33

SARGNON, A.: Ten years' experience with radium therapy of cancer of larynx. J. de radiol. et d'electrol. *10:*553–555, Dec '26

SARGNON, A.: Treatment of old and recent nasal fractures. Arch. internat. de laryngol. *33:*129–148, Feb '27

SARGNON, A.: Treatment of recent nasal fractures. Rev. de chir. plastique, pp. 111–130, July '31

SARGNON, A.: Endonasal free graft in therapy of old fractures of nose. Rev. de chir. structive, pp. 185–204, Oct '37

SARGNON, A. AND BERTEIN, P.: Paralysis of intrapetrosal portion of facial nerve; clinical forms, treatment. J. de med. de Lyon *10:*539–560, Sept 5, '29

SARKAR, K. D.: Burns and treatment of third degree. Antiseptic *43:*126–130, Feb '46

SARNAT, B. G. (see BYARS, L. T.) Nov '45

SARNAT, B. G. (see BYARS, L. T.) Jan '46

SARNOFF, J.: Plastic surgery, what to expect. M. Rec. *144:*58–62, July 15, '36

SARNOFF, J.: Procedure of choice in correction of saddle nose. M. Rec. *151:*155–156, March 6, '40

SARNOFF, J.: Simplified plastic operation for hump, hook and twist of nose. Surgery *7:*908–909, June '40

SARNOFF, J. AND SARNOFF, S. J.: Surgery of congenital anomalies of female genitals. J. Internat. Coll. Surgeons *6:*36–47, Jan–Feb '43

SARNOFF, S. J. (see SARNOFF, J.) Jan–Feb '43

SARRADON, P. (see POINSO, R. *et al*) Jan '35

SARROSTE: Technic of surgical therapy of hand injuries. Arch. de med. et pharm. mil. *97:*24–43, July '32

SARRU, P.; RIGA, I. T. AND STEFANESCU, G.: Maxillofacial surgery during campaign in Poland. Rev. san. mil., Bucuresti *39:*277–281, May '40

SARTORI, C.: Implants of embryonic tissues. Arch. ital. di chir. *15:*339–349, '26 abstr: J.A.M.A. *87:*67, July 3, '26

SARTORIUS, K.: Fractures involving frontal air sinuses, due to localized violence; 30 cases. South African M. J. *20:*202–203, April 27, '46

SARTORIUS, K.: Fractures involving frontal air sinuses due to localized violence; 30 cases. South African M. J. *20:*234–237, May 11 '46

SARTRE. (see LÉRI, L) May '24

SARTRE. (see LÉRI, A.) Dec '24

SASAKI, M. AND SUEMITSU, S.: New method of plastic surgery for septal defects; case. Otorhino-laryng. *12:*834, Oct '39

SASAKI, S.: Denudation of scrotum and its plastic repair by skin graft. Taiwan Igakkai Zasshi *34:*455, April '35

SASSARD, P.: Treatment of burns of face without dressings; 2 cases. Lyon med. *147:*43, Jan 11, '31

SATANOWSKY, P.: Sarcoma of eyelid. Semana med. *2:*169–177, July 23, '25 abstr: J.A.M.A. *85:*1264, Oct 17, '25

SATANOWSKY, P.: Partial cryptophthalmus with epicanthus and congenital ptosis of upper eyelid; author's technic for surgical correction; 2 cases. Semana med. *1:*1953–1958, June 15, '33 abstr: Rev. Asoc. med. argent. *47:*2718–2724, June '33

SATANOWSKY, P.: Partial cryptophthalmos with epicanthus and congenital ptosis of upper eyelid; author's technic for surgical correction; 2 cases. Arch. de oftal. hispano-am. *33:*643–652, Nov '33

SATANOWSKY, S.: Late results of imperforate anus operation. Arch. argent. de pediat. *4:*25–29, Jan '33

SATANOWSKY, S.: Incomplete membranous syndactylia of all fingers; author's surgical technic; case. Rev. ortop. y traumatol. *7:*187–192, Oct '37

SATANOWSKY, S.: Surgical therapy of clubhand due to spastic paralysis of cerebral origin; cases. Rev. ortop. y traumatol. *9:*19–25, July '39

SATANOWSKY, S.: Skin grafting in therapy of large ulcerations, with report of cases. Semana med. *2:*1216–1223, Nov 20, '41

SATHAYE, V. D.: Ptosis of eyelids. Indian J. Ophth. *4:*54–55, July '43

SATTA, F.: Evolution of bone implants. Chir. d. org. di movimento *7:*345–366, June '23 (illus.)

SATTLER, C. H.: Operations on lacrimal ducts. Ztschr. f. Augenh. *75:*237–239, Oct '31

SATULLO, R.: Burn therapy. Policlinico (sez. prat.) *39:*1947–1950, Dec 12, '32

SAUER, W. E.: Dacryocystorhinostomy; combined methods. Ann. Otol., Rhin. & Laryng. *32:*25–43, March '23 (illus.)

SAUERBRUCH, F. AND VON DANCKELMAN, A.: Technic for surgical therapy of Dupuytren's contracture. Arch. ital. di chir. *54:*502–507, '38

Sauerbruch Operation

Transplantation of leg; Sauerbruch's plastic operation. NISSEN, R. Umschau *31:*526, June 25, '27

SAUNDERS, J. B. DE C. M. (see ABBOTT, L. C.) Dec '39

SAUTOT, J. (see CREYSSEL, J.) Jan–Feb '46

SAUVAIN, Y.: Indications for nasal surgery. Paris med. *2:*434–436, Sept 21–28, '40

SAVAGE, R. (see PAVLOVSKY, A. J.) June '29

SAVATARD, L.: Cancerous and precancerous conditions of the skin. Brit. M. J. *2:*460–463, Sept 13, '24

DE SAVITSCH, E.: Surgical treatment of elephantiasis of scrotum and penis. J. Urol. *45:*216–222, Feb '41

SAWYER, E. J. (see COTTON, F. J.) Feb '22

SAXENA, K. N.: Management and treatment of surgical shock. Antiseptic *39:*741–747, Nov '42

SAXL, A.: Surgical and physical therapy of contractures. Wien. klin. Wchschr. *42:*1266–1267, Sept 26, '29

SAXL, A.: Surgical treatment and physiotherapy of contractures. Wien. med. Wchnschr. *80:*203–207, Feb 1, '30

SAXL, A.: Splint bandage with lever in treatment of rupture of extensor aponeurosis of terminal digital phalanx. Zentralbl. f. Chir. *63:*394–395, Feb 15, '36

SAXL, N. T.: Burns en masse (at Pearl Harbor). U.S. Nav. M. Bull. *40:*570–576, July '42

SAYER, B. AND SCULLY, J. B.: Fissural cysts of jaws. Am. J. Orthodontics (Oral Surg. Sect.) *29:*320–327, June '43

SAYPOL, G. M.: Technic for repair of "baseball" finger. Am. J. Surg. *61:*103–104, July '43

SAYPOL, G. M.: Splint for treatment of fractured fingers requiring traction. Mil. Surgeon *95:*226–228, Sept '44

SAYPOL, G. M. AND SLATTERY, L. R.: Displaced fractures of hand. Surg., Gynec. & Obst. *79:*522–525, Nov '44

SAYRE, B. E.: Treatment of burns. Illinois M. J. *48:*325–327, Oct '25

SAZAVSKY, K.: Collapse and shock. Casop. lek. cesk. *80:*126–129, Jan 24, '41

SCADUTO, G.: Roentgentherapy in inoperable epithelioma of face. Urol. & Cutan. Rev. *33:*28–35, Jan '29

SCALORI, G.: Congenital fistula of ear lobe; case. Valsalva *11:*606–622, Oct 1, '35

Scalp

Avulsion of scalp and its treatment. LENORMANT, C., J. de chir. *17:*9, '21 abstr: J.A.M.A. *76:*553, Feb 19, '21

Scalp flaps in reconstruction of face. MOURE, P. Presse med. *29:*1021–1022, Dec 4, '21 (illus.) Abstr: J.A.M.A. *78:*470, Feb 11, '22

Avulsion of scalp; review of literature and report of a case. PORTER, C. A. AND SHEDDEN, W. M. Boston M. & S. J. *186:*727–730, June 1, '22 (illus.)

Scalp – Cont.

Congenital scalp defects. WALZ, W. Monatschr. f. Geburtsch. u. Gynak. *65:*167–178, Jan '24

Congenital scalp defects. NEUMANN, H. O. Zentralbl. f. Gynak. *48:*628–634, March 15, '24

Principles of 4 types of skin grafting; with an improved method of treating total avulsion of scalp. MCWILLIAMS, C. A., J.A.M.A. *83:*183–189, July 19, '24

Restoration of scalp; management of skin grafts. HOIMAN, E., J.A.M.A. *84:*350–352, Jan 31, '25

Treatment of extensive injuries of scalp. MELAND, O. N. Minnesota Med. *8:*116–120, Feb '25

Congenital defect of scalp. HIRSHLAND, H. Atlantic M. J. *28:*684–685, July '25

Avulsion of scalp; skin grafting; with report of unusual case. NORTHCUTT, J. D. Kentucky M. J. *23:*493–497, Oct '25

Method of repair of scalp defects (grafts). COLEMAN, E. P. Illinois M. J. *49:*40–43, Jan '26

Case of complete avulsion of scalp. BROOKES, W. L. Indian M. Gaz. *61:*128, March '26

Two cases of interest; septic dementia; avulsion of scalp. DOUGLASS, R. China M. J. *40:*463–464, May '26

Treatment of fungus cerebri by skin graft with report of case. KUMM, C. China M. J. *40:*1126–1132, Nov '26

Traumatic removal of entire scalp. MORRISON, O. C. Surg. J. *33:*93–96, March–April '27

Avulsion of scalp; with report of 3 cases. NUZUM, T. W. Surg. J. *33:*117–119, May–June '27

Avulsion of scalp; treatment by dermo-epidermic grafts; case. MOURE, P. Bull. et mem. Soc. nat. de chir. *53:*1040–1043, July 16, '27

Avulsion of scalp. BANKS, A. G. Brit. M. J. *2:*893–894, Nov 17, '28

Avulsion of scalp, skin grafting for complete. HAGGARD, W. D., S. Clin. N. Amer. *10:*719–723, Aug '30

Burns of scalp in women. KINDLAY, R. T. Am. J. Surg. *8:*389–396, Feb '30

Skin-grafting in complete avulsion of scalp. MALLIK, K. L. B. Indian M. Gaz. *66:*86–88, Feb '31

Facial injuries and scalp. RHEA, B. S., J. Tennessee M. A. *24:*41–42, Feb '31

Plastic operation for avulsion of scalp. EHLER, F. Casop. lek. cesk. *70:*1525; 1555; 1578, '31

Scalp – Cont.

Plastic method of repairing defects in soft coverings of cranium due to trauma. FLICK, K. AND TRAUM, E. Zentralbl. f. Chir. *59:*908–909, April 2, '32

Plastic repair of avulsion of scalp. MEYER-BURGDORFF, H. Zentralbl. f. Chir. *59:*1209–1211, May 14, '32

Total avulsion of scalp; new method of restoration. MITCHELL, G. F. Brit. M. J. *1:*13–14, Jan 7, '33

Removal of wens – simple technic. WARING, J. B. H. Virginia M. Monthly *59:*607–608, Jan '33

Large scalp wound treated by total homoplastic graft of large cellulocutaneous flap. DUFOURMENTEL, L. Bull. et mem. Soc. d. chirurgiens de Paris *25:*724–726, Dec 15, '33

Therapy of lupus by transplantation of tubular grafts from scalp. MOURE, P. AND BARRAYA. Bull. Soc. franc. de dermat. et syph. *41:*136–137, Jan '34

Replacement of tissues of forehead and scalp. NEW, G. B. *et al.* S. Clin. North America *14:*607–613, June '34

Congenital absence of skin on skull. KOLBE, L. Orvosi hetil. *78:*1039–1040, Nov 10, '34

Congenital absence of skin above small fontanelle in new-born infant. FROMMOLT, G. Ztschr. f. Geburtsch. u. Gynak. *108:*178–179, '34

Therapy of scalping wounds (head). SOLOVEV, A. G. Sovet. khir. (no. 6) *6:*805–813, '34

Avulsion of scalp treated without grafting. OTTO, T. O. Ann. Surg. *102:*315–317, Aug '35

Restoration of scalp avulsion. FLYNN, R. M. J. Australia *2:*525–526, Sept 25, '37

Plastic repair of scalp. ZHOLONDZ, A. M. Khirurgiya, no. 9, pp. 151–152, '37

Complete avulsion of scalp and loss of right ear; reconstruction by pedunculated tube grafts and costal cartilage. CAHILL, J. A. JR. AND CAULFIELD, P. A. Surg., Gynec. and Obst. *66:*459–465, Feb (no. 2A) '38

Traumatic alopecias of scalp; different types. RABUT, R. Presse med. *46:*379–380, March 9, '38

Value of delayed single pedicle skin flaps in plastic repair of scalp. DAVIS, W. B. Surg., Gynec. & Obst. *66:*899–901, May '38

Massive angioma of scalp; rapid growth; case. PAUTRIER, L. M. AND ROEDERER, J. Bull. Soc. franc. de dermat. et syph. (Reunion dermat., Strabourg) *45:*692–694, May '38

Complete avulsion of scalp (case in operator

Scalp—Cont.

of buttercutting machine). WILKER, W. F. Wisconsin M. J. *37:*900–903, Oct '38

Augustin Belloste and treatment for avulsion of scalp; old history of operation in head surgery. STRAYER, L. M. New England J. Med. *220:*901–905, June 1, '39

Rare congenital malformation of eyelid, eyebrow, scalp and of eyeball; case. VALERIO, M. Ann. di ottal. e clin. ocul. *67:*704–714, Sept '39

Use of flaps from avulsed scalp and skin grafts in repair of total avulsion. ECKHARDT, G. Zentralbl. f. Chir. *66:*2337–2340, Oct 28, '39

Etiology and treatment of common diseases of face and scalp (acne). BARBER, H. W. Guy's Hosp. Gaz. *53:*397–399, Dec 16, '39 *53:*382, Dec 2, '39

Total avulsion of scalp; case. TOMILIN, A. I. Vestnik khir. *59:*375, April '40

Therapy of wounds associated with avulsion of scalp. ZHURAVLEVA, E. P. Vestnik khir. *59:*373–375, April '40

Late sequels of roentgen depilation of scalp. PROPPE, A. AND GAHLEN, W. Arch. f. Dermat. u. Syph. *108:*155–164, '40

Avulsion of scalp; case. SANTILLAN, J. S. *et al*. Rev. filipina de med. y farm. *32:*1–5; 10, Jan '41

Extensive mole of face and scalp; excision and full thickness skin graft. FIGI, F. A. Proc. Staff Meet., Mayo Clin. *16:*280–282, April 30, '41

Free graft of scalp in repair of alopecia of eyebrows. SILVEIRA, L. M. Arq. de cir. clin. e exper. *6:*689–692, April–June '42

Successful modern plastic surgery in serious disfiguration due to scalping; reconstruction of eyelids and eyebrows and replacement of total skin of forehead and temples. VON SEEMEN, H. Zentralbl. f. Chir. *69:*1280–1287, Aug 1, '42

Avulsion of scalp; case. RYLANDER, C. M. AND KISNER, W. H. Am. J. Surg. *58:*150–151, Oct '42

Scalping treated with free skin grafts. COVARRUBIAS ZENTENO, R. Arch. Soc. cirujanos hosp. *13:*115–118, Sept '43

Hair-bearing scalp flap for repair of unilateral scalp defects. NEW, G. B. AND ERICH, J. B., S. Clin. North America *24:*741–750, Aug '44

Closure of wounds of the scalp. GILLIES, H. Lancet *2:*310–311, Sept 2, '44

Complete avulsion of scalp; review of literature and case report. EISENSTRODT, L. W. Am. J. Surg. *68:*376–382, June '45

Scalp—Cont.

Total avulsion of scalp; review of problem with presentation of case of skin graft in which thrombin plasma fixation was used. STRAITH, C. L. AND MCEVITT, W. G. Occup. Med. *1:*451–462, May '46

Two cases avulsion of scalp. KELLY, M. W. Am. J. Surg. *72:*103–109, July '46

Scalp, Avulsion

Surgical removal and pathological study of massive squamous cell epithelioma associated with angioma of scalp. PULFORD, D. S. AND ADSON, A. W. Surg., Gynec. & Obst. *42:*846–848, June '26

Coexistence of basal celled epithelioma of temporal region and spinocellular epithelioma of lip; case. MARIN, A. Union med. du Canada *61:*770–772, June '32

Avulsion of scalp, treated by large free skin flaps by "grate" or "sieve" method; case. DIAZ INFANTE, A. Medicina, Mexico *17:*107–114, March 10, '37

Total avulsion of scalp with comment on treatment of wound; case. HARTTUNG, H. Zentralbl. f. Chir. *66:*951–953, April 22, '39

Reconstruction of scalp following excision for malignancy. STEISS, C. F. Am. J. Surg. *52:*378–380, May '41

Total avulsion of scalp; therapy of case. DUFRESNE, E. Union med. du Canada *70:*825–829, Aug '41

SCARCELLA PERINO, G.: Complications of unilateral harelip. Stomatol. *33:*56–62, Jan '35

SCARFF, J. E.: Surgical treatment of injuries of brain, spinal cords, peripheral nerves. Surg. Gynec. & Obst. *81:*405–424, Oct '45

SCARFF, R. W. (see PATEY, D. H.) July '44

SCARFF, R. W. (see Patey, D. H.) Feb '45

SCARLETT, H. W.: Operation according to Shoemaker method for ptosis. Am. J. Ophth. *11:*779–780, Oct '28

Scars

Cicatricial contractures. VAN NECK, M. Arch. franco-belges de chir. *26:*245–257, March '23 (illus.) abstr: J.A.M.A. *80:*1813, June 16, '23

Disfiguring scars; prevention and treatment. DORRANCE, G. M. AND BRANSFIELD, J. W. Am. J. M. Sc. *165:*562–567, April '23 (illus.)

Surgery of head without scars. DUFOURMENTEL, L. Medecine *5:*52, Oct '23

Typical cicatricial bridges between fingers of dairymaids. PICHLER, K. Wien. klin. Wchnschr. *36:*850–851, Nov 29, '23 (illus.)

Successful radiotherapy of cicatrices and ke-

Scars – Cont.
loids with case report. Du Bois, C. Rev. med. de la Suisse Rom. *44:*705–713, Nov '24
Iontophoresis in treatment of deforming or adherent scars. Bourguignon, G. Paris med. *2:*515-520, Dec 20, '24 abstr: J.A.M.A. *84:*404, Jan 31, '25
Therapeutic softening of scar tissue. Stoeltzner, W. Munchen. med. Wchnschr. *72:*2133-2135, Dec 11, '25 abstr: J.A.M.A. *86:*384, Jan 30, '26
Therapeutic softening of scar tissue. Stoye, W. Munchen. med. Wchnschr. *72:*2135–2138, Dec 11, '25 abstr: J.A.M.A. *86:*384, Jan 30, '26
Liquefaction of fatty tissue and softening of scars; experimental studies on action of pepsin. Roos, J. Zentralbl. f. Chir. *53:*2136-2144, Aug 21, '26.
Practical experiences with some "scar dissolving" substances. Kurtzahn, H. and v. Bülow, W. Deutsche Ztschr. f. Chir. *198:*43–52, '26
Scars; new triple technic for reducing disfiguring cicatrices to degree of invisibility amounting to practical removal. Grattan, J. F., J.A.M.A. *88:*638–641, Feb 26, '27
Plastic surgery; removal of scars by stages. Sistrunk, W. E. Ann. Surg. *85:*185-187, Feb '27
Surgical correction of cervicofacial scars of dental origin. Maurel, G., J. de med. de Paris *46:*577–583, July 21, '27
Treatment of facial scars, with remarks on their psychological aspects. Hunt, H. L. Am. J. Surg. *4:*313-320, March '28
Cosmetic treatment of facial scars. Eitner, E. Urol. & Cutan. Rev. *32:*282, May '28
Repair of faulty, postoperative cicatrices of mastoid region. Grivot, M. Ann. d. mal. de l'oreille, du larynx *48:*666–670, June '29
Plastic surgery in retractile cicatrices or extensive loss of skin; cases. Mirizzi, P. L. Rev. de cir. *8:*337-348, Aug '29
Removal of wide scars and large disfigurements of skin by gradual partial excision with closure. Davis, J. S. Ann. Surg. *90:*645-653, Oct '29
Plastic surgery of cicatrices. Sanvenero-Rosselli, G. Igiene e vita *12:*406-410, Oct '29
Eliminating facial scars. Bames, H. O., M. J. & Rec. *131:*348–350, April 2, '30
Removal of large scars or blemishes (nevi) by graduated partial removal. Packard, G. B. Jr. Colorado Med. *28:*289–292, July '31
Full-thickness skin graft in correction of soft tissue deformities (cicatrices). Padgett, E. C., Tr. Sect. Surg., Gen. & Abd., A.M.A.,

Scars – Cont.
pp. 304–319, '31 also: J.A.M.A. *98:*18–23, Jan 2, '32
X-ray treatment of keloidal and hypertrophic scars. Sherman, B. H. Radiology *18:*754–757, April '32
Correction of cicatrices from smallpox and acne necrotica. Halle, M. Fortschr. d. Therap. *8:*505-506, Aug 25, '32
Therapy of scars after variola and acne necrotica. Halle, M. Rev. de chir. plastique, pp. 293–294, Oct '32
Plastic surgery of cicatrical contractures of skin. Karfík, V. Casop. lek. cesk. *71:*1289–1292, Oct 7, '32
Traumatic facial scarring; removal. Figi, F. A., S. Clin. North America *13:*882–884, Aug '33
Adherent scars; their treatment (with skin grafts.). Kiskadden, W. S. California & West. Med. *39:*109–113, Aug '33
Paraffin therapy of burns produced by heat and cold and for cicatrices. Jouan, S. *et al.* Rev. med. latino-am. *18:*1424–1427, Sept '33
Cicatrization and scars. Dantrelle. Rev. de chir. plastique, pp. 301–319, Jan '34
Retractile scars. Dufourmentel, L. Bull. med., Paris *48:*85, Feb 10, '34
Radium treatment of cicatricial keloids. Fuhs, H. Med. Klin. *30:*160–161, Feb 2, '34
Use of radium in traumatic and postoperative scars. Keith, D. Y. Radiol. Rev. & Chicago M. Rec. *56:*61–63, March '34
Postoperative cicatrices in otorhinolaryngologic surgery. Dufourmentel, L. Prat. med. franc. *15:*243-247, April (B) '34
Cosmetic therapy of facial cicatrices. Eitner, E. Wien. med. Wchnschr. *84:*555–556, May 12, '34
Skin grafts in correction of deforming scars. Weichherz, I. Budapesti orvosi ujsag *32:*796–798, Aug 30, '34
Treatment of head scars in Japan. Mayeda, T. Ztschr. d. japan. chirurg. Gesellsch. *35:*59–60, '34
Surgical treatment of smallpox scars. Gurvich, M. O. Sovet. vrach. gaz., pp. 421–422, March 15, '35
Deforming scars; causes, prevention and treatment. Webster, J. P. Pennsylvania M. J. *38:*929–938, Sept '35
Study of favorable conditions for cicatrix formation; practical application in skin grafting. Dufourmentel, L. Bull. et mem. Soc. d. chirurgiens de Paris *28:*401–423, June 19, '36
Causes of abnormal cicatrization. Gery, L. Bull. et mem. Soc. d. chirurgiens de Paris

Scars—Cont.
*28:*405–417, June 19, '36
Cicatrix in reparative surgery of breast. CLAOUE, C. AND BERNARD, MME. I., J. de med. de Bordeaux *113:*695–697, Oct 10, '36
Scars of facial wounds. STRAITH, C. L. Am. J. Surg. *36:*88–90, April '37
Concealment of scars (with covermark). TAMERIN, J. A. Am. J. Surg. *36:*91–92, April '37
Repair of depressed disfiguring scars by means of rib cartilage implant. TRUSLER, H. M., J. Indiana M.A. *30:*194–196, April '37
Disfiguring scars in industrial and civil accidents. SEGRE, G. Minerva med. *1:*61–65, Jan 20, '38
Removal of accidental vaccination scar by blistering doses of ultraviolet rays. FISHER, A. A., J.A.M.A. *110:*642–643, Feb 26, '38
Use of relaxation incision in treatment of scars. DAVIS, J. S. Pennsylvania M. J. *41:*565–572, April '38
Medicamentous cosmetics for plastic covering of grave cicatrices left by various diseases. DAUBRESSE-MORELLE, E. Rev. Franc. de dermat. et de venereol. *14:*355–362, Sept–Oct '38
Human oil (from omental fat) in treatment of adherant scars. WAKELEY, C. P. G. Brit. M. J. *2:*618–619, Sept 17, '38
Cyrotherapy (with mixture containing carbon dioxide snow) for acne and its scars. KARP, F. L. *et al.* Arch. Dermat. & Syph. *39:*995–998, June '39
Significance of subcutaneous scar tissue. MOSIMAN, R. E. West. J. Surg. *47:*397–401, July '39
Facial scars; evaluation in medicolegal expertise. DOMENICI, F. Boll. d. Soc. med.-Chir., Pavia *53:*41–55, '39
Plastic surgery in therapy of facial scars (grafts). DUJARDIN, E. Ugesk. f. laeger *102:*222, Feb 29, '40
Spectral analysis of eschars. MAYER, F. X. AND PESTA, H. Wien. klin. Wchnschr. *53:*397–399, May 17, '40
Surgical therapy of scars. GONZALEZ ULLOA, M. Rev. mex. de cir., ginec. y cancer *8:*321–329, Aug '40
Retractile scars of cervicofacial region; biologic fundamentals for plastic reconstruction. ZENO, L. Bol. Soc. de cir. de Rosario *7:*446–454, Nov '40 also: An. de cir. *6:*341–349, Dec '40 also: Dia med. *13:*264–266, April 14, '41
Correction of scars. MAY, H. Am. J. Surg. *50:*754–760, Dec '40
Wound closure, with particular reference to avoidance of scars. UPDEGRAFF, H. L. Am. J. Surg. *50:*749–753, Dec '40
Esthetic surgery for elimination of sequels of smallpox of face in girl 18 years old. KANKAT, C. T. Turk tib cem. mec. *6:*260–266, '40
Skin peeling and scarification in treatment of pitted scars, pigmentations and certain facial blemishes. ELLER, J. J. AND WOLFF, S. J.A.M.A. *116:*2208, May 10, '41
Determination of real defect in plastic repair of cicatrix. GABARRO, P. Rev. san. mil., Buenos Aires *40:*923–926, Oct '41
Evaluation of cryotherapy of post-acne scars. HOLLANDER, L. AND SHELTON, J. M. Pennsylvania M. J. *45:*226–228, Dec '41
Blue scar formation; 2 cases. BARBIERI PALMIERI, C. Boll. Soc. med.-chir. Modena *42:*613–618, '41–'42
Plasticity of cicatricial tissue; application to reparative surgery. ZENO, L. An. de cir. *8:*40–47, March–June '42
Paraffinoma, harelip, cicatrices, auricular prosthesis in plastic surgery. GONCALVES, G. Arq. de cir. clin. e exper. *6:*307–316, April–June '42
Cicatricial tissue as element of plastic repair; tissular reversibility. ZENO, L. Arq. de cir. clin. e exper. *6:*597–608, April–June '42
Plasticity of cicatricial tissue; application to reparative surgery. ZENO, L. Bol. Soc. de cir. de Rosario *9:*5–12, April '42
Cutaneous cicatrix. CORA ELISEHT, F. Prensa med. argent. *29:*1648–1654, Oct 14, '42
Failure with cryotherapy (using carbon dioxide slush) in treatment of acne scars. FRIEDLANDER, H. M. Arch. Dermat. & Syph. *46:*734–736, Nov '42
Free full thickness skin graft; case in cicatrix. MALBEC, E. F. Prensa med. argent. *30:*1576–1577, Aug 18, '43
Fibrokeloid cicatrix after attempted removal of pilous nevus; free full thickness skin graft; case. MALBEC, E. F. Dia med. *15:*1100, Sept. 13, '43
Plastic surgery of cicatrix; case. MARINO, H. Prensa med. argent. *30:*2502–2505, Dec 29, '43
Plastic repair of scar contractures. GREELEY, P. W. Surgery *15:*224–241, Feb '44
Plastic surgery of retractile cicatrix of hand. ZENO, L. An. de cir. *10:*183–185, Sept–Dec '44 also: Bol. Soc. de cir. de Rosario *11:*451–454, Nov '44
Retractile cicatrix causing pes planopronatovalgus; plastic surgery in therapy of case. ZENO, L. An. de cir. *10:*179–182, Sept–Dec '44

Scars – Cont.
Defective ulcerated cicatrices; plastic correction. ZENO, L. Bol. Soc. de cir. de Rosario *10:*354-366, Oct-Nov '43 also: An. de cir. *10:*76-88, March-June '44
Adherent scars of lower extremity. WEBSTER, G. V., U.S. Nav. M. Bull. *43:*878-888, Nov '44
Antireticular cytotoxic serum in therapy of ulcerating cicatrix BEREZOV, Y. E. Med. zhur. *13:*101-103, '44
Scar problem in compound injuries of lower leg. WEBSTER, G. V. Stanford M. Bull. *3:*109-113, Aug '45
Cicatrix preventation and treatment; general considerations. PASSALACQUA, L. A. Bol. Asoc. med. de Puerto Rico *37:*355-360, Sept '45
Influence of pH on cicatrization. DESAULNIERS, L. AND DUGAL, L. P. Rev. canad. de biol. *4:*325-333, '45
Fibrous tumor developing on laparotomy cicatrix; case. CREYSSEL, J. AND SAUTOT, J. Lyon chir. *41:*67-68, Jan-Feb '46
Cicatrization of wounds and treatment of cicatrices by massage. LEROY, R. Monde med., Paris *56:*11-26, Jan-Feb '46
Use of x-rays in treatment of indurations due to scars and chronic inflammation. RHYS-LEWIS, R. D. S. Proc. Roy. Soc. Med. *39:*150-151, Feb '46
Formula for cryotherapy (with carbon dioxide slush) for acne and postacne scarring. ZUGERMAN, I. Arch. Dermat. & Syph. *54:*209-210, Aug '46

Scars, Hypertrophic (See also Keloids)
Treatment of hypertrophic cicatrices. NEUMANN, B. I. Vestnik khir. (no. 47) *16:*65-76, '29
Therapy of extensive hypertrophic cutaneous scars by application of mud and injection of turpentine. LANDA, G. I. Klin. med. *16:*99-102, '38
Zinc iontophoresis (ion transfer) in hypertrophic scars. KRICHEVSKIY, A. M. Sovet. med. (no. 1) *7:*7-9, '43

SCAVUZZO, R.: Esthetic surgery; criteria or artistic precepts (nose). Semana med. *1:*144-146, Jan 19, '39
SCEVOLA, P.: Mast cells as system of local and general defense in burns of mammals. Arch. ital. di otol. *50:*169-199, April '38
SCHAAF, R. A.: Burns. J. M. Soc. New Jersey *40:*128-133, April '43
SCHABADASCH, A.: Principles of and method for compensating for nerve deficiency by grafting prepared nervous tissue. Compt. rend. Acad. d. sc. URSS *43:*40-42, April 10, '44
SCHACHTER, M. (see KREINDLER, A.) Aug '34
SCHACHTER, R. J.: Use of cholinesterase (and plasma) in shock. Am. J. Physiol. *143:*552-557, April '45
SCHAEFER, A. A.: Therapy of thermal burns. Marquette M. Rev. *4:*101-106, March '40
SCHAEFER, A. A.: Burn therapy. Wisconsin M. J. *40:*391-393, May '41
SCHAEFER, A. A.: Modern burn treatment. Marquette M. Rev. *8:*93-97, Aug '43
SCHAEFER, A. A.: Burn therapy. Wisconsin M. J. *42:*1052-1054, Oct '43
SCHAEFER, A. A. AND SAKAGUCHI, S.: Report of 2 patients with exstrophy of bladder operated upon at 2 months of age. J. Pediat. *26:*492-500, May '45
SCHAEFER, A. A. (see SEEGER, S. J.) Nov-Dec '34
SCHAEFER, F. (see HOEDE, K.) 1940
SCHAEFER, J. E.: Osteomyelitis of jaws. J. Am. Dent. A. *16:*2188-2216, Dec '29
SCHAEFER, J. E.: Oral and plastic surgery. J. Indiana M. A. *33:*60-66, Feb '40
SCHAEFER, V.: Importance of predisposition, chronic trauma and accident in genesis of Dupuytren's contracture. Zentralbl. f. Chir. *63:*1712-1716, July 18, '36
SCHAEFFER, G. C.: Plastic surgery, its relation to general surgery. Ohio State M. J. *21:*11-14, Jan '25
SCHAEFFER, G. C.: Saddle nose; unfortunate result of too thorough operation for deflected septum. Ohio State M. J.: *23:*989, Dec '27
SCHAFER, D. P. H.: Facial hemiatrophy. M. J. Australia *1:*901-902, June 29, '40
SCHALIT, A.: Nasal voice; treatment by obturator. Wien. med. Wchnschr. *78:*964-966, July 14, '28
SCHALIT, A.: New obturator (meatus obturator) for preventing nasal speech in cleft palate. Ztschr. f. Stomatol. *26:*888-898, Sept '28
SCHALIT, A.: Obturator of choice for congenital cleft palate. Am. J. Orthodontics (Oral Surg. Sect.) *32:*688-713, Nov '46
SCHALIT, A. (see FRÖSCHELS, E.) Nov '29
SCHALIT, H. (see FRÖSCHELS, E.) June '28
SCHAMBERG, J. F.: Basal-cell carcinoma of face. S. Clin. N. Amer. *7:*113-115, Feb '27
SCHAMBYE, G. (see UHLMANN, E.) '35
SCHAPIRO, I. E., WALDEN, A. AND CARMAN, G. A.: Obturator (acrylic) for newborn infant with cleft palate. J. Pediat. *27:*288-290, Sept '45
SCHARAPO, M.: Snegiroff's method of formation of artificial vagina; case. Zentralbl. f. Gynak. *51:*1131-1133, April 30, '27
SCHARF, J.: Familial eyelid and ophthalmoplegia of supranuclear type. Klin. Monatsbl. f.

Augenh. *101:*71–76, July '38

SCHARFE, E. E.: Value of speech training in cleft palate. Tr. Sect. Laryng., Otol. & Rhin., A.M.A., pp. 116–128, '35

SCHARFE, E. E.: Value of speech training in cleft palate. Arch. Oto-laryng. *22:*585–596, Nov '35 also: Canad. M. A. J. *33:*641–647, Dec '35

SCHARFE, E. E.: Method of fixation in fractures involving maxillary antrum. Canad. M. A. J. *50:*435–437, May '44

SCHARNAGEL, I. M.: Melanoma of skin. J. Am. M. Women's A. *1:*76–83, June '46

SCHARNAGEL, I. M. (see PACK G. T. *et al*) June '45

SCHATTNER, A.: Skin isograft transplants in identical twins. Arch. Otolaryng. *39:*521–522, June '44

SCHATTNER, A. (see GRIFFITH, C. M.) April '33

SCHATZKI, P.: Heredity of concealed syndactylic polydactylia. Arch. f. orthop. u. Unfall-Chir. *36:*613, '36

SCHAUBEL, H. J. AND SMITH, E. W.: Splint for treatment of mallet finger. J. Bone & Joint Surg. *28:*394–395, Apr '46

SCHAUBEL, H. J. (see ROBERTS, W. M.) Jan '45

SCHAXEL, J.: Regeneration and transplantation of tissue. Zool. Anz. *78:*153–157, Sept 1, '28

SCHECK, M.: New method (transplantation of flexor pollicis longus tendon) for relief of paralysis of opponens pollicis. Indian M. Gaz. *75:*464–466, Aug '40

SCHEEL, P. F.: Muscle transplantation. Deutsche Ztschr. f. Chir. *192:*136–142, '25

SCHEFFELAAR KLOTS, T. (see VAN DER LEE, H. S.) Dec '29

SCHEGGI, S.: Cause of irreducibility of metacarpophalangeal joint of index finger in palmar luxation; 6 cases. Chir. d. org. di movimento *20:*142–148, July '35

SCHEGGI, S.: Technic for surgical reduction of palmar metacarpophalangeal luxation of thumb and index finger. Chir. d. org. di movimento *22:*281–284, Aug '36

SCHEIN, A. J. (see SELIG S.) April '40

SCHELLING, V. (see HARTMAN, F. W.) Dec '39

SCHENA, A. T.: Metacarpophalangeal luxation of index finger; case. Dia med. *11:*267–269, April 3, '39

SCHENK, P.: Angiomas of parotid region. Mitt. a. d. Grenzgeb. d. Med. u. chir. *37:*51–55, '23

SCHEPETINSKY, A.: Baldwin operation for artificial vagina. Monatschr. f. Geburtsh. u. Gynak. *95:*270–273, Oct '33

SCHEPPOKAT: Frequent occurrence of scarlet fever following cleft palate operations. Deutsche Ztschr. f. Chir. *218:*383–386, '29

SCHER, S. L.: Nasal deformities. Arch. Otolaryng. *34:*307–320, Aug '41

SCHER, S. L.: Deformed chin and lower jaw. Ann. Surg. *115:*869–879, May '42

SCHERB, R.: Functional adaption of muscles after transplantation of muscle tendons. Ztschr. f. orthop. Chir. *48:*582–592, Nov 18, '27

SCHERB, R.: Functional adaptability, inhibition and repair of antagonistic muscles in poliomyelitis; role in tendon transplantation; biologic aspect. Ztschr. f. orthop. Chir. *50:*470–493, Nov. 13, '28

SCHERB, R.: Tendon transplantation in therapy of poliomyelitic paralysis; cases. Schweiz. med. Wchnschr. *68:*354–360, April 2, '38

SCHERER, F.: Reverdin mosaic grafts. Deutsche Ztschr. f. Chir. *258:*42, '43

SCHERWITZ, K.: Surgical therapy of local gigantism of one leg resulting from congenital vascular abnormality. Chirurg. *15:*263, May 1, '43

SCHETTINO, M.: De Quervain's stenosing tendovaginitis (Winterstein's styloidalgia radii); 8 cases. Riforma med. *48:*1142–1145, July 23, '32

SCHIE, E.: Traumatic exophthalmos and its treatment. Nord. med. (Norsk mag. f. laegevidensk.) *7:*1275–1283, July 27, '40

SCHIEBEL, H. M. (see SHANDS, A. R. JR.) April '37

SCHIESS, EMILE: *Considerations sur les fractures du maxillaire inferieur*. Hans Huber, Berne, '32

SCHIESSL, M.: Incision in natural folds of hand; contribution to treatment of cellulitis of sheaths of tendons and calluses. Munchen. med. Wchnschr. *72:*1728–1730, Oct 9, '25 abstr: J.A.M.A. *85:*1681, Nov 21, '25

SCHIEVERS, J. (see HELDERWEIRT, G. *et al*) Dec '38

SCHIFFMANN, H.: Pseudarthroses in fractures of terminal phalanx. Rontgenpraxis *9:*394–399, June '37

SCHILDT, E.: Fractures of upper jaw, malar bone and zygomatic arch. Nord. med. (Hygiea) *16:*3700–3705, Dec 26, '42

SCHILLING, B.: Plastic surgery of artificial vagina. Orvosi hetil. *79:*863–866, Aug 10, '35

SCHILLING, F.: Low position of right breast. Arch. f. Verdauungskr. *32:*81–82, Sept '23

SCHILOWZEFF, S. P. (see SHILOVTSEV, S. P.)

SCHIRESON, HENRY J.: *As Others See You: The Story of Plastic Surgery*. Macauley, New York, '38

SCHJØTH-IVERSEN, I.: Syndactylia operated on according to Klapp method. Norsk mag. f. laegevidensk. *97:*700–704, July '36

SCHLAEPFER, K.: Plastic operations on face. Schweiz. med. Wchnschr. *52:*383–386, April 20, '22

SCHLAEPFER, K.: Closure of granulating wounds with Reverdin-Halsted grafts. Bull. Johns Hopkins Hosp. *34:*114–118, April '23 (illus.) also: Beitr. z. klin. Chir. *129:*162–174, '23 abstr: J.A.M.A. *80:*1884, June 23, '23
SCHLAEPFER, K.: Antagonistic effect of metrazol in shock. Anesth. and Analg. *15:*202–206, July–Aug '36
SCHLAMPP, H. (see MORAL, H.) Nov '29
SCHLAMPP, H. (see MORAL, H.) Nov '30
SCHLAMPP, H. (see MORAL, H.) Nov '31
SCHLANDER, E.: Surgical correction of abnormally protruding ears. Chirurg *2:*699–704, Aug 1, '30
SCHLÄPFER, H.: Correction of entropion according to Vogt method. Klin. Monatsbl. f. Augenh. *94:*610–611, May '35
SCHLEICHER, R. (see CAMERER, J. W.) Feb '35
SCHLEIPEN, C.: Value of cardiazol (metrazol) as analeptic in surgery to prevent shock. Munchen. med. Wchnschr. *77:*1101–1103, June 27, '30
SCHLESINGER: Comment on Kromayer's article on removal of facial wrinkles. Deutsche med. Wchnschr. *55:*1512–1513, Sept 6, '29
SCHLESINGER, E.: Technic of plastic surgery of breast. Zentralbl. f. Gynak. *57:*440–442, Feb 18, '33
SCHLESSELMAN, J. T.: Nasal splint. Arch. Otolaryng. *29:*988–989, June '39
SCHLEUSS, W.: Speech training of children with cleft palate. Eos *21:*29–38, '29
SCHLITTLER, E.: Trophic postencephalitic ulcerations of outer nose and of cheek. Schweiz. med. Wchnschr. *59:*1121–1122, Nov 9, '29
SCHLOFFER, H.: Treatment of torn extensor tendons of terminal phalanges. Zentralbl. f. Chir. *57:*1053–1055, April 26, '30
SCHLOSSER: Dupuytren's contracture, development favored by existence of diabetes mellitus; case. Munchen. med. Wchnschr. *79:*1238, July 29, '32
SCHMELEW, W.: Artificial vagina formed from rectum; 2 cases. Med. Welt *2:*403–405, March 17, '28
SCHMELKES, F. C. (see ANDRUS, W. DEW. *et al*) Jan '43
SCHMERZ, H.: Operative correction of paralysis of lower lip. Arch. f. klin. Chir. *131:*353–360, '24 abstr: J.A.M.A. *83:*1464, Nov 1, '24
SCHMID, B.: Plastic surgery in therapy of irreparable facial paralyses; Lexer-Rosenthal method. Zentralbl. f. Chir. *65:*1296–1297, June 4, '38
SCHMID, H. H.: Artificial vagina from bladder. Monatschr. f. Geburtsh. u. Gynak. *72:*330–336, March '26
SCHMID, R.: Useful prostheses for nasal and facial defects due to destructive lesions. Munchen. med. Wchnschr. *85:*1784–1786, Nov 18, '38 comment by Moncorps *86:*252–253, Feb 17, '39
SCHMID, R.: Practical elastic permanent prosthesis for facial defects. Munchen. med. Wchnschr. *91:*183, April 7, '44
SCHMID, W.: Surgical therapy of facial furuncle. Chirurg *6:*447–456, June 15, '34
SCHMIDHUBER, K. F.: Treatment of military facial injuries. Deut. Militararzt *5:*418–419, Oct '40
SCHMIDT, A.: Surgical treatment of hermaphroditism. Orvosi hetil. *80:*719–722, Aug 1, '36
SCHMIDT, A.: Surgical therapy of hermaphroditism. Ztschr. f. Urol. *35:*152–169, '41
SCHMIDT, B.: Rare malformation of nose; case. Monatschr. f. Ohrenh. *72:*880–893, Sept '38
SCHMIDT, C.: Plastic reconstruction of larynx and trachea. Schweiz. med. Wchnschr. *52:*539–540, May 25, '22
SCHMIDT, C.: Tamponing nose (after surgery). Schweiz. med. Wchnschr. *52:*540–541, May 25, '22 (illus.)
SCHMIDT, E. R.: Burn therapy. Am. J. Surg. *8:*274–276, Feb '30
SCHMIDT, G.: Surgical correction of prognathism; 7 cases. Deutsche Ztschr. f. Chir. *215:*212–225, '29
SCHMIDT, G.: Surgical therapy of ordinary dislocations of lower jaw. Deutsche Ztschr. f. Chir. *233:*536–542, '31
SCHMIDT, G.: Surgical approach in operations on temporomaxillary articulation and on upper portion of ascending ramus of maxilla. Deutsche Ztschr. f. Chir. *236:*260–265, '32
SCHMIDT, G. AND REICHENBACH, E.: "Open bite"; surgical and prosthetic treatment. Deutsche Ztschr. f. Chir. *237:*167–176, '32
SCHMIDT, L.: Extension apparatus for crooked fingers. Deutsche med. Wchnschr. *47:*564, May 19, '21
SCHMIDT, P.: Sound for dilating strictures of naso-lacrimal duct. Klin. Monatsbl. f. Augenh. *80:*390, March 23, '28
SCHMIDT, W.: Keloid on tip of tongue in trumpeter; case. Dermat. Wchnschr. *99:*1341–1342, Oct 13, '34
SCHMIDT, W. H.: Treatment of precancerous and cancerous lesions in mouth. New York M. J. *118:*732–737, Dec 19, '23 (illus.)
SCHMIDT, W. T.: Successful grafting of hypoglossal on facial nerve. Munchen. med. Wchnschr. *69:*708–709, May 12, '22 (illus.)
SCHMIDT, W. T.: Successful plastic operation for vaginal atresia, using portion of ileum for new wall; case. Monatschr. f. Geburtsch. u. Gynak. *97:*50–52, April '34
SCHMIEDEN, V,: Radical surgical therapy of lupus (grafting). Zentralbl. f. Chir. *61:*790–793,

April 7, '34
SCHMIEGELOW, E.: Surgical treatment of chronic cicatricial stenosis of larynx; Semon lecture. J. Laryng. & Otol. *53:*1-14, Jan '38
SCHMIER, A. A.: Fracture of zygomatic bone and arch; postoperative headgear. Am. J. Surg. *70:*27-37, Oct '45
SCHMORELL, H.: Surgical treatment of injuries of hand and finger, with exception of fractures. Med. Klin. *29:*1382, Oct 6; 1414, Oct 13, '33
SCHMORELL, H.: Surgical treatment of injuries of hand and fingers, with exception of bone fractures. Med. Klin. *29:*1449-1450, Oct 20, '33
SCHMUZIGER, P.: Jaw fractures treated by Swiss accident insurance, 1923-1926; 178 cases. Schweiz. Monatschr. f. Zahnh. *39:*234-260, April '29
SCHMUZIGER, P.: Principles of treatment of fractures of superior and inferior maxillae. Schweiz. med. Wchnschr. *60:*101-104, Feb 1, '30
SCHMUZIGER, P.: Fracture of zygomatic arch; 2 cases with cicatricial closure of jaws. Schweiz. med. Wchnschr. *65:*721-722, Aug 10, '35
SCHMUZIGER, P.: Surgical therapy of prognathism. Helvet. med. acta *3:*834-839, Dec '36
SCHMUZIGER, P.: Immediate care of war wounds of face and jaw. Helvet. med. acta *8:*49-53, April '41
SCHNEDORF, J. G. AND ORR, T. G.: Beneficial effects of oxygen therapy in experimental traumatic shock. Surg., Gynec. and Obst. *73:*79-83, July '41
SCHNEDORF, J. G. AND ORR, T. G.: Oxygen therapy in shock due to hemorrhage. Surg., Gynec. and Obst. *73:*495-497, Oct '41
SCHNEIDER, C. C.: Stenosing fibrous tendovaginitis over radial styloid (de Quervain). Surg., Gynec. and Obst. *46:*846-850, June '28
SCHNEIDER, E. (see FOHL, T.) '29
SCHNEIDER, P.: Medicolegal aspects in plastic surgery. Wien. klin. Wchnschr. *52:*1029-1031, Nov 17, '39
SCHNEIDER, R.: Palliative operation for eyelid ptosis. Ber. u. d. Versamml. d. deutsch. ophth. Gesellsch. (1928) *47:*274-277, '29
SCHNEIDER, R. C. (see WEBSTER, J. E. *et al*) July '46
SCHNEK, F.: Use of splints in wounds of fingers. Munchen. med. Wchnschr. *74:*977-979, June 10, '27
SCHNEK, F.: Severe hand injury restored to complete function. Arch. f. Orthop. *26:*308-314, March 22, '28
SCHNEK, F.: Harmful effects of hot water in open finger and hand injuries. Munchen. med. Wchnschr. *76:*57-58, Jan 11, '29
SCHNEPP, K. H. (see ZELLE, O. L.) Aug '36
SCHNETZ, H.: Late gangrene of finger after electrical injuries; case. Ztschr. f. klin. Med. *132:*120-127, '37
SCHMINCKE, A. (see ELIMER, G.) March '25
SCHNITKER, M. T.: Peripheral nerve injuries; principles of treatment. Northwest Med. *43:*5-9, Jan '44 also: Bull. U. S. Army M. Dept. (no. 73) pp. 53-61, Feb '44
SCHNITZLER, O.: Significance of occupational and sport injuries in etiology of Dupuytren's contracture. Munchen. med. Wchnschr. *82:*248-249, Feb 14, '35
SCHOEMAKER, J.: Suture technic of palate. Chirurg *1:*1012, Oct 1, '29
SCHOEMAKER, J.: Uranostaphylorrhaphy with Donati suture. Arch. ital. di chir. *54:*513-515, '38
SCHOFIELD, J. E.: Non-filarial elephantiasis therapy (Kondoleon operation). Brit. M. J. *1:*795, May 9, '31
SCHOLE, M. L. AND KATZ, T.: Cleft palate prosthesis. Bull. U.S. Army M. Dept. (no. 84) pp. 90-93, Jan '45
SCHOLL, A. J. JR.: Potential malignancy in exstrophy of bladder. Ann. Surg. *75:*365-371, March '22 (illus.)
SCHOLLE, W.: Dupuytren's contracture; etiology, especially in young adults. Deutsche Ztschr. f. Chir. *223:*328-339, '30
SCHOLLE, W.: Dislocation of 2 joints on same finger. Munchen. med. Wchnschr. *78:*1337-1338, Aug 7, '31
SCHOLONDZ, A. M. (see ZHOLONDZ, A. M.)
SCHOLTZ, A.: Multiple deformities of hand. Ztschr. f. Orthop. *72:*231-237, '41
SCHOLZ. (see BLUME) Feb '29
SCHOMAKER, T. P. (see MEHERIN, J. M.) April '39

Schönborn Operation

Schönborn operation (velopharyngorrhaphy) for correction of defective speech. SEEMANN, M. Casop. lek. cesk. *70:*1570-1574, Nov 20, '31 also: Otolaryng. slavica *4:*24-25, Jan '32
Schönborn-Rosenthal operation for cleft palate. FRÜND, H. Zentralbl. f. Chir. *54:*3206-3210, Dec 10, '27

SCHÖNE, G.: "Biochemical" individuality; experiments with homeoplastic transplants. Zentralbl. f. Chir. *68:*1523-1546, Aug 9, '41
SCHÖNFELD, M.: Atresia of urethral orifice with penoscrotal hypospadias. Casop. lek. cesk. *70:*921-923, June 26, '31
SCHÖRCHER, F.: Dislocations of 2 joints of same finger; case. Chirurg *4:*150-151, Feb 15, '32

SCHÖRCHER, F.: Shock, collapse and electrosurgery. Deutsche Ztschr. f. Chir. *243:*225–273, '34
SCHÖRCHER, F.: Phlegmon of tendon sheaths. Med. Klin. *34:*1647–1649, Dec 16, '38
SCHÖRCHER, F.: Traumatic edema of hand. Beitr. z. klin. Chir. *171:*176–194, '40
SCHÖRCHER, F.: Snapping of finger joints due to injury to tendons. Zentralbl. f. chir. *67:*627–628, April 6, '40
SCHORK, C. J.: Prosthetic appliance for comminuted fracture of nose; case. J. Oral Surg. *2:*324–328, Oct '44
SCHORK, C. J. (see MAXWELL, M. M. *et al*) Oct '46
SCHORNSTEIN, T.: Question of congenital fistula of lacrimal gland; case. Arch. f. Augenh. *109:*86–102, '35
SCHORSTEIN, J.: Erosion of ala nasi following trigeminal denervation. J. Neurol. and Psychiat. *6:*46–51, Jan-April '43
SCHORSTEIN, J.: Compound fronto-orbital fractures; 8 cases. Brit. J. Surg. *31:*221–230, Jan '44
SCHORSTEIN, J.: Gunshot wounds of fronto-orbital region. Lancet *1:*44–47, Jan 8, '44
SCHORSTEIN, J. (see CLARKSON, P.) Sept '45
SCHOSSERER, W.: Primary plastic operations on fingers. Deutsche Ztschr. f. Chir. *233:*434–440, '31
SCHRADER, E.: Three-jointed thumbs; case. Fortschr. a. d. Geb. d. Rontgenstrahlen *40:*693, Oct '29
SCHREIBER, F.: Rhinoplasty; 3 cases. Beitr. z. klin. Chir. *144:*307, '28
SCHREIBER, F.: Operation for pendulous breast. Beitr. z. klin. Chir. *147:*56–59, '29
SCHREIBER, F.: Plastic surgery of face. Ztschr. f. Laryng., Rhin. *20:*1–9, Oct '30
SCHREIBER, F.: Surgical therapy of pendulous breasts. An. Fac. de med. de Montevideo *26:*251–271, '41
SCHREINER, B. F. AND CHRISTY, C. J.: Results of irradiation treatment for cancer of lips; analysis of 636 cases from 1926–1936. Radiology *39:*293–297, Sept '42
SCHREINER, B. F. AND KRESS, L. C.: Contribution to treatment of cancer of lip by irradiation; report on 136 cases. J. Cancer Research *8:*221–233, July '24
SCHREINER, B. F. AND MATTICK, W. L.: Study of 66 cases of salivary gland tumors. Am. J. Roentgenol. *21:*541–546, June '29
SCHREINER, B. F. AND MATTICK, W. L.: Five-year end-results obtained by radiation treatment of cancer of lips. Am. J. Roentgenol. *30:*67–74, July '33
SCHREINER, B. F. AND SIMPSON, B. T.: End-results of irradiation of cancer of lips; based on study of 173 cases, January 1914 to January 1924. Radiol. Rev. and Chicago M. Rec. *51:*235–245, June '29
SCHREINER, B. F. AND SIMPSON, B. T.: Five year end-results of radiation treatment of cancer of oral cavity, nasopharynx and pharynx, based on study of 309 cases, 1912–1923. Radiol. Rev. and Chicago M. Rec. *51:*327–332, Aug '29
SCHREINER, B. F. AND WEHR, W. H.: Primary new growths involving hand. Am. J. Roentgenol. *32:*516–523, Oct '34
SCHREINER, K.: Prevention of deaths from burns by treatment with medicaments, particularly vasano (scopolamine preparation). Med. Klin. *25:*706–708, May 3, '29
SCHREINER, K.: Burn therapy. Wien. klin. Wchnschr. *43:*871–876, July 10, '30
SCHREINER, K. AND STOCKER, H.: Tetanus after burns. Wien. med. Wchnschr. *79:*1020–1022, Aug 3, '29
SCHREINER, K. AND WENDLBERGER, J.: Reaction of reticulo-endothelial system in severe burns. Wien. med. Wchnschr. *83:*891–894, Aug 5, '33
SCHREINER, P. K.: Burns. Med. Klinik *21:*1187–1189, Aug 7; 1231–1233, Aug 14, '25
SCHREK, R.: Skin carcinoma; analysis of 20 cases in Negroes. Cancer Research *4:*119–127, Feb '44
SCHRIDDE, H.: Keloid in man. Klin. Wchnschr. *7:*582–584, March 25, '28
SCHROCK, R. D. AND JOHNSON, H. F.: Free full-thickness skin transplant. Nebraska M. J. *19:*91–93, March '34
SCHRÖDER, C. H.: Hereditary aspect of cleft lip and palate. Arch. f. Rassen-u. Gesellsch. Biol. *25:*369–394, Nov 25, '31
SCHRÖDER, C. H.: Dupuytren's contracture and its relation to trauma and occupation. Deutsche Ztschr. f. Chir. *244:*140–149, '34 abstr.: Arch. f. orthop. u. Unfall-Chir. *35:*125–127, '34
SCHRÖDER, C. H.: Heredity of Dupuytren's contracture. Zentralbl. f. Chir. *61:*1056–1059, May 5, '34
SCHRÖDER, C. H.: Studies on heredity of harelip and cleft palate with particular regard to mode of transmission. Arch. f. klin. Chir. *182:*299–330, '35
SCHRÖDER, C. H.: Hereditary relations between harelip and cleft palate and other malformations, especially of spine. Beitr. z. klin. Chir. *169:*402–413, '39
SCHRÖDER, C. H.: Harelip and cleft palate in uniovular twins. Zentralbl. f. Chir. *66:*2299–2308, Oct 21, '39
SCHRÖDER, C. H. AND HILLENBRAND, H. J.: Significance of occult spina bifida in hered-

ity of harelip and cleft palate. Arch. f. klin. Chir. *203:*328-342, '42

SCHROEDER, E.: Formation of vagina by Schubert method, with fatal result. Zentralbl. f. Gynak. *47:*842–844, May 26, '23 abstr: J.A.M.A. *81:*869, Sept 8, '23

SCHROEDER, H.: Present status of prostheses, etc., for jaws. Arch. f. klin. Chir. *118:*275–297, '21 (illus.)

SCHTARKMAN, (see JOUAN, S. *et al*) Sept '33

SCHUBERT, A.: Etiology of Dupuytren's contracture. Deutsche Ztschr. f. Chir. *177:*362–377, '23

SCHUBERT, A.: Trauma and Dupuytren's contracture. Med. Klin. *23:*549–551, April 15, '27

SCHUBERT, G.: Construction of an artificial vagina. Zentralbl. f. Gynak. *45:*229, Feb. 19, '21

SCHUBERT, G.: Technic for artificial vagina with menstruating uterus. Monatschr. f. Geburtsh. u. Gynak. *65:*45–60, Dec '23

SCHUBERT, G.: Construction of artificial vagina from rectum, with presence of uterus. Beitr. z. klin. Chir. *134:*421–425, '25 abstr: J.A.M.A. *85:*1844, Dec 5, '25

SCHUBERT, G.: Schubert's method for formation of artificial vagina; 20 cases. Zentralbl. f. Gynak. *51:*80–88, Jan 8, '27

SCHUBERT, G.: Artificial vagina justified by subsequent conception and childbirth. Med. Klin. *23:*1334–1336, Sept 2, '27

SCHUBERT, G.: Treatment of persistent tubular urogenital sinus by formation of vagina from rectum; case. Arch. f. Gynak. *141:*228–236, '30

SCHUBERT, G.: Permanent results in Schubert plastic operation for artificial vagina (transplantion of piece of colon). Chirurg *3:*796–801, Sept 15, '31

SCHUBERT, G.: Surgical formation of artificial vagina; review of literature. Ber. u. d. ges. Gynak. u. Geburtsh. *23:*241–268, Dec 27, '32

Schubert Operation

Construction of vagina (Schubert method). KEYSERLINGK, R. Zentralbl. f. Gynak. *46:*380–381, March 11, '22

Artificial vagina made from rectum (Schubert's method). HARTTUNG, H. Zentralbl. f. Gynak. *46:*1610–1612, Oct 7, '22

Formation of vagina by Schubert method, with fatal result. SCHROEDER, E. Zentralbl. f. Gynak. *47:*842–844, May 26, '23 abstr: J.A.M.A. *81:*869, Sept 8, '23

Schubert's method of formation of artificial vagina; cases. WAGNER, G. A. Zentralbl. f. Gynak. *51:*1300–1304, May 21, '27

Schubert's operation for artificial vagina. HILLE, K. Monatschr. f. Geburtsh. u. Gynak. *76:*288–293, June '27

Schubert Operation – Cont.

Schubert's method of plastic construction of vagina; 2 cases. MALUSCHEW, D. Zentralbl. f. Gynak. *53:*428–430, Feb 16, '29

Defective vagina and formation of artificial vagina by Schubert-Grigoriu's method. IUBAS, C. Cluj. med. *10:*404–408, Aug 1, '29

Plastic formation of artificial vagina by Schubert operation; 4 cases. NOVAK, J. Zentralbl. f. Gynak. *53:*2902–2908, Nov 16, '29

Cure of complete incontinentia alvi following Schubert's operation for plastic formation of vagina; case. HEYER, E. Zentralbl. f. Gynak. *54:*1238–1240, May 17, '30

Success of Schubert's operation in aplasia of vagina; 3 cases. WICHMANN, S. E. Acta obst. et gynec. Scandinav. *9:*661–683, '30

Formation of artificial vagina from rectum (Schubert operation) in congenital vaginal defect; preliminary report. STARCK, H. Zentralbl. f. Gynak. *57:*2562–2565, Oct 28, '33

Late cancer of artificial vagina formed from rectum (Schubert operation); case. LAVAND'HOMME, P. Bruxelles-med. *19:*14–15, Nov 6, '38

Schubert operation for artificial vagina; case. COTTE, G. Mem. Acad. de chir. *64:*1365–1374, Dec 14, '38

Histologic and biologic value of Schubert operation for vaginal reconstruction after one year; report of case with peritonitis as sequel. KLIMKO, D. Zentralbl. f. Gynak. *63:*1150-1161, May 20, '39

SCHUBERTH, O.: Shock and blood transfusion at front. Nord. med. (Hygiea) *3:*2442–2444, Aug 5, '39

SCHUBERTH, O.: Blood transfusion in shock. Svenska lak.-tidning. *37:*900–907, May 17, '40

SCHUCHARDT, K.: Plastic reconstruction of ear lobe with circular pedicled flap from neck. Zentralbl. f. Chir. *69:*345, Feb 28, '42

SCHUCHARDT, K.: New intraoral spring mouth opener for treatment of lockjaw. Ztschr. f. Stomatol. *40:*677–680, Sept 25, '42

SCHÜCK: Reply to article by Joseph on shock therapy. Also one by Stejskal. Zentralbl. f. Chir. *60:*634–635, March 18, '33

SCHÜCK, F.: Intravenous injection of hypertonic solutions in shock. Zentralbl. f. Chir. *59:*2027–2029, Aug 20, '32 (Comment on Schük's article). STEJSKAL, K. Zentralbl. F. Chir. *59:*2896, Nov 26, '32

SCHÜLE, A.: Cautery pencil in treatment of furunculosis. Med. Welt *8:*407, March 24, '34

SCHÜLLER, J.: Heredity of fistula auris congenita. Munchen. med. Wchnschr. *76:*160–162, Jan 25, '29

SCHÜPPEL, A.: Perineal hypospadias; surgical treatment. Ztschr. f. Urol. *23:*753–761, '29

SCHÜRCH, O.: Necessity of early diagnosis and early treatment of cancer of mouth for effective therapy; 202 cases treated in hospitals of Eastern Switzerland from 1919–1928. Schweiz. med. Wchnschr. *60:*96–101, Feb 1, '30

SCHÜRCH, O.: Homoplastic transplantation of epithelium; case. Zentralbl. f. Chir. *58:*451–453, Feb 21, '31. Comment by Mannheim. Zentralbl. f. Chir. *58:*789–790, March 28, '31

SCHÜRCH, O.: Plastic reconstruction after therapy for facial cancer. Plast. chir. *1:*60–70, '39

SCHÜRCH, O.: Amputation–plastic surgery with bone reversal. Helvet. med. acta *6:*874, March '40

SCHÜRCH, O.: Covering defects of popliteal space with skin grafts. Schweiz. med. Wchnschr. *76:*1040–1041, Oct 5, '46

SCHÜRCH, O. AND FEHR, A.: Surgical therapy of metastases in cervical lymph nodes from cancer of mouth. Deutsche Ztschr. f. Chir. *251:*641–672, '39

SCHÜRCH, O. (see CLAIRMONT, P.) '30

SCHUERMANN, H.: Prognosis and therapy of blue nevi. Med. Welt *12:*1102–1104, July 30, '38

SCHUESSLER, W. W.: New technic for repair of facial paralysis with tantalum wire. Surgery *15:*646–652, April '44

SCHULENBURG, C. A. R.: Maxillofacial surgery. South African M. J. *18:*225–226, July 8, '44

SCHULLINGER, R. N. (see CROCE, E. J. *et al*) Jan '46

SCHULTZ, A. AND JAECKLE, C. E.: Plastic surgical repair about eyes with free grafts. Arch. Ophth. *34:*103–106, Aug '45

SCHULTZ, L. W.: Bilateral resection of mandible for prognathism. Surg., Gynec. and Obst. *45:*379–384, Sept '27

SCHULTZ, L. W.: Radical uranoplasty (Limberg): new operation (for closure of cleft palate). J. Am. Dent. A. *23:*407–415, March '36

SCHULTZ, L. W.: Treatment for subluxation of temporomandibular joint. J.A.M.A. *109:*1032–1035, Sept 25, '37

SCHULTZ, L. W.: Curative treatment for subluxations of temporomandibular joint (injections of sodium psylliate). J. Am. Dent. A. *24:*1947–1950, Dec '37

SCHULTZ, L. W.: Cleft palate surgery. Illinois M. J. *75:*127–131, Feb '39

SCHULTZ, L. W.: Bilateral cleft lip reconstruction. J. Am. Dent. A. *29:*248–250, Feb '42

SCHULTZ, L. W.: Care of cleft lip and palate in babies. Illinois M. J. *86:*138–159, Sept '44

SCHULTZ, L. W.: Harelip – urgent maxillofacial surgery. M. Times, New York *74:*33, Feb; 63, Mar '46

SCHULTZ, L. W. (see GLASER, K. *et al*) June '46

SCHULZ, F. (see RABL, R.) '39

SCHULZE, H. A.: Treatment of fracture-dislocations of proximal interphalangeal joints of fingers. Mil. Surgeon *99:*190–191, Sept '46

SCHULZE, W.: Transplantation of tissues. Klin. Wchnschr. *1:*793–797, April 15, '22

SCHUM, H.: Pathology, prognosis and treatment of fractures of phalanges and metacarpal bones. Deutsche Ztschr. f. Chir. *188:*234–272, '24

SCHUM, H.: Fractures of bones of hand and fingers. Deutsche Ztschr. f. Chir. *193:*132–139, '25

SCHUMANN, H.: Pregnancy in woman 25 years old after Maydl operation in childhood for exstrophy of bladder and cleft pelvis; review of clinical aspects of exstrophy. Geburtsh. u. Frauenh. *4:*318–333, Aug '42

SCHÜTZ, F.: Experimental research on cutaneous burns; trials of serotherapy; preliminary report. Boll. d. Ist. sieroterap. milanese *13:*253–262, April '34

SCHÜTZ, W.: Practice model for plastic surgery of auditory canal. Ztschr. f. Hals-, Nasen-u. Ohrenh. *47:*388–389, '41

SCHUYLER, C. H.: Effect of abnormalities of occlusion upon temporomandibular joint and associated structures. Proc. Dent. Centen. Celeb., pp. 303–308, '40

SCHWAB, W. J. AND FOLEY, F. A.: Simple treatment for hemorrhage into nail bed. U. S. Nav. M. Bull. *43:*371, Aug '44

SCHWARTZ, A.: Exercise after burns. Paris med. *2:*175–176, Aug 30, '24

SCHWARTZ, A.: Bone transplantation. Bull. et mem. Soc. nat. de chir. *53:*767–775, June 4, '27

SCHWARTZ, A. A.: Post-operative complications of submucous resection and their treatment. Am. J. Surg. *36:*133–136, June '22

SCHWARTZ, A. A. AND ISAACS, H. J.: Congenital atresia of posterior nares; 2 cases. Arch. Otolaryng. *35:*603–612, April '42

SCHWARTZ, A. B. AND ABBOTT, T. R.: Rational treatment of labial frenum. Am. J. Dis. Child. *52:*1061–1064, Nov '36

SCHWARTZ, A. B. AND ABBOTT, T. R.: Effect of growth and development on abnormal labial frenum. Am. J. Dis. Child. *71:*248–251, March '46

SCHWARTZ, H. G. AND PARKER, J. M.: Early nerve and bone repair in war wounds. J. Neurosurg. *2:*510–515, Nov '45

SCHWARTZ, H. G. AND ROULHAC, G. E.: Symposium: medicine and surgery in 21st General

Hospital; brain and nerve injuries. Washington Univ. M. Alumni Quart. *9:*69–73, Jan '46
SCHWARTZ, L. JR.: Branchial cyst. New York State J. Med. *31:*1376–1377, Nov 15, '31
SCHWARTZ, L. L.: Development of treatment for fractured jaw. J. Oral Surg. *2:*193–221, July '44
SCHWARTZ, M.: Unreduced unilateral dislocation of jaw; operative correction after 4 years. J. Bone and Joint Surg. *22:*176–181, Jan '40
SCHWARTZ, M.: Tensor and digital tractor (Ferres). Dia. med. *12:*433–434, May 20, '40
SCHWARTZ, V. J.: Simple rules for management of recent nasal fractures in general practice. Minnesota Med. *18:*101–106, Feb '35
SCHWARTZMAN, J.; GROSSMAN, L. AND DRAGUTSKY, D.: True total hemihypertrophy; case. Arch. Pediat. *59:*637–645, Oct '42
SCHWARZ, R.: Deformities of lips from maxillary abnormalities. Schweiz. Monatschr. f. Zahnh. *39:*331–344, June '29
SCHWARZ, R. (see HENSCHEN, C.) Nov '28
SCHWARZ, E.: Outcome of plastic operations on tendons. Deutsche Ztschr. f. Chir. *173:*301–385, '22 (illus.) abstr: J.A.M.A. *79:*1726, Nov 11, '22
SCHWARZ, E. G.: Case of club-hand associated with congenital syphilis. South. M. J. *19:*105–106, Feb '26
SCHWARZELL, H. H. (see DRURY, R. B.) Feb '35
SCHWARZMANN, E.: Technic of plastic operations of breast. Chirurg *2:*932–943, Oct 15, '30
SCHWARZMANN, E.: Technic of plastic surgery of breasts. Dia med. *3:*830, May 25, '31
SCHWARZMANN, E.: (comment on article by Claoue on plastic reduction of breast volume). Wien. med. Wchnschr. *86:*100–102, Jan 25, '36
SCHWARZMANN, E.: Avoidance of nipple necrosis by preservation of corium in one-stage plastic surgery of breast. Rev. de chir. structive, pp. 206–209, Oct '37
SCHWARZMANN, E.: Prophylaxis of cicatricial keloid in plastic surgery of pendulous breasts. Rev. de chir. structive *8:*93–98, Aug '38
SCHWARZMANN, E. AND POLLACZEK, K. F.: Prophylaxis of cicatricial keloid in plastic surgery of breast. Wien. med. Wchnschr. *87:*1248–1253, Nov 27, '37
SCHWARZWELLER, F.: Etiology of acrocephalosyndactylia. Ztschr. f. menschl. Vererb. -u. Konstitutionslehre *20:*341–349, '37
SCHWECKENDIEK, H.: Transpalatinal therapy of congenital choanal atresia. Ztschr. f. Hals-, Nasen-u. Ohrenh. *42:*367–373, '37
SCHWERDTFEGER, H.: Complete tearing of right thumb from joint by electric hand drill; rare case. Zentralbl. f. Chir. *64:*741–742, March 27, '37
SCHWERS, H.: Branchiogenous cyst with postoperative recurrence; recovery after iodine injection; case. Liege med. (supp.) *24:*1–4, Feb 8, '31
SCHWIEGK, H.: Shock and collapse; functional pathology and therapy. Klin. Wchnschr. *21:*741, Aug 22, '42; 765, Aug 29, '42
SCHWOERER, M.: Particular form of congenital median fissure of nose; independence of pars lacrimalis of nasal process. Frankfurt. Ztschr. f. Path. *34:*48–64, '26
SCIANDRA, A.: Improved surgical technic for subperichondrial resection used in Colonial Hospital of National Railroads of Mexico, Federal District. Cir. y cirujanos *7:*389–394, Sept 30–Oct 31, '39

Scleroderma

Progressive hemiatrophies combined with scleroderma; pathogenic study. ALVAREZ, G. Arch. argent. de pediat. *21:*83–94, Feb '44

SCOBIE, W. H.: Crush fracture of sesamoid bone of thumb. Brit. M. J. *2:*912, Dec 27, '41
SCOLLO, G.: Therapy of deep phlegmon of hand by intraarterial injection of colloidal silver. (Comment on Bonoli's article.) Policlinico (sez. prat.) *37:*546–548, April 14, '30 (Reply to Scollo.) BONOLI, U. Policlinico (sez. prat.) *37:*949–950, June 30, '30
SCOLLO, G.: Reply to article by Bonoli on hand infections. Policlinico (sez. prat.) *37:*1103, July 28, '30
SCOTT, A. C. JR.: Melanomas; 5 year cures. Surg., Gynec. and Obst. *60:*465–466, Feb (no. 2A) '35
SCOTT, J. F.: Simple treatment of extensive burns. Northwest Med. *27:*347–348, July '28
SCOTT, M. AND WYCIS, H. T.: Experimental observations on use of stainless steel for cranioplasty; comparison with tantalum. J. Neurosurg. *3:*310–317, July '46
SCOTT, P. G. (see HUNT, J. H.) Oct '32
SCOTT, R. K.: Treatment of epitheliomatous glands of neck following cancer of lips. M. J. Australia *2:*505–512, Oct 24, '31
SCOTT, R. T.: Tenosynovitis and fascial space abscesses. Northwest Med. *28:*317–322, July '29
SCOTT, W.: Syndactylism with variations. J. Hered. *24:*241–243, June '33
SCOTT, W. J. M. (see YOUNG, F.) June'43

Scrotum

Avulsion of scrotum, left testicle and sheath of penis. COTTLE, G. F., U.S. Nav. M. Bull. *20:*457–460, April '24
Unusually extensive injury of scrotum, avul-

Scrotum–Cont.
sion. SPROAT, S. M. California and West. Med. *23:*1318–1319, Oct '25
Operative treatment of elephantiasis of scrotum and penis. NÄGELSBACH, E. Arch. f. Schiffs-u. Tropen-Hyg. *31:*282–291, June '27
Plastic surgery for extensive atrophy of scrotum with fissure; case. SVIRIDOFF, K. Vrach. dielo *10:*1178, Sept 1, '27
Plastic surgery of penis and scrotum; case. CORNEJO SARAVIA, E. Rev. de cir. *6:*662–670, Dec '27
Unsuccessful attempt at plastic surgery of pedunculated scrotal flap. KOCH, K. Zentralbl. f. Chir. *55:*587–590, March 10, '28
Plastic reconstruction of scrotum; case. KONIG, E. Arch. f. klin. Chir. *150:*244–250, '28
Skin grafts derived from scrotum. CANAVERO, G. Policlinico (sez. chir.) *36:*61–69, Feb '29
Genitoplasty; restitution of skin of penis and of scrotum by autograft; restitution of function after trauma. KENNY, T. B. AND MERELLO, M. Prensa med. argent. *15:*1549–1560, May 30, '29
Avulsion of skin of penis and scrotum. COUNSELLER, V. S. AND PALMER, B. M., S. Clin. N. Amer. *9:*993–996, Aug '29
Plastic operation; avulsion of skin of penis; good functional results of graft of scrotum. VADI, E. Bol. Asoc. med. de Puerto Rico *22:*25–26, Sept–Oct '29
Avulsion of skin of scrotum and reconstruction. ROBERTSON, J. F. South. Med. and Surg. *93:*527–528, July '31
Double penis and scrotum (diphallus); case. HARRENSTEIN, R. J. Beitr. z. klin. Chir. *154:*308–314, '31
Traumatic avulsion of skin of penis and scrotum. TÜRSCHMID, W. Polska gaz. lek. *11:*373–374, May 15, '32
Denudation of penis and scrotum; case. DEXELMANN, J. Zentralbl. f. Chir. *59:*2760–2761, Nov 12, '32
Denudation of scrotum and its plastic repair by skin graft. SASAKI, S. Taiwan Igakkai Zasshi *34:*455, April '35
Plastic reconstruction of skin of scrotum by Filatov grafts. FROLOV, V. I. Vestnik khir. *46:*251–252, '36
Urethroplasty using scrotal grafts; review of various methods. GODARD, H., J. d'urol. *43:*201–232, March '37
Autoplastic restoration of scrotum by so-called Hindu method, using flap taken from psterointernal section of thigh; cases. GONZALEZ HURTADO, R. Cir. y cirujanos

Scrotum–Cont.
*6:*359–366, Aug '38
Total loss of skin of external male genitals due to unusual industrial trauma; plastic repair; case. PLACITELLI, G. Arch. ital. di urol. *15:*423–428, Aug '38
Discussion of subject of hypospadias from viewpoint of reconstructive surgery and report of use of depilated scrotal flap. RITCHIE, H. P. Surgery *5:*911–931, June '39
Phalloplasty; technic of skin grafting in avulsion of skin of penis and scrotum; review of literature and report of case. AGOSTINELLI, E. Policlinico (sez. prat.) *46:*1303–1306, July 17, '39
Surgical treatment of elephantiasis of scrotum and penis. DE SAVITSCH, E., J. Urol. *45:*216–222, Feb '41
Operation on huge scrotal elephantiasis performed by Casimiro Saez y Garcia in 1882. MULLER, F. Rev. de med. y cir. Habana *46:*373–383, Aug 31, '41
Transplants from scrotum for repair of urethral defects. DODSON, A. I. Tr. Am. A. Genito-Urin. Surgeons (1940) *33:*211–220, '41
Biologic scrotal flaps–new approach. ESSER, J. F. S., J. Internat. Coll. Surgeons *5:*168–170, March–April '42
Reconstruction for traumatic denudation of penis and scrotum; case. OWENS, N. Surgery *12:*88–96, July '42
Avulsion of scrotum and skin of penis; technic of delayed and immediate repair (using skin grafts). BYARS, L. T. Surg., Gynec. and Obst. *77:*326–329, Sept '43
Traumatic avulsion of skin of penis and scrotum. JUDD, E. S. JR. AND HAVENS, F. Z. Am. J. Surg. *62:*246–252, Nov '43
Reconstruction following complete avulsion of skin of penis and scrotum; case. SUTTON, L. E. New York State J. Med. *43:*2279–2282, Dec 1, '43
Elephantiasis of penis and scrotum; study apropos of case treated surgically. FOSSATI, A. Bol. Soc. cir. d. Uruguay *14:*355–364, '43
Elephantiasis of penis and scrotum; clinical study of case treated surgically. FOSSATI, A. Arch. urug. de med., cir. y especialid. *24:*285–294, March '44
Repair of avulsed scrotum. WHELAN, E. P. Surg., Gynec. and Obst. *78:*649–652, June '44
Traumatic avulsion of skin of penis and scrotum. ROTH, R. B. AND WARREN, K. W. J. Urol. *52:*162–168, Aug '44
Plastic repair of scrotum following gangrene; case. O'CONNOR, G. B., U.S. Nav. M. Bull. *44:*1060–1062, May '45

Scrotum – Cont.
Traumatic avulsion of penis and scrotum. LYONS, B. H. Canad. M. A. J. *52:*610, June '45
Total avulsion of skin of male genital organs; therapy of case. MAZZINI, O. F. Bol. y trab., Acad. argent. de cir. *30:*591–594, July 31, '46
Avulsion of skin of penis and scrotum; reparative genitoplasty. TORRES, G. A. AND OSACAR, E. M. Bol. y trab., Soc. de cir. de Cordoba *7:*225–237, '46

SCUDDER, J.: Blood studies as guides to therapy of shock. Tr. Am. Proct. Soc. *40:*249–256, '39
SCUDDER, J.: Blood studies as guide to shock therapy. J. Med. *21:*519–521, Feb '41
SCUDDER, J.: Blood studies in shock as guide to therapy; defense mechanism of kidney. New York State J. Med. *42:*1146–1149, June 15, '42
SCUDDER, J. AND ELLIOTT, R. H. E. JR.: Controlled fluid therapy in burns; case report illustrating severe hemoconcentration, electrolyte changes and futility of formulas in replacement therapy. South. Med. and Surg. *104:*651–658, Dec '42
SCUDDER, J. (see MCDONALD, J. J. *et al*) Aug '46
SCUDERI, R.: Malignant tumors of rhinopharynx with metastases; 15 cases. Arch. ital. di otol. *54:*273–316, Aug '42
SCULL, C. W. AND EIMAN, J.: Physiologic and clinical basis of shock treatment. Clinics *1:*43–58, June '42
SCULLY, J. B. (see SAYER, B.) June '43
SCULLY, J. C.: Glomus tumor or glomangioma of fingers; case. J. Michigan M. Soc. *42:*118–121, Feb '43
SCULLY, J. H. (see PUTZKI, P. S.) July '46
SDRAWOMYSLOW, W. I.: Technic and results of Popoff's method of formation of artificial vagina; 7 cases. Monatschr. f. Geburtsh. u. Gynak. *82:*182–204, June '29
SEABRA, D. DOS S.: Burn therapy. Bahia med. *14:*45–53, '43
SEARA, P.: Lesions of hands of bakers. Prensa med. argent. *24:*580–583, March 17, '37
SEARA, P.: Cutting wound of wrist with section of tendon and radial artery; functional restitution. Prensa med. argent. *32:*674–675, April 13, '45
SEARBY, H.: Tumors of neck. M. J. Australia *2:*406–408, Sept 20, '30
SEARCY, H. B.; CARMICHAEL, E. B. AND WHEELOCK, M. C.: Implant material; production of fibrous tissue around fibers of cottón and other foreign material implanted subcutaneously in rats. South. M. J. *37:*149–150, March '44
SEARS, N. P.: Congenital absence of vagina; features simplifying procedure for reconstruction. New York State J. Med. *39:*2019–2021, Nov 1, '39
SEAVER, E. P. JR.: Neuromuscular control of mandible. Am. J. Orthodontics *28:*222–229, April '42

Sebaceous Cysts
Cystic disease of pilosebaceous system of face. FAVRE, M., Bull. Soc. Franc. de dermat. et syph. (Reunion dermat.) *39:*93–96, Jan '32
Bygone operations in surgery; removal of sebaceous cyst from King George IV. POWER, D'A. Brit. J. Surg. *20:*361–365, Jan '33
Removal of wens – simple technic. WARING, J. B. H. Virginia M. Monthly *59:*607–608, Jan '33
Extirpation of small sebaceous cysts. BOZZINI, M. Rev. med. del Rosario *25:*800–805, July '35
Simplified method of local anesthesia for removal of sebaceous cysts. HAVENS, F. Z., S. Clin. North America *15:*1230–1232, Oct '35
Plastic surgery of sebaceous cysts. DE ANGELIS, H. Semana med. *1:*1176–1177, April 9, '36
Procedure for removing sebaceous cysts of face with conservative excision. UGGERI, C. Gazz. d. osp. *59:*456–458, May 1, '38
Cysts; sebaceous, mucous, dermoid and epidermoid. ERICH, J. B. Am. J. Surg. *50:*672–677, Dec '40
Flap operation for treatment of multiple sebaceous cysts (steatomata). MARSHALL, W. J. Invest. Dermat. *5:*299–302, Dec '42
Sebaceous cysts of face; extirpation. FINOCHIETTO, R. Prensa med. argent. *30:*1876–1877, Sept 29, '43
Treatment of sebaceous cysts by electrosurgical marsupialization. DANNA, J. A. Ann. Surg. *123:*952–956, May '46

SEBASTIANO, M.: Reaction to homoplastic skin grafts. Arch. per le sc. med. *49:*193–200, April '27
SEBENING, W.: Flexion contracture of fingers. Zentralbl. f. Chir. *53:*2526–2527, Oct 2, '26
SEBENING, W.: Plastic surgery of pendulous breasts. Chirurg *3:*510–515, June 1, '31
SEBILEAU, P.: Flap autoplasty; adherent skin anaplasty. Rev. de chir. *64:*207–258, '26 abstr: J.A.M.A. *87:*1074, Sept 25, '26
SEBILEAU, P.: Rights and duties of surgeon in plastic surgery. Ann. d. mal. de l'oreille, du larynx *49:*1–9, Jan '30
SEBILEAU, P. AND DUFOURMENTEL, L.: Surgical correction of congenital and acquired deform-

ities of nasal pyramid; with 105 illustrations. Ann. d. mal. de l'oreille, du larynx *46:*753, Aug '27

SEBILEAU, PIERRE, AND DUFOURMENTEL, LÉON: *Correction chirurgicale des difformités congenitales et acquises de la pyramide nasale.* Arnette, Paris, 1927

SEBILEAU, P. AND DUFOURMENTEL, L.: Surgical correction of congenital and acquired deformities of nasal pyramid. Ann. d. mal. de l'oreille, du larynx *46:*753, Aug; 853, Sept. '27

Secretan Syndrome: See Ledderhose-Secretan Syndrome

SECRIST, D. L.: Surgical shock. Southwestern Med. *22:*391–393, Oct '38

SEDAM, M. S.: Present-day therapy of burns. M. Woman's J. *49:*129–133, May '42

SEDAN, J.: Pigmented basocellular epithelioma of palpebral skin. Bull. Soc. d'opht. de Paris, pp. 341–348, April '36

SEDDON, H. J.: Peripheral nerve injuries (John Burns Trust lecture). Glasgow M. J. *139:*61–75, March '43

SEDDON, H. J.: Peripheral nerve injuries; early management. Practitioner *152:*101–107, Feb '44

SEDDON, H. J. AND HOLMES, W.: Late condition of nerve homografts in man. Surg., Gynec. and Obst. *79:*342–351, Oct '44

SEDDON, H. J. AND MEDAWAR, P. B.: Fibrin suture of human nerves. Lancet *2:*87–88, July 25, '42

SEDDON, H. J., MEDAWAR, P. B. AND SMITH, H.: Rate of peripheral nerve regeneration in man. J. Physiol. *102:*191–215, Sept. 30, '43

SEDDON, H. J., YOUNG, J. Z. AND HOLMES, W.: Histologic condition of autograft of nerve in man. Brit. J. Surg. *29:*378–384, April '42

SEED, L.: Branchial cyst. S. Clin. N. Amer. *6:*1029–1031, Aug '26

SEED, L.: Dermoid cyst of neck. S. Clin. N. Amer. *6:*1033–1035, Aug '26

SEEGER, S. J.: Tannic acid in burns. Wisconsin M. J. *27:*1–6, Jan '28

SEEGER, S. J.: Hydrogen-ion concentration value of tannic acid solutions in burn therapy. Surg., Gynec. and Obst. *55:*455–463, Oct '32

SEEGER, S. J.: Burn therapy with report of 278 cases (tannic acid in 158 cases). Wisconsin M. J. *31:*755–759, Nov '32

SEEGER, S. J.: Burn therapy. Texas State J. Med. *31:*488–494, Dec '35

SEEGER, S. J.: Burns. J. Michigan M. Soc. *38:*133–138, Feb '39 also: Wisconsin M. J. *38:*279–282, April '39

SEEGER, S. J. AND SCHAEFER, A. A.: Burn therapy. Physiotherapy Rev. *14:*174–176, Nov-Dec '34

SEELIG, M. G.: Midline congenital cervical fistula of tracheal origin. Arch. Surg. *2:*338, March '21

SEELIG, M. G.: Rhinophyma. S. Clin. N. America *5:*1381–1386, Oct '25

SEELER, E.: Submucous cleft palate with impairment of hearing; case. Beitr. z. Anat., Physiol., Path. u. Therap. d. Ohres *28:*427–430, Jan '31

SEELEY, R. C.: Correction of congenital protruding ear; new surgical concept. Am. J. Surg. *72:*12–15, July '46

SEEMANN, M.: Training the speech after operations for cleft palate. Cas. lek. cesk. *61:*811–815, Sept 2, '22

SEEMANN, M.: Submucous fissure of palate. Cas. lek. cesk. *62:*641–646, June 16, '23 (illus.) abstr: J.A.M.A. *81:*1734, Nov 17, '23

SEEMANN, M.: Schönborn operation (velopharyngorrhaphy) for correction of defective speech. Casop. lek. cesk. *70:*1570–1574, Nov. 20 '31 also: Otolaryng. slavica *4:*24–25, Jan '32

SEGAL, G. I. AND UZDIN, Z. M.: Treatment of burns with blood and serum of convalescents. Sovet. vrach. zhur. *44:*835–840, Dec '40

SEGALE, G. C.: Results of treatment of cancer in mouth in 82 cases. Arch. ed atti d. Soc. ital. di chir. *36:*770, '30

Segond Operation

Late results of Segond operation for exstrophy of bladder. DOTTI, E. Gior. vensto di sc. med. *8:*730–739, July '34

SEGRE, G.: Disfiguring scars in industrial and civil accidents. Minerva med. *1:*61–65, Jan 20, '38

SEGRÈ, R.: Cleft palate and rhinopharyngeal functions; case. Arch. ital. di otol. *40:*633–643, Oct '29

SEGRÈ, R.: Submucous clefts of palate. Monatschr. f. Ohrenh. *67:*649–670, June '33

SEGRÈ, R.: Tubal (eustachian) function in cleft palate. Valsalva *9:*856–875, Nov '33

SEGRÈ, R.: Prosthetic therapy for cleft palate. Monatschr. f. Ohrenh. *70:*865–884, July '36

SEGRÈ, R.: Submucosal palatoschisis. Valsalva *14:*356–363, July '38

SEGRÈ, R.: Functional surgical therapy of cleft palate. Rev. Asoc. med. argent. *55:*89–91, Feb 15–28, '41

SEGRÈ, R.: (see MELA, B.) Sept '32

SEIBERLING, J. D.: Fracture of frontal sinus and ethmoid through dura, orbit and maxillary sinus; case; phenomenal recovery. Laryngoscope *41:*93–96, Feb '31

SEIDMAN M.: Sulfanilamide (sulfonamide)

ointment in local therapy of burns (in Hebrew). Harefuah *27:*6-8, July 2, '44

SEIFERT, E.: Micrognathia. Arch. f. klin. Chir. *135:*726-735, '25

SEIFERT, E.: So-called fistula auris congenita. Deutsche Ztschr. f. Chir. *209:*118-124, '28

SEIFERT, E.: Tannic acid treatment of fresh burns; erroneous methods of application. Zentralbl. f. Chir. *60:*1051-1055, May 6, '33

SEIFERT, E.: Surgery of jaws; review of literature. Chirurg *6:*489-493, July 1, '34

SEIFERTH, L. B.: Roentgenologic studies of closure of oropharynx against nasopharynx and position of tongue during blowing up of cheeks in persons with cleft palate; function tests of soft palate. Klin. Wchnschr. *14:*897-899, June 22, '35

SEIFFERT, K.: Plastic surgery of fingers and hand. Arch. f. Orthop. *28:*370-375, May 6, '30

SEIFFERT, L.: Successful primary suture of nerves in seriously infected wounds. Zentralbl. f. Chir. *63:*1890-1892, Aug 8, '36

SEIGALL, H. A. AND MANCOLL, M. M.: Fractures involving nasal bones. M. J. and Rec. *134:*328-329, Oct 7, '31

SEKULIĆ, B.: Autoplasty of nasal septal perforations. Otolaryng. slavica *4:*40, Jan '32

SELDON, T. H.: First aid treatment of shock. Proc. Staff Meet., Mayo Clin. *15:*742-743, Nov 20, '40

SELDON, T. H. AND LUNDY, J. S.: Supportive measures in care of surgical patients (transfusion of blood and plasma, parenteral administration of solutions and stimulants). Southwestern Med. *25:*236-240, Aug '41

SELDON, T. H. (see LUNDY, J. S. *et al*) Aug '44

SELETSKIY, V. V.: Therapy of decubitus ulcer. Klin. Med. *15:*241-246, '37

SELETZ, E.: Peripheral nerve surgery; review of incisions for operative exposure; preliminary report. J. Neurosurg. *3:*135-147, March '46

SELFRIDGE, G.: Cosmetic surgery of nose. Laryngoscope *31:*337, June '21

SELIG, S.: Surgical treatment of chronic arthritis. New York State J. Med. *39:*2114-2117, Nov 15, '39

SELIG, S. AND SCHEIN, A.: Irreducible buttonhole dislocations of fingers. J. Bone and Joint Surg. *22:*436-441, April '40

SELIGMAN, A. M. (see FINE, J.) March '43

SELIGMAN, A. M. (see FINE, J. *et al*) Oct '45

SELIGMAN, A. M. (see FRANK, H. A. *et al*) July '45

SELKIRK, T. K.: Congenital aural fistula. Am. J. Dis. Child. *49:*431-447, Feb '35

SELLECK, G. A. (see DAVIS, A. D.) April '44

SELLEI, J.: Treatment of decubitus ulcers with epithelin. Dermat. Wchnschr. *89:*1911-1916, Nov 30, '29

SELLERA CASTRO, R. (see DEL CAMPO, R. M.) Jan '32

SELLERS, E. A. AND GORANSON, E. S.: Closed plaster method of burn therapy in prevention of shock. Canad. M. A. J. *51:*111-114, Aug '44

SELLERS, E. A. AND GORANSON, E. S.: Closed plaster method in prevention of shock after burns. J. Canad. M. Serv. *2:*431-437, May '45

SELLERS, E. A. AND WILLARD, J. W.: Effect of plaster bandages and local cooling on hemoconcentration and mortality rate in burns. Canad. M. A. J. *49:*461-464, Dec '43

SELLERS, E. D. (see HYDE, T. L. *et al*) Feb '44

SELLHEIM, H.: Care, preservation and repair of female breasts; review of Erna Glaesmer's "Die Formfehler und die plastischen Operationen de weiblichen Brust," and H. Biesenberger's "Deformitaten und Operationen de weiblichen Brust". Deutsche med. Wchnschr. *58:*1414-1417, Sept 2, '32

SELTSOVSKIY, P. L.: Shock and its therapy. Khirurgiya, no. 10, pp. 25-27, '44

SELTZER, A. P.: History of plastic surgery. Laryngoscope *51:*256-262, March '41

SELTZER, A. P.: New medicated gauze for use in nasal operations. Eye, Ear, Nose and Throat Monthly *24:*189, April '45

SELTZER, A. P.: Improved method of narrowing the nose. Ann. Otol., Rhin. and Laryng. *52:*460-472, June '43

SELTZER, A. P.: Plastic repair of deviated septum associated with deflected nasal tip. Arch. Otolaryng. *40:*433-444, Dec '44

SELTZER, A. P.: New nasal tissue clamp used in new method of narrowing columella. J. Internat. Coll. Surgeons *8:*154-159, March-April '45

SELTZER, A. P.: Fixity of facial expression following undermining of skin over nose; modified method by which it is avoided. Am. J. Surg. *68:*326-335, June '45

SELTZER, A. P.: Plastic repair of hereditary and developmental anomalies. Arch. Pediat. *62:*248-254, June '45

SELYE, H; DOSNE, C.; BASSETT, L. AND WHITTAKER, J.: Therapeutic value of adrenal cortical hormones in traumatic shock and allied conditions. Canad. M. A. J. *43:*1-8, July '40

SELYE, H. AND DOSNE, C.: Treatment of wound shock with corticosterone (suprarenal preparation). Lancet *2:*70-71, July 20, '40

SEMON, H. C.: Treatment of warts and moles. Lancet *1:*1359-1360, June 27, '25

SEMON, H. C.: Treatment of angiomas with carbon dioxide snow pencil. Lancet *1:*1167-1169, June 2, '34

SEMRAU, J.: Traumatic origin of late angioneurotic condition in region of nose and cheek; 3 cases. Hals-, Nasen-u. Ohrenarzt (Teil 1)

*27:*363-370, '36

SENÁ, J. A.: Autoplastic skin grafts in therapy of cicatricial ectropion; 5 cases. Rev. Asoc. med. argent. *48:*298-306, March-April '34 also: Semana med. *2:*489-498, Aug 16, '34

SENDRAIL, M.: Familial aplasia of upper jaw, new type of facial dysostosis. Prat. med. franc. *15:*127-130, Feb (B) '34

SÉNÈQUE, J.: Pathogenic and therapeutic considerations of Volkmann's contracture. Presse med. *34:*133-135, Jan 30, '26

SÉNÈQUE, J.: Volkmann syndrome. Prat. med. franc. *17:*427-435, Oct (A-B) '36

SÉNÈQUE, J. (see CUNÉO, B.) Aug '31

SENGER, F. L. AND MORGAN, E. K.: Case of hermaphroditism; operation and end result. J. Urol. *48:*658-664, Dec '42

SENTENAC, E. AND KOEFF, G.: Bimaxillary blockage in jaw fractures; compared advantages of 2 orthodontic apparatuses. J. de med. de Bordeaux *115:*90-96, Jan 29, '38

SEPP, E. K.: Peripheral nerve injuries; early therapy. Klin. med. (no. 8-9) *20:*7-11, '42

SERAFINI, G. AND ANTONIOLI, G. M.: Autoplastic bone transplants in man. Arch. ital. di chir. *16:*273-293, '26

SERAFINI, G. AND ANTONIOLI, G. M.: Carcinoma of mucosa of cheek treated surgically; 10 cases. Gior. d. r. Accad. di med. di Torino *91:*51-56, Jan-March '28 also: Minerva med. (pt. 2) *8:*599-610, Sept 15, '28

ŠERCER, A.: Postoperative perforations of nasal septum. Cas. lek. cesk. *63:*842-845, May 31, '24 abstr: J.A.M.A. *83:*161, July 12, '24

ŠERCER, A.: Complete absence (anotia) of ear with tonsillar aplasia. Ztschr. f. Hals-, Nasen-u. Ohrenh. *22:*75-78, June 16, '28

ŠERCER, A.: Experiences in rhinoplasty. Otolaryng. slavica *3:*415-435, Oct '31

ŠERCER, A.: Technic of therapy (palatopharyngorrhaphy) of rhinolalia aperta due to too short palate. Rev. de chir. structive, pp. 5-18, July '35

ŠERCER, A.: Histologic study of development of septal deformities. Acta oto-laryng. *28:*529-547, '40

ŠERCER, A.: Congenital ptosis of ear. Arch. f. Ohren-, Nasen-u. Kehlkopfh. *149:*298-308, '41

SERGI, G.: Method of determination of prognathism. Riv. di antropol. *28:*271-279, '28-'29

SERGIEVA, M.: Modification of Millingen-Sapezhko operation for trachomatous entropion. Sovet. vestnik oftal. *8:*244-245, '36

SEROICZKOWSKI, A.: Symmetrical malformation (cleft) of hands and feet. Ztschr. f. d. ges. Anat. (Abt. 1) *89:*145-155, March 25, '29

SERRA, A.: Experiments with free transplantation of entire muscle. Arch. ital. di chir. *12:*355-370, '25

SERRÃO, B.: Differential diagnosis and treatment of obstetric shock. Folha med. *9:*365, Nov 5, '28

SERT, D. (see LADEWIG, P.) 1944

SERTA, S. L.: Plastic surgery; case of hypertrophy of breast. Hospital, Rio de Janeiro *25:*877-887, June '44

SERFATY, M. (see VALLINO, M. T.) Dec '34

SEVERIN, E.: Tannic acid in therapy of burns in children. Nord. med. tidskr. *14:*1787-1789, Oct 30, '37

SEWELL, S. A.: Rational treatment of burns. M. J. Australia *2:*590-592, Dec 2, '44

SEXTON, W. G.: Epispadias in women; case report. J.Urol. *18:*663-666, Dec '27

SEYEWETZ, A.: Chemical burns. Avenir med. *37:*27, Jan '40

SEYNSCHE, K.: Epispadias as cause of incontinence in woman; case. Zentralbl. f. Gynak. *55:*3585-3591, Dec 12, '31

SÉZARY, A.; DUCOURTIOUX, M. AND BARBARA, G.: Therapy of cutaneous angiomas with sclerosing injections of quinine and urea hydrochloride associated with cryotherapy with carbon dioxide snow. Presse med. *41:*260, Feb 15, '33

SGROSSO, J. A.: Rare trauma of hand; tearing off of part of index finger with 20 cm. of flexor tendon; case. Bol. Soc. de cir. de Rosario *10:*172-174, June '43

SHAAR, C. M.: Preservation of facial nerve in excision of parotid tumors; 2 cases. U. S. Nav. M. Bull. *27:*351-360, April '29

SHAAR, C. M.; FERGUSON, L. K. AND NOVA, P. L.: Microcrystalline sulfathiazole (sulfanilamide derivative) in superficial burns. U. S. Nav. M. Bull. *40:*954-957, Oct '42

SHACKELFORD, J. G.: Fracture of mandible. Southwestern Med. *21:*96-98, March '37

SHACKELFORD, J. H. (see ROGERS, L. *et al*) Jan '32

SHACKLETON, R. P. W.: Anesthesia in fractures of jaws. Lancet *1:*396-398, March 25, '44

SHACKLETON, R. P. W. (see GORDON, R. A.) March '43

SHAFIROFF, B. G. P.: Instrument for skin grafts. Ann. Surg. *101:*814-815, Feb '35

SHAMBAUGH, G. E. JR.: Minor surgery of nose and throat. S. Clin. North America *21:*21-36, Feb '41

SHAMBAUGH, G. E. JR.: New plastic flap for use in endaural radical mastoidectomy. Ann. Otol., Rhin. and Laryng. *51:*117-121, March '42

SHANDS, A. R. JR. AND SCHIEBEL, H. M.: Hand fractures; incidence over 5 year period. Indust. Med. *6:*210-213, April '37

SHANIN, A. P.: Malignant tumors of upper and

lower lip treated at Oncologic Institute of Leningrad in past 10 years. Vestnik khir. *57:*43–62, Jan '39

SHANK, R. A.: Harelip. J. Med. *8:*434–437, Nov '27

SHANKS, J.: Plastic surgery of eyelids. M. Rec. *152:*408, Dec 4, '40

SHAPIRO, S. E.: Blood transfusion in treatment of decubitus. Klin. med. (nos. 4–5) *21:*66, '43

SHARGORODSKAY, I. I.: Rational way of bandaging palmar arches. Vestnik khir. (nos. 37–38) *13:*150–157, '28

SHARMAN, A.: Intersexuality; case. Glasgow M. J. *142:*40–44, Aug '44

SHARP, G. S. AND FREEMAN, R. G.: Cancer of lips. Eye, Ear, Nose and Throat Monthly *23:*17–26, Jan '44

SHARP, G. S. AND SMITH, H. D.: Treatment of cancer of lips. West. J. Surg. *47:*695–705, Dec '39

SHARPEY-SCHAFER, E. P. (see HILL, D. K. *et al*) Dec '40

SHARPLESS, D. H. (see MACKENZIE, C. M.) Oct '41

SHATKINSKY, M. P.: Problem of rhinoplasty. Klin. j. saratov. Univ. *5:*463–471, April '28

SHATKINSKY, M. P.: Further observations on rhinoplasty. Vestnik khir. (no. 52) *18:*77–84, '29

SHATUNOVSKIY, L. Y.: Surgical therapy of dorsal luxation of thumb. Ortop. i. travmatol. (no. 1) *11:*58–63, '37

SHAW, C. E. W.: How they treat burn cases aboard U. S. S. Solace. Mod. Hosp. *63:*72–75, Nov '44

SHAW, D. T.: Open abdominal flaps for repair of surface defects of upper extremity. S. Clin. North America *24:*293–308, April '44

SHAW, D. T. AND PAYNE, R. L., JR.: Repair of surface defects of upper extremity. Tr. South. S. A. (1945) *57:*243–268, '46

SHAW, D. T. AND PAYNE, R. L. JR.: Repair of surface defects of arms. Ann. Surg. *123:*705–730, May '46

SHAW, D. T. AND PAYNE, R. L., JR.: One stage tubed abdominal flaps; single pedicle tubes. Surg. Gynec. and Obst. *83:*205–209, Aug '46

SHAW, J. J. M.: Plastic repair of face and hand. Brit. J. Surg. *10:*47–51, July '22 (illus.)

SHAW, J. J. M.: Plastic repair of face and limbs. Tr. Medico-Chir. Soc. Edinburgh, pp. 110–116, '22–'23 (illus.); in Edinburgh M. J., June '23

SHAW, J. J. M.: Plastic repair of extremities and face. Tr. Roy. Med.-Chir. Soc., Glasgow (1927–1928) *22:*151, '29

SHAW, J. J. M.: War injuries to face and jaw. War and Doctor, pp. 41–46, '42

SHAW, M. H.: Military plastic surgery. M. Press *214:*312–317, Nov 14, '45

SHAWVER, J. R.: Severe burn therapy. M. Bull. Vet. Admin. *17:*319–321, Jan '41

SHCHEKINA, A. N.: Blaskovics operation for eyelid ptosis. Sovet. vestnik oftal. *8:*551–558, '36

SHCHERBINA, I. A.: Primary suture in finger injuries, and hand. Sovet. khir., no. 3, pp. 22–27, '35

SHEA, J. J.: Fractures of bones of face; management. Tri-State M. J. *5:*1160, Sept '33 also: J.M.A. Alabama *3:*125–128, Oct '33

SHEA, J. J.: Open treatment of facial bone fractures. J. Tennessee M. A. *27:*15–21, Jan '34

SHEA, J. J.: Management of facial fractures. Mississippi Doctor *18:*498–502, Feb '41 also: Memphis M. J. *16:*75–76, May '41

SHEA, J. J.: Management of facial fractures involving paranasal sinuses. J.A.M.A. *120:*745–749, Nov 7, '42

SHEA, J. J.: Management of fractures into nasal sinuses. Laryngoscope *56:*22–25, Jan '46

SHEARER, T. P.; WIPER, T. B. AND MILLER, J. M.: Battle injuries of urethra with urinary fistula. Texas State J. Med. *41:*137–140, July '45

SHEARER, T. P. (see CROCE, E. J. *et al*) Jan '46

SHEARER, W. L.: Cleft palate and harelip. Minnesota Med. *4:*293, May '21

SHEARER, W. L.: Cleft palate and cleft lip cases. Nebraska M. J. *9:*160–164, May '24

SHEARER, W. L.: Cleft palate. Nebraska M. J. *11:*462–468, Dec '26

SHEARER, W. L.: Cleft palate. J. Am. Dent. A. *15:*2135–2140, Nov '28

SHEARER, W. L.: Cleft palate. Nebraska M. J. *17:*66–70, Feb '32

SHEARER, W. L.: Cleft palate and cleft lip. J. Am. Dent. A. *21:*1446–1454, Aug '34

SHEARER, W. L.: Intraoral open reduction for management of certain difficult fractures of jaw. J. Am. Dent. A. *30:*833–834, June 1, '43

SHEARER, W. L.: Cleft palate and cleft lip. Nebraska M. J. *30:*125–126, April '45

SHEARON, C. G. (see MASON, M. L.) Oct '32

SHEDDEN, W. M.: Results of surgical treatment of epithelioma of lip from Massachusetts General Hospital and Cancer Commission of Harvard University. Boston M. and S. J. *196:*262–270, Feb 17, '27

SHEDDEN, W. M.: Cysts and fistulae (branchial). New England J. Med. *205:*800–811, Oct 22, '31

SHEDDEN, W. M. (see PORTER, C. A.) June '22

SHEEHAN. (see DANTRELLE) Dec '28

SHEEHAN, J. E.: Gillies new method in giving support to depressed nasal bridge and columella. New York M. J. *113:*448, March 16, '21

SHEEHAN, J. E.: New instruments used in nose

and throat and plastic surgery. New York M. J. *115:*493–494, April 19, '22 (illus.)
Sheehan, J. E.: Thiersch graft in radical cure of frontal sinus and maxillary antrum diseases; its further application to tonsil and gingival sulci. Surg., Gynec. and Obst. *35:*358–360, Sept '22 (illus.)
Sheehan, J. E.: New surgical procedure for relief of depression of nasal bridge and columella; its further application for relief of hump and deflected noses; plastic treatment of syphilitic nose. Laryngoscope *32:*709–718, Sept '22 (illus.)
Sheehan, J. E.: Correction of nasal deformities. Brit. M. J. *2:*981–982, Nov 24, '23
Sheehan, J. E.: Plastic surgery of face and neck. New York M. J. *118:*676–678, Dec 5, '23 (illus.)
Sheehan, J. E.: Case of rhinophyma and its cure. M. J. and Rec. *119:*94–95, Jan 16, '24
Sheehan, J. E.: Recommended procedure for relief of ala deformity in certain cases in adult associated with harelip and its mechanical counterpart. M. J. and Rec. *120:*72–73, July 16, '24
Sheehan, J. E.: Repair of syphilitic nose. M. J. and Rec. (supp.) *120:*81–84, Sept 17, '24
Sheehan, J. Eastman: *Plastic Surgery of the Nose*. P. Hoeber, New York, 1925
Sheehan, J. E.: Plastic repair of syphilitic nose. Laryngoscope *35:*22, Jan '25
Sheehan, J. E.: Phenol burns of left eyelids, eyeball, upper face and temporal area. Laryngoscope *35:*55, Jan '25
Sheehan, J. E.: Case after operation for extensive burn of left lids, eyeball, upper face and temporal area. M. J. and Rec. *121:*291–292, March 4, '25
Sheehan, J. E.: Plastic surgery. Am. J. Surg. *39:*88–90, April '25
Sheehan, J. E.: Repair of inoperable cleft of soft palate by utilizing faucial tonsils. M. J. and Rec. *122:*185–188, Aug 19, '25
Sheehan, J. E.: General review of field of plastic surgery. J. M. Soc. New Jersey *22:*338–341, Sept '25
Sheehan, J. E.: Plastic surgery. Arch. Otolaryng. *4:*427–429, Nov '26
Sheehan, J. Eastman: *Plastic Surgery of the Orbit*. Macmillan Co., New York, 1927
Sheehan, J. E.: Correction of nasal disfigurements by readjustment of nasal tissues. M. J. and Rec. *125:*585, May 4; 664, May 18, '27
Sheehan, J. E.: Correction of nasal deformities (including skin grafts). Virginia M. Monthly *54:*138–141, June '27
Sheehan, J. E.: Utilization of skin of upper eyelid for repair of small facial defects. Arch. Otolaryng. *6:*107–111, Aug '27
Sheehan, J. E.: Plastic surgery. Arch. Otolaryng. *6:*385–389, Oct '27
Sheehan, J. E.: Functional restoration in repair of facial injuries; value of color photography in this work. J. M. Soc. New Jersey *24:*618–621, Nov '27
Sheehan, J. E.: Progress in reparative surgery of face. Arch. franco-belges de chir. *31:*122–125, Feb '28
Sheehan, J. E.: Functional restoration as element in facial repair and nose. Bull. New York Acad. Med. *4:*416–421, March '28
Sheehan, J. E.: Reparative facial surgery. M. J. and Rec. *127:*245–246, March 7, '28
Sheehan, J. E.: Dermatologist's interest in reconstructive surgery—skin grafting. M. J. and Rec. *127:*326, March 21, '28
Sheehan, J. E.: Plastic surgery. Arch. Otolaryng. *7:*299–311, April '28
Sheehan, J. E.: Functional restoration as chief concern in repair of facial defects. S. Clin. N. Amer. *8:*293–307, April '28
Sheehan, J. E.: Functional restoration as element in facial repair. Am. J. Surg. *5:*164–166, Aug '28
Sheehan, J. E.: Treatment of X-ray and radium burns. Laryngoscope *38:*612–617, Sept '28
Sheehan, J. E.: Plastic surgery. Arch. Otolaryng. *8:*448–451, Oct '28
Sheehan, J. E.: Reconstructive surgery in relation to cancer defects. Internat. J. Med. and Surg. *42:*177–180, April '29
Sheehan, J. E.: Replacement of thumb nail. J.A.M.A. *92:*1253–1255, April 13, '29
Sheehan, J. E.: Capillary drainage in treatment of keloidal scars. M. J. and Rec. *129:*548–549, May 15, '29
Sheehan, J. E.: Plastic surgery. Arch. Otolaryng. *10:*426–428, Oct '29
Sheehan, J. E.: Skin grafting in reparative surgery. Actas y trab. del primer Cong. de la Asoc. med. Panamericana, pp. 527–535, '30
Sheehan, J. E.: Plastic surgery, summary of material available in field of otolaryngology. Arch. Otolaryng. *12:*527–530, Oct '30
Sheehan, J. E.: Correction of disfigurements of nose by readjustment of frame-work and tissues. Arch. Otolaryng. *13:*584–596, April '31
Sheehan, J. E.: Plastic surgery. Arch. Otolaryng. *14:*377–379, Sept '31
Sheehan, J. E.: Variety in plastic surgery. Rev. de chir. plastique, pp. 161–181, Oct '31
Sheehan, J. E.: Keloid therapy; clinic in reparative surgery. Unilateral facial paralysis. S. Clin. North America *12:*341–356, April '32
Sheehan, J. E.: Correction of unilateral facial paralysis. J. M. Soc. New Jersey *29:*556–560, July '32

SHEEHAN, J. E.: Plastic surgery; summary of bibliographic material available in field of otolaryngology. Arch. Otolaryng. *16:*867–870, Dec '32

SHEEHAN, J. E.: Progress in plastic and reconstructive surgery. Union med. du Canada *62:*639–643, July '33

SHEEHAN, J. E.: Plastic surgery; summary of bibliographic material available in field of otolaryngology. Arch. Otolaryng. *18:*531–533, Oct '33

SHEEHAN, J. E.: Problems of plastic and reconstructive surgery. Bruxelles-med. *14:*39–48, Nov 12, '33

SHEEHAN, J. E.: Reparative surgery. M. Rec. *139:*647–653, June 20, '34

SHEEHAN, J. E.: Plastic surgery; summary of bibliographic material available in field of otolaryngology. Arch. Otolaryng. *20:*577–582, Oct '34

SHEEHAN, J. E.: Muscle-nerve graft. S. Clin. North America *15:*471–482, April '35

SHEEHAN, J. E.: Reparative and reconstructive surgery. Guy's Hosp. Gaz. *49:*327–336, Aug 31, '35

SHEEHAN, J. EASTMAN: *Plastic Surgery of the Nose*. Paul Hoeber Co., New York, 1925. Second Edition, 1936

SHEEHAN, J. E.: Variety in reparative surgery. M. Rec. *146:*307–310, Oct 6, '37

SHEEHAN, J. EASTMAN: *General and Plastic Surgery with Emphasis on War Injuries*. Paul Hoeber Co., New York, 1938

SHEEHAN, J. EASTMAN: *A Manual of Reparative Plastic Surgery*. Paul Hoeber Co., New York, 1938

SHEEHAN, J. E.: Free full thickness skin grafts. J.A.M.A. *112:*27–29, Jan 7, '39

SHEEHAN, J. E.: Application of mucous membrane grafts to congenital and acquired states. M. Rec. *152:*404–408, Dec 4, '40

SHEEHAN, J. E.: Use of iliac bone in facial and cranial repair. Am. J. Surg. *52:*55–61, April '41

SHEEHAN, J. E.: Burns treated as war wounds. Am. J. Surg. *61:*331–338, Sept '43

SHEEHAN, J. E.: Tissue grafting. Am. J. Surg. *61:*339–349, Sept '43

SHEEHAN, J. E.: Plasma fixation of skin grafts. Am. J. Surg. *65:*74–78, July '44, also: Lancet *2:*363–365, Sept 16, '44

SHEEHAN, J. E. AND JENNEY, J.: Continuous epithelization on large denuded areas. Lancet *1:*123–124, Jan 26, '46

SHEEHAN, J. E.: Unilateral facial paralysis; correction with tantalum wire; preliminary report on 8 cases. Lancet *1:*263–264, Feb 23, '46

SHEEHAN, J. E. AND BARSKY, A. J.: Reparative surgery in relation to face. Proc. Internat. Assemb. Inter-State Post-Grad. M. A., North America (1930) *6:*434–437, '31

Sheehan Operation

Sheehan's method of plastic surgery of nose. DELLEPIANE RAWSON, R. Rev. med. latino-am. *15:*1055–1090, May '30

SHELDEN, C. H. (see WEBSTER, G. V. *et al*) July '45

SHELDON, W. P. H. (see LIGHTWOOD, R. C.) June '28

SHELMIRE, B.: Diseases of vermillion borders of lips. Dallas M. J. *14:*82–91, June '28, also: Internat. J. Orthodontia *14:*817–832, Sept '28

SHELTON, J. M.: "Thimble forceps" for epilation (during electrolysis). Arch. Dermat. and Syph. *44:*260, Aug '41

SHELTON, J. M. (see HOLLANDER, L.) Aug '39

SHELTON, J. M. (see HOLLANDER, L.) Dec '41

SHELTON, J. M. (see HOLLANDER, L.) Jan '44

SHEMELEY, W. G.: Case of miacrotia, with occlusion of left external auditory canal; operated with satisfactory results. Laryngoscope *33:*841–844, Nov '23 (illus.)

SHEN, J. K.: Tea in treatment of burns. China M. J. *41:*150–153, Feb '27

SHEN, S. C. AND HAM, T. H.: Studies on destruction of red blood cells; mechanism and complications of hemoglobinuria in patients with thermal burns; spherocytosis and increased osmotic fragility of red blood cells. New England J. Med. *229:*701–713, Nov 4, '43

SHEPARD, G. W.: Extensive superficial burns. U. S. Nav. M. Bull. *20:*697–701, June '24

SHEPARD, J. H. (see COSTELLO, M. J.) April '39

SHEPHARD, J. H.: Squamous-cell epithelioma of lip, its surgical indications. Surg., Gynec. and Obst. *35:*107–109, July '22 (illus.)

SHEPHERD, J. A.: Osteochondromata of tendon sheaths; case arising from flexor sheath of index finger. Brit. J. Surg. *30:*179–180, Oct '42

SHEPHERD, P. R. (see PARFITT, G. J. *et al*) Feb '43

SHERIDAN, W. J.: Principles in treatment of fractures of small bones of hand. J. Tennessee M. A. *31:*263–271, July '38

SHERMAN, B. H.: X-ray treatment of keloidal and hypertrophic scars. Radiology *18:*754–757, April '32

SHERRILL, J. D.: Wrist bone injuries. South. M. J. *38:*306–312, May '45

SHERRILL, J. G.: Carcinoma of cheek, case report. Kentucky M. J. *20:*284–285, April '22

SHERRILL, W. P.: Two case reports of extensive burns in children; both recovered; one with

Curling ulcer. Southwestern Med. *21:*135–138, April '37
SHERSHEVSKAYA, O. I.: Congenital coloboma of eyelids. Vestnik oftal. *13:*822–828, '38
SHERWIN, C. F.: Surgical management of carcinoma of larynx. S. Clin. North America *24:*1089–1099, Oct '44
SHEVELEV, M. M.: Vertical section and flat incisions of cartilage of eyelids in therapy of trachomatous entropion. Vestnik oftal. *11:*383–386, '37
SHEYNKMAN, S. S.: Therapy at the front for burns. Khirurgiya, no. 12, pp. 41–46, '44
SHIH, H. E.: Reverdin grafts, with report of 2 cases. Nat. M. J., China *16:*563–571, Oct '30
SHIH, H. E.: Volkmann's contracture with report of case. Nat. M. J., China *17:*315–322, June '31
SHILLITO, L.: Ionized silver in burns. Brit. M. J. *2:*668, Oct 12, '29
SHILOVTSEV, S. P.: Operative treatment of extensive angioma of head. Arch. f. klin. Chir. *184:*179–182, '35
SHILOVTSEV, S. P.: Surgical therapy of extensive angioma of head. Vestnik khir. *45:*236–239, '36
SHILOVTZEFF, S. P.: Transplantation of ureters into rectum by Mirotvortzeff's method in exstrophy of bladder. Lancet *2:*412–415, Aug 19, '39
SHIMANKO, I. I.: Drying of burns by means of heliotherapy. Sovet. khir., no. 6, pp. 226–230, '35
SHIMKIN, N.: Autoplastic operation on lower margin of tarsus for ingrown eyelash. Klin. Monatsbl. f. Augenh. *77:*538–546, Oct 30, '26
SHIMKIN, N.: Spastic entropion after total tarsectomy of upper lid cured by tarsal homoplasty; 3 cases. Klin. Monatsbl. f. Augenh. *82:*360–364, March 22, '29
SHIMKIN, N.: Entropion spasticum after tarsectomia totalis of upper eyelid cured by homoplastica tarsi; 3 cases. Cong. internat. de med. trop. et d'hyg., Compt. rend. (1928) *3:*743–751, '31
SHIMKIN, N. I.: Transplanted conchae auriculae as new method of correcting spastic entropion of upper eyelid following total tarsectomy. Rev. internat. du trachome *15:*15–20, Jan '38, also: Brit. J. Ophth. *22:*282–287, May '38
SHIMKIN, N. I.: Two rare cases of homoplastic surgery of eyelids. Brit. J. Ophth. *29:*363–369, July '45
SHIMKIN, N. I.: Ectropion due to ichthyosis of both upper and lower lids on child corrected by homoplastic grafting of skin from child's mother. Harefuah *29:*155, Oct 1, '45
SHIMOZUMA, T.: Plastic operation for correction of saddle nose. Sei-I-Kwai M. J. *44:*13–24, Oct '25
SHINKAI, T.: Amyloid formation caused by intraabdominal implantation of organ tissue. Tr. Jap. Path. Soc. *18:*235, '28
SHINOI, K.: Fate of homoplastic flaps. Mitt. d. med. Gesellsch. zu Tokio *46:*324–325; 369, Feb '32
SHINOI, K.: Immunologic reactions and acid-base equilibrium of flaps in homoplastic skin grafts. Mitt. d. med. Gesellsch. zu Tokio *46:*1913–1914, Nov '32
SHIPLEY, A. M.: Plastic operation on chest. Ann. Surg. *84:*246–250, Aug '26
SHIPMON, T. H.: External skeletal fixation of jaw fractures in dental office. Am. J. Orthodontics (Oral Surg. Sect.) *31:*486–492, Aug '45
SHIPOV, A. K.: Restoration of thumb from carpal bone. Sovet. khir., no. 8, p. 163, '35
SHIRAZY, E. (see DORRANCE, G. M.) July '35
SHIRLEY, C. (see COGSWELL, H. D.) Sept '39
SHIROKOV, B. A.: Phalangization of first metacarpal bone in plastic restoration of thumb; anatomic basis of author's method. Khirurgiya, no. 7, pp. 115–122, '39
SHKUROV, B. I.: Therapy of traumatic dislocations of digital phalanges. Ortop. i travmatol. (no. 3) *9:*99–103, '35
SHLEPOV, A. V. (see KHEYFETS, A. B.) 1934
SHNAYERSON, N.: Finger splint for extension or flexion. J.A.M.A. *110:*2070–2071, June 18, '38
SHNEYDER, S. L.: Symmetric polydactylia and macromelia of upper and lower extremities. Sovet. khir. (no. 6) *6:*889–894, '34

Shock

Modern conception and treatment of shock. LEE, B. J., Am. J. Surg. *36:*166–169, July '22
Nitroglycerin in surgery for shock. FRANKE, F. Zentralbl. f. Chir. *50:*1325–1328, Aug 25, '23
Paralysis of parasympathetics as basis for shock treatment. GAUTRELET, J. Medecine *5:*204–206, Dec '23, abstr: J.A.M.A. *82:*424, Feb 2, '24
Shock and its treatment. RUTHERFORD, A. G. W. Virginia M. J. *18:*298–302, Dec '23
Ideas of Dr. Crile on operative shock and their clinical application. DE NECKER, J. Arch. franco-belges de chir. *27:*411–421, May '24
Anesthesia and shock. DE WAELE, H. Compt. rend. Soc. de biol. *91:*909–910, Oct 24, '24
Treatment of shock with glucose infusions and insulin. FISHER, D. AND SNELL, M. W. J.A.M.A. *83:*1906–1908, Dec 13, '24
Glucose and insulin in treatment of shock. LEVY, W. E. AND MACHECA, H. New Or-

Shock – Cont.
leans M. and S. J. *77:*478–480, May '25
Non-specific stimulation of natural antibody in treatment of shock. MACKIE, T. J., J. Hygiene *24:*176–188, Oct '25
Obstetrical shock. AKERMAN, J., South. M. J. *19:*134–136, Feb '26
Phenomena of shock in obstetrics. RIVIERE, M. Arch. franco-belges de chir. *29:*106–109, Feb '26
Shock in pregnant and puerperal woman. BAILEY, H. AND DRISCOLL, W. P., Am. J. Obst. and Gynec. *11:*287–304, March '26
Obstetric shock. STONE, E. L., Am. J. Obst. and Gynec. *11:*650–660, May '26
Insulin-glucose treatment of shock. FISHER, D. Surg., Gynec. and Obst. *43:*224–229, Aug '26
Shall we wait for shock to pass before operating? PORTER, M. F., J. Indiana M. A. *19:*401–402, Oct '26
Diathermy in treatment of shock. CRADDOCK, F. H. AND WHETSTONE, G. South. M. J. *19:*812–813, Nov '26
Case of obstetric shock. RIVIÈRE, M. Bull. Soc. d'obst. et de gynec. *16:*225–228, March '27
Diathermy in shock; case. COTTLE, G. F. U. S. Nav. M. Bull. *25:*340–343, April '27
Intravenous use of solutions of gum arabic (acacia). HUFFMAN, L. D. Proc. Staff Meet., Mayo Clin. *2:*84, April 20, '27
Intravenous injections of salt-gum solutions in shock from hemorrhage. BUCCI, P. Boll. d. Soc. ital. di biol. Sper. *2:*965–972, Nov '27
Observations on insulin-glucose method in obstetric shock. GREEN-ARMYTAGE, V. B. Indian M. Gaz. *62:*675–680, Dec '27
Hemorrhages during pregnancy; obstetrical shock; death. VORON, AND BROCHIER, A. Bull. Soc. d'obst. et de gynec. *17:*60, Jan '28
Shock in pregnancy and labor. DRISCOLL, W. P., Anesth. and Analg. *7:*113–120, March–April '28
Epinephrine; method of prolonging its effect in asthma and depression of shock; preliminary note. LILIENTHAL, H. J.A.M.A. *90:*1192–1193, April 14, '28
Glucose and insulin in shock. LEVY, W. E. AND MACHECA, H. Anesth. and Analg. *7:*161–164, May–June '28
Dextrose-insulin therapy of shock. WADE, P. A., J.A.M.A. *90:*1859–1860, June 9, '28
Postpartum shock; case. FALSÍA, M. V. Folha med. *9:*269–273, Aug 15, '28, Semana med. *2:*625–631, Sept 6, '28
Diathermia for prevention and treatment of shock. PORTMANN, U. V. Arch. Physical Therapy *9:*385–388, Sept '28

Shock – Cont.
Shock therapy. RIBAS Y RIBAS, E. Arch. de med., cir. y espec. *29:*393–398, Oct 6, '28
Further observations on prevention with insulin-glucose in shock. ANDERSON, C. M. Anesth. and Analg. *7:*346–353, Nov–Dec '28
Differential diagnosis and treatment of obstetric shock. SERRÃO, B. Folha med. *9:*365, Nov 5, '28
Treatment of collapse; drug modifiers of tonus, and excitors of arterial contractility. TREMONTI, P. Arch. di farmacol. sper. *46:*119; 129; 145, 1928–1929
Normet's citrated solution in shock; cases. NORMET. Bull. et mem. Soc. nat. de chir. *55:*848–853, June 22, '29
Normet's citrated solution in shock. BARTHÉLEMY, M. Bull. et mem. Soc. nat. de chir. *55:*1050–1052, July 20, '29
Treatment of obstetric shock with intravenous injections of acacia. RANDALL, L. M. J.A.M.A. *93:*845–847, Sept 14, '29
Present status of glucose-insulin in shock. WADE, P. A., Anesth. and Analg. *8:*298–301, Sept–Oct '29
Solution of acacia and sodium chloride; effects of intravenous administration in shock. HUFFMAN, L. D., J.A.M.A. *93:*1698–1702, Nov 30, '29
Shock in childbirth and sudden death following labor. MANDELSTAMM, A. Arch. f. Gynak. *138:*543–557, '29
Obstetric shock; treatment with intravenous injections of acacia. RANDALL, L. M., Tr. Sect. Obst., Gynec. and Abd. Surg., A. M. A., pp. 141–148, '29
Significance and management of shock. RUTHERFORD, A. G. West Virginia M. J. *26:*26–28, Jan '30
Value of cardiazol (metrazol) as analeptic in surgery to prevent shock. SCHLEIPEN, C. Munchen. med. Wchnschr. *77:*1101–1103, June 27, '30
Obstetric shock, case. PINSONNEAULT, G. Union med. du Canada *59:*477–482, Aug '30
Treatment of shock in rattlesnake bites. CRIMMINS, M. L. Texas State J. Med. *26:*449–450, Oct '30
Nature, diagnosis, clinical aspects, pathogenesis and treatment of obstetric shock. ALDERS, N. Wien. klin. Wchnschr. *43:*1562–1565, Dec 18, '30
Effects of loss of whole blood, of blood plasma and of red blood cells in experimental shock. JOHNSON, G. S. AND BLALOCK, A. Arch. Surg. *22:*626–637, April '31
Use of Normet's citrated solution in shock. BRESSOT, E. Cron. med. mex. *30:*207–209, May '31

Shock – Cont.
Obstetric shock. PHILLIPS, M. H. Brit. M. J. *1:*833–837, May 16, '31
Present conception of shock and its treatment. WENGER, H. L. Am. J. Surg. *13:*307–310, Aug '31
Ephedrine and its compounds in treatment of shock in spinal anesthesia. DESPLAS, B. Rev. crit. de path. et de therap. *2:*669–674, Sept '31
Grave postoperative hemorrhages; pathogenesis of late hemorrhages and their treatment by shock. ANTONETTI, H. Presse med. *39:*1766–1768, Dec 2, '31
Surgical method of nasal surgery which does not cause shock. WOJATSCHEK. Acta otolaryng. *15:*327–341, '31
Closure of lymph vessels in electrocoagulation; significance in prevention of shock. ZSCHAU, H. Deutsche Ztschr. f. Chir. *233:*109–120, '31
Ephedrine and its compounds in treatment of shock in spinal anesthesia. DESPLAS, B. Bull. et mem. Soc. nat. de chir. *58:*158–162, Feb 6, '32
Intravenous use of acacia solution in shock. GOOD, R. W. AND BOYER, B. E., J. Med. *12:*630–636, Feb '32
Normet's citrated solution in shock. NISSEL, W. Chirurg *4:*363–369, May 1, '32
Intravenous injection of hypertonic solutions in shock. SCHÜCK, F. Zentralbl. f. Chir. *59:*2027–2029, Aug 20, '32
Intravenous injections of hypertonic solutions in shock. (Comment on Schück's article). STEJSKAL, K. Zentralbl. f. Chir. *59:*2896, Nov 26, '32
Intravenous injections of hypertonic solutions in shock. (Comment on Schück's article). JOSEPH, E. Zentralbl. f. Chir. *59:*2934, Dec 3, '32
Reply to article by Joseph on shock therapy; also, one by Stejskal. SCHÜCK, F. Zentralbl. f. Chir. *60:*634–635, March 18, '33
Reviten in prophylaxis and therapy of shock. FAUST, H. Monatschr. f. Unfallh. *40:*282–286, June '33
Shock and collapse. EWIG, W. Zentralbl. f. inn. Med. *54:*690–704, Aug 5, '33
Fresh embryonal juices in shock after surgical therapy of peptic ulcers; 2 cases. PAUCHET, V. *et al.* Compt. rend. Acad. d. sc. *197:*1470–1472, Dec 4, '33
Acacia solution in treatment of shock; analysis of 111 case histories. GOOD, R. W. *et al.* Am. J. Surg. *25:*134–139, July '34
Physiological considerations related to infusion treatment of shock. MACFEE, W. F. AND BALDRIDGE, R. R. Ann. Surg. *100:*266–278, Aug '34
Metrazol-ephedrine in prevention of shock. IONESCU-MILTIADE, I. Romania med. *12:*233–234, Sept 15, '34
Differential diagnosis between hemorrhage and shock following abdominal surgery. KENNEDY, J. W., M. Rec. *140:*420–421, Oct 17, '34
Autotransfusion of blood to counteract shock. DOSHOYANTS, S. L. Sovet. khir. (no. 1) *6:*57–58, '34
Shock, collapse and electrosurgery. SCHÖRCHER, F. Deutsche Ztschr. f. Chir. *243:*225–273, '34
Problems illustrating importance of knowledge of biochemistry by surgeon (including shock). RAVDIN, I. S. AND RHOADS, J. E. S. Clin. North America *15:*85–100, Feb '35
Blood transfusion in shock. MOSCOSO, A. Rev. med.-cir. do Brasil *43:*125–139, April '35
Modern treatment of shock. FRAZIER, C. H. J.A.M.A. *105:*1731–1734, Nov 30, '35
Shock therapy. KÖNIG, W. Zentralbl. f. Chir. *62:*2862–2873, Nov 30, '35, Abstr: Med. Welt *9:*1693–1696, Nov 23, '35
Shock and its therapy by gum acacia. CORREIA NETTO, A. AND ETZEL, E. Rev. de cir. de Sao Paulo *2:*137–148, Dec '35
Gum acacia in shock; 80 cases. ETZEL, E. Rev. de cir. de Buenos Aires *14:*691–705, Dec '35
Action of slow continuous injections of epinephrine in shock. BAUDOUIN, A. *et al.* Compt. rend. Soc. de biol. *119:*474–476, '35
Shock therapy by warmed air (use of Sweetland castdryer). HITCHCOCK, H. H. AND REYNOLDS, T. E. California and West. Med. *44:*98–99, Feb '36
Therapy of shock. ELLIS RIBEIRO, F. Rev. brasil. de cir. *5:*171–174, April '36
Antagonistic effect of metrazol in shock. SCHLAEPFER, K. Anesth. and Analg. *15:*202–206, July–Aug '36
Present day conception of therapy of shock. MEEK, W. J., Northwest. Med. *35:*325–334, Sept '36
Inversion of inhibition phenomenon by tetanus toxin; application to therapy of shock; experimental study. LEON, A. P. Medicina, Mexico *16:*505–513, Nov 10, '36
General norms in shock therapy. STAJANO, C. Arch. urug. de med., cir. y especialid. *9:*634–644, Nov '36
Blood transfusion in shock therapy. LINDENBAUM, I. S. AND DEPP, M. E. Vestnik khir. *46:*189–198, '36

Shock – Cont.
Effect of vasotonic drugs in various types of shock. WAHREN, H. Ztschr. f. d. ges. exper. Med. *99:*306-319, '36
Shock and postoperative hypotension. STAJANO, C. Arch. urug. de med., cir. y especialid. *10:*373-380, March '37
Syncope, collapse and shock; medical significance and treatment. WEISS, S. AND WILKINS, R. W., M. Clin. North America *21:*481-510, March '37
Shock therapy. MAKEL, H. P. Mil. Surgeon *80:*436-447, June '37
Intravenous injection of caffeine in therapy of shock. FERRANNINI, L. Policlinico (sez. prat.) *44:*1648-1650, Aug 30, '37
Physiologic availability of fluids in secondary shock. DAVIS, H. A. Arch. Surg. *35:*461-477, Sept '37
Prevention and treatment of shock. TRIMBLE, I. R. South. M. J. *30:*876-880, Sept '37
Shock and some associated factors. CLEMENT, F. W. Anesth. and Analg. *16:*271-274, Sept-Oct '37
Therapy of sudden circulatory failure (collapse and shock). LIEBMANN, E. Schweiz. med. Wchnschr. *67:*1086-1089, Nov 13, '37
Clinical application of salt solutions in shock. ANDRIEVSKIY, B. Y. Novy khir. arkhiv *37:*580-588, '37
Treatment of shock and collapse. VON BERGMANN, G. Ztschr. f. arztl. Fortbild. *35:*125-131, March 1, '38
Treatment of shock or peripheral circulatory failure. BLALOCK, A. South. Surgeon *7:*150-156, April '38
Human ascitic fluid as blood substitute in secondary shock. DAVIS, H. A. AND WHITE, C. S. Proc. Soc. Exper. Biol. and Med. *38:*462-465, May '38
Use of ascitic fluid in primary shock. CHOISSER, R. M. AND RAMSEY, E. M. Proc. Soc. Exper. Biol. and Med. *38:*651-652, June '38
Acute adrenal cortex exhaustion and its relationship to shock. REED, F. R. Am. J. Surg. *40:*514-528, June '38
Secondary vascular shock. LAWSON, H. Kentucky M. J. *36:*281-284, July '38
Veritol therapy of shock. NOGUEIRA, N. G. Ann. brasil. de gynec. *6:*123-126, Aug '38
Shock and circulatory collapse. BÜSSEMAKER, J. Jahresk. f. arztl. Fortbild. *30:*20-27, Feb '39
Clinical types of circulatory failure and their treatment. HARRISON, W. G. JR. J. M. A. Alabama *8:*305-309, March '39
Prevention and treatment of shock. COWELL, E. M. Brit. M. J. *1:*883-885, April 29, '39
Symposium on shock. (Various authors.) Med. Klin. *35:*493-499, April 14, '39
Pressure infusion; method of treating persistent shock. HEDIN, R. F. AND KARP, M. Anesth. and Analg. *18:*148-149, May-June '39
Importance of rhythmic injection of blood or its substitutes (preserved blood, human plasma and Bayliss, Normet or physiologic serum) in acute hemorrhage and shock. BECART, A. Presse med. *47:*1681-1682, Dec 27-30, '39
Blood studies as guides to therapy of shock. SCUDDER, J. Tr. Am. Proct. Soc. *40:*249-256, '39
High traumatic amputation of thigh and treatment of shock. DELANEY, W. E. JR. Indust. Med. *9:*28-29, Jan '40
Early recognition and management of shock. MOON, V. H., Urol. and Cutan. Rev. *44:*5-12, Jan '40
Direct arterial and venous pressure measurements in man as affected by anesthesia, operation and shock. VOLPITTO, P. P. *et al.* Am. J. Physiol. *128:*238-245, Jan '40
Syncope, collapse and shock. WEISS, S. Proc. Inst. Med. Chicago *13:*2-12, Jan 15, '40
Prevention of shock by cortical hormone (desoxycorticosterone acetate and cortin) and saline. PERLA, D. *et al.* Proc. Soc. Exper. Biol. and Med. *43:*397-404, Feb '40
Shock – circulatory failure of capillary origin. MOON, V. H., J.A.M.A. *114:*1312-1318, April 6, '40
Use of citrated plasma in treatment of secondary shock. STRUMIA, M. M. *et al.* J.A.M.A. *114:*1337-1341, April 6, '40
Shock therapy. DUJOVICH, A. Dia med. *12:*418-421, May 20, '40
Therapy of Cook County Hospital; therapy of acute peripheral circulation failure; syncope, shock and collapse, in collaboration with L. Seed. FANTUS, B., J.A.M.A. *114:*2010-2015, May 18, '40
Solutions of acacia in shock. RAIA, A. Rev. de cir. de Sao Paulo *5:*463-476, May-June '40
Blood transfusion in shock. SCHUBERTH, O. Svenska lak.-tidning. *37:*900-907, May 17, '40
Intravenous injection of morphine in therapy of shock; case. FUNCK-BRENTANO, P. Mem. Acad. de chir. *66:*615-616, June 5-26, '40
Shock and collapse. GOLDHAHN, R. Med. Welt. *14:*573, June 8, '40; 597, June 15, '40
Question of using preserved whole blood or blood plasma. MALMROS, H. AND WILANDER, O. Svenska lak.-tidning. *37:*1026-1029, June 14, '40
Pathology of shock in man; visceral effects of

Shock-Cont.
burns–trauma, hemorrhage and surgical operat. DAVIS, H. A., Arch. Surg. *41:*123-146, July '40
Preparation and use of human serum for blood transfusion. CLEGG, J. W. AND DIBLE, J. H. Lancet *2:*294-296, Sept 7, '40
Shock therapy. MEAKINS, J. C. Canad. M. A. J. *43:*201-205, Sept '40
Study of shock and therapeutic deductions. BINET, L. AND STRUMZA, M. V. Presse med. *48:*825-828, Oct 16-19, '40
Shock and its treatment. LOUGHRIDGE, J. S. Ulster M. J. *9:*127-131, Oct '40
Plasma loss in severe dehydration, shock and other conditions as affected by therapy. MINOT, A. S. AND BLALOCK, A. Ann. Surg. *112:*557-567, Oct '40
Human ascitic fluid and starch-Ringer solution in shock therapy. SANTOS, H. A. *et al.* U. S. T. J. Med. *1:*75-85, Nov '40
Effects of serum and saline infusions in shock; quantitative studies in man. HILL, D. K. *et al.* Lancet *2:*774-776, Dec 21, '40
Diagnosis and treatment of secondary shock; 24 cases. KEKWICK, A. *et al.* Lancet *1:*99-103, Jan 25, '41
Evaluation of various intravenous medications in shock therapy (use of blood serum and plasma). MCFARLAND, O. W. AND CONNELL, J. H. New Orleans M. and S. J. *93:*353-357, Jan '41
Collapse and shock. SAZAVSKY, K. Casop. lek. cesk. *80:*126-129, Jan 24, '41
Desiccated plasma in shock therapy. HILL, J. M. *et al.* J.A.M.A. *116:*395-402, Feb 1, '41
Blood studies as guide to shock therapy. SCUDDER, J., J. Med. *21:*519-521, Feb '41
Shock therapy. JORGE, J. M. *et al.* Rev. Asoc. med. argent. *55:*182-204, March 15-30, '41
Pathogenesis and treatment of shock. ASHWORTH, C. T. Tri-State M. J. *13:*2735-2738, April '41
Adrenal cortical hormone (preoperative administration in prevention of shock). CORRADO, P. C., M. Times, New York *69:*155-162, April '41
Plasma therapy in shock. DIGGS, L. W. Memphis M. J. *16:*58-61, April '41
Physiologic pathology as applied to treatment of shock. GIORDANO, A. S., J. Indiana M. A. *34:*197-200, April '41
Shock. LINDGREN, S. Svenska lak.-tidning. *38:*933-939, April 25, '41
Blood plasma in shock therapy. ELLIOTT, J. South. Med. and Surg. *103:*252-254, May '41
Quantitative aspects of transfusion in shock. HARRISON, G. A. AND PICKEN, L. E. R. Lancet *1:*685-686, May 31, '41
Use of concentrated pooled human serum and pooled lyophile serum in shock therapy. ROSE, B. *et al.* Canad. M. A. J. *44:*442-448, May '41
Treatment of circulatory collapse and shock. STEAD, E. A. JR. Am. J. M. Sc. *201:*775-782, May '41
Analysis of 50 cases of shock treated with plasma. WHITE, C. S. *et al.* South. Med. and Surg. *103:*250-251, May '41
Use of pooled human serum for treatment of hemorrhage and shock. BICK, M. AND DREVERMANN, E. B., M. J. Australia *1:*750-754, June 21, '41
Shock, collapse and hemorrhage. NEUMANN, B. Harefuah *20:*71, June 1, '41
Shock, Blood transfusion and supportive treatment. ADAMS, R. C. Mil. Surgeon *89:*34-41, July '41
Review of current literature on classification, etiology and treatment of shock. BAIRD, C. L., Mil. Surgeon *89:*24-34, July '41
Shock treatment, with particular reference to use of blood plasma. BLALOCK, A. J. Tennessee M. A. *34:*254-257, July '41
Value of hemoconcentration in shock phenomena; therapeutic deductions. ISELIN, M. Presse med. *49:*836-838, July 30-Aug 2, '41
Present conception of cause and treatment of shock. RILEY, J. G. Lahey Clin. Bull. *2:*154-160, July '41
Role of adrenal glands in shock; value of desoxycorticosterone acetate (adrenal preparation) in prevention of operative shock. BESSER, E. L. Arch. Surg. *43:*249-256, Aug '41
Pectin solution as blood substitute in shock therapy. HARTMAN, F. W. *et al.* Ann. Surg. *114:*212-225, Aug '41
Plasma protein; physiologic action and therapeutic application in shock. MARSH, F. B. Indust. Med. *10:*352-359, Aug '41
Supportive measures in care of surgical patients (transfusion of blood and plasma, parenteral administration of solutions and stimulants). SELDON, T. H. AND LUNDY, J. S., Southwestern Med. *25:*236-240, Aug '41
Stored dextrose-citrate plasma in treatment of operative shock. BESSER, E. L. Arch. Surg. *43:*451-457, Sept '41
Enema of concentrated coffee in shock therapy; study from 1916-1941. STAJANO, C. Arch. urug. de med., cir. y especialid. *19:*241-260, Sept '41
Treatment of circulatory collapse and shock. STEAD, E. A. JR. Rev. Asoc. med. argent.

Shock – Cont.
*55:*710-713, Sept 15-30, '41
New concepts of postoperative secondary shock and its therapy; physiology and general pathology. GOMEZ DE ROSAS, N. Vida nueva *48:*283-297, Nov '41
Controlled fluid administration in shock. Lindgren, S. AND WILANDER, O. Nord. med. (Hygiea) *12:*3099-3106, Nov 1, '41
Review of literature on shock. NORES, A. JR. Rev. med. de Cordoba *29:*629-643, Nov '41
Shock and syncope in postoperative period. COSSIO, P. Dia med. *13:*1309-1313, Dec 15, '41
Similarities and distinctions between shock and effects of hemorrhage. MOON, V. H. *et al.* J.A.M.A. *177:*2024-2030, Dec 13, '41
Prophylactic and therapeutic use of adrenal cortical substances in shock; preliminary report. DALY, R. F. Rev. M. Progr., pp. 33-35, '41
Plasma and its clinical use in shock. BULMER, J. W., M. Times, New York *70:*3-8, Jan '42
Crushing of extremities with resulting shock. CARVALHO LUZ, F. Brasil-med. *56:*35-41, Jan 17, '42
Intravenous administration of bovine serum albumin as blood substitute in experimental secondary shock. DAVIS, H. A. AND EATON, A. G. Proc. Soc. Exper. Biol. and Med. *49:*20-22, Jan '42
Cortical extract in treatment of shock; preliminary report. HELFRICH, L. S. *et al.* Am. J. Surg. *55:*410-426, Feb '42
Advantages and clinical uses of desiccated plasma in shock prepared by adtevac process. MUIRHEAD, E. E. AND HILL, J. M. Ann. Int. Med. *16:*286-302, Feb '42
Emergency care of wounds, hemorrhage and shock. THOMPSON, L. M. New York State J. Med. *42:*355-356, Feb 15, '42
Shock and concussion. TOMB, J. W., M. J. Australia *1:*250-256, Feb 28, '42
Comparative effects of horse serum, horse serum albumin and horse serum globulin in experimental shock. DAVIS, H. A. AND EATON, A. G. Proc. Soc. Exper. Biol. and Med. *49:*359-361, March '42
Early recognition and treatment of shock. DREW, C. R. Anesthesiology *3:*176-194, March '42
Postshock metabolic response (Arris and Gale lecture). CUTHBERTSON, D. P. Lancet *1:*433-436, April 11, '42
Discussion on methods of resuscitation in shock. GRANT, R. T. *et al.* Proc. Roy. Soc. Med. *35:*445-454, April '42
Human serum albumin (concentrated); clinical indications and dosage. NEWHOUSER, L. R. AND LOZNER, E. L., U. S. Nav. M. Bull. *40:*277-279, April '42
Brief review of etiology of shock. ROOT, G. T. Proc. Staff Meet., Mayo Clin. *17:*218-221, April 8, '42
Shock therapy. LAIRES, L. Amatus *1:*463-480, May '42
Transfusions of blood and plasma in shock. TAIANA, J. A. Bol. d. Inst. clin. quir. *18:*282-283, May '42
Methyl cellulose solution as plasma substitute in shock. HUEPER, W. C. *et al.* Am. J. Surg. *56:*629-635, June '42
Discussion of use of blood and plasma transfusion in shock; method of influencing pH and prothrombin of plasma, intra-marrow injection of concentrated plasma. JONES, H. W. *et al.* Delaware State M. J. *14:*137-146, June '42
Shock and collapse. LIEBAU, G. Munche. med. Wchnschr. *89:*577, June 26, '42 also: Bull. War Med. *3:*274-275, Jan '43 (abstract)
Use of human plasma protein solutions in shock. MUIRHEAD, E. E. *et al.* South. Surgeon *11:*414-431, June '42
Blood studies in shock as guide to therapy; defense mechanism of kidney. SCUDDER, J. New York State J. Med. *42:*1146-1149, June 15, '42
Physiologic and clinical basis of shock treatment. SCULL, C. W. AND EIMAN, J. Clinics *1:*43-58, June '42
Shock and its treatment (with special reference to hemoconcentration and hemodilution). WEIL, P. G. AND MEAKINS, J. C. Clinics *1:*59-67, June '42 also: Dallas M. J. *28:*147-149, Nov '42 (abstr).
Shock therapy. COOPER, R. N. Indian Physician *1:*305-314, July '42
Shock. DEVINE, H., M. J. Australia *2:*19-26, July 11, '42
Symptoms, recognition and treatment of severe shock. ROBERTSON, F. Newcastle M. J. *21:*67-77, July '42
Present concepts of origin and treatment of traumatic shock; collective review. ANDRUS, W. DEW. Internat. Abstr. Surg. *75:*161-175, '42; in Surg., Gynec. and Obst. Aug '42
Adjuvant secondary therapy in shock. CULLEN, S. C. West. J. Surg. *50:*392-395, Aug '42
Shock produced by crush injury; effects of administration of plasma and local application of cold. DUNCAN, G. W. AND BLALOCK, A. Arch. Surg. *45:*183-194, Aug '42

Shock – Cont.

Shock and collapse; functional pathology and therapy. SCHWIECK, H. Klin. Wchnschr. *21:*741, Aug 22 '42; 765, Aug 29, '42

Shock and anesthesia. HARKINS, H. N. Anesth. and Analg. *21:*273–279, Sept–Oct '42

Technic of administering blood and other fluids via bone marrow; further experiences. O'NEILL, J. F. *et al.* North Carolina M. J. *3:*495–500, Sept '42

Shock. YOUNG, C. T. Hawaii M. J. *2:*22–25, Sept–Oct '42

Shock. BOVE, C., M. Rec. *155:*463–466, Oct '42

Shock; prevention and treatment. PRICE, P. B., S. Clin. North America *22:*1297–1310, Oct '42

Treatment of shock by direct action on vegetative nerve centers (injection of potassium ions into lateral ventricles or cisterna magna). STERN, L. S. Brit. M. J. *2:*538–540, Nov 7, '42 also: Lancet *2:*572–573, Nov 14, '42

Shock treatment. VAUGHN, A. M. Illinois M. J. *82:*365–368, Nov '42

Concentrated plasma; use in treatment of shock. HILL, J. M. AND MUIRHEAD, E. E. Tri-State M. J. *15:*2844–2849, Dec '42

Shock and its treatment. YODH, B. B. Indian Physician *1:*547–554, Dec '42

Gordon Wilson lecture; shock or peripheral circulatory failure. BLALOCK, A. Tr. Am. Clin and Climatol. A. (1941) *57:*2–11, '42

4X concentrated blood plasma intrasternally in treatment of shock. JONES, H. W. *et al.* Tr. A. Am. Physicians *57:*88–92, '42

Shock. KHAN, B., J. Indian M. A. *11:*311–316, July '42

Plasma therapy in shock; importance. DE AZEVEDO, M. Rev. clin. de Sao Paulo *13:*6–16, Jan '43

Diagnosis and treatment of shock. HILL, R. H., J. M. Soc. New Jersey *40:*51–54, Feb '43

Clinical aspects of shock therapy. MAHONEY, E. B. AND HOWLAND, J. W. Surgery *13:*188–198, Feb '43

Recent advances in use of human serum and plasma in shock. HARDGROVE, M. Wisconsin M. J. *42:*298–302, March '43

Prevention and treatment of secondary shock. YOW, E. M., J. Bowman Gray School Med. *1:*31–37, March '43

Relative value of pectin solution in shock therapy. HARTMAN, F. W. *et al.* J.A.M.A. *121:*1337–1342, April 24, '43

Treatment of shock and fresh wounds. RITTER, H. H. Am. J. Surg. *60:*112–114, April '43

Shock – Cont.

Shock therapy. CONROY, C. F. Wisconsin M. J. *42:*498–500, May '43

Form of bovine serum suitable for plasma substitute in treatment of shock. EDWARDS, F. R. Proc. Roy. Soc. Med. *36:*337, May '43

Treatment of shock. HARKINS, H. N. Illinois M. J. *83:*325–331, May '43

Shock; new needle for treatment by sternal infusion. JONES, R. M. Surg., Gynec. and Obst. *76:*587–588, May '43

Shock therapy and observations. KATZ, L. N. *et al.* J.A.M.A. *122:*197, May 15, '43

Recognition and treatment of shock. VAUGHN, A. M. AND MCCARTHY, M. J. Illinois M. J. *83:*331–336, May '43

Use of concentrated and normal plasma in shock therapy. WESTON, R. E. *et al.* J.A.M.A. *122:*198, May 15, '43

Theory and therapy of shock; reduced temperatures. ALLEN, F. M. Am. J. Surg. *60:*335–348, June '43

Shock therapy. REA, C. E. Minnesota Med. *26:*531–534, June '43

Plasmotherapy in shock. VALLE ANTELO, J. Prensa med., La Paz *3:*37–40, June–July '43

Theory and therapy of shock; excessive fluid administration. ALLEN, F. M. Am. J. Surg. *61:*79–92, July '43

Present views of shock therapy; address in medicine before Royal College of Physicians and Surgeons of Canada. MEAKINS, J. C. Canad. M. A. J. *49:*21–29, July '43

Modern concept of shock therapy. PRESNO ALBARRAN, J. A. Rev. de med. y cir. Habana *48:*295–313, July 31, '43

Plasma bank in shock therapy. WILEY, A. R. J. Oklahoma M. A. *36:*285–287, July '43

Clinical aspects of acute shock. PARSONS, W. H., Mississippi Doctor *21:*70–74, Aug '43

Practical approach to shock therapy. KENDRICK, D. B. JR. AND REICHEL, J. JR. Anesthesiology *4:*497–507, Sept '43

Recent advances in vascular physiology and their therapeutic implications (shock). WILKINS, R. W., M. Clin. North America *27:*1397–1408, Sept '43

Theory and therapy of shock; varied fluid injections. ALLEN, F. M. Am. J. Surg. *62:*80–104, Oct '43

Present status of problem; "problem on shocks." BLALOCK, A. Surgery *14:*487–508, Oct '43

Use of isinglass (ishthyocolla) as blood substitute in shock therapy. TAYLOR, N. B. AND MOORHOUSE, M. S. Canad. M. A. J. *49:*251–262, Oct '43

Shock – Cont.
Physiology and treatment of shock. LANDS, A. M., Mod. Hosp. *61:*110, Nov '43
Present concept of shock syndrome and its treatment. STANDARD, S. Hebrew M. J. *1:*170, '43
Effect of dialyzed serum proteins and serum dialysates in shock. VOLKERT, M. AND ASTRUP, T. Acta med. Scandinav. *115:*537-541, '43
Shock; resuscitation in surgery. BOLOT, F. AND DAUSSET. Afrique franc. chir. *2:*39-43, Jan-March '44
Oral sodium lactate in burn shock. FOX, C. L. JR. J.A.M.A. *124:*207-212, Jan 22, '44
Pectin solutions in treatment of shock. MEYER, K. A. *et al.* Surg., Gynec. and Obst. *78:*327-332, March '44
Substitutes for human plasma in combatting shock. FOA, C. Resenha clin.-cient. *13:*157-169, April 1, '44
Successful treatment of so-called "irreversible" shock by whole blood supplemented with sodium bicarbonate and glucose. LEVINE, R. *et al.* Am. J. Physiol. *141:*209-215, April '44
Physiopathogenesis and therapy of shock. LAIRES, L. Amatus *3:*265-299, May '44
Gelatin and saline as plasma substitutes (in prevention of shock). SWINGLE, W. W. *et al.* Am. J. Physiol. *141:*329-337, May '44
Use of pectin (as substitute for whole blood or plasma) and other agents in shock prevention. FIGUEROA, L. AND LAVIERI, F. J. Surg., Gynec. and Obst. *78:*600-605, June '44
Clinic use of concentrated human serum albumin; comparison with whole blood and with rapid saline infusion. COURNAND, A. *et al.* J. Clin. Investigation *23:*491-505, July '44
Concentrated human serum albumin, safety of albumin, in shock. JANEWAY, C. A. *et al.* J. Clin. Investigation *23:*465-490, July '44
Concentrated human serum albumin in shock; preliminary report. WARREN, J. V. *et al.* J. Clin. Investigation *23:*506-509, July '44
Gelatin solutions (as plasma substitute) in human shock. KOZOLL, D. D. *et al.* Am. J. M. Sc. *208:*141-147, Aug '44
Shock therapy; biochemical aspects (hematocrit and plasma protein determinations as guide to intravenous infusions). KRETCHMAR, H. H., M. J. Australia *2:*305-309, Sept 16, '44
Intravenous pectin solution in prophylaxis and treatment of shock. MCCLURE, R. D. *et al.* Canad. M. A. J. *51:*206-210, Sept '44

Shock – Cont.
Shock; new method for treatment. ASRATYAN, E. A. Am. Rev. Soviet Med. *2:*37-43, Oct '44
Vascular collapse and its therapy. GIMENEZ, A. LEON. Dia med. *16:*1322-1325, Oct 30, '44
Etiopathogenesis and therapy of shock. MONTEIRO FILHO, A. Rev. med. brasil. *17:*489-500, Oct '44
General anesthesia in shock. CROOKE, A. C. *et al.* Brit. M. J. *2:*683-686, Nov 25, '44
Shock and hemorrhage; rapid replacement of fluid. GRAHAM, J. D. P. Brit. M. J. *2:*623-625, Nov 11, '44
Present status of problem of shock. HUNTER, A. R., M. Press *212:*350-351, Nov 29, '44
Clinical use of products of human plasma fractionation; albumin in shock and hypoproteinemia. JANEWAY, C. A. J.A.M.A. *126:*674-680, Nov 11, '44
Rational therapy of shock. KLEIMAN, M. Arch. Soc. cirujanos hosp. *14:*596-600. Dec '44
Shock and its therapy. TAGNON, H. J. *et al.* Union med. du Canada *73:*1498-1507, Dec '44
Comparative study of effects of human plasma, physiologic saline, pectin and gelatin (4% and 5%) on plasma volume in man. JACOBSON, S. D. AND SMYTH, C. J. Proc. Central Soc. Clin. Research *17:*45-46, '44
Excretion of intravenously injected gelatin. KOZOLL, D. D. AND HOFFMAN, W. S. Proc. Central Soc. Clin. Research *17:*47-48, '44
Pathologic anatomy and pathogenesis of shock. KRAEVSKIY, N. A. Khirurgiya, no. 9, pp. 7-12, '44
Intra-arterial blood transfusion in irreversible form of shock and hemorrhage. RADUSHKEVICH, V. P. Khirurgiya, no. 8, pp. 38-40, '44
The adrenals and shock. HONAN, M. S., M. Press *213:*13-14, Jan 3, '45
Evaluation of gelatin and pectin solutions as substitutes for plasma; histologic changes produced in human beings. POPPER, H. *et al.* Arch. Surg. *50:*34-45, Jan '45 also: abst., Proc. Central Soc. Clin. Research *17:*9-10, '44 abst., J. Lab. and Clin. Med. *30:*352-354, April '45
Venopressor mechanism in production of shock (role of muscle tonus); treatment with nikethamide. GUNTHER, L., U.S. Nav. M. Bull. *44:*300-307, Feb '45
Pervitin (d-desoxyephedrine) therapy in shock. HUDON, F. AND PARADIS, B. Laval med. *10:*110-128, Feb '45

Shock – Cont.

Physiopathology of shock. GUNTHER, B. Arch. Soc. cirujanos hosp. *15:*369–377, March '45

"Shock"; second thoughts. WHITBY, L. Middlesex Hosp. J. *45:*7–9, March '45

Mechanism and management of shock. PHEMISTER, D. B., J.A.M.A. *127:*1109–1112, April 28, '45

Use of cholinesterase (and plasma) in shock. SCHACHTER, R. J. Am. J. Physiol. *143:*552–557, April '45

Plasma administration in severe shock. SZYLEJKO, H. W., U.S. Nav. M. Bull. *44:*857–859, April '45

Peripheral circulation during anesthesia, shock and hemorrhage; digital plethysmograph as clinical guide. FOSTER, A. D. JR. *et al.* Anesthesiology *6:*246–257, May '45

Shock and refrigeration; newer developments. ALLEN, F. M., J. Internat. Coll. Surgeons *8:*438–452, Sept–Oct, '45

Shock following injuries of extremities; procaine hydrochloride block of vagus nerve. ERMOLAEV, P. E. Khirurgiya, no. 6, pp. 45–46, '45

Present status of clinical problem of "shock." MCMICHAEL, J. Brit. M. Bull. *3:*105–107, '45

Comparison of efficacy of different infusion media in shock. HAMILTON, J. I. *et al.* Canad. J. Research, Sect. E, *24:*31–35, Feb '46

Peripheral circulatory insufficiency with shock; present status of theories on physiopathogenesis and treatment. NOGUEIRA, A. JR. Med. cir. farm., pp. 242–276, May '46

Concentrated human albumin in treatment of shock. STEAD, E. A. JR. *et al.* Arch. Int. Med. *77:*564–575, May '46

Shock, Burn (See also Burns, Shock)

Experimental shock; composition of fluid that escapes from blood stream after burns. BEARD, J. W. AND BLALOCK, A. Arch. Surg. *22:*617–625, April '31

Experimental shock; importance of local loss of fluid in production of low blood pressure after burns. BLALOCK, A. Arch. Surg. *22:*610–616, April '31

Use of fluids in burns and shock. BRANDSON, B. J. AND HILLSMAN, J. A. Canad. M. A. J. *26:*689–698, June '32

Burns; treatment of shock and toxemia; healing wound; reconstruction. BETTMAN, A. G., Am. J. Surg. *20:*33–37, April '33

Tannic acid-silver nitrate in burns; method of minimizing shock and toxemia and shortening convalescence. BETTMAN, A. G.

Shock, Burn – Cont.

Northwest Med. *34:*46–51, Feb '35

Collapse following burns. EWIG, W. Verhandl. d. deutsch. Gesellsch. f. Kreislaufforsch., pp. 148–157, '38

Blood plasma in therapy of burn case with severe shock. ST-ONGE, G., J. de l'Hotel-Dieu de Montreal *10:*396–408, Nov–Dec '41

Treatment of shock of burns. DAVISON, G. Newcastle M. J. *21:*78–82, July '42

Shock, without or with hemorrhage, and burns. FENNEL, E. A. Hawaii M. J. *1:*385–389, July '42

Experimental chemotherapy of burns and shock; effects of systemic therapy on early mortality. ROSENTHAL, S. M. Pub. Health Rep. *58:*513–522, March 26, '43

Failure of plasma and serum transfusion prolonged during 8 days in extensive burns. LOMBARD, P. Afrique franc. chir. *1:*375–378, Nov–Dec '43

Treatment of burn shock. COONEY, E. A. Bull. New England M. Center *5:*248–256, Dec '43

Adrenal cortical extract in burn shock; further experiences. RHOADS, J. E. *et al.* Ann. Surg. *118:*982–987, Dec '43

Treatment of burn shock with continuous hypodermoclysis of physiologic saline solution into burned area; experimental study. BERMAN, J. K. *et al.* Surg., Gynec. and Obst. *78:*337–345, April '44

Plasma and blood in treatment of shock in burns. LUNDY, J. S. *et al.* S. Clin. North America *24:*798–807, Aug '44

Closed plaster method of burn therapy in prevention of shock. SELLERS, E. A. AND GORANSON, E. S. Canad. M. A. J. *51:*111–114, Aug '44

Principle from liver effective against shock due to burns. PRINZMETAL, M.; *et al.* J. Clin. Investigation *23:*795–806, Sept '44

Comparison of therapeutic effectiveness of serum and sodium chloride in scald shock. HECHTER, O. *et al.* Am. Heart J. *29:*484–492, April '45

Role of renal pressor system in shock of burns. HECHTER, O. *et al.* Am. Heart J. *29:*493–498, April '45

Liver principle which is effective against burn shock; further studies. HECHTER, O. *et al.* Am. Heart J. *29:*499–505, April '45

Closed plaster method of prevention of shock after burns. SELLERS, E. A. AND GORANSON, E. S., J. Canad. M. Serv. *2:*431–437, May '45

Blood changes in shock following burns. GORDIENKO, A. N. Bull. War Med. *6:*473, July '46 (abstract)

Shock, Experimental

Mechanism of production and treatment of shock. BLALOCK, A., J. M. A. Alabama *1:*94–99, Sept '31

Therapy in experimental shock. BLALOCK, A. *et al.* J.A.M.A. *97:*1794–1797, Dec 12, '31

Experimental shock; production and treatment. BLALOCK, A. *et al.* Tr. Sect. Surg., Gen. and Abd., A. M. A. pp. 294–303, '31

Experimental shock, with special reference to anesthesia. (Arris and Gale lecture). McDOWALL, R. J. S. Brit. M. J. *1:*690–693, April 22, '33

Factors in treatment of shock; experimental study (Davidson lecture abstract). DAVIS, H. A., M. Ann. District of Columbia *6:*344–349, Dec '37

Experimental and clinical shock, with special reference to its treatment by intravenous injection of preserved plasma. MAHONEY, E. B. Ann. Surg. *108:*178–193, Aug '38

Transfusion of blood stabilized with magnesium sulfate in experimental shock. ABRAMSON, B. P. Vestnik khir. *56:*659–670, Nov '38

Intra-arterial hypertonic saline solution in experimental shock. KENDRICK, D. B. JR. AND WAKIM, K. G. Proc. Soc. Exper. Biol. and Med. *40:*114–116, Jan '39

Intravenous injections of diluted blood; experimental study in shock. BINET, L. AND STRUMZA. Bull. Acad. de med., Paris *123:*592–595, Aug 6–27, '40

Effects of inhalation of high concentration of oxygen in experimental shock. WOOD, G. O. *et al.* Surgery *8:*247–256, Aug '40

Methods of fluid administration in treatment of shock; experimental comparison. KING, R. A., Brit. M. J. *2:*485–487, Oct 12, '40

Shock toxin; pharmacologic effects of perfusate flowing through crushed muscle tissue. SUZUKI, K. Jap. J. M. Sc., IV, Pharmacol. *13:*117*–119*, Oct '40

Comparison of effects of heat and cold in shock therapy. BLALOCK, A. AND MASON, M. F. Arch. Surg. *42:*1054–1059, June '41

Physiologic effects of high concentrations of oxygen in experimental secondary shock. DAVIS, H. A. Arch. Surg. *43:*1–13, July '41

Effect of replacement therapy (especially with plasma or saline) in experimental shock. DUNPHY, J. E. AND GIBSON, J. G. JR. Surgery *10:*108–118, July '41

Desoxycorticosterone (adrenal preparation) as prophylactic foretreatment for prevention of circulatory failure following hemorrhage and surgical trauma in adrenalectomized dog. PARKINS, W. M. *et al.* Am. J. Physiol. *134:*426–435, Sept '41

Shock, Experimental – Cont.

Treatment of experimental shock by intravenous injection of dilute, normal and concentrated plasma. MAHONEY, E. B. *et al.* Surg., Gynec. and Obst. *74:*319–325, Feb (no. 2A) '42

Procaine hydrochloride anesthesia of carotid sinus in treatment of shock; experimental study. PIULACHS, P. Med. clin., Barcelona *3:*223–236, Sept '44

The heart in experimental shock. PRINZMETAL, M. AND BERGMAN, H. C., J. Mt. Sinai Hosp. *12:*579–583, May–June '45

Shock, Surgical

Surgical shock. O'CONNOR, D. C. Journal-Lancet *41:*287, May 15, '21

Observation on nature and treatment of surgical shock. DAVISON, T. C., J. M. A. Georgia *10:*779, Nov '21

Use of gum-glucose solution in major urological surgery. LOWSLEY, O. S. *et al.* J. Urology *6:*381, Nov '21

Rational treatment of surgical shock based on proven physiological data. MUNROE, A. R., Canad. M. A. J. *12:*136–138, March '22

Surgical shock. MALCOLM, J. D. Proc. Roy. Soc. Med. (Sect. Obst. and Gynec.) *15:*71–80, July '22

Postoperative shock. MISRACHI. Presse med. *31:*565–567, June 23, '23

Surgical shock. ADAMS, J. L. AND GRAVES, J. Q. New Orleans M. and S. J. *76:*291–295, Dec '23

Operation shock. FRASER, J. Brit. J. Surg. *11:*410–425, Jan '24

Shockless surgery; Crile's contribution to humanity and to the medical profession; with simple and dependable method of preparation of patient for same; and remarks. SMYTHE, F. D., J. Tennessee M. A. *16:*313–317, Jan '24

Surgical shock. KÁLALOVÁ, V. Cas. lek. cesk. *63:*1867–1878, Dec 22, '24

Insulin-glucose treatment of surgical shock and nondiabetic acidosis. FISHER, D. AND MENSING, E. Surg., Gynec. and Obst. *40:*548–555, April '25

Insulin-dextrose treatment of surgical shock. BERESOW, S. L. Zentralbl. f. Chir. *53:*3214–3217, Dec 18, '26

Use of glucose and insulin in prevention of surgical shock. ANDERSON, C. M. California and West. Med. *27:*56–61, July '27

Insulin-glucose in surgical shock, with observations on 2 cases. TUASON, M. N., J. Philippine Islands M. A. *7:*283–286, Aug '27

Treatment of surgical and traumatic shock. BAUMANN, E. Schweiz. med. Wchnschr.

Shock, Surgical–Cont.
*57:*1045-1047, Oct 29, '27
Surgical shock. VALDES, U. Rev. Asoc. med. mex., no. 14, p. 25, Feb; no. 15, p. 5, March '29
Treatment of surgical shock with ephetonin(synthetic ephedrine). HOLZBACH, E. Zentralbl. f. Gynak. *53:*1106-1110, May 4, '29
Surgical shock. SOHLBERG, O. I. Minnesota Med. *12:*360-361, June '29
Surgical shock. MCSWAIN, G., J. Tennessee M. A. *22:*135-137, Aug '29
Nature and prevention of surgical shock. FOHL, T. AND SCHNEIDER, E. Deutsche Ztschr. f. Chir. *220:*179-195, '29
Post-operative shock and shock-like conditions; treatment by infusion (physiologic sodium chloride solution with or without dextrose) in large volume. MACFEE, W. F. AND BALDRIDGE, R. R. Ann. Surg. *91:*329-341, March '30
Toxemia producing shock after operation; report of case. CRISP, N. W. Proc. Staff Meet., Mayo Clin. *5:*128, May 7, '30
Acapnia as factor in post-operative shock. HENDERSON, Y., J.A.M.A. *95:*572-575, Aug 23, '30
Intravenous therapy for postoperative shock. HOWLETT, H. Internat. Clin. *3:*26-29, Sept '30
Experimental study of surgical shock. METZLER, F. Deutsche Ztschr. f. Chir. *228:*340-348, '30
Postoperative shock. EPPINGER, H. Wien. klin. Wchnschr. *44:*65-71, Jan 16, '31
Nature and treatment of surgical shock and postoperative collapse. HOLZBACH, E. Fortschr. d. Therap. *7:*169-172, March 25, '31
Surgical shock. FOSTER, G. S., J. Missouri M. A. *28:*424-427, Sept '31
Treatment of surgical shock (blood transfusion and intravenous drip). RANSOHOFF, J. L. AND MENDELSOHN, S. N., J. Med. *12:*637-641, Feb '32
Postoperative syndrome (shock and collapse). EPPINGER, H. Klin. Wchnschr. *11:*618-622, April 9, '32
Therapy of postoperative circulatory shock. VON BERGMANN, G. Deutsche med. Wchnschr. *58:*519-523, April 1, '32
Postoperative shock. EWIG, W. AND KLOTZ, L. Deutsche Ztschr. f. Chir. *235:*681-710, '32 also: Klin. Wchnschr. *11:*932-936, May 28, '32
Postoperative shock following splenectomy for chronic thrombocytopenic purpura. LEWISOHN, R. Ann. Surg. *96:*447-450, Sept '32

Shock, Surgical–Cont.
Postoperative shock interpreted as secondary hemorrhage following subtotal hysterectomy. MATERZANINI, A. Clin. ostet. *34:*593-596, Sept '32
Therapy of circulatory insufficiency following surgical interventions. JAGIĆ, N. Wien. klin. Wchnschr. *45:*1241-1244, Oct 7, '32
Anuria and symptoms of uremia in clinical picture of postoperative shock. PUHL, H. Deutsche Ztschr. f. Chir. *235:*393-413, '32
Acacia therapy in surgical shock. CORRÊA NETTO, A. AND ETZEL, E. Rev. Assoc. paulista de med. *3:*244-264, Nov '33
Surgical shock. REHN, E. Arch. f. klin. Chir. *177:*360-370, '33 also: Internat. Clin. *2:*57-65, June '34 abstr: Ztschr. f. Urol. *27:*709-710, '33
Circulating blood volume and operative trauma; experimental studies. AIKAWA, T. Arch. f. klin. Chir. *181:*330-336, '34
Treatment of postoperative shock in gastrointestinal diseases. STAROSHKLOVSKAYA, R. M. Novy khir. arkhiv *32:*351-364, '34
Surgical shock. CLARK, A. Glasgow M. J. *123:*1-7, Jan '35
Prophylaxis of surgical shock. JONES, W. C. South. M. J. *28:*166-168, Feb '35
Surgical shock. ANDREWS, E. Northwest Med. *34:*122-126, April '35
Energy background of genesis of gallstones and of prevention of immediate postoperative shock. CRILE, G. Surg., Gynec. and Obst. *60:*818-825, April '35
Prevention and treatment of surgical shock. HINTON, J. W., S. Clin. North America *15:*287-293, April '35
Causation and treatment of surgical shock. MILLER, I. D., M. J. Australia *1:*522-523, April 27, '35
Shock syndrome in surgery. MOON, V. H. Ann. Int. Med. *8:*1633-1648, June '35
Crampton test (blood pressure and pulse re2cording in recumbent and erect positions) and surgical shock. IRWIN, J. H., J. M. Soc. New Jersey *32:*416-418, July '35
Intravenous use of hypertonic glucose in gynecology; experimental and clinical study of surgical shock. MATTHEWS, H. B. AND MAZZOLA, V. P. Surg., Gynec. and Obst. *62:*781-790, May '36
Surgical shock. RIDDOCH, J. W. Birmingham M. Rev. *11:*131-143, June '36
Lethal factors in bile peritonitis; "surgical shock." HARKINS, H. N. *et al.* Arch Surg. *33:*576-608, Oct '36
Surgical shock from burns, freezing and similar traumatic agents. HARKINS, H. N. Colorado Med. *33:*871-876, Dec '36
Shock and postoperative hypotension. STA-

Shock, Surgical – Cont.
JANO, C. Arch. urug. de med., cir. y especialid. *10:*373-380, March '37
Mechanism and treatment of surgical shock. AUSTIN, T. R., U. S. Nav. M. Bull. *35:*426-434, Oct '37
Plasma exudation; loss of plasma-like fluid in various conditions resembling surgical shock; experimental study. HARKINS, H. N. AND HARMON, P. H. Ann. Surg. *106:*1070-1083, Dec '37
Postoperative shock. GRIGOROVSKIY, I. M. Vestnik khir. *55:*129-132, Feb '38
Surgical shock. KIRSCHNER, M. Chirurg *10:*249, April 15, '38; 314, May 1, '38
Review of acute postoperative circulatory disturbances. DEVINE, H. Australian and New Zealand J. Surg. *8:*145-155, Oct '38
Surgical shock. SECRIST, D. L. Southwestern Med. *22:*391-393, Oct '38
Shock, surgical. GRAY, H. K. AND CHAUNCEY, L. R., U. S. Nav. M. Bull. *37:*1-10, Jan '39
Coramin therapy of preoperative and postoperative shock. FERRO, G. Sett. med. *27:*361-364, March 23, '39
Method of raising venous pressure (stimulation of voluntary muscles by faradic current), to be used in surgical and traumatic shock (preliminary report). ORNSTEIN, G. G. *et al.* Quart. Bull., Sea View Hosp. *4:*333-338, April '39
Symposium on surgical shock. (Various authors.) Med. Klin. *35:*842-844, June 23, '39
Mechanism and management of surgical shock. FREEMAN, N. E. Pennsylvania M. J. *42:*1449-1452, Sept '39
Prevention and treatment of surgical shock. CRESSMAN, R. D. AND BLALOCK, A. Am. J. Surg. *46:*417-425, Dec '39
Treatment of shock in urologic surgery. ANDRE, R. H., S. Clin. North America *20:*431-438, April '40
Surgical shock. McMillan, W. O. Indust. Med. *9:*567-569, Nov '40
Surgical shock. CHRISTMANN, F. E. Dia med. *12:*1175-1180, Dec 23, '40
Surgical shock treatment with blood plasma. WHITE, C. S. *et al.* South. M. J. *34:*38-42, Jan '41
Surgical shock. McCURDY, G. A. Bull. Vancouver M. A. *17:*131-138, Feb '41
Surgical shock – practical aspects; medical progress. DUNPHY, J. E. New England J. Med. *224:*903-908, May 22, '41
Treatment of surgical shock. McMICHAEL, J. Practitioner *147:*526-530, Aug '41
Surgical shock, review of literature. NORES, A. JR. Rev. med. de Cordoba *29:*474, Aug; 545-553, Sept; 558-560, Oct '41

Shock, Surgical – Cont.
Present status of intravenous fluid treatment of traumatic and surgical shock. HARKINS, H. N. AND McCLURE, R. D. Ann. Surg. *114:*891-906, Nov '41
Treatment of surgical and traumatic shock with citrated plasma-saline mixture. WHITE, C. S. *et al.* Am. J. Surg. *54:*701-710, Dec '41
Present concept of surgical shock. PARKER, E. F., J. South Carolina M. A. *38:*12-15, Jan '42
Surgical shock. ARGIL, G. Medicina, Mexico *22:*259-268, June 25, '42
Effect of desoxycorticosterone acetate (adrenal preparation) in postoperative shock. KOSTER, H. AND KASMAN, L. P. Arch. Surg. *45:*272-285, Aug '42
Pholedrine (veritol) in prevention of operative shock. LANDAU, E. *et al.* Lancet *2:*210-212, Aug 22, '42
Clinical aspects and therapy of surgical shock. STARUP, U. Nord. med. (Hospitalstid.) *15:*2526-2531, Sept 12, '42
Modern conceptions and biologic therapy of shock in surgery. ST-ONGE, G., J. de l'Hotel-Dieu de Montreal *11:*355-406, Sept-Oct '42
Management and treatment of surgical shock. SAXENA, K. N. Antiseptic *39:*741-747, Nov '42
Surgical shock. PEDLOW, W. L. West. J. Surg. *51:*81-84, Feb '43
Clinical considerations of surgical shock. COLE, W. H. Illinois M. J. *83:*162-165, March '43
Prevention and treatment of shock during surgical procedures. KENDRICK, D. B. JR. Mil. Surgeon *92:*247-253, March '43
Clinical aspect of surgical shock. LAMONTAGNE, H. Manitoba. M. Rev. *23:*119-122, May '43
Problem of surgical shock. CALVER, G. W., U. S. Nav. M. Bull. *42:*358-380, Feb '44
Surgical shock. HAUN, E., J. Tennessee M. A. *37:*57-61, Feb '44
Surgical shock. ROOF, C. S. Rocky Mountain M. J. *41:*100-103, Feb '44
Substitutes for human blood and plasma in treatment of surgical shock. GERALD, H. F. Nebraska M. J. *29:*77-80, March '44
Surgical shock. CRAIG, W. M., J. Internat. Coll. Surgeons *7:*103-106, March-April '44
Treatment of surgical shock and embolism. ALLEN, F. M., J. Internat. Coll. Surgeons *7:*423-434, Nov-Dec '44
Use of polyvinyl pyrrolidine as blood substitute in therapy of postoperative shock. RICHARD, A. *et al.* Lyon chir *40:*110-113, Jan-Feb '45

Shock, Surgical – Cont.

Clinical evolution of traumatic and surgical shock. CHAVEZ TRUJILLO, A. Medicina, Mexico *25:*54-56, Feb 25, '45

Recent advances in surgical shock. WEIL, P. G., McGill M. J. *14:*179-183, April '45

Treatment of surgical shock. ALLEN, F. M. Dia med. *17:*996-1000, Sept 3, '45

Use of solution of sodium chloride, bicarbonate and thiosulfate in prevention of surgical shock. AMELINE, A. Presse med. *54:*174-175, March 16, '46

Shock, Traumatic

Report of the British Medical Research Committee on traumatic shock. KROGH, A. Ugesk. f. Laeger *83:*333, March 10, '21

Indications for infusion of blood substitutes and transfusion of blood in cases of traumatic hemorrhage and shock. BUTLER, E. California State J. Med. *19:*145, April '21

Present status of traumatic shock and hemorrhage. BILLET, H. Arch. de med. et pharm. mil. *74:*473-486, May '21

Diagnosis of traumatic shock. GUYOT, J. AND JEANNENEY, G. Progres med. *36:*199, May 7, '21 abstr: J.A.M.A. *77:*73, July 2, '21

Prevention and treatment of wound shock in theatre of army operations. MACRAE, D. JR. J. Iowa M. Soc. *11:*394, Oct '21

Traumatic shock. GUYOT, J. AND JEANNENEY, G. Paris med. *11:*157, Aug 27, '21

Pathogenesis of traumatic shock. JEANNENEY, G. Progres med. *36:*425, Sept 10, '21

Studies in experimental traumatic shock; evidence of toxic factor in wound shock. CANNON, W. B. Arch. Surg. *4:*1-22, Jan '22

Research of Fenton B. Turck on traumatic shock. QUÉNU. Bull. Acad. de med., Par. *87:*92-97, Jan 24, '22

Studies in experimental traumatic shock; critical level in a falling blood pressure. CANNON, W. B. AND CATTELL, McK. Arch. Surg. *4:*300-323, March '22 (illus.)

Present status of traumatic shock. KNORR, H. Klin. Wchnschr. *1:*1115-1117, May 27, '22

Studies in experimental traumatic shock; liberation of epinephrine in traumatic shock. RAPPORT, D. Am. J. Physiol. *60:*461-475, May '22

Recent evidence as to nature of wound shock. CANNON, W. B. Northwest Med. *21:*351-355, Sept '22

Studies in experimental traumatic shock; action of ether on circulation in traumatic shock. CATTELL, McK. Arch. Surg. *6:*41-84, (pt. 1), Jan '23

Prognosis of traumatic shock. JEANNENEY, G. Paris med. *13:*129-133, Feb 10, '23 abstr: J.A.M.A. *80:*1737, June 9, '23

Shock, Traumatic – Cont.

Treatment of traumatic shock. JEANNENEY, G. Arch. franco-belges de chir. *26:*157-175, Feb '23

Traumatic shock; some experimental work on crossed circulation. MCIVER, M. A. AND HAGGART, W. W. Surg., Gynec. and Obst. *36:*542-546, April '23 (illus.)

Studies in experimental traumatic shock; influence of morphine on blood pressure and alkali reserve in traumatic shock. CATTELL, McK. Arch. Surg. *7:*96-110, July '23 (illus.)

Traumatic shock due to war wound. BARUCH, D., J. de chir. *23:*354-372, April '24

Traumatic shock. OLTRAMARE, J. H. AND OLTRAMARE, H. Schweiz. med. Wchnschr. *54:*420, May 1, '24 abstr: J.A.M.A. *82:*1997, June 14, '24

Traumatic shock and inspissation of blood. OLTRAMARE, J. H. AND OLTRAMARE, H. Schweiz. med. Wchnschr. *54:*912-914, Oct 2, '24 abstr: J.A.M.A. *83:*1625, Nov 15, '24

Circulatory changes in wounded soldiers (shock), with special reference to influence of drugs used for production of anesthesia. MARSHALL, G. Guy's Hosp. Rep. *75:*98-111, Jan '25

Traumatic shock. WELLER, C. A., J. Indiana M. A. *18:*253-257, July '25

Traumatic abdominal shock. ROSSELLO, H. J. AND BENATTI, D. An. de Fac. de med., Montevideo *11:*295-302, May '26 abstr: J.A.M.A. *87:*2131, Dec 18, '26

Therapy of traumatic shock (insulin and dextrose). RANDALL, H. E., J. Michigan M. Soc. *26:*19-20, Jan '27

Treatment of surgical and traumatic shock. BAUMANN, E. Schweiz. med. Wchnschr. *57:*1045-1047, Oct 29, '27

Insulin-glucose treatment of traumatic shock; discussion with experimental report. PADGETT, E. C. AND ORR, T. G. Surg., Gynec. and Obst. *46:*783-788, June '28

Pathology and treatment of traumatic (wound) shock. COWELL, E. Proc. Roy. Soc. Med. (War Sect.) *21:*39-46, July '28 also: J. Roy. Army M. Corps *51:*81-102, Aug '28

Traumatic shock. MICHAEL, P. R. Nederl. tijdschr. v. geneesk. *2:*5415-5426, Nov 16, '29

Immediate treatment of severely injured; general traumatism – shock. HILL, L. V., J. Kansas M. Soc. *31:*119-121, April '30

Traumatic shock. REED, T. G. West Virginia M. J. *26:*205-207, April '30

Ephedrine sulphate in acute shock from

Shock, Traumatic – Cont.
trauma or hemorrhage; clinical use. JOHNSON, C. A., J.A.M.A. *94:*1388-1390, May 3, '30
Traumatic shock; mechanism, symptomatology and treatment. PETROVITCH, G. AND YOVANOVITCH, I. Voj. san. glasnik *1:*192-206, July-Dec '30
Traumatic shock; newer aspects and treatment. RHODES, G. K. AND MCKENNEY, C. California and West. Med. *33:*665-670, Sept '30
Grave postoperative hemorrhages; pathogenesis of late hemorrhages and their treatment by shock. ANTONETTI, H. Presse med. *39:*1766-1768, Dec 2, '31
Present concept of traumatic shock and its treatment. WANGENSTEEN, O. H. Journal-Lancet *51:*711-718, Dec 1, '31
Traumatic shock. FREELANDER, S. O. AND LENHART, C. H. Arch. Surg. *25:*693-708, Oct '32
Cortin (hormone from suprarenal cortex) and traumatic shock. FREEMAN, N. E. Science *77:*211-212, Feb 24, '33
Causes of shock associated with injury to tissues. BLALOCK, A. Internat. Clin. *1:*144-161, March '33
Traumatic shock syndrome following rupture of aorta and multiple fractures. WILSON, H. AND ROOME, N. W. Am. J. Surg. *22:*333-334, Nov '33
Experimental studies on traumatic shock. HERBST, R. Arch. f. klin. Chir. *176:*98-122, '33
Traumatic shock and hemorrhage. BLALOCK, A. South. M. J. *27:*126-130, Feb '34
Digitalis therapy of cardiac insufficiency in primary and secondary traumatic shock. SALAS GONZÁLEZ, J. Rev. espan. de med. y cir. *17:*489-490, Oct '34
Influence of epinephrine on shock caused by removal of hemostatic bandage; clinical and experimental study. PANNELLA, P. Ann. ital. di chir. *14:*1-14, Jan '35
Traumatic and hemorrhagic shock; experimental and clinical study. COONSE, G. K.; *et al.* New England J. Med. *212:*647-663, April 11, '35
Traumatic slow intraperitoneal hemorrhage with delayed shock; 3 cases. REID, W. L. Southeastern Med. *19:*160-162, May '35
Rate of fluid shift and its relation to onset of shock in severe experimental burns. HARKINS, H. N. Arch. Surg. *31:*71-85, July '35
Discussion on traumatic shock. HOLT, R. L.; *et al.* Proc. Roy. Soc. Med. *28:*1473-1496, Sept '35
Traumatic shock. PERKINS, P. A., J. Tennessee M. A. *28:*461-464, Nov '35
Effect of procaine hydrochloride block of nerve trunks in traumatic shock. POMOSOV, V. N. Novy khir. arkhiv. *35:*109-113, '35
Use of ah-chiao (donkey skin glue) for circulatory failure encountered in severe hemorrhage and shock. NI, T. G. Chinese J. Physiol. *10:*125-132, Feb 15, '36
Traumatic shock. STANBRO, G. E., J. Oklahoma M. A. *29:*199-202, June '36
Neo-synephrin hydrochloride in acute shock from trauma or hemorrhage. JOHNSON, C. A., Surg., Gynec. and Obst. *63:*35-42, July '36
Traumatic shock. MARCY, G. H. Indust. Med. *5:*493-497, Oct '36
Trauma; occupational diseases and hazards; shock and hemorrhage. BLALOCK, A. Bull. New York Acad. Med. *12:*610-622, Nov '36
Experimental data on pathogenesis of traumatic shock; toxic action of products of muscular disintegration. VESELKIN, P. N.; *et al.* Vestnik khir. *44:*176-186, '36
Traumatic shock. FENKNER, W. Med. Welt *10:*1869-1872, Dec 26, '36
Traumatic shock. CANNON, W. B. Sovet. khir., no. 1, pp. 3-9, '36
Active surgical therapy of traumatic shock. GUSYNIN, V. A. Novy khir. arkhiv. *35:*566-572, '36
Experimental data on pathogenesis of traumatic shock; role of fat embolism. VESELKIN, P. N. *et al.* Vestnik khir. *44:*198-203, '36
Concealed hemorrhage into tissues and its relation to traumatic shock. HARKINS, H. N. AND ROOME, N. W. Arch. Surg. *35:*130-139, July '37
Neo-synephrin hydrochloride in treatment of hypotension and shock from trauma or hemorrhage. JOHNSON, C. A. Surg., Gynec. and Obst. *65:*458-463, Oct '37
Therapy of traumatic shock according to experimental data. BUBNOV, M. A. Khirurgiya, no. 9, pp. 38-45, '37
Ephedrine therapy of traumatic shock; experimental study. LEPUKALN, A. F. Khirurgiya, no. 9, pp. 46-53, '37
Experimental and clincial contributions to question of alcohol therapy of traumatic shock. OBRAZTSOV, G. D. Vestnik khir. *53:*123-129, '37
Experimental data on pathogenesis of traumatic shock. VESELKIN, P. N. *et al.* Vestnik khir. *51:*211-229, '37
Therapy of primary shock due to burns; 2 cases. WANDERLEY FILHO, E. AND GALVAO,

Shock, Traumatic—Cont.
H. Arq. brasil. de cir. e ortop. *5:*308–318, March '38
Treatment of hemorrhage and traumatic shock by intravenous use of lyophile serum. BOND, D. D. AND WRIGHT, D. G. Ann. Surg. *107:*500–510, April '38
Traumatic shock and burns. HILLSMAN, J. A. AND GUNN, J. A. Manitoba M. A. Rev. *18:*65–68, April '38
Symptoms and control of traumatic shock. MAHAFFEY, H. Kentucky M. J. *36:*137–142, April '38
Traumatic shock. JOHANSSON, S. Nord. med. tidskr. *16:*1767–1771, Nov 12, '38
Intravenous drop infusion of ephedrine in therapy of traumatic shock. LEPUKALN, A. F., Vrach. delo *20:*353–358, '38
Shock in burns. STAJANO, C. An. Fac. de med. de Montevideo *23:*923–941, '38
Theories of shock and their relation to burns. DEVINE, J. B., M. J. Australia *1:*14–17, Jan 7, '39
Air raids; wound shock, hemorrhage and blood transfusion. MITCHINER, P. H. AND COWELL, E. M. Lancet *1:*228–231, Jan 28, '39
Experimental traumatic shock; further studies with particular reference to role of nervous system. BLALOCK, A. AND CRESSMAN, R. D. Surg., Gynec. and Obst. *68:*278–287, Feb (no. 2A) '39
Method of raising venous pressure (stimulation of voluntary muscles by faradic current), to be used in surgical and traumatic shock (preliminary report). ORNSTEIN, G. G. *et al.* Quart. Bull., Sea View Hosp. *4:*333–338, April '39
Symptoms and control of traumatic shock. MAHAFFEY, H. Anesth. and Analg. *18:*196–205, July–Aug '39
Traumatic shock. BALCH, F. G. JR. J. Maine M. A. *30:*216–218, Sept '39
Post-traumatic shock and gas gangrene successfully treated with several massive blood transfusions and sulfanilamide. WIELENGA, D. K. Nederl. tijdschr. v. geneesk. *83:*4740–4746, Sept 30, '39
Results of intravenous and intra-arterial administration of fluids in traumatic shock produced experimentally. KENDRICK, D. B. JR. Surgery *6:*520–523, Oct '39
Therapy of hemorrhages and states of traumatic shock in armies in wartime. NORMET, L. Bruxelles-med. *19:*1474–1482, Oct 8, '39
Transfusion of plasma instead of whole blood in massive hemorrhages; use in war. BRODIN, P. AND SAINT-GIRONS, F. Bull. et mem. Soc. d. hop. de Paris *55:*1224–1226, Nov 10, '39
General principles of treatment of high explosive and bomb injuries and shock hemorrhage, and of resuscitation. HURLEY, T. E. V., M. J. Australia *2:*740–742, Nov 11, '39
Importance of rhythmic injection of blood or its substitutes (preserved blood, human plasma and Bayliss, Normet or physiologic serum) in acute hemorrhage and shock. BECART, A. Presse med. *47:*1681–1682, Dec 27–30, '39
Traumatic shock and its therapy, with special reference to blood transfusion; importance of rhythmic injection. BECART, A. Monde med., Paris *49:*859–862, Dec '39
Burn shock; question of water intoxication as complicating factor; blood chemical studies and report of extensive burn treated by repeated transfusions of blood and blood plasma. TRUSLER, H. M. *et al.* J.A.M.A. *113:*2207–2213, Dec 16, '39
Pathology of collapse following burns. GÜNTHER, G. W. Arch. f. klin. Chir. *194:*539–557, '39
Pathogenesis and therapy of traumatic shock. SHRAYBER, M. G. Sovet. vrach. zhur. *44:*7–14, Jan 30, '40
Traumatic shock and suprarenal cortical hormone; etiologic and therapeutic studies of shock and experiments with suprarenalectomy. VARANGOT, J. Presse med. *48:*103–107, Jan 31–Feb 3, '40
Human serum as blood substitute in treatment of hemorrhage and shock. LEVINSON, S. O. *et al.* J.A.M.A. *114:*455–461, Feb 10, '40
Task of internist in treatent of war injuries; posttraumatic (secondary) shock. BORST, J. G. G. AND VEENING, H. P. Nederl. tijdschr. v. geneesk. *84:*914–922, March 9, '40
Traumatic shock of war wounded. CREYSSEL, J. AND SUIRE, P., J. de med. de Lyon *21:*83–96, March 5, '40
New therapeutic methods in traumatic shock. JEANNENEY, G. AND JUSTIN-BESANCON, L. Mem. Acad. de chir. *66:*337–358, March 13–April 3, '40
Shock toxin; pharmacologic effects of perfusate flowing through crushed muscle tissue. SUZUKI, K. Jap. J. M. Sc., IV, Pharmacol. *12:*115–116, March '40
Syndrome of traumatic shock. RAVEN, R. W. Post-Grad. M. J. *16:*118–124, April '40
Concentrated serum in treatment of traumatic shock in experimental animals. BEST, C. H. AND SOLANDT, D. Y. Brit. M. J.

Shock, Traumatic – Cont.
*1:*799–802, May 18, '40
Investigation of traumatic shock bearing on toxemia theory. KENDRICK, D. B. JR *et al.* Surgery *7:*753–762, May '40
Therapeutic value of adrenal cortical hormones in traumatic shock and allied conditions. SELYE, H. *et al.* Canad. M. A. J. *43:* 1–8, July '40
Treatment of wound shock with corticosterone (suprarenal preparation). SELYE, H. AND DOSNE C. Lancet *2:*70–71, July 20, '40
Reduction of mortality from experimental traumatic shock with adrenal cortical substances. WEIL, P. G. *et al.* Canad. M. A. J. *43:*8–11, July '40
Etiology and treatment of traumatic shock. WILSON, H. South. M. J. *33:*754–756, July '40
Pathogenesis of functional disturbances in traumatic shock and significance of blood transfusion in therapy. PETROV, I. R. Vestnik khir. *60:*119–126, Sept '40
Pressor response in adrenalin in course of traumatic shock. FREEDMAN, A. M. AND KABAT, H. Am. J. Physiol. *130:*620–626, Oct '40
Nervous factor in traumatic shock. LORBER, V. *et al.* Surg., Gynec. and Obst. *71:*469–477, Oct '40
Death due to shock after scalding of pharynx and larynx. TANAKA, H. Oto-rhino-laryng. (Abstr. Sect.) *13:*45–46, Oct '40
Treatment of burn shock with plasma and serum. BLACK, D. A. K. Brit. M. J. *2:*693–697, Nov 23, '40
Traumatic shock of war wounded; bilateral procaine hydrochloride infiltration of carotid sinus; case. CREYSSEL, J. AND SUIRE, P. Mem. Acad. de chir. *66:*762–765, Nov 6–20, '40
Traumatic shock. DO AMARAL, A. C. Rev. med.-cir. do Brasil *48:*667–680, Nov '40
Traumatic shock. GRODINS, F. S. AND FREEMAN, S. Internat. Abstr. Surg. *72:*1–8, '41; in Surg., Gynec. and Obst., Jan '41
Physiologic principles in treatment of traumatic shock. MCDOWALL, R. J. S. Practitioner *146:*21–26, Jan '41
Traumatic shock; review. OPIZZI, J. Rev. san. mil., Buenos Aires *40:*76–78, Jan '41
Recent advances in study and management of traumatic shock. HARKINS, H. N. Surgery *9:*231, Feb; 447, March; 607, April '41
Circulatory collapse and wound shock (Honyman Gillespie lecture). MCMICHAEL, J. Edinburgh M. J. *48:*160–172, March '41
Traumatic shock and sympathetic overstimulation. TOMB, J. W. South African M. J.

Shock, Traumatic – Cont.
*15:*109–111, March 22, '41
Modern concept of traumatic shock. GOMEZ DURAN, M. Semana med. espan. *4:*673–681, June 14, '41
Management of shock and toxemia in severe burns. LEE, W. E. *et al.* Pennsylvania M. J. *44:*1114–1117, June '41
Use of adrenal cortical extract in treatment of traumatic shock of burns. RHOADS, J. E. *et al.* Ann. Surg. *113:*955–968, June '41
Beneficial effects of oxygen therapy in experimental traumatic shock, SCHNEDORF, J. G. AND ORR, T. G. Surg., Gynec. and Obst. *73:*79–83, July '41
Laboratory aids of value in diagnosis of traumatic shock and internal hemorrhage with brief reference to use of blood plasma as therapeutic agent. WILLIAMSON, C. S. Wisconsin M. J. *40:*570–574, July '41
Memorandum on observations required in cases of wound shock. GRANT, R. T. Brit. M. J. *2:*332–336, Sept 6, '41
Aspects of wound shock with experiences in treatment. MAYCOCK, W. D'A. AND WHITBY, L. E. H., J. Roy. Army M. Corps *77:*173–187, Oct '41
Wound shock with experiences in treatment. MAYCOCK, W. D'A. AND WHITBY, L. E. H. J. Roy. Nav. M. Serv. *27:*358–371, Oct '41
Oxygen therapy in shock due to hemorrhage. SCHNEDORF, J. G. AND ORR, T. G. Surg., Gynec. and Obst. *73:*495–497, Oct '41
Modern treatment of traumatic shock. HANELIN, H. A., J. Michigan M. Soc. *40:*876–881, Nov '41
Present status of intravenous fluid treatment of traumatic and surgical shock. HARKINS, H. N. AND MCCLURE, R. D. Ann. Surg. *114:*891–906, Nov '41
Collapse (of circulation in traumatic shock) and renal failure. TOMB, J. W., M. J. Australia *2:*569–570, Nov 15, '41
Similarities and distinctions between shock and effects of hemorrhage. MOON, V. H. *et al.* J.A.M.A. *117:*2024–2030, Dec 13, '41
Infusions of blood and other fluids via bone marrow in traumatic shock and other forms of peripheral circulatory failure. TOCANTINS, L. M. *et al.* Ann. Surg. *114:*1085–1092, Dec '41
Treatment of surgical and traumatic shock with citrated plasma-saline mixture. WHITE, C. S. *et al.* Am. J. Surg. *54:*701–710, Dec '41
Blood transfusion in traumatic shock. KAZANSKIY, V. I. Sovet. med. (nos. 17–18) *5:*13, '41
Burn shock; consideration of its mechanism

Shock, Traumatic – Cont.
and management. WILSON, H. Memphis M. J. *17:*3–5, Jan '42
Chemical research on traumatic shock. CREMER, H. D. Deut. Militararzt *7:*79, Feb '42 also: Bull. War Med. *3:*150–151, Nov '42 (abstract)
So-called wound shock; physiopathology of posthemorrhagic states. DUESBERG, R. Deut. Militararzt *7:*69, Feb '42 also: Bull. War Med. *3:*149–150, Nov '42 (abstract)
Traumatic shock. JURASZ, A. Lek. wojsk. *34:*80–86, Feb–April '42
Nervous factor in etiology of shock in burns. KABAT, H. AND HEDIN, R. F. Surgery *11:*766–776, May '42 also: Proc. Soc. Exper. Biol. and Med. *49:*114–116, Feb '42 (abstract)
Emergency care of wounds, hemorrhage and shock. THOMPSON, L. M. New York State J. Med. *42:*355–356, Feb 15, '42
Comparison of effects of local application of heat and of cold in prevention and treatment of experimental traumatic shock. BLALOCK, A. Surgery *11:*356–359, March '42
Panel discussions; traumatic shock; early signs, prevention and treatment. BLALOCK, A. AND PRICE, P. B. Bull. Am. Coll. Surgeons *27:*102–105, April '42
Shock due to extensive superficial burns; case. LABRECQUE, R. Ann. med.-chir. de l'Hop. Sainte-Justine, Montreal *4:*131–140, May '42
Use of plasma in treatment of burn shock. RHOADS, J. E. *et al.* Clinics *1:*37–42, June '42
Shock, without or with hemorrhage, and burns. FENNEL, E. A. Hawaii M. J. *1:*385–389, July '42
Effect of adrenal cortical hormones in hemorrhage and shock. FINE, J. *et al.* Surgery *12:*1–13, July '42
Rationale of use of concentrated plasma protein solutions in treatment of hematogenic shock. MUIRHEAD, E. E. *et al.* Texas State J. Med. *38:*199–207, July '42
Burns of thermal origin (with shock). HULL, H. C. Arch. Surg. *45:*235–252, Aug '42
Use of blood and blood substitutes in shock and hemorrhage. LEVINSON, S. O. West. J. Surg. *50:*388–391, Aug '42
Blood and blood substitutes in hemorrhage and shock. BURDESHAW, H. B., J.M.A. Alabama *12:*79–81, Sept '42
Traumatic shock – consideration of several types of injuries (Donald C. Balfour lecture). BLALOCK, A. AND DUNCAN, G. W. Surg., Gynec. and Obst. *75:*401–409, Oct '42

Shock, Traumatic – Cont.
Role of transfusion and infusion in treatment of wound shock. RANGANATHAN, K. S. Antiseptic *39:*646–654, Oct '42
Acute protein deficiency (hypoproteinemia) in shock due to severe hemorrhage and in burns, intestinal obstruction and general peritonitis, with special reference to use of plasma and hydrolized protein (amigen). ELMAN, R. J.A.M.A. *120:*1176–1180, Dec 12, '42
War medicine series; practical management of wound shock. MCMICHAEL, J. Brit. M. J. *2:*671–673, Dec 5, '42
Experimental chemotherapy of burns; effects of local therapy upon mortality from shock. ROSENTHAL, S. M. Pub. Health Rep. *57:*1923–1935, Dec 18, '42
Bilateral procaine hydrochloride infiltration of carotid sinus region in therapy of traumatic shock. CREYSSEL, J. AND SUIRE, P. Lyon chir. *37:*101–104, '41–'42
Shock and hemorrhage. FRASER, J. War and Doctor, pp. 25–40, '42
Traumatic shock. LANG, G. F. Klin. med. (nos. 5–6) *20:*3; (no. 7) *20:*3, '42
Therapy of traumatic shock. PETROV, I. R. Klin. med. (no. 10) *20:*3–9, '42
Failure of intravenous injection of plasma in severe traumatic shock; case. LOMBARD, P. Afrique franc. chir. *1:*17–18, Jan–Feb '43
Traumatic shock. VER BRUGGHEN, A. H. Pennsylvania M. J. *46:*319–326, Jan '43
Traumatic shock. EBERBACH, C. W. Wisconsin M. J. *42:*225–228, Feb '43
Traumatic shock; study of problem of "lost plasma" in hemorrhagic shock by use of radioactive plasma protein. FINE, J. AND SELIGMAN, A. M., J. Clin. Investigation *22:*285–303, March '43
Experimental chemotherapy of burns and shock; effects of systemic therapy on early mortality. ROSENTHAL, S. M. Pub. Health Rep. *58:*513–522, March 26, '43
Traumatic shock; prevention and treatment. CHILD, C. G., III. S. Clin. North America *23:*321–332, April '43
Traumatic shock and hemorrhage. ALESEN, L. A., California and West. Med. *58:*265–269, May '43
Shock and hemorrhage. SUPERNAW, J. S. Wisconsin M. J. *42:*501–504, May '43
Etiology and treatment of traumatic or secondary shock. WILHELMJ, C. M., J. Arkansas M. Soc. *39:*257–260, May '43
Traumatic shock; physiopathology and therapy. ALMOYNA, C. M. Medicina, Madrid (pt. I) *11:*518–527, June '43
Hematogenic shock; recent advances in early recognition and treatment. BLUM, L. L.

Shock, Traumatic—Cont.
Urol. and Cutan. Rev. *47:*401-409, July '43
Shock factor in burns and its treatment. McCLURE, R. D. AND LAM, C. R. Univ. Hosp. Bull., Ann Arbor *9:*62-64, July '43
Occurrence of vasoconstrictor substance in blood during shock induced by trauma, hemorrhage and burns. PAGE, I. H. Am. J. Physiol. *139:*386-398, July '43
Intensive human serum treatment of burn shock; modified formula for calculating amount of infusion. PRESMAN, D. L. *et al.* J.A.M.A. *122:*924-928, July 31, '43
Principle from liver effective against shock due to burns; preliminary report. PRINZMETAL, M. *et al.* J.A.M.A. *122:*720-723, July 10, '43
Recent observations on value of adrenal cortex preparations in hemorrhagic shock. WIGGERS, C. J. Univ. Hosp. Bull., Ann Arbor *9:*61, July '43
Gelatin infusion (as blood substitute) in hemorrhagic shock. JANOTA, M. *et al.* Exper. Med. and Surg. *1:*298-303, Aug '43
Hemorrhagic hypotension and its treatment by intraarterial and intravenous infusion of blood. KOHLSTAEDT, K. G. AND PAGE, I. H., Arch. Surg. *47:*178-191, Aug '43
Vasopressor effect of thermal trauma. OLSON, W. H. AND NECHELES, H. Am. J. Physiol. *139:*574-582, Aug '43
Gelatin as plasma substitute, with particular reference to burn shock. PARKINS, W. M. *et al.* Ann. Surg. *118:*193-214, Aug '43
Potassium and cause of death in traumatic shock. WINKLER, A. W. AND HOFF, H. E. Am. J. Physiol. *139:*686-692, Sept '43
Biologic properties of blood and spinal fluid in traumatic shock complicated by burns. GROMAKOVSKAYA, M. M. AND KAPLAN, L. E., Byull. eksper. biol. i med. (no. 6) *15:*12-16, '43
Therapy of traumatic shock according to method of I. R. Petrov. GUGEL-MOROZOVA, T. P. Klin. med. (no. 9) *21:*60-63, '43
Treatment of burns (including shock). PENBERTHY, G. C. AND WELLER, C. N. Am. Acad. Orthop. Surgeons, Lect., pp. 188-198, '43
Therapy of traumatic shock complicated by burns. SHTERN, L. S. *et al.* Byull. eksper. biol. i med. (no. 6) *15:*6-9, '43
Modern treatment of traumatic shock. DE GOWIN, E. L., J. Iowa M. Soc. *34:*1-7, Jan '44
Principles of prophylaxis and therapy of surgical shock. DRESSLER, L. Harefuah *26:*5, Jan 1, '44; 24, Jan 16, '44 (in Hebrew)
Another failure of transfusion in severe burns; case. LOMBARD, P. Afrique franc.

Shock, Traumatic—Cont.
chir. *2:*77-79, Jan-March '44
Pathogenesis and treatment of shock resulting from crushing of muscle. PRINZMETAL, M. *et al.* War Med. *5:*74-79, Feb '44
Traumatic shock; restoration of blood volume in. EVANS, E. I. *et al.* Surgery *15:*420-431, March '44
Traumatic shock and its interpretation. DOSNE, C. Rev. de med. y aliment. *6:*107-114, April-July '44
Traumatic shock. GALVAO, L. Hora med., Rio de Janeiro *2:*33-44, Aug '44
Shock associated with deep muscle burns. ANTOS, R. J. *et al.* Proc. Soc. Exper. Biol. and Med. *57:*11-13, Oct '44
Demonstration of 2 types of shock in burns. PRINZMETAL, M. *et al.* Surgery *16:*906-913, Dec '44
Purified gelatin solution as blood plasma substitute (for treatment of hemorrhagic shock). WENNER, W. F. Ann. Otol., Rhin. and Laryng. *53:*635-643, Dec '44
Intracisternal injection of potassium phosphate according to Shtern method in therapy of traumatic shock at the front. BERKOVICH, E. M. Khirurgiya, no. 7, pp. 8-12, '44
Transfusion of hypertonic plasma in therapy of shock following acute blood loss. KEVDIN, N. A. AND GENDLER, A. V. Klin. med. (nos. 10-11) *22:*20-22, '44
Physiologic bases of traumatic shock. ORBELI, L. A. Voen.-med. sborn. *1:*5-13, '44
Intra-arterial blood transfusion in irreversible form of shock and hemorrhage. RADUSHKEVICH, V. P. Khirurgiya, no. 8, pp. 38-40, '44
Circulation in traumatic shock in man. RICHARDS, D. W. JR. Harvey Lect. (1943-1944) *39:*217-253, '44
Hemorrhage, shock and their treatment (including teaching principles for naval personnel). HORNBAKER, R. W. Hosp. Corps Quart. (no. 1) *18:*27-31, Jan '45
Clinical evolution of traumatic and surgical shock. CHAVEZ TRUJILLO, A. Medicina, Mexico *25:*54-56, Feb 25, '45
Effects of environmental temperature on traumatic shock produced by ischemic compression of extremities. GREEN, H. D. AND BERGERON, G. A. Surgery *17:*404-412, March '45
Shock induced by hemorrhage; hemoglobin solutions as blood substitutes in therapy. LAMSON, P. D. *et al.* J. Pharmacol. and Exper. Therap. *83:*225-234, March '45
Effect of short-term nutritional stress upon resistance to scald shock. BERGMAN, H. C.; *et al.* Am. Heart J. *29:*513-515, April '45

Shock, Traumatic – Cont.

Ineffectiveness of adrenocortical hormones, thiamine, ascorbic acid, nupercaine and post-traumatic serum in shock due to scalding burns. BERGMAN, H. C. *et al.* Am. Heart J. *29:*506–512, April '45

Influence of environmental temperature on shock in burns. BERGMAN, H. C. AND PRINZMETAL, M. Arch. Surg. *50:*201–206, April '45

Traumatic shock; treatment of clinical shock with gelatin (as plasma substitute). EVANS, E. I. AND RAFAL, H. S. Ann. Surg. *121:*478–494, April '45

Symposium on traumatic surgery; management of shock and hemorrhage. KOOP, C. E. Clinics *3:*1586–1617, April '45

Blood circulation in traumatic shock in man. RICHARDS, D. W. JR. Nord. med. *26:*1069–1080, May 25, '45

Mechanism of shock from burns and trauma traced with radiosodium. FOX, C. L. JR. AND KESTON, A. S. Surg., Gynec. and Obst. *80:*561–567, June '45

Traumatic shock; recent physiopathologic data. CHICHE, P. Presse med. *53:*407–409, July 28, '45

Traumatic shock; treatment of hemorrhagic shock irreversible to replacement of blood volume deficiency. FRANK, H. A. *et al.* J. Clin. Investigation *24:*435–444, July '45

Shock due to tissue trauma; diagnosis and assessment. WILKINSON, A. W. Edinburgh M. J. *52:*306–316, Sept '45

Traumatic shock incurable by volume replacement therapy; summary of further studies including observations on hemodynamics, intermediary metabolism and therapeutics. FINE, J. *et al.* Ann. Surg. *122:*652–662, Oct '45

Metabolic changes in shock after burns. HARKINS, H. N. AND LONG, C. N. H. Am. J. Physiol. *144:*661–668, Oct '45

Electrolyte changes and chemotherapy in experimental burn and traumatic shock and hemorrhage (use of isotonic sodium chloride solution). ROSENTHAL, S. M. AND TABOR, H. Arch. Surg. *51:*244–252, Nov–Dec, '45

Nature of circulatory changes in burn shock. PRINZMETAL, M. AND BERGMAN, H. C. Clin. Sc. *5:*205–227, Dec '45

Traumatic shock; treatment of clinical shock with gelatin. EVANS, E. I. AND RAFAL, H. S., Tr. South. S. A. (1944) *56:*94–110, '45

Traumatic shock and its therapy. PETROV, I. R. Voen.-med. sborn, *2:*61–97, '45

Extent and cause of blood volume reduction in traumatic, hemorrhagic and burn shock. NOBLE, R. P. AND GREGERSEN, M. I., J. Clin. Investigation *25:*172–183, Mar '46

Therapy of traumatic shock. HISSINK, L. A. G., Nederl. tijdschr. v. geneesk. *90:*335–336, April 20, '46

Traumatic shock in war wounded; blood transfusion therapy. MORIN, E. Union med. du Canada *75:*400–404, April '46

Antishock action of certain drugs in burned mice. BERGMAN, H. C. AND PRINZMETAL, M., J. Lab. and Clin. Med. *31:*663–671, June '46

Antishock action of ethanol (ethyl alcohol) in burned mice; effect of edema formation and capillary atony. BERGMAN, H. C. AND PRINZMETAL, M., J. Lab. and Clin. Med. *31:*654–662, June '46

Burn shock; treatment with continuous hypodermoclysis of isotonic solution of sodium chloride into burned areas; clinical studies in 2 cases. BERMAN, J. K. *et al.* Arch. Surg. *53:*577–587, Nov '46

Burns and shock in children; Mentana Street disaster in Montreal, September 1945. BISSON, C. AND ROYER, A. Ann. med.-chir. de l'Hop. Sainte-Justine, Montreal *5:*5–19, '46

SHOR, A. M.: Modification of operation for artificial vagina from sigmoid. Novy khir. arkhiv *45:*252–253, '40

SHORE, L. R.: Case of multiple anomaly of phalanges of hands in girl aged 15. J. Anat. *60:*420–425, July '26

SHRAYBER, M. G.: Pathogenesis and therapy of traumatic shock. Sovet. vrach. zhur. *44:*7–14, Jan 30, '40

SHREVES, H. B. AND HAWKINS, G.: Nerve regeneration; clinical test. Bull. U. S. Army M. Dept. *5:*110–111, Jan '46

SHTERN, L. S. *et al:* Therapy of traumatic shock complicated by burns. Byull. eksper. biol. i med. (no. 6) *15:*6–9, '43

Shugrue Operation

Cavernous hemangioma of orbit successfully removed by Shugrue operation. PAUL, M. Brit. J. Ophth. *30:*35–41, Jan '46

SHULTS, V. A. (see BURSUK, G. G.) 1940

SHUMACKER, H. B. JR.: Congenital hypertrophy of lower extremity associated with elephantiasis; case. Am. J. Surg. *58:*258–263, Nov '42

SHUMACKER, H. B. JR.: Improved cutting edge for Padgett dermatome. Surgery *15:*457–459, March '44

SHUMAN, G. H.: Paraffin film treatment of burns of eyelids. Pennsylvania M. J. *42:*907–

909, May '39
SHUTTLEWORTH, C. B.: Repair of bony defects of cranium. Canad. M. A. J. *11*:562, Aug '21
SIBBALD, D. AND O'FARRELL, G.: Toti-Mosher operation; dacryocystorhinostomy; combined endonasal and external technic. Rev. Soc. argent. de Oftal. *1*:79–82, '25
SIBBALD, D. AND O'FARRELL, G.: Toti-Mosher operation; dacryocystorhinostomy. Rev. de especialid. *1*:568–573, '26
SIBBALD, D. (see ARGANARAZ, R. *et al*) 1938
SIBILLA, C. E.: Thyroglossal cysts and fistulas; 8 cases. Rev. Asoc. med. argent. *58*:888–891, Oct 15, '44
SIBILLA, C. E. Thyroglossal cysts and fistulas; 8 cases. Bol. y trab., Soc. argent. de cirujanos *5*:543–553, '44
SIBILLA, C. E. AND CATALANO, F. E.: Total parotidectomy; cases. Bol. y trab., Soc. argent. de cirujanos *6*:142–150, '45 also: Rev. Asoc. med. argent. *59*:698–700, June 30, '45
SIBILLA, C. E. (see CATALANO, F. E.) May '45
SIBLEY, K.: Alopecia and its treatment. Post-Grad. M. J. *8*:110–113, April '32
SICARD, A.: Dupuytren's contracture. Ann. d'anat. path. *7*:745–746, June '30
SICARD, A. AND FAUREL: Metallic tube for nerve suture. Mem. Acad. de chir. *72*:393, July 3–10, '46
SICARD, J. A.: Prosthesis to correct facial paralysis. Bull. et mem. Soc. med. d. hop. de Paris *45*:612, May 6, '21 abstr: J.A.M.A. *76*:1862, June 25, '21
SICARD, J. A.: Intramuscular injection of alcohol in treatment of recurring luxation of jaw. Bull. Acad. de med., Par. *89*:271–274, Feb 20, '23
SICHER, H. AND POHL, L.: Development of human lower jaw; study of development of fistula of lower lip. Ztschr. f. Stomatol. *32*:552–560, May 25, '34
SICILIANI, G.: Fate of free muscular transplants. Morgagni *70*:329–353, Feb 19, '28
SIDORENKO, V. I.: Jaw fractures. Sovet. med. (no. 6) *5*:23–24, '41
SIE BOEN LIAN: Transplantation of conjunctiva of cadaver; clinical and histologic aspects. Geneesk. tijdschr. v. Nederl.-Indie *81*:2097–2101, Sept 30, '41
SIE BOEN LIAN: Tubed pedicle skin graft to eyelids. Geneesk. tijdschr. v. Nederl.-Indie *81*:2781–2784, Dec 30, '41

Sie Boen Lian Operation

Sie Boen Lian operation in entropion. KANTOR, D. V. Sovet. vestnik oftal. *2*:292–295, '33
Author's modification of Sie Boen Lian operation for trachomatous entropion and its

Sie Boen Lian Operation – Cont.
late results. KANTOR, D. V. Vestnik oftal. *18*:301–305, '41

SIEGEL, R.: Buccal mucous membrane grafts in treatment of burns of eye. Arch. Ophth. *32*:104–108, Aug '44
SIEGEL, S. A.; MARRONE, L. V. AND GORDON, D.: Practical aspects of burn therapy. Surgery *18*:298–305, Sept '45
SIEGLING, J. A. AND FAHEY, J. J.: Fate of transplanted cow's horn in treatment of bone fractures. J. Bone and Joint Surg. *18*:439–444, April '36
SIEMENS, H. W.: Elastic prosthesis for nasal defects. Munchen. med. Wchnschr. *85*:1987–1988, Dec 23, '38 comment by Zinsser *86*:252, Feb 17, '39 comment by Moncorps *86*:252–253, Feb 17, '39 comment by Bering *86*:253–254, Feb 17, '39 reply by Siemens *86*:254, Feb 17, '39
SIEMERLING, E.: Facial paralysis; causes, symptoms and treatment. Deutsche med. Wchnschr. *53*:1467–1470, Aug 26, '27
SIEVERS, R.: Hypospadias, relation to abnormalities of penis. Deutsche Ztschr. f. Chir. *199*:286–306, '26
SIGAL, E.: Case of syndactylia and gigantonychia. Casop. lek. cesk. *71*:329–331, March 11, '32
SIGERIST, H. E.: Ambroise Pare's onion treatment of burns. Bull. Hist. Med. *15*:143–149, Feb '44

Sigmoid

Ectopia vesicae successfully treated by transplantation of trigone into the sigmoid. BROWN, H. H. Brit. M. J. *1*:15, Jan 1, '21
Operation for concealed prolapse of rectum and sigmoid. HIRSCHMAN, L. J., J. Michigan M. Soc. *24*:345–347, July '25
Construction of artificial vagina from sigmoid flexure in case of congenital aplasia. RUGE, E. Monatschr. f. Geburtsh. u. Gynak. *78*:313–326, March '28
Pregnancy terminated by caesarean section after ureteral transplantation into sigmoid for exstrophy of bladder. EBERBACH, C. W. AND PIERCE, J. M. Surg., Gynec. and Obst. *47*:540–542, Oct '28
Vaginal formation from sigmoid flexure; case. FAEHRMANN, J. Zentralbl. f. Chir. *56*:1989–1993, Aug 10, '29
Artificial vagina formation from sigmoid flexure. RUGE, E. Zentralbl. f. Chir. *56*:2958, Nov 23, '29
Artificial vagina formed from sigmoid. FRANKENBERG, B. Arch. f. Gynak. *140*:226–252, '30

Sigmoid – Cont.
Artificial vagina from sigmoid. HEJDUK, B. Casop. lek. cesk. *70:*1458–1461, Oct 30, '31
Transplantation of ureters to rectosigmoid and cystectomy in exstrophy; 76 cases. WALTERS, W. Am. J. Surg. *15:*15–22, Jan '32
Transplantation of ureters into sigmoid in exstrophy of bladder. NORTHROP, H. L., J. Am. Inst. Homeop. *26:*33–34, Jan '33
Construction of artificial vagina from loop of sigmoid. CARLING, E. R. Brit. M. J. *1:*375–376, March 3, '34
Construction of vagina with loop from sigmoid. HEJDUK, B. Bratisl. lekar. listy *15:*241–251, March '35
Reconstruction of vagina from portion of sigmoid; case. PITTS, H. C. New England J. Med. *213:*1136–1137, Dec 5, '35
Reconstruction of vagina from portion of sigmoid; case. PITTS, H. C. Tr. New England S. Soc. *18:*273–275, '35
Plastic replacement of vagina with portion of sigmoid flexure (Ruge operation) after Wertheim operation for total extirpation; case. BALKOW, E. Deutsche med. Wchnschr. *62:*586–588, April 10, '36
Artificial vagina formation from sigmoid. BALKOW, E. Ztschr. f. Geburtsh. u. Gynak. *112:*256–260, '36
Exstrophy of bladder (treated by ureterosigmoidostomy). LADD, W. E. AND LANMAN, T. H. New England J. Med. *216:*637–645, April 15, '37
Transplantation of ureters into sigmoid in therapy of urinary incontinence due to grave congenital malformation; case (exstrophy of bladder). BUFALINI, M. Policlinico (sez. prat.) *44:*880–883, May 3, '37
Transplantation of ureters into rectosigmoid in young children and infants with exstrophy of bladder; preliminary report. LOWER, W. E., J. Mt. Sinai Hosp. *4:*650–653, March–April '38
Plastic surgery of vaginal aplasia, using portion of sigmoid flexure; review of literature and report of 2 personal cases. HEJDUK, B. Zentralbl. f. Gynak. *63:*1298–1309, June 10, '39
Transplantation of ureters into sigmoid and cystectomy in radical therapy of exstrophy; late results in case. AREZZI, G. Arch. ital. di urol. *16:*384–405, Dec '39
Modification of operation for artificial vagina from sigmoid. SHOR, A. M. Novy khir. arkhiv. *45:*252–253, '40

SIGNORIS, E.: Medical and surgical technic in therapy of furunculosis. Riv. med. *36:*146–148, Oct '28

SIGWART, W.: Congenital vaginal and anal atresia. Geburtsh. u. Frauenh. *2:*628–635, Dec '40
SILBER, W.: Peripheral nerve surgery. South African M. J. *20:*601, Oct 12, '46; 634, Oct 26, '46
SILER, V. E.: Surgical treatment of burns. Cincinnati J. Med. *22:*451–456, Dec '41
SILER, V. E.: Primary cleansing, compression and rest in burn treatment. Surg., Gynec. and Obst. *75:*161–164, Aug '42 also: Am. J. Nursing *42:*994–1000, Sept '42
SILER, V. E.: Management of acute hand infections. Ohio State M. J. *38:*922–924, Oct '42
SILER, V. E.: Trend in burns. Cincinnati J. Med. *24:*163–167, June '43
SILER, V. E.: Prevention and treatment of hand infections. J. Indiana M. A. *36:*334–339, July '43
SILER, V. E.: Management of injuries and infections of upper extremities. J.A.M.A. *124:*408–412, Feb 12, '44
SILER, V. E.: Management of heat burns. J.A.M.A. *124:*486–487, Feb 19, '44
SILER, V. E.: Surgical reconstruction following serious burns. South. M. J. *37:*187–195, April '44
SILER, V. E. AND REID, M. R.: Clinical and experimental studies with Koch method in heat burns. Ann. Surg. *115:*1106–1117, June '42
SILFVERSKIÖLD, N.: Transplantation of tendons of flexor pollicis longus for paralysis of flexor opponens pollicis. Acta chir. Scandinav. *64:*296–299, '28
SILFVERSKIÖLD, N.: Tenoplasty for ulnar paralysis. Acta chir. Scandinav. *64:*300–302, '28
SILFVERSKIÖLD, N.: Traumatic luxation of some extensor tendons of hand. Acta chir. Scandinav. *64:*305–310, '28
SILFVERSKIÖLD, N.: Treatment of rupture of extensor tendons of phalanges of hand. Zentralbl. f. Chir. *56:*3210, Dec 21, '29
SILLMAN, J. H.: Feeding infant with cleft palate with aid of dental plate; 5 cases. Am. J. Dis. Child. *56:*1055–1058, Nov '38
SILTEN, A. M. (see STOLOFF, I. A.) Jan '39
SILVA, D. (see SANCHEZ BULNES, L.) 1945
SILVA, F.: Dupuytren's contracture. Brazil-med. *2:*269–272, Nov 8, '24 abstr: J.A.M.A. *84:*557, Feb 14, '25
DA SILVA, G.: Restoration of subseptum and lower lip by process of tubular autoplasty; case. Arq. de cir. clin. e exper. *6:*287–299, April–June '42
DA SILVA, S. C.: Present status of plastic surgery of nose and face. Brazil-med. *2:*96–97, Aug 12, '22
DA SILVA, CANDIDO: Complications of burns. Amatus *1:*781–798, Nov '42

da Silva Costa, A.: Surgical technic for construction of pituitary conjunctival canal (artificial lacrimal canal). Bull. Soc. d'opht. de Paris *51:*385–388, June '39

Silvani, H. (see McCorkle, H. J.) March '45

Silveira, L. M.: Surgical correction of superciliary alopecia in leprosy. Rev. brasil. de leprol. (num. espec.) *7:*277–281, '39

Silveira, L. M.: Surgical correction of hypertrophy of auricular lobe in leprosy. Rev. brasil. de leprol. *8:*1–3, March '40

Silveira, L. M.: Problem of nasal deformity in leprosy. Arq. de cir. clin. e exper. *6:*531–535, April–June '42

Silveira, L. M.: Plastic surgery in exeresis of epitheliomas of dorsum of nose. Arq. de cir. clin. e exper. *6:*573–577, April–June '42

Silveira, L. M.: Plastic correction of deformities of ear lobe in leprosy. Arq. de cir. clin. e exper. *6:*485–488, April–June '42

Silveira, L. M.: Free graft of scalp in repair of alopecia of eyebrows. Arq. de cir. clin. e exper. *6:*689–692, April–June '42

Silveira, L. M.: Direction for therapy of hand wounds. Rev. paulista de med. *22:*41–52, Jan '43

Silveira, R.: Indications for operations and operations most commonly performed on nasal septum. Rev. de med. y cir. de la Habana *38:*428–436, June 30, '33

Silver, D.: Role of capsule in joint contractures; with especial reference to subperiosteal separation. J. Bone and Joint Surg. *9:*96–105, Jan '27

Silver, E. I. (see Perkins, H. W.) Sept '42

Silverman, I.: Cancer and malignant tumors of neck; with special reference to incidence, pathology and prognosis. Long Island M. J. *22:*651–656, Nov '28

Silverman, S. L.: Reasons for operations in early infancy on cleft-lip and cleft palate. J. M. A. Georgia *12:*143–147, April '23 (illus.)

Silverman, S. L.: *Principles and Practice of Oral Surgery*. Blakiston Co., Phila., 1926

Silvestri, G.: Therapy of keloids. Minerva chir. *1:*21–22, March '46

Silvis, R. S.: Immediate transfer of pedunculated flap graft to palm; case. U. S. Nav. M. Bull. *41:*821–824, May '43

Simarro Puig, J.; Otero Sanchez, A. and Lluch Caralps, J.: Error in determination of sex; study on pseudohermaphroditism based on case with perineal hypospadias. Rev. clin. espan. *6:*39–42, July 15, '42

Simeon. (see Roger, H. *et al*) April '28

Simeoni, V.: Statistics on 1,323 operations on mouth, pharynx and esophagus for cancer. Valsalva *5:*86–89, Feb '29

Simmons, C. C.: Cancer of mouth; results of treatment by operation and radiation; 376 cases observed at Massachusetts General and Collis P. Huntington Memorial Hospitals in three-year period, 1918–1920. Surg., Gynec. and Obst. *43:*377–382, Sept '26

Simmons, C. C.: Adamantinoma (14 cases with illustrations). Tr. Am. S. A. *46:*383–394, '28

Simmons, C. C.: Results of treatment of cancer of jaws by operation and radiation. Ann. Surg. *92:*681–693, Oct '30

Simmons, C. C. and Daland, E. M.: Results of operations for cancer of lip at Massachusetts General Hospital from 1909 to 1919. Surg., Gynec. and Obst. *35:*766–771, Dec '22

Simmons, H. T. (see Telford, E. D.) April '38

Simmons, H. T. (see Telford, E. D.) Nov '41

Simmons, J. W.: Compound and multiple fractures of lower jaw; (case report). J. M. A. Georgia *13:*22–23, Jan '24

Simon, H.: Demonstrations of cosmetic surgery. Beitr. z. klin. Chir. *154:*174–177, '31

Simon, H.: Modern therapy of extensive burns. Therap. d. Gegenw. *81:*295–298, Aug '40

Simon, H. E. and Alban, H.: Ring injuries to fingers. Mil. Surgeon *97:*506–508, Dec '45

Simon, H. E. and Kaye, B.: Progressive hemiatrophy of face. Arch. Neurol. and Psychiat. *53:*437–438, June '45

Simon, J.: Treatment of epithelioma of lower jaw. Marseille med. *1:*629, May 15, '27

Simon, L.: Incendiary air raids; incendiary bombs, extinction of fires and treatment of burns. Strasbourg med. *98:*175–179, May 15, '38

Simon, L. G.: Finger surgery; analysis of 1000 cases. Indust. Med. *11:*517–518, Nov '42

Simon, R.: Grafts of bone tissue. Rev. de chir. *60:*207–286, '22 (illus.) abstr: J.A.M.A. *79:*1276, Oct. 7; 2122, Dec 16, '22

Simon, R.: Therapy of arthritis from point of view of surgeon. Strasbourg med. *98:*484–488, Dec 5, '38

Simon, R. and Aron, M.: Grafts of bones of embryos. Arch. franco-belges de chir. *25:*869–883, July '22 (illus.) abstr: J.A.M.A. *80:*65, Jan 6, '23

Simon, R., Stulz, E. and Fontaine, R.: Fistulae and congenital cysts of lateral region of neck; 3 personal cases. Arch. franco-belges de chir. *28:*203–258, March '25

Simon, S. (see Cogniaux, P.) May '37

Simon, W. V.: Late rupture of tendon of extensor pollicis longus following fracture of radius. Zentralbl. f. Chir. *58:*1298–1301, May 23, '31

Simonart, A. (see Helderweirt, G. *et al*) Dec '38

Simoncini, M.: Effects of benzopyrene on speed of regeneration of skin. Tumori *14:*394–411, Sept–Dec '40

Simonetta, B.: Origin of congenital fistula of

dorsum of nose. Boll. d. mal. d. orecchio, d. gola. d. naso *51:*503–512, Dec '33
SIMONETTA, B.: Rare congenital malformation of nose (transverse duplication of fossa); case. Boll. d. mal. d. orecchio, d. gola. d. naso *54:*361–366, Oct '36
SIMONETTI, G.: Ozone in burns; preliminary report. Osp. maggiore *20:*287–290, May '32
SIMONIN, J. (see RICHON *et al*) March '33
SIMONS, A.: Treatment of keloids and hypertrophic scars by introduction of radio-active substances into tissue. Strahlentherapie *37:*89–123, '30
SIMONS, R. D. G. P.: Technic of making artificial noses. Nederl. tijdschr. v. geneesk. *81:*1421–1425, April 3, '37
SIMONSON, S. G. (see ROCHLIN, D. G.) Aug '32
SIMONT, D.: Plastic operation for saddle nose. Zentralbl. f. Chir. *56:*910–912, April 13, '29
SIMPSON, B. T. (see SCHREINER, B. F.) June '29
SIMPSON, B. T. (see SCHREINER, B. F.) Aug '29
SIMPSON, C. A.: Treatment of epithelioma of face and eyelid. Virginia M. Monthly *52:*337–340, Sept '25
SIMPSON, D.: Use of cautery in plastic operations of eyelids. Brit. M. J. *2:*424–425, Sept 29, '45
SIMPSON, F. E. AND FLESHER, R. E.: Radium emanation in treatment of intra-oral cancer; with report of 141 cases. Tr. Sect. Dermat. and Syphil., A.M.A., pp. 120–129, '25
SIMPSON, F. E. AND FLESHER, R. E.: Radium in removal of "birthmarks." Clin. Med. and Surg. *34:*605–607, Aug '27
SIMPSON, F. E. AND FLESHER, R. E.: Radium and radon in treatment of epithelioma of lips. Arch. Physical Therapy *9:*207–208, May '28
SIMPSON, F. E. AND FLESHER, R. E.: Radium and radon in treatment of epithelioma of lips. Illinois M. J. *54:*48–50, July '28
SIMPSON, H. L.: Method of holding septal membranes in apposition after a submucous resection without use of packing, description and demonstration of instruments and method of use. J. Michigan M. Soc. *23:*64–67, Feb '24
SIMPSON, R. K.: Needle and needle holder for intranasal use. Am. J. Ophth. *25:*1368–1369, Nov '42
SIMPSON-SMITH, A. AND GRAVES-MORRIS, W. M.: Treatment of maxillary fractures. Brit. M. J. *2:*632, Oct 6, '34
SIMSA, J. (see NEUWIRT, F.) July '37
SINAIKO, E. S.: Skin transposition in incisional defects; modification of Z plastic for primary skin closure following extensive breast surgery. Surgery *18:*650–652, Nov '45
SINBERG, S. E.: Fractures of sesamoid of thumb. J. Bone and Joint Surg. *22:*444–445, April '40
SINCLAIR, J. G.: Intestinal hernia with eversion and exstrophic bladder. J. Pediat. *26:*78–81, Jan '45
SINCLAIR, J. G. AND MCKAY, J.: Median harelip, cleft palate and glossal agenesis. Anat. Rec. *91:*155–160, Feb '45
SINGLETON, A. O.: Developmental anomalies of face and neck and their surgical significance (also cleft palate). Texas State J. Med. *25:*659–663, Feb '30
SINGLETON, A. O. AND DUREN, N.: Salivary gland tumors. Texas State J. Med. *36:*784–792, April '41
SINISCAL, A. A. (see SMITH, J. E.) April '43
SINITSKIY, A. A. (see POLISADOVA, K. I.) 1934
SISTO HONTAN, E.: Congenital implantation of penis with hypospadias in perineum between scrotum and anus; case. Pediatria espan. *24:*344–347, Sept '35
SISTRUNK, W. E.: Mixed tumors of parotid. Minnesota Med. *4:*155, March '21
SISTRUNK, W. E.: Results of surgical treatment of epithelioma of lip. Ann. Surg. *73:*521, May '21
SISTRUNK, W. E.: Report of end results of Kondoleon operation for elephantiasis. Southern M. J. *14:*619, Aug '21
SISTRUNK, W. E.: Cysts of thyroglossal tract. S. Clin. N. Amer. *1:*1509, Oct '21
SISTRUNK, W. E.: Elephantiasis. S. Clin. N. Amer. *1:*1523, Oct '21
SISTRUNK, W. E.: Results obtained in elephantiasis through Kondoleon operation. Minnesota Med. *6:*173–177, March '23 (illus.)
SISTRUNK, W. E.: Plastic surgery; removal of scars by stages. Ann. Surg. *85:*185–187, Feb '27
SISTRUNK, W. E.: Plastic surgery; certain modifications of Kondoleon operation for elephantiasis. Ann. Surg. *85:*190–193, Feb '27

Sistrunk Operation

Sistrunk operation (parotid); case. ZAVALETA, D. E. Prensa med. argent. *32:*1331–1334, July 13, '45

SITKOVSKY, P.: Method of closing extensive skin defects. Vestnik Khir. (no. 30) *10:*176–178, '27
SITTENAUER, L.: Treatment of facial furuncles. Med. Klin. *36:*1385–1388, Dec 13, '40
SITTERLI, A.: Cicatricial adhesive contracture of thumb with surface of hand; surgical therapy. Ztschr. f. orthop. Chir. *59:*142–144, '33
SITTIG, O. AND BAUMRUCK, K. O.: Acrocephalosyndactylia; case. Med. Klin. *34:*502–505, April 14, '38
SIURKUS, T.: Plastic surgery of face. Medicina, Kaunas *22:*90–96, Jan '41

SJÖVALL, H.: Case of delayed death following lightning burns. Acta chir. Scandinav. *85:*455-472, '41

Skin

Surgery of skin without disfigurement; esthetic surgery. GIMENO Y RODRÍGUEZ JAÉN, V. AND PULIDO, A. Siglo med. *71:*503-506, May 26; 532-534, June 2; 555-558, June 9; 582-585, June 16; 603-607, June 23; 629-632, June 30, '23

Die Chirurgie: . . . Band II, Pp. 393-602, Die plastischen Operationen der Haut, by K. Tiesenhausen. Edited by M. Kirschner and O. Nordmann. Urban, Berlin, 1927

Method of closing extensive skin defects. SITKOVSKY, P. Vestnik Khir. (no. 30) *10:*176-178, '27

Plastic surgery in retractile cicatrices or extensive loss of skin; cases. MIRIZZI, P. L. Rev. de cir. *8:*337-348, Aug '29

Repair of cutaneous defects. HAYWARD. Med. Klin. *25:*1365, Aug 30; 1397, Sept 6, '29

Removal of wide scars and large disfigurements of skin by gradual partial excision with closure. DAVIS, J. S. Ann. Surg. *90:*645-653, Oct '29

Excision of unsightly skin folds. GUMPERT, M. Med. Welt. *4:*219, Feb 15, '30

Treatment of late injuries of skin with radium ointment; 3 cases. UHLMANN, E. Dermat. Wchnschr. *91:*1825-1828, Dec 13, '30

Therapy of late injuries of skin with ointment containing radium emanations. ROST, G. A. AND UHLMANN, E. Deutsche med. Wchnschr. *58:*655-656, April 22, '32

Reconstructive surgery; repair of superficial injuries. GILLIES, H. Surg., Gynec. and Obst. *60:*559-567, Feb. (no. 2A) '35

Epidermolysis bullosa dystrophica; etiopathogenic study of case following burn in tuberculous child. CIACCIO, I. Arch. ital. di dermat., sif. *12:*326-344, May '36

Surgical treatment of congenital webbed skin across joints. MATOLCSY, T. Orvosi hetil. *80:*1159-1161, Dec 5, '36

Surgical therapy of congenital webbed skin. MATOLCSY, T. Arch. f. klin. Chir. *185:*675-681, '36

Treatment of traumatic avulsion of skin. RUBASHEV, S. M. Vestnik. khir. *47:*87-88, '36

Repair of traumatic defects of skin (grafts). KALMANOVSKIY, S. M. AND ZHAK, E. Vestnik khir. *55:*375-379, April '38

Plastic surgical repair of unusual dermatologic conditions. BARSKY, A. J., S. Clin. North America *19:*459-466, April '39

Significance of subcutaneous scar tissue. MOSIMAN, R. E. West. J. Surg. *47:*397-401,

Skin – Cont.

July '39

Therapy of traumatic exfoliation of skin. ELKIN, M. A. Khirurgiya, no. 1, pp. 60-62, '39

Birth-marks; relationship to skin cancer. TRAUB, E. F. Hygeia *18:*513, June '40

Effects of benzopyrene on speed of regeneration of skin. SIMONCINI, M. Tumori *14:*394-411, Sept-Dec '40

Treatment of common disfigurements of skin. CANNON, A. B. New York State J. Med. *40:*1567-1572, Nov 1, '40

Dermatologic esthetics; pigmentation, freckles, etc. of exposed parts; means of preventing, improving and curing them. SAINZ DE AJA, E. A. Actas dermo-sif. *32:*145-151, Nov '40

Substances promoting formation of skin. SAINZ DE AJA, E. A. Actas dermo-sif. *32:*229-233, Dec '40

Principles of treatment of avulsion of skin. STEVENSON, T. W. JR. S. Clin. North America *21:*555-564, April '41

Local supracutaneous serotherapy used in skin diseases and surgery for esthetic results. DE CAMPOS, A. Rev. paulista de med. *20:*12-19, Jan '42

Diagnosis of skin diseases of hand and fingers. KRANTZ, W. Med. Klin. *38:*29, Jan 9, '42; 54, Jan 16, '42; 98, Jan 30, '42

Effects of pregnancy hormones on healing process; experimental and clinical studies (of skin). VURCHIO, G. Ginecologia *8:*237-246, June '42

Extensive skin detachment; therapy. GAXIOLA GANDARA, J. Prensa med. mex. *7:*178-179, Dec 15, '42

Precancerous conditions of skin and adjacent mucosa. MIESCHER, G. Schweiz. med. Wchnschr. *73:*1072, Sept 4, '43

Effect of different agents on rate of epithelial regeneration; use of dermatome donor area in obtaining clinical data. BAXTER, H. *et al.* Canad. M. A. J. *50:*411-415, May '44

Surface repair of compound injuries of extremities. BROWN, J. B., J. Bone and Joint Surg. *26:*448-454, July '44

Origin of elasticity of skin and its significance in plastic surgery. SOMALO, M. Prensa med. argent. *31:*1313-1316, July 12, '44

Healing of surface cutaneous wounds (donor areas); analogy with healing of superficial burns. CONVERSE, J. M. AND ROBB-SMITH, A. H. T. Ann. Surg. *120:*873-885, Dec '44

Skin defects of extremities. LEWIS, G. K. Am. Acad. Orthop. Surgeons, Lect., pp. 229-245, '44

Skin – Cont.

Regeneration of skin after experimental removal in man. BISHOP, G. H. Am. J. Anat. *76:*153–181, March '45

Plastic operations for covering cutaneous defects following soft tissue wounds. ANTELAVA, N. V. Khirurgiya, no. 6, pp. 40–43, '45

Spontaneous gangrene (Fournier's gangrene). MANSFIELD, O. T. Brit. J. Surg. *33:*275–277, Jan '46

Surgical treatment of ichthyosis hystrix. KAZANJIAN, V. H. Plast. and Reconstruct. Surg. *1:*91–97, July '46

Treatment of loss of skin substance in surgery of extremities. DUCHET, G. Semaine d. hop. Paris *22:*1671–1680, Sept 21, '46

Common precanceroses of skin. DUNCAN, C. S., West Virginia M. J. *42:*299–301, Dec '46

Healing of skin defects; experimental study on white rat. LINDQUIST, G. Acta chir. Scandinav. (supp. 107) *94:*1–163, '46

Skin, Cancer (See also Cancer, Basal Cell; Cancer, Skin; Melanoma)

Squamous-cell epithelioma of skin. BRODERS, A. C. Ann. Surg. *73:*141, Feb '21

Surgical treatment of extensive basal cell carcinoma. HORSLEY, J. S. J.A.M.A. *78:*412–416, Feb 11, '22 (illus.)

Basal-cell carcinoma of skin. HORSLEY, J. S. S. Clin. N. America *2:*1247–1257, Oct '22

Relationship of cellular differentiation, fibrosis, hyalinization, and lymphocytic infiltration to postoperative longevity of patients with squamous-cell epithelioma of skin and lip. POWELL, L. D., J. Cancer Research *7:*371–378, Oct '22 (illus.)

Treatment of skin cancer. PFAHLER, G. E. New York M. J. *116:*553–555, Nov 15, '22

Statistic and technique in treatment of malignant disease of skin by radiation. MORROW, H. AND TAUSSIG, L. R. Am. J. Roentgenol. *10:*212–218, March '23; *10:*867–871, Nov '23

Unusual type of skin cancer with remarks on its genesis. ELIASSOW, A. Dermat. Wchnschr. *78:*365–370, March 29, '24

Multiple malignant skin epitheliomas in the young. PICCARDI, G. Gior. ital. d. mal. ven. *65:*338–343, April '24

Precancerous eruptions of skin. KNOWLES, F. C., J. Iowa M. Soc. *14:*403–407, Sept '24

Cancerous and precancerous conditions of the skin. MACCORMAC, H. Brit. M. J. *2:*457–460, Sept 13, '24

Cancerous and precancerous conditions of the skin. SAVATARD, L. Brit. M. J. *2:*460–463, Sept 13, '24

Skin, Cancer – Cont.

Precancerous dermatoses, report of case. FUKAMACHI, T. Arch. Dermat. and Syph. *10:*714–721, Dec '24

Superficial epitheliomas of skin. MARTINOTTI, L. Arch. ital. di chir. *10:*471–556, '24

Transplantation of distant skin flaps for cure of intractable basal-cell carcinoma. HORSLEY, J. S. Ann. Surg. *82:*14–29, July '25

Electrocoagulation and desiccation of surface malignancies. PLANK, T. H. Physical Therap. *44:*363–367, July '26

Cancer of skin and mouth. KING, J. M., J. Tennessee M. A. *19:*115–121, Sept '26

Cases of cancer after skin transplantation. KORKHOV, V. Vestnik khir. (no. 41) *14:*137–142, '28

Spreading epitheliomas, recurring after radium therapy; cure by surgical treatment (face). BÉRARD, L., AND DUNET. Lyon chir. *26:*562–565, Aug–Sept '29

Review of cases of squamous cell carcinoma at New Haven Hospital from Janaury 1, 1920, to November 1, 1931. ROBERTS, F. W. Yale J. Biol. and Med. *4:*187–198, Dec '31

Old and new facts about Chaoul method of close exposure (plesioroentgenotherapy) for cancer of skin and lip; 42 cases. LIEBMANN, G. Dermat. Wchnschr. *104:*293–300, March 6, '37

Cancer of lip and oral cavity and skin. HOLLANDER, L. Pennsylvania M. J. *40:*749–750, June '37

Transplantation of skin cancer by use of superficial grafts of epidermis covering epithelioma. CROSTI, A. Gior. ital. di dermat. e sif. *79:*1091–1108, Dec '38

Treatment of large protruding carcinomas of skin and lip by irradiation and surgery. HUNT, H. B. Am. J. Roentgenol. *44:*254–264, Aug '40

Treatment of persistent recurrent basal cell carcinoma. YOUNG, F. Surg., Gynec. and Obst. *73:*152–162, Aug '41

"Field-fire" and invasive basal cell carcinoma – basal-squamous type. BROWN, J. B. AND MCDOWELL, F. Surg., Gynec. and Obst. *74:*1128–1132, June '42

Therapy of nevi; relationship to skin malignancies. TRAUB, E. F., J. Michigan M. Soc. *42:*297–300, April '43

Free grafts and pedicle flaps in treatment of recurring basal cell epitheliomas; cases. WEAVER, D. F. Laryngoscope *53:*336–342, May '43

Skin carcinoma; analysis of 20 cases in Negroes. SCHREK, R. Cancer Research *4:*119–127, Feb '44

Cancer of skin, lip and tongue. MARTIN, H.

Skin—Cont.
Bull. Am. Soc. Control Cancer *26:*82–83, July '44
Closure of defects of skin after surgery for cancer. MAY, H. Clinics *4:*53-62, June '45
Common precanceroses of skin. DUNCAN, C. S., West Virginia M. J. *42:*299–301, Dec '46

Skin Flaps

Sensibility of flap in remote plastic operations. LEHMANN, W. AND JUNGERMANN, E. Mitt. a. d. Grenzgeb. d. Med. u. Chir. *32:*653–658, '20
Pedunculated flaps without skin pedicle in plastic surgery. ESSER, J. F. S. Arch. f. klin. Chir. *177:*477-491, '21 (illus.) abstr: J.A.M.A. *78:*1009, April 1, '22
Pedicled flaps aided by free fat transplantation in plastic surgery. VAN HOOK, W. Med. Rec. *101:*625-626, April 15, '22
Transplantation of skin flaps. TAKAHASHI, N. AND MIYATA, R. Arch. f. klin. Chir. *120:*170–205, '22 (illus.)
Long curve and small triangle flap (plastic surgery). KREIKER, A. AND ORSÓS, J. Deutsche Ztschr. f. Chir. *179:*145–159, '23 (illus.) addendum *182:*118, '23 abstr: J.A.M.A. *81:*866, Sept 8, '23
Transplantation of distant skin flaps for cure of intractable basal-cell carcinoma. HORSLEY, J. S. Ann. Surg. *82:*14–29, July '25
Skin flap cover for projecting intestine. STEINBERG, M. E. Ann. Surg. *83:*123-125, Jan '26
Flap autoplasty; adherent skin anaplasty. SEBILEAU, P. Rev. de chir. *64:*207-258, '26 abstr: J.A.M.A. *87:*1074, Sept 25, '26
Pedicled skin grafts. BETTMAN, A. G. Northwest Med. *27:*78-86, Feb '28
Use of pedicle grafts in traumatic surgery. COLP, R. Internat. Clin. *1:*189-206, March '28
Autoplasty by flap; cases. BURTY. Bull. et mem. Soc. de chir. de Paris *20:*848-850, '28
Contractures due to burns; treatment with free full thickness grafts and pedunculated flaps. KOCH, S. L. AND KANAVEL, A. B. Tr. Sect. Surg, General and Abd., A.M.A., pp. 208–227, '28
Contracture due to burns; treatment with free full thickness grafts and pedunculated flaps. KOCH, S. L. AND KANAVEL, A. B. J.A.M.A. *92:*277-281, Jan 26, '29
Two-stage pedicle graft to replace unsatisfactory scar. COTTON, F. J. AND BERG, R. New England J. Med. *201:*981-982, Nov 14, '29
Free and pediculated skin grafts. POGGI, J. Folha med. *10:*403-406, Nov 25, '29
Autotransplantation of fascia by cutaneous

Skin Flaps—Cont.
flaps with tubulate pedicles. MOURE, P. Rev. odont. *51:*5-10, Jan '30
Use of pedicled skin flaps to cover skin defects. TIESENHAUSEN, K. Zentralbl. f. Chir. *57:*1985–1988, Aug 9, '30
Attempt at nephropexy by means of pedicled cutaneous-subcutaneous flap (Sokolow method). PAWLONSKY, J. M. Zentralbl. f. Chir. *58:*1306–1312, May 23, '31
Grafting of hairy skin with aid of pedunculated flap for formation of eyebrows, mustache and beard. PARIN, V. N. Vestnik khir. (nos. 73–74) *24:*10–12, '31
Design of direct pedicle flaps. GILLIES, H. D. Brit. M. J. *2:*1008, Dec 3, '32
Biological skin flaps for pronounced scars. ESSER, J. F. S. Zentralbl. f. Chir. *60:*1639-1641, July 15, '33
Back as source for pedicled grafts. BETTMAN, A. G. Northwest Med. *32:*453-456, Nov '33
Dermo-subcutaneous flaps; management in reconstructive surgery. O'CONNOR, G. B. AND PIERCE, G. W. California and West. Med. *40:*151-156, March '34
Changes in cutaneous localization in pedicle flap. DOUGLAS, B. AND LANIER, L. H. Arch. Neurol. and Psychiat. *32:*756-762, Oct '34
General sensations in pedunculated skin flaps. DAVIS, J. S. AND KITLOWSKI, E. A. Arch. Surg. *29:*982–1000, Dec '34
Transplantation of thick skin flap in plastic surgery of face. DUBOV, M. D. Sovet. khir. (nos. 3–4) *6:*489–502, '34
Failures, hazards and unforeseen complications involved in use of pedicled flap in plastic operations. LINDENBAUM, J. Arch. f. klin. Chir. *181:*529-547, '35
Management of large skin flaps. UPDEGRAFF, H. L. Am. J. Surg. *33:*104-107, July '36
Resorption in pedunculated skin grafts. WITTE, G. Arch. f. klin. Chir. *184:*689-707, '36
Use of pedicle graft for chronic osteomyelitis. BEEKMAN, F., S. Clin. North America *17:*185-190, Feb '37
Simple method of measuring skin for flaps. MALONE, J. Y. Ann. Surg. *105:*303-304, Feb '37
Autoplastic restoration of scrotum by so-called Hindu method, using flap taken from posterointernal section of thigh; cases. GONZALEZ HURTADO, R. Cir. y cirujanos *6:*359-366, Aug '38
Fistulized tuberculous trochanteritis with extensive bone loss; immediate transplantation of pedicled cutaneous flap into residual cavity; case with recovery. INGIANNI,

Skin Flaps – Cont.

G. Arch. ed atti d. Soc. ital. di chir. *44:*873-875, '38

Autoplastic therapy of tuberculous and nontuberculous trochanteritis using free and pedicled flaps; cases. INGIANNI, G. Accad. med., Genova *54:*446-453, May '39

Treatment of avulsed flaps. FARMER, A. W. Ann. Surg. *110:*951-959, Nov '39

Surgical therapy of cryptorchidism with pedicled flap from thigh. HILD, J. Beitr. z. klin. Chir. *170:*387-397, '39

Transplantation of skin and subcutaneous tissue to hand. KOCH, S. L. Surg., Gynec. and Obst. *72:*157-177, Feb '41

Free skin grafts versus flaps in surface defects of face and neck. MALINIAC, J. W. Am. J. Surg. *58:*100-109, Oct '42

Flap operation for treatment of multiple sebaceous cysts (steatomata). MARSHALL, W. J. Invest. Dermat. *5:*299-302, Dec '42

Endocutaneous (Eloesser) flap; application in various types of intrathoracic lesions. BROWN, A. L. Brunn, Med.-Surg. Tributes, pp. 73-79, '42

New type of relaxing incision – dermatome-flap method. HARKINS, H. N. Am. J. Surg. *59:*79-82, Jan '43

Repair of limb wounds by use of direct skin flaps. BROWN, D. O. Brit. J. Surg. *30:*307-314, April '43

Circulation in pedicle flaps; accurate test ("temperature-return test") for determining its efficiency. DOUGLAS, B. AND BUCHHOLZ, R. R. Ann. Surg. *117:*692-709, May '43

Sacrococcygeal dermoid cysts; Lahey plastic repair using bipedicled flap. BAILA, A. E. Bol. y trab., Soc. argent. de cirujanos *4:*292-293, '43 also: Rev. Asoc. med. argent. *57:*495, July 30, '43

Application of dermatome-flap method; use in case of recurrent incisional hernia. SWENSON, S. A. JR. AND HARKINS, H. N. Arch. Surg. *47:*564-570, Dec '43

Evaluation of pedicle flaps versus skin grafts in reconstruction of surface defects and scar contractures of chin, cheeks and neck. AUFRICHT, G. Surgery *15:*75-84, Jan '44

Grafts of pedicled soft tissue flaps in therapy of osseous fistulas following gunshot fractures. HUNDEMER, W. Munchen. med. Wchnschr. *91:*154, March 24, '44

Pedicled grafts versus free grafts. FARINA, R. Sao Paulo med. *2:*125-132, Aug '44

Choice of pedicle flaps for plastic and reconstructive surgery. WEBSTER, G. V., S. Clin. North America *24:*1472-1482, Dec '44

Use of skin flaps in repair of scarred defects over bone and tendons. PADGETT, E. C. AND GASKINS, J. H. Surgery *18:*287-298, Sept '45

Pedicle grafts. ALDUNATE PHILLIPS, E. Arch. Soc. cirujanos hosp. *15:*758-764, Dec '45

Full thickness flap closure of large thoracotomy due to chemical destruction of chest wall (by injection of nitric acid). PRIOLEAU, W. H., J. Thoracic Surg. *14:*433-437, Dec '45

Use of skin flaps in repair of scarred or ulcerative defects over bone and tendons. PADGETT, E. C. AND GASKINS, J. H. Tr. West. S. A. (1944) *52:*195-211. '45

Use of flaps. RIVAS, C. I. Dia med. *18:*946-955, July 15, '46

Total laryngectomy with right hemipharyngectomy; plastic surgery to reconstruct pharynx using laryngeal flap from left vestibular zone. LEYRO DIAZ, J. Bol. y trab., Acad. argent. de cir. *30:*815-833, Sept 11, '46

Repair of avulsion wounds by flap graft technic. RUBIN, L. R. Am. J. Surg. *72:*373-384, Sept '46

Skin Flaps from Arm

Plastic surgery of nose by Italian method using tubular grafts. BURIAN, F. Presse med. *39:*1418-1420, Sept 26, '31

Autoplastic graft on elbow by Italian method; case. MAKSUD. Cong. internat. de med. trop. et d'hyg., Compt. rend (1928) *3:*385, '31

Autoplastic graft of flap by Italian method in reconstructive surgery of mouth; case. REBELO NETO, J. Bol. Soc. de med. e cir. de Sao Paulo *16:*94-108, Nov '32

Pedicle grafts from arm for reconstructions about face. JENKINS, H. P., S. Clin. North America *26:*20-32, Feb '46

Skin Flaps, Arterial

Arterial flaps and epithelial inserts in plastic surgery. ESSER, J. F. S. Munchen. med. Wchnschr. *69:*669-671, May 5, '22 (illus.)

Biological or artery flaps; general observations and technic. ESSER, J. F. S. Rev. de chir. plastique, pp. 275-286, Jan '34

Frontal flaps of lips; special practice of biological or artery flaps. ESSER, J. F. S. Rev. de chir. plastique, pp. 288-294, Jan '34

Skin Flaps to Breast

Abdominal flap to cover defect after mammectomy. SOUPAULT, R. Presse med. *31:*177-178, Feb 24, '23 (illus.)

Skin Flaps to Breast—Cont.

Abdominal skin flap after amputation of breast. HEIDENHAIN, L. Zentralbl. f. Gynak. *48:*2649-2650, Nov 29, '24

Artificial breasts formed by union of 3 flaps following mammectomy for adenofibroma; case. ZORRAQUÍN, G. AND BOIX POU, M. Rev. de cir de Buenos Aires *13:*244-248, April '34

Use of skin flaps for cosmetic plastic surgery of breast. EITNER, E. Zentralbl. f. Chir. *62:*625-627, March 16, '35

Transplantation of nipple, most complicated form of pedicle graft. BAMES, H. O. Rev. de chir. structive, pp. 93-96, June '37

Skin Flaps, Compound

Transplantation of skin together with implanted bone to cover defects of soft tissues and bones. KLEINSCHMIDT, O. Chirurg *14:*737-742, Dec 15, '42

Ability of bone tissue (including "os novum") to survive in pedicled grafts. HELLSTADIUS, A. Acta chir. Scandinav. *86:*85-109, '42

Musculocutaneous graft and its importance in war surgery. PRUDENTE, A. Rev. paulista de med. *22:*435-436, June '43

Skin Flaps, Cross-Lip

Cheiloplasty; using upper lip to make new lower lip. PÓLYA, E. Zentralbl. f. Chir. *48:*262, Feb 26, '21

Switching of vermilion-bordered lip flaps. BROWN, J. B. Surg., Gynec. and Obst. *46:*701-704, May '28

Split vermilion-bordered lip flap in cleft lip. CANNON, B. Surg., Gynec. and Obst. *73:*95-97, July '41

Use of vermilion bordered flaps in surgery about mouth. CANNON, B. Am. J. Orthodontics (Oral Surg. Sect) *28:*423-430, July '42

Use of vermilion bordered flaps in surgery about mouth. CANNON, B. Surg., Gynec. and Obst. *74:*458-462, Feb (no. 2A) '42

Simplified method of rotating skin and mucous membrane flaps for complete reconstruction of lower lip. OWENS, N. Am. J. Orthodontics (Oral Surg. Sect.) *30:*340-349, June '44

Skin Flaps, Delayed

Scar excision; two-stage flap-graft. COTTON, F. J., S. Clin. N. Amer. *1:*904, June '21

Delayed transfer of long pedicle flaps in plastic surgery (face). BLAIR, V. P. Surg., Gynec. and Obst. *33:*261, Sept '21

Uses of dermal graft and delayed flap. RITCHIE, H. P., S. Clin. America *3:*1371-1387, Oct '23 (illus.)

Skin Flaps, Delayed—Cont.

Two-stage pedicle graft to replace unsatisfactory scar. COTTON, F. J. AND BERG, R. New England J. Med. *201:*981-982, Nov 14, '29

Value of delayed single pedicle skin flaps in plastic repair of scalp. DAVIS, W. B. Surg., Gynec. and Obst. *66:*899-901, May '38

Skin Flaps to Ear

Plastic reconstruction of ear with pedunculated tube flap. VAN DIJK, J. A. Nederl. Tijdschr. v. Geneesk. *1:*895-900, Feb 21, '25

Reconstruction of totally lost ear by "tubed pedicle flap" method. VAN DIJK, J. A. Acta oto-laryng. *10:*121-129, '26

Technic of reparation of ear lobe by tubular skin grafts. GONZALEZ ULLOA, M. Rev. mex. de cir., ginec. y cancer *5:*33-41, Jan '37

Plastic reconstruction of ear lobe with circular pedicled flap from neck. SCHUCHARDT, K. Zentralbl. f. Chir. *69:*345, Feb 28, '42

Skin Flaps to Eyelids

Plastic repair of eyelids by pedunculated skin grafts. CROSS, G. H., J.A.M.A. *77:*1233, Oct 15, '21

Transplantation flap repair of lower eyelid following removal of epithelioma. MINCHEW, B. H., J. M. A. Georgia *11:*110-111, March '22

Cancer in right eye; unsuccessful radium therapy; extended exeresis and graft of medio-frontal, pediculated flap; 2 photographs. NIDA. Bull. Soc. d'opht. de Paris, no. 9, pp. 532-536, '27

Machine for shaping skinflaps in anaplasty of eyelids. LÉNÁRD, E. Klin. Monatsbl. f. Augenh. *83:*526-530, Oct-Nov '29

Plastic surgery of eyelid using cervical flap with tubular pedicle; case. DUPUY-DUTEMPS, L. Ann. d'ocul. *167:*895-907, Nov '30 also: Bull. et mem. Soc. franc. d'opht. *43:*451-458, '30

Pedicled flap in plastic surgery of eyelids. SPAETH, E. B. Pennsylvania M. J. *35:*560-562, May '32

Eyelid flaps. ESSER, J. F. S. Rev. de chir. plastique, pp. 295-297, Jan '34

Biologic flap to form 2 eyelids at same time; case. ESSER, J. F. S. Rev. espan. de cir. *17:*1-3, Jan-Feb '35

New method for construction of artificial conjunctival sac by transplantation of skin flap divided into 2 parts. VON CSAPODY, I. Ztschr. f. Augenh. *87:*114-130, Sept '35

Skin Flaps to Eyelids – Cont.

Plastic surgery of eyelids; use of pedicled flaps with handle. von Seemen, H. Deutsche Ztschr. f. Chir. *248:*411–419, '37

New experiences with plastic construction of artificial conjunctival sac, using flaps. von Csapody, I. Ztschr. f. Augenh. *94:*23–33, Jan '38

Pedicled dermomuscular blepharoplasty; 12 cases. Charamis, J. S. Arch. d'opht. *2:*206–218, March '38

Biologic frontal flaps in eyelid surgery. Esser, J. F. S. Am. J. Ophth. *21:*963–967, Sept '38

Eyelid surgery; about sliding-flap, known also as Hungarian plastic. Czukrasz, I. Tr. Ophth. Soc. U. Kingdom (pt. 2) *58:*561–575, '38

Tubed pedicle skin graft to eyelids. Sie Boen Lian. Geneesk. Tijdschr. v. Nederl.-Indie *81:*2781–2784, Dec 30, '41

"Pocket-flap" as method for total restoration of eyelid; preliminary report. Kurlov, I. N., Vestnik oftal. (nos. 1–2) *20:*12–19, '42

Tarsoconjunctival sliding-graft technics for reconstruction of eyelids. Sugar, H. S. Am. J. Ophth. *27:*109–123, Feb '44

Skin Flaps to Face

Restoration of cheek and temporal region by pedicled and sliding grafts of skin and muscle. Whitham, J. D., J.A.M.A. *76:*448, Feb 12, '21

Scalp flaps in reconstruction of face. Moure, P. Presse med. *29:*1021–1022, Dec 4, '21 (illus.) Abstr: J.A.M.A. *78:*470, Feb 11, '22

Rotation of cheek in plastic surgery. Esser, J. F. S. Munchen. med. Wchnschr. *69:*780–781, May 26, '22 (illus.)

Correction of facial defects with special reference to nutrition of skin flaps and planning of repair. Coleman, C. C. Virginia M. Monthly *49:*301–306, Sept '22 (illus.)

Delayed pedicle flap in plastic surgery of face and neck. New, G. B. Minnesota Med. *6:*721–724, Dec '22 (illus.)

New method of resection of upper maxillary with lower facial flap. Lauwers, E. E. Surg., Gynec. and Obst. *39:*499–502, Oct '24

Gersuny's pedunculated flaps for reconstruction of face. Moszkowicz, L. Arch. f. klin. Chir. *130:*796–798, '24

Reconstruction of lower lip according to round pedicle method. Woloschinow, W. Arch. f. klin. Chir. *135:*770–775, '25

Epithelialized flap from forehead to reconstruct lower lip and cheek. New, G. B., S. Clin. N. Amer. *7:*1481–1483, Dec '27

Plastic covering of defects of jaws. Lindemann, A. Chirurg *1:*817–829, Aug 1, '29

Use of double skin flap in restoration of lip defects. von Czeyda-Pommersheim, F. Zentralbl. f. Chir. *56:*2381–2382, Sept 21, '29

Reparation of loss of facial substance with tubular graft; case. Kroeff, M. Folha med. *11:*325–327, Oct 5, '30

Restoration of lower lip by means of Filatov's tubular skin flap. Kartaschew, S. Deutsche Ztschr. f. Chir. *229:*395–400, '30

Tube flaps in reconstructive surgery of face. Peer, L. A., J. M. Soc. New Jersey *28:*86–89, Feb '31

Use of pedicled flaps in reconstructive surgery of face. New, G. B. Tr. Am. Laryng., Rhin. and Otol. Soc. *37:*485–491, '31

Lined pedicled flaps in reconstructive surgery of face; modification of technic. Havens, F. Z., S. Clin. North America *12:*955–957, Aug '32

Syphilitic origin of perforation of palate and destruction of nose; uranoplasty; reconstruction of nose by tubular grafts with cartilaginous support of costal origin. Rocher, H. L. Bull. et mem. Soc. de chir. de Bordeaux et du Sud-Ouest, pp. 150–152, '32

Extensive cicatrix of face; reconstruction of both eyelids and of both lips by tubular grafts. Rocher, H. L. Bull. et mem. Soc. de chir. de Bordeaux et du Sud-Ouest, pp. 154–156, '32

Transplantation of pedicled skin flap to face; case. Kanematsu, T. Okayama-Igakkai-Zasshi *45:*2099–2100, Sept '33

Transplantation of thick skin flap in plastic surgery of face. Dubov, M. D. Sovet. khir. (nos. 3–4) *6:*489–502, '34

Possibility of reconstructing whole face by full thickness, free cutaneous grafts, using several flaps. Coelst. Rev. de chir. structive, pp. 105–125, Dec '35

Rhinoplasty using cutaneous flap from abdomen via forearm. Claoue. Bull. et mem. Soc. de med. de Paris *140:*208–209, March 28, '36

Rotation of cheek to remake face; case. Esser, J. F. S. Tech. chir. *28:*293–296, Dec '36

Rotation of cheek in ophthalmology. Esser, J. F. S. Arch. Ophth. *20:*410–416, Sept '38

Tumor of lower lip and right cheek; extirpation followed by pedicled skin graft from head. Porumbaru, I. Rev. de chir., Bucuresti *41:*714–721, Sept-Oct '38

Use of tubular flap for transplantation of cartilage (ear) in surgical restoration of alae nasi. Novoshinova, E. N. Zhur. ush., nos. i gorl. bolez. *15:*164–168, '38

Skin Flaps to Face – Cont.

Surgery of face; graft by bipedicled flaps. DUFOURMENTEL. Oto-rhino-laryng. internat. *3:*528–529, Oct '39

Apparatus for fixation of skin flap during epithelization of wound cavity after resection of upper jaw. KHARI, A. P. Novy khir. arkhiv *43:*328–330, '39

Plastic repair of defects of lips and corner of mouth by means of Filatov's tubular flaps. GNILORYBOV, T. E. Vestnik khir. *59:*592–599, June '40

Tubed pedicle graft in facial reconstruction; superiority when subcutaneous loss is present. WILMOTH, C. L. Am. J. Surg. *53:*300–305, Aug '41

Restoration of subseptum and lower lip by process of tubular autoplasty; case. DA SILVA, G. Arq. de cir. clin. e exper. *6:*287–299, April–June '42

New forehead flap for nasal reconstruction. CONVERSE, J. M. Proc. Roy. Soc. Med. *35:*811–812, Oct '42 also: J. Laryng. and Otol. *57:*508–509, Nov '42

Use of tubular flaps in repair of defects of face. RAPIN, M. Helvet. med. acta *9:*787–792, Dec '42

Care of military and civilian injuries; use of remote flaps in repairing defects of face and mouth. CANNON, B. Am. J. Orthodontics (Oral Surg. Sect.) *29:*77–85, Feb '43

Plastic surgery of upper lip with skin flaps from chin. FREY, S. Zentralbl. f. Chir. *70:*539, April 10, '43

Use of one flap to restore extensive losses of middle third of face. BARSKY, A. J. Ann. Surg. *118:*988–999, Dec '43

Use of one flap to restore extensive losses of middle third of face. BARSKY, A. J. Tr. Am. Soc. Plastic and Reconstructive Surg. *12:*29–41, '43

Simplified method of rotating skin and mucous membrane flaps for complete reconstruction of lower lip. OWENS, N. Surgery *15:*196–206, Jan '44

Sickle flap for nasal reconstruction. NEW, G. B., Surg., Gynec. and Obst. *80:*497–499, May '45

Sickle flap for reconstruction of nose. NEW, G. B. Proc. Staff Meet., Mayo Clin. *20:*353–356, Oct 3, '45

Pedicle grafts from arm for reconstructions about face. JENKINS, H. P., S. Clin. North America *26:*20–32, Feb '46

Skin Flaps to Foot

Plantar warts, flaps and grafts. BLAIR, V. P.; *et al.* J.A.M.A. *108:*24–27, Jan 2, '37

Pedicle graft of sole of foot. WHITE, W. C. Ann. Surg. *105:*472–473, March '37

Skin Flaps to Foot – Cont.

Total loss of skin and subcutaneous cellular tissue of heel; monopedicled graft; case. PEDEMONTE, P. V. Arch. urug. de med., cir. y especialid. *23:*154–157, Aug '43

Total loss of skin and of subcutaneous cellular tissue of heel; monopedicled graft; case. PEDEMONTE, P. V. Bol. Soc. cir. d. Uruguay *14:*57–60, '43

Use of untubed pedicle grafts in repair of deep defects of foot and ankle; technic and results. GHORMLEY, R. K. AND LIPSCOMB, P. R., J. Bone and Joint Surg. *26:*483–488, July '44

Skin Flaps, Free

Free transplantation of flaps. WITTMOSER, R. Beitr. z. klin. Chir. *174:*387, '43

Skin Flaps to Hand

Skin flap methods in upper extremity deformities. STEINDLER, A., J. Bone and Joint Surg. *7:*512–527, July '25

Hyperextension of hand and fingers from burn; correction by single pedicled skin and fascial flap from anterior abdominal wall. JACKSON, C. AND BABCOCK, W. W., S. Clin. North America *10:*1285–1286, Dec '30

Extensive burns on both forearms and back of hand; remote results of resection of retractile scar and pedicled graft from thigh. MIRIZZI, P. L. Bull. et mem. Soc. nat. de chir. *59:*694–695, May 6, '33

Palmar contracture of hand as sequel of burn received in infancy; therapy with Gillies tubular graft at age 17 years. LLUESMA URANGA, E. Cron. med., Valencia *38:*11–14, Jan 15, '34

Autoplasty using digital flap in therapy of stubborn ulcers resulting from burns received in childhood. CHAUVENET, A. Bordeaux chir. *6:*18–25, Jan '35

Glove flap method of dorsal repair in hand surgery. O'CONNOR, G. B. Am. J. Surg. *32:*445–447, June '36

Glove flap method of dorsal hand repair. O'CONNOR, G. B. Rev. de chir. structive, pp. 384–389, Dec '36

Pedicle flap patterns for reconstruction of hand. PIERCE, G. W. AND O'CONNOR, G. B. Rev. de chir. structive, pp. 85–90, June '37 also: Surg., Gynec. and Obst. *65:*523–527, Oct '37

Immediate flap grafts following trauma (of fingers). DAY, H. F. New England J. Med. *218:*758–759, May 5, '38

Technic of pedicled flaps in plastic surgery of skin; use in treating cicatricial contracture of hand. ZENO, L. Semana med.

Skin Flaps to Hand – Cont.

*2:*1058–1061, Nov 7, '40 also: Bol. y trab., Acad. argent. de cir. *24:*886–890, Sept 18, '40

Technic of application of Filatov flaps in plastic operations on amputation-stumps of hands and fingers. YUSEVICH, M. S. Ortop. i travmatol. (no. 3) *14:*50–56, '40

Fat formation in abdominal skin flap on hand 23 years after grafting. VON MEZÖ, B. Chirurg *13:*18–19, Jan 1, '41

Preservation of tendon function in hand by use of skin flaps. KITLOWSKI, E. A. Am. J. Surg. *51:*653–661, March '41

Operative correction of Dupuytren's contracture by use of tunnel skin graft. SKINNER, H. L. Surgery *10:*313–317, Aug '41

Immediate transfer of pedunculated flap graft to palm; case. SILVIS, R. S., U.S. Nav. M. Bull. *41:*821–824, May '43

Plastic surgery; advantages and inconveniences of tubular transplants in grave cicatrices of hand. PEDEMONTE, P. V. Bol. Soc. cir. d. Uruguay *14:*114–122, '43 also: Arch. urug. de med., cir. y especialid. *23:*453–461, Nov '43

Open abdominal flaps for repair of surface defects of upper extremity. SHAW, D. T., S. Clin. North America *24:*293–308, April '44

Use of flaps and pedicles in repair of hand and arm defects. KISKADDEN, W. S. Am. Acad. Orthop. Surgeons, Lect., pp. 180–183, '44

Direct flap repair of defects of arm and hand; preparation of gunshot wounds for repair of nerves, bones and tendons. BROWN, J. B. *et al.* Ann. Surg. *122:*706–715, Oct '45

Skin Flaps, Homoplastic (Parabiosis)

Homio transplantation of skin flaps. RABINOVITCH, P. Proc. Soc. Exper. Biol. and Med. *25:*798–799, June '28

Fate of homoplastic flaps. SHINOI, K. Mitt. d. med. Gesellsch. zu Tokio *46:*324–325; 369, Feb '32

Immunologic reactions and acid-base equilibrium of flaps in homoplastic skin grafts. SHINOI, K. Mitt. d. med. Gesellsch. zu Tokio *46:*1913–1914, Nov '32

Large scalp wound treated by total homoplastic graft of large cellulocutaneous flap. DUFOURMENTEL, L. Bull. et mem. Soc. d. chirurgiens de Paris *25:*724–726, Dec 15, '33

Dangers in pedicled graft in homeoplasty; case of serious blood changes in patient and donor. REINHARD, W. AND LAUER, A. Deutsche Ztschr. f. Chir. *254:*661–668, '41

Skin Flaps, Inverted

Use of inverted flaps in plastic surgery. KUNZE, W. Zentralbl. f. Chir. *56:*1099–1102, May 4, '29

New method of tube pedicle grafting. MALTZ, M. Am. J. Surg. *43:*216–222, Feb '39

Skin Flaps, Jump

Jump method or interrupted tube flap; new technic in fashioning tube flaps for skin grafts. DE RIVER, J. P., J.A.M.A. *87:*662–663, Aug 28, '26

Replacement of scar over tibia and os calcis by tube pedicle transplant from abdomen. JONES, H. T., S. Clin. N. Amer. *9:*936–938, Aug '29

Covering defects of face by double skin transplantation from abdomen to forearm and face. IVANITZKYI, G. Ukrain. m. visti *5:*41–42, '29

Covering disfiguring cuts on face by method of skin transplantation from abdomen to forearm and face. KHARTZIEFF. Ukrain. m. visti *5:*42–46, '29

Skin Flaps to Leg

Replacement of scar over tibia and os calcis by tube pedicle transplant from abdomen. JONES, H. T., S. Clin. N. Amer. *9:*936–938, Aug '29

Anemic ulcer of leg treated by pedicle graft. JONES, H. T., S. Clin. N. Amer. *9:*933–935, Aug '29

Covering of recurrent crural ulcers by means of plastic use of skin flap from thigh of other leg. PETERS, A. Deutsche med. Wchnschr. *55:*1458–1461, Aug 30, '29

Circulation of skin and muscle flaps of osteoplastic amputations on lower extremity. CHASIN, A. Arch. f. klin. Chir. *155:*630–648, '29

Treatment of chronic ulcer of leg by means of skin flap taken from dorsum of foot. KARTASCHEW, S. Zentralbl. f. Chir. *57:*2472–2475, Oct 4, '30

Pedicle breast flap for amputation-stump; structive surgery applied to amputation stump at knee. ESSER, J. F. S. Ann. Surg. *105:*469–472, March '37

Use of muscular flap to fill cavitations of bones in chronic osteomyelitis. STOTZ, W. Zentralbl. f. Chir. *66:*352–355, Feb 18, '39

Sequestrectomy and autoplasty with skin flaps in therapy of subacute and chronic nonspecific osteomyelitis. PARODI, L. Ann. ital. di chir. *21:*307–314, May '42

Italian method of plastic repair of denuded areas followed by mermaid cast immobilization. MURPHY, F. G. Surgery *12:*294–

Skin Flaps to Leg – Cont.

301, Aug '42

Contiguous skin flaps for wounds of extremities. Rubin, L. R. Am. J. Surg. *71:*36–54, Jan '46

Use of pedicled flaps in surgical treatment of chronic osteomyelitis resulting from compound fractures. Stark, W. J., J. Bone and Joint Surg. *28:*343-350, April '46

Guillotine amputation modified to preserve skin flaps. Meyer, N. C., U.S. Nav. Bull. *46:*1844-1847, Dec '46

Skin Flaps to Mastoid Area

New and simple plastic-flap method in radical mastoid operation. Dintenfass, H. Atlantic M. J. *30:*426-428, April '27

Plastic surgery with bridge flap for correction of retroauricular defects. Claus, G. Deutsche med. Wchnschr. *57:*1779–1780, Oct 16, '31

Use of periosteal flap with skin graft in radical mastoid surgery. Ziegelman, E. F. Laryngoscope *42:*170–176, March '32

Closure of persistent retro-auricular opening by means of Hungarian method of using semicircular flaps. Szokolik, E. Monatschr. f. Ohrenh. *66:*1058–1059, Sept '32

Variation of pedicle flap for epithelization of radical mastoidectomy cavity. Ersner, M. S. and Myers, D. Arch. Otolaryng. *23:*469–474, April '36

New plastic flap for use in endaural radical mastoidectomy. Shambaugh, G. E. Jr. Ann. Otol., Rhin. and Laryng. *51:*117-121, March '42

Skin Flaps to Mouth

Surgical restoration of lining of mouth. Blair, V. P. Surg., Gynec. and Obst. *40:*165–174, Feb '25

Skin Flaps to Neck

Wry-neck following burns, relieved by skin flaps; case report. Miller, O. R. Kentucky M. J. *26:*190-192, April '28

Tubular skin graft in therapy of extensive contracture of neck. Kartashev, Z. I. Sovet. khir., no. 11, pp. 22–30, '35

Skin Flaps, Nerve Regeneration in (See also Skin Grafts, Nerve Regeneration in)

Sensibility of flap in remote plastic operations. Lehmann, W. and Jungermann, E. Mitt. a. d. Grenzgeb. d. Med. u. Chir. *32:*653-658, '20

Recovery of sensation in denervated pedicle and free skin grafts. Kredel, F. E. and Evans, J. P. Arch. Neurol. and Psychiat. *29:*1203-1221, June '33

Changes in cutaneous localization in pedicle flap. Douglas, B. and Lanier, L. H. Arch. Neurol. and Psychiat. *32:*756-762, Oct '34

General sensations in pedunculated skin flaps. Davis, J. S. and Kitlowski, E. A. Arch. Surg. *29:*982-1000, Dec '34

Skin Flaps to Nose

Restoration of nose by transplantation of skin from forehead in year 1881. Teale, T. P., Brit. J. Surg. *9:*449, Jan '22 (illus.)

Rhinoplasty with flap from patient's chest. Steinthal, K. Zentralbl. f. Chir. *50:*508-509, March 31, '23 (illus.)

Idiopathic perforation of nasal septum; autoplasty with pedunculated flap of mucous membrane; cure. Roy, J. N. Ann. Otol., Rhin. and Laryng. *32:*554-560, June '23

Rhinoplasty by rotation of flaps from cheek. d'Agata, G. Policlinico (sez. prat.) *34:*168, Jan 31, '26

Enfolding flap in correction of nasal deformities. Réthi, A. Acta oto-laryng. *11:*443-452, '27

Closure of large nasal breach by grafts of frontal and cervicothoracic flaps placed side by side; case. Dupuy-Dutemps, L. and Bourguet. Bull. Soc. d'opht. de Paris, pp. 435-442, Oct '30

Formation of end, ala and cutaneous partition of nose by transplanting auricle on round stem. Limberg, A. A. Vestnik khir. (no. 55) *20:*151-159, '30

Use of tubular stem in transplantation from ear to defect of ala. Vetchtomoff, A. A. Vestnik khir. (no. 55) *20:*143-150, '30

Use of pedicled flaps in reconstruction of nose. New, G. B. and Figi, F. A. Surg., Gynec. and Obst. *53:*780-787, Dec '31

Surgical correction of syphilitic saddle nose by Joseph operation and Filatov graft; case. Rebelo Neto, J. Bol. Soc. de med. e cir. de Sao Paulo *16:*123-130, Dec '32

Technic of rhinoplasty by tubular grafts. Claoue, C., J. de med. de Bordeaux *113:*633-635, Sept 10-30, '36

Partial rhinoplasty using tissue from auricle on round Filatov pedicle. Khrizman, I. A. Sovet. Khir., no. 6, pp. 975-980, '36

Rhinoplasty using cutaneous flap from abdomen via forearm. Claoue. Bull. et mem. Soc. de med. de Paris *141:*278-280, April 24, '37

Rhinoplasty by frontal flap; case. Peri. Rev. de chir. structive *8:*216-217, '38

Partial nasal defects; new modification of

Skin Flaps to Nose – Cont.

"French" method of restoration with sliding flaps of adjoining tissue. TWYMAN, E. D., West. J. Surg. *48:*106–109, Feb '40

Reconstruction of nasal tip and subseptum by means of tubular graft. ZENO, L. An. de cir. *7:*183–190, Sept '41

Reconstruction of nasal tip and subseptum by means of tubular graft; case. ZENO, L. Bol. y trab., Acad. argent. de cir. *25:*1028–1033, Sept 10, '41

Reconstruction of nasal septum by tubular skin graft; cases. ZENO, L. AND RECALDE, J. F. Arq. de cir. clin. e exper. *6:*185–194, April–June '42

Uses of transplanted pedicle flaps for restoration or correction of nose. BLAIR, V. P. Tr. Am. Soc. Plastic and Reconstructive Surg. *12:*23–24, '43

Technic of total rhinoplasty by method of double frontal flap. VIRENQUE, M. Ann. d'oto-laryng., pp. 45–47, April–June '44

"Hits, strikes and outs" in use of pedicle flaps for restoration or correction of nose. BLAIR, V. P. AND BYARS, L. T. Surg., Gynec. and Obst. *82:*367–385, April '46

Repair of nasal defects with median forehead flap; primary closure of forehead wound. KAZANJIAN, V. H. Surg., Gynec. and Obst. *83:*37–49, July '46

Skin Flaps to Palate

Use of delayed flap in secondary operations on palate and antrum. NEW, G. B. Minnesota Med. *6:*214–220, April '23 (illus.)

Pedicled grafts in therapy of defects of hard palate. PUTSCHKOWSKY, A. Ztschr. f. Laryng., Rhin., Otol. *22:*98–102, '31

Plastic closure of palate defects by means of tube-pedicle flap. SMYRNOFF, S. A. Am. Med. *39:*115, March '33

Closure of defect in hard palate by pedicled tube graft. BURNELL, G. H., M. J. Australia *2:*484, Oct 7, '33

Plastic closure of defective hard palate by means of round pedicled flap (Filatov). FRANKENBERG, B. E. Sovet. khir. *4:*591–595, '33

Palatoplasty using extra-oral tissues. DAVIS, A. D. Ann. Surg. *99:*94–100, Jan '34

Two cases illustrating elastic traction in plastic surgery; pedicle flap to close large opening in hard palate. MOOREHEAD, F. B., S. Clin. North America *14:*745–749, Aug '34

Skin Flaps to Scalp

Complete avulsion of scalp and loss of right ear; reconstruction by pedunculated tube grafts and costal cartilage. CAHILL, J. A. JR. AND CAULFIELD, P. A. Surg., Gynec. and Obst. *66:*459–465, Feb (no. 2A) '38

Alopecia prematura and its surgical treatment (flap-method of plastic surgery). TAUBER, H., J. Ceylon Br., Brit. M. A. *36:*237–242, July '39

Use of flaps from avulsed scalp and skin grafts in repair of total avulsion. ECKHARDT, G. Zentralbl. f. Chir. *66:*2337–2340, Oct 28, '39

Hair-bearing scalp flap for repair of unilateral scalp defects. NEW, G. B. AND ERICH, J. B., S. Clin. North America *24:*741–750, Aug '44

Plastic closure of defect of cranium; case report illustrating use of tantalum plate and pedicle-tube graft. HARRIS, M. H. AND WOODHALL, B. Surgery *17:*422–428, March '45

Skin Flaps from Scrotum

Unsuccessful attempt at plastic surgery of pedunculated scrotal flap. KOCH, K. Zentralbl. f. Chir. *55:*587–590, March 10, '28

Biologic scrotal flaps – new approach. ESSER, J. F. S., J. Internat. Coll. Surgeons *5:*168–170, March-April '42

Skin Flaps, Tubed

Plastic surgery, tube skin-flap in plastic surgery of face. PICKERILL, H. P. AND WHITE, J. R. Brit. J. Surg. *9:*321–333, Jan '22 (illus.)

Laryngectomy for cancer of larynx with modified technique and attempted formation of skin tube in place of larynx. GOLDTHWAITE, R. H. Laryngoscope *32:*446–450, June '22

Rhinoplasty and cheek, chin, and lip plastics with tubed, temporal-pedicled, forehead flaps. MCWILLIAMS, C. A. AND DUNNING, H. S. Surg., Gynec. and Obst. *36:*1–10, Jan '23 (illus.)

Combined satchel handle or tubed pedicle and large delayed whole skin pedicle flaps in case of plastic surgery of face, neck and chest. ALDEN, B. F. Surg., Gynec. and Obst. *41:*493–496, Oct '25

Plastic with round pedicle. DIBAN, P. AND DIENERMANN, J. Deutsche Ztschr. f. Chir. *191:*164–169, '25

Plastic surgery with tissue pedicles (Filatov's method). BAKKAL, T. S. Vestnik Khir. (no. 25) *9:*144–146, '27

Round movable pedicles in complicated plastic operations on eyelids and face. FILA-

Skin Flaps, Tubed – Cont.
TOV, W. P. Arch. f. klin. Chir. 146:609–614, '27
Use of tubular skin grafts. IVANISSEVICH, O. Bol. y trab. de la Soc. de cir. de Buenos Aires *13:*144–145, May 22, '29
Tubular skin transplants. BURIAN, F. Casop. lek. cesk. *70:*741–743, May 22, '31
Tubed pedicle flap in reconstructive surgery; cases. PIERCE, G. W. AND O'CONNOR, G. B. California and West. Med. *35:*94–97, Aug '31
Result of transplantations of blood vessels in Filatov cutaneous pedicle; experiments. BELOSOR, I. Arch. f. klin. Chir. *168:*199–208, '31
Plastic repair of tip of nose, alae and septum with T-shaped round skin flap (Limberg method); case. FALTIN, R. Acta chir. Scandinav. *68:*254–265, '31
Transplantation of large pieces of skin with aid of Filatov cutaneous pedicle. PARIN, B. Arch. f. klin. Chir. *168:*191–198, '31
Technic of Filatov's tubular pedicle. PARIN, B. Sovet. khir. *1:*141–144, '31
Method of shortening healing process in Filatov graft. PARIN, B. V. Vestnik khir. (no. 67) *23:* 90–95, '31
Filatov grafts in large ulcers due to X-ray burns. SOKOLOFF, A. P. Vestnik khir. (nos. 70–71) *24:*237–241, '31
Rare complications in osteomyelitis of lower jaw; Filatov's grafts in defects of oral cavity. STEPANOFF, N. M. Vestnik khir. (nos. 70–71) *24:*233–236, '31
Lesions of jaw, nose and cheek; cleft lip and palate; cartilage transplant; tube graft. MOOREHEAD, F. B., S. Clin. North America *12:*57–66, Feb '32
Actinodermatitis (roentgen-ray burn) of entire neck; replacement with tubed flap from thorax. FIGI, F. A., S. Clin. North America *12:*947–949, Aug '32
Establishment of circulation in tubed skin flaps; experimental study. GERMAN, W. Arch. Surg. *26:*27–40, Jan '33
Arm-chest adhesions and their plastic reconstruction by tube flap method. KULOWSKI, J. Ann. Surg. *97:*683–692, May '33
Chondrosarcoma of ethmoid; surgical therapy, radiotherapy and autoplasty with tubular flap. LARROUDÉ, C. Rev. de chir. plastique, pp. 239–245, Oct '33
Tubed pedicle flap for scar contracture. NASSAU, C. F., S. Clin. North America *14:*13–18, Feb '34
Failures and hazards of Filatov's circular pedicled flap. LINDENBAUM, I. Beitr. z. klin. Chir. *160:*359–368, '34

Skin Flaps, Tubed – Cont.
Closure of esophageal defect after laryngectomy with help of movable flap (Filatov operation). SOLOWJEW, L. M. Acta oto-laryng. *21:*219–221, '34
Experiences with tubed pedicle flaps. GILLIES, H. Surg., Gynec. and Obst. *60:*291–303, Feb (no. 2A) '35
Use of movable tubular skin graft; 2 cases. CORACHÁN, M. Rev. de cir. de Barcelona *10:*36–41, July-Aug '35
Errors and dangers of graft with round pedicle flap according to Filatov method. LINDENBAUM, I. S. Sovet. khir., no. 3, pp. 126–131, '35
Transplantation of large pieces of skin by Filatov-Parin method. VILESOV, S. P. Sovet. khir., no. 3, pp. 132–134, '35
Method of tubed flap formation. DAVIS, J. S. AND KITLOWSKI, E. A. South. M. J. *29:*1169–1174, Dec '36
Plastic reconstruction of skin of scrotum by Filatov grafts. FROLOV, V. I. Vestnik khir. *46:*251–252, '36
Thoraco-epigastric tubed pedicles. WEBSTER, J. P., S. Clin. North America *17:*145–184, Feb '37
Tubular graft in autoplastic therapy of burn cicatrix; case. TECQMENNE, C. Liege med. *30:*818–820, July 11, '37
Viability of tube pedicle graft. SPARROW, T. D. Am. J. Surg. *41:*92–95, July '38
Tube-pedicle skin graft's usefulness to general surgeon. (concerning cicatrix). SPARROW, T. D. South. Med. and Surg. *100:*514–523, Nov '38
New technical procedure for preparation of tubular cutaneous graft for plastic surgery; experimental study. CAMINITI MANGANARO, E. Rinasc. med. *16:*11–12, Jan 15, '39
Practical uses of tubed pedicle flap. GILLIES, H. Am. J. Surg. *43:*201–215, Feb '39
Gillies-Filatov tubal graft used to replace loss of substance of thigh; case. COVARRUBIAS ZENTENO, R. Rev. med. de Chile *67:*903–907, Aug '39
Transplantation of conserved skin according to Filatov method in therapy of chronic crural ulcers; preliminary report. BROVER, B. I. Vrach. delo *21:*105–110, '39
Dermo-epidermal grafts and pedicled tubular grafts in surgical therapy of osteomyelitis. INGIANNI, G. Arch. ed atti d. Soc. ital. di chir. *45:*724–730, '39
Tubular graft (Gillies-Filatov Anglo-Russian graft) in repair of facial defects; cases. CODAZZI AGUIRRE, J. A. Rev. med. de Rosario *30:*208–218, Feb '40
Esthetic results of grafts of Anglo-Russian

Skin Flaps, Tubed – Cont.
type in facial burn; case. CODAZZI AGUIRRE, J. A. Semana med. *1:*651-655, March 14, '40
Tubular flaps transferred by dermal inclusion (leech method). CLAOUE. Monde med., Paris *50:*149-152, May '40
Use of tubed pedicle flaps for study of wound healing in human skin. SUTTON, L. E. New York State J. Med. *40:*852-859, June 1, '40
New method of tube pedicle grafting. MALTZ, M., J. Internat. Coll. Surgeons *3:*526-531, Dec '40
Tubular skin flaps. CACCIALANZA, P. Boll. Soc. med.-chir. Modena *42:*455-460, '41-'42
Tubular grafts. CACCIALANZA, P. Boll. Soc. ital. biol. sper. *17:*94, Feb '42
Axillary-iliac tubed flap in neck surgery. HAVENS, F. Z. AND DIX, C. R. Proc. Staff Meet., Mayo Clin. *17:*167-169, March 18, '42
Tubular graft in therapy of ulcers of legs. DUARTE CARDOSO, A. Arq. de cir. clin. e exper. *6:*251-260, April-June '42
Tubed pedicle graft. RECALDE, J. F. JR. Rev. med. d. Paraguay *5:*24-28, April-June '42
Skin transplantation with tubular flap. ROSSELLI, D. Pathologica *34:*209-225, July '42
Fluorescein test in management of tubed (pedicle) flaps. DINGWALL, J. A. III AND LORD, J. W. JR. Bull. Johns Hopkins Hosp. *73:*129-131, Aug '43
Recovery of function with autoplastic bone graft and tubular skin flaps. JENTZER, A. Schweiz. med. Wchnschr. *73:*1023, Aug 21, '43
Tubed pedicle graft in therapy of burn cicatrix; resulting keloids. PEDEMONTE, P. V. Bol. Soc. cir. d. Uruguay *14:*106-108, '43 also: Arch. urug. de med., cir. y especialid. *23:*296-298, Sept '43
New design for raising tubed pedicle flap. GABARRO, P. Surgery *18:*732-741, Dec '45
Use of tubular flap in amputations of extremities. KUKIN, N. I. Khirurgiya No. 6, pp. 83-86, '45
Tubular graft in laryngotracheal fistula. VIANA ROSA, A. Rev. med. Rio Grande do Sul *2:*167-172, Jan-Feb '46
Reflex vasodilatation in tubed pedicle grafts. GORDON, S. AND WARREN, R. F. Ann. Surg. *123:*436-446, March '46
Tubular grafts in plastic repair. SUSONI, A. H. Bol. y trab., Soc. argent. de cirujanos *7:*368-379, '46 also: Rev. Asoc. med. argent. *60:*601-605, July 15, '46
One stage tubed abdominal flaps; single pedicle tubes. SHAW, D. T. AND PAYNE, R. L., JR. Surg. Gynec. and Obst. *83:*205-209, Aug '46

Skin Flaps, Visor
Visor scalp flap reconstruction of face. PERTHES, G. Arch. f. klin. Chir. *127:*165-177, '23 (illus.) abstr: J.A.M.A. *81:*2155, Dec 22, '23
Case of extensive plastic repair of face and neck with "visor flap." GOLDSCHMIDT, T. Zentralbl. f. Chir. *52:*688-691, March 28, '25
Use of visor flaps from chest in plastic operations upon neck, chin and lip. FREEMAN, L. Ann. Surg. *87:*364-368, March '28

Skin Grafts
Hypertrophic capillary angioma of cheek; removal; plastic replacement of skin, case. WEICHERT, M. Beitr. z. klin. Chir. *145:*718-720, '20
Skin grafts. BRAUN, W. Med. Klin. *17:*398, April 3, '21
Braun's skin grafts. DE SANSON, R. D. Brazil-med. *35:*299, June 11, '21 abstr: J.A.M.A. *77:*977, Sept 17, '21
Method of skin-grafting. SAMUEL, S. Brit. M. J. *2:*632, Oct 22, '21
Method of skin grafting. NEVE, E. F. Brit. M. J. *2:*987, Dec 10, '21
Preparing a wound for skin grafting. KILGORE, A. R., S. Clin. N. America *2:*521-524, April '22
An improved method of skin grafting. PARCE, A. D. Ann. Surg. *75:*658-662, June '22 (illus.)
Bloodless transplantation of skin. WOLF, W. Munchen. med. Wchnschr. *69:*1217, Aug 18, '22
Braun's skin grafting. WILDEGANS, Arch. f. klin. Chir. *120:*415-440, '22 (illus.) abstr: J.A.M.A. *79:*1887, Nov 25, '22
Skin grafting by exact pattern, a report of cosmetic results obtained without employment of sutures. DOUGLAS, B. Ann. Surg. *77:*223-227, Feb '23 (illus.)
Epithelization of skin grafts with roentgen rays. HABERLAND, H. F. O. Klin. Wchnschr. *2:*353-354, Feb 19, '23
Preliminary serum treatment before skin grafting. LAQUA, K. Klin. Wchnschr. *2:*1360-1362, July 16, '23 abstr: J.A.M.A. *81:*1478, Oct 27, '23
Subcutaneous skin transplants. RUEF, H. Arch. f. klin. Chir. *125:*366-377, '23 (illus.) abstr: J.A.M.A. *81:*1322, Oct 13, '23
Principles of 4 types of skin grafting; with an improved method of treating total avulsion of scalp. MCWILLIAMS, C. A., J.A.M.A. *83:*183-189, July 19, '24
Ultimate outcome of skin grafts. BRAUN, W. Med. Klinik *20:*1383-1385, Oct 5, '24 abstr: J. A. M. A. *83:*1628, Nov 15, '24

Skin Grafts – Cont.

Transplantation of fibrous tissues in repair of anatomical defects. GALLIE, W. E. AND LE MESURIER, A. B. Brit. J. Surg. *12:*289–320, Oct '24

Epithelium pulp in epithelium grafting. HILAROWICZ, H. Zentralbl. f. Chir. *51:*2192–2193, Oct 4, '24

Skin grafting in general practice. BERTWISTLE, A. P. Practitioner *113:*440–441, Dec '24

Plea for skin-grafting. WOODWARD, C. S. Texas State J. Med. *20:*445–446, Dec '24

Skin grafts. BERTOCCHI, A. Arch. ital. di chir. *11:*445–482, '25 abstr: J.A.M.A. *85:*1096, Oct 3, '25

Growth energy of implanted epithelium. KURTZAHN, H. Arch. f. klin. Chir. *138:*534–551, '25

Rope (skin) grafts. LAHEY, F. H. Boston M. and S. J. *194:*1–5, Jan 7, '26

Skin transplantation. VON WEDEL, C., J. Oklahoma M. A. *19:*7–11, Jan '26

Rational management of skin grafts. SMITH, F. Surg., Gynec. and Obst. *42:*556–562, April '26

Skin grafts and conditions which favor their vitality and attachment; experimental research. CECCARELLI, G. Arch. ital. di chir. *15:*353–412, '26 abstr: J.A.M.A. *87:*284, July 24, '26

Action of periarterial sympathectomy on skin grafts. DALGER, J. Lyon chir. *23:*451–452, July–Aug '26

Skin grafts; effect of emulsion of pyogenic bacteria. TINOZZI, F. P. Ann. ital. di chir. *5:*981–1000, Oct 30, '26

Skin grafting of extensive areas. VENABLE, C. S. Texas State J. Med. *22:*381–382, Oct '26

Braun's skin grafting after amputations. LIHOTZKY, Med. Klin. *22:*1757–1758, Nov 12, '26

Skin grafts; effect of cervical sympathectomy; experiments. TINOZZI, F. P. Rassegna internaz. di clin. e terap. *7:*585–604, Nov 10, '26

Relative reaction within mammalian tissues; factors determining reaction of skin grafts; study by indicator method of conditions within ischemic tissue. ROUS, P., J. Exper. Med. *44:*815–834, Dec '26

Surgical grafts. MAUCLAIRE. Rev. med. franc. *8:*9–30, Jan '27

Transplantation of skin. DAVIS, J. S. Surg., Gynec. and Obst. *44:*181–189, Feb '27

Periarterial decortication as aid to skin grafting. BERTOCCHI, A. Gior. d. r. Accad. di med. di Torino *33:*129–134, March '27

"Godets" method of dermo-epidermic graft. COULLAUD. Bull. et mem. Soc. nat. de chir.

Skin Grafts – Cont.

*53:*389–405, March 19, '27

Dermo-epidermic grafts. ALGLAVE, P., J. de chir. *29:*659–667, June '27

Cutaneous plastics; their scientific basis. URKOV, J. Illinois M. J. *51:*469–471, June '27

Experimental skin grafting. NAVA, V. Boll. d. Soc. ital. di biol. sper. *2:*858–860, July '27

Three cases of skin grafting. BROWN, C. P. Surg. J. *34:*20, Sept–Oct '27

Influence of insufficient nutrition on taking of skin grafts. MORPURGO, B. AND MILONE, S. Arch. per le sc. med. *49:*648–664, Nov '27

New method of covering denuded areas with surrounding skin. HIGHSMITH, E. D. Surg., Gynec. and Obst. *45:*823–824, Dec '27

Grafting of fixed skin. NAVA, V. Boll. d. Soc. med. chir. di Pavia *2:*369–372, '27

Grafting or transplantation of tissues. PERRONCITO, A. Tratt. di anat. patol. no. 5, pp. 79–155, '27

Regeneration and grafts. PERRONCITO, A. Tratt. di anat. patol., no. 5, pp. 3–148, '27

Repair of nerves and tendons of hand, and grafting. BUNNELL, S., J. Bone and Joint Surg. *10:*1–26, Jan '28 abstr: Arch. franco-belges de chir. *30:*93–97, Feb '27

Lack of taking of autoplastic skin-grafts. PAOLUCCI, F. Ann. ital. di chir. *7:*41–64, Jan '28

Skin grafts in herpes recurrens. NICOLAU, S. AND POINCLOUX, P. Compt. rend. Soc. de biol. *98:*360–363, Feb 10, '28

Case of skin grafting. MAXEINER, S. R. Minnesota Med. *11:*185, March '28

Dermatologist's interest in reconstructive surgery – skin grafting. SHEEHAN, J. E., M. J. and Rec. *127:*326, March 21, '28

Skin grafting method favoring epidermic and dermo-epidermic growth. PAGANI, M. Boll. d'ocul. *7:*442–444, May '28

Technic for ideal skin-graft, with report of extensive lymphangioma pigmentosa verrucosa. EMERSON, C. Nebraska M. J. *13:*214–216, June '28

General principles of plastic surgery; cutaneous graft, sutures; cases. LEWIS, D. Bull. et mem. Soc. de chir. de Paris *20:*476–487, June 1, '28

"Transport" plastic operations of face. MATTI, H. Schweiz. med. Wchnschr. *58:*669–673, July 7, '28

Skin grafting upon dry bone. BABCOCK, W. W., S. Clin. N. Amer. *8:*773–775, Aug '28

Successful use of disinfecting agents in skin grafts. KAMEYA, K. Zentralbl. f. Chir. *55:*2316–2317, Sept 15, '28

Regeneration and transplantation of tissue. SCHAXEL, J. Zool. Anz. *78:*153–157, Sept 1,

Skin Grafts – Cont.
'28
Anaplasty of skin; case. DORE, R. Union med. du Canada *57:*710–713, Dec '28
Types of skin grafts and indications. MECHTENBERG, W. R. Nebraska M. J. *13:*454–457, Dec '28
Various uses of transplanted twisted skin in surgery. BOGOLJUBOFF, W. L. Arch. f. klin. Chir. *149:*412–414, '28
Effect of thyroid injection and skin grafts in sensitized animals. CARMONA, L. Arch. ital. di chir. *21:*436–456, '28
Life and growth processes in explanted normal and malignant human tissue. HEIM, K. Arch. f. Gynak. *134:*250–309, '28
Effect of periarterial sympathectomy on growth of autoplastic skin grafts; experiments. MAGLIULO, A. Sperimentale, Arch. di biol. *82:*685–705, '28
Use and uses of large split-skin grafts of intermediate thickness. BLAIR, V. P., AND BROWN, J. B. Tr. South. S. A. *41:*409–424, '28 Also: Surg., Gynec., and Obst. *49:*82–97, July '29
Free transplants of skin in plastic surgery of face. and neck. SANVENERO-ROSSELLI, G. Arch. ital. di chir. *21:*245–265, '28
Contracture due to burns; treatment with free full thickness grafts and pedunculated flaps. KOCH, S. L. AND KANAVEL, A. B. J.A.M.A. *92:*277–281, Jan 26, '29
Skin grafts derived from scrotum. CANAVERO, G. Policlinico (sez. chir.) *36:*61–69, Feb '29
Skin grafts. CHANG CHI. Nat. M. J., China *15:*20–27, Feb '29
Skin grafts. HULLSIEK, H. E. Am. Mercury *17:*456–459, Aug '29
Free and pediculated skin grafts. POGGI, J. Folha med. *10:*403–406, Nov 25, '29
Use of pieces of skin in deep plastic operations. LOEWE, O. Munchen. med. Wchnschr. *76:*2125–2128, Dec 20, '29
Treatment of electric burns by immediate resection and skin graft. WELLS, D. B. Ann. Surg. *90:*1069–1078, Dec '29
Clinical experiences with Braun's epidermal grafts. MANNHEIM, H. Arch. f. Klin. Chir. *154:*98–113, '29
Biology of skin transplants. MELCHIOR, E. Beitr. z. klin. Chir. *147:*45–52, '29
Treatment of electric burns by immediate resection and skin graft. WELLS, D. B. Proc. Connecticut M. Soc. *137:*138–147, '29
Technique and Results of Grafting Skin, by H. KENRICK CHRISTIE. H. K. Lewis and Co., London, '30
Transplantation of skin, fat, blood vessels,

Skin Grafts – Cont.
nerves, etc. EISELSBERG, A. Wien. med. Wchnschr. *80:*50–55, Jan 4, '30
Part played by transplanted skin in regeneration. TAUBE, E. Arch. f. Entwckngsmechn. d. Organ. *121:*204–209, Jan 6, '30
Use of ultraviolet light in preparation of infected granulation tissue for grafting; value of very thick Thiersch grafts. GATCH, W. D. AND TRUSLER, H. M. Surg., Gynec. and Obst. *50:*478–482, Feb '30
Skin grafts; uses of various types. KIRKHAM, H. L. D., M. Rec. and Ann. *24:*554, May '30
Skin grafts, use in plastic surgery. MASSIE, F. M. Kentucky M. J. *28:*238–246, May '30
Ten years of tunnel graft of skin. KELLER, W. L. Ann. Surg. *91:*924–936, June '30
Influence of ablation of sympathetic ganglions on evolution of different forms of skin grafts; experimental study. DOBRZANIECKI, W. Lyon chir. *27:*537–578, Sept-Oct '30
Buried skin grafts of burned children; new use of old method of grafting. HENSON, E. B. West Virginia M. J. *26:*557–559, Sept '30
Problem of skin grafting, with description of newer technique. UPDEGRAFF, H. L. California and West. Med. *33:*679–681, Sept '30
Transplantation of epithelium by Braun method. DE WAARD, Geneesk. tijdschr. v. Nederl. Indie *70:*1050, Oct 1, '30
Technic for epithelisation with grafts in cases of skin defects. LANG, M. Dermat. Wchnschr. *91:*1478–1483, Oct 4, '30
Use of Thiersch skin flaps in treatment of recent wounds of arms. FLICK, K. Deutsche Ztschr. f. Chir. *222:*331–334, '30
Plastic surgery by Rehn's method of shifting soft parts to cover defect of face. FOHL, T. AND KILLIAN, H. Deutsche Ztschr. f. Chir. *222:*309–320, '30
Skin grafting in reparative surgery. SHEEHAN, J. E. Actas y trab. del primer Cong. de la Asoc. med. Panamericana, pp. 527–535, '30
Immediate skin graft contraction and its cause. DAVIS, J. S. AND KITLOWSKI, E. A. Arch. Surg. *23:*954–965, Dec '31
Comparative value of surgical procedures in repair of skin defects (including grafts). MALINIAK, J. W., M. J. and Rec. *133:*82–84, Jan 21, '31
Physiology and technic of free skin transplant. BURIAN, F. Casop. lek. cesk. *70:*667, May 8; 714, May 15, '31
Braun method of skin grafting; 2 cases. KROEFF, M. Folha med. *12:*145–148, May 5, '31

Skin Grafts—Cont.
Colpopoiesis by means of transplantation according to Thiersch method. OSTRČIL, A. Zentralbl. f. Gynak. *55:*1900–1901, June 13, '31
Use of tannic acid dressing for Ollier-Thiersch graft beds. MADDOCK, W. G., J.A.M.A. *97:*102, July 11, '31
Treatment of extensive granulating areas, with special reference to use of physical therapy measures in burns and skin grafts. POTTER, E. B. AND PECK, W. S. Am. J. Surg. *14:*472–476, Nov '31
Factors of resistance and receptivity in skin transplanted in epitheliomatous regions. PERAZZO, G. Arch. ital. di dermat., sif. *7:*573–584, Dec '31
Skin grafting with reference to extensive burns. SUTTON, H. T. Ohio State M. J. *27:*943–949, Dec '31
New method of skin grafting, "à godet." CAFORIO, L. Rinasc. med. *9:*84–86, Feb 15, '32
Grafts and implantations of tissue and organs in man and in animals. MAUCLAIRE, P. Medecine (supp.) *13:*1–67, Feb '32
Free skin grafts. DANTRELLE. Rev. de chir. plastique, pp. 3–15, April '32
Forceps for skin grafts. WRIGHT, A. D. Lancet *1:*840, April 16, '32
Treatment of ulcers with skin grafts. ANDERSON, T. F. AND ROBERTS, M. A. W. East African M. J. *9:*79–83, June '32
Plant and animal grafts. RETTERER, E. Progres med., pp. 1041–1050, June 11, '32
Plastic surgery in therapy of trichiasis and free skin graft for hemangioma. DESELAERS, H. Rev. espan. de med. y cir. *15:*353–355, July '32
Transplantation of active epithelium. KOHN, K. W. Zentralbl. f. Chir. *59:*1748–1750, July 16, '32
Forceps for skin grafts. WRIGHT, A. D. Indian M. Gaz. *67:* 479–480, Aug '32
Thiocresol in wound healing and in skin grafting. BIRNBAUM, I. R. Ann. Surg. *96:*467–470, Sept '32
Comment on article by Kohn on skin grafting. NEUHÄUSER, H. Zentralbl. f. Chir. *59:*2532, Oct 15, '32
Plastic surgery (skin grafts). VON WEDEL, C. Southwestern Med. *16:*409–411, Oct '32
Tropical ulcers; quick and successful method of treatment by excision and skin graft. JAMES, C. Lancet *2:*1095–1101, Nov 19, '32
Surgical grafts. BLANC Y FORTACÍN, J. Rev. ibero-am. de cien. med. *7:*193–204, Dec '32 also: Siglo med. *90:*641–645, Dec 17, '32
New method of skin grafting. RUSSELL, C. V. J. Michigan M. Soc. *31:*804, Dec '32

Skin Grafts—Cont.
Skin grafts for great loss of skin. BORDEIANU, I. Bucuresti med. *4:*1–2, '32
Technic of autoplastic grafts. PALMÉN, A. J. Duodecim *48:*36–39, '32
Clinical aspects of plastic use of skin, especially for repair of postoperative hernia. POLANO, H. Beitr. z. klin. Chir. *154:*551–562, '32
Effect of periarterial sympathectomy on autoplastic grafts (including bone); experimental study. SANTI, E. Arch. ital. di chir. *31:*209–227, '32
Elephantiasis of plastic skin graft on thumb. WICHMANN, F. W. Arch. f. klin. Chir. *169:*783–788, '32
Autoplasties (grafts). HAMANT, A., *et al.* Bull. Soc. franc. de dermat. et syph. (Reunion dermat.) *40:*28–30, Jan '33
Treatment of old unhealed *burns (grafts).* DAVIS, J. S. AND KITLOWSKI, E. A. Ann. Surg. *97:*648–669, May '33
Recovery of sensation of denervated pedicle and free skin grafts. KREDEL, F. E. AND EVANS, J. P. Arch. Neurol. and Psychiat. *29:*1203–1221, June '33
Experiments with skin grafts in plastic surgery of tendons. BONACCORSI, A. Clin. chir. *36:*839–853, July-Aug '33
Basal skin grafts. CORACHAN, M. Bull. et mem. Soc. nat. de chir. *59:*1185–1192, July 22, '33
Autoplastic skin grafts in man; histologic study. IMPERATI, L. Riforma med. *49:*1133–1134, July 29, '33
Question of fixed grafts in relation to probable regenerative processes of host. IMPERATI, L. Ann. ital. di chir. *12:*903–914, July 31, '33
Surgical importance of skin grafts. MARTÍNEZ, E. Rev. med. peruana *5:*964–968, July '33
Multiple cutaneous horns; removal and skin graft. FIGI, F. A., S. Clin. North America *13:*880–881, Aug '33
Adherent scars; their treatment (with skin grafts). KISKADDEN, U. S., California and West. Med. *39:*109–113, Aug '33
Corachan method of making basal skin grafts for rapid epidermization. VAN GRAEFSCHEPE, C., J. de chir. et ann. Soc. belge de chir. *32-30:*353–355, Dec '33
Plastic surgery (grafts) in pathology and in clinical conditions. BERDICHEVSKIY, G. A. Novy khir. arkhiv *28:*79–87, '33
Skin grafts. ZAMKOV, A. A. Sovet. khir. *4:*51–57, '33
Dermo-epidermal grafts; history, technic and indications. VERRIÈRE, AND BARNEVILLE.

Skin Grafts – Cont.
Arch. de med. et pharm. mil. *100:*173–192, Feb '34
Plastic repair of face by means of skin transplantation; case. BARROS LIMA. Arq. de cir. e ortop. *1:*386–394, June '34
Skin grafts in correction of deforming scars. WEICHHERZ, I. Budapesti orvosi ujsag *32:*796–798, Aug 30, '34
Plastic surgery of soft parts of chin, with report of case treated by scalp graft. FINOCHIETTO, R. AND MARINO, H. Prensa med. argent. *21:*1672–1685, Sept 5, '34
Indications, limitations and uses of various types of skin grafts. OWENS, N. New Orleans M, and S. J. *87:*158–165, Sept '34
Skin grafts. BURTON, J. F., J. Oklahoma M. A. *27:*363–367, Oct '34
Grafts and transplants. BEEKMAN, F. Am. J. Surg. *26:*528–532, Dec '34
Skin-grafting of arm wound; successful outcome despite unusual difficulties. SALVIN, A. A. Am. J. Surg. *26:*572–574, Dec '34
Autoplastic osseous and cutaneous grafts in destruction of lower jaw. DUFOURMENTEL. Bull. et mem. Soc. d chirurgiens de Paris *27:*82–85, Feb 1, '35
Treatment (with skin grafts) of deformities from burns. MILLER, O. L. AND ROBERTS, W. M. South. Surgeon *4:*52–62, March '35
Fundamental principles of plastic surgery (face) including grafts. FORD, J. F. Texas State J. Med. *30:*761–763, April '35
New principle for skin grafting. GOLYANITSKIY, I. A. Sovet. vrach. gaz., pp. 588–590, April 15, '35
Free transplantation of skin. POTTER, E. B. Univ. Hosp. Bull., Ann Arbor *1:*5–6, April '35
Denudation of scrotum and its plastic repair by skin graft. SASAKI, S. Taiwan Igakkai Zasshi *34:*455, April '35
Surgical restoration by means of grafts in severe burns of face with cicatrix. SANVENERO-ROSSELLI, G. Bull. et mem. Soc. d. chirurgiens de Paris *27:*391–403, July 5, '35
Skin grafting in relation to general surgery. OWENS, N., J. M. A. Alabama *5:*41–46, Aug '35
Skin grafts. PEER, L. A., J. M. Soc. New Jersey *32:*484–487, Aug '35
Immediate transplantation of bone, cartilage and soft tissues in accident cases. CARTER, W. W. Laryngoscope *45:*730–738, Sept '35
Technic for covering defects after extirpation of malignant melanoma of skin (grafts). ORBACH, E. Wien. med. Wchnschr. *85:*1112–1113, Oct 5, '35
Skin grafts. GRINDA, M. Presse med.

Skin Grafts. – Cont.
*43:*2053–2055, Dec 18, '35
Free transplantation of skin; evaluation of methods. POTTER, E. B. Surg., Gynec. and Obst. *61:*713–720, Dec '35
Value of primary skin grafts in fresh cutaneous wounds. BRZHOZOVSKIY, A. A. Sovet. khir., no. 7, pp. 72–73, '35
Behavior of lymphatic vessels in autoplastic skin grafts. CAVALLI, M. Sperimentale, Arch. di biol. *89:*504–508, '35
Skin grafts in cutaneous wounds. VAYNSHTEYN, V. G. Sovet. khir., no. 9, pp. 62–65, '35
Burn therapy (skin grafts). RITTER, H. H. Am. J. Surg. *31:*48–55, Jan '36
Method of dealing with chronic osteomyelitis by saucerization followed by skin grafting. ARMSTRONG, B. AND JARMAN, T. F., J. Bone and Joint Surg. *18:*387–396, April '36
Plastic surgery of elbow after transplantation of skin in ankylosis with cicatricial contracture; case. VON SEEMEN, H. Zentralbl. f. Chir. *63:*946–950, April 18, '36
Free skin grafts. DUFOURMENTEL, L. Oto-rhino-laryng. internat. *20:*354–355, June '36
Study of favorable conditions for cicatrix formation; practical application in skin grafting. DUFOURMENTEL, L. Bull. et mem. Soc. d. chirurgiens de Paris *28:*401–423, June 19, '36
Importance of prickle cell layer in skin grafting. GRACE, E. J. Am. J. Surg. *32:*498, June '36
Branchioma of right parotid in young girl; extracapsular extirpation and closure of resulting defect by Thiersch graft. GOUFAS, G. Ann. d'oto-laryng., pp. 677–685, July '36
Technical details of skin grafting. CONWAY, J. H. Surg., Gynec. and Obst. *63:*369–371, Sept '36
Dermo-epidermal grafts in delayed healing of burn wounds; 2 cases. CLEMENTE, D. Policlinico (sez. prat.) *43:*1861–1863, Oct 19, '36
Process of healing after free transplantation of skin. DUJARDIN, E. Ugesk. f. laeger *98:*1073, Oct 29, '36
The fate of free grafts. DUFOURMENTEL, L. Rev. de chir. structive, pp. 371–383, Dec '36
Repair of contractures resulting from burns (grafts). KAZANJIAN, V. H. New England J. Med. *215:*1104–1120, Dec 10, '36
Autoplastic grafts in rabbits whose skin had been frozen previously. DEL GENIO, F. Sperimentale, Arch. di biol. *90:*75–85, '36
Value of reparative surgery, inclusive of free transplantations. REHN, E. Arch. f. klin. Chir. *186:*244–266, '36

Skin Grafts – Cont.
Cutaneous and subcutaneous grafts in therapy of rectal prolapse. VOSKRESENSKIY, N. V. Sovet. khir., no. 6, pp. 1011–1014, '36
Plastic surgery for general practitioner (grafts). BARSKY, A. J. Radiol. Rev. and Mississippi Valley M. J. *59:*13–15, Jan '37
Replacement of large amounts of skin. EHALT, W. Zentralbl. f. Chir. *64:*70–73, Jan 9, '37
Presentation of cases requiring plastic repair (grafts). PEER, L. A., J. M. Soc. New Jersey *34:*15–20, Jan '37
Comparison of 2 methods of skin grafting (in ulcers). CAROTHERS, J. C. East African M. J. *13:*345, Feb '37
Applications of cavity grafting with skin. McINDOE, A. H. Surgery *1:*535–557, April '37
Perifemoral sympathectomy associated with dermoepidermal grafts in therapy of varicose ulcers; 7 cases. ARDOINO, A. Policlinico (sez. prat.) *44:*1265–1267, June 28, '37
The different application of free grafts in oto-rhino-laryngology. DUFOURMENTEL, L. Prat. med. franc. *18:*187–195, June '37
Technic of skin grafting. MAYNARD, A. DE L. Am. J. Surg. *37:*92–105, July '37
Care of severely burned, with special reference to skin grafting. PADGETT, E. C. Arch. Surg. *35:*64–86, July '37
Foreskins as skin grafts. ASHLEY, F. Ann. Surg. *106:*252–256, Aug '37
Plastic operation (skin grafting); case (tendon grafting). BLACK, J. R. AND MACEY, H. B. Proc. Staff Meet., Mayo Clin. *12:*497–500, Aug 11, '37
Total free skin grafts; indications and operative technic. GALTIER, M., J. de chir. *50:*322–335, Sept '37
Experimental studies in skin grafting. MEYER, R. Wien. klin. Wchnschr. *50:*1424–1425, Oct 15, '37
Skin graft use in reparation of tendinous lesions with loss of substance. MOSKOFF, G. J. de chir. *50:*607–620, Nov '37
Free skin grafts. CLAIRMONT, P. Rev. de chir. structive, p. 268, Dec '37
Topographic varieties of free skin grafts. DUFOURMENTEL, L. Rev. de chir. structive, pp. 259–263, Dec '37
Free skin grafts; classification. SANCHEZ-ARBIDE, A. Rev. de chir. structive, pp. 270–272, Dec '37
Skin grafts for plastic surgery of face. SANCHEZ ARBIDE, A. Semana med. *2:*1281–1286, Dec 2, '37
Skin grafts in certain cutaneous diseases and corneal transplants. FILATOV, V. P. Med. zhur. *7:*743–753, '37 also: Vestnik oftal. *11:*295–310, '37

Skin Grafts – Cont.
Grafts as method of primary therapy of wounds. GOFREN, A. G. Khirurgiya, no. 12, pp. 3–14, '37
Replacement of almost entire skin of upper extremity by skin graft; case. REYNBERG, G. A. Khirurgiya, no. 12, pp. 144–145, '37
Plastic surgery as allied with treatment of cancer (grafts). OWENS, N. New Orleans M. and S. J. *90:*417–424, Jan '38
Use of prepuce to epithelialize tract in treatment of imperforate anus. DAVISON, T. C. South. Surgeon *7:*68–70, Feb '38
Value of skin grafts in traumatic lesions. PARTRIDGE, G. T., M. Press *196:*132–135, Feb 16, '38
Skin grafts in protection of exposed area after extirpation of cancer. PRUDENTE, A. Arch. urug. de med., cir. y especialid. *12:*196–209, Feb '38
Wringer arm; report of 26 cases (with special reference to technic of razor skin graft). MACCOLLUM, D. W. New England J. Med. *218:*549–554, March 31, '38
Simple method of skin grafting. MCMAHON, J. E., J. Malaya Br., Brit. M. A. *1:*334–335, March '38
Repair of traumatic defects of skin (grafts). KALMANOVSKIY, S. M. AND ZHAK, E. Vestnik khir. *55:*375–379, April '38
Transcorium tegumental graft; value in case. MARRO, A. Chir. plast. *4:*49–59, April-June '38
Skin grafts for ambulatory patient. SMITH, F. L. Am. J. Surg. *41:*67–69, July '38
Recurrent epithelioma of arm; method of covering defect after radical excision illustrating 2 useful types of skin transplantation. GARLOCK, J. H., J. Mt. Sinai Hosp. *5:*75–78, July-Aug '38
Skin graft covering of raw surfaces. BROWN, J. B. Internat. Abstr. Surg. *67:*105–116, '38; in Surg., Gynec. and Obst. Aug '38
Extensive resection and graft in therapy of recidivating radioresistant tumors. COGNIAUX, P., J. de chir. et ann. Soc. belge de chir. *37-35:*270–275, Oct '38
Skin grafts in évidement cavity with proud flesh; case. LEMOINE, J. Ann. d'oto-laryng., pp. 1085–1088, Nov '38
Advantages of split graft following tonsillectomy. HARRIS, H. I. Ann. Otol., Rhin. and Laryng. *47:*1045–1048, Dec '38
Free graft in reparation of extensive axillary wound after burns. ALICH, S. Turk. tib cem. mec *4:*183–187, '38
Extensive cerebral changes in case of "sudden" death following plastic transfer of

Skin Grafts – Cont.
skin on neck under local anesthesia. CAMMERMEYER, J. Acta path. et microbiol. Scandinav. *15:*307-329, '38
Therapeutic transplantation of tissue. FILATOV, V. P. Acta med. URSS *1:*412-439, '38
Vrach. delo *20:*813-822, '38
Flat skin graft in restoration of extensive facial defects. NIKANOROV, A. M. Novy khir. arkhiv *40:*255-258, '38
Technical results of grafting skin into cavity of bone after surgical therapy of osteomyelitis. INGIANNI, G. Accad. med., Genova *54:*25-33, Jan '39
Skin grafts in plastic operations. UIHLEIN, A. JR. Arch. Surg. *38:*118-130, Jan '39
Skin grafts in certain cutaneous diseases. FILATOV, V. P. Gaz. clin. *37:*61-64, Feb '39
Skin grafts. MARINO, H. Dia med. *11:*143-146, Feb 20, '39
Skin grafting in severe burns. PADGETT, E. C. Am. J. Surg. *43:*626-636, Feb '39
Dermigraft. DEAN, S. R. Surg., Gynec. and Obst. *68:*930-931, May '39
Types of grafts and their individual application. GREELEY, P. W. Illinois M. J. *75:*436-441, May '39
Skin defects repaired with grafts. CONNOLLY, E. A. AND JENSEN, W. P. Nebraska M. J. *24:*253-256, July '39
Modern treatment of soft tissue injuries (skin grafts). MOWLEM, R. Clin. J. *68:*271-276, July '39
Autoplastic skin grafts for covering defects on extremities. BEREZKIN, N. F. Vestnik khir. *58:*196-204, Sept '39
Skin grafts in casualty department. MATTHEWS, D. N. Lancet *2:*597-598, Sept 9, '39
Plastic surgery and transplantations in dermatology. TAPPEINER, S. Wien. klin. Wchnschr. *52:*1140-1143, Dec 22, '39
Visor-like method of cutaneous grafts in open wounds of bones and joints. BEREZKIN, N. F. Ortop. i travmatol. (no. 2) *13:*38-41, '39
Therapeutic transplantation of tissues. FILATOV, V. P. Probl. tuberk., no. 6, pp. 8-13, '39
Fixation of movable kidney by implantation of skin. GNILORYBOV, T. E. Khirurgiya, no. 11, pp. 114-116, '39
Modified Alglav method of skin grafting. KRIKENT, R. K. Khirurgiya, no. 6, pp. 58-63, '39
Skin and fascia grafting. BRENIZER, A. G. Am. J. Surg. *47:*265-279, Feb '40
Dermo-epidermoid graft in third degree burns. CANIZARES, RAUL AND CANIZARES, RAFAEL. Vida nueva *45:*113-118, Feb '40
Plastic surgery in therapy of facial scars

Skin Grafts – Cont.
(grafts). DUJARDIN, E. Ugesk. f. laeger *102:*222, Feb 29, '40
Graft in situ of skin completely avulsed (case). KEYES, E. L., J. Missouri M. A. *37:*75-76, Feb '40
Application of sollux lamp in skin grafting in plastic surgery. KOTSUBEY, L. A. Vestnik khir. *59:*637-639, June '40
Epithelization of granulating and fresh wounds with skin from blisters. JENSEN, W. Zentralbl. f. Chir. *67:*1399-1401, July 27, '40
Skin grafting and reconstructive surgery. THUSS, C. J., J. M. A. Alabama *10:*77-83, Sept '40
Skin grafting for spina bifida with meningocele or myelomeningocele. PINHEIRO CAMPOS, O., J. Internat. Coll. Surgeons *3:*438-440, Oct '40
Spontaneous and surgical covering (grafts) of raw surfaces. BROWN J. B. AND BYARS, L. T. Journal-Lancet *60:*503-512, Nov '40
Accidental skin transplantation in Tschmarke brushing therapy of severe burns. MATYAS, M. Zentralbl. f. Chir. *67:*2245-2246, Nov 30, '40
Indications, results and reasons for use of different types of skin grafts. ELLIS, S. S. AND VON WEDEL, C., J. Oklahoma M. A. *33:*8-14, Dec '40
Early skin grafts in burns. KRIKENT, R. K. Ortop. i travmatol. (no. 2) *14:*26-28, '40
New studies on brephroplastic grafts. MAY, R. M. Arch. d'anat. micr. *35:*147-199, '40
Choice of skin grafts in plastic surgery. GERRIE, J. W. Canad. M. A. J. *44:*9-13, Jan '41
Dermoepidermal grafts; autostabilizing retractor. MARINO, H. AND ESPERNE, P. Rev. med.-quir. de pat. fem. *17:*137-140, Feb '41
Use of skin grafts in general surgery. GONZALEZ ULLOA, M. Rev. mex. de cir., ginec. y cancer *9:*91-113, March '41
Persistence of function of skin grafts through long periods of growth. BROWN, J. B. AND McDOWELL, F. Surg., Gynec., and Obst., *72:*848, May '41. Also in J. Iowa State Med. Soc., *31:*457, Oct '41
Regeneration of epithelium in grafts. LEVANDER, G. Nord. med. (Hygiea) *10:*1489-1492, May 10, '41
Rehn method of skin grafting. VON BRANDIS, H. J. Chirurg *13:*418-425, July 15, '41
Improved method for experimental grafting. BARKER, D. E. Arch. Path. *32:*425-428, Sept '41
New skin for burns. MILLER, L. M. Hygeia *19:*884-885, Nov '41
Skin grafting in therapy of large ulcerations,

Skin Grafts – Cont.
with report of cases. SATANOWSKY, S. Semana med. *2:*1216–1223, Nov 20, '41
Preparation of superficial wounds for grafting by local use of sulfanilamide and sulfanilamide-allantoin ointment. VEAL, J. R.; *et al.* Am. J. Surg. *54:*716–720, Dec '41
Cutaneous cone (artifically produced closed necrobiotic focus) as method of nonspecific therapy replacing grafts; preliminary report. SKOSOGORENKO, G. F. Vrach. delo (no. 2) *23:*113–118, '41
Skin Grafting from a Personal and Experimental Viewpoint, by PADGETT, EARL C., C C Thomas Co., Springfield, Ill., 1942
Therapy of furunculosis by means of Thiersch graft. HOELZ, P. Arq. de cir. clin. e exper. *6:*550–558, April–June '42
Physiologic integration of skin grafts. PRUDENTE, A. AND ARIE, G. Arq. de cir. clin. e exper. *6:*577–586, April-June '42
Epithelial healing and the transplantation of skin. BROWN, J. B. AND McDOWELL, F. Ann. Surg., *115:*1166, June '42. Also in Trans. American Surgical Assn., *60:*1166, June '42. Also in Digest of Treatment, *6:*481, Jan. '43. Also in Anales de Cirugia, pp. 272, 1942.
Plastic repair with free skin grafts in burns. BROWN, J. B. AND McDOWELL, F. Clinics *1:*25–36, June '42
Immediate skin grafting in burns; preliminary report. YOUNG, F. Ann. Surg. *116:*445–451, Sept '42
Free grafts in plastic surgery. DELLEPIANE RAWSON, R. Prensa med argent. *29:*1643–1648, Oct 14, '42
Therapy of burns (coagulation therapy; saline regime; skin grafting). RANK, B. K. Australian and New Zealand J. Surg. *12:*103–110, Oct '42
Skin graft technic. POTH, E. J. Surg., Gynec. and Obst. *75:*779–784, Dec '42
Indications, technic and results of skin grafting in third degree frostbite of foot. MARZIANI, R. Boll. e mem. Soc. piemontese chir. *12:*277–279, '42
Skin Grafting of Burns, by BROWN, J. B. AND McDOWELL, F., J. B. Lippincott Co., Phila., 1943
Skin transplantation; uses in surgery. CANNADAY, J. E. Am. J. Surg. *59:*409–419, Feb '43
Dermoepidermal grafts. GARCIA CAPURRO, R. Arch. urug. de med., cir. y especialid. *22:*406–418, April '43
Skin transplantation. ORTNER, A. B. Kentucky M. J. *41:*176–178, May '43
Comparison of effects of tanning agents (especially tannic acid) and of vaseline gauze on fresh wounds of man (donor sites for skin grafts). HIRSHFELD, J. W. *et al.* Surg., Gynec. and Obst. *76:*556–561, May '43
Free grafts and pedicle flaps in treatment of recurring basal cell epitheliomas; cases. WEAVER, D. F. Laryngoscope *53:*336–342, May '43
New method of skin grafting. GABARRO, P. Brit. M. J. *1:*723–724, June 12, '43
Verrucous hairy nevus of interciliary region; extirpation and free skin graft; case with recovery. IVANISSEVICH, O. AND FERRARI, R. C. Bol. y trab., Acad. argent. de cir. *27:*422–424, June 30, '43
Skin grafting in plastic surgery. PRUDENTE, A. Rev. paulista de med. *22:*439–441, June '43
Radical operation for intractable pruritis ani (skin transplantation). YOUNG, F. AND SCOTT, W. J. M. Surgery *13:*911–915, June '43
New method of skin grafting based on principles of tissue culture. SANO, M. E. Am. J. Surg. *61:*105–106, July '43
Tissue grafting. SHEEHAN, J. E. Am. J. Surg. *61:*339–349, Sept '43
Free grafts in plastic surgery. HARRIS, M. M. Semana med. *2:*841–844, Oct 7, '43
Skin grafts in treatment of wounds. McINDOE, A. H. Proc. Roy. Soc. Med. *36:*647–656, Oct '43
Biologic recovery of skin grafts doomed to necrosis, by means of histamine; preliminary report. PRUDENTE, A. Rev. paulista de med. *23:*262–265, Nov '43
Behavior of skin grafts under experimental avitaminosus, C. BARBERA, G. Bull. War Med. *4:*211–212, Dec '43
Dermatome pattern graft and its use in reconstruction (after burns). KANTHAK, F. F. Surg., Gynec. and Obst. *77:*610–614, Dec '43
Transplantation tissue therapy in certain diseases. FILATOV, V. P. Sovet. med. (no. 10) *7:*1–3, '43
Dental arch of upper jaw as support for apparatus during surgical interventions on head in cases of nasal fractures and corrections, skin grafts of face and mobilization of maxillary ankylosis. KUNZENDORF, W. Deutsche Ztschr. f. Chir. *258:*348, '43
Early treatment of war wounds, with emphasis on prevention of deformities (grafting). MALINIAC, J. W. Hebrew M. J. *1:*183, '43
Plastic surgery in dermatology; large free grafts. MARINO, H. Rev. argent. dermatosif. *27:*458–461, '43

Skin Grafts – Cont.

Improved methods of skin grafting. PADGETT, E. C. Proc. Interst. Postgrad. M. A. North America (1942) pp. 32–34, '43

Skin transplantation in surgical after-treatment of amputation-stumps following frostbite of foot. STUDEMEISTER, A. Deutsche Ztschr. f. Chir. *258:*49, '43

Skin grafting in operations of the frontal sinus. BRADBEER, W. H., J. Laryng. and Otol. *59:*36–37, Jan '44

Vascular prerequisites of successful grafting; new method (using fluorescein) for immediate determination of adequacy of circulation in ulcers, skin grafts and flaps. LANGE, K. Surgery *15:*85–89, Jan '44

Skin graft restoration after exicision for malignant disease. PICKERILL, H. P. Australian and New Zealand J. Surg. *13:*147–154, Jan '44

Skin grafts. THOMASON, T. H. Texas State J. Med. *39:*476–477, Jan '44

Large skin grafts in surgery. COVARRUBIAS ZENTENO, R. Arch. Soc. cirujanos hosp. *14:*303–305, March '44

Surgical repair of burns. MCDOWELL, F. AND BROWN, J. B. Wisconsin Med. J., *43:*310, Mar '44

Discussion on modern methods of skin grafting. MOWLEM, R. *et al.* Proc. Roy. Soc. Med. *37:*215–225, March '44

Scrape method of skin grafting. GLASSER, B. F. AND RICHLIN, P. Am. J. Surg. *64:*131–134, April '44

Role of free grafts in surface defects. STRAATSMA, C. R., S. Clin. North America *24:*309–318, April '44

Sulfonamide-impregnated membranes; further experience. ANDRUS, W. DEW. AND DINGWALL, J. A. III. Ann. Surg. *119:*694–699, May '44

Ethyl chloride spray for freezing donor area for skin grafting. GASTON, J. H., J. M. A. Georgia *33:*151, May '44

Modified technic in skin grafting of extensive deep burns. SALTONSTALL, H. AND LEE, W. E. Ann. Surg. *119:*690–693, May '44

Indications and results of immediate free grafts to repair extensive loss of substance. GARAVANO, P. H. Dia med. (sup.) *1:*33–40, July 3, '44

Pedicled grafts versus free grafts. FARINA, R. Sao Paulo med. *2:*125–132, Aug '44

Penicillin and skin grafting in burns. HIRSHFELD, J. W. *et al.* J.A.M.A. *125:*1017–1019, Aug 12, '44

Skin grafts in general surgery, orthopedic surgery and gynecology. CANNADAY, J. E. West Virginia M. J. *40:*277–282, Sept '44

Skin Grafts – Cont.

Free graft; special technic. POTH, E. J. Texas State J. Med. *40:*290–294, Sept '44

Therapy of external cancer by extirpation and Padgett grafts. FERRARI, R. C. AND VIACAVA, E. P. Bol. y trab., Acad. argent. de cir. *28:*959–970, Oct 18, '44

Use of preputial skin in "structive" surgery. ESSER, J. F. S., J. Internat. Coll. Surgeons *7:*469–470, Nov-Dec '44

Color matching of skin grafts and flaps with permanent pigment injection. BROWN, J. B., BYARS, L. T., MCDOWELL, F. AND HANCE, G. Surg., Gynec. and Obst., *79:*624, Dec '44

Healing of surface cutaneous wounds (donor areas); analogy with healing of superficial burns. CONVERSE, J. M. AND ROBB-SMITH, A. H. T. Ann. Surg. *120:*873–885, Dec '44

Skin grafts to cover defects of stumps after frostbite. GEKTIN, F. L. Khirurgiya, no. 4, pp. 23–27, '44

Transplantation tissue therapy. KRYMOV, A. P. Sovet. med. (no. 9) *8:*15–16, '44

Penicillin as adjunct in skin grafting of severe burns. LAM, C. R. AND MCCLURE, R. D. Proc. Am. Federation Clin. Research *1:*56, '44

Immediate and late results of free transplantation in form of perforated flap; preliminary report. PARIN, B. V. Khirurgiya, no. 12, pp. 21–29, '44

Biopsy as accurate guide to decision of early skin grafting. PRITCHARD, J. E. Ann. Surg. *121:*164–171, Feb '45

Free skin grafts; clinical and technical study. ARESPACOCHAGA, F. L. Dia med. *17:*186–188, March 5, '45

Selection of time for grafting of skin to extensive defects resulting from deep thermal burns. MCCORKLE, H. J. AND SILVANI, H. Ann. Surg. *121:*285–290, March '45

Closure of orifices of tracheotomy; Aubry procedure (graft). CARDIN, M. Ann. d'oto-laryng. *12:*305–314, April-June '45

Symposium on traumatic surgery; principles of grafting. IVY, R. H. Clinics *3:*1623–1640, April '45

Skin grafting by general surgeon. URKOV, J. C. Am. J. Surg. *68:*195–207, May '45

Skin graft in hemophilia with preparation of thrombin and sulfanilamide (sulfonamide). DAVIDSON, C. S. AND LEVENSON, S. M., J.A.M.A. *128:*656–657, June 30, '45

Technical details in dermatome grafting. WALLACE, F. T. South. M. J. *38:*380–381, June '45

Immediate grafting following injuries. KING, M. K. Surg., Gynec. and Obst. *81:*75–78,

Skin Grafts – Cont.
July '45
Technical aspects of skin transplantation. POTH, E. J., M. Rec. and Ann. *39:*1081–1088, July '45
Skin grafting in moribund patients. EISENSTODT, L. W. Am. J. Surg. *69:*168–176, Aug '45
Autoplastic grafts in cicatricial deformities due to burns. PASSALACQUA, L. A. Bol. Asoc. med. de Puerto Rico *37:*285–295, Aug '45
Skin transplantation. KOSTRUBALA, J. G. Mil. Surgeon *97:*203–208, Sept '45
Skin transplantation. MACPHERSON, N. S., J. Christian M. A. *20:*136–140, Sept '45
Skin transplantation. GORDON, S. D. Bull. Vancouver M. A. *22:*9–11, Oct '45
Surgical obliteration of cavities following traumatic osteomyelitis (by bone and skin transplantation). KNIGHT, M. P. AND WOOD, G. O., J. Bone and Joint Surg. *27:*547–556, Oct '45
Use of free grafts in surgical therapy of frontal sinusitis. MOULONGUET. Ann. d'oto-laryng. *12:*501–503, Oct-Dec '45
Principles of skin grafting. IVY, R. H., J. Internat. Coll. Surgeons. *8:*520–524, Nov-Dec '45
Critique of free graft. PICK, J. F. South M. J. *38:*827–831, Dec '45
Routine for early skin grafting of deep burns. RAWLES, B. W. JR. Surgery *18:*696–706, Dec '45
Plastic operations for covering cutaneous defects following soft tissue wounds. ANTELAVA, N. V. Khirurgiya, no. 6, pp. 40–43, '45
Tattooing of free grafts and pedicle flaps. BYARS, L. T. Tr. South. S. A. (1944) *56:*260–264, '45
Review of results in skin grafting; additional cases. CANNADAY, J. E. Tr. South. S. A. (1944) *56:*372–386, '45
Transplantation tissue therapy. FILATOV, V. P. Vrach. delo (nos. 11–12) *25:*499–510, '45
Experimental study of skin transplantation. MEDAWAR, P. B. Brit. M. Bull. *3:*79–81, '45
Effect of experimental sleep on healing of skin defects in man. POLYAKOV, K. L. Voen.-med. sborn. *2:*223–233, '45
Continuous epithelization on large denuded areas. SHEEHAN, J. E. AND JENNEY, J. Lancet *1:*123–124, Jan 26, '46
Osteomyelitis treated by radical saucerization and early grafting (skin). McCLINTOCK, J. A., J. Indiana M. A. *39:*9–14, Jan '46
Burns and their sequels; therapy with free

Skin Grafts – Cont.
skin grafts. PAVLOWSKY, A. J. *et al.* Rev. Asoc. med. Argent. *60:*78–83, Feb 15–28, '46
Advantages of early skin grafting. PICKERILL, H. P. New Zealand M. J. *45:*45–49, Feb '46
Surface defects of skin; treatment by controlled exfoliation. URKOV, J. C. Illinois M. J. *89:*75–81, Feb'46
Management and surgical resurfacing of serious burns. CARKSON, P. AND LAWRIE, R. S. Brit. J. Surg. *33:*311–323, Apr '46
Use of acetic acid-glycerin-saline solution in skin grafting. LUDWIG, F. E. Surgery *19:*492–497, Apr '46
Activation of skin grafts. ROUS, P., J. Exper. Med. *83:*383–400, May '46
Problem of skin grafts in severe burns DEL-RIO, J. M. A. Bol. y trab. Acad. argent. de cir. *30:*363–376, Jun 26 '46
Free grafts. DICK, A., M. Ann. District of Columbia *15:*262, June '46
Dermoepidermal grafts in grave traumas of upper extremity; case. BULFARO, J. A. H. Bol. y trab. Soc. argent. de cirujanos *7:*340–343, '46 also: Rev. Asoc. med. argent. *60:*605–606, July 15 '46
Technic of free skin grafts; indications. HUMPLIK, H. Wien. med. Wchnschr. *96:*265–269, July 15, '46
Surgical treatment of ichthyosis hystrix. KAZANJIAN, V. H. Plast. and Reconstruct. Surg. *1:*91–97, July '46
Skin dressings (split grafts) in treatment of debrided wounds. GAY, E. C. Am. J. Surg. *72:*212–218, Aug '46
Methods and indications for skin transplantation. NEW, G. B. AND DEVINE, K. D., S. Clin. North America *26:*890–905, Aug '46
Fundamental principles of skin grafting. BYARS, L. T., BROWN, J. B. AND McDOWELL, F. The Interne, *12:*558, Sept '46
Reconstructive surgery following treatment of osteomyelitis by saucerization and early grafting. McCLINTOCK, J. A., J. Indiana M. A. *39:*436–439, Sept '46
Hair growth in skin transplanted under skin and into peritoneal cavity in rat. BUTCHER, E. O. Anat. Rec. *96:*101–109, Oct '46
Source of autografts in clinical surgery; technic for their suture. TARLOV, I. M. *et al.* Am. J. Surg. *72:*700–710, Nov '46

Skin Grafts to Breast
Plastic covering of large defects following breast amputation. GRUCA, A. Zentralbl. f. Chir. *54:*1293–1297, May 21, '27

Skin Grafts to Breast—Cont.

Breast surgery with graft of areolar region; 2 cases. DARTIGUES, L. Monde med., Paris *38:*75–85, Feb 1, '28

Excision of breast combined with autoplastic areolomammary graft. DARTIGUES, L. Paris chir. *21:*11–19, Jan-Feb '29

Use of skin of female breast in plastic surgery. ESSER, J. F. S. Brit. M. J. *2:*1256–1257, Dec 17, '38

Method for closure of operative wound in cancer of breast; skin grafting. KOROLEV, B. A. Novy khir. arkhiv. *46:*48–51, '40

Derma-fat-fascia transplants used in building up breasts. BERSON, M. I. Surgery *15:*451–456, March '44

Skin Grafts, Cancer Transplantation with

Cases of cancer after skin transplantation. KORKHOV, V. Vestnik khir. (no. 41) *14:*137–142, '28

Accidental autogenous transplantation of mammary carcinoma to thigh during skin graft operation; case. SPIES, J. W. *et al.* Am. J. Cancer *20:*606–609, March '34

Transplantation of skin cancer by use of superficial grafts of epidermis covering epithelioma. CROSTI, A. Gior. ital. di dermat. e sif. *79:*1091–1108, Dec '38

Autogenous transplantation of fibrosarcoma during application of full-thickness skin graft. HARRELL, G. T. AND VALK, A. DET. Ann. Surg. *111:*285–291, Feb '40

Accidental transplantation of cancer (in skin of donor site) in operation room, with case report. BRANDES, W. W. *et al.* Dia med. *18:*153–154, Feb 25, '46 also: Surg. Gynec. and Obst. *82:*212–214, Feb '46

Recidivation of vulvar cancer in arm, due to graft to prevent local recurrence; case. PIULACHES, P. AND PLANAS-GUASCH, J. Med. clin., Barcelona *6:*334–336, May '46

Skin Grafts, Contraction of

Immediate skin graft contraction and its cause. DAVIS, J. S. AND KITLOWSKI, E. A. Arch. Surg. *23:*954–965, Dec '31

Contracted dense scar of neck despite use of many Thiersch grafts. BABCOCK, W. W. S. Clin. North America *12:*1405–1407, Dec '32

Skin Grafts, Cysts in

Fate of free transplants of epidermis into deep-lying tissues; relation to epithelial cysts. ZIMCHES, J. L. Frankfurt, Ztschr. f. Path. *42:*203–227, '31

Mechanism of development of epithelial cysts; behavior of autogenous skin particle implanted subcutaneously. ŌKUMA, M. Nagasaki Igakkwai Zassi *14:*94–96, Jan 25, '36

Skin Grafts, Cysts in—Cont.

Cysts of skin graft into rectovaginal septum; case. ROSSI, D. Clin. ostet. *38:*464–470, Sept '36

Cysts; fate of buried skin grafts in man. PEER, L. A. Arch. Surg. *39:*131–144, July '39

Skin Grafts, Dressings for

Simple protection for newly placed skin grafts. SMYTHE, F. W., J.A.M.A. *78:*1963, June 24, '22 (illus.)

Use of paraffin as primary dressing for skin grafts. COLLER, F. A. Surg., Gynec. and Obst. *41:*221–225, Aug '25

Pressure bags for skin grafting. SMITH, F. Surg., Gynec. & Obst. *43:*99, July '26

Immobilizing cage in burn therapy and skin grafts. HOSMER, A. J. Am. J. Surg. *3:*23–30, July '27

Postoperative care of Ollier-Thiersch skin grafts; advisability of daily surgical dressings. RULISON, E. T. Surg., Gynec. and Obst. *45:*708–710, Nov '27

Simpler technic for promoting epithelization and protecting skin grafts (oxyquinoline sulphate scarlet R ointment). BETTMAN, A. G., J.A.M.A. *97:*1879–1881, Dec 19, '31

New technic of bandaging of epidermic grafts; application in therapy of ulcers of leg. RIOU, M. Bull. Soc. path. exot. *26:*1296–1301, '33

Effects of moist-heat medication on free autoplastic skin transplants. CARDIA, A. AND LIGAS, A. Riv. di pat. sper. *12:*475–484, '34

Ambulatory method of grafting small areas of skin by use of elastic adhesive. BRONAUGH, W. West Virginia M. J. *32:*180–181, April '36

Pressure bag in skin grafting. TAYLOR, F. Am. J. Surg. *33:*328–329, Aug '36

Paraffin dressing for transplanted grafts. TRUEBLOOD, D. V. West. J. Surg. *44:*578, Oct '36

Skin grafts with film bandage. OLESEN, M. Ugesk. f. laeger *101:*144–147, Feb 2, '39

Thiersch skin grafting; use of collodion-gauze technic. SZUTU, C. AND CHEN, C. Y. Chinese M. J. *57:*535–545, June '40

Preoperative and postoperative care in skin grafts. HAVENS, F. Z., S. Clin. North America *20:*1087–1092, Aug '40

Immovable bandage in free cutaneous graft (extremities). VORONCHIKHIN, S. I. Novy khir. arkhiv. *45:*244–247, '40

Collodion as dressing for skin grafting of granulating wounds. ELLIS, S. S. AND VON

Skin Grafts, Dressings for – Cont.
WEDEL, C., J. Oklahoma M. A. *34:*103-105, March '41
"Transplantation Microtome" new apparatus for obtaining uniformly thick epidermal and cutaneous grafts. SACHARIEW, G. Chirurg. *15:*94, Feb 1, '43
Coagulum-contact method as applied to human grafts. SANO, M. E. Surg., Gynec. and Obst. *77:*510-513, Nov '43
Use of coagulum-contact method in surgery for grafting. SANO, M. E. *et al.* S. Clin. North America *23:*1673-1695, Dec '43
Fibrin fixation of skin transplants. TIDRICK, R. T. AND WARNER, E. D. Surgery *15:*90-95, Jan '44
Skin grafting with "human glue" (coagulum-contact method); supplementary note on some technical details. FENNEL, E. A. Proc. Staff. Med. Clin., Honolulu *10:*19-22, Feb '44
Fixation of skin grafts by thrombin-plasma adhesion. YOUNG, F. AND FAVATA, B. V. Surgery *15:*378-386, March '44
Use of thrombin and fibrinogen in skin grafting; preliminary report. CRONKITE, E. P. *et al.* J.A.M.A. *124:*976-978, April 1, '44
Use of small pieces of film-covered skin grafts. HARDY, S. B. AND MCNICHOL, J. W. S. Clin. North America *24:*281-292, April '44
New method of skin grafting (coagulum-contact method). SANO, M. E. Delaware State M. J. *16:*51-52, April '44
Film-cemented skin grafts. WEBSTER, J. P., S. Clin. North America *24:*251-280, April '44
Simplification of split skin grafts; gum acacia technic. RUBIN, L. R., M. Bull. North African Theat. Op. (no. 6) *1:*14-15, June '44
New coagulum-contact method of skin grafting; further simplifications in technic. SANO, M. E. Am. J. Surg. *64:*359-360, June '44
Plasma fixation of skin grafts. SHEEHAN, J. E. Am. J. Surg. *65:*74-78, July '44 also: Lancet *2:*363-365, Sept 16, '44
Fixation of skin grafts by plasmathrombin adhesion. YOUNG, F. Ann. Surg. *120:*450-462, Oct '44
Possibilities and advantages of gluing grafts in place (coagulum-contact method). SANO, M. E. Am. Acad. Orthop. Surgeons, Lect. pp. 224-225, '44
Fixation of skin grafts by plasma-thrombin adhesion. YOUNG, F. Tr. Am. S. A. *62:*450-462, '44
Modification of plasma fixation method (Sano) by use of bobbinet and mirror attachment-skin grafts. JENNY, J. A. Am. J. Surg. *67:*3-7, Jan '45
Vaseline gauze contact fixation of split thickness (Padgett) skin grafts. ROBERTS, W. M. AND SCHAUBEL, H. J. Am. J. Surg. *67:*16-22, Jan '45
Fixation of grafts with human plasma and thrombin. CLARK, A. M. *et al.* Lancet *1:*498-499, April 21, '45
Device for fixation of Wolfe graft. MICHAELSON, I. C. Brit. M. J. *2:*49, July 14, '45
Tape method of skin grafting. BERKOW, S. G. U. S. Nav. M. Bull. *45:*1-13, July '45
GREEN, R. W. *et al.* Nylon backing for dermatome grafts. New England J. Med. *233:*268-270, Aug 30, '45
Sano tissue glue skin grafting. EVANS, J. G. J. Internat. Coll. Surgeons *8:*424-425, Sept-Oct '45
Fibrin fixation methods of skin grafting; clinical evaluation. MCEVITT, W. G., J. Michigan M. Soc. *44:*1347-1351, Dec '45
Simplification of split grafting; gum acacia technic. RUBIN, L. R. Am. J. Surg. *70:*302-307, Dec '45
Coagulum-contact method of skin graft fixation; present status. MACGREGOR, M. W. Permanente Found. M. Bull. *4:*42-46, Feb '46
Coagulum-contact method (Sano) of skin grafting. BRANCH, C. D. *et al.* Surgery *19:*460-466, April '46
Free graft in form of cutaneous "bandage"; use in severe burns. MARINO, H. Bol. y trab. Acad. argent. de cir. *30:*451-459, July 17 '46
Use of thromboplastin fixation in skin grafts. HEATLY, M. D. Texas State J. Med. *42:*275-278, Aug '46

Skin Grafts to Ear
Experimental transplantation of cartilage and skin for repair of concha. GUSSIO, S. Valsalva *3:*58-77, Feb '27
Autoplastic surgery of ear. OMBRÉDANNE, L. Presse med. *39:*982-983, July 4, '31
Reconstruction of pavilion using skin grafts (ear); case. DUFOURMENTEL, L. Rev. de laryng. *59:*517-518, May '38 also: Oto-rhino-laryng. internat. *22:*395-396, July '38
Free full thickness graft in restoration of loss of substance of auricle; case. COELST. Rev. de chir. structive *8:*111-112, Aug '38
Use of full thickness free grafts in surgical therapy of microtia; case. COELST, M. Rev. de chir. structive *8:*155-159, '38
Ear reconstruction (graft). MACOMBER, D. Rocky Mountain M. J. *36:*37-40, Jan '39

Skin Grafts to Ear – Cont.

Auriculoplasty for hypoplasia of pavilion using tubular skin graft; case. ZENO, L. Bol. y trab., Acad. argent. de cir. *26:*807–812, Sept 16, '42

Skin Grafts to Eyelids (See also Blepharoplasty; Eyelids; Skin Grafts to Orbit)

Use of epidermic graft in plastic eye surgery. WHEELER, J. M. Internat. Clinics *3:*292–302, '22 (illus.)

Autoplastic skin implant in blepharoplasty. D'ALESSANDRO, A. Semana med. *2:*1531–1534, Dec 17, '25

Skin-grafting in acute symblepharon (eyelids). BALL, J. M. Lancet *1:*863, April 24, '26

Skin grafting in 2 cases of epithelioma of eyelids. MORAX, V. Ann. d'ocul. *164:*6–15, Jan '27

Restoration of completely destroyed eyelid by cutaneous and tarso-conjunctival grafts from other lid; 3 cases. DUPUY-DUTEMPS, L. Ann. d-ocul. *164:*915–926, Dec '27

Transplantation of eyelid tissue. VON GERNET, R. Klin. Monatsbl. f. Augenh. *80:*496, April 27, '28

Repair of conjunctival fornix by Reverdin-Thiersch graft. SALVATI, G. Gior. di ocul. *9:*56, May '28

Regeneration of destroyed eyelid by cutaneous and tarsoconjunctival graft taken from other lid; case. DUPUY-DUTEMPS, L. Monde med., Paris *38:*705–711, Sept 1, '28

Plastic restoration of all 4 eyelids, with use of skin from arm in 3 cases. PAYR, E. Arch. f. klin. Chir. *152:*532–540, '28

Repair of cicatricial ectropion by free dermic graft. TAYLOR, J. W. South. M. J. *22:*634–637, July '29

Symblepharon of eyelids; treatment by Thiersch and mucous membrane grafting. GILLIES, H. D. AND KILNER, T. P. Tr. Ophth. Soc. U. Kingdom *49:*470–479, '29

Autoplastic graft of conjunctiva and of eyelid; 2 cases. DÉJEAN, C. Arch. Soc. d. sc. med. et biol. de Montpellier *12:*23–25, Jan '31

Skin grafts in repair of ocular lesions from pemphigus (eyelids). TERRIEN, F. *et al.* Arch. d'opht. *48:*275–281, April '31

Epithelioma of face secondary to extensive epithelioma of eyelids; three-stage operation; removal of tumor, skin graft and restoration of eyelids. TIXIER, L. AND BONNET, P. Lyon chir. *28:*719–722, Nov-Dec '31

Reconstruction of conjunctival sac with Thiersch grafts. GLOVER, D. M. AND JACOBY, M. W. Arch. Surg. *26:*617–622, April '33

Skin Grafts to Eyelids – Cont.

Good esthetic and functional results in correction of cicatricial ectropion by means of plastic graft operation. ORZALESI, F. Boll. d'ocul. *12:*906–931, Sept '33

Autoplastic skin grafts in therapy of cicatricial ectropion; 5 cases. SENÁ, J. A. Rev. Asoc. med. argent. *48:*298–306, March-April '34 also: Semana med. *2:*489–498, Aug 16, '34

Closure of defects of lower eyelid on side nearest to nose by means of skin grafts from nose. KRAUPA, E. Ztschr. f. Augenh. *84:*216–217, Oct '34

New method of blepharoplastic operation for cicatricial ectropion using free transplant from ear flap. GOLDFEDER, A. E. Sovet. vestnik. oftal. *6:*173–177, '35

Application of grafts early in burns of eye. O'CONNOR, G. B. Rev. de chir. structive, pp. 273–277, June '36

Sources of grafts for plastic surgery about eyes. WHEELER, J. M. New York State J. Med. *36:*1372–1376, Oct 1, '36

Autoplasty of eyelids. LEONARDI. Bull. et mem. Soc. franc. d'opht. *50:*20–24, '37

Blepharoplasty by means of free transplants of skin. LEVITSKIY, M. A. Vestnik oftal. *11:*798–802, '37

Reconstruction of 4 eyelids for ectropion resulting from cicatrix of severe facial burn, by means of free cutaneous grafts; case. DE LIETO VOLLARO, A. Arch. ital. di chir. *51:*588–595, '38

Blepharoplasty with free skin flap from auricle. BULACH, K. Vestnik oftal. (no. 6) *14:*46–48, '39

Paralysis of lower eyelid and scleral scars and grafts. BLAIR, V. P. AND BYARS, L. T. Surg., Gynec. and Obst. *70:*426–437, Feb (no. 2A) '40

Free full-thickness grafts of skin to eyelids; cases. ZENO, L. Bol. Soc. de cir. de Rosario *7:*127–135, May '40 also: An. de cir. *6:*156–164, June '40

Cicatricial ectropion; therapy by free grafts; case. MARINO, H. Rev. med.-quir.de pat. fem. *16:*231–236, Sept '40

Elimination of cicatricial ectropion by free Thiersch graft. MÜLLER, P. Schweiz. med. Wchnschr. *71:*5–6, Jan 4, '41

Conservative autoplasty for malignant melanoma of upper eyelid; case. BADEAUX, F. AND PERRON, L. Union med. du Canada *70:*1065–1066, Oct '41

Skin autoplasty by Hungarian method. AUBRY, M. Semaine d. hop. Paris *21:*488–491, May 14 '45

Full-thickness skin grafts from neck for func-

Skin Grafts to Eyelids – Cont.

tion and color in eyelid. BROWN, J. B. AND CANNON, B. Ann. Surg. *121:*639-643, May '45

Plastic surgical repair about eyes with free grafts. SCHULTZ, A. AND JAECKLE, C. E. Arch. Ophth. *34:*103-106, Aug '45

Full-thickness skin grafts from neck for function and color in eyelid. BROWN, J. B. AND CANNON, B. Tr. South. S. A. (1944) *56:*255-259, '45

Skin Grafts to Face

Use of pedicled flaps and skin grafts in reconstructive surgery of (face) head and neck. FIGI, F. A. Nebraska M. J. *17:*361-365, Sept '32

Possibility of reconstructing whole face by full thickness, free cutaneous grafts, using several flaps. COELST. Rev. de chir. structive, pp. 105-125, Dec '35

Preoperative and postoperative prosthesis in application of skin, cutaneomucosal, cartilage and bone grafts and in improvement of cicatrix of face. DARCISSAC, M. Bull. et mem. Soc. d. chirurgiens de Paris *28:*424-433, June 19, '36

Repair of facial defects with special reference to source of skin grafts. MALINIAK, J. W. Rev. de chir. structive, pp. 431-439, Dec '36 also: Arch. Surg. *34:*897-908, May '37

Skin, cartilage and bone grafts to face. NEW, G. B. Proc. Staff Meet., Mayo Clin. *11:*791-794, Dec 9, '36

Skin grafts and suspension of labial commissure by skin sutures for facial paralysis. ZENO, L. An. de cir. *4:*187-189, Sept '38 Also: Bol. Soc. de cir. de Rosario *5:*412-414, Oct '38

Experiences in reconstruction in surgical treatment of malignant diseases of face with skin grafts. KILNER. Rev. de chir. structive *8:*170-180, '38

Repair of deformities following surgical removal of malignant tumors of face with grafting. MCINDOE, A. H. Rev. de chir. structive *8:*181-186, '38

Surgical therapy of extensive facial tumors, and plastic restoration (grafts). VON SEEMEN, H. Arch. f. klin. chir. *200:*553-566, '40

Surgical removal of hemangioma of face with grafting. BERSON, M. I. Am. J. Surg. *51:*362-365, Feb '41

Extensive mole of face and scalp; excision and full thickness skin graft. FIGI, F. A. Proc. Staff Meet., Mayo Clin. *16:*280-282, April 30, '41

Facial autoplasty; cases. KROEFF, M. Hospital, Rio de Janeiro *19:*559-570, April '41

Free skin grafts versus flaps in surface defects of face and neck. MALINIAC, J. W. Am. J. Surg. *58:*100-109, Oct '42

Primary skin graft for repair of traumatic skin loss of face; case. OBERDORFER, A. Z., U. S. Nav. M. Bull. *42:*695-696, March '44

Esthetic repair of face (after burn) by free grafts of skin; case. ROCHER, H. L. Bordeaux chir. *3-4:*98-100, July-Oct '44

Surgical cure of acne rosacea and rhinophyma with skin grafting. MACOMBER, D. W. Rocky Mountain M. J. *43:*466-467, June '46

Skin Grafts to Foot

Transplantation of skin in amputations of foot. BLENCKE, A. Zentralbl. f. Chir. *56:*2050-2054, Aug 17, '29

Loss of substance of sole of foot; treatment by autoplastic grafts from ischiatic region. COSTANTINI, H. AND CURTILLET, É. Rev. de chir., Paris *67:*515-539, '29

Plastic reparation of heel by grafts. FERRÉ, R. L. Semana med. *2:*2049-2053, Dec 27, '34

Plantar warts, flaps and grafts. BLAIR, V. P.; *et al.* J.A.M.A. *108:*24-27, Jan 2, '37

Late evolution in case of "scalping" of heel (with skin grafting). LANDIVAR, A. F. AND LEONI IPARRAGUIRRE, C. A. Dia med. *14:*202-203, March 16, '42

Ulcer of dorsum pedis; free graft on granulation tissue. FERNANDEZ, L. L. Prensa med. argent. *32:*1601-1604, Aug 17, '45

Skin Grafts, Full-Thickness

Full thickness skin graft. BLAIR, V. P. Ann. Surg. *80:*298-324, Sept '24

Use of full thickness skin grafts. NEW, G. B. AND FIGI, F. A. Minnesota med. *7:*714-716, Nov '24

Origin and development of blood supply of whole-thickness skin grafts; experimental study. DAVIS, J. S. AND TRAUT, H. F. Ann. Surg. *82:*871-879, Dec '25

Extended use of whole thickness skin graft. COLE, P. P. Practitioner *116:*311-313, April '26

Method of obtaining greater relaxation with whole thickness skin grafts. DAVIS, J. S. AND TRAUT, H. F. Surg., Gynec. and Obst. *42:*710-711, May '26

Free, full-thickness skin grafts. MCWILLIAMS, C. A. Ann. Surg. *84:*237-245, Aug '26

Free full-thickness skin transplantation. PADGETT, E. C., J. Kansas M. Soc. *27:*145-148, May '27

Skin Grafts, Full Thickness—Cont.
Therapy of contractures with aid of free full thickness skin-grafts and pedunculated flaps. KOCH, S. L., S. Clin. North America *7:*611–626, June '27
Utilization of skin of upper eyelid for repair of small facial defects. SHEEHAN, J. E. Arch. Otolaryng. *6:*107–111, Aug '27
Whole skin grafted on dura mater in case of cancer of parietal bone. ROUX-BERGER, J. L. Bull. et mem. Soc. nat. de chir. *53:*1305–1308, Dec 3, '27
Contractures due to burns; treatment with free full thickness grafts and pedunculated flaps. KOCH, S. L. AND KANAVEL, A. B. Tr. Sect. Surg, General and Abd., A.M.A., pp. 208–227, '28
Whole-skin method of grafting. YOUNG, A. Proc. Internat. Assemb. Inter-State Post-Grad. M. A., North America (1928), pp. 217–233, '29
Full-thickness skin graft in correction of soft tissue deformities (cicatrices). PADGETT, E. C. Tr. Sect. Surg., Gen. and Abd., A.M.A., pp. 304–319, '31 also: J.A.M.A. *98:*18–23, Jan 2, '32
Full-thickness graft; field of applicability and technical considerations. GARLOCK, J. H. Ann. Surg. *97:*259–273, Feb '33
Free full-thickness skin transplant. SCHROCK, R. D. AND JOHNSON, H. F. Nebraska M. J. *19:*91–93, March '34
Full-thickness skin graft. KILNER, T. P. Post-Grad. M. J. *11:*279–282, Aug '35
New method of transfer of full-thickness skin; grille graft. SAMMIS, G. F. Am. J. Surg. *36:*46–49, April '37
Free full thickness skin grafts. DUFOURMENTEL, L. Bull. et mem. Soc. d. chirurgiens de Paris *29:*306–317, June 18, '37
Free full thickness skin grafts. TIERNY, A. Gaz. med. de France *44:*795–797, Oct 1, '37
Experiences of Prague Institute for Plastic Surgery with free whole thickness grafts. BURIAN, F. Rev. de chir. structive, pp. 264–266, Dec '37
Method of free whole thickness skin graft. COELST, M. Rev. de chir. structive, pp. 253–258, Dec '37
Total free skin grafts. DUFOURMENTEL, L. Rev. de chir., Paris *76:*37–53, Jan '38
Cutaneous full thickness graft in therapy of cicatrix due to burn of elbow fold; case. COELST. Rev. de chir. structive *8:*124–126, Aug '38
Free full thickness skin grafts. SHEEHAN, J. E., J.A.M.A. *112:*27–29, Jan 7, '39
Whole-thickness grafts in correction of contractures due to burn scars; 3 cases. CONWAY, H. Ann. Surg. *109:*286–290, Feb '39
Immediate full thickness grafts to finger tips. REED, J. V. AND HARCOURT, A. K. Surg., Gynec. and Obst. *68:*925–929, May '39
Advantages, inconveniences and limits of free grafts of whole skin. DUFOURMENTEL, L. Presse med. *47:*1336–1337, Sept 13, '39
Technic of full thickness free grafts for cicatricial contracture of hand. ZENO, L. Semana med. *2:*829–831, Oct 12, '39
Free full-thickness skin grafts; indications and technic. ZENO, L. An. de cir. *5:*279–289, Dec '39
Indications and technic of full thickness free grafts of total skin. ZENO, L. Dia med. *12:*214–215, March 18, '40 abstr: Rev. med. de Rosario *29:*1310–1314, Dec '39
Free full-thickness skin graft for relief of burn contracture of neck. BLOCKER, T. G., JR. South. Surgeon *10:*849–857, Dec '41
Full thickness skin grafts in injured fingers; 2 cases. ANDERSON, W. S. Memphis M. J. *17:*23–24, Feb '42
Physiology of free full thickness skin graft. RECALDE, J. F. Arq. de cir. clin. e exper. *6:*547–549, April–June '42
Free full thickness grafts; principles involved and technic of application. BYARS, L. T. Surg., Gynec. and Obst. *75:*8–20, July '42
Free full thickness graft in case of lupus erythematosus. MALBEC, E. F. Dia med. *14:*1119–1120, Oct 26, '42
Free full thickness skin graft in nasal cancer; case. MALBEC, E. F. Semana med. *2:*1489–1491, Dec 17, '42
Free graft of full thickness skin in case of lupus erythematosus of nose. MALBEC, E. F. Semana med. *1:*1232–1235, June 3, '43
Free full thickness skin graft; case in cicatrix. MALBEC, E. F. Prensa med. argent. *30:*1576–1577, Aug 18, '43
Fibrokeloid cicatrix after attempted removal of pilous nevus; free full thickness skin graft; case. MALBEC, E. F. Dia med. *15:*1100, Sept 13, '43
Whole skin removal and replacement; operative procedure of value for salvage of skin undermined by trauma, or for recovering areas from which resection of extensive subcutaneous tissue has been necessary. FARMER, A. W., S. Clin. North America *23:*1440–1447, Oct '43
Fibrokeloid cicatrix after attempted removal of pilous nevus; free full thickness skin graft; case. MALBEC, E. F. Semana med. *2:*1416–1417, Dec 23, '43
Free grafts of whole skin. BEZERRA, M. Arq. brasil. de cir. e ortop *12:*165–174, '44

Skin Grafts, Full Thickness – Cont.

Free transplant of full thickness graft. KHITROV, F. M. Khirurgiya, no. 9, pp. 31–34, '44

Free full thickness skin grafts in children; cases. RUIZ MORENO, V. Semana med. *1:*1089-1097, June 28, '45

Use of whole skin grafts as substitute for fascial sutures in treatment of hernias; preliminary report. MAIR, G. B. Am. J. Surg. *69:*352-365, Sept '45

Analysis of series of 454 inguinal hernias, with special reference to morbidity and recurrence after whole skin graft method. MAIR, G. B. Brit. J. Surg. *34:*42–48, July '46

Skin Grafts, Growth of

Skin grafting and its compensatory growth. HILZE, A. Latvijas Arstu z., no. 3-4, pp. 61–66, March-April '27

Persistence of function of skin grafts through long periods of growth. BROWN, J. B. AND McDOWELL, F. Surg., Gynec. and Obst. *72:*848-853, May '41

Persistence of function of grafts through long periods of growth. BROWN, J. B. AND McDOWELL, F., J. Iowa M. Soc. *31:*457-462, Oct '41

Skin Grafts to Hand (See also: Hand)

Skin plastics in treatment of traumatic lesions of hand and forearm. LYLE, H. H. M. Ann. Surg. *83:*537-542, April '26

Covering of raw surfaces with particular reference to hand. KOCH, S. L. Surg., Gynec. and Obst. *43:*677-686, Nov '26

Burns on both forearms and back of hand; treatment by graft from thigh. MIRIZZI, P. L. Bull. et mem. Soc. nat. de chir. *55:*780-785, June 8, '29

Contracture of right hand treated by full-thickness skin grafts. JONES, H. T., S. Clin. N. Amer. *9:*939-940, Aug '29

Thiersch's skin grafting in fresh industrial mutilations of fingers. STOLZE, M. AND MELTZER, H. Chirurg *1:*1068-1072, Oct 15, '29

Skin transplantation in fresh wounds of fingers. BAGER, B. Chirurg *2:*169–171, Feb 15, '30

Reconstruction of burned hand (grafts). VON WEDEL, C., J. Oklahoma M. A. *24:*164-165, May '31

Syndactylizing fingers preliminary to skin grafting. BETTMAN, A. G. Northwest. Med. *31:*70-71, Feb '32

Plastic reconstruction of fingers by Italian method of skin graft; case. FERRARI, R. C.

Skin Grafts to Hand – Cont.

Semana med. *2:*1104-1105, Oct 12, '33

Treatment of chronically recurring paronychias and related ungual diseases by excision and by Thiersch grafts. RUDOFSKY, F. Med. Klin. *30:*198, Feb 9, '34

Epithelial inlay in therapy of syndactylia. ESSER, J. F. S. AND RAOUL. Rev. de chir. plastique, pp. 21–32, May '34

Full thickness skin grafts in finger amputations. O'MALLEY, T. S. Wisconsin M. J. *33:*337-340, May '34

Skin grafts in changing of fingerprints. UPDEGRAFF, H. L. Am. J. Surg. *26:*533-534, Dec '34

Primary skin graft in fresh injuries of hand and fingers. BASS, Y. M. AND ZHOLONDZ, A. M. Sovet. khir. (nos. 3-4) *6:*350-357, '34

New plastic operation for avulsion of skin of thumb; utilization of scrotal skin. MAYANTS, I. A. Arch. f. klin. Chir. *181:*303-310, '34 abstr.: Novy khir. arkhiv. *32:*180-184, '34

Technic of Italian graft in hand injuries. BIAILLE DE LANGIBAUDIERE, M. Bull. Soc. med.-chir. de l'Indochine *13:*387-396, May '35

Reconstruction of left thumb by skin and osteoperiosteal grafts; case. DESPLAS, B. Mem. Acad. de chir. *62:*1292-1296, Nov 25, '36

Dupuytren's contracture, covering palmar defects with skin from little finger. FRANKENTHAL, L. Zentralbl. f. Chir. *64:*211-214, Jan 23, '37

Restoration of thumb using bone and skin grafts. HUARD, P. AND LONG, M. Bull. Soc. med.-chir. de l'Indochine *15:*855-860, Aug-Sept '37

Skin grafts in surgical correction of defective cicatrix of hand causing contracture; 2 cases. BARBERIS, J. C. Bol. Soc. de cir. de Rosario *5:*469-477, Nov '38

Dupuytren's contracture; plastic surgery of hands (grafts). MASON, M. L., S. Clin. North America *19:*227-248, Feb '39

Finger tip reconstruction; new operation (using bone and skin grafts). LAUTEN, W. F. Indust. Med. *8:*99-100, March '39

Treatment of syndactylias by total free skin grafts. BOPPE, M. AND FAUGERON, P. Paris med. *1:*522-527, June 17, '39

Free full thickness skin grafts in hand contracted by cicatrix; technical problems in case. ZENO, L. Rev. ortop. y traumatol. *9:*73-77, July '39

Technic of free graft of whole skin for cicatricial contracture of hand. ZENO, L. Bol. y trab., Soc. de cir. de Buenos Aires *23:*525-

Skin Grafts to Hand–Cont.
531, July 26, '39
- Clawhand; Morestin plastic surgery with free full-thickness skin graft. ZENO, L. Bol. Soc. de cir. de Rosario *7:*308–315, Aug '40 also: An. de cir. *6:*315–321, Sept '40
- Covering cutaneous defect after avulsion of skin of thumb. ZAMOSHCHIN, M. B. Novy khir. arkhiv *46:*260–262, '40
- Transplantation of skin and subcutaneous tissue to hand. KOCH, S. L. Surg., Gynec. and Obst. *72:*157–177, Feb '41
- Rigid hand caused by fibrous cicatrix; free graft of full-thickness skin. ZENO, L. An. de cir. *7:*52–56, March–June '41 also: Bol. Soc. de cir. de Rosario *8:*53–58, April '41
- Skin and tendon transplantation in severe injury to back of right hand by polishing machine. HILLEBRAND, H. Chirurg *13:*521–523, Sept 1, '41
- Method for closing traumatic defect of finger tip (graft). JONES, R. A. Am. J. Surg. *55:*326–338, Feb '42
- Treatment of injuries to hand requiring skin grafting. HAWKINS, T. L. Am. J. Surg. *59:*383–391, Feb '43
- Immediate skin grafting for traumatic amputation of finger tips. ZADIK, F. R. Lancet *1:*335–336, March 13, '43
- Immediate skin grafts on finger injuries. READ, F. L. AND HASLAM, E. T., U. S. Nav. M. Bull. *42:*183–186, Jan '44
- Immediate application of free full-thickness skin graft for traumatic amputation of finger. MCCARROLL, H. R., J. Bone and Joint Surg. *26:*489–494, July '44
- Skin graft of dorsum of hand; use of large size dermatome to obtain one-piece pattern. CONVERSE, J. M. Ann. Surg. *121:*172–174, Feb '45
- Conservation of metacarpus by skin and bone grafting in 3 patients. MORONEY, P. B. Brit. J. Surg. *32:*464–466, April '45
- Dermoplasty of healed burned dorsum of hand. PICK, J. F., J. Internat. Coll. Surgeons *8:*217–223, May–June '45
- Therapy of cicatrices of fingers by "pocket-book" graft. CASCO, C. M. Dia med. *18:*788–789, June 24, '46
- Skin grafting burned dorsum of hand. WEBSTER, G. V. AND ROWLAND, W. D. Ann. Surg. *124:*449–462, Aug '46
- Split thickness graft as covering following removal of fingernail. HANRAHAN, E. M. Surgery *20:*398–400, Sept '46

Skin Grafts, Homografts and Heterografts
- Homoplastic transplantation of adult frog skin. GASSUL, R. Deutsche med.

Skin Grafts, Homografts and Heterographs–Cont.
Wchnschr. *48:*1163–1164, Sept 1, '22 (illus.)
- Protein sensitization in iso-skin grafting; is the latter of practical value? HOLMAN, E. Surg., Gynec. and Obst. *38:*100–106, Jan '24
- Grafts of embryonal tissue. FALDINO, G. Chir. d. org. di movimento *9:*1–27, Dec '24 abstr: J.A.M.A. *84:*786, March 7, '25
- Free homeoplastic skin grafting. DEUCHER, W. G. AND OCHSNER, A. E. W. Arch. f. klin. Chir. *132:*470–479, '24
- Blood grouping as guide in skin grafting. KUBÁNYI, A. Arch. f. klin. Chir. *129:*644–647, '24 abstr: J.A.M.A. *82:*2090, June 21, '24
- Free homeoplastic skin grafting; comment on Deucher and Ochsner's article. ASCHER, K. W. Arch. f. klin. Chir. *137:*198, '25
- Implants of embryonic tissues. SARTORI, C. Arch. ital. di chir. *15:*339–349, '26 abstr: J.A.M.A. *87:*67, July 3, '26
- Reaction of skin in homoplastic grafts studied by means of phenol red (phenol sulphon-phthalein). MILONE, S. Gior. d. r. Accad. di med. di Torino *33:*147–150, March '27
- Reaction to homoplastic skin grafts. SEBASTIANO, M. Arch. per le sc. med. *49:*193–200, April '27
- Deep homoplastic grafts and successive superficial grafts. MORPURGO, B. AND MILONE, S. Arch. per le sc. med. *49:*306–309, May '27
- Influence of inanition on homoplastic skin-grafts. MORPURGO, B. AND MILONE, S. Boll. d. Soc. ital. di biol. sper. *2:*709–712, July '27
- Influence of inanition on homeoplastic transplantations. MORPURGO, B. Centralbl. f. allg. Path. u. path. Anat. *40:*1–3, July 1, '27
- Autoplastic, homoplastic and heteroplastic skin grafts. CARMONA, L. Ann. ital. di chir. *6:*1234–1256, Dec '27
- Behavior of autoplastic and homoplastic grafts placed in subcutaneous tissue; experiments on rabbits. RIGANO-IRRERA, D. AND SACERDOTE, G. Arch. ital. di chir. *20:*190–198, '27
- Homeoplastic skin transplantation after reticulo-endothelial storage. TAMMANN, H. AND PATRIKALAKIS, M. Beit. z. klin. Chir. *139:*550–568, '27
- Experiments to improve survival of homoplastic transplants. NIGRISOLI, P. Arch. per sc. med. *52:*65–75, Feb '28
- Experiments on taking of homoplastic skin-grafts. VELO, C. A. Ann. ital. di chir. *7:*97–

Skin Grafts, Homografts and Heterographs – Cont.

112, Feb '28

Nasal reconstruction by means of auto and iso-grafts. METZENBAUM, M. Ohio State M. J. *24:*196–200, March '28 also: Laryngoscope *38:*197–205, March '28

Importance of local immunity in elimination of homoplastic skin grafts. TINOZZI, F. P. Ann. ital. di chir. *7:*660–683, July 31, '28

Comparative effects on skin of homo- and heteroplastic grafts. MORPURGO, B. AND MILONE, S. Arch. ed atti d. Soc. ital. di chir (1927) *34:*lxxxiv, '28

Effect of insufficient nutrition on growth of homoplastic skin grafts. MORPURGO, B. AND MILONE, S. Arch. ed atti d. Soc. ital. di chir. (1927) *34:*lxxxv, '28

Homotransplantation based on blood-group determination with special regard to skin transplantation. KETTEL, K. Bibliot. f. Laeger *121:*204–230, May '29

Homotransplantation and several blood groups; epidermal grafts made by Thiersch method. DOBRZANIECKI, W. Ann. Surg. *90:*926–938, Nov '29

Homoplastic and heteroplastic transplantation of skin in man. MANNHEIM, H. Arch. f. klin. Chir. *162:*551–560, '30

Homoplastic transplantation of epithelium; case. SCHÜRCH, O. Zentralbl. f. Chir. *58:*451–453, Feb 21, '31

Comment on article by Schürch on homoplastic transplantation of epithelium. MANNHEIM, H. Zentralbl. f. Chir. *58:*789–790, March 28, '31

Effect of removal of sympathetic ganglia on cutaneous autoplastic and homoplastic transplants (skin). DOBRZANIECKI, W. Polska gaz. lek. *10:*262, April 5; 287, April 12, '31

Plastic repair of vagina by graft of 2 prepuces; case. PETIT, R. Rev. franc. de gynec. et d'obst. *26:*605–607, Nov '31

Periarterial decortication by Leriche method and autoplastic and homoplastic grafts. BERTOCCHI, A. Arch. ital. di chir. *29:*1–36, '31

Homeoplastic skin grafts. ERKES, F. Deutsche Ztschr. f. Chir. *234:*852–854, '31

Partial cheiloplasty by transplantation from one person to another. DUJARDIN, E. Ugesk. f. laeger *94:*382–383, April 14, '32

Possibility of transmission of biologic properties of skin from animal to animal by means of transplantation. BERNUCCI, F. Gior. ital. di dermat. e sif. *73:*1373–1379, Aug '32

Is iso-skin grafting practicable? PADGETT, E. C. South. M. J. *25:*895–900, Sept '32

Skin Grafts, Homografts and Heterographs – Cont.

Autoplastic and homoplastic implantation of epidermis. LOEFFLER. Deutsche Ztschr. f. Chir. *236:*169–190, '32

Respective value of autografts, homografts and heterografts. DUFOURMENTEL, L. Bull. med., Paris *47:*175–176, March 11, '33

Application of auto-, homo- and heterografts in reconstructive surgery. DUFOURMENTEL, L. Bull. et mem. Soc. d. chirurgiens de Paris *25:*269–282, May 5, '33

Effect of removal of cervical ganglion of sympathetic nerve on growth of autoplastic and homoplastic skin transplants. VASILEV, A. A. AND ZHOLONDZ, A. M. Arch. f. klin. Chir. *178:*148–169, '33 also: Novy khir. arkhiv *29:*3–20, '33

Homotransplantation of skin in relation to blood groups. ISHCHENKO, I. M. Med. zhur. *4:*59–68, '34

Question of homoplastic grafting of skin. TRUSLER, H. M. AND COGSWELL, H. D. J.A.M.A. *104:*2076–2077, June 8, '35

Results of homologous skin transplantation in lepers. FLARER, F. AND GRILLO, V. Arch. ital. di dermat., sif. *12:*309–325, May '36

Homografting, with report of success in identical twins. BROWN, J. B. Surgery *1:*558–563, April '37

Fate and activity of autografts and homografts in white rats. BUTCHER, E. O. Arch. Dermat. and Syph. *36:*53–56, July '37

Experimental study upon prevention of adhesions about repaired nerves and tendons (especially by use of allantoic and amniotic membranes). DAVIS, L. AND ARIES, L. J. Surgery *2:*877–888, Dec '37

Influence of sympathectomy on homoplastic grafts. LEXER, E. W. Deutsche Ztschr. f. Chir. *249:*337–370, '37

Homogenous Thiersch grafting as life saving measure in burns. BETTMAN, A. G. Am. J. Surg. *39:*156–162, Jan '38

Homoplastic transplantations of human skin, with special consideration of blood characteristics. BINHOLD. Deutsche Ztschr. f. Chir. *252:*183–196, '39

Artificial vagina construction using fetal membranes. MARSALEK, J. Casop. lek. cesk. *79:*1075–1078, Dec 6, '40

Homotransplantation of skin of rabbit embryo into bone marrow. YANO, S. Tr. Soc. path. jap. *30:*746–747, '40

Regenerative power and possibilities of homograft. VILLAFANE, I. Z. Semana med. *1:*1197–1200, May 22, '41

Late results of double heterogenous graft performed in 1911. DUROUX, E. AND DUROUX, P. E. Progres med. *70:*140–145, March 7,

Skin Grafts, Homografts and Heterographs—Cont.

'42

Massive repairs with thick split-skin grafts; emergency "dressing" with homografts in burns. BROWN, J. B. AND McDOWELL, F. Ann. Surg. *115:*658-674, April '42

Epithelial healing and transplantation. BROWN, J. B. AND McDOWELL, F. Ann. Surg. *115:*1166-1181, June '42

Behavior of embryonic tissue transplanted into adult organism. SPEMANN, H. Arch. f. Entwckingsmechn. d. Organ. *141:*693-769, '42

Foreskin isografts. SACHS, A. E. AND GOLDBERG, S. L. Am. J. Surg. *60:*255-259, May '43

Fate of skin homografts in man. GIBSON, T. AND MEDAWAR, P. B., J. Anat. *77:*299-310, July '43

Problem of skin homografts. MEDAWAR, P. B. Bull. War Med. *4:*1-4, Sept '43

Heterologous transplantation of embryonic mammalian tissues. GREENE, H. S. N. Cancer Research *3:*809-822, Dec '43

Skin isograft transplants in identical twins. SCHATTNER, A. Arch. Otolaryng. *39:*521-522, June '44

Heterogenous grafts by coagulum contact method. HARRIS, H. I. Am. J. Surg. *65:*315-320, Sept '44

Experiments on heterotropic transplantation of skin. BRAUN, A. A. AND ORLOVA, G. N. Compt. rend. Acad. d. sc. URSS *47:*138-139, April 20, '45

Two rare cases of homoplastic surgery of eyelids. SHIMKIN, N. I. Brit. J. Ophth. *29:*363-369, July '45

Graft of cadaver skin; preliminary report. BIANCHI, R. G. Dia med. *17:*1168, Oct 8, '45 also: Prensa med. argent. *32:*1997, Oct 12, '45

Ectropion due to ichthyosis of both upper and lower lids on child corrected by homoplastic grafting of skin from child's mother. SHIMKIN, N. I. Harefuah *29:*155, Oct 1, '45

Homotransplantation of skin on denervated area. KUCHERENKO, Y. G. Med. zhur. *14:*283-285, '45

Immunity to homologous grafted skin; suppression of cell division in grafts transplanted to immunized animals. MEDAWAR, P. B. Brit. J. Exper. Path. *27:*9-14, Feb '46

Immunity to homologous grafted skin; relationship between antigens of blood and skin. MEDAWAR, P. B. Brit. J. Exper. Path. *27:*15-24, Feb '46

Relationship between antigens of blood and skin (grafts). MEDAWAR, P. B. Nature, London *157:*161-162, Feb 9, '46

Skin Grafts, Homografts and Heterographs—Cont.

Experiments with "cuto-omentopexy" and skin homotransplantation. MANDL, F. AND RABINOVICI, N. J. Internat. Coll. Surgeons *9:*525-530, Sept-Oct '46

Skin Grafts, Implantation

Implantation method of skin grafts. WANGENSTEEN, O. H. Surg., Gynec. and Obst. *50:*634-638, March '30

Skin grafting by implantation. CONNOLLY, E. A. Nebraska M. J. *15:*323-324, Aug '30

Implantation method of skin grafting. MACDERMOTT, E. N. Irish J. M. Sc., pp. 613-614, Nov '31

Implantation of skin grafts into muscular tissue. IMAKITA, T. Acta dermat. *20:*137-139, '32

Skin grafting by seed implantation. McPHEETERS, H. O. Minnesota Med. *17:*360-361, June '34

Histologic studies on fate of deeply implanted skin grafts; observations on sections of implants buried from one week to one year. PEER, L. A. AND PADDOCK, R. Arch. Surg. *34:*268-290, Feb '37

Use of implantation grafts in healing of infected ulcers. MARCKS, K. M. Am. J. Surg. *51:*354-361, Feb '41

Implant skin grafting; case in burns. HORTON, W. S. S. Am. J. Surg. *55:*597-599, March '42

Skin Grafts, Inlay

Arterial flaps and epithelial inserts in plastic surgery. ESSER, J. F. S. Munchen. med. Wchnschr. *69:*669-671, May 5, '22 (illus.)

Application of dental molding compound for maintenance of skin grafts in middle ear and mastoid cavities. ISRAEL, J. Ann. Otol. Rhinol. and Laryngol. *31:*543-545, June '22

Inlays in plastic nasal operations. ESSER, J. F. S. Munchen. med. Wchnschr. *69:*1154-1155, Aug 4, '22

Reconstruction of face by Esser's method of Thiersch flaps fitted on dentist's cast. ESSER, J. F. S. Zentralbl. f. Chir. *49:*1217-1219, Aug 19, '22 (illus.)

Use of dental stent in skin grafts of middle ear and mastoid cavities. DE RIVER, J. P., M. J. and Rec. *122:*63-64, July 15, '25

Use of moulages in application of skin grafts; 2 cases. ESSER, J. F. S. Presse med. *43:*1286-1288, Aug 14, '35

Value of epithelial inlays in general surgery. ESSER, J. F. S. Tech. chir. *27:*125-129, Aug-Sept '35

Difficulties in technic of epithelial inlay. Es-

Sking Grafts, Inlay – Cont.

SER, J. F. S. Rev. de chir. structive, pp. 127-132, Dec '35

Epithelial inlay in cases of refractory ectropion. ESSER, J. F. S. Arch. Ophth. *16:*55-57, July '36

Epithelial inlay graft in dentistry. ESSER, J. F. S. Am. J. Orthodontics *24:*1083-1090, Nov '38

Use of biologic flaps and Esser inlay to form chin and lip. PENHALE, K. W. AND ESSER, J. F. S., J. Am. Dent. A. *29:*1417-1420, Aug 1, '42

Esser inlays as practical auxiliary operation. ESSER, J. F. S., J. Internat. Coll. Surgeons *6:*208-211, May-June '43

Use of stents in skin grafting in mouth. BEDER, O. E., J. Oral Surg. *2:*32-38, Jan '44

Skin Grafts, Instruments for Cutting

Dermatome. HAGEN, G. L., J.A.M.A. *82:*1933, June 14, '24

New Thiersch graft razor. BETTMAN, A. G. J.A.M.A. *89:*451, Aug 6, '27

New instrument for use in skin grafting. BORS, E. Zentralbl. f. Chir. *54:*2890-2891, Nov 12, '27

New method of cutting large skin grafts (instrument). JOYNT, R. L. Lancet *1:*816, April 21, '28

Subcutaneous plates and knives for cutting large Thiersch grafts for plastic surgery. JOYNT, R. L. Irish J. M. Sc., pp. 700-702, Nov '28

Use and uses of large split-skin grafts of intermediate thickness. BLAIR, V. P., AND BROWN, J. B. Tr. South. S. A. *41:*409-424, '28 also: Surg., Gynec. and Obst. *49:*82-97, July '29

Technic for securing large flaps of epidermis. FLICK, K. Deutsche Ztschr. f. Chir. *222:*302-305, '30

New instrument for taking skin grafts. ALTRUDA, J. B., M. J. and Rec. *133:*348, April 1, '31

Instrument for skin grafts. SHAFIROFF, B. G. P. Ann. Surg. *101:*814-815, Feb '35

Instrument for obtaining Thiersch grafts. EYMER, H. Deutsche med. Wchnschr. *61:*1954-1955, Dec 6, '35

Instrument for pinch grafting. HAGGLAND, P. B. Am. J. Surg. *39:*171, Jan '38

New technic for cutting skin grafts, including description of new instruments. POTH, E. J. Surgery *6:*935-939, Dec '39

Double-edged knife for removing mucous membrane and skin grafts. BERENS, C. Tr. Sect. Ophth., A.M.A., p. 291, '40

Skin transplantation by injection; effect on

Skin Grafts, Instruments for Cutting – Cont.

healing of granulating wounds. BARBER, C. G. Arch. Surg. *43:*21-31, July '41

Three-fourths graft and other thicknesses cut with dermatome. PADGETT, E. C. AND SODERBERG, N. B. Dia med. *14:*8-11, Jan 5, '42

Simple instrument for cutting Thiersch flaps. MULLER-MEERNACH, O. Munchen. med. Wchnschr. *89:*591, June 26, '42

Use of Padgett dermatome to obtain grafts. ZENO, L. AND VERDAGUER, J. F. Bol. Soc. de cir. de Rosario *9:*211-214, July '42

Dermoepidermal grafts using Padgett dermatome; detail of technic. MARINO, H. Dia med. *14:*912-914, Sept 7, '42

Free grafts (called intermediate or transchorionic) using Padgett dermatome. PAVLOVSKY, A. J. AND HARRIS, M. M. Semana med. *2:*709-713, Sept 24, '42

Modified calibrated grafting knife. MARCKS, K. M. Mil. Surgeon *92:*653-654, June '43

Dermatome for cutting small grafts. WEBSTER, G. V., U. S. Nav. M. Bull. *41:*1145-1151, July '43

Grafts using Padgett dermatome. COVARRUBIAS ZENTENO, R. Rev. med. de Chile *71:*729-741, Aug '43

Free graft; advantages and inconveniences of dermatome. ZENO, L. Bol. y trab., Acad. argent. de cir. *28:*690-698, Aug 23, '44

New cement for use in cutting skin grafts. GERRIE, J. W. Canad. M. A. J. *51:*465-466, Nov '44

Instrument for obtaining split skin grafts. MCCALLA, L. H., J. South Carolina M. A. *40:*228, Nov '44

Board for cutting grafts of definite width. GABARRO, P. Lancet *2:*788, Dec 16, '44

Modified calibrated knife in skin grafting; further observations. MARCKS, K. M. Surgery *17:*109-115, Jan '45

Resplitting split-thickness skin grafts with dermatome; method for increasing yield of limited donor sites. ZINTEL, H. A. Ann. Surg. *121:*1-5, Jan '45

Lamination with dermatome and "split" grafts; method for increasing yield of limited donor regions. ZINTEL, H. A. Salud y belleza (no. 5) *1:*10-11; 39, Oct-Dec '45

Simple knife for skin grafts for general use. WEBSTER, G. V. Am. J. Surg. *67:*569-571, March '45

Instruments for dermoepidermal grafts. DELRIO, J. M. A. AND BULFARO, J. A. Bol. y trab., Soc. argent. de cirujanos *6:*745-748, '45 also: Rev. Asoc. med. argent. *59:*1328-1329, Nov 30, '45

New method for cutting full thickness or split thickness grafts. RITT, A. E. Minnesota Med. *29:*437, May '46

Skin Grafts, Instruments for Cutting – Cont.

Dermatape; new method for management of split grafts. REESE, J. D. Plast. and Reconstruct. Surg. *1:*98–105, July '46

Dermatome. TAULLARD, J. C. Bol. y trab., Soc. argent. de circjanos *7:*30–38, '46 also: Rev. Asoc. med. argent. *60:*248–251, April 30, '46

Skin Grafts to Larynx

Stenosis of larynx; laryngofissure and skin graft. FIGI, F. A., S. Clin. North America *11:*837–840, Aug '31

Traumatic stenosis of trachea treated by skin grafting. HARRISON, W. J. Brit. M. J. *2:*811, Oct 24, '36

Treatment of chronic laryngeal stenosis, with special reference to skin grafting. NEGUS, V. E. Ann. Otol., Rhin. and Laryng. *47:*891–901, Dec '38

Treatment of chronic laryngeal stenosis, with special reference to skin grafting. NEGUS, V. E. Tr. Am. Laryng. A. *60:*82–92, '38

Chronic laryngeal stenosis, with special consideration of skin grafting. FIGI, F. A. Ann. Otol., Rhin. and Laryng. *49:*394–409, June '40

Excision of amyloid tumor of larynx and skin graft; case. FIGI, F. A. Proc. Staff Meet., Mayo Clin. *17:*239–240, April 15, '42

Plastic procedure in correction of laryngotracheostenosis with dermoepidermic skin grafts. RAPIN, M. Pract. oto-rhino-laryng. *4:*88–91, '42

Skin grafting in case of chronic laryngeal stenosis. MOORE, P. M. Cleveland Clin. Quart. *11:*5–8, Jan '44

Skin Grafts to Leg (See also Burns; Leg Ulcer)

Skin grafts in treatment of chronic leg ulcer. TIXIER, L. AND BIZE, P. R. Monde med., Paris *37:*449–455, April 1, '27

Repair of large wound of calf by means of graft taken from thigh. L'HEUREUX, M. Bull. et mem. Soc. nat. de chir. *53:*722, May 28, '27

Contracture from burn with extensive ulcer in popliteal space; excision and full-thickness skin graft. JONES, H. T., S. Clin. N. America *7:*1447–1449, Dec '27

Skin grafts on extremities. PIERI, G. Arch. ital. di chir. *18:*607–621, '27

Good results of combined periarterial sympathectomy and skin grafts on leg; 24 cases. LERICHE, R. AND FONTAINE, R. Strasbourgh-med. (pt. 2) *86:*101–105, April 20, '28

Extensive chronic ulceration on leg; success-

Skin Grafts to Leg – Cont.

ful treatment by autoplastic skin grafts. SANTY, P. Lyon chir. *26:*456–457, May-June '29

Radical repair of large skin defects with particular reference to leg ulcers (grafts). DOUGLAS, B., South. M. J. *24:*53–58, Jan '31

Histological verification of efficacy of free transplantation of nipple. THOREK, M., M. J. and Rec. *134:*474–476, Nov 18, '31

Phagedenic ulcer of lower leg with subjacent osteitis and extensive tissue loss; cure by autodermic graft and later anesthesia of articular ligaments according to Leriche; case. DUMAS, J. M. R. Marseille-med. *1:*553–556, April 25, '32

Therapy of slowly-healing crural ulcers by "circumcision," i.e. by transplantation of active epithelium. BÜTTNER, G. Zentralbl. f. Chir. *59:*2530–2531, Oct 15, '32

Therapy of slowly-healing crural ulcers by "circumcision," i.e., by transplantation of active epithelium. BÜTTNER, G. Zentralbl. f. Chir. *59:*3092, Dec 29, '32 (Addendum)

Therapy of so-called varicose syndrome, with special reference to sympathectomy and grafts. JENTZER, A. Rev. med. de la Suisse Rom. *53:*482–532, June 25, '33

Surgical treatment of trophic ulcers of leg and foot; autoplastic operation by Italian method, periarterial sympathectomy, lumbar sympathetic ganglionectomy and ramisection. ROMITI, C. Tr. Roy. Soc. Trop. Med. and Hyg. *27:*185–194, July '33

Ulcer of leg, resistant to therapy, cured by cutaneous autotransplant; case. RODRÍGUEZ DE MATA. Actas Soc. de cir. de Madrid *3:*53–56, Oct-Dec '33

Traumatic ulcer of leg resisting all therapy, finally cured by autoplastic skin graft; case. RODRÍGUEZ DE MATA. Rev. espan. de cir. *16:*105–108, March-April '34

Therapy of large ulcers of leg with Thiersch grafts. ORTHNER, F. Wien. klin. Wchnschr. *47:*1047–1048, Aug 24, '34

Late results of therapy of leg ulcers by sympathectomy combined with skin grafts; study based on 52 cases. LERICHE, R. *et al.* J. de chir. *45:*689–710, May '35

Perifemoral sympathectomy and skin grafts in therapy of leg ulcers; cases. LEFRANCOIS, C. Union med. du Canada *65:*214–219, March '36

Repair of ulcerations of lower extremity with thick split skin grafts. BROWN, J. B. *et al.* Surg., Gynec. and Obst. *63:*331–340, Sept '36

Treatment of chronic varicose ulcers of lower

Skin Grafts to Leg—Cont.

extremities (grafting). OWENS, N. New Orleans M. and S. J. *89:*483–491, March '37

Periarterial sympathectomy and Thiersch graft in therapy of varicose veins. AREL, F. Turk tib cem. mec. *3:*394–395, '37

Therapy of inveterate ulcers of leg by excision followed by immediate dermo-epidermic graft; cases. GOINARD, P. Algerie med. (Ed. chir.) *42:*75–81, Feb '38

Total excision of skin of leg in elephantiasis and closure of defect with Thiersch graft. GERGENREDER, F. A. Vestnik khir. *55:*603–609, May '38

Ulceration of lower extremities and grafts. BROWN, J. B. *et al.* Am. J. Surg. *43:*452–457, Feb '39

Plastic repair of leg ulcers (skin grafting). BURSTEIN, T., M. Rec. *150:*307–308, Nov 1, '39

Early skin grafting in war wounds of extremities. CONVERSE, J. M. Ann. Surg. *115:*321–335, March '42

Braun graft in therapy of varicose ulcers; histopathologic evolution of graft. DE OLIVEIRA MATOS, J. Arq. de cir. clin. e exper. *6:*653–669, April–June '42

Trophic necrosis, skin grafting and vitamin C (in 2 cases of leg ulcers). EVANS, G. Brit. M. J. *1:*788, June 26, '43

Giant epithelioma of lower extremity; roentgenotherapy and Reverdin grafts; case. CAMPOS MARTIN, R. AND USUA MARINE, J. Actas dermo-sif. *34:*747–750, June '43

Dermoepidermal grafts in therapy of ulcers of legs. ALARCON, C. J. AND GENATIOS, T. Rev. san. y asist. social *8:*783–796, Aug '43

Giant nevus of thigh successfully treated by complete excision and primary grafting. PICKRELL, K. L. AND CLAY, R. C. Arch. Surg. *48:*319–324, April '44

Skin graft to cover defects in short stump of leg; modified technic. SMIRNOVA, L. A. Khirurgiya, No. 1, pp. 27–28, '45

Penicillin for ulcers of leg treated by pinch grafts. NOMLAND, R. AND WALLACE, E. G. J.A.M.A. *130:*563–564, March 2, '46

Severe septic wound of left lower leg treated with small deep grafts; case. HUMPHRIES, S. V. South African M. J. *20:*472–473, Aug 24, '46

Treatment of loss skin substance in surgery of extremities. DUCHET, G. Semaine d. hop. Paris *22:*1671–1680, Sept 21, '46

Covering defects of popliteal space with skin grafts. SCHURCH, O. Schweiz. med. Wchnschr. *76:*1040–1041, Oct 5, '46

Venous surgery (skin transplantation for stasis ulcers). CARROLL, W. W. Quart. Bull., Northwestern Univ. M. School *20:*373–379, '46

Skin Grafts of Mastoid

New method for skin grafting mastoid cavity; new method for closing off Eustachian tube at its tympanic end in radical mastoid operation. KAHN, A. Laryngoscope *37:*889–893, Dec '27

Favorable results with primary skin transplantation in radical operation of middle ear. TEMKIN, J. Ztschr. f. hals-, Nasen-u. Ohrenh. *22:*467–474, Feb 16, '29

End-results in 20 cases of primary skin grafts in radical mastoidectomies. CUNNING, D. S. Laryngoscope *41:*484–486, July '31

Radical mastoid graft. ROBISON, J. T. Texas State J. Med. *29:*525–528, Dec '33

Repair of postauricular fistula following radical mastoidectomy (grafting). STRAATSMA, C. R. Arch. Otolaryng. *19:*616–618, May '34

Transplantation of epidermal flaps by Pontoppidan method in radical surgery in otitis media. VON MAGNUS, R. Ztschr. f. Laryng., Rhin., Otol. *25:*48–52, '34

Series of cases of radical mastoidectomy with skin graft. CUNNING, D. S. Laryngoscope *45:*76–781, Oct '35

Primary Thiersch grafting in radical mastodectomies, with description of new modified technic. LIU, J. H. AND HSU, Y. H. Chinese M. J. *55:*343–356, April '39

Skin graft in closure of retro-auricular fistulas. MATIS, I. Medicina, Kaunas *21:*1027–1031, Dec '40

Secondary endaural grafting of cavity resulting from radical mastoidectomy. HAGAN, C. E., JR. Arch. Otolaryng. *34:*1029–1033, Nov '41

Skin Grafts to Mouth

Skin-grafting in buccal cavity. KILNER, T. P. AND JACKSON, T. Brit. J. Surg. *9:*148, July '21

Case of skin plastic operation for mucous membrane replacement in mouth. SMYTHE, G. J. C., S. African M. Rec. *24:*408–409, Sept 25, '26

Ankylosis of mandible due to scarring of cheek; restoration of cheek lining with skin graft. KIRCH, W. Proc. Staff Meet., Mayo Clin. *5:*339–341, Nov 26, '30

Skin grafting in mouth; 2 cases. FIGI, F. A. Proc. Staff Meet., Mayo Clin. *9:*740–742, Dec 5, '34

Free skin grafts in restoration of defects of conjunctiva, oral mucous membranes and cutaneous defects of nasal fossae. LIM-

Skin Grafts to Mouth—Cont.
BERG, A. A. Sovet. khir. (nos. 3–4) *6:*462–482, '34
Transplantation of skin into oral cavity. ZHAKOV, M. P. Novy khir. arkhiv. *35:*573–577, '36
Use of stents in skin grafting in mouth. BEDER, O. E., J. Oral Surg. *2:*32–38, Jan '44
Covering extensive defects of chin and floor of mouth following gunshot wounds. LINDENBAUM, L. M. Vrach. delo (nos. 7–8) *26:*469–474, '46

Skin Grafts to Neck
Evaluation of pedicle flaps versus skin grafts in reconstruction of surface defects and scar contractures of chin, cheeks and neck. AUFRICHT, G. Surgery *15:*75–84, Jan '44
Epithelial inlay for scars in neck dragging lower jaw downwards. ESSER, J. F. S. Am. J. Surg. *45:*148–149, July '39
Use of abdominal skin to correct cervical defect due to burn. GABARRO, P. Rev. Fac. de med., Bogota *10:*339–342, Oct '41

Skin Grafts, Nerve Regeneration in
Histologic observations on regeneration of sensory nerve fibres in skin transplantations. KADANOFF, D. Klin. Wchnschr. *4:*1266, June 25, '25
Recuperation of innervation in skin transplants. POLISSADOWA, X. Zentralbl. f. Chir. *52:*2166–2168, Sept 26, '25
Processes of regeneration in nerve fibers of transplanted skin. MASUMOTO, K. Tr. Jap. Path. Soc. *22:*876–877, '32
Regeneration of nerve fibers in transplanted skin; experimental study. MASUMOTO, K. Mitt. a. d. med. Akad. zu Kioto *7:*1036–1038, '33
Regeneration of nerves in grafts and flaps. DAVIS, J. S. AND KITLOWSKI, E. A. Am. J. Surg. *24:*501–545, May '34
Return of sensation to transplanted skin. DAVIS, L. Surg., Gynec. and Obst. *59:*533–543, Sept '34
Regeneration of sensation in transplanted skin. MCCARROLL, H. R. Ann. Surg. *108:*309–320, Aug '38
Recovery of sympathetic nerve function in skin transplants. KREDEL, F. E. AND PHEMISTER, D. B. Arch. Neurol. and Psychiat. *42:*403–412, Sept '39

Skin Grafts to Nose
Correction of nasal deformities (including skin grafts). SHEEHAN, J. E. Virginia M. Monthly *54:*138–141, June '27

Skin Grafts to Nose—Cont.
Traumatic loss of substance of nostril; rhinoplasty with dermo-epidermic graft. ROY, J. N. Arch. Otolaryng. *7:*601–605, June '28 also: J. Laryng. and Otol. *43:*490–495, July '28
Loss of substance in nostril; rhinoplasty with skin graft; case. ROY, J. N., Ann. d. mal. de l'oreille, du larynx *47:*571–576, June '28 also: Union med. du Canada *57:*505–510, Sept '28
Technic of total rhinoplasty in which portions of abdominal skin are used. TROFIMOW, A. M. Arch. f. klin. Chir. *163:*681–692, '31
Reconstruction of nasal tip, wings and septum by T-shaped graft from neck. LIMBERG, A. A. Novy khir. arkhiv *28:*147–163, '33
Pilous verrucous pigmentary nevus of nose; autoplasty using Thiersch graft. ROY, J. N. Union med. du Canada *66:*945–948, Sept '37
Pilous verrucous pigmented nevus of nose; autoplasty using Thiersch graft; case. ROY, J. N. Rev. argent. de oto-rhino-laring. *7:*53–57, March–April '38
Reconstruction of nasal lobule, using skin graft. BAMES, H. O. An. de cir. *4:*224–229, Sept '38
Loss of cutaneous substance of nasal pyramid; skin grafts in therapy. RIVAS, C. I. Rev. Asoc. med. argent. *54:*167–169, March 15–30, '40
Free graft of closely sutured skin in small rhinoplasties. ZENO, L. Bol. Soc. de cir. de Rosario *8:*361–365, Oct '41 also: An. de cir. *7:*295–299, Dec '41
Epithelioma of nose; free graft of whole skin; case. MALBEC, E. F. Prensa med. argent. *29:*1763–1765, Nov 4, '42

Skin Grafts to Orbit
Plastic surgery of orbital cavity with dermo-epidermal grafts. WORMS, G. Bull. Soc. d'opht. de Paris, pp. 358–361, June '32
Construction of artificial conjunctival sac by free transplantation of epidermis as preliminary to prosthesis. HERSCHENDÖRFER, A. Ztschr. f. Augenh. *84:*284–292, Nov '34
Fixation of artificial eye in conjunctival sac made of skin graft. CSAPODY, I. Budapesti orvosi ujsag *33:*337–43, April 11, '35
Restoration of orbit and repair of conjunctival defects, with grafts from prepuce and labia minora. CLAY, G. E. AND BAIRD, J. M. J.A.M.A. *107:*1122–1125, Oct 3, '36
Restoration of eye socket with Thiersch graft; 6 cases. LIN, C. K. Chinese M. J. *50:*1335–1344, Oct '36

Skin Grafts to Orbit—Cont.

Restoration of orbit and repair of conjunctival defects, with grafts from prepuce and labia minora. CLAY, G. E. AND BAIRD, J. M. Tr. Sect. Ophth., A.M.A., pp. 252–259, '36

Skin grafting after enucleation of eye; case. MOERS. Rev. de chir. structive, pp. 119–120, June '37

Plastic construction of artificial conjunctival sac using skin flaps. CSAPODY, I. Orvosi hetil. *81:*1217–1219, Dec 4, '37

Total symblepharon after enucleation of eye; remaking of orbital cavity for ocular prosthesis by means of dermo-epidermic graft; case. JEANDELIZE, P. AND THOMAS, C. Bull. Soc. d'opht. de Paris *50:*272, May '38

Epithelial inlay with Kerr-material to form eye socket. CZUKRASZ, I. Brit. J. Ophth. *23:*343–347, May '39

Use of ocular prosthesis during plastic reconstruction of conjunctival sac with free cutaneous or mucous graft. NEYMAN, V. N. Vestnik oftal. (no. 5) *14:*45–46, '39

Eye socket reconstruction; new form and method of handling skin graft. HUGHES, W. L. Arch. Ophth. *26:*965–968, Dec '41

New method and appliance for grafting eye sockets. PICKERILL, H. P. Brit. M. J. *1:*596, April 28, '45

Choice of grafts for orbital reconstruction MACKENZIE, C. M. Am. J. Ophth. *29:*867–869, July '46

Skin Grafts to Penis

Genitoplasty; restitution of skin of penis and of scrotum by autograft; restitution of function after trauma. KENNY, T. B. AND MERELLO, M. Prensa med. argent. *15:*1549–1560, May 30, '29

Phalloplasty after traumatic loss of skin of penis. MEYER, H. Arch. f. Orthop. *27:*437–442, July 18, '29

Plastic operation; avulsion of skin of penis; good functional results of graft of scrotum. VADI, E. Bol. Asoc. med. de Puerto Rico *22:*25/26, Sept-Oct '29

Plastic repair of penis by autografts. NEUMANN, A. G. Rev. med. del Rosario *22:*292–299, May '32

Complete removal of foreskin by factory machine; plastic replacement; case. TAKASHIMA, R. AND KUSANO, M. Zentralbl. f. Chir. *63:*84–86, Jan 11, '36

Restoration of the entire skin of the penis. BROWN, J. B. Surg., Gynec., and Obst. *65:*362–365, '37

Phalloplasty; technic of skin grafting in avulsion of skin of penis and scrotum; review of literature and report of case. AGOSTINELLI, E. Policlinico (sez. prat.) *46:*1303–1306, July 17, '39

Avulsion of scrotum and skin of penis; technic of delayed and immediate repair (using skin grafts). BYARS, L. T. Surg., Gynec. and Obst. *77:*326–329, Sept '43

Skin Grafts, Pigmentation of

Pigmentation and transplantation of skin. FESSLER, A. Brit. J. Dermat. *53:*201–214, July '41

Skin graft pigment studies in experimental animals. LEWIN, M. L. AND PECK, S. M., J. Invest. Dermat. *4:*483–504, Dec '41

Skin Grafts, Pinch (Reverdin)

Successful skin graft with a slight modification of Reverdin method. WEHLE, F. Med. Rec. *101:*587–588, April 8, '22

Closure of granulating wounds with Reverdin-Halsted grafts. SCHLAEPFER, K. Bull. Johns Hopkins Hosp. *34:*114–118, April '23 (illus.) also: Beitr. z. klin. Chir. *129:*162–174, '23 abstr: J.A.M.A. *80:*1884, June 23, '23

Small deep graft (skin); experiences and results of last 3 years. CASSEGRAIN, O. C. Surg., Gynec. and Obst. *38:*557–559, April '24

Case of Reverdin skin grafting exhibited in Dr. Halsted's clinic on wound healing. BRÖDEL, M. Bull. Johns Hopkins Hosp. *36:*60, Jan '25

Reverdin's method of skin grafting; case. FRASER, N. D. China M. J. *41:*364–365, April '27

Halsted-Davis skin grafts; indications and results. DEGIRARDIER, J. Lyon med. *140:*117, Aug. 7; 145, Aug 14, '27

Small deep graft; development; relationship to true Reverdin graft; technic. DAVIS, J. S. Tr. South. S. A. *41:*395–408, '28

Small deep graft; relationship to true Reverdin graft. DAVIS, J. S. Ann. Surg. *89:*902–916, June '29

Small deep skin graft. DAVIS, J. S. Ann. Surg. *91:*633–635, April '30

Reverdin grafts, with report of 2 cases. SHIH, H. E. Nat. M. J., China *16:*563–571, Oct '30

Loss of cutaneous substance in ulceration of thigh cured by Davies graft. DESJACQUES, R. AND MILLET. Lyon med. *152:*222–223, Aug 27, '33

Modified technic of application of Davis grafts in extensive burns. DANTLO, R. Rev. de chir. plastique, pp. 219–237, Oct '33

Reverdin-Ollier-Davis method of skin grafting. IVANOV, S. Vestnik khir. *34:*107–112,

Skin Grafts, Pinch (Reverdin) – Cont.
'34
Possible uses of Reverdin skin flap for plastic surgery, primarily for covering skin defects, and secondarily for scar contractures. EHALT, W. Munchen. med. Wchnschr. *82:*669-671, April 25, '35
New technic for obtaining small deep grafts. ZEE, Z. U. Chinese M. J. *50:*935-938, July '36
Use of small skin grafts for treating recent injuries of nail bed. RÖPER, W. Zentralbl. f. Chir. *64:*2679-2681, Nov 20, '37
Carcinoma developing on extensive scars; inefficiency of pinch grafts as prophylactic measure. DANZIS, M. *et al.* Am. J. Surg. *41:*304-306, Aug '38
Pinch graft. VOKOUN, F. J. Mil. Surgeon *83:*442-443, Nov '38
Use of small deep grafts in repair of surface defects. DAVIS, J. S. Am. J. Surg. *47:*280-298, Feb '40
Reverdin grafts in therapy of extensive defects. KRATOCHVIL, K. Deutsche Ztschr. f. Chir. *256:*309-358, '42
Rare case of horny epithelioma on burn cicatrix; surgical extirpation and plastic repair of residual defect by free skin graft of Davis type. HALLEY MIRALLES, G. Bol. Liga. contra el cancer *18:*41-46, Feb '43
Treatment of large stasis ulcers by pinch grafts. RINGROSE, E. J., J. Iowa M. Soc. *33:*175-178, April '43
Reverdin mosaic grafts. SCHERER, F. Deutsche Ztschr. f. Chir. *258:*42, '43
Davis grafts in reparative surgery of face. FERRIE, J. Ophthalmologica *110:*292-299, Nov-Dec '45
Microscopically verified success of pinch homografting in human case. MANDL, F. AND RABINOVICI, N., J. Internat. Coll. Surgeons *9:*439-446, July-Aug '46
Postage stamp grafts; technic and results. BEAUX, A. R. Bol. y trab., Soc. argent. de cirujanos *7:*355-362, '46 also: Rev. Asoc. med. argent. *60:*587-589, July 15, '46

Skin Grafts, Preservation of

Transplantation of skin preserved in fluids. NAVA VERA. Arch. per le sc. med. *52:*236-242, May '28
Experimental and clinical study of transplantation of tissues preserved in alcohol or formalin solution. HOSOMI, K. Deutsche Ztschr. f. Chir. *209:*14-30, '28
Transplantation of preserved skin in experimental cutaneous tuberculosis. GLEYBERMAN, E. Y. Med. zhur. *10:*269-275, '40
Further data on therapeutic value of preserved tissue, especially in ocular diseases; transplantation of tissues and use of placental microclysters; preliminary report. FILATOV, V. P. Gaz. clin. *39:*292-295, Aug '41
Autoimplantation of preserved skin in therapy of trachomatous pannus. KOTELNIKOV, F. S. AND MELNIK, D. A. Vestnik oftal. *18:*390-393, '41
Grafts of refrigerated skin; Filatov graft. DELLEPIANE RAWSON, R. Dia med. *15:*1150-1151, Oct 4, '43
Successful grafting of frozen and thawed mouse skin. BRIGGS, R. AND JUND, L. Anat. Rec. *89:*75-85, May '44
Refrigerated skin grafts. WEBSTER, J. P. Ann. Surg. *120:*431-449, Oct '44
Refrigerated grafts of skin. WEBSTER, J. P. Tr. Am. S. A. *62:*431-449, '44
Storage of skin for autogenous grafts (Hunterian lecture, abridged). MATTHEWS, D. N. Lancet *1:*775-778, June 23, '45
Frozen skin grafts (human). STRUMIA, M. M. AND HODGE, C. C. Ann. Surg. *121:*860-865, June '45

Skin Grafts to Scalp

Restoration of scalp; management of skin grafts. HOLMAN, E., J.A.M.A. *84:*350-352, Jan 31, '25
Avulsion of scalp; skin grafting; with report of unusual case. NORTHCUTT, J. D. Kentucky M. J. *23:*493-497, Oct '25
Method of repair of scalp defects (grafts). COLEMAN, E. P. Illinois M. J. *49:*40-43, Jan '26
Treatment of fungus cerebri by skin graft with report of case. KUMM, C. China M. J. *40:*1126-1132, Nov '26
Avulsion of scalp; treatment by dermo-epidermic grafts; case. MOURE, P. Bull. et mem. Soc. nat. de chir. *53:*1040-1043, July 16, '27
Avulsion of scalp, skin grafting for complete. HAGGARD, W. D., S. Clin. N. Amer. *10:*719-723, Aug '30
Skin-grafting in complete avulsion of scalp. MALLIK, K. L. B. Indian M. Gaz. *66:*86-88, Feb '31
Avulsion of scalp, treated by large free skin flaps by "grate" or "sieve" method; case. DIAZ INFANTE, A. Medicina, Mexico *17:*107-114, March 10, '37
Hernia cerebri treated by Thiersch grafts. WRIGHT, A. D. Proc. Roy. Soc. Med. *32:*213-214, Jan '39
Treatment of major cranial wounds; cerebral fungus; skin grafting. HYNDMAN, O. R.

Skin Grafts to Scalp—Cont.
Surgery *11:*466–471, March '42
Immediate covering of denuded area of skull. DORRANCE, G. M. AND BRANSFIELD, J. W. Am. J. Surg. *58:*236–239, Nov '42
Scalping treated with free skin grafts. COVARRUBIAS ZENTENO, R. Arch. Soc. cirujanos hosp. *13:*115–118, Sept '43
Total avulsion of scalp; review of problem with presentation of case of skin graft in which thrombin plasma fixation was used. STRAITH, C. L. AND MCEVITT, W. G. Occup. Med. *1:*451–462, May '46

Skin Grafts, Sieve

Sieve graft—stable transplant for covering large skin defects. DOUGLAS, B. Surg., Gynec. and Obst. *50:*1018–1023, June '30
Full thickness grafts (with special reference to Douglas "sieve graft"). HORSLEY, J. S. JR. Internat. S. Digest *16:*67–82, Aug '33
Modified sieve graft; full thickness graft for covering large defects. DRAGSTEDT, L. R. AND WILSON, H. Surg., Gynec. and Obst. *65:*104–106, July '37
Immediate and late results of free transplantation in form of perforated flap; preliminary report. PARIN, B. V. Khirurgiya, no. 12, pp. 21–29, '44

Skin Grafts, Split (Thiersch)

Correction of scar tissue deformities by epithelial grafts, report of 5 cases (including eyelids). SPAETH, E. B. Arch. Surg. *2:*176, Jan '21
Case for Thiersch skin-grafting. MEYER, H. W., S. Clin. N. Amer. *1:*1650, Dec '21
Thiersch graft in radical cure of frontal sinus and maxillary antrum diseases; its further application to tonsil and gingival sulci. SHEEHAN, J. E. Surg., Gynec. and Obst. *35:*358–360, Sept '22 (illus.)
New technique in application of Thiersch skin grafts. MCLELLAN, D. Canad. M. A. J. *15:*908–910, Sept '25
Thiersch grafts; 2 technical points. HOFFMANN, R. Schweiz. med. Wchnschr. *56:*816–817, Aug 21, '26
Whole thickness dermo-epidermal grafts. NEWLAND, H. S., J. Coll. Surgeons, Australasia *1:*62–64, July '28
End-result in Thiersch graft; case observed after 30 years. WILLIAMS, G. A. Arch. Surg. *16:*938–941, April '28
Technic and value of Thiersch's method of skin grafting. HAYWARD. Med. Klin. *25:*1435–1437, Sept 13, '29
Use and uses of large split-skin grafts of intermediate thickness. BLAIR, V. P. AND

Skin Grafts, Split (Thiersch)—Cont.
BROWN, J. B. Tr. South. S. A. *41:*409–424, '28 also: Surg., Gynec. and Obst. *49:*82–97, July '29
Thiersch grafts. ESAU, P. Zentralbl. f. Chir. *57:*1780–1783, July 19, '30
Use of Thiersch skin flaps in treatment of recent wounds of arms. FLICK, K. Deutsche Ztschr. f. Chir. *222:*331–334, '30
Method of drying surface of wound before application of Thiersch grafts. LAPP, F. W. AND NEUFFER, H. Zentralbl. f. Chir. *58:*1634–1635, June 27, '31
Newer methods of Thiersch grafting. KISKADDEN, W. S. West. J. Surg. *39:*758–762, Oct '31
Free skin grafts of less than full thickness; causes for failure or success. WOOLSEY, J. H. California and West. Med. *36:*334–337, May '32
Transplantation of epidermis (Thiersch grafts). KIRSCHNER. Acta chir. Scandinav. *72:*21–35, '32
Technic for care of Ollier-Thiersch grafts. LEITHAUSER, D. J. Ann. Surg. *97:*311–313, Feb '33
Thiersch grafts. EISELSBERG, A. Wien. klin. Wchnschr. *46:*1179, Sept 29, '33
Secondary Thiersch grafting of radical mastoid cavity through meatus. DAGGETT, W. I. AND BATEMAN, G. H., J. Laryng. and Otol. *49:*169–174, March '34
Thiersch graft; preparation and uses. KILNER, T. P. Post-Grad. M. J. *10:*176–181, May '34
Thiersch method of skin grafting. OMAR BEY, T., J. Egyptian M. A. *17:*654, July '34
Application of Thiersch graft to special areas. KILNER, T. P. Post-Grad. M. J. *10:*317–322, Sept '34
Repair of surface defects, from burns and other causes, with thick split skin grafts. BROWN, J. B. *et al.* South. M. J. *28:*408, May; 529, June '35
Cosmetic results obtained by use of Thiersch technic of skin grafting. HSU, H. A. Chinese M. J. *40:*939–944, July '36
Split skin graft. HAMM, W. G., J. M. A. Georgia *26:*495–500, Oct '37
Pigmentary verrucous pilous nasal nevus; autoplasty by means of Thiersch graft; case. ROY, J. N. Rev. de chir. structive, pp. 180–184, Oct '37
Advantage of production and fixation of nearly full thickness skin graft. HUMBY, G. Rev. de chir. structive, pp. 274–276, Dec '37
Calibrated intermediate skin grafts. PADGETT, E. C. Surg., Gynec. and Obst. *69:*779–

Skin Grafts, Split (Thiersch) – Cont.
793, Dec '39
Eudermic grafts in plastic surgery. COMEL, M. Plast. chir. *1:*78–88, '39
Use of Thiersch graft. RANK, B. K. Brit. M. J. *1:*846–849, May 25, '40
Skin grafting and "three quarter" thickness skin graft for prevention and correction of cicatricial formation. PADGETT, E. C. Ann. Surg. *113:*1034–1049, June '41
Blanket split skin graft for covering large granulating areas. MCPHEETERS, H. O. AND NELSON, H., J.A.M.A. *117:*1173–1174, Oct 4, '41
Improved skin graft according to Thiersch. ZIELKE Deut. Militararzt *9:*51, Jan '44
Skin transplantation with especial reference to split thickness graft. CARMICHAEL, J. L. J. M. A. Alabama *14:*11–13, July '44
Dermatome skin grafts in patients prepared with dry dressings and with and without penicillin. LEVENSON, S. M. AND LUND, C. C. New England J. Med. *233:*607–612, Nov 22, '45
Surgical principles of split thickness grafts LEVETON, A. L., J. Bone and Joint Surg. *28:*699–715, Oct '46
Indications for determination of thickness for split grafts. PADGETT, E. C. Am. J. Surg. *72:*683–693, Nov '46

Skin Grafts, Sweating of

Reestablishment of function of sweat glands in grafted skin. GUTTMANN, L. Dermat. Ztschr. *77:*73–77, Feb '38
Sweating function of transplanted skin. CONWAY, H. Surg., Gynec. and Obst. *69:*756–761, Dec '39

Skin Graft to Vagina: See Vagina

Skin Tumors

Research on melanomas of skin. HALKIN, H. Ann. de med. *12:*189–225, Sept '22 (illus.) abstr: J.A.M.A. *79:*1722, Nov 11, '22
Indications for technic of radium treatment of cutaneous angiomas. WALLON, E. Presse med. *37:*803–804, June 19, '29
Pigmented growths of skin; their significance and treatment. CANNON, A. B. New York State J. Med. *29:*857–864, July 15, '29
Present opinion about malignant melanotic tumors of skin and their most suitable treatment. FRANKENTHAL, L. Arch. f. klin. Chir. *166:*678–693, '31
Cavernous hemangioma of skin; radium therapy in infants. RATTI, A. Gior. ital. di dermat. e sif. *73:*1430–1436, Aug '32
Angiomas of skin; therapy. PÉRIN, L. Rev.

Skin Tumors – Cont.
franc. de dermat. et de venereol. *10:*27–39, Jan '34
Angiomas of skin in infants; therapy. HARRENSTEIN, R. J. Maandschr. v. kindergeneesk. *3:*388–395, July '34
Melanoma of skin. BECKER, S. W. Am. J. Cancer *22:*17–40, Sept '34
Nevocarcinoma of skin and mucous membranes. WILLIAMS, I. G. AND MARTIN, L. C. Lancet *1:*135–138, Jan 16, '37
Cutaneous melanoma; 2 cases alive 30 and 38 years after operation. PRINGLE, J. H. Lancet *1:*508–509, Feb 27, '37
Rare case of cornu cutaneum humanum of forehead. EMILIADIS, K. Zentralbl. f. Chir. *64:*727–728, March 27, '37
Treatment of hemangiomas of skin in children by carbon dioxide snow. WRONG, N. M. Canad. M. A. J. *41:*571–572, Dec '39
Radiation treatment of hemangioma of skin. SPENCER, J. Am. J. Roentgenol. *46:*220–223, Aug '41
Clinical problems of tumors of skin. ROUSSY, G. *et al.* Presse med. *50:*193–196, Feb 24, '42
Treatment of congenital hemangiomata of skin. JOHNSON, G. S. AND LIGHT, R. A. Ann. Surg. *117:*134–139, Jan '43

SKINNER, H. G. AND WAUD, R. A.: Plastic film (containing sulfonamides) in treatment of experimental burns. Canad. M. A. J. *48:*13–18, Jan '43
SKINNER, H. L.: Operative correction of Dupuytren's contracture by use of tunnel skin graft. Surgery *10:*313–317, Aug '41
SKINNER, H. L. AND ROBINSON, R. L.: Nonunion in fracture of mandible, with report of case. J. Oral Surg. *1:*162–167, April '43
SKINNER, M.: Surgical treatment of harelip and cleft palate. J. M. A. Alabama *2:*253–259, Jan '33
SKOSOGORENKO, G. F.: Cutaneous cone (artificially produced closed necrobiotic focus) as method of nonspecific therapy replacing grafts; preliminary report. Vrach. delo (no. 2) *23:*113–118, '41
SKUBISZEWSKI, L.: Growth of transplanted embryonal tissue and origin of neoplasms. Compt. rend. Soc. de biol. *93:*1398–1400, Dec 4, '25
SKUBISZEWSKI, L.: Growth of transplanted embryonal tissue and its significance with regard to origin of tumors. Ztschr. f. Krebsforsch. *26:*308–329, '28
SKUES, K. F.: Complications associated with treatment of fractures of mandible. Roy. Melbourne Hosp. Clin. Rep. *10:*123–126, Dec '39

SLATTERY, L. R. (see SAYPOL, G. M.) Nov '44
SLAUGHTER, W. B. AND WONG, W.: Early management of facial injuries. S. Clin. North America *26:*2-19, Feb '46
SLAUGHTER, W. B. (see STRAITH, C. L.) May '41
SLO-BODKIN, S. G.: Ocular hypertelorism. Arch. Pediat. *53:*191-196, March '36
SLOCUM, D. B.: Stabilization of articulation of greater multangular and first metacarpal. J. Bone and Joint Surg. *25:*626-630, July '43
SLOCUM, D. B. AND PRATT, D. R.: Principles of amputations of fingers and hand. J. Bone and Joint Surg. *26:*535-546, July '44
SLOCUM, H. C. AND ALLEN, C. R.: Orotracheal anesthesia for cheiloplasty. Anesthesiology *6:*355-358, July '45
SLOME, D. (see HOLT, R. L. *et al*) Sept '35
SLOT, G. M. J.: Ammonia gas burns; account of 6 cases. Lancet *2:*1356-1357, Dec 10, '38
SLUDER, F. S. (see COUNSELLER, V. S.) Aug '44
SMALL, J. M. AND GRAHAM, M. P.: Acrylic resin (methyl methacrylate) for closure of defects; preliminary report. Brit. J. Surg. *33:*106-113, Oct '45
SMART, F. P.: Wounds of eye, ear, nose and throat. U. S. Nav. M. Bull. *44:*1231-1233, June '45
SMERETCHINSKY, T. M. (see KORNMAN, I. E.) 1929
SMILLIE, I. S.: Mallet finger. Brit. J. Surg. *24:*439-445, Jan '37
SMIRNOV, A. A.: Plastic surgery of nose. Russk. oto-laring. *24:*356-358, '31
SMIRNOV, V. I.: Leukoplast for bandaging burns. Khirurgiya, no. 1, pp. 54-59, '39
SMIRNOVA, L. A.: Skin graft to cover defects in short stump of leg; modified technic. Khirurgiya, No. 1, pp. 27-28, '45
SMITAL, W.: Plastic surgery of chin and mouth mucosa; case. Zentralbl. f. Chir. *55:*142-145, Jan 21, '28
SMITH, A. D.: Modern burn therapy. M. J. Australia *2:*335-337, Oct 10, '42
SMITH, A. E.: Reconstructive plastic and oral surgery. J. Am. Dent. A. *21:*2190-2200, Dec '34
SMITH, A. E.: Reconstructive plastic and oral surgery. California and West. Med. *42:*432-438, June '35
SMITH, A. E. AND JOHNSON, J. B.: Reconstructive plastic and oral surgery. J. Am. Dent. A. *24:*1142-1153, July '37
SMITH, A. E. AND JOHNSON, J. B.: Surgery of cleft palate. Am. J. Surg. *45:*93-103, July '39
SMITH, A. E. AND JOHNSON, J. B.: Surgical treatment of mandibular deformities. J. Am. Dent. A. *27:*689-700, May '40
SMITH, A. K.: Treatment of acid and alkali burns. Mod. Med. *3:*232, April '21
SMITH, B.: Use of Padgett dermatome in ophthalmic plastic surgery. Arch. Ophth. *28:*484-489, Sept '42
SMITH, B.; CORNELL, C. AND NEILL, C. L.: Principles in early reconstructive surgery of severe thermal burns of hand. Brit. J. Surg. *33:*155-159, Oct '45
SMITH, C.: Removal of nasal septum. Arch. Otolaryng. *20:*709-710, Nov '34
SMITH, C. H.: Compound fracture of fingers. Ann. Surg. *119:*266-273, Feb '44
SMITH, C. K.: Surgical procedure for correction of hypospadias. J. Urol. *40:*239-247, July '38
SMITH, E. M. JR. (see ROSENBERG, W. A.) May '43
SMITH, E. O.: Keloid of penis. J. Urology *11:*515-524, May '24
SMITH, E. W. (see SCHAUBEL, H. J.) Apr '46
SMITH, F.: Surgical treatment of saddle nose and malignancies. J. Michigan M. Soc. *20:*413, Oct '21
SMITH, F.: Rational management of skin grafts. Surg., Gynec. and Obst. *42:*556-562, April '26
SMITH, F.: Pressure bags for skin grafting. Surg., Gynec. and Obst. *43:*99, July '26
SMITH, F.: Total rhinoplasty. Warthin Ann. Vol., pp. 601-612, '27
SMITH, F.: Three new instruments for fronto-ethmo-sphenoid operation. Ann. Otol., Rhin. and Laryng. *40:*198-200, March '31
SMITH, F.: Five year cures in cancer of mouth, lip, nose, etc. Surg., Gynec. and Obst. *56:*470-471, Feb (no. 2A) '33
SMITH, F.: Surgical management of cancer of lips. Surg., Gynec. and Obst. *56:*782-785, April '33
SMITH, F.: Refinements in reconstructive surgery of face. J.A.M.A. *120:*352-358, Oct 3, '42
SMITH, F.: Symposium on plastic surgery; planning the reconstruction of the face. Surgery *15:*1-15, Jan '44
SMITH, F. H.: Penetration of tissue (of finger) by grease under pressure of 7,000 pounds. J.A.M.A. *112:*907-908, March 11, '39
SMITH, F. L.: Skin grafts for ambulatory patient. Am. J. Surg. *41:*67-69, July '38
SMITH, F. L. AND RIDER, D. L.: Healing of 100 consecutive phalangeal fractures. J. Bone and Joint Surg. *17:*91-109, Jan '35
SMITH, G. C.: Reduction of faciocranial fractures. J. Missouri M. A. *39:*178-180, June '42
SMITH, G. W.: Symposium on automobile fractures (including facial). Rocky Mountain M. J. *36:*238-240, April '39
SMITH, G. W.: Mandibular fractures, malocclusion and osteomyelitis. Rocky Mountain M.

J. *38:*794–798, Oct '41
SMITH, H. (See SEDDON, H. J. *et al*) Sept '43
SMITH, H. D. (see SHARP, G. S.) Dec '39
SMITH, J. E. AND SINISCAL, A. A.: Modified Ewing operation for cicatricial entropion. Am. J. Ophth. *26:*382–389, April '43
SMITH, K. D. AND MASTERS, W. E.: Dupuytren's contracture among upholsterers. J. Indust. Hyg. and Toxicol. *21:*97–100, March '39
SMITH, L. D.: Operation for correction of recurrent dislocation of jaw. Arch. Surg. *46:*762–763, May '43
SMITH, L. M. (see HUGHES, R. P.) June '39
SMITH, L. W. (see LEECH, J. V. *et al*) Sept '28
SMITH, N. D.: Perianal actinodermatitis; treatment by excision and pedicle graft. Proc. Staff Meet., Mayo Clin. *14:*113–115, Feb. 22, '39
SMITH, N. F.: Two cases of congenital deformities of hands and feet. Lancet *1:*802, April 19, '24
SMITH, P. E.: Case of serious burns; problem of reconstructive surgery. Mississippi Doctor *22:*258–262, March '45
SMITH, R. M. AND MANGES, W. F.: Roentgen treatment of infection from human bite of hand. Am. J. Roentgenol. *38:*720–725, Nov '37
SMITH, R. R. AND TORGERSON, W. R.: Congenital salivary fistula of neck. Surg., Gynec. and Obst. *41:*318–319, Sept '25
SMITH, S.; RISK, R. AND BECK, C.: Warm moist air therapy in burns. Arch. Surg. *39:*686–690, Oct '39
SMITH-PETERSEN, M. N.; AUFRANC, O. E. AND LARSON, C. B. Useful surgical procedures for rheumatoid arthritis involving joints of upper extremity. Arch. Surg. *46:*764–770, May '43
SMITHERS, D. W.: Treatment of carcinoma of lip (and involved lymph nodes). Post-Grad. M. J. *15:*376–381, Nov '39
SMORODINTZEFF, A. A. AND TOGUNOVA, E. F.: Course of infectious process in burns. Microbiol. J. *13:*27–35, '31
SMYRNOFF, S. A.: Plastic closure of palate defects by means of tubed pedicle flap. Am. Med. *39:*115, March '33
SMYRNOFF, S. S.: Plastic operation of face following noma. M. Rec. *143:*186–188, March 4, '36
SMYTH, C. J. (see JACOBSON, S. D.) 1944
SMYTH, C. M. JR: Modern burn treatment; review. Clinics *2:*201–217, June '43
SMYTH, G. J. C.: Plastic repair of face; case. South African M. J. *8:*181–182, March 10, '34
SMYTHE, F. D.: Shockless surgery; Crile's contribution to humanity and to the medical profession; with simple and dependable method of preparation of patient for same; and remarks. J. Tennessee M. A. *16:*313–317, Jan '24
SMYTHE, F. W.: Simple protection for newly placed skin grafts. J.A.M.A. *78:*1963, June 24, '22 (illus.)
SMYTHE, G. J. C.: Case of skin plastic operation for mucous membrane replacement in mouth. S. African M. Rec. *24:*408–409, Sept 25, '26

Snakebite

Therapy of shock in rattlesnake bites. CRIMMINS, M. L. Mil. Surgeon *69:*42–44, July '31

SNEAD, L. O. (see HODGES, F. M. *et al*) May '39
SNEDECOR, S. T.: Burn therapy. J. M. Soc. New Jersey *32:*535–537, Sept '35
SNEDECOR, S. T.: Reconstructive surgery of war injuries. Delaware State M. J. *16:*39–41, March '44
SNEDECOR, S. T.: Reconstructive surgery in patients with war fractures of ankle and foot. J. Bone and Joint Surg. *28:*332–342, Apr '46
SNEDECOR, S. T.: Hand, bone surgery in war injuries Am. J. Surg. *72:*363–372, Sept '46
SNEDECOR, S. T. AND HARRYMAN, W. K.: Surgical problems in hereditary polydactylism and syndactylism. J. M. Soc. New Jersey *37:*443–449, Sept '40

Snegiroff Operation

Snegiroff's method of formation of artificial vagina; case. SCHARAPO, M. Zentralbl. f. Gynak. *51:*1131–1133, April 30, '27

SNELL, M. W.(see FISHER, D.) Dec '24

Snellen Operation

Comparison of immediate and late results of Panas, Snellen and Millingen-Sapezhko eyelid operations. AVGUSHEVICH, P. L. Vestnik oftal. *11:*557–563, '37

SNELLMAN, A.: Tannin in burns. Duodecim *51:*579–603, '35
SNODGRASS, T. J.: Infections of hand and surgery. Wisconsin M. J. *44:*503–507, May '45
SNOKE, P. O. (see BRADLEY, R. A.) Feb '27
SNYDER, C. D.: Salivery gland tumors. J. Kansas M. Soc. *41:*389–390, Sept '40
SNYDER, M. H. AND SNYDER, W. H. JR.: Traumatic thrombosis of deep palmar vein (case). J.A.M.A. *111:*2007–2008, Nov 26, '38
SNYDER, W. H. JR. (see SNYDER, M. H.) Nov '38
SNYDER, W. S. JR.: Submucous resection of sep-

tum of nose. Kentucky M. J. *40:*59-62, Feb '42

SOBATIER, J. A. (see COX, F. J. *et al*) Dec '44

SOBOL, I.: Technic of plastic repair of cranium. Rev. oto-neuro-oftal. *8:*351-355, Oct '33

SØBYE, P.: Treatment of fracture of corpus mandibulae ad modum Ipsen (introduction of Kirschner nails). Acta chir. Scandinav. *83:*445-477, '40

SODERBERG, N. B.: Maxillofacial reconstruction. Mil. Surgeon *92:*268-276, March '43

SODERBERG, N. B. (see PADGETT, E. C.) Jan '42

SÖDERLUND, S.: Familial congenital aural fistula; case. Finska lak.-sallsk. handl. *80:*71-77, Jan '37

SODRE FILHO, L.: Plasty surgery of nose; case of rhinophyma. Arq. de cir. clin. e exper. *6:*692-695, April-June '42

SOER, J. J.: Mandibular hypoplasia with atresia of esophagus; case. Maandschr. v. kindergeneesk. *1:*309-310, March '32

SOHIER, H. (see ROQUES, P.) May '39

SOHLBERG, O. I.: Surgical shock. Minnesota Med. *12:*360-361, June '29

SOHMA, T. AND IMAMURA, T.: Surgical therapy of facial paralysis; case. Mitt. a. d. med. Akad. zu Kioto *16:*1403-1404, '36

SOILAND, A. AND MELAND, O. N.: Intraoral cancer and its treatment. California and West. Med. *33:*559-562, Aug '30

SOIVIO, A.: Surgical correction of prognathism. Duodecim *51:*702-712, '35

SOIVIO, A.: Surgical technic in cleft palate. Duodecim *52:*723-735, '36

SOIVIO, A.: Optimal age for operations in cases of cleft palate and harelip. Duodecim *53:*335-344, '37

SOIVIO, A.: Cleft palate. Duodecim *55:*607-620, '39

SOIVIO, A.: Cleft palate therapy in Finland. Acta Soc. med. fenn. duodecim (Ser. B, Fasc. 1-2, art. 25) *27:*1-8, '39

SOIVIO, A.: Harelip and cleft palate. Nord. med. (Duodecim) *4:*3705-3709, Dec 23, '39

SOKOLOFF, A. P.: Filatov grafts in large ulcers due to X-ray burns. Vestnik khir. (nos. 70-71) *24:*237-241, '31

SOKOLOV, N. N.: Total restoration of lower half of face. Novy khir. arkhiv *40:*426-437, '38

SOKOLOV, S.: Treatment of suppurations of fingers and hands. Arch. f. klin. Chir. *161:*89-116, '30

SOKOLOV, V.: Technic of temporary craniectomy and of plastics in cranium defects. Vestnik khir. (no. 32) *11:*115-116, Nov 5, '27

SOKOLOW, N. N.: Beresowski method in surgical treatment of ankylosis of lower jaw. Deutsche Ztschr. f. Chir. *231:*294-298, '31

SOKOLOWSKI, M.: Lymphangioplastic treatment of elephantiasis of lower extremities. Zentralbl. f. Chir. *52:*2583-2586, Nov. 14, '25

SOKOVNINA, R.: Burn therapy. Vrach. Gaz. *31:*524, April 15, '27

SOLANDT, D. Y. (see BEST, C. H.) May '40

SOLCARD: Remote results in radial paralysis after tendon transplantation; 4 cases. Bull. et mem. Soc. nat. de chir. *58:*677-682, May 7, '32

SOLCARD, AND MORVAN: Unusual cicatrix following burn. Ann. d'anat. path. *8:*530, May '31

SOLDANO, H. A. O.: Total bimaxillary necrobiosis; case with recovery after surgical therapy aided especially by extract of calf jawbone (vaduril). Prensa med. argent. *30:*1945-1947, Oct 6, '43

SOLÉ, R.: Repair of radialis through grafting of dead calf nerve according to Nageotte's method. Semana med. *2:*452-454, Aug 19, '26

SOLENTE, (see TOURAINE, A.) Feb '34

SOLENTE, (see TOURAINE, *et al*) March '36

SOLER JULIÁ, J.: Technic of formation of artificial vagina. Ann. de Hosp. de Santa Creu i Sant Pau *7:*332-334, Sept 15, '33

SOLER JULIÁ, J.: Formation of artificial vagina by transplantation of muscular flap. Rev. de cir. de Barcelona *7:*194-198, March '34

SOLLA, L.: Diathermic depilation in hypertrichosis. Actas dermo-sif. *26:*445-449, March '34

SOLO, A.: New splint for nasal septum. Arch. Otolaryng. *27:*343-346, March '38

SOLONCOV, N.: Cosmetic surgery of nose and ear. Cas. lek. cesk. *63:*833-839, May 31, '24

SOLOVEV, A. G.: Therapy of scalping wounds (head). Sovet. khir. (no. 6) *6:*805-813, '34

SOLOWJEW, L. M.: Closure of esophageal defect after laryngectomy with help of movable flap (Filatov operation). Acta oto-laryng. *21:*219-221, '34

SOMALO, M.: Circular dermolipectomy of trunk in obesity. Arq. de cir. clin. e exper. *6:*540-543, April-June '42

SOMALO, M.: Origin of elasticity of skin and its significance in plastic surgery. Prensa med. argent. *31:*1313-1316, July 12, '44

SOMALO, M.: Cruciform ventral dermolipectomy; swallow-shaped incision. Prensa med. argent. *33:*75-83, Jan 11 '46

SOMERVELL, T. H.: Cancer of mouth and jaws (with emphasis on therapy). Indian J. Surg. (no. 2) *5:*5-28, June '43

SOMERVELL, T. H.: Recent advances in treament of carcinoma of jaw. Brit. J. Surg. *32:*35-43, July '44

SOMMER, G. N. J. JR.; CONLEY, J. J. AND DUNLAP, H. J. Cervical lesions of branchial origin. Am. J. Surg. *61:*266-270, Aug '43

Sommer, R.: Subcuticular suture. Zentralbl. f. Chir. *56:*2265-2266, Sept 7, '29

Sonnenschein, H. D.: Repair of lacerated nerves at wrist. S. Clin. North America *23:*487-496, April '43

Sonnenschein, H. D. (see Eisberg, H. B.) Dec '27

Sonntag: Treatment of rupture of extensor tendon of third phalanx. Munchen. med. Wchnschr. *69:*1333-1334, Sept 15, '22 (illus.)

Sonntag: Unusual cases of jaw surgery. Deutsche Ztschr. f. Chir. *223:*236-260, '30

Sonntag, A.: Local anesthesia in nasal septal surgery. Ztschr. f. Laryng., Rhin. *21:*32-36, June '31

Sonntag, E.: Rupture of extensor tendon at terminal phalanx of finger (comment on Glass' article). Zentralbl. f. Chir. *55:*410, Feb 18, '28

Sonntag, E.: Plastic surgery by Holländer's operation for breasts. Arch. f. klin. Chir. *164:*812-824, '31

Sonntag, E.: Jaw fractures. Monatschr. f. Unfallh. *43:*369-387, Aug '36

Soraluce, J. A.: Reparative plastic surgery; loss of thumb and methods of substitution. Cir. ortop. y tramatol., Madrid *1:*247-254, '36

Soraluce, J. A.: Plastic surgery of nose. Semana med. espan. *2:*782-789, Dec 30, '39

Soraluce, J. A.: Transplantation of large toe to replace thumb; case. Semana med. espan. *3:*81-84, Jan 20, '40

Soraluce, J. A.: Plastic surgery of breast; present status of problems. Actas Soc. de cir. de Madrid *5:*137-153, Jan-Mar '46

Sorensen, F.: Hemangioma of hand muscles. Klin. Wchnschr. *20:*222-224, March 1, '41

Soret: Radium treatment of burns. Paris med. *1:*534, June 9, '28

Soria: Twenty-five years of dacryorhinostomy (1919-1944). Arch. Soc. oftal. hispano-am. *4:*807-812, Sept-Oct '44

Soriano, F. S. (see Santillan, J. S. *et al*) Jan '41

Sorrel,E.: Volkmann syndrome; new technic of resection of bones of forearm (chevron osteotomy). Paris med. *1:*569-573, June 15, '35

Sorrel, E.: Voluminous angioma of upper lip; treatment by intratumoral quinine injections followed by extirpation of tumor. Bull. Soc. de pediat. de Paris *34:*210-215, April '36

Sorrel, E.; Guichard, and Gigon: Cleansing and painting extensive burns with mercurochrome; therapy without use of bandages. Bull. Soc. de pediat. de Paris *33:*564-568, Nov '35

Sorrel, E. and Sorrel-Dejerine, Mme. Nerves; management of war injuries. Rev. neurol. *72:*649-660, '39-'40

Sorrel, E. and Sorrel-Dejerine, Mme: Peripheral nerve suture; 13 cases. Mem. Acad. de chir. *68:*448-452, Dec 9-16, '42

Sorrel, E. (see Thomas, A. *et al*) April '35

Sorrel-Dejerine, Mme. (see Sorrel, E.) 1939-1940

Sorrel-Dejerine, Mme. (see Sorrel, E.) Dec '42

Sorrel-Dejerine, Mme. (see Thomas, A. *et al*) April '35

Sorrels, T. W.: First aid appliance for treatment of jaw fractures. Am. J. Orthodontics, *27:*714-716, Dec '41

Sorrentino, M.: Hypospadias in girl 4 years old. Rinasc. med. *18:*65-66, Feb 15, '41

Sorsby, A. (see Blaine, G. *et al*) 1945

Sorton. (see Roussy, *et al*) June '27

Soru, S. *et al:* Persistence of thyroglossal duct; median cervical fistula; 2 cases. Rev. de chir., Bucuresti *41:*48-56, Jan-Feb '38 also: Ann. d'oto-laryng., pp. 318-324, April '38

Sosodoro-Djatikoesoemo, R.: Trypaflavine (acridine dye) compresses in burns. Geneesk. tijdschr. v. Nederl.-Indie *74:*759-760, June 5, '34

Soto, M. (see Jorge, J. M. *et al*) March '41

Soubeiran, M.: Congenital lymphoid cysts in lateral portion of neck. Arch. franco-belges de chir. *29:*514-521, June '26

Soubeiran, M.: Cervicofacial branchiomas. Arch. franco-belges de chir. *33:*542-554, June '32

Soubiran: Wrist-drop; graft of 15 cm. of rabbit's spinal cord and infiltration of stellate ganglion followed by rapid recovery; case. J. de med. de Bordeaux *116:*353-354, Nov 4-25, '39

Soubiran, (see Jeanneney, G.) Aug '38

Soubrane: Therapy of injuries of hands and fingers. J. de med. et chir. prat. *110:*533-542, Oct 10-25, '39

Soudakoff, P. S.: Lagrange's law of indirect ocular war injuries (facial fractures). Am. J. Ophth. *26:*293-296, March '43

Soulairac, A. (see Chatagnon, P. *et al*) July '38

Soupault, R.: Abdominal flap to cover defect after mammectomy. Presse med. *31:*177-178, Feb. 24, '23 (illus.)

de Sousa Dias, A.: Therapy of first, second and third degree burns with biologic pomade; case. Hospital, Rio de Janeiro *14:*1415-1417, Dec '38

de Sousa Dias, A. Goncalo: Congenital malformations of hands and feet. Amatus *3:*325-329, May '44

de Sousa Dias, J. V.: Huge paradental cyst of left upper jaw (giant cell sarcoma with gigantic cystic cavity); surgical therapy of case. Amatus *2:*552–558, July '43

Southworth, J. L. (see Palmer, L. A.) June '45

Souttar, H. S.: Burns and scalds. Lancet *1:*142–143, Jan 17, '25

Souttar, H. S.: War injuries to radial nerve; treatment. M. Press *210:*345–347, Dec 1, '43

Souttar, H. S. (see Muecke, F. F.) Jan '24

de Souza, A. R.: Furuncle of face; modification of continuous sutures. Folha med. *25:*60, April 25, '44

Souza Cunha, A.: Osteoplasty of mandibular arch and complementary surgical prosthesis. Arq. de cir. clin. e exper. *6:*587–593, April–June '42

Souza Mendes, J.: New method for plastic operations in bony frame of nose. Brazil-med. *2:*100–102, Aug 21, '26

de Souza Ramos, R.: Immediate repair by means of free total graft in flat (guillotine) mutilation of fingers. Med. cir. Farm. pp. 339–341, June '46

Sowles, H. K.: Plastic operation for correction of breast hypertrophy. New England J. Med. *218:*253–257, Feb 10, '38

Spaeth, E. B.: Correction of scar tissue deformities by epithelial grafts, report of 5 cases (including eyelids). Arch. Surg. *2:*176, Jan '21

Spaeth, Edmund B.: *Newer Methods of Ophthalmic Plastic Surgery*. Blakiston Co., Phila., 1925

Spaeth, E. B.: Mosher-Toti dacryocystorhinostomy. Arch. Ophth. *4:*487–496, Oct '30

Spaeth, E. B.: Pedicled flap in plastic surgery of eyelids. Pennsylvania M. J. *35:*560–562, May '32

Spaeth, E. B.: Biological principles which underlie plastic surgery of eyelids. Am. J. Ophth. *15:*589–603, July '32

Spaeth, E. B.: Use of mucous membrane in ophthalmic surgery. Am. J. Ophth. *20:*897–907, Sept '37

Spaeth, E. B.: Eyelid ptosis and its surgical correction. J.A.M.A. *109:*1889–1894, Dec 4, '37

Spaeth, E. B.: Eyelid ptosis and its surgical correction. Tr. Sect. Ophth., A. M. A., pp. 66–89, '37

Spaeth, E. B.: Review of some modern methods for plastic surgery of eyes. Am. J. Surg. *42:*89–100, Oct '38

Spaeth, E. B.: Plastic surgery about eye and orbit. Tr. Indiana Acad. Ophth. and Otolaryng. *23:*81–83, '39

Spaeth, E. B.: Correction of massive defects of both eyelids. Pennsylvania M. J. *43:*663–668, Feb '40

Spaeth, E. B.: Congenital colobomata of lower eyelid. Am. J. Ophth. *24:*186–190, Feb '41

Spaeth, E. B.: Congenial blepharoptosis – classification; principles of surgical correction. Tr. Am. Acad. Ophth. (1942) *47:*285–301, March–April '43

Spaid, J. D.: Anesthesia for harelip surgery during infancy. J. Indiana M. A. *34:*143–145, March '41

Spalding, J. E.: Fascial spaces of palm; surgical anatomy. Guy's Hosp. Rep. *88:*432–439, Oct '38

Spangler, P. C.: Plan for larger numbers of burns. Hawaii M. J. *2:*40–41, Sept–Oct '42

Spanier, F.: Elastic bandage in fracture of mandible. Chirurg *3:*891–893, Oct 15, '31

Spanier, F.: Simple plastic method of covering palatal defects. Deutsche Ztschr. f. Chir. *231:*284–293, '31

Spanier, F.: Substitute for implantation prosthesis and for osteoplasty in resection of jaw. Deutsche Ztschr. f. Chir. *231:*456–469, '31

Spanier, F.: Alloplastic and heteroplastic grafts in reconstruction of facial defects; use of ivory and cartilage. Rev. de chir. structive, pp. 391–401, Dec '36

Spanier, F.: Optimum age for operation of cleft palate, with special reference to normal speech development. J. Internat. Coll. Surgeons *4:*338–343, Aug '41

Spanier, F.: First aid splinting of jaw fractures. M. Rec. *155:*377, July '42

Sparer, W.: Plastic operation to correct large hump with deviation of nasal axis; modified technic. M. Rec. *153:*92–94, Feb 5, '41

Sparer, W.: Simplified method of removing triangular wedge of nasal bone in plastic correction of lateral deviation. Arch. Otolaryng. *33:*666–667, April '41

Sparrow, T. D.: Viability of tube pedicle graft. Am. J. Surg. *41:*92–95, July '38

Sparrow, T. D.: Tube-pedicle skin graft's usefulness to general surgeon (concerning cicatrix). South. Med. and Surg. *100:*514–523, Nov '38

Specht, F.: Specialists' experiences with wounds of facial portion of skull in war and peace. Munchen. med. Wchnschr. *89:*391, May 1, '42

Specklin, P. and Stoeber, R.: Contracture of aponeurosis of palms and soles plus neuralgia treated with X-ray. Presse med. *30:*743–745, Aug 30, '22 abstr: J.A.M.A. *79:*1368, Oct 14, '22

Speech Defects

Some mouth and jaw conditions responsible for defects in speech. Greene, J. S. Med. Rec. *100:*8, July 2, '21

Speech Defects – Cont.
Training the speech after operations for cleft palate. SEEMANN, M. Cas. lek. cesk. *61:*811–815, Sept 2, '22
Training of speech in children with cleft palate. RUPPE, L. AND RUPPE, C. Arch. de med. d. enf. *26:*19–35, Jan '23 (illus.)
Necessity of speech and voice re-education, with special reference to nasality. GIFFORD, M. F. Laryngoscope *35:*317–323, April '25
Speech complications involved in certain types of inadequate palate, especially congenital short palate, with exhibition of patients. KENYON, E. L. Ann. Otol., Rhin. and Laryng. *34:*887–900, Sept '25
Preliminary paper on improvement of speech in cleft palate cases. KIRKHAM, H. L. D. Surg., Gynec. and Obst. *44:*244–246, Feb '27
Peripheral expressive or articular speech defects; cleft palate. VAN BAGGEN, N. Y. P., M. J. and Rec. *125:*535–537, April 20, '27
Cleft palate and re-education of speech. WARD, W. K. Brit. J. Dent. Sc. *72:*1–4, Jan '28
Nasal speech and cleft palate. BURGER, H. Nederl. Tijdschr. v. Geneesk. *1:*1563–1571, March 31, '28
Obturators in treatment of rhinolalia aperta. FRÖSCHELS, E. AND SCHALIT, H. Wien. med. Wchnschr. *78:*840, June 23, '28
Nasal voice; treatment by obturator. SCHALIT, A. Wien. med. Wchnschr. *78:*964–966, July 14, '28
Phonetic result of surgical treatment of cleft palate; case. VEAU, V. AND BOREL, S. Bull. et mem. Soc. nat. de chir. *54:*1017, July 14, '28
Form of new obturator (meatus obturator) for preventing nasal speech in cleft palate. FRÖSCHELS, E. Ztschr. f. Stomatol. *26:*882–888, Sept '28
New obturator (meatus obturator) for preventing nasal speech in cleft palate. SCHALIT, A. Ztschr. f. Stomatol. *26:*888–898, Sept '28
Correction of cleft-palate speech by phonetic instruction. BERRY, M. F. Quart. J. Speech Educ. *14:*523–529, Nov '28
Surgical and phonetic results of late cleft palate operations. HALLE. Med. Klin. *24:*1976–1979, Dec 21, '28
Rhinolalia aperta. STEPOWSKA, A. Polska gaz. lek. *8:*183–185, March 10, '29
Phonetic results of 100 staphylorrhaphies. VEAU, V. AND BOREL, S. Bull. et mem. Soc. nat. de chir. *55:*894–909, June 29, '29
Re-educating cleft palate speech. WARD, W. K. Practitioner *123:*147–152, Aug '29
New obturator to combat nasalization in patients with cleft of hard palate. FRÖSCHELS, E. AND SCHALIT, A. Wien. klin. Wchnschr. *42:*1442–1444, Nov 7, '29
Surgical and phonetic results of late operations for cleft palate. HALLE, M. Verhandl. d. Berl. med. Gesellsch. (1928) *59:*267–276, '29
Speech training of children with cleft palate. SCHLEUSS, W. Eos *21:*29–38, '29
Speech training without obturator in children with cleft palate who have not had operations. HELWIG, K. Ztschr. f. Kinderforsch. *36:*178–194, Jan 18, '30
Correction of congenital cleft-palate speech by appliances. FITZ-GIBBON, J. J. Dental Cosmos *72:*231–238, March '30
Pathology and treatment of rhinolalia. STEIN, L. Wien. klin. Wchnschr. *43:*1068–1069, Aug. 21, '30
Speech exercises after cleft palate operation. GUTZMANN, H. Chirurg *2:*1019–1027, Nov 15, '30
Cleft palate speech. GLASSBURG, J. A. Arch. Otolaryng. *12:*820–821, Dec '30
Correction of nasal speech from congenital defects of palate by obturators. REICHENBACH, E. Vrtljsschr. f. Zahnh. *46:*418–434, '30
Rhinolalia clausa palatina functionalis. DAITÔ, T. Fukuoka-Ikwadaigaku-Zasshi *24:*87–90, Sept '31
Schönborn operation (velopharyngorrhaphy) for correction of defective speech. SEEMANN, M. Casop. lek. cesk. *70:*1570–1574, Nov 20, '31 also: Otolaryng. slavica *4:*24–25, Jan '32
Phonation after operations for palatal division. VEAU, V. AND BOREL, S. Rev. franc. de pediat. *7:*333–342, '31
Handicap of cleft-palate speech. WOLDSTAD, D. M. Ment. Hyg. *16:*281–288, April '32
Perfect phonetic results of uranostaphylorrhaphy (Langenbeck-Trelat method). ROCHER. J. de med. de Bordeaux *109:*402–403, May 20, '32
Nasal lisping and speech in palatoschisis; palatographic study. GUMPERTZ, F. Wien. med. Wchnschr. *82:*901–903, July 9, '32
Surgical contraction of pharynx in therapy of rhinolalia aperta. RÉTHI, A. Monatschr. f. Ohrenh. *66:*842–848, July '32
Rhinolalia aperta; further studies. POE, D. L. Arch. Pediat. *50:*147–157, March '33
Lengthening of velum and shortening of pharynx for amelioration of voice after uranoplasty. MEISSNER, A. Rev. de stomatol.

Speech Defects – Cont.
*35:*405-411, July '33
Study of improvement of speech after operation for cleft hard palate; case. LAMBECK, A. Ztschr. f. Kinderforsch. *42:*369-384, '33
Phonetic education of patients with palatal fissures. FIORINI, J. M. Semana med. *1:*1985-1997, June 21, '34
Phonetic results in 200 cases of staphylorrhaphy. VEAU, V. Helvet. med. acta *1:*99-103, June '34
Speech training for cleft palate patients. PARSONS, F. Proc. Roy. Soc. Med. *27:*1301-1303, July '34
Palatographic researches on phonation in cleft palate. RICHERI, S. Arch. ital. di otol. *45:*487-509, July '34
Comment on phonetic education in palatal fissures in article by Fiorini. FIKH, E. Semana med. *2:*735-738, Sept 6, '34
Rhinolalia aperta caused by velopalatine insufficiency; case. VARGA, V. Cluj. med. *15:*576-578, Oct 1, '34
Correcting deformities of velum and mesopharynx to insure better speech following cleft palate surgery. BOYNE, H. N. Nebraska M. J. *19:*407-409, Nov '34
Therapeutic technic for staphylolalia (so-called short palate speech). VOELKER, C. H.) Arch. Otolaryng. *21:*94-96, Jan '35
Technic of therapy (palatopharyngorrhaphy) of rhinolalia aperta due to too short palate. SERCER, A. Rev. de chir. structive, pp. 5-18, July '35
Value of speech training in cleft palate. SCHARFE, E. E. Arch. Oto-laryng. *22:*585-596, Nov '35 also: Canad. M. A. J. *33:*641-647, Dec '35
Value of speech training in cleft palate. SCHARFE, E. E. Tr. Sect. Laryng., Otol. and Rhin., A. M. A., pp. 116-128, '35
Effect of suture of cleft palate on phonation. VEAU, V. AND BOREL-MAISONNY, S. Monatschr. f. Ohrenh. *70:*858-864, July '36
Phonation and staphylorraphy. VEAU, V. AND BOREL-MAISONNY, S. Rev. franc. de phoniatrie *4:*133-141, July '36
Claims of various obturators, from standpoint of correction of speech defects in cleft palate. REICHENBACH, E. Hals-, Nasen-. u. Ohrenarzt (Teil 1) *28:*29-33, Feb '37
Mechanism of speech in cleft palates. WARDILL, W. E. M. Monatschr. f. Ohrenh. *71:*424-429, April '37
Treatment of cleft-palate speech. WARD, W. K. South African M. J. *11:*433-435, June 26, '37
Surgical and phonetic problems of harelip and cleft palate. BERNDORFER, A. Gyogyaszat *77:*433, July 18-25; 452, Aug 1-8, '37

Speech Defects – Cont.
Cleft palate repair technic affording better speech results. HYSLOP, V. B. Wisconsin M. J. *36:*540-543, July '37
Phonetic results obtained after cleft palate therapy. BOREL-MAISONNY, MME. Rev. de stomatol. *39:*733-754, Oct '37
Pedagogic therapy of speech disturbances in congenital palatoschisis. LIISBERG, H. B. Valsalva *14:*346-351, July '38
Phonetic reeducation for velopalatine division; conditions necessary for improving speech. FROMENT, AND FEYEUX, A. Lyon chir. *36:*201-207, March-April '39
Reeducation of speech in ablation of lower jaw; case. FREUD, E. Rev. franc. de phoniatrie *7:*119-121, April '39
Speech rehabilitation following excision of tip of tongue. BACKUS, O. Am. J. Dis. Child. *60:*368-370, Aug '40
Skin grafting for spina bifida with meningocele or myelomeningocele. PINHEIRO CAMPOS, O., J. Internat. Coll. Surgeons *3:*438-440, Oct '40
Unusual case of submucosal cleft palate in conjunction with deformity of soft palate and nasal speech. ARNOLD, G. E. Arch. f. Ohren-, Nasen-u. Kehlkopfh. *147:*173-176, '40
Physiopathology of phonetic formation and education of cleft palate patients treated surgically. LIMA, J. Rev. med. Bahia *9:*74-85, March '41
Optimum age for operation of cleft palate, with special reference to normal speech development. SPANIER, F., J. Internat. Coll. Surgeons *4:*338-343, Aug '41
Cleft palate and mechanism of speech. (Arris and Gale lecture). OLDFIELD, M. C. Brit. J. Surg. *29:*197-227, Oct '41
Correction of phonetic disorders in cleft palate lacking timely surgical therapy. ROVIRALTA, E. Rev. clin. espan. *4:*48-49, Jan 15, '42
Speech re-education following palatal reconstruction. HUBER, M. Canad. M.A.J. *46:*325-326, April '42
Speech function following 300 palate operations. AXHAUSEN, G. Zentralbl. f. Chir. *69:*770, May 9, '42
Facial reconstruction and speech. HIGLEY, L. B., J. Am. Dent. A. *30:*1716-1725, Nov 1, '43
Speech reeducation in cleft palate. RUMSEY, H. ST. J. Guy's Hosp. Gaz. *58:*6-8, Jan 8, '44
Attempt to correct congenital rhinolalia aperta by plastic operation. WODAK, E.

Speech Defects – Cont.
Harefuah *27:*8, July 2, '44
Speech training center for cleft palate children. WELLS, C. G. Quart. J. Speech *31:*68–73, Feb '45
Improving speech of cleft palate child. WELLS, C. G., J. Speech Disorders *10:*162–168, June '45
Methods of exaination of dysarthria and dyslalia in World War II. PEACHER, W. G. AND PEACHER, G. M., J. Nerv. and Ment. Dis. *103:*484–493, May '46
Speech defects in relation to oral defects. OLINGER, N. A. Am. J. Orthodontics (Oral Surg. Sect.) *32:*469–471, July '46
Present status of speech training of patients who wear speech correction appliances. BAKES, F. P. Am. J. Orthodontics (Oral Surg. Sect.) *32:*718–723, Nov '46
Responsibility of speech correctionist in treatment of patient who has received surgical or prosthetic treatment. KOEPP-BAKER, H. Am. J. Orthodontics (Oral Surg. Sect.) *32:*714–717, Nov '46

SPEED, K.: Injuries of carpal bones. S. Clin. North America *25:*1-13, Feb '45
SPEIGEL, I. J.: Problems in late management of craniocerebral injuries, with special reference to repair of defects with tantalum plate; analysis of 170 cases. Am. J. Surg. *72:*448–467, Sept '46
SPEIRS, R. E.: Immediate repair of flexor tendons. J. Kansas M. Soc. *41:*370–373, Sept '40
SPEKTOR, I. Z. (see NEGLO, L. G.) 1942
SPEMANN, H.: Behavior of embryonic tissue transplanted into adult organism. Arch. f. Entwckingsmechn. d. Organ. *141:*693–769, '42
SPENCER, J.: Radiation treatment of hemangioma of skin. Am. J. Roentgenol. *46:*220–223, Aug '41
SPENCER, J. A.: Treatment of hand injuries. J. Michigan M. Soc. *37:*515–521, June '38
SPERANSKI, A. D.: Post traumatic contractures. Am. Rev. Soviet Med. *4:*22–24, Oct '46
SPERRY, R. W.: Transplantation of motor nerves and muscles in forelimb of rat. J. Comp. Neurol. *76:*283–321, April '42
SPERRY, R. W.: Restoration of vision after crossing of optic nerves and after contralateral transplantation of eye. J. Neurophysiol. *8:*15–28, Jan '45
SPERRY, R. W.: Problem of central nervous reorganization after nerve regeneration and muscle transposition. Quart. Rev. Biol. *20:*311-369, Dec '45
SPIES, J. W.; ADAIR, F. E. AND JOBE, M. C.: Accidental autogenous transplantation of mammary carcinoma to thigh during skin graft operation; case. Am. J. Cancer *20:*606–609, March '34
SPIESMAN, M. G.: Decubitus. Am. J. Surg. *36:*17–21, April '37
SPILLMANN, L.; HAMANT, A. AND WATRIN, J.: Surgical therapy of rhinophyma; case. Bull. Soc. franc. de dermat. et syph. (Reunion dermat., Nancy) *41:*813–815, June '34
SPINA, V.: Female pseudohermaphroditism with hypospadias limited to glans; anomaly due to cessation of development; plastic correction of case. Rev. de obst. e ginec. de Sao Paulo *7:*195–208, June–Aug '45
SPINELLI, C. A. (see OTTOLENGHI, C. E.) Oct '36
SPINELLI, F.: Diathermic recanalization of lacrimonasal canal. Klin. Monatsbl. f. Augenh. *91:*202–207, Aug '33
ŠPIŠIĆ, B.: Successful therapy of severe contractures of fingers and hand by cotton redressments. Ztschr. f. orthop. Chir. *57:*195–202, '32
ŠPIŠIĆ, B.: Surgical therapy of trigger finger. Zentralbl. f. Chir. *67:*157–159, Jan 27, '40
ŠPIŠIĆ, B.: Tendovaginitis stenosans of finger. Lijecn. vjes. *62:*246–248, May '40
ŠPIŠIĆ, B.: Tendon transplantation in radial paralysis. Lijecn. vjes. *63:*12–13, Jan '41
ŠPIŠIĆ, B.: Bilateral symmetric contractures of hand and phalanges; case. Ztschr. f. Orthop. *75:*33, '44
SPITZY: Implantation of silk in plastic repair of tissues. Wien. med. Wchnschr. *77:*394–396, March 19, '27
SPITZY, M.: Results of electrocoagulation therapy of congenital fistulas of neck. Zentralbl. f. Chir. *65:*114–117, Jan 15, '38

Splints, Facial Paralysis
Preservation of muscle function in Bell's palsy with splint. LEWIN, P. J.A.M.A. *112:*2273, June 3, '39
Facial paralysis; intraoral splint. ALLEN, A. G. AND NORTHFIELD, D. W. C. Lancet *2:*172–173, Aug 5, '44
Intraoral splint for facial palsy. ALLEN, A. G. AND NORTHFIELD, D. W. C. Brit. Dent. J. *79:*213–215, Oct 19, '45
Facial splint for treatment of Bell's palsy. PRACY, J. P. Brit. M. J. *1:*528, April 6, '46

Splints, Finger
Extension apparatus for crooked fingers. SCHMIDT, L. Deutsche med. Wchnschr. *47:*564, May 19, '21
Traction splint for fractured metacarpals and phalanges. HAWK, G. W., J.A.M.A. *78:*106, Jan 14, '22 (illus.)
Simple finger splint. FRANKE, F. Munchen. med. Wchnschr. *69:*468, March 31, '22 (il-

Splints, Finger – Cont.
lus.)
Apparatus for treatment of fractures of fingers. VALLET, E. Presse med. *33:*590–591, May 6, '25 abstr: J.A.M.A. *84:*1966, June 20, '25
Simple splint for baseball finger. LEWIN, P. J.A.M.A. *85:*1059, Oct 3, '25
Useful appliances in treatment of common finger injury. WEGEFORTH, H. M. AND WEGEFORTH, A. California and West Med. *23:*1590, Dec '25
Splint for overcoming contractures of fingers. MONTGOMERY, A. H. Surg., Gynec. and Obst. *44:*404–405, March '27
Use of splints in wounds of fingers. SCHNEK, F. Munchen. med. Wchnschr. *74:*977–979, June 10, '27
Metal splint for injuries of extensor tendons of fingers. GLASS, E. Zentralbl. f. Chir. *54:*3027–3028, Nov 26, '27
New traction finger splint for fractures. DAVIDOFF, R. B. New England J. Med. *198:*79–80, March 1, '28
Metal finger splints for injuries received in athletic games. GLASS, E. Zentralbl. f. Chir. *55:*601–602, March 10, '28
Metal splint for injuries of extensor tendons of fingers (reply to Glass). FRANKE, F. Zentralbl. f. Chir. *55:*852–853, April 7, '28
Improved splint for baseball finger. LEWIN, P., J.A.M.A. *90:*2102, June 30, '28
Practical metal finger splint for injured finger. GLASS, E. Deutsche med. Wchnschr. *54:*1121, July 6, '28
Coaptation splint for immobilization of thumb in abduction. LESTER, C. W. J.A.M.A. *91:*96–97, July 14, '28
New splint for finger tip fractures. ELLIS, J. D. Am. J. Surg. *5:*508, Nov '28
Thomas finger splint for fractures. MILCH, H. M. J. and Rec. *128:*473, Nov 7, '28
Value of Böhler's wire-finger-splint in treatment of severe injuries of fingers. FELSENREICH, F. Wien. klin. Wchnschr. *42:*1046–1048, Aug 8, '29
Curved metal finger splint. GLASS, E. Zentralbl. f. Chir. *56:*2459–2460, Sept 28, '29
Simplified method of traction for finger fractures. ROBINSON, W. H. Am. J. Surg. *8:*791–792, April '30
Splint for fractures of phalanges. KNOWLES, J. R., J.A.M.A. *94:*2065, June 28, '30
New finger splint. MYERS, T. Minnesota Med. *13:*840, Nov '30
Extension treatment for fractures of fingers. ADAMS, B. S. Journal-Lancet *51:*283–284, May 1, '31
Safetypin "tongs" for fractured fingers, with

Splints, Finger – Cont.
report of case. FOWLER, E. B. Illinois M. J. *59:*438–439, June '31
New splint for finger traction in fractures. LANGAN, A. J. California and West. Med. *35:*377, Nov '31
Traction with rustless steel wire in finger fractures. HALL, E. S. Maine M. J. *23:*11, Jan '32
Apparatus for treatment of finger fractures by skeletal traction. PAGE, C. M. Lancet *1:*986, May 7, '32
Wire extension treatment of fractures of fingers. MELTZER, H. Surg., Gynec. and Obst. *55:*87–89, July '32
Modification of extension treatment in fractures of fingers. CHRISTOFFERSEN, A. K. Ugesk. f. laeger *95:*1239–1240, Nov 16, '33
Finger and hand fractures treated by skeletal traction. HAGGART, G. E., S. Clin. North America *14:*1203–1210, Oct '34
Correction appliance for contracture of fingers and wrist. HOWITT, F. Lancet *2:*1394–1395, Dec 22, '34
Practical and easily prepared finger splint. ANDERSSON, O. J. Svenska lak.-tidning. *32:*1776–1777, Dec 20, '35
Splint bandage with lever in treatment of rupture of extensor aponeurosis of terminal digital phalanx. SAXL, A. Zentralbl. f. Chir. *63:*394–395, Feb 15, '36
Splint for extension and immobilization of digital fractures. LESER, A. J. Zentralbl. f. Chir. *63:*795–797, April 4, '36
Method of splinting septic fingers. HUNT, A. H. Lancet *2:*370–371, Aug 15, '36
Simple and efficient finger splint. HART, V. L., J. Bone and Joint Surg. *19:*245, Jan '37
Instrument for insertion of Kirschner wire in phalanges for skeletal traction. MEEKISON, D. M., J. Bone and Joint Surg. *19:*234, Jan '37
Splint for correction of finger contracture. OPPENHEIMER, E. D., J. Bone and Joint Surg. *19:*247–248, Jan '37
Simple pliable finger splint. BURCH, J. E. J.A.M.A. *108:*2036–2037, June 12, '37
New type of finger splints (for fractures). MIKKELSEN, O. Ugesk. f. laeger *99:*790–791, July 22, '37
New splint with surface for supporting injured fingers. BOECKER, P. Zentralbl. f. Chir. *64:*2134–2137, Sept 11, '37
Splint for therapy of lesions of extension tendons of fingers. ROZOV, V. I. Ortop. i travmatol. (no. 2) *11:*98–100, '37
Simple wire extension for use in therapy of metatarsal and metacarpal fractures and in fractures of fingers and toes. STEBER, F.

Splints, Finger – Cont.
Munchen. med. Wchnschr. *85:*480–481, March 31, '38
Technic of wire extension in fractures of fingers. THOMSEN, W. Chirurg *10:*145–148, March 1, '38
Method for skeletal traction to digits. TAYLOR, G. M. AND NEUFELD, A. J., J. Bone and Joint Surg. *20:*496–497, April '38
Finger splint for extension or flexion. SHNAYERSON, N., J.A.M.A. *110:*2070–2071, June 18, '38
Pin and stirrup for finger and toe traction. REED, E. N., J. Bone and Joint Surg. *20:*786, July '38
New banjo splint (for extension of contractures of metacarpophalangeal and interphalangeal joints). COZEN, L. Mil. Surgeon *85:*67–68, July '39
Splints for fingers and thumb. WHEELER, W. I. DEC. Lancet *2:*546–547, Nov 2, '40
Tautening arch for wire traction in therapy of fractures of phalanges. URRUTIA, J. M. Bol. y trab., Soc. de cir. de Cordoba (no. 1) *1:*54–58, '40
Two small wire splints for treatment by traction of fractures and deformities of fingers and metacarpal bones. LYFORD, J. III, J. Bone and Joint Surg. *24:*202–203, Jan '42
Extension splint for fingers. MADSEN, E. Nord. med. (Hospitalstid.) *14:*1650, May 30, '42
Modification of banjo splint for finger fractures. WILSON, C. S. Canad. M.A.J. *46:*585–586, June '42
Opponens thumb wire splint. HORWITZ, T. Am. J. Surg. *58:*460, Dec '42
Splint for control of ulnar deviation of fingers in rheumatoid arthritis. BODENHAM, D. C. Lancet *2:*354–355, Sept 18, '43
Celluloid splint in traumatic amputation of distal phalanges. O'TOOLE, J. B. JR. U. S. Nav. M. Bull. *42:*460–461, Feb '44
Splint for treatment of fractured fingers requiring traction. SAYPOL, G. M. Mil. Surgeon *95:*226–228, Sept '44
Improvised finger splint. PALMEN, A. J. Nord. med. *27:*1960, Sept 28, '45
Metal finger splint. PACKARD, J. W. JR. U. S. Nav. M. Bull. *45:*769–770, Oct '45
Improved finger splint. CHARBONNEAU, L. O. Hosp. Corps Quart. (no. 12) *18:*57, Dec '45
Small type skeletal traction apparatus (fingers). BOND, B. J., U. S. Nav. M. Bull. *46:*124–126, Jan '46
Corrective splint for paralysis of thenar muscles. NAPIER, J. R. Brit. M. J. *1:*15, Jan 5, '46
Knuckle bender splint. BUNNELL, S. Bull. U.

Splint, Finger – Cont.
S. Army M. Dept. *5:*230–231, Feb '46
Finger traps for banjo splint. ALDRED-BROWN, G. R. P. Brit. M. J. *1:*652, Apr 27, '46
Splint for treatment of mallet finger. SCHAUBEL, H. F. AND SMITH, E. W., J. Bone and Joint Surg. *28:*394–395, Apr '46
Novel method of digital traction in fractures. MACLEOD, K. M. Brit. M. J. *2:*614, Oct 26, '46

Splints, Hand: See Fingers, Splints; Hands, Splints

Splints, Jaw
Improvised emergency apparatus for fractured jaw. CANALE, A. Semana med. *2:*1189–1193, Dec 7, '22 (illus.)
Splint for unusual break of face. BOYCE, W. A., Laryngoscope *36:*266–269, April '26
Apparatus for treatment of jaw fractures, with loss of substance. DUCHANGE. Rev. d'hyg. *49:*608–613, Oct '27
Value of orthodontic appliances to immobilize jaw fractures. FEDERSPIEL, M. N. Internat. J. Orthodontia *14:*185–196, March '28
Fractures of upper and lower jaw and their correction with dental splint. MOREMEN, C. W., J. Florida M. A. *15:*207–209, Oct '28
Extra-oral splinting to support jaw after resection of middle portion of lower jaw. STAHNKE, E. Deutsche Ztschr. f. Chir. *215:*234–239, '29
Splint for fractures of inferior maxilla. MASLAND, H. C., M. Times, New York *58:*75, March '30
Methods of immobilization with mouth open and closed in fracture of lower jaw. RIDARD, L. Rev. gen. de clin. et de therap. *44:*454–456, July 12, '30
Operative treatment of losses of substance of mandible, with special reference to fixation of edentulous fragments. IVY, R. H. AND CURTIS, L. Surg., Gynec. and Obst. *52:*849–854, April '31
Metal splint for fractures of mandible. LISTER, C. S., U. S. Vet. Bur. M. Bull. *7:*498, May '31
Use of splints in complicated maxillary fracture. WUHRMANN, H. Schweiz. med. Wchnschr. *62:*767–769, Aug 20, '32
Use of cranial supports in reduction of fractures of mandibular angle. CROCQUEFER. Rev. de stomatol. *34:*347–351, June '32
Fracture of maxilla through left optic foramen; reduction with Kingsley splint, with restoration of vision. LANGDON, H. M.

Splints, Jaw – cont.

Arch. Ophth. *9:*980-981, June '33

Osteosynthesis by external fixation apparatus in fractures of lower jaw; technic and description of apparatus. BERCHER, J. AND GINESTET, G. Rev. de stomatol. *36:*294-300, May '34

Mandibular automobilizer; use in therapy of postoperative temporomaxillary ankylosis. DARCISSAC, M. Bull. et mem. Soc. d. chirurgiens de Paris *26:*561-568, Oct 19, '34

Splint for fractures of maxillary bones. MORGAN, W. M., J. Am. Dent. A. *21:*1736-1746, Oct '34

Extension method of Faltin for fractures of lower jaw. FALTIN, R. Vestnik khir. *35:*221-223, '34

Mistaken application of Faltin extension in case of fracture of lower jaw. KALINEYKO, I. P. Vestnik khir. *35:*219-220, '34

Preparation of splint for extra-oral extension in jaw fractures. NIRENBERG, B. B. AND FUKS, B. I. Sovet khir. (no. 4) *7:*732-734, '34

Disadvantages of Vorschütz method of treating complicated fractures and defects of lower jaw with plaster of paris bandage fastened to each side of jaw by screw arm. WASSMUND, M. Zentralbl. f. Chir. *62:*914-921, April 20, '35

Wire extension in treatment of mandibular fractures. BROOKE, R. Brit. M. J. *2:*498-499, Sept 14, '35

Therapy and prophylaxis of maxillary deformities by immobilization with monobloc. LASSERRE, C. AND MARRONEAUD, P. Arch. franco-belges de chir. *35:*131-134, Feb '36

Laterally displaced mandible; treatment simplified by aid of splint. LUSSIER, E. F. Internat. J. Orthodontia *22:*139-146, Feb '36

Disadvantages of Vorschütz method of treating complicated fractures and defects of lower jaw with plaster of paris bandage fastened to each side of jaw by screw arm (Reply to Vorschütz). WASSMUND, M. Zentralbl. f. Chir. *63:*444-445, Feb 22, '36 Further comment by Vorschütz; *63:*446, Feb 22, '36

Therapy of fractures of condyles of jaw; advantages of perifacial arc. LEBOURG, L. Presse med. *44:*360-361, March 4, '36

Fractures of upper jaw; reduction apparatus with pneumatic cushion. HAMON, J. Rev. de stomatol. *38:*518-521, July '36

Fractures of upper part of face necessitating cranial support; author's device. DUBECQ, X. J., J. de med. de Bordeaux *113:*817-820, Nov 30, '36

Splints, Jaw – Cont.

Simplified splinting of jaw fractures. FRANKL, Z. Gyogyaszat *77:*686, Dec 5; 714, Dec 12, '37

New apparatus for producing mechanical movements in cases of ankylosis of jaws. KOCHEV, K. N. Khirurgiya, no. 9, pp. 160-161, '37

Bimaxillary blockage in jaw fractures; compared advantages of 2 orthodontic apparatuses. SENTENAC, E. AND KOEFF, G., J. de med. de Bordeaux *115:*90-96, Jan 29 ('38)

Kirschner traction in treatment of maxillary fractures. MAJOR, G., J.A.M.A. *110:*1252-1254, April 16, '38

Reduction of double fracture of lower jaw by combined action of intermaxillary forces and transosseous loop. GINESTET, G. Rev. de stomatol. *40:*289-294, May '38

Fractured maxillae; description of appliance for reduction and fixation with case report. RALPH, H. G. AND MAXWELL, M. M., U.S. Nav. M. Bull. *36:*507-511, Oct '38

Methods of immobilization of fractured mandible. RICHARDS, R. L. Am. J. Orthodontics *24:*973-979, Oct '38

Technic of preparation and fixation of wire splints with intermaxillary traction. TARNOPOLSKIY, A. I. Ortop. i. travmatol. (no. 6) *12:*71-77, '38

Case of zygomatic fracture cured by direct skeletal traction applied with screw. GIORGI, C. Riv. di chir. *5:*34-39, Jan-Feb '39

Emergency treatment and primary apparatus for war fractures (of jaws). WEDDELL, J. M. Internat. Cong. Mil. Med. and Pharm *1:*237-249, '39

Suggestions for war surgery of facial injuries; use of wire cradle and fixation of tongue, facial flaps and bone fragments by means of safety pin in patients with jaw fractures. HENSCHEN, C. Schweiz. med. Wchnschr. *70:*711-715, July 30, '40

Wire grating chin cap in military surgery of jaw fractures. ROOS, W. Schweiz. med. Wchnschr. *70:*770, Aug 10, '40

Orthopedic therapy of fractures of lower jaw; new apparatuses. DE COSTER, L. Rev. de stomatol. *41:*933-947, '40

Facial fractures; pericranial anchorage utilizing lining of French soldier's helmet; model B.B.V. 236. FREIDEL, C. Rev. de stomatol. *41:*867-872, '40

Choice of apparatus for reduction and bandaging in maxillary fractures. PONROY, AND PSAUME. Rev. de stomatol. *41:*782-789, '40

New method of treatment of depressed frac-

Splints, Jaw – Cont.

ture of zygomatic bone (splint). BAXTER, H. Canad. M.A.J. *44:*5-9, Jan '41

Wire screen chin cap; suggestion for first aid for jaw injuries in field. Roos, W. Schweiz. med. Wchnschr. *71:*719-720, June 7, '41

Treating fractures of mandible by skeletal fixation. GRIFFIN, J. R. Am. J. Orthodontics (Oral Surg. Sect) *27:*364-376, July '41

Therapy of fractures of edentulous mandibles by external skeletal fixation, with report of case. INCLAN, A. Cir. ortop. y traumatol., Habana *9:*158-164, Oct-Dec '41

External pin fixation for mandible fractures. MOWLEM, R.; *et al.* Lancet *2:*391-393, Oct 4, '41

Extra-oral splinting of edentulous mandible in fractures. POHL, L. Lancet *2:*389-391, Oct 4, '41

Treating fractures of mandible by skeletal fixation. GRIFFIN, J. R. Rev. san. mil., Buenos Aires *40:*1006-1010, Nov '41

External skeletal fixation in fractures of mandibular angle. CONVERSE, J. M. AND WAKNITZ, F. W., J. Bone and Joint Surg. *24:*154-160, Jan '42

Stretcher head support in cases of smashed jaw. PAISLEY, J. C. Brit. M. J. *1:*16, Jan 3, '42

Fractures of maxillae and mandible; 2 cases (with description of apparatus). YANDO, A. H. AND TAYLOR, R. W., U. S. Nav. M. Bull. *40:*155-157, Jan '42

Internal wire fixation of jaw fractures; preliminary report. BROWN, J. B. AND McDOWELL, F. Surg., Gynec. and Obst. *74:*227-230, Feb '42

Experiences with various methods of skeletal fixation in jaw fractures. MOWLEM, R. Proc. Roy. Soc. Med. *35:*415-426, April '42

Plastic correction of depressed deformities of facial bones, especially by means of traction apparatus. REGO, G. Arq. de cir. clin. e exper. *6:*200-234, April-June '42

Care of military and civilian injuries; mandibular fractures treated by pin fixation; 21 cases. RUSHTON, M. A. AND WALKER, F. A. Am. J. Orthodontics (Oral Surg. Sect) *28:*307-315, May '42

Fractures of mandible, with special reference to reduction of complicated displacements and subsequent immobilization. WALDRON, C. W. Journal-Lancet *62:*228-240, June '42

Compact splints with new fixation method for maxillary fractures. DIMEG, O. Ztschr. f. Stomatol. *40:*485-504, July '42

First aid splinting of jaw fractures. SPANIER, F., M. Rec. *155:*377, July '42

Splints, Jaw – Cont.

New intraoral spring mouth opener for treatment of lockjaw. SCHUCHARDT, K. Ztschr. f. Stomatol. *40:*677-680, Sept 25, '42

Facial fractures; internal wiring fixation. ADAMS, W. M. Surgery *12:*523-540, Oct '42

Immobilization of wartime, compound, comminuted fractures of mandible. KAZANJIAN, V. H. Am. J. Orthodontics (Oral Surg. Sect) *28:*551-560, Oct '42

Treatment of facial fractures (description of extraoral fixation appliance). ADAMS, W. M., J. Tennessee M. A. *35:*469-475, Dec '42

External splint for use in derangements of temporomandibular joint. TREGARTHEN, G. G. T. Bull. War Med. *3:*271-272, Jan '43 (abstract)

Skeletal fixation in treatment of fractures of mandible; review. WALDRON, C. W., J. Oral Surg. *1:*59-83, Jan '43

Care of military and civilian injuries; external traction appliance for jaw fractures. BISNOFF, H. L. Am. J. Orthodontics (Oral Surg. Sect) *29:*96-101, Feb '43

Notes from maxillofacial centers; intraoral methods of immobilizing mandibular fractures. DALLING, E. J. Bull. War Med. *3:*555, June '43 (abstract)

Combined intraoral and dental fixation in fracture of mandibular angle with considerable displacement. FERBER, E. W., J. Am. Dent. A. *30:*906-910, June 1, '43

External skeletal fixation of mandibles. CONVERSE, J. M., J. Oral Surg. *1:*210-214, July '43

Use of ordinary small brass hinge as locking device for splints in multiple fractures of jaws. GOODSELL, J. O., J. Oral Surg. *1:*250-251, July '43

Extraoral skeletal fixation of mandibular fractures; cases. GROSS, P. P. Am. J. Orthodontics (Oral Surg. Sect.) *29:*392-400, July '43

Correlated fixation of mandibular fractures. KAMRIN, B. B., J. Oral Surg. *1:*235-240, July '43

Tie-loop wiring of fractured jaws. PETERSON, R. G., J. Oral Surg. *1:*246-249, July '43

New method of intermaxillary fixation in patients wearing artificial dentures. THOMA, K. H. Am. J. Orthodontics (Oral Surg. Sect) *29:*433-441, Aug '43

Simple skeletal fixation method for quick repair in war surgery (jaws). BERRY, H. C., J. Am. Dent. A. *30:*1377-1378, Sept 1, '43

Extraoral splinting of mandible. BOURGOYNE, J. R., J. Am. Dent. A. *30:*1390-1392, Sept 1, '43

Mandibular fractures; report of 50 applica-

Splints, Jaw – Cont.
tions of Roger Anderson skeletal fixation appliance. WINTER, L. Am. J. Surg. *61:*367–379, Sept '43
Acrylic resin splints for jaw fractures. HENDERSON, R. L. V., J. Roy. Nav. M. Serv. *29:*268, Oct '43
Recent experiences with skeletal fixation in fractures of mandible. IVY, R. H. AND CURTIS, L., J. Oral Surg. *1:*296–308, Oct '43
Extraoral utilization of screws or pins in immobilization of mandibular fractures. LOGSDON, C. M., J. Am. Dent. A. *30:*1529–1540, Oct 1, '43
Horizontal pin fixation for fractures of mandible using pin guide. PINCOCK, D. F. Surg., Gynec. and Obst. *77:*493–496, Nov '43
Dental arch of upper jaw as support for apparatus during surgical interventions on head in cases of nasal fractures and corrections, skin grafts of face and mobilization of maxillary ankylosis. KUNZENDORF, W. Deutsche Ztschr. f. Chir. *258:*348, '43
Extraoral plaster splint fixation in treatment of fractures of mandible. GODWIN, J. G., J. Am. Dent. A. *31:*76–85, Jan 1, '44
Acrylic half-splint for jaw injuries. MACKTA, L. Bull. U. S. Army M. Dept. (no. 72) pp. 81–83, Jan '44
Technic for building head cast fracture appliances from coat hangers for facial fractures. VAN ZILE, W. N., U. S. Nav. M. Bull. *42:*200–207, Jan '44
Removable plaster headcap for facial fractures. WOODARD, D. E., J. Oral Surg. *2:*23–31, Jan '44
Horizontal pin fixation for fractures of mandible using pin guide. PINCOCK, D. F. Am. J. Orthodontics (Oral Surg. Sect.) *30:*67–72, Feb '44
Fractures of mandible; review of experience in 52 patients with particular reference to use of external skeletal fixation. WIESENFELD, I. H. AND MEADOFF, N. Permanente Found. M. Bull. *2:*49–63, March '44
Arteriovenous aneurysm resulting from application of Roger Anderson splint for fractured jaw. GREELEY, P. W. AND THRONDSON, A. H., J.A.M.A. *124:*1128, April 15, '44
Skeletal fixation in treatment of fractures of mandible. PARKER, D. B., S. Clin. North America *24:*381–391, April '44
Skeletal fixation splint in mandibular fractures as aid to early denture construction. RICHISON, F. A. AND KENNEDY, J. T., J. Am. Dent. A. *31:*646–648, May 1, '44
Treatment of multiple fractures of face with

Splints, Jaw – Cont.
external pin fixation splint. ELVIDGE, A. AND BAXTER, H. McGill M. J. *13:*469–475, Dec '44
Modified maxillary fracture splint for jaw. BLAUSTEN, S. Bull. U. S. Army M. Dept. (no. 84) pp. 119–121, Jan '45
Appliances for external fixation of mandible and cranial fixation of maxilla. CONVERSE, J. M. Am. J. Orthodontics (Oral Surg. Sect.) *31:*111–112, Feb '45
Uses of screw-pin in maxillofacial cases. RUSHTON, M. A. AND WALKER, F. A. Brit. Dent. J. *78:*289–292, May 18, '45
Screw-pin for use in connection with mandibular fractures and grafts. WALKER, F. A. Brit. Dent. J. *78:*266–267, May 4, '45
Extraoral pin fixation for fractures of mandible. MACGREGOR, A. B. Lancet *1:*816, June 30, '45
Haynes splint in case of bone graft of lower jaw. INCLAN, A. JR. Cir. ortop. y traumatol. Habana *12:*132–137, July–Sept '45
Method of facilitating insertion of pins in skeletal fixation of jaw fractures. PETERSON, R. G. *et al.* J. Oral Surg. *3:*258–262, July '45
Modified traction and fixation splint for fractures of facial bones. WACHSBERGER, A. Arch. Otolaryng. *42:*53–55, July '45
Fixation of pathologic fractures of mandible. BOURGOYNE, J. R. Am. J. Orthodontics (Oral Surg. Sect.) *31:*492–500, Aug '45
Open reduction vs. skeletal fixation in jaw fractures. BOURGOYNE, J. R. Am. J. Orthodontics (Oral Surg. Sect.) *31:*519–532, Aug '45
Mandibular fractures at King County Hospital treated by Roger Anderson skeletal fixation. GRAHAM, J. W. Northwest Med. *44:*250–252, Aug '45
Headpiece for face wounds and fractures. JORDAN, C. E., U. S. Nav. M. Bull. *45:*330, Aug '45
Fracture of zygomatic bone and arch; postoperative headgear. SCHMIER, A. A. Am. J. Surg. *70:*27–37, Oct '45
Surgical therapy of mandibular fracture by Kirschner nails; case. CAUDENAT *et al.* Rev. de stomatol. *46:*130–133, Oct–Dec '45
Skeletal fixation of mandibular fractures; 5 cases with 9 fractures. BURKE, H. S. *et al.* Arch. Surg. *51:*279–282, Nov–Dec '45
Advances in construction and use of splints in treatment of jaw fractures. FICKLING, B. W. Brit. Dent. J. *80:*8–13, Jan 4, '46
Control of mandibular fragments by external fixation. ROBERTS, W. R. Brit. Dent. J. *80:*257, April 18, '46; 291, May 3, '46

Splints, Jaw – Cont.

Fractures of lower jaw; indications for new surgical method of pin fixation. MARONNEAUD, P. L., J. de med. de Bordeaux *123:*201-205, June '46

Fractures of mandible; Mowlem method of external pin fixation. MARINO, H. AND CRAVIOTTO, M. Prensa med. argent. *33:*1823-1827, Sept 6, '46

Preparation of screw lock sectional splint with mechanical retention for fracture of jaw. McCARTHY, W. D. AND BURNS, S. R., J. Oral Surg. *4:*343-352, Oct '46

Splints, Nasal

Nasal septum splint. VERDIER, R. A. Am. J. Surg. *36:*44, Feb '22 (illus.)

Apparatus for restoring shape to sunken nose. FREUND. Deutsche med. Wchnschr. *48:*1422, Oct 20, '22

Nasal fractures; treatment of same by new adjustable splint. SALINGER, S. Ann. Otol. Rhin. and Laryng. *33:*413-416, June '24

New nasal splint. WHITE, F. W. Laryngoscope *35:*76, Jan '25

Adjustable splint for fractures of nose. SALINGER, S. Illinois M. J. *48:*304-306, Oct '25

Splint for treatment of wide depressed nasal bridges. WATKINS, A. B. K., M. J. Australia *2:*556-557, Oct 23, '26

New nasal brace. SAFIAN, J. Arch. Otolaryng. *8:*566-568, Nov '28

Treatment of severer cases of nasal fractures (splint). WATKINS, A. B. K. Brit. M. J. *2:*917-918, Nov 18, '33

Copper molded nasal splint; new method of application. SALINGER, S. Arch. Otolaryng. *20:*211-214, Aug '34

New type of plaster of paris protector for use in therapy of nasal fractures. GAUS, W. Hals-, Nasen-u. Ohrenarzt (Teil 1) *28:*94-97, April '37

New splint for nasal septum. SOLO, A. Arch. Otolaryng. *27:*343-346, March '38

Lateral pressure splint in nasal fractures. KAZANJIAN, V. H. Arch. Otolaryng. *27:*474-475, April '38

Plaster cast in therapy of nasal fractures. ZENO, L. An. de cir. *4:*124-127, June '38 also: Bol. Soc. de cir. de Rosario *5:*269-272, July '38

Technic of making plaster of paris cast for nasal fractures and deformities. RODE, B. Ztschr. f. Hals-, Nasen-u. Ohrenh. *43:*294-295, '38

Nasal splint. SCHLESSELMAN, J. T. Arch. Otolaryng. *29:*988-989, June '39

Dental molding compound cast and adhesive strapping in rhinoplastic procedure. AUFRICHT, G. Arch. Otolaryng. *32:*333-338, Aug '40

Splints, Nasal – Cont.

Improved instruments and postoperative splint for nasal plastic operations; combined chisel and periosteal elevator. PEARLMAN, L. M. Arch. Otolaryng. *32:*338-340, Aug '40

Simple nasal splint. MATIS, E. I., J. Laryng. and Otol. *55:*425-426, Sept '40

New traction and fixation apparatus for fractured nose. GONZALEZ ULLOA, M. Rev. mex. de cir., ginec. y cancer *10:*65-74, Feb '42 also: Rev. brasil. de cir. *11:*215-218, May '42

Plaster splint for fractured noses. PARSONS, H. H. Mil. Surgeon *91:*212, Aug '42

SPOONER, E. T. C.: "Hospital infection" in plastic surgery ward. J. Hyg. *41:*320-329, Nov '41

SPRAGUE, E. W.: Management of cleft-lip and palate cases. S. Clin. N. Amer. *6:*1481-1496, Dec '26

SPRATT, C. N.: Improved nasofrontal rasp. Arch. Otolaryng. *11:*783, June '30

SPRENGER, W.: Keloid formation in ear lobe. Monatschr. f. Ohrenh. *70:*188-194, Feb '36

SPRINGER, C.: Plastic operation for epispadias by means of temporary suturing into scrotum; case. Zentralbl. f. Chir. *58:*1047-1051, April 25, '31

SPROAT, S. M.: Unusually extensive injury of scrotum, avulsion. California and West. Med. *23:*1318-1319, Oct '25

SPROGIS, G.: Theory of heredity of Dupuytren's contracture. Deutsche Ztschr. f. Chir. *194:*259-263, '26

SPROGIS, G.: Problem of heredity of Dupuytren's contracture. Compt. rend. Soc. de biol. *94:*631-632, March 12, '26 abstr: J.A.M.A. *87:*131, July 10, '26

SPURLING, R. G.: Symposium on war surgery; use of tantalum wire and foil in repair of peripheral nerves. S. Clin. North America *23:*1491-1504, Dec '43

SPURLING, R. G.: Peripheral nerve surgery; technical considerations. Am. Acad. Orthop. Surgeons, Lect. pp. 259-269, '44

SPURLING, R. G.: Peripheral nerve injuries in European Theater of Operations; management, with special reference to early nerve surgery. J.A.M.A. *129:*1011-1014, Dec 8, '45 abst., Bull. U. S. Army M. Dept. *4:*557-559, Nov '45

SPURLING, R. G. *et al*: Failure of whole fresh homogenous nerve grafts in man. J. Neurosurg. *2:*79-101, March '45

SPURLING, R. G. AND WOODHALL, B.: Peripheral nerve injuries; experience with early

nerve surgery. Ann. Surg. *123:*731–748, May '46
SPURLING, R. G. AND WOODHALL, B.: Peripheral nerve injuries; early surgery. Tr. South. S. A. (1945) *57:*269–286, '46
SQUIRE, C. M.: Contractures of fingers and toes after war wounds. Proc. Roy. Soc. Med. *36:*665–666, Oct '43
SQUIRRU, C. M.: Dentists and first surgical care of face and jaw injuries on battlefield. Rev. san. mil., Buenos Aires *41:*457–469, July '42
SQUIRRU, C. M.: New technic in therapy of temporomandibular ankylosis. Rev. san. mil., Buenos Aires *42:*789–799, Nov '43
SRIBMAN, I.: Cystic lymphangioma, with report of case (neck). Dia med. *15:*175–178, March 1, '43
SROUB, W. E. (see COLE, H. N.) Aug '36
ST-ONGE, G.: Blood plasma in therapy of burn case with severe shock. J. de l'Hotel-Dieu de Montreal *10:*396–408, Nov–Dec '41
ST-ONGE, G.: Modern conceptions and biologic therapy of shock in surgery. J. de l'Hotel-Dieu de Montreal *11:*355–406, Sept–Oct '42
STACEY, R. S.: Rare hand malformation. J. Anat. *72:*456–457, April '38
STACY, H. S.: Fractures of maxillary zygomatic region and their treatment. M. J. Australia *1:*779–780, June 27, '31
STACY, H. S.: Carcinoma of mouth and its treatment. M. J. Australia *1:*549–550, May 6, '33
STACY, H. S.: Role of surgery in carcinoma of buccal cavity. M. J. Australia *1:*712–717, June 2, '34
STAFNE, E. C. (see MILLHON, J. A.) Nov '41
STAGMAN, J.: Device for cutting cartilage isografts. Arch. Otolaryng. *42:*284, Oct '45
STAHEL, W.: Injury of hand tendons. Schweiz. med. Wchnschr. *67:*51–54, Jan 16, '37
STAHL, F.: Ankylosing operations in therapy of hallux rigidus; after-examination. Acta orthop. Scandinav. *14:*97–126, '43
STAHL, O.: Ultimate results of Langenbeck's operation for cleft palate. Arch. f. klin. Chir. *123:*271–316, '23 (illus.) abstr: J.A.M.A. *80:*1421, May 12, '23
STAHLMAN, T. M.: Use of paraffin and wax in ear and nose surgery. Pennsylvania M. J. *24:*875, Sept '21
STAHNKE, E.: Dupuytren's contracture treated with humanol injections. Zentralbl. f. Chir. *54:*2438–2442, Sept 24, '27
STAHNKE, E.: Extra-oral splinting to support jaw after resection of middle portion of lower jaw. Deutsche Ztschr. f. Chir. *215:*234–239, '29
STAJANO, C.: General norms in shock therapy. Arch. urug. de med., cir. y especialid. *9:*634–644, Nov '36
STAJANO, C.: Shock and postoperative hypotension. Arch. urug. de med., cir. y especialid. *10:*373–380, March '37
STAJANO, C.: Shock in burns. An. Fac. de med. de Montevideo *23:*923–941, '38
STAJANO, C.: Enema of concentrated coffee in shock therapy; study from 1916-1941. Arch. urug. de med., cir. y especialid. *19:*241–260, Sept '41
STAJANO, C. (see JORGE, J. M. *et al*) March '41
STALKER, L. K. (see PEMBERTON, J. DEJ.) May '39
STALKER, L. K. (see PEMBERTON, J. DEJ.) June '40
STALLARD, H. B.: Cavernous hemangioma of orbit successfully removed by Krönlein's operation. Lancet *1:*131–133, Jan 15, '38
STALLARD, H. B.: Modified Brigg's retractor for dacryocystorhinostomy. Brit. J. Ophth. *22:*361, June '38
STAMM, T. T.: Method of grafting long bones. Proc. Roy. Soc. Med. *31:*461–464, March '38
STAMM, T. T.: Excision of proximal row of carpus. Proc. Roy. Soc. Med. *38:*74–75, Dec '44
STAMMERS, F. A. R.: Pre-auricular fistulae. Brit. J. Surg. *14:*359–363, Oct '26
STANBRO, G. E.: Traumatic shock. J. Oklahoma M. A. *29:*199–202, June '36
STANČIUS, P.: Plastic operation of cleft palate according to Ernst method. Medicina, Kaunas *18:*558–562, July '37
STANDARD, S.: Lymphedema of arm following radical mastectomy for carcinoma of breast; new operation for its control. Ann. Surg. *116:*816–820, Dec '42
STANDARD, S.: Present concept of shock syndrome and its treatment. Hebrew M. J. *1:*170, '43
STANHOPE, E. D.: Points on treatment of maxillofacial injuries. East African M. J. *20:*399–408, Dec '43
STANLEY-BROWN, M.: Extensive burns. M. Clin. North America *17:*1393–1405, March '34
STANLEY-BROWN, M.: Extensive burns. S. Clin. North America *15:*375–385, April '35
STANLEY-BROWN, M.: Modified Kondoleon operation for chronic leg ulcers. S. Clin. North America *21:*617–623, April '41
STANLEY-BROWN, M. (see BANCROFT, F. W. *et al*) May '40
STAPLER, D.: Technical details of esthetic surgery. Ann. paulist. de med. e cir. *38:*101–108, Aug '39
STARCK, H.: Formation of artificial vagina from rectum (Schubert operation) in congenital vaginal defect; preliminary report. Zentralbl. f. Gynak. *57:*2562–2565, Oct 28, '33
STARK, W. J.: Use of pedicled flaps in surgical treatment of chronic osteomyelitis resulting

from compound fractures. J. Bone and Joint Surg. *28:*343–350, April '46
STARKENSTEIN, E.: Hereditary transmission of branchial fistulas; case. Med. Klin. *24:*701, May 4, '28
STAROSHKLOVSKAYA, R. M.: Treatment of postoperative shock in gastro-intestinal diseases. Novy khir. arkhiv *32:*351–364, '34
STARR, C. L.: Reconstruction surgery and its application to civilian practice. Surg., Gynec. and Obst. *32:*311, April '21
STARR, C. L.: Army experiences with tendon transference. J. Bone and Joint Surg. *4:*3–21, Jan '22 (illus.)
STARR, F. N. G.: Late result in ectopia vesicae. Brit. J. Surg. *15:*328, Oct '27
STARR, K. W.: Successful suture of facial nerve trunk. Australian and New Zealand J. Surg. *14:*53–57, July '44
STARUP, U.: Clinical aspects and therapy of surgical shock. Nord. med. (Hospitalstid.) *15:*2526–2531, Sept 12, '42
STAUB, H. A.: Splint for tendon of extensor digitorum. Munchen. med. Wchnschr. *69:*119–120, Jan 27, '22 (illus.)
STAUFFER, H.: Cancer forming in inflamed tissue following burns; case. Ztschr. f. Krebsforsch. *28:*418–430, '29
STEAD, E. A. JR.: Treatment of circulatory collapse and shock. Am. J. M. Sc. *201:*775–782, May '41
STEAD, E. A. JR.: Treatment of circulatory collapse and shock. Rev. Asoc. med. argent. *55:*710–713, Sept 15–30, '41
STEAD, E. A. JR.; *et al*: Concentrated human albumin in treatment of shock. Arch. Int. Med. *77:*564–575, May '46
STEADMAN, F. ST. J.: Jaw fractures, with special reference to treatment. Brit. Dent. J. *50:*824–838, July 15, '29
STEBER, F.: Simple wire extension for use in therapy of metatarsal and metacarpal fractures and in fractures of fingers and toes. Munchen. med. Wchnschr. *85:*480–481, March 31, '38
STECHER, L.: Aplasia of joints in fingers. Arch. f. klin. Chir. *134:*818–825, '25
STECHER, W. R.: Genealogical study of case of symmetrical congenital brachydactylia. M. Rec. *144:*5–8, July 1, '36
STEEL, J. P.: Cod liver oil in burns. Lancet *2:*290–292, Aug 10, '35
STEEL, W. A.: Hot air mineral oil treatment of extensive burns. New York M. J. *116:*418–419, Oct 4, '22
STEENROD, E. J.; GHORMLEY, R. K. AND CRAIG, W. M.: Hand injuries due to shattered porcelain handles of water faucets. Surg., Gynec. and Obst. *64:*950–955, May '37
STEFANESCU, G. (see SARRU, P. *et al*) May '40
STEFANI, F.: Nonoperative treatment in mandibular fracture. Stomatol. *29:*128–134, Feb '31
STEFANI, F.: Reconstruction of upper and middle portions of nose by author's technic; case. Riv. di chir. *3:*433–439, Sept '37
STEFANI, F.: Rare congenital malformation of face; median harelip with dissociation without deformation of 2 halves of nose (double nose); case. Plast. chir. *1:*162–166, '40
STEFANINI, P.: Free autoplastic graft of gastric mucosa to replace urinary bladder tissue loss. Arch. ed atti d. Soc. ital. di chir. *43:*951–967, '37
STEGEMANN, H.: Surgical treatment of large contraction scars of burns according to Morestin's plastic operations. Zentralbl. f. Chir. *53:*1880–1884, July 24, '26
STEHR, L.: Ulnar-volar bayonet hand as typical deformity in chrondrodysplasia. Fortschr. a. d. Geb. d. Rontgenstrahlen *57:*587–604, June '38
STEIDL, H.: Clinical sequelae of injury to inferior alveolar nerve following fractures of mandible. Deutsche Ztschr. f. Chir. *230:*129–146, '31
STEIGER-KAZAL, D.: Paraffin in burns. Orvosi hetil. (mell.) *76:*2–3, Jan 9, '32
STEIN, C.: Faulty anlage and defects of ear. Handb. d. Neurol. d. Ohres (Teil 1) *2:*113–150, '28
STEIN, G.: Bone transplantation. Ztschr. f. Stomatol. *26:*284–309, March '28
STEIN, H. C. AND BETTMANN, E. H.: Rare malformation of arm; double humerus with 3 hands and 16 fingers. Am. J. Surg. *50:*336–343, Nov '40
STEIN, J. C. (see GRADLE, H. S.) May '24
STEIN, J. J.: Burn therapy in the field. Hosp. Corps Quart. *16:*113–115, July '43
STEIN, L.: Pathology and treatment of rhinolalia. Wien. klin. Wchnschr. *43:*1068–1069, Aug 21, '30
STEIN, R.: Modification of Lowenstein clamp used in transplantation of lip mucosa. Klin. Monatsbl. f. Augenh. *88:*370–371, March '32
STEIN, R. O.: Cosmetic paraffin injections in facial surgery. Wien. klin. Wchnschr. *40:*830, June 23, '27
STEIN, R. O.: Removal of folds and wrinkles of face; indications and technic. Wien. klin. Wchnschr. *40:*1168–1172, Sept 15, '27
STEIN, R. O.: Excision of oval pieces of skin in treatment of facial wrinkles. Arch. f. Dermat. u. Syph. *155:*304–307, '28
STEIN, R. O.: Keloid therapy. Wien. klin. Wchnschr. *45:*996–998, Aug 5, '32
STEINBERG, C. L.: New method of treatment

(vitamin E) of Dupuytren's contracture, form of fibrositis. M. Clin. North America *30:*221-231, Jan '46

STEINBERG, M. E.: Skin flap cover for projecting intestine. Ann. Surg. *83:*123-125, Jan '26

STEINDEL, S. (see BAUMGARTNER, C. J.) Jan '43

STEINDL, H.: Treatment of injuries of fingers. Wien. klin. Wchnschr. *42:*1631-1636, Dec 19, '29

STEINDLER, A.: Skin flap methods in upper extremity deformities. J. Bone and Joint Surg. *7:*512-527, July '25

STEINDLER, A.: Orthopedic reconstruction work on hand; early and late results. Surg., Gynec. and Obst. *45:*476-481, Oct '27

STEINDLER, A.: Pill roller hand deformities due to imbalance of intrinsic muscles; relief by ulnar resection. J. Bone and Joint Surg. *10:*550-553, July '28

STEINDLER, A.: Flexor plasty of thumb in thenar palsy. Surg., Gynec. and Obst. *50:*1005-1007, June '30

STEINDLER, A.: Reconstructive surgery following traumatic deformities of upper extremity. Am. Acad. Orthop. Surgeons, Lect., pp. 268-279, '43

STEINDLER, A.: Tendon transplantation at elbow. Am. Acad. Orthop. Surgeons, Lect., pp. 276-283, '44

STEINER, A.: Congenital fistula of external ear; 2 cases. Dermat. Wchnschr. *86:*325-328, March 10, '28

STEINER, F.: Heredity of hypospadias. Munchen. med. Wchnschr. *83:*1271, July 31, '36

STEINIGER, F.: Effect of certain experimental conditions on development of hereditary harelip in mice. Ztschr. f. menschl. Vererb. -u. Konstitutionslehre *24:*1-12, '39

STEINIGER, F.: Embryologic study of harelip cysts. Ztschr. f. menschl. Vererb.-u. Konstitutionslehre *25:*1-27, '41

STEINIGER, F. AND VEIT, G.: "Heteropenetration" and twin discordance in hereditary harelip and cleft palate. Ztschr. f. menschl. Vereb. -u. Konstitutionslehre *26:*75-92, '42

STEINKAMM, J.: Application of Vorschutz lever screw in fractures of lower jaw. Chirurg *7:*820-824, Dec 1, '35

STEINMANN, B.: Injuries of thumb. Casop. lek. cesk. *76:*963-965, June 11, '37

STEINMETZ, E. P.: Formation of artificial vagina. West. J. Surg. *48:*169-180, March '40

STEINREICH, O. S. (see THIESSEN, N. W.) Aug '42

STEINTHAL, K.: Rhinoplasty with flap from patient's chest. Zentralbl. f. Chir. *50:*508-509, March 31, '23 (illus.)

STEISS, C. F.: Reconstruction of scalp following excision for malignancy. Am. J. Surg. *52:*378-380, May '41

Stejskal

Reply to article by Joseph on shock therapy; also, one by Stejskal. SCHÜCK. Zentralbl. f. Chir. *60:*634-635, March 18, '33

STEJSKAL, K.: Intravenous injections of hypertonic solutions in shock. (Comment on Schück's article). Zentralbl. f. Chir. *59:*2896, Nov 26, '32

STENHOUSE, H. M.: Kondoleon operation and filariasis. U. S. Nav. M. Bull. *20:*715-716, June '24

Stent: See Skin Grafts, Dressings for; Skin Grafts, Inlay

STEOPOE, V.: Neotonocain (procaine preparation) in surgery of fingers. Romania med. *7:*245, Nov 15, '29

STEPANOFF, N. M.: Rare complications in osteomyelitis of lower jaw; Filatov's grafts in defects of oral cavity. Vestnik khir. (nos. 70-71) *24:*233-236, '31

STEPANOVA, E. N.: Thiersch graft in therapy of syndactylia. Novy khir. arkhiv *32:*101-104, '34

STEPHAN, H.: Surgical therapy of syndactylia. Zentralbl. f. Chir. *66:*794-796, April 8, '39

STEPHENS, H. D.: Harelip. Brit. M. J. *1:*5-8, Jan 4, '36 also: M. J. Australia *1:*494-498, April 11, '36

STEPHENS, R.: "Baseball finger" cured by operation. J. Bone and Joint Surg. *6:*469-470, April '24

STEPHENSON, K. L. (see ROBINSON, D. W. *et al*) July '46

STEPLEANU-HORBATZKY: Extensive loss of substance in subhyoid region; recovery after fat transplantation. Rev. de chir., Bucuresti *41:*512-515, July-Aug '38

STEPOWSKA, A.: Rhinolalia aperta. Polska gaz. lek. *8:*183-185, March 10, '29

STERN, E. L.: New operative procedure for Dupuytren's contracture. Am. J. Surg. *54:*711-715, Dec '41

STERN, L. S.: Treatment of shock by direct action on vegetative nerve centers (injection of potassium ions into lateral ventricles or cisterna magna). Brit. M. J. *2:*538-540, Nov 7, '42 also: Lancet *2:*572-573, Nov 14, '42

STERN, W. G.: Report of cured case of ankylosis of jaw. Ohio State M. J. *19:*248-249, April '23 (illus.)

STERNBERG, H.: Morphological genesis of cleft of abdomen and bladder (ectopia vesicae). Urol. and Cutan. Rev. *31:*475-479, Aug '27

STERNBERG, H. (see FRÜHMANN, P.) 1930

STETTEN, DEW.: Plastic reconstruction of hand with phalangealization of thumb. Ann. Surg. *97:*290–296, Feb '33

STEUDING, O.: Formation of artificial vagina. Zentralbl. f. Gynak. *46:*61–63, Jan 14, '22

STEVENS, J. T.: Cancer of lip; its treatment by means of electrothermic coagulation, radium and roentgen rays. Radiology *4:*372–377, May '25

STEVENS, J. T.: Electrothermic surgery of cancer of lips. Am. J. Surg. *7:*831–835, Dec '29

STEVENS, R. H.: Treatment of naevi. J. Radiol. *2:*33, Nov '21

STEVENSON, G. H.: Tendon transplantations for musculo-spiral paralysis. Glasgow M. J. *99:*225–230, April '23

STEVENSON, G. H.: Treatment of ununited fractures and other bone defects by bone grafts and bone comminution. Glasgow M. J. *101:*274–286, May '24

STEVENSON, H. N.: Elimination of intranasal pack by topical use of thrombin. Ann. Otol., Rhin. and Laryng. *53:*159–162, March '44

STEVENSON, H. N.: Instrument for anchoring fractures of face. Arch. Otolaryng. *40:*503, Dec '44

STEVENSON, H. N. AND TUOTI, F. A.: Reduction of complete transverse fracture of edentulous maxilla. U. S. Nav. M. Bull. *45:*910–913, Nov '45

STEVENSON, T. W.: Release of circular constricting scar by Z flaps. Plastic and Reconstruct. Surg. *1:*39–42, July '46

STEVENSON, T. W. (see WEBSTER, J. B. *et al*) April '44

STEVENSON, T. W. JR.: Principles of treatment of avulsion of skin. S. Clin. North America *21:*555–564, April '41

STEVENSON, W. B.: Maxillary fractures. Am. J. Orthodontics *29:*331–332, June '43

STEWART, C. B.: Report of 88 cases of cancer of lips from Steiner Clinic. Surg., Gynec. and Obst. *53:*533–535, Oct '31

STEWART, C. B.: Care of cervical glands in intra-oral carcinoma. Am. J. Roentgenol. *29:*234–236, Feb '33

STEWART, C. B.: Management of tumors of the parotid. Am. J. Surg. *30:*18–20, Oct '35

STEWART, C. P. (see HARKINS, H. N. *et al*) March '35

STEWART, C. P. (see WILSON, W. C.) April '38

STEWART, C. P. (see WILSON, W. C.) Nov '39

STEWART, J. D. AND WARNER, F.: Shock in severely wounded in forward field hospitals, with special reference to wound shock. Ann. Surg. *122:*129–146, Aug '45

STEWART, J. E.: Experimental study of transplantation of nerve supply of muscles. J. Bone and Joint Surg. *7:*948–956, Oct '25

STEWART, M. B. AND CONLEY, J. J.: Fractures of malar-zygomatic compound; treatment by improved methods and myoplasty. Arch. Otolaryng. *44:*443–451, Oct '46

STEWART, R. L.: Treatment of minor burns by amyl salicylate and other salicyl esters. Brit. M. J. *1:*380–383, Feb 20, '37

STEWART, W. J.: Experimental bone regeneration using lime salts and autogenous grafts as source of available calcium. Surg., Gynec. and Obst. *59:*867–871, Dec '34

STEWART, W. J.: Congenital median cleft of chin. Arch. Surg. *31:*813–815, Nov '35

STIBBE, F. H. (see BENJAMINS, C. E.) Dec '26

STIBBE, F. H. (see BENJAMINS, C. E.) 1927

STIEF, ALEXANDER (SANDOR): (see STIEF, S.)

STIEF, S.: Facial hemiatrophy; autopsy findings; case. Ztschr. f. d. ges. Neurol. u. Psychiat. *147:*573–593, '33

STIEFLER, G.: Bilateral progressive facial hemiatrophy. Jahrb. f. Psychiat. u. Neurol. *51:*277–292, '34

STILES, K. A. AND WEBER, R. A.: Pedigree of symphalangism. J. Hered. *29:*199–202, May '38

STILMAN, I.: Burn therapy based on etiopathogenesis. Semana med. *1:*882–883, April 30, '42

STINSON, W. D.: Perforation of nasal septum occurring in manufacture of calcium arsenate. J. Tennessee M. A. *24:*65, Feb '31

STINSON, W. D.: Osseous atresia of posterior choanae. Arch. Otolaryng. *15:*101–103, Jan '32

STOCK, F. E.: Artificial vagina; bicornate uterus and absence of vagina; case. M. Press *211:*365–366, June 7, '44

STOCK, W.: Result of surgical therapy of suppuration of lacrimal sac after implantation of lower end of lacrimal sac into nose; modified Toti operation. Klin. Monatsbl. f. Augenh. *92:*433–435, April '34

STOCKER, H. (see SCHREINER, K.) Aug '29

STOCKTON, A. B.: Local treatment of war burns. Stanford M. Bull. *2:*71–73, May '44

STOEBER, R. (see SPECKLIN, P.) Aug '22

STOECKEL, W.: Technic of formation of artificial vagina; 4 cases. Monatschr. f. Geburtsh. u. Gynak. *90:*23–33, Jan '32

Stoeckel Operation: See Goebell-Stoeckel Operation

STOELTZNER, W.: Therapeutic softening of scar tissue. Munchen. med. Wchnschr. *72:*2133–2135, Dec 11, '25 abstr: J.A.M.A. *86:*384, Jan 30, '26

STOFT, W. E.: Tailor-made chin retractor (for mandibular protrusion). Am. J. Orthodontics *25:*461–466, May '39

STÖHR, F. J.: Unilateral symbrachydactylia with defect of thoracic wall and amastia; case. Ztschr. f. Morphol. u. Anthrop. *26:*384–390, '27

STOIAN, C. (see BUTOIANU, S.) Sept '29

STOKES, J. H.: Differential diagnosis of lesion on lip. M. Clin. N. America *8:*894–898, Nov '24

STOKES, W. H.: Refinements in tear sac surgery. Nebraska M. J. *20:*388-393, Oct '35

STOKES, W. H.: Transplantation (implantation) of lacrimal sac in chronic dacryocystitis. Arch. Ophth. *22:*193–210, Aug '39

STOLERU, D. (see BART, C. *et al*) June '40

STOLOFF, I. A. AND SILTEN, A. M.: Hand injuries. Indust. Med. *8:*16–18, Jan '39

STOLZE, M. AND MELTZER, H.: Thiersch's skin grafting in fresh industrial mutilations of fingers. Chirurg *1:*1068–1072, Oct 15, '29

STONE, D. (see GILLIES, H. D. *et al*) April '27

STONE, E. L.: Obstetric shock. Am. J. Obst. and Gynec. *11:*650–660, May '26

STONE, H. B.: Defense of human body against living mammalian cells; address of president. Ann. Surg. *115:*883-891, June '42

STONE, H. B. AND MCLANAHAN, S.: Results with fascia plastic operation for incontinence of anus. Ann. Surg. *114:*73–77, July '41

STONE, M. J. (see GARB, J.) Dec '42

STONEY, R. A.: Case of facio-hypoglossal anastomosis for facial palsy. Irish J. M. Soc., pp. 404–408, Nov '22

STONEY, R. A.: Peripheral nerve suture; forty years' experience. Irish J. M. Sc., pp. 85–92, March '44

STONHAM, F. V.: Surgery of hand. Indian M. Gaz. *80:*597–601, Dec '45

STONHAM, F. V.: Surgery of divided digital tendons. Indian M. Gaz. *81:*225–227, June–July '46

STOOKEY, B. P.: Insidious paralysis of intrinsic muscles of hand and its operative relief. S. Clin. N. America *3:*465–488, April '23 (illus.)

STOPFORD-TAYLOR, R.: Perforated oiled silk in burns. Brit. M. J. *1:*403–404, March 15, '41

STOPPANY, G. A.: Personal reminiscences of men and methods in field of prosthesis in jaw surgery. Ztschr. f. Stomatol. *35:*525–531, April 23, '37

STORCK, H.: Tendovaginitis and tendon nodules, ganglion, hygroma and bursitis. Med. Welt *10:*522–525, April 11, '36

STOTTER, A. L. (see STOTTER, J.) June '21

STOTTER, J. AND STOTTER, A. L.: Correction of nasal deformities with autogenous transplants. Ohio State M. J. *17:*384, June '21

STOTZ, W.: Use of muscular flap to fill cavitations of bones in chronic osteomyelitis. Zentralbl. f. Chir. *66:*352–355, Feb 18, '39

STOTZ, W.: Use of muscular flap to fill bone cavities in osteomyelitis due to gunshot wounds. Zentralbl. f. Chir. *69:*427, March 14, '42

STOUT, A. P.: Pigmented mole of hand. Texas State J. Med. *41:*579–580, Mar '46

STOUT, A. P. (see CARP, L.) Feb '28

STOUT, A. P. (see CIESLAK, A. K.) Dec '46

STOUT, A. P. (see WEBSTER, J. B. *et al*) April '44

STOUT, P. S.: Bovine cartilage in correction of nasal deformities. Laryngoscope *43:*976–979, Dec '33

STOUT, R. A.: Gunshot wounds of face and jaws; first aid treatment, field service. Mil. Surgeon *87:*247–250, Sept '40

STOUT, R. A. (see IVY, R. H.) June '41

STOYE, W.: Therapeutic softening of scar tissue. Munchen. med. Wchnschr. *72:*2135–2138, Dec 11, '25 abstr: J.A.M.A. *86:*384, Jan 30, '26

STRAATSMA, C. R.: Plastic repair of severe radium burns and angioma of face. New York J. Med. *30:*9–10, Jan 1, '30

STRAATSMA, C. R.: Congenital deformities of external ear; their mental effect. Arch. Otolaryng. *11:*609–613, May '30

STRAATSMA, C. R.: Plastic repair of partial losses of nasal tip. Ann. Surg. *91:*792–794, May '30

STRAATSMA, C. R.: Uses and limitations of plastic surgery. New York State J. Med. *32:*253–257, March 1, '32

STRAATSMA, C. R.: Plastic preparation of nose; preliminary report on new local anesthetic. M. J. and Rec. *135:*399–400, April 20, '32

STRAATSMA, C. R.: Method for repair of syphilitic nose. Arch. Otolaryng. *15:*906–909, June '32

STRAATSMA, C. R.: Simplification of nasal plastic surgery. New York State J. Med. *32:*871–872, July 15, '32

STRAATSMA, C. R.: Use of dermal graft in repair of small saddle defects (nose). Arch. Otolaryng. *16:*506–509, Oct '32

STRAATSMA, C. R.: Repair of postauricular fistula following radical mastoidectomy (grafting). Arch. Otolaryng. *19:*616–618, May '34

STRAATSMA, C. R.: Plastic repair of frontal deformity using hump from nose. Tr. Am. Acad. Ophth. *41:*625–626, '36

STRAATSMA, C. R.: Plastic reconstruction for facial paralysis. Laryngoscope *49:*482–483, June '39

STRAATSMA, C. R.: Problems in plastic surgery of nose. Laryngoscope *50:*1092–1099, Nov '40

STRAATSMA, C. R.: Role of free grafts in surface defects. S. Clin. North America *24:*309–318, April '44

STRAATSMA, C. R.: Plastic and reconstructive

surgery in military. Mil. Surgeon *96:*255-257, March '45
STRAATSMA, C. R. AND PEER, L. A.: Repair of postauricular fistula by means of free fat graft. Arch. Oto-laryng. *15:*620-621, April '32
STRACHAN, J. G.: "Saddle-nose" deformity in children. Canad. M.A.J. *17:*324-326, March '27
STRACKER, O.: Thumb contractures in children. Wien. klin. Wchnschr. *44:*197-199, Feb 6, '31
STRACKER, O.: Treatment of rupture of extensor tendon of terminal phalanx of finger. Zentralbl. f. Chir. *58:*727-730, March 21, '31
STRACKER, O.: Which finger deformities are more amenable to surgical than to conservative therapy? Wien. klin. Wchnschr. *45:*1541-1542, Dec 9, '32
STRAITH, C. L.: Correction of some facial disfigurements. J. Michigan M. Soc. *26:*506-515, Aug '27
STRAITH, C. L.: Treatment of traumatic and acquired deformities of face. J. Michigan M. Soc. *28:*431-443, June '29
STRAITH, C. L.: Psychological aspects of plastic surgery. J. Michigan M. Soc. *31:*13-18, Jan '32
STRAITH, C. L.: Method of rhinoplasty. Rev. de chir., Plastique, pp. 109-115, Aug '33
STRAITH, C. L.: Treatment of facial wounds in automobile accidents. J. Michigan M. Soc. *34:*64-70, Feb '35
STRAITH, C. L.: Management of facial injuries in automobile accidents. J.A.M.A. *108:*101-105, Jan 9, '37 also: Rev. de chir. structive, pp. 403-412, Dec '36
STRAITH, C. L.: Scars of facial wounds. Am. J. Surg. *36:*88-90, April '37
STRAITH, C. L.: New profilometer (instrument for plastic surgery of nasal deformities). Rev. de chir. structive, pp. 156-157, June '37
STRAITH, C. L.: Automobile injuries (face). J.A.M.A. *109:*940-945, Sept 18, '37
STRAITH, C. L.: Reconstructions about nasal tip. Am. J. Surg. *43:*223-236, Feb '39
STRAITH, C. L.: Injury to nose. Tr. Indiana Acad. Ophth. and Otolaryng. *26:*88-99, '42
STRAITH, C. L.: Treatment of wounds to face due to explosions. J. Michigan M. Soc. *41:*484-487, June '42
STRAITH, C. L.: Treatment of crushing injuries of face. Proc. Interst. Postgrad. M. A. North America (1942) pp. 292-294, '43
STRAITH, C. L.: Elongation of nasal columella; new operative technic. Plast. and Reconstruct. Surg. *1:*79-86, July '46
STRAITH, C. L. AND DE KLEINE, E. H.: Modern management of nasal fractures; collective review. Internat. Abstr. Surg. *66:*9-15, '38; in Surg., Gynec. and Obst. Jan '38
STRAITH, C. L. AND DE KLEINE, E. H.: Plastic surgery in children; medical and psychologic aspects of deformity. J.A.M.A. *111:*2364-2370, Dec 24, '38
STRAITH, C. L. AND MCEVITT, W. G.: Total avulsion of scalp; review of problem with presentation of case of skin graft in which thrombin plasma fixation was used. Occup. Med. *1:*451-462, May '46
STRAITH, C. L. AND PATTON, H. S.: Three generations of mucous cysts occurring with harelip and cleft palate. J.A.M.A. *123:*693-694, Nov 13, '43
STRAITH, C. L. AND SLAUGHTER, W. B.: Grafts of preserved cartilage in restorations of facial contour. J.A.M.A. *116:*2008-2013, May 3, '41

Strakhov

Extirpation of lacrimal sac. (Comment on Strakhov's article). POLYAK, B. L. Vestnik oftal. *10:*448-450, '37

STRAKHOV, V. P.: Extirpation of lacrimal sac. (Reply to comment by Polyak). Vestnik oftal. *10:*450-451, '37
STRAKOSCH, E. A. (see CLARK, W. G. *et al*) Dec '42
STRAND, S.: Keloids and their treatment. Acta radiol. *26:*397-408, '45
STRANDQVIST, M.: Radium treatment of cutaneous cavernous haemangiomas, using surface application of radium tubes in glass capsules. Acta radiol. *20:*185-211, '39
STRANGE, W. W. AND MOUROT, A. J.: Late treatment of flash burns. U. S. Nav. M. Bull. *41:*953-960, July '43
STRASSMANN, G.: Fat embolism after injury from blunt force and after burns; 130 cases. Deutsche Ztschr. f. d. ges. gerichtl. Med. *22:*272-298, '33
STRAUB, G. F.: Anatomical survival, growth and physiological function of epiphyseal bone transplant. Surg., Gynec. and Obst. *48:*687-690, May '29
STRAUS, F. H.: Luxation of extensor tendons. Ann. Surg. *111:*135-140, Jan '40
STRAUSS: Replacement of nose and ear by gelatin prosthesis. Schweiz. med. Wchnschr. *56:*464-465, May 15, '26
STRAUSS, A.: Burns and their treatment; review of 352 cases. Ohio State M. J. *28:*101-106, Feb '32
STRAUSS, J. F. (see FRANK, I.) Sept '21
STRAYER, L. M.: Augustin Belloste and treatment for avulsion of scalp; odd history of operation in head surgery. New England J. Med. *220:*901-905, June 1, '39
STRECKFUSS, H.: Bag bandage for hand burns. Chirurg *13:*96, Feb 1, '41

STREICHER, C. J. AND ROSEDALE, R. S.: Maxillofacial injuries. Ohio State M. J. *40:*38–40, Jan '44

STROCK, A. E.: Inert metals in direct fixation of mandibular fractures. Surg., Gynec. and Obst. *78:*527–532, May '44

STROCK, M. S.: Fractures of mandible. Surg., Gynec. and Obst. *72:*1047–1051, June '41

STROCK, M. S. (see KAZANJIAN, V. H.) Jan '42

STRODE, J. E.: Imperforate anus, intrinsic congenital malformations. Proc. Staff Meet. Clin., Honolulu *7:*1–7, March (pt. 2) '41

STRODE, J. E.: Papillary tumors of lateral aberrant thyroid origin; discussion and report of 4 cases. Proc. Staff Meet. Clin., Honolulu *9:*103–113, Nov '43

STRÖER, W. F. H.: Familial occurrence of deformities of hands and feet in 5 generations. Genetica *17:*299–312, '35

STRÖER, W. F. H.: Harelip in human embryo of 18 mm. Ztschr. f. Anat. u. Entwckingsgesch. *109:*339–343, '39

STRØM, R.: Late rupture of extensor pollicis longus tendon; rare and peculiar complication of trauma of wrist. Norsk mag. f. laegevidensk. *98:*346–359, April '37

STROMBECK, J. P.: Primary bone grafting in resected tumor of mandible. Acta chir. Scandinav. *86:*554–560, '42

STRÖMBERG, N.: Fracture of jaw with luxation of collum mandibulae; surgical treatment. Acta chir. Scandinav. *74:*379–404, '34

STROTHER, W. H.: Elephantiasis. Kentucky M. J. *19:*175, April '21

STROUD, H. A. (see LUTTERLOH, P. W.) Jan '31

STRUCHKOV, V. I.: Blood transfusion in extensive burns. Khirurgiya, no. 6, pp. 53–57, '39

STRUCHKOV, V. I. (see RUDANOVSKAYA, V. A.) 1937

STRUMIA, M. M. AND HODGE, C. C.: Frozen skin grafts (human). Ann. Surg. *121:*860–865, June '45

STRUMIA, M. M.; WAGNER, J. A. AND HAYLLAR, B. L.: Symposium on military medicine, burn and shock therapy. M. Clin. North America *25:*1813–1827, Nov '41

STRUMIA, M. M.; WAGNER, J. A. AND MONAGHAN, J. F.: Use of citrated plasma in treatment of secondary shock. J.A.M.A. *114:*1337–1341, April 6, '40

STRUMZA, M. V. (see BINET, L.) Aug '40

STRUMZA, M. V. (see BINET, L.) Oct '40

STRYKER, G. V.: Radium treatment of vascular nevi in infants. J. Missouri M. A. *25:*417–421, Sept '28

STUART, F. A. (see MCDONALD, J. E.) Oct '39

STUBINGER, K.: Decubitus ulcers. Med. Klin. *38:*913–916, Sept 25, '42

STUCK, W. G. (see GHORMLEY, R. K.) April '34

STUCK, W. G. (see GHORMLEY, R. K.) April '34

STUDEMEISTER, A.: Skin transplantation in surgical after-treatment of amputation-stumps following frostbite of foot. Deutsche Ztschr. f. Chir. *258:*49, '43

STUDEMEISTER, A.: Osteotomy of ascending ramus of lower jaw in therapy of ankylosis. Deutsche Ztschr. f. Chir. *258:*358, '43

STÜHMER, A. AND WUCHERPFENNIG, V.: Treatment of roentgen ray ulcers. Ztschr. f. arztl. Fortbild. *27:*689–695, Nov 1, '30

STULZ, E. (see SIMON, R. *et al*) March '25

STUMPF, F. W.: Laceration of face with traumatic avulsion of entire maxilla; case. J. Am. Dent. A. *22:*1206–1208, July '35

STUMPF, F. W.: Cleft-lip correction (and palate). J. Am. Dent. A. *25:*1196–1201, Aug '38

STUMPF, F. W.: Jaw fractures. J. Am. Dent. A. *29:*1615–1628, Sept 1, '42

STUMPFEGGER, L.: Substitute tenoplasties according to Perthes in therapy of radial paralysis. Chirurg. *15:*430, July 15, '43

STUMPKE, G.: Prosthesis for lupus and other facial defects. Dermat. Wchnschr. *109:*1058–1061, Sept 2, '39

STUPKA, W.: Plastic method for correcting depression after external operations of frontal sinus; celluloid plates. Monatschr. f. Ohrenh. *65:*39–56, Jan '31

STUPKA, W.: Histology and pathogenesis of some marked abnormalities of nose. Acta otolaryng. *19:*1–5, '33

STUPKA, W.: New mouth gag with interchangeable and adjustable tongue depressors and anesthetizing tube. Laryngoscope *43:*585–588, July '33

STUPKA, W.: Celluloid prosthesis in cosmetic correction after disfiguring surgery of frontal sinus. Arch. f. Ohren-Nasen-u. Kelkopfh. *138:*79–86, '34

STUPKA, W.: Atypical cartilage in nose, upper lip and palate in cheilognathopalatoschisis. Monatschr. f. Ohrenh. *71:*1333–1344, Nov '37

STURGIS, S. H.: Physiology and metabolism of severe burn. Mil. Surgeon *97:*215–224, Sept '45

STURGIS, S. H. AND HOLLAND, D. J. JR.: Maxillofacial surgery. M. Bull. North African Theat. Op. (no. 1) *1:*13–14, Jan '44

STURGIS, S. H. AND HOLLAND, D. J. JR.: Treatment of maxillofacial wounds and injuries. M. Bull. North African Theat. Op. (no. 3) *1:*8–11, March '44

STURGIS, S. H. AND HOLLAND, D. J. JR.: Observations of 200 jaw fracture cases admitted to 6th General Hospital. Am. J. Orthodontics (Oral Surg. Sect.) *32:*605–634, Oct '46

STURGIS, S. H. AND HOLLAND, D. J. JR.: Case reports from maxillofacial team, 6th General

Hospital. Am. J. Orthodontics (Oral Surg. Sect) *32:*635–664, Oct '46

STURGIS, S. H. AND LUND, C. C.: Leukoplakia buccalis and keratosis labialis (precancerous lesions). New England J. Med. *210:*996–1006, May 10, '34

STURGIS, S. H. AND LUND, C. C.: Leukoplakia buccalis and cancer of mouth. New England J. Med. *212:*7–9, Jan 3, '35

STURGIS, S. H. (see KAZANJIAN, V. H.) Aug '40

STURM, F. P.: Local anaesthesia in submucous resection of nasal septum. Brit. M. J. *1:*720, April 16, '27

SUAREZ, A. R. (see FREYTES, M. V.) 1941

SUAREZ VILLAFRANCA, M. R.: Plastic surgery of eyelids. Arch. Soc. oftal. hispano-am. *4:*816–838, Sept–Oct '44

Subbotin's Operation

Late results of Subbotin's operation for complete epispadias with urinary incontinence; 2 cases. PETROV, N. Arch. f. klin. Chir. *149:*762–768, '28

SUBILEAU, J. M.: Hemo-aspiration and trephining with aid of electric apparatus in dacryocystorhinostomy. Ann. d'ocul. *167:*301–306, April '30

Submucous Resection

Submucous resection of nasal septum. DUNNING, W. M., Am. J. Surg. *35:*1, Jan '21

Submucous replacement for external deviation of nose. OERTEL, T. E. Ann. Otol. Rhinol. and Laryng. *30:*147, March '21

Use of hollow tube following submucous resection of nasal septum. GOODYEAR, H. M. J.A.M.A. *77:*1103, Oct 1, '21

Submucous resection of nasal septum. BROWN, K. T., J. Indiana M. A. *14:*339, Oct '21

Modification of submucous resection operation. NOTHENBERG, O. J. Illinois M. J. *40:*385, Nov '21

New perichondrium elevator for resection of nasal septum. CAMPBELL, C. A. Laryngoscope *31:*973, Dec '21 (illus.)

Fatal meningitis following submucous resection of nasal septum, post-mortem discovery of latent sphenoidal sinusitis. POWELL, W. E., J. Laryngol. and Otol. *37:*39–40, Jan '22

After-treatment of submucous resection. JONES, D. H. New York M. J. *115:*494, April 19, '22

Post-operative complications of submucous resection and their treatment. SCHWARTZ, A. A. Am. J. Surg. *36:*133–136, June '22

Submucous Resection – Cont.

Submucous resection of nasal septum. NOTTAGE, H. P. China M. J. *36:*469–473, Nov '22

Indications and contraindications for submucous resection of nasal septum. HOFFMANN, J. N. Laryngoscope *33:*13–15, Jan '23

General anesthesia in submucous and other nasal operations. POE, J. G. Am. J. Surg. (Anesthesia supp.) *37:*56–57, April '23

Submucous resection; complications and after-results. WEINBERGER, N. S. Ann. Otol., Rhin. and Laryng. *32:*387–393, June '23

Method of holding septal membranes in apposition after a submucous resection without use of packing, description and demonstration of instruments and method of use. SIMPSON, H. L., J. Michigan M. Soc. *23:*64–67, Feb '24

Submucous resection in children. WHITE, F. W. Ann. Otol., Rhin. and Laryng. *33:*526–533, June '24

New elevator for submucous resection. MYERSON, M. C. Laryngoscope *34:*660, Aug '24

Submucous resection of nasal septum; simple flap suture. WILSON, W. F. Brit. M. J. *2:*814, Nov 1, '24

Submucosa dissector. GRAHAM, A. J. Surg., Gynec. and Obst. *40:*709, May '25 also: M. J. and Rec. *122:*527, Nov 4, '25

Technic for submucous resection, with presentation of membrane elevator. JONES, M. F. Laryngoscope *35:*406–408, May '25

Depressed nose following submucous resection. BABCOCK, W. W., S. Clin. N. Amer. *6:*48–52, Feb '26

Submucous resection of nasal septum. WAHRER, F. L., J. Iowa M. Soc. *16:*371–372, Aug '26

Evolution of submucous resection with new technic. ATKINSON, D. T. Laryngoscope *37:*132–136, Feb '27

Local anaesthesia in submucous resection of nasal septum. STURM, F. P. Brit. M. J. *1:*720, April 16, '27

Local anaesthesia in submucous resection of nasal septum. MCKELVIE, B. Brit. M. J. *1:*920, May 21, '27

Prevention and correction of nasal deformities following submucous resection; presentation of cases. MALINIAK, J. W. Arch. Otolaryng. *6:*320–329, Oct '27

Double-end arrow elevator for nasal plastic operations and submucous resections. FISHBEIN, J. N. Laryngoscope *38:*97, Feb '28

Submucous Resection – Cont.
Submucous resection followed by complications of acute otitis, mastoiditis and sinus thrombosis. HOUSER, K. M. Arch. Otolaryng. *7:*631–634, June '28
Submucous resection in children. WINDHAM, R. E. Eye, Ear, Nose and Throat Monthly *7:*307–311, July '28 Also: Northwest Med. *27:*392–396, Aug '28
Prevention of nasal deformity following submucous resection. CARTER, W. W. Arch. Otolaryng. *8:*555–563, Nov '28
Prevention of deformities following submucous resection. CARTER, W. W. Tr. Am. Laryng., Rhin. and Otol. Soc. *34:*123–131, '28 also: Laryngoscope *39:*52–57, Jan '29
Replacement of lower end of dislocated septal cartilage versus submucous resection of dislocated end of septal cartilage. METZENBAUM, M. Tr. Sect. Laryng., Otol. and Rhin., A.M.A., pp. 236–251, '28 also: Arch. Otolaryng. *9:*282–296, March '29
Submucous resection in children. WHITE, F. W. Tr. Sect. Laryng., Otol. and Rhin., A.M.A., pp. 123–134, '29 also: Arch. Otolaryng. *11:*415–425, April '30
Submucous resection of nasal castration symbol. OBERNDORF, C. P. Internat. J. Psycho-Analysis *10:*228–241, April–July '29
Complications following resections of submucous septum. CLAUS, G. Ztschr. f. Hals-, Nasen-u. Ohrenh. *23:*444–449, Sept 10, '29
High submucous excision of nasal septum. TAKAHASHI, K. Ztschr. f. Laryng., Rhin. *19:*22–40, Nov '29
Method of correcting lax, boggy septa following submucous resection. PRATT, J. A. Ann. Otol., Rhin. and Laryng. *38:*1156–1157, Dec '29
Suggestions for modification of operative procedure and postoperative treatment of submucous resection. McGIVERN, C. S., J. M. Soc. New Jersey *27:*28–31, Jan '30
Indications for resection of nasal septum. RICHTER, H. Ztschr. f. Laryng., Rhin. *19:*399–402, July '30 also: Munchen. med. Wchnschr. *77:*1354–1356, Aug 8, '30
Submucous septum punch. REAVES, R. G. Tr. Am. Acad. Ophth. *35:*475, '30
Submucous resection. BALDENWECK, L. Medecine *12:*75–79, Jan '31
Submucous resection from technical, respiratory and esthetic viewpoints. TEMPEA, V. Spitalul *51:*98–99, March '31
Technic of resection of nasal septum. ZAMBRINI, A. R. Semana med. *1:*1153–1155, April 30, '31
Method of nasal packing following submucous resection which allows free nasal respiration. ROTH, E. Arch. Otolaryng. *13:*732, May '31
Development of nose; dynamic relation to traumatic injuries and to submucous resection. CARTER, W. W. Laryngoscope *42:*189–194, March '32
Retrobulbar abscess complicating submucous resection. MAHONEY, P. L. Laryngoscope *42:*199–200, March '32
Submucous resection in children. WINDHAM, R. E. Texas State J. Med. *27:*859–862, April '32
Sinking of nasal bone following submucous resection. DUFOURMENTEL, L. Oto-rhino-laryng. internat. *16:*233–234, May '32
Technic of submucous resection. HUTTER, F. Monatschr. f. Ohrenh. *66:*584–585, May '32
Otological sepsis following submucous resection. MENGER, L. C. Laryngoscope *42:*371–375, May '32
New instruments for submucous resection of nasal septum. GAMMAGE, F. V. Arch. Otolaryng. *16:*573–574, Oct '32
Submucous resection in children. YEARSLEY, M. Practitioner *129:*581–583, Nov '32
Indications for operations and operations most commonly performed on nasal septum. SILVEIRA, R. Rev. de med. y cir. de la Habana *38:*428–436, June 30, '33
Knife for submucous resection. MILLER, A. Lancet *1:*1395, June 30, '34
Ways of treating most anterior portions during submucous resection. BEHRMAN, W. Acta oto-laryng. *21:*248–255, '34
Submucous resection. BERMAN, H. L. Laryngoscope *45:*184–187, March '35
Behavior of cartilage in submucous resection; histopathologic study. GIANNI, O. Arch. ital. di otol. *47:*487–498, July '35
Injection anesthesia for submucous resection. LIEBERMANN, T. Budapesti orvosi ujsag *34:*831–832, Oct 1, '36
Direct incision in submucous resection; modification of Killian operation. TEMPEA, V. Rev. san. mil., Bucuresti *35:*1077–1079, Oct '36
Practical points on submucous resection; pitfalls and corrections. LASZLO, A. F. Laryngoscope *46:*840–847, Nov '36
New postoperative pack for submucous resection. DIXON, O. J. Ann. Otol., Rhin. and Laryng. *45:*1184–1185, Dec '36
Complications of submucosal resection (Killian operation). CARANDO, V. *et al.* Semana med. *1:*225–227, Jan 21, '37
Submucous resection in relation to nasal plastic surgery. WOLFE, M. M. Laryngoscope *47:*281–285, April '37

Submucous Resection-Cont.
Indications and technic for submucous resection. MOORE, P. M., S. Clin. North America *17:*1437-1448, Oct '37
Evaluation of submucous resection; points as to technic. FRANK, P., M. Rec. *146:*469-470, Dec 1, '37
Deviation of septum with insufficient nasal respiration as indication for submucous resection; preliminary report. AMERSBACH, K. Arch. f. Ohren- Nasen-u. Kehl Kopfh. *143:*241-245, '37
Method for maintaining apposition of mucosal flaps after submucous resection. KEARNEY, H. L. Tr. Am. Laryng., Rhin. and Otol. Soc. *43:*109-110, '37
Transitory conditions contraindicating resection of nasal septum. LEWIS, E. R. Tr. Am. Laryng., Rhin. and Otol. Soc. *43:*402-403, '37
Injection anesthesia for submucous resection. LIEBERMANN, T. Ztschr. f. Hals-, Nasen-u. Ohrenh. *41:*290, '37
Direct incision in submucous resection; modification of Killian operation. TEMPEA, V. Ztschr. f. Hals-, Nasen-u. Ohrenh. *40:*548-552, '37
Combined nasal reconstruction and submucous resection. TAMERIN, J. A. New York State J. Med. *38:*1129-1133, Aug 15, '38
Hemorrhage in nasal septal resection. HARTUNG, F. Rev. oto-laring. de Sao Paulo *6:*379-382, Sept-Oct '38
Essential points in submucous resection. YEARSLEY, M., M. Press *197:*518-520, Dec 7, '38
Submucous resection; methods of preventing post-operative fluttering and perforation. DÖDERLEIN, W. Hals-, Nasen-u. Ohrenarzt (Teil 1) *30:*273-275, July '39
Prevention of hematoma after submucous resection. CHAMBERLIN, W. B. Tr. Am. Laryng. A. *61:*21-28, '39
Complementary turbinotomy in submucosal resection of septum. RESENDE, E. Acta med., Rio de Janeiro *6:*166-167, Sept '40
Nasal obstruction and impairment of hearing; 46 cases of submucous resection with audiometric studies. JOHNSON, M. R. Arch. Otolaryng. *33:*536-549, April '41
Submucous elevator. METZENBAUM, M. F. Arch. oto-laryng. *34:*847, Oct '41
Submucous resection of septum of nose. SNYDER, W. S. JR. Kentucky M. J. *40:*59-62, Feb '42
Dressings after submucous resection of septum. PRUVOT, M. Rev. de laryng. *63:*196-199, June-July '42
Complications of plastic surgery of nasal septum. COHEN, S. Dis. Eye, Ear, Nose and Throat *2:*235-243, Aug '42
Pitfalls in submucous resection. MALIS, S. Dis. Eye, Ear, Nose and Throat *2:*343-347, Nov '42
Use of diathermy in submucous resection. JONES, A. C. Tr. Am. Laryng., Rhin. and Otol. Soc. *48:*331-332, '42
Priority of Murray-Nelson-Hulsman original method for avoiding perforation in submucous resection. NELSON, R. M., J. M. A. Georgia *32:*338-339, Oct '43
Use of diathermy in submucous resection. JONES, A. C. Arch. Otolaryng. *38:*445-446, Nov '43
Cerebral infarction following submucous resection and turbinectomy. KERN, E. C. Eye, Ear, Nose and Throat Monthly *23:*29, Jan '44
Extranasal block anesthesia for submucous resection. FRED, G. B. Ann. Otol., Rhin. and Laryng. *53:*127-132, March '44
Reconstruction of deformed septum; critical evaluation of orthodox submucous resection from anatomophysiologic standpoint. ERSNER, M. S. Arch. Otolaryng. *39:*476-484, June '44

SUDECK: Surgery of jaw in ununited fractures and defects from operation. Deutsche med. Wchnschr. *53:*47, Jan 1, '27
SUDECK, P.: Plastic surgery in radial paralysis. Chirurg *15:*665, Nov 15, '43
SUDECK, P.: Plastic operations in radial nerve paralysis. Bull. War Med. *4:*627-628, July '44 (abstract)
SUDECK, P. AND RIEDER, W.: Operations suitable for defects and lack of continuity of inferior maxilla. Beitr. z. klin. Chir. *146:*493-518, '29
SUDECK, P. AND RIEDER, W.: Malignant tumors of mandible; review of literature. Ergebn. d. Chir. u. Orthop. *22:*585-678, '29
SUDLER, M. T.: Cleft palate and harelip. J. Kansas M. Soc. *24:*18-20, Jan '24
SUEMITSU, S. (see SASAKI, M.) Oct '39
SUERMONDT, W. F.: Rare case of tendon rupture of thumb. Deutsche Ztschr. f. Chir. *201:*400-402, '27
SUERMONDT, W. F.: Bilateral ankylosis of jaws; case. Nederl. tijdschr. v. geneesk. *75:*249, Jan 10, '31
SUERMONDT, W. F.: Fistulas and cysts of neck. Nederl. tijdschr. v. geneesk. *81:*1528-1535, April 10, '37
SUGAR, H. S.: Tarsoconjunctival sliding-graft technics for reconstruction of eyelids. Am. J. Ophth. *27:*109-123, Feb '44

SUGGIT, S.: Bleeding from external auditory meatus following fracture of mandible. J. Laryng. and Otol. *56:*364–367, Oct '41
SUGGIT, S.: Repair of depressed nasal bridge. J. Laryng. and Otol. *40:*501–503, Dec '45
SUGGIT, S. C. (see UNGLEY, H. G.) Oct '44
SUIRE, P. (see CREYSSEL, J.) March '40
SUIRE, P. (see CREYSSEL, J.) Nov '40
SUIRE, P. (see CREYSSEL, J.) 1941–1942
SULLIVAN, J. A.: Surgical treatment of facial paralysis by autoplastic nerve graft. Canad. M.A.J. *31:*474–479, Nov '34
SULLIVAN, J. A.: Modification of Ballance-Duel technic in treatment of facial paralysis. Tr. Am. Acad. Ophth. *41:*282–299, '36
SULLIVAN, J. A.: Nerve transplantation in mastoid surgery. Arch. Otolaryng. *37:*845–851, June '43
SULLIVAN, J. M.: Shock and hemorrhage. M. Bull. North African Theat. Op. (no. 6) *1:*2–3, June '44
SULLIVAN, J. M.: Shock in forward areas. Wisconsin M. J. *45:*213–216, Feb '46
SUMERMAN, S.: Extirpation of hyoid bone in therapy of thyroglossal cyst; 3 cases. Turk tib cem. mec. *5:*265–271, '39
SUMMERILL, F. (see YACHNIN, S. C.) March '41
SUN, K. S.: Eyelid ptosis operations. Nat. M. J. China *27:*245–246, April '41
SUNDARANADANAM, B. M.: Burn therapy. Indian M. Rec. *56:*129–131, June '36
SUNDBERG, S. (see FRENCKNER, P.) 1939
SUNDERLAND, S.: Flexion of distal phalanx of thumb in lesions of median nerve. Australian and New Zealand J. Surg. *13:*157–159, Jan '44
SUNDERLAND, S.: Significance of hypothenar elevation in movements of opposition of thumb. Australian and New Zealand J. Surg. *13:*155–156, Jan '44
SUNDERLAND, S.: Peripheral nerve injuries; simple compression injuries of radial nerve. Brain *68:*56–72, March '45
SUNDERLAND, S.: Radial nerve lesions; course and rate of regeneration of motor fibers. Arch. Neurol. and Psychiat. *56:*133–157, Aug '46
SUNSHINE, L.: New instruments in rhinoplastic surgery. Am. J. Surg. *71:*434–435, March '46
SUPERNAW, J. S.: Shock and hemorrhage. Wisconsin M. J. *42:*501–504, May '43
SURACI, A. J.: Plastic reconstruction of acquired defects of external ear, with case reports. Am. J. Surg. *66:*196–202, Nov '44
SURAT, W. S.: Facial hemiatrophy. Monatschr. f. Psychiat. u. Neurol. *77:*202–216, Oct '30
SUSONI, A. H.: Tubular grafts in plastic repair. Bol. y trab., Soc. argent. de cirujanos *7:*368–379, '46 also: Rev. Asoc. med. argent. *60:*601–605, July 15, '46
SÜSS, H.: Case of hemihypertrophy of face with buphthalmos. Ztschr. f. Kinderh. *41:*404–408, '26
SUTTON, H. T.: Skin grafting with reference to extensive burns. Ohio State M. J. *27:*943–949, Dec '31
SUTTON, J. B. (see BRANDES, W. W. *et al*) Feb '46
SUTTON, L. E.: Use of tubed pedicle flaps for study of wound healing in human skin. New York State J. Med. *40:*852–859, June 1, '40
SUTTON, L. E.: Plastic surgery in treatment of war casualties. Am. J. Surg. *61:*239–243, Aug '43
SUTTON, L. E.: Reconstruction following complete avulsion of skin of penis and scrotum; case. New York State J. Med. *43:*2279–2282, Dec 1, '43
SUTTON, L. E.: Reconstruction of contracted axilla. Plast. and Reconstruct. Surg. *1:*43–48, July '46
SUTTON, R. L.: Clinical study of carcinoma of nose. J.A.M.A. *77:*1561, Nov 12, '21

Sutures

Technic of suture of divided tendons. Zentralbl. f. Chir. *48:*338, March 12, '21
Methods to secure end-to-end suture of peripheral nerves. NAFFZIGER, H. C. Surg., Gynec. and Obst. *32:*193, March '21
Use of living sutures in operative surgery. GALLIE, W. E. AND LE MESURIER, A. B. Canad. M.A.J. *11:*504, July '21
New intra-nasal suture set. ISRAEL, S. Laryngoscope *31:*633, Aug '21
Use of living sutures in treatment of eyelid ptosis. WRIGHT, W. W. Arch. Ophth. *51:*99–102, March '22 (illus.)
Simple knot for intranasal sutures. JOHNSTON, W. Ann. Otol., Rhin. and Laryng. *32:*201–209, March '23 (illus.)
Tendon suture which permits immediate motion. LAHEY, F. H. Boston M. and S. J. *188:*851–852, May 31, '23 (illus.)
Wiring method of treatment for fractures of mandible. TENNENT, E. H., U.S. Nav. M. Bull. *19:*38–42, July '23 (illus.)
Living suture in tendon transplantation. ROYLE, N. D., M. J. Australia *1:*333–334, April 5, '24
Submucous resection of nasal septum; simple flap suture. WILSON, W. F. Brit. M. J. *2:*814, Nov 1, '24
Implantation of silk in plastic repair of tissues. SPITZY. Wien. med. Wchnschr. *77:*394–396, March 19, '27
Tendon sutures. MOSER, E. Zentralbl. f. Chir. *54:*1606, June 25, '27

Sutures—Cont.

General principles of plastic surgery; cutaneous graft, sutures; cases. Lewis, D. Bull. et mem. Soc. de chir. de Paris *20:*476–487, June 1, '28

New instrument for intranasal suture. Takahashi, K. Ztschr. f. Laryng., Rhin. *17:*211–216, Sept '28

A new procedure for execution of intra-dermal suture. Dobrzaniecki, W. Paris chir. *21:*19–23, Jan–Feb '29

Treatment of fractures of lower jaw by bone suture with silver wire; cases. Dieulafé, L. Rev. de stomatol. *31:*330–336, June '29

Subcuticular suture. Sommer, R. Zentralbl. f. Chir. *56:*2265–2266, Sept 7, '29

New method of tendon suture; preliminary report. Tschalenko, G. Zentralbl. f. Chir. *56:*2388–2389, Sept 21, '29

Fascia as suture material. Wolfsohn, G. Chirurg *2:*475–477, May 15, '30

Bone suture in treatment of jaw fractures. Greve, K. Beitr. z. klin. Chir. *152:*310–322, '31

Interpretation of suture of tendons. Banet, V. An. de cir. *4:*352–354, May '32

Technic of sutures in cosmetic surgery. Kapp, J. F. Fortschr. d. Med. *50:*967–968, Nov 11, '32

Further studies and experiences with transfixion suture technic (technic 3) for transplantation of ureters into large intestine. Coffey, R. C. Northwest Med. *32:*31–34, Jan '33

Technic of incisions and sutures in plastic surgery (face). Dantrelle. Rev. de chir. plastique, pp. 75–108, Aug '33

On-end or vertical mattress suture. Davis, J. S., Ann. Surg. *98:*941–951, Nov '33

Reconstruction of crucial ligaments of knee with kangaroo tendons; late results. Micheli, E. Boll. e mem. Soc. piemontese di chir. *3:*874–883, '33

Supporting suture in ptosis operations. Frost, A. D. Am. J. Ophth. *17:*633, July '34

Primary bone suture in fracture of lower jaw. Dubov, M. D. Novy khir. arkhiv *31:*89–95, '34

Esthetic sutures. Karfík, V. Rozhl. v chir. a gynaek. (cast chir.) *13:*207–219, '34

Two new methods of tendon suture. Dykhno, A. M. Novy khir. arkhiv. *37:*403–416, '36

Comparative value of different sutures in tendon surgery, with presentation of 2 new technics. Dychno, A. Lyon chir. *34:*290–303, May–June '37

New suture for tendon and fascia repair. Gratz, C. M. Surg., Gynec. and Obst.

Sutures—Cont.

*65:*700–701, Nov '37

Simplified intranasal suture. Childrey, J. H. Arch. Otolaryng. *27:*618, May '38

Massive prolapse of rectum and its treatment by elastic ligature; criticism. Emerson, M. L. Tr. Am. Proct. Soc. *39:*138–140, '38

Uranostaphylorrhaphy with Donati suture. Schoemaker, J. Arch. ital. di chir. *54:*513–515, '38

Application of general principles in tendon suture. Huber, H. S., S. Clin. North America *19:*499–518, April '39

Bone ligation and suture in relation to functional defects and tissue losses in mandible; collective review. Weisengreen, H. H. Internat. Abstr. Surg. *68:*450–460, '39; in Surg., Gynec. and Obst., May '39

Correction of eyelid ptosis by means of buried sutures. Askalonova, T. M. and Zakharov, A. P. Vestnik oftal. (no. 6) *14:*64–66, '39

Primary repair of severed tendons; use of stainless steel wire. Bunnell, S. Am. J. Surg. *47:*502–516, Feb '40

Wire reposition in linear fractures of lower jaw. Reichenbach, E. Ztschr. f. Stomatol. *38:*347–357, May 24, '40

Method for suturing of nasal mucous membrane. Matis, E. I. Acta oto-laryng. *29:*80–82, '41 also: Medicina Kaunas *21:*1031–1034, Dec '40

Use of various materials for isolation of suture to prevent adhesion in tendon surgery; experimental study. Nikolaev, G. F. Ortop. i travmatol. (no. 4) *14:*18–26, '40

Suturing of flexor tendons (transfixation) in hand. Bove, C., M. Rec. *153:*94, Feb 5, '41

Use of stainless steel wire in operation for hypospadias. Coe, H. E. Urol. and Cutan. Rev. *45:*297–298, May '41

Use of kangaroo tendon for muscle and tendon suture. Trethewie, E. R. and Williams, E. Australian and New Zealand J. Surg. *11:*207–208, Jan '42

Facial fractures; treatment by wiring fixation. Adams, W. M. Mississippi Doctor *19:*427–435, Feb '42

Autologous plasma clot suture of nerves. Tarlov, I. M. and Benjamin, B. Science *95:*258, March 6, '42

Fibrin suture of human nerves. Seddon, H. J. and Medawar, P. B. Lancet *2:*87–88, July 25, '42

Surgical repair of recent lacerations of eyelids; intramarginal splinting suture. Minsky, H. Surg., Gynec. and Obst. *75:*449–456, Oct '42

Experiments on cadaver nerve graft and

Sutures – Cont.
"glue" suture of divided nerves. DE REZENDE, N. New York State J. Med. *42:*2124-2128, Nov 15, '42
Use of silk in musculotendinous and ligamentary reparative surgery. BOPPE. Mem. Acad. de chir. *68:*452-456, Dec 9-16, '42
Use of buttons with wire suture in gunshot wounds of face and jaw. PERWITZSCHKY, R. Ztschr. f. Hals-, Nasen-u. Ohrenh. *48:*270; 458, '42
Care of military and civilian injuries; internal wiring fixation of facial fractures. ADAMS, W. M. Am. J. Orthodontics (Oral Surg. Sect.) *29:*111-130, Feb '43
Care of military and civilian injuries; internal wire fixation of jaw fractures; preliminary report. BROWN, J. B. AND McDOWELL, F. Am. J. Orthodontics (Oral Surg. Sect.) *29:*86-91, Feb '43
Plasma clot and silk suture of nerves; experimental study of comparative tissue reaction. TARLOV, I. M. AND BENJAMIN, B. Surg., Gynec. and Obst. *76:*366-374, March '43
New instrument with needle continuously threaded for suturing. GONZALEZ ULLOA, M. Rev. mex. de cir., ginec. y cancer *11:*123-135, April '43
Experimental study on nerve suture with various suture materials. GUTTMANN, L. Brit. J. Surg. *30:*370-375, April '43
Wire suturing in treatment of facial fractures. GORDON, S. D. Canad. M.A.J. *48:*406-409, May '43
Technique of good suturing. GILLIES, H. St. Barth. Hosp. J. *47:*170-173, July '43
Tie-loop wiring of fractured jaws. PETERSON, R. G., J. Oral Surg. *1:*246-249, July '43
Plasma clot suture of peripheral nerves; experimental technic. TARLOV, I. M. *et al.* Arch. Surg. *47:*44-58, July '43
New needle holder for plastic surgery. WEBSTER, G. V., U. S. Nav. M. Bull. *41:*1434-1439, Sept '43
Sutures, use of human fibrinogen in reconstructive surgery. MICHAEL, P. AND ABBOTT, W. D., J.A.M.A. *123:*279, Oct 2, '43
Coagulum-contact method as applied to human grafts. SANO, M. E. Surg., Gynec. and Obst. *77:*510-513, Nov '43
Nerve reunion with sleeves of frozen-dried artery in rabbits, cats and monkeys. WEISS, P. Proc. Soc. Exper. Biol. and Med. *54:*274-277, Dec '43
Tendon repair by transfixion. GEBHARD, U. E., Indust. Med. *13:*38-39, Jan '44
Fibrin fixation of skin transplants. TIDRICK, R. T. AND WARNER, E. D. Surgery *15:*90-95, Jan '44

Sutures – Cont.
Repair of severed tendons; new tendon suture. REES, C. E. Arizona Med. *1:*12-15, Jan-Feb '44
Fixation of skin grafts by thrombin-plasma adhesion. YOUNG, F. AND FAVATA, B. V. Surgery *15:*378-386, March '44
Film-cemented skin grafts. WEBSTER, J. P., S. Clin. North America *24:*251-280, April '44
Sutureless reunion of severed nerves with elastic cuffs of tantalum. WEISS, P., J. Neurosurg. *1:*219-225, May '44
Closure of granulating wounds of face by means of button sutures. ENTIN, D. A. Am. Rev. Soviet. Med. *1:*351-354, April '44
Autologous plasma clot suture of nerves; use in clinical surgery. TARLOV, I. M. J.A.M.A. *126:*741-748, Nov 18, '44
Secondary suture of granulating wounds of face. FELDMAN, S. P. AND GROSSMAN, S. Y. Sovet. med. (no. 6) *8:*22-23, '44
Fixation of skin grafts by plasma-thrombin adhesion. YOUNG, F. Tr. Am. S. A. *62:*450-462, '44
New device for suturing skin. DA ROCHA, J. Dia med. *17:*77, Jan 22, '45
Modification of plasma fixation method (Sano) by use of bobbinet and mirror attachment. JENNEY, J. A. Am. J. Surg. *67:*3-7, Jan '45
Palatoplasty; procedure for immobilization of mucosa and sutures. MARINO, H. Prensa med. argent. *32:*436-438, March 9, '45
Fixation of grafts with human plasma and thrombin. CLARK, A. M.; *et al.* Lancet *1:*498-499, April 21, '45
Metal anastomosis tubes in suture of tendons. McKEE, G. K. Lancet *1:*659-660, May 26, '45
Use of whole skin grafts as substitute for fascial sutures in treatment of hernias; preliminary report. MAIR, G. B. Am. J. Surg. *69:*352-365, Sept '45
New uses of tantalum in suture and control of neuroma formation; illustration of technical procedures. WHITE, J. C. AND HAMLIN, H., J. Neurosurg. *2:*402-413, Sept '45
Sano tissue glue skin grafting. EVANS, J. G. J. Internat. Coll. Surgeons *8:*424-425, Sept-Oct '45
Instrument to facilitate multiple loop wiring in jaw fractures. KLEIN, D. Bull. U. S. Army M. Dept. *4:*479, Oct '45
Fibrin fixation methods of skin grafting; clinical evaluation. McEVITT, W. G., J. Michigan M. Soc. *44:*1347-1351, Dec '45
Use of cheek wires in treatment of fractures

Sutures—Cont.
of maxilla. HOLLAND, N. W. A. Brit. Dent. J. *79:*333-340, Dec 21, '45
Secondary sutures and skin transplantations at front line hospitals. TABORISSKIY, M. G. Khirurgiya, no. 2, pp. 23-30, '45
Suture in crushing injuries of finger nails. HAMRICK, W. H., U. S. Nav. M. Bull. *46:*225-228, Feb '46
Coagulum contact method of skin graft fixation; present status. MACGREGOR, M. W. Permanente Found. M. Bull. *4:*42-46, Feb '46
Fistula of penile urethra; method of repair utilizing stainless steel "pull-out" sutures. CORDONNIER, J. J., J. Urol. *55:*278-286, Mar '46
Coagulum contact method (Sano) of skin grafting. BRANCH, C. D.; *et al.* Surgery *19:*460-466, April '46
Fixation of ligaments by Bunnell's pull-out wire suture. KEY, J. A. Ann. Surg. *123:*656-663, April '46
Technic of suture of peripheral nerves. LIVINGSTON, K. E.; *et al.* J. Neurosurg. *3:*270-271, May '46
"Islet" method of wiring fractures of mandible. HUMPHRIES, S. V. Clin. Proc. *5:*154-160, June '46
Metallic tube for nerve suture. SICARD, A. AND FAUREL. Mem. Acad. de chir. *72:*393, July 3-10, '46
Removal suture method of repair of peripheral nerves. POTTER, S. E., J. Neurosurg. *3:*354-357, July '46
Dermatape; new method for management of split grafts. REESE, J. D. Plast. and Reconstruct. Surg. *1:*98-105, July '46
Cotton sutures in vaginal plastic operations about bladder and urethra. COLLINS, C. G. S. Clin. North America *26:*1221-1229, Oct '46
Fixation of tendons, ligaments and bone by Bunnell's pull-out suture. KEY, J. A. (St. Louis) Tr. South. S. A. (1945) *57:*187-194, '46

SUZUKI, K.: Shock toxin; pharmacologic effects of perfusate flowing through crushed muscle tissue. Jap. J. M. Sc. IV, Pharmacol. *12:*115-116, March '40
SUZUKI, K.: Shock toxin; pharmacologic effects of perfusate flowing through crushed muscle tissue. Jap. J. M. Sc., IV, Pharmacol. *13:*117*-119*, Oct '40
SUZUKI, S.: Homeotransplantation. Fukuoka acta med. (Abstr. Sect.) *32:*1-5, Jan '39
SUZUKI, T.: Congenital ectopia vesicae with recovery after operation. Okayama-Igakkai-Zasshi *45:*2615, Nov '33
SVERDLICK, J. AND FERNANDEZ, L. L.: Reconstruction of orbit by Esser-Wheeler technic. Semana med. *2:*142-144, July 26, '45
SVERDLOV, D. G.: New method for formation of stump after enucleation by transplantation of cadaver's cartilage into Tenon's capsule of eye. Vestnik oftal. (nos. 5-6) *19:*45-50, '41
SVERDLOV, D. G. AND GOLDIN, L. B.: Fracture of upper maxilla associated with extensive trauma of left half of forehead, injury to right optic canal and blindness of right eye; case. Vestnik oftal. *12:*515-516, '38
SVIRIDOFF, K.: Plastic surgery for extensive atrophy of scrotum with fissure; case. Vrach. dielo *10:*1178, Sept 1, '27
SVYADOSHCH, B. I. (see BALTIN, M. M.) 1941
SWART, H. A. AND HENDERSON, M. S.: Tendon transplants for paralytic wrist drop; presentation of patient. Proc. Staff Meet., Mayo Clin. *9:*377-379, June 27, '34
SWEET, P. W.: Alcoholized nerve graft; experimental study. Ann. Surg. *89:*191-198, Feb '29
SWEET, P. W.: Branchial anomalies. Tr. A. Resid. and ex-Resid. Physicians, Mayo Clin. (1928) *9:*94-103, '29
SWEET, R. H.: Pectus excavatum; 2 cases successfully operated upon. Ann. Surg. *119:*922-934, June '44
SWEEZEY, E.; BAXTER, H. AND COPEMAN, R.: Use of acrylic and elastic resin prosthesis for deformities of face. Canad. M.A.J. *50:*16-21, Jan '44
SWENSON, S. A. JR. AND HARKINS, H. N.: Application of dermatome-flap method; use in case of recurrent incisional hernia. Arch. Surg. *47:*564-570, Dec '43
ŚWIATLOWSKI, B.: Congenital median fistula of neck; pathogenesis and histology. Monatschr. f. Ohrenh. *68:*1096-1106, Sept '34
SWINGLE, W. W.; KLEINBERG, W. AND HAYS, H. W.: Gelatin and saline as plasma substitutes (in prevention of shock). Am. J. Physiol. *141:*329-337, May '44
SWINTON, N. W. AND WARREN, S.: Salivary gland tumors. Surg., Gynec. and Obst. *67:*424-435, Oct '38
SYDOW, A. F. (see GLOVER, D. M.) March '41
SYLVESTRE BEGNIS, C. AND PICENA, J. P.: Darier's fibrosarcoma on scar of human bite on male breast; case. Rev. med. de Rosario *36:*233-239, May '46
SYME, W. S.: Deflection of nasal septum. Brit. M. J. *2:*656-657, Sept 24, '38

Syndactylism

2 interesting cases of ectrosyndactyly. YAP, S. E. AND PINEDA, E. V. Philippine J. Sc. *20:*1-13, Jan '22 (illus.)
Rare malformation of hands, polydactylia, syndactylia and thumb with 3 phalanges.

Syndactylism – Cont.
DHALLUIN, A. Arch. franco-belges de chir. *25:*931-933, July '22 (illus.)
Web fingers. RÖMER, H. Deutsche Ztschr. f. Chir. *174:*1-9, '22 (illus.) abstr: J.A.M.A. *79:*2124, Dec 16, '22
Treatment of webbed fingers, congenital or acquired. DORRANCE, G. M. AND BRANSFIELD, J. W. Ann. Surg. *78:*532-533, Oct '23 (illus.)
Acrocephalosyndactylia. APERT. Bull. et mem. Soc. med. d. hop. de Par. *47:*1669-1672, Dec 7, '23
Coexistence of congenital amputations and syndactylism. COLEMAN, H. A., J.A.M.A. *83:*1164-1165, Oct 11, '24
Acrocephaly associated with syndactylism, with report of case. LANGMANN, A. G. Arch. Pediat. *41:*699-706, Oct '24
Acrocephalosyndactylia. DE BRUIN, J. Nederl. Tijdschr. v. Geneesk. *2:*2380-2393, Nov 28, '25 also: Acta Paediat. *5:*280-293, '26 abstr: J.A.M.A. *86:*456, Feb 6, '26
Ectrodactylia and syndactylia; case. ANDREUCCI, A. Monitore zool. ital. *37:*289-296, Dec 30, '26
Acrocephalosyndactylia; case. DE TONI, G. Pediatria *34:*1305-1309, Dec 1, '26
Syndactylia with acrocephaly; case. BIANCHINI, A. Radiol. med. *14:*1-12, Jan '27
Combined acrocephaly and syndactylism occurring in mother and daughter; case report. WEECH, A. A. Bull. Johns Hopkins Hosp. *40:*73-76, Feb '27
Technic of surgical treatment of syndactylia. VILLECHAISE, AND JEAN, G. Rev. d'orthop. *14:*241-243, May '27
Rare variety of congenital syndactylia. BUSULENGA, A. Cluj. med. *8:*219-222, June '27
Acrocephalosyndactylia; 2 cases. REUSS, A. Wien. med. Wchnschr. *77:*1208, Sept 3, '27
Syndactylia and synectrodactyly. TOMESKU, I. Fortschr. a. d. Geb. d. Rontgenstrahlen *36:*629-631, Sept '27
Congenital web fingers; addition to Didot's operation for syndactylism. JONES, H. T., S. Clin. N. Amer. *7:*1450-1452, Dec '27
Peculiarities of hereditary polydactylia and syndactylia. THOMSEN, O. Acta med. Scandinav. *65:*609-644, '27 also: Hospitalstid. *70:*789-819, Aug 25, '27
Peculiarities of hereditary polydactylia and syndactylia; supplement to author's original article. THOMSEN, O. Acta med. Scandinav. *66:*588-590, '27
Roentgen ray findings in case of acrocephaly with syndactylia. ROVIDA, F. Gazz. med. lomb. *87:*49-56, April 10, '28
Acrocephaly with associated syndactylism. BOSTOCK, J., M. J. Australia *1:*572-574, May 12, '28
Syndactylism in 4 generations. PERKOFF, D. Brit. M. J. *2:*341-342, Aug 25, '28
Syndactylism; case. ETIENNE. Arch. Soc. d. sc. med. et biol. de Montpellier *9:*409, Sept '28
Familial syndactylia. BONNETT, L. Bull. et mem. Soc. de chir. de Paris *20:*677-681, Oct 19, '28
Peculiarites concerning hereditary polydactylism and syndactylism. THOMSEN, O. Acta path. et microbiol. Scandinav. (supp) *5:*148-149, '28
Acrocephalosyndactylia in brother and sister. NØRVIG, J. Hospitalstid. *72:*165-178, Feb 14, '29
Bilateral syndactylism, case. PORTER, C. P. Brit. M. J. *1:*502, March 16, '29
New pedigrees of hereditary disease; polydactylism and syndactylism. BELL, J. Ann. Eugenics *4:*41-48, April '29
Megalosyndactylia; case. ABRAMOVIČS, H. Munchen. med. Wchnschr. *76:*921, May 31, '29
Syndactylia; cases. CARCASSONNE. Lyon med. *143:*778, June 23, '29
Surgical treatment of syndactylia. HASS, J. Zentralbl. f. Chir. *56:*1413-1416, June 8, '29
Hereditary polysyndactylia; case. LEGORBURU, R. Arch. de med., cir. y espec. *30:*745-752, June 29, '29
Acrocephalic dysostosis; study of cranium of patient with acrocephalosyndactylia. APERT, AND REGNAULT, F. Bull. et mem. Soc. med. d. hop. de Paris *53:*832-835, July 1, '29
Acrocephalosyndactylia; 2 cases. CAUSSADE, L. AND NICOLAS. Paris med. *2:*399-402, Nov 2, '29
Acrocephalo-syndactylia, a general malformation of bony system. EDLING, L. Acta radiol., supp. 3, pars 2, pp. 70-71, '29
Acrocephalosyndactylia; case. ROMAGNA MANOIA, A. Riv. di antropol. *28:*165-188, '28-'29
Webbed fingers. WOOLSEY, J. H. Am. J. Surg. *8:*307-309, Feb '30
Syndactylism. DAVIS, J. S. AND GERMAN, W. J., Arch. Surg. *21:*32-75, July '30
Symphalangism. MUSSER, J. H. New Orleans M. and S. J. *83:*325-326, Nov '30
Syndactylia and hypophalangism of spoon-shaped hand; case. BRITES, G. Folia anat. univ. conimb. (nos. 7-8) *5:*1-5, '30
Pathogenic theories in typical case of acrocephalosyndactylia; case. VALENTINI, P. Clin. pediat. *13:*211-222, March '31
Simple method of plastic surgery in syndactylia. MEYER-BURGDORFF, H. Zentralbl. f.

Syndactylism – Cont.
Chir. *58:*998-1000, April 18, '31
Case of syndactylia and gigantonychia. SIGAL, E. Casop. lek. cesk. *71:*329-331, March 11, '32
Serrated plastic surgery; one of several beneficial methods of treating syndactylia and Dupuytren's. PALMÉN, A. J. Zentralbl. f. Chir. *59:*1377-1379, May 28, '32
Familial syndactylia. ČÍPEK, J. Casop. lek. cesk. *71:*806-811, June 24, '32
Acrocephalo-syndactylism; case. JOHNSTONE, G. G. Lancet *2:*15-16, July 2, '32
Unusual form of brachyphalangy and syndactylia, with double proximal phalanx in middle fingers. COCKAYNE, E. A., J. Anat. *67:*165-167, Oct '32
Unusual familial developmental disturbance of face, (acrocephalosyndactylia, craniofacial dysostosis and hypertelorism). CHOTZEN, F. Monatschr. f. Kinderh. *55:*97-122, '32
Syndactylia. GOURDON, J. Bull. et mem. Soc. med. et chir. de Bordeaux, pp. 252-255, '32
Hereditary deformities of hand and foot in members of one family; polydactylia and syndactylia. KEMP, T. AND RAVN, J. Acta psychiat. et neurol. *7:*275-296, '32
General skeletal changes in acrocephalosyndactylia. WIGERT, V. Acta psychiat. et neurol. *7:*701-718, '32
Ectrodactylia with syndactylia; case. BOURGEOIS, P., *et al.* Bull. et mem. Soc. med. d. hop. de Paris *49:*320-322, March 13, '33
Craniofacial dysostosis (dyscephaly, Crouzon's disease) associated with syndactylia of 4 extremities (dyscephalodactylia). VOGT, A. Klin. Monatsbl. f. Augenh. *90:*441-454, April '33
Syndactylism with variations. SCOTT, W., J. Hered. *24:*241-245, June '33
Therapy of syndactylia. GRISANTI, S. Riv. san. siciliana *21:*1304-1308, Sept 1, '33
Anatomic examination of human hemicephalic fetus 10 months old with harelip, cleft palate, hyperdactylia, syndactylia, etc. IKEDA, Y. Arb. a. d. anat. Inst. d. kaiserlich-japan. Univ. zu Sendai, Hft. 15, pp. 61-212, '33
Operation for syndactylia. KLAPP, R. Arch. f. klin. Chir. *177:*688-690, '33
Syndactylia combined with macrodactyly in patient with fibrolipoma of right foot. YOKOTA, K. Taiwan Igakkai Zasshi (Abstr. Sect.) *33:*5, Feb '34
Oxycephalosyndactylia; case. DE CASTRO, A. Rev. neurol. *1:*359-367, March '34
Epithelial inlay in therapy of syndactylia. ESSER, J. F. S. AND RAOUL. Rev. de chir. plastique, pp. 21-32, May '34

Syndactylism – Cont.
Heredity of syndactylia in one family during period of 100 years. FINCKH. Med. Welt *8:*705, May 19, '34
Roentgen study of polydactylia and syndactylia in 3 generations of family. JAUBERT DE BEAUJEU, A. Bull. et mem. Soc. de radiol. med. de France *22:*339-342, June '34
Peculiar form of craniofacial malformation (acrocephalosyndactylia with facial asymmetry and ophthalmoplegia); case. KREINDLER, A. AND SCHACHTER, M. Paris med. *2:*102-105, Aug 4, '34
Modifications of Zeller operation in therapy of syndactylia. PALMA, R. Ann. ital. di chir. *13:*1068-1074, Sept 30, '34
Syndactylia; therapy of case. FIESCHI, D. Arch. ital. di chir. *37:*204-208, '34
Question of double malformations; acrocephalosyndactylia and dysencephalia splanchnocystica. GRUBER, G. B. Beitr. z. path. Anat. u. z. allg. Path. *93:*459-476, '34
Thiersch graft in therapy of syndactylia. STEPANOVA, E. N. Novy khir. arkhiv. *32:*101-104, '34
Question of surgical intervention in syndactylia. TSVETKOV, A. A. Sovet. khir. (no. 6) *6:*876-877, '34
Acrocephalosyndactylia (Apert syndrome); case. NOVIS FILHO, A. Brasil-med. *49:*28-32, Jan 12, '35
Cranial deformities due to premature synostoses of sutures with particular reference to Crouzon's disease (craniofacial dysostoses) and Apert syndrome (acrocephaly and syndactylia). MASTROMARINO, A. Arch. di ortop. *51:*233-304, June 30, '35
Surgical therapy of syndactylia; case. POLYA, J. Riv. di chir. *1:*469-472, Aug '35
Surgical therapy of syndactylia. LAUBER, H. J., Chirurg *7:*598-599, Sept 1, '35
Surgical therapy of syndactylia. POLYA, J. Orvosi hetil. *80:*38-40, Jan 11, '36
Family tree showing hereditary syndactylia. KIRCHMAIR, H. Munchen. med. Wchnschr. *83:*605-606, April 10, '36
Congenital syndactylia; study of 3 generations. NICITA, A. Minerva med. *1:*346-352, April 14, '36
Syndactylia operated on according to Klapp method. SCHJØTH-IVERSEN, I. Norsk mag. f. laegevidensk. *97:*700-704, July '36
Congenital malformation of hand with syndactylia and hypoplasia of fourth metacarpal bone; case. CARDI, G. Arch. di ortop. *52:*427-434, Sept 30, '36
Syndactyly. MEHTA, K. B. AND MODI, N. J. Indian J. Pediat. *3:*241-243, Oct '36
Complete syndactylia of hands and feet with other deformities in heredosyphilitic; case.

Syndactylism – Cont.
LICEAGA, F. J. Semana med. *2:*1685-1691, Dec 17, '36
Heredity of concealed syndactylic polydactylia. SCHATZKI, P. Arch. f. orthop. u. Unfall-Chir. *36:*613, '36
Syndactylia and its therapy. HARRENSTEIN, R. J. Maandschr. v. kindergeneesk. *6:*131-147, Jan '37
Complete syndactylia of hands and feet associated with other deformities; case. LICEAGA, F. J. Arch. de med. d. enf. *40:*448-452, July '37 abstr: Bull. Soc. de pediat. de Paris *35:*141-146, Feb '37
Acrocephalosyndactylia (Apert syndrome) in new-born infant; case. ALANTAR, I. H. Arch. de med. d. enf. *40:*171-172, March '37
Modified Agnew operation for syndactylism. COGSWELL, H. D. AND TRUSLER, H. M. Surg., Gynec. and Obst. *64:*793, April '37
Etiologic study of multiple congenital malformations, with report of case of acrocephalosyndactylia. BERARIU, A. Rev. pediat. si puericult. *1:*314-318, May-Aug '37
Acrocephalosyndactylia; evolution of case. CAUSSADE, L. *et al.* Rev. med. de Nancy *65:*576-586, July 1, '37
Constructive surgical therapy of syndactylia; case. Also: nasal deform. LLUESMA URANGA, E. Cron. med., Valencia *41:*201-207, Sept-Oct '37
Incomplete membranous syndactylia of all fingers; author's surgical technic; case. SATANOWSKY, S. Rev. ortop. y traumatol. *7:*187-192, Oct '37
Pedigree of syndactyly. WIGHTMAN, J. C., J. Hered. *28:*421-423, Dec '37
Genesis of genopathic syndrome (Bardet-Biedl acrocephalosyndactylia). POOL, F. L. Wien. Arch. f. inn. Med. *31:*187-200, '37
Complete syndactylia of hands and feet and other deformities; case. LICEAGA, F. J. Pediatria prat., Sao Paulo *8:*72-83, March-July '37 also: Monatschr. f. Kinderh. *72:*179-186, '38
Local gigantism involving webbed fingers. LEVI, D. Proc. Roy. Soc. Med. *31:*764-765, May '38
Pedigree of symphalangism. STILES, K. A. AND WEBER, R. A., J. Hered. *29:*199-202, May '38
Aspects of so-called symbrachydactylia. ECKINGER, W. Arch. f. orthop. u. Unfall-Chir. *38:*662-669, '38
Study of family with syndactylia. LUEKEN, K. G. Ztschr. f. menschl. Vererb.-u. Konstitutionslehre *22:*152-159, '38
Treatment of webbed fingers; syndactylism; case. DICKSON, J. A. Cleveland Clin. Quart. *6:*72-74, Jan '39

Syndactylism – Cont.
Surgical therapy of syndactylia. STEPHAN, H. Zentralbl. f. Chir. *66:*794-796, April 8, '39
Treatment of syndactylias by total free skin grafts. BOPPE, M. AND FAUGERON, P. Paris med. *1:*522-527, June 17, '39
Syndactylia and symphalangism; case. GLASNER, J. Arq. brasil. de cir. e ortop. *7:*338-344, Dec '39
Syndactylism with absence of pectoralis major. BROWN, J. B. AND MCDOWELL, F. Surgery *7:*599-601, April '40
Polydactylia and syndactylia; case. CATALANO, F. E. Prensa med. argent. *27:*1081-1082, May 22, '40
Megalodactylia and megalosyndactylia. DE ARAUJO, A. Rev. brasil. de orthop. e traumatol. *1:*341-368, May-June '40
Modern views on etiology and therapy of syndactylia. HEIM, W. Med. Welt *14:*481-483, May 11, '40
Hereditary etiology of syndactylia; remarkable association of polydactylia and syndactylia in case. DE LUCA, R. Minerva med. *2:*324-327, Sept 29, '40
Surgical problems in hereditary polydactylism and syndactylism. SNEDECOR, S. T. AND HARRYMAN, W. K., J. M. Soc. New Jersey *37:*443-449, Sept '40
Bilateral complete syndactylism of all fingers. HAAS, S. L. Am. J. Surg. *50:*363-366, Nov '40
Acrocephalosyndactyly; case. ROUDINESCO, MME. Bull. et mem. Soc. med. d. hop. de Paris *56:*624-627, Nov 25, '40
Webbed fingers. MACCOLLUM, D. W. Surg., Gynec. and Obst. *71:*782-789, Dec '40
Acrocephalosyndactylia with cleft hand in one of a pair of uniovular twins. GOLL, H. AND KAHLICH-KOENNER, D. M. Ztschr. f. menschl. Vererb.-u. Konstitutionslehre *24:*516-535, '40
Unilateral microphthalmia with congenital anterior synechiae and syndactyly. BERLINER, M. L. Arch. Ophth. *26:*653-660, Oct '41
Syndactylia; solution to problem. GONZALEZ ULLOA, M. Rev. mex. de cir., ginec. y cancer *10:*157-167, April '42
Congenital unilateral absence of pectoral muscles often associated with syndactylism. RESNICK, E., J. Bone and Joint Surg. *24:*925-928, Oct '42
Syndactylism; correction. CRONIN, T. D. Tri-State M. J. *15:*2869, Jan '43

Syndactylism with Absence of Pectoral Muscles (See also Syndactylism)

Syndactylism with absence of pectoralis major. BROWN, J. B. AND MCDOWELL, F. Sur-

Syndactylism with Absence of Pectoral Muscles—Cont.
gery *7:*599-601, April '40
Congenital unilateral absence of pectoral muscles often associated with syndactylism. RESNICK, E., J. Bone and Joint Surg. *24:*925-928, Oct '42

SZÁNTÓ, M.: Davidson method of burn therapy. Gyogyaszat *74:*555-556, Sept 23, '34
SZCZAWINSKA, W.: Congenital absence of pectoralis muscles and of right mammary gland. Nourrisson *11:*187-190, May '23 (illus.)
SZÉKELY, L.: Rare case of pseudohermaphroditism of internal male type subjected to surgical treatment. Zentralbl. f. Chir. *57:*3168-3171, Dec 20, '30
SZÉKELY, L.: Congenital ectopy of bladder cured by operation 15 years previously. Zentralbl. f. Chir. *64:*464-467, Feb 20, '37
SZÉKELY, L.: Ectopia vesicae, surgically treated 15 years ago; case. Budapesti orvosi ujsag *35:*221-223, March 4, '37
SZENDE, B.: Fistulas of nasal entrance. Orvosi hetil. *83:*112, Feb 4, '39
SZILI, E.: Transplantation of rectum in defective vagina. Verhandl. d. ungar. arztl. Gesellsch. *1:*149, June '29
SZOKOLIK, E.: Hungarian method of forming lower eyelid. Klin. Monatsbl. f. Augenh. *80:*652-655, May 25, '28
SZOKOLIK, E.: Closure of persistent retro-auricular opening by means of Hungarian method of using semicircular flaps. Monatschr. f. Ohrenh. *66:*1058-1059, Sept '32
SZUTU, C. AND CHEN, C. Y.: Thiersch skin grafting; use of collodion-gauze technic. Chinese M. J. *57:*535-545, June '40
SZYLEJKO, H. W.: Plasma administration in severe shock. U. S. Nav. M. Bull. *44:*857-859, April '45

Szymanowsky Operation: See Kuhnt-Szymanowsky Operation

T

TABANELLI, M.: Frostbite in wartime. Arch. ital. chir. *68:*111-195, '46
TABAR, F.: Fractures of lower jaw; necessity of extracting teeth at point of fracture. Practicien du Nord de l'Afrique *5:*422-428, July 15, '32
TABERSHAW, I. R. (see RUBENSTEIN, A. D. *et al*) Nov '45
TABOR, H. (see ROSENTHAL, S. M.) Nov-Dec '45
TABORISSKIY, M. G.: Secondary sutures and skin transplantations at front line hospitals. Khirurgiya, no. 2, pp. 23-30, '45
TAGGART, H. J.: Modification of Motais' operation for ptosis of eyelid. Tr. Ophth. Soc. U. Kingdom *53:*417-421, '33
TAGNON, H. J.; LEVERSON, S. M. AND TAYLOR, F. H. L.: Shock and its therapy. Union med. du Canada *73:*1498-1507, Dec '44
TAIANA, J. A.: Transfusions of blood and plasma in shock. Bol. d. Inst. clin. quir. *18:*282-283, May '42
TAILHEFER, A.: Primitive suture of 2 flexor tendons of fourth finger in palmar region; suture of deep flexor of index in same region; case. Bull. et mem. Soc. nat. de chir. *54:*827-829, June 16, '28
TAILHEFER, A. (see BLOCH, J. C.) Jan '29
TAILHEFER, A. (see ISELIN, M.) July '27
TAILHEFER, ANDRÉ: *Les techniques et les résultats actuals de la réparation des tendons de la main et des doigts*. Arnette, Paris, 1928
TAISNY, E. (see HENNEBERT, P.) Dec '33
TAKAHARA, T. AND WATANABE, D.: Congenital lateral neck cyst; case. Oto-rhino-laryng. *12:*44-45, Jan '39
TAKAHASHI, K.: Modified nasal septal forceps. Ztschr. f. Hals-, Nasen-u. Ohrenh. *22:*130, June 16, '28
TAKAHASHI, K.: New instrument for intranasal suture. Ztschr. f. Laryng., Rhin. *17:*211-216, Sept '28
TAKAHASHI, K.: High submucous excision of nasal septum. Ztschr. f. Laryng., Rhin. *19:*22-40, Nov '29
TAKAHASHI, N. AND MIYATA, R.: Transplantation of skin flaps. Arch. f. klin. Chir. *120:*170-205, '22 (illus.)
TAKASHIMA, R. AND KUSANO, M.: Complete removal of foreskin by factory machine; plastic replacement; case. Zentralbl. f. Chir. *63:*84-86, Jan 11, '36
TAKEDA: Complete median fistula of neck. Deutsche med. Wchnschr. *48:*1649-1650, Dec 8, '22
TAKEZAWA, N. AND NAKAJIMA, K.: Angioma of auricle; case. Oto-rhino-laryng. *11:*406, May '38
TALAMO, P.: Exstrophy of bladder with genital malformations; case in new-born infant. Clin. ostet. *38:*516-520, Oct '36
TAMAI, T.: Combined burn therapy with rivanol (acridine dye) and cod liver oil. Bull. Nav. M. A., Japan (Abstr. Sect.) *27:*15, March 15, '38
TAMERIN, J. (see ROTHMAN, M. *et al*) Nov '42
TAMERIN, J. A.: Concealment of scars (with covermark). Am. J. Surg. *36:*91-92, April '37
TAMERIN, J. A.: New operations for correction of external deviations of lower end of nose. Ann. Otol., Rhin. and Laryng. *47:*235-239, March '38

TAMERIN, J. A.: Combined nasal reconstruction and submucous resection. New York State J. Med. *38:*1129–1133, Aug 15, '38

TAMIYA, C. AND KOYAMA, M.: Roentgen treatment of thermal and chemical burns of skin. Strahlentherapie *34:*808–812, '29

TAMMANN, H.: Metabolism in transplanted tissues. Klin. Wchnschr. *10:*1858–1859, Oct 3, '31

TAMMANN, H. AND PATRIKALAKIS, M.: Homeoplastic skin transplantation after reticulo-endothelial storage. Beit. z. klin. Chir. *139:*550–568, '27

TAMMANN, H. (see LEHMANN, W.) 1925

TANAKA, H.: Death due to shock after scalding of pharynx and larynx. Oto-rhino-laryng. (Abstr. Sect.) *13:*45–46, Oct '40

TANAKAYA, K.: Technic and results of suture of ulnar nerve in gunshot injury; case. Okayama-Igakkai-Zasshi *45:*2677, Nov '33

TANCREDI, G.: Mommsen's bloodless treatment of Volkmann's contracture. Arch. di ortop. *43:*362–377, '27

TANCREDI, G.: Operative treatment in Madelung deformity of hand; case. Bull. e atti. d. r. Accad. med. di Roma *57:*153–158, June '31

TANER, F.: Exstrophy of bladder; case. J. d'urol. *44:*340–342, Oct '37

TANGUY, R.: Enormous angioma of bones of hand; case. Gaz. med. de France (supp. Cah. radiol.) *45:*371–373, Feb 15, '38

Tansley Operation: See Hunt-Tansley Operation

TANZER, R. C.: Bacteremia due to Staphylococcus aureus and Streptococcus hemolyticus arising from hand infection. Clin. Misc., Mary I. Bassett Hosp. *2:*69–74, '35

TAPPEINER, S.: Plastic surgery and transplantations in dermatology. Wien. klin. Wchnschr. *52:*1140–1143, Dec 22, '39

TARABUCHIN, M.: Hypospadias scrotalis. Vrach. dielo *10:*442, March 30, '27

TARLOV, I. M.: Plasma clot suture of peripheral nerves; illustrated technic. Surgery *15:*257–269, Feb '44

TARLOV, I. M.: Autologous plasma clot suture of nerves; use in clinical surgery. J.A.M.A. *126:*741–748, Nov 18, '44

TARLOV, I. M. AND BENJAMIN, B.: Autologous plasma clot suture of nerves. Science *95:*258, March 6, '42

TARLOV, I. M. AND BENJAMIN, B.: Plasma clot and silk suture of nerves; experimental study of comparative tissue reaction. Surg., Gynec. and Obst. *76:*366–374, March '43

TARLOV, I. M.; *et al*: Plasma clot suture of peripheral nerves; experimental technic. Arch. Surg. *47:*44–58, July '43

TARLOV, I. M. AND EPSTEIN, J.: Importance of adequate blood supply in nerve transplantation. J. Neurosurg. *2:*49–71, Jan '45

TARLOV, I. M.; HOFFMAN, W. AND HAYNER, J. C.: Source of autografts in clinical surgery; technic for their suture. Am. J. Surg. *72:*700–710, Nov '46

TARNOPOLSKIY, A. I.: Technic of preparation and fixation of wire splints with intermaxillary traction. Ortop. i travmatol. (no. 6) *12:*71–77, '38

TARTAKOVSKIY, B. S.: Reconstruction of axillary space in cases of cicatricial contracture of shoulder. Novy khir. arkhiv *44:*201–204, '39

TARTAKOWSKY, A.: Congenital facial malformation; case. Folia oto-laryng. orient. *2:*46–51, Jan '35

TASCH, H.: Surgical therapy of aplasia of vagina. Wien. klin. Wchnschr. *54:*883–888, Oct 24, '41

TASKER, D. G. C. (see ROBERTSON, D.) 1929

TATAFIORE, E.: Rare type of congenital deformity of right hand; case. Pediatria *40:*829–834, Aug 1, '32

TATAFIORE, E.: Congenital macrodactyly; case. Pediatria *42:*405–412, April '34

TATO, J. M. (see MASSA, D.) April-May '29

TATRALLYAY, Z.: Unusual possible injuries of facial nerves. Monatschr. f. Ohrenh. *76:*30–37, Jan '42

Tattooing of Skin Grafts

- Color matching of skin grafts and flaps with permanent pigment injection. HANCE, G.; *et al.* Surg., Gynec. and Obst. *79:*624–628, Dec '44
- Tattooing of free grafts and pedicle flaps. BYARS, L. T. Ann. Surg. *121:*644–648, May '45
- Tattooing of free grafts and pedicle flaps. BYARS, L. T. Tr. South. S. A. (1944) *56:*260–264, '45

Tattoos, Commercial

- Excision of tattoo marks. MILLER, C. C. Am. J. Surg. *39:*121, May '25

Tattoos, Dirt

- Tattooing of nose and face following automobile injuries. CARTER, W. W. New York State J. Med. *35:*573–575, June 1, '35
- Accidental tattooing by fall; removal by potassium permanganate method; case. LACASSAGNE, J. AND ROUSSET, J. Bull. Soc. franc. de dermat. et syph. (Reunion dermat., Lyon) *42:*1518–1520, July '35
- Pigmentation of cutaneous scars in coal

Tattoos, Dirt–Cont.
miners. LEVINE, J. M. Dermat. Ztschr. *73:*135-136, April '36
Removal of powder tattoo of face by minor surgery. LINDSAY, H. C. L. J.A.M.A. *109:*1530, Nov 6, '37
Abrasions and accidental tattoos, scars, keloids and scar contractures, and nasal deformities. GREELEY, P. W., S. Clin. North America *22:*253-276, Feb '42

TAUB. (see GRIMAUD, *et al*) July '33
TAUBE, E.: Part played by transplanted skin in regeneration. Arch. f. Entwckingsmechn. d. Organ. *121:*204-209, Jan 6, '30
TAUBER, E. B.: Modern concepts and theories of burn therapy. Arch. de med. int. *4:*210-219, '38
TAUBER, E. B. AND GOLDMAN, L.: Hemiatrophia faciei progressiva. Arch. Dermat. and Syph. *39:*696-704, April '39
TAUBER, H.: Alopecia prematura and its surgical treatment (flap-method of plastic surgery). J. Ceylon Br., Brit. M. A. *36:*237-242, July '39
TAUBER-HRADSKY, H. T.: Nasal mutilation in India and new rhinoplasty. J. Internat. Coll. Surgeons *6:*27-34, Jan-Feb '43
TAULLARD, J. C.: Spontaneous cicatrization of section of tendon of extensor pollicis longus (biologic therapy); cases. Bol. y trab., Soc. argent. de cirujanos *4:*772-776, '43 also: Rev. Asoc. med. argent. *57:*1018-1019, Nov 30, '43
TAULLARD, J. C.: Dermatome. Bol. y trab., Soc. argent. de cirujanos *7:*30-38, '46 also: Rev. Asoc. med. argent. *60:*248-251, April 30, '46
TAULLARD, J. C. (see RODRIGUEZ VILLEGAS, R.) April '37
TAULLARD, J. C. (see RODRIGUEZ VILLEGAS, R.) July '37
TAUSSIG, L. R.: Radium treatment of carcinoma of lip. M. Clin. N. America *6:*1579-1586, May '23 (illus.)
TAUSSIG, L. R.: Treatment of keloids with radium. California State J. Med. *21:*520-522, Dec '23
TAUSSIG, L. R. AND TORREY, F. A.: Malignant melanoma; statistical and pathological review of 35 cases. California and West. Med. *52:*15-18, Jan '40
TAUSSIG, L. R. (see KILGORE, A. R.) Oct '31
TAUSSIG, L. R. (see MORROW, H.) Jan '22
TAUSSIG, L. R. (see MORROW, H.) March '23
TAUSSIG, L. R. (see MORROW, H.) Nov '23
TAUSSIG, L. R. (see MORROW, H. *et al*) May '37
TAVANI, E.: Keloid of nose; case. Boll. d. mal. d. orecchio, d. gola, d. naso *52:*281-288, June '34
TAVARES, A.: Cavernous hemangioma of upper lip. Ann. d'anat. path. *3:*147-150, Feb '26
TAVERNIER, L.: Immediate results of operations for facial paralysis. Bull. et mem. Soc. nat. de chir. *52:*992-994, Nov 20, '26
TAVERNIER, L.: Bone graft with dead bone. Lyon chir. *27:*233-236, March-April '30
TAVERNIER, L.: Paralysis of brachial plexus; rupture of superior roots in supraclavicular fossa; nerve graft; beginning of functional restoration 3 years later. Lyon chir. *29:*110-112, Jan-Feb '32
TAVERNIER, L.: Makkas operation for exstrophy of bladder in child; case. Lyon chir. *29:*587-591, Sept-Oct '32
TAVERNIER, L.: Most favorable age for harelip operation in infants. Lyon chir. *36:*345-346, May-June '39
TAVERNIER, L. AND DECHAUME, J.: Initial lesions in Volkmann paralysis; 2 cases. Lyon chir. *34:*117-122, Jan-Feb '37
TAVERNIER, L., DECHAUME, J. AND POUZET, F.: Muscular infarct and necrotic lesions of nerves in Volkmann syndrome; biopsy study. J. de med. de Lyon *17:*815-826, Dec 20, '36
TAVERNIER, L. AND POUZET, F.: So-called congenital temporomandibular ankyloses. Lyon chir. *35:*328-332, May-June '38
TAYLOR, A. B.: New instrument for use in long-standing dislocations of jaws. J. M. A. South Africa *4:*326, June 14, '30
TAYLOR, A. C. (see WEISS, P.) April '43
TAYLOR, A. C. (see WEISS, P.) Sept '46
TAYLOR, E. E. T.: Fracture of zygomatic tripod; method of fixation. M. Press *214:*158-159, Sept 5, '45
TAYLOR, F.: Misuse of tannic acid in burns. J.A.M.A. *106:*1144-1146, April 4, '36
TAYLOR, F.: Pressure bag in skin grafting. Am. J. Surg. *33:*328-329, Aug '36
TAYLOR, F. H. L.: Nitrogen requirement of patients with thermal burns. J. Indust. Hyg. and Toxicol. *26:*152-155, May '44
TAYLOR, F. H. L.; DAVIDSON, C. S. AND LEVENSON, S. M.: Problem of nutrition in presence of excessive nitrogen requirement in seriously ill patients, with particular reference to thermal burns. Connecticut M. J. *8:*141-148, March '44
TAYLOR, F. H. L.; *et al*: Abnormal nitrogen metabolism in patients with thermal burns. New England J. Med. *229:*855-859, Dec 2, '43
TAYLOR, F. H. L. *et al*: Problems of protein nutrition in burn patients. Ann. Surg. *118:*215-224, Aug '43
TAYLOR, F. H. L. (see TAGNON, H. J. *et al*) Dec '44
TAYLOR, G. M. AND NEUFELD, A. J.: Method for

skeletal traction to digits. J. Bone and Joint Surg. *20:*496–497, April '38

Taylor, G. W.: Analysis of cases at Pondville Hospital; cancer of lip and mouth. Am. J. Cancer (supp.) *15:*2380–2385, July '31

Taylor, G. W.: Carcinoma of buccal mucosa; analysis of cases observed at Massachusetts General Hospital in 3 year period 1924–1926. Surg., Gynec. and Obst. *58:*914–916, May '34

Taylor, G. W. and Nathanson, I. T.: Evaluation of neck dissection in cancer of lips. Surg., Gynec. and Obst. *69:*484–492, Oct '39

Taylor, H. P.: Congenital cleft palate and harelip in infants; mode of nutrition in preoperative period. Brit. Dent. J. *78:*1–7, Jan 5, '45

Taylor, J.: Treatment of facial wounds and cut throat. Brit. M. J. *1:*792–795, April 9, '38

Taylor, J.: Surgical treatment of pain (painful fingers). Lancet *2:*1151–1154, Nov 19, '38

Taylor, J. W.: Repair of cicatricial ectropion by free dermic graft. South. M. J. *22:*634–637, July '29

Taylor, M. M.: Soft tissues of hand in infection; microscopic study of pathologic changes produced by deep cellulitis complicated by osteomyelitis. Indust. Med. *5:*187–192, April '36

Taylor, N. B. and Moorhouse, M. S.: Use of isinglass (ishthyocolla) as blood substitute in shock therapy. Canad. M.A.J. *49:*251–262, Oct '43

Taylor, R. C.: Exstrophy of bladder; case. Memphis M. J. *10:*43–44, July '35

Taylor, R. F. (see Bancroft, F. W. *et al*) May '40

Taylor, R. T.: Reconstruction of hand, a new technic in tenoplasty. Surg., Gynec. and Obst. *32:*237, March '21

Taylor, R. W. (see Hook, F. R.) Jan '42

Taylor, R. W. (see Welch, C. C.) Oct '38

Taylor, R. W. (see Yando, A. H.) Jan '42

Tcharkviani, I. I.: Baldwin operation in case of congenital absence of vagina. J. akush. i zhensk. boliez. *41:*477–481, '30

Tchernigovsky, N. N.: Popoff method of formation of artificial vagina. Vrach. gaz. *34:*216–218, Feb 15, '30

Teale, T. P.: Restoration of nose by transplantation of skin from forehead in year 1881. Brit. J. Surg. *9:*449, Jan '22 (illus.)

Tecqmenne, C.: Tubular graft in autoplastic therapy of burn cicatrix; case. Liege med. *30:*818–820, July 11, '37

Teece, L.: Treatment of hand injuries (with special reference to tendons). M. J. Australia *2:*532–534, Oct 7, '39

Tees, F. J.: Primary repair of injuries to parotid duct. Canad. M.A.J. *16:*145–146, Feb '26

Tejera Lorenzo, F.: Utilization of Haynes splint (hand). Vida nueva *56:*29–34, July '45

Tejerina Fotheringham, W.: Grave burns; physiopathology and therapy. Dia med. *15:*1255–1259, Nov 15, '43

Teleky, L.: Paralysis of extensors of hand and fingers in persons working with lead. Deutsche med. Wchnschr. *59:*723–724, May 12, '33

Teleky, L.: Dupuytren's contracture as occupational disease. J. Indust. Hyg. and Toxicol. *21:*233–235, Sept '39

Telford, E. D. and Simmons, H. T.: Chronic lymphoedema. Brit. J. Surg. *25:*765–772, April '38

Telford, E. D. and Simmons, H. T.: Kondoleon operation for chronic lymphedema. Lancet *2:*667, Nov 29, '41

Temkin, J.: Favorable results with primary skin transplantation in radical operation of middle ear. Ztschr. f. Hals-, Nasen-u. Ohrenh. *22:*467–474, Feb 16, '29

Tempea, V.: Submucous resection from technical, respiratory and esthetic viewpoints. Spitalul *51:*98–99, March '31

Tempea, V.: Direct incision in submucous resection; modification of Killian operation. Rev. san. mil., Bucuresti *35:*1077–1079, Oct '36

Tempea, V.: Direct incision in submucous resection; modification of Killian operation. Ztschr. f. Hals-, Nasen-u. Ohrenh. *40:*548–552, '37

Tempestini, O.: Recurrent dislocation of temporomaxillary joint; therapy with intramuscular alcohol injections. Stomatol. *33:*901–912, Oct '35

Temporomandibular Joint

Treatment of ankylosis of temporomaxillary articulation. Imbert, L. Lyon chir. *18:*572–578, Sept–Oct '21 (illus.)

Old ankylosis of temporomaxillary articulation. Fasano, M. Arch. ital. di chir. *8:*575–588, Dec '23

Arthroplasty upon temporomandibular joint. Dorrance, G. M.; *et al.* Ann. Surg. *79:*485–487, April '24

Two cases of ankylosis of left temporo-mandibular joint. Crymble, P. T. Brit. M. J. *1:*996–997, June 7, '24

Prosthetic restoration of portion of mandible, including temporo-mandibular articulation on one side. Mitchell, V. E. Am. J. Surg. *38:*274–276, Nov '24

Arthroplasty of temporomaxillary joint. Ris-

Temporomandibular Joint—Cont.
DON, F., J.A.M.A. *85:*2011–2013, Dec 26, '25
Resection and arthroplasty in case of lockjaw from old osseous ankylosis of temporomaxillary articulation. DE GAETANO, L. Arch. ital. di chir. *12:*673–712, '25
New points of view in arthroplasty of jaw; comment on Haas's article. KOFMANN, S. Zentralbl. f. Chir. *53:*1125–1126, May 1, '26
Exposure of articulation of jaw. MERMINGAS, K. Zentralbl. f. Chir. *53:*1510–1511, June 12, '26
Chronic temporomaxillary subluxation. MORRIS, J. H. Am. J. Surg. *1:*288, Nov '26
Bilateral temporo-maxillary ankylosis with pleuropneumonia; death; autopsy; case. MALLET-GUY, P. AND JOUVE, P. Ann. d'anat. path. *4:*19–24, Jan '27
Temporo-maxillary ankylosis; case. FISCHER, H. Ann. d'anat. path. *4:*223, Feb '27
Continual dislocation of jaw at temporomaxillary articulation. BERCHER, J.; *et al.* Rev. d'hyg. *49:*605–607, Oct '27
Meniscus injuries of temporomaxillary joint resulting in so-called anterior dislocation. LOTSCH, F. Arch. f. klin. Chir. *149:*40–54, '27
Chirurgie de l'articulation temporomaxillaire, by LÉON DUFOURMENTEL. Masson et Cie, Paris, 1928
Surgery of temporomaxillary joint in its relation to odontostomatology. DUFOURMENTEL, L. Odontologie *66:*330–338, May '28
Loose cartilages in temporo-mandibular articulation. KNAPP, H. B., J. Michigan M. Soc. *27:*798–801, Dec '28
Orthopedic treatment of contracture of temporomaxillary joint. KNORR, H. Zentralbl. f. Chir. *56:*1229–1232, May 18, '29
Causation and treatment of displaced mandibular cartilage. WAKELEY, C. P. G. Lancet *2:*543–545, Sept 14, '29
Treatment of habitual luxation and so-called habitual subluxation of lower jaw and snapping of temporomaxillary joint. KONJETZNY, G. E. Zentralbl. f. Chir. *56:*3018–3023, Nov 30, '29
Clicking of temporomaxillary joint and habitual dislocations; cases. VON STAPELMOHR, S. Acta chir. Scandinav. *65:*1–68, '29
Curative and plastic surgery in different deformities of temporomaxillary joint. BOURGUET, J. Monde med., Paris *40:*109–114, Feb 15, '30
Chronic recurring temporomaxillary subluxation; surgical consideration of "snapping jaw" with report of successful operative result. MORRIS, J. H. Surg., Gynec. and Obst. *50:*483–491, Feb '30

Temporomandibular Joint—Cont.
New operative method in habitual temporomaxillary dislocations; case. MOCZAR, L. Rev. de stomatol. *32:*129–143, March '30
Therapy of temporomandibular ankylosis. ROCCIA, B. Boll. e mem. Soc. piemontese di chir. *2:*502–518, April 30, '32
Temporomaxillary ankylosis of obstetric origin. DUFOURMENTEL, L. Bull. et mem. Soc. de chir. de Paris *22:*502–507, July 4, '30
Temporomaxillary ankylosis; case. CANALS MAYNER, R. Rev. med. de Barcelona *15:*3–21, Jan '31
Pathology and therapy of temporomandibular joint. AXHAUSEN, G. Fortschr. d. Zahnh. *7:*199–215, March '31
Treatment of fractures of temporomaxillary joint. DUFOURMENTEL, L. Rev. odont. *52:*517–526, July–Aug '31
Exposure of temporomaxillary joint. AXHAUSEN, G. Chirurg *3:*713–716, Aug 15, '31
Three cases of snapping temporomaxillary joint. GUTIERREZ, A. Bol. y trab. de la Soc. de cir. de Buenos Aires *16:*65–74, April 20, '32
Arthroplasty of temporomandibular joint; case. BLACKBURN, J. D., J. M. A. Georgia *21:*314–315, Aug '32
Postpuerperal ankylosing polyarthritis; subluxation of atlas and axis; temporomaxillary and articulatory ankylosis; radiologic and etiologic study. ROCHER, H. L. Bull. et mem. Soc. med. et chir. de Bordeaux, pp. 279–293, '32
Surgical approach in operations on temporomaxillary articulation and on upper portion of ascending ramus of maxilla. SCHMIDT, G. Deutsche Ztschr. f. Chir. *236:*260–265, '32
Les luxations habituelles sans blocage de l'articulation temporo-maxillaire, by PIERRE FRIEZ. Le François, Paris, 1933
Surgery of articulation of jaws; 3 cases. JIRÁSEK, A. Casop. lek. cesk. *73:*169–170, Feb 16, '34
Complete ankylosis of temporomaxillary joint; surgical therapy; 2 cases. TRANQUILLI-LEALI, E. Rassegna d. previd. sociale *21:*8–45, Sept '34
Unusual localization of arthropathies (mandibulotemporal and metacarpophalangeal ankylosis), in postencephalitic parkinsonian syndrome and their pathogenesis. GORDON, A., M. Rec. *140:*351–353, Oct 3, '34
Surgical therapy of temporomaxillary ankylosis; 100 cases. DUFOURMENTEL, L. AND

Temporomandibular Joint—Cont.
DARCISSAC, M. Bull. et mem. Soc. d. chirurgiens de Paris *27:*149-161, March 15, '35
Recurrent dislocation of temporomaxillary joint; therapy with intramuscular alcohol injections. TEMPESTINI, O. Stomatol. *33:*901-912, Oct '35
Frequency of bilateral ankylosis of temporomaxillary joint. DUBOV, M. D. Sovet. khir., no. 9, pp. 106-113, '35
Habitual temporomaxillary luxation; cure of 3 years duration after meniscopexy; case. CONTIADES, X. J. Mem. Acad. de chir. *62:*18-21, Jan 15, '36
Recurrent dislocation of jaw; bilateral ablation of temporomaxillary menisci; case. SANTY, P. AND BERARD, M. Lyon chir. *33:*75-76, Jan-Feb '36
Osteotomy and arthroplasty for bony ankylosis of left temporo-mandibular joint of 20 years' duration. LOOP, F. A., J. Indiana M. A. *29:*70-72, Feb '36
Congenital bony temporomandibular ankylosis and facial hemiatrophy; review of literature and report of case. BURKET, L. W. J.A.M.A. *106:*1719-1722, May 16, '36
Surgical therapy of temporomaxillary ankylosis followed by prosthesis of dental arches. VARGAS SALCEDO, L. AND ILABACA L., L. Bol. y trab. de la Soc. de cir. de Buenos Aires *20:*1071-1082, Oct 21, '36
Morphologic, physiologic and clinical study of mandibular meniscus; habitual luxation and temporomaxillary cracking. DUBECQ, X. J., J. de med. de Bordeaux *114:*125-178, Jan 30, '37 also: Rev. d'odonto-stomatol. *1:*1-54, Jan '37
Double exposed fracture of lower jaw with luxation of one of temporomaxillary articulations; recovery of case after surgical therapy. VES LOSADA, C. AND BRAMBILLA, A. Semana med. *1:*1012-1019, April 8, '37
Recidivating temporomaxillary subluxation; surgical therapy of case. RODRIGUEZ VILLEGAS, R. AND TAULLARD, J. C. Bol. y trab. de la Soc. de cir. de Buenos Aires *21:*484-492, July 21, '37
Recidivating temporomaxillary luxation; author's experience with therapy. CAMES, O. AND MAROTTOLI, O. R. An. de cir. *3:*274-279, Sept '37
Treatment for subluxation of temporomandibular joint. SCHULTZ, L. W., J.A.M.A. *109:*1032-1035, Sept 25, '37
Curative treatment for subluxations of temporomandibular joint (injections of sodium psylliate). SCHULTZ, L. W., J. Am. Dent.

Temporomandibular Joint—Cont.
A. *24:*1947-1950, Dec '37
Bayonet incision for temporomandibular arthrotomy. MILCH, H. Am. J. Orthodontics *24:*287-288, March '38
Temporomandibular ankylosis. MARFORT, A. AND EMILIANI, C. M. Rev. oto-neuro-oftal. *13:*103-105, April '38
Stabilization of mandibular joint by injection of sclerosing solution (sodium psylliate). GINGRASS, R. P. Wisconsin M. J. *37:*383-384, May '38
Pathogenesis and surgical therapy of ankylosis of temporomandibular joint. MELA, B. Minerva med. *1:*553-556, May 26, '38
So-called congenital temporomandibular ankyloses. TAVERNIER, AND POUZET, F. Lyon chir. *35:*328-332, May-June '38
Recurrent temporomaxillary luxation; osteoplastic abutment (Elbim method); case. POLLOSSON, E. AND FREIDEL. Lyon chir. *35:*460-463, July-Aug '38
Ankylosis of temporomandibular joint. KAZANJIAN, V. H. Surg., Gynec. and Obst. *67:*333-348, Sept '38
New route of approach to temporomaxillary articulation; case. DUFOURMENTEL, L. Bull. et mem. Soc. d. chirurgiens de Paris *30:*420-424, Nov 4-18, '38
Right osseous temporomaxillary ankylosis; surgical therapy; case. BIANCHERI, A. Arch. ital. di chir. *50:*396-403, '38
Surgery and orthopedics of temporomaxillary joint. LINDEMANN, A. Rev. de stomatol. *41:*65-77, Feb '39
Temporomaxillary arthroplasty (Lindemann operation); results in 2 cases. MARFORT, A.; *et al.* Rev. Asoc. med. argent. *53:*88-90, Feb 15-28, '39
Ankylosis of temporomandibular joints; cure by Esmarch operation. MILLER, I. D. Australian and New Zealand J. Surg. *8:*406-407, April '39
Surgery of temporomandibular joint. WAKELEY, C. P. G. Surgery *5:*697-706, May '39
Orthopedic surgery of temporomaxillary joint; cases. GINESTET, G. *et al.* Rev. de stomatol. *41:*520-532, July '39
Mechanism of temporomaxillary fractures. BECK, H. Ztschr. f. Stomatol. *38:*201-221, March 22, '40
Temporomaxillary ankylosis. MARIN, G. M. Med. espan. *3:*406-428, May '40
Temporomandibular ankylosis and its surgical correction. BELLINGER, D. H., J. Am. Dent. A. *27:*1563-1568, Oct '40
Bilateral osseous ankylosis of temporomaxillary joints with marked facial deformity;

Temporomandibular Joint—Cont.
therapy of case. Ivy, R. H. An. de cir. *6:*383–387, Dec '40
Method of reduction of luxation of temporomaxillary joint. Ognev, B. V. Sovet. med. (no. 4) *4:*17–18, '40
Effect of abnormalities of occlusion upon temporomandibular joint and associated structures. Schuyler, C. H. Proc. Dent. Centen. Celeb., pp. 303–308, '40
Extra-articular bony ankylosis of temporomandibular joint. Berger, A. Bull. Hosp. Joint Dis. *2:*27–33, Jan '41
Traumatic internal derangement of temporomandibular joint. Kleinberg, S. Am. J. Orthodontics (Oral Surg. Sect.) *27:*328–332, June '41
Arthroplasty of jaws. Axhausen, G. Munchen. med. Wchnschr. *88:*776–779, July 11, '41
Pseudoankylosis of temporomandibular joint of cicatricial origin; surgical therapy of case. Loza Diaz, F. A. Cir. ortop. y traumatol., Habana *9:*129–136, July–Sept '41
Problem of anesthesia in surgery of temporomaxillary joint. Mondadori, E. C. F. An. paulist. de med. e cir. *42:*227–230, Sept '41
Approach to rational study and treatment of temporomandibular joint problems. Block, L. S. and Harris, E., J. Am. Dent. A. *29:*349–358, March '42
Procedure for treating habitual or recidivating luxation of temporomaxillary joint. Bertola, V. J. Prensa med. argent. *29:*536–542, April 1, '42
Treatment of temporomandibular dysfunction accompanied by severe pain syndrome. Kohn, S. I. Am. J. Orthodontics *28:*302–310, May '42
External splint for use in derangements of temporomandibular joint. Tregarthen, G. G. T. Bull. War Med. *3:*271–272, Jan '43 (abstract)
Gag for dysfunction of temporomandibular joint following mandibular injury. Hallum, J. W. Brit. M. J. *1:*569, May 8, '43
Temporomandibular joint. Willis, L. L., U. S. Nav. M. Bull. *41:*681–691, May '43
Temporomandibular articulation. Vaughan, H. C., J. Am. Dent. A. *30:*1501–1507, Oct 1, '43
Temporomandibular ankylosis; surgical therapy in cases. de Andrade, M. A. Med. cir. pharm., pp. 45–58, Jan '44
Bilateral ankylosis of temporomandibular joints with retrusion deformity; case. Dingman, R. O., J. Oral Surg. *2:*71–76, Jan '44

Temporomandibular Joint—Cont.
Temporomandibular ankylosis. Pettersson, G. Nord. med. (Hygiea) *23:*1521–1523, Aug 18, '44
Surgical treatment for dysfunction of temporomandibular joint. Percival, R. T. New York State J. Med. *45:*186–189, Jan 15, '45
Traumatic temporomandibular articulation syndrome. Vaughan, H. C., U. S. Nav. M. Bull. *44:*841–843, April '45
Traumatic lesions of head of mandible; treatment. Wakeley, C. P. G., M. Press *214:*166–168, Sept 12, '45
Retro-auricular route of access to temporomaxillary joint. Aubry, M. and Bourdon, E. Ann. d'oto-laryng. *12:*465–476, Oct–Dec '45
Arthroplasty of temporomandibular joint in children with interposition of tantalum foil; preliminary report. Eggers, G. W. N. J. Bone and Joint Surg. *26:*603–606, July '46
Sclerosing treatment (using sylnasol, fatty acid solution) for subluxation of temporomandibular joint. Rosenbaum, W. Am. J. Orthodontics *32:*551–571, Oct '46

Tendler, M. J.: Anatomy, pathology and treatment of infections of finger tip and nail. Memphis M. J. *15:*139–140. Sept '40

Tendon

Postoperative treatment of tendon injuries. Lewis, D. Boston M. and S. J. *194:*913–920, May 20, '26
Regeneration of tendons and treatment of ruptures of tendons, especially in region of synovial sheaths. Närvi, E. J. Acta chir. Scandinav. *60:*1–54, '26 abstr: J.A.M.A. *86:*1670, May 22, '26
Repair processes in wounds of tendons and in tendon grafts. Garlock, J. H. Ann. Surg. *85:*92–103, Jan '27
Pathologic anatomy and therapy of wounds of flexor tendons of hands. Iselin, M. Presse med. *40:*606–610, April 20, '32
Process of tendon repair; experimental study of tendon suture and tendon graft. Mason, M. L. and Shearon, C. G. Arch. Surg. *25:*615–692, Oct '32
Therapy of lesions of extensor tendons of fingers. Pedotti, F. Helvet. med. acta *3:*161–165, May '36
Athletic injuries to tendons. Deaver, G. G. S. Clin. North America *16:*753–761, June '36
Tendon regeneration after plastic operations;

Tendon – Cont.
experimental study. KRIVOROTOV, I. A. Novy khir. arkhiv *35:*357-367, '36
Surgery of muscle and tendon in relation to paralysis and injury. DUNN, N. Post-Grad. M. J. *13:*374-380, Oct '37
Skin graft use in reparation of tendinous lesions with loss of substance. MOSKOFF, G. J. de chir. *50:*607-620, Nov '37
Hematoma of flexor tendon sheaths following penetrating wounds (hand). DEVENISH, E. A. Lancet *1:*447-448, Feb 25, '39
Tendon transplantation in lower extremity. LEVINTHAL, D. H., S. Clin. North America *19:*79-100, Feb '39
Tenotomy; indications and technic. RUGH, J. T. Am. J. Surg. *44:*272-278, April '39
Tensor and digital tractor (Ferres). SCHWARTZ, M. Dia med. *12:*433-434, May 20, '40
Surgical principles in repair of divided nerves and tendons. KOCH, S. L. Quart. Bull., Northwestern Univ. M. School *14:*1-8, '40
Significance of early resumption of function following plastic repair of tendons according to Bunnell. NIKOLAEV, G. F. Novy khir. arkhiv. *45:*327-331, '40
Lesions of tendons and their prognosis with respect to hand function. FLEISCHER-HANSEN, C. C. Nord. med. (Hospitalstid.) *9:*88-98, Jan 11, '41
Osteochondromata of tendon sheaths; case arising from flexor sheath of index finger. SHEPHERD, J. A. Brit. J. Surg. *30:*179-180, Oct '42
Post-traumatic hematoma of tendon sheaths. PIULACHS, P. AND ARANDES, R. Rev. clin. espan. *8:*435-436, March 30, '43
Spontaneous cicatrization of section of tendon of extensor pollicis longus (biologic therapy); cases. TAULLARD, J. C. Bol. y trab., Soc. argent. de cirujanos *4:*772-776, '43 also: Rev. Asoc. med. argent. *57:*1018-1019, Nov 30, '43
Functional significance of insertions of extensor communis digitorum in man. KAPLAN, E. B. Anat. Rec. *92:*293-303, July '45
Surgical anatomy of flexor tendons of wrist. KAPLAN, E. B., J. Bone and Joint Surg. *27:*368-372, July '45
Musculotendinous surgery in treatment of sequels of poliomyelitis. NOE, M. Rev. chilena de pediat. *17:*20-22, Jan '46

Tendon, Dislocation of (See also Fingers, Boutonniere Deformity of)

Luxation of tendons of extensor digitorum. LEVY, W. Zentralbl. f. Chir. *48:*482, April 9, '21
Luxation of tendons of extensores digitorum. HABERERN, J. P. Zentralbl. f. Chir. *48:*1080, July 30, '21
Traumatic luxation of some extensor tendons of hand. SILFVERSKIÖLD, N. Acta chir. Scandinav. *64:*305-310, '28
Traumatic dislocation of extensor tendon of second finger. RAZEMON, P. Ann. d'anat. path. *7:*238-241, Feb '30
Traumatic dislocation of extensor tendons of fingers; case. RAZEMON, P. Echo m. du nord *34:*213-216, May 3, '30
Buttonhole rupture of extensor tendon of finger at point of insertion into terminal phalanx. KALLIUS, H. U. Zentralbl. f. Chir. *57:*2432-2435, Sept 27, '30
Subcutaneous ruptures of extensor tendons of fingers in buttonhole dislocation of first interphalangeal joint. EILERS. Deutsche Ztschr. f. Chir. *223:*317-327, '30
Button-hole rupture of extensor tendon of finger. MILCH, H. Am. J. Surg. *13:*244-245, Aug '31
"Buttonholed" extensor expansion of finger. BINGHAM, D. L. C. AND JACK, E. A. Brit. M. J. *2:*701-702, Oct 9, '37
Rupture and luxation of dorsal (extensor) tendons of fingers at first interphalangeal articulation; physiologic and clinical study. MONTANT, R. AND BAUMANN, A. Rev. d'orthop. *25:*5-22, Jan '38
Habitual dislocation of digital extensor tendons. FITZGERALD, R. R. Ann. Surg. *110:*81-83, July '39
Lateral luxation of portion of extensor tendon of finger. DE ROUGEMONT, J. Presse med. *47:*1197, Aug 2, '39
Luxation of extensor tendons. STRAUS, F. H. Ann. Surg. *111:*135-140, Jan '40
Irreducible buttonhole dislocations of fingers. SELIG, S. AND SCHEIN, A., J. Bone and Joint Surg. *22:*436-441, April '40
Buttonhole rupture-luxation of extensor tendon of fingers. CASANUEVA DEL C., M. AND CROQUEVIELLE, G. A. Rev. med. de Chile *70:*57-63, Jan '42
Traumatic luxation of extensor tendon of middle finger. MOUCHET, A. Presse med. *50:*455, July 11, '42

Tendon Infections (See also Fingers, Infections; Hands, Infections)

Incision in natural folds of hand; contribution to treatment of cellulitis of sheaths of tendons and calluses. SCHIESSL, M. Munchen.

Tendon Infections – Cont.
med. Wchnschr. *72:*1728–1730, Oct 9, '25 abstr: J.A.M.A. *85:*1681, Nov 21, '25
Treatment of phlegmonous tendovaginitis. HORWITZ, A. Munchen. med. Wchnschr. *73:*1987–1989, Nov 19, '26
Tendovaginitis and bursitis. ZOLLINGER, F. Arch. f. Orthop. *24:*456–467, Jan 26, '27
Phlegmon of tendon sheaths; operation. MOURE, P. Bull. et mem. Soc. nat. de chir. *54:*572–576, April 28, '28
Infections of tendon sheaths. CURTIS, J. F. Univ. Toronto M. J. *7:*16–22, Nov '29
Traumatic tendovaginitis crepitans; case. HAUSER, G. Deutsche Ztschr. f. d. ges. gerichtl. Med. *15:*242–245, May 18, '30
Anatomic grounds for clinical treatment of tendovaginitis of palm. KHAITZISS, G. M. Vestnik khir. (nos. 56–57) *19:*356–362, '30
Operative treatment in inflammation of digital tendon sheaths. CADENAT, F. M. Bull. et mem. Soc. nat. de chir. *57:*522, April 25, '31
Operative technic in inflammation of digital tendon sheaths. ISELIN, M. Bull. et mem. Soc. nat. de chir. *57:*456–465, April 4, '31
Tenosynovitis. CONN, H. R. Ohio State M. J. *27:*713–716, Sept '31
Surgical treatment of tendovaginitis crepitans and abscesses of sheaths. HAYWARD. Med. Klin. *27:*1321–1322, Sept 4, '31
Treatment of gonorrhea of tendon sheaths. HAYWARD. Med. Klin. *27:*1683–1684, Nov 13, '31
Acute suppurative synovitis of tendon sheath following wound of right index finger; excellent function after surgical therapy; case. TIXIER, L.; *et al.* Lyon chir. *28:*714–717, Nov–Dec '31
Digital tendovaginitis. ISELIN, M. Schweiz. med. Wchnschr. *62:*1159–1163, Dec 10, '32
Suppurative tenosynovitis; treatment and ultimate outcome. DEICKE, H. Beitr. z. klin. Chir. *158:*461–480, '33
Lateral incisions in phlegmons of tendon sheaths of hand. ORY, M. Ann. Soc. med.-chir. de Liege, no. 1, pp. 30–35, '33 abstr: Liege med. *27:*384–387, March 18, '34
Tenosynovitis; cases. COIMBRA, A. Arq. de cir. e ortop. *2:*159–168, Dec '34
Acute suppurative gonoccoccic tenosynovitis. BIRNBAUM, W. AND CALLANDER, C. L. J.A.M.A. *105:*1025–1028, Sept 28, '35
Acute suppurative tenosynovitis of flexor tendon sheaths; review of 125 cases. GRINNELL, R. S. Ann. Surg. *105:*97–119, Jan '37
Phlegmon of tendon sheaths. SCHÖRCHER, F. Med. Klin. *34:*1647–1649, Dec 16, '38
Tendon sheath infections. COLONNA, P. C. Am. J. Surg. *50:*509–511, Dec '40
Etiology and therapy of paronychia of tendon sheath. WELCKER, E. R. Zentralbl. f. Chir. *68:*1564–1568, Aug 9, '41
Infection of tendons and tendon sheaths. HANDFIELD-JONES, R. M. M. Press *211:*53–57, Jan 26, '44

Tendon Injuries (See also: Hands, Tendon Injuries)
Technic of suture of divided tendons. LINNARTZ, M. Zentralbl. f. Chir. *48:*338, March 12, '21
Suture of tendon in hand or finger. KAUFMANN, C. Schweiz. med. Wchnschr. *51:*601, June 30, '21 abstr: J.A.M.A. *77:*653, Aug 20, '21
Fate of sutured tendons. SALOMON, A. Zentralbl. f. Chir. *49:*74–76, Jan 21, '22 abstr: J.A.M.A. *78:*1769, June 3, '22
Repair of tendons in fingers. BUNNELL, S. Surg., Gynec. and Obst. *35:*88–97, July '22 (illus.)
Functional prognosis of suture of tendons. LANG, K. Med. Klinik *19:*530–533, April 22, '23 (illus.)
Tendon suture which permits immediate motion. LAHEY, F. H. Boston M. and S. J. *188:*851–852, May 31, '23 (illus.)
Suture of tendons. JUST, E. Arch. f. klin. Chir. *124:*165–177, '23 (illus.) abstr: J.A.M.A. *81:*1647, Nov 10, '23
Technic of primary suture of tendons. PORGES, H. Wien. klin. Wchnschr. *37:*285–286, March 20, '24 abstr: J.A.M.A. *82:*1486, May 3, '24
Injury, regeneration and suture of tendons. HAUCK, G. Arch. f. klin. Chir. *128:*568–585, '24
To improve outcome of suture of tendon in hand. RUEF, H. Arch. f. klin. Chir. *130:*757–762, '24 abstr: J.A.M.A. *83:*1379, Oct 25, '24
Laceration of tendons of thumb. MOORHEAD, J. J., S. Clin. N. America *5:*170–173, Feb '25
Repair of wounds of flexor tendons of hand. GARLOCK, J. H. Ann. Surg. *83:*111–122, Jan '26
Tendon suture after injuries. BAUMANN, E. Zentralbl. f. Chir. *53:*3037–3038, Nov 27, '26
Suture of tendons; technic and outcome in 101 cases. MÜLLER, O. Beitr. z. klin. Chir. *128:*754–765, '23
Suture of superficial sectioned tendon. DUPUY DE FRENELLE. Hopital *15:*198–200, March (B) '27

Tendon Injuries – Cont.
Loop operation for paralysis of adductors of thumb. MAYER, L. Am. J. Surg. *2:*456–458, May '27
Treatment of wounds of tendons of hand and fingers. ISELIN, M. AND TAILHEFER, A. Gaz. d. hop. *100:*961–964, July 20, '27
Tendon sutures. MOSER, E. Zentralbl. f. Chir. *54:*1606, June 25, '27
Repair of cut flexor tendons of fingers. ISELIN, M., J. de chir. *30:*531–540, Nov '27
Primary repair of lacerated tendons and nerves. EISBERG, H. B. AND SONNENSCHEIN, H. D. Am. J. Surg. *3:*582–587, Dec '27
Tendon suture; location of proximal end of tendon. BONIKOWSKY, H. Arch. f. klin. Chir. *145:*598, '27
Repair of nerves and tendons of hand and grafting. BUNNELL, S., J. Bone and Joint Surg. *10:*1–26, Jan '28 abstr: Arch. francobelges de chir. *30:*93–97, Feb '27
Primitive suture of 2 flexor tendons of fourth finger in palmar region; suture of deep flexor of index in same region; case. TAILHEFER, A. Bull. et mem. Soc. nat. de chir. *54:*827–829, June 16, '28
Tenoplasty for ulnar paralysis. SILFVERSKIÖLD, N. Acta chir. Scandinav. *64:*300–302, '28
Repairs of severed tendons without suture. ZANUSO, F. Osp. maggiore *17:*44, Feb 28, '29
Treatment of section of tendons of fingers. CHATON, M. Rev. gen. de clin. et de therap. *43:*289–296, May 4, '29
Traumatic wounds of tendons. BONA, T. Cluj. med. *10:*435–439, Sept 1, '29
New method of tendon suture; preliminary report. TSCHALENKO, G. Zentralbl. f. Chir. *56:*2388–2389, Sept 21, '29
Evolution and treatment in wounds of tendons of hands and fingers. CAZIN, M. Paris chir. *21:*179–190, Sept–Oct '29
Injuries of tendons of hand; surgical repair. BLOCH, J. C. AND BONNET, P., J. de chir. *34:*456–474, Oct '29
Evolution and treatment of wounds of tendons of hand. BLOCH, J. J. AND BONNET, P. Gaz. d. hop. *102:*1581, Nov 6, '29
Wound of flexor tendon of thumb; perfect functional cure. BONNET, P. AND MICHON, L. Lyon chir. *26:*849–852, Nov–Dec '29
Suture of tendon of flexor digitorum profundus; case. RIVARD, J. H. Union med. du Canada *59:*28–30, Jan '30
Treatment of cuts of flexor tendons of fingers by tendinous graft. ALBERT, F. Liege med. *23:*1069–1077, Aug 10, '30 also: Ann. Soc.

Tendon Injuries – Cont.
med.-chir. de Liege *63:*18–21, Sept '30
Results of suture of flexor tendon of thumb after healing of wound; case. BONNET, P. AND DELAYE. Lyon chir. *28:*189–190, March–April '31
Section of flexor tendons and ulnar nerve in injury to wrist; good results from secondary tendon and nerve sutures. POUZET, F. Lyon chir. *28:*203–206, March–April '31
Functional results of section of extensor tendons of third and fourth fingers; 2 cases. FOGLIANI, U. Policlinico (sez. prat.) *38:*1431–1433, Sept 28, '31
Treatment of open tendon injuries. SALOMON, A. Ztschr. f. arztl. Fortbild. *28:*559–562, Sept 1, '31
Invalidism after cutting of tendons of hand. KIAER, S. Acta orthop. Scandinav. *2:*202–220, '31
Interpretation of suture of tendons. BANET, V. An. de cir. *4:*352–354, May '32
Suture of flexor tendon in therapy of hand injury; case. LASSERRE, C., J. de med. de Bordeaux *109:*357–358, May 10, '32
Section of flexor tendons of middle finger of left hand through palmar wound; primary suture and cure. ANDREASEN, A., J. Bone and Joint Surg. *14:*700–701, July '32
Successful suture of extensor tendons of hand sectioned by wounds; case. JARAMILLO ARANGO, J. Repert. de med. y cir. *23:*289–320, July '32
Recovery after late suture of flexor tendon of index finger. CORNET, J. Scalpel *85:*1296–1297, Oct 22, '32
Section of flexor tendons of index and middle fingers in palm of hand. DE LEEUW, E. Scalpel *85:*1269–1271, Oct 15, '32
Division of nerves and tendons of hand, with discussion of surgical treatment and its results. KOCH, S. L. AND MASON, M. L. Surg., Gynec. and Obst. *56:*1–39, Jan '33
Injuries of nerves and tendons of hand (surgical therapy). KOCH, S. L., J. Oklahoma M. A. *26:*323–327, Sept '33
Tendons in hand injuries. SALSBURY, C. R. Am. J. Surg. *21:*354–357, Sept '33
Primary suture of accidentally sectioned flexor tendons of fingers. DE LA MARNIERRE. Bull. et mem. Soc. nat. de chir. *59:*1314–1317, Nov 18, '33
Successful suture of tendon. KLAPP, R. Sovet. khir. (nos. 1–3) *5:*69–71, '33
Suture of tendon with central filament. KLAPP, R. Arch. f. klin. Chir. *177:*690–691, '33
Injuries to nerves and tendons of hand. KOCH, S. L. Pennsylvania M. J. *37:*555–

Tendon Injuries – Cont.
557, April '34
Injuries of nerves and tendons of hand. KOCH, S. L. Wisconsin M. J. *33:*655–661, Sept '34
Repair of severed tendons. ROCKEY, E. W., S. Clin. North America *14:*1497–1499, Dec '34
Instruments for restoration of severed flexor tendons of fingers according to Bunnell method. Rozov, V. I. Sovet. khir. (nos. 3–4) *6:*458–461, '34
Therapy of section of tendons of hand in industrial accidents; 50 cases. ROGERS, S. P. AND ESPINOSA ROBLEDO, M. Cir. ortop. y traumatol. *3:*177–181, July–Sept '35
Technic for repair of flexor tendons of fingers. INTROINI, L. A. Rev. med. del Rosario *25:*1191–1200, Nov '35
Immediate and delayed tendon repair. MASON, M. L. Surg., Gynec. and Obst. *62:*449–457, Feb. (no. 2A) '36
Late sequels of finger tendon sutures. VON ZWEIGBERGK, J. O. Chirurg *8:*243–247, April 1, '36
Section of flexor tendons of hand; suture with recovery after physiopathic phenomena; case. FIGARELLA, J. Marseille-med. *1:*725–727, May 25, '36
Instrument for grasping ends of ruptured tendon during suture. HIRSCHBERG, O. Schweiz. med. Wchnschr. *66:*514–515, May 23, '36
Primary tenorrhaphy in therapy of section of tendons during cane cutting. OLIVERAS GUERRA, A. Bol. Asoc. med. de Puerto Rico *28:*114–118, June '36
Nerve and tendon suture: illustrative case. WHELAN, H. M., J. Roy. Nav. M. Serv. *22:*234–237, July '36
Industrial accidents; management of injuries of tendons and nerve of hand. GARLOCK, J. H. New York State J. Med. *36:*1740–1748, Nov 15, '36
Two new methods of tendon suture. DYKHNO, A. M. Novy khir. arkhiv. *37:*403–416, '36
Suture of tendons of hand. DZHANELIDZE, Y. Y. Novy khir. arkhiv. *36:*497–507, '36
Injury of hand tendons. STAHEL, W. Schweiz. med. Wchnschr. *67:*51–54, Jan 16, '37
Comparative value of different sutures in tendon surgery, with presentation of 2 new technics. DYCHNO, A. Lyon chir. *34:*290–303, May–June '37
Repair of flexor tendons of fingers. THATCHER, H. V. Northwest Med. *36:*259–263, Aug '37
Repair of laceration of flexor pollicis longus tendon (by faucet handle). MURPHY, F. G. J. Bone and Joint Surg. *19:*1121–1123, Oct '37
New suture for tendon and fascia repair. GRATZ, C. M. Surg., Gynec. and Obst. *65:*700–701, Nov '37
Treatment of acute tendon injuries. KENDRICK, J. I., S. Clin. North America *17:*1469–1474, Oct '37
Injuries of extensor tendons of fingers and their therapy. Rozov, V. I. Vestnik khir. *54:*95–105, '37
End results of early and delayed suture of tendon wounds. FORRESTER, C. R. G. Am. J. Surg. *39:*552–556, March '38
Management of recent wound of tendons of fingers. ISELIN, M. Presse med. *46:*499–500, March 30, '38
Principles of management of tendon injuries (hand). MASON, M. L. Physiotherapy Rev. *18:*119–123, May–June '38
Late results of surgical therapy in injuries to tendons of hand. DERRA, E. AND RUBERG, G. Monatschr. f. Unfallh. *45:*305–315, June '38
Cut tendon. CAULFIELD, P. A., M. Ann. District of Columbia *7:*207–211, July '38
Bunnell operation to repair loss of grasping power of thumb (paralysis of opponens pollicis) after infantile paralysis; case (transplantation of tendon). INCLAN, A. AND RODRIGUEZ, R. Cir. ortop. y traumatol., Habana *6:*140–145, July–Sept '38
Elective traumatism of extensor digitorum and flexor digitorum profundus in injury to forearm; reflex inhibition of extension; infiltration of stellate ganglion; Volkmann contracture; tendinous transmutation. FROMENT, J. AND MALLET-GUY, P. Lyon chir. *35:*623–629, Sept–Oct '38
Repair of severed tendons in hand. MAYER, L. Am. J. Surg. *42:*714–722, Dec '38
Late results of sutures of tendons of arm and hand. HECK, F. Arch. f. orthop. u. Unfall-Chir. *39:*21–28, '38
Restoration of function of injured tendons of upper extremities. NIKOLAEV, G. F. Ortop. i travmatol. (no. 2) *12:*3–17, '38
Primary and secondary suture of flexor tendons of wrist and fingers. Rozov, V. I. Novy khir. arkhiv *41:*490–504, '38
Surgical therapy of tendon wounds; experimental study. BASSI, P. Ann. ital. di chir. *18:*33–48, Jan–Feb '39
Unusual tendon injuries to fingers; 3 cases. LEVIN, J. J. South African M. J. *13:*29–33, Jan 14, '39
Treatment and results of 870 severed tendons

Tendon Injuries – Cont.
and 57 severed nerves of hand and forearm (in 362 patients). O'SHEA, M. C. Am. J. Surg. *43:*346–366, Feb '39
Application of general principles in tendon suture. HUBER, H. S., S. Clin North America *19:*499–518, April '39
Personal restorative technic of section of flexor tendons of fingers. MONTANT, R. J. de chir. *53:*768–774, June '39
Principles of tendon suture. COUCH, J. H. Canad. M.A.J. *41:*27–30, July '39
Extensive primary nerve and tendon suture at wrist; 2 cases. HOWARD, R. N., M. J. Australia *2:*322–323, Aug 26, '39
Treatment of hand injuries (with special reference to tendons). TEECE, L., M. J. Australia *2:*532–534, Oct 7, '39
Repair of tendons of hand. CLEVELAND, H. E. Journal-Lancet *59:*524–525, Dec '39
Injuries of tendons in glass workers and their treatment. ATANOV, V. A. Khirurgiya, no. 1, pp. 46–53, '39
Plastic surgery of flexor tendon of hand, with special reference to paralysis of opponens pollicis. PACHER, W. Arch. f. orthop. u. Unfall-Chir. *40:*93–101, '39
Primary repair of severed tendons; use of stainless steel wire. BUNNELL, S. Am. J. Surg. *47:*502–516, Feb '40
Primary and secondary suture of tendons; discussion of significance of technic. MASON, M. L. Surg., Gynec. and Obst. *70:*392–402, Feb (no. 2A) '40
Immediate repair of flexor tendons. SPEIRS, R. E., J. Kansas M. Soc. *41:*370–373, Sept '40
Injuries of flexor tendons of hand. BETTS, L. O., M. J. Australia *2:*457–460, Nov 9, '40
Luxated and severed tendons. ROUNTREE, C. R. Am. J. Surg. *50:*516–518, Dec '40
Significance of function in repair of tendons. MASON, M. L. Arch. Phys. Therapy *22:*28–34, Jan '41
Suturing of flexor tendons (transfixation) in hand. BOVE, C., M. Rec. *153:*94, Feb 5, '41
Injuries to nerves and tendons of hand. MASON, M. L., J.A.M.A. *116:*1375–1379, March 29, '41
Treatment of tendons in compound injuries to hand. BUNNELL, S., J. Bone and Joint Surg. *23:*240–250, April '41
Primary repair of tendons; end-results in 207 cases. DEBENHAM, M. California and West. Med. *54:*273–276, May '41
Hand tendon injuries; study of 116 cases. HOOKER, D. H. AND LAM, C. R. Am. J. Surg. *54:*412–416, Nov '41

Tendon Injuries – Cont.
Plastic repair of flexor tendons of fingers. DUBROV, Y. G. Ortop. i travmatol. (no. 1) *15:*66–74, '41
Late results of primary suture of tendons. KHORANOV, V. M. Novy khir. arkhiv. *48:*195–199, '41
Use of kangaroo tendon for muscle and tendon suture. TRETHEWIE, E. R. AND WILLIAMS, E. Australian and New Zealand J. Surg. *11:*207–208, Jan '42
Nerve and tendon injuries of hand. MASON, M. L. Indust. Med. *11:*61–66, Feb '42
Tendon suturing. KOCH, S. L. Indust. Med. *11:*327–328, July '42
Tendon and nerve injuries. KOCH, S. L. New York State J. Med. *42:*1819–1823, Oct 1, '42
New method of tendon repair. WILLIAMS, E. R. P., J. Roy. Nav. M. Serv. *28:*384–386, Oct '42
Repair of severed tendons of hand and wrist; statistical analysis of 300 cases. MILLER, H. Surg., Gynec. and Obst. *75:*693–698, Dec '42
Nerve and tendon injuries. KOCH, S. L. Bull. Am. Coll. Surgeons *28:*125–126, June '43
Results of repair of flexor tendons of wrist, hand and fingers. IVANISSEVICH, O. AND RIVAS, C. I. Bol. y trab., Acad. argent. de cir. *27:*576–583, July 28, '43
Primary and secondary repair of flexor tendons. BUNNELL, S. Tr. Am. Soc. Plastic and Reconstructive Surg. *12:*65–67, '43
Suturing tendons. BUNNELL, S. Am. Acad. Orthop. Surgeons, Lect., pp. 1–5, '43
Early and late repair of extensor tendons. CUTLER, C. W. JR. Tr. Am. Soc. Plastic and Reconstructive Surg. *12:*69–77, '43
Divison of flexor tendons within digital sheath. KOCH, S. L. Surg., Gynec. and Obst. *78:*9–22, Jan '44
Repair of severed tendons; new tendon suture. REES, C. E. Arizona Med. *1:*12–15, Jan–Feb '44
Myotomy in repair of divided flexor tendons. BLUM, L., U. S. Nav. M. Bull. *42:*1317–1322, June '44
Successful sutre of finger flexor tendon. JONES, R. M. Lancet *2:*111, July 22, '44
Plastic repair of section of flexor tendons of hand and of median nerve; case. MARINO, H. Prensa med. argent. *31:*1305–1308, July 12, '44
Tendon repair. COLE, T. C., U. S. Nav. M. Bull. *43:*241–244, Aug '44
Treatment of wounds of tendons. FROMM, G. A. Dia med. *16:*1182–1187, Oct 2, '44
Wounds of hand tendons; analysis of 168

Tendon Injuries – Cont.
cases. CASANUEVA DEL C., M. AND FLUHMANN D., G. Rev. med. de Chile *72:*1044–1048, Dec '44
Cut tendons of fingers, with special reference to flexor tendon cut within its digital sheath. KINMONTH, J. B. St. Thomas's Hosp. Gaz. *42:*154–158, Dec '44
Occupational injury of hand (palmar tendon injury of agricultural workers). CHAN, L. F. Caribbean M. J. (no. 5) *6:*341–342, '44
Cutting wound of wrist with section of tendon and radial artery; functional restitution. SEARA, P. Prensa med. argent. *32:*674–675, April 13, '45
Metal anastomosis tubes in suture of tendons. MCKEE, G. K. Lancet *1:*659–660, May 26, '45
Radial paralysis; tenoplasty of extensors. POINOT, J. Bordeaux chir. *3-4:*148–149, July–Oct '45
Wounds and injuries of tendons. IOAN-JONES, D. Practitioner *156:*262–266, April '46
Fixation of ligaments by Bunnell's pull-out wire suture. KEY, J. A. Ann. Surg. *123:*656–663, April '46
Treatment of injuries, with particular reference to nerve and tendon repair in hand. MASON, M. L. Indust. Med. *15:*323–325, May '46
Trauma to hand; with particular reference to indications for primary and secondary nerve and tendon repair. MASON, M. L., J. Oklahoma M. A. *39:*246–251, June '46
Surgery of divided digital tendons. STONHAM, F. V. Indian M. Gaz. *81:*225–227, June–July '46
Treatment of injuries of tendons of hand. HERTZBERG, J. Nord med. *31:*1893–1897, Aug 23, '46
Injuries of nerves and tendons of hand. KOCH, S. L. Cincinnati J. Med. *27:*515–521, Aug '46
Fixation of tendons, ligaments and bone by Bunnell's pull-out wire suture. KEY, J. A. Tr. South. S. A. (1945) *57:*187–194, '46

Tendon, Reconstructive Surgery (See also Hands, Reconstructive Surgery of)
Reconstruction of hand, a new technic in tenoplasty. TAYLOR, R. T. Surg., Gynec. and Obst. *32:*237, March '21
Reconstruction of muscles and tendons. CHARBONNEL. J. de med. de Bordeaux *92:*437, Aug 10, '21 abstr: J.A.M.A. *77:*1210, Oct 8, '21
Tendon reconstruction. BRADBURN, M., S. Clin. N. America *2:*1363–1365, Oct '22 (illus.)

Tendon, Reconstructive Surgery – Cont.
Outcome of plastic operations on tendons. SCHWARZ, E. Deutsche Ztschr. f. Chir. *173:*301–385, '22 (illus.) abstr: J.A.M.A. *79:*1726, Nov 11, '22
Tendon transplants in forearm. KENNEDY, R. An. de Fac. de med., Montevideo *8:*558, May–June '23
Complete disability of hand by relaxed articulation of first metacarpus and trapezium, and slipping of tendon and extensor brevis pollicis; postoperative result. GODDU, L. A. O. Boston M. and S. J. *192:*666–667, April 2, '25
Surgery of flexor tendons of hand. GARLOCK, J. H. Am. J. Surg. *40:*68–69, March '26
Treatment of old extensive destruction of tendons (hand). CHIANELLO, C. Cultura med. mod. *6:*104–106, March 1, '27
Technic of tendon surgery. LANGE, F. Tungchi, Med. Monatschr. *2:*462–469, Aug '27
Experimental researches on grafting cartilage on to tendons. BORGHI, M. Arch. per. le sc. med. *50:*437–465, '27
Importance of tendinous union in lesion of extensor tendons of fingers. PRATI, M. Arch. ital. di chir. *17:*597–610, '27
Silk tendons and joint ligaments; results of plastic operations. LANGE, F. Munchen. med. Wchnschr. *75:*39–42, Jan 6, '28
Prevention of adhesions to tendons in hand and wrist, with report of 2 cases. MARSHALL, G. D., J. Bone and Joint Surg. *10:*816–818, Oct '28
Use of rubber in plastic operations on tendons and nerves, in repairing defects in abdominal wall, in hernia and in fractures with loss of substance. DELBET, P. Rev. de chir. *66:*181–213, '28
Section of 2 extensor tendons of fingers; delayed suture; case. BLANC, H. Bull. et mem. Soc. de chir. de Paris *21:*42, Jan 4, '29
Plastic operations on tendon flexors of fingers; technic. BLOCH, J. C. AND TAILHEFER, A. Gaz. d. hop. *102:*5, Jan 2, '29
Modification of incision for reparation of flexor tendons on fingers. ISELIN, M. Presse med. *37:*124–126, Jan 26, '29
Subcutaneous transplantation for ruptured tendons; cases. KRAFT, R. Arch. f. Orthop. *28:*532–540, July 23, '30
Method in exposure of flexor tendons of hand. KHAITZISS, G. M. Vestnik khir. (no. 64) *22:*115–120, '30
Reparative surgery of flexor tendons of fingers. ISELIN, M. Bull. et mem. Soc. nat. de chir. *57:*1227–1231, Oct 31, '31
Use of silk in plastic construction of tendons

Tendon, Reconstructive Surgery – Cont.
of fingers. COENEN, H. Deutsche Ztschr. f. Chir. *234:*699–709, '31
Plastic replacement of flexor tendons of finger. LEXER, E. Deutsche Ztschr. f. Chir. *234:*688–698, '31
Nerve suture and muscle repair; primary suture of ulnar nerve and secondary reconstruction of extensor tendons of forearm. HORGAN, E. Ann. Surg. *95:*93–100, Jan '32
Plastic surgery of tendons and nerves of hand. CHIARIELLO, A. G. Policlinico (sez. prat.) *39:*520–525, April 4, '32
Treatment of injuries of tendons within synovial sheaths in palm of hand and flexor tendons of finger by insertion of foreign substance. HESSE, F. Arch. f. klin. Chir. *170:*772–789, '32
Experiments with skin grafts in plastic surgery of tendons. BONACCORSI, A. Clin. chir. *36:*839–853, July–Aug '33
Restoration of digital portion of flexor tendon and sheath. CLEVELAND, M., J. Bone and Joint Surg. *15:*762–765, July '33
Technic and results of tendon translocations. FABER, A. Verhandl. d. deutsch. orthop. Gesellsch., Kong. 27, pp. 331–333, '33
Section of flexor tendons of finger treated by reinsertion; case. LYONNET, J. H. AND MOREDA, J. J. Rev. Asoc. med. argent. *48:*260–264, March–April '34
Surgery of muscles and tendons for contracture. GILL, A. B., S. Clin. North America *15:*203–212, Feb '35
Plastic surgery of flexor tendons of hand. DUBROV, Y. G. Ortop. i travatol. (no. 5) *9:*109–120, '35
Physiological method of repair of damaged finger tendons; preliminary report on reconstruction of destroyed tendon sheath. MAYER, L. AND RANSOHOFF, N. S. Am. J. Surg. *31:*56–58, Jan '36
Late results of secondary plastic operations on tendons and nerves of hand. KALALOVA-DI LOTTIOVA, V. Bratisl. lekar. listy *16:*162–174, April '36
Sutures or reconstruction (using fascia lata) of sectioned hand tendons; 3 cases. MASMONTEIL, F. Bull. et mem. Soc. d. chirurgiens de Paris *28:*379–384, June 5, '36
Reconstruction of digital tendon sheath; contribution to physiological method of repair of damaged finger tendons. MAYER, L. AND RANSOHOFF, N., J. Bone and Joint Surg. *18:*607–616, July '36
Tendinoplasty of flexor tendons of hand; use of tunica vaginalis in reconstructing tendon sheaths. WILMOTH, C. L., J. Bone and Joint Surg. *19:*152–156, Jan '37

Tendon, Reconstructive Surgery – Cont.
Severed tendons and nerves of hand and forearm. O'SHEA. M. C. Ann. Surg. *105:*228–242, Feb '37
"Tendon stretcher" for pulling forward muscle for tenotomy. (Comment on Streiff's article). GUTZEIT, R. Klin. Monatsbl. f. Augenh. *98:*671, May '37
Experimental study upon prevention of adhesions about repaired nerves and tendons (especially by use of allantoic and amniotic membranes). DAVIS, L. AND ARIES, L. J. Surgery *2:*877–888, Dec '37
Tendoplasty according to Bunnell method. KRINITSKIY, Y. M. Ortop. i travmatol. (no. 5) *11:*149–151, '37
Experimental data on plastic surgery of tendons according to Bunnell. NIKOLAEV, G. F. Ortop. i travmatol. (no. 6) *11:*3–11, '37
Joining dorsal aponeurosis and tendons in therapy of injuries to extensor tendons of fingers; cases. JOHNER, T. Schweiz. med. Wchnschr. *68:*111–113, Jan 29, '38
Restoration of function of injured tendons of upper extremities. NIKOLAEV, G. F. Ortop. i travmatol. (no. 2) *12:*3–17, '38
Use of stainless steel rods to canalize flexor tendon sheaths. THATCHER, H. V. South. M. J. *32:*13–18, Jan '39
Use of cellophane as permanent tendon sheath. WHEELDON, T. F., J. Bone and Joint Surg. *21:*393–396, April '39
Pathology and operative correction of finger deformities due to contractures of extensor digitorum tendon. KAPLAN, E. B. Surgery *6:*451, Sept '39
Reconstruction of tendons of fingers. NIKIFOROVA, E. K. Vestnik khir. *58:*255–260, Sept '39
Celloidin tube reconstruction of extensor digitorum communis sheath. MAYER, L. Bull. Hosp. Joint Dis. *1:*39–45, July '40
New instrument for grasping tendons. DUSCHL, L. Chirurg *12:*756, Dec 15, '40
Use of various materials for isolation of suture to prevent adhesion in tendon surgery; experimental study. NIKOLAEV, G. F. Ortop. i travmatol. (no. 4) *14:*18–26, '40
Preservation of tendon function in hand by use of skin flaps. KITLOWSKI, E. A. Am. J. Surg. *51:*653–661, March '41
Use of myotomy in repair of divided flexor tendons. BLUM, L. Ann. Surg. *116:*461–469, Sept '42
Use of silk in musculotendinous and ligamentary reparative surgery. BOPPE. Mem. Acad. de chir. *68:*452–456, Dec 9–16, '42
Post-traumatic neuralgia as serious complication of section of tendons of hand in culti-

Tendon, Reconstructive Surgery – Cont.
vators of sugar cane. OLIVERAS GUERRA, A. Bol. Asoc. med. de Puerto Rico *35:*47-51, Feb '43
Substitute tenoplasties according to Perthes in therapy of radial paralysis. STUMPFEGGER, L. Chirurg. *15:*430, July 15, '43
Tendon repair by transfixion. GEBHARD, U. E. Indust. Med. *13:*38-39, Jan '44
Use of nylon sheath in secondary repair of torn finger flexor tendons. BURMAN, M. S. Bull. Hosp. Joint Dis. *5:*122-133, Oct '44
Tendon surgery of hand. MOBERG, E. Nord. med. (Hygiea) *25:*535-539, March 23, '45
Use of skin flaps in repair of scarred defects over bone and tendons. PADGETT, E. C. AND GASKINS, J. H. Surgery *18:*287-298, Sept '45
Generalities and fundamentals of tendon surgery. MAYER, L. Medicina, Mexico *25:*468-474, Nov 10, '45
Use of skin flaps in repair of scarred or ulcerative defects over bone and tendons. PADGETT, E. C. AND GASKINS, J. H. Tr. West. S. A. (1944) *52:*195-211, '45
Late repair of tendons of hand. WEBSTER, G. V. Am. J. Surg. *72:*171-178, Aug '46
Use of tantalum in tendon reconstruction of hand. PEARLMAN, R. C., U. S. Nav. M. Bull. *46:*1647-1650, Nov '46

Tendon, Rupture of (See also Hands, Tendon Ruptures)
Rupture of extensor longus pollicis tendon. DYKES, S. N. Brit. M. J. *1:*387-388, March 11, '22
Rupture of extensor longus pollicis tendon. GARDNER, F. G. Brit. M. J. *1:*476, March 25, '22
Rupture of tendon of extensor longus pollicis following a Colles' fracture. ASHHURST, A. P. C. Ann. Surg. *78:*398-400, Sept '23
Operation for rupture of thumb tendon and fracture of radius. HAUCK, G. Arch. f. Klin. Chir. *124:*81-91 '23 (illus.)
Tardy rupture of tendon with fracture of radius. AXHAUSEN, G. Beitr. z. Klin. Chir. *133:*78-88, '25
Rupture of tendon of long extensor of thumb occurring late after injury. HONIGMANN, F. Med. Klin. *22:*728-731, May 7, '26 abstr: J.A.M.A. *87:*133, July 10, '26
Spontaneous rupture of extensor pollicis longus. BARNES, C. K., J.A.M.A. *87:*663, Aug 28, '26
Subcutaneous ruptures of extensor tendons of fingers. DURBAN, K. Zentralbl. f. Chir. *53:*2773-2774, Oct 30, '26
Rupture of tendon of thumb cured by tendon-

Tendon, Rupture of – Cont.
ous graft. DUJARIER, C. AND BOURGUIGNON. Bull. et mem. Soc. nat. de chir. *53:*532-535, April 9, '27
Rare case of tendon rupture of thumb. SUERMONDT, W. F. Deutsche Ztschr. f. Chir. *201:*400-402, '27
Late rupture of extensor pollicis longus tendon; case. LÜLSDORF, F. Ztschr. f. orthop. Chir. *51:*191-199, Jan 11, '29
Late rupture of extensor pollicis longus tendon after fracture of radius. LASSEN, E. Hospitalstid. *72:*460-464, April 25, '29
Rupture of subcutaneous tendon of thumb; case. NUBOER, J. F. Nederl. tijdschr. v. geneesk. *2:*5645-5649, Nov 30, '29
Treatment of rupture of extensor tendons of phalanges of hand. SILFVERSKIÖLD, N. Zentralbl. f. Chir. *56:*3210, Dec 21, '29
Spontaneous rupture of extensor pollicis longus tendon. VAN DER LEE, H. S. AND SCHEFFELAAR KLOTS, T. Geneesk. gids *7:*1141, Dec 13; 1171, Dec 20, '29
Explanation of late rupture of extensor pollicis longus following fracture of radius. KLEINSCHMIDT, K. Beitr. z. Klin. Chir. *146:*530-535, '29
Treatment of rupture of extensor tendons of fingers. EWALD, P. Zentralbl. f. Chir. *57:*714-715, March 22, '30
Cause of rupture of extensor pollicis longus tendon in typical fracture of radius. COENEN, H. Arch. f. Orthop. *28:*193-206, May 6, '30
Comment on article by Horwitz on rupture of extensor tendons of fingers. GLASS, E. Zentralbl. f. Chir. *57:*2063, Aug 16, '30
Late rupture of tendon of extensor pollicis longus. KHURGIN, M. A. Ortop. i travmatol. (nos. 5-6) *4:*47-50, '30
Late rupture of tendon of extensor pollicis longus following fracture of radius. SIMON, W. V. Zentralbl. f. Chir. *58:*1298-1301, May 23, '31
Rupture of extensor longus of thumb in fractures of lower extremity of radius; case. FROELICH, M. Rev. d'orthop. *18:*584-597, Sept '31
Late subcutaneous rupture of tendon of extensor pollicis longus after fracture of radius and other bone changes in region of injury. HORWITZ, A. Deutsche Ztschr. f. Chir. *234:*710-722, '31
Subcutaneous rupture of extensor pollicus longus simulating partial radial paralysis; case. CROUZON, O. *et al.* Bull. et mem. Soc. med. d. hop. de Paris *48:*1043-1046, June 27, '32
Pathologic rupture of tendon of extensor pol-

Tendon, Rupture of—Cont.
licus longus. BIZARD, G. *et al.* Echo med. du nord. *36:*368-369, July 30, '32
Functional prognosis in rupture of tendons of fingers. VON ZWEIGBERGK, J. O. Svenska lak.-tidning. *32:*1064-1070, July 26, '35
Spontaneous healing of subcutaneous rupture of tendons in terminal phalanx of finger. LINDENSTEIN, L. Zentralbl. f. Chir. *62:*2961, Dec 14, '35
Bilateral rupture of extensor aponeurosis of terminal phalanx of finger and its treatment. GOLLA, F. Beitr. z. klin. Chir. *162:*594-600, '35
So-called late rupture of tendon of extensor pollicis longus in connection with wrist fractures. VON STAPELMOHR, S. Nord. med. tidskr. *11:*174-178, Jan 31, '36
Spontaneous rupture of extensor pollicis longus tendon associated with Colles' fracture. MOORE, T. Brit. J. Surg. *23:*721-726, April '36
Subcutaneous rupture of tendon of long extensor of thumb; case. AIMES, A. Progres med., pp. 1533-1534, Oct 3, '36
Late rupture of extensor pollicis longus tendon; rare and peculiar complication of trauma of wrist. STRØM, R. Norsk mag. f. laegevidensk. *98:*346-359, April '37
Avulsion of so-called extensor aponeurosis of thumb. GOLLA, F. Zentralbl. f. Chir. *65:*1803-1807, Aug 13, '38
Late rupture of extensor pollicis longus tendon following Colles' fracture. BLOUNT, W. P. Wisconsin M. J. *37:*912-916, Oct '38
Subcutaneous rupture of long extensor tendon of thumb; case. CORRET, P. Rev. med. de Nancy *66:*867-870, Oct 15, '38
Late rupture of tendon of extensor pollicis longus after fracture of radius; case. CLEMETSEN, N. Norsk mag. f. laegevidensk. *99:*1322-1328, Dec '38
Subcutaneous rupture of tendon of extensor pollicis longus; case. ROQUES, P. AND SOHIER, H. Rev. d'orthop. *26:*230-235, May '39
So-called late rupture of extensor pollicis longus tendon after fracture of radius. ARONSSON, H. Nord. med. (Hygiea) *2:*1985-1987, June 30, '39
Late rupture of tendon of extensor pollicis longus 10 years after fracture of lower end of radius; case. MOUCHET, A. Presse med. *48:*1007-1008, Dec 11-14, '40
Rupture of tendon of extensor pollicis longus as sequel of fracture of lower end of radius; case. CAGNOLI, H. Arch. urug. de med., cir. y especialid. *19:*598-603, Dec '41
High "late rupture" of tendon of extensor

Tendon, Rupture of—Cont.
pollicis longus. VON STAPELMOHR, S. Acta chir. Scandinav. *86:*110-128, '42
Subcutaneous rupture of tendon of extensor pollicis longus after fracture of inferior epiphysis of radius; case. MICHANS, J. R. AND GARCIA FRUGONI, A. Prensa med. argent. *30:*1221-1235, July 7, '43 also: Bol. y trab., Acad. argent. de cir. *27:*288-298, June 9, '43 (abstr)

Tendon Rupture, Baseball Finger (See also Fingers, Baseball Injuries)
Fracture of terminal phalanx of finger with rupture of common extensor tendon. BURNHAM, C. Brit. M. J. *1:*141, Jan 28, '22
Fracture of end phalanx of finger with rupture of common extensor tendon. LAIRD, J. N. Brit. M. J. *1:*101, Jan 21, '22
Splint for tendon of extensor digitorum. STAUB, H. A. Munchen. med. Wchnschr. *69:*119-120, Jan 27, '22 (illus.)
Mallet finger. FOSTER, W. J. Brit. M. J. *1:*226, Feb 11, '22
Treatment of rupture of extensor tendon of third phalanx. SONNTAG. Munchen. med. Wchnschr. *69:*1333-1334, Sept 15, '22 (illus.)
"Baseball finger" cured by operation. STEPHENS, R., J. Bone and Joint Surg. *6:*469-470, April '24
Typical finger injuries in baseball. MANDL, F. Wien. med. Wchnschr. *77:*965, July 16, '27
Metal splint for injuries of extensor tendons of fingers. GLASS, E. Zentralbl. f. Chir. *54:*3027-3028, Nov 26, '27
Rupture of extensor tendon at terminal phalanx of finger (comment on Glass' article). SONNTAG, E. Zentralbl. f. Chir. *55:*410, Feb 18, '28
Metal splint for injuries of extensor tendons of fingers (reply to Glass). FRANKE, F. Zentralbl. f. Chir. *55:*852-853, April 7, '28
Improved splint for baseball finger. LEWIN, P., J.A.M.A. *90:*2102, June 30, '28
Treatment of rupture of extensor tendons of fingers. KAEFER, N. Zentralbl. f. Chir. *56:*389, Feb 16, '29
Suture of avulsion of extension tendon of last phalanx. HAUCK, G. J. Med. Welt. *3:*1657, Nov 16, '29
Rupture of tendons of hand; with study of extensor tendon insertions in fingers. MASON, M. L. Surg., Gynec. and Obst. *50:*611-624, March '30
Treatment of torn extensor tendons of terminal phalanges. SCHLOFFER, H. Zentralbl. f. Chir. *57:*1053-1055, April 26, '30

Tendon Rupture, Baseball Finger—Cont.

Treatment of rupture of extensor tendons of fingers. HORWITZ, A. Zentralbl. f. Chir. *57:*1463-1464, June 14, '30

Surgical or nonsurgical treatment of rupture of extensor tendons of terminal phalanx of finger. HORWITZ, A. Deutsche med. Wchnschr. *57:*445-448, March 13, '31

Treatment of rupture of extensor tendon of terminal phalanx of finger. STRACKER, O. Zentralbl. f. Chir. *58:*727-730, March 21, '31

Subcutaneous rupture of tendon in finger injuries. ROMBACH, K. A. Nederl. tijdschr. v. geneesk. *77:*2938-2939, June 24, '33

Treatment of disrupted extensor tendon from terminal phalanx of finger by means of simple splint. DALSGAARD, S. Ugesk. f. laeger *96:*273-274, March 8, '34 abstr: Acta chir. Scandinav. *74:*429, '34

Splint bandage with lever in treatment of rupture of extensor aponeurosis of terminal digital phalanx. SAXL, A. Zentralbl. f. Chir. *63:*394-395, Feb 15, '36

Treatment of subcutaneous rupture of extensor tendons of distal phalanges of fingers. VAN REE, A. Nederl. tijdschr. v. geneesk. *80:*1999-2000, May 9, '36

Treatment of subcutaneous rupture of extensor tendons of terminal phalanges of fingers. KANTALA. J. Duodecim *52:*31-45, '36

Complete tearing of ungual phalanx of ring finger and of its extensor tendon; case. RAFFO, J. M. AND ARCONE, R. Rev. ortop. y traumatol. *7:*29-31, July '37

Splint for therapy of lesions of extension tendons of fingers. ROZOV, V. I. Ortop. i travmatol. (no. 2) *11:*98-100, '37

Mallet or baseball finger. KAPLAN, E. B. Surgery *7:*784-791, May '40

Technic for repair of "baseball" finger. SAYPOL, G. M. Am. J. Surg. *61:*103-104, July '43

Bloodless treatment of avulsion of extensor tendon of finger. LEDERGERBER, E. Schweiz. med. Wchnschr. *75:*1088-1089, Dec 8, '45

Tendon, Snapping Finger (See also Finger, Trigger)

Etiology and mechanism of snapping finger. KÖNIG, E. Med. Klin. *17:*434, April 10, '21

Snapping finger. HOOGVELD, W. P. J. Nederlandsch Tijdschr. v. Geneesk. *1:*2663, May 14, '21 abstr: J.A.M.A. *77:*416, July 30, '21

Tendovaginitis and snapping finger. HAUCK, G. Arch. f. klin. Chir. *123:*233-258, '23 (illus.)

Snapping finger in polyarthritis. HELWEG, J.

Tendon, Snapping Finger—Cont.

Ugesk. f. Laeger *86:*546-547, July 17, '24 abstr: J.A.M.A. *83:*1042, Sept 27, '24

Snapping finger in polyarthritis. HELWEG, J. Klin. Wchnschr. *3:*2383-2384, Dec 23, '24 abstr: J.A.M.A. *84:*560, Feb 14, '25

Snapping finger and its treatment. MONBERG, A. Hospitalstid. *68:*295-300, April 2, '25

Contracture of thumb in infants following symptoms of snapping finger. GÖHLER, W. Deutsche med. Wchnschr. *51:*1200, July 17, '25

Snapping finger and stenosis from tendovaginitis of flexor tendons. KROH, F. Arch. f. klin. Chir. *136:*240-276, '25

Snapping finger. PEIPER, H. Arch. f. klin. Chir. *150:*496-505, '28

Treatment of snapping thumb. OTTENDORF, Zentralbl. f. Chir. *57:*1273, May 24, '30

Snapping hand. HINRICHSMEYER, C. Zentralbl. f. Chir. *58:*834-837, April 4, '31

Bilateral snapping thumbs. COMPERE, E. L. Ann. Surg. *97:*773-777, May '33

Snapping thumb in childhood; 8 cases. HUDSON, H. W. JR. New England J. Med. *210:*854-857, April 19, '34

Snapping finger (intermittent reflex contraction) in electric welders. VEGER, A. M. Novy khir. arkhiv *30:*321-325, '34

Etiology of "snapping finger"; simultaneous appearance in uniovular twins. CAMERER, J. W. AND SCHLEICHER, R. Med. Klin. *31:*245-246, Feb 22, '35

Snapping thumb; tendovaginitis stenosans. ZELLE, O. L. AND SCHNEPP, K. H. Am. J. Surg. *33:*321-322, Aug '36

Trigger finger in children. JAHSS, S. A. J.A.M.A. *107:*1463-1464, Oct 31, '36

Snapping thumb in young children. HARRENSTEIN, R. J. Nederl. tijdschr. v. geneesk. *81:*1237-1241, March 20, '37

Blocking of tendons of both thumbs; comparison with syndrome described by Notta (trigger finger). Dreyfus, J. R. Schweiz. med. Wchnschr. *68:*650-654, May 28, '38

Surgical therapy of trigger finger. SPISIC, B. Zentralbl. f. Chir. *67:*157-159, Jan 27, '40

Snapping of finger joints due to injury to tendons. SCHÖRCHER, F. Zentralbl. f. Chir. *67:*627-628, April 6, '40

Tendovaginitis stenosans of finger. SPISIC, B. Lijecn. vjes. *62:*246-248, May '40

Snapping fingers due to tendosynovitis; case. SANDBERG, I. R. Nord. med. (Hygiea) *9:*707-709, March 8, '41

Blockage of tendon of flexor pollicis longus. FEVRE, M. Presse med. *50:*754-755, Dec 12, '42

Tendon, Snapping Finger – Cont.

Stenosing tenosynovitis of flexors; treated cases (hand). ALJAMA, V. Rev. espan. cir., traumatol. y ortop. *1:*373–374, Nov '44

Trigger finger; surgical therapy of case. DE FARIA VOZ, J. Arq. brasil. de cir. e ortop. *(12):*157–163, '44

Bilateral trigger thumb in infants. ROSE, T. F., M. J. Australia *1:*18–20, Jan 5, '46

Tendon, Spring Fingers (See also Fingers, Spring)

Spring fingers and flexion contracture due to blockage of digital tendons. FEVRE, M. Rev. d'orthop. *23:*137–142, March '36

Congenital bilateral flexion contracture of thumb (spring finger) in children. REGELE, H. Munchen. med. Wchnschr. *83:*391–392, March 6, '36

Spring finger and Dupuytren's contracture; case in woman. RUIZ MORENO, A. Semana med. *1:*939–946, March 19, '36

Congenital nodules of tendons; etiology of spring thumbs. VAN NECK, M. Arch. franco-belges de chir. *29:*924–927, Oct '26

Blockage of digital tendons causing spring fingers; 4 cases. GRINDA, J. P. Mem. Acad. de chir. *68:*34–38, Jan 14–21, '42

Spring finger due to partial hernia of flexor tendon. BEAUX, A. R. Prensa med. argent. *29:*1694–1698, Oct 21, '42

Simple treatment of spring finger. LASSERRE, C., J. de med. de Bordeaux *121-122:*375–376, July '45

Tendon Transplantation

Tendon transplantation for radial paralysis. RIOSALIDO. Arch. espan. de pediat. *5:*210, April '21 abstr: J.A.M.A. *77:*497, Aug 6, '21

Implantation of tendons. GALLIE, W. E. Am. J. Surg. *35:*268, Sept '21

Free transplantation of tendons. MAYER, L. Am. J. Surg. *35:*271, Sept '21

Tendon transplant for intrinsic hand muscle paralysis. NEY, K. W. Surg., Gynec. and Obst. *33:*342, Oct '21

Physiological method of tendon transplantation. MAYER, L. Surg., Gynec. and Obst. *33:*528, Nov '21

Clinical aspect of tendon transposition. BERNSTEIN, M. A. Surg., Gynec. and Obst. *34:*84–90, Jan '22 (illus.)

Army experiences with tendon transference. STARR, C. L., J. Bone and Joint Surg. *4:*3–21, Jan '22 (illus.)

Tendon substitution to restore function of extensor muscles of fingers and thumb. MERRILL, W. J., J.A.M.A. *78:*425–426, Feb 11, '22 (illus.)

Tendon Transplantation – Cont.

Tendon transplantation in forearm. KENNEDY, R. D. Southwestern Med. *6:*153–154, April '22

Tendon transplantation. SANDES, T. L., M. J. South Africa *17:*217–220, June '22

Tendon transplantation for musculospiral (radial) nerve injury. BILLINGTON, R. W., J. Bone and Joint Surg. *4:*538–547, July '22 (illus.)

Clinical and experimental study of free transplantation of fascia and tendon. GALLIE, W. E. AND LE MESURIER, A. B., J. Bone and Joint Surg. *4:*600–612, July '22 (illus.)

Tendon transplantation. OLLERENSHAW, R. Brit. M. J. *2:*77–78, July 15, '22

Results of tendon transplantation for intrinsic hand paralysis (Ney's operation). JOHNSTONE, J. G., J. Bone and Joint Surg. *5:*278–283, April '23 (illus.)

Tendon transplantations for musculo-spiral paralysis. STEVENSON, G. H. Glasgow M. J. *99:*225–230, April '23

Tendon transplants in forearm. KENNEDY, R. An. de Fac. de med., Montevideo *8:*558, May–June '23

Tendon and fascial autografts drawn through channel in bone or joint. BERTOCCHI, A. AND BIANCHETTI, C. F. Chir. d. org. di movimento *7:*225–243, June '23 (illus.) abstr: J.A.M.A. *81:*964, Sept 15, '23

Treatment of paralysis by dead tendon grafting. REGARD, G. L. Rev. med. de la Suisse Rom. *43:*364–374, June '23

Tendon transplantation. ROBERTS, W. S. Southern M. J. *16:*545–550, July '23

Living suture in tendon transplantation. ROYLE, N. D., M. J. Australia *1:*333–334, April 5, '24

Transplantation of preserved tendons; comment on Weidenreich's article. BUSACCA, A. Virchows Arch. f. path. Anat. *258:*238–245, '25

Tendon transplantations for division of extensor tendon of fingers. MAYER, L., J. Bone and Joint Surg. *8:*383–394, April '26

Grafts of fresh tendon unite with tissue of host later than grafts of devitalized tendon. NAGEOTTE, J. Compt. rend. Soc. de biol. *95:*669–672, Sept 21, '26

Tendon transplantation for radial paralysis. COMBAULT, A. Clinique, Paris *21:*315–320, Nov '26

Remote effects of grafting of dead tissue (tendon injury). NAGEOTTE, J. Compt. rend. Soc. de biol. *95:*1552–1554, Dec 31, '26

Treatment of radial paralysis by tendon anastomosis. DUPUY DE FRENELLE. Paris

Tendon Transplantation – Cont.
chir. *19:*20–27, Jan '27
Repair processes in wounds of tendons and in tendon grafts. GARLOCK, J. H. Ann. Surg. *85:*92–103, Jan '27
Rupture of tendon of thumb cured by tendinous graft. DUJARIER, C. AND BOURGUIGNON. Bull. et mem. Soc. nat. de chir. *53:*532–535, April 9, '27
Tendon transplantation. LANGE, F. Surg., Gynec. and Obst. *44:*455–462, April (pt. 1) '27
Tendon shifting and tendon transplantation. FRANCISCO, C. B., J. Kansas M. Soc. *27:*274–275, Aug '27
Functional adaptation of muscles after transplantation of muscle tendons. SCHERB, R. Ztschr. f. orthop. Chir. *48:*582–592, Nov 18, '27
Original technique in transplantation of tendons. ROYLE, N. D., J. Coll. Surgeons, Australasia *1:*115–119, July '28
Functional adaptability, inhibition and repair of antagonistic muscles in poliomyelitis; role in tendon transplantation; biologic aspect. SCHERB, R. Ztschr. f. orthop. Chir. *50:*470–493, Nov 13, '28
Transplantation of tendons of flexor pollicis longus for paralysis of flexor opponens pollicis. SILFVERSKIÖLD, N. Acta chir. Scandinav. *64:*296–299, '28
Transplantation of tendons in paralysis of radial nerve. HASS, J. Wien. klin. Wchnschr. *42:*642–644, May 9, '29
Practical results of tendon transplantation. HERZ, M. Chirurg *1:*555–559, May 1, '29
Technic of tendon transplantation. LANGE, F. Wien. med. Wchnschr. *79:*927–929, July 13, '29
Flexor plasty of thumb in thenar palsy. STEINDLER, A. Surg., Gynec. and Obst. *50:*1005–1007, June '30
Subcutaneous transplantation for ruptured tendons; cases. KRAFT, R. Arch. f. Orthop. *28:*532–540, July 23, '30
Tendon transplantation by physiologic method with cinematographic projection. ZENO, L. O. Rev. med. del Rosario *29:*310–313, July '30
Treatment of cuts of flexor tendons of fingers by tendinous graft. ALBERT, F. Liege med. *23:*1069–1077, Aug 10. '30 also: Ann. Soc. med.-chir. de Liege *63:*18–21, Sept '30
Tendon transplantation for irreparable musculo-spiral injury (radial nerve). KRIDA, A. Am. J. Surg. *9:*331–332, Aug '30
Further observation upon compensatory use of live tendon strips in facial paralysis.

Tendon Transplantation – Cont.
BLAIR, V. P. Ann. Surg. *92:*694–703, Oct '30
Free tendon grafts in fingers; case. MORRIS, K. A., J. Florida M. A. *17:*161–164, Oct '30
Compensatory use of live tendon strips; further observations in facial paralysis. BLAIR, V. P. Tr. Am. S. A. *48:*369–378, '30
Late results of tendon transplantation. COHN, M. Deutsche Ztschr. f. Chir. *230:*220–238, '31
Unfortunate results of tendon transplantation. PORT, K. Deutsche Ztschr. f. Chir. *232:*12–18, '31
Two grafts on flexor tendons. BARANGER, J., J. de med. de Bordeaux *109:*203–204, March 10, '32
Suture of ulnar nerve and reconstruction of brachial triceps tendon by grafting. ROCHER, H. L. Bordeaux chir. *3:*133–136, April '32
Remote results in radial paralysis after tendon transplantation; 4 cases. SOLCARD. Bull. et mem. Soc. nat. de chir. *58:*677–682, May 7, '32
Use of plantaris tendon in certain types of plastic surgery of hand. GLISSAN, D. J. Australian and New Zealand J. Surg. *2:*64–67, July '32
Process of tendon repair; experimental study of tendon suture and tendon graft. MASON, M. L. AND SHEARON, C. G. Arch. Surg. *25:*615–692, Oct '32
Suture of ulnar nerve and reconstruction of brachial triceps tendon by grafting. ROCHER, H. L. Bull. et mem. Soc. de chir. de Bordeaux et du Sud-Ouest, pp. 247–254, '32
Tendon transplantation; case. DELCHEF, J. Scalpel *86:*1099–1100, July 15, '33
Complicated contractures of hand; their treatment by freeing fibrosed tendons and replacing destroyed tendons with grafts. KOCH, S. L. Ann. Surg. *98:*546–580, Oct '33
Technic and results of tendon translocations. FABER, A. Verhandl. d. deutsch. orthop. Gesellsch., Kong. 27, pp. 331–333, '33
Reconstruction of crucial ligaments of knee with kangaroo tendons; late results. MICHELI, E. Boll. e mem. Soc. piemontese di chir. *3:*874–883, '33
Tendon transplants for paralytic wrist drop; presentation of patient. SWART, H. A. AND HENDERSON, M. S. Proc. Staff Meet., Mayo Clin. *9:*377–379, June 27, '34
Factors in success and failure of tendon transplants; especially in therapy of sequels of poliomyelitis. BASTOS ANSART, M.

Tendon Transplantation – Cont.
Bol. y trab. de la Soc. de cir. de Buenos Aires *18:*848-868, Sept 12, '34
Factors of success and failure in tendon transplantation. BASTOS ANSART, M. Rev. de cir. de Buenos Aires *13:*657-683, Nov '34
Result of graft of extensor tendon of left index finger in repair of flexor tendon of same finger. BURTY. Bull. et mem. Soc. d. chirurgiens de Paris *26:*659-660, Dec 7, '34
Therapy of paralysis in poliomyelitis (tendon transplantation). TRUETA RASPALL, J. Ars med., Barcelona *11:*418-423, Oct '35
Tenoplasty of flexor muscles of fingers for clawhand (pseudo-Volkmann contracture); results in case. DIAMANT-BERGER, L. Bull. et mem. Soc. d. chirurgiens de Paris *27:*541-545, Nov 22, '35
Favorable results of surgical therapy of aplasia of opponens muscle of thumb by transplantation of tendons of flexor digitalis sublimis V; survey of methods. GÖBELL, R. AND FREUDENBERG, K. Arch. f. orthop. u. Unfall-Chir. *35:*675-677, '35
Tendon transplantation in therapy of sequels of infantile paralysis. SOROKINA. Ortop. i travmatol. (no. 6) *9:*130-135, '35
Therapy of digital wounds of flexor tendons; St. Bünnell operation using tendon graft; technic and results; 14 cases. BLOCH, J. C. AND ZAGDOUN, J., J. de chir. *47:*376-391, March '36
Tendon transplantation in therapy of inveterate radial paralysis; physiologic aims, technic and results. BONOLA, A. Chir. d. org. di movimento *22:*239-254, Aug '36
Successful and unsuccessful tendon transplants. BASTOS ANSART, M. Cir. ortop. y traumatol., Madrid *1:*5-26, '36
Tendon transplantation in therapy of complete paralysis of radial nerve; case. GIULIANI, G. M. Arch. ital. di chir. *42:*613-616, '36
Plastic operation (skin grafting); case. (Tendon grafting.) BLACK, J. R. AND MACEY, H. B. Proc. Staff Meet., Mayo Clin. *12:*497-500, Aug 11, '37
Tendon transplantation in therapy of inveterate radial paralysis. (Comment on Bonola's article.) GIULIANI, G. M. Chir. d. org. di movimento *23:*102, Oct '37
Further experiences with tendon transplantation. GALLIE, W. E. Tr. West. S. A. (1936) *46:*47-57, '37
Tendon transplantation, end-result study. PEABODY, C. W., J. Bone and Joint Surg. *20:*193-205, Jan '38
Tendon transplantation in therapy of poliomyelitic paralysis; cases. SCHERB, R. Schweiz. med. Wchnschr. *68:*354-360, April 2, '38
Correction of sequels of infantile paralysis; technic of osteoperiosteal incision in tendinous transplants. DE GAETANO, L. Riforma med. *54:*887-895, June 11, '38
Tendon transplants in surgical therapy of radial paralysis; case. VEZINA, C. *et al.* Laval med. *3:*181-186, June '38
Transplantation of tendons in therapy of paralytic clubfoot. DEBELUT, J. Semaine d. hop. de Paris *14:*353-354, July 15, '38
Operation for paralysis of intrinsic muscles of thumb. ROYLE, N. D., J.A.M.A. *111:*612-613, Aug 13, '38
Surgery for opposition of thumb. BUNNELL, S., J. Bone and Joint Surg. *20:*1072, Oct '38
Tendon transplantation in therapy of permanent radial paralysis; case. MAROTTOLI, O. R. Bol. Soc. de cir. de Rosario *5:*434-435, Oct '38
Late results of tendon transplantation; study based on 95 cases. ZANOLI, R. Arch. ital. di chir. *54:*907-914, '38
Recurrent pseudoarthrosis of humerus complicated by irreparable paralysis of radial nerve; curative osteoplasty and functional reconstruction of hand by means of tendon transplants. INCLAN, A. Cir. ortop. y traumatol., Habana *7:*43-53, April-June '39
Use of grafts of devitalized connective tissue (tendon and nerve) in reparative surgery. NAGEOTTE, J. Presse med. *47:*1365-1366, Sept 27, '39
End-result study of 458 tendon transplantations. CARPENTER A. R., J. Bone and Joint Surg. *21:*921-932, Oct '39
Instrument for transplantation of tendons. GUSEV, B. P. Vestnik khir. *58:*590-591, Dec '39
Surgical repair of extensive tendon loss by tendon transplantation; 7 cases. MORGANTI, R. Chir. d. org. di movimento *25:*182-188, Dec '39
Tendon transplantation for radial nerve paralysis. YOUNG, H. H. Proc. Staff Meet., Mayo Clin. *15:*26-28, Jan 10, '40
New instrument for passing portions of tendons and fasciae latae. MACEY, H. B. Am. J. Surg. *47:*686, March '40
Tendon transplantation. COMPERE, E. L. Physiotherapy Rev. *20:*131-133, May-June '40
Tendon transplantation for paralysis of radial nerve. GHORMLEY, R. K. AND CAMERON, D. M. Proc. Staff Meet., Mayo Clin.

Tendon Transplantation – Cont.
*15:*537-539, Aug 21, '40
New method (transplantation of flexor pollicis longus tendon) for relief of paralysis of opponens pollicis. SCHECK, M. Indian M. Gaz. *75:*464-466, Aug '40
Restoration of function of paralyzed arm following poliomyelitis by transplantation of epitrochlear muscles and arthrodesis of shoulder. VECCHIONE, F. Arch. ortop. *56:*145-156, Sept '40
Tendon transplantation for paralysis of external rectus muscle of eye; further report. GIFFORD, S. R. Arch. Ophth. *24:*916-923, Nov '40
Tendon transplantation in radial paralysis. SPISIC, B. Lijecn. vjes. *63:*12-13, Jan '41
Tendon transplantation, in therapy of inveterate radial paralysis. ARGUELLES LOPEZ, R. Rev. clin. espan. *2:*319-323, April 1, '41
Anatomy and physiology in relation to tendon transplantation. CASTILLO ODENA, I. Dia med. *13:*246-249, April 7, '41
Skin and tendon transplantation in severe injury to back of right hand by polishing machine. HILLEBRAND, H. Chirurg *13:*521-523, Sept 1, '41
Transplants to thumb to restore function of opposition; end results. IRWIN, C. E. South. M. J. *35:*257-262, March '42
Device for measuring length of tendon graft in flexor tendon surgery. KAPLAN, E. B. Bull. Hosp. Joint Dis. *3:*97-99, July '42
Transplantation of flexor carpi ulnaris for pronation-flexion deformity of wrist. GREEN, W. T. Surg., Gynec. and Obst. *75:*337-342, Sept '42
Substitute tenoplasties in therapy of radial paralysis. D'HARCOURT, J. Pasteur *1:*121-127, June 15, '43
Tendon transplant for complete radial paralysis; case. CHARBONNEL AND BARROUX, R. Bordeaux chir. *1-2:*55, Jan-Apr '44
Reconstructive orthopedic surgery (tendon transplantation and arthrodesis of wrist) for disabilities resulting from irreparable injuries to radial nerve. ABBOTT, L. C., J. Nerv. and Ment. Dis. *99:*466-474, May '44
Value of tendon transplantation for rapid restoration of function of wrist following injuries. LOMAZOV, M. G. Vrach. delo *24:*51-54, Dec 1, '44
Tendon transplantation at elbow. STEINDLER, A. Am. Acad. Orthop. Surgeons, Lect. pp. 276-283, '44
Functional reeducation of transplanted tendons. ZAUSMER, E. Physiotherapy Rev. *25:*160-164, July-Aug '45
Bandage for Perthes operation (tendon transplant). NIKIFOROVA, E. K. Khirurgiya, no. 6, p. 94, '45
Tendon transplant in paralysis of extensors of hand and fingers; case in boy 5 years old. GUILLEMINET, M. AND DUBOST, T. Rev. d'orthop. *32:*72-75, Jan-Apr '46
Tendon transplant method in definitive paralysis of peroneal nerve and of sciatic-external popliteal nerve. TENEFF, S. Minerva chir. *1:*1-3, March '46
Tendon transplant for radial paralysis. ZACHARY, R. B. Brit. J. Surg. *33:*358-364, April '46
Tendon transplant in treatment of post-traumatic radial paralysis. MERLE D'AUBIGNE, R. AND LANCE, P. Semaine d. hop. Paris *22:*1666-1671, Sept 21, '46
Tendon transplantation in hand. MAY, H. Surg. Gynec. and Obst. *83:*631-638, Nov '46

Tendon, Tumors of

Cavernous angioma of tendon sheaths; case. DELLA MANO, N. Policlinico (sez. chir.) *39:*593-612, Oct '32
Cavernous angiomas of tendons of hands. BOTTO MICCA, A. Riv. san. siciliana *22:*568-577, April 15, '34
Synoviomas of tendon sheaths and of serous bursae. ZWAHLEN, P. Bull. Assoc. franc. p. l'etude du cancer *24:*682-707, Dec '35
Hemangioma of tendon or tendon sheath; report of case with study of 24 cases from literature. HARKINS, H. N. Arch. Surg. *34:*12-22, Jan '37
Tumors of synovia, tendons and joint capsules (hand). BRUNSCHWIG, A. Surgery *5:*101-111, Jan '39
Ganglia of tendon sheaths (bursae). NELSON, H. Minnesota Med. *26:*734-737, Aug '43

TENEFF, S.: Tendon transplant method in definitive paralysis of peroneal nerve and of sciatic-external popliteal nerve. Minerva chir. *1:*1-3, March '46
TENERY, J. H. (see TENERY, W. C.) Oct '41
TENERY, R. M.: Extensive cutaneous burns. Surg., Gynec. and Obst. *72:*1018-1027, June '41
TENERY, R. M.: Cutaneous burns. Am. J. M. Sc. *203:*293-300, Feb '42
TENERY, W. C. AND TENERY, J. H.: Emergency treatment of burns. South. Surgeon *10:*759-764, Oct '41
TEN HORN, C.: Operative lymph drainage in elephantiasis. Zentralbl . f. Chir. *51:*233, Feb 9, '24
TEN KATE, J.: Surgical impressions from Eng-

land; burns and plastic surgery. Geneesk. gids. *24:*25, Jan 31, '46; 52, Feb 28, '46

TENNANT, R. (see OUGHTERSON, A. W.) Jan '39

TENNENT, E. H.: Wiring method of treatment for fractures of mandible. U. S. Nav. M. Bull. *19:*38–42, July '23 (illus.)

Tenosynovitis, Stenosing, De Quervain's

Tendovaginitis or tendinitis stenosans. HANSON, R. Acta chir. Scandinav. *60:*281–286, '26 (in English)

Stenosing tendovaginitis on styloid process of radius (styloidalgia). WINTERSTEIN, O. Munchen. med. Wchnschr. *74:*12–15, Jan 7, '27

Stenosing tendovaginitis of long abductor and of short extensor of thumb. LAROYENNE, AND BOUYSSET. Arch. franco-belges de chir. *30:*98–104, Feb '27 also: Lyon med. *140:*573–575, Nov 27, '27

Styloidalgia radii and some other cases of tendovaginitis stensans. JAGERINK, T. A. Nederl. Tijdschr. v. Geneesk. *1:*3227, June 30, '28

Stenosing fibrous tendovaginitis over radial styloid (de QUERVAIN). SCHNEIDER, C. C. Surg., Gynec. and Obst. *46:*846–850, June '28

Stenosis of tendon sheath of wrist. WINTERSTEIN, O. Schweiz. med. Wchnschr. *58:*746–748, July 28, '28

Strangulation of long abductor and short extensor of thumb; treatment. LAROYENNE, AND TREPOZ. Lyon med. *142:*394, Sept 30, '28

Stenosing tendovaginitis of first portion of styloid process of radius; its nature and treatment. LASSEN, E. Ugesk. f. laeger *91:*837–840, Oct 3, '29

Stenosing tendovaginitis of DeQuervain; case. WATKINS, J. T. AND PITKIN, H. C. California and West. Med. *32:*101–102, Feb '30

Causes, pathology, diagnosis and therapy of stenosing tendovaginitis of thumb. LANDOIS, F. Med. Klin. *26:*927–929, June 20, '30

Stenosing tendovaginitis at radial styloid process. FINKELSTEIN, H., J. Bone and Joint Surg. *12:*509–540, July '30

Stenosing tendovaginitis at radial styloid process. HOFFMANN, P., J. Bone and Joint Surg. *13:*89–90, Jan '31

Diagnosis of deQuervain's chronic stenosing inflammation of tendons. WEISSENBACH, R. J. AND FRANÇON, F. Bull. med., Paris *45:*378–382, May 30, '31

DeQuervain's chronic stenosing tendovaginitis; 3 cases. LAMY, L. Bull. et mem. Soc. d.

Tenosynovitis, Stenosing, De Quervain's—Cont.

chirurgiens de Paris *24:*373–377, June 3, '32

DeQuervain's stenosing tendovaginitis (Winterstein's styloidalgia radii); 8 cases. SCHETTINO, M. Riforma med. *48:*1142–1145, July 23, '32

Acute forms of de Quervain's stenosing tendovaginitis; 2 cases. LAROYENNE, L. AND BRUN, M. Lyon med. *151:*3–9, Jan 1, '33

De Quervain's disease; stenosing tendovaginitis at radial styloid. PATTERSON, D. C. New England J. Med. *214:*101–103, Jan 16, '36

Stenosing tenosynovitis; surgical therapy of 2 cases. OTTOLENGHI, C. E. AND SPINELLI, C. A. Rev. ortop. y traumatol. *6:*196–202, Oct '36

Tendovaginitis stenosans of extensor pollicis longus sinister. POHL, H. Med. Klin. *32:*1596–1597, Nov 20, '36

Stenosing tendovaginitis at radial styloid process (de Quervain's disease). KEYES, H. B. Ann. Surg. *107:*602–606, April '38

De Quervain's disease; radial styloid tendovaginitis. COTTON, F. J. *et al.* New England J. Med. *219:*120–123, July 28, '38

Stenosing tendovaginitis at radial styloid process (de Quervain's disease). McDONALD, J. E. AND STUART, F. A., J. Bone and Joint Surg. *21:*1035, Oct '39

De Quervain's disease; frequently missed diagnosis. DIACK, A. W. AND TROMMALD, J. P. West. J. Surg. *47:*629–633, Nov '39

Stenosing tendovaginitis at radial styloid process (de Quervain's disease). WOOD, C. F. South. Surgeon *10:*105–110, Feb '41

Chronic stenosing tenosynovitis (de Quervain's disease); symptoms, diagnosis and therapy. WEISSENBACH, R. J. AND FRANCON, F. Rev. argent. de reumatol. *5:*299–305, March '41

TEOPACO, R. L.: Use of insulin in second-degree burn developing hyperglycemia and glycosuria. J. Philippine Islands M. A. *10:*162–165, April '30

TERCERO, M.: Pseudo-unilocular serous cyst of neck in infant; case. Arch. espan. de pediat. *16:*306–309, July '32

TERHUNE, S. R.: Volkmann contracture. J. M. A. Alabama *4:*116–117, Sept '34

TERHUNE, S. R. AND CAMP, M. N.: Traumatic amputation of finger tips (with special reference to tank door accident; value of skin grafts). South. Surgeon *11:*646–651, Sept '42

TERNOVSKIY, S. D.: Burn in children and their therapy with powdered chalk dressings. Vestnik khir. *39:*3–8, '35

TERRELL, T. C.: Comparative study of foille with tannic acid and tannic acid preparations. Texas State J. Med. *34:*409–415, Oct '38

TERRIEN, F.: Reconstruction of orbit. Paris med. *12:*157–159, Feb 25, '22

TERRIEN, F.; GOUGEROT, AND HASSON: Skin grafts in repair of ocular lesions from pemphigus (eyelids). Arch. d'opht. *48:*275–281, April '31

TESCOLA, C.: Rare congenital osseous abnormalities of hands and feet in same patient; case. Riv. di radiol. e fis. med. *5:*570–576, '31

TESONE, J. D. (see FINOCHIETTO, E. *et al*) July '40

Testicles

Testicular transplantation; successful autoplastic graft following accidental castration. KEARNS, W. M. Ann. Surg. *114:*886–890, Nov '41

Tetanus

Tetanus after burn from high power current. FÖRSTER, W. Munchen. med. Wchnschr. *68:*1655, Dec 23, '21

Tetanus after burns. SCHREINER, K. AND STOCKER, H. Wien. med. Wchnschr. *79:*1020–1022, Aug 3, '29

Prophylaxis of tetanus following burns. FASAL, P. Wien. klin. Wchnschr. *48:*181–182, Feb 8, '35

Rare case of tetanus following burn. MUKHIN, M. V. Sovet. vrach. zhur., pp. 1820–1821, Dec 15, '36

Tetanus after burns. KUDRINSKIY, A. A. Sovet. khir., no. 9, pp. 522–524, '36

Fatal tetanus in burn; case. MAZZINI, O. F. Prensa med. argent. *25:*554–556, March 16, '38

Tetanus after burns. MAURER, G. Zentralbl. f. Chir. *65:*2771–2772, Dec 10, '38

Gas bacillus infections, burns and tetanus. BURNETT, J. H. Am. J. Orthodontics (Oral Surg. Sect.) *27:*698–700, Dec '41

TETU, I. AND DUMITRESCU, J.: Correction of saddle nose by autograft from costal cartilage. Spitalul *55:*65–66, Feb '35

THACKER NEVILLE, W. S.: Morphine-scopolamine narco-anaesthesia in nasal surgery. Proc. Roy. Soc. Med. (Sect. Laryng.) *22:*61–64, Sept '29

THACKER NEVILLE, W. S.: Postoperative hemorrhage in nose and throat operations; treatment with clauden. Lancet *2:*624–625, Sept 17, '32

THALHEIMER, M. AND BLONDIN-WALTHER, M.: Section of radial nerve and heterograft of dog's fresh nerve into man; case. Bull. et mem. Soc. nat. de chir. *57:*535–543, April 25, '31

THATCHER, H. V.: Repair of flexor tendons of fingers. Northwest Med. *36:*259–263, Aug '37

THATCHER, H. V.: Use of stainless steel rods to canalize flexor tendon sheaths. South. M. J. *32:*13–18, Jan '39

THELEN, W. P.: Burn therapy. Surg. J. *34:*146–149, July–Aug '28

THEN BERGH, H.: Dupuytren's contracture; concordant occurrence in fingers of 3 sets of twins. Allg. Ztschr. f. Psychiat. *112:*327–336, '39

THEODORESCO, D.: Mandibular macrognathia and its correction. Rev. de chir., Bucuresti *38:*22–34, March–April '35

THEODORESCO, D.: Badly consolidated fracture of upper jaw; reduction by osteotomy and elastic traction apparatus. Rev. de chir., Bucuresti *41:*918–926, Nov–Dec '38

THEODORESCO, D.: Deformation of lower jaw corrected by surgical intervention and prosthesis. Rev. de chir., Bucuresti *41:*926–930, Nov–Dec '38

THEODORESCO, D.: New data on surgical therapy of cleft palate. Rev. de chir., Bucuresti *42:*126–134, Jan–Feb '39

THEODORESCO, D.: Plastic surgery of face. Rev. de chir., Bucuresti *42:*365–372, May–June '39

THEODORESCO, D.: Surgical therapy of zygoma fractures. Ztschr. f. Stomatol. *40:*359–363, May 22, '42

THEODORESCO, D.: Maxillofacial war wounds; principles of therapy and results. J. de chir. *62:*171–183, '46

THEODORESCO, D. AND CRISTODULO: Technic of reduction of fracture of upper jaw; case. Rev. de chir., Bucuresti *41:*496–499, July–Aug '38

THEODORESCO, D. AND HOFER, O.: Cancer of cheek, with special reference to results of surgical therapy. Presse med. *42:*2040–2043, Dec 19, '34

THEODORESCO, D. (see TOPA, P.) March–April '38

THÉVENARD: Late results of surgical therapy of traumatic lesions of peripheral nerves. Bull. et mem. Soc. d. chirurgiens de Paris *28:*479–485, Nov 6, '36

THÉVENARD, A. (see LÉCHELLE, *et al*) Feb '33

THEVENET, V.: Use of alevolate rubber in preventive and curative therapy of sacral eschar. Lyon med. *157:*709–711, June 14, '36

THEVENIN, J.: Intolerance of cartilage grafts. Rev. de chir. structive *8:*7–12, May '38

THEVENIN, J.: Arterial vascularization of nose; relation to certain plastic reactions after corrective interventions. Plast. chir. *1:*155–161, '40

THÉVENON, J. A. (see GATÉ, J. *et al*) Dec '32

THEVENOT, AND GAYET, R.: Traumatic rupture of urethra in child; reconstruction of canal by means of cutaneous graft; dysuria resulting from cicatricial stricture and urethral calculus 33 years later. Lyon chir. *35:*592–595, Sept–Oct '38

THIBONNEAU: Fracture of finger; bone cyst. Bull. et mem. Soc. de radiol. med. de France *14:*197, Dec '26

THIEL, R.: Reconstruction of lacrimal ducts. Klin. Monatsbl. f. Augenh. *108:*576–583, Sept–Oct '42

THIELEMANN: Results of implantations of porous gold in plastic surgery of nose. Ztschr. f. Laryng., Rhin., Otol. *24:*175–180, '33

THIERS, H. (see FROMENT, J. *et al*) Oct '36

Thiersch Operation: See Wagner-Thiersch Operation

THIES, O.: Favorable results of iridectomy in case of ammonia burn of eyes. Klin. Monatsbl. f. Augenh. *79:*534–536, Oct 28, '27

THIES, O.: Ammonia burns of eyes. Zentralbl. f. Gewerbehyg. *5:*83–88, March '28

THIES, O.: Early plastic operation (transplantation of oral mucosa) in caustic injuries of eye. Arch. f. Ophth. *123:*165–170, '29

THIES, O.: Osteochondritis deformans juvenilis of fingers with brachyphalangia; case. Chirurg *8:*807–813, Oct 15, '36

THIES, O.: Reasons for early operation in cases of severe burns of eyes. Arch. f. Ophth. *138:*686–692, '38

THIES, O.: Severe chemical burns to eyes. Klin. Monatsbl. f. Augenh. *106:*47–56, Jan '41

THIESSEN, N. W.: Local burn treatment. South. Med. and Surg. *105:*1–3, Jan '43

THIESSEN, N. W. AND STEINREICH, O. S.: Local burn treatment (with sulfathiazole, sulfanilamide derivative, and cod liver oil ointment) in the Army. Mil. Surgeon *91:*208–211, Aug '42

THILENIUS: Therapy of furunculosis by fan-shaped section. Deutsche med. Wchnschr. *55:*618, April 12, '29

THOLEN, E. F. (see KISKADDEN, W. S.) Aug '32

THOMA, K. H.: Progressive atrophy of facial bones with complete atrophy of mandible; case. J. Bone and Joint Surg. *15:*494–501, April '33

THOMA, K. H.: Facial cleft or fissural cysts. Internat. J. Orthodontia *23:*83–89, Jan '37

THOMA, K. H.: Traumatic injury of condyloid process of mandible. New England J. Med. *218:*63–71, Jan 13, '38

THOMA, K. H.: Traumatic injury of condyloid process of mandible. Am. J. Orthodontics *24:*774–790, Aug '38

THOMA, K. H.: Cancer of mandible. Am. J. Orthodontics *24:*995–999, Oct '38

THOMA, K. H.: Jaw tumors; collective review. Internat. Abstr. Surg. *67:*522–545, '38; in Surg., Gynec. and Obst., Dec '38

THOMA, KURT H.: *Traumatic Surgery of the Jaws, Including First-Aid Treatment.* C. V. Mosby Co., St. Louis, 1942

THOMA, K. H.: Adenocarcinoma of maxilla. Am. J. Orthodontics (Oral Surg. Sect.) *28:*65–85, Feb '42

THOMA, K. H.: Care of military and civilian injuries; fractures of maxilla. Am. J. Orthodontics (Oral Surg. Sect.) *28:*275–291, May '42

THOMA, K. H.: New method of intermaxillary fixation in patients wearing artificial dentures. Am. J. Orthodontics (Oral Surg. Sect.) *29:*433–441, Aug '43

THOMA, K. H.: Y-shaped osteotomy for correction of open bite in adults. Surg., Gynec. and Obst. *77:*40–50, July '43 also: Am. J. Orthodontics (Oral Surg. Sect.) *29:*465–479, Sept '43

THOMA, K. H.: History and treatment of fractured jaws from World War I to World War II; collective review. Internat. Abstr. Surg. *78:*281–312, '44; in Surg., Gynec. and Obst. April '44

THOMA, K. H.: Historical review of methods advocated for treatment of fractured jaw; 10 commandments for modern treatment. Am. J. Orthodontics (Oral Surg. Sect.) *30:*399–504, Aug '44

THOMA, K. H.: Fracture-dislocations of mandibular condyle; method for open reduction and internal wiring and one for skeletal fixation, with report of thirty-two cases. J. Oral Surg. *3:*3–59, Jan '45

THOMA, K. H.: Three fractures at angle of jaw; one treated by internal wiring, two by internal clamp fixation. Am. J. Orthodontics (Oral Surg. Sect.) *31:*206–220, Apr '45

THOMA, K. H.: Comparison of 2 methods of treating apertognathia. Am. J. Orthodontics (Oral Surg. Sect.) *31:*248–259, Apr '45

THOMA, K. H.: Ankylosis of mandibular joint. Am. J. Orthodontics (Oral Surg. Sect.) *32:*259–272, May '46

THOMA, K. H.: Surgical treatment of jaw deformity. Am. J. Orthodontics *32:*333–339, June '46

THOMA, K. H.; HOWE, H. D. AND WENIG, M.: Fractures of condyle of mandible. Am. J. Orthodontics (Oral Surg. Sect.) *31:*220–226, Apr '45

THOMA, K. H.; HOWE, H. D. AND WENIG, M.: Fractures of middle third of face. Am. J. Orthodontics (Oral Surg. Sect.) *31:*226–234,

Apr '45
THOMA, K. H.; HOWE, H. D. AND WENIG, M.: Osteomyelitis of jaw. Am. J. Orthodontics (Oral Surg. Sect.) *31:*235–244, Apr '45
THOMA, K. H.; HOWE, H. D. AND WENIG, M.: Ankylosis of jaws. Am. J. Orthodontics (Oral Surg. Sect.) *31:*244–248, April '45
THOMA, K. H.; HOWE, H. D. AND WENIG, M.: Tumors of jaws. Am. J. Orthodontics (Oral Surg. Sect.) *31:*260–288, Apr '45
THOMA, K. H.; WENIG, M. AND KAPLAN, S. I.: Further uses for peripheral bone clamp in jaw fractures. Am. J. Orthodontics (Oral Surg. Sect.) *31:*607–618, Oct '45
THOMA, K. H.; WENIG, M. AND KAPLAN, S. I.: Clinic of Dental Department of Massachusetts General Hospital and Department of Oral Surgery of Harvard School of Dental Medicine; miscellaneous case reports of jaw tumors. Am. J. Orthodontics (Oral Surg. Sect.) *31:*619–636, Oct '45
THOMAS, A.: Sympathetic disturbances in course of facial hemiatrophy; case. Presse med. *43:*1339–1340, Aug 24, '35
THOMAS, A. AND DE AJURIAGUERRA: Anastomosis between hypoglossal and facial nerves; case. Rev. neurol. *74:*308–310, Nov–Dec '42
THOMAS, A. AND HUC, G.: Syndrome characterized by bilateral clubfoot and clubhand associated with special type of amyotrophy of upper and lower extremities, dating from birth; case. Rev. neurol. *64:*918–925, Dec '35
THOMAS, A. *et al*: Nerves; management of war injuries. Rev. neurol. *72:*639–677, '39–'40
THOMAS, A. AND PETIT-DUTAILLIS: Sensory-motor restoration after section of nerves of arm; suture of radial nerve with subsequent graft of median and ulnar nerves. Rev. neurol. *1:*56–60, Jan '30
THOMAS, A.; SORREL, E. AND SORRELL-DEJERINE, MME.: Volkmann syndrome; therapeutic measures; 4 cases in children. Rev. neurol *63:*505–528, April '35
THOMAS, A. K.: Unusual developmental abnormalities (including imperforate anus, epispadias). Brit. M. J. *2:*985–986, Nov 26, '27
THOMAS, C. (see JEANDELIZE, P.) May '38
THOMAS, C. H.: Repair for partial loss of auricle. J. Laryng. and Otol. *53:*259–260, April '38
THOMAS, E. H.: Osteomyelitis of bones of face; diagnosis and treatment. J. Am. Dent. A. *20:*614–621, April '33
THOMAS, E. H.: Symposium on industrial surgery; fractures of jaws and injuries of face, mouth and teeth. S. Clin. North America *22:*1029–1048, Aug '42
THOMAS, F. B. Splint for radial (musculospiral) nerve palsy. J. Bone and Joint Surg. *26:*602–605, July '44

Thomas, H. O.

Purposeful splinting of hand following injuries (including sketch on Hugh Owen Thomas). KOCH, S. L. AND MASON, M. L. Surg., Gynec. and Obst. *68:*1–16, Jan '39

THOMASON, T. H.: Skin grafts. Texas State J. Med. *39:*476–477, Jan '44
THOMASSEN, C.: Treatment of roentgen burn of elbow with salicylic acid solution and skin graft. Nederl. tijdschr. v. geneesk. *78:*1621–1624, April 14, '34
THOMPSON, A. R.: Case of epispadias associated with complete incontinence treated by rectus transplantation. Brit. J. Child. Dis. *20:*146–151, July–Sept '23
THOMPSON, A. R.: Extroversion of bladder with control of micturition. Brit. M. J. *2:*3–5, July 3, '37
THOMPSON, A. R.: Effects, symptoms and treatment of hypospadias; review of 101 cases. Lancet *2:*429–432, Aug 21, '37
THOMPSON, A. R.: Clinical anatomy of cases of epispadias and extroversion of bladder. Brit. J. Child. Dis. *35:*36–43, Jan–March '38
THOMPSON, C. F.: Extensive burn of arms. J. Indiana M. A. *25:*301–302, July '32
THOMPSON, C. F.: Fusion of metacarpals of thumb and index finger to maintain functional position of thumb. J. Bone and Joint Surg. *24:*907–911, Oct '42
THOMPSON, C. M.: Danger of finger rings in injuries. U. S. Nav. M. Bull. *46:*1273–1274, Aug '46
THOMPSON, F. G. JR. (see PEARMAN, R. O.) Nov '42
THOMPSON, H. A.: Sprains and injuries of fingers. Am. J. Surg. *6:*522–523, April '29
THOMPSON, H. A.: Prevention of contracture deformities following burns by use of Padgett dermatome. South. Med. and Surg. *105:*51–55, Feb '43
THOMPSON, H. L. (see JUDD, E. S.) Oct '28
THOMPSON, I. M.: Some anatomical points relative to infections of hand. Canad. M.A.J. *14:*683–686, Aug '24
THOMPSON, J. E.: Atypical plastic operations for congenital fissures of lip and palate. S. Clin. N. America *2:*1387–1401, Oct '22 (illus.)
THOMPSON, J. E.: Use of septal flap in closure of unilateral clefts of palate. J.A.M.A. *87:*1384–1388, Oct 23, '26
THOMPSON, J. E. AND KEILLER, V. H.: Lymphangioma of neck. Ann. Surg. *77:*385–396, April '23 (illus.)
THOMPSON, J. F.: Simplification of technique in operations for hare-lip and cleft palate. Ann. Surg. *74:*394, Oct '21

THOMPSON, L. M.: Emergency care of wounds, hemorrhage and shock. New York State J. Med. *42:*355–356, Feb 15, '42

THOMPSON, M. R. (see HUEPER, W. C. *et al*) June '42

THOMPSON, T. C.: Modified operation for opponens paralysis. J. Bone and Joint Surg. *24:*632–640, July '42

THOMPSON, T. C. AND ALLDREDGE, R. H.: Amputation surgery and plastic repair. J. Bone and Joint Surg. *26:*639–644, Oct '44

THOMPSON, W. D. JR. (see WHELAN, C. S.) Dec '44

THOMSEN, O.: Peculiarities of hereditary polydactylia and syndactylia; supplement to author's original article. Acta med. Scandinav. *66:*588–590, '27

THOMSEN, O.: Peculiarities of hereditary polydactylia and syndactylia. Acta med. Scandinav. *65:*609–644, '27 also: Hospitalstid. *70:*789–819, Aug 25, '27

THOMSEN, O.: Peculiarities concerning hereditary polydactylism and syndactylism. Acta path. et microbiol. Scandinav. (supp) *5:*148–149, '28

THOMSEN, W.: Diagnosis and treatment of contractures of fingers. Arch. f. orthop. u. Unfall-Chir. *39:*201–205, '38

THOMSEN, W.: Technic of wire extension in fractures of fingers. Chirurg. *10:*145–148, March 1, '38

THOMSEN, W.: Therapeutic technic in Bennett fracture of thumb. Chirurg *12:*520–522, Sept 1, '40

THOMSEN, W.: Two small supplementary devices for author's extension apparatus for fractured fingers. Chirurg. *15:*311, May 15, '43

THOMSON, D.; CLAYTON, W. AND HOWARD, A. J.: Physical chemistry of oils in burn treatment. Lancet *1:*341–343, March 15, '41

THOMSON, J. L. *et al.*: Peripheral nerve injuries overseas; plan for care. Arch. Surg. *52:*557–570, May '46

THOMSON, J. W.: Branchial cyst; case. Lancet *1:*76, Jan 8, '27

THOMSON, ST. C.: Intrinsic cancer operated on by laryngo-fissure; immediate and ultimate results. Eye, Ear, Nose and Throat Monthly *7:*266–270, June '28 also: Arch. Otolaryng. *8:*377–385, Oct '28

THOMSON, ST. C.: Intrinsic laryngeal cancer; lasting cure in 76 per cent of cases by laryngo-fissure. Canad. M.A.J. *21:*4–8, July '29

THOMSON, ST. C.: Intrinsic laryngeal cancer; lasting recovery in 76 per cent of cases of laryngo-fissure. Ann. d. mal. de l'oreille, du larynx *48:*1079–1088, Nov '29 also: Union med. du Canada *59:*5–16, Jan '30

THOREK, M.: Possibilities in reconstruction of human form. New York M. J. *116:*572–575, Nov 15, '22 (illus.)

THOREK, M.: Tumors of fingers; with report of cases. M. J. and Rec. *122:*443–446, Oct 21, '25

THOREK, M.: Esthetic surgery of pendulous breast, abdomen and arms in female. Illinois M. J. *58:*48–57, July '30

THOREK, M.: Possibilities of esthetic remodeling of human form. Tri-State M. J. *3:*621–622, July '31

THOREK, M.: Histological verification of efficacy of free transplantation of nipple. M. J. and Rec. *134:*474–476, Nov 18, '31

THOREK, M.: Simplicity versus complicated methods in reconstruction of pendulous breasts. Illinois M. J. *69:*338–456, April '36

THOREK, M.: Plastic reconstruction of female breasts. Am. J. Surg. *43:*268–278, Feb '39

THOREK, MAX: *Plastic Surgery of the Breast and Abdominal Wall.* C. C Thomas Co., Springfield, Ill., 1942

THOREK, M.: Twenty-five years' experience with plastic reconstruction of breast and transplantation of nipple. Am. J. Surg. *67:*445–466, March '45

THOREK, M.: Plastic reconstruction of breast and free transplantation of nipple (author's one-stage operation; microscopic proof of survival of transplanted nipple). J. Internat. Coll. Surgeons *9:*194–224, Mar–Apr '46

THORNTON, H. L. AND ROWBOTHAM, S.: Anesthesia in maxillofacial surgical unit with British Liberation Army. Anesthesiology *6:*580–596, Nov '45

THORSON, J. A.: Intratracheal anesthesia for surgery of head. J. Iowa M. Soc. *31:*465–472, Oct '41

THOUREN, G.: Jaw fractures in war; treatment. Nord. med. (Hygiea) *3:*2642–2656, Aug 26, '39

Throat

General versus local anesthesia in operations on nose and throat. WATSON, W. R. New York M. J. *113:*444, March 16, '21

Pulmonary complications following nose and throat operations. BORDEN, C. R. C. Laryngoscope *31:*851, Nov '21

A new local anesthetic for nose and throat work. BULSON, A. E. JR. Ann. Otol., Rhin. and Laryng. *31:*131–136, March '22

New instruments used in nose and throat and plastic surgery. SHEEHAN, J. E. New York M. J. *115:*493–494, April 19, '22 (illus.)

Fatalities following operations upon nose and throat not dependent upon anesthesia–study of 332 hitherto unreported cases. LOEB, H. W. Ann. Otol., Rhin. and Laryng. *31:*273–296, June '22

Throat—Cont.

Surgery of throat, nose and ear. Dundas-Grant, J. Practitioner *110:*11–25, Jan '23

Surgery in cancer of mouth and throat. Heidrich, L. Beitr. z. klin. Chir. *128:*310–347, '23 abstr: J.A.M.A. *80:*1348, May 5, '23

Further studies of fatalities following operations on nose and throat. Loeb, H. W. Ann. Otol., Rhin. and Laryng. *32:*1103-1107, Dec '23

Tumors of nose, throat and ear; review of literature. New, G. B. Arch. Otolaryng. *1:*545–552, May '25

Electrocoagulation and radiation therapy in malignant disease of ear, nose and throat. Pfahler, G. E., J.A.M.A. *85:*344–347, Aug 1, '25

Tumors of nose and throat. New, G. B. Arch. Otolaryng. *3:*461–465, May '26

Tumors of nose and throat; review of literature. New, G. B. Arch. Otolaryng. *5:*352–356, April '27

Peroral endoscopy; its use in complications following operations on nose and throat. Tucker, G. Arch. Otolaryng. *5:*321–333, April '27

Use of foreign bodies in ear, nose and throat surgery. Pollock, H. L. Ann. Otol., Rhin. and Laryng. *36:*463–471, June '27

Treatment of malignant tumors of mouth and throat. Figi, F. A. Am. J. Roentgenol. *23:*648–653, June '30

Personal and practical experiences with neoplasms about head and neck, with special reference to ear, nose and throat. Beck, J. C. Pennsylvania M. J. *34:*467–469, April '31

Tumors of nose and throat; summary of bibliographic material available in field of otolaryngology. New, G. B. and Kirch, W. Arch. Otolaryng. *15:*623–633, April '32

Postoperative hemorrhage in nose and throat operations; treatment with clauden. Thacker Neville, W. S. Lancet *2:*624–625, Sept 17, '32

Diagnosis and treatment of cancer of lip, mouth and throat. Christie, A. C. Fortschr. a. d. Geb. d. Rontgenstrahlen *53:*529–534, March '36

Recent advances in plastic and reconstructive surgery (of ears, nose and throat). Guttman, M. R. Am. J. M. Sc. *196:*875–882, Dec '38

Tumors of nose and throat; summaries of bibliographic material available in field of otolaryngology. New, G. B. *et al.* Arch. Otolaryng. *30:*283–297, Aug '39

War injuries of ear, nose and throat. Voss, O. Med. Klin. *35:*1589–1591, Dec 15, '39

Throat—Cont.

Progress of surgery of head (including face, ear, nose, mouth, etc.) and throat (esophagus and larynx); review of literature for 1940. Rebelo Neto, J. Rev. brasil. de oto-rino-laring. *9:*37–46, Jan–Feb '41

Minor surgery of nose and throat. Shambaugh, G. Jr. S. Clin. North America *21:*21–36, Feb '41

Surgical progress; head and throat; review of literature for 1941. Rebelo Neto, J. Rev. brasil. de oto-rino laring. *10:*347–357, May–June '42

Local regional anesthesia in nose and throat operations. Martin, G. E., J. Laryng. and Otol. *59:*38–43, Jan '44

Wounds of eye, ear, nose and throat. Smart, F. P., U.S. Nav. M. Bull. *44:*1231–1233, June '45

Throndson, A. H. (see Greeley, P. W.) April '44

Thumb: See Fingers, Various Categories

Thumb, Reconstruction of (See also: Fingers, Transplantation of Toe to Finger or Thumb)

Use of index finger for thumb, some interesting points in hand surgery. Dunlop, J., J. Bone and Joint Surg. *5:*99–103, Jan '23 (illus.)

Big toe as substitute for thumb. Troell, A. Hygiea *86:*407–413, June 30, '24

Cleft-thumb operated on by Cloquet's method. van Neck, M. Arch. franco-belges de chir. *28:*607–608, July '25

Transformation of middle finger into thumb; report of case. Jepson, P. N. Minnesota Med. *8:*552, Aug '25

Successful thumb plasty from big toe from opposite side 4½ years after unsuccessful transplantation. Porzelt, W. Arch. f. klin. Chir. *135:*340–355, '25

Supernumerary phalanx in thumbs; hyperphalangia pollicis. Kristjansen, A. Hospitalstid. *69:*109–119, Feb 4, '26

Autotransplantation of toe for traumatic loss of finger. Fuld, J. E., J.A.M.A. *86:*1281–1282, April 24, '26

Plastic reconstruction of thumb. Pieri, G. Chir. d. org. di movimento *11:*89–93, Sept '26

Reconstruction of thumb after total loss. Pierce, G. W. Surg., Gynec. and Obst. *45:*825–826, Dec '27

Treatment of finger injuries; plastic replacement of parts of thumb lost in industrial accident. Baumann, R. Schweiz. med. Wchnschr. *58:*918–925, Sept 15, '28

Thumb, Reconstruction of–Cont.
Results of new operation for substitution of thumb. JOYCE, J. L. Brit. J. Surg. *16:*362-369, Jan '29
Technic of restoration of thumb. GUEULLETTE, R., J. de chir. *36:*1-23, July '30
Construction of thumb from first metacarpal in case of absence of all fingers. KRAFT, R. Deutsche Ztschr. f. Chir. *226:*426-430, '30
Physiological reconstruction of thumb after total loss. BUNNELL, S. Surg., Gynec. and Obst. *52:*245-248, Feb '31
Anatomic restoration of injured thumb by graft of mutilated and useless index finger. BONNET, P. AND CARCASSONNE, F. Lyon chir. *28:*247-248, March-April '31
Phalangization of first metacarpal bone; technic, indications and results. BONNET, P. AND CARCASSONNE, F. Rev. de chir., Paris *50:*341-355, May '31
Anatomic restoration of thumb by graft of functionally useless index finger; case. BONNET, P. AND CARCASSONNE, F. Lyon chir. *28:*529-540, Sept-Oct '31
Autoplastic operations on thumb. PACHNER, E. Arch. di ortop. *48:*817-828, Dec 31, '32
Reconstruction of thumb from mutilated index finger with preservation and extension of skin fold from thumb to middle finger. PORZELT, W. Chirurg. *5:*61-65, Jan 15, '33
Plastic reconstruction of hand with phalangization of thumb. STETTEN, DEW. Ann. Surg. *97:*290-296, Feb '33
Phalangization of first metacarpal bone in surgical therapy of thumb injuries; 2 cases. FROSTE, N. Svenska lak.-tidning. *30:*337-341, April 7, '33
Phalangization of first metacarpal bone in surgical therapy of thumb injuries. NASTA, T. *et al.* Rev. de chir., Bucuresti *37:*234-237, March-April '34
Transplantation of toes for fingers. LABUNSKAYA, O. V. Ann. Surg. *102:*1-4, July '35
Transplantation of forefinger as substitute for lost thumb; preservation of fold dividing forefinger from middle finger and new formation of ball of thumb by transplantation of pedicled flap of abdominal skin. PORZELT, W. Zentralbl. f. Chir. *62:*2248-2253, Sept 21, '35
Transplantation of toes for fingers. BORISOV, M. V. Sovet. khir., no. 10, pp. 136-140, '35
Restoration of thumb from carpal bone. SHIPOV, A. K. Sovet. khir., no. 8, p. 163, '35
Transplantation of toe according to method of Nicoladoni; case. KUSLIK, M. I. Arch. Surg. *32:*123-130, Jan '36
Replacement of thumb with portion of index finger. GABRIEL, E. Munchen. med.

Thumb, Reconstruction of–Cont.
Wchnschr. *83:*1391-1393, Aug 21, '36
Reconstruction of left thumb by skin and osteoperiosteal grafts; case. DESPLAS, B. Mem. Acad. de chir. *62:*1292-1296, Nov 25, '36
Plastic transposition of index finger to replace entire thumb. BUZELLO, A. Zentralbl. f. Chir. *63:*2945-2952, Dec 12, '36
Plastic surgery of thumb and of thenar region. ANGLESIO, B. Boll. e mem. Soc. piemontese di chir. *6:*64-72, '36
Reparative plastic surgery; loss of thumb and methods of substitution. SORALUCE, J. Cir. ortop. y tramatol., Madrid *1:*247-254, '36
Usefulness of single finger; justifiability of using uninjured index finger to replace lost thumb. PORZELT, W. Zentralbl. f. Chir. *64:*550-551, March 6, '37
Restoration of thumb by transposition of second metacarpal; indications and technic; 2 cases. ISELIN, M. AND MURAT, J. Presse med. *45:*1099-1102, July 28, '37
Restoration of thumb using bone and skin grafts. HUARD, P. AND LONG, M. Bull. Soc. med.-chir. de l'Indochine *15:*855-860, Aug-Sept '37
Reconstruction of thumb. KINDERSLEY, C. E. Proc. Roy. Soc. Med. *30:*1260-1262, Aug '37
Plastic replacement of thumb by index finger; case. TIERNY, A. AND ISELIN, M. Mem. Acad. de chir. *63:*1007-1012, Oct 13, '37
Late results of transplantation of large toe to replace lost thumb. OEHLECKER, F. Arch. f. klin. Chir. *189:*674-680, '37
Plastic operation for congenital absence of thumb. LAMBRINUDI, C. Proc. Roy. Soc. Med. *31:*181-183, Jan '38
Plastic transposition of index finger to replace thumb. ZSULYEVICH, I. Orvosi hetil. *82:*153-154, Feb 12, '38
Use of first metacarpus in plastic restoration of thumb; case. BOLTE, R., J. de l'Hotel-Dieu de Montreal *7:*359-365, Nov-Dec '38
Plastic operations in loss of thumb. KÖSTER, K. H. Acta orthop. Scandinav. *9:*115-131, '38
Reconstruction of thumb after traumatic amputation. DIAL, D. E., J. Bone and Joint Surg. *21:*98-100, Jan '39
Total transplantation of large toe to replace thumb. NOVITSKIY, S. T. Vestnik khir. *57:*352-361, Feb-March '39
Phalangization of first metacarpal bone combined with round stylus plastic surgery in case of loss of thumb and skin on both hands. FALTIN, R. Nord. med. (Finska lak.-sallsk. handl.) *2:*1412-1415, May 13, '39

Thumb, Reconstruction of–Cont.
Plastic operations on great toe and thumb. PITZEN, P. Ztschr. f. Orthop. *70:*93–98, '39
Plastic reconstruction of fingers by means of transplantation of toes. APETROSYAN, K. A. Ortop. i travmatol. (no. 1) *13:*74–78, '39
Phalangization of first metacarpal bone in plastic restoration of thumb; anatomic basis of author's method. SHIROKOV, B. A. Khirurgiya, no. 7, pp. 115–122, '39
Plastic surgery to restore function after loss of thumb. MEYER-WILDISEN, R. Helvet. med. acta *6:*872–873, March '40
Conservation of useful thumb after complete phalangeal necrosis. HENRY, A. K. Lancet *1:*1123, June 22, '40
Toe to finger transplant. BLAIR, V. P. AND BYARS, L. T. Ann. Surg. *112:*287–290, Aug '40
Transplantation of toe for missing finger; end-result. NEUHOF, H. Ann. Surg. *112:*291–293, Aug '40
Successful substitution of second metacarpal bone for missing thumb; case. WITTEK, A. Chirurg *13:*577–581, Oct 1, '41
Reconstruction of thumb; new technic. MALTZ, M. Am. J. Surg. *58:*429–433, Dec '42
Phalangization of first metacarpus to substitute for thumb, with report of case. GIOIA, T. Semana med. *1:*490–497, March 4, '43
Plastic reconstruction of thumb. PETERSEN, N. South African M. J. *17:*137–138, May 8, '43
Simultaneous osteocutaneous graft in reconstruction of thumb. LABOK, D. M. Khirurgiya, no. 2, pp. 73–75, '44
Reconstruction of thumb; indications and results of 15 cases. MORANDI, G. Chir. d. org. di movimento *30:*41–51, Jan–Mar '46
Reconstruction of thumb. BEARDSLEY, J. M. AND ZECCHINO, V. Am. J. Surg. *71:*825–827, June '46
Reconstruction of thumb. GREELEY, P. W. Ann. Surg. *124:*60–70, July '46
Refrigeration in treatment of trauma (lacerated and almost detached thumb) KANAAR, A. G. Anesth. and Analg. *25:*177–190, Sept–Oct '46 *25:*228, Nov–Dec '46
Functional restoration of thumb; pollicization of the index. KELIKIAN, H. AND BINTCLIFFE, E. W. Surg. Gynec. and Obst. *83:*807–814, Dec '46

THUREL, R. (see GARCIN, R. *et al*) Nov '32
THUREL, R. (see GARCIN, R. *et al*) June '33
THUSS, C. J.: Skin grafting and reconstructive surgery. J. M. A. Alabama *10:*77–83, Sept '40
THUSS, C. J.: Simplified chin support. J. M. A. Alabama *13:*387–388, June '44

Thyroglossal Cysts and Fistulas

Cysts and fistulae of thyroglossal duct. GILMAN, P. K. Surg., Gynec. and Obst. *32:*141, Feb '21
Cysts of thyroglossal tract. SISTRUNK, W. E. S. Clin. N. Amer. *1:*1509, Oct '21
Congenital median and lateral fistulas in neck. BLAESEN, C. Deutsche Ztschr. f. Chir. *167:*60–64, '21
Thyroglossal cyst and fistula. GESSNER, H. B. Southern M. J. *17:*428–430, June '24
Case of true congenital thyroglossal fistula. BAILEY, H. Proc. Roy. Soc. Med. (Clin. Sect.) *18:*6–7, Jan '25
Thyroglossal cysts and fistulae. BAILEY, H. Brit. J. Surg. *12:*579–589, Jan '25
Study of thyroglossal tract. BERTWISTLE, A. P. AND FRAZER, J. E. Brit. J. Surg. *12:*561–578, Jan '25
Results of operations on thyroglossal tract and a note on thyroid secretions. BERTWISTLE, A. P. Canad. M.A.J. *15:*400–401, April '25
Congenital cysts and fistulae of neck; review of 42 thyroglossal cysts and fistulae. KLINGENSTEIN, P. AND COLP, R. Ann. Surg. *82:*854–864, Dec '25
Median cervical fistulae. HLAVÁČEK, V. Casop. lek. Cesk. *66:*511–514, March 28, '27
Persistent or patent thymic duct. COMER, M. C. Southwestern Med. *11:*308–309, July '27
Thyroglossal fistula, four times recurrent; case. BIDART MALBRÁN, J. C. Bol. y trab. de la Soc. de cir. de Buenos Aires *12:*491–498, Sept 5, '28
Aberrant thyroid glands in neck. LEECH, J. V. *et al*. Am. J. Path. *4:*481–492, Sept '28
Cysts and fistulae; thyroglossal; with notes of case. ARMSTRONG, H. G. St. Michael's Hosp. M. Bull. *3:*90–93, Dec '28
Congenital median fistula of neck. DE MARCHI, E. Arch. ital. di chir. *22:*91–100, '28
Thyroglossal fistula; classification, clinical aspects, surgical treatment; cases. EGÜES, A. Bol. Inst. de clin. quir. *4:*313–367, '28
Cysts and fistulae of median cervical line. MAGLIULO, A. Sperimentale. Arch. di biol *82:*455–504. '28
Lateral and internal cysts and fistula of neck. TOMILOFF, N. L. Vestnik khir. (nos. 43–44) *14:*234–237, '28
Congenital cyst of thymic origin in neck. PEZCOLLER, A. Clin. chir. *32:*272–284, March '29

Thyroglossal Cysts and Fistulas – Cont.
Cyst of ductus thymopharyngeus; case. BRECHET, J. Zentralbl. f. alig. Path. u. path. Anat. *69:*353-357, March 30, '38
Formation of medial cysts of neck. KORKHOFF, U. Vrach. gaz. *34:*779-781, May 31, '30
Fistula in center of neck; recidivation because of inflammation of Boyer's bursa; case. CIEZA RODRIGUEZ, M. Semana med. *1:*552-554, Feb 26, '31
Thyroglossal cysts and fistulae. JARVIS, H. G. New England J. Med. *205:*987-991, Nov 19, '31
Thyroglossal fistula; medical therapy; case. BERGARA, R. AND BERGARA, C. Rev. Asoc. med. argent. *47:*1983-1986, Jan '33
Thyroglossal fistula with submental opening (case). PARSONS, W. B. JR. Ann. Surg. *97:*143, Jan '33
Thyroglossal fistula in children; surgical therapy; 2 cases. NOGUEIRA, P. Rev. Assoc. paulista de med. *2:*206-212, April '33
Branchial cysts and fistulas in children; also thyroglossal duct cysts and fistulas. BAUMGARTNER, C. J. Surg., Gynec. and Obst. *56:*948-955, May '33
Medial cervical fistula probably of thyroglossal origin; recovery after surgical intervention. BÉRARD. *et al*. Lyon med. *151:*611-613, May 13, '33
Cystic tumors of neck; branchial and thyroglossal cysts. MCNEALY, R. W., S. Clin. North America *13:*1083-1100, Oct '33
Congenital median fistula of neck; pathogenesis and histology. ŚWIATLOWSKI, B. Monatschr. f. Ohrenh. *68:*1096-1106, Sept '34
Thyroglossal fistulae. BASTOS, E. Rev. otolaring. de Sao Paulo *3:*227-238, May-June '35
Branchial and thyroglossal duct cysts and fistulas. BROWN, J. M. Ann. Otol., Rhin. and Laryng. *44:*644-652, Sept '35
Congenital median cysts and fistulae of neck. IONESCU, N. V. Rev. san. mil., Bucuresti *35:*71-80, Jan '36
Management of cysts and fistulas (thyroglossal). HENDRICK, J. W. Texas State J. Med. *32:*34-36, May '36
Anatomy of subhyoid region with reference to diagnosis of mid-line swellings of neck. MEKIE, D. E. C. Malayan M. J. *11:*178-179, Sept '36
Complete thyroglossal fistula; case. PASQUALINO, G. Riv. san. siciliana *25:*586-593, May 15, '37
Persistence of thyroglossal duct; median cervical fistula; 2 cases. SORU, S. *et al*. Rev. de

Thyroglossal Cysts and Fistulas – Cont.
chir., Bucuresti *41:*48-56, Jan-Feb '38 also: Ann. d'oto-laryng., pp. 318-324, April '38
Avoiding postoperative recurrence of thyroglossal fistula in surgical therapy; necessity of resection of hyoid bone. CHIAROLANZA, R. Arch. ital. di chir. *51:*331-336, '38
Medial cervical fistula due to persistence of thyroglossal tract; case. RASTELLI, E. Gior. med. d. Alto Adige *11:*3-14, Jan '39
Complete thyroglossal fistulas. KINSELLA, V. J., Brit. J. Surg. *26:*714-720, April '39
Injection treatment of chronic sinuses; case of infected thyroglossal duct cured by copper sulfate injections. HUGHES, R. P. AND SMITH, L. M. Southwestern Med. *23:*187, June '39
Thyroglossal fistulas and cysts. OTTOBRINI COSTA, M. AND LABATE, F. Pediatria prat., Sao Paulo *10:*287-300, July-Aug '39
Technic for extirpation of thyroglossal fistulas. FINOCHIETTO, R. AND VEPPO, A. A. Prensa med. argent. *26:*1920-1926, Oct 4, '39
Extirpation of hyoid bone in therapy of thyroglossal cyst; 3 cases. SUMERMAN, S. Turk tib cem. mec. *5:*265-271, '39
Thyroglossal cysts, sinuses and fistulae; results in 293 surgical cases. PEMBERTON, J. DEJ. AND STALKER, L. K. Ann. Surg. *111:*950-957, June '40
Thyroglossal fistula due to persistence of thyroglossal tract; cases. ALTAVISTA, A. E. Rev. otorrinolaring. d. litoral *1:*232-241, March '42
Thyroglossal fistula, with report of case. CASANUEVA DEL C., M. AND VILLARROEL, E. Arch. Soc. cirujanos hosp. *12:*79-84, May-Aug '42
Cystic tumors; branchial and thyroglossal cysts. MCNEALY, R. W., J. Am. Dent. A. *29:*1808-1818, Oct 1, '42
Differential diagnosis between thymic duct fistulas and branchial cleft fistulas; case of bilateral aural fistulas and bilateral thymic duct fistulas. BAUMGARTNER, C. J. AND STEINDEL, S. Am. J. Surg. *59:*99-103, Jan '43
Lymphoepithelial papilliferous cystomas of branchial, thyroglossal and thyropharyngeal origin. LUPPI, J. E. Rev. med. de Rosario *33:*608-623, July '43
Papillary tumors of lateral aberrant thyroid origin; discussion and report of 4 cases. STRODE, J. E. Proc. Staff Meet. Clin., Honolulu *9:*103-113, Nov '43
Complete thyroglossal fistula; 2 cases. COU-

Thyroglossal Cysts and Fistulas – Cont.

Dane, R. and Fabre, A. Ann. d'oto-laryng., pp. 93-99, July-Sept '44

Thyroglossal cysts and fistulas; 8 cases. Sibilia, C. E. Rev. Asoc. med. argent. *58:*888-891, Oct 15, '44

Thyroglossal cysts and fistulas; 8 cases. Sibilla, C. E. Bol. y trab., Soc. argent. de cirujanos *5:*543-553, '44

Salivary fistula of submaxillary gland following excision of thyroglossal cyst. Jenkins, H. B. Am. J. Surg. *70:*118-120, Oct '45

Thyrotomy

Two-stage thyrotomy in cases considered bad risks. New, G. B. Arch. Otolaryng. *9:*538-542, May '29

Tice, L. F. (see Flack, H. L. *et al*) July '45

Tichonovich, A.: Formation of artificial vagina by Baldwin method with Constantini's modification. J. Akush. i Zhensk. Boliez. *38:*301-305, May-June '27

Tickle, T. G.: Nerve transplant for facial paralysis. Laryngoscope *49:*475-481, June '39

Tickle, T. G.: Facial nerve surgery in 300 cases. Laryngoscope *55:*191-195, May '45

Tickle, T. G. (see Duel, A. B.) March '36

Tidrick, R. T. and Warner, E. D.: Fibrin fixation of skin transplants. Surgery *15:*90-95, Jan '44

Tieck, G. J. E. and Hunt, H. L.: Plastic and cosmetic surgery of head, neck and face (including keloids). Am. J. Surg. *35:*173, June '21; 355, Nov '21

Tieck, G. J. E. and Hunt, H. L.: Plastic and cosmetic surgery of head, face and neck; correction of nasal deformities. Am. J. Surg. *35:*234, Aug '21

Tieck, G. J. E.; Hunt, H. L. and Maxeiner, S. R.: Plastic surgery of head, face and neck, local anesthesia in operations upon head, face and neck. Am. J. Surg. *36:*29-42, Feb '22 (illus.)

Tierny, A.: Free full thickness skin grafts. Gaz. med. de France *44:*795-797, Oct 1, '37

Tierny, A. and Iselin, M.: Plastic replacement of thumb by index finger; case. Mem. Acad. de chir. *63:*1007-1012, Oct 13, '37

Tiesenhausen, K.: Use of pedicled skin flaps to cover skin defects. Zentralbl. f. Chir. *57:*1985-1988, Aug 9, '30

Tikanadse, I.: Congenital absence of vagina and its artificial formation with Amann's method. Zentralbl. f. Gynak. *50:*547-549, Feb 27, '26

Tikhomirov, P. E.: Operation for correction of eversion of inferior lacrimal point. Vestnik oftal. *11:*216-217, '37

Tikhonovich, A. V.: Transplantation of muscles in paralysis of radial nerve following gunshot wounds. Khirurgiya, no. 3, pp. 72-73, '44

Tikhova, V. A.: Local application of cod liver oil in therapy of burns of eyes. Vestnik oftal. *17:*396-397, '40

Tilk, G. U.: Surgical therapy of exstrophy of bladder, with special reference to Maydl and Coffey operations. Deutsche Ztschr. f. Chir. *257:*287, '43

Tillier, R.: Cranioplasty with osseous grafts for large loss of substance of frontal bone; case. Bull. et mem. Soc. nat. de chir. *56:*1277-1282, Nov 29, '30

Tillier, R. (see Curtillet, J.) Nov-Dec '25

Tillmann, G.: Statistics for years 1936-1940 in clinic for dentistry and maxillary injuries at University of Kiel. Ztschr. f. Stomatol. *40:*61-75, Jan 30, '42

Tillotson, R. S.: Fractures of bones of face. California and West. Med. *57:*137-141, Aug '42

Timofeev, S. L.: Clinical aspects of burns. Sovet. vrach. zhur., pp. 416-420, March 30, '36

Timoney, F. X.: Macrodactyly; case. Ann. Surg. *119:*144-147, Jan '44

Tinel Sign

Value of Tinel sign (in relation to regeneration of peripheral nerve lesions). Nathan, P. W. and Rennie, A. M. Lancet *1:*610-611, April 27, '46

Tinker, M. B. and Tinker, M. B. Jr.: Repair of peripheral nerve injuries. Ann. Surg. *106:*943-951, Nov '37

Tinker, M. B. Jr. (see Tinker, M. B.) Nov '37

Tinozzi, F. P.: Skin grafts; effect of emulsion of pyogenic bacteria. Ann. ital. di chir. *5:*981-1000, Oct 30, '26

Tinozzi, F. P.: Skin grafts; effect of cervical sympathectomy; experiments. Rassegna internaz. di clin. e terap. *7:*585-604, Nov 10, '26

Tinozzi, F. P.: Importance of local immunity in elimination of homoplastic skin grafts. Ann. ital. di chir. *7:*660-683, July 31, '28

Tippett, G. O.: Orthopedic surgery in treatment of rheumatism and rheumatoid arthritis. Practitioner *139:*271-278, Sept '37

Tirelli, G.: Congenital fistulas of lacrimal sac. Rassegna ital. d'ottal. *1:*66-75, Jan-Feb '32

Tirelli, G.: Congenital eyelid ptosis; cases. Rassegna ital. d'ottal. *4:*224-236, March-April '35

Tiscornia, A.: Histophilic asepsis (in plastic

surgery). Minerva med. *1:*481-485, June 16, '42

TISALE, A. A.: The more common hand fractures. New Orleans M. and S. J. *92:*356-359, Jan '40

TISSANDIÉ. (see GUILLERMO) Dec '36

Tissue Banks

Transplantation and vital storage. LEHMANN, W. AND TAMMANN, H. Beitr. z. klin. Chir. *135:*259-302, '25 abstr: Klin. Wchnschr. *4:*2342-2343, Dec 3, '25 abstr: J.A.M.A. *86:*316, Jan 23, '26

Provisional storage of tissues to be transplanted (experiments with surviving tissues). KUBANYL, E. Arch. f. klin. Chir. *161:*502-510, '30

Refrigerated cartilage isografts; source, storage and use. O'CONNOR, G. B. California and West. Med. *52:*21-23, Jan '40

Therapy of trachomatous pannus by transplantation of lip mucosa preserved at low temperature. KIPARISOV, N. M. Vestnik oftal. *17:*227-229, '40

Refrigerated cartilage for use in plastic surgery. ADLER, D. Arq. de cir. clin. e exper. *6:*608-611, April–June '42

Peripheral nerve repair by grafts of frozen-dried nerve. WEISS, P. AND TAYLOR, A. C. Proc. Soc. Exper. Biol. and Med. *52:*326-328, April '43

Cadaver cailage banks. NUNN, L. L. Bull. U. S. Army M. Dept. (no. 74) pp. 99-101, March '44

Storage of skin for autogenous grafts (Hunterian lecture, abridged). MATTHEWS, D. N. Lancet *1:*775-778, June 23, '45

TITONE, M.: Spinofacial anastomosis for facial paralysis. Lyon chir. *18:*601-605, Sept-Oct '21 (illus.) abstr: J.A.M.A. *78:*249, Jan 21, '22

TITOV, E. S.: Atomizer for burn therapy with vitaderm (carotene preparation). Ortop. i. travmatol. (no. 2) *14:*24-25, '40

TITTERINGTON, P. F.: Facial bone fractures. Radiology *11:*207-212, Sept '28

TITZE, L. O. (see JOHNSTON, B.) Nov '44

TIXIER, L. AND BIZE, P. R.: Skin grafts in treatment of chronic leg ulcer. Monde med., Paris *37:*449-455, April 1, '27

TIXIER, L. AND BONNET, P.: Epithelioma of face secondary to extensive epithelioma of eyelids; three-stage operation; removal of tumor, skin graft and restoration of eyelids. Lyon chir. *28:*719-722, Nov–Dec '31

TIXIER, L.; DE ROUGEMONT, J. AND CARCASSONNE, F.: Acute suppurative synovitis of tendon sheath following wound of right index finger; excellent function after surgical therapy; case. Lyon chir. *28:*714-717, Nov–Dec '31

TJIONG NJAN HAN: Veau operation for correction of harelip. Geneesk. tijdschr. v. Nederl. - Indie *79:*3034-3045, Nov 28, '39

TOBECK, A.: Neurogenic tumors of nose. Ztschr. f. Hals-, Nasen-u. Ohrenh. *23:*329-339, Sept 10, '29

TOBECK, A.: Postoperative disturbances in nasal surgery. Med. Klin. *30:*629-631, May 11, '34

TOBECK, A.: Surgical therapy of perichondritis of auricle. Ztschr. f. Hals-, Nasen-u. Ohrenh. *44:*368-373, '38

TOBIÁŠEK: Tobiášek's method of operation for Dupuytren's disease. Casop. lek. cesk. *69:*421, March 14; 459, March 21, '30

TOCANTINS, L. M.; O'NEILL, J. F. AND PRICE, A. H.: Infusions of blood and other fluids via bone marrow in traumatic shock and other forms of peripheral circulatory failure. Ann. Surg. *114:*1085-1092, Dec '41

TOCANTINS, L. M. (see O'NEILL, J. R. *et al*) Sept '42

TOD, M. C.: Tragedy of malignant melanoma. Lancet *2:*532-534, Oct 21, '44

TOD, M. C. (see PATERSON, R.) Nov '39

TODD, I. P.: Labial adhesions in children. Brit. M. J. *2:*13-14, July 6, '46

TODD, J. P. (see CLARK, A. M. *et al*) April '45

TODD, J. P. (see COLEBROOK, L. *et al*) April '44

TODD, M. C.: Extensive burns. Illinois M. J. *81:*329-331, April '42

TODD, T. W.: Prognathism; study in development of face. J. Am. Dent. A. *19:*2172-2184, Dec '32

Toe-to-Finger Transplants: See Fingers, Transplantation of Toe to; Thumb, Reconstruction of

TOGUNOVA, E. F. (see SMORODINTZEFF, A. A.) 1931

TOKAREVA, B. A. (see KLYKOVA, A. L.) 1938

TOLAND, J. J. JR. AND KORNBLUEH, I. H.: Industrial injuries to fingers. Pennsylvania M. J. *47:*466-473, Feb '44

TOLMACH, J. A. (see TRAUB, E. F.) July '33

TOLOSA, A.: Dupuytren's contracture; case, probably of medullary origin complicating sensory disturbances of syringomyelic type. Bol. Soc. de med. e cir. de Sao Paulo *16:*158-162, Jan '33

TOMÁNEK, F.: Radium therapy of Dupuytren's contracture. Casop. lek. cesk. *74:*46-47, Jan 11, '35

TOMB, J. W.: Case of minor surgery of hand; accidental amputation of finger with preservation of terminal phalanx. Lancet *2:*930, Oct 27, '23

TOMB, J. W.: Linimentum calcis chlorinatae in treatment of burns. Brit. M. J. *1:*711, April 19, '24

TOMB, J. W.: Chlorinated carron oil for burns. M. Press *125:*99, Feb 1, '28

TOMB, J. W.: Traumatic shock and sympathetic overstimulation. South African M. J. *15:*109–111, March 22, '41

TOMB, J. W.: Collapse (of circulation in traumatic shock) and renal failure. M. J. Australia *2:*569–570, Nov 15, '41

TOMB, J. W.: Shock and concussion. M. J. Australia *1:*250–256, Feb 28, '42

TOMESKU, I.: Syndactylia and synectrodactyly. Fortschr. a. d. Geb. d. Rontgenstrahlen *36:*629–631, Sept '27

TOMESKU, I.: Congenital contractures of fingers and clinodactyly; 4 cases. Arch. f. Orthop. *26:*126–137, '28

TOMILIN, A. I.: Total avulsion of scalp; case. Vestnik khir. *59:*375, April '40

TOMILOFF, N. L.: Lateral and internal cysts and fistula of neck. Vestnik khir. (nos. 43–44) *14:*234–237, '28

TOMIRDIARO, O.: Extension treatment of fractures of mandible by combined method (Darcissac-Bruhn-Petroff). Deutsche Monatschr. f. Zahnh. *49:*1112–1116, Nov 15, '31

TOMKEVICH, A. I.: Late results of external dacryocystorhinostomy. Vestnik oftal. *13:*388–396, '38

TOMOFF, W.: Preventing formation of painful neuromas after amputations by direct implantation of nerves into muscle (neurotization). Ztschr. f. d. ges. exper. Med. *84:*287–300, '32

TOMOFF, W.: Therapy of cleft lip, jaw and palate with protruding intermaxillary bone. Zentralbl. f. Chir. *63:*2535–2538, Oct 24, '36

Tongue

Two rare congenital anomalies; 1. hydro-encephalocele; 2. intra-uterine adhesion of tip of tongue to hard palate. ESAU, P. Arch. f. klin. Chir. *118:*817–820, '21

Plastic reconstruction of larynx and trachea. SCHMIDT, C. Schweiz. med. Wchnschr. *52:*539–540, May 25, '22

Carcinoma of jaws, tongue, cheek and lips; general principles involved in operations and results obtained at Cleveland Clinic. CRILE, G. W. Surg., Gynec. and Obst. *36:*159–162, Feb '23 (illus.)

Automatic gag and tongue holder. SAMENGO, L. Semana med. *1:*734–738, April 19, '23 (illus.)

Carcinoma of tongue; general principles involved in operations and results obtained at Mayo Clinic. JUDD, E. S. AND NEW, G. B. Surg., Gynec. and Obst. *36:*163–169, Feb '23 (illus.)

Tongue – Cont.

Resection of lower jaw for removal of cancer of tongue. KRASSIN, P. M. Zentralbl. f. Chir. *53:*3095–3100, Dec 4, '26

Glandular involvement following cancer of lips, tongue and floor of mouth. REGAUD, C. *et al.* Paris med. *1:*357–372, April 16, '27 also: Strahlentherapie *26:*221–251, '27

Experience in treatment of epitheliomata of tongue with glandular involvement. ROUX-BERGER, J. L. AND MONOD, O. Bull. et mem. Soc. nat. de chir. *53:*648–659, May 14, '27

Glossoptosis and facial deformity. LAUMONIER, J. Gaz. d. hop. *100:*848–850, June 25, '27

Surgical treatment of invasion of cervical glands in lingual cancer. ROUX-BERGER, J. L. Presse med. *35:*881, July 13, '27

Radium therapy of cancer of tongue; 143 cases. CAPIZZANO, N. Rev. med. latino-am. *13:*464–470, Dec '27

Early clinical and therapeutic study of invasion of lymphatic nodes in pavement epitheliomas of lips and tongue; 8 cases. LECÈNE, P. Prat. med. franc. *7:*219–227, May (A) '28

Adjustable mouthgag tongue depressor. LEWIS, E. R. Arch. Otolaryng. *7:*636, June '28

Cancer of tongue and floor of mouth. DORRANCE, G. M. AND MCSHANE, J. K. Ann. Surg. *88:*1007–1021, Dec '28

Tumors of lips, tongue, gums and alveolar processes. MITTERMAIER, R. Handb. d. Hals-, Nasen-, Ohrenh. *5:*582–618, '29

Osteoplastic partial resection of lower jaw by Krassin's method for removal of lingual cancer; 5 cases. NASAROW, N. N. AND KUSCHEWA, M. N. Deutsche Ztschr. f. Chir. *215:*145–146, '29

Leukoplakia of mouth and labial and lingual cancer in smokers. HAASE, G. Deutsche Monatschr. f. Zahnh. *49:*881, Sept 15; 929, Oct 1, '31

Tumors of tonsil and pharynx; 357 cases. NEW, G. B. Tr. Am. Laryng. A. *53:*277–309, '31

Highly malignant tumors of pharynx and base of tongue; identification and treatment. NEW, G. B. *et al.* Surg., Gynec. and Obst. *54:*164–174, Feb '32

Massive electrical burns with destruction of part of larynx and trachea. BABCOCK, W. W., S. Clin. North America *12:*1415–1417, Dec '32

Analysis of 138 cases of cancer of tongue

Tongue—Cont.
treated at Instituto del Cancer in Havana. MARTÍNEZ, E. Bol. Liga contra el cancer *8:*12–21, Jan '33
Treatment of neck glands in cancer of lip, tongue and mouth; study of present-day practice (questionnaire report of Cancer Commission of California Medical Association). PFLUEGER, O. H. California and West. Med. *39:*391–397, Dec '33
Keloid on tip of tongue in trumpeter; case. SCHMIDT, W. Dermat. Wchnschr. *99:*1341–1342, Oct 13, '34
Two instruments for modelling transplanted cartilage in closure of laryngeal and tracheal defects. MAYER, F. J. Monatschr. f. Ohrenh. *69:*1193–1196, Oct '35
Cancer of tongue and lower jaw. NEW, G. B. Tr. Am. Laryng., Rhin. and Otol. Soc. *41:*610–613, '35
Combined congenital malformation of tongue and hard palate; case. KOLESOV, G. G. Sovet. khir., no. 9, pp. 524–526, '36
Five year end-results in treatment of cancer of tongue, lip and cheek. MARTIN, H. E. Surg., Gynec. and Obst. *65:*793–797, Dec '37
Results of surgical therapy and radiotherapy of epitheliomas of mouth, tongue and larynx. CHERYSSICOS, J. AND LAMBADARIDIS, A. Ztschr. f. Hals-, Nasen-u. Ohrenh. *40:*410–413, '37
Tracheotomy for grave subcutaneous emphysema following cervicofacial trauma; cases. CASTELNAU, M. Oto-rhino-Laryng. internat. *22:*195–196, April '38
Analysis of 73 consecutive cases of tongue cancer; preliminary report. TURNER, J. W. AND RIFE, C. S. Univ. Hosp. Bull., Ann Arbor *4:*33–35, May '38
Treatment of cancer of tongue. BLAIR, V. P. *et al.* S. Clin. North America *18:*1255–1274, Oct '38
Injuries to tongue and palate; therapy. ROCHETTE, M. Hospital *27:*281–282, May '39
Lesions of tongue; collective review. BROWN, J. B. AND HAFFNER, H. Am. J. Orthodontics *25:*1213–1223, Dec '39
Speech rehabilitation following excision of tip of tongue. BACKUS, O. Am. J. Dis. Child. *60:*368–370, Aug '40
Angioma arteriale racemosum of face and tongue; surgical therapy; case. PAVLOVSKY, A. J. Bol. y trab., Acad. argent. de cir. *26:*670–672, Aug 19, '42
Tongue wounds. MIKHELSON, N. M. Sovet. med. (no. 1) *7:*6–7, '43
Tongue wounds. MICHAELSON, N. M. Am. Rev. Soviet Med. *1:*216–219, Feb '44 also:

Tongue—Cont.
Sovet. med., no. 1, pp. 6–7, '43
Epithelioid giant cell tumor of tongue, locally malignant; report of case. DINGMAN, R. O. J. Oral Surg. *2:*77–80, Jan '44
Cancer of skin, lip and tongue. MARTIN, H. Bull. Am. Soc. Control Cancer *26:*82–83, July '44
Congenital lymphangiomatous macroglossia with cystic hygroma of neck. LIERLE, D. M. Ann. Otol., Rhin. and Laryng. *53:*574–575, Sept '44
Congenital lymphangiomatous macroglossia with cystic hygroma. LIERLE, D. M. Tr. Am. Laryng. A. *66:*194–196, '44
Median harelip, cleft palate and glossal agenesis. SINCLAIR, J. G. AND MCKAY, J. Anat. Rec. *91:*155–160, Feb '45

DE TONI, G.: Acrocephalosyndactylia; case. Pediatria *34:*1305–1309, Dec 1, '26
TONNIS, W. AND GOTZE, W.: Surgical therapy of gunshot wounds of peripheral nerves; outlook for its success. Deut.Militararzt *7:*245–253, April '42
TÖNNIS, W. AND GÖTZE, W.: Operative treatment of gunshot wounds of peripheral nerves. Bull. War Med. *3:*196–197, Dec '42 (abstract)
TOPA, P.: Infra-red light in burns. Rev. de chir., Bucuresti *42:*718–721, Sept–Oct '39
TOPA, P. AND THEODORESCO, D.: Surgical therapy of zygomatic fracture; case. Tech. chir. *30:*45–50, March–April '38
TOPROWER, G. S.: Forced method of total rhinoplasty. Wien. klin. Wchnschr. *45:*1015–1017, Aug 12, '32
TORCHIANA, L.: Congenital cystic lymphangioma of neck. Arch. ital. di chir. *16:*173–192, '26
TORCHIANA, L.: Duodenal ulcer following burns; medicolegal importance, with report of case following industrial accident. Policlinico (sez. prat.) *43:*2105–2112, Nov 23, '36
TORELLÓ CENDRA, M.: Auricular dyschondrogenesis; technic of surgical correction. But. Soc. catalana de pediat. *6:*193–198, July–Aug '33
TORGERSON, W. R.: Auchincloss operation in elephantiasis; preliminary report. Porto Rico J. Pub. Health and Trop. Med. *6:*411–418, June '31
TORGERSON, W. R. (see SMITH, R. R.) Sept '25
TORMEY, A.: Diagnosis and treatment of hand infections. Wisconsin M. J. *30:*176–182, March '31
DEL TORO, J.; PONS, J. A. AND RODRÍGUEZ MOLINA, R.: Case report of 12 Auchincloss or modified Auchincloss operations for filariasis elephantiasis; preliminary report. Porto Rico

J. Pub. Health and Trop. Med. *7:*3–10, Sept '31

TORRACA, L.: Total necrosis of mandible from acute osteomyelitis. Arch. ital. di chir. *12:*653–672, '25

TORRE, D.: Urethroplasty in penoscrotal hypospadias using Passaggi-Galliera technic. Ann. ital. di chir. *16:*841–854, Oct '37

DELLA TORRE, P. L.: Postoperative facial paralysis treated with Leriche operation, excision of upper cervical sympathetic ganglion; case. Cervello *9:*299–312, Nov 15, '30

TORRES, G. A. AND OSACAR, E. M.: Avulsion of skin of penis and scrotum; reparative genitoplasty. Bol. y trab. Soc. de cir. de Cordoba *7:*225–237, '46

TORRES ESTRADA, A.: Technic in external dacryocystorhinostomy. Gac. med. de Mexico *62:*339–360, Aug '31

TORRES ESTRADA, A.: Technic of external dacryocystorhinostomy. An. Soc. mex. de oftal. y oto-rino-laring. *9:*131–157, April–June '32

TORRES ESTRADA, A.: Simplification of classic technic of external dacryocystorhinostomy. Cir. y cirujanos *5:*219–250, May–June '37

TORRES ESTRADA, A.: Spasmodic entropion; new surgical technic in therapy. Bol. d. Hosp. oftal. de Ntra. Sra. de la Luz *1:*265–272, Nov–Dec '41

TORRES ESTRADA, A.: New surgical technic for treating spasmodic entropion. Cir. y cirujanos *9:*559–569, Dec 31, '41

TORRES ESTRADA, A.: Simplified technic for dacryocystorhinostomy. J. Internat. Coll. Surgeons *7:*147–158, March–April '44

TORRES ESTRADA, A.: Importance of repositioning of lacrimal openings in treating senile ectropion. Gac. med. de Mexico *75:*336–351, Oct 31, '45

Torres Estrada Operation

External dacryocystorhinostomy by Torres Estrada technic. GURRIA URGELL, D. Gac. med. de Mexico *69:*336–340, Oct 30, '39

TORRES LUQUIN, P.: Nasal septal autoplasty in therapy of perforation; cases. An. Soc. mex. de oftal. y oto-rino-laring. *10:*47–54, March–June '33

TORRES POSSE, A.: Surgical therapy of harelip. Bol. Soc. de cir. de Rosario *12:*88–107, June '45

TORRES TORIJA, J.: Mediosocial problem of false hermaphroditism; case with hypospadias and ectopic testicles. Gac. med. de Mexico *64:*534–542, Dec '33

TORREY, F. A. (see TAUSSIG, L. R.) Jan '40

TORTI, D. D. (see CABALLERO, A.) July '46

TORTI, M.: Congenital fistula of lacrimal sac; 2 cases. Rassegna ital. d'ottal. *15:*69–76, Jan–Feb '46

Torticollis

Congenital torticollis with unilateral facial atrophy; case. DE VESTEA, D. Rassegna internaz. de clin. e terap. *9:*16–29, Jan '28

Causes of facial asymmetry in muscular wryneck and jaw dislocations. BECK, O. Ztschr. f. orthop. Chir. *49:*424–449, May 18, '28

TORTOLONE, V.: Cicatricial stenosis of choannae narium. Arch. ital. di otol. *43:*265–276, May '32

TORVISO, R. E.: Mendez biologic method of burn therapy. Semana med. *2:*732–734, Sept 6, '34

TOSTIVINT, R. (see DESPLAS, B.) Oct '45

TOTI: Results of anastomotic method of treatment of lacrimal obstruction. Proc. Roy. Soc. Med. (Sect. Ophth.) *14:*59, Aug. '21

Toti Operation (See also Mosher-Toti Operation)

Toti-Mosher operation; dacryocystorhinostomy; combined endonasal and external technic. SIBBALD, D. AND O'FARRELL, G. Rev. Soc. argent. de Oftal. *1:*79–82, '25

Historical observation on improvement of Toti's operation (dacryocystorhinostomy). OHM, J. Klin. Monatsbl. f. Augenh. *77:*825–832, Dec '26

Toti-Mosher operation; dacryocystorhinostomy. SIBBALD, AND O'FARRELL. Rev. de especialid. *1:*568–573, '26

Toti's dacryocystorhinostomy. WISSELINK, G. W. Klin. Monatsbl. f. Augenh. *78:*550, April '27

Simplified dacryocystorhinostomy, modification of Toti's method. DE LIETO VOLLARO, A. Boll. d'ocul. *8:*561–574, June '29

Modification of Toti's dacryocystorhinostomy. POLJAK, G. D. Klin. Monatsbl. f. Augenh. *83:*510–515, Oct–Nov '29

New instruments for Toti operation (dacryocystorhinostomy). GUTZEIT, R. Klin. Monatsbl. f. Augenh. *84:*92, Jan '30

Toti-Mosher operation (lacrimal ducts) and its end results. MARTIN, R. C. Tr. Pacific Coast Oto-Ophth. Soc. *21:*50–58, '33

Result of surgical therapy of suppuration of lacrimal sac after implantation of lower end of lacrimal sac into nose; modified Toti operation. STOCK, W. Klin. Monatsbl. f. Augenh. *92:*433–435, April '34

Use of mucosa of lips in Toti operation on lacrimal ducts. JANCKE, G. Ber. u. d. Versamml. d. deutsch. ophth. Gesellsch. *51:*478–479, '36

TOTIS, B.: Cosmetic surgery of breast. Gyogyaszat *73:*467–468, July 23–30, '33

TOURAINE, A.: Therapy of elephantiasis of extremities by lymphatic drainage by buried tubes (Walther operation); 2 cases. Bull. Soc. franc. de dermat. et syph. *42:*1771–1775, Dec '35

TOURAINE, A. AND RENAULT, P.: Therapy of tuberous angiomas with sclerosing injections of sodium salicylate. Presse med. *41:*259, Feb 15, '33

TOURAINE, A. AND SOLENTE: Glandular cheilitis, precancerous state of lower lip. Presse med. *42:*191–194, Feb 3, '34

TOURAINE, A.; SOLENTE AND VIALATTE: Craniofacial dysostosis with hypertelorism in congenital syphilis; case. Bull. Soc. franc. de dermat. et syph. *43:*612–618, March '36

TOURNEUX, J. P.: Hypertrophy of breasts at puberty. Rev. franc. de gynec. et d'obstet. *18:*454–459, July 10–25, '23

TOURNEUX, J. P.: Cancer of back of hand. Progres med., pp. 149–158, Jan 24, '31

TOUSSAINT ARAGON, E.: Left total congenital hemihypertrophy; case. Rev. mex. de pediat. *12:*343–356, Oct 10, '42

TOWBIN, B. G.: Histologic changes in membrane transplanted from lip to trachomatous eye (Denig's method). Arch. f. Ophth. *125:*643–651, '31

TOWBIN, B. G.: Surgical therapy of flow of tears after removal of lacrimal sac. Arch. f. Ophth. *135:*579–580, '36

TOWN, A. E. (see KIRBY, D. B.) April '43

TOYOSHIMA, Y.: Congenital aural fistula in marines; statistical study. Oto-rhino-laryng. *9:*825, Sept '36

TOZER, F. H. W.: Hypertelorism, case. Roy. Berkshire Hosp. Rep., pp. 17–21, '33

TRABUE, C. C.: Triple dyes in burn therapy. J. Tennessee M. A. *36:*13–19, Jan '43

Trachea

Midline congenital cervical fistula of tracheal origin. SEELIG, M. G. Arch. Surg. *2:*338, March '21

Plastic correction of defects in larynx and trachea. PFEIFFER, C. Zentralbl. f. Chir. *48:*965, July 9, '21

Plastic closure of tracheostomic fistula. JACKSON, C. AND BABCOCK, W. W., S. Clin. North America *14:*199–202, Feb '34

Plastic closure of laryngostomic fistulas and enlargement of lumen of trachea or larynx by implantatiion of chondrocutaneous flap. BABCOCK, W. W. Arch. Otolaryng. *19:*585–589, May '34

Experimental studies on transplantation of cartilage (ear) to cover tracheal defect. MORI, S. Okayama-Igakkai-Zasshi *48:*516, March '36

Traumatic stenosis of trachea treated by skin grafting. HARRISON, W. J. Brit. M. J. *2:*811, Oct 24, '36

Plastic closure of tracheal fistula. KÖNIG, E. Hals-, Nasen-u. Ohrenarzt (Teil 1) *28:*279–282, July '37

Laryngotracheal reconstruction with free autoplastic cartilaginous grafts. GIUSSANI, M. Arch. ital. di chir. *52:*472–483, '38

Wounds of neck and lesions of larynx, trachea and esophagus in war surgery. DE ANDRADE MEDICIS, J. Arq. brasil. de cir. e ortop. *10:*155–179, '42

Plastic procedure in correction of laryngotracheostenosis with dermoepidermic skin grafts. RAPIN, M. Pract. oto-rhino-laryng. *4:*88–91, '42

Emergency treatment of smashed-in face; value of tracheotomy and laryngotomy. PATEY, D. H. AND RICHES, E. W. Lancet *2:*161–162, Aug 7, '43

Closure of orifices of tracheotomy; Aubry procedure (graft). CARDIN, M. Ann. d'oto-laryng. *12:*305–314, April–June '45

Tubular graft in laryngotracheal fistula. VIANA ROSA, A. Rev. med. Rio Grande do Sul *2:*167–172, Jan–Feb '46

TRAINOR, M. E.: Eyelid ptosis operation. Tr. Sect. Ophth., A. M. A., pp. 93–97, '35

TRAKHTENBERG, K. I.: Trophic ulcers and their surgical therapy in injuries of sciatic nerve. Vopr. neyrokhir. (no. 4) *5:*61, '41

TRAMPNAU: Dermoid cyst of nose; case. Ztschr. f. Hals-, Nasen-u. Ohrenh. *28:*163–165, March 3, '31

TRAMSEN, H.: Preparation of concentrated or dry serum and plasma and its application in treatment of shock (especially in war surgery). Ugesk. f. laeger *103:*1357–1362, Oct 23, '41

TRANQUILLI-LEALI, E.: Complete ankylosis of temporomaxillary joint: surgical therapy; 2 cases. Rassegna d. previd. sociale *21:*8–45, Sept '34

Transplantation

Leukocytic and fibroblastic reactions about transplanted tissues. FLEISHER, M. S. J. M. Research *42:*163, Nov '20–Jan '21

Unsuccessful trials with alloplasty in vascular wounds. HABERLAND, H. F. O. Zentralbl. f. Chir. *49:*542–543, April 22, '22

Transplantation of tissues. SCHULZE, W. Klin. Wchnschr. *1:*793–797, April 15, '22

Use of tissues for various plastic purposes. ESSER, J. F. S. Munchen. med. Wchnschr. *69:*1186–1187, Aug 11, '22

Transplantation – Cont.
Research on autoplastics. IMBERT, L., J. de chir. *18:*113–129, Aug '21 (illus.) abstr: J.A.M.A. *78:*688, March 4, '22
Parabiosis and organ transplantation. KROSS, I. Surg., Gynec. and Obst. *35:*495–496, Oct '22
Transplantation of tissues and organs. GOODMAN, C. Internat. Clinics *3:*54–72, '22
Experimental growth of bone and cartilage. POLETTINI, B. Arch. ital. di chir. *6:*179–191, Nov '22 (illus.) abstr: J.A.M.A. *80:*360, Feb 3, '23
Transplantation and vital storage. LEHMANN, W. AND TAMMANN, H. Beitr. z. klin. Chir. *135:*259–302, '25, abstr: Klin. Wchnschr. *4:*2342–2343, Dec 3, '25, abstr: J.A.M.A. *86:*316, Jan 23, '26
Growth energy of implanted epithelium. KURTZAHN, H. Arch. f. klin. Chir. *138:*534–551, '25
Twenty years of transplantation research. LEXER, E. Arch. f. klin. Chir. *138:*251–302, '25
Relative reaction within mammalian tissues; factors determining reaction of skin grafts; study by indicator method of conditions within ischemic tissue. ROUS, P., J. Exper. Med. *44:*815–834, Dec '26
Surgical grafts. MAUCLAIRE. Rev. med. franc. *8:*9–30, Jan '27
Biologic stdy of tissue transplantation. KUBÁNYI, E. AND JAKOB, M. Orvosi hetil. *71:*365–370, April 3, '27
Transplantation of leg; Sauerbruch's plastic operation. NISSEN, R. Umschau *31:*526, June 25, '27
Experimental implantation of cartilage into kidney and transplantation of cartilage into bone defects. NIGRISOLI, P. Arch. per le sc. med. *49:*689–703, Dec '27
Experimental researches on grafting cartilage on to tendons. BORGHI, M. Arch. per. le sc. med. *50:*437–465, '27
Surgical organotherapy by grafts. BREITNER, B. Wien. klin. Wchnschr. (Sonderbeil. 32) *40:*4–5, '27
Regeneration and grafts. PERRONCITO, A. Tratt. di anat. patol., no. 5, pp. 3–148, '27
Grafting or transplantation of tissues. PERRONCITO, A. Tratt. di anat. patol. no. 5, pp. 79–155, '27
Role of allergy in degeneration of tissues transplanted into peritoneal cavity. PAGEL, W. Krankheits-forschung *6:*337–377, Aug '28
Regeneration and transplantation of tissue. SCHAXEL, J. Zool. Anz. *78:*153–157, Sept 1, '28

Transplantation – Cont.
Transplantation of organs. KOPPÁNYI, T. Scient. Monthly *27:*502–505, Dec '28
Life and growth processes in explanted normal and malignant human tissue. HEIM, K. Arch. f. Gynak. *134:*250–309, '28
Experimental and clinical study of transplantation of tissues preserved in alcohol or formalin solution. HOSOMI, K. Deutsche Ztschr. f. Chir. *209:*14–30, '28
Amyloid formation caused by intraabdominal implantation of organ tissue. SHINKAI, T. Tr. Jap. Path. Soc. *18:*235, '28
Effect of radium rays on transplanted tissues. KRONTOVSKY, A. A. Vranch. dielo *12:*669–671, May 31, '29
Metaplastic formation of bone in transplanted connective tissue. LEXER, E. Deutsche Ztschr. f. Chir. *217:*1–32, '29
Atypical epithelial proliferation of transplanted mammary tissue. POLISSADOWA, X. AND BJELOSOR, I. Virchows Arch. f. path. Anat. *272:*759–762, '29
Transplantation of skin, fat, blood vessels, nerves, etc. EISELSBERG, A. Wien. med. Wchnschr. *80:*50–55, Jan 4, '30
Age factor in transplantation. DANCHAKOFF, V. AND DANCHAKOFF, V. E. Contrib. Embryol. (no. 124) *21:*125–140, June '30
Composition of embryonal tissue fluid; significance for growth of transplanted tissue. GUILLERY, H. Virchows Arch. f. path. Anat. *275:*181–192, '30
Provisional storage of tissues to be transplanted (experiments with surviving tissues). KUBANYL, E. Arch. f. klin. Chir. *161:*502–510, '30
Metabolism in transplanted tissues. TAMMANN, H. Klin. Wchnschr. *10:*1858–1859, Oct 3, '31
Amyloid degeneration of transplanted tissues (in Japanese). FUZII, M. AND MURATA, M. Tr. Jap. Path. Soc. *21:*84–88, '31
Grafts and implantations of tissue and organs in man and in animals. MAUCLAIRE, P. Medecine (supp.) *13:*1–67, Feb '32
Plant and animal grafts. RETTERER, E. Progres med., pp. 1041–1050, June 11, '32
Surgical grafts. BLANC Y FORTACÍN, J. Rev. ibero-am.de cien. med. *7:*193–204, Dec '32, also: Siglo med. *90:*641–645, Dec 17, '32
Significance of mitosis of epithelial cells of implanted tissue. IMAKITA, T. Acta dermat. *20:*138–139, '32
Grafts of organs. MANN, F. C. Libman Anniv. Vols. *2:*757–771, '32
Technic of autoplastic grafts. PALMÉN, A. J. Duodecim *48:*36–39, '32
Autoplasties (grafts). HAMANT, A.; *et al.*

Transplantation – Cont.
Bull. Soc. franc. de dermat. et syph. (Reunion dermat.) *40:*28–30, Jan '33
Therapy of cancer by means of transplantation of normal organs; review. NYKA, W. AND LAVEDAN, J. Paris med. *1:*229–240, March 18, '33
Grafts and transplants. BEEKMAN, F. Am. J. Surg. *26:*528–532, Dec '34
Immediate transplantation of bone, cartilage and soft tissues in accident cases. CARTER, W. W. Laryngoscope *45:*730–738, Sept '35
Mechanism of development of epithelial cysts; behavior of autogenous skin particle implanted subcutaneously. ŌKUMA, M. Nagasaki Igakkai Zasshi *14:*94–96, Jan 25, '36
Fate of transplanted cow's horn in treatment of bone fractures. SIEGLING, J. A. AND FAHEY, J. J., J. Bone and Joint Surg. *18:*439–444, April '36
Autoplastic grafts in rabbits whose skin had been frozen previously. DEL GENIO, F. Sperimentale, Arch. di biol. *90:*75–85, '36
Late results after transplantation of mammary gland in closure of facial defect. IGNATEV, S. S. Vestnik khir. *47:*103, '36
Successful application of regeneration theory (plastic surgery). VON ERTL, J. Arch. f. klin. Chir. *189:*398–400, '37
Buried grafts used to repair depressions in brow, eye socket, skull and nose. PEER, L. A., J. M. Soc. New Jersey *35:*601–605, Oct '38
Therapeutic transplantation of tissue. FILATOV, V. P. Acta med. URSS *1:*412–439, '38, Vrach. delo *20:*813–822, '38
History of transplantation in general and orthopedic surgery. ORR, H. W. Am. J. Surg. *43:*547–553, Feb '39
Transplantation of conserved skin according to Filatov method in therapy of chronic crural ulcers; preliminary report. BROVER, B. I. Vrach. delo *21:*105–110, '39
Therapeutic transplantation of tissues. FILATOV, V. P. Probl. tuberk., no. 6, pp. 8–13, '39
Reconstruction of hand and 4 fingers by transplantation of middle part of foot and 4 toes. ESSER, J. F. S. AND RANSCHBURG, P. Ann. Surg. *111:*655–659, April '40
History of total transplantation of eyeball. AYRES, F. Arq. brasil. de oftal. *3:*305–310, Dec '40
General principles of tissue transplantation. ZSCHAU, H. Sitzungsb. d. phys.-med. Soz. zu Erlangen (1939) *71:*255–256, '40
Skin transplantation by injection; effect on healing of granulating wounds. BARBER,

Transplantation – Cont.
C. G. Arch. Surg. *43:*21–31, July '41
Testicular transplantation; successful autoplastic graft following accidental castration. KEARNS, W. M. Ann. Surg. *114:*886–890, Nov '41
Transplantation and regeneration of tissue. MAY, H. Pennsylvania M. J. *45:*130–135, Nov '41
Revival of "slumbering cells" theory; criticism of Busse-Grawitz' experiments claiming vitality of various tissues in subcutaneous implantations. HÖRA, J. Ztschr. f. d. ges. exper. Med. *108:*757–771, '41
Reactions in tissues of mummies following implantation. BUSSE-GRAWITZ, P. Arch. f. exper. Zellforsch. *24:*320–358, '42
Method of fractional implantation and other systematic implantation experiments. BUSSE-GRAWITZ, P. Ztschr. d. d. ges. exper. Med. *111:*1–19, '42 (Reply to Hora)
Question of "cellular tissue decomposition" or wandering of leukocytes; testing of Busse-Grawitz experiments. HEINEMANN, K. Beitr. z. path. Anat. u. z. allg. Path. *106:*525–534, '42
Tissue grafting. SHEEHAN, J. E. Am. J. Surg. *61:*339–349, Sept '43
Free grafts in plastic surgery. HARRIS, M. M. Semana med. *2:*841–844, Oct 7, '43
Inhibition of coagulation necrosis of implants by means of oxalate and enzyme poisons. CAIN, H. Frankfurt. Ztschr. f. Path. *58:*171, '43
Transplantation tissue therapy in certain diseases. FILATOV, V. P. Sovet. med. (no. 10) *7:*1–3, '43
Whole upper extremity transplant for human beings; general plans of procedure and operative technic. HALL, R. H. Ann. Surg. *120:*12–23, July '44
Subcutaneous implantation of chemically treated tissues. KRAUZE, N. I. Khirurgiya, no. 10, pp. 16–25, '44
Transplantation tissue therapy. KRYMOV, A. P. Sovet. med. (no. 9) *8:*15–16, '44
Characteristics of local reaction following implantation of tissues preserved in formalin (solution of formaldehyde). LEBEDINSKAYA, S. I. Khirurgiya, no. 4, pp. 18–23, '44
Restoration of vision after crossing of optic nerves and after contralateral transplantation of eye. SPERRY, R. W., J. Neurophysiol. *8:*15–28, Jan '45
Therapy of nonhealing wounds, ulcers and contractures by transplantation of chemically treated tissues according to Krauze. BLOKHIN, V. N. Khirurgiya No. 6, pp. 3–

Transplantation—Cont.
10, '45
Transplantation tissue therapy. FILATOV, V. P. Vrach. delo (nos. 11–12) *25:*499–510, '45
Tissue reactions induced by series of fibrogen plastics implanted in abdominal wall of guinea pigs. BAILEY, O. T. AND FORD, R. Arch. Path. *42:*535–542, Nov '46

Transplantation, Cancer in

Growth of transplanted embryonal tissue and origin of neoplasms. SKUBISREWSKI, L. Compt. rend. Soc. be biol. *93:*1398–1400, Dec 4, '25
Possibility of producing tumors by subcutaneous inoculation of normal, particularly embryonal tissue; experimental study. LÖWENTHAL, K. Med. Klin. *24:*1263–1268, Aug 17, '28
Growth of transplanted embryonal tissue and its significance with regard to origin of tumors. SKUBISZEWSKI, L. Ztschr. f. Krebsforsch. *26:*308–329, '28
Production of malignant tumors by transplantation of embryonal tissues. KLEE-RAWIDOWWICZ, E. Deutsche med. Wchnschr. *58:*1439–1440, Sept 9, '32

Transplantation of Conjunctiva

Homotransplantation of mucous membrane in ophthalmic surgery. MITSKEVICH, L. D. Sovet. vestnik oftal. *3:*299–302, '33
Experimental studies on transplantation of conjunctiva from eye of cadaver; preliminary report. ROZENTSVEYG, M. G. Vestnik oftal. *11:*311–316, '37
Transplantation of conjunctiva from cadaver. ROZENTSVEYG, M. G. Vestnik oftal. (nos. 2–3) *14:*26–36, '39
Transplantation of conjunctiva of cadaver; clinical and histologic aspects. SIE BOEN LIAN. Geneesk. tijdschr. v. Nederl.-Indie *81:*2097-2101, Sept 30, '41

Transplantation, Connective Tissue

Transplantation of fibrous tissues in repair of anatomical defects. GALLIE, W. E. AND LE MESURIER, A. B. Brit. J. Surg. *12:*289–320, Oct '24
Transplantation of dead connective tissue. NAGEOTTE, J. Virchow's Arch. f. path. Anat. *263:*69–88, '27
Use of grafts of devitalized connective tissue (tendon and nerve) in reparative surgery. NAGEOTTE, J. Presse med. *47:*1365–1366, Sept 27, '39

Transplantation of Cornea

Further data on therapeutic value of preserved tissue, especially in ocular diseases; transplantation of tissues and use of placental microclysters; preliminary report. FILATOV, V. P. Gaz. clin. *39:*292–295, Aug '41

Transplantation of Embryonic Tissues

Grafts of bones of embryos. SIMON, R. AND ARON, M. Arch. franco-belges de chir. *25:*869–883, July '22 (illus.), abstr: J.A.M.A. *80:*65, Jan 6, '23
Grafts of embryonal tissue. FALDINO, G. Chir. d. org. di movimento *9:*1–27, Dec '24, abstr: J.A.M.A. *84:*786, March 7, '25
Implants of embryonic tissues. SARTORI, C. Arch. ital. di chir. *15:*339–349, '26, abstr: J.A.M.A. *87:*67, July 3, '26
Experimental study upon prevention of adhesions about repaired nerves and tendons (especially by use of allantoic and amniotic membranes). DAVIS, L. AND ARIES, L. J. Surgery *2:*877–888, Dec '37
Therapy of fresh wounds by transplantation of chemically treated tissues (skin and fetal membranes). PIKIN, K. I. Sovet. med. (no. 9) *6:*15–16, '42
Behavior of embryonic tissue transplanted into adult organism. SPEMANN, H. Arch. f. Entwckingsmechn. d. Organ. *141:*693–769, '42
Heterologous transplantation of embryonic mammalian tissues. GREENE, H. S. N. Cancer Research *3:*809–822, Dec '43

Transplantation, Homografts and Heterografts

Immunity in relation to transplanted tissue. FLEISHER, M. S., J. M. Research *43:*145–153, April–May '22
Homoplastic transplantation of adult frog skin. GASSUL, R. Deutsche med. Wchnschr. *48:*1163–1164, Sept 1, '22 (illus.)
Experiments on implantation of dead preserved tissue. REGOLI, G. Policlinico (sez. chir.) *29:*559–574, Oct '22 (illus.)
Preliminary serum treatment before skin grafting. LAQUA, K. Klin. Wchnschr. *2:*1360–1362, July 16, '23, abstr: J.A.M.A. *81:*1478, Oct 27, '23
Protein sensitization in isoskingrafting; is the latter of practical value? HOLMAN, E. Surg., Gynec. and Obst. *38:*100–106, Jan '24
Blood grouping as guide in skin grafting. KUBÁNYI, A. Arch. f. klin. Chir. *129:*644–647, '24, abstr: J.A.M.A. *82:*2090, June 21, '24

Transplantatin, Homografts and Heterografts – Cont.
Free homeoplastic skin grafting. DEUCHER, W. G. AND OCHSNER, A. E. W. Arch. f. klin. Chir. *132:*470–479, '24
Attempts to overcome difficulties in healing of homoplastic transplants. ROHDE, C. Beitr. z. klin. Chir. *134:*111–127, '25
Autotransplantation and homoiotransplantation of cartilage and bone in rat. LOEB, L. Am. J. Path. *2:*315–333, July '26
Heterotransplantation of cartilage and fat tissue and reaction against heterotransplants in general. LOEB, L. AND HARTER, J. S. Am. J. Path. *2:*521–537, Nov '26
New experiments with homoplastic transplantation of organs. CASTIGLIONI, G. Atti d. Soc. di sc. med. e biol. *16:*34–49, Jan–Feb '27
Reaction of skin in homoplastic grafts studied by means of phenol red (phenol sulphon-phthalein). MILONE, S. Gior. d. r. Accad. di med. di Torino *33:*147–150, March '27
Reaction to homoplastic skin grafts. SEBASTIANO, M. Arch. per le sc. med. *49:*193–200, April '27
Deep homoplastic grafts and successive superficial grafts. MORPURGO, B. AND MILONE, S. Arch. per le sc. med. *49:*306–309, May '27
Significance of specific immunity of organs during growth of homoplastic grafts. BAUDOLINO, M. Gior. di batteriol. e immunol. *2:*381–389, June '27
Influence of inanition on homeoplastic transplantations. MORPURGO, B. Centralbl. f. allg. Path. u. path. Anat. *40:*1–3, July 1, '27
Influence of inanition on homoplastic skin-grafts. MORPURGO, B. AND MILONE, S. Boll. d. Soc. ital. di biol. sper. *2:*709–712, July '27
Experimental researches on homoplastic transplantation of striated muscle preserved in vitro. BERTOCCHI, A. AND BIANCHETTI, C. F. Gior. d. r. Accad. di med. di Torino *90:*434–438, Aug '27
Autoplastic, homoplastic and heteroplastic skin grafts. CARMONA, L. Ann. ital. di chir. *6:*1234–1256, Dec '27
Homeotransplants in uniovular twins. BAUER, K. H. Beitr. z. klin. Chir. *141:*442–447, '27
Grafting of fixed skin. NAVA V. Boll. d. Soc. med. chir. di Pavia *2:*369–372, '27
Behavior of autoplastic and homoplastic grafts placed in subcutaneous tissue; experiments on rabbits. RIGANO-IRRERA, D. AND SACERDOTE, G. Arch. ital. di chir.

Transplantation, Homografts and Heterografts – Cont.
*20:*190–198, '27
Homeoplastic skin transplantation after reticulo-endothelial storage. TAMMANN, H. AND PATRIKALAKIS, M. Beit. z. klin. Chir. *139:*550–568, '27
Experiments to improve survival of homoplastic transplants. NIGRISOLI, P. Arch. per sc. med. *52:*65–75, Feb '28
Experiments on taking of homoplastic skin-grafts. VELO, C. A. Ann. ital. di chir. *7:*97–112, Feb '28
New operative technic of animal grafts in women. DARTIGUES. Rev. espan. de med. y chir. *11:*271–275, May '28
Transplantation of skin preserved in fluids. NAVA VERA. Arch. per le sc. med. *52:*236–242, May '28
Homio transplantation of skin flaps. RABINOVITCH, P. Proc. Soc. Exper. Biol. and Med. *25:*798–799, June '28
Heteroplasties and autoplasties. DORDU, F. Arch. franco-belges de chir. *31:*601–608, July '28
Importance of local immunity in elimination of homoplastic skin grafts. TINOZZI, F. P. Ann. ital. di chir. *7:*660–683, July 31, '28
Application to study of human constitution, of biological laws discovered by transplantation of extremities. BRANDT. Verhandl. d. anat. Gesellsch. *37:*38–41, '28
Comparative effects on skin of homo- and heteroplastic grafts. MORPURGO, B. AND MILONE, S. Arch. ed atti d. Soc. ital. di chir (1927) *34:*lxxxiv, '28
Effect of insufficient nutrition on growth of homoplastic skin grafts. MORPURGO, B. AND MILONE, S. Arch. ed atti d. Soc. ital. di chir (1927) *34:*lxxxv, '28
Spastic entropion after total tarsectomy of upper lid cured by tarsal homoplasty; 3 cases. SHIMKIN, N. Klin. Monatsbl. f. Augenh. *82:*360–364, March 22, '29
Homotransplantation based on blood-group determination with special regard to skin transplantation. KETTEL, K. Bibliot. f. Laeger *121:*204–230, May '29
Homotransplantation and several blood groups; epidermal grafts made by Thiersch method. DOBRZANIECKI, W. Ann. Surg. *90:*926–938, Nov '29
Heteroplastic implantation of tissues. HERZBERG, E. AND GUTTMANN, E. Munchen. med. Wchnschr. *76:*1922–1923, Nov 15, '29
Experimental studies on homeotransplantation. FISCHER, H. Arch. f. klin. Chir. *156:*224–250, '29
Experimental transplantation of cartilage fixed in bone. BLAVET DI BRIGA, C. Arch.

Transplantation, Homografts and Heterografts – Cont.
ital. de biol. *83:*26–33, July 30, '30
Transplantation and individuality. LOEB, L. Physiol. Rev. *10:*547–616, Oct '30
Homeoplasty and reticulo-endothelial system; effect of injuries of reticulo-endothelial system on rapidity with which transplanted tissue heals. BRÜDA, B. E. AND KREINER, W. Deutsche Ztschr. f. Chir. *222:*285–301, '30
Homoplastic and heteroplastic transplantation of skin in man. MANNHEIM, H. Arch. f. klin. Chir. *162:*551–560, '30
Homoplastic transplantation of epithelium; case. SCHÜRCH, O. Zentralbl. f. Chir. *58:*451–453, Feb 21, '31
Comment on article by Schurch on homoplastic transplantation of epithelium. MANNHEIM, H. Zentralbl. f. Chir. *58:*789–790, March 28, '31
Effect of removal of sympathetic ganglia on cutaneous autoplastic and homoplastic transplants (skin). DOBRZANIECKI, W. Polska gaz. lek. *10:*262, April 5; 287, April 12, '31
Further observation on transplantation of epiphyseal cartilage plate. HAAS, S. L. Surg., Gynec. and Obst. *52:*958–963, May '31
Homotransplantation and heterotransplantation in man with reference to blood groups. ROLLO, S. Riforma med. *47:*1190–1192, Aug 3, '31
Periarterial decortication by Leriche method and autoplastic and homoplastic grafts. BERTOCCHI, A. Arch. ital. di chir. *29:*1–36, '31
Homeoplastic skin grafts. ERKES, F. Deutsche Ztschr. f. Chir. *234:*852–854, '31
Possibility of transmission of biologic properties of skin from animal to animal by means of transplantation. BERNUCCI, F. Gior. ital. di dermat. e sif. *73:*1373–1379, Aug '32
Is iso-skin grafting practicable? PADGETT, E. C. South. M. J. *25:*895–900, Sept '32
Free homoplastic and heteroplastic grafts of periosteum and of bone in sensitized animals. GAGLIO, V. Ann. ital. di chir *11:*2017–2030, Oct 31, '32
Immunologic reactions and acid-base equilibrium of flaps in homoplastic skin grafts. SHINOI, K. Mitt. d. med. Gesellsch. zu Tokio *46:*1913–1914, Nov '32
Autoplastic and homoplastic implantation of epidermis. LOEFFLER, Deutsche Ztschr. f. Chir. *236:*169–190, '32
Respective value of autografts, homografts and heterografts. DUFOURMENTEL, L. Bull. med., Paris *47:*175–176, March 11, '33
Is grafting with isografts or homografts practicable? PADGETT, E. C. West. J. Surg. *41:*205–212, April '33
Application of auto-, homo- and heterografts in reconstructive surgery. DUFOURMENTEL, L. Bull. et mem. Soc. d. chirurgiens de Paris *25:*269–282, May 5, '33
Question of fixed grafts in relation to probable regenerative processes of host. IMPERATI, L. Ann. ital. di chir. *12:*903–914, July 31, '33
Large scalp wound treated by total homoplastic graft of large cellulocutaneous flap. DUFOURMENTEL, L. Bull. et mem. Soc. d. chirurgiens de Paris *25:*724–726, Dec 15, '33
Bovine cartilage in correction of nasal deformities. STOUT, P. S. Laryngoscope *43:*976–979, Dec '33
Effect of removal of cervical ganglion of sympathetic nerve on growth of autoplastic and homoplastic skin transplants. VASILEV, A. A. AND ZHOLONDZ, A. M. Arch. f. klin. Chir. *178:*148–169, '33, also: Novy khir. arkhiv *29:*3–20, '33
Homotransplantation of skin in relation to blood groups. ISHCHENKO, I. M. Med. zhur. *4:*59–68, '34
Question of homoplastic grafting of skin. TRUSLER, H. M. AND COGSWELL, H. D. J.A.M.A. *104:*2076–2077, June 8, '35
Why homotransplantation fails. BOGOMOLETS, O. Med. zhur. *5:*137–141, '35
Formation of antibodies following homotransplantation and heterotransplantation. KUCHERENKO, Y. G. Med. zhur. *5:*287–294, '35
Alloplastic and heteroplastic grafts in reconstruction of facial defects; use of ivory and cartilage. SPANIER, F. Rev. de chir. structive, pp. 391–401, Dec '36
Homografting, with report of success in identical twins. BROWN, J. B. Surgery *1:*558–563, April '37
Fate and activity of autografts and homografts in white rats. BUTCHER, E. O. Arch. Dermat. and Syph. *36:*53–56, July '37
Cartilage homografts. DUFOURMENTEL, L. Oto-rhino-laryng. internat. *21:*461–462, Aug '37
Reconstruction of external ear with special reference to use of maternal ear cartilage as supporting structure (cases). GILLIES, H. Rev. de chir. structive, pp. 169–179, Oct '37
Local metabolism and tissue reaction; effect

Transplantation, Homografts and Heterografts –Cont.
of transplantation into heterogenic tissue and of application of salt solution and of organ extract on growth of transplanted cartilage. BINGEL, K. Beitr. z. path. Anat. u. z. allg. Path. *99:*205–223, '37
Influence of sympathectomy on homoplastic grafts. LEXER, E. W. Deutsche Ztschr. f. Chir. *249:*337-370, '37
Cartilage transplanted beneath skin of chest in man; experimental studies with sections of cartilage preserved in alcohol and buried from 7 days to 14 months. PEER, L. A. Arch. Otolaryng. *27:*42–58, Jan '38
Refrigerated cartilage isografts in facial surgery. O'CONNOR, G. B. AND PIERCE, G. W. Surg., Gynec. and Obst. *67:*796–798, Dec '38
Homeotransplantation. SUZUKI, S. Fukuoka acta med. (Abstr. Sect.) *32:*1–5, Jan '39
Merthiolate (mercury compound): tissue preservative and antispetic (for "refrigerated cartilage isografts"). O'CONNOR, G. B. Am. J. Surg. *45:*563-565, Sept '39
Homoplastic transplantations of human skin, with special consideration of blood characteristics. BINHOLD. Deutsche Ztschr. f. Chir. *252:*183-196, '39
Further data on therapeutic value of transplantation of preserved tissue; preliminary report. FILATOV, V. P. Sovet. med. (nos. 13–14) *4:*5–8, '40
Transplantation of preserved skin in experimental cutaneous tuberculosis. GLEYBERMAN, E. Y. Med. zhur. *10:*269–275, '40
Homotransplantation of skin of rabbit embryo into bone marrow. YANO, S. Tr. Soc. path. jap. *30:*746-747, '40
Grafts of preserved cartilage in restorations of facial contour. STRAITH, C. L. AND SLAUGHTER, W. B., J.A.M.A. *116:*2008–2013, May 3, '41
Regenerative power and possibilities of homograft. VILLAFANE, I. Z. Semana med. *1:*1197–1200, May 22, '41
Actual growth of young cartilage transplants in rabbits; experimental studies. DUPERTUIS, S. M. Arch. Surg. *43:*32–63, July '41
"Biochemical" individuality; experiments with homeoplastic transplants. SCHÖNE, G. Zentralbl. f. Chir. *68:*1523–1546, Aug 9, '41
Preserved human cartilage in reconstructive surgery of face. IGLAUER, S. Ann. Otol., Rhin. and Laryng. *50:*1072–1078, Dec '41
Late results of double heterogenous graft performed in 1911. DUROUX, E. AND DUROUX, P. E. Progres med. *70:*140–145, March 7,

Transplantation, Homografts and Heterografts –Cont.
'42
Massive repairs with thick split-skin grafts; emergency "dressing" with homografts in burns. BROWN, J. B. AND McDOWELL, F. Ann. Surg. *115:*658–674, April '42
Defense of human body against living mammalian cells; address of president. STONE, H. B. Ann. Surg. *115:*883-891, June '42
Pathogenesis of allergic eczema elucidated by transplantation experiments on identical twins. HAXTHAUSEN, H. Acta dermat.-venereol. *23:*438–454, Jan '43
Role of humoral antagonism (due to cytotoxins) in heteroplastic transplantation in mammals. HARRIS, M., J. Exper. Zool. *93:*131–145, June '43
Fate of skin homografts in man. GIBSON, T. AND MEDAWAR, P. B., J. Anat. *77:*299-310, July '43
Problem of skin homografts. MEDAWAR, P. B. Bull. War Med. *4:*1–4, Sept '43
Skin isograft transplants in identical twins. SCHATTNER, A. Arch. Otolaryng. *39:*521–522, June '44
Breast tissue as new source for heterogenous implants; preliminary report. LA ROE, E. K. Am. J. Surg. *66:*58–67, Oct '44
Experiments on heterotropic transplantation of skin. BRAUN, A. A. AND ORLOVA, G. N. Compt. rend. Acad. d. sc. URSS *47:*138–139, April 20, '45
Graft of cadaver skin; preliminary report. BIANCHI, R. G. Dia med. *17:*1168, Oct 8, '45, also: Prensa med. argent. *32:*1997, Oct 12, '45
Ectropion due to ichthyosis of both upper and lower lids on child corrected by homoplastic grafting of skin from child's mother. SHIMKIN, N. I. Harefuah *29:*155, Oct 1, '45
Utilization of cadaver cartilage in surgery. GONZALEZ ULLOA, M. Medicina, Mexico *25:*495–503, Dec 10, '45
Use of cadaver cartilage in surgery. GONZALEZ ULLOA, M. Rev. brasil. de cir. *14:*663–670, Dec '45; also: Prensa med. argent. *33:*705–709, April 5, '46
Homotransplantation of skin on denervated area. KUCHERENKO, Y. G. Med. zhur. *14:*283–285, '45
Immunity to homologous grafted skin; suppression of cell division in grafts transplanted to immunized animals. MEDAWAR, P. B. Brit. J. Exper. Path. *27:*9–14, Feb '46
Immunity to homologous grafted skin; relationship between antigens of blood and skin. MEDAWAR, P. B. Brit. J. Exper. Path. *27:*15–24, Feb '46

Transplantation, Homografts and Heterografts – Cont.

Relationship between antigens of blood and skin (grafts). Medawar, P. B. Nature, London *157:*161–162, Feb 9, '46

Experiments with "cuto-omentopexy" and skin homotransplantation. Mandl, F. and Rabinovici, N., J. Internat. Coll. Surgeons *9:*525–530, Sept–Oct. '46

Transplantation of Joints

Grafts of long bones and joints. Fieschi, D. Chir. d. org. di movimento *5:*359, Aug '21; abstr: J.A.M.A. *77:*1373, Oct 22, '21

Joint transplantations and arthroplasty. Lexer, E. Surg., Gynec. and Obst. *40:*782–809, June '25

Regeneration of joint transplants and intracapsular fragments. May, H. Ann. Surg. *116:*297–310, Aug '42

Transplantation of Nails

Cosmetic autotransplantation of nails. Ko, G. Taiwan Igakkai Zasshi *35:*1072, May '36

Transplantation of Toe to Nose

Plastic surgery of saddle nose (transplantation of toe). Linberg, B. E. Vestnik khir. (no. 52) *18:*70–76, '29

Trapl, J.: Plastic reconstruction of vagina with total defect. Cas. lek. cesk. *62:*197–202, Feb 24, '23

Tratman, E. K.: Treatment of fractured jaws. J. Malaya Br., Brit. M. A. *3:*357–373, March '40

Traub, E. F.: Should vascular nevi be treated? Arch. Pediat. *50:*272–278, April '33

Traub, E. F.: Burns. Hygeia *16:*1064, Dec '38

Traub, E. F.: Birth-marks; relationship to skin cancer. Hygeia *18:*513, June '40

Traub, E. F.: Therapy of nevi; relationship to skin malignancies. J. Michigan M. Soc. *42:*297–300, April '43

Traub, E. F.: Treatment of nevi. Clinics *3:*974–981, Dec '44

Traub, E. F. and Keil, H.: "Common mole"; clinicopathologic relations and question of malignant degeneration. Arch. Dermat. and Syph. *41:*241–252, Feb '40

Traub, E. F. and Tolmach, J. A.: Squamous cell epitheliomata of face; 26 cases. New York State J. Med. *33:*875–881, July 15, '33

Traum, E. (see Flick, K.) April '32

Trauner, F.: Restoration of width of lower jaw following loss of both condyles; case. Zentralbl. f. Chir. *56:*1986–1989, Aug 10, '29

Trauner, R.: Heredity of congenital fossette of lip in conjunction with clefts of upper jaw. Wien. klin. Wchnschr. *54:*427–429, May 16, '41 addendum: *54:*454, May 23, '41

Trauner, R.: Review of recent literature on technic of surgical therapy of cleft palate. Beitr. z. klin. Chir. *174:*599, '43

Trauner, R.: Oral and maxillary tumors; experience at First Surgical Clinic of Vienna University during years 1930–1940. Wien. klin. Wchnschr. *57:*192, April 21, '44

Traut, H. F. (see Davis, J. S.) Dec '25

Traut, H. F. (see Davis, J. S.) May '26

Travers, M. P.: Treatment of hand injuries. J. Florida M. A. *28:*66–71, Aug '41

Traversa Gaudioso, E.: Experiments on transplants of fresh and preserved bone. Policlinico (sez.prat.) *31:*735–740, June 9, '24 abstr: J.A.M.A. *83:*227, July 19, '24

Traynham, W. H. Jr.: Osteotomy of rami of lower jaw (for prognathism). Bull. U. S. Army M. Dept. (no. 74) pp. 115–118, March '44

Traynham, W. H. Jr.: Bilateral osteotomy of rami for marked protrusion of lower jaw; case. J. Am. Dent. A. *31:*1025–1029, Aug 1, '44

Traynor Operation

Bilateral congenital ptosis of eyelids treated by Traynor operation. Duran Rodriguez, C. Vida nueva *53:*245–249, May '44

Tregarthen, G. G. T.: External splint for use in derangements of temporomandibular joint. Bull. War Med. *3:*271–272, Jan '43 (abstract)

Trelat Operation: See Langenbeck-Trelat Operation

Tremonti, P.: Treatment of collapse; drug modifiers of tonus, and excitors of arterial contractility. Arch. di farmacol. sper. *46:*119; 129; 145, 1928–1929

Trendelenburg Operation

Fate of patient in whom exstrophy of bladder was cured by Trendelenburg operation (synchondroseotomy). Heinsius, F. Zentralbl. f. Gynak. *55:*322–332, Feb 7, '31 abstr.: Ztschr. f. Geburtsh. u. Gynak. *99:*187–191, '30

Trendtel: Dangers of Whitehead mouth-gag used on young children. Klin. Wchnschr. *6:*2436–2437, Dec 17, '27

Trépagne, D.: Keloids, radium therapy; case, with suggestions of other physiotherapeutic methods (electrolysis, electropuncture, ionization, cryotherapy, electrocoagulation and roentgenotherapy). Ann. de med. phys. *25:*291–297, '32

TREPOZ. (see LAROYENNE) Sept '28

TRETHEWIE, E. R. AND WILLIAMS, E.: Use of kangaroo tendon for muscle and tendon suture. Australian and New Zealand J. Surg. *11:*207–208, Jan '42

TRÈVES, A.: Role of periosteum in bone grafts. Arch. franco-belges de chir. *31:*213–219, March '28

TRÈVES, A.: Role of periosteum in osseous grafts. Bull. et mem. Soc. de chir. de Paris *20:*550, June 15, '28

TREVOR, D.: Dislocations and fractures of thumb and fingers. Brit. M. J. *2:*461, Aug 27, '38; 583, Sept 10, '38

TRICAULT, G. (see POMMÉ, B. *et al*) May '31

TRIER, K.: Treatment of angiomas with carbon dioxide snow and electrolysis. Hospitalstid. *68:*117–118, Feb 5, '25

Trigger Thumb (or Finger): See Finger, Trigger

TRIMBLE, I. R.: Prevention and treatment of shock. South. M. J. *30:*876–880, Sept '37

TRINDER, J. H.: Congenital perforated soft palate and double uvula, with repair of perforation. J.A.M.A. *80:*914, March 31, '23 (illus.)

TRINTIGNAC, P. (see ENSELME, J.) July–Aug '39

TROCMAIER, C. (see COVALI, N.) March–April '38

TROELL, A.: Autoplastic and heteroplastic bone grafts. Hygiea *85:*79–92, Feb 15, '23 (illus.) abstr: J.A.M.A. *80:*1112, April 14, '23

TROELL, A.: Bone grafting. Acta chir. Scandinav. *56:*59–72, '23 (illus., in English) abstr: J.A.M.A. *81:*1062, Sept 22, '23

TROELL, A.: Big toe as substitute for thumb. Hygiea *86:*407–413, June 30, '24

TROELL, A.: Operation of case of bulbo-scrotal hypospadias. Ztschr. f. urol. Chir. *22:*372–376, '27

TROELL, A.: Pharyngo-staphylo-uranoplasty, operation in older children and adults. Svenska lak.-tidning. *34:*521–524, April 9, '37

TROFIMOW, A. M.: Technic of total rhinoplasty in which portions of abdominal skin are used. Arch. f. klin. Chir. *163:*681–692, '31

TROITSKIY, V. V.: Ligature for prevention of terminal neuromas. Khirurgiya, no. 2, pp. 61–65, '45

TROMMALD, J. P. (see DIACK, A. W.) Nov '39

TROTOT, R.: War lesions due to toxic gases and incendiary projectiles (burns). Tunisie med. *29:*293–304, July–Aug '35

TROTT, R. H. (see ALTMAN, H.) July '46

TROXELL, E. L.: Thumb of man. Scient. Monthly *43:*148–150, Aug '36

Truc Operation

Truc operation in ectropion; technic and review of cases. DELORD, E. *et al.* Arch. d'opht. *51:*763–774, Dec '34

TRUEBLOOD, D. V.: Paraffin treatment for burns and denuded areas. Northwest Med. *25:*255–258, May '26

TRUEBLOOD, D. V.: Severe burns. West. J. Surg. *39:*543–546, July '31

TRUEBLOOD, D. V.: Surgery for cancer of face and lip. West. J. Surg. *40:*401–404, Aug '32

TRUEBLOOD, D. V.: Paraffin dressing for transplanted grafts. West. J. Surg. *44:*578, Oct '36

TRUEBLOOD, D. V.: Tumors of lip and oral cavity. West. J. Surg. *46:*395–411, Aug '38

TRUEBLOOD, D. V.: Parotid tumors; clinical observations and surgical experiences. West. J. Surg. *52:*109–118, March '44

Truehart, M.: Radium treatment of cancer of face. J. Kansas M. Soc. *25:*70–73, March '25

TRUEHEART, M.: Cancer of lip; report of 25 cases treated with radium. J. Kansas M. Soc. *26:*311–313, Oct '26

TRUEHEART, M.: Superficial cancer of lip. J. Kansas M. Soc. *40:*419, Oct '39

TRUFFERT, P.: Diagnosis of tumors of neck. Bull. med., Paris *41:*726–731, June 18, '27

TRUFFERT, P.: Cervical branchioma; 3 cases. Bull. et mem. Soc. nat. de chir. *60:*602–611, May 5, '34

TRUFFI, G.: Hemiatrophy on left side of face with circumscribed scleroderma; case. Dermosifilografo *8:*90–99, Feb '33

TRUMBLE, H. C.: Nerve (hypoglossal-facial) anastomosis in treatment of facial paralysis. M. J. Australia *1:*300–302, Feb. 25, '39

TRUMPER, W. A.: Dupuytren's contracture; case. Lancet *2:*17, July 4, '31

Trunk

Circular dermolipectomy of trunk in obesity. SOMALO, M. Arq. de cir. clin. e exper. *6:*540–543, April–June '42

TRUSLER, H. M.: Extensive cutaneous burns; ultraviolet light as adjunct to the repair of defects. J. Indiana M. A. *28:*113–118, March '35

TRUSLER, H. M.: Repair of depressed disfiguring scars by means of rib cartilage implant. J. Indiana M. A. *30:*194–196, April '37

TRUSLER, H. M. AND COGSWELL, H. D.: Question of homoplastic grafting of skin. J.A.M.A. *104:*2076–2077, June 8, '35

TRUSLER, H. M.; EGBERT, H. L. AND WILLIAMS, H. S.: Burn shock; question of water intoxication as complicating factor; blood chemical studies and report of extensive burn treated by repeated transfusions of blood and blood plasma. J.A.M.A. *113:*2207-2213, Dec 16, '39

TRUSLER, H. M. (see COGSWELL, H. D.) April '37

TRUSLER, H. M. (see GATCH, W. D.) Feb '30

TRÝB, A.: Cystic tuberous lymphangioma of skin with hypertrichosis. Arch. f. Dermat. u. Syph. *158:*468-479, '29

TSANOV, A. I.: Plugging of tuberculous cavities with transplants of fatty tissue. Kazanskiy med. j. *28:*203-206, Feb-March '32

TSCHALENKO, G.: New method of tendon suture; preliminary report. Zentralbl. f. Chir. *56:*2388-2389, Sept 21, '29

TSCHIASSNY, K.: Endonasal plastic operation on alar cartilages of nose. Wien. klin. Wchnschr. *34:*120, March 17, '21

Tschmarke

Tschmarke's antiseptic treatment of burns. RESCHKE, K. Arch. f. klin. Chir. *146:*763-776, '27

Tschmarke method of burn therapy. RESCHKE, K. Med. Welt *5:*444, March 28, '31

TSCHMARKE, G.: Operative treatment of cleft palate. Arch. f. klin. Chir. *144:*697-722, '27

TSCHMARKE, G.: Diphallism; case. Beitr. z. klin. Chir. *151:*631-637, '31

TSHERNOFF, L.: New technic of operation in case of hypertrophy of tarsal plate, with trichiasis as complication. Hebrew Physician *2:*55, '33

TSITOVSKIY, M. L.: Correction of eyelid ptosis by transplantation of fascia lata. Vestnik oftal. *11:*373-377, '37

*T*SOUCANELIS, A.: Therapy of superior pro-alveolism (superior alveolar prognathism). Stomatol., Athenes *1:*77-90, '38

TSUNODA, E.: Plastic operation of mandibular region by Clapp's method; case. Mitt. a. d. med. Akad. zu Kioto *8:*131-132, '33

TSVETKOV, S. A.: Question of surgical intervention in syndactylia. Sovet. khir. (no. 6) *6:*876-877, '34

TSYPIN, M. Y.: New instrument for conservative operations on nasal septum. Zhur. ush., nos. i gorl. bolez. *16:*141-145, '39

TUASON, M. N.: Insulin-glucose in surgical shock, with observations on 2 cases. J. Philippine Islands M. A. *7:*283-286, Aug '27

TUBBY, A. H.: Dupuytren's contraction of palmar fascia and some other deformities. Practitioner *110:*214-220, March '23

TUCHEL, V. (see CONSTANTINESCO, M. *et al*) Jan '38

TUCHEL, V. (see CONSTANTINESCO, M.) Sept-Oct '40

TUCKER, G.: Peroral endoscopy; its use in complications following operations on nose and throat. Arch. Otolaryng. *5:*321-333, April '27

TUCKER, G.: Observations in 200 consecutive cases of cancer of larynx. Arch. Otolaryng. *21:*1-8, Jan '35

TUCKER, G.: Diagnosis and surgical cure of cancer of larynx. Delaware State M. J. *8:*80-82, May '36

TULASNE, R.: *De la prosthèse immédiate des maxillaires*. LeGrand, Paris, 1928

TŮMA, V.: Attempt to culture tissue from Dupuytren's contracture in adults. Arch. f. exper. Zellforsch. *15:*173-178, '34

TUMARKIN, I. A.: Problem of facial paralysis. J. Laryng. and Otol. *52:*107-115, Feb '37

TUNG, P. C.: Cleft palate. Chinese M. J. *49:*22-41, Jan '35

TUNG, P. C. AND CHEN, H. I.: Ankylosis of jaws. Chinese M. J. *49:*101-110, Feb '35

TUNG, P. C. (see BROWN, J. B.) March '35

TUNG, P. C. (see BROWN, J. B.) Jan '36

TUNGER: Burn treatment. Deutsche med. Wchnschr. *48:*95, Jan 19, '22

TUOMIKOSKI, V.: Primary plastic surgery in injuries of fingers, hands and forearms. Duodecim *48:*393-411, '32

TUOMIKOSKI, V.: Technic of plastic surgery for correction of microstomia resulting from Estlander cheiloplasty. Duodecim *48:*691-698, '32

TUOMIKOSKI, V.: Plastic method of correcting microstomia, particularly of type following Estlander cheiloplastic operation. Acta chir. Scandinav. *70:*353-362, '33

TUOTI, F. A. (see STEVENSON, H. N.) Nov '45

TUPINAMBA, J.: Congenital unilateral partial blepharoptosis; case. Rev. de oftal. de Sao Paulo *6:*29-32, Jan.-March '38

TURAI, I. (see COSTESCU, P.) May-June '40

Turck, F. B.

Research of Fenton B. Turck on traumatic shock. QUÉNU. Bull. Acad. de med., Par. *87:*92-97, Jan 24, '22

TURCO, N. B.: Osteomyelitis of jaw; mandibular operation; buccal operation. Prensa Med. argent. *30:*2209-2210, Nov 17, '43

TURCO, N. B. (see FINOCHIETTO, R.) March '36

TURCO, N. B. (see FINOCHIETTO, R. *et al*) 1944

TURENNE, A.: Operative formation of vagina in patient with congenital absence of vagina;

case. An. de Fac. de med., Montevideo *15:*725–749, Sept-Oct '30

TURENNE, A.: Artificial vagina in case of congenital absence of vagina. Rev. de med., Rosario *6:*291–303, Aug '31

TURNBULL, F.: Nerve injuries; management in late stages. Canad. M. A. J. *53:*438–443, Nov '45

TURNER, A. C.: Contribution to treatment of burns (use of mercurochrome). Brit. M. J. *2:*995–996, Nov 23, '35

TURNER, G. G.: Cleft palate. Proc. Internat. Assemb. Inter-State Post-Grad. M. A., North America (1930) *6:*255–260, '31

TURNER, G. G.: Fistula of penile urethra after gunshot wound. Lancet *2:*649, Nov 23, '40

TURNER, G. I.: Finger injuries with injury of peripheral nerves. Vestnik khir. (nos. 65–66) *22:*49–55, '31

TURNER, J. W. AND RIFE, C. S.: Analysis of 73 consecutive cases of tongue cancer; preliminary report. Univ. Hosp. Bull., Ann Arbor *4:*33–35, May '38

TURNER, O. A.: Tantalum cranioplasty. Ohio State M. J. *42:*604–607, June '46

TURNER, O. A.: Repair of defects (using tantalum), with special reference to periorbital structures and frontal sinus. Arch. Surg. *53:*312–326, Sept '46

TURNER, R. H.: Influence of trauma of small portion of finger pad on rate of blood flow in distal segment of finger. Tr. A. Am. Physicians *57:*182–183, '42

TÜRSCHMID, W.: Traumatic avulsion of skin of penis and scrotum. Polska gaz. lek. *11:*373–374, May 15, '32

TURTUR, G.: Benign tumors of external ear: condyloma, hemangioma; cases. Valsalva *6:*97–104, Feb '30

TVEDT, A.: Acute spontaneous infectious gangrene. Nord. med. (Norsk mag. f. laegevidensk.) *27:*1750–1753, Sept 7, '45

Twins, Lesions in

Tripartite cleft palate and double harelip in identical twins. DAVIS, A. D. Surg., Gynec. and Obst. *35:*586–592, Nov '22 (illus.)

Homeotransplants in uniovular twins. BAUER, K. H. Beitr. z. klin. Chir. *141:*442–447, '27

Study of twins with cleft lip, jaw, and palate from standpoint of pathologic heredity. BIRKENFELD, W. Beitr. z. klin. Chir. *141:*257–267, '27

Harelip in univitelline twins; case. LÉVY, G. Bull. Soc. d'obst. et de gynec. *17:*661, July '28

Congenital pendulous hypertrophic breasts

Twins, Lesions in – Cont.

in female twins; case. BIRKENFELD, W. Arch. f. klin. Chir. *168:*568–576, '32

Cleft palate found in only one of identical twins. WRIGHT, H. B. Internat. J. Orthodontia *20:*649–657, July '34

Homografting, with report of success in identical twins. BROWN, J. B. Surgery *1:*558–563, April '37

Identical Dupuytren's contracture in identical twins. COUCH, H. Canad. M. A. J. *39:*225–226, Sept '38

Harelip and cleft palate in uniovular twins. SCHRÖDER, C. H. Zentralbl. f. Chir. *66:*2299–2308, Oct 21, '39

Heredopathology of fissures of lips, jaws and palate; report on unselected series of 41 pairs of twins. IDELBERGER, A. AND IDELBERGER, K. Ztschr. f. menschl. Vererb.-u. Konstitutionslehre *24:*417–479, '40

Pathogenesis of allergic eczema elucidated by transplantation experiments on identical twins. HAXTHAUSEN, H. Acta dermat.-venereol. *23:*438–454, Jan '43

Exstrophy of bladder in twins. HIGGINS, C. C. Cleveland Clin. Quart. *11:*25, Jan '44

TWYMAN, E. D.: Epithelioma of lip. J.A.M.A. *78:*348–349, Feb 4, '22

TWYMAN, E. D.: Modification of Estlander's operation for lip defect. Surg., Gynec. and Obst. *38:*824–825, June '24

TWYMAN, E. D.: Partial nasal defects; new modification of "French" method of restoration with sliding flaps of adjoining tissue. West. J. Surg. *48:*106–109, Feb '40

TYLER, A. F.: New technic designed for electrocoagulation of vascular tumors. Nebraska M. J. *18:*6–9, Jan '33

TYLER, A. F.: Radium treatment of angiomas. Radiol. Rev. and Chicago M. Rec. *55:*51–54, March '33

TYLER, A. F. AND HOLMES, W. E.: Enlarged thymus (especially in relation to cleft palate operations and roentgenotherapy). Nebraska M. J. *24:*121–125, April '39

TYLER, E. A. Nitrous oxide-oxygen anesthesia; endotracheal technic in oromaxillofacial surgery. Anesth. and Analg. *22:*177–179, May-June '43

TYNICKI, M.: Burns. Polska gaz. lek. *17:*653–657, Aug 7, '38; 679–682, Aug 21, '38

TZAÏCO, A.: Reconstruction of lower lip. Presse med. *29:*723, Sept 10, '21 abstr: J.A.M.A. *77:*1606, Nov 12, '21

TZUKERMANN, M. A.: Corrective plastic surgery of nose. Vrach. dielo *12:*1020–1023, Aug 31, '29

U

UDINE, S.S.: Unusual case of jaw ankylosis. Vestnik khir. (no. 35–36) *12:*134–136, '28

UEBERMUTH, H.: Harelip and cleft palate from eugenic point of view. Arch. f. klin. Chir. *193:*224–229, '38

UEBERMUTH, H.: Care of fresh wounds of face and jaws. Arch. f. klin. Chir. *200:*546–552, '40

UFFENORDE, W.: Plastic operation on auditory canal after complete opening of middle ear with chisel. Ztschr. of Hals-, Nasen-u. Ohrenh. *23:*317, Sept 10, '29

UFFENORDE, W.: Surgery of choanal atresia; roentgenography with iodipin (iodized oil). Hals-, Nasen-u. Ohrenarzt (Teil 1) *28:*174–175, May '37

UGGERI, C.: Procedure for removing sebaceous cysts of face with conservative excision. Gazz. d. osp. *59:*456–458, May 1, '38

UHLMANN, E.: Treatment of late injuries of skin with radium ointment; 3 cases. Dermat. Wchnschr. *91:*1825–1828, Dec 13, '30

UHLMANN, E.: Treatment of injuries produced by roentgen rays and radioactive substances. Am. J. Roentgenol. *41:*80–90, Jan '39

UHLMANN, E. AND SCHAMBYE, G.: Successful therapy of injuries of skin from roentgen and radium rays. Strahlentherapie *52:*282–298, '35

UHLMANN, E. (see ROST, G. A.) April '32

UIHLEIN, A. JR.: Skin grafts in plastic operations. Arch. Surg. *38:*118–130, Jan '39

Ulcers

Treatment of burns and ulcers with Veroform and Epithelan. LINDEN. Deutsche med. Wchnschr. *50:*719–720, May 30, '24

Necrotic ulcer from cocaine-epinephrine injections; 2 cases. QUINTARELLI, L. Ann. di med. nav. *1:*67–75, Jan–Feb '27

Treatment of ulcers of thigh and burns with polysan (magnesium hydroxide preparation). JANOUŠEK, B. Ceska dermat. *9:*154–159, '28

Trophic postencephalitic ulcerations of outer nose and of cheek. SCHLITTLER, E. Schweiz. med. Wchnschr. *59:*1121–1122, Nov 9, '29

Treatment of ulcers with skin grafts. ANDERSON, T. F. AND ROBERTS, M. A. W. East African M. J. *9:*79–83, June '32

Tropical ulcers; quick and successful method of treatment by excision and skin graft. JAMES, C. Lancet *2:*1095–1101, Nov 19, '32

Surgical treatment of trophic ulcers of leg and foot; autoplastic operation by Italian method, periarterial sympathectomy, lumbar sympathetic ganglionectomy and ramisection. ROMITI, C. Tr. Roy. Soc. Trop. Med. and Hyg. *27:*185–194, July '33

Loss of cutaneous substance in ulceration of thigh cured by Davies graft. DESJACQUES, R. AND MILLET. Lyon med. *152:*222–223, Aug 27, '33

Tumors and ulcers of palate and fauces (Semon lecture, abstract). HOWARTH, W. Lancet *2:*1139–1142, Nov 14, '36

Comparison of 2 methods of skin grafting (in ulcers). CAROTHERS, J. C. East African M. J. *13:*345, Feb '37

New method for slowly healing ulcers. ADLER, S. Gyogyaszat *77:*376–377, June 20, '37

Therapy of slowly healing ulcers. KESSEL, F. K. Vrach. delo *20:*311–314, '37

Perforating ulcer of septum (Hajek's ulcer), with report of case. MOREIRA, E. Rev. brasil. de oto-rino-laring. *8:*265–267, July–Aug '40

Use of implantation grafts in healing of infected ulcers. MARCKS, K. M. Am. J. Surg. *51:*354–361, Feb '41

Skin grafting in therapy of large ulcerations, with report of cases. SATANOWSKY, S. Semana med. *2:*1216–1223, Nov 20 '41

Bone drilling in resistant chronic ulcers; new principle. ALBEE, F. H. Am. J. Surg. *54:*605–608, Dec '41

Therapy of neuropathic ulcers of foot (mal perforant) by implantation of sensory nerves. NORDMANN, O. Chirurg *14:*116–122, Feb 15, '42

Treatment of perforating ulcer of foot. MUIR, E. Leprosy Rev. *14:*49, July '43

Defective ulcerated cicatrices; plastic correction. ZENO, L. Bol. Soc. de cir. de Rosario *10:*354–366, Oct–Nov '43 also: An. de cir. *10:*76–88, March–June '44

Vascular prerequisites of successful grafting; new method (using fluorescein) for immediate determination of adequacy of circulation in ulcers, skin grafts and flaps. LANGE, K. Surgery *15:*85–89, Jan '44

Antireticular cytotoxic serum in therapy of ulcerating cicatrix. BEREZOV, Y. E. Med. zhur. *13:*101–103, '44

Secondary closure of ulcers with aid of penicillin. LAMON, J. D. AND ALEXANDER, E. JR. J.A.M.A. *127:*396, Feb 17, '45

Ulcer of dorsum pedis; free graft on granulation tissue. FERNANDEZ, L. L. Prensa med. argent. *32:*1601–1604, Aug 17, '45

Use of desiccated red blood cells in treatment of ulcers of skin. HOLMES, R. L. JR. AND MIMS, A. T. Dallas M. J. *31:*138–144, Nov '45

Ulcers – Cont.

Therapy of nonhealing wounds, ulcers and contractures by transplantation of chemically treated tissues according to Krauze. BLOKHIN, V. N. Khirurgiya No. 6, pp. 3-10, '45

Recurrent aphthous ulceration of oral mucous membrane and genitals associated with recurrent hypopyon iritis (Behcet syndrome); 3 cases. KATZENELLENBOGEN, I. Brit. J. Dermat. *58:*161-172, Jul-Aug '46

ULLIK, R.: Kostecka operation for prognathism; follow up studies on 21 cases. Ztschr. f Stomatol. *40:*255, April 10, '42; 294, April 24, '42

ULLIK, R.: Therapy, especially of gunshot fractures of lower jaw. Wien. klin. Wchnschr. *55:*913-915, Nov 13, '42

ULLMANN, S.: Accidents in conduction anesthesia of sphenopalatine ganglion; 4 cases. Ztschr. f. Hals-, Nasen-u. Ohrenh. *21:*587-595, May 10, '28

ULLRICH, G.: Glossoptosis in micrognathia; 2 cases. Deutsche med. Wchnschr. *61:*1033-1036, June 28, '35

Ultraviolet Therapy

Removal of accidental vaccination scar by blistering doses of ultraviolet rays. FISHER, A. A., J.A.M.A. *110:*642-643, Feb 26, '38

UNDERHILL, F. P.: Changes in blood concentration with special reference to treatment of extensive superficial burns. Ann. Surg. *86:*840-849, Dec '27

UNDERHILL, F. P. *et al*: Blood concentration changes in extensive superficial burns, and their significance for systemic treatment. Arch. Int. Med. *32:*31-49, July '23

UNGER, E. (see CASSIRER, R.) May '21

UNGER, L. J. (see MOORHEAD, J. J.) Jan '43

UNGLEY, C. C.: Immersion hand (peripheral vasoneuropathy after chilling). Bull. War Med. *4:*61-65, Oct '43

UNGLEY, H. G. AND SUGGIT, S. C.: Fractures of zygomatic tripod. Brit. J. Surg. *32:*287-299, Oct '44

UNGUREÀNU, V.: Dupuytren's contracture, clinical case. Cluj. med. *10:*522-524, Nov 1, '29

UPDEGRAFF, H. L.: Problem of rhinoplasty. Ann. Surg. *90:*961-973, Dec '29

UPDEGRAFF, H. L.: Problem of skin grafting, with description of newer technique. California and West. Med. *33:*679-681, Sept '30

UPDEGRAFF, H. L.: Reconstructive surgery in progressive facial hemiatrophy. Am. J. Surg. *10:*439-443, Dec '30

UPDEGRAFF, H. L.: Problem of cartilage implant (face). Am. J. Surg. *14:*492-498, Nov '31

UPDEGRAFF, H. L.: Reconstructive surgery and old facial burns. J.A.M.A. *101:*1138-1140, Oct 7, '33

UPDEGRAFF, H. L.: Skin grafts in changing of fingerprints. Am. J. Surg. *26:*533-534, Dec '34

UPDEGRAFF, H. L.: Reconstruction of columella nasi. Am. J. Surg. *29:*29-31, July '35

UPDEGRAFF, H. L.: Management of large skin flaps. Am. J. Surg. *33:*104-107, July '36

UPDEGRAFF, H. L.: Reconstruction in hypertrophy of breast. California and West. Med. *46:*28-31, Jan '37

UPDEGRAFF, H. L.: Emergency plastic surgery. Mil. Surgeon *82:*315-321, April '38

UPDEGRAFF, H. L.: Fall and rise of plastic surgery. Am. J. Surg. *43:*637-656, Feb '39

UPDEGRAFF, H. L.: Reparative surgery. Australian and New Zealand J. Surg. *9:*237-258, Jan '40

UPDEGRAFF, H. L.: Wound closure, with particular reference to avoidance of scars. Am. J. Surg. *50:*749-753, Dec '40

UPDEGRAFF, H. L. AND MENNINGER, K. A.: Psychoanalytic aspects of plastic surgery. Am. J. Surg. *25:*554-558, Sept '34

UPSON, W. O. (see DUGAN, W. M.) July '30

URBAN, W. G.: Treatment of complications arising from cleft palate. Am. J. Orthodontics *24:*87-89, Jan '38

URBANEK, J.: Indications for dacryocystorhinostomy. Wien. med. Wchnschr. *77:*1109, Aug 20, '27

URECHIA, C. I. AND DRAGOMIR, L.: Retraction of palmar aponeurosis with syringomelic dissociation of sensitivity; 2 cases. Paris med. *2:*274-276, Oct 5, '35

URECHIA, C. I. AND RETEZEANU, MME.: Right facial hemiatrophy with muscular atrophy of left upper extremity; case. Bull. et mem. Soc. med. d. hop. de Paris *52:*398-402, March 16, '36

Urethra (See also Epispadias; Hypospadias; Urethral Fistula; Urethral Stricture)

Case of plastic operation including urethra, bladder and vagina. JORGE, J. M. Semana med. *2:*499-502, Sept 13, '23 (illus)

Muscle transplantation, method for cure of urinary incontinence in male. PLAYER, L. P. AND CALLANDER, C. L., J.A.M.A. *88:*989-991, March 26, '27

Imperforate anus, with exit through prostatic urethra; 3 cases. HELWIG, F. C. Am. J. Dis. Child. *38:*559-561, Sept '29

Reconstruction of urethra and penis follow-

Urethra – Cont.

ing extensive gangrene. MALLARD, R. S. J.A.M.A. *95:*332–335, Aug 2, '30

Traumatic removal of entire external cutaneous covering of penis with subsequent partial necrosis of urethra; plastic repair; case. VON RIHMER, B. Ztschr. f. Urol. *26:*369–373, '32

Abnormalities and plastic surgery of lower urogenital tract (Ramon Guiteras lecture). YOUNG, H. H., J. Urol. *35:*417–480, April '36

Urethroplasty for congenital strictures; method of temporary graft of penis to scrotum; case. GODARD, H. Rev. de chir., Paris *74:*374–386, May '36

Urethroplasty using scrotal grafts; review of various methods. GODARD, H., J. d'urol. *43:*201–232, March '37

Reconstruction of extensive urethral defects by transplantation of pedicled flap. BONA, T. Rev. de chir., Bucuresti *41:*347–352, May–June '38

Traumatic rupture of urethra in child; reconstruction of canal by means of cutaneous graft; dysuria resulting from cicatricial stricture and urethral calculus 33 years later. THEVENOT, AND GAYET, R. Lyon chir. *35:*592–595, Sept–Oct '38

Transplants from scrotum for repair of urethral defects. DODSON, A. I. Tr. Am. A. Genito-Urin. Surgeons (1940) *33:*211–220, '41

New plastic operation for male urethra. LACHMANN, O. Bull. War Med. *4:*393, March '44 (abstract)

Urethra; repair of complete tear of membranous portion; case report and suggested new technic for operation. LEADBETTER, W. F., M. Bull. North African Theat. Op. (no. 4) *2:*70–74, Oct '44

Loss of coverage of penis, scrotum and urethra. ROBINSON, D. W. *et al.* Plast. and Reconstruct. Surg. *1:*58–68, July '46

Cotton sutures in vaginal plastic operations about bladder and urethra COLLINS, C. G. S. Clin. North America *26:*1221–1229, Oct '46

Repair of war wounds of bulbous and membranous urethra using split thickness grafts and penicillin. MACLEAN, J. T. AND GERRIE, J. W., J. Urol. *56:*485–497, Oct '46

Urethral Fistula

Treatment of fistulas into male urethra by inversion of skin. SALLERAS PAGÉS, J. Semana med. *28:*602, May 26, '21 Abstr: J.A.M.A. *77:*580, Aug 13, '21

Urethral Fistula – Cont.

Correction of urethroperineal fistula. JUNGANO, M., J. d'urol. *15:*459–462, June '23 (illus.)

Urethral fistulas in women. CRESCENZI, G. Policlinico (sez. chir.) *30:*497–502, Oct '23

Congenital case of recto-urethral fistula with imperforate anus. DOTTI, S. Gazz. med. lomb. *86:*41–44, March 25, '27

Therapy of para-urethral fistulas with glacial acetic acid. FIGUEROA ALCORTA, L. Rev. de especialid. *6:*1125–1137, Nov '31 also: Med. argent. *11:*1239–1243, Feb '32

Urethroperineal fistulas; surgical therapy; technic and results in 4 cases. ISNARDI, U. Semana med. *1:*1668–1672, May 18, '33

Urethropubic fistula; surgical therapy of case. PINI, R. AND ZERBINI, C. Semana med. *2:*639–641, Aug 31, '33

Congenital fistula of penile urethra; case in boy 9 years old. AFFONSO, J. Arq. de cir. e ortop. *2:*81–83, Sept '34

Urethroperineal fistula, cure by pedicled graft; urethroplasty without preliminary cystostomy; case. GUILLERMO, AND TISSANDIE. Bull. Soc. franc. d'urol. pp. 322–326, Dec 21, '36

Urethral fistula. ROCHAT, R. L. Helvet. med. acta *4:*67–69, Feb '37

Treatment of urethral fistula. HAYES, B. A. J. Oklahoma M. A. *31:*33–35, Feb '38

Repair of fistula of penile urethra. ATTWATER, H. L. AND HUGHES, J. R. Lancet *2:*569–570, Sept 3, '38

Fistula of penile urethra after gunshot wound. TURNER, G. G. Lancet *2:*649, Nov 23, '40

Landerer-Bidder operation in cure of large urethral fistula; case. GRIMALDI, F. E. AND BERNARDI, R. Rev. argent. de urol. *10:*535–539, Sept–Oct '41

Urethral fistula cured by Landerer-Bidder procedure; case. GRIMALDI, F. E. AND BERNARDI, R. Prensa med. argent. *28:*1886–1888, Sept 24, '41

Rare case of urethral fistula. DE GOUVEIA, G. S. Hospital, Rio de Janeiro *21:*195–199, Feb '42

Sectional urethrectomy in therapy of fistulas of perineobulbar portion of urethra. CABANIE, G., J. d'urol. *50:*124–126, March–April '42

Technic and indications for sectional urethrectomy in urethroperineal fistula. CABANIE, G., J. d'urol. *52:*66–73, May–June '44

Battle injuries of urethra with urinary fistula. SHEARER, T. P. *et al.* Texas State J. Med. *41:*137–140, July '45

Urethral Fistula – Cont.
Fistula of penile urethra; method of repair utilizing stainless steel "pull-out" sutures. CORDONNIER, J. J., J. Urol. *55:*278-286, Mar '46

Urethral Stricture
Urethroplasty for congenital strictures; method of temporary graft of penis to scrotum; case. GODARD, H. Rev. de chir., Paris *74:*374-386, May '36
Impassable stricture of urethra; resection of 8 cm. with plastic repair; case (graft). CARTELLI, N. AND ALBORNOZ, I. Rev. argent. de urol. *6:*242-249, May-June '37

URIBURU, J. V. JR.: Lipoma of forehead; surgical therapy of case. Prensa med. argent. *30:*2451-2452, Dec 22, '43
URKOV, J. C.: Cutaneous plastics; their scientific basis. Illinois M. J. *51:*469-471, June '27
URKOV, J. C.: Skin grafting by general surgeon. Am. J. Surg. *68:*195-207, May '45
URKOV, J. C.: Surface defects of skin; treatment by controlled exfoliation. Illinois M. J. *89:*75-81, Feb '46
URKOV, J. C.: The critically burned patient. Am. J. Surg. *71:*242-252, Feb '46
URRUTIA, J. M.: Tautening arch for wire traction in therapy of fractures of phalanges. Bol. y trab., Soc. de cir. de Cordoba (no. 1) *1:*54-58, '40
URRUTIA, J. M. (see MIRIZZI, P. L.) 1940
URZUA, R.: Plastic surgery. Dia med. *11:*556-558, June 26, '39 also: Arq. de cir. clin. e exper. *3:*103-105, April '39
URZUA, R.: Concept of plastic surgery. Rev. med. brasil. *4:*41-44, June '39
URZUA, R.: Grafts of adipose tissue and their use in correction of depressed cicatrices of face. Rev. Asoc. med. argent. *53:*647-649, July 30, '39
URZUA, R. (see JOHOW, A.) Nov '40
URZUA C. C., R.: Correction of depressed cicatrices with grafts of fatty tissue. Arq. de cir. clin. e exper. *6:*269-272, April-June '42
URZUA C. C., R.: New classification of congenital auricular malformations. Arq. de cir. clin. e exper. *6:*479-484, April-June '42
URZUA C. C., R. (see RIVAS, C. I. *et al*) April-June '42
USPENSKIY, A. A.: Burn therapy with vitaderm (carotene preparation). Ortop. i travmatol. (no. 2) *14:*12-23, '40
USUA MARINE, J. (see CAMPOS MARTIN, R. *et al*) April '43
USUA MARINE, J. (see CAMPOS MARTIN, R.) June '43
UTRATA-BANYAI, J.: Intramural tumors of soft palate. Ztschr. f. Hals-, Nasen-u. Ohrenh. *48:*113-116, '41

Uvula, Bifid
Bifid uvula. DUCUING, L. Rev. de laryng. *52:*76-80, Jan 31, '31
Bifid uvula in school children; statistical study. BENVENUTO, E. Valsalva *15:*492-494, Nov '39

UZDIN, Z. M. (see SEGAL, G. I.) Dec '40

V

VACCAREZZA, R. A.: Cause of death from burns. Rev. Asoc. med. argent. *35:*48-53, Jan-April '22 abstr: J.A.M.A. *79:*859, Sept 2, '22
DE VADDER, A. (see JOLY, P.) Feb '40
VADI, E.: Plastic operation; avulsion of skin of penis; good functional results of graft of scrotum. Bol. Asoc. med. de Puerto Rico *22:*25-26, Sept-Oct '29

Vagina
Case of plastic operation including urethra, bladder and vagina. JORGE, J. M. Semana med. *2:*499-502, Sept 13, '23 (illus)
Plastic repair of vagina by graft of 2 prepuces; case. PETIT, R. Rev. franc. de gynec. et d'obst. *26:*605-607, Nov '31
Local anesthesia in plastic surgery of vagina. DE ARAGON, E. R. Vida nueva *39:*272-275, April 15, '37
Technic of plastic repair in wound of vagina. BUCHANAN, J. M. Australian and New Zealand J. Surg. *8:*300-307, Jan '39
New operation for atresia ani vaginalis. MURDOCH, R. L. Tr. Am. Proct. Soc. (1941) *42:*274-285, '42
Surgery of congenital anomalies of female genitals. SARNOFF, J. AND SARNOFF, S. J. J. Internat. Coll. Surgeons *6:*36-47, Jan-Feb '43
Cotton sutures in vaginal plastic operations about bladder and urethra. COLLINS, C. G. S. Clin. North America *26:*1221-1229, Oct '46

Vagina, Artificial
Plastic construction of artificial vagina. MOSZKOWICZ, L. Zentralbl. f. Gynak. *45:*80, Jan 15, '21
Artificial vagina. BRENNER, M. Monatschr. f. Geburtsh. u. Gynak. *54:*112, Feb '21 abstr: J.A.M.A. *76:*1436, May 21, '21
Construction of an artificial vagina. SCHUBERT, G. Zentralbl. f. Gynak. *45:*229, Feb 19, '21

Vagina, Artificial –Cont.

Artificial vagina in case of external male pseudohermaphroditism. GRUSS, J. Deutsche med. Wchnschr. *47:*509, May 5, '21

Operative formation of vagina. BROSSMANN, H. Zentralbl. f. Gynak. *45:*789, June 4, '21

Method of constructing artificial vagina. GRAVES, W. P., S. Clin. N. Amer. *1:*611, June '21

Formation of vagina from rectum. NEMES, A. Zentralbl. f. Gynak. *45:*787, June 4, '21

Artificial vagina in case of external male pseudohermaphroditism. FRANK, M. Monatschr. f. Geburtsh. u. Gynak. *55:*5, July '21 abstr: J.A.M.A. *77:*1215, Oct 8, '21

Construction of artificial vagina. BENTHIN, W. Zentralbl. f. Gynak. *45:*1330, Sept 17, '21

Construction of artificial vagina; mortality rate. FOHR, O. Zentralbl. f. Gynak. *45:*1332, Sept 17, '21 abstr: J.A.M.A. *77:*2154, Dec 31, '21

Artificial vagina made from intestine. FÜTH, H. Monatschr. f. Geburtsh. u. Gynak. *55:*262–266, Sept '21

Artificial vagina made from intestine. MARTENS, M. Deutsche med. Wchnschr. *47:*1226, Oct 13, '21

Two cases of artificial vagina. WALLERSTEIN. Zentralbl. f. Gynak. *45:*1492–1494, Oct 15, '21

Formation of artificial vagina. MICHAEL, H. Zentralbl. f. Gynak. *45:*1665–1667, Nov 19, '21

Formation of artificial vagina. STEUDING, O. Zentralbl. f. Gynak. *46:*61–63, Jan 14, '22

Construction of vagina (Schubert method). KEYSERLINGK, R. Zentralbl. f. Gynak. *46:*380–381, March 11, '22

Construction of vagina from small intestine. NEUGEBAUER, F. Zentralbl. f. Gynak. *46:*381–384, March 11, '22

Congenital absence of vagina, accompanied by marked nervous symptoms; Baldwin's operation and removal of ovarian tissue. WRIGHT, T. Am. J. Surg. *36:*114–115, May '22

Congenital non-existence of vagina and its treatment; 2 cases. DHALLUIN, A. Arch. franco-belges de chir. *25:*808–816, June '22 (illus.) abstr: J.A.M.A. *79:*2039, Dec 9, '22

Artificial vagina from intestine; 2 cases. ROSENSTEIN. Monatschr. f. Geburtsh. u. Gynak. *58:*176–183, July '22 abstr: J.A.M.A. *79:*1372, Oct 14, '22

Artificial vagina made from small intestine. ROSENTHAL. Zentralbl. f. Gynak. *46:*1102–1104, July 8, '22

Vagina, Artificial–Cont.

Artificial vagina made from rectum (Schubert's method). HARTTUNG, H. Zentralbl. f. Gynak. *46:*1610–1612, Oct 7, '22

Construction of vagina; 2 cases. LAMAS, A. An. de Fac. de med., Montevideo *8:*1–6, Jan '23

Construction of artificial vagina from small intestine, 4 cases. HORTOLOMEI, N. Zentralbl. f. Chir. *50:*259–262, Feb 17, '23 abstr: J.A.M.A. *80:*1110, April 14, '23

Plastic reconstruction of vagina with total defect. TRAPL, J. Cas. lek. cesk. *62:*197–202, Feb 24, '23

Formation of vagina by Schubert method, with fatal result. SCHROEDER, E. Zentralbl. f. Gynak. *47:*842–844, May 26, '23 abstr: J.A.M.A. *81:*869, Sept 8, '23

Formation of an artificial vagina to remedy congenital defect. PAUNZ, A. Zentralbl. f. Gynak. *47:*883–888, June 2, '23

Artificial vagina made from loop of small intestine. VILLETTE, J. Arch. franco-belges de chir. *26:*1047–1055, Nov '23

Technic for artificial vagina with menstruating uterus. SCHUBERT, G. Monatschr. f. Geburtsh. u. Gynak. *65:*45–60, Dec '23

Artificial vagina made from skin. FRAENKEL, L. Zentralbl. f. Gynak. *48:*193–197, Feb 9, '24

Artificial vagina; comment on Paunz's article. MORI, M. Zentralbl. f. Gynak. *48:*859, April 19, '24 abstr: J.A.M.A. *83:*77, July 5, '24

Artificial vagina made from intestine; 13 cases. DANIEL, C. Rev. franc. de gynec. et d'obst. *19:*305–321, May 25, '24

Construction of vagina from intestine. BRUSKIN, J. Zentralbl. f. Gynak. *48:*1597–1599, July 19, '24

Construction of an artificial vagina, with report of case. MILLER, C. J. Am. J. Obst. and Gynec. *8:*333–334, Sept '24

Technic for artificial vagina. HAIM, E. Zentralbl. f. Gynak. *48:*2382–2387, Oct 25, '24

Modified technic for artificial vagina. COSTANTINI, H. Presse med. *32:*798, Oct 4, '24 abstr: J.A.M.A. *83:*1543, Nov 8, '24

Artificial vagina made from rectum. KAKUSCHKIN, N. Zentralbl. f. Gynak. *48:*2702–2704, Dec 6, '24

Formation of an artificial vagina. PEMBERTON, F. A. Am. J. Obst. and Gynec. *10:*294–303, Aug '25

Construction of artificial vagina from rectum, with presence of uterus. SCHUBERT, G. Beitr. z. klin. Chir. *134:*421–425, '25 abstr: J.A.M.A. *85:*1844, Dec 5, '25

Formation of artificial vagina from rectum in

Vagina, Artificial—Cont.
deficiency of vagina. FRANZ, R. Zentralbl. f. Gynak. *50:*545–547, Feb 27, '26
Revision of vagina formed according to Mori after 3 years. PARSAMOW, O. S. Zentralbl. f. Gynak, *50:*550–551, Feb 27, '26
Congenital absence of vagina and its artificial formation with Amann's method. TIKANADSE, I. Zentralbl. f. Gynak. *50:*547–549, Feb 27, '26
Artificial vagina from bladder. SCHMID, H. H. Monatschr. f. Geburtsh. u. Gynak. *72:*330–336, March '26
Artificial vagina made by Baldwin's method for congenital defect in vagina. RABINOWITSCH, K. N. Zentralbl. f. Gynak *50:*1851–1864, July 10, '26 abstr: J.A.M.A. *87:*1081, Sept 25, '26
Construction of vagina from loop of small bowel. HOLBROOK, J. S. Minnesota med. *10:*55, Jan '27
Artificial vagina formed from intestinal segment. KOCH, C. F. Nederl. Tijdschr. v. Geneesk. *1:*214–225, Jan 8, '27
Schubert's method for formation of artificial vagina; 20 cases. SCHUBERT, G. Zentralbl. f. Gynak. *51:*80–88, Jan 8, '27
Functions of isolated fascia of jejunum tenue used in operation for artificial vagina by Baldwin's method. VAKAR, A. A. Russk. Klin. *7:*19–34, Jan '27
Complete absence of vagina in two sisters and operation of artificial formation by fasciae method. DEENETZ, B. J. Vrach. Gaz. *31:*362–365, March 15, '27
Formation of artificial vagina from segment of small intestine. VAN DER HOFF, H. Nederl. Tijdschr. v. Geneesk. *1:*1538–1546, March 26, '27
Artificial vagina formation from Meckel's diverticulum; case. WASSILIEW, B. N. Zentralbl. f. Gynak. *51:*806–808, March 26, '27
Baldwin operation for formation of artificial vagina; report of 6 cases. JUDIN, S. Surg., Gynec. and Obst. *44:*530–539, April (pt. 1) '27
Popoff's method of formation of artificial vagina; 2 cases. MANDELSTAMM, A. Zentralbl. f. Gynak. *51:*1058–1063, April 23, '27
Snegiroff's method of formation of artificial vagina; case. SCHARAPO, M. Zentralbl. f. Gynak. *51:*1131–1133, April 30, '27
Formation of artificial vagina by Baldwin method with Constantini's modification. TICHONOVICH, A., J. Akush. i Zhensk. Boliez. *38:*301–305, May–June '27
Schubert's method of formation of artificial vagina; cases. WAGNER, G. A. Zentralbl. f. Gynak. *51:*1300–1304, May 21, '27

Vagina, Artificial—Cont.
Schubert's operation for artificial vagina. HILLE, K. Monatschr. f. Geburtsh. u. Gynak. *76:*288–293, June '27
Formation of artificial vagina from segment of small intestine. LEBEDEFF, V. Monatschr. f. Geburtsh. u. Gynak. *76:*294–296, June '27
Artificial vagina justified by subsequent conception and childbirth. SCHUBERT, G. Med. Klin. *23:*1334–1336, Sept 2, '27
Artificial vagina formation by new plastic technic. FRANK, R. T. AND GEIST, S. H. Am. J. Obst. and Gynec. *14:*712–718, Dec '27
Successful plastic operation for aplasia of vagina. KÖHLER, M. Wein. klin. Wchnschr. *40:*1577–1578, Dec 15, '27
Artificial vagina formation by Baldwin's method. GAMBAROW, G. Monatschr. f. Geburtsh. u. Gynak. *78:*106–108, Jan '28
Two cases of absence of vagina treated by plastic operations. DAVIS, C. H. AND CRON, R. S. Am. J. Obst. and Gynec. *15:*196–201, Feb '28
Construction of artificial vagina from sigmoid flexure in case of congenital aplasia. RUGE, E. Monatschr. f. Geburtsh. u. Gynak. *78:*313–326, March '28
Artificial vagina formed from rectum; 2 cases. SCHMELEW, W. Med. Welt *2:*403–405, March 17, '28
New method of formation of artificial vagina. VON JASCHKE, R. T. Zentralbl. f. Gynak. *52:*735–736, March 24, '28
Artificial vagina—plastic surgery; Abalos' method. ABALOS, J. B. AND NATALE, A. M. Rev. de chir. *7:*551–557, Dec '28
Baldwin's operation in case of complete absence of vagina. AKHVLEDYANI, A. V., J. akush. i zhensk. boliez. *39:*912–916, '28
Artificial vagina formation by transplantation of piece of ileum. CHERNIGOVSKY, N. N., J. akush. i zhensk. boliez. *39:*329–332, '28
Baldwin's operation with Constantini's modification for artificial vagina; case. LAMPRECHT, V. L., J. akush. i zhensk. boliez. *39:*916–918, '28
Artificial vagina formation from large intestine (S. Romanum). MARCHENKO, E. Mosk. med. j. (no. 2) *8:*61–65, '28
Artificial vagina formation by grafting tissue from small intestine. RODIONOV, F. I. Vestnik khir. (nos. 37–38) *13:*342–345, '28
Artificial vagina formation by Popoff's method and its remote results. ZDRAVOMYSLOFF, V. I., J. akush. i zhensk. boliez. *39:*333–344, '28

Vagina, Artificial – Cont.
Schubert's method of plastic construction of vagina; 2 cases. MALUSCHEW, D. Zentralbl. f. Gynak. *53:*428–430, Feb 16, '29
Plastic formation of vagina with bladder. MARKOFF, N. Gynec. et Obst. *19:*182–190, March '29
Intestinal obstruction simulated by segregated closed loop of bowel; case following Baldwin operation for artificial vagina. QUIGLEY, R. A. Northwest Med. *28:*122–123, March '29
Technic and results of Popoff's method of formation of artificial vagina; 7 cases. SDRAWOMYSLOW, W. I. Monatschr. f. Geburtsh. u. Gynak. *82:*182–204, June '29
Transplantation of rectum in defective vagina. SZILI, E. Verhandl. d. ungar. arztl. Gesellsch. *1:*149, June '29
Vagina formation from sigmoid flexure; case. FAEHRMANN, J. Zentralbl. f. Chir. *56:*1989–1993, Aug 10, '29
Defective vagina and formation of artificial vagina by Schubert-Grigoriu's method. IUBAS, C. Cluj. med. *10:*404–408, Aug 1, '29
Obliteration of orifice of artificial vagina with subsequent suppuration and perforation of blind sac of intestine used in formation of vagina; case. MALINOWSKY, N. N. Monatschr. f. Geburtsh. u. Gynak. *83:*77–81, Sept '29
Formation of artificial vagina. RUSHMORE, S. Am. J. Obst. and Gynec. *18:*427–429, Sept '29
Function of isolated section of small intestine three and one-half years after Baldwin's operation (artificial vagina). VAKAR, A. A. Russk. klin. *12:*565–575, Oct–Nov '29
Plastic formation of artificial vagina by Schubert operation; 4 cases. NOVAK, J. Zentralbl. f. Gynak. *53:*2902–2908, Nov 16, '29
Artificial vagina formation from sigmoid flexure. RUGE, E. Zentralbl. f. Chir. *56:*2958, Nov 23, '29
Primary carcinoma of vagina following Baldwin reconstruction operation for congenital absence of vagina. RITCHIE, R. N. Am. J. Obst. and Gynec. *18:*794–799, Dec '29
Technic of Popoff method of formation of artificial vagina. MANDELSTAMM, A. Arch. f. Gynak. *138:*739–746, '29
Artificial vagina; formation from double coil of small intestine. GALAKHOFF, E. V. Vrach. gaz. *34:*127–130, Jan 31, '30
Popoff method of formation of artificial vagina. TCHERNIGOVSKY, N. N. Vrach. gaz. *34:*216–218, Feb 15, '30

Vagina, Artificial – Cont.
Artificial vagina formation in case of normal uterus. ZUBRZYCHI, J. Polska gaz. lek. *9:*105–106, Feb 9, '30
Cure of complete incontinentia alvi following Schubert's operation for plastic formation of vagina; case. HEYER, E. Zentralbl. f. Gynak. *54:*1238–1240, May 17, '30
Formation of artificial vagina. FELSTEAD, R. J. Coll. Surgeons, Australasia *3:*112–114, July '30
Comment on Heyer's article about formation of vagina. MELZNER, E. Zentralbl. f. Gynak. *54:*2072–2075, Aug 16, '30
Operative formation of vagina in patient with congenital absence of vagina; case. TURENNE, A. An. de Fac. de med., Montevideo *15:*725–749, Sept–Oct '30
Baldwin operation for formation of vagina closely resembling normal one, from vagina septa (bipartite vagina). FRANKENBERG, B. E. Zentralbl. f. Chir. *57:*2792–2796, Nov 8, '30
Surgical construction of vagina; 2 cases. FALTIN, R. Acta obst. et gynec. Scandinav. *9:*124–131, '30
Artificial vagina formed from sigmoid. FRANKENBERG, B. Arch. f. Gynak. *140:*226–252, '30
Baldwin operation for artificial vagina; 7 cases. GITELSON, U. E., J. akush. i. zhensk. boliez. *41:*467–476, '30
New procedure for formation of artificial vagina. KIRSCHNER, M. AND WAGNER, G. A. Deutsche Ztschr. f. Chir. *225:*242–264, '30 abstr: Zentralbl. f. Gynak. *54:*2690–2696, Oct 25, '30
New principle in formation of artificial vagina. OGNEFF, B. V. Vestnik khir. (no. 64) *22:*105–110, '30
Treatment of persistent tubular urogenital sinus by formation of vagina from rectum; case. SCHUBERT, G. Arch. f. Gynak. *141:*228–236, '30
Baldwin operation in case of congenital absence of vagina. TCHARKVIANI, I. I., J. akush. i zhensk. boliez. *41:*477–481, '30
New method of formation of artificial vagina. WAGNER, G. A. Ztschr. f. Geburtsh. u. Gynak. *98:*412–421, '30
Success of Schubert's operation in aplasia of vagina; 3 cases. WICHMANN, S. E. Acta obst. et gynec. Scandinav. *9:*661–683, '30
New procedure for formation of artificial vagina. (Comment on Kirschner and Wagner's article.) MÜLLER, P. Zentralbl. f. Gynak. *55:*201–203, Jan 24, '31
Operative methods in formation of artificial

Vagina, Artificial – Cont.
vagina. Ostrčil, A. Casop. lek. cesk. *70:*596–599, April 24, '31
Formation of artificial vagina by Kirschner-Wagner operation. Vogt, E. Zentralbl. f. Gynak. *55:*1634–1639, May 16, '31
Colpopoiesis by means of transplantation according to Thiersch method. Ostrčil, A. Zentralbl. f. Gynak. *55:*1900–1901, June 13, '31
Formation of artificial vagina by Kirschner-Wagner operation; case. Kraul, L. Zentralbl. f. Gynak. *55:*2102–2104, July 4, '31
Artificial vagina in case of congenital absence of vagina. Turenne, A. Rev. de med., Rosario *6:*291–303, Aug '31
Advantages of Kirschner-Wagner operation for artificial vagina. Miländer, J. Zentralbl. f. Gynak. *55:*2746–2749, Sept 12, '31
Formation of artificial vagina; contribution to 25th anniversary of Baldwin operation. Rabinovitch, C. N. Am. J. Surg. *13:*480–483, Sept '31
Permanent results in Schubert plastic operation for artificial vagina (transplantation of piece of colon). Schubert, G. Chirurg *3:*796–801, Sept 15, '31
Artificial vagina from sigmoid. Hejduk, B. Casop. lek. cesk. *70:*1458–1461, Oct 30, '31
Grigoriu modification of Schubert method in aplasia vaginae. Iubas, C. Zentralbl. f. Gynak. *55:*3379–3384, Nov 21, '31
Plastic repair of vagina by graft of 2 prepuces; case. Petit, R. Rev. franc. de gynec. et d'obst. *26:*605–607, Nov '31
Plastic methods of construction of vagina; 10 cases. Bazala, W. Ztschr. f. Geburtsh. u. Gynak. *100:*85–114, '31
Methods of formation of artificial vagina. Graf, P. Deutsche Ztschr. f. Chir. *232:*364–374, '31
Formation of artificial vagina from tubular portion of skin; case. Lichtenauer, K. Deutsche Ztschr. f. Chir. *232:*375–380, '31
Formation of artificial vagina and bladder from sigmoid. Rudolf, A. Beitr. z. klin. Chir. *153:*103–109, '31
Formation of artificial vagina with use of skin flaps. Müller, P. Vereinsbl. d. pfalz. Aerzte *44:*21, Jan 15, '32, Feb 1, '32
Technic of formation of artificial vagina; 4 cases. Stoeckel, W. Monatschr. f. Geburtsh. u. Gynak. *90:*23–33, Jan '32
Additional reports on satchel handle operation for artificial vagina. Frank, R. T. and Geist, S. H. Am. J. Obst. and Gynec. *23:*256–258, Feb '32
Technic of formation of artificial vagina.

Vagina, Artificial – Cont.
Grad, H. Surg., Gynec. and Obst. *54:*200–206, Feb '32
Surgical construction of artificial vagina by Wagner-Kirschner operation and Krause method of using skin flaps. Warnecke, K. Zentralbl. f. Gynak. *56:*416–418, Feb 13, '32
Formation of artificial vagina (Frank-Geist method). Frank, R. T., S. Clin. North America *12:*305–310, April '32
Construction of artificial vagina. Glatzel, J. and Zubrzycki, J. Ginek. polska *11:*580, April–June '32
Formation of artificial vagina from epidermis. Maczewski, S. and Gruca, A. Ginek. polska *11:*577–579, April–June '32
Construction of artificial vagina. Gilmer, L. Monatschr. f. Geburtsh. u. Gynak. *91:*48–56, May '32
Formation of artificial vagina. Hartmann, H. Gynec. et obst. *25:*401–403, May '32
Formation of artificial vagina by Kirschner-Wagner operation. Kayser, K. Zentralbl. f. Gynak. *56:*1633–1635, July 2, '32
Formation of artificial vagina from epidermis. Müller, P. Chirurg *4:*527–533, July 1, '32
Formation of artificial vagina by use of labial tissue. Santi, E. Clin. ostet. *34:*517–520, Aug '32
Formation of artificial vagina by Wagner-Kirschner operation; case. Heller, P. Zentralbl. f. Gynak. *56:*2491–2494, Oct 8, '32
Congenital absence of vagina and its treatment. Masson, J. C. Am. J. Obst. and Gynec. *24:*583–591, Oct '32
Solid double rudimentary uterus with absence of cervix and vagina. Ronka, E. K. F. New England J. Med. *207:*945–946, Nov 24, '32
Surgical formation of artificial vagina; review of literature. Schubert, G. Ber. u. d. ges. Gynak. u. Geburtsh. *23:*241–268, Dec 27, '32
Construction of artificial vagina with aid of Thiersch transplants. Henkel, M. Ztschr. f. Geburtsh. u. Gynak. *104:*36–45, '32
Technic and some unsuccessful results of various methods of plastic repair of congenital absence of vagina; case. Landois, F. Arch. f. klin. Chir. *170:*178–187, '32
Formation of artificial vagina by skin flap (Ostrčil method); case. Müller, G. Rozhl. v chir. a gynaek. (cast gynaek.) *11:*55–59, '32
Total and partial absence of vagina; 2 cases. Pérez Olivares, C. Bol. an. clin. ginec. *2:*124–136, '32

Vagina, Artificial –Cont.

Baldwin operation in congenital absence of vagina; result after 11 years. BROHEE, G. J. de chir. et ann. Soc belge de chir. *30–32:*13–16, Jan '33

Artificial vagina formation by Kirschner-Wagner operation; case. ALFEROW, M. W. Zentralbl. f. Gynak. *57:*884–885, April 15, '33

Artificial vagina in case of total absence of uterus and vagina. BUENO RODRIGO, L. Siglo med. *91:*549–550, May 27, '33

Formation of artificial vagina by Kirschner-Wagner operation. KÖHLER, H. Zentralbl. f. Gynak. *57:*1182–1186, May 20, '33

Baldwin operation in congenital absence of vagina; result after 11 years. BROHEE, C. Scalpel *86:*825–829, June 3, '33

Kirschner-Wagner operation for artificial vagina. GLATZEL, J. AND ZUBRZYCKI, J. Polska gaz. lek. *12:*577–579, July 29, '33

Baldwin-Mori operation for artificial vagina; case. GUTIÉREZ, A. Bol. y trab. de la Soc. de cir. de Buenos Aires *17:*739–742, Aug 2, '33

Technic of formation of artificial vagina. SOLER JULIÁ, J. Ann. de Hosp. de Santa Creu i Sant Pau *7:*332–334, Sept 15, '33

Simple method of construction of artificial vagina. GAMBAROW, G. Zentralbl. f. Gynak. *57:*2559–2562, Oct 28, '33

Formation of artificial vagina by Kirschner-Wagner operation. MACZEWSKI, S. Polska gaz. lek. *12:*829–830, Oct 22, '33

Baldwin operation for artificial vagina. SCHEPETINSKY, A. Monatschr. f. Geburtsh. u. Gynak. *95:*270–273, Oct '33

Formation of artificial vagina from rectum (Schubert operation) in congenital vaginal defect; preliminary report. STARCK, H. Zentralbl. f. Gynak. *57:*2562–2565, Oct 28, '33

Construction of artificial vagina with aid of Thiersch transplants. JUNG, J. Rozhl. v chir. a gynaek. (cast gynaek.) *12:*104–109, '33

Cure of vaginal aplasia by Kirschner-Wagner operation. WESTMAN, A. Acta obst. et gynec. Scandinav. *13:*269–273, '33

Surgical therapy of total absence of vagina. FAVREAU, M. Gynecologie *33:*5–14, Jan '34 also: J. d'obst. et de gynec. prat. *5:*3–16, Jan '34

Formation of artificial vagina by Mandelshtam modification of rectal method (Popoff); report of 8 additional cases. MANDELSHTAM, A. E. Zentralbl. f. Gynak. *58:*222–228, Jan 27, '34

Vagina, Artificial–Cont.

Construction of artificial vagina from loop of sigmoid. CARLING, E. R. Brit. M. J. *1:*375–376, March 3, '34

Formation of artificial vagina by transplantation of muscular flap. SOLER JULIÁ, J. Rev. de cir. de Barcelona *7:*194–198, March '34

Successful plastic operation for vaginal atresia, using portion of ileum for new wall; case. SCHMIDT, W. T. Monatschr. f. Geburtsh. u. Gynak. *97:*50–52, April '34

Formation of artificial vagina with membrane from fetus at term; case. BRINDEAU, A. Gynec. et obst. *29:*385–392, May '34

Reconstruction of vagina; employment of flap transplantation method in one stage with favorable anatomical result. DOUGLASS, M. D. Surg., Gynec. and Obst. *58:*982–985, June '34

New plastic operation in case of uterovaginal aplasia. KREIS, J. Rev. franc. de gynec. et d'obst. *29:*898–903, Aug '34

Creation of vagina by autoplasty; case. LAFFONT, AND BONAFOS. Bull. Soc. d'obst. et de gynec. *23:*637–640, Nov '34

Formation of vagina by means of modified skin graft method. MATWEJEW, F. P. Zentralbl. f. Gynak. *58:*2727–2736, Nov 17, '34 also: Rev. franc. de gynec. et d'obst. *30:*57–71, Feb '35

Question of advantages of use of loop of small intestine, of segment of rectum or Thiersch grafts in colpoplasty for congenital absence of vagina. FORGUE, E. Paris med. *2:*479–486, Dec 15, '34

Surgical correction of vaginal aplasia. WESTMAN, A. Nord. med. tidskr. *8:*1688–1692, Dec 15, '34

Use of modified Kirschner-Wagner operation in aplasia of vagina and atresia of cervix; case. WESTMAN, A. Zentralbl. f. Gynak. *58:*2843–2845, Dec 1, '34

Plastic operation for vaginal defect ad modum Kirschner-Wagner. NEILSEN, M. Acta obst. et gynec. Scandinav. *14:*314–320, '34

Neoplasty of vagina by Wagner-Thiersch method (grafts). RISMONDO, P. Lijecn. vjes. *56:*312–313, '34

Formation of artificial vagina. ESAT, A. Turk tip cem. mec. *1:*15–20, Jan 1, '35

Congenital absence of vagina; surgical therapy. RIBAS, G. Ann. de Hosp. de Santa Creu i Sant Pau *9:*66–83, Jan 15, '35

Surgical technic for formation of artificial vagina. PŘÍBRSKÝ, J. Zentralbl. f. Gynak. *59:*403–406, Feb 16, '35

Vagina, Artificial–Cont.

Construction of vagina with loop from sigmoid. HEJDUK, B. Bratisl. lekar. listy *15:*241-251, March '35

Use of vernix caseosa in formation of artificial vagina; histologic examination of vagina some time after operation. KLEITSMAN, R. AND POSKA-TEISS, L. Zentralbl. f. Gynak. *59:*755-760, March 30, '35

Technics of formation of artificial vagina; case. CASU, C. Rassegna d'ostet. e ginec. *44:*208-228, April 30, '35

Creation of artificial vagina; value of use of vernix caseosa; case. KLEITSMAN, R. Gynec. et obst. *31:*725-728, May '35

Vaginal aplasia (with ectopic kidney) and creation of artificial vagina. ISRAEL, S. L. Am. J. Obst. and Gynec. *30:*273-276, Aug '35

Plastic surgery of artificial vagina. SCHILLING, B. Orvosi hetil. *79:*863-866, Aug 10, '35

Plastic operation for congenital absence of vagina. WELLS, W. F. Am. J. Surg. *29:*253-255, Aug '35

Construction of artificial vagina according to Grigoriu method in case of aplasia. IUBAS, C. Rev. de chir., Bucuresti *38:*170-175, Sept-Dec '35

Congenital absence of vagina; simplified operation with report of one case. KANTER, A. E. Am. J. Surg. *30:*314-316, Nov '35

Reconstruction of vagina from portion of sigmoid; case. PITTS, H. C. New England J. Med. *213:*1136-1137, Dec 5, '35

Formation of artificial vagina by using Thiersch transplants (Henkel modification of Kirschner-Wagner operation). FRIEDL-MEYER, M. Deutsche Ztschr. f. Chir. *244:*379-386, '35

Reconstruction of vagina from portion of sigmoid; case. PITTS, H. C. Tr. New England S. Soc. *18:*273-275, '35

Artificial vagina; Kirschner-Wagner operation. BARROWS, D. N. Am. J. Obst. and Gynec. *31:*156-158, Jan '36

Artificial vagina. ANDERSON, G. V. W. East African M. J. *12:*377-378, March '36

Formation of artificial vagina. BECK, H. Orvosi hetil. *80:*207-209, March 7, '36

New method of surgical therapy of acquired vaginal stenosis. REMZI, T., J. Egyptian M. A. *19:*137-139, March '36

Plastic replacement of vagina with portion of sigmoid flexure (Ruge operation) after Wertheim operation for total extirpation; case. BALKOW, E. Deutsche med. Wchnschr. *62:*586-588, April 10, '36

Vagina, Artificial–Cont.

Plastic operations for construction of artificial vagina. FLYNN, C. W. AND DUCKETT, J. W. Surg., Gynec. and Obst. *62:*753-756, April '36

Colpoplasty for congenital absence of vagina by modified method of Thiersch grafts mounted on rigid supports. MONOD, R. AND ISELIN, M. Mem. Acad. de chir. *62:*997-1002, June 24, '36

Congenital absence of vagina; reconstruction according to Italian method by grafts from genitocrural fold on each side; case in girl 21 years old. VIOLET, H. Lyon med. *158:*277-282, Sept 13, '36

Colpoplasty by modified Baldwin technic for congenital absence of vagina; case. COSTANTINI, AND FERRARI. Mem. Acad. de chir. *62:*1213-1215, Oct 28, '36

Baldwin-Mori operation for artificial vagina; case. GRIDNEW, A. Gynec. et obst. *34:*312-314, Oct '36

New technic for formation of artificial vagina. MACHADO, L. M. Rev. de gynec. e d'obst. *30:*782-789, Oct '36

Late results of surgical formation of artificial vagina. WARGASSOWA, W. G. Zentralbl. f. Gynak. *60:*2623-2631, Oct 31, '36

Artificial vagina obtained by section of urethro-vesico-rectal septum. MÜLLER, G. Casŏp. lek. cesk. *75:*1393-1399, Nov 6, '36

Operation for vaginal aplasia and malformation of cervix uteri. WESTMAN, A. Svenska lak.-tidning. *33:*1721-1725, Nov 27, '36

Plastic method in construction of artificial vagina. ASTRAKHANSKIY, V. A. Sovet. khir., no. 9, pp. 497-500, '36

Artificial vagina formation from sigmoid. BALKOW, E. Ztschr. f. Geburtsh. u. Gynak. *112:*256-260, '36

Evaluation of formation of artificial vagina by Baldwin-Mori operation. GRIDNEV, A. Arch. f. Gynak. *162:*397-402, '36

Formation of artificial vagina according to Baldwin technic. LEBEDEV, V. F. Sovet. khir., no. 2, pp. 351-354, '36

Plastic formation of artificial vagina by Kirschner-Wagner operation; case. NIELSEN, M. Acta obst. et gynec. Scandinav. *16:*179-188, '36

Formation of artificial vagina. PORTUGALOV, S. O. Vestnik khir. *44:*261-270, '36

Artificial vagina construction from fetal membranes; 2 cases. PODVINEC, J. Casop. lek. cesk. *76:*48-49, Jan 15, '37

Artificial vagina construction by Kirschner method. ZURALSKI, T. Ginek. polska *16:*64-70, Jan-Feb '37

Vagina, Artificial–Cont.

Congenital absence of vagina; creation of new vagina by perieotomy; failure of amniotic graft; excellent functional and anatomic results; case. LAFARGUE, P. AND RIVIERE, M. Bull. Soc. d'obst. et de gynec. *26:*278–280, April '37

Congenital absence of vagina; creation of artificial vagina by autoplastic graft. PAVLOVSKY, A. J. Bol. y trab. de la Soc. de cir. de Buenos Aires *21:*307–328, June 9, '37 also: Rev. de cir. de Buenos Aires *16:*344–362, July '37

New method of construction of artificial vagina. BURGER, K. Orvosi hetil. *81:*788–790, July 31, '37

Artificial vagina constructed from peritoneum. GLOWINSKI, M. Ginek. polska *16:*683–687, July–Aug '37

Artificial vagina, plastic formation in uterovaginal aplasia, with report of case. PALAZZO, O. R. Semana med. *2:*189–200, July 22, '37

Use of fetal membranes in formation of artificial vagina. BURGER, K. Zentralbl. f. Gynak. *61:*2437–2440, Oct 16, '37

Artificial vagina constructed from Douglas pouch. GLOWINSKI, M. Zentralbl. f. Gynak. *61:*2440–2442, Oct 16, '37

Artificial vagina, formation from urethra. KNAUS, H. Zentralbl. f. Gynak. *61:*2540–2545, Oct 30, '37

Artificial vagina constructed from Douglas pouch; question of priority. MACHADO, L. M. Rev. de gynec. e d'obst. *31:*500–501, Dec '37

Creation of artificial vagina in congenital absence. BORRAS, P. E. Bol. Soc. de cir. de Rosario *4:*24–34, '37

Operation for aplasia of vagina. DE RAAD, H. Nederl. tijdschr. v. verlosk. en gynaec. *40:*153–158, '37

Results and indications for Kirschner-Wagner operation in connection with 2 cases of vaginal aplasia. PELKONEN, E. Duodecim *53:*1003–1017, '37

Frank-Geist operation for congenital absence of vagina (skin graft). DANNREUTHER, W. T. Am. J. Obst. and Gynec. *35:*452–468, March '38

Construction of artificial vagina by tube graft method. DOUGLASS, M. Am. J. Obst. and Gynec. *35:*675–680, April '38

Artificial vagina construction using transplanted amniotic membrane as lining. CAFFIER, P. Zentralbl. f. Gynak. *62:*1186–1192, May 28, '38

Simple method of construction of vagina; 4 cases. WHARTON, L. R. Ann. Surg. *107:*842–854, May '38

Artificial vagina formation without operation. FRANK, R. T. Am. J. Obst. and Gynec. *35:*1053–1055, June '38

Operation for cure of congenital absence of vagina. MCINDOE, A. H. AND BANISTER, J. B., J. Obst. and Gynaec. Brit. Emp. *45:*490–494, June '38

Congenital absence of vagina, treated by means of indwelling skin-graft. BANISTER, J. B. AND MCINDOE, A. H. Proc. Roy. Soc. Med. *31:*1055–1056, July '38

Congenital anomalies with particular reference to cryptorchidism, hypospadias and congenital absence of vagina (surgical treatment). COUNSELLER, V. S., J. Michigan M. Soc. *37:*689–697, Aug '38

Artificial vagina. KRAUL, L. Zentralbl. f. Gynak. *62:*2099–2102, Sept 17, '38

Congenital absence and traumatic obliteration of vagina and its treatment with inlaying Thiersch grafts. COUNSELLER, V. S. Am. J. Obst. and Gynec. *36:*632–638, Oct '38

Late cancer of artificial vagina formed from rectum (Schubert operation); case. LAVAND'HOMME, P. Bruxelles-med. *19:*14–15, Nov 6, '38

Schubert operation for artificial vagina; case. COTTE, G. Mem. Acad. de chir. *64:*1365–1374, Dec 14, '38

Indications for artificial vagina. KRAATZ, H. Ztschr. f. Geburtsh. u. Gynak. *117:*168–174, '38

Baldwin-Mori operation for congenital absence of vagina. HORTOLOMEI, N. Rev. de chir., Burcuresti *42:*136–138, Jan–Feb '39

Construction of artificial vagina from vesicourethro-rectal septum; late results. MÜLLER, G. Casop. lek. cesk. *78:*169–171, Feb 17, '39

Use of fetal membranes in vaginal reconstruction. BURGER, K. Geburtsh. u. Frauenh. *1:*183–187, March '39

Biologic significance of fetal membranes (including use as grafts); Joseph Price oration (artificial vagina). BURGER, K. Am. J. Obst. and Gynec. *37:*572–584, April '39

Creation of artificial vagina from intraperitoneal hematocolpos in atresia, with subsequent normal childbirth; case. LOSSEN, W. Zentralbl. f. Gynak. *63:*844–847, April 15, '39

Creation of artificial vagina by perineal autoplasty in case of congenital aplasia. PASCALIS, G. Rev. de chir., Paris *77:*304–306,

Vagina, Artificial – Cont.

April '39

Vaginal aplasia; modern trends in therapy. Colmeiro Laforet, C. Rev. med. cubana *50:*423–427, May '39

Histologic and biologic value of Schubert operation for vaginal reconstruction after one year; report of case with peritonitis as sequel. Klimko, D. Zentralbl. f. Gynak. *63:*1150–1161, May 20, '39

Congenital vaginal absence; surgical therapy of case. Abreu e Lima, A. Ann. brasil. de gynec. *7:*478–484, June '39

Plastic surgery of vaginal aplasia, using portion of sigmoid flexure; review of literature and report of 2 personal cases. Hejduk, B. Zentralbl. f. Gynak. *63:*1298–1309, June 10, '39

New surgical treatment for congenital absence and traumatic obliteration of vagina (skin grafting). Counseller, V. S., S. Clin. North America *19:*1047–1052, Aug '39

Construction of artificial vagina by formation of pedicled skin flap. Grossmann, H. Zentralbl. f. Gynak. *63:*1810–1814, Aug 12, '39

Construction of artificial vagina by Kirschner-Wagner operation. Colombino, C. and Sanvenero Rosselli, G. Atti Soc. ital. di ostet. e ginec. *35:*460–464, Sept–Oct '39

Artificial vagina. Block, F. B. Am. J. M. Sc. *198:*567–576, Oct '39

Artificial vagina in case of aplasia. Ismail, M., J. Egyptian M. A. *22:*583–586, Oct '39

Congenital absence of vagina; creation of artificial vagina by author's autoplastic procedure. Pavlovsky, A. J. Bol. Soc. de cir. de Rosario *6:*453–458, Nov '39

Congenital absence of vagina; features simplifying procedure for reconstruction. Sears, N. P. New York State J. Med. *39:*2019–2021, Nov 1, '39

Various methods for construction of artificial vagina in correction with 7 cases. Pachner, F. Gynaekologie *18:*142–150, '39

Formation of artificial vagina without operation by Frank method. Holmes, W. R. and Williams, G. A. Am. J. Obst. and Gynec. *39:*145–146, Jan '40

Agenesis of vagina (surgical treatment). Cowles, A. G. Texas State J. Med. *35:*685–688, Feb '40

Artificial vagina; plastic surgery according to Baldwin-Mori. Constantinescu, M. and Covali, N. Rev. de chir., Bucuresti *43:*296–298, March–April '40

Formation of artificial vagina. Steinmetz, E. P. West. J. Surg. *48:*169–180, March '40

Vagina, Artificial – Cont.

Construction of artificial vagina; modification of Wharton operation; 3 cases. Word, B. South. M. J. *33:*293–301, March '40

Congenital absence of vagina; creation of artificial vagina by autoplastic procedure. Arenas, N. and Bolla, I. Semana med. *1:*841–845, April 4, '40

Further experiences in construction of artificial vagina; 12 cases. Wharton, L. R. Ann. Surg. *111:*1010–1020, June '40

Silver-plated vaginal prosthesis for construction of artificial vagina. Word, B. Am. J. Obst. and Gynec. *39:*1071, June '40

Creation of artificial vagina by Baldwin-Mori operation. Goni Moreno, I. Bol. y trab., Acad. argent. de cir. *24:*453–460, July 3, '40

Single kidney and congenital absence of uterus and vagina; vaginoplasty. Constantinesco, M. M. *et al.* Rev. de chir., Bucuresti *43:*713–714, Sept–Oct '40

Simple method for construction of artificial vagina. Falls, F. H. Am. J. Obst. and Gynec. *40:*906–917, Nov '40

Formation of artificial vagina without operation (by intubation method). Frank, R. T. New York State J. Med. *40:*1669–1670, Nov 15, '40

Artificial vagina; Baldwin-Mori procedure; surgical technic. Goni Moreno, I. Prensa med. argent. *27:*2579–2583, Dec 11, '40

Artificial vagina construction using fetal membranes. Marsalek, J. Casop. lek. cesk. *79:*1075–1078, Dec 6, '40

Congenital vaginal and anal atresia. Sigwart, W. Geburtsh. u. Frauenh. *2:*628–635, Dec '40

Modification of operation for artificial vagina from sigmoid. Shor, A. M. Novy khir. arkhiv. *45:*252–253, '40

Case of genital aplasia; artificial vagina successfully constructed by Baldwin operation. Bodenheimer, M. and Goldman, M. L., J. Mt. Sinai Hosp. *7:*310–315, Jan–Feb '41

Evolution of treatment for absent vagina. Frank, R. T., J. Mt. Sinai Hosp. *7:*259–262, Jan–Feb '41

Creation of artificial vagina in girl before marriage. Gomez Navarro, A. C. Semana med. *1:*221–224, Jan 23, '41

Construction of artificial vagina. Heymann, J. A. Texas State J. Med. *37:*30–33, May '41

Artificial vagina, creation before marriage; case. Gomez Navarro, A. C. Rev. Asoc. med. argent. *55:*484–486, June 15–30, '41

Plastic construction of artificial vagina. Blocker, T. G. Jr. Texas State J. Med.

Vagina, Artificial – Cont.
*37:*345–348, Sept '41
Management of congenital absence of vagina. SADLER, L., J. Oklahoma M. A. *34:*382–385, Sept '41
Surgical therapy of aplasia of vagina. TASCH, H. Wien. klin. Wchnschr. *54:*883–888, Oct 24, '41
Absence of vagina; successful treatment without operation. CAMPBELL, K., M. J. Australia *2:*650, Dec 6, '41
Imperforate vagina; case. GUIMARAES, N. A. Med. cir. pharm., pp. 40–41, Jan '42
Simplified method for formation of artificial vagina by split graft; case. OWENS, N. Surgery *12:*139–150, July '42
Aplasia of vagina. BUENO PLEMONT, I. Rev. med.-cir. do Brasil *50:*899–906, Sept '42
Technic in creation of artificial vagina from rectum. POPOFF, D. Rev. franc. de gynec. et d'obst. *37:*225–236, Oct '42
Construction of artificial vagina in case of congenital absence. BITTENCOURT, J. Rev. med. de Pernambuco *12:*315–325, Dec '42
Partial congenital aplasia of vagina (transplantation of fetal membranes for artificial vagina in one case). DANNREUTHER, W. T. Am. J. Obst. and Gynec. *44:*1063–1073, Dec '42 also: Tr. Am. Gynec. Soc. (1942) *67:*35–45, '43.
Congenital absence of vagina and its construction. ADAMS, W. M. Memphis M. J. *18:*3–5, Jan '43
Construction of artificial vagina. ADAMS, W. M. Surg., Gynec. and Obst. *76:*746–751, June '43
Congenital absence of vagina; choice of operative procedure. ESSER, E., J. Internat. Coll. Surgeons *6:*496–499, Sept–Oct '43
Congenital absence of vagina treated successfully by Baldwin technic. O'NEILL, T. Brit. M. J. *2:*746–747, Dec 11, '43
Artificial vagina in congenital absence. REEL, P. J. Ohio State M. J. *39:*1117–1119, Dec '43
Artificial vagina, creation in congenital absence. DIONISI, H. AND YORNET, H. Bol. y trab., Soc. de cir. de Cordoba *4:*40–59, '43
Unique constructive operation in artificial vagina. BONNEY, V. AND McINDOE, A. H. J. Obst. and Gynaec. Brit. Emp. *51:*24–29, Feb '44
Surgical treatment of congenital (stricture) absence of vagina. READ, C. D. Irish J. M. Sc., pp. 52–57, Feb '44
Artificial vagina formation; experiences with 3 different corrective procedures. MARSHALL, H. K. West. J. Surg. *52:*245–255, June '44

Vagina, Artificial – Cont.
Artificial vagina; bicornate uterus and absence of vagina; case. STOCK, F. E., M. Press *211:*365–366, June 7, '44
Artificial vagina in treatment for congenital absence. COUNSELLER, V. S. AND SLUDER, F. S., S. Clin. North America *24:*938–942, Aug '44
Artificial vagina; biologic changes in squamous epithelium transplanted to pelvic connective tissue. WHITACRE, F. E. AND WANG, Y. Y. Surg., Gynec. and Obst. *79:*192–194, Aug '44
Cyclic ovarian changes in artificial vaginal mucosa. AYRE, J. E. Am. J. Obst. and Gynec. *48:*690–695, Nov '44
Construction of artificial vagina. PICKERILL, H. P. New Zealand M. J. *44:*37–40, Feb '45
Methods of constructing vagina. BRADY, L. Ann. Surg. *121:*518–529, April '45
Spontaneous perforation of rectovaginal septum, 5 weeks after construction of vagina; cases. WHARTON, L. R. Ann. Surg. *121:*530–533, April '45
Artificial vagina covered with dermoepidermal graft. PALAZZO, O. R. Bol. Soc. de obst. y ginec. de Buenos Aires *24:*183–192, June 21, '45
Construction of artificial vagina in case of aplasia. WESTERBORN, A. Nord. med. (Hygiea) *26:*1194–1195, June 8, '45
Surgical treatment of absence of vagina; 2 cases. WHITACRE, F. E. AND CHEN, C. Y. Am. J. Obst. and Gynec. *49:*789–796, June '45
Formation of artificial vagina without operation. DAWSON, J. B. New Zealand M. J. *44:*132–133, June '45
Wharton operation in case of partial aplasia of vagina. CABRAL JUNIOR, A. An. brasil. de ginec. *20:*87–107, Aug '45
Surgical correction of congenital aplasia of vagina; evaluation of operative procedures, end result and functional activity of transplanted epithelium. MILLER, N. F.; *et al.* Am. J. Obst. and Gynec. *50:*735–747, Dec '45
Surgical correction of congenital aplasia of vagina; evaluation of operative procedures, end result and functional activity of transplanted epithelium. MILLER, N. F.; *et al.* Am. J. Obst. and Gynec. *50:*735–747, Dec '45
Methods of construction of artificial vagina. BRADY, L. Tr. South. S. A. (1944) *56:*134–145, '45
Spontaneous perforation of rectovaginal septum, 5 weeks after construction of vagina; case. WHARTON, L. R. Tr. South. S. A.

Vagina, Artificial – Cont.
(1944) *56:*146–148, '45
Difficulties and accidents encountered in construction of artificial vagina. WHARTON, L. R. Am. J. Obst. and Gynec. *51:*866–875, June '46
Urologic complications following operation for imperforate hymen (use of bladder to form artificial vagina). CRIGLER, C. M., J. Urol. *56:*211–222, Aug '46

VAKAR, A. A.: Functions of isolated fascia of jejunum tenue used in operation for artificial vagina by Baldwin's method. Russk. Klin. *7:*19–34, Jan '27
VAKAR, A. A.: Function of isolated section of small intestine three and one-half years after Baldwin's operation (artificial vagina). Russk. klin. *12:*565–575, Oct–Nov '29
VAKULENKO, M. V.: Restoration of function of hand after loss of 4 fingers. Sovet. khir., no. 8, p. 135, '35
VALCARCEL, A. G.: Dupuytren's contracture and retraction of connective tissue fibers. Zentralbl. f. Chir. *65:*2506–2508, Nov 5, '38
VALDES, G. Nasal septal deviations and their results. Rev. mex. de cir., ginec. y cancer *6:*559–569, Oct '38
VALDES, U.: Surgical shock. Rev. Asoc. med. mex., no. 14, p. 25, Feb; no. 15 p. 5, March '29
VALENTINI, P.: Pathogenic theories in typical case of acrocephalosyndactylia; case. Clin. pediat. *13:*211–222, March '31
VALERIO, A.: Exstrophy of bladder. Brazil-med. *2:*295–298, Nov 22, '24
VALERIO, M.: Surgical therapy of eyelid ptosis with special reference to Nida technic; results in cases. Rassegna ital. d'ottal. *8:*62–83, Jan–Feb '39
VALERIO, M.: Rare congenital malformation of eyelid, eyebrow, scalp and of eyeball; case. Ann. di ottal. e clin. ocul. *67:*704–714, Sept '39
VALERIO, M. (see FRANCESCHETTI, A.) 1945
VALK, A. (see HARRELL, G. T.) Feb '40
VALLE, D.: Dacryostomy and canaliculorhinostomy. Arq. brasil. de oftal. *5:*236–251, Oct '42
VALLE, S.: Eyelid paralysis; lagophthalmos in leprosy and its surgical correction. Arq. Inst. Penido Burnier *5:*238–264, Dec '39

Valle Operation

Valle operation (lacrimal), Brazilian contribution. CATALAO, P. V. B. Brasil-med. *57:*213, May 1–15, '43

VALLE ANTELO, J.: Plasmotherapy in shock. Prensa med., La Paz *3:*37–40, June–July '43
VALLEBONA, A.: Value and dangers of radium therapy of tumors of jaws; osteonecrosis; cases. Minerva med. (pt. 2) *8:*422–440, Aug 25, '28
VALLET, E.: Apparatus for treatment of fractures of fingers. Presse med. *33:*590–591, May 6, '25 abstr: J.A.M.A. *84:*1966, June 20, '25
VALLINO, M. T. AND SERFATY, M.: Success of surgical therapy of angiomas on face of nurslings; 2 cases. Rev. Asoc. med. argent. *48:*1463–1465, Dec '34
VALONE, J. A.: Modern treatment of burns. Mississippi Doctor *23:*610–614, Apr '46
VAN BAGGEN, N. Y. P.: Peripheral expressive or articular speech defects; cleft palate. M. J. and Rec. *125:*535–537, April 20, '27
VAN BRAAM HOUCKGEEST, A. Q.: Dupuytren's contracture. Nederlandsch Tijdschr. v. Geneesk. *2:*1032–1034, Sept 8, '23
VAN CANEGHEM, D.: Branchial cysts of lateral cervical region. Belg. tijdschr. geneesk. *2:*236–246, May '46
VAN CAPPELLEN, D.: Urethroplasty in hypospadias. Nederl. Tijdschr. v. Geneesk. *1:*356–358, Jan 21, '28
VAN DIJK, J. A.: Plastic reconstruction of ear with pedunculated tube flap. Nederl. Tijdschr. v. Geneesk. *1:*895–900, Feb 21, '25
VAN DIJK, J. A.: Reconstruction of totally lost ear by "tubed pedicle flap" method. Acta otolaryng. *10:*121–129, '26
VAN GELDEREN, D. N.: Burns from splashing of molten metal; advantages of picric acid treatment. Nederlandsch Tijdschr. v. Geneesk. *2:*2793–2794, Dec 3, '21
VAN GRAEFSCHEPE, C.: Corachan method of making basal skin grafts for rapid epidermization. J. de chir. et ann. Soc. belge de chir. *32–30:*353–355, Dec '33
VAN HARREVELD, A. (see BILLIG, H. E. JR.) March '43
VAN HOOK, W.: Pedicled flaps aided by free fat transplantation in plastic surgery. Med. Rec. *101:*625–626, April 15, '22
VAN LINT, A. AND HENNEBERT, P.: Congenital atrophy of lower eyelids, both auricles and lower jaw; case. Bull. Soc. belge d'opht., no. 73, pp. 51–61, '36
VAN LINT, A. AND HENNEBERT, P.: Congenital atrophy of lower eyelids, both auricles and lower jaw; case. Bruxelles-med. *17:*1065–1070, May 16, '37

van Millingen Operation

Author's modification of van Millingen-Sapejko operation for ectropion and trichiasis. LOSEV, N. A. Vestnik oftal. *12:*573–579, '38

van Millingen Operation–Cont.
New knife for van Millingen grafting operation (ingrown eyelashes). KAMEL, S. Bull. Ophth. Soc. Egypt *32:*73–78, '39

VAN NECK, M.: Cicatricial contractures. Arch. franco-belges de chir. *26:*245–257, March '23 (illus.) abstr: J.A.M.A. *80:*1813, June 16, '23
VAN NECK, M.: Case of macrodactylia. Arch. franco-belges de chir. *26:*895–898, Sept '23 (illus.)
VAN NECK, M.: Cleft-thumb operated on by Cloquet's method. Arch. franco-belges de chir. *28:*607–608, July '25
VAN NECK, M.: Congenital nodules of tendons; etiology of spring thumbs. Arch. franco-belges de chir. *29:*924–927, Oct '26
VAN OMMEN, B.: Jaw fractures. Nederl. tijdschr. v. geneesk. *83:*3888–3892, Aug 5, '39
VAN PUTTE, P. J.: Permanent destruction of hair by diathermy in facial hypertrichosis. Nederl. Tijdschr. v. Geneesk. *1:*924–928, Feb 19, '27
VAN REE, A.: Treatment of subcutaneous rupture of extensor tendons of distal phalanges of fingers. Nederl. tijdschr. v. geneesk. *80:*1999–2000, May 9, '36
VAN ROMUNDE, L. H. (see BENJAMINS, C. E) July '22
VAN SETERS, W. H.: Family of eighteenth century with eyelid ptosis; hereditary aspect. Nederl. tijdschr. v. geneesk. *74:*1775–1779, April 5, '30
VAN STUDDIFORD, M. T.: Radium treatment of cancer of lips. New Orleans M. and S. J. *84:*252–259, Oct '31
VAN THAL, J. H.: *Cleft Palate Speech*. George Allen and Unwin, Ltd., London, 1934
VAN VOORTHUYSEN, D. G. W.: Hypertelorism, case with unusual congenital malformation of external portion of nose, double overlapping external parts. Acta oto-laryng. *22:*540–544, '35
VAN ZILE, W. N.: Technic for building head cast fracture appliances from coat hangers for facial fractures. U. S. Nav. M. Bull. *42:*200–207, Jan '44
VAN DEN BERG, W. J.: Ganglion (of wrist); case (treated with sylnasol, fatty acid solution). California and West Med. *60:*24, Jan '44
VAN DEN BOSSCHE, P.: Acute pulmonary edema in course of local anesthesia for deviation of nasal septum; case. Ann. d. mal. de l'oreille, du larynx *49:*983–995, Oct '30
VAN DEN BRANDEN, J.: Technic of plastic surgery of face and nose. Bruxelles-med. *7:*917–920, May 15, '27
VAN DEN BROEK, A. J. P.: Bilateral absence of thumb; case. Nederl. Tijdschr. v. Geneesk. *1:*1452–1456, March 19, '27
VAN DEN WILDENBERG: Congenital anomalies in otorhinolaryngology. Bull. Soc. belge d'otol., rhinol., laryng., pp. 282–292, '37
VAN DEN WILDENBERG: Diathermy applied to facial lymphangiomas; cases. Oto-rhino-laryng. internat. *22:*5–10, Jan '38
VAN DEN WILDENBERG, L.: Tumors of hyothryo-pharyngeal region; laryngocele and branchial cyst. Scalpel *85:*265–271, Feb 27, '32
VANDER ELST: Homoplastic bone graft in tibia. Arch. franco-belges de chir. *26:*181–183, Feb '23 (illus.)
VAN DER GHINST, J.: Therapy and evolution of comminuted fractures of mandible; 2 cases. Arch. med. belges *85:*780–784, Nov '32
VAN DER HOEVEN, J.: Harelip operation in 1808. Nederl. Tidjschr. v. Geneesk. *1:*44–51, Jan 3, '25
VAN DER HOEVEN, L.: Local and general use of melted paraffin at 54°–60° C. in burns. Geneesk. Gids *6:*176–182, Feb 24, '28
VAN DER HOEVEN, LEONHARD J.: Cutting hook and inverse hammer for nasal surgery. Oto-rhino-laryng. internat. *17:*27–31, Jan '33
VAN DER HOFF, H.: Formation of artificial vagina from segment of small intestine. Nederl. Tijdschr. v. Geneesk. *1:*1538–1546, March 26, '27
VAN DER HOFF, H. L. M.: Surgical therapy of cleft palate. Chirurg *13:*396–403, July 1, '41
VAN DER LEE, H. S. AND SCHEFFELAAR KLOTS, T.: Spontaneous rupture of extensor pollicis longus tendon. Geneesk. gids *7:*1141, Dec 13; 1171, Dec 20, '29
VAN DER SPEK JSZN., J.: Freshly prepared tannic acid solution in burns. Nederl. tijdschr. v. geneesk. *75:*873–877, Feb 21, '31
VAN DER STRAETEN, AND APPELMANS, M.: Tooth in eyelid and palpebral coloboma; case. Arch. d'opht. *51:*417–425, July '34
VANDER VELDE, K. M.: Surgical technic for lacerations of face. U. S. Nav. M. Bull. *46:*1451–1452, Sept '46
VANCE, C. L.: Burns and their treatment. U. S. Nav. M. Bull. *42:*1129–1133, May '44
VANCEA, P.: Dacryocystorhinostomy according to plastic procedure of Bourguet-Dupuy-Dutemps. Rev. san. mil., Bucuresti *35:*393–395, April '36
VANDORY, W.: Therapy of malposition of healed jaw fractures; 2 cases. Ztschr. f. Stomatol. *35:*866–871, July 9, '37
VAQUERO, L.: New technic for dacryocystorhinostomy. Rev. med. d. Hosp. gen. *3:*244–253, Dec 15, '40

VAQUERO, L.: Surgical intervention on second and third portions of seventh cranial nerves in therapy; preliminary report. An. Soc. mex. de oftal. y oto-rino-laring. *16:*264–272, Sept–Oct '41
VARA LÓPEZ, R.: Congenital megalodactylia; case. Progresos de la clin. *42:*96–99, Feb '34
VARAMISARA, P. (see CONGDON, E. D. *et al*) Nov '32
VARANGOT, J.: Traumatic shock and suprarenal cortical hormone; etiologic and therapeutic studies of shock and experiments with suprarenalectomy. Presse med. *48:*103–107, Jan 31–Feb 3, '40
VARGA, V.: Rhinolalia aperta caused by velopalatine insufficiency; case. Cluj. med. *15:*576–578, Oct 1, '34
VARGAS, R. (see ALESSANDRINI, I. *et al*) Dec '31
VARGAS MOLINARE, R. AND CORREA CASTILLO, H.: Therapy of elephantiasis and lymphangiectasia of lower extremities. Arch. Soc. cirujanos hosp. *15:*594–596, June '45 also: Rev. med. de Chile *73:*703–708, Aug '45
VARGAS SALCEDO, L. AND ILABACA L., L.: Surgical therapy of temporomaxillary ankylosis followed by prosthesis of dental arches. Bol. y trab. de la Soc. de cir. de Buenos Aires *20:*1071–1082, Oct 21, '36
VARIOT, G.: Dissemblance of external ear in uniovular male twins of 17 years. Bull. et mem. Soc. d'anthrop. de Paris *9:*94, '28
VARIOUS AUTHORS: Plastic operations on face, in region of eye. Proc. Roy. Soc. Med. (sect. Ophth.) *19:*14–38, June '26
VARIOUS AUTHORS: Cosmetic results of treatment of facial wrinkles. (Wie sind die kosmetischen Erfolge bei operativer Behandlung der Runzein?) Wien. med. Wchnschr. *77:*1320, Sept 24, '27
VARIOUS AUTHORS: Discussion on treatment of cleft palate by operation. Proc. Roy. Soc. Med. (Sect. Surg.) *20:*127–183, Oct '27
VARIOUS AUTHORS: Symposium on question of permanent epilation of excessive hair for cosmetic purposes (Dauerepilation an kosmetisch wichtigen Korperstellen). Dermat. Wchnschr. *98:*275–287, March 3, '34
VARIOUS AUTHORS: Problem of inclusions in surgical therapy of saddle nose; answers to questionnaire (Le probleme des inclusions). Rev. de chir., plastique, pp. 132–141, Oct '34
VARIOUS AUTHORS: Problem of inclusions in surgical therapy of saddle nose; answers to questionnaire (Le probleme des inclusions). Rev. de chir. structive, pp. 59–64, July '35
VARIOUS AUTHORS: Symposium on shock. Med. Klin. *35:*493–499, April 14, '39
VARIOUS AUTHORS: Symposium on surgical shock. Med. Klin. *35:*842–844, June 23, '39
VARIOUS AUTHORS: Symposium on practical management of acne vulgaris. J. Invest. Dermat. *3:*143–157, April '40
VARIOUS AUTHORS: Symposium on management of Cocoanut Grove burns at Massachusetts General Hospital. Ann. Surg. *117:*801–975, June '43
VARSHAVSKAYA, A. D. (see MAZEL, Z. A. *et al*) 1935
VASCONCELLOS ALVARENGA, E.: Plastic surgery of face and neck to remove cicatricial adhesions caused by burns; case. Rev. brasil. de med. e pharm. *7:*334–337, '31
DE VASCONCELOS MARQUES, A.: Plastic surgery in case of severe wound of cranium and face. Amatus *1:*612–615, July '42
VASILE, D.: Hand infections and their therapy. Cluj. med. *13:*317–321, June 1 '32
VASILEV, A. A. AND ZHOLONDZ, A. M.: Effect of removal of cervical ganglion of sympathetic nerve on growth of autoplastic and homoplastic skin transplants. Arch. f. klin. Chir. *178:*148–169, '33 also: Novy khir. arkhiv *29:*3–20, '33
VASILEVSKIY, M. V.: Progressive hemiatrophy of face, shoulder girdle and hand; case. Sovet. nevropat. psikhiat. i psikhogig. (no. 7) *2:*78–79, '33
VASILIU. (see MARINESCO, G. *et al*) May '28
VASILKOVAN, V. Y.: Primary treatment of burns. Novy khir. arkhiv *38:*456–464, '37
VASILKOVAN, V. Y.: Primary burn treatment. Khirurgiya, no. 10, pp. 29–36, '37
VASSILIEFF, A. I.: Branchial cysts. Vestnik khir. (nos. 58–60) *20:*181–187, '30
VASTINE, J. H. (see PFAHLER, G. E.) Feb '34
VATTEONE, A. L.: Constriction of mandible; report of case and presentation of new dilator apparatus. Dia med. *13:*688–692, July 21, '41
VAUGHAN, H. C.: Temporomandibular articulation. J. Am. Dent. A. *30:*1501–1507, Oct 1, '43
VAUGHAN, H. C.: Traumatic temporomandibular articulation syndrome. U. S. Nav. M. Bull. *44:*841–843, April '45
VAUGHAN, H. S.: Important factors in treatment of cleft lip and palate. Ann. Surg. *84:*223–232, Aug '26
VAUGHAN, H. S.: Surgical correction of maxillary and palatal defects in cooperation with orthodontist and prosthodontist. Dental Cosmos *69:*63–67, Jan '27
VAUGHAN, H. S.: Surgery of cleft palate. Am. Med. *39:*149–154, April '33 abstr: Eye, Ear, Nose and Throat Monthly *12:*25–27, Feb '33
VAUGHAN, H. S.: Cleft palate – surgical repair;

with special reference to lengthening soft palate. Am. J. Surg. *31:*5–9, Jan '36

Vaughan, Harold S.: *Congenital Cleft Lip, Cleft Palate, and Associated Nasal Deformities*. Lea and Febiger Co., Phila., 1940

Vaughan, H. S.: Wide nostril in unilateral cleft lip. Tr. Am. Soc. Plastic and Reconstructive Surg. *12:*117–123, '43

Vaughan, H. S.: Surgical correction of congenital cleft palate. S. Clin. North America *24:*370–380, April '44

Vaughn, A. M.: Cystic hygroma of neck; report of case and review of literature. Am. J. Dis. Child. *48:*149–158, July '34

Vaughn, A. M.: Shock treatment. Illinois M. J. *82:*365–368, Nov '42

Vaughn, A. M. and McCarthy, M. J.: Recognition and treatment of shock. Illinois M. J. *83:*331–336, May '43

Vaynshteyn, V. G.: Skin grafts in cutaneous wounds. Sovet. khir., no. 9, pp. 62–65, '35

Vaza, D. L.: Anterior thoracic esophagoplasty by means of skin graft; case. Klin. med. (no. 1) *12:*121–124, '34

Vázquez Rodríguez, A.: Case of facial hemiatrophy. Pediat. espan. *16:*135–138, May '27

Veal, J. R.; Klepser, R. G. and DeVito, M. P.: Preparation of superficial wounds for grafting by local use of sulfanilamide and sulfanilamide-allantoin ointment. Am. J. Surg. *54:*716–720, Dec '41

Veal, J. R. and McFetridge, E. M.: Exstrophy of bladder (persistent cloaca) associated with intestinal fistulas, with brief analysis of 36 cases of anal and rectal anomalies from records of Charity Hospital in New Orleans. J. Pediat. *4:*95–103, Jan '34

Veau

(Reply to Veau's comments on Axhausen's book.) Axhausen, G. Deutsche Ztschr. f. Chir. *247:*582–589, '36

Veau, V.: Operative treatment of complete double harelip. Ann. Surg. *76:*143–156, Aug '22 (illus.)

Veau, V.: Staphylorrhaphy. Medecine *5:*21–25, Oct '23

Veau, V.: Role of median nasal process in development of face; study of hare-lip. Ann. d'anat. path. *3:*305–348, April '26 abstr: J.A.M.A. *87:*1160, Oct 2, '26

Veau, V.: Anatomy of total, unilateral harelip. Ann. d'anat. path. *5:*601–632, June '28

Veau, V.: Technic of staphylorrhaphy in simple division of palate. J. de chir. *35:*1–21, Jan '30

Veau, Victor, and Borel, S.: *Division palatine, anatomie, chirurgie, phonetique*. Masson et Cie, Paris, 1931

Veau, V.: Phonetic results in 200 cases of staphylorrhaphy. Helvet. med. acta *1:*99–103, June '34

Veau, V.: Clinical forms of unilateral harelip. Deutsche Ztschr. f. Chir. *244:*595–610, '35

Veau, V.: Clinical forms of unilateral harelip. Deutsche Ztschr. f. Chir. *244:*595–610, '35

Veau, V.: Skeletal malformations in total unilateral and bilateral harelip. Ann. d'anat. path. *11:*873–904, Dec '34 abstr: Schweiz. med. Wchnschr. *65:*99–101, Jan 26, '35

Veau, V.: Hypothesis on initial malformation in harelip; role of skeleton and muscles. Ann. d'anat. path. *12:*389–424, April '35

Veau, V.: Initial malformation in harelip. Bull. et mem. Soc. nat. de chir. *61:*496–502, April 6, '35

Veau, V.: Principles of plastic operation for cleft palate (Langenbeck-Axhausen). Deutsche Ztschr. f. Chir. *247:*300–316, '36 also: J. de chir. *48:*465–481, Oct '36 (comment on Axhausen's book).

Veau, V.: Basic trends in surgical therapy of harelip. Chirurg *8:*1–12, Jan 1, '36

Veau Victor, and Récamier, Jacques: *Bec-de lièvre*. Masson et Cie, Paris, 1938

Veau, V.: Harelip of human embryo 21–23 mm. long. Ztschr. f. Anat. u. Entwcklngsgesch. *108:*459–493, '38

Veau, V.: Harelip in relation to embryology of face. Arch. ital. di chir. *54:*824–845, '38

Veau, V.: Embryology of face in relation to harelip. Bull. Acad. de med., Paris *120:*227–233, Oct 18, '38

Veau, V.: Surgical therapy of harelip. Plast. chir. *1:*29–33, '39

Veau, V.: Surgical therapy of harelip. Salud y belleza *1:*10–11; 42, April–May '45

Veau, V. and Borel, S.: Phonetic result of surgical treatment of cleft palate; case. Bull. et mem. Soc. nat. de chir. *54:*1017, July 14, '28

Veau, V. and Borel, S.: Phonetic results of 100 staphylorrhaphies. Bull. et mem. Soc. nat. de chir. *55:*894–909, June 29, '29

Veau, V. and Borel, S.: Phonation after operations for palatal division. Rev. franc. de pediat. *7:*333–342, '31

Veau, V. and Borel-Maisonny, Mme.: Functional results of 200 staphylorrhaphies. Bull. et mem. Soc. nat. de chir. *59:*1372–1382, Nov 25, '33

Veau, V.; Borel-Maisonny, Mme. and Misset: Functional results of plastic surgery of cleft palate as shown in roentgenograms. Ztschr. f. Stomatol. *35:*597–606, May 14, '37

VEAU, V. AND BOREL-MAISONNY, S.: Effect of suture of cleft palate on phonation. Monatschr. f. Ohrenh. *70:*858–864, July '36

VEAU, V. AND BOREL-MAISONNY, S.: Phonation and staphylorraphy. Rev. franc. de phoniatrie *4:*133–141, July '36

VEAU, V. AND LASCOMBE, J.: Treatment of complex bilateral harelip. J. de chir. *19:*113–136, Feb '22 (illus.) abstr: J.A.M.A. *78:*1168, April 15, '22

VEAU, V. *et al:* Discussion on treatment of harelip. Proc. Roy. Soc. Med. (sect. Surg.) *21:*100–120, Oct '28

VEAU, V. AND PLESSIER, P.: Operative methods in unilateral harelip. Bull. et mem. Soc. nat. de chir. *57:*861–863, June 13, '31

VEAU, V. AND PLESSIER, P.: Operation for total bilateral harelip; technic and results. J. de chir. *40:*321–357, Sept '32 abstr: Bull. et mem. Soc. nat. de chir. *56:*1079–1082, July 16, '32

VEAU, V. AND POLITZER, G.: Normal and anomalous formation of primary palate; embryology of harelip. Ann. d'anat. path. *13:*275–326, March '36

VEAU, V. AND RUPPE, C.: Median upper harelip. Arch. de med. d. enf. *24:*241, April '21

VEAU, V. AND RUPPE, C.: Correction of unilateral harelip. Presse med. *29:*321, April 23, '21 abstr: J.A.M.A. *76:*1712, June 11, '21

VEAU, V. AND RUPPE, C.: Results of treatment of cleft palate. Rev. de chir. *60:*81–99, '22 (illus.) abstr: J.A.M.A. *78:*1998, June 24, '22

VEAU, V. AND RUPPE, C.: Surgical anatomy of palate. J. de chir. *20:*1–30, July '22 (illus.) abstr: J.A.M.A. *79:*687, Aug 19, '22

VEAU, V. AND RUPPE, C.: Correction of cleft palate. J. de chir. *20:*113–144, Aug '22 (illus.) abstr: J.A.M.A. *79:*1179, Sept 30, '22

Veau Operation

Veau operation for cleft palate. RUPPE, C. Ann. d'oto-laryng., pp. 1029–1043, Oct '31

Uranostaphylorrhaphy according to method of Victor Veau. RUPPE, C. French M. Rev. *2:*259–275, May '32

Cleft palate procedures in surgery; experiences with Veau and Dorrance technic. IVY, R. H. AND CURTIS, L. Ann. Surg. *100:*502–511, Sept '34

Veau operation for correction of harelip. TJIONG NJAN HAN. Geneesk. tijdschr. v. Nederl.-Indie *79:*3034–3045, Nov 28, '39

Surgical therapy of harelip in Denmark; results of 4 years of using Veau method. ANDERSEN, V. F. Plast. chir. *1:*35–38, '39

Therapy of palatine fissure by combined Veau and Axhausen technics. CASTELLANO, J. L. AND GIGANTI, I. J. Semana med. *2:*887–889, Oct 14, '43

Veau Operation – Cont.

Surgical therapy of cleft palate by Veau technic. DE SANSON, R. D. Rev. oto-laring. de Sao Paulo *4:*349–364, July–Aug '36

VECCHIONE, F.: Vaginal fistula with anal atresia; case. Gazz. internaz. med.-chir. *37:*255–260, April 30, '29

VEENING, H. P. (see BORST, J. G. G.) March '40

VEGER, A. M.: Snapping finger (intermittent reflex contraction) in electric welders. Novy khir. arkhiv *30:*321–325, '34

VEIL, P.: Eyelid ptosis. Rev. gen. de clin. et de therap. *47:*310–311, May 13, '33

VEIL, P.: Nevocarcinoma of eyelids and conjunctiva. Bull. med., Paris *51:*371–375, May 29, '37

VEINTEMILLAS, F.: Autoplastic methods for surgical restoration of congenital agenesis of ear. Rev. brasil. de oto-rino-laring. *8:*413–418, Nov–Dec '40

VEINTEMILLAS, F.: Recent cases of agenesis of ears. Prensa med. La Paz (nos. 7–8) *6:*1–6, Jul–Aug '46

VEIT, G. (see STEINIGER, F.) 1942

VELASCO L., R.: Congenital cysts of neck, with report of cases. Rev. otorrinolaring. *1:*27–30, Sept '41

VELASCO, S., A. (see CASANUEVA DEL C., M.) June '42

VELASCO BLANCO, L. AND WAISBEIN, S.: Congenital hemiatrophy of face with Claude Bernard-Horner syndrome; case. Arch. am. d. *14:*74–76, '38

VELEZ DIEZ CANSECO, J. B. (see IVANISSEVICH, O. *et al*) June '41

VELLOSO VIANNA, E.: New set of automatic retractors for nasal surgery. Rev. brasil. de oto-rino-laring. *10:*533–550, Sept–Oct '42

VELO, C. A.: Experiments on taking of homoplastic skin-grafts. Ann. ital. di chir. *7:*97–112, Feb '28

VENABLE, C. S.: Skin grafting of extensive areas. Texas State J. Med. *22:*381–382, Oct '26

VENCO, L.: Dacryocystorhinostomy by external route; technic. Rassegna ital. d'ottal. *7:*593–612, Sept–Oct '38

VENCO, L.: Dacryocystorhinostomy; criteria of operability, indications, complications and results. Riv. oto-neuro-oftal. *15:*510–531, Nov–Dec '38

VENETIANER, P.: Present status of therapy of hemangioma. Gyogyaszat *73:*499–500, Aug 13, '33

VENETIANER, P.: Noël technic in plastic surgery of nipple. Gyogyaszat *73:*553-555, Sept 3, '33

VENEZIAN, E.: Phalangization of metacarpals for functional restoration of hand of workman deprived of all fingers. Rassegna d. previd. sociale *20:*38-46, Nov '33

VENGEROVSKIY, I. S.: Harelip and its therapy at surgical clinic of children's hospital during 14 years. Novy khir. arkhiv *44:*302-305, '39

VENTURELLI, G.: Carbon dioxide snow in treatment of angiomas. Riforma med. *42:*1039-1041, Nov 1, '26

VENTURINO, H. (see RUA, L.) April '43

VEPPO, A. A. (see FINOCHIETTO, R.) Oct '39

VERAART, B.: Therapy of injuries in fingernail region. Nederl. tijdschr. v. geneesk. *90:*743-745, June 29, '46

VERBRUGGHEN, A.: Treatment of facial paralysis. S. Clin. North America *16:*223-229, Feb '36

VER BRUGǴHEN. A. H.: Traumatic shock. Pennsylvania M. J. *46:*319-326, Jan '43

VERDAGUER, J. F. (see ZENO, L.) July '42

VERDERAME, F.: Methods of surgical treatment of congenital ptosis; case. Rev. gen. d'opht. *41:*277-288, July '27

VERDERAME, F.: Surgical correction of traumatic epicanthus. Klin. Monatsbl. f. Augenh. *103:*436-441, Oct-Nov '39

VERDIER, R. A.: Nasal septum splint. Am. J. Surg. *36:*44, Feb '22 (illus.)

VEREBELY, T. JR.: Value of immediate treatment of hand injuries. Orvosi hetil. *84:*647-651, Dec 21, '40

VERESHCHAKOVSKIY, I. I.: Prevention of decubitus ulcers during therapy of contracture by Mommsen cast method. Ortop. i travmatol. (no. 1) *9:*100, '35

VERGARA, R. G.: Fractures of fingers in work accidents. Arch. Soc. cirujanos hosp., num. espec. pp. 50-56, Dec '41

VERGER: *Epithelioma du Maxillaire Superieur.* Doin, Paris, 1925

VERGER, G. (see HAUTANT, A. *et al*) Sept '26

VERMEL, S. S.: Pathogenesis and etiology of Dupuytren's contracture. Novy khir. arkhiv *36:*249-252, '36

VERMEULEN, B. S.: Congenital fistulae and dermoid cysts on dorsum of nose. Geneesk. gids *7:*1117-1126, Dec 6, '29

VERMEULEN, B. S.: Congenital fistulae and dermoid cysts on dorsum of nose. Acta otolaryng. *16:*48-56, '31

VERMOOTEN, V.: Ball of hair in urethra; late complication of Bucknall operation for hypospadias. New England J. Med. *202:*658-660, April 3, '30

VERNAZA, F.: Maneuvers for reducing fractures of the nasal pyramid with luxation or simple luxations of bones. Colombia med. *2:*70-73, March-April '40

VERNE, J. AND ISELIN, M.: Nerve repair in man; studies on 2 cases, 10 weeks and 6 months after operation; evaluations of grafts and tubular prosthesis. Presse med. *49:*789-791, July 22, '41

VERNON, E. L.: Technic of total ectropion operation. Am. J. Ophth. *9:*598-600, Aug '26

VERNON, S.: Fracture of proximal phalanx of thumb. Am. J. Surg. *39:*130-132, Jan '38

VERRIER, E.: New surgical technic for restoration of pendulous breasts. Rev. espan. de med. y cir. *18:*68-70, Feb '35

VERRIÈRE AND BARNEVILLE: Dermo-epidermal grafts; history, technic and indications. Arch. de med. et pharm. mil. *100:*173-192, Feb '34

VES LOSADA, C. AND BRAMBILLA, A.: Double exposed fracture of lower jaw with luxation of one of temporomaxillary articulations; recovery of case after surgical therapy. Semana med. *1:*1012-1019, April 8, '37

VESEEN, L. L. AND O'NEILL, C. P.: Plastic operation of penis; case. J. Urol. *30:*375-377, Sept '33

VESELKIN, P. N.; *et al*: Experimental data on pathogenesis of traumatic shock; toxic action of products of muscular disintegration. Vestnik khir. *44:*176-186, '36

VESELKIN, P. N.; *et al*: Experimental data on pathogenesis of traumatic shock; role of fat embolism. Vestnik khir. *44:*198-203, '36

VESELKIN, P. N.; *et al*: Experimental data on pathogenesis of traumatic shock. Vestnik khir. *51:*211-229, '37

VESTAL, P. W.: Plastic operation of breast with flexible adaptation. Am. J. Surg. *39:*614-616, March '38

DI VESTEA, D.: Congenital torticollis with unilateral facial atrophy; case. Rassegna internaz. di clin. e terap. *9:*16-29, Jan '28

DI VESTEA, D.: Congenital malformation of nose; case. Valsalva *5:*214-219, April '29

VETCHTOMOFF, A. A.: Use of tubular stem in transplantation from ear to defect of ala. Vestnik khir. (no. 55) *20:*143-150, '30

Vestibuloplasty

Restoration of buccal sulcus by intraoral skin grafting. PICKERILL, H. P., M. J. and Rec. *126:*671-674, Dec 7, '27

Lowering floor of mouth; new operation to provide additional support for lower denture; case. IGLAUER, S., J. Med. *14:*507-509, Dec '33

Cleft palate and harelip; adolescent case treated orthodontically in conjunction with

Vestibuloplasty – Cont.
lip-stretching device and skin grafting of labial sulcus. HARDY, E. A. Internat. J. Orthodontia *20:*750–758, Aug '34
Vestibulo-alveolar adhesions; destruction by plastic reconstruction of gingivo-jugo-labial groove. CLAOUE, C. Oto-rhino-laryng. internat. *24:*41–45, Feb '40 also: Rev. gen. de clin. et de therap. *54:*95–96, Feb 24, '40
Creation of mandibular ridge by deepening labial sulcus and lining it with graft. GORNEY, H. S.; *et al.* J. Am. Dent. A. *29:*751–754, May '42
Severe retrusion of mandible treated by buccal inlay and dental prosthesis. FICKLING, B. W. Proc. Roy. Soc. Med. *37:*7–10, Nov '43
Epithelial inlays to labial sulcus of mandible. HARDY, E. A. Proc. Roy. Soc. Med. *38:*645–646, Sept '45 (Comment on Fickling's article)

VEYRASSAT, J.: Treatment of serious injuries of fingers. Rev. med. de la Suisse Rom. *51:*193–211, March 25, '31
VEZINA, C.; GARNEAU, P. AND ROY, L. P.: Tendon transplants in surgical therapy of radial paralysis; case. Laval med. *3:*181–186, June '38
VIACAVA, E. P. (see FERRARI, R. C.) Oct '44
VIALATTE (see TOURAINE, A. *et al*) March '36
VIALE DEL CARRIL, A.: Unilateral choanal imperforation, with report of case. Rev. Asoc. med. argent. *52:*977–979, Sept 30, '38
VIALLE, P.: Therapy of phlegmons of digitopalmar tendon sheaths. Arch. med. -chir. de Province *21:*412–423, Dec '31
VIALLE, P.: Surgical removal followed by radiotherapy of cicatricial keloids. Arch. med. -chir. de Province *23:*429–432, Dec '33
VIANA, F.: Congenital cystic lymphangioma, with recurrence after surgical therapy; case in newborn infant (neck). Pediat. prat., Sao Paulo *13:*91–98, March–June '42
VIANA ROSA, A.: Tubular graft in laryngotracheal fistula. Rev. med. Rio Grande do Sul *2:*167–172, Jan–Feb '46
VIANNA, J. B.: Repair of extensive loss of substance of lower lip (due to cancer). Hospital, Rio de Janeiro *23:*69–79, Jan '43
VIANNA, J. B.: Plastic repair after electrothermal operations (cancer). Med. cir. farm., pp. 598–606, Nov '44
VIANNA, J. B.: Sclerosing injections in therapy of hemangiomas. Med. cir. farm. pp. 139–150, Feb–Mar '46
VIANNA DE PAULA, G. (see VIANNA DE PAULA, H.) June '41
VIANNA DE PAULA, H. AND VIANNA DE PAULA, G.: General norms of surgical conduct; case of gynandroid with clitoris-penis. Rev. de ginec. e d'obst. *1:*402–414, June '41
VICENTE CARCELLAR, M.: Pathogenesis of exstrophy of bladder; embryological study; case. Clin. y lab. *12:*115–122, Aug '28
VICTORIA, M.: Acrodystonia following injury to thumb; case. Rev. oto-neur-oftal. *10:*180–183, July '35
VIDAL, J. (see EUZIÈRE, J. *et al*) Aug '34
VIDAL-NAQUET, G. (see MASSART, R.) Nov '34
VIDAL-NAQUET, G. (see MASSART, R.) Jan '35
DE VIDAS, J. AND MCEACHERN, A. C.: Biochemical investigation of tannic acid and sulfanilamide in burns. M. J. Australia *2:*470–474, Oct 25, '41
VIDEMAN, G. K.: Plastic surgery of cicatricial contractures of underarm. Vestnik khir. (nos. 56–57) *19:*323–328, '30
VIEIRA FILHO, O. (see AMARAL, O.) July '42
VIÉLA, A. AND ESCAT, M.: Vulnerability of sphenopalatine artery in deep endonasal surgery. Ann. d. mal. de l'oreille, du larynx *47:*980–985, Nov '28
VIGLIANI, E. C.: Mechanism and therapy of electric injuries. Rassegna di med. indust. *10:*143–158, March '39
VIGNARD: Surgical therapy of bilateral harelip and total cleft palate; case. Avenir med. *29:*41, Feb '32
VIGNARD: Cleft palate. Avenir med. *33:*240–241, Sept–Oct '36
VIGNE, P.: Spinocellular epithelioma of cheek in patient with old lupus. Marseille med. *2:*369–371, Dec 15, '30
VIGNOLO, Q.: Reconstruction of nose, lid region and cheek following shell wound. Arch. ital. di chir. *3:*649, July '21 abstr: J.A.M.A. *77:*1290, Oct 15, '21
VILA ORTIZ, J. J. JR.: Congenital bilateral palpebral coloboma complicated by corneal ulcer with hypopyon; case. Arch. de oftal. hispano-am. *34:*315–319, June '34
VILAFANE, A. R. (see DE NICOLA, C. P.) 1942
VILARDOSA LLUBES, E.: Facial and nasal plastic surgery from esthetic point of view. Rev. de cir. de Barcelona *8:*1, July–Aug; 99, Sept–Dec '34
VILESOV, S. P.: Transplantation of large pieces of skin by Filatov-Parin method. Sovet. khir., no. 3, pp. 132–134, '35
VILLAFANE, I. Z.: Regenerative power and possibilities of homograft. Semana med. *1:*1197–1200, May 22, '41
VILLANUEVA, A.: Burn therapy. Arch. am. de med. *15:*43–44, '39
VILLARAN, C. AND SALAS, N. E.: Reconstruc-

tion of lower jaw after resection for neoplasm (epulis); medico-odontologic collaboration; case. An. clin. quir. *1:*40–49, May '39
VILLARD: Entire resection of lower jaw. Lyon chir. *26:*618–621, Aug–Sept '29
VILLARD, H.: Epithelioma of eyelids; indications for radium treatment and surgical intervention. Medecine *11:*19–23, Jan '30
VILLARROEL, E. (see CASANUEVA DEL C., M.) May–Aug '42
VILLATA, G.: Survival of bone marrow and bone in homoplastic grafting. Gior. d. r. Accad. di med. di Torino *93:*167–174, July–Sept '30
VILLATA, I.: Malignant tumors of nasopharynx; anatomicopathologic study. Oro-rino-laring. ital. *10:*106–151, March '40
DE VILLAVERDE, J. M.: Supposed pathogenesis; case of polyneuritis with retraction of palmar aponeurosis. Med. ibera *2:*213–222, Aug 31, '29
VILLECHAISE AND JEAN, G.: Technic of surgical treatment of syndactylia. Rev. d'orthop. *14:*241–243, May '27
VILLETTE, J.: Artificial vagina made from loop of small intestine. Arch. franco-belges de chir. *26:*1047–1055, Nov '23
DE VILLIERS, R.: Plastic surgery of nose. Rev. san. mil., Habana *4:*27–40, Jan–March '40
VINAŘ, J.: Facial hemiatrophy (Romberg's disease). Casop. lek. cesk. *73:*865–867, Aug 3, '34
VINCENT, C. (see CANTONNET, A.) Nov '26
VINCENT, R. W. (see OWENS, N.) Nov '41

Vincent's Infection

Vincent's ulceration of soft palate. HOUSER, K. M. Tr. Am. Laryng. A. *64:*141–143, '42

VINOGOROV, D. R. AND KOPIT, R. Z.: Alkali burns to eyes; experimental study. Sovet. vestnik oftal. *8:*333–347, '36
VIOLATO, A.: Experiments with adrenalin in burn therapy. Umbria med. *7:*1237–1239, May '27
VIOLE, P.: Facial nerve; experiences in surgery. Laryngoscope *54:*455–466, Sept '44
VIOLET, H.: Painting burns with methylthionine chloride; case. Lyon med. *157:*308–310, March 15, '36
VIOLET, H.: Congenital absense of vagina; reconstruction according to Italian method by grafts from genitocrural fold on each side; case in girl 21 years old. Lyon med. *158:*277–282, Sept 13, '36
VIRANO, G. (see MAIRANO, M.) Dec '29
VIRCHOW, H.: Facial deformities of mid face. Ztschr. f. d. ges. Anat. (abt. 1) *84:*555–596, Dec 28, '27
VIRENQUE, M.: *Chirurgie esthétique; le sein.* Maloine, Paris, 1928
VIRENQUE, M.: *Chirurgie réparatrice maxillo-faciale.* Maloine, Paris, 1940
VIRENQUE: New ideas in reconstructive maxillofacial surgery. Rev. de stomatol. *43:*149–158, Sept–Oct '42
VIRENQUE, M.: Technic of total rhinoplasty by method of double frontal flap. Ann. d'otolaryng., pp. 45–57, April–June '44
VISCONTI, C.: Neoprontosil (sulfonamide); local therapy of second degree burn. Semana med. *2:*1017, Oct 28, '43
VISHNYAKOV, S. L.: Therapy of gunshot wounds of fingers (and hand). Khirurgiya, no. 5, pp. 76–78, '44
VITALE, F.: Margino-tarsal graft in treatment of trichiasis and cicatricial entropion of both eyelids. Gior. di ocul. *9:*61–65, June '28
VITALE, F.: Marginotarsal graft in correction of cicatricial entropion of lower eyelid. Cultura med. mod. *9:*588–592, July 31, '30
VIVIANI, J. E. (see GAREISO, A. *et al*) Aug '38
VIVOLI, D. (see DELLEPIANE RAWSON, J.) May '29
VIVONE, R. A. (see JORGE, J. M.) May '44
VLAD, V. (see POPESCU, A.) March '41
VLADESCU, V. (see NASTA, T. *et al*) March–April '34
VOELKER, C. H.: Therapeutic technic for staphylolalia (so-called short palate speech). Arch. Otolaryng. *21:*94–96, Jan '35
VOGEL, K.: Depression fracture of root of nose. Ztschr. f. Laryng., Rhin. Otol. *25:*426–428, '34
VOGEL, K.: Surgical correction of too large auricles. Ztschr. f. Hals-, Nasen-u. Ohrenh. *44:*366–367, '38
VOGELER, K.: Therapy of injuries to fingers and hands. Med. Welt. *7:*1097–1100, Aug 5, '33
VOGT, A.: Craniofacial dysostosis (dyscephaly, Crouzon's disease) associated with syndactylia of 4 extremities (dyscephalodactylia). Klin. Monatsbl. f. Augenh. *90:*441–454, April '33
VOGT, E.: Formation of artificial vagina by Kirschner-Wagner operation. Zentralbl. f. Gynak. *55:*1634–1639, May 16, '31
VOGT, L. G.: Plastic surgery in gynecomastia. Chirurg *13:*322–324, May 15, '41

Vogt Syndrome

Correction of entropion according to Vogt method. SCHLÄPFER, H. Klin. Monatsbl. f. Augenh. *94:*610–611, May '35
Dyscephalodactylia (Vogt) and developmental abnormalities of uvea. INCZE, K. Arch. f. Augenh. *109:*562–566, '36

VOHWINKEL, K. H.: Burn therapy. Therap. d.

Gegenw. *77:*313–315 July '36

VOIGT, H. W.: Therapy of so-called ganglia of wrist. Ztschr. f. arztl. Fortbild. *39:*55–57, Feb 1, '42

VOKOUN, F. J.: Pinch graft. Mil. Surgeon *83:*442–443, Nov '38

VOLAVSEK, W.: Dupuytren's contracture, relation to plastic induration of penis. Ztschr. f. Urol. *35:*173–178, '41

VOLKERT, M. AND ASTRUP, T.: Effect of dialyzed serum proteins and serum dialysates in shock. Acta med. Scandinav. *115:*537–541, '43

VOLKERT, M. AND ASTRUP, T.: Effect of dialyzed serum proteins and serum dialysates in shock treatment. Bull. War Med. *4:*640, July '44 (abstract)

VOLKMANN, J.: Chylocystic lymphangioma of neck; 3 cases. Beitr. z. klin. Chir. *146:*654–667, '29

VOLKMANN, J.: Prevention of hand and finger injuries in industry. Monatschr. f. Unfallh. *43:*417–425, Sept '36

Volkmann's Contracture: See Contracture, Volkmann's

VOLOSHCHENKO, D. L.: Fatal facial wounds difficult to diagnose. Khirurgiya. No. 6, pp. 89–90, '45

VOLPITTO, P. P.; WOODBURY, R. A. AND HAMILTON, W. F: Direct arterial and venous pressure measurements in man as affected by anesthesia, operation and shock. Am. J. Physiol. *128:*238–245, Jan '40

VON BARTHA, E.: Congenital entropion; case. Klin. Monatsbl. f. Augenh. *88:*517–520, April '32

VON BERGMANN, G.: Treatment of shock and collapse. Ztschr. f. arztl. Fortbild. *35:*125–131, March 1, '38

VON BERGMANN, G.: Therapy of postoperative circulatory shock. Deutsche med. Wchnschr. *58:*519–523, April 1, '32

VON BLASKOVICS, L.: Formation of folding lid in ptosis operation. Ber. u. d. Versamml. d. deutsch. ophth. Gesellsch. (1928) *47:*277–283, '29

VON BLASKOVICS, L.: Treatment of ptosis; formation of fold in eyelid and resection of levator and tarsus. Arch. Ophth. *1:*672–680, June '29

VON BRANDIS, H. J.: Plastic surgery of corner of mouth (Rehn operation). Deutsche Ztschr. f. Chir. *241:*479–482, '33

VON BRANDIS, H. J.: Free fat transplants in facial plastic surgery. Deutsche Ztschr. f. Chir. *244:*228–232, '34

VON BRANDIS, H. J.: Rehn method of skin grafting. Chirurg *13:*418–425, July 15, '41

VON CSAPODY, I.: New method for construction of artificial conjunctival sac by transplantation of skin flap divided into 2 parts. Ztschr. f. Augenh. *87:*114–130, Sept '35

VON CSAPODY, I.: New experiences with plastic construction of artificial conjunctival sac, using flaps. Ztschr. f. Augenh. *94:*23–33, Jan '38

VON CZEYDA-POMMERSHEIM, F.: Use of double skin flap in restoration of lip defects. Zentralbl. f. Chir. *56:*2381–2382, Sept 21, '29

VON DANCKELMAN, A. (see SAUERBRUCH, F.) 1938

VON DOELINGER DA GRACA: Biologic aspects of cancer of face in view of results of treatment. Folha med. *10:*384–386, Nov 5, '29

von Eicken Operation

Permanent results of von Eicken operation for choanal atresia. LABHARDT, E. Schweiz. med. Wchnschr. *66:*1153–1154, Nov 21, '36

VON ERTL, J.: Successful application of regeneration theory (plastic surgery). Arch. f. klin. Chir. *189:*398–400, '37

VON ERTL, J.: Flexible bone transplants. Zentralbl. f. Chir. *64:*362–371, Feb 6, '37

VON GELDERN, C. E.: Etiology of exstrophy of bladder. Arch. Surg. *8:*61–99, (pt. 1) Jan '24

VON GERNET, R.: Modification of Maher's operation (entropion). Klin. Monatsbl. f. Augenh. *78:*73, Jan '27

VON GERNET, R.: Transplantation of eyelid tissue. Klin. Monatsbl. f. Augenh. *80:*496, April 27, '28

VON GERNET, R.: Blaskovics operation for eyelid ptosis. Klin. Monatsbl. f. Augenh. *101:*422–423, Sept '38

VON GROLMAN, G.: Mucosal graft in therapy of corneoconjunctival burns. Arch. de oftal. de Buenos Aires *15:*429–434, Sept '40 also: Rev. med. y cien. afines *2:*629–632, Sept 30, '40

VON GROLMAN, G.: Conjunctival burn due to ammonia treated by Denig method (excision of tissue and graft of buccal mucosa); case. Prensa med. argent. *28:*839–840, April 16, '41

von Hacker Operation

Von Hacker's operation for hypospadias. MAYET, H. Bull. et mem. Soc. de chir. de Paris *21:*394–403, May 17, '29 also: Paris chir. *21:*149–154, July–Aug '29

VON HEDRY, N.: New method of surgical therapy of angioma racemosum capitis. Zentralbl. f. Chir. *64:*22–26, Jan 2, '37

VON HEREPEY-CSÁBÁNYI, G.: Bilateral lym-

phangioma of neck. Zentralbl. f. Chir. *54:*1672, July 2, '27
VON JASCHKE, R. T.: New method of formation of artificial vagina. Zentralbl. f. Gynak. *52:*735-736, March 24, '28
VON JASCHKE, R. T.: Treatment of total ectopy in adults. Zentralbl. f. Gynak. *56:*322-326, Feb 6, '32

von Langenbeck Operation

Ultimate results of Langenbeck's operation for cleft palate. STAHL, O. Arch. f. klin. Chir. *123:*271-316, '23 (illus.) abstr: J.A.M.A. *80:*1421, May 12, '23

von Langenbeck-Axhausen Operation

Principles of plastic operation for cleft palate (Langenbeck-Axhausen). VEAU, V. Deutsche Ztschr. f. Chir. *247:*300-316, '36 also: J. de chir. *48:*465-481, Oct '36 (comment on Axhausen's book)
Principles of plastic operation (Langenbeck-Axhausen) of cleft palate. (Reply to Veau). AXHAUSEN, G., J. de chir. *49:*47-53, Jan '37

von Langenbeck-Trelat Operation

Perfect phonetic results of uranostaphylorrhaphy (Langenbeck-Trelat method). ROCHER, J. de med. de Bordeaux *109:*420-403, May 20, '32

von Liebermann

Question of tamponade after nasal operations. (Comment on von Liebermann's article). KREBS, G. Ztschr. f. Hals-, Nasen-u. Ohrenh. *30:*684-685, '32

VON LIEBERMANN, T.: Surgical therapy of cleft palate. Ztschr. f. Hals-, Nasen-u. Ohrenh. *30:*556-559, '32
VON LIEBERMANN, T.: New method of surgical correction of nasal deformities. Ztschr. f. Hals-, Nasen-u. Ohrenh. *30:*560-566, '32
VON LOBMAYER, G.: Development of keloids from trifling causes (case following puncture of ear during delivery). Zentralbl. f. Chir. *61:*253, Feb 3, '34
VON LUCADOU, W.: Problem of shock and collapse as observed at the front. Deutsche med. Wchnschr. *69:*652, Sept 17, '43
VON MADARASZ, E.: Therapy of jaw fractures. Ztschr. f. Stomatol. *33:*838-848, July 26, '35
VON MAGNUS, R.: Transplantation of epidermal flaps by Pontoppidan method in radical surgery in otitis media. Ztschr. f. Laryng., Rhin., Otol. *25:*48-52, '34
VON MADARASZ, E.: Extension of uniform system of therapy of jaw fractures. Ztschr. f. Stomatol. *35:*799-804, June 25, '37
VON MATOLCSY, T.: Practical significance and uses of bone grafts. Arch. f. klin. Chir. *176:*319-334, '33
VON MATOLCSY, T.: Function of breast following plastic surgery for hypertrophy. Arch. f. klin. Chir. *201:*791-795, '41
VON MEZÖ, B.: Fat formation in abdominal skin flap on hand 23 years after grafting. Chirurg *13:*18-19, Jan 1, '41
VON OPPOLZER, R.: Avulsion fracture of terminal phalanx due to pull on flexor tendon. Zentralbl. f. Chir. *62:*2907-2910, Dec 7, '35
VON RIHMER, B.: Traumatic removal of entire external cutaneous covering of penis with subsequent partial necrosis of urethra; plastic repair; case. Ztschr. f. Urol. *26:*369-373, '32
VON SEEMEN, H.: Operation for Dupuytren's contracture. Deutsche Ztschr. f. Chir. *246:*693-696, '36
VON SEEMEN, H.: Plastic surgery of elbow after transplantation of skin in ankylosis with cicatricial contracture; case. Zentralbl. f. Chir. *63:*946-950, April 18, '36
VON SEEMEN, H.: Plastic surgery of eyelids; use of pedicled flaps with handle. Deutsche Ztschr. f. Chir. *248:*411-419, '37
VON SEEMEN, H.: General principles and application of plastic surgery. Jahresk. f. arztl. Fortbild. *29:*31-42, Dec '38
VON SEEMEN, H.: Surgical therapy of extensive facial tumors, and plastic restoration (grafts). Arch. f. klin. Chir. *200:*553-566, '40
VON SEEMEN, H.: Successful modern plastic surgery in serious disfiguration due to scalping; reconstruction of eyelids and eyebrows and replacement of total skin of forehead and temples. Zentralbl. f. Chir. *69:*1280-1287, Aug 1, '42
VON SEEMEN, H.: Surgical therapy of facial paralysis. Arch. f. klin. Chir. *205:*598, '44
VON SOUBIRON, N.; GERCHUNOFF, G. AND EMILIANI, C. M.: Cricoid perichondritis due to decubitus ulcer; case. Rev. Asoc. med. argent. *52:*529-530, June 15, '38
VON SOUBIRON, N. (see MARFORT, A. *et al*) Feb '39
VON STAPELMOHR, S.: Clicking of temporomaxillary joint and habitual dislocations; cases. Acta chir. Scandinav. *65:*1-68, '29
VON STAPELMOHR, S.: Cavities of hand from surgical point of view. Nord. med. tidskr. *10:*1341-1344, Aug 31, '35
VON STAPELMOHR, S.: So-called late rupture of tendon of extensor pollicis longus in connec-

tion with wrist fractures. Nord. med. tidskr. *11:*174-178, Jan 31, '36
von Stapelmohr, S.: High "late rupture" of tendon of extensor pollicis longus. Acta chir. Scandinav. *86:*110-128, '42
von Stapelmohr, S.: Operation for habitual luxation of thumb. Acta chir. Scandinav. *94:*379-382, '46
von Wedel, C.: Harelip and cleft palate. Southwest J. Med. and Surg. *29:*148-149, Nov '21 (illus.)
von Wedel, C.: Congenital deformities of mouth and face. J. Oklahoma M. A. *15:*46-49, Feb '22 (illus.)
von Wedel, C.: Skin transplantation. J. Oklahoma M. A. *19:*7-11, Jan '26
von Wedel, C.: Plastics of external nose. J. Oklahoma M. A. *20:*44-45, Feb '27
von Wedel, C.: Hand deformities. J. Oklahoma M. A. *22:*38-42, Feb '29
von Wedel, C.: Newer methods in plastic surgery. J. Oklahoma M. A. *24:*75-76, March '31
von Wedel, C.: Reconstruction of burned hand (grafts). J. Oklahoma M. A. *24:*164-165, May '31
von Wedel, C.: Plastic surgery (skin grafts). Southwestern Med. *16:*409-411, Oct '32
von Wedel, C.: Crippled hand. J. Oklahoma M. A. *26:*320-323, Sept '33
von Wedel, C.: Operative procedures for cosmetic purposes (nose). J. Oklahoma M. A. *30:*249-252, July '37
von Wedel, C.: Role of plastic surgery in facial injuries. South. M. J. *32:*1118-1120, Nov '39
von Wedel, C. (see Ellis, S. S.) Dec '40
von Wedel, C. (see Ellis, S. S.) March '41
von Zwehl, W.: Etiology of postoperative anginas in nasal surgery. Beitr. z. Anat., Physiol., Path. u. Therap. d. Ohres *28:*311-325, Oct '30
von Zweigbergk, J. O.: Functional prognosis in rupture of tendons of fingers. Svenska lak.-tidning. *32:*1064-1070, July 26, '35
von Zweigbergk, J. O.: Late sequels of finger tendon sutures. Chirurg *8:*243-247, April 1, '36
Vonachen, H. A. (see Baker, W. B.) Nov '37
Vondracek, V. and Nedved, M.: Spurious biglandular hermaphroditism. Casop. lek. cesk. *80:*293-295, Feb 28, '41
Voorhees, I. W.: Bucco-antral fistula; plastic operation. Internat. J. Surg. *40:*19, Jan '27
Voorhees, I. W.: Management of abscess of nasal septum. Laryngoscope *39:*652-654, Oct '29
Voorhees I. W.: Cleft palate procedures; experiences and observations. Arch. Pediat. *50:*73-80, Feb '33
Voorhees, I. W.: Causes of surgical failure in cleft palate repair. Am. J. Surg. *40:*588-595, June '38
Vordenbäumen: Special cases of jaw fractures. Arch. f. orthop. u. Unfall-Chir. *32:*608-611, '33
Vorhaus, M. G.; Gompertz, M. L. and Feder, A.: Clinical experiments with riboflavin (in decubital ulcer). Am. J. Digest Dis. *10:*45-48, Feb '43
Voris, H. C.: Repair of defects with special reference to use of tantalum in cranium. S. Clin. North America *26:*33-55, Feb '46
Voron and Brochier, A.: Hemorrhages during pregnancy; obstetrical shock; death. Bull. Soc. d'obst. et de gynec. *17:*60, Jan '28
Voronchikhin, S. I.: Immovable bandage in free cutaneous graft (extremities). Novy khir. arkhiv. *45:*244-247, '40
Voronoff, S.: Study on transplantation of organs. Siglo med. *68:*1172-1176, Dec 3, '21
Vorschütz, I. (see Vorschütz, J.)
Vorschütz, J.: Therapy of complicated fractures of lower jaw. Med. Welt *8:*1474-1475, Oct 20, '34
Vorschütz, J.: Therapy of complicated fractures of lower jaw (comment on Wassmund's article). Zentralbl. f. Chir. *62:*2624-2625, Nov 2, '35
Vorschütz, J.: (Comment to article by Wassmund on Vorschutz method of treatment of jaw fractures.) Zentralbl. f. Chir. *63:*446, Feb 22, '36

Vorschütz Operation

Disadvantages of Vorschütz method of treating complicated fractures and defects of lower jaw with plaster of paris bandage fastened to each side of jaw by screw arm. Wassmund, M. Zentralbl. f. Chir. *62:*914-921, April 20, '35

Vorstoffel, E.: Congenital absence of one vas deferens with aplasia of left kidney and hypospadias. Zentralbl. f. Chir. *64:*2825-2826, Dec 11, '37
Voskresenskiy, N. V.: First bandage in hand injuries. Sovet. khir. (no. 1) *7:*171-172, '34
Voskresenskiy, N. V.: Needles in hands and method of extraction. Khirurgiya, no. 12, pp. 86-91, '39
Voss, O.: War injuries of ear, nose and throat. Med. Klin. *35:*1589-1591, Dec 15, '39
Votta, E. A.: Fibroid osteitis of phalanx; therapy of case. Rev. Asoc. med. argent. *54:*299-302, April 15-30, '40
Voûte, P. A.: Hypospadias of penis in uniovu-

lar twins. Nederl. tijdschr. v. geneesk. *77:*2431–2433, May 27, '33

VOZNESENSKIY, V. P.: Plastic surgery of urethra and penis in total epispadias. Novy khir. arkhiv *47:*281–283, '40

VRAA-JENSEN, G. F.: Progressive hemiatrophy of face. Nord. med. (Hospitalstid.) *14:*1861–1865, June 20, '42

VREDEN R. R.: Surgical treatment of facial deformity due to paralysis. Vestnik khir. (nos. 43–44) *14:*11–13, '28

Vreden Operation

Modification of Vreden operation in therapy of paralytic facial deformity. KORSUNSKIY, P. D. Khirurgiya, no. 10, pp. 35–38, '39

DE VRIES, J. J.: Blocking nerve for lower jaw surgery. Nederlandsch Tijdschr. f. Geneesk. *1:*197–200, Jan 14, '22

VULLIET, M.: Removal of blood from mouth by suction during operations (staphylorrhaphy). Zentralbl. f. Chir. *55:*1996–1997, Aug 11, '28

Vulva

Double penis and double vulva. MACLENNAN, A. Glasgow M. J. *101:*287–288, May '24

VURCHIO, G.: Effects of pregnancy hormones on healing process; experimental and clinical studies (of skin). Ginecologia *8:*237–246, June '42

W

DE WAAL, H. L.: Wound infection; preliminary note on combined clinical and bacteriologic investigation of 708 wounds (and burn). Edinburgh M. J. *50:*577–588, Oct '43

WAAR, C. A. H.: Technic for correcting deformities of ears among natives of Dutch East Indies acquired from wearing heavy things in ear lobes. Nederlandsch Tijdschr. v. Geneesk. *2:*32–35, July 7, '23 (illus.)

DE WAARD: Transplantation of epithelium by Braun method. Geneesk. tijdschr. v. Nederl. Indie *70:*1050, Oct 1, '30

WAARDENBURG, P. J.: Anomalies of eye and orbit in acrocephalosyndactylia (Apert sy drome). Maandschr. v. kindergeneesk. *3:*196–212, Feb '34

WACHSBERGER, A.: Endonasal surgery with aid of new instrument; simplified technic. Arch. Otolaryng. *8:*712–714, Dec '28

WACHSBERGER, A.: Modified traction and fixation splint for fractures of facial bones. Arch. Otolaryng. *42:*53–55, July '45

WADE, P. A.: Dextrose-insulin therapy of shock. J.A.M.A. *90:*1859–1860, June 9, '28

WADE, P. A.: Present status of glucose-insulin in shock. Anesth. and Analg. *8:*298–301, Sept–Oct '29

WADE, R.: Improved gag. Lancet *2:*1220, Dec 3, '32

WADE, R.: Operation for harelip. Australia and New Zealand J. Surg. *10:*75–76, July '40

WADE, R. B.: Treatment of hypospadias. Australian and New Zealand J. Surg. *2:*417–418, April '33

DE WAELE, H.: Anesthesia and shock. Compt. rend. Soc. de biol. *91:*909–910, Oct 24, '24

WÄNGLER, K.: Familial bilateral eyelid ptosis. Arch. f. Kinderh. *114:*102–107, '38

WAFFLE, E. B. AND FOWLER, F. E.: Lymphatic cysts of neck with report of case. Northwest Med. *25:*142–144, March '26

WAGENHALS, F. C.: Progressive facial hemiatrophy. Ohio State M. J. *27:*217–219, March '31

WAGERS, A. J.: Projecting or lop ear; case corrected by operation. M. J. and Rec. *128:*623–624, Dec 19, '28

WAGNER, G. A.: Schubert's method of formation of artificial vagina; cases. Zentralbl. f. Gynak. *51:*1300–1304, May 21, '27

WAGNER, G. A.: New method of formation of artificial vagina. Ztschr. f. Geburtsh. u. Gynak. *98:*412–421, '30

WAGNER, G. A. (see KIRSCHNER, M.) 1930

WAGNER, J. A. (see STRUMIA, M. M. *et al*) April '40

WAGNER, J. A. (see STRUMIA, M. M. *et al*) Nov '41

WAGNER, W.: Surgical therapy of Dupuytren's contracture. Beitr. z. klin. Chir. *155:*271–274, '32

Wagner-Kirschner

Formation of artificial vagina by Wagner-Kirschner operation; case. HELLER, P. Zentralbl. f. Gynak. *56:*2491–2494, Oct 8, '32

Surgical construction of artificial vagina by Wagner-Kirschner operation and Krause method of using skin flaps. WARNECKE, K. Zentralbl. f. Gynak. *56:*416–418, Feb 13, '32

Neoplasty of vagina by Wagner-Thiersch method (grafts). RISMONDO, P. Lijecn. vjes. *56:*312–313, '34

WAGONER, G. W. (see DORRANCE, G. M.) Oct '26

WAHL, J. P.: Fractures of mandible; their treatment. New Orleans M. and S. J. *85:*900–906, June '33

WAHL, S.: Simple method for reducing abnormally protruding nasal tip. Rev. de chir. structive, pp. 315–318, June '36

WAHLGREN, F. (see LINDVALL, S.) April '36

WAHREN, H.: Effect of vasotonic drugs in various types of shock. Ztschr. f. d. ges. exper. Med. *99:*306–319, '36

WAHRER, F. L.: Submucous resection of nasal septum. J. Iowa M. Soc. *16:*371–372, Aug '26

WAINWRIGHT, J. M.: Cancer of lip, breast and cervix; end result study. Bull. Moses Taylor Hosp. *1:*9–14, May '27

WAINWRIGHT, L.: Dupuytren's contracture. Practitioner *117:*263–265, Oct '26

WAISBEIN, S. (see VELASCO BLANCO, L.) 1938

WAKELEY, C. P. G.: Inflammations and fistulae of salivary glands and their treatment. Lancet *2:*7–10, July 7, '28

WAKELEY, C. P. G.: Clinical manifestations of branchial cysts. Clin. J. *58:*109–111, March 6, '29

WAKELEY, C. P. G.: Tumors of salivary glands. Surg., Gynec. and Obst. *48:*635–638, May '29

WAKELEY, C. P. G.: Burns in children. M. Press *128:*32, July 10, '29

WAKELEY, C. P. G.: Causation and treatment of displaced mandibular cartilage. Lancet *2:*543–545, Sept 14, '29

WAKELEY, C. P. G.: Diffuse hypertrophy of breasts in girl aged 17. Tr. M. Soc. London *54:*146–148, '31

WAKELEY, C. P. G.: Infant with deformed ears (case). Proc. Roy. Soc. Med. *25:*421, Feb '32

WAKELEY, C. P. G.: Old-standing facial paralysis treated by removal of inferior cervical ganglion of sympathetic (case). Proc. Roy. Soc. Med. *25:*795, April '32

WAKELEY, C. P. G.: Massive diffuse breast hypertrophy in girls; 4 cases. Practitioner *132:*608–613, May '34

WAKELEY, C. P. G.: Human oil (from omental fat) in treatment of adherant scars. Brit. M. J. *2:*618–619, Sept 17, '38

WAKELEY, C. P. G.: Surgery of temporomandibular joint. Surgery *5:*697–706, May '39

WAKELEY, C. P. G.: War burns and their treatment. Practitioner *146:*27–37, Jan '41

WAKELEY, C. P. G.: War burns. J. Roy. Nav. M. Serv. *27:*20–34, Jan '41 also: Surgery *10:*207–232, Aug '41

WAKELEY, C. P. G.: First aid in burns. M. Press *205:*93–96, Jan 29, '41

WAKELEY, C. P. G.: Electrical burns and their treatment. M. Press *206:*482–484, Dec 31, '41

WAKELEY, C. P. G.: Late end-results of war burns. Lancet *1:*410–412, April 4, '42

WAKELEY, C. P. G.: Therapy of chemical burns. M. Press *208:*360–363, Dec 2, '42

WAKELEY, C. P. G.: Rehabilitation of burns. M. Press *209:*173–175, March 17, '43

WAKELEY, C. P. G.: War wounds of hands. M. Press *211:*61–62, Jan 26, '44

WAKELEY, C. P. G.: Traumatic lesions of head of mandible; treatment. M. Press *214:*166–168, Sept 12, '45

WAKELEY, C. P. G.; GILLIES, H. AND HUDSON, R. V.: Late end-results of war burns. Tr. M. Soc. London (1940–1943) *63:*129–142, '45

WAKELEY, C. P. G. *et al*: Burn therapy. Proc. Roy. Soc. Med. *34:*43–72, Nov '40

WAKELEY, C. P. G. *et al*: Discussion on burns of eyelids and conjunctiva. Proc. Roy. Soc. Med. *37:*29–33, Nov '43

WAKIM, K. G. (see KENDRICK, D. B. JR.) Jan '39

WAKNITZ, F. W. (see CONVERSE, J. M.) Jan '42

WALD, A. H. (see WEINER, L.) June '46

WALDAPFEL, R.: Complications following nasal surgery. Wien. med. Wchnschr. *83:*1431–1433, Dec 16, '33

WALDAPFEL, R.: Rhinocanalicular anastomosis. Arch. Ophth. *31:*432–433, May '44

WALDAPFEL, R. (see RIGG, J. P.) July '39

WALDE, I.: Plastic correction of saddle nose. Monatschr. f. Ohrenh. *69:*850–863, July '35

WALDEN, A. (see SCHAPIRO, I. E. *et al*) Sept '45

WALDHEIM C., E.: Surgical therapy of cleft palate. Salubridad *1:*538, July–Sept '30

WALDRON, C. A. (see WALDRON, C. W. *et al*) Jan '46

WALDRON, C. W.: Plastic surgery of eyelids and orbit. Minnesota Med. *4:*504, Aug '21

WALDRON, C. W.: Jaw fractures. Journal-Lancet *53:*317, June 15; 351, July 1, '33

WALDRON, C. W.: Cystic tumors of jaws; conservative and 2 stage operative procedures to prevent deformity and loss of useful teeth. Am. J. Orthodontics (Oral Surg. Sect) *27:*313–322, June '41

WALDRON, C. W.: Nasal fractures. Minnesota Med. *25:*258–267, April '42

WALDRON, C. W.: Fractures of mandible, with special reference to reduction of complicated displacements and subsequent immobilization. Journal-Lancet *62:*228–240, June '42

WALDRON, C. W.: Skeletal fixation in treatment of fractures of mandible; review. J. Oral Surg. *1:*59–83, Jan '43

WALDRON, C. W. AND BALKIN, S. G.: Fractures of maxilla; simplified appliance for craniomaxillary support and fixation. Surgery *11:*183–194, Feb '42

WALDRON, C. W.; BALKIN, S. G. AND PETERSON, R. G.: Fractures of jaw in children. J. Oral Surg. *1:*215–234, July '43

WALDRON, C. W.; PETERSON, R. G. AND WALDRON, C. A.: Surgical treatment of mandibular

prognathism. J. Oral Surg. *4:*61–85, Jan '46
WALDRON, C. W. (see BALKIN, S. G.) Jan '44
WALDRON, C. W. (see PETERSON, R. G. *et al*) July '45
WALDRON, C. W. (see WORMAN, H. G. *et al*) Jan '46
WALKER, A. E. (see WOOLF, J. I.) Jan–Feb '46
WALKER, D. G.: Aid to prosthetic restorations of maxilla after excision. Lancet *1:*1209–1210, May 27, '39
WALKER, D. G.: Should teeth and comminuted bone be removed in jaw fractures? Proc. Roy. Soc. Med. *35:*663–682, Aug '42
WALKER, D. G.: Fractures of ramus, condyloid and coronoid processes of mandible. Bull. War Med. *3:*147–148, Nov '42 (abstract)
WALKER, F. A.: Screw-pin for use in connection with mandibular fractures and grafts. Brit. Dent. J. *78:*266–267, May 4, 1945
WALKER, F. A. (see RUSHTON, M. A.) Nov '36
WALKER, F. A. (see RUSHTON, M.A.) May '42
WALKER, F. A. (see RUSHTON, M. A.) May '45
WALKER, J. B.: Study of series of bone graft cases operated in U. S. Army Hospitals. Ann. Surg. *73:*1, Jan '21
WALKER, R. H.: Hand injuries and infections. W. Virginia M. J. *22:*456–460, Sept '26
WALL, C. K.: Cancer of lip, its treatment by radium and surgery combined. J. M. A. Georgia *12:*67–69, Feb '23
WALLACE, A. B.: Burn therapy. Practitioner *145:*180–187, Sept '40
WALLACE, A. B.: *The Treatment of Burns*. Oxford Press, London, 1941
WALLACE, A. B.: First aid treatment in burns. Practitioner *147:*513–517, Aug '41
WALLACE, A. B. (see LEARMONTH, J. R.) Jan '43
WALLACE, A. B. (see ROBSON, J. M.) March '41
WALLACE, E. G. (see NOMLAND, R.) March '46
WALLACE, F. T.: Technical details in dermatome grafting. South. M. J. *38:*380–381, June '45
WALLACE, F. T.: Primary repair of parotid duct. Am. J. Surg. *70:*412–413 Dec '45
WALLENTIN Y SPRINGER, R.: Modern therapy of burns. Rev. med. y cien. afines. Mexico *4:*409–444, Jan '46
WALLER, J. B.: Makkas operation in case of exstrophy of bladder. Zentralbl. f. Chir. *51:*1841–1842, Aug 23, '24
WALLERSTEIN: Two cases of artificial vagina. Zentralbl. f. Gynak. *45:*1492–1494, Oct 15, '21
WALLIN, C. C.: Fracture of articular process of lower jaw. Northwest Med. *26:*214, April '27
WALLISCH, W.: Patient with only one mandibular condyle. Ztschr. f. Stomatol. *25:*621–626, July '27
WALLON, E.: Angioma of nose following erysipelas; radium therapy proposed; case. Bull. Soc. franc. de dermat. et syph. *35:*406–408, May '28
WALLON, E.: Indications for technic of radium treatment of cutaneous angiomas. Presse med. *37:*803–804, June 19, '29
WALRATH, C. H. (see PETTIT, J. A.) Dec '32
WALRATH, C. H. (see PETTIT, J. A.) Jan '34
WALSH, F. B.: Hemiatrophy of face; 2 cases. Am. J. Ophth. *22:*1–10, Jan '39
WALSH, J. N.: Treatment of severe cutaneous burns. J. South Carolina M. A. *31:*189–194, Oct '35
WALSH, T. E. AND BOTHMAN, L.: Results of intranasal dacryocystorhinostomy. Am. J. Ophth. *20:*939–941, Sept '37
WALSH, T. F. P. AND NUTINI, L. G.: Burn therapy founded on cellular stimulation. South. Med. and Surg. *105:*341–350, Aug '43
WALTER, E. L.: Typical mandibular fracture. U. S. Nav. M. Bull. *18:*88–89, Jan '23
WALTER, E. V. (see HANNS *et al*) Dec '28
WALTERS, W.: Transplantation of ureters into rectosigmoid portion of intestines in exstrophy, with extirpation of bladder; 76 cases. Arch. f. klin. Chir. *167:*589–600, '31
WALTERS, W.: Transplantation of ureters to rectosigmoid and cystectomy in exstrophy; 76 cases. Am. J. Surg. *15:*15–22, Jan '32
WALTERS, W.: Transplantation of ureters into sigmoid colon for exstrophy of bladder incontinence (unilateral versus simultaneous bilateral transplantation). Proc. Staff Meet., Mayo Clin. *7:*470–472, Aug 10, '32
WALTERS, W.: Transplantation of ureters to sigmoid colon for exstrophy of bladder and other ureteral abnormalities with urinary incontinence. Minnesota Med. *16:*416–419, June '33
WALTERS, W.: Ombredanne-Lyle operation for hypospadias; case. Proc. Staff Meet., Mayo Clin. *8:*467–469, Aug 2, '33
WALTERS, W.: Ureterosigmoidal transplantation for exstrophy and complete epispadias with absent urinary sphincters. Am. J. Surg. *24:*776–792, June '34
WALTERS, W.: Transplantation of solitary ureter to sigmoid colon for exstrophy of bladder; case. Proc. Staff Meet., Mayo Clin. *9:*485–486, Aug 15, '34
WALTERS, W.: Successful operations for hypospadias. Ann. Surg. *103:*949–958, June '36
WALTERS, W. AND BRAASCH, W. F.: Ureteral transplantation to rectosigmoid for exstrophy of bladder, complete epispadias and other urethral abnormalities with total urinary incontinence; 85 cases operated. Am. J. Surg. *23:*255–270, Feb '34
WALTERS, W.; PRIESTLEY, J. B. AND GRAY, H.

K.: Ureterosigmoidal transplantation and plastic operations on penis in exstrophy of bladder. S. Clin. North America *11:*823–828, Aug '31
WALTERS, W. (see CABOT, H. *et al.*) April '35
WALTERS, W. (see MAYO, C. H.) Feb '24

Walters Operation: See Mayo-Walters Operation

WALTHER, E.: Nature and significance of keloids. Med. Welt *9:*1006–1008, July 13, '35

Walther Operation

Therapy of elephantiasis of extremities by lymphatic drainage by buried tubes (Walther operation); 2 cases. TOURAINE, A. Bull. Soc. franc. de dermat. et syph. *42:*1771–1775, Dec '35

WALTON, F. E.: Burn management. Surgery *15:*547–552, April '44
WALZ, W.: Congenital scalp defects. Monatschr. f. Geburtsh. u. Gynak. *65:*167–178, Jan '24
WANAMAKER, F. H.: Acute osteomyelitis of jaw and its complications. Eye, Ear, Nose and Throat Monthly *14:*56–58, March '35
WANAMAKER, F. H.: Care of burn casualty. U. S. Nav. M. Bull. *44:*1239–1244, June '45
WANDERLEY FILHO, E. AND GALVAO, H.: Therapy of primary shock due to burns; 2 cases. Arq. brasil. de cir. e ortop. *5:*308–318, March '38
WANG, Y. Y. (see WHITACRE, F. E.) Aug '44
WANGENSTEEN, O. H.: Implantation method of skin grafts. Surg., Gynec. and Obst. *50:*634–638, March '30
WANGENSTEEN, O. H.: Differentiation of branchial from other cervical cysts by X-ray examination. Ann. Surg. *93:*790–792, March '31
WANGENSTEEN, O. H.: Present concept of traumatic shock and its treatment. Journal-Lancet *51:*711–718, Dec 1, '31
WANGENSTEEN, O. H.: Abdominal surgery in old age; mechanism of development of "bedsores." Journal-Lancet *64:*178–183, June '44
WANGENSTEEN, O H. AND RANDALL, O. S.: Treatment and results of cancer of lips; 130 cases. Am. J. Roentgenol. *30:*75–81, July '33
WANGERMEZ. (see PETGES.) May '36

War Burns

Burn therapy in army medical department. CLAVELIN, C. AND CARILLON, R. J., Rev. serv. de san. mil. *106:*571–596, April '37
Incendiary air raids; incendiary bombs, extinction of fires and treatment of burns. SIMON, L. Strasbourg med. *98:*175–179, May 15, '38

War Burns–Cont.

Death resulting from burns on military field. LEYVA PEREIRA, L. Rev. Fac. de med., Bogota *7:*149–154, Oct '38
Burn therapy under war conditions. MITCHINER, P. H., M. Press *202:*26–31, July 12, '39
First aid in burns, with special consideration of conditions prevailing in air raids. FICK. Ztschr. f. arztl. Fortbild. *36:*584–592, Oct 1, '39
First aid for thermal war injuries. HOCHE, O. Med. Klin. *35:*1532, Dec 1; 1563, Dec 8, '39 *36:*39, Jan 12; 67, Jan 19; 94, Jan 26; 154, Feb 9; 239, March 1; 265, March 8; 291, March 15, '40
Skin injuries from incendiary bombs and war chemicals. FUHS, H. Wien. klin. Wchnschr. *53:*40–44, Jan 12, '40
War burns. FLÖRCKEN, H. Chirurg *12:*89–92, Feb 15, '40
Local first aid treatment of burns during naval combat. GUISO, L. Ann. di med. nav. e colon *46:*151–154, March–April '40
Experience in treatment of war burns. COHEN, S. M. Brit. M. J. *2:*251–254, Aug 24, '40
War burns. KENDALL, A. W., M. Press *205:*42–45, Jan 15, '41
War burns and their treatment. WAKELEY, C. P. G. Practitioner *146:*27–37, Jan '41
War burns. WAKELEY, C. P. G., J. Roy. Nav. M. Serv. *27:*20–34, Jan '41 also: Surgery *10:*207–232, Aug '41
Treatment of 100 war wounds and burns. ROSS, J. A. AND HULBERT, K. F. Brit. M. J. *1:*618–621, April 26, '41
Suggestions for first aid of burns at front. WESTERMANN, H. H. Deut. Militärarzt *6:*209–211, April '41
Injuries due to burns from point of view of naval surgery. KOCH, F. Svenska lak. -tidning. *38:*1351–1356, June 13, '41
Burn therapy in wartime. DENNISON, W. M. AND DIVINE, D., J. Roy. Army M. Corps *77:*14–18, July '41
Burn therapy in wartime. OLDFIELD, M. C., J. Roy. Army M. Corps *77:*1–13, July '41
Management of war burns. HALFORD, F. J. Hawaii M. J. *1:*191–192, Jan '42
War burns; survey of treatment and results in 100 cases. MAITLAND, A. I. L., J. Roy. Nav. M. Serv. *28:*3–17, Jan '42
Care of military and civilian injuries (burns). HICKEY, M. J. Am. J. Orthodontics (Oral Surg. Sect.) *28:*177–182, April '42
Wartime burns. PASSALACQUA, L. A. Bol. Asoc. med. de Puerto Rico *34:*140–146, April '42
Late end-results of war burns. WAKELEY, C.

War Burns—Cont.
P. G. Lancet *1:*410-412, April 4, '42
Burn therapy in wartime. (Ernest Edward Irons lecture) HARKINS, H. N., J.A.M.A. *119:*385-390, May 30, '42
War surgery; management of burns. ATKINS, H. J. B. Brit. M. J. *1:*704, June 6, '42; 729, June 13, '42
War burns. LINDSAY, H. C. L. Urol. and Cutan. Rev. *46:*386-390, June '42
War burns. BOVE, C. New York State J. Med. *42:*1366-1370, July 15, '42
"Solace" (hospital ship) in action (burns). ECKERT, G. A. AND MADER, J. W., U. S. Nav. M. Bull. *40:*552-557, July '42
Newer concepts, with suggestions for management of wartime thermal injuries. FOX, T. A., U. S. Nav. M. Bull. *40:*557-570, July '42
Military burns; analysis of 308 cases. KNOEPP, L. F. Am. J. Surg. *57:*226-230, Aug '42
War burns. PALMER, E. P. AND PALMER, E. P. JR. Southwestern Med. *26:*251-255, Aug '42
War burns; varieties according to method of production. DE ARAGON, E. R. Rev. med. -social san. y benef. mumic. *2:*309-314, Oct-Dec '42
War burns and their treatment. RAU, U. M. Antiseptic *39:*655-665, Oct '42
Burns, various types; treatment and prognosis from military as well as civilian viewpoint. WIDMEYER, R. S., J. Florida M. A. *29:*165-168, Oct '42
War burns. GONCALVES BOGADO, L. Rev. med.-cir. do Brasil *50:*1087-1098, Dec '42
Infected burns in naval personnel. HEGGIE, R. M. AND HEGGIE, J. F. Lancet *2:*664-667, Dec 5, '42
Newer concepts, with suggestions for management of wartime thermal injuries. FOX, T. A., J. Lab. and Clin. Med. *28:*474-484, Jan '43
Burn therapy in war. YEMM, W. A. Physiotherapy Rev. *23:*13-16, Jan-Feb '43
Forum on therapy of wartime injuries (burns). HOUCK, J. S. New York State J. Med. *43:*226-228, Feb 1, '43
Most recent advances in burn therapy; question of therapy used in present war. PETIT ODDO. Publ. med., Sao Paulo *14:*43-56, March-April '43
Burn cases off the U. S. S. Wasp. JACOBS, R. G., J. Oklahoma M. A. *36:*235-236, June '43
Local therapy of war burns. DESJARDINS, E. Union med. du Canada *72:*790-792, July '43

War Burns—Cont.
Sulfonamides in war wounds and burns. FOX, C. L. Spec. Libraries *34:*244-247, July-Aug '43
Burn therapy in warfare. MACEY, H. B. Proc. Staff Meet., Mayo Clin. *18:*241-246, July 28, '43
Burn therapy in the field. STEIN, J. J. Hosp. Corps Quart. *16:*113-115, July '43
War burns and their therapy. COUTINHO, A. Rev. med. de Pernambuco *13:*175-190, Aug '43
War burns; traumatologic study on action of flame throwers and explosives. PARANAGUA, C. Imprensa med., Rio de Janeiro *19:*57-72, Aug '43
Burns treated as war wounds. SHEEHAN, J. E. Am. J. Surg. *61:*331-338, Sept '43
Discussion of burns based on experience with 360 cases seen on board a U. S. hospital ship. KERN, R. A. *et al.* U. S. Nav. M. Bull. *41:*1654-1678, Nov '43
Therapy of war burns. MARQUES PORTO, E. Rev. med.-cir. do Brasil *51:*585-608, Nov '43
Therapy of war burns. HAMILTON, J. E. AND BARNETT, L. A., S. Clin. North America *23:*1575-1588, Dec '43
Discussion based on experience with 360 burn cases seen on board a U. S. hospital ship. KERN, R. A. *et al.* U. S. Nav. M. Bull. *42:*59-81, Jan '44
Burns incident to war (treatment). BERKOW, S. G. Clinics *2:*1265-1294, Feb '44
Therapy of war burns. RANKIN, F. W. *et al.* Clinics *2:*1194-1218, Feb '44
Treatment of burns incident to war; Wellcome prize essay. RODDIS, L. H. Mil. Surgeon *94:*65-75, Feb '44
Burn therapy at sea. CZWALINSKI, P. F., U. S. Nav. M. Bull. *42:*838-840, April '44
Burn therapy experience from South Pacific area. YANDELL, H. R., U. S. Nav. M. Bull. *42:*829-837, April '44
Burn therapy in forward areas. JOHNSTON, C. C. Bull. U. S. Army M. Dept. (no. 76) pp. 109-113, May '44
Local treatment of war burns. STOCKTON, A. B. Stanford M. Bull. *2:*71-73, May '44
Burn therapy in warfare. LOGIE, N. J. Lancet *2:*138-140, July 29, '44
How they treat burn cases aboard U. S. S. Solace. SHAW, C. E. W. Mod. Hosp. *63:*72-75, Nov '44
Sulfonamides in treatment of war burns. FOX, C. L. JR. Smithsonian Inst. Annual Rep. (1943) pp. 569-574, '44
Plastic surgery in burns among naval personnel; current experiences. GREELEY, P. W.

War Burns—Cont.
Am. J. Surg. *67:*401-411, Feb '45
Dermoepidermal grafts in early treatment of severe war burns. HUBER, J. P. Semaine d. hop. Paris *21:*741-747, July 21, '45 also: Bull. internat. serv. san. *18:*197-209, Aug '45
Late end-results of war burns. WAKELEY, C. P. G.; *et al.* Tr. M. Soc. London (1940-1943) *63:*129-142, '45
Short review of treatment of service burns during the war. HILL. M. Bull. Bombay *14:*13-15, Jan 28, '46
Major burns in naval warfare. McLAUGHLIN, C. W. JR. Nebraska M. J. *31:*11-19, Jan '46
Therapy of burns in last war. BERMUDEZ, E. Gac. med. Lima *2:*275-281, March '46
Modern therapy of burns in war. DRIESSEN, H. E. Nederl. tijdschr. v. geneesk. *90:*497-500, May 18, '46

War Injuries
Study of series of bone graft cases operated in U. S. Army Hospitals. WALKER, J. B. Ann. Surg. *73:*1, Jan '21
Plastic surgery in relation to armed forces; past, present and future (Kober lecture). JOHNSON, L. W. Mil. Surgeon *79:*90-102, Aug '36
War lesions due to toxic gases and incendiary projectiles (burns). TROTOT, R. Tunisie med. *29:*293-304, July-Aug '35
Centers for restorative surgery and prosthesis after war wounds. LEMAITRE. Mem. Acad. de chir. *65:*1143-1147, Oct 25-Nov 8, '39
Therapy of skin lesions due to war gases. GRZHEBIN, Z. N. Klin. med. (no. 6) *17:*83-86, '39
Maxillofacial surgery during campaign in Poland. SARRU, P. *et al.* Rev. san. mil., Bucuresti *39:*277-281, May '40
Cooperation between maxillofacial surgeon and other surgeons in treatment of soldiers with multiple wounds. BERCHER. Rev. de stomatol. *41:*759-760, '40
Principles of reconstructive surgery in war wounds. REHN, E. Beitr. z. klin. Chir. *171:*1-24, '40
Symposium on sequelae to war wounds; scarring and contracture. MOWLEM, R., M. Press *205:*384-387, May 7, '41
Plastic surgery in war; preparedness of profession at large. MALINIAC, J. W., M. Rec. *154:*325-326, Nov 5, '41
Scope of plastic surgery in war. MALINIAC, J. W. Bol. d. Hosp. policia mac. *2:*65-68, April 1, '43
Musculocutaneous graft and its importance

War Injuries—Cont.
in war surgery. PRUDENTE, A. Rev. paulista de med. *22:*435-436, June '43
Corrective surgery in war; progress, advantages and possibilities. HERNANDEZ RAMIREZ, S. Pasteur *2:*15-18, July 15, '43
Plastic surgery in treatment of war casualties. SUTTON, L. E. Am. J. Surg. *61:*239-243, Aug '43
Plastic surgery and war. PRUDENTE, A. Imprensa med., Rio de Janeiro *19:*39-58, Sept '43
Plastic surgery as related to war surgery. KIRKHAM, H. L. D.; *et al.* S. Clin. North America *23:*1603-1611, Dec '43
(Plastic) surgery heals scars of war. BROWN, D. AND LUMSDEN, R. Hygeia *22:*26, Jan '44
Ear wounds and injuries among battle casualties of Western Desert. COLLINS, E. G. J. Laryng. and Otol. *59:*1-15, Jan '44
Symposium on war medicine; plastic and reconstruction surgery. IVY, R. H. *et al.* Clinics *2:*1165-1193, Feb '44
Plastic surgery in combat and civilian casualities. IVY, R. H., M. Ann. District of Columbia *13:*45-49, Feb '44
Plastic surgery of war wounds. ASCHAN, P. E. Deut. Militararzt *9:*142, March '44
Reparative surgery in the war. COVARRUBIAS ZENTENO, R. Arch. Soc. cirujanos hosp. *14:*49-56, March '44
Reconstructive surgery of war injuries. SNEDECOR, S. T. Delaware State M. J. *16:*39-41, March '44
Plastic surgery in treatment of war wounds. ASCHAN, P. E. Nord. med. (Finska lak. -sallsk. handl.) *22:*933-939, May 19, 1944
Reconstruction surgery of Imperial and Union Defense Force. FOUCHE, F. P. Am. Acad. Orthop. Surgeons, Lect. pp. 542-546, '44
Reconstructive surgery of war wounded. WILSON, P. D. Rocky Mountain M. J. *42:*267-274, April '45
Plastic and reconstructive surgery in military. STRAATSMA, C. R. Mil. Surgeon *96:*255-257, March '45
War wounds of spinal cord; surgical treatment of decubitus ulcers. BARKER, D. E. J.A.M.A. *129:*160, Sept 8, '45
Reconstructive surgery of war wounded. WILSON, P. D. New England J. Med. *233:*492-497, Oct 25, '45
Military plastic surgery. SHAW, M. H., M. Press *214:*312-317, Nov 14, '45
Reconstructive surgery of war wounds. WILSON, P. D. Medicina, Mexico *25:*475-491, Nov 25, '45
Plastic surgery in war; recent advances in

War Injuries – Cont.
United States and Great Britain. MARINO, H. Bol. y trab., Soc. argent. de cirujanos *6:*778–788, '45 also: Rev. Asoc. med. argent. *59:*1373–1376, Dec 15, '45
Plastic surgery in present war. MARINO, H. Bol. Soc. cir. d. Uruguay *16:*311–321, '45
Plastic surgery in second World War. MARINO, H. Arch. urug. de med., cir. y especialid. *28:*197–207, Feb '46
Frostbite in wartime. TABANELLI, M. Arch. ital. chir. *68:*111–195, '46

War Injuries, Face
Reconstruction of nose, lid region and cheek following shell wound. VIGNOLO, Q. Arch. ital. di chir. *3:*649, July '21 abstr: J.A.M.A. *77:*1290, Oct 15, '21
Maxillo-facial centers. LEMAITRE, F. Mil. Surgeon *57:*242–255, Sept '25
Treatment of war wounds of face and jaws. BERCHER, J. Mil. Surgeon *58:*130–132, Feb '26
Organization of department for maxillary-facial surgery among war wounded. WATRY. Arch. med. belges *80:*457–461, Sept '27
Social sequels of maxillo-facial wounds received in war. REGNART, R. L. F. Rev. odont. *51:*372–378, Sept–Oct '30
Maxillo-Facial Injuries, Report of Army Standing Ctte., by War Office of Great Britain. H. M. Stationery Office, London, 1935
Fracture of lower jaw due to gunshot wounds in face during Waziristan operations, 1937; 3 cases. GOLDING, H. S., J. Roy. Army M. Corps *71:*50–54, July '38
Fractures of bones of face in war-time; president's address. PARROTT, A. H. Proc. Roy. Soc. Med. *32:*53–58, Nov '38
Air-raid injuries to face. MITCHINER, P. H. AND COWELL, E. M. Lancet *1:*601–602, March 11, '39
Basic principles of therapy of gunshot wounds of face in military surgery. AXHAUSEN, G. Ztschr. f. Stomatol. *37:*436–440, April 28, '39
War injuries of nose and nasal sinuses; 5 cases. NISHIYAMA, A. Oto-rhino-laryng. *12:*476–477, June '39
War wounds of face. RUPPE, C. Presse med. *47:*1334–1336, Sept 13, '39
Therapy of wounds of face and jaws at battalion or regiment first aid stations, in army corps field hospital and in evacuation hospital. ROCHETTE, M. Hopital *27:*521–527, Nov '39
Surgical therapy of war wounds of jaws and

War Injuries, Face – Cont.
face. AXHAUSEN, G. Chirurg *11:*801–807, Dec 1, '39
War wounds of face and jaws. PEYRUS, J. J. Rev. serv. de san. mil. *111:*1017–1030, Dec '39
War injuries of ear, nose and throat. VOSS, O. Med. Klin. *35:*1589–1591, Dec 15, '39
Surgical therapy of war wounds to face due to projectile. DUBECQ, X. J. AND BOIVIN, J. Progres med. *68:*56–58, 63, Jan 20, '40
Therapy of maxillofacial war lesions in teritorial hospitals. CALABRO, N. Stomatol. ital. *2:*297–302, April '40
Maxillofacial surgery during campaign in Poland. SARRU, P. *et al.* Rev. san. mil., Bucuresti *39:*277–281, May '40
War injuries of jaws and face. COLE, P. P. Post-Grad. M. J. *16:*233–244, July '40
Suggestions for war surgery of facial injuries; use of wire cradle and fixation of tongue, facial flaps and bone fragments by means of safety pin in patients with jaw fractures. HENSCHEN, C. Schweiz. med. Wchnschr. *70:*711–715, July 30, '40
Care and therapeutic provisions for maxillofacial wounds on battlefield; limits and possibilities of aid in dressing stations of troops, battalions and regiments and in advanced posts of sanitary service. PALAZZI, S. Gior. di med. mil. *88:*500–508, July '40
Sinusofacial wounds in war surgery with report of cases. ESCAT, M. Oto-rhino-laryng. internat. *24:*241–252, Sept '40
Gunshot wounds of face and jaws; first aid treatment, field service. STOUT, R. A. Mil. Surgeon *87:*247–250, Sept '40
Treatment of military facial injuries. SCHMIDHUBER, K. F. Deut. Militararzt *5:*418–419, Oct '40
Cooperation between maxillofacial surgeon and other surgeons in treatment of soldiers with multiple wounds. BERCHER. Rev. de stomatol. *41:*759–760, '40
Facial and maxillary injuries in war. CUPAR, I. Voj.-san. glasnik *11:*457–471, '40
Treatment of war injuries to face. KILNER, T. P., M. Press *205:*26–29, Jan 8, '41
Immediate care of war wounds of face and jaw. SCHMUZIGER, P. Helvet. med. acta *8:*49–53, April '41
Emergency treatment of war injuries to face. IVY, R. H. AND STOUT, R. A. Ann. Surg. *113:*1001–1009, June '41
Symposium on military surgery; plastic and maxillofacial surgery. IVY, R. H., S. Clin. North America *21:*1583–1592, Dec '41
Migraine due to war injury to nose, with

War Injuries, Face – Cont.
recovery following resection of cicatrix. LEBOURG, L. Rev. de stomatol. *43:*27–28, Jan–Feb '42
Care of face and jaw casualties in United States Army. FAIRBANK, L. C. War Med. *2:*223–229, March '42
Care of military and civilian injuries of face and jaws. PADGETT, E. C. Am. J. Orthodontics (Oral Surg. Sect.) *28:*213–221, April '42
Face injuries in war. CONVERSE, J. M. Tr. Am. Acad. Ophth. (1941) *46:*250–255, May–June '42
War surgery of face and head. GERMAN, W. J., Yale J. Biol. and Med. *14:*453–462, May '42
Early and late treatment of face and jaws as applied to war injuries. IVY, R. H. South. Surgeon *11:*366–373, May '42
Specialists' experiences with wounds of facial portion of skull in war and peace. SPECHT, F. Munchen. med. Wchnschr. *89:*391, May 1, '42
Chemotherapy (with sulfanilamide and its derivatives) in gunshot wounds of face, neck and jaws. OGLE, M. W. Mil. Surgeon *90:*650–655, June '42
Practical points in anesthesia at maxillofacial unit. HUNTER, J. T. Anesth. and Analg. *21:*223–228, July–Aug '42
Results of front line plastic surgery of face; experiences with the Army at Eastern Front, I. REICHENBACH, E. Zentralbl. f. Chir. *69:*1333–1350, Aug 15, '42
Permanent therapy of maxillofacial wounds in war surgery. IVY, R. H. AND CURTIS, L. Rev. san. mil., Buenos Aires *41:*638–650, Sept '42
Use of buttons with wire suture in gunshot wounds of face and jaw. PERWITZSCHKY, R. Ztschr. f. Hals-, Nasen-u. Ohrenh. *48:*270; 458, '42
War injuries to face and jaw. SHAW, J. J. M. War and Doctor, pp. 41–46, '42
Plastic surgery applied to war wounds of face. ALFREDO, J. Rev. med. de Pernambuco *13:*1–10, Jan '43
Care of military and civilian injuries; use of remote flaps in repairing defects of face and mouth. CANNON, B. Am. J. Orthodontics (Oral Surg. Sect.) *29:*77–85, Feb '43
Relation of early care to final outcome of major wounds of face in war surgery. BLAIR, V. P. Mil. Surgeon *92:*12–17, Jan '43 also: Cincinnati J. Med. *24:*121–127, May '43
Early treatment of war wounds of face. CASHMAN, C. J. Rev. san. mil., Buenos Aires

War Injuries, Face – Cont.
*42:*291–298, May '43
Surgical treatment of war injuries of nasal accessory sinuses. ESCHER, F. Schweiz. med. Wchnschr. *73:*715, May 29, '43 abstr. Bull. War Med. *4:*278, Jan '44
Rehabilitation in maxillofacial and plastic center. MCINDOE, A. H. Post-Grad. M. J. *19:*161–167, July '43
Early treatment of war wounds of upper part of face. OLDFIELD, M. C. Brit. M. J. *2:*163–165, Aug 7, '43
Emergency plastic surgery in war injuries of face. CONVERSE, J. M. Ann. Otol., Rhin. and Laryng. *52:*637–654, Sept '43
Ophthalmic injuries (including burns) of war. MATTHEWS, J. L. War Med. *4:*247–261, Sept '43
Facial bone fractures as seen in naval service. LIPSCOMB, T. H. South. M. J. *36:*665–668, Oct '43
Maxillofacial injuries produced by gunshot wounds in modern warfare. MEYER, G. E. J. Am. Dent. A. *30:*1576–1583, Oct 1, '43
Therapy of war wounds of eyelids and their surrounding area. HEESCH, K. Deut. Militararzt *8:*699, Dec '43
Therapy of wounds of maxillofacial region; later experiences with war wounded who were first treated at field hospitals. PIERITZ, G. Deut. Militararzt *8:*693, Dec '43
Plastic surgery in wartime; how to manage head and neck wounds. REBELO NETO, J. Rev. paulista de med. *23:*345–346, Dec '43
Points on treatment of maxillofacial injuries. STANHOPE, E. D. East African M. J. *20:*399–408, Dec '43
Facial war surgery. DOS SANTOS, F. Arq. brasil. de cir. e ortop. *11:*24–35, '43
Present status of therapy of maxillofacial war wounds. RAUER, A. E. Sovet. med. (nos. 7–8) *7:*22–24, '43
Symposium on plastic surgery; treatment of battle casualties and street or industrial wounds (face). BLAIR, V. P. Surgery *15:*16–21, Jan '44
Prosthesis in relation to war wounds of face. CLARKE, C. D., M. Bull. North African Theat. Op. (no. 1) *1:*17–24, Jan '44 also: J. Lab. and Clin. Med. *29:*667–672, June '44
Symposium on plastic surgery; early treatment of gunshot wounds of face and jaws; case histories of patients treated during World War I. KAZANJIAN, V. H. Surgery *15:*22–42, Jan '44
Early treatment of war wounds of upper part of face. OLDFIELD, M. C. Rev. san. mil., Buenos Aires. *43:*11–17, Jan '44
Gunshot wounds of fronto-orbital region.

War Injuries, Face – Cont.
Schorstein, J. Lancet *1:*44-47, Jan 8, '44
Primary skin graft for repair of traumatic skin loss of face; case. Oberdorfer, A. Z. U. S. Nav. M. Bull. *42:*695-696, March '44
Early care of facial wounds. Myers, S. A. U. S. Nav. M. Bull. *42:*1019-1020, May '44
Recuperation of war wounded with orbital-ocular injuries. Paiva Goncalves. Hospital, Rio de Janeiro *26:*429-444, Sept '44
Recommendations for treatment of maxillofacial cases in forward areas. Clarkson, P. and Wilson, T. H. H. Brit. Dent. J. *77:*229-234, Oct 20, '44
Reparative surgery of face in Middle East, with short review of 1,200 cases treated during last 2 years. Oldfield, M. C. Brit. J. Surg. *32:*237-246, Oct '44
Relation of transport speed to type and treatment of facial injuries. Mowlem, R. M. Press *212:*310-312, Nov 15, '44
Maxillofacial traumatology in military medicine. Morayta, M. An. med. d. Ateneo Ramon y Cajal (no. 4) *2:*45-46, Dec '44
Treatment of penetrating war wounds of neck. Drobyshev, G. I. Khirurgiya, no. 2, pp. 49-54, '44
Salivary fistulas following gunshot wounds to face, and their therapy. Gutner, Y. I. Khirurgiya, no. 7, pp. 54-58, '44
Penicillin in oral and maxillofacial surgery. Christiansen, G. W. Mil. Surgeon *96:*51-54, Jan '45
Maxillofacial surgical unit mobile dental laboratory. Dalling, E. J. Brit. Dent. J. *78:*10-12, Jan 5, '45
Severe faciomaxillary injury treated at sea. Kennedy, R. L. and Lewis, F. C. R., J. Roy. Nav. M. Serv. *31:*36-39, Jan '45
Facial traumatisms in war surgery. Castro O'Connor, R. Bol. d. Inst. clin. quir. *21:*95-98, Feb '45
First aid and preliminary treatment of maxillofacial injuries. Fuller, W. H. A. Brit. Dent. J. *78:*106-108, Feb 16, '45
Treatment of maxillofacial casualties in B. L. A. Holland, N. Brit. Dent. J. *78:*78-80, Feb 2, '45
Therapy of war trauma of facial region. Rivas, C. I. Bol. d. Inst. clin. quir. *21:*90-95, Feb '45
Course of instruction in treatment of maxillofacial injuries, Ballochmyle E. M. S. Hospital. Inglis, J. V. Brit. Dent. J. *78:*242-243, April 20, '45
Primary closure of battle wounds of face. Lawrie, R. Lancet *1:*625-626, May 19, '45
Facial nerve lesions due to war injuries and

War Injuries, Face – Cont.
their repair. Lathrop, F. D., J. Laryng. and Otol. *60:*257-266, June '45
Treatment of gunshot wounds of face. Gordon, S. D. Bull. Acad. Med., Toronto *18:*185-187, July '45
Nose and sinuses; primary war injuries. Canfield, N. Proc. Roy. Soc. Med. *38:*627-628, Sept '45
Facial nerve lesions due to war injuries and their repair. Lathrop, F. D. Proc. Roy. Soc. Med. *38:*629-634, Sept '45
Maxillofacial bandage. Kincaid, C. J. Bull. U. S. Army M. Dept. *4:*475-477, Oct '45
Primary war injuries involving nose and sinuses. Canfield, N., J. Laryng. and Otol. *60:*458-460, Nov '45
War wounds of lips and cheek. Webster, G. V., U. S. Nav. M. Bull. *45:*819-826, Nov '45
Report from maxillofacial center at Royal Air Force casualty clearing station in England. Badenoch, A. W. and Holms, S. Brit. Dent. J. *79:*346-348, Dec 21, '45
Fatal facial wounds difficult to diagnose. Voloshchenko, D. L. Khirurgiya, No. 6, pp. 89-90, '45
Symposium on military medicine aboard U. S. S. Samaritan; injuries of face in war casualties. Wiser, H. J. and McAfee, M. F., U. S. Nav. M. Bull. *46:*57-66, Jan '46
Plastic reconstruction following gunshot wound of lip; case. Chambers, J. V. U. S. Nav. M. Bull. *46:*588-590, April '46
Facial nerve; repair of traumatic lesions secondary to war wounds. Lathrop, F. D., S. Clin. North America *26:*763-773, June '46
Headpiece for face wounds and fractures. Jordan, C. E., U. S. Nav. M. Bull. *45:*330, Aug '45
Repair of defects (using tantalum), with special reference to periorbital structures and frontal sinus. Turner, O. A. Arch. Surg. *53:*312-326, Sept '46
Management of plastic maxillofacial wounds in evacuation hospital. Leech, C. H. *et al.* Surg. Gynec. and Obst. *83:*462-473, Oct '46
War injuries to mastoid and facial nerve. Myers, D. Arch. Otolaryng. *44:*392-405, Oct '46
Case reports from maxillofacial team, 6th General Hospital. Sturgis, S. H. and Holland, D. J. Jr. Am. J. Orthodontics (Oral Surg. Sect.) *32:*635-664, Oct '46
Proper time and principles of primary treatment of gunshot wounds of face. Frankenberg, B. E. Vrach. delo (nos. 7-8) *26:*465-470, '46
Maxillofacial war wounds; principles of ther-

War Injuries, Face – Cont.
apy and results. THEODORESCO, D., J. de chir. *62:*171–183, '46

War Injuries, Hand

War wounds of fingers. OLDHAM, J. B. M. Press *204:*476–480, Dec 18, '40
Urgent surgery for hand. BEACH, W. V. J. Roy. Nav. M. Serv. *27:*258–267, July '41
Traumatic amputation of finger tips (with special reference to tank door accident; value of skin grafts). TERHUNE, S. R. AND CAMP, M. N. South. Surgeon *11:*646–651, Sept '42
Care of injured hand. REQUARTH, W. H. U. S. Nav. M. Bull. *41:*1329–1335, Sept '43
Contractures of fingers and toes after war wounds. SQUIRE, C. M. Proc. Roy. Soc. Med. *36:*665–666, Oct '43
Principles governing design and details of first aid Stannard glove. HUDSON, R. V. Bull. War Med. *4:*193–195, Dec '43 (abstract)
Symposium on war surgery; rehabilitation of burned hand. MEHERIN, J. M. AND GREELEY, P. W., S. Clin. North America *23:*1651–1665, Dec '43
War wounds of hands. WAKELEY, C. P. G. M. Press *211:*61–62, Jan 26, '44
New type of hand dressing to improve function. COX, F. J. *et al.* M. Bull. Mediterranean Theat. Op. *2:*168–169, Dec '44
Lessons learned from review of cases of hand wounds evacuated from South Pacific. AITKEN, G. T. Am. Acad. Orthop. Surgeons, Lect., pp. 202–208, '44
Contracture of fingers and hand following gunshot wounds. FRIDLAND, M. O. Khirurgiya, no. 8, pp. 56–61, '44
Skin and soft tissue war wounds of hand and forearm. IVERSON, P. C. Am. Acad. Orthop. Surgeons, Lect., pp. 184–187, '44
Therapy of gunshot wounds of fingers (and hand). VISHNYAKOV, S. L. Khirurgiya, no. 5, pp. 76–78, '44
Direct flap repair of defects of arm and hand; preparation of gunshot wounds for repair of nerves, bones and tendons. BROWN, J. B. *et al.* Ann. Surg. *122:*706–715, Oct '45
Therapy of osteomyelitis of hand and fingers at evacuation hospitals. KONONENKO, I. F. Vrach. delo (nos. 7–8) *25:*341–346, '45
Metacarpal defects due to gunshot wounds; tenon and mortise grafts. MORRIS, H. D. Surgery *20:*364–372, Sept '46
Hand, bone surgery in war injuries. SNEDECOR, S. T. Am. J. Surg. *72:*363–372, Sept '46

War Injuries, Hand – Cont.
Hand; treatment of war injuries in U. S. Army. BRUNER, J. M., J. Iowa M. Soc. *36:*509–511, Dec '46

War Injuries, Jaws

Use of modified Baker anchorage in naval dental service for fractured jaw. DARNALL, W. L., U. S. Nav. M. Bull. *19:*42–45, July '23 (illus.)
Maxillo-facial centers. LEMAITRE, F. Mil. Surgeon *57:*242–255, Sept '25
Treatment of war wounds of face and jaws. BERCHER, J. Mil. Surgeon *58:*130–132, Feb '26
Organization of department for maxillary-facial surgery among war wounded. WATRY. Arch. med. belges *80:*457–461, Sept '27
Social sequels of maxillo-facial wounds received in war. REGNART, R. L. F. Rev. odont. *51:*372–378, Sept–Oct '30
Gunshot fracture of mandible; case. WEISENGREEN, H. H. Am. J. Surg. *39:*133–134, Jan '38
Fracture of lower jaw due to gunshot wounds in face during Waziristan operations, 1937; 3 cases. GOLDING, H. S., J. Roy. Army M. Corps *71:*50–54, July '38
Treatment of maxillomandibular fractures at aid station and at base hospital. GILKISON, C. C. Mil. Surgeon *84:*441–451, May '39
Jaw fractures in war; treatment. THOUREN, G. Nord. med. (Hygiea) *3:*2642–2656, Aug 26, '39
Care of jaw wounds in wartime. ZEMAN, J. Ztschr. f. Stomatol. *37:*1169–1173, Aug 25, '39
Therapy of wounds of face and jaws at battalion or regiment first aid stations, in army corps field hospital and in evacuation hospital. ROCHETTE, M. Hopital *27:*521–527, Nov '39
Surgical therapy of war wounds of jaws and face. AXHAUSEN, G. Chirurg *11:*801–807, Dec 1, '39
War wounds of face and jaws. PEYRUS, J. J. Rev. serv. de san. mil. *111:*1017–1030, Dec '39
Emergency treatment and primary apparatus for war fractures of jaw (reports of various countries). DEDONCKER *et al.* Internat. Cong. Mil. Med. and Pharm. *2:*206–218, '39
Emergency treatment and primary apparatus for war fractures (of jaws). WEDDELL, J. M. Internat. Cong. Mil. Med. and Pharm. *1:*237–249, '39
Gunshot wounds of face and jaws. MACLURE, F., M. J. Australia *1:*62–64, Jan 13, '40

War Injuries, Jaws—Cont.
Therapy of bullet wounds of jaw at Vienna Surgical Clinic. PICHLER, H. Wien. klin. Wchnschr. *53:*22–24, Jan 5, '40
Emergency treatment and primary apparatus for jaw fractures in warfare. FAIRBANK, L. C. AND IVY, R. H. Mil. Surgeon *86:*124–134, Feb '40
Therapy of maxillofacial war lesions in teritorial hospitals. CALABRO, N. Stomatol. ital. *2:*297–302, April '40
Surgical therapy of war wounds of jaws; 2 cases. GRANDI, E. Stomatol. ital. *2:*391–397, May '40
Maxillofacial surgery during campaign in Poland. SARRU, P.; *et al.* Rev. san. mil., Bucuresti *39:*277–281, May '40
Experiences in therapy of maxillary injuries during Russian-Finnish war. DAHL, G. M. Acta odont. Scandinav. *2:*1–18, June '40
Gunshot wounds of jaws. FRY, W. K. M. Press *203:*524–527, June 26, '40
Therapy of war injuries to jaws. LINK, K. H. Zentralbl. f. Chir. *67:*994–998, June 1, '40
War injuries of jaws and face. COLE, P. P. Post-Grad. M. J. *16:*233–244, July '40
Experiences in therapy of maxillary injuries during Russian-Finnish war. DAHL, G. M. Acta odont. Scandinav. *2:*1–18, June '40
Suggestions for war surgery of facial injuries; use of wire cradle and fixation of tongue, facial flaps and bone fragments by means of safety pin in patients with jaw fractures. HENSCHEN, C. Schweiz. med. Wchnschr. *70:*711–715, July 30, '40
Care and therapeutic provisions for maxillofacial wounds on battlefield; limits and possibilities of aid in dressing stations of troops, battalions and regiments and in advanced posts of sanitary service. PALAZZI, S. Gior. di med. mil. *88:*500–508, July '40
Wire grating chin cap in military surgery of jaw fractures. ROOS, W. Schweiz. med. Wchnschr. *70:*770, Aug 10, '40
Gunshot wounds of face and jaws; first aid treatment, field service. STOUT, R. A. Mil. Surgeon *87:*247–250, Sept '40
War injuries to jaws. GANZER, H. Deut. Militararzt *5:*419–426, Oct '40
Gunshot wounds to jaws; therapy and prognosis. HAUENSTEIN, K. Med. Welt *14:*1189–1193, Nov 23, '40
Surgical therapy of war wounds of jaws and face. AXHAUSEN, G. Chirurg *11:*801–807, Dec 1, '39
Cases of gunshot wounds of jaws treated 1914–1918. DOUBLEDAY, F. N. Guy's Hosp. Gaz. *54:*358–360, Dec 14, '40

War Injuries, Jaws—Cont.
Cooperation between maxillofacial surgeon and other surgeons in treatment of soldiers with multiple wounds. BERCHER. Rev. de stomatol. *41:*759–760, '40
Facial and maxillary injuries in war. CUPAR, I. Voj.-san. glasnik *11:*457–471, '40
First aid for maxillary injuries. ENTIN, D. A. Vrach. delo (nos. 11–12) *22:*727–730, '40
Therapy of maxillary gunshot wounds, with special reference to war wounds. HAMMER, H. Therap. d. Gegenw. *82:*100–106, March '41
Surgical and dental treatment of fractures of upper and lower jaws in wartime; review of 119 cases. McINDOE, A. H. Proc. Roy. Soc. Med. *34:*267–288, March '41
Therapy of gunshot wounds to jaws. HAMMER, H. Therap. d. Gegenw. *82:*174–177, April '41
Immediate care of war wounds of face and jaw. SCHMUZIGER, P. Helvet. med. acta *8:*49–53, April '41
Wire screen chin cap; suggestion for first aid for jaw injuries in field. ROOS, W. Schweiz. med. Wchnschr. *71:*719–720, June 7, '41
First aid and emergency treatment of gunshot wounds to jaws. IVY, R. H. Rev. san. mil., Habana *5:*105–109, July-Dec '41
Emergency therapy of gunshot wounds of lower jaw. RODRIGUEZ SEGADE. Med. espan. *6:*59–69, July '41
Responsibility of orthodontist in treatment of traumatic injuries of face and jaws. FAIRBANK, L. C. Am. J. Orthodontics *27:*414–422, Aug '41
First aid and emergency treatment of gunshot wounds of jaws. IVY, R. H. Mil. Surgeon *89:*197–201, Aug '41
Initial treatment of jaw injuries (with special reference to air raid casualties). FICKLING, B. W., M. Press *206:*203–208, Sept 10, '41
Symposium on military surgery; plastic and maxillofacial surgery. IVY, R. H., S. Clin. North America *21:*1583–1592, Dec '41
Fractures of maxillae and mandible; 2 cases (with description of apparatus). YANDO, A. H. AND TAYLOR, R. W., U. S. Nav. M. Bull. *40:*155–157, Jan '42
Care of face and jaw casualties in United States Army. FAIRBANK, L. C. War Med. *2:*223–229, March '42
Maxillofacial injuries. FOX, C. Mil. Surgeon *90:*61–72, Jan '42; Also: Am. J. Orthodontics (Oral Surg. Sect) *28:*202–212, April '42
Surgical and dental treatment of jaw fractures in wartime; review based on 119 cases. McINDOE, A. M. Rev. san. mil., Habana *6:*178–180, April–June '42

War Injuries, Jaws – Cont.

Care of military and civilian injuries; implantation method of setting fractured mandibles. BERRY, H. C. Am. J. Orthodontics (Oral Surg. Sect) *28:*292–306, May '42

Care of military and civilian injuries; conservative treatment of simultaneous fractures through necks of both mandibular condyles associated with multiple fractures of other parts of mandible. GRUBER, L. W. AND LYFORD, J. III. Am. J. Orthodontics (Oral Surg. Sect) *28:*258–264, May '42

Early and late treatment of face and jaws as applied to war injuries. IVY, R. H. South. Surgeon *11:*366–373, May '42

Outline of treatment of extensive comminuted fractures of mandible (based chiefly on experience gained during last war). KAZANJIAN, V. H. Am. J. Orthodontics (Oral Surg. Sect) *28:*265–274, May '42

Chemotherapy (with sulfanilamide and its derivatives) in gunshot wounds of face, neck and jaws. OGLE, M. W. Mil. Surgeon *90:*650–655, June '42

Care of military and civilian injuries; mandibular fractures treated by pin fixation; 21 cases. RUSHTON, M. A. AND WALKER, F. A. Am. J. Orthodontics (Oral Surg. Sect) *28:*307–315, May '42

Care of military and civilian injuries; fractures of maxilla. THOMA, K. H. Am. J. Orthodontics (Oral Surg. Sect) *28:*275–291, May '42

Dentists and first surgical care of face and jaw injuries on battlefield. SQUIRRU, C. M. Rev. san. mil., Buenos Aires *41:*457–469, July '42

Treatment of gunshot fractures of jaw at advanced first aid posts. LEHNER, R. Deut. Militararzt *7:*98, Feb '42; also: Rev. san. mil., Buenos Aires *41:*542–549, Aug '42; also: Bull. War Med. *3:*146–147, Nov '42 (abstract)

Jaw injuries; work and therapeutic aims of front line specialized unit; results in the Army on Eastern Front IV. CHRIST, H. G. Munchen. med. Wchnschr. *89:*832, Sept 25, '42

Permanent therapy of maxillofacial wounds in war surgery. IVY, R. H. AND CURTIS, L. Rev. san. mil., Buenos Aires *41:*638–650, Sept '42

Immobilization of wartime, compound, comminuted fractures of mandible. KAZANJIAN, V. H. Am. J. Orthodontics (Oral Surg. Sect) *28:*551–560, Oct '42

Plastic surgery and jaw injuries center somewhere in England. MARTINDALE, L. M. Woman's J. *49:*299, Oct '42

War Injuries, Jaws – Cont.

Chemotherapy (with sulfonamides) in gunshot wounds of face, neck and jaws. OGLE, M. W. Rev. san. mil., Habana *6:*312–317, Oct–Dec '42

Simple device for temporary support of fractured mandible. ROMMEL, R. W., U. S. Nav. M. Bull. *40:*977, Oct '42

Therapy, especially of gunshot fractures of lower jaw. ULLIK, R. Wien. klin. Wchnschr. *55:*913–915, Nov 13, '42

Use of buttons with wire suture in gunshot wounds of face and jaw. PERWITZSCHKY, R. Ztschr. f. Hals-, Nasen-u. Ohrenh. *48:*270; 458, '42

Organizational problem of nutrition in maxillofacial trauma. PYATNITSKIY, F. A. Klin. med. (nos. 3–4) *20:*22–28, '42

War injuries to face and jaw. SHAW, J. J. M. War and Doctor, pp. 41–46, '42

Emergency therapy of gunshot wounds of face with fracture of lower jaw. BROGGI, M. AND DOMENECH-ALSINA, F. Med. espan. *9:*70–74, Jan '43

Care of military and civilian injuries; external traction appliance for jaw fractures. BISNOFF, H. L. Am. J. Orthodontics (Oral Surg. Sect) *29:*96–101, Feb '43

Emergency therapy of gunshot wounds of face with fracture of lower jaw. BROGGI, M. AND DOMENECH-ALSINA, F. Med. espan. *9:*70–74, Jan '43

Care of military and civilian injuries; internal wire fixation of jaw fractures; preliminary report. BROWN, J. B. AND McDOWELL, F. Am. J. Orthodontics (Oral Surg. Sect.) *29:*86–91, Feb '43

Care of military and civilian injuries; problem of teeth in line of fracture of mandible. JACOBS, M. H. Am. J. Orthodontics (Oral Surg. Sect.) *29:*102–110, Feb '43

Care of military and civilian injuries; fractures of mandible, maxilla, zygoma and other facial bones; statistical study of 1,149 cases. LYONS, D. C. Am. J. Orthodontics (Oral Surg. Sect.) *29:*67–76, Feb '43

Maxillofacial reconstruction. SODERBERG, N. B. Mil. Surgeon *92:*268–276, March '43

Gunshot wounds of maxillofacial region with spinal complications. ARONOVICH, G. D. Am. Rev. Soviet Med. *1:*344–350, April '44; also: Khirurgiya, no. 1, pp. 14–22, '43

Moulages as aid to maxillofacial restorations. JACOBSEN, H. H. AND BARRON, J. B. Mil. Surgeon *92:*511–520, May '43

Notes from maxillofacial centers; intraoral methods of immobilizing mandibular fractures. DALLING, E. J. Bull. War Med. *3:*555, June '43 (abstract)

War Injuries, Jaws—Cont.
Rehabilitation in maxillofacial and plastic center. McIndoe, A. H. Post-Grad. M. J. *19:*161–167, July '43
Simple skeletal fixation method for quick repair in war surgery. (Jaws) Berry, H. C. J. Am. Dent. A. *30:*1377–1378, Sept 1, '43
Physical medicine in maxillofacial injuries. Weisengreen, H. H. Mil. Surgeon *93:*294–298, Sept '43
Maxillofacial injuries produced by gunshot wounds in modern warfare. Meyer, G. E. J. Am. Dent. A. *30:*1576–1583, Oct 1, '43
Therapy of wounds of maxillofacial region; later experiences with war wounded who were first treated at field hospitals. Pieritz, G. Deut. Militararzt *8:*693, Dec '43
Points on treatment of maxillofacial injuries. Stanhope, E. D. East African M. J. *20:*399–408, Dec '43
Maxillofacial wounds; prophylaxis and therapy of pulmonary complications. Badyikes, S. O. Sovet. med. (no. 10) *7:*15–16, '43
Present status of therapy of maxillofacial war wounds. Rauer, A. E. Sovet. med. (nos. 7–8) *7:*22–24, '43
Practical suggestions on therapy of maxillary wounds at front. Leix, R. Deut. Militararzt *9:*48, Jan '44
Symposium on plastic surgery; early treatment of gunshot wounds of face and jaws; case histories of patients treated during World War I. Kazanjian, V. H. Surgery *15:*22–42, Jan '44
Acrylic half-splint for jaw injuries. Mackta, L. Bull. U. S. Army M. Dept. (no. 72) pp. 81–83, Jan '44
Maxillofacial injuries. Streicher, C. J. and Rosedale, R. S. Ohio State M. J. *40:*38–40, Jan '44
Maxillofacial surgery. Sturgis, S. H. and Holland, D. J., M. Bull. North African Theat. Op. (no. 1) *1:*13–14, Jan '44
Prosthetic appliance for war injury (maxillofacial injuries). Jeffreys, F. E., U. S. Nav. M. Bull. *42:*711–714, March '44
Treatment of maxillofacial wounds and injuries. Sturgis, S. H. and Holland, D. J. M. Bull. North African Theat. Op. (no. 3) *1:*8–11, March '44
Compound fracture of mandible due to gunshot wound. Cal, C. and Cambiaggi, J. E. Rev. san. mil., Buenos Aires *43:*873–875, June '44
Comminuted fractures of mandible; 25 consecutive cases from plastic and jaw unit, Emergency Medical Service. Cuthbert, J. B. Lancet *1:*748–750, June 10, '44

War Injuries, Jaws—Cont.
Maxillofacial injuries; extracts from case histories. Graham, M. P. Brit. Dent. J. *76:*339–341, June 16, '44
Maxillofacial surgery. Schulenburg, C. A. R. South African M. J. *18:*225–226, July 8, '44
Notes from maxillofacial centers, Warwick, October, 1942. Brown, O. F. Brit. Dent. J. *77:*195–197, Oct 6, '44
Recommendations for treatment of maxillofacial cases in forward areas. Clarkson, P. and Wilson, T. H. H. Brit. Dent. J. *77:*229–234, Oct 20, '44
Comminuted fractures of mandible; 25 consecutive cases from plastic and jaw unit, Emergency Medical Service. Cuthbert, J. B. Dia med. *16:*1395–1397, Nov 13, '44
Management of mandibular bone loss. Kulick, L. R., M. Bull. North African Theat. Op. *2:*128–132, Nov '44
Maxillofacial traumatology in military medicine. Morayta, M. An. med. d. Ateneo Ramon y Cajal (no. 4) *2:*45–46, Dec '44
Therapy of maxillofacial gunshot wounds. Faltin, R. Acta chir. Scandinav. *91:*434–447, '44
Modified maxillary fracture splint for jaw. Blausten, S. Bull. U. S. Army M. Dept. (no. 84) pp. 119–121, Jan '45
Penicillin in oral and maxillofacial surgery. Christiansen, G. W. Mil. Surgeon *96:*51–54, Jan '45
Maxillofacial surgical unit mobile dental laboratory. Dalling, E. J. Brit. Dent. J. *78:*10–12, Jan 5, '45
Severe faciomaxillary injury treated at sea. Kennedy, R. L. and Lewis, F. C. R. J. Roy. Nav. M. Serv. *31:*36–39, Jan '45
Maxillofacial injuries. Christiansen, G. W. M. Ann. District of Columbia *14:*76–77, Feb '45
First aid and preliminary treatment of maxillofacial injuries. Fuller, W. H. A. Brit. Dent. J. *78:*106–108, Feb 16, '45
Treatment of maxillofacial casualties in B. L. A. Holland, N. Brit. Dent. J. *78:*78–80, Feb 2, '45
Jaws, early and late treatment of gunshot wounds in French battle casualties in North Africa and Italy. Converse, J. M. J. Oral. Surg. *3:*112–137, April '45
Course of instruction in treatment of maxillofacial injuries, Ballochmyle E. M. S. Hospital. Inglis, J. V. Brit. Dent. J. *78:*242–243, April 20, '45
Management of mandibular bone loss. Kulick, L. R., J. Am. Dent. A. *32:*866–871, July 1, '45

War Injuries, Jaws—Cont.

Fractures of upper jaw; 150 cases in overseas maxillofacial center. CLARK, H. B. JR. J. Oral Surg. *3:*286–303, Oct '45

Treatment of gunshot fractures of mandible. COOK, T. J. *et al.* J. Oral Surg. *3:*326–335, Oct '45

Maxillofacial bandage. KINCAID, C. J. Bull. U. S. Army M. Dept. *4:*475–477, Oct '45

Anesthesia in maxillofacial surgical unit with British Liberation Army. THORNTON, H. L. AND ROWBOTHAM, S. Anesthesiology *6:*580–596, Nov '45

Report from maxillofacial center at Royal Air Force casualty clearing station in England. BADENOCH, A. W. AND HOLMS, S. Brit. Dent. J. *79:*346–348, Dec 21, '45

Maxillofacial injuries. BLOCKER, T. G. JR. AND WEISS, L. R., J. Indiana M. A. *39:*60–63, Feb '46

Treatment of 1,000 fractures (in British army) of jaw. CLARKSON, P. *et al.* Ann. Surg. *123:*190–208, Feb '46; also: Brit. Dent. J. *80:*69, Feb 1, '46; 107, Feb 15, '46

Therapy of acute maxillofacial wounds. HENDERSON, J. A. Dia med. *18:*183–184, March 4, '46

Ankylosis and trismus resulting from war wounds involving coronoid region of mandible; 3 cases. BROWN, J. B. AND PETERSON, L. W., J. Oral Surg. *4:*258–266, July '46

Temporary prosthesis as aid in treatment of war injuries of face. EMORY, L. Mil. Surgeon *99:*105–109, Aug '46

Oral prosthesis in repair of war injuries. POUND, E. Am. J. Orthodontics (Oral Surg. Sect) *32:*435–439, Aug '46

Management of plastic maxillofacial wounds in evacuation hospital. LEECH, C. H.; *et al.* Surg. Gynec. and Obst. *83:*462–473, Oct '46

Case reports from maxillofacial team, 6th General Hospital. STURGIS, S. H. AND HOLLAND, D. J. JR. Am. J. Orthodontics (Oral Surg. Sect) *32:*635–664, Oct '46

Observations of 200 jaw fracture cases admitted to 6th General Hospital. STURGIS, S. H. AND HOLLAND, D. J. JR. Am. J. Orthodontics (Oral Surg. Sect.) *32:*605–634, Oct '46

Covering extensive defects of chin and floor of mouth following gunshot wounds. LINDENBAUM, L. M. Vrach. delo (nos. 7–8) *26:*469–474, '46

Maxillofacial war wounds; principles of therapy and results. THEODORESCO, D., J. de chir. *62:*171–183, '46

War Injuries, Neck

Chemotherapy (with sulfanilamide and its derivatives) in gunshot wounds of face, neck and jaws. OGLE, M. W. Mil. Surgeon *90:*650–655, June '42

Chemotherapy (with sulfonamides) in gunshot wounds of face, neck and jaws. OGLE, M. W. Rev. san. mil., Habana *6:*312–317, Oct–Dec '42

Wounds of neck and lesions of larynx, trachea and esophagus in war surgery. DE ANDRADE MEDICIS, J. Arq. brasil. de cir. e ortop. *10:*155–179, '42

Gunshot wounds of neck. GREIFENSTEIN. Bull. War Med. *3:*441, April '43 (abstract)

Plastic surgery in wartime; how to manage head and neck wounds. REBELO NETO, J. Rev. paulista de med. *23:*345–346, Dec '43

Treatment of penetrating war wounds of neck. DROBYSHEV, G. I. Khirurgiya, no. 2, pp. 49–54, '44

Neck wounds; clinical and roentgenologic analysis. IGAMBERDIEV, Z. Khirurgiya, no. 8, pp. 65–68, '44

War Injuries, Nerve

Gunshot injuries of nerves during war; general considerations, regeneration and transplants. DEBEYRE, A. Echo. med. du Nord *7:*769–783, June 13, '37

Nerves; management of war injuries. THOMAS, A. *et al.* Rev. neurol. *72:*639–677, '39–'40

Nerves; management of war injuries. SOREL, E. AND SORREL-DEJERINE, MME. Rev. neurol. *72:*649–660, '39–'40

Nerves; management of war injuries. THOMAS, A. *et al.* Rev. neurol. *72:*639–677, '39–'40

War injuries of nerves of arm. GERLACH, J. Med. Klin. *38:*173, Feb 20, '42

Surgical therapy of gunshot wounds of peripheral nerves; outlook for its success. TONNIS, W. AND GOTZE, W. Deut. Militararzt *7:*245–253, April '42

Peripheral nerve injuries in war; diagnosis and therapy. ZULCH, K. J. Med. Klin. *38:*985, Oct 16, '42; 1016, Oct 23, '42

Operative treatment of gunshot wounds of peripheral nerves. TÖNNIS, W. AND GÖTZE, W. Bull. War Med. *3:*196–197, Dec '42 (abstract)

Peripheral nerve injuries in war; transplantation of nerves. GRASHCHENKOV, N. I. P. Sovet. med. (no. 9) *6:*8–10, '42

War wounds of peripheral nerves. CRAIG, W. M., U. S. Nav. M. Bull. *41:*613–624, May '43

Operative eperiences on wounds of peripheral nerves from Pacific combat area; preliminary report based on 50 cases. NOR-

War Injuries, Nerve – Cont.

CROSS, N. C. Bull. Am. Coll. Surgeons *28:*127-128, June '43

War injuries to radial nerve; treatment. SOUTTAR, H. S., M. Press *210:*345-347, Dec 1, '43

Symposium on war surgery; use of tantalum wire and foil in repair of peripheral nerves. SPURLING, R. G., S. Clin. North America *23:*1491-1504, Dec '43

Nerve gunshot wounds; surgical therapy. OSTERMANN, F. A. Deut. Militararzt *9:*42, Jan '44

Nerve regeneration in end to end sutures, grafts and gunshot nerve injuries. DAVIS, L. AND HILLER, F. Tr. Am. Neurol. A. *70:*178-179, '44

Peripheral nerves; missile injuries. CAMPBELL, E. H. JR. M. Bull. Mediterranean Theat. Op. *3:*246-251, June '45

Plastic technic in surgery of peripheral nerves. WEBSTER, G. V. *et al.* U. S. Nav. M. Bull. *45:*22-31, July '45

Direct flap repair of defects of arm and hand; preparation of gunshot wounds for repair of nerves, bones and tendons. BROWN, J. B. *et al.* Ann. Surg. *122:*706-715, Oct '45

Peripheral nerve injuries in European Theater of Operations; management, with special reference to early nerve surgery. SPURLING, R. G., J.A.M.A. *129:*1011-1014, Dec 8 '45; abst., Bull. U. S. Army M. Dept. *4:*557-559, Nov '45

Peripheral nerves; reconstructive surgery following gunshot wounds. CHIBUKMAKHER, N. B. Khirurgiya, no. 5, pp. 45-50, '45

Surgical therapy of injuries of nerve trunks at front. MARGOLIN, G. S. Khirurgiya, no. 5, pp. 68-73, '45

Symposium: medicine and surgery in 21st General Hospital; brain and nerve injuries. SCHWARTZ, H. G. AND ROULHAC, G. E. Washington Univ. M. Alumni Quart. *9:*69-73, Jan '46

Nerve regeneration; clinical test. SHREVES, H. B. AND HAWKINS, G. Bull. U. S. Army M. Dept. *5:*110-111, Jan '46

Peripheral nerve lesions; experience in South Pacific area. FULCHER, O. H., U. S. Nav. M. Bull. *46:*325-334, March '46

Peripheral nerve injuries overseas; plan for care. THOMSON, J. L. *et al.* Arch. Surg. *52:*557-570, May '46

Peripheral nerves; treatment of war wounds. MERLE D'AUBIGNE, R. AND ZIMMER, M. Semaine d. hop. Paris *22:*1652-1657, Sept 21, '46

Peripheral nerves; surgical therapy of gunshot wounds. ISHCHENKO, I. N. Vrach delo. (nos. 7-8) *26:*429-436, '46

War Injuries, Nose

Reconstruction of nose, lid region and cheek following shell wound. VIGNOLO, Q. Arch. ital. di chir. *3:*649, July '21; abstr: J.A.M.A. *77:*1290, Oct 15, '21

War injuries of nose and nasal sinuses; 5 cases. NISHIYAMA, A. Oto-rhino-laryng. *12:*467-477, June '39

War injuries of ear, nose and throat. VOSS, O. Med. Klin. *35:*1589-1591, Dec 15, '39

Migraine due to war injury to nose, with recovery following resection of cicatrix. LEBOURG, L. Rev. de stomatol. *43:*27-28, Jan-Feb '42

Nasal plastic operations; proper uses in military practice. WEBSTER, G. V. Arch. Otolaryng. *41:*170-174, March '45

Wounds of eye, ear, nose and throat. SMART, F. P., U. S. Nav. M. Bull. *44:*1231-1233, June '45

Nose and sinuses; primary war injuries. CANFIELD, N. Proc. Roy. Soc. Med. *38:*627-628, Sept '45

Primary war injuries involving nose and sinuses. CANFIELD, N., J. Laryng. and Otol. *60:*458-460, Nov '45

Rhinoplastic operations following gunshot wounds. NATANZON, A. M. Vrach. delo (nos. 1-2) *25:*61-66, '45

War Injuries, Shock

Prevention and treatment of wound shock in theatre of army operations. MACRAE, D. JR. J. Iowa M. Soc. *11:*394, Oct '21

Traumatic shock due to war wound. BARUCH, D., J. de chir. *23:*354-372, April '24

Circulatory changes in wounded soldiers (shock), with special reference to influence of drugs used for production of anesthesia. MARSHALL, G. Guy's Hosp. Rep. *75:*98-111, Jan '25

Shock and blood transfusion at front. SCHUBERTH, O. Nord. med. (Hygiea) *3:*2442-2444, Aug 5, '39

Therapy of hemorrhages and states of traumatic shock in armies in wartime. NORMET, L. Bruxelles-med. *19:*1474-1482, Oct 8, '39

Shock and surgical collapse in war wounded. REHN. Deutsche med. Wchnschr. *65:*1594-1598, Oct 27 '39

Transfusion of plasma instead of whole blood in massive hemorrhages; use in war. BRO-

War Injuries, Shock – Cont.
DIN, P. AND SAINT-GIRONS, F. Bull. et mem. Soc. d. hop. de Paris *55:*1224-1226, Nov 10, '39
Task of internist in treatment of war injuries; postraumatic (secondary) shock. BORST, J. G. G. AND VEENING, H. P. Nederl. tijdschr. v. geneesk. *84:*914-922, March 9, '40
Traumatic shock of war wounded. CREYSSEL, J. AND SUIRE, P., J. de med. de Lyon *21:*83-96, March 6, '40
States of shock; form for clinical and therapeutic records of military cases. JEANNENEY, C. AND JUSTIN-BESANCON, L. Presse med. *48:*423-424, April 17-20, '40
Traumatic shock of war wounded; bilateral procaine hydrochloride infiltration of carotid sinus; case. CREYSSEL, J. AND SUIRE, P. Mem. Acad. de chir. *66:*762-765, Nov 6-20,'40
Prevention and treatment of shock in combat zone. KENDRICK, D. R. JR. Mil. Surgeon *88:*97-113, Feb '41
Discussion of prevention and treatment of shock in combat zone. MATTISON, J. A. Mil. Surgeon *88:*114-118, Feb '41
Shock in air raid casualties. GRANT, R. T. Guy's Hosp. Gaz. *55:*90-95, April 19, '41
Nature and treatment of shock. BOWERS, W. F. Mil. Surgeon *89:*41-48, July '41
Treatment of shock in wartime (Theodore A. McGraw memorial lecture). HARKINS, H. N. War Med. *1:*520-535, July '41
Shock; prevention and treatment in combat zone. KENDRICK, D. B. JR. Army M. Bull. (no. 58) pp. 38-60, Oct '41
Preparation of concentrated or dry serum and plasma and its application in treatment of shock (especially in war surgery). TRAMSEN, H. Ugesk. f. laeger *103:*1357-1362, Oct 23, '41
Symposium on military medicine, burn and shock therapy. STRUMIA, M. M. *et al.* M. Clin. North American *25:*1813-1827, Nov '41
Prevention and treatment of shock; symposium on military surgery. BLALOCK, A., S. Clin. North America *21:*1663-1683, Dec '41
Intravenous fluid therapy in shock; symposium on military surgery. FREEMAN, N. E. S. Clin. North America *21:*1769-1781, Dec '41
Use of plasma in hospital ship for burns. WOLFE, H. R. I. AND CLEGG, H. W. Lancet *1:*191-193, Feb 14, '42
Shock from war injuries. HARKINS, H. N. J. Michigan M. Soc. *41:*287-293, April '42
Shock treatment in air raid casualties. EDWARDS, F. R., M. Press *208:*3-5, July 1, '42
Prevention and treatment of shock in military medicine. BLALOCK, A. Dia med. *14:*1063-1066, Oct 12, '42
Shock treatment in war medicine. CANOSA, F. Rev. med.-social san. y benef. munic. *2:*282-290, Oct-Dec '42
Shock in war medicine. RODRIGUEZ BAZ, L. Rev. med.-social san. y benef. munic. *2:*272-281, Oct-Dec '42
War medicine series; practical management of wound shock. MCMICHAEL, J. Brit. M. J. *2:*671-673, Dec 5, '42
Shock in war surgery. PINHEIRO GUIMARAES, U. Rev. med.-cir. do Brasil *50:*1043-1078, Dec '42
Nature and therapy of shock. WHEELER, D. W., U. S. Nav. M. Bull. *41:*93-106, Jan '43
Forum on therapy of wartime injuries; shock. BARNARD, M. A. New York State J. Med. *43:*228-230, Feb 1, '43
Use of human albumin in military medicine; theoretic and experimental basis for use (shock). HEYL, J. T. AND JANEWAY, C. A. Army M. Bull. (no. 68) pp. 227-233, July '43
Use of human albumin in military medicine; clinical evaluation. WOODRUFF, L. M. AND GIBSON, S. T. Army M. Bull. (no. 68) pp. 234-240, July '43
Shock in war traumatology. PINHEIRO GUIMARAES, U. Imprensa med., Rio de Janeiro *19:*73-92, Aug '43
Shock; treatment during Tunisian campaign of 1942-1943. CURTILLET, E. Afrique franc. chir. *1:*297-303, Sept-Oct '43
Problem of shock and collapse as observed at the front. VON LUCADOU, W. Deutsche med. Wchnschr. *69:*652, Sept 17, '43
Shock in military medicine. FREITAS, G. DA C. Rev. med. brasil. *16:*337-351, March '44
Shock; treatment in the field. FORMBY, R. H. M. J. Australia *1:*357-368, April 22, '44
Shock and hemorrhage; management in evacuation hospital. RIFE, C. S., M. Bull. North African Theat. Op. (no. 6) *1:*3-4, June '44
Shock and hemorrhage. SULLIVAN, J. M. M. Bull. North African Theat. Op. (no. 6) *1:*2-3, June '44
Effect of dialyzed serum proteins and serum dialysates in shock treatment. VOLKER, M. AND ASTRUP, T. Bull. War Med. *4:*640, July '44 (abstract)
Shock and its therapy. SELTSOVSKIY, P. L. Khirurgiya, no. 10, pp. 25-27, '44
Shock in war surgery. SANTAS, A. A. Bol. d. Inst. clin. quir. *21:*55-61, Feb '45

War Injuries, Shock—Cont.

Possible role of whole blood transfusions in military medicine (shock). DE GOWIN, E. L., J.A.M.A. *127:*1037–1039, April 21, '45

Shock, therapy, lessons from military surgery. DUNPHY, J. E. Post-Grad. M. J. *21:*111–116, April '45

Shock; medical treatment and surgical intervention in war wounded. ROYER AND BARBIZET. Med. Acad. de chir. *71:*334–335, July 4–11, '45

Shock in severely wounded in forward field hospitals, with special reference to wound shock. STEWART, J. D. AND WARNER, F. Ann. Surg. *122:*129–146, Aug '45

Shock; treatment in 32nd Field Hospital, Nov 22, 1944 to March 22, 1945, Brazilian Expeditionary Forces, North American Fifth Army. CORREIA NETO, A. AND MONTEIRO, J. Rev. med.-cir. do Brasil (nos. 9–10) *53:*349–357, Sept–Oct, '45

Shock; problem in war and laboratory. DOSNE DE PASQUALINI, C. Rev. san. mil., Buenos Aires *44:*1405–1417, Oct '45

Shock in battle casualties; measurements of blood volume changes occurring in response to therapy. EMERSON, C. P. JR. AND EBERT, R. V. Ann. Surg. *122:*745–772, Nov '45

Shock following war wounds; changes of blood in. BOROVSKAYA, V. M. Byull. eksper. biol. i. med. (nos. 1–2) *19:*33–36, '45

Resuscitation and transfusion service during offensives in Italy from May 11 to July 27, 1944. RICARD AND FANJEAUX. Bull. internat. serv. san. *19:*7–22, Jan '46

Shock in forward areas. SULLIVAN, J. M. Wisconsin M. J. *45:*213–216, Feb '46

Traumatic shock in war wounded; blood transfusion therapy. MORIN, E. Union med. du Canada *75:*400–404, April '46

War Injuries, Skin Grafting for

Skin grafting in therapy of paraffinomas due to self-mutilation during World War. CAFORIO, L. Riforma med. *52:*1414–1417, Oct 17, '36

Orthopedic aspects of plastic surgery; early replacement of skin losses in war injuries to extremities. CONVERSE, J. M. Proc. Roy. Soc. Med. *34:*791–799, Oct '41

Base hospital management of soft tissue injuries (including skin grafts). RANK, B. K. Australian and New Zealand J. Surg. *11:*171–184, Jan '42

Early skin grafting in war wounds of extremities. CONVERSE, J. M. Ann. Surg. *115:*321–335, March '42

War Injuries, Skin Grafting for—Cont.

Therapy of fresh wounds by transplantation of chemically treated tissues (skin and fetal membranes). PIKIN, K. I. Sovet. med. (no. 9) *6:*15–16, '42

Skin grafts in military surgery. PETERSEN, O. H. Zentralbl. f. Chir. *70:*1624, Nov 6, '43

Early treatment of war wounds, with emphasis on prevention of deformities (grafting). MALINIAC, J. W. Hebrew M. J. *1:*183, '43

Factors influencing choice of skin grafts. GREELEY, P. W., U.S. Nav. M. Bull. *42:*659–663, March '44

Early skin grafting of war wounds. LAMONT, H. A., U.S. Nav. M. Bull. *42:*654–658, March '44

Skin plastic procedures in war injuries. BLOCKHIN, N. N. Am. Rev. Soviet Med. *2:*104–107, Dec '44

Skin grafting and secondary closure in war wounds; preliminary report. WHELAN, C. S. AND THOMPSON, W. D. JR. Surg., Gynec. and Obst. *79:*584–588, Dec '44

Problems of surface restoration in Royal Canadian Air Force. FARMER, A. Am. Acad. Orthop. Surgeons, Lect. pp. 226–229, '44

Skin grafts in reconstructive surgery at base hospitals. GEKTIN, F. L. Khirurgiya, no. 2, pp. 26–35, '44

Problems of surface restoration (in Navy). GREELEY, P. W. Am. Acad. Orthop. Surgeons, Lect. pp. 250–253, '44

Skin grafts in war wounded. PARIN, B. V. Sovet. med. (nos. 7–8) *8:*4–8, '44

Dermoepidermal grafts in early treatment of severe war burns. HUBER, J. P. Semaine d. hop. Paris *21:*741–747, July 21, '45; also: Bull. internat. serv. san. *18:*197–209, Aug '45

Dermoplasty of war wounds of lower leg. PICK, J. F. Am. J. Surg. *69:*25–38, July '45

Secondary sutures and skin transplantations at front line hospitals. TABORISSKIY, M. G. Khirurgiya, no. 2, pp. 23–30, '45

Reconstructive surgery in patients with war fractures of ankle and foot. SNEDECOR, S. T., J. Bone and Joint Surg. *28:*332–342, Apr '46

Split skin grafts in early closure of wounds. HARBISON, S. P. AND ODEN, L. H., JR. Bull. U. S. Army M. Dept. *6:*88–90, July '46

Skin grafting in treatment of osteomyelitic war wounds. KELLY, R. P., J. Bone and Joint Surg. *28:*681–691, Oct '46

Repair of war wounds of bulbous and membranous urethra using split thickness grafts and penicillin. MACLEAN, J. T. AND GERRIE, J. W., J. Urol. *56:*485–497, Oct '46

WARBURTON, G. B.: Hare-lip and its treatment. Brit. M. J. *1:*732–734, April 19, '30
WARD, W. K.: Cleft palate and re-education of speech. Brit. J. Dent. Sc. *72:*1–4, Jan '28
WARD, W. K.: Re-educating cleft palate speech. Practitioner *123:*147–152, Aug '29
WARD, W. K.: Treatment of cleft-palate speech. South African M. J. *11:*433–435, June 26, '37
WARDILL, W. E. M.: Cleft palate. Brit. J. Surg. *16:*127–148, July '28
WARDILL, W. E. M.: Results of surgical therapy in cleft palate. Arch. f. klin. Chir. *177:*504–509, '33
WARDILL, W. E. M.: Fascia lata grafts in facial paralysis. Newcastle M. J. *13:*35–38, Jan '33
WARDILL, W. E. M.: Hunterian lecture; cleft palate. Brit. J. Surg. *21:*347–369, Oct '33
WARDILL, W. E. M.: Cleft palate. Lancet *1:*1435–1437, June 22, '35
WARDILL, W. E. M.: Mechanism of speech in cleft palates. Monatschr. f. Ohrenh. *71:*424–429, April '37
WARDILL, W. E. M.: Technic of operation for cleft palate. Brit. J. Surg. *25:*117–130, July '37
WARGASSOWA, W. G.: Late results of surgical formation of artificial vagina. Zentralbl. f. Gynak. *60:*2623–2631, Oct 31, '36
WARING, J. B. H.: Removal of wens—simple technic. Virginia M. Monthly *59:*607–608, Jan '33
WARNECKE, K.: Surgical construction of artificial vagina by Wagner-Kirschner operation and Krause method of using skin flaps. Zentralbl. f. Gynak. *56:*416–418, Feb 13, '32
WARNER, E. D. (see TIDRICK, R. T.) Jan '44
WARNER, F. (see STEWART, J. D.) Aug '45
WARNEYER: Medicolegal responsibility for failures in plastic surgery; case. Chirurg *7:*294–298, May 1, '35
WARREN, E. D.: New operation for fractures into maxillary sinus and antrum. Dis. Eye, Ear, Nose and Throat *2:*304–305, Oct '42
WARREN, K. W. (see MCCLURE, R. D. *et al*) Sept '44
WARREN, J. V.; STEAD, E. A. JR.; MERRILL, A. J. AND BRANNON, E. S.: Concentrated human serum albumin in shock; preliminary report. J. Clin. Investigation 23:506–509, July '44
WARREN, K. W. (see ROTH, R. B.) Aug '44
WARREN, R. F. (see GORDON, S.) March '46
WARREN, S. (see SWINTON, N. W.) Oct '38

Warren Operation: See Dieffenbach-Warren Operation

WARSCHAWSKI, J.: Removal of cartilage in trachomatous entropion. Klin. Monatsbl. f. Augenh. *87:*378–382, Sept '31
WARTENBERG, R.: Progressive hemiatrophy (facial). Arch. Neurol. and Psychiat. *54:*75–96, Aug '45
WARTER, J. (see WEISS, A. G.) July '43
WARTHEN, H. J. AND JORDAN, W. R.: Complications in diabetic; nodular thyroid and branchial cleft fistulas. South. M. J. *36:*536–537, July '43
WARTHEN, H. J. AND WILLIAMS, P.: True hermaphrodite, case with necropsy. Ann. Surg. *103:*402–409, March '36
WARTHEN, H. J. JR.: Treatment of burns complicated by fractures of extremities. Tr. South. S. A. (1943) *55:*237–243, '44
WARTHEN, H. J. JR.: Recent advances in burn therapy. Virginia M. Monthly *60:*30–36, April '33
WARTHEN, H. J. JR.: Treatment of burns complicated by fractures of extremities. Ann. Surg. *119:*526–532, April '44

Warts

Treatment of warts and moles. SEMON, H. C. Lancet *1:*1359–1360, June 27, '25
Simultaneous appearance of acuminate condylomata and warts on face with keloid. MÜHLPFORDT, H. Dermat. Wchnschr. *84:*463–466, April 2, '27
Plantar warts, flaps and grafts. BLAIR, V. P. *et al.* J.A.M.A. *108:*24–27, Jan 2, '37
Moles, warts and keloids. MORSE, J. L. Am. J. Surg. *36:*137–144, April '37

WARWICK, M.: Model of carcinoma of lip reconstructed from serial section. J.A.M.A. *82:*1119–1120, April 5, '24
WASHBURN, B. A.: Palm abscess. Kentucky M. J. *27:*529–531, Nov '29
WASHBURN, S. L.: Effect of facial paralysis on growth of skull of rat and rabbit. Anat. Rec. *94:*163–168, Feb '46
WASHBURNE, A. C.: Congenital atresia of anterior nares; 2 cases in sisters. Arch. Otolaryng. *16:*789–790, Dec '32
WASSILIEW, B. N.: Artificial vagina formation from Meckel's diverticulum; case. Zentralbl. f. Gynak. *51:*806–808, March 26, '27
WASSILJEFF, A. A.: See VASILEV, A. A.
WASSINK, W. F.: Treatment of cancer of lip. Nederl. Tijdschr. v. Geneesk. *2:*1059–1069, Sept 4, '26; abstr: J.A.M.A. *87:*1524, Oct 30, '26
WASSMUND, M.: Plastic surgery of jaw deformities and mouth. Med. Welt *4:*327, March 8, '30
WASSMUND, M.: Surgical therapy of cleft lip and palate. Deutsche med. Wchnschr.

*58:*445–448, March 18, '32
WASSMUND, M.: Methods of transplanting bone into lower jaw. Deutsche Ztschr. f. Chir. *244:*704–735, '35
WASSMUND, M.: Disadvantages of Vorschütz method of treating complicated fractures and defects of lower jaw with plaster of paris bandage fastened to each side of jaw by screw arm. Zentralbl. f. Chir. *62:*914–921, April 20, '35
WASSMUND, M.: Disadvantages of Vorschütz method of treating complicated fractures and defects of lower jaw with plaster of paris bandage fastened to each side of jaw by screw arm. (Reply to Vorschütz) Zentralbl. f. Chir. *63:*444–445, Feb 22, '36 Further comment by Vorschütz; *63:*446, Feb 22, '36
WASSMUND, M.: Surgical therapy of unilateral cleft palate. Zentralbl. f. Chir. *66:*994–999, April 29, '39
WASSMUND, M. AND LABAND, F.: Fractures of toothless mandibles; treatment; 2 cases. Deutsche Monatschr. f. Zahnh. *45:*1009–1015, Dec 15, '27
WATANABE, D. (see TAKAHARA, T.) Jan '39
WATHEN, J. R.: Imperforate anus; case report. Kentucky M. J. *19:*827, Dec '21
WATKINS, A. B. K.: Splint for treatment of wide depressed nasal bridges. M. J. Australia *2:*556–557, Oct 23, '26
WATKINS, A. B. K.: Treatment of severer cases of nasal fractures (splint). Brit. M. J. *2:*917–918, Nov 18, '33
WATKINS, A. B. K.: Plastic surgery of nose. J. Laryng. and Otol. *48:*809–820, Dec '33
WATKINS, A. B. K.: Dovetail joint simplified for bone graft purposes. M. J. Australia *1:*430–431, March 31, '34
WATKINS, A. B. K.: Treatment of depressed fractures of zygoma. Brit. M. J. *1:*326–327, Feb 13, '37
WATKINS, A. L.: Symposium on management of Cocoanut Grove burns at Massachusetts General Hospital; note on physical therapy (hands). Ann. Surg. *117:*911–914, June '43
WATKINS, A. L. (see MARBLE, H. C. *et al*) Feb '42
WATKINS, D. E.: Gastroschisis, with case report. Virginia M. Monthly *70:*42–44, Jan '43
WATKINS, J. T. AND PITKIN, H. C.: Stenosing tendovaginitis of DeQuervain; case. California and West. Med. *32:*101–102, Feb '30
WATRIN, J. (see SPILLMANN, L. *et al*) June '34
WATRY: Organization of department for maxillary-facial surgery among war wounded. Arch. med. belges *80:*457–461, Sept '27
WATRY: Facial deformities caused by congenital syphilis. Bruxelles-med. *14:*471–484, Feb 4, '34
WATSON, O. A.: Fractures of nose. J. Oklahoma M. A. *39:*337–340, Aug '46
WATSON, R. G.: Treatment of jaw fractures. M. Press *206:*458–460, Dec 17, '41
WATSON, W. R.: General versus local anesthesia in operations on nose and throat. New York M. J. *113:*444, March 16 '21
WATSON-WILLIAMS, E.: Method of nasal plastic repair by cartilage graft. Brit. M. J. *2:*987–988, Nov 28, '25
WATSON-WILLIAMS, E.: Glossopharyngeal-facial nerve anastomosis. Proc. Roy. Soc. Med. (Sect. Otol.) *20:*59–63, July '27 also: J. Laryng. and Otol. *42:*516–519, Aug '27
WATSON-WILLIAMS, E.: Congenital abnormalities of external ear. Bristol Med.-Chir. J. *48:*273–274, '31
WATSON-WILLIAMS, E.: Nasal fractures. Brit. M. J. *2:*791–794, Oct 31, '31
WAUD, R. A. AND RAMSAY, A.: Diffusion of sulfonamides (sulfathiazole and sulfanilamide) out of certain bases in burn therapy. Canad. M. A. J. *48:*121–123, Feb '43
WAUD, R. A. (see SKINNER, H. G.) Jan '43
WAUGH, J. M. (see NEW, G. B.) May '34
WEARN, W. J.: Immediate dental treatment of cleft palate babies. Australia J. Dent. *34:*423–435, Dec '30
WEAVER, D.: Burn therapy. California and West. Med. *41:*222–226, Oct '34
WEAVER, D. D.: Burn wounds; their treatment. California and West. Med. *57:*9–12, July '42
WEAVER, D. F.: Plastic surgery of nose; cases. J. Michigan M. Soc. *41:*229–232, March '42
WEAVER, D. F.: Free grafts and pedicle flaps in treatment of recurring basal cell epitheliomas; cases. Laryngoscope *53:*336–342, May '43
WEAVER, D. F.: Preauricular congenital sinuses. Laryngoscope *56:*246–251, May '46
WEAVER, D. F.: Keloid formation in both ear lobes. Arch. Otolaryng. *44:*212–213, Aug '46
WEAVER, D. F. AND BELLINGER, D. H.: Bifid nose associated with midline cleft of upper lip. Arch. Otolaryng. *44:*480–482, Oct '46
WEAVER, J. B. AND RUMOLD, M. J.: Amputation of buttock for eradication of cavernous hemangioma. Am. J. Surg. *60:*149–150, April '43
WEBB, A. JR.: Physiologic treatment of burns. North Carolina M. J. *3:*220–223, May '42
WEBB, C. C. (see MOCK, A. E.) Dec '40
WEBER, A.: Regeneration and reconstitution of severed nerves. Lyon chir. *41:*129–137, Mar–Apr '46
WEBER, F. P.: Note on Dupuytren's contracture, camptodactylia and knuckle-pads. Brit. J. Dermat. *50:*26–31, Jan '38
WEBER, H.: Unguentolan (cod liver oil oint-

ment) in therapy of decubitus and postoperative fistula and wound infection; 15 cases. Wien. med. Wchnschr. *87:*219–221, Feb 20, '37

WEBER, M. L. (see WOLFE, M. O.) May '40

WEBER, M. L. (see WOLFE, M. O.) Jan '41

WEBER, R. A. (see STILES, K. A.) May '38

WEBSTER, D. (see DORRANCE, G. M. *et al*) April '24

WEBSTER, D. R. (see FARMER, A. W. *et al*) March '43

WEBSTER, G. V.: Dermatome for cutting small grafts. U. S. Nav. M. Bull. *41:*1145–1151, July '43

WEBSTER, G. V.: New needle holder for plastic surgery. U. S. Nav. M. Bull. *41:*1434–1439, Sept '43

WEBSTER, G. V.: Adherent scars of lower extremity. U. S. Nav. M. Bull. *43:*878–888, Nov '44

WEBSTER, G. V.: Choice of pedicle flaps for plastic and reconstructive surgery. S. Clin. North America *24:*1472–1482, Dec '44

WEBSTER, G. V.: Treatment of tendons in finger amputations and description of new instrument. Surgery *17:*102–108, Jan '45

WEBSTER, G. V.: Simple knife for skin grafts for general use. Am. J. Surg. *67:*569–571, March '45

WEBSTER, G. V.: Nasal plastic operations; proper uses in military practice. Arch. Otolaryng. *41:*170–174, March '45

WEBSTER, G. V.: Scar problem in compound injuries of lower leg. Stanford M. Bull. *3:*109–113, Aug '45

WEBSTER, G. V.: Care of injured ear. Surgery *18:*515–521, Oct '45

WEBSTER, G. V.: War wounds of lips and cheek. U. S. Nav. M. Bull. *45:*819–826, Nov '45

WEBSTER, G. V.: Late repair of tendons of hand. Am. J. Surg. *72:*171–178, Aug '46

WEBSTER, G. V. AND ROWLAND, W. D.: Skin grafting burned dorsum of hand. Ann. Surg. *124:*449–462, Aug '46

WEBSTER, G. V.; SHELDEN, C. H. AND PUDENZ, R. H.: Plastic technic in surgery of peripheral nerves. U. S. Nav. M. Bull. *45:*22–31, July '45

WEBSTER, J. B.; STEVENSON, T. W. AND STOUT, A. P.: Symposium on reparative surgery; treatment of malignant melanomas. S. Clin. North America *24:*319–339, April '44

WEBSTER, J. E.; SCHNEIDER, R. C. AND LOFSTROM, J. E.: Management of orbitocranial wounds. J. Neurosurg. *3:*329–336, July '46

WEBSTER, J. E. (see GURDJIAN, E. S.) April '44

WEBSTER, J. P.: Operation for epithelioma of lips. Am. J. Roentgenol. *30:*82–88, July '33

WEBSTER, J. P.: Deforming scars; causes, prevention and treatment. Pennsylvania M. J. *38:*929–938, Sept '35

WEBSTER, J. P.: Thoraco-epigastric tubed pedicles. S. Clin. North America *17:*145–184, Feb '37

WEBSTER, J. P.: Plastic surgery of amputation stumps. S. Clin. North America *18:*441–466, April '38

WEBSTER, J. P.: Refrigerated grafts of skin. Tr. Am. S. A. *62:*431–449, '44

WEBSTER, J. P.: Film-cemented skin grafts. S. Clin. North America *24:*251–280, April '44

WEBSTER, J. P.: Refrigerated skin grafts. Ann. Surg. *120:*431–449, Oct '44

WEBSTER, J. P.: Mastectomy for gynecomastia through semicircular intra-areolar incision. Ann. Surg. *124:*557–575, Sept '46

WEBSTER, J. P. (see MCDONALD, J. J.) July '46

Webster Operation

Webster's operation for entropion of upper lid. MACRAE, A. Brit. J. Ophth. *12:*25–30, Jan '28

WEDDELL, J. M.: Emergency treatment and primary apparatus for war fractures (of jaws). Internat. Cong. Mil. Med. and Pharm *1:*237–249, '39

WEECH, A. A.: Combined acrocephaly and syndactylism occurring in mother and daughter; case report. Bull. Johns Hopkins Hosp. *40:*73–76, Feb '27

WEEKERS, L.: Therapy of spasmodic entropion with palpebral injections of alcohol associated with canthotomy. Bull. Soc. belge d'opht., no. 64, pp. 34–38, '32 also: Arch. d'opht. *49:*427–430, July '32

WEEKERS, L.: Dacryocystorhinostomy; easy and sure method. Arch. d'opht. *52:*241–246, April '35

WEEKERS, L. AND LAPIERE, S.: Angiomas of eyelids; therapy by sclerosing injections. Bull. Soc. belge d'opht., no. 68, pp. 23–36, '34

WEEKERS, L. AND LAPIERRE, S.: Angiomas of eyelids; therapy by sclerosing injections; technic, indications and results; 4 cases. Arch. d'opht. *52:*14–22, Jan '35

Weeker's Operation

Treatment of spastic entropion by Weeker's method. ZBOROWSKY, W. F. Klin. Monatsbl. f. Augenh. *80:*648–651, May 25, '28

WEEKS, W. W.: Technique of Motais operation for ptosis. Am. J. Ophth. *11:*879–883, Nov '28

WEEKS, W. W.: Technic of dacryocystorhinostomy. Arch. Ophth. *7:*443–447, March '32

WEEKS, W. W.: Surgical treatment of exophthalmos. New York State J. Med. *33:*78–83, Jan 15, '33

WEEKS, W. W.: Ectropion and entropion of eyelids. Am. J. Surg. *42:*78–82, Oct '38

WEGEFORTH, A. (see WEGEFORTH, H. M.) Dec '25

WEGEFORTH, H. M. AND WEGEFORTH, A.: Useful appliances in treatment of common finger injury. California and West. Med. *23:*1590, Dec '25

WEHLE, F.: Successful skin graft with a slight modification of Reverdin method. Med. Rec. *101:*587–588, April 8, '22

WEHR, W. H. (see SCHREINER, B. F.) Oct '34

WEHRBEIN, H. L.: Congenital ventral curvature of penis and its surgical correction. Urol. and Cutan. Rev. *45:*359–360, June '41

WEHRBEIN, H. L.: Hypospadias. J. Urol. *50:*335–340, Sept '43

WEICHERT, M.: Hypertrophic capillary angioma of cheek; removal; plastic replacement of skin, case. Beitr. z. klin. Chir. *145:*718–720, '20

WEICHHERZ, I.: Skin grafts in correction of deforming scars. Budapesti orvosi ujsag *32:*796–798, Aug 30, '34

WEICHHERZ, I.: Possibilities and principles of plastic surgery of nose. Budapesti orvosi ujsag *38:*134–136, March 21, '40

Weidenreich

Transplantation of preserved tendons; comment on Weidenreich's article. BUSACCA, A. Virchows Arch. f. path. Anat. *258:*238–245, '25

WEIL, A. I.: Corrective rhinoplasty, with presentation of case. New Orleans M. & S. J. *73:*507, June '21

WEIL, P. G.: Recent advances in surgical shock. McGill M. J. *14:*179–183, April '45

WEIL, P. G. AND MEAKINS, J. C.: Shock and its treatment (with special reference to hemoconcentration and hemodilution). Clinics *1:*59–67, June '42 also: Dallas M. J. *28:*147–149, Nov '42 (abstr.)

WEIL, P. G.; ROSE, B. AND BROWNE, J. S. L.: Reduction of mortality from experimental traumatic shock with adrenal cortical substances. Canad. M. A. J. *43:*8–11, July '40

WEIL, P. G. (see ROSE, B. *et al*) May '41

WEIL, S.: Surgical treatment of so-called paralysis of opponens muscle. Klin. Wchnschr. *5:*650–651, April 9, '26

WEILER, H. G.: Bilateral bony ankylosis of jaws. West Virginia M. J. *33:*117–120, March '37

WEILL, J. AND MAIRE, R.: Association of retraction of palmar aponeurosis and scleroderma; relation to diseases of endocrine glands and of sympathetic nervous system. Paris med. *1:*263–268, March 24, '34

WEILL, R.: Surgical and radium therapy of keloids. Bull. et mem. Soc. de med. de Paris *139:*340–343, May 10, '35

WEILLE, F. L. AND DE BLOIS, E.: Use of T tube for drainage of septal abscess in nose. Arch. Otolaryng. *39:*85–86, Jan '44

WEINBERG, J. A.: Hand infections; involvement of tendon sheaths and fascial spaces. Nebraska M. J. *11:*144–146, April '26

WEINBERGER, M.: Bilateral fracture of angles of lower jaw; case. Rev. med. -cir. do Brasil *46:*1112–1118, Nov '38

WEINBERGER, N. S.: Submucous resection; complications and after-results. Ann. Otol., Rhin. & Laryng. *32:*387–393, June '23

WEINER, D. O.; ROWLETTE, A. P. AND ELMAN, R.: Significance of loss of serum protein in therapy of severe burns. Proc. Soc. Exper. Biol. & Med. *34:*484–486, May '36

WEINER, L. AND WALD, A. H.: Fibrin foam and thrombin as used in surgical removal of large fibromyxoma of mandible. J. Am. Dent. A. *33:*731–735, June '46

WEINGOTT, L.: Plastic operation for cicatricial ectropion of eyelids resulting from burn. Arch. d'opht. *48:*505–507, July '31

WEINGROW, S. M.: Supernumerary distal phalanx of thumb; case. Am. J. Roentgenol. *23:*206–207, Feb '30

WEINMANN, J. AND KRONFELD, R.: Traumatic injuries to jaws in infants. J. Dent. Research *19:*357–366, Aug '40

WEINSHEIMER, K. (see FLESCH-THEBESIUS, M.) Oct '31

WEINSHEL, L. R.: Burn therapy at an Army Air Forces advanced flying school. Mil. Surgeon *93:*389–399, Nov '43

WEINSHEL, L. R. AND DEMAKOPOULOS, N.: Supernumerary breasts, with special reference to pseudomamma type (case of large breast in inguinal region). Am. J. Surg. *60:*76–80, April '43

WEINSTEIN, J. J. (see WHITE, C. S. *et al*) Jan '41

WEINSTEIN, J. J. (see WHITE, C. S. *et al*) May '41

WEINSTEIN, J. J. (see WHITE, C. S. *et al*) Dec '41

WEINSTEIN, M.: Elephantiasis of lower extremities successfully treated by Kondoleon's operation. Am. J. Surg. *7:*704–710, Nov '29

WEISENGREEN, H. H.: Selection of anesthetic in cases of jaw fracture. J. Bone & Joint Surg. *18:*1005–1007, Oct '36

WEISENGREEN, H. H.: Evaluation of physiotherapeutic modalities in jaw and associated

fractures. West. J. Surg. *45:*537-539, Oct '37
WEISENGREEN, H. H.: Gunshot fracture of mandible; case. Am. J. Surg. *39:*133-134, Jan '38
WEISENGREEN, H. H.: Bone ligation and suture in relation to functional defects and tissue losses in mandible; collective review. Internat. Abstr. Surg. *68:*450-460 '39; in Surg., Gynec. & Obst., May '39
WEISENGREEN, H. H.: Physical medicine in maxillofacial injuries. Mil. Surgeon *93:*294-298, Sept '43
WEISENGREEN, H. H. AND LEVIN, W. N.: Fractures of jaw and allied traumatic lesions of facial structures. Ann. Surg. *103:*428-437, March '36
WEISKITTEL, R. (see GOOD, R. W. *et al*) July '34
WEISS, A. G. AND WARTER, J.: Role of neuroma in evolution of wounds. Bull. War Med. *3:*607, July '43 (abstract)
WEISS, A. S.: New therapeutic procedure in trichiasis. Folia ophth. orient. *2:*143-147, '36
WEISS, B.; LENTZ, M. J. AND NEWMAN, J.: Correction of severe mandibular protrusion by osteotomy of rami and orthodontics. Am. J. Orthodontics *27:*1-8, Jan '41
WEISS, J.: Cosmetic surgery of nose. Semana med. *1:*1779-1783, May 25, '33
WEISS, L. R.: Control of bone fragments in maxillofacial surgery. J. Oral Surg. *3:*271-285, Oct '45
WEISS, L. R. (see BLOCKER, T. G. JR) 1946
WEISS, L. R. (see BLOCKER, T. G.) Feb '46
WEISS, L. R. (see BLOCKER, T. G.) April '46
WEISS, P.: Experiments on repair of peripheral nerves. Tr. Am. Neurol. A. *69:*42-45, '43
WEISS, P.: Nerve reunion with sleeves of frozen-dried artery in rabbits, cats and monkeys. Proc. Soc. Exper. Biol. & Med. *54:*274-277, Dec '43
WEISS, P.: Sutureless reunion of severed nerves with elastic cuffs of tantalum. J. Neurosurg. *1:*219-225, May '44
WEISS, P.: Technology of regeneration; review; sutureless tubulation and related methods of nerve repair. J. Neurosurg. *1:*400-450, Nov '44
WEISS, P. AND TAYLOR, A. C.: Peripheral nerve repair by grafts of frozen-dried nerve. Proc. Soc. Exper. Biol. & Med. *52:*326-328, April '43
WEISS, P. AND TAYLOR, A. C.: Guides for regeneration of peripheral nerves across gaps. J. Neurosurg. *3:*375-389, Sept '46
WEISS, S.: Syncope, collapse and shock. Proc. Inst. Med. Chicago *13:*2-12, Jan 15, '40
WEISS, S. AND WILKINS, R. W.: Syncope, collapse and shock; medical significance and treatment. M. Clin. North America *21:*481-510, March '37
WEISSENBACH, R. J.: Surgical therapy of chronic rheumatism; indications and results. Monde med., Paris *45:*40-52, Jan 1-15, '35
WEISSENBACH, R. J.; DREYFUS, G. AND PERLES, L.: Modern surgical therapy of chronic progressive rheumatism. Hospital *23:*287-289, April (B) '35
WEISSENBACH, R. J. AND FRANÇON, F.: Diagnosis of de Quervain's chronic stenosing inflammation of tendons. Bull. med., Paris *45:*378-382, May 30, '31
WEISSENBACH, R. J. AND FRANÇON, F.: Chronic stenosing tenosynovitis (de Quervain's disease); symptoms, diagnosis and therapy. Rev. argent. de reumatol. *5:*299-305, March '41
WEISSENFELS, G.: Transplantation of bone and tissues in reconstruction of lower jaw. Deutsche Zahnh., Hft. 79, pp. 1-30, '31
WELBORN, M. B.: Burn therapy. J. Indiana M. A. *35:*363-364, July '42
WELBORN, M. B.: Sulfanilamide (sulfonamide); absorption from burned surfaces. J. Indiana M. A. *36:*447-448, Sept '43
WELCH, C. C. AND TAYLOR, R. W.: Healing time in fractures of mandible. U. S. Nav. M. Bull. *36:*513-517, Oct '38
WELCH, C. E.: Human bite infections of hand. New England J. Med. *215:*901-908, Nov 12, '36
WELCH, C. E. AND NATHANSON, I. T.: Life expectancy and incidence; carcinoma of lip and oral cavity. Am. J. Cancer *31:*238-252, Oct '37
WELCHMAN, W.: Notes on use of bone graft with illustrated cases. M. J. South Africa *17:*224-228, June '22
WELCKER, E. R.: Etiology and therapy of paronychia of tendon sheath. Zentralbl. f. Chir. *68:*1564-1568, Aug 9, '41
WELEMINSKY, J.: Causes and operative treatment of deformities of nasal septum. Monatschr. f. Ohrenh. *63:*530-535, May '29
WELLER, C. A.: Traumatic shock. J. Indiana M. A. *18:*253-257, July '25
WELLER, C. N. (see PENBERTHY, G. C.) Oct '34
WELLER, C. N. (see PENBERTHY, G. C.) Dec '39
WELLER, C. N. (see PENBERTHY, G. C.) Feb '42
WELLER, C. N. (see PENBERTHY, G. C. *et al*) Aug '42
WELLER, C. N. (see PENBERTHY, G. C.) 1943
WELLER, C. N. (see PENBERTHY, G. C. *et al*) May '43
WELLMAN, J. M. (see POTTER, E. B.) Feb '33
WELLS, C. G.: Speech training center for cleft palate children. Quart. J. Speech *31:*68-73, Feb '45

Wells, C. G.: Improving speech of cleft palate child. J. Speech Disorders *10:*162–168, June '45
Wells, D. B.: Treatment of electric burns by immediate resection and skin graft. Proc. Connecticut M. Soc. *137:*138–147, '29
Wells, D. B.: Treatment of electric burns by immediate resection and skin graft. Ann. Surg. *90:*1069–1078, Dec '29
Wells, D. B.: Aseptic tannic acid treatment of diffuse superficial burns. J.A.M.A. *101:*1136–1138, Oct 7, '33
Wells, D. B.: Burn therapy. Connecticut M. J. *6:*704–708, Sept '42
Wells, D. B.; Humphrey, H. D. and Coll, J. J.: Relation of tannic acid to liver necrosis in burns. New England J. Med. *226:*629–636, April 16, '42
Wells, W. F.: Plastic operation for congenital absence of vagina. Am. J. Surg. *29:*253–255, Aug '35
Welte, E. J. (see Lorber, V. *et al*) Oct '40
Welti, H. and Offret, G.: Decompressive trephining for malignant basedowian exophthalmos. Mem. Acad. de chir. *68:*379–384, Oct 28–Nov 4, '42
Wen, I. C. (see Jones, F. W.) July '34
Wendlberger, J.: Nevi, review of literature. Dermat. Ztschr. *78:*95–111, July '38
Wendlberger, J. (see Schreiner, K.) Aug '33
Wendt, H.: Therapy of nevi with thorium X; case. Dermat. Wchnschr. *108:*10–14, Jan 7, '39
Wenger, H. L.: Present conception of shock and its treatment. Am. J. Surg. *13:*307–310, Aug '31
Wenger, H. L.: Transplantation of epiphysial cartilage. Arch. Surg. *50:*148–151, March '45
Wenig, M. (see Thoma, K. H. *et al*) April '45
Wenig, M. (see Thoma, K. H. *et al*) Oct '45
Wenner, W. F.: Purified gelatin solution as blood plasma substitute (for treatment of hemorrhagic shock). Ann. Otol., Rhin. and Laryng. *53:*635–643, Dec '44
Werba, D. H.: Facial hemiatrophy. M. Bull. Vet. Admin. *17:*291–292, Jan '41
Wereschinski, A.: Fate of bone transplants. Arch. f. klin. Chir. *136:*545–567, '25
Werhatzky, N. P.: Complete inversion of bladder; case. Zentralbl. f. Gynak. *58:*1543–1546, June 30, '34
Werneck, C.: Reduction of jaw dislocations. Rev. brasil. med. *1:*598–599, July '44
Werneck, C.: Luxation of thumb; therapy in rural practice. Rev. brasil med. *1:*782–783, Sept '44
Werner, H. (see Kerr, A. B.) Oct '44
Werner, H. (see Kerr, A. B.) April '45
Werner, S.: Double blepharostat of varying widths for entropion operation. Acta ophth. *12:*149–152, '34
Werner, S.: Double blepharostat of varying width for entropion operation. Finska lak. -sallsk. handl. *76:*275–277, March '34
Wertheim, W.: New type of splint for hand fractures. J.A.M.A. *92:*2171, June 29, '29
Wertheimer, P.: Surgical therapy of facial paralysis. Lyon chir. *28:*111–113, Jan–Feb '31
Wertheimer, P.: Therapy of peripheral facial paralysis by resection of superior cervical sympathetic ganglion. Bull. et mem. Soc. nat. de chir. *59:*4–7, Jan 14, '33
Wertheimer, P. and Carcassonne, F.: Surgical therapy of peripheral facial paralysis. Lyon chir. *28:*560–570, Sept–Oct '31
Werthemann, A.: Brucella abortus infection of hand after injury; fatal case. Schweiz. med. Wchnschr. *66:*333–335, April 4, '36
Wessely, E.: Two atypical methods for plastic closure of pharynx. Monatschr. f. Ohrenh. *66:*423–430, April '32
West, B. S.: Technic for producing facial masks and models. Ann. Surg. *109:*474–478, March '39
West, C. M.: Well marked hypospadias; case. Irish J. M. Sc. pp. 29–33, Jan '27
West, C. O.: Immediate treatment of severely injured (including burn). J. Kansas M. Soc. *31:*129–131, April '30
West, J. M.: Clinical results of intranasal tear sac operation. Tr. Sect. Ophth., A.M.A. pp. 69–81, '31
West, W. T. (see Coloviras, G. J. Jr. *et al*) Dec '42

West Operation

West operation (endonasal dacryocystostomy). McArthur, G. A. D., M. J. Australia *1:*508–510, April 13, '46
Results of intranasal dacryocystorhinostomy (West operation). Henry, L. M. J. Brit. J. Ophth. *17:*550–552, Sept '33
West's dacryocystorhinostomy in 300 cases. Alcaino, A. and Rodríguez D., M. Arch. de oftal. hispano-am. *31:*65–79, Feb '31
Dacryocystorhinostomy by nasal route (West operation) and its results. Arganaraz, R. *et al*. Cong. argent. de oftal. (1936) *2:*491–496, '38

Westendorff, E. G.: Arachnodactylia in children; 3 cases. Kinderarztl. Praxis *7:*393–399, Sept '36
Westerborn, A.: Construction of artificial vagina in case of aplasia. Nord. med. (Hygiea) *26:*1194–1195, June 8, '45
Westermann, H. H.: Suggestions for first aid

of burns at front. Deut. Militärarzt *6:*209-211, April '41

WESTHUES, H.: Half suspension of pelvis (to prevent bedsores). Chirurg. *14:*489-493, Aug 15, '42

WESTHUES, H.: Half suspension of pelvis (to prevent bedsores). Bull. War Med. *3:*440-441, April '43 (abstract)

WESTMAN, A.: Cure of vaginal aplasia by Kirschner-Wagner operation. Acta obst. et gynec. Scandinav. *13:*269-273, '33

WESTMAN, A.: Use of modified Kirschner-Wagner operation in aplasia of vagina and atresia of cervix; case. Zentralbl. f. Gynak. *58:*2843-2845, Dec 1, '34

WESTMAN, A.: Surgical correction of vaginal aplasia. Nord. med. tidskr. *8:*1688-1692, Dec 15, '34

WESTMAN, A.: Operation for vaginal aplasia and malformation of cervix uteri. Svenska lak.-tidning. *33:*1721-1725, Nov 27, '36

WESTON, R. E.; LEVINSON, S. O.; JANOTA, M. AND NECHELES, H.: Use of concentrated and normal plasma in shock therapy. J.A.M.A. *122:*198, May 15, '43

WETHERBY, M.: Procedures in chronic rheumatoid disease. Journal-Lancet *61:*414-417, Oct '41

WETSCHTOMOW, A. A.: Use of ferric chloride solution as hemostatic during operative treatment of rhinophyma; 2 cases. Zentralbl. f. Chir. *57:*333-335, Feb 8, '30

WETTE, W.: Bilateral fissure of navicular bone of hand from injury; question of aseptic necrosis. (Comment on Reich's article.) Arch. f. orthop. u. Unfall-Chir. *33:*194-199, '33

WETTE, W.: Dupuytren's contracture and industrial accident; case. Monatschr. f. Unfallh. *44:*195-197, April '37

WETZEL, J. O.: Epithelioma of face and buccal cavity. New York State J. Med. *26:*634-639, July 15, '26

WEVE, H.: Euroblepharon; case. Nederl. tijdschr. v. geneesk. *80:*1213-1217, March 21, '36

WEVE, H. J. M. AND KENTGENS, S. K.: Dacryocystorhinostomy; technic and results. Klin. Monatsbl. f. Augenh. *98:*195-205, Feb '37

WEYER, S. M.: Case report of severe burn, with special reference to tannic acid treatment. Nebraska M. J. *22:*23-25, Jan '37

WHALMAN, H. F.: Reconstruction of ablated lower eyelid. Arch. Ophth. *32:*66-67, July '44

WHARTON, L. R.: Simple method of construction of vagina; 4 cases. Ann. Surg. *107:*842-854, May '38

WHARTON, L. R.: Further experiences in construction of artificial vagina; 12 cases. Ann. Surg. *111:*1010-1020, June '40

WHARTON, L. R.: Spontaneous perforation of rectovaginal septum, 5 weeks after construction of vagina; case. Tr. South. S. A. (1944) *56:*146-148, '45

WHARTON, L. R.: Spontaneous perforation of rectovaginal septum, 5 weeks after construction of vagina; cases. Ann. Surg. *121:*530-533, April '45

WHARTON, L. R.: Difficulties and accidents encountered in construction of artificial vagina. Am. J. Obst. and Gynec. *51:*866-875, June '46

Wharton Operation

Wharton operation in case of partial aplasia of vagina. CABRAL JUNIOR, A. An. brasil. de ginec. *20:*87-107, Aug '45

Construction of artificial vagina; modification of Wharton operation; 3 cases. WORD, B. South. M. J. *33:*293-301, March '40

WHEELDON, T. F.: Use of cellophane as permanent tendon sheath. J. Bone and Joint Surg. *21:*393-396, April '39

WHEELER, D. W.: Nature and therapy of shock. U. S. Nav. M. Bull. *41:*93-106, Jan '43

WHEELER, J. M.: Use of epidermic graft in plastic eye surgery. Internat. Clinics *3:*292-302, '22 (illus.)

WHEELER, J. M.: Ectropion; problem for eye surgeons. South. M. J. *29:*377-382, April '36

WHEELER, J. M.: Sources of grafts for plastic surgery about eyes. New York State J. Med. *36:*1372-1376, Oct 1, '36

WHEELER, J. M.: Correction of eyelid ptosis by attachment of strips of orbicularis muscle to superior rectus muscle. Tr. Sect. Ophth., A. M. A., pp. 130-137, '38 Also: Arch. Ophth. *21:*1-7, Jan '39

WHEELER, J. M.: Use of orbicularis palpebrarum muscle in eyelid surgery. Am. J. Surg. *42:*7-9, Oct '38

WHEELER, J. M.: Spastic entropion correction by orbicularis transplantation. Am. J. Ophth. *22:*477-483, May '39

WHEELER, R. H.: Treatment of fractures of metacarpals and phalanges of fingers. J.A.M.A. *78:*422-423, Feb 11, '22 (illus.)

WHEELER, W. I. DE C.: Bennett fracture of thumb. J. Bone and Joint Surg. *19:*520-521, April '37

WHEELER, W. I. DE C.: Splints for fingers and thumb. Lancet *2:*546-547, Nov 2, '40

Wheeler Operation: See Esser-Wheeler Operation

WHEELOCK, M. C. (see SEARCY, H. B. *et al*) March '44

WHELAN, C. S. AND THOMPSON, W. D. JR.: Skin grafting and secondary closure in war wounds; preliminary report. Surg., Gynec. and Obst. *79:*584–588, Dec '44

Whelan, E. P.: Repair of avulsed scrotum. Surg., Gynec. and Obst. *78:*649–652, June '44

Whelan, H. M.: Nerve and tendon suture: illustrative case. J. Roy. Nav. M. Serv. *22:*234–237, July '36

Whelchel, H. C.: Burns, a case report. J. M. A. Georgia *10:*239, Jan '21

Whetstone, G. (see Craddock, F. H.) Nov '26

Whigham, J. R. M.: Severe burns associated with duodenal ulceration. Brit. J. Surg. *30:*178–179, Oct '42

Whipple, A. O.: Basic principles in thermal burns. Ann. Surg. *118:*187–192, Aug '43

Whipple, A. O. (see Meleney, F. L.) March '45

Whitacre, F. E. and Chen, C. Y.: Surgical treatment of absence of vagina; 2 cases. Am. J. Obst. and Gynec. *49:*789–796, June '45

Whitacre, F. E. and Wang, Y. Y.: Artificial vagina; biologic changes in squamous epithelium transplanted to pelvic connective tissue. Surg., Gynec. and Obst. *79:*192–194, Aug '44

Whitaker, L. W. (see Parish, B. B.) Feb '31

Whitby, L.: "Shock"; second thoughts. Middlesex Hosp. J. *45:*7–9, March '45

Whitby, L. E. H. (see Maycock, W. d'A.) Oct '41

Whitcomb, B. B.: Separation at suture site as cause of failure in regeneration of peripheral nerves. J. Neurosurg. *3:*399–406, Sept '46

Whitcomb, C. A.: Study of 56 5-year cases of cancer of lips. Am. J. Surg. *63:*304–315, March '44

White, C.: Treatment of portwine birthmarks (nevus flammeus) by grenz (infra-roentgen) rays. Illinois M. J. *76:*449–451, Nov '39

White, C. S.; Collins, J. L. and Weinstein, J. J.: Surgical shock treatment with blood plasma. South. M. J. *34:*38–42, Jan '41

White, C. S.; Collins, J. L. and Weinstein, J.: Analysis of 50 cases of shock treated with plasma. South. Med. and Surg. *103:*250–251, May '41

White, C. S.; Collins, J. L. and Weinstein, J. J.: Treatment of surgical and traumatic shock with citrated plasma-saline mixture. Am. J. Surg. *54:*701–710, Dec '41

White, C. S. (see Davis, H. A.) May '38

White, F. W.: Submucous resection in children. Ann. Otol., Rhin. and Laryng. *33:*526–533, June '24

White, F. W.: New nasal splint. Laryngoscope *35:*76, Jan '25

White, F. W.: Submucous resection in children. Tr. Sect. Laryng., Otol. and Rhin., A. M. A., pp. 123–134, '29 also: Arch. Otolaryng. *11:*415–425, April '30

White, F. W.: Plea for early treatment of nasal fractures. Laryngoscope *41:*253–256, April '31

White, J. C.: Painful injuries of nerves and their surgical treatment. Am. J. Surg. *72:*468–488, Sept '46

White, J. C. and Hamlin, H.: New uses of tantalum in suture and control of neuroma formation; illustration of technical procedures. J. Neurosurg. *2:*402–413, Sept '45

White, J. C.; Hudson, H. W. and Kennard, H. E.: Treatment of bedsores by total excision with plastic closure. U. S. Nav. M. Bull. *45:*454–463, Sept '45

White, J. R. (see Pickerill, H. P.) Jan '22

White, M. F. (see Coakley, W. A.) Oct '43

White, W. C.: Pedicle graft of sole of foot. Ann. Surg. *105:*472–473, March '37

White, W. C. (see Brandes, W. W. *et al*) Feb '46

Whitehead Operation

Plastic surgery of anal canal after unsuccessful Whitehead operation. Fischer, A. W. Zentralbl. f. Chir. *61:*157–159, Jan 20, '34

Whitehill, N. M.: Diagnosis of cancer of lips. J. Iowa M. Soc. *22:*533–534, Nov '32

Whitehill, N. M.: Burn therapy. J. Iowa M. Soc. *24:*481–482, Sept '34

Whitham, J. D.: Restoration of cheek and temporal region by pedicled and sliding grafts of skin and muscle. J.A.M.A. *76:*448, Feb 12, '21

Whitham, J. D.: Plastic repair of soft tissues injuries of face. Mil. Surgeon *48:*65, Jan '21

Whitham, J. D.: Reduction of old fractures of nose. Laryngoscope *31:*620, Aug '21

Whitham, J. D.: Operation for correction of elongated and humped noses. Laryngoscope *34:*271–273, April '24

Whitham, J. D.: Treatment of facial fractures and nose. Laryngoscope *49:*394–400, May '39

Whitney, D. D.: Three generations of ear pits. J. Hered. *30:*323–324, Aug '39

Whitney, L. F.: Inheritance of doublejointedness in thumb. J. Hered. *23:*425–426, Oct '32

Whittaker, R.: Wounds in ear and mastoid region. J. Laryng. and Otol. *59:*205–217, June '44

Whyte, D.: Nasal prosthesis. Australian and New Zealand J. Surg. *3:*74–75, July '33

Wiberg, G.: De Quervain's tendovaginitis as sequel to hand injury. Nord. med. (Hygiea) *10:*1929–1933, June 21, '41

Wible, L. E. and Howard, J. C. Jr.: Traumatic palatine fistula. Arch. Otolaryng. *44:*159–165, Aug '46

Wichmann, F. W.: Elephantiasis of plastic skin graft on thumb. Arch. f. klin. Chir. *169:*783–788, '32

WICHMANN, F. W.: Unguentolan (cod liver oil ointment) and plaster casts in industrial burns. Zentralbl. f. Chir. *66:*655-662, March 25, '39

WICHMANN, S. E.: Success of Schubert's operation in aplasia of vagina; 3 cases. Acta obst. et gynec. Scandinav. *9:*661-683, '30

WIDMEYER, R. S.: Burns, various types; treatment and prognosis from military as well as civilian viewpoint. J. Florida M. A. *29:*165-168, Oct '42

WIEDHOPF, O.: Reposition of dislocated mandible after injection of local anesthetics into muscles of mastication. Munchen. med. Wchnschr. *72:*2007, Nov 20, '25 abstr: J.A.M.A. *86:*78, Jan 2, '26

WIEDHOPF, O.: Surgical therapy of cancer of lips. Deutsche Ztschr. f. Chir. *238:*741-744, '33

WIEL, P.: Fractures of mandible; treatment by so-called maxillary block. Stomatol. ital. *2:*112-126, Feb '40

WIELAGE, M. F.: New method in reducing fracture of zygomatic arch. J. Am. Dent. A. *15:*1228-1230, July '28

WIELENGA, D. K.: Post-traumatic shock and gas gangrene successfully treated with several massive blood transfusions and sulfanilamide. Nederl. tijdschr. v. geneesk. *83:*4740-4746, Sept 30, '39

WIENECKE, H.: Tannin ointment in burns. Med. Welt *7:*1643-1644, Nov 18, '33

WIENER, A.: Simple procedure for relief of entropin (device attached to spectacle frame). Arch. Ophth. *29:*634, April '43

WIENER, E.: Multiple epitheliomata of face developed from keratoma senile. Nederl. Tijdschr. v. Geneesk. *1:*614-616, Feb 4, '28

WIENER, M.: Correction of ocular disfigurements. Surg., Gynec. and Obst. *58:*390-394, Feb (no. 2A) '34

WIER, C. K.: Fractures of phalanges. J. Kansas M. Soc. *39:*501-504, Dec '38

WIESENFELD, I. H. AND MEADOFF, N.: Fractures of mandible; review of experience in 52 patients with particular reference to use of external skeletal fixation. Permanente Found. M. Bull. *2:*49-63, March '44

WIGERT, V.: Acrocephalosyndactylia; clinical study with description of recent case (roentgen examination by Prof. Lars Edling). Svenska Lak.-Sallsk. Handl. *53:*91-112, '27

WIGERT, V.: General skeletal changes in acrocephalosyndactylia. Acta psychiat. et neurol. *7:*701-718, '32

WIGGERS, C. J.: Recent observations on value of adrenal cortex preparations in hemorrhagic shock. Univ. Hosp. Bull., Ann Arbor *9:*61, July '43

WIGHTMAN, J. C.: Pedigree of syndactyly. J. Hered. *28:*421-423, Dec '37

WILANDER, O. (see LINDGREN, S.) Nov '41

WILANDER, O. (see MALMROS, H.) June '40

WILDE, A. G.: Plastic surgery of orbit. Texas State J. Med. *24:*336-344, Sept '28

WILDE, A. G.: Plastic surgery of orbit. New Orleans M. and S. J. *83:*239-244, Oct '30

WILDEGANS: Braun's skin grafting. Arch. f. klin. Chir. *120:*415-440, '22 (illus.) abstr: J.A.M.A. *79:*1887, Nov 25, '22

WILE, U. J. AND HAND, E. A.: Results of therapy in four hundred and twenty-five cases of cancers of lips followed from one to ten years. J.A.M.A. *108:*374-382, Jan 30, '37

WILEY, A. R.: Plasma bank in shock therapy. J. Oklahoma M. A. *36:*285-287, July '43

WILGIS, H. E. (see DAVIS, J. S.) April '34

WILHELMJ, C. M.: Etiology and treatment of traumatic or secondary shock. J. Arkansas M. Soc. *39:*257-260, May '43

WILKER, W. F.: Complete avulsion of scalp (case in operator of buttercutting machine). Wisconsin M. J. *37:*900-903, Oct '38

WILKERSON, W. V. (see LAIRD, W. R.) March '31

WILKEY, J. L. (see MEYER, K. A.) Sept '38

WILKIE, D. P. D.: Septic hand. Brit. M. J. *2:*1127-1130, Dec 3, '38

WILKIE, D. P. D. *et al*: Treatment of acute primary infections of hand. Brit. M. J. *2:*1025-1032, Dec 1, '23

WILKINS, G. F. (see BRANCH, C. D. *et al*) Apr '46

WILKINS, R. W.: Recent advances in vascular physiology and their therapeutic implications (shock). M. Clin. North. America *27:*1397-1408, Sept '43

WILKINS, R. W. (see WEISS, S.) March '37

WILKINSON, A. W.: Shock due to tissue trauma; diagnosis and assessment. Edinburgh M. J. *52:*306-316, Sept '45

WILKINSON, A. W. (see RAE, S. L.) March '44

WILKINSON, B.: Jaw fractures. Tri-State M. J. *7:*1503-1504, Aug '35

WILKINSON, D. E.: Plastic surgery. Vet. Rec. *9:*579-588, July 13, '29

WILKINSON, G.: Bifid nose. J. Laryngol. and Otol. *37:*560-563, Nov '22 (illus.)

WILLARD, J. W. (see SELLERS, E. A.) Dec '43

WILLCUTTS, M. D.: Treatment of irreducible dislocated lower jaw of 98 days' duration; case. U. S. Nav. M. Bull. *25:*331-336, April '27

WILLEMS, J. D.: Amputation of fingers. Surg., Gynec. and Obst. *62:*892-894, May '36

WILLEMS, J. D. AND KUHN, L. P.: Statistical study of 1206 burn cases. Am. J. Surg. *34:*254-258, Nov '36

WILLETT, R. C.: Surgical-orthodontic correction of macro-mandibular deformity; case report.

Internat. Orthodont. Cong. *1:*458–473, '27
WILLETT, R. C.: Interdental fixation appliance for jaw fractures. Dental Items Interest *50:*788–799, Oct '28
WILLIAMS, E. (see TRETHEWIE, E. R.) Jan '42
WILLIAMS, E. R. P.: New method of tendon repair. J. Roy. Nav. M. Serv. *28:*384–386, Oct '42
WILLIAMS, G. A.: End-result in Thiersch graft; case observed after 30 years. Arch. Surg. *16:*938–941, April '28
WILLIAMS, G. A. (see HOLMES, W. R.) Jan '40
WILLIAMS, H. L. (see PASTORE, P. N.) Oct '39
WILLIAMS, H. S. (see TRUSLER, H. M. *et al*) Dec '39
WILLIAMS, H. W. (see GURDJIAN, E. S.) Dec '28
WILLIAMS, I. G. AND MARTIN, L. C.: Nevocarcinoma of skin and mucous membranes. Lancet *1:*135–138, Jan 16, '37
WILLIAMS, J. L. D. AND HILL, B. G.: Simplified external dacryocystorhinostomy. Brit. J. Ophth. *28:*407–410, Aug '44
WILLIAMS, J. R. F. (see BUTLER, E. C. B. *et al*) Jan '45
WILLIAMS, L. R.: Hypospadias. Bull. Vancouver M. A. *18:*348–349, Aug '42
WILLIAMS, P. E.: Facial injuries; care and treatment. Mil. Surgeon *91:*650–659, Dec '42
WILLIAMS, P. (see WARTHEN, H. J.) March '36
WILLIAMS, P. E. AND MARCKS, K. M.: Ameloblastoma of mandible; case. J. Oral Surg. *4:*133–144, April '46
WILLIAMS, R. E. O. AND MILES, A. A.: Bacterial flora of wounds and septic lesions of hand. J. Path. and Bact. *57:*27–36, Jan '45
WILLIAMS, V. T.: Physiologic management of burns. J. Missouri M. A. *41:*205–206, Oct '44
WILLIAMSON, C. S.: Laboratory aids of value in diagnosis of traumatic shock and internal hemorrhage with brief reference to use of blood plasma as therapeutic agent. Wisconsin M. J. *40:*570–574, July '41
WILLIS, A. M.: Value of debridement in treatment of burns. J.A.M.A. *84:*655–658, Feb 28, '25
WILLIS, D. A.: Localization and removal of metallic bodies in hand. Surg., Gynec. and Obst. *65:*698–699, Nov '37
WILLIS, L. L.: Temporomandibular joint. U. S. Nav. M. Bull. *41:*681–691, May '43
WILLIS, R. A.: Unusual case of cancer of face. J. Coll. Surgeons, Australasia *2:*417–421, March '30
WILLSON, J. R. (see MILLER, N. F. *et al*) Dec '45
WILSON, A. K.: Nasal deformities and their correction. J. Florida M. A. *10:*270–273, April '24
WILSON, C. A.: Coloboma of eyelid; cases. California and West. Med. *44:*484–486, June '36
WILSON, C. H. (see NOLAND, L.) Nov '40
WILSON, C. S.: Modification of banjo splint for finger fractures. Canad. M. A. J. *46:*585–586, June '42
WILSON, G. (see ACKMAN, D.) July '42
WILSON, G. E.: Hand infections. Canad. M. A. J. *15:*715–718, July '25
WILSON, G. E.: Hand infections. St. Michael's Hosp. M. Bull. *3:*43–49, Aug '28
WILSON, H.: Management of cancer of lips. Memphis M. J. *15:*80–82, May '40
WILSON, H.: Etiology and treatment of traumatic shock. South. M. J. *33:*754–756, July '40
WILSON, H.: Burn shock; consideration of its mechanism and management. Memphis M. J. *17:*3–5, Jan '42
WILSON, H. AND ROOME, N. W.: Traumatic shock syndrome following rupture of aorta and multiple fractures. Am. J. Surg. *22:*333–334, Nov '33
WILSON, H. (see DRAGSTEDT, L. R.) July '37
WILSON, H. C.: Physical therapy in plastic surgery unit. Physiotherapy Rev. *25:*3–21, Jan–Feb, '45
WILSON, J. A. AND EGEBERG, B.: Burns of skin due to molten magnesium. Indust. Med. *11:*436–437, Sept '42
WILSON, P. D.: Surgical reconstruction of rheumatoid cripple. M. Clin. North America *21:*1623–1639, Nov '37
WILSON, P. D.: Reconstructive surgery of war wounded. Rocky Mountain M. J. *42:*267–274, April '45
WILSON, P. D.: Reconstructive surgery of war wounded. New England J. Med. *233:*492–497, Oct 25, '45
WILSON, P. D.: Reconstructive surgery of war wounds. Medicina, Mexico *25:*475–491, Nov 25, '45
WILSON, P. D. AND OSGOOD, R. B.: Reconstructive surgery in chronic arthritis. New England J. Med. *209:*117–125, July 20, '33
WILSON, S. J.: Malignancy of lower lip complicated by mouth infections. South. M. J. *24:*359–363, April '31
WILSON, T. E.: Burn therapy. M. J. Australia *1:*131–133, Jan 31, '42
WILSON, T. H. H. (see CLARKSON, P.) Oct '44
WILSON, T. H. H. (see CLARKSON, P. *et al*) Feb '46
WILSON, W. C.: Treatment of burns and scalds by tannic acid. Brit. M. J. *2:*91–94, July 21, '28
WILSON, W. C.: Modern treatment (tannic acid) of burns and scalds. Practitioner *129:*183–193, July '32

WILSON, W. C.: Extensive burns and scalds. Tr. Med.-Chir. Soc. Edinburgh, pp. 177-192, '34-'35; in Edinburgh M. J. Oct '35

WILSON, W. C.: Modern methods of burn therapy. Practitioner *136:*394-403, April '36

WILSON, W. C.: Burn therapy. J. Roy. Nav. M. Serv. *26:*352-361, Oct '40

WILSON, W. C.: Cause and treatment of lethal factors in burns (Honyman Gillespie lecture). Edinburgh M. J. *48:*85-93, Feb '41

WILSON, W. C.; MACGREGOR, A. R. AND STEWART, C. P.: Clinical course and pathology of burns and scalds under modern methods of treatment. Brit. J. Surg. *25:*826-865, April '38

WILSON, W. C. AND STEWART, C. P.: Changes in blood chemistry after burning injuries; with reference to treatment by desoxycorticosterone acetate (suprarenal preparation). Tr. Med.-Chir. Soc. Edinburgh, pp. 153-173, '38-'39; in Edinburgh M. J., Nov '39

WILSON, W. C. (see HARKINS, H. N. *et al*) March '35

WILSON, W. F.: Submucous resection of nasal septum; simple flap suture. Brit. M. J. *2:*814, Nov 1, '24

WILSON, W. R.: Detoxication in treatment of burns. Brit. M. J. *1:*54-55, Jan 8, '27

WILMOTH, C. L.: Tendinoplasty of flexor tendons of hand; use of tunica vaginalis in reconstructing tendon sheaths. J. Bone and Joint Surg. *19:*152-156, Jan '37

WILMOTH, C. L.: Tubed pedicle graft in facial reconstruction; superiority when subcutaneous loss is present. Am. J. Surg. *53:*300-305, Aug '41

WINCKLER, E.: Pagnelin cautery in therapy of furunculosis. Munchen. med. Wchnschr. *80:*1974-1975, Dec 15, '33

WINDEYER, B. W.: Malignant tumors of upper jaw; Skinner lecture, 1943. Brit. J. Radiol. *16:*362, Dec '43; *17:*18, Jan '44

WINDHAM, R. E.: Submucous resection in children. Eye, Ear, Nose and Throat Monthly *7:*307-311, July '28 Also: Northwest Med. *27:*392-396, Aug '28

WINDHAM, R. E.: Submucous resection in children. Texas State J. Med. *27:*859-862, April '32

WINFIELD, J. M.: Anatomic diagnosis of hand injuries. J.A.M.A. *116:*1367-1370, March 29, '41

WINFIELD, J. M. (see MILLER, H.) Feb '42

WINKLER, A.: Phenol burns of both eyes and their general sequels; therapy of chemical burns. Klin. Monatsbl. f. Augenh. *102:*810-815, June '39

WINKLER, A. W. AND HOFF, H. E.: Potassium and cause of death in traumatic shock. Am. J. Physiol. *139:*686-692, Sept '43

WINTER, L.: Differential diagnosis of swellings of face and neck. Am. J. Orthodontics *25:*1087-1116, Nov '39

WINTER, LEO: *Operative Oral Surgery*. C. V. Mosby Co., St. Louis, 1941

WINTER, L.: Mandibular fractures; report of 50 applications of Roger Anderson skeletal fixation appliance. Am. J. Surg. *61:*367-379, Sept '43

WINTER, L.; LIFTON, J. C. AND MCQUILLAN, A. S.: Embedment of vitallium mandibular prosthesis as integral part of operation for removal of adamantinoma. Am. J. Surg. *69:*318-324, Sept '45

WINTERSTEIN, O.: Stenosing tendovaginitis on styloid process of radius (styloidalgia). Munchen. med. Wchnschr. *74:*12-15, Jan 7, '27

WINTERSTEIN, O.: Stenosis of tendon sheath of wrist. Schweiz. med. Wchnschr. *58:*746-748, July 28, '28

WIPER, T. B. (see SHEARER, T. P. *et al*) July '45

WIRTH, J. E.: Radical inferior cheiloplasty for advanced carcinoma of lower lip; 2 cases. Northwest Med. *37:*109-112, April '38

WIRZ, F.: Comment on article by Eiger on keloid therapy by iodine iontophoresis. Munchen. med. Wchnschr. *76:*1515, Sept 6, '29

WIRZ, S. (see PICHON, E.) June '36

WISE, B. T.: Transplantation of ureters in exstrophy; case. J. M. A. Georgia *21:*100-103, March '32

WISE, R. A.: Unusual fracture of terminal phalanx. J. Bone and Joint Surg. *21:*467-469, April '39

WISER, H. J. AND MCAFEE, M. F.: Symposium on military medicine aboard U.S.S. Samaritan; injuries of face in war casualities. U. S. Nav. M. Bull. *46:*57-66, Jan '46

WISSELINK, G. W.: Toti's dacryocystorhinostomy. Klin. Monatsbl. f. Augenh. *78:*550, April '27

WITHERS, S.: Carcinoma of eyelids treated with radium. Am. J. Ophth. *4:*8, Jan '21

WITHERS, S. AND RANSON, J. R.: Treatment of malignant growths about the face. Colorado Med. *21:*92-97, April '24

WITTE, G.: Resorption in pedunculated skin grafts. Arch. f. klin. Chir. *184:*689-707, '36

WITTEK, A.: Successful substitution of second metacarpal bone for missing thumb; case. Chirurg *13:*577-581, Oct 1, '41

WITTMER, J. J.: Industrial burn. New York State J. Med. *37:*1931-1937, Nov 15, '37

WITTMOSER, R.: Free transplantation of flaps. Beitr. z. klin. Chir. *174:*387, '43

Wodak

Defects of tip of nose; surgical correction. (Comment on Wodak's article.) Halla, F. Med. Klin. *28:*50, Jan 8, '32

Defects of tip of nose; surgical correction. (Comment on Wodak's article.) Eitner, E. Med. Klin. *28:*49–50, Jan 8, '32

Wodak, E.: Cosmetic surgery of nose and ear. Med. Klinik *20:*1042–1044, July 27, '24

Wodak, E.: Corrective plastic operations on nose. Med. Klinik *21:*1573–1575, Oct 16, '25

Wodak, E.: Defects of tip of nose; surgical correction. Med. Klin. *27:*1606–1608, Oct 30, '31

Wodak, E.: Reply to Eitner's comments on article about nasal tip defects and Halla's comments. Med. Klin. *28:*50, Jan 8, '32

Wodak, E.: Plastic surgery of nasal deformities. Rev. de chir. plastique, pp. 157–169, July '32

Wodak, E.: Psychologic aspects of relationship between surgeon and patient (plastic surgery). Med. Klin. *33:*833–835, June 18, '37

Wodak, E.: Esthetic and psychologic principles of plastic surgery (ear, face, nose). Monatschr. f. Ohrenh. *72:*288–303, March '38

Wodak, E.: Esthetic and psychologic principles of plastic surgery of nose, ears and face. Monatschr. f. Ohrenh. *72:*424, April; 490, May '38

Wodak, E.: Nasal fractures and their treatment. Harefuah *25:*211, Dec 1, '43

Wodak, E.: Attempt to correct congenital rhinolalia aperta by plastic operation. Harefuah *27:*8, July 2, '44

Wodak, E.: Congenital anteflexion accompanied by swelling of soft palate; correction by plastic methods. Ann. Otol., Rhin. and Laryng. *53:*581–582, Sept '44

Wodak, E. M.: Surgical treatment of harelip and cleft palate. Acta oto-laryng. orient. *1:*13–17, '45

Wodak, E. M.: Surgical treatment of harelip and cleft palate. Acta oto-laryng. orient. *1:*42–45, '45

Wodon: Dacryocystorhinostomy. Arch. med. belges *87:*95–97, June '34

Wojatschek: Surgical method of nasal surgery which does not cause shock. Acta oto-laryng. *15:*327–341, '31

Wojatschek, W. I.: Technic of cosmetic operations of nose. Monatschr. f. Ohrenh. *64:*1066–1070, Sept '30

Wojatschek, W. I.: New nasal septum operation. Monatschr. f. Ohrenh. *60:*910–914, Oct '26

Woldstad, D. M.: Handicap of cleft-palate speech. Ment. Hyg. *16:*281–288, April '32

Wolf, C.: True (lateral) hermaphroditism; complete restoration of masculine habitus after removal of female organs; case. Endokrinologie *15:*225–232, '35

Wolf, G. D.: Mouth gag and tongue depressor combination. Tr. Sect. Laryng. Otol. and Rhin., A. M. A. p. 287, 1921

Wolf, G. D.: Rhinoplasty; facts and fiction. Tr. Sect. Laryng., Otol. and Rhin., A. M. A., pp. 174–189, '29 also: Arch. Otolaryng. *11:*322–335, March '30

Wolf, G. D.: End results in nasal surgery. M. J. and Rec. *133:*178–182, Feb 18, '31

Wolf, G. D.: What plastic surgery is doing for deformed and badly proportioned noses. Hygeia *9:*1005–1006, Nov '31

Wolf, G. D.: Correction of saddle nose. Arch. Otolaryng. *22:*304–311, Sept '35

Wolf, G. D.: Rhinoplasty and its relation to rhinology. Tr. Sect. Laryng., Otol. and Rhin., A. M. A., pp. 81–95F, '41

Wolf, G. D.: Rhinoplasty and its relation to rhinology. Am. J. Surg. *62:*216–224, Nov '43

Wolf, G. D.: Receded chin; correction with preserved cartilage. Am. J. Surg. *72:*74–77, July '46

Wolf, H.: Use of gnathotome in resection of lower jaw. Zentralbl. f. Chir. *56:*452–455, Feb 23, '29

Wolf, H.: Plastic operations on cheeks and nose for cancer. Arch. f. klin. Chir. *160:*105–117, '30

Wolf, H.: Secondary operations for structural and functional correction of post-traumatic deformities of jaws. Ztschr. f. Stomatol. *39:*157–184, March 14, '41

Wolf, J.: Slow screw extension in contractures of fingers. Monatschr. f. Unfallh. *36:*447–451, Oct '29

Wolf, J.: Dislocation of hand. Vereinsbl. d. pfalz. Aerzte *44:*1–5, Jan 1, '32

Wolf, M.: Familial occurrence of keloids. Wien. med. Wchnschr. *86:*722–723, June 27, '36

Wolf, W.: Bloodless transplantation of skin. Munchen. med. Wchnschr. *69:*1217, Aug 18, '22

Wolfe, H. R. I. and Clegg, H. W.: Use of plasma in hospital ship for burns. Lancet *1:*191–193, Feb 14, '42

Wolfe, J. J.: Osteomyelitis of mandible; observations on etiology, pathogenesis and diagnosis. Chinese M. J. *49:*422–428, May '35

Wolfe, J. J. (see Miltner, L. J.) Aug '34

Wolfe, M. M.: Plastic surgery of saddle nose. Laryngoscope *43:*897–904, Nov '33

Wolfe, M. M.: Protruding ears; psychological effect and plastic correction. M. Rec. *144:*306–307, Oct 7, '36

Wolfe, M. M.: Submucous resection in relation

to nasal plastic surgery. Laryngoscope *47:*281-285, April '37
WOLFE, M. M.: Etiology of saddle nose; preliminary report (syphilis). Ann. Otol., Rhin. and Laryng. *46:*504–509, June '37
WOLFE, M. M.: Technic of ivory implant for correction of saddle nose. Arch. Surg. *37:*800–807, Nov '38
WOLFE, M. M.: Story (historical sketch) of plastic surgery. Ann. Otol., Rhin. and Laryng. *48:*473-483, June '39
WOLFE, M. M.: Partial saddle nose; simplified technic without use of implant or transplant. Ann. Otol., Rhin. and Laryng. *49:*700–708, Sept '40
WOLFE, M. M.: Rhinophyma with new etiologic and therapeutic considerations (case with ascorbic acid deficiency). Laryngoscope *53:*172–180, March '43
WOLFE, M. O. AND WEBER, M. L.: Progressive facial hemiatrophy; case with attacks of syncope and gynandromorphism. J. Nerv. and Ment. Dis. *91:*595–607, May '40
WOLFE, M. O. AND WEBER, M. L.: Progressive facial hemiatrophy; case with attacks of syncope and gynandromorphism. M. Bull. Vet. Admin. *17:*283–290, Jan '41
WOLFER, J. A.: Burn wounds and their therapy. Northwest Med. *35:*339–342, Sept '36
WOLFER, J. A.: Tumors of head and face. Indust. Med. *10:*59–60, Feb '41
WOLFER, J. A.: Tumors of head, face and neck. Indust. Med. *11:*528–529, Nov '42
WOLFF, E.: Treatment of lime burns of cornea by 10 per cent neutral ammonium tartrate. Brit. J. Ophth. *10:*196–197, April '26
WOLFF, E.: Relative ptosis of eyelids. Tr. Ophth. Soc. U. Kingdom *53:*317–319, '33
WOLFF, H. G.: Progessive facial hemiatrophy; case with other signs of disease of central nervous system. Arch. Otolaryng. *7:*580–582, June '28
WOLFF, H. G.: Progressive facial hemiatrophy; case with convulsions and anisocoria. J. Nerv. and Ment. Dis. *69:*140–144, Feb '29
WOLFF, H. G. AND EHRENCLOU, A. H.: Trophic disorders of central origin; report of case of progressive facial hemiatrophy, associated with lipodystrophy and other metabolic derangements. J.A.M.A. *88:*991–994, March 26, '27
WOLFF, S. (see ELLER, J. J.) May '41
WOLFF, W. A.; RHOADS, J. E. AND LEE, W. E.: Recent developments in severe third degree burns. Nebraska M. J. *27:*369–374, Nov '42
WOLFF, W. A. (see ELKINTON, J. R. *et al*) July '40
WOLFF, W. A. (see LEE, W. E. *et al*) June '41
WOLFF, W. A. (see RHOADS, J. E. *et al*) June '41
WOLFF, W. A. (see RHOADS, J. E. *et al*) Oct '42

Wolff's Law

Application of Wolff's law to bone transplants. PUYO VILLAFANE, E. Semana med. *2:*840–843, Oct 8, '42
Evaluation of Wolff's law of bone formation as related to transplantation. KUSHNER, A. J. Bone and Joint Surg. *22:*589–596, July '40

WOLFRAM, S.: Plastic surgery for general practitioner. Wien. klin. Wchnschr. *55:*878–879, Oct 30, '42
WOLFRAM, S.: Treatment of burns. Wien. klin. Wchnschr. *57:*142, March 24, '44
WOLFSOHN, G.: Operative treatment of pendulous breast. Med. Welt *2:*477, March 31, '28
WOLFSOHN, G.: Fascia as suture material. Chirurg *2:*475–477, May 15, '30
WOLLESEN, J. M.: Tannic acid in burns. Ugesk. f. laeger *92:*487–491, May 22, '30
WOLLESEN, J. M.: Tannic acid in burns. Chirurg *8:*732–740, Sept 15, '36
WOLLESEN, J. M.: Tannic acid and silver nitrate in burns. Ugesk. f. laeger *99:*405–409, April 15, '37
WOLOSCHINOW, W.: Reconstruction of lower lip according to round pedicle method. Arch. f. klin. Chir. *135:*770–775, '25
WOMACK, D. R.: Nasal fracture device. U. S. Nav. M. Bull. *41:*852–856, May '43
WOMACK, N. A. (see BLAIR, V. P. *et al*) 1928
WOMACK, N. A. (see BLAIR, V. P. *et al*) Oc '28
WOMACK, N. A. (see BLAIR, V. P. *et al*) Feb '30
WONG, W. (see SLAUGHTER, W. B.) Feb '46
WOOD, C. F.: Stenosing tendovaginitis at radial styloid process (de Quervain's disease). South. Surgeon *10:*105–110, Feb '41
WOOD, G. O.; MASON, M. F. AND BLALOCK, A.: Effects of inhalation of high concentration of oxygen in experimental shock. Surgery *8:*247–256, Aug '40
WOOD, G. O. (see KNIGHT, M. P.) Oct '45
WOODARD, D. E.: Healing time of fractures of jaw in relation to delay before reduction, infection, syphilis and blood calcium and phosphorus content. J. Am. Dent. A. *18:*419–442, March '31
WOODARD, D. E.: Removable plaster headcap for facial fractures. J. Oral Surg. *2:*23–31, Jan '44
WOODBURN, J. J.: Use of packing in postoperative treatment in nasal surgery. M. J. Australia *2:*390–392, Sept 26, '31
WOODBURY, R. A. (see VOLPITTO, P. P. *et al*) Jan '40

WOODEN, W. AND HUTCHENS, D. K.: Bilateral complete cervical fistulae. Am. J. Surg. *3:*377–378, Oct '27
WOODHALL, B. AND CRAMER, F. J.: Extradural pneumatocele following tantalum cranioplasty. J. Neurosurg. *2:*524–529, Nov '45
WOODHALL, B. AND LYONS, W. R.: Peripheral nerve injuries; results of "early" nerve suture; preliminary report. Surgery *19:*757–789, June '46
WOODHALL, B. (see HARRIS, M. H.) March '45
WOODHALL, B. (see SPURLING, R. G.) 1946
WOODHALL, B. (see SPURLING, R. G.) May '46
WOODMAN, E. M.: Plastic repair after operations on upper jaw. Proc. Roy. Soc. Med. (Sect. Laryng.) *24:*11–14, Feb '31 also: J. Laryng. and Otol. *46:*405–409, June '31
WOODRUFF, L. M. AND GIBSON, S. T.: Human albumin in military medicine; clinical evaluation (burns). U. S. Nav. M. Bull. *40:*791–796, Oct '42
WOODRUFF, L. M. AND GIBSON, S. T.: Use of human albumin in military medicine; clinical evaluation. Army M. Bull. (no. 68) pp. 234–240, July '43
WOODS, R.: Aids to palatal sufficiency after cleft palate operations. Brit. M. J. *1:*371–372, Feb 26, '27
WOODS, S. H.: Jaw fractures; types, causes, locations and treatment of 76 recent cases. J. Roy. Army M. Corps *68:*366–378, June '37
WOODSON, L. M.: Hand infections. J. Tennessee M. A. *18:*112–114, Aug '25
WOODSON, W. H. (see GRISWOLD, R. A.) Feb '43
WOODWARD, C. M.: Surgical and prosthetic interference for correction of excessive protrusion of maxilla. Dental Digest *37:*213–218, April '31
WOODWARD, C. M.: New devices for reduction of maxillary fractures. Mil. Surgeon *87:*525–531, Dec '40
WOODWARD, C. S.: Plea for skin-grafting. Texas State J. Med. *20:*445–446, Dec '24
WOODWARD, F. D.: Management of recent fractures of nose and sinuses. Ann. Otol., Rhin. and Laryng. *44:*264–273, March '35
WOODWARD, F. D. AND ARCHER, V. W.: Results of treatment of malignant tumors of larynx and hypopharynx. Virginia M. Monthly *67:*751–755, Dec '40
WOODWARD, F. D. AND FITZ-HUGH, G. S.: Management of recent faciomaxillary and mandibular fractures. Virginia M. Monthly *69:*612–619, Nov '42
WOOLF, J. I. AND WALKER, A. E.: Cranioplasty; metallic inserts Rev. oto-neuro-oftal. *21:*16–18, Jan–Feb '46
WOOLHOUSE, F. M.: Reconstruction of hand; early surfacing of burns. Am. Acad. Orthop. Surgeons, Lect., pp. 187–190, '44
WOOLHOUSE, F. M. (see FARMER, A. W. *et al*) March '43
WOOLHOUSE, F. M. (see FARMER, A. W.) July '45
WOOLSEY, J. H.: Traumatic fracture of mandible, preoperative preparation; type of bone-graft; adaption of bone-graft. S. Clin. N. America *2:*333–340, April '22 (illus.)
WOOLSEY, J. H.: Congenital cleft lip and palate. California and West. Med. *26:*633–636, May '27
WOOLSEY, J. H.: Webbed fingers. Am. J. Surg. *8:*307–309, Feb '30
WOOLSEY, J. H.: Free skin grafts of less than full thickness; causes for failure or success. California and West. Med. *36:*334–337, May '32
WOOLSEY, R. D. (see KLEMME, R. M. *et al*) Oct '43
WOOLSTON, W. H. (see MASON, M. L.) Oct '27
WORD, B.: Construction of artificial vagina; modification of Wharton operation; 3 cases. South. M. J. *33:*293–301, March '40
WORD, B.: Silver-plated vaginal prosthesis for construction of artificial vagina. Am. J. Obst. and Gynec. *39:*1071, June '40
WORKMAN, J. B.: Treatment of burns. J. S. Carolina M. A. *17:*176, July '21
WORMAN, H. G.; WALDRON, C. W. AND RADUSCH, D. F.: Osteoma of mandibular condyle with deviation and prognathic deformity; case. J. Oral Surg. *4:*27–32, Jan '46
WORMS, G.: Plastic surgery of orbital cavity with dermo-epidermal grafts. Bull. Soc. d'opht. de Paris, pp. 358–361, June '32
WORMS, G.: Atypical facial hemiatrophy of sympathetic origin. Rev. d'oto-neuro-opht. *11:*99–103, Feb '33
WORONYTSCH, N.: Internal plastic surgery of tarsus in posttrachomatous entropion and trichiasis. Ztschr. f. Augenh. *84:*58–72, Aug '34

Wound

Influence of nasal bacteria on healing process of surgical wounds. LAKOS, T. Z. Ztschr. f. Hals-, Nasen-u. Ohrenh. *23:*426–435, Sept 10, '29
Repair of cutaneous defects. HAYWARD. Med. Klin. *25:*1365, Aug 30; 1397, Sept 6, '29
Technic for epithalisation with grafts in cases of skin defects. LANG, M. Dermat. Wchnschr. *91:*1478–1483, Oct 4, '30
Method of drying surface of wound before application of Thiersch grafts. LAPP, F. W. AND NEUFFER, H. Zentralbl. f. Chir. *58:*1634–1635, June 27, '31

Wound—Cont.
Value of primary skin grafts in fresh cutaneous wounds. Brzhozovskiy, A. A. Sovet. khir., no. 7, pp. 72–73, '35
Skin grafts in cutaneous wounds. Vaynshteyn, V. G. Sovet. khir., no. 9, pp. 62–65, '35
Good dressing for wounds produced by electrocoagulation. Hollander, L. Arch. Dermat. and Syph. *33:*730, April '36
Skin grafts in évidement cavity with proud flesh; case. Lemoine, J. Ann. d'oto-laryng., pp. 1085–1088, Nov '38
Epithelization of granulating and fresh wounds with skin from blisters. Jensen, W. Zentralbl. f. Chir. *67:*1399–1401, July 27, '40
Combination of burns and wounds; treatment. Flemming, C. Proc. Roy. Soc. Med. *34:*53, Nov '40
Wound closure, with particular reference to avoidance of scars. Updegraff, H. L. Am. J. Surg. *50:*749–753, Dec '40
Dressing of open wounds and burns with tulle gras. Matthews, D. N. Lancet *1:*43–44, Jan 11, '41
Collodion as dressing for skin grafting of granulating wounds. Ellis, S. S. and von Wedel, C., J. Oklahoma M. A. *34:*103–105, March '41
Treatment of 100 war wounds and burns. Ross, J. A. and Hulbert, K. F. Brit. M. J. *1:*618–621, April 26, '41
Italian method of plastic repair of denuded areas followed by mermaid cast immobilization. Murphy, F. G. Surgery *12:*294–301, Aug '42
Treatment of raw surfaces. Koch, S. L. J. Iowa M. Soc. *32:*445–450, Oct '42
Wound infection; preliminary note on combined clinical and bacteriologic investigation of 708 wounds (and burns). de Waal, H. L. Edinburgh M. J. *50:*577–588, Oct '43
Prevention of infection in wounds, fractures and burns (report on 1500 cases, especially evaluation of sulfonamides). Meleney, F. L. Bull. U. S. Army M. Dept. (no. 72) pp. 41–46, Jan '44
Healing of surface cutaneous wounds (donor areas); analogy with healing of superficial burns. Converse, J. M. and Robb-Smith, A. H. T. Ann. Surg. *120:*873–885, Dec '44
Initial care of wounds from reconstructive viewpoint. Gallagher, J. L. Rev. san. mil., Buenos Aires *43:*1629–1636, Dec '44
Rayon, ideal surgical dressing for surface wounds. Owens, N. Surgery *19:*482–485, April '46
Split skin grafts in early closure of wounds. Harbison, S. P. and Oden, L. H., Jr. Bull. U. S. Army M. Dept. *6:*88–90, July '46
Use of cellophane in treatment of wounds. Chistyakov, N. L. Am. Rev. Soviet Med. *3:*490–493, Aug '46
Skin dressings (split grafts) in treatment of debrided wounds. Gay, E. C. Am. J. Surg. *72:*212–218, Aug '46

Wound Healing
Influence of mechanical pressure on wound healing. Blair, V. P. Illinois M. J. *46:*249–252, Oct '24
Case of Reverdin skin grafting exhibited in Dr. Halsted's clinic on wound healing. Brödel, M. Bull. Johns Hopkins Hosp. *36:*60, Jan '25
Repair processes in wounds of tendons and in tendon grafts. Garlock, J. H. Ann. Surg. *85:*92–103, Jan '27
Simpler technic for promoting epithelization and protecting skin grafts (oxyquinoline sulphate scarlet R ointment). Bettman, A. G., J.A.M.A. *97:*1879–1881, Dec 19, '31
Thiocresol in wound healing and in skin grafting. Birnbaum, I. R. Ann. Surg. *96:*467–470, Sept '32
Healing of surface wounds for prevention of deformities. Beekman, F. and O'Connell, R. J. Jr. Ann. Surg. *98:*394–407, Sept '33
Conservative and radical measures for treatment of ulcer of leg; critical study of healing in experimental and human wounds under elastic adhesive plaster. Douglas, B. Arch. Surg. *32:*756–775, May '36
Successful application of regeneration theory (plastic surgery). von Ertl, J. Arch. f. klin. Chir. *189:*398–400, '37
Use of tubed pedicle flaps for study of wound healing in human skin. Sutton, L. E. New York State J. Med. *40:*852–859, June 1, '40
Substances promoting formation of skin. Sainz de Aja, E. A. Actas dermo-sif. *32:*229–233, Dec '40
Skin transplantation by injection; effect on healing of granulating wounds. Barber, C. G. Arch. Surg. *43:*21–31, July '41
Speed of repair of wounds of mucosa in mouth. Maj, G. Boll. Soc. ital. biol. sper. *17:*322, May '42
Epithelial healing and transplantation. Brown, J. B. and McDowell, F. Ann. Surg. *115:*1166–1181, June '42
Effects of pregnancy hormones on healing process; experimental and clinical studies (of skin). Vurchio, G. Ginecologia *8:*237–246, June '42

Wound Healing – Cont.

Rate of epithelial regeneration; clinical method of measurement, and effect of various agents recommended in treatment. CANNON, B. AND COPE, O. Ann. Surg. *117:*85-92, Jan '43

Role of neuroma in evolution of wounds. WEISS, A. G. AND WARTER, J. Bull. War Med. *3:*607, July '43 (abstract)

Effect of different agents on rate of epithelial regeneration; use of dermatome donor area in obtaining clinical data. BAXTER, H. *et al*. Canad. M. A. J. *50:*411-415, May '44

Clinical value of growth-promoting substance (H. E. P.) in treatment of indolent wounds. KERR, A. B. AND WERNER, H. Brit. J. Surg. *32:*281-287, Oct '44

Clinical value of growth-promoting substance (H. E. P.) in treatment of indolent wounds. KERR, A. B. AND WERNER, H. Rev. san. mil., Buenos Aires *44:*461-475, April '45

Plastic trend in wound therapy. ZENO, L. Salud y belleza *1:*25-31, April-May '45

Effect of experimental sleep on healing of skin defects in man. POLYAKOV, K. L. Voen.-med. sborn. *2:*223-233, '45

Healing of skin defects; experimental study on white rat. LINDQUIST, G. Acta chir. Scandinav. (supp. 107) *94:*1-163, '46

WREDE, L.: Late results of fat transplantation in breast surgery. Deutsche Ztschr. f. Chir. *203-204:*672-685, '27

WRETE, M.: Congenital absence of fifth finger. Upsala Lakaref. Forh. *32:*285-294, March '27

WRIGHT, A. D.: Forceps for skin grafts. Lancet *1:*840, April 16, '32

WRIGHT, A. D.: Forceps for skin grafts. Indian M. Gaz. *67:*479-480, Aug '32

WRIGHT, A. D.: Hernia cerebri treated by Thiersch grafts. Proc. Roy. Soc. Med. *32:*213-214, Jan '39

WRIGHT, A. D. (see HARRIS, W.) March '32

WRIGHT, C. B.: Fractures of mandible. West Virginia M. J. *29:*525-526, Dec '33

WRIGHT, C. F.: Occlusal reduction in management of jaw fractures. Angle Orthodontist *7:*67-80, April '37

WRIGHT, D. G. (see BOND, D. D.) April '38

WRIGHT, H. B.: Cleft palate found in only one of identical twins. Internat. J. Orthodontia *20:*649-657, July '34

WRIGHT, H. W. S.: Peripheral nerve injuries; treatment. M. Press *211:*228-230, April 12, '44

WRIGHT, I. S. (see PRATT, G. H.) Feb '41

WRIGHT, R. E.: Buediner's modification of Dieffenbach's operation for early epithelioma of lower lid. Brit. J. Ophth. *8:*58-61, Feb '24

WRIGHT, R. E.: Dacrocystorhinostomy. Lancet *2:*250-251, July 31, '37

WRIGHT, T.: Congenital absence of vagina, accompanied by marked nervous syptoms; Baldwin's operation and removal of ovarian tissue. Am. J. Surg. *36:*114-115, May '22

WRIGHT, W. A.: Burn therapy. Journal-Lancet *57:*449-450, Oct '37

WRIGHT, W. W.: Use of living sutures in treatment of eyelid ptosis. Arch. Ophth. *51:*99-102, March '22 (illus.)

WRIGHT-SMITH, R. J.: Epithelioma of lip with visceral metastases. J. Coll. Surgeons, Australasia *2:*421-424, March '30

Wringer Injuries

Wringer arm; report of 26 cases (with special reference to technic of razor skin graft). MACCOLLUM, D. W. New England J. Med. *218:*549-554, March 31, '38

Wrist Drop

Tendon transplants for paralytic wrist drop; presentation of patient. SWART, H. A. AND HENDERSON, M. S. Proc. Staff Meet., Mayo Clin. *9:*377-379, June 27, '34

Wrist drop, case of posterior interosseous paralysis. HOBHOUSE, N. AND HEALD, C. B. Brit. M. J. *1:*841, April 25, '36

Temporary wrist drop, operation and prompt recovery. YOHANNAN, J. I., U. S. Nav. M. Bull. *15:*547, July '21

Wrist-drop; graft of 15 cm. of rabbit's spinal cord and infiltration of stellate ganglion followed by rapid recovery; case. SOUBIRAN. J. de med. de Bordeaux *116:*353-354, Nov 4-25, '39

Easily made "drop-wrist" splint. ELLIOT, H. Canad. M. A. J. *47:*363, Oct '42

New elastic splint for wrist drop. MAYFIELD, F. H. Bull. U. S. Army M. Dept. (no. 73) pp. 96-97, Feb '44

WRONG, N. M.: Treatment of hemangiomas of skin in children by carbon dioxide snow. Canad. M. A. J. *41:*571-572, Dec '39

WUCHERPFENNIG, V.: Permanent epilation of hair for cosmetic purposes. (Reply to Zoon). Dermat. Wchnschr. *99:*933-934, July 14, '34

WUCHERPFENNIG, V. (see STÜHMER, A.) Nov '30

WUEHRMANN, A. H. (see LAZANSKY, J. P.) March '46

WUEHRMANN, A. H. (see LAZANSKY, J. P. *et al*) March '46

WUHRMANN, H.: Use of splints in complicated maxillary fracture. Schweiz. med. Wchnschr. *62:*767-769, Aug. 20, '32

WULFF, H.: Traumatic lesions of frequent occurrence to fingers and their treatment, especially after-treatment. Ugesk. f. laeger *97:*405–411, April 4, '35
WULLE, H.: Authorization of physician to perform plastic, and particularly cosmetic operations. Med. Welt *8:*132, Jan 27; 171, Feb 3, '34
WUSTROW, P.: Functional therapy of jaw fractures. Ztschr. f. Stomatol. *36:*1171–1190, Oct 28, '38
WYBURN, G. M. (see BARNES, R. *et al*) Oct '45
WYCIS, H. T. (see SCOTT, M.) July '46
WYMER, I.: Surgical correction of prognathism; 2 cases. Deutsche Ztschr. f. Chir. *215:*226–233, '29
WYNNE, F. E.: Non-operative treatment of fractures of forearm and hand. J. M. A. S. Africa *1:*582–584, Nov 26, '27

X

Xanthomas

Isolated giant cell xanthomatic tumors of fingers and hand. MASON, M. L. AND WOOLSTON, W. H. Arch. Surg. *15:*499–529, Oct '27

XICLUNA, R. (see CABANES, E.) July '39

Y

YACHNIN, S. C. AND SUMMERILL, F.: Traumatic implantation of epithelial cyst in phalanx. J.A.M.A. *116:*1215–1218, March 22, '41
YADAROLA, D. (see BERTOLA, V. *et al*) Oct '36
YAMANAKA, K.: "Pocket ear"; case. Oto-rhino-laryng. (abstr. sect) *13:* n.p., Feb '40
YAMASAKI, Y.: Acute purulent parotitis caused by facial trauma; case. Oto-rhino-laryng. *10:*1027, Nov '37
YAMBAO, C. V. (see AYUYAO, C. D.) Aug '41
YANDELL, H. R.: Burn therapy experience from South Pacific area. U. S. Nav. M. Bull. *42:*829–837, April '44
YANDO, A. H. AND TAYLOR, R. W.: Fractures of maxillae and mandible; 2 cases (with description of apparatus). U. S. Nav. M. Bull. *40:*155–157, Jan '42
YANES, T. R.: Paradoxic monocular ptosis. Arch. Ophth. *23:*1169–1172, June '40
YANES, T. R.: Dacryocystorhinostomy; interesting points on operation. Arch. Ophth. *26:*12–20, July '41
YANES, T. R.: Dacryocystorhinostomy versus dacryocystectomy. Vida nueva *49:*132–136, April '42
YANO, S.: Homotransplantation of skin of rabbit embryo into bone marrow. Tr. Soc. path. jap. *30:*746–747, '40
YAP, S. E. AND PINEDA, E. V.: 2 interesting cases of ectrosyndactyly. Philippine J. Sc. *20:*1–13, Jan '22 (illus.)
YARITSYN, A. A.: Muscle-nerve graft in paralysis of facial nerve. Vestnik-khir. *39:*132–134, '35
YATER, W. M. AND CAVANAGH, J. R.: Progressive facial hemiatrophy; case. M. Ann. District of Columbia *1:*236–239, Sept '32
YAVLINSKIY, A. L.: Principles governing first aid of facial injuries. Ortop. i travmatol. (no. 1) *7:*43–45, '33
YEARSLEY, M.: Essentials of nasal septal operations. Practitioner *121:*178–182, Sept '28
YEARSLEY, M.: Submucous resection in children. Practitioner *129:*581–583, Nov '32
YEARSLEY, M.: Essential points in submucous resection. M. Press *197:*518–520, Dec 7, '38
YEMM, W. A.: Burn therapy in war. Physiotherapy Rev. *23:*13–16, Jan–Feb '43
YGLESIAS, L. (see COLLER, F. A.) Feb '35
YMAZ, J. I. (see IMAZ, J. I.)
YODH, B. B.: Shock and its treatment. Indian Physician *1:*547–554, Dec '42
YOEL, J.: Therapy of shortness of frenum of penis. Prensa med. argent. *32:*2539–2540, Dec 21, '45
YOHANNAN, J. I.: Temporary wrist drop, operation and prompt recovery. U. S. Nav. M. Bull. *15:*547, July '21
YOKOTA, K.: Syndactylia combined with macrodactyly in patient with fibrolipoma of right foot. Taiwan Igakkai Zasshi (Abstr. Sect.) *33:*5, Feb '34
YOKOTA, K. AND HASAMA, T.: Hypospadias, case. Mitt. a. d. med. Akad. zu Kioto *15:*906, '35
YONIS, Z.: Burns in childhood. Harefuah *15:*ii–iii, July–Aug '38
YORNET, H. (see DIONISI, H.) 1943
YOSHIDA, S.: New suction elevator for otorhinolaryngologic operations. Oto-rhino-laryng. *11:*651, July '38
YOUNG, A.: Whole-skin method of grafting. Proc. Internat. Assemb. Inter-State Post-Grad. M. A., North America (1928), pp. 217–233, '29
YOUNG, C. T.: Shock. Hawaii M. J. *2:*22–25, Sept–Oct '42
YOUNG, EDNA H.: *Overcoming Cleft Palate Speech.* Hill-Young School, Minneapolis, 1928
YOUNG, F.: Problems of unilateral harelip repair. Surg., Gynec. and Obst. *65:*348–354, Sept '37
YOUNG, F.: Surgical repair of long-disabled hand. Surg., Gynec. and Obst. *67:*73–81, July '38

YOUNG, F.: Principle to be considered in transplanting costal cartilage for repairing deficiencies of nasal skeleton. Ann. Surg. *108:*1113–1117, Dec '38

YOUNG, F.: Autogenous cartilage grafts; experimental study. Surgery *10:*7–20, July '41

YOUNG, F.: Treatment of persistent recurrent basal cell carcinoma. Surg., Gynec. and Obst. *73:*152–162, Aug '41

YOUNG, F.: Function of lower jaw following partial resection. Surgery *11:*966–982, June '42

YOUNG, F.: Immediate skin grafting in burns; preliminary report. Ann. Surg. *116:*445–451, Sept '42

YOUNG, F.: Function of lower jaw following partial resection. Am. J. Orthodontics (Oral Surg. Sect.) *28:*581–598, Oct '42

YOUNG, F.: Fixation of skin grafts by plasma-thrombin adhesion. Tr. Am. S. A. *62:*450–462, '44

YOUNG, F.: Correction of abnormally prominent ears. Surg., Gynec. and Obst. *78:*541–550, May '44

YOUNG, F.: Cast and precast cartilage grafts; use in restoration of contour of face. Surgery *15:*735–748, May '44

YOUNG, F.: Fixation of skin grafts by plasma-thrombin adhesion. Ann. Surg. *120:*450–462, Oct '44

YOUNG, F.: Homogenous cartilage grafts; experimental study. Surgery *17:*616–621, April '45

YOUNG, F.: Transplantation of toes for fingers. Surg. *20:*117–123, July '46

YOUNG, F.: Repair of nasal losses. Surgery *20:*670–683, Nov '46

YOUNG, F. AND FAVATA, B. V.: Fixation of skin grafts by thrombin-plasma adhesion. Surgery *15:*378–386, March '44

YOUNG, F. AND SCOTT, W. J. M.: Radical operation for intractable pruritis ani (skin transplantation). Surgery *13:*911–915, June '43

YOUNG, G.: An operation for congenital eyelid ptosis. Brit. J. Ophth. *8:*272–275, June '24

YOUNG, H. A. (see KAZANJIAN, V. H. *et al*) Oct '32

YOUNG, H. H.: Operation for cure of incontinence associated with epispadias. J. Urology *7:*1–32, Jan '22

YOUNG, H. H.: Nasal drill for removal of septal spur. J.A.M.A. *80:*1216, April 28, '23 (illus.)

YOUNG, H. H.: Screw curet; use in curettage and in excision of fistulous tracts. J.A.M.A. *93:*110–113, July 13, '29

YOUNG, H. H.: Abnormalities and plastic surgery of lower urogenital tract (Ramon Guiteras lecture). J. Urol. *35:*417–480, April '36

YOUNG, H. H.: Imperforate anus, bowel opening into urethra; hypospadias; presentation of new plastic methods. J.A.M.A. *107:*1448–1451, Oct 31, '36

YOUNG, H. H.: Treatment of hypospadias. J. Urol. *42:*470–473, Sept '39

YOUNG, H. H.: Tendon transplantation for radial nerve paralysis. Proc. Staff Meet., Mayo Clin. *15:*26–28, Jan 10, '40

YOUNG, H. H.: Operative treatment of true hermaphroditism and new technic for curing hypospadias. Arch. Surg. *41:*557–568, Aug '40

YOUNG, H. H.: Plastic operations for exstrophy of bladder. Proc. Interst. Postgrad. M. A. North America (1941) pp. 241–244, '42

YOUNG, H. H.: First case of exstrophy of bladder in which normal bladder and urinary control have been obtained by plastic operation. Surg., Gynec. and Obst. *74:*729–737, March '42

YOUNG, H. H.: Surgical treatment of elephantiasis. Tr. Am. A. Genito-Urin. Surgeons (1943) *36:*169–173, '44

YOUNG, H. H. AND CASH, J. R.: Case of pseudohermaphrodismus masculinus, showing hypospadias, greatly enlarged utricle, abdominal testis and absence of seminal vesicles. J. Urology *5:*405, May '21

YOUNG, J. Z.: Effect of delay on success of suture of peripheral nerves. Proc. Roy. Soc. Med. *37:*551–552, Aug '44

YOUNG, J. Z.; HOLMES, W. AND SANDERS, F. K.: Nerve regeneration; importance of peripheral stump and value of nerve grafts. Lancet *2:*128–130, Aug 3, '40

YOUNG, J. Z. (see HOLMES, W.) Oct '42

YOUNG, J. Z. (see SANDERS, F. K.) Jan '42

YOUNG, J. Z. (see SANDERS, F. K.) July–Aug '43

YOUNG, J. Z. (see SEDDON, H. J. *et al*) April '42

YOUNG, W. J.: Treatment of basal epithelioma of face. Kentucky M. J. *19:*154, April '21

YOUNG, W. J.: Epithelioma of face and ear. Kentucky M. J. *20:*367–368, May '22

Young Operation

Operative treatment of anal stricture (modification of Young operation). JOSEPH, E. S. Acta med. orient. *4:*312–313, Sept '45

Young's Operation

Young's operation for eyelid ptosis; case. BUTLER, T. H. Tr. Ophth. Soc. U. Kingdom *47:*387, '27

YOVANOVICH, B. Y.: Surgical therapy of Dupuytren's contracture. Voj.-san. glasnik *7:*331–347, '36

YOVANOVITCH, I. (see PETROVITCH, G.) July–

Dec '30
Yovtchitch, J.: Coffey operation in exstrophy of bladder; case. Mem. Acad. de chir. *65:*368-369, March 8, '39
Yow, E. M.: Prevention and treatment of secondary shock. J. Bowman Gray School Med. *1:*31-37, March '43
Yudilevich, S. L. (see Mazel, Z. A. *et al*) 1935
Yuhara, K.: Experimental studies on influence of previous fractures on behavior of transplants of bone. Tr. Soc. path. jap. *30:*738-741, '40
Yusevich, M. S.: Technic of application of Filatov flaps in plastic operations on amputation-stumps of hands and fingers. Ortop. i. travmatol. (no. 3) *14:*50-56, '40

Z

Z-Plasty
Correction of burn scar deformity by Z-plastic method. McCurdy, S. L., J. Bone and Joint Surg. *6:*683-688, July '24
Relaxation of scar contractures by means of Z-, or reversed Z-type incision; stressing use of scar infiltrated tissues. Davis, J. S. Ann. Surg. *94:*871-884, Nov '31
Z plastic or web splitting operation for relief of scar contractures of extremities. Jones, H. T. Surg., Gynec. and Obst. *58:*178-182, Feb '34
Theory and practical use of Z-incision for relief of contractures. Davis, J. S. and Kitlowski, E. A. Ann. Surg. *109:*1001-1015, June '39
Z-shaped incision in plastic surgery for cicatricial contracture. Marino, H. Rev. Assoc. med. argent. *55:*208-211, March 15-30, '41
Roentgenograms of mandibular condyle and zygomatic arch in jaw fractures. McGrail, F. R. and Doherty, J. A. Am. J. Roentgenol. *45:*637-639, April '41
Deficiency of malar bones with defect of lower eyelids. Johnstone, I. L. Brit. J. Ophth. *27:*21-23, Jan '43
Skin transposition in incisional defects; modification of Z plastic for primary skin closure following extensive breast surgery. Sinaiko, E. S. Surgery *18:*650-652, Nov '45
Present evaluation of merits of Z-plastic operation (for scar contractures). Davis, J. S. Plast. and Reconstruct. Surg. *1:*26-38, July '46
Release of circular constricting scar by Z flaps. Stevenson, T. W. Plastic and Reconstruct. Surg. *1:*39-42, July '46

Zaaijer, J. H.: Modified operation for ectopia vesicae. Zentralbl. f. Chir. *50:*114-115, Jan 27, '23 (illus.)
Zaaijer, J. H.: Surgical treatment of protruding ears. Nederl. tijdschr. v. geneesk. *74:*5572-5575, Nov 15, '30
Zacharinas, B.: Treatment of lacerated wounds of hands. Medicina, Kaunas *11:*39-41, Jan '30
Zachary, R. B.: Tendon transplant for radial paralysis. Brit. J. Surg. *33:*358-364, April '46
Zacher, K. (see Löhr, W.) Jan '39
Zadik, F. R.: Immediate skin grafting for traumatic amputation of finger tips. Lancet *1:*335-336, March 13, '43
Zagami, A.: Surgical therapy of hand injuries. Riv. san. siciliana *24:*295-312, March 15, '36
Zagdoun, J. (see Bloch, J. C.) March '36
Zagni, L.: Plastic operation for ulcerative epithelioma of upper lip and cheek. Stomatol. *25:*591-594, July '27
Zahradniček, J.: Surgical treatment of prognathism and of lack of articulation of incisors. Cas. lek. cesk. *62:*1361-1368, Dec 15, '23
Zahradniček, J.: Treatment of funnel-shaped chest. Cas. lek. cesk. *64:*1814-1817, Dec 12, '25 abstr: J.A.M.A. *86:*456, Feb 6, '26
Zahradniček, J.: Surgical treatment of facial paralysis. Casop. lek. cesk. *66:*592-594, March 28, '27
Zahumenszky, E.: Extension apparatus for therapy of fractures of phalangeal and metacarpal bones. Orvosi hetil. *76:*629-630, July 16, '32
Zakharov, A. P.: Late results of Snellen and Millingen-Sapezhko operations for correction of trachomatous entropion. Sovet. vestnik oftal. *4:*491-497, '34
Zakharov, A. P. (see Askalonova, T. M.) 1939
Zalewski, F.: Extensive X-ray burns; repeated blood transfusions. Rev. de chir., Paris *68:*75-79, '30
Zambrini, A. R.: Technic of resection of nasal septum. Semana med. *1:*1153-1155, April 30, '31
Zambrini, A. R., and Casterán, E.: Sequestra and suppurative mucocele in frontal sinus following fracture; operation; case. Rev. Asoc. med. argent. *46:*788-789, Aug '32
Zamkov, A. A.: Skin grafts. Sovet. khir. *4:*51-57, '33
Zamoshchin, M. B.: Covering cutaneous defect after avulsion of skin of thumb. Novy khir. arkhiv *46:*260-262, '40
Zampa, G.: Bifid and supernumerary fingers. Chir. d. org. di movimento *13:*195-212, Dec '28
Zampa, G.: Lateral cyst of neck of thyroid ori-

gin. Policlinico (sez. chir.) *36:*51-60, Jan '29
ZANGE, J.: Plastic covering of large defects in laryngeal tube; case. Ztschr. f. Hals-, Nasen-u. Ohrenh. *21:*638-651, May 10, '28
ZANOLI, R.: Late results of tendon transplantation; study based on 95 cases. Arch. ital. di chir. *54:*907-914, '38
ZANUSO, F.: Repairs of severed tendons without suture. Osp. maggiore *17:*44, Feb 28, '29
ZARAZAGA, J.: Bettman therapy in burns; results in 5 cases. Dia med. *10:*1316-1317, Dec 19, '38
ZARENKO, P. P.: Compression treatment of fracture of superior maxilla resulting from blow; case. Arch. f. klin. Chir. *153:*161-169, '28
ZARZYCKI, P.: Technic of dacryocystostomy. Bull. Soc. d'opht. de Paris *49:*9-12, Jan '37
ZARZYCKI, P.: Lacrimal laminaria in surgical therapy of stricture of nasal canal. Bull. Soc. d'opht. de Paris *50:*306-310, June '38
ZATLOUKAL, F.: Facial hemiatrophy and its therapy. Casop. lek. cesk. *76:*553-563, May 7, '37
ZATS, L. B.: Imre operation for ectropion of lower eyelid. Vestnik oftal. *13:*554-557, '38
ZATSEPIN, T. S.: Operation for irreducible contractures of fingers. Khirurgiya, No. 5, pp. 81-83, '45
ZAUSMER, E.: Functional reeducation of transplanted tendons. Physiotherapy Rev. *25:*160-164, July-Aug '45
ZAVALETA, D. E.: Clinical study of burns. Dia med. *11:*162-168, Feb 27, '39
ZAVALETA, D. E.: Diagnosis and surgical therapy of parotid tumors. Rev. med. y cien. afines *2:*422-424, June 30, '40
ZAVALETA, D. E.: Sistrunk operation (parotid); case. Prensa med. argent. *32:*1331-1334, July 13, '45
ZAVALETA, D. E. (see AGUILAR, H.) Jan '34
ZAVALETA, D. E. (see FINOCHIETTO, R.) May '40
ZAVALETA, D. E. (see FINOCHIETTO, R. *et al*) Dec '41
ZAYCHENKO, I. L.: Fractures of digital phalanges. Ortop. i travmatol. (no. 2) *7:*34-48, '33
ZAYTSEV, G. P.: Classification of acute inflammatory processes in hand. Novy khir. arkhiv *31:*394-399, '34
ZAYTSEV, G. P.: Symptoms and therapy of acute purulent diseases of hands and fingers. Sovet. vrach. zhur., pp. 422-428, March 30, '36
ZBOROWSKY, W. F.: Treatment of spastic entropion by Weeker's method. Klin. Monatsbl. f. Augenh. *80:*648-651, May 25, '28
ZDRAVOMYSLOFF, V. I.: Artificial vagina formation by Popoff's method and its remote results. J. akush, i zhensk. boliez. *39:*333-344, '28
ZEBOLD, A.: Resection of phalanges as method of treating skin defects of fingers. Vestnik khir. *39:*204-205, '35
ZECCHINO, V. (see BEARDSLEY, J. M.) June '46
ZECHEL, G.: Hypospadias operation. Arch. f. klin. Chir. *153:*491-494, '28
ZEE, Z. U.: New technic for obtaining small deep grafts. Chinese M. J. *50:*935-938, July '36
ZEEMAN, W. P. C.: Ptosis of eyelids. Nederl. tijdschr. v. geneesk. *83:*2714-2720, June 10, '39
ZEISS, C. R.: Burn treatment (with paraffin dressing). Illinois M. J. *78:*540-544, Dec '40
ZELLE, O. L. AND SCHNEPP, K. H.: Snapping thumb; tendovaginitis stenosans. Am. J. Surg. *33:*321-322, Aug '36
ZELLER, O.: Replacement of missing urethra in patient with scrotal hypospadias by pedicled flaps from bladder wall; case. Med. Welt *9:*565-567, April 20, '35
ZELLER, W. E. (see JOYCE, T. M. *et al*) Feb '41

Zeller Operation

Modifications of Zeller operation in therapy of syndactylia. PALMA, R. Ann. ital. di chir. *13:*1068-1074, Sept 30, '34

ZEMAN, J.: Care of jaw wounds in wartime. Ztschr. f. Stomatol. *37:*1169-1173, Aug, 25, '39
ZENKER, R.: Results of surgical therapy of severe forms of hypospadias by means of plastic transplantation of epidermis. Chirurg *6:*576-578, Aug 15, '34
ZENKINA, L. V.: Therapy of ocular burns by transplantation of conjunctiva from cadaver. Vestnik oftal. (no. 2) *15:*28-29, '39
ZENO, L. O.: Tendon transplantation by physiologic method with cinematographic projection. Rev. med. del Rosario *20:*310-313, July '30
ZENO, L.: Biologic therapy of burns; rest and immobilization with plaster of paris bandaging. An. de cir. *3:*228-232, Sept '37
ZENO, L.: Corrective rhinoplasty. An. de cir. *3:*357-363, Dec '37
ZENO, L.: Plastic surgery of nose. An. de otorino-laring. d. Uruguay *8:*225-235, '38
ZENO, L.: Plastic surgery of double lip. An. de cir. *4:*11-13, March '38
ZENO, L.: Plastic surgery of cutaneous lesion of leg due to amniotic adhesions. An. de cir. *4:*14-15, March '38
ZENO, L.: Plastic surgery in loss of bone substance of cranium. An. de cir. *4:*16-18, March '38
ZENO, L.: Plastic surgery. An. de cir. *4:*65-74, June '38
ZENO, L.: Saddle nose, flattened nose and lat-

eral deviation; surgical therapy. An. de cir. *4:*128–133, June '38
ZENO, L.: Facial asymmetry; plastic surgery (including jaws). An. de cir. *4:*134–136, June '38
ZENO, L.: Plaster cast in therapy of nasal fractures. An. de cir. *4:*124–127, June '38 also: Bol. Soc. de cir. de Rosario *5:*269–272, July '38
ZENO, L.: Technic of surgical correction of nasal deformities. Bol. Soc. de cir. de Rosario *5:*345–348, Aug '38
ZENO, L.: Plastic surgery (nose). Rev. Asoc. med. argent. *52:*902–907, Sept 15, '38
ZENO, L.: Plaster casts in simple and complicated burns. Bol. y trab. de la Soc. de cir. de Buenos Aires *22:*712–722, Sept 28, '38
ZENO, L.: Biologic therapy in burns; rest and immobilization in plaster cast. Arq. brasil. de cir. e ortop. *6:*295–300, Sept–Dec '38
ZENO, L.: Skin grafts and suspension of labial commissure by skin sutures for facial paralysis. An. de cir. *4:*187–189, Sept '38 Also: Bol. Soc. de cir. de Rosario *5:*412–414, Oct '38
ZENO, L.: Lop ear; psychologic importance of early surgical correction. An. de cir. *4:*190–192, Sept '38 also: Bol. Soc. de cir. de Rosario *5:*429–431, Oct '38
ZENO, L.: Corrective plastic surgery of nasal lobe. An. de cir. *5:*3–14, March '39
ZENO, L.: Plastic surgery; progress in Argentina. An. de cir. *5:*82–84, March '39
ZENO, L.: Therapy of simple and complicated burns by means of plaster casts. Arch. urug. de med., cir. y especialid. *14:*322–324, March '39
ZENO, L.: Traumatic tear of ala nasi and of tip; surgical repair in case. An. de cir. *5:*15–16, March '39 also: Bol. Soc. de cir. de Rosario *6:*8–9, April '39
ZENO, L.: Marble prosthesis in correction of saddle nose. Bol. y trab. de la Soc. de cir. de Buenos Aires *23:*332–338, June 21, '39 also: An. de cir. *5:*111–122, June '39
ZENO, L.: Free full thickness skin grafts in hand contracted by cicatrix; technical problems in case. Rev. ortop. y traumatol. *9:*73–77, July '39
ZENO, L.: Technic of free graft of whole skin for cicatricial contracture of hand. Bol. y trab., Soc. de cir. de Buenos Aires *23:*525–531, July 26, '39
ZENO, L.: Plastic surgery and esthetic feeling. An. de cir. *5:*199–211, Sept '39
ZENO, L.: Technic of full thickness free grafts for cicatricial contracture of hand. Semana med. *2:*829–831, Oct 12, '39
ZENO, L.: Plastic surgery in Italy. Bol. Soc. de cir. de Rosario *6:*430–438, Nov '39
ZENO, L.: Marble prosthesis in correction of saddle nose. Dia med. (Ed. espec., no. 9), pp. 170–171, Nov '39
ZENO, L.: Free full-thickness skin grafts; indications and technic. An. de cir. *5:*279–289, Dec '39
ZENO, L.: Plastic surgery in Italy. An. de cir. *5:*311–319, Dec '39
ZENO, L.: Indications and technic of full thickness free grafts of total skin. Dia med. *12:*214–215, March 18, '40 abstr: Rev. med. de Rosario *29:*1310–1314, Dec '39
ZENO, L.: Insertion "OSEO" in inferior maxilla. Bol. y trab., Acad. argent. de cir. *24:*248–258, May '40
ZENO, L.: Free full-thickness grafts of skin to eyelids; cases. Bol. Soc. de cir. de Rosario *7:*127–135, May '40 also: An. de cir. *6:*156–164, June '40
ZENO, L.: Clawhand; Morestin plastic surgery with free full-thickness skin graft. Bol. Soc. de cir. de Rosario *7:*308–315, Aug '40 also: An. de cir. *6:*315–321, Sept '40
ZENO, L.: Grave wounds of hands; biologic therapy. Bol. y trab., Acad. argent. de cir. *24:*639–652, Aug 7, '40
ZENO, L.: Nasal deformity in harelip; technic of plastic correction. Bol. Soc. de cir. de Rosario *7:*408–414, Oct '40 also: An. de cir. *6:*388–394, Dec '40
ZENO, L.: Paraffinoma of nose; surgical therapy of case. Bol. Soc. de cir. de Rosario *7:*415–418, Oct '40
ZENO, L.: Retractile scars of cervicofacial region; biologic fundamentals for plastic reconstruction. Bol. Soc. de cir. de Rosario *7:*446–454, Nov '40 also: An. de cir. *6:*341–349, Dec '40 also: Dia med. *13:*264–266, April 14, '41
ZENO, L.: Technic of pedicled flaps in plastic surgery of skin; use in treating cicatricial contracture of hand. Bol. y trab., Acad. argent. de cir. *24:*886–890, Sept 18, '40 also: Semana med. *2:*1058–1061, Nov 7, '40
ZENO, L.: Grave hand wounds and their biologic therapy. Dia med. *12:*1138–1141, Dec 9, '40
ZENO, L.: Biologic orientation in burn therapy in plastic surgery. Bol. y trab., Soc. argent. de cirujanos *2:*904–961, '41
ZENO, L.: Medical responsibility in plastic surgery. Rev. med. leg. y jurisp. med. *5:*17–24, Jan–June '41
ZENO, L.: Correction of asymmetric chins. Semana med. *1:*674–679, March 20, '41
ZENO, L.: Paraffinoma of nose; surgical therapy; cases. An. de cir. *7:*41–45, March–June '41
ZENO, L.: Graft of fat in correction of cicatricial depressions. An. de cir. *7:*47–51, March–June '41 also: Bol. Soc. de cir. de Rosario *8:*1–5, April '41
ZENO, L.: Rigid hand caused by fibrous cicatrix;

free graft of full-thickness skin. An. de cir. *7:*52–56, March–June '41 also: Bol. Soc. de cir. de Rosario *8:*53–58, April '41

Zeno, L.: Plastic surgery; medical responsibility. An. de cir. *7:*57–62, March–June '41

Zeno, L.: Prosthetic inclusions. Bol. Soc. de cir. de Rosario *8:*158–169, June '41

Zeno, L.: Transplantation of fat in correction of cicatricial depressions. Semana med. *1:*1324–1327, June 5, '41

Zeno, L.: Prosthetic inclusions in plastic surgery. An. de cir. *7:*108–118, Sept '41

Zeno, L.: Reconstruction of nasal tip and subseptum by means of tubular graft. An. de cir. *7:*183–190, Sept '41

Zeno, L.: Reconstruction of nasal tip and subseptum by means of tubular graft; case. Bol. y trab., Acad. argent. de cir. *25:*1028–1033, Sept 10, '41

Zeno, L.: Free graft of closely sutured skin in small rhinoplasties. Bol. Soc. de cir. de Rosario *8:*361–365, Oct '41 also: An. de cir. *7:*295–299, Dec '41

Zeno, L.: Plastic orientation in treatment of wounds. Arq. de cir. clin. e exper. *5:*97–123, Oct '41

Zeno, L.: Plastic surgery of face, with report of cases. Bol. Soc. de cir. de Rosario *8:*469–476, Nov '41 also: An. de cir. *7:*287–294, Dec '41

Zeno, L.: Sir Harold Gillies, surgeon examplatory. An. de cir. *7:*315–320, Dec '41 also: Semana med. *2:*1543–1546, Dec 25, '41

Zeno, L.: Hemiatrophy of face; graft of fat in therapy. An. de cir. *8:*52–57, March–June '42

Zeno, L.: Hypertelorism; case with median nasal fissure. An. de cir. *8:*37–39, March–June '42 also: Bol. Soc. de cir. de Rosario *9:*59–62, May '42

Zeno, L.: Plasticity of cicatricial tissue; application to reparative surgery. An. de cir. *8:*40–47, March–June '42

Zeno, L.: Anomalies of maxillary angle; Albrecht's lemurine apophysis. An. de cir. *8:*48–51, March–June '42

Zeno, L.: Plasticity of cicatricial tissue; application to reparative surgery. Bol. Soc. de cir. de Rosario *9:*5–12, April '42

Zeno, L.: Prosthetic inclusions in plastic surgery. Arq. de cir. clin. e exper. *6:*523–531, April–June '42

Zeno, L.: Cicatricial tissue as element of plastic repair; tissular reversibility. Arq. de cir. clin. e exper. *6:*597–608, April–June '42

Zeno, L.: Plastic repair of baggy eyelids. Bol. Soc. de cir. de Rosario *9:*131–133, June '42

Zeno, L.: Plastic surgery of face. An. de cir. *8:*139–151, Sept '42

Zeno, L.: Bone transplantation with report of cases. An. de cir. *8:*216–232, Sept '42

Zeno, L.: Auriculoplasty for hypoplasia of pavilion using tubular skin graft; case. Bol. y trab., Acad. argent. de cir. *26:*807–812, Sept 16, '42

Zeno, L.: Burn therapy with special reference to use of casts. An. de cir. *8:*265–280, Dec '42

Zeno, Lelio: *Cirugía plástica*. El Ateñeo Press, Buenos Aires, 1943

Zeno, L.: Postoperative immobilization and holding of sutured flaps in harelips. Bol. y trab., Soc. argent. de cirujanos *4:*648–653, '43 also: An. de cir. *9:*236–241, Sept–Dec '43 also: Rev. Asoc. med. argent. *57:*945–947, Nov 15, '43

Zeno, L.: Hypertelorism associated with median nasal cleft; case. An. argent. de oftal. *4:*3–5, Jan–March '43

Zeno, L.: Plastic surgery. An. de cir. *9:*52–57, March–June '43

Zeno, L.: Congenital eyelid ptosis; simple useful corrective operation; case. Bol. y trab., Acad. argent. de cir. *27:*930–935, Oct 6, '43

Zeno, L.: Biologic fundamentals of immobilization and exposure to air. Rev. Asoc. med. argent. *57:*854–862, Oct 30, '43

Zeno, L.: Biologic fundamentals of immobilization and exposure to air, burns. Rev. Asoc. med. argent. *57:*854–862, Oct 30, '43

Zeno, L.: Defective ulcerated cicatrices; plastic correction. Bol. Soc. de cir. de Rosario *10:*354–366, Oct–Nov '43 also: An. de cir. *10:*76–88, March–June '44

Zeno, L.: Psychosomatic clinical study of case of lupus of nose treated by plastic surgery. Rev. med. de Rosario *33:*1041–1058, Nov '43 also: An. de cir. *9:*125–142, Sept–Dec '43 also: Dia med. *16:*264–268, March 20, '44

Zeno, L.: Grave trauma of hand and forearm; biologic therapy of case. Bol. y trab., Soc. argent. de cirujanos *5:*583–595, '44

Zeno, L.: Congenital ptosis of eyelids; simple useful corrective operation. An. de chir. *10:*38–42, March–June '44

Zeno, L.: Postoperative immobilization and holding of sutured flaps in harelip. Pediat. Americas *2:*238–240, April 15, '44

Zeno, L.: Grave trauma of hand and forearm; biologic therapy. Bol. Soc. de cir. de Rosario *11:*221–224, Aug '44 also: Rev. Asoc. med. argent. *58:*938–942, Oct 30, '44

Zeno, L.: Free graft; advantages and inconveniences of dermatome. Bol. y trab., Acad. argent. de cir. *28:*690–698, Aug 23, '44

Zeno, L.: Retractile cicatrix causing pes planopronatovalgus; plastic surgery in therapy of case. An. de cir. *10:*179–182, Sept–Dec '44

Zeno, L.: Plastic surgery of retractile cicatrix of hand. An. de cir. *10:*183–185, Sept–Dec '44 also: Bol. Soc. de cir. de Rosario *11:*451–454,

Nov '44
ZENO, L.: Free transplant of areola preliminary to amputation of breast for benign tumor; free fat graft; case. An. de cir. *10:*190-194, Sept-Dec '44
ZENO, L.: Plastic trend in wound therapy. Salud y belleza *1:*25-31, April-May '45
ZENO, L. AND BARENBOYM, S.: Plaster of paris bandage in therapy of burns of extremities.
ZENO, L. AND KAPLAN, A. V.: Plaster of paris bandages in treatment of burns of extremities. Vestnik khir. *51:*16-18, '37
ZENO, L. AND MAROTTOLI, O. R.: Orthopedic surgical therapy of elephantiasis of leg; case. Bol. Soc. de cir. de Rosario *6:*10-18, April '39 also: An. de cir. *5:*167-175, June '39
ZENO, L. AND PELUFFO, A.: Insertion "OSEO" in inferior maxilla. An. de cir. *6:*148-155, June '40
ZENO, L. AND PIZARRO CRESPO, E.: Plastic surgery and psychology. An. de cir. *6:*1-22, March '40 also: Semana med. *2:*231-244, Aug 1, '40
ZENO, L. AND RECALDE, J. F.: Reconstruction of nasal septum by tubular skin graft; cases. Arq. de cir. clin. e exper. *6:*185-194, April-June '42
ZENO, L. AND VERDAGUER, J. F.: Use of Padgett dermatome to obtain grafts. Bol. Soc. de cir. de Rosario *9:*211-214, July '42
ZERBINI, C. (see PINI, R.) Aug '33
ZHAK, E. (see KALMANOVSKIY, S. M.) April '38
ZHAKOV, M. P.: Transplantation of skin into oral cavity. Novy khir. arkhiv. *35:*573-577, '36
ZHOLONDZ, A. M.: Plastic repair of scalp. Khirurgiya, no. 9, pp. 151-152, '37
ZHOLONDZ, A. M. (see BASS, Y. M.) 1934
ZHOLONDZ, A. M. (see VASILEV, A. A.) 1933
ZHURAVLEVA, E. P.: Therapy of wounds associated with avulsion of scalp. Vestnik khir. *59:*373-375, April '40
ZIEGELMAN, E. F.: Use of periosteal flap with skin graft in radical mastoid surgery. Laryngoscope *42:*170-176, March '32
ZIEGLER, E.: Complications of local anesthesia in surgery of nasal septum. Ztschr. f. Hals-, Nasen-u. Ohrenh. *32:*476-479, '33
ZIELKE: Improved skin graft according to Thiersch. Deut. Militararzt *9:*51, Jan '44
ZIMCHES, J. L.: Fate of free transplants of epidermis into deep-lying tissues; relation to epithelial cysts. Frankfurt, Ztschr. f. Path. *42:*203-227, '31
ZIMMER, M. (see MERLE D'AUBIGNE, R. *et al*) Sept '46
ZIMMERN, A. AND CHAVANY, J. A.: Classification of peripheral facial paralyses. Medecine *11:*453-457, June '30
ZINCK, K. H.: Circulatory histopathology following burns. Verhandl. d. deutsch. Gesellsch. f. Kreislaufforsch., pp. 263-275, '38
ZINSSER, F. (see SIEMENS, H. W.) Dec '38

Zinsser Operation: See Hennig-Zinsser Operation

ZINTEL, H. A.: Resplitting split-thickness skin grafts with dermatome; method for increasing yield of limited donor sites. Ann. Surg. *121:*1-5, Jan '45
ZINTEL, H. A.: Lamination with dermatome and "split" grafts; method for increasing yield of limited donor regions. Salud y belleza (no. 5) *1:*10-11, 39, Oct-Dec '45
ZLATOVEROV, A. I.: Encephalitic blepharospasm and its therapy. Nevropat. i psikhiat. (nos. 1-2) *9:*160-163, '40
ZÖLLNER, F.: Erroneous diagnoses in cases of aural and cervical fistulas and cysts. Ztschr. f. Hals-, Nasen-u. Ohrenh. *32:*54-61, '32
ZOLLINGER, A.: Plastic reconstruction of fingers with particular regard to formation of cleft hand. Deutsche Ztschr. f. Chir. *196:*271-287, '26
ZOLLINGER, F.: Tendovaginitis and bursitis. Arch. f. Orthop. *24:*456-467, Jan 26, '27
ZONDEK, B.: Artificial vagina. Harefuah *30:*7, Jan 1, '46
ZONDEK, L. H.: Congenital hemiatrophy. Arch. Dis. Childhood *20:*35-43, March '45
ZOON, J. J.: Comment on article by various authors on permanent epilation for cosmetic purposes. Dermat. Wchnschr. *98:*501, April 21, '34
ZORRAQUÍN, G. AND BOIX POU, M.: Topography of burns of normal man who catches on fire; therapy with gutta-percha. Pressa med. argent. *18:*995-999, Dec 30, '31
ZORRAQUÍN, G. AND BOIX POU, M.: Artificial breasts formed by union of 3 flaps following mammectomy for adenofibroma; case. Rev. de cir. de Buenos Aires *13:*244-248, April '34
ZORRAQUÍN, G. AND ZORRAQUÍN, G. F.: Local therapy including facial, interdigital and perineal burns; preliminary report. Dia med. *17:*329-331, April 16, '45
ZORRAQUÍN, G. F. (see ZORRAQUÍN, G.) April '45
ZSCHAU, H.: Closure of lymph vessels in electrocoagulation; significance in prevention of shock. Deutsche Ztschr. f. Chir. *233:*109-120, '31
ZSCHAU, H.: Use of pedicled muscular flaps in surgical therapy of residual empyema and indirect bronchial fistula. Zentralbl. f. Chir. *66:*2529-2534, Dec 2, '39

ZSCHAU, H.: General principles of tissue transplantation. Sitzungsb. d. phys.-med. Soz. zu Erlangen (1939) *71:*255–256, '40

ZSULYEVICH, I.: Plastic transposition of index finger to replace thumb. Orvosi hetil. *82:*153–154, Feb 12, '38

ZUBIZARRETA, H.: External, traumatic deformity of nose with total destruction of both fossae; surgical treatment. Rev. de cir. *7:*380–384, Aug '28 also: Rev. de especialid. *3:*646–652, Nov '28

ZUBRZYCHI, J.: Artificial vagina formation in case of normal uterus. Polska gaz. lek. *9:*105–106, Feb 9, '30

ZUBRZYCKI, J. (see GLATZEL, J.) April–June '32

ZUBRZYCKI, J. (see GLATZEL, J.) July '33

ZUGERMAN, I.: Formula for cryotherapy (with carbon dioxide slush) for acne and postacne scarring. Arch. Dermat. and Syph. *54:*209–210, Aug '46

ZUGSMITH, G. S.: Roentgen burns, with report of 9 cases from University Hospital, Philadelphia, 1907–1933. Radiology *23:*36–44, July '34

ZUGSMITH, G. S. (see MARCKS, K. M.) July '46

ZULCH, K. J.: Peripheral nerve injuries in war; diagnosis and therapy. Med. Klin. *38:*985, Oct 16, '42; 1016, Oct 23, '42

ZUPPA, A.: Congenital malformations of hands and feet; roentgen study of 12 cases. Pediatria *42:*943–966, Aug '34

ZUR VERTH, M.: Fracture at base of terminal phalanx of finger. Arch. f. klin. Chir. *118:*630–644, '21 (illus.) abstr: J.A.M.A. *78:*852, March 18, '22

ZUR VERTH, M.: Useful splints for hand and finger. Zentralbl. f. Chir. *62:*2270–2274, Sept 21, '35

ZUR VERTH, M.: Indications for amputation of fingers. Deutsche med. Wchnschr. *65:*1795–1797, Dec 15, '39

ZURALSKI, T.: Artificial vagina construction by Kirschner method. Ginek. polska *16:*64–70, Jan–Feb '37

ZWAHLEN, P.: Synoviomas of tendon sheaths and of serous bursae. Bull. Assoc. franc. p. l'etude du cancer *24:*682–707, Dec '35

ZWANCK, T.: Chronic radiodermatitis and plastic surgery. Semana med. *1:*471–476, March 15, '45

Zygoma, Fractures

Study and treatment of fractures of malar bone and zygoma. DUCHANGE, R., J. de med. de Bordeaux *95:*557–561, Aug 10, '23 (illus.)

Depression fracture of zygomatic arch. LEHMANN, J. C. Zentralbl. f. Chir. *51:*2016 2017, Sept 13, '24 abstr: J.A.M.A. *83:*1629, Nov 15, '24

Fractures of malar-zygomatic compound, with description of new X-ray position. GILLIES, H. D. *et al.* Brit. J. Surg. *14:*651–656, April '27

Fractures of zygoma. HODGSON, N. Newcastle M. J. *9:*227–230, July '29

New method in reducing fracture of zygomatic arch. WIELAGE, M. F., J. Am. Dent. A. *15:*1228–1230, July '28

Fracture of malar zygomatic arch; review of literature; simplified operative technic; case reports. ROBERTS, S. E. Ann. Otol. Rhin. and Laryng. *37:*826–838, Sept '28

Zygoma fractures; diagnosis and treatment. BRONNER, H. Chirurg *2:*606–611, July 1, '30

Fractures of maxillary zygomatic region and their treatment. STACY, H. S., M. J. Australia *1:*779–780, June 27, '31

Fractures of upper jaw and malar bone. IVY, R. H. AND CURTIS, L. Ann. Surg. *94:*337–346, Sept '31

Relaxation of scar contractures by means of Z-, or reversed Z-type incision; stressing use of scar infiltrated tissues. DAVIS, J. S. Tr. Am. S. A. *49:*381–394, '31

Fractures of zygoma as result of collision with device on automobile which gives signal for turning; case. MICHAËLIS, L. Beitr. z. klin. Chir. *154:*252–253, '31

Traumatic scarring and depressed fracture of right malar bone and orbital border; cartilage implant. FIGI, F. A., S. Clin. North America *12:*949–951, Aug '32

Fractures of zygoma. HUDSON, O. C., J. Bone and Joint Surg. *14:*958–962, Oct '32

Depressed fractures of zygoma. BALYEAT, F. S. California and West. Med. *37:*315, Nov '32

Diagnosis of depressed zygomatic fracture. MACLURE, F. Australian and New Zealand J. Surg. *2:*415–416, April '33

Zygoma fractures; five cases. MORIOKA, K. Taiwan Igakkai Zasshi (Abstr. Sect.) *33:*108, July '34

Operation for elevation of depressed zygomatic fractures. DAVIS, G. G. AND HUEY, W. B. Indust. Med. *4:*404–408, Aug '35

Fracture of zygomatic arch; 2 cases with cicatricial closure of jaws. SCHMUZIGER, P. Schweiz. med. Wchnschr. *65:*721–722, Aug 10, '35

Zygoma fractures; with report of 2 cases. FINOCHIETTO, R. AND MARINO, H. Prensa med. argent. *22:*2101–2110, Oct 30, '35

Fractures of nasal and malar bones. NEW, G. B., S. Clin. North America *15:*1241–1250, Oct '35

Zygoma, Fractures – Cont.
Treatment of depressed fractures of zygomatic (malar) bone and zygomatic arch. PATTERSON, R. F., J. Bone and Joint Surg. *17:*1069–1071, Oct '35
Fracture of zygomatic arch; case. DUBOV, M. D. Vestnik khir. *41:*189–190, '35
Zygoma fractures. IVY, R. H. AND CURTIS, L. S. Clin. North America *16:*587–594, April '36
Diagnosis and therapy of fresh fractures of zygoma. HAMMEL, H. Chirurg *8:*964–966, Dec 15, '36
Orthopedic surgery in treatment of simple fractures of zygomatic arch. GERKE, J. Deutsche Ztschr. f. Chir. *247:*398–403, '36
Treatment of depressed fractures of zygoma. WATKINS, A. B. K. Brit. M. J. *1:*326–327, Feb 13, '37
Gillies operation for correction of depressed fracture deformities of zygomatic-malar bones. GREELEY, P. W. Illinois M. J. *71:*419–420, May '37
Healing of fractures of mandible and zygoma. GRIMSON, K. S., J. Am. Dent. A. *24:*1458–1469, Sept '37
Apparatus for reducing fractures of zygomatic arch. LIMBERG, A. A. Vestnik khir. *50:*194–197, '37
Surgical therapy of zygomatic fracture; case. TOPA, P. AND THEODORESCO, D. Tech. chir. *30:*45–50, March–April '38
Fracture of maxillary zygomatic compound. GERRIE, J. W. Canad. M. A. J. *38:*535–538, June '38
Isolated fracture of zygomatic arch; case. PAIS, C. Gior. veneto di sc. med. *12:*685–690, Nov '38
Therapy of dislocation fractures of zygoma. AKERMAN, N. Acta chir. Scandinav. *80:*359–364, '38
Case of zygomatic fracture cured by direct skeletal traction applied with screw. GIORGI, C. Riv. di chir. *5:*34–39, Jan–Feb '39
Zygomatic fractures. DOHERTY, J. L. AND DOHERTY, J. A., J. Am. Dent. A. *26:*730–733, May '39
Diplopia in fracture of upper and lower maxillary and of malar bones; case. PAOLI, M. Rev. de stomatol. *41:*548–552, July '39
Fractures of malar bone and zygoma with eye, ear, nose and throat complications. MEYER, M. F. New Orleans M. and S. J. *92:*90–94, Aug '39
Treatment of malar and zygomatic fractures. RICHISON, F. A., U. S. Nav. M. Bull. *37:*566–571, Oct '39
Zygoma fractures. KANTHAK, F. F. Surgery *7:*796–805, May '40
Fractures in zygomatic region. BRAENDSTRUP, P. Nord. med. (Hospitalstid.) *7:*1527–1534, Sept 14, '40
New method of treatment of depressed fracture of zygomatic bone (splint). BAXTER, H. Canad. M. A. J. *44:*5–9, Jan '41
Early care of depressed fractures of malar bone. JOHNSON, V. E., J. M. Soc. New Jersey *38:*113–117, March '41
Fractures of malar and zygoma. CORBIN, F. R. Mil. Surgeon *89:*750–754, Nov '41
Zygoma fractures and their therapy; cases. INCLAN, A. Cir. ortop. y traumatol., Habana *10:*14–29, Jan–March '42
Surgical therapy of zygoma fractures. THEODORESCU, D. Ztschr. f. Stomatol. *40:*359–363, May 22, '42
Fractures of malar bone; cases. CHILDREY, J. H. Laryngoscope *52:*473–479, June '42
Fractures of malar-zygomatic compound. BALKIN, S. G. Journal-Lancet *62:*267–270, July '42
Isolated fractures of zygomatic arch. MONTANARI-REGGIANI, M. Arch. ortop. *57:*431–450, Dec '42
Fractures of upper jaw, malar bone and zygomatic arch. SCHILDT, E. Nord. med. (Hygiea) *16:*3700–3705, Dec 26, '42
Care of military and civilian injuries; fractures of mandible, maxilla, zygoma and other facial bones; statistical study of 1,149 cases. LYONS, D. C. Am. J. Orthodontics (Oral Surg. Sect.) *29:*67–76, Feb '43
Fractures of malar bone. MACINDOE, P. H. M. J. Australia *1:*317–319, April 10, '43
Report of 72 consecutive cases of zygoma fractures. COAKLEY, W. A. AND WHITE, M. F. Surg., Gynec. and Obst. *77:*360–366, Oct '43
Fractures of malar bone and of zygomatic arch. REGGI, J. P. Bol. y trab., Soc. argent. de cirujanos *4:*905–914, '43 also: Rev. Assoc. med. argent. *58:*21–24, Jan–Feb '44
Fractures of zygoma. GONZALEZ ULLOA, M. Rev. mex. de cir., ginec. y cancer *12:*171–177, June '44
Fractures of zygomatic tripod. UNGLEY, H. G. AND SUGGIT, S. C. Brit. J. Surg. *32:*287–299, Oct '44
Fractures of zygoma. NESBITT, B. E. AND LEEDS, C. R. D. Brit. M. J. *1:*512–513, April 14, '45
Treatment of depressed fracture of zygomatic arch by Gillies method. CHRISTIANSEN, G. W. AND BRADLEY, J. L., U. S. Nav. M. Bull. *44:*1066–1068, May '45
Bilateral depressed zygomatic fractures.

Zygoma, Fractures – Cont.
CHRISTIANSEN, G. W. AND BRADLEY, J. L. U. S. Nav. M. Bull. *45:*153–155, July '45
Fracture of zygomatic tripod; method of fixation. TAYLOR, E. E. T., M. Press *214:*158–159, Sept 5, '45
Fracture of zygomatic bone and arch; postoperative headgear. SCHMIER, A. A. Am. J. Surg. *70:*27–37, Oct '45
Fractures of malar-zygomatic compound. GONZALEZ ULLOA, M. Vida nueva *56:*190–

Zygoma, Fractures – Cont.
194, Dec '45
Zygomatic fracture; case. LARSON, A. B. U. S. Nav. M. Bull. *45:*1151–1154, Dec '45
Fractures of malar-zygomatic compound; treatment by improved methods and myoplasty. STEWART, M. B. AND CONLEY, J. J., Arch. Otolaryng. *44:*443–451, Oct '46

ZYPKIN, B. (see MANNHEIM, A.) 1926
ZYPKIN, B. (see MANNHEIM, A.) 1927

SUBJECT HEADINGS USED IN THIS INDEX

Abdomen, Defect of ... 1
Abdominal Flap ... 1
Abdominoplasty ... 1
Acne ... 2
Acne Scars ... 2
Anatomy ... 8
Anesthesia ... 10
Anesthesia Complications ... 13
Anus ... 14
Anus, Imperforate ... 14
Apert's Syndrome ... 15
Arteries ... 18
Arthritis ... 18
Ascher Syndrome ... 20
Auchincloss Operation ... 21
Axhausen Operation (*See also Von Langenbeck-Axhausen Operation*) ... 22
Axillary Contracture ... 23
Back Flap ... 24
Baker Operation ... 25
Baldwin Operation ... 26
Baldwin-Mori Operation ... 26
Ballance-Duel Operation (*See also Duel-Ballance Operation*) ... 27
Bandages ... 28
Banjo Splint ... 29
Bardet-Biedl Syndrome ... 29
Barg Operation ... 29
Beaumetz Operation: *See Dujardin-Beaumetz Operation* ... 33
Beck Operation ... 33
Beck-Von Hacker Operation ... 34
Behcet Syndrome ... 34
Belloste, Augustin ... 35
Bell's Palsy: *See Facial Paralysis* ... 35
Bennett Fracture ... 36
Beresowski Operation ... 37
Bergenhem Operation ... 38
Bidder Operation: *See Landerer-Bidder Operation* ... 42
Bipp Operation ... 43
Bisi Operation ... 44
Bite, Human ... 44
Bladder ... 45
Bladder, Exstrophy ... 45
Bladder, Exstrophy – Cancer ... 51
Blair Operation ... 53
Blair-Brown Operation ... 53
Blaskovics Operation ... 54
Blepharoplasty ... 54
Blepharoplasty, Cosmetic ... 57
Blepharoplasty for Ectropion ... 57
Blepharoplasty for Entropion ... 58
Blepharoptosis ... 59
Blepharospasm ... 63
Bohler Operation ... 65
Bohler's Splint ... 65
Bone ... 65
Bone Derivatives, Grafting ... 66
Bone Formation by Grafts of Bladder Mucosa ... 66
Bone Grafts ... 66
Bone Grafts, Pedicled ... 71
Bone Grafts, Preserved ... 71
Bone Grafts to Face ... 71
Bone Grafts to Hand ... 72
Bone Grafts to Mandible ... 72
Bone Grafts to Nose ... 73
Bone Grafts to Skull ... 74
Bone Heterografts ... 74
Bone Homografts ... 75
Bone Infections ... 75
Books (*Alphabetically by First Author*) ... 77
Borchers Operation: *See Nové-Josserand-Borchers Operation* ... 80
Borelius Operation (*See also Maydl Operation*) ... 81
Bourguet Operation ... 82
Boyer Operation: *See Heitz-Boyer-Hovelacque Operation; Marion-Heitz-Boyer Operation* ... 83
Branchial Cysts and Fistulas (*See also Lateral Cervical Fistula*) ... 84
Braun's Operation ... 87
Breasts (*See also Gynecomastia; Mammaplasty, Mastopexy*) ... 87
Breasts, Atrophy ... 88
Breasts, Augmentation: *See Mammaplasty, Augmentation* ... 88
Breasts, Cancer ... 88
Breasts, Deformity ... 88
Breasts, Hypertrophy ... 89
Breasts, Hypoplasia ... 89
Breasts, Nipple Operations ... 89
Breasts, Pendulous (*See also Mammaplasty, Mastopexy*) ... 89
Breasts, Reconstruction ... 90
Breasts, Reduction: *See Mammaplasty, Reduction* ... 90
Breasts, Supernumerary ... 90
Breasts, Suspension: *See Mammaplasty, Mastopexy* ... 90
Bronchial Fistula ... 92
Brown-Blair Operation ... 95
Brown Operation (*See also Blair-Brown Operation*) ... 95
Bruhn Operation: *See Darcissac-Bruhn-Petroff Operation* ... 96
Bucknall Operation ... 97
Bucknall Operation, Complications ... 97
Buediner-Dieffenbach Operation ... 97
Bunnell Operation ... 99
Bunnell Suture ... 99
Burns ... 100
Burns, Anesthesia for ... 104
Burns, Bones, and Fractures with ... 104

Burns, Cancer in ... 104
Burns, Chemical ... 105
Burns, Complications ... 106
Burns, Contractures ... 109
Burns, Debridement ... 111
Burns, Electrical ... 111
Burns, Experimental Work ... 112
Burns, Eyes and Eyelids ... 113
Burns, History ... 113
Burns, Radiation: *See Radiation Injuries* ... 113
Burns, Scars (*See also Burns, Contractures; Burns, Skin Grafting*) ... 113
Burns, Shock ... 114
Burns, Skin Grafting ... 117
Burns, Topical Therapy ... 119
Burns, Treatment ... 131
Burns, War ... 141
Busse-Grawitz Experiments ... 144
Buttocks ... 145
Cadaver ... 146
Cadenat Operation ... 147
Caldwell-Luc Operation ... 147
Cancer ... 149
Cancer, Antrum ... 150
Cancer in Artificial Vagina ... 151
Cancer, Basal Cell ... 151
Cancer, Basal-Squamous ... 151
Cancer, Burns, Scars: *See Burns, Cancer in* . 151
Cancer, Cheek: *See Cancer, Mouth* ... 151
Cancer, Ear ... 152
Cancer in Exstrophied Bladders ... 152
Cancer, Eyelid ... 152
Cancer, Face ... 153
Cancer, Hand ... 154
Cancer, Jaws ... 154
Cancer, Larynx ... 155
Cancer, Lip ... 157
Cancer, Lupus ... 161
Cancer, Lymph Nodes: *See Neck Dissections* 161
Cancer, Metastases: *See Neck Dissections* ... 161
Cancer, Mouth ... 161
Cancer, Neck: *See Neck Dissections* ... 162
Cancer, Nevi ... 162
Cancer, Nose ... 163
Cancer, Parotid ... 163
Cancer, Pharynx ... 164
Cancer, Radiation Dermatitis ... 164
Cancer, Skin (*See also Cancer, Basal Cell; Skin, Cancer*) ... 164
Cancer, Tongue ... 165
Cancer, Transplantation of by Skin Grafting 165
Carbon Dioxide Freezing ... 166
Cartilage Grafts ... 169
Cartilage Grafts, Cadaver: *See Cartilage Grafts, Preserved* ... 172
Cartilage Grafts, Ear ... 172
Cartilage Grafts, Experimental ... 172
Cartilage Grafts, Preserved ... 173
Cartilage Heterografts ... 173
Cartilage Homografts (*See also Cartilage Grafts, Preserved; Homografts*) ... 174
Cerebral Fungus, Skin Grafting ... 176
Cheiloplasty ... 177
Chemical Peeling ... 180
Chest ... 180
Chin ... 181
Chronis Operation ... 183
Clapp's Operation ... 184
Clawhand ... 185
Cleft Hand ... 186
Cleft Lip ... 186
Cleft Lip, Bilateral ... 194
Cleft Lip, Median ... 195
Cleft Lip, Secondary Deformity ... 195
Cleft Palate ... 197
Cleft Palate, Age for Operation ... 206
Cleft Palate, Associated Anomalies ... 206
Cleft Palate, Bilateral (*See also Cleft Palate*) 206
Cleft Palate, Complications ... 207
Cleft Palate, Ear Problems ... 207
Cleft Palate, Elongation of ... 207
Cleft Palate, Etiology ... 207
Cleft Palate, Extra-Oral Flaps for ... 208
Cleft Palate Growth: (*See also Cleft Palate*) . 208
Cleft Palate Incidence ... 208
Cleft Palate Obturators ... 209
Cleft Palate Operations, Anesthesia for ... 209
Cleft Palate Orthodontia ... 210
Cleft Palate, Pediatric Care ... 210
Cleft Palate, Pharyngeal Flap ... 210
Cleft Palate Pushback: *See Cleft Palate, Elongation* ... 210
Cleft Palate, Secondary Operations ... 210
Cleft Palate, Social Problems ... 211
Cleft Palate, Speech ... 211
Cleft Palate, Submucous ... 212
Cleft Palate, Traumatic ... 212
Cleft Palate, X-ray Studies ... 212
Cloquet Operation ... 213
Club Hand ... 213
Coffey's Operation ... 215
Composite Flaps ... 218
Composite Grafts ... 219
Constantini Operation ... 220
Contracture ... 220
Contracture, Burn (*See also Burns, Contractures*) ... 223
Contracture, Dupuytren's ... 224
Contracture, Volkmann's ... 230
Cosmetics ... 234
Craniofacial Deformity (*See also Apert's Syndrome; Crouzon's Syndrome; Hypertelorism*) ... 237
Craniofacial Injuries ... 238
Cranioplasty (*See also Bone Grafts to Skull*) 238
Cranium, Osteomyelitis of ... 240
Cranium, Tumors of ... 240
Crile, G. ... 241
Crouzon's Syndrome ... 242
Cryotherapy ... 242

Cuenod-Saunders Operation 243
Curling's Ulcer 243
Cystic Hygroma (*See also Lymphangiomas*) . 245
Cysts and Fistulas 245
Cysts and Fistulas, Branchial 248
Cysts and Fistulas, Thyroglossal (*See also Cysts and Fistulas*) 252
Cysts, Implantation 253
Cysts, Sebaceous (*See also Cysts and Fistulas; Dermoid Cysts*) 253
Cysts, Thymic 253
Dacryocystorhinostomy 253
Darcissac-Bruhn-Petroff Operation 259
Deformities (*See also Anatomical Area and Plastic Surgery*) 264
Delorme-Juvara Operation 265
Denig Operation 266
Denker Operation: *See Rouge-Denker Operation* 266
De Quervain's Syndrome 266
Dermal Grafts 267
Dermoid Cysts 268
D'Espine Operation 269
Dickey Operation 270
Didot's Operation 270
Dieffenbach-Warren Operation 270
Dorrance Operation 274
Dressings 275
Duel-Ballance Operation 280
Duel Operation: *See Ballance-Duel Operation* 280
Dufourmentel Operation 282
Dujardin-Beaumetz Operation 282
Duplay Operation 283
Dupuy-Dutemps Operation 284
Dupuy Operation: *See Bourguet Operation* .. 284
Dupuytren's Contracture: *See Contracture, Dupuytren's* 284
Dutemps Operation: *See Bourguet Operation; Dupuy-Dutemps Operation* 285
Duval Operation 285
Earlobes 285
Ears (*See also Otoplasty; Earlobes*) 285
Ears, Avulsion 287
Ears, Cancer (*See also Cancer, Basal Cell; Cancer, Basal-Squamous; Skin Cancer*) ... 287
Ears, Cauliflower 287
Ears, Cryptotia (*See also Ears, Deformity*) .. 287
Ears, Cysts and Fistulas 288
Ears, Deformity (*See also Ears, Cryptotia; Ears, Reconstruction; Otoplasty*) 289
Ears, Electrical Injuries 291
Ears, Injuries 291
Ears, Prostheses 291
Ears, Reconstruction 292
Ears, Tumors 293
Eiger 295
Eitner 297
Elbim Operation 297
Electrotherapy 297
Elephantiasis: *See Lymphedema* 301
Embryonal Tissue Grafts, Cancer in 302
Enophthalmos 302
Epicanthus 302
Epidermolysis Bullosa 303
Epilation 303
Epispadias (*See also Bladder, Exstrophy*) ... 303
Erich Operation: *See New-Erich Operation* .. 305
Ernst Operation 306
Esmarch Operation 306
Esophagus 306
Esser-Wheeler Operation 308
Esthetic Surgery 308
Estlander Operation 311
Ewing Operation 312
Exophthalmos 312
Extremities (*See also Burns; Contractures; Hands; Leg Ulcers; Lymphedema; War Injuries; Wringer Injuries*) 312
Eye, Burns of 314
Eye Prostheses 316
Eyebrows 316
Eyelids (*See also Blepharoplasty; Blepharoptosis; Blepharospasm; Enophthalmos; Epicanthus; Exophthalmos; Lacrimal Apparatus; Lagophthalmos*) 317
Eyelids, Cancer 320
Eyelids, Canthoplasty 321
Eyelids, Colobomas of 321
Eyelids, Congenital Deformities 322
Eyelids, Deformity 322
Eyelids, Ectropion 322
Eyelids, Entropion 324
Eyelids, Injuries of 327
Eyelids, Reconstruction 327
Eyelids, Symblepharon 328
Eyelids, Tumors 328
Face; *See Facial* 329
Face, Anatomy of 329
Face, Burns (*See also Burns*) 329
Face, Cancer of (*See also Cancer; Melanoma; etc.*) 330
Face, Congenital Deformities (*See also Cleft Lip; Facial Clefts; and Other Specific Deformities*) 333
Face, Infections of 333
Face, Surgery of 333
Face, Tumors of (*See also Specific Tumor; Face, Cancer of; Face, Surgery of*) 340
Facial (*See also Face*) 342
Facial Bones, Fractures of (*See also Jaws, Fractures of*) 342
Facial Bones, Osteomyelitis 344
Facial Clefts 345
Facial Deformities (*See also Face, Congenital Deformities; Facial Hemiatrophy; Facial Hypertrophy; Facial Lesions; Hypertelorism*) 345
Facial Deformities, Medicolegal Aspects 346

Facial Deformities, Psychological Aspects ... 346
Facial Hemiatrophy (*See also Facial Hypertrophy*) ... 347
Facial Hypertrophy (*See also Facial Hemiatrophy*) ... 350
Facial Injuries ... 350
Facial Injuries, Tracheotomy in ... 353
Facial Lesions ... 353
Facial Paralysis ... 353
Facial Prostheses: *See Prostheses* ... 359
Facial Spasm ... 359
Facial Surgery, Anesthesia for ... 359
Facial Surgery, Dental Aspects of ... 359
Facial Surgery, Reviews of ... 359
Farrell Operation: *See Lyman-Farrell Operation* ... 362
Fascia ... 362
Fat Grafts ... 364
Fingernails ... 370
Fingertips ... 371
Finger, Trigger ... 372
Fingers, Amputations of ... 373
Fingers, Ankylosis ... 373
Fingers, Arachnodactylia ... 374
Fingers, Avulsion Injuries ... 374
Fingers, Baseball Injuries (*See also Fingers, Splints*) ... 375
Fingers, Boutonniere Deformity of ... 375
Fingers, Burns of (*See also Burns, Contractures*) ... 375
Fingers, Camptodacylism ... 376
Fingers, Contractures ... 376
Fingers, Deformity: *See Specific Deformities and also Fingers, Reconstructive Surgery of; Syndactylism* ... 376
Fingers, Dislocations ... 379
Fingers, Dressings for ... 380
Fingers, Drumstick ... 380
Fingers, Fractures ... 380
Fingers, Grease Gun Injuries ... 383
Fingers, Infections ... 383
Fingers, Injuries of (*See also Fingers, Amputations of; Fingers, Avulsion Injuries; Fingers, Baseball Injuries; Fingers, Boutonniere Deformity of; Fingers, Burns of; Fingers, Dislocations of; Fingers, Fractures of; Fingers, Grease Gun Injuries; Fingers, Injuries, Immediate Skin Grafting for; Fingers, Ring Injuries; Fingers, Tendon Ruptures in; Fingers, Tendon Surgery; Fingers, Vascular Injuries*) ... 384
Fingers, Injuries, Immediate Skin Grafting for ... 386
Fingers, Mallet: *See Fingers, Baseball Injuries* ... 386
Fingers, Miscellaneous Topics ... 387
Fingers, Paralysis of ... 387
Fingers, Reconstructive Surgery of ... 388
Fingers, Ring Injuries ... 389
Fingers, Splints for (*See also Fingers, Baseball Injuries*) ... 389
Fingers, Spring ... 390
Fingers, Tendon Ruptures in ... 392
Fingers, Tendon Surgery (*See also Fingers, Injuries of; Fingers, Tendon Ruptures; Fingers, Avulsion Injuries*) ... 392
Fingers, Transplantation of Toe to Finger or Thumb ... 393
Fingers, Tumors ... 394
Fingers, Vascular Injuries ... 394
Flaps: *See Composite Flaps; Skin Flaps* ... 397
Fogh-Andersen, Poul ... 398
Foot ... 399
Fournier's Syndrome ... 401
Foville Syndrome ... 401
Frank Operation ... 402
Frank-Geist Operation ... 402
Frostbite (*See also War Injuries*) ... 405
Furuncles ... 406
Galliera Operation: *See Passaggi-Galliera Operation* ... 408
Ganglions ... 409
Gas Gangrene ... 410
Geist Frank Operation ... 412
Genetics: *See Heredity* ... 412
Genitalia (*See also Bladder, Exstrophy; Epispadias; Hypospadias; Penis; Scrotum; Urethra; Vagina*) ... 412
Gensoul ... 412
Gersuny Operation ... 413
Gillies, H.D. ... 415
Gillies Operation ... 416
Glaesmer, E. ... 417
Glass ... 418
Glomus Tumors ... 418
Goebell-Stoeckel Operation ... 419
González-Loza Operation ... 422
Graefe's Apparatus ... 425
Grafts: *See Bone Grafts; Cartilage Grafts; Composite Grafts; Dermal Grafts; Fascia; Fat Grafts; Homografts; Mucosal Grafts; Muscle Grafts, Free; Nerves, Grafts; Skin Grafts; Tendon Transplantation* ... 425
Grawitz Experiments: *See Busse-Grawitz Experiments* ... 426
Grigoriu Operation (*See also Schubert Operation*) ... 428
Gunn's Phenomenon ... 431
Gunshot Wounds (*See also War Injuries*) ... 431
Gutzeit Operation ... 433
Gynecomastia ... 433
Hair ... 435
Halle Operation ... 438
Hands, Amputations ... 439
Hands, Anatomy of ... 439
Hands, Burns (*See also Burns, War Injuries, Hand*) ... 440
Hands, Cancer (*See also Radiation Injuries*) 441

Hands, Congenital Deformities (*See also Clubhand; Syndactylism*) ... 441
Hands, Cysts of ... 442
Hands, Deformities, Acquired ... 442
Hands, Dislocations ... 443
Hands, Dressings for (*See also War Injuries, Hand*) ... 444
Hands, Fractures ... 444
Hands, Grease Gun Injuries (*See also Fingers, Grease Gun Injuries*) ... 445
Hands, Infections ... 445
Hands, Injuries of (*See also Hands, Nerve Injuries in; Hands, Reconstructive Surgery of; Hands, Tendon Injuries in; War Injuries, Hand*) ... 451
Hand, Miscellaneous ... 454
Hands, Nerve Injuries in (*See also Hands, Injuries of; Hands, Tendon Injuries in*) ... 456
Hands, Reconstructive Surgery of ... 457
Hands, Skin Grafts and Flaps to ... 459
Hands, Splints ... 460
Hands, Tendon Injuries in (*See also Hands, Injuries of; Hands, Nerve Injuries in*) ... 461
Hands, Tendon Ruptures in ... 463
Hands, Tumors of ... 463
Hands, Vascular Injuries of ... 463
Head ... 469
Heitz-Boyer-Hovelacque Operation ... 471
Heitz Operation: *See Marion-Heitz-Boyer Operation* ... 471
Hemangiomas ... 471
Henkel Operation ... 476
Henle Operation ... 476
Hennig-Zinsser Operation ... 476
Heredity ... 477
Hermaphrodism (*See also Hypospadias*) ... 480
Hess Operation ... 482
Hidradenitis ... 483
Hippocrates ... 484
History of Plastic Surgery ... 484
Holländer's Operation ... 487
Homografts ... 488
Hotz Operation ... 490
Hovelacque Operation: *See Heitz-Boyer-Hovelacque Operation* ... 491
Hughes Operation ... 492
Hulsman Operation: *See Murray-Nelson-Hulsman Operation* ... 493
Human Bite Injuries ... 493
Hungarian Operation for Eyelid ... 493
Hunt-Tansley Operation ... 494
Hutchinson Syndrome ... 494
Hygroma: *See Cystic Hygroma* ... 494
Hyperhidrosis ... 494
Hypertelorism ... 494
Hypospadias ... 495
Ichthyosis ... 500
Implants ... 501
Imre Operation ... 506
Infection ... 506
Instruments ... 507
Ipsen Operation ... 514
Italian Arm Flap ... 515
Ivy Operation ... 518
Jaws, Ankylosis (*See also Jaws, Ankylosis, Fibrous; Temporomandibular Joint* ... 520
Jaws, Ankylosis, Fibrous (*See also Jaws, Ankylosis; Temporomandibular Joint*) ... 523
Jaws, Bone Grafts to ... 523
Jaws, Cancer of (*See also Cancer; Jaws, Tumors of; Jaws, Surgery of; Mouth Cancer; Tongue Cancer*) ... 524
Jaws, Cysts ... 526
Jaws, Deformity ... 526
Jaws, Dislocation ... 527
Jaws, Enlarged Condyle ... 529
Jaws, Fractured, Edentulous Fragments ... 529
Jaws, Fractures ... 531
Jaws, Fractures, Complications (*See also Jaws, Fractures, Infections; Jaws, Fractures, Malunion of; Jaws, Fractures, Non-Union*) ... 535
Jaws, Fractures, First-Aid ... 535
Jaws, Fractures in Children ... 535
Jaws, Fractures, Infections in ... 536
Jaws, Fractures, Malunion of ... 536
Jaws, Fractures, Mandible ... 536
Jaws, Fractures, Mandibular Condyle ... 539
Jaws, Fractures, Maxilla ... 540
Jaws, Fractures, Non-Union of (*See also Jaws, Bone Grafts to*) ... 542
Jaws, Fractures, Spontaneous ... 542
Jaws, Fractures, Teamwork ... 542
Jaws, Gunshot Injuries (*See also War Injuries, Jaws*) ... 542
Jaws, Infection ... 542
Jaws, Injuries of ... 544
Jaws, Laterognathia (*See also Jaws, Deformity; Jaws, Enlarged Condyle; Jaws, Miscellaneous; Jaws, Surgery of*) ... 544
Jaws, Micrognathia of ... 545
Jaws, Miscellaneous ... 545
Jaws, Osteomyelitis: *See Jaws, Infection* ... 546
Jaws, Prognathism ... 546
Jaws, Surgery of ... 548
Jaws, Surgery, Anesthesia for ... 551
Jaws, Surgery, Prostheses in ... 551
Jaws, Tumors of (*See also Jaws, Cancer of; Jaws, Surgery of*) ... 551
Joint Transplantation ... 555
Joseph ... 557
Joseph, Jacques ... 557
Josserand Operation: *See Nove-Josserand Operation; Nove-Josserand-Borchers Operation* ... 557
Juvara Operation: *See Delorme-Juvara Operation* ... 558
Kankrov Operation ... 560

Keloids: (*See also Scars, Hypertrophic*) 564
Keysser 568
Kilian Operation 569
Killian Operation 569
Kirschner Operation 571
Kirschner-Wagner Operation 571
Klapp Operation 573
Kocher Operation 576
Kohn 576
Kondoleon Operation 576
Kostecka Operation 578
Krause Operation 579
Krauze 579
Kroenlein Operation 580
Kromayer 580
Krukenberg Operation: *See Putti-Krukenberg Operation* 581
Kuhnt-Szymanowsky Operation 581
Lacrimal Apparatus 583
Lagley's Operation 588
Lagophthalmos 588
Lagrange's Law 588
Lahey Operation 589
Landerer-Bidder Operation 590
Larynx, Cancer of 592
Larynx, Miscellaneous 594
Larynx, Stenosis of 595
Larynx, Tumors of 595
Lateral Cervical Fistula (*See also Branchial Cysts and Fistulas*) 595
Ledderhose-Secretan Syndrome 598
Leech Method 598
Leg Ulcers (*See also Ulcers*) 599
Legal Aspects 600
Lengemann Operation: *See Makkhas-Lengemann Operation* 602
Leprosy 602
Leriche Operation 603
Leukoplakia 604
Lexer Operation 606
Limberg Operation 608
Lindemann Operation 608
Lip, Frenum of 609
Lip Pits, Congenital 609
Lips, Cancer 610
Lips, Cancer, Cure Rates 613
Lip, Cancer, Distant Metastases 614
Lips, Cancer, Neck Metastases 614
Lips, Cancer, Radiation Therapy 614
Lips, Cross-Lip Flaps (*See also Lips, Reconstruction of*) 615
Lips, Deformity of (*See also Cleft Lip; Facial Clefts*) 616
Lips, Esthetic Surgery of 617
Lips, Infections of 617
Lips, Lesions of 617
Lips, Miscellaneous Procedures 617
Lips, Mucosal Grafts from 617
Lips, Paralysis of 617
Lips, Reconstruction of (*See also Lips; Cross-Lip Flaps*) 618
Lips, Tumors of 619
Loop Operation 621
Luc Operation: *See Caldwell-Luc Operation* . 623
Lupus 624
Lyman-Farrell Operation 625
Lymph 625
Lymph Nodes 625
Lymphangiomas (*See also Cystic Hygroma; Hemangiomas*) 626
Lymphedema 627
McIndoe Operation 634
Machek Operation 637
Madelung's Syndrome 637
Maher Operation 638
Makkas Operation 639
Makkas-Lengemann Operation 639
Malbec Operation 640
Mammaplasty after Amputation 643
Mammaplasty, Arterial Supply for 643
Mammaplasty, Augmentation 643
Mammaplasty, Complications 643
Mammaplasty, Dermal Pedicle 643
Mammaplasty, Free Graft of Areola in 643
Mammaplasty for Inverted Nipples 643
Mammaplasty, Lactation After 643
Mammaplasty, Local Anesthesia for 643
Mammaplasty, Mastopexy: (*See also Mammaplasty, Reduction*) 643
Mammaplasty, Physiology After 646
Mammaplasty, Reduction (*See also Mammaplasty, Mastopexy*) 647
Mandible, Ankylosis: *See Jaws, Ankylosis* .. 650
Mandible, Bone Grafting: *See Jaws, Bone Grafts to* 650
Mandible, Cancer: *See Jaws, Cancer of* 650
Mandible, Cysts: *See Jaws, Cysts* 650
Mandible, Deformity: *See Jaws, Deformity* . 650
Mandible, Dislocation: *See Jaws, Dislocation* 650
Mandible, Fractures: *See Jaws, Fractures* ... 651
Mandible, Micrognathia: *See Jaws, Micrognathia of* 651
Mandible, Prognathism: *See Jaws, Prognathism* 651
Mandible, Resection of: *See Jaws, Bone Grafts to; Jaws, Cancer of; Jaws, Surgery, Prostheses in; Jaws, Tumors of* 651
Marcus-Gunn Phenomenon 652
Marfan Syndrome 652
Marion Operation 654
Marion-Heitz-Boyer Operation 654
Mastopexy: *See Mammaplasty, Mastopexy* ... 659
Matti Operation: *See Reich-Mattie Operation* 660
Maxilla, Cancer (*See also Jaws, Cancer of*) .. 661
Maxilla, Fractures (*See also Jaws, Fractures; War Injuries, Jaws*) 661
Maxilla, Infections (*See also Jaws, Frac-*

tures, Infections; Jaws, Infections) 664
Maxilla, Tumors (*See also Jaws, Tumors of; Maxilla, Cancer*) 664
Maxillary Resection (*See also Jaws, Cancer of; Maxilla, Cancer*) 664
Maxillofacial Deformities (*See also Specific Deformities; Jaws, Deformity*) 664
Maxillofacial Injuries (*See also Jaws, Fractures; Jaws, Injuries of; Maxilla, Fractures; War Injuries, Jaws*) 665
Maxillofacial Prostheses (*See also Jaws, Prostheses*) 665
Maxillofacial Surgery (*See also Face, Surgery of; Facial Bones, Fractures of; Facial Injuries; Jaws, Fractures; Jaws, Injuries of; Jaws, Surgery of; Maxillofacial Injuries; War Injuries, Jaws*) 666
Maxillofacial Surgery, Anesthesia for (*See also Jaws, Surgery, Anesthesia for; War Injuries, Jaws*) 666
Maxillofacial Surgery, Dental Aspects (*See also Jaws, Fractures, Teamwork; War Injuries, Jaws*) 667
Maydl Operation: (*See also Borelius*) 668
Mayo Operation: *See Coffey's Operation* 669
Mayo-Walters Operation 669
Melanomas 670
Meloplasty: *See Rhytidectomy* 672
Metzenbaum Operation 674
Micrognathia: *See Jaws, Micrognathia of* 676
Microtia: *See Otoplasty* 676
Mikhelson Operation 676
Military Surgery: *See War Injuries* 676
Millingen-Sapezhko Operation 677
Mirault Operation 678
Mirotvortzeff Operation 678
Mommsen Procedure 680
Mora Operation 683
Morestin Operation 683
Mori Operation 683
Mosher-Toti Operation 685
Moskovits 685
Motais Operation 685
Moulages 686
Mouth, Cancer 687
Mouth, Deformities (*See also Jaws, Deformity; Maxillofacial Deformities*) 690
Mouth, Infections (*See also Jaws, Infection; Maxilla, Infections*) 690
Mouth, Injuries of (*See also Burns, Chemical; Burns, Electrical; Maxillofacial Injuries*) 690
Mouth, Miscellanous 691
Mouth, Prostheses (*See also Jaws, Prostheses*) 691
Mouth, Surgery of (*See also Jaws, Surgery of; Maxillofacial Surgery*) 691
Mouth, Surgery, Anesthesia for (*See also Jaws, Surgery, Anesthesia for; Maxillofacial Surgery, Anesthesia for; War Injuries, Jaws*) 692
Mouth, Surgery, Instruments for 692
Mouth, Tumors (*See also Jaws, Tumors of; Maxilla, Tumors*) 693
Mowlem Operation 693
Mucosal Grafts 694
Mucous Membrane 694
Mucous Membranes, Tumors 696
Murphy's Operation 698
Murray-Nelson-Hulsman Operation 698
Muscles 698
Muscle Grafts, Free 698
Muscle, Transposition of 699
Nagel 700
Nageotte Operation 700
Nasopharynx, Cancer 701
Nasopharynx, Tumors 701
Nataf-Saunders Operation 701
Neck 702
Neck, Cancer of (*See also Neck Dissections*) 702
Neck, Cystic Hygroma (*See also Cystic Hygroma*) 703
Neck Dissections 703
Neck Surgery 704
Neck Surgery, Anesthesia for 706
Neck, Tumors (*See also Cystic Hygroma, Neck; Cysts and Fistulas*) 706
Neck Wounds 706
Nelson Operation: *See Murray-Nelson-Hulsman Operation* 707
Nerves, Dupuytren's Contracture and 707
Nerves, Effects of Sympathectomy on Skin Grafts 707
Nerves, Facial Hemiatrophy 708
Nerves, Facial 708
Nerves, Grafts 711
Nerves, Injuries (*See also Nerves, Grafts; Nerves, Injuries, Hand; War Injuries, Nerve*) 715
Nerves, Injuries, Hand (*See also Nerves, Median; Nerves, Radial; Nerves, Ulnar*) 718
Nerves, Median 719
Nerves, Miscellaneous Items 719
Nerves, Neuromas 720
Nerves, Radial 720
Nerves, Recovery of Sensation in Skin Grafts and Flaps 722
Nerves, Sympathectomy for Facial Paralysis 722
Nerves, Ulnar 722
Nevi, Giant 724
Nevi, Pigmented 724
Nevi, Pigmented, Malignancy in (*See also Nevi, Giant*) 725
Nevi, Vascular 725
New-Erich Operation 729
Ney Operation 729
Nicoladoni Operation 729
Nida Operation 730

Nieden's Operation 730
Nissen Operation 731
Noël Operation 731
Noma 732
Nose, Anterior Atresia (*See also Nose, Choanal Atresia*) 732
Nose, Atrophic Rhinitis of 733
Nose, Bone and Cartilage Autografts to 733
Nose, Bone and Cartilage Heterografts to 735
Nose, Cancer 735
Nose, Cartilage Homografts to 736
Nose, Choanal Atresia (*See also Nose, Anterior Atresia*) 736
Nose, Cleft Lip Deformities of 737
Nose, Deformity 738
Nose, Dermoid Cyst 740
Nose, Fractures 741
Nose, Infections of 743
Nose, Injuries of 743
Nose, Leishmaniasis of 745
Nose, Leprosy of 745
Nose, Lupus of 745
Nose, Miscellaneous 745
Nose, Polyps of 745
Nose, Prostheses 745
Nose, Rat Bite of 746
Nose, Septal Abscess of 746
Nose, Septal Obstruction in Children 746
Nose, Septal Perforations 746
Nose, Septal Resection 747
Nose, Septal Resection, Complications of 750
Nose, Septal Resection Instruments 750
Nose, Septum, Dislocation of 751
Nose, Septum, Excision of 751
Nose, Septum, Miscellaneous 751
Nose, Sinuses 753
Nose, Surgery, Complications: See *Rhinoplasty, Complications* 754
Nose, Syphylitic Deformity of 754
Nose, Toe Transplants to 755
Nose, Tumors 755
Nove-Josserand Operation 756
Nove-Josserand-Borchers Operation 756
Nursing 757
Nutrition 757
Ollier Operation 760
Ombredanne Operation 761
Oral Surgery (*See also Maxillofacial Surgery, Mouth, Etc.*) 761
Orbit 762
Orbit, Fracture 764
Orbit, Infections 764
Orbit, Tumors 765
Orell Operation 765
Oroantral Fistula 765
Orthodontia 766
Orthopedics 766
Ostrcil Method 766
Otoplasty 767
Otorhinolaryngology 771
Palate (*See also Cleft Palate*) 775
Palate, Cancer (*See also Jaws, Cancer of; Mouth, Cancer*) 778
Palate, Tumors 778
Panas Operation 779
Pare, Ambroise 779
Parotid, Cancer 780
Parotid Gland 780
Parotid Tumors 782
Passaggi-Galliera Operation 783
Pectoralis Muscle, Absence of 785
Penis 787
Perthes Operation 791
Peters Operation 792
Petroff Operation: See *Darcissac-Bruhn-Petroff Operation* 792
Pharynx 794
Pharynx, Cancer 794
Pharynx, Tumors 795
Photography 795
Physical Therapy 795
Pierre Robin Syndrome (*See also Cleft Palate; Micrognathia*) 798
Plastic Surgery 799
Plastic Surgery Articles, Reviews of 805
Plastic Surgery Books: *See Books* 805
Plastic Surgery, History: *See History of Plastic Surgery* 805
Plastic Surgery, Medicolegal Aspects 805
Plastic Surgery, Military (*See also War Injuries*) 806
Plastic Surgery, Psychology of 807
Pontoppidan Operation 810
Popoff Operation 811
Port-Wine Stains (*See also Hemangiomas; Nevi*) 812
Preauricular Cysts and Sinuses 814
Pressure Sores 814
Prince D. 816
Prostheses 817
Psychology: *See Plastic Surgery, Psychology of* 824
Putti-Krukenberg Operation 824
Radial Nerve: *See Nerves, Radial* 825
Radiation Injuries 825
Radiation Treatment of Benign Conditions 827
Radiation Treatment of Cancer 829
Radiation Treatment of Keloids 832
Ranula 834
Rectum 837
Rehn's Operation 838
Reich-Matti Operation 838
Replantation 839
Rhinolalia (*See also Cleft Palate*) 841
Rhinophyma 841
Rhinoplasty (*See also Nose, Various Categories*) 842
Rhinoplasty, Alar Collapse 842

Rhinoplasty, Anesthesia for 842
Rhinoplasty, Chin Corrections with 843
Rhinoplasty, Complications 843
Rhinoplasty, Corrective 845
Rhinoplasty, Deviated Nose 850
Rhinoplasty, Function in 851
Rhinoplasty, History of (*See also History of Plastic Surgery*) 851
Rhinoplasty, Implants in 851
Rhinoplasty, Instruments for 853
Rhinoplasty, Miscellaneous 853
Rhinoplasty, Planning 854
Rhinoplasty, Postoperative Care 855
Rhinoplasty, Postoperative Packing 855
Rhinoplasty, Psychology of 856
Rhinoplasty, Reconstructive 856
Rhinoplasty, Reduction 860
Rhinoplasty, Results 861
Rhinoplasty, Reviews of 862
Rhinoplasty, Saddle Nose 862
Rhinoplasty, Tip Corrections 863
Rhytidectomy 864
Rib Grafts (*See also Bone Grafts; Cranioplasty; Jaws, Bone Grafts to*) 865
Riedel Operation 867
Romanum, S. 873
Rosenthal 874
Rosenthal Operation (*See also Lexer-Rosenthal Operation; Schonborn-Rosenthal Operation*) 875
Rouge-Denker Operation 876
Ruge Operation 879
Salivary Fistula 882
Salivary Glands, Cancer (*See also Cancer, Jaws; Neck; Parotid, Cancer*) 882
Salivary Glands, Stone 882
Salivary Glands, Tumors 883
Sapejko Operation: *See Van Millingen Operation* 886
Sapezhko Operation: *See Millingen-Sapezhko Operation* 886
Sapozhkov Operation 886
Sauerbruch Operation 887
Scalp 887
Scalp, Avulsion 889
Scars 889
Schonborn Operation 895
Schubert Operation 897
Scleroderma 899
Scrotum 899
Sebaceous Cysts 901
Secretan Syndrome: *See Ledderhose-Secretan Syndrome* 902
Segond Operation 902
Sheehan Operation 907
Shock 908
Shock, Burn (*See also Burns, Shock*) 916
Shock, Experimental 917
Shock, Surgical 917
Shock, Traumatic 920
Shugrue Operation 926
Sie Boen Lian Operation 927
Sigmoid 927
Sistrunk Operation 930
Skin 931
Skin, Cancer (*See also Cancer, Basal Cell; Cancer (region); Cancer, Skin; Melanoma*) . 932
Skin Flaps 933
Skin Flaps from Arm 934
Skin Flaps, Arterial 934
Skin Flaps to Breast 934
Skin Flaps, Compound 935
Skin Flaps, Cross-Lip 935
Skin Flaps, Delayed 935
Skin Flaps to Ear 935
Skin Flaps to Eyelids 935
Skin Flaps to Face 936
Skin Flaps to Foot 937
Skin Flaps, Free 937
Skin Flaps to Hand 937
Skin Flaps, Homoplastic (Parabiosis) 938
Skin Flaps, Inverted 938
Skin Flaps, Jump 938
Skin Flaps to Leg 938
Skin Flaps to Mastoid Area 939
Skin Flaps to Mouth 939
Skin Flaps to Neck 939
Skin Flaps, Nerve Regeneration in (*See also Skin Grafts, Nerve Regeneration in*) 939
Skin Flaps to Nose 939
Skin Flaps to Palate 940
Skin Flaps to Scalp 940
Skin Flaps from Scrotum 940
Skin Flaps, Tubed 940
Skin Flaps, Visor 942
Skin Grafts 942
Skin Grafts to Breast 951
Skin Grafts, Cancer Transplantation with .. 952
Skin Grafts, Contraction of 952
Skin Grafts, Cysts in 952
Skin Grafts, Dressings for 952
Skin Grafts to Ear 953
Skin Grafts to Eyelids (*See also Blepharoplasty; Eyelids; Skin Grafts to Orbit*) 954
Skin Grafts to Face 955
Skin Grafts to Foot 955
Skin Grafts, Full Thickness 955
Skin Grafts, Growth of 957
Skin Grafts to Hand (*See also Hands, Skin Grafts and Flaps to*) 957
Skin Grafts, Homografts and Heterografts .. 958
Skin Grafts, Implantation 960
Skin Grafts, Inlay 960
Skin Grafts, Instruments for Cutting 961
Skin Grafts to Larynx 962
Skin Grafts to Leg (*See also Burns; Leg Ulcers*) 962
Skin Grafts to Mastoid 963

Skin Grafts to Mouth 963
Skin Grafts to Neck 964
Skin Grafts, Nerve Regeneration in 964
Skin Grafts to Nose 964
Skin Grafts to Orbit 964
Skin Grafts to Penis 965
Skin Grafts, Pigmentation of 965
Skin Grafts, Pinch (Reverdin) 965
Skin Grafts, Preservation of 966
Skin Grafts to Scalp 966
Skin Grafts, Sieve 967
Skin Grafts, Split (Thiersch) 967
Skin Grafts, Sweating of 968
Skin Graft to Vagina (*See Vagina*) 968
Skin Tumors 968
Snakebite 970
Snegiroff Operation 970
Snellen Operation 970
Speech Defects 973
Splints, Facial Paralysis 976
Splints, Finger 976
Splints, Hand: *See Fingers, Splints for; Hands, Splints* 978
Splints, Jaw 978
Splints, Nasal 982
Stejskal 985
Stent: *See Skin Grafts, Dressings for; Skin Grafts, Inlay* 985
Stoeckel Operation: *See Goebell- Stoeckel Operation* 986
Strakhov 988
Subbotin's Operation 990
Submucous Resection 990
Sutures 993
Syndactylism 996
Syndactylism with Absence of Pectoral Muscles (*See also Syndactylism*) 999
Szymanowsky Operation: *See Kuhnt-Szymanowsky Operation* 1000
Tansley Operation: *See Hunt-Tansley Operation* 1001
Tattooing of Skin Grafts 1001
Tattoos, Commercial 1001
Tattoos, Dirt 1001
Temporomandibular Joint 1003
Tendon 1006
Tendon, Dislocation of (*See also Fingers, Boutonniere Deformity of*) 1007
Tendon, Infections (*See also Fingers, Infections; Hands, Infections*) 1007
Tendon Injuries (*See also Hands, Tendon Injuries in*) 1008
Tendon, Reconstructive Surgery (*See also Hands, Reconstructive Surgery of*) 1012
Tendon, Rupture of (*See also Hands, Tendon Ruptures in*) 1014
Tendon Rupture, Baseball Finger (*See also Fingers, Baseball Injuries*) 1015
Tendon, Snapping Finger (*See also Finger, Trigger*) 1016
Tendon, Spring Fingers 1017
Tendon Transplantation 1017
Tendon, Tumors of 1020
Tenosynovitis, Stenosing, De Quervain's 1021
Testicles 1022
Tetanus 1022
Thomas, H. O. 1024
Throat 1025
Thumb: *See Fingers* 1026
Thumb, Reconstruction of (*See also Fingers, Transplantation of Toe to Finger or Thumb*) 1026
Thyroglossal Cysts and Fistulas 1028
Thyrotomy 1030
Tinel Sign 1030
Tissue Banks 1031
Toe-to-Finger Transplants: *See Fingers, Transplantation of Toe to; Thumb, Reconstruction of* 1031
Tongue 1032
Torres Estrada Operation 1034
Torticollis 1034
Toti Operation (*See also Mosher-Toti Operation*) 1034
Trachea 1035
Transplantation 1035
Transplantation, Cancer in 1038
Transplantation of Conjunctiva 1038
Transplantation, Connective Tissue 1038
Transplantation of Cornea 1038
Transplantation of Embryonic Tissues 1038
Transplantation, Homografts and Heterografts 1038
Transplantation of Joints 1042
Transplantation of Nails 1042
Transplantation of Toe to Nose 1042
Traynor Operation 1042
Trelat Operation: *See von Langenbeck-Trelat Operation* 1042
Trendelenburg Operation 1042
Trigger Thumb (or Finger): *See Finger, Trigger* 1043
Truc Operation 1043
Trunk 1043
Tschmarke 1044
Turck, F. B. 1044
Twins, Lesions in 1045
Ulcers 1046
Ultraviolet Therapy 1047
Urethra (*See also Epispadias; Hypospadias; Urethral Fistula; Urethral Stricture*) 1047
Urethral Fistula 1048
Urethral Stricture 1049
Uvula, Bifid 1049
Vagina 1049
Vagina, Artificial 1049
Valle Operation 1059
Van Millingen Operation 1059
Veau 1062

Veau Operation 1063
Vestibuloplasty 1064
Vincent's Infection 1066
Vogt Syndrome 1066
Volkmann's Contracture: *See Contracture, Volkmann's* 1067
Von Eiken Operation 1067
Von Hacker Operation 1067
Von Langenbeck Operation 1068
Von Langenbeck-Axhausen Operation 1068
Von Langenbeck-Trelat Operation 1068
Von Liebermann 1068
Vorschütz Operation 1069
Vreden Operation 1070
Vulva 1070
Wagner-Kirschner Operation 1070
Walters Operation: *See Mayo-Walters Operation* 1073
Walther Operation 1073
War Burns 1073
War Injuries 1075
War Injuries, Face 1076
War Injuries, Hand 1079
War Injuries, Jaws 1079
War Injuries, Neck 1083
War Injuries, Nerve 1083
War Injuries, Nose 1084
War Injuries, Shock 1084
War Injuries, Skin Grafting for 1086
Warren Operation: *See Dieffenbach-Warren Operation* 1087
Warts 1087
Webster Operation 1089
Weeker's Operation 1089
Weidenreich 1090
West Operation 1092
Wharton Operation 1093
Wheeler Operation: *See Esser-Wheeler Operation* 1093
Whitehead Operation 1094
Wodak 1098
Wolff's Law 1099
Wound 1100
Wound, Healing of 1101
Wringer Injuries 1102
Wrist Drop 1102
Xanthomas 1103
Young Operation 1104
Young's Operation 1104
Z-Plasty 1105
Zeller Operation 1106
Zinsser Operation: *See Hennig-Zinsser Operation* 1109
Zygoma, Fractures 1110